CARDIAC ARRHYTHMIAS

CARDIAC ARRHYTHMIAS

Their Mechanisms, Diagnosis, and Management

Third Edition

William J. Mandel, M.D.

Professor of Medicine
University of California, Los Angeles School of Medicine
Clinical Director of Electrophysiology
Cedars-Sinai Medical Center
Los Angeles, California

With 102 Contributors

J. B. Lippincott Company
Philadelphia

Acquisitions Editor: Richard H. Lampert
Sponsoring Editor: Kimberley J. Cox
Project Editor: Bridget C. Hannon
Indexer: Alexandra Nickerson
Design Coordinator: Melissa G. Olson
Interior Designer: Joan Jacobus
Cover Designer: Larry Pezzato
Production Manager: Caren Erlichman
Production Coordinator: David Yurkovich
Compositor: Circle Graphics
Printer/Binder: Quebecor/Kingsport
Pre-Press: Jay's Publishers Services, Inc.

Third Edition

6 5 4 3 2 1

Library of Congress Cataloging in Publication Data

Cardiac arrhythmias : their mechanisms, diagnosis, and management /
    William J. Mandel ; with 102 contributors. — 3rd ed.
        p.   cm.
    Includes bibliographical references and index.
    ISBN 0-397-51185-X (alk. paper)
    1. Arrhythmia.   I. Mandel, William J., 1937–
    [DNLM: 1. Arrhythmia.   WG 330 C2685 1995]
RC685.A65C283   1995
616.1'28–dc20
DNLM/DLC
for Library of Congress   94-33853
                                                   CIP

♾ This Paper Meets the Requirements of ANSI/NISO 239.48-1992
(Permanence of Paper).

The authors and publisher have exerted every effort to ensure
that drug selection and dosage set forth in this text are in accord
with current recommendations and practice at the time of publication. However, in view of ongoing research, changes in government regulations, and the constant flow of information relating to drug therapy and drug reactions, the reader is urged to
check the package insert for each drug for any change in indications and dosage and for added warnings and precautions. This is
particularly important when the recommended agent is a new or
infrequently employed drug.

Dedication

This edition is dedicated to all my mentors who have helped me develop the skills needed to bridge the gap between clinical electrophysiologist and research scientist. I am indebted specifically to Dr. Ludwig Eichna, who expanded my horizons, and to Dr. Mario Vassale, who introduced me to basic research. My research skills could not have been developed without the nurturing of Drs. J. A. Abildskov, Brian Hoffman and J. Thomas Bigger, Jr. Their patience, understanding and intellect have been a guiding light to me throughout my career. Finally, Dr. H. J. C. Swan has helped me hone my abilities to evaluate my own and other's research. These research skills have enhanced my abilities as a clinician and, therefore, have aided all my patients.

I have a special note of gratitude to my wife, Dede, and my children, Stacey and Jay, whose love and understanding have allowed me to complete this project.

Contributors

Stuart W. Adler, MD
Assistant Professor of Medicine
Department of Medicine
Cardiovascular Division
University of Minnesota Hospitals
Director of Electrocardiography Laboratory
Co-Director, The Cardiac Arrhythmia Center
Minneapolis, Minnesota

Maurits A. Allesie, MD, PhD
Professor of Physiology
University of Limburg
Maastricht
The Netherlands

Mark H. Anderson, MD, MRCP
Senior Registrar in Cardiology
St. Mary's Hospital
London
United Kingdom

Robert H. Anderson, BSc, MD, FRCPath
Joseph Levy Professor of Paediatric Cardiac Morphology
Department of Paediatrics
Honorary Consultant
Royal Brompton National Heart and Lung Institute
London
United Kingdom

Elliott Antman, MD
Associate Professor of Medicine
Harvard Medical School
Director, Samuel A. Levine Cardiac Unit
Brigham and Women's Hospital
Boston, Massachusetts

P. Aouate, MD
Staff Member
Centre Medico-Chirurgical
Villiers Saint Denis
France

Robert A. Bauernfeind, MD
Clinical Associate Professor
University of Illinois College of Medicine at Peoria
Cardiac Electrophysiologist
St. Francis Medical Center
Peoria, Illinois

Anton E. Becker, MD, PhD
Professor of Cardiovascular Pathology
University of Amsterdam
Academic Medical Center
The Netherlands

David G. Benditt, MD
Professor of Medicine
Director, Cardiac Arrhythmia Service
University of Minnesota
Minneapolis, Minnesota

Selvyn B. Bleifer, MD
Associate Clinical Professor of Medicine
University of California, Los Angeles
School of Medicine
Los Angeles, California
Chairman, Division of Cardiology
Brotman Medical Center
Culver City, California

Felix I. M. Bonke, MD, PhD
Professor of Physiology
Medical Faculty
University of Limburg
Maastricht
The Netherlands

Martin Borggrefe, MD
Consultant Cardiologist
University of Munster
Medizinische Klinik und Poliklinik
Munster
Germany

Günter Breithardt, MD
Professor of Medicine (Cardiology)
Department of Cardiology and Angiology
University of Munster
Medizinische Klinik und Poliklinik
Munster
Germany

David S. Buckles, PhD
Assistant Professor of Pediatrics
South Carolina Children's Heart Center
Medical University of South Carolina
Charleston, South Carolina

A. John Camm, MD
Professor of Clinical Cardiology
St. George's Hospital Medical School
Consultant Cardiologist
St. George's Hospital
London
United Kingdom

Christopher L. Case, DMD, MD
Associate Professor of Pediatrics
Director of Pediatric Electrophysiology Laboratory
Medical University of South Carolina
Charleston, South Carolina

Agustin Castellanos, MD
Professor of Medicine
University of Miami School of Medicine
Director, Clinical Electrophysiology
University of Miami/Jackson Memorial Medical Center
Miami, Florida

Peng-Sheng Chen, MD
Associate Professor of Medicine
University of California, Los Angeles
Staff Cardiologist
Cedars-Sinai Medical Center
Los Angeles, California

Jacques Clémenty, MD
University of Bordeaux
Hopital Cardiologique du Haut Leveque
Bordeaux-Pessac
France

Howard C. Cohen, MD
Clinical Associate Professor of Medicine
University of Illinois
Attending Physician in Cardiology
Illinois Masonic Hospital
Director of Electrophysiology Laboratory
Michael Reese Hospital
Chicago, Illinois

James L. Cox, MD
Evarts A. Graham Professor of Surgery
Washington University School of Medicine
Chief, Division of Cardiothoracic Surgery
Barnes Hospital
St. Louis, Missouri

Paul V. L. Curry, MD, FRCP
Consultant Cardiologist
Guy's Hospital
London
England

Mary L. Dohrmann, MD
Associate Clinical Professor of Medicine
University of California, San Francisco
Director of Cardiac Clinic
San Francisco General Hospital
San Francisco, California

Leonard S. Dreifus, MD
Professor of Medicine
Hahnemann University
Hahnemann University Hospital
Philadelphia, Pennsylvania

Nabil El-Sherif, MD
Professor of Medicine and Physiology
Director, Electrophysiology Program
State University of New York Health Science Center
Chief, Cardiology Division
Veterans Affairs Medical Center
Brooklyn, New York

Jeronimo Farre, MD, FESC
Associate Professor of Medicine
Madrid Autonomous University
Director, Coronary Care and Arrhythmia Units
Fundacion Jimenez Diaz
Madrid
Spain

T. Bruce Ferguson Jr., MD
Associate Professor of Surgery
Division of Cardiothoracic Surgery
Washington University School of Medicine
St. Louis, Missouri

Pedro R. Fernandez, MD
Assistant Professor of Medicine
Director of Arrhythmia and Pacemaker Clinics
Division of Cardiology
University of Miami School of Medicine
Miami, Florida

Thomas Fetsch, MD
Westfalische Wilhelms-Universitat
Department of Cardiology and Angiology
Munster
Germany

Bruno Fischer, MD
Universite de Bordeaux II
Hopital Cardiologique Haut Leveque
Bordeaux Pessac
France

Guy Fontaine, MD, PhD
Director of Clinical Electrophysiology
and Cardiac Pacing Department
Hopital Jean-Rostand
Paris
France

Robert Frank, MD
Medecin des Hopitaux
Director of the Clinical Electrophysiology
and Pacemaker Departments
Hopital Jean-Rostand
Paris
France

Derek A. Fyfe, MD, PhD
Associate Professor
Medical University of South Carolina
Charleston, South Carolina

David C. Gadsby, PhD
Professor and Head
Laboratory of Cardiac/Membrane Physiology
The Rockefeller University
New York, New York

John D. Gallagher, MD
Associate Professor of Anesthesiology
Dartmouth Medical School
Hanover, New Hampshire
Attending Anesthesiologist
Department of Anesthesiology
Dartmouth-Hitchcock Medical Center
Lebanon, New Hampshire

Yves Gallais, MD
Member of the Staff
Hopitaux de Paris
Hopital Jean-Rostand
Paris
France

Eli S. Gang, MD
Associate Professor of Clinical Medicine
University of California, Los Angeles School of Medicine
Cardiologist
Cedars-Sinai Medical Center
Director of Pacemaker Clinic
St. Vincent Medical Center
Los Angeles, California

Annette Geibel, MD
Innere Medizin III
Universitatklinik Freiburg
Freiburg
Germany

Paul C. Gillette, MD
Professor and Director
Pediatric Cardiology
Medical University of South Carolina
Professor and Director
Pediatric Cardiology
South Carolina Children's Heart Center
Charleston, South Carolina

Nora Goldschlager, MD
Professor of Clinical Medicine
University of California, San Francisco
Director, Coronary Care Unit
Director, ECG Laboratory and Pacemaker Clinic
San Francisco General Hospital
San Francisco, California

MaryAnn Goldstein, MD
Attending Physician
Minneapolis Children's Hospital
Minneapolis, Minnesota

Jeffrey S. Goodman, MD
Clinical Instructor
University of California, Los Angeles School of Medicine
Division of Cardiology/Electrophysiology
Cedars-Sinai Medical Center
Los Angeles, California

Anton P. M. Gorgels, MD, PhD
Assistant Professor
University of Limburg
Academic Hospital Maastricht
Maastricht
The Netherlands

Richard J. Gray, MD
Professor and Chairman
Department of Internal Medicine
University of North Dakota School of Medicine
Grand Forks, North Dakota

H. Leon Greene, MD
Professor of Medicine
University of Washington
Harborview Medical Center
Seattle, Washington

Michel Haissaguerre, MD
Universite de Bordeaux II
Hopital Cardiologique Haut Leveque
Bordeaux Pessac
France

Siew Yen Ho, PhD, MRCPath
Senior Lecturer
Royal Brompton National Heart and Lung Institute
London
United Kingdom

Shoei K. Stephen Huang, MD
Professor of Medicine
University of Massachusetts Medical School
Director, Section of Cardiac Electrophysiology and Pacing
University of Massachusetts Medical Center
Worcester, Massachusetts

Alberto Interian, Jr., MD
Associate Professor of Medicine
University of Miami School of Medicine
Director, Electrophysiology Laboratory
Jackson Memorial Hospital
Miami, Florida

Jay L. Jordan, MD
Assistant Clinical Professor of Medicine
University of California, Los Angeles
Attending Cardiologist
Cedars-Sinai Medical Center
Los Angeles, California

Hanjörg Just, MD, PhD
Medizinische Klinik
Kardiologie und Angiologie
Universitatsklinik Freiburg
Freiburg
Germany

Hrayr S. Karagueuzian, PhD
Professor of Medicine
University of California, Los Angeles School of Medicine
Director, Cardiac Electrophysiology Research
Cedars-Sinai Medical Research Institute
Los Angeles, California

Dirar S. Khoury, PhD
Section of Cardiology
Department of Medicine
Baylor College of Medicine
Houston, Texas

Dennis M. Krikler, MD, RFCP
Senior Lecturer in Cardiology
Royal Postgraduate Medical School
Consultant Cardiologist
Hammersmith Hospital
London
United Kingdom

G. Lascault, MD
Staff Member
Hopitaux de Paris
Hopital Jean-Rostand
Paris
France

Keith G. Lurie, MD
Assistant Professor of Medicine
University of Minnesota
Director of Clinical Electrophysiology Laboratory
University of Minnesota Hospital and Clinics
Minneapolis, Minnesota

Markku Mäkijärvi, MD
First Department of Medicine
Helsinki University Central Hospital
Helsinki
Finland

James D. Maloney, MD
Professor of Medicine
Director, Center for Cardiac Arrhythmia Services
* and Electrophysiology*
Baylor College of Medicine
Houston, Texas

William J. Mandel, MD
Professor of Medicine
University of California, Los Angeles School of Medicine
Clinical Director of Electrophysiology
Cedars-Sinai Medical Center
Los Angeles, California

Frank I. Marcus, MD
Distinguished Professor of Internal Medicine (Cardiology)
Director of Electrophysiology
Section of Cardiology
University of Arizona Health Sciences Center
Tucson, Arizona

Melinda L. Marks, MD
Assistant Professor
University of Utah School of Medicine
University of Utah Health Sciences Center
Salt Lake City, Utah

Antoni Martínez-Rubio, MD
Resident of Cardiology and of Internal Medicine
University Hospital of Munster
Munster
Germany

Todor Mazgalev, PhD
Research Associate Professor
Director of Basic Electrophysiology Laboratories
University of Pittsburgh
Pittsburgh, Pennsylvania

Thomas Meinertz, MD
Professor of Medicine
Chief, Division of Cardiology
University Hospital Eppendorf Hamburg
Hamburg
Germany

Holly R. Middlekauff, MD
Assistant Professor of Medicine
University of California, Los Angeles School of Medicine
Los Angeles, California

Fred Morady, MD
Professor of Medicine
University of Michigan
Director, Clinical Electrophysiology Laboratory
University of Michigan Medical Center
Ann Arbor, Michigan

Morton M. Mower, MD
Visiting Associate Professor of Medicine
The Johns Hopkins University School of Medicine
Baltimore, Maryland

Robert J. Myerburg, MD
Professor of Medicine and Physiology
Director, Division of Cardiology
University of Miami School of Medicine
Miami, Florida

Onkar S. Narula, MD
Clinical Professor of Medicine
University of Miami School of Medicine
Cedars Medical Center
Miami, Florida

J. Elias Neto, MD
Foreign Resident
Hopitaux de Paris
Hopital Jean-Rostand
Paris
France

S. Bertil Olsson, MD, PhD, FESC
Professor of Cardiology
Department of Cardiology
University Hospital
Lund
Sweden

Michael Perelman, MD
Honorary Fellow
Division of Cardiovascular Disease
Royal Postgraduate Medical School
Hammersmith Hospital
London
United Kingdom

C. Thomas Peter, MD
Professor of Medicine in Residence
University of California, Los Angeles School of Medicine
Director, Electrocardiography and Electrophysiology
Division of Cardiology
Cedars-Sinai Medical Center
Los Angeles, California

Sergio L. Pinski, MD
Attending Staff
Department of Cardiology
Section of Cardiac Pacing and Electrophysiology
Cleveland Clinic Foundation
Cleveland, Ohio

Francois Poulain, MD
Member of the Staff
Hopitaux de Paris
Hopital Jean-Rostand
Paris
France

Lutz Reinhardt, MSc
Medizinische Klinik und Poliklinik
Munster
Germany

Leon Resnekov, MD, FRCP[†]
Rawson Professor of Medicine (Cardiology)
University of Chicago Pritzker School of Medicine
University of Chicago Medical Center
Chicago, Illinois

Thomas F. Ross, MD
St. Luke's Medical Center
Phoenix, Arizona

Edward Rowland, MD
Senior Lecturer and Consultant Cardiologist
St. George's Hospital Medical School
St. George's Hospital
London
United Kingdom

Scott Sakaguchi, MD
Assistant Professor of Medicine
University of Minnesota
Attending Physician
University Hospital
Minneapolis, Minnesota

Joseph J. Sarmiento, Jr., MD
Clinical Assistant Professor
University of Illinois
College of Medicine at Peoria
Saint Francis Medical Center
Peoria, Illinois

Edward Shapiro, MD
Clinical Professor of Medicine, Emeritus
University of Southern California School of Medicine
Attending Cardiologist
Cedars-Sinai Medical Center
Los Angeles, California

Hossein Shenasa, MD
Fellow, Electrophysiology Laboratory
Division of Cardiology
Department of Medicine
Duke University Medical Center
Durham, North Carolina

Mohammad Shenasa, MD
Attending Physician
Department of Medicine
Cardiovascular Disease Section
O'Connor Hospital
San Jose, California

Donald H. Singer, MD
Professor of Clinical Medicine
University of Illinois College of Medicine
Department of Medicine
Division of Cardiology
Chicago, Illinois
Associate Attending Physician
Department of Medicine
Division of Cardiology
Alexian Brothers Medical Center
Elk Grove Village, Illinois

Joep L.R.M. Smeets, MD, PhD
Assistant Professor in Cardiology
Director, Laboratory of Clinical Electrophysiology
Academic Hospital Maastricht
University of Limburg
Maastricht
The Netherlands

[†] Deceased.

Thomas Woodward Smith, AB, MD
Professor of Medicine
Harvard Medical School
Chief, Cardiovascular Division
Brigham and Women's Hospital
Boston, Massachusetts

William G. Stevenson, MD
Associate Professor of Medicine
Harvard Medical School
Co-Director of Cardiac Arrhythmia Service and
  Cardiac Electrophysiology Laboratory
Brigham and Women's Hospital
Boston, Massachusetts

Borys Surawicz, MD
Professor Emeritus
Indiana University School of Medicine
Senior Research Associate
Krannert Institute of Cardiology
Indiana University School of Medicine
Indianapolis, Indiana

Ashby B. Taylor, III, MD
Associate Professor of Pediatrics
Medical University of South Carolina
South Carolina Children's Hospital
Charleston, South Carolina

Joelli Tonet, MD, FCCP
Member of the Staff
Hopitaux de Paris
Hopital Jean-Rostand
Paris
France

Gioia Turitto, MD
Assistant Professor of Medicine
Director, Coronary Care Unit
  and Electrophysiology Laboratory
State University of New York
Health Science Center at Brooklyn
Brooklyn, New York

Gabriel Vanerio, MD
Doctor in Medicine
Electrophysiology Department
British Hospital
Montevideo
Uruguay

G. Michael Vincent, MD
Professor of Medicine
University of Utah School of Medicine
Chairman, Department of Medicine
LDS Hospital
Salt Lake City, Utah

Alan B. Wagshal, MD
Assistant Professor of Medicine
Department of Cardiology
Assistant Director of Electrophysiology Laboratory
University of Massachusetts Medical Center
Worcester, Massachusetts

Yoshio Watanabe, MD, FACC
Professor of Medicine
Director, Cardiovascular Institute
Fujita Health University School of Medicine
Toyoake, Aichi
Japan

Hein J. J. Wellens, MD
Professor and Chairman
Department of Cardiology
Academic Hospital Maastricht
Maastricht
The Netherlands

John Wharton, BSc, PhD
Senior Lecturer
Histochemistry Department
Royal Postgraduate Medical School
Hammersmith Hospital
London
United Kingdom

Henry B. Wiles, MD
Associate Professor of Pediatrics
South Carolina Children's Heart Center
Medical University of South Carolina
Charleston, South Carolina

Andrew L. Wit, PhD
Professor of Pharmacology
Columbia University
College of Physicians and Surgeons
New York, New York

Shiwen Yuan, MD
Research Fellow
Department of Cardiology
University Hospital of Lund
Lund
Sweden

Manfred Zehender, MD
Assistant Professor
Innere Medizin III
Universitatsklinik Freiburg
Freiburg
Germany

Vicki L. Zeigler, RN, MSN
Pediatric Arrhythmia Case Manager
Division of Cardiovascular Nursing
South Carolina Children's Heart Center
Medical University of South Carolina
Charleston, South Carolina

Preface

The third edition of this textbook comes at a time when electrophysiology is at a crossroads. In the early days of clinical electrophysiology invasive studies were of diagnostic importance. Then came the era of therapeutic interventions so that therapy was guided by the results of electrophysiologic studies. This era changed significantly with the advent of the CAST Study and the introduction of radiofrequency ablation techniques.

This present edition has combined information on clinical, noninvasive electrophysiology with material on invasive and interventional electrophysiology.

The development of interventional electrophysiology is in its formative years and is expected to expand both in terms of indications and technology. Nevertheless, significant data is covered in this edition concerning present methodologic considerations as well as indications and techniques.

Of equal importance is the expansion of our knowledge in noninterventional areas such as the evaluation of patients with possible QT abnormalities, the use of the signal averaged electrocardiogram, tests for heart rate variability, tilt table studies, evaluation for possible proarrhythmia, etc. Data in areas of additional interest, such as the effects of anesthesia in patients with arrhythmias and arrhythmias in athletes, complement the material presented.

Therefore, this textbook is intended to serve the reader in all areas of electrophysiology, blending the old and the new, noninvasive and invasive, as well as interventional electrophysiology. It is hoped that this third edition will serve the clinician's needs in all areas.

I would like to specifically thank Brenda Williams, Shantel Brown and Elaine Lebowitz for their skillful secretarial assistance. I owe a special debt of gratitude to Bridget Hannon, Kim Cox and Richard Lampert from J. B. Lippincott, whose support and advice were the major thrust for completing this project.

William J. Mandel, MD

Preface to Previous Edition

The second edition of this textbook on cardiac arrhythmias has come about because of the continued expansion of our knowledge concerning the mechanisms, diagnosis, and management of rhythm disorders in man.

In the time span between these two editions, there has been a significant increase in data concerning cellular electrophysiologic mechanisms of arrhythmias, which can be expected to enhance the understanding and management of clinical arrhythmias. Pharmacologically, the armamentarium of clinically available antiarrhythmic drugs has expanded dramatically. This increase in drug availability has been associated with an increase in basic electrophysiologic-pharmacologic data concerning drug mechanisms. The latter is essential to the clinician in the management of patients with cardiac arrhythmias.

This edition also addresses noninvasive assessment of the propensity for ventricular arrhythmias with the use of late potential recordings, as well as alteration of autonomic tone for assessment of the types and location of AV block.

New therapeutic approaches have been emphasized in this edition, including the use of lasers and other ablation techniques, new modes of pacemaker therapy, and the use of the automatic implantable defibrillator.

An extensive new section has been added on the techniques of general electrophysiologic testing, with a separate chapter on ventricular tachycardia evaluation. A chapter on the evaluation of patients with unexplained syncope has also been added.

Finally, significant changes have been made in the chapters on cardiac surgery for atrial arrhythmias, the WPW syndrome, and ventricular tachycardia.

In total, there has been updating and expansion of the electrophysiologic material in this textbook, so that the clinician with a keen interest in clinical electrophysiology may have a ready reference source of basic and clinical electrophysiologic material.

The editor wishes to acknowledge the important contributions made by his colleagues: Doctors C. Thomas Peter, Eli Gang, Daniel Oseran, and Hrayr Karagueuzian. He would also particularly like to acknowledge the essential contribution of Ms. Brenda Williams, without whose assistance in all areas of preparation this text could not have been completed.

The support of my family, Dede, Stacey, and Jay, was essential to the completion of this manuscript.

Finally, to the staff of J. B. Lippincott Company and, especially, Richard Winters, I am most grateful.

William J. Mandel, MD

Table of Contents

CARDIAC ARRHYTHMIAS

Cardiac Arrhythmias, 3rd edition, edited by William J. Mandel.
J. B. Lippincott Company, Philadelphia © 1995.

1

Edward Shapiro

The Electrocardiogram and the Arrhythmias: Historical Insights

I compare myself to a scavenger: with my hook in my hand and my pack on my back, I go about the domain of science picking up what I can find.

Francois Magendie[1]

Although the electrocardiograph is the Rosetta stone of arrhythmias, it should not be assumed that only ignorance existed in the realm of cardiac irregularities before Willem Einthoven developed the earliest electrocardiogram. Twenty-two years earlier, in 1902, James Mackenzie published *The Study of the Pulse*, a compilation of his studies of arterial and venous pulsations using his improved clinical ink-writing polygraph (Fig. 1-1). The reliable tracings of this instrument were used as guides to correct the inexact interpretations of the early electrocardiograms. Basically, for the diagnosis of arrhythmias, the electrocardiogram is searched for P and QRS complexes and their relationship to each other. The polygraph's a and v waves gave the same information, not from electrical activation, but from the consequent contraction of the atria and ventricles as reflected in the jugular and radial pulses.

The laddergram that is used today to aid the analysis of complex arrhythmias was devised by Engelmann in 1896 to explain tracings inscribed by the polygraph.[2] In

1903, Wenckebach published *Die Arrhythmie, als Ausdruck bestimmter Funktionsstörungen des Herzens*, also based on the ink-writing polygraph. The Wenckebach phenomenon, the name ascribed to recurrent dropped beats, was discovered in 1899 by using the polygraph, not the electrocardiogram, to record the radial arteriogram.

Before the electrocardiograph was invented in 1903, the ink-writing polygraph allowed the accurate graphic diagnosis of the following:

1. Sinus arrhythmia
2. Sinus tachycardia and bradycardia
3. Atrial fibrillation
4. First, second, and third degree heart block
5. Wenckebach phenomenon
6. Junctional rhythm
7. Pulsus alternans
8. Paroxysmal atrial tachycardia
9. Atrial tachycardia with block

The polygraph, however, could not clearly distinguish flutter from paroxysmal atrial tachycardia.

In 1897, Cushny described a clashing double rhythm in myographic tracings of rabbits, cats, and dogs poisoned

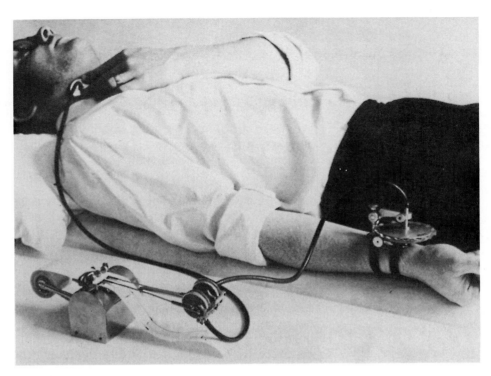

Figure 1-1. Mackenzie's ink-writing polygraph inscribing the radical arterial and jugular venous pulsations. (Courtesy of the Wellcome Trustees.)

with digitalis.[3] Mobitz ascribed the name of *interference-dissociation* to this arrhythmia in 1923.[4]

Because the electrocardiogram is merely the graphic inscription of electrophysiologic events, it is germane to read what was known of electrophysiology circa 1900, as collated by Wiggers.[5] DuBois-Reymond had recognized that action-currents reflected potential difference between the interior and the exterior of the skeletal muscle cell. As early as 1899, Samojloff, Einthoven's Russian colleague, estimated that 60 to 80 mV was 60% of the actual transmembrane potential difference. In 1902, Overton postulated that excitation of the skeletal muscle cell depends on a shift of sodium and potassium ions; he was perplexed that, by the age of 70 years, a human heart had contracted a quarter of a billion times, yet the ionic balance in the cardiac cell was unchanged. Julius Bernstein wrote a monograph on the membrane theory. Augustus D. Waller clearly perceived that electrical activity in the heart preceded mechanical contraction.

In 1876, Marey had established the existence of the refractory period of cardiac muscle.[6] He invented the term and learned that after the heart contracted, the refractory period lasted longer than that of skeletal muscle or nerve. Burn states that this long action potential of cardiac muscle serves "to prevent fibrillation among fibers which are out of phase."[7] A. J. Carlson first used the terms *absolute* and *relative frequency period*.[8] Both Gaskell (1883) and Engelmann (1897) recognized that conduction in the hearts of warm-blooded animals was myogenic. By 1893,

Wilhelm His, Jr., had described the atrioventricular (AV) bundle and postulated that it ferried AV conduction. Purkinje assigned his pupil Palicke to study the unusual muscle cells seen in the sheep's heart; by 1845, they had described the fine ramifications of the conduction system. By 1900, Engelmann, Wenckebach, and Bowditch had promulgated the axioms of cardiac muscle, characterizing it by (1) automaticity, (2) a refractory period, (3) an all-or-none reactivity to stimuli of diverse strengths, and (4) the treppe phenomenon after excitation.[5]

Ventricular fibrillation (VF) was first recognized by Erichsen in 1842, and Oskar Langendorff had watched it in his isolated, perfused-heart preparation in 1898. Atrial fibrillation was studied clinically as early as 1827. In 1903, Cushny learned that poisonous doses of digitalis could provoke VF. Hering demonstrated in 1900 that excess potassium in the perfusate of the isolated heart preparation arrested VF. By following the potassium with Locke's solution, sinoatrial (SA) rhythm was reinstituted. Sidney Ringer proved that calcium ion was needed for cardiac contraction.

EXTRASYSTOLES

Even though the extrasystole is brief, it was detected before the introduction of the electrocardiogram. In 1876, Marey showed that the ventricle was excitable by artificial stimuli during diastole but refractory during systole.[6] In 1872, Knoll delineated the compensatory pause of premature ventricular contractions (PVCs) as equal to twice the original cardiac cycle.[9] But it was Engelmann, working with the frog's heart, who explained that the next atrial impulse falls during the refractory period set up by the PVC, making the ventricle await the next atrial stimulus.[10] Engelmann coined the term *extrasystole* and demonstrated that atrial extrasystoles reset SA rhythm. Wenckebach as well as Cushny noted atrial extrasystoles in humans.[11,12]

Kraus and Nicolai first registered extrasystoles with the electrocardiograph.[13] They explained the premature beat as being caused by the contraction of a single ventricle, later called *hemisystole*. Mackenzie accepted this concept. Lewis quashed this error by producing simultaneous tracings of the venous pulse and the electrocardiogram, which bridged the difference between Mackenzie's and Einthoven's studies.[14] Junctional extrasystoles shown in venous pulse tracings were published by Pan in 1904.[15]

Extrasystoles, considered in Lewis' time to be an active usurpative arrhythmia, are today believed to be forced by the preceding SA contraction. Despite the frequency of extrasystoles recorded, Langendorf, Pick, and Winternitz did not enunciate their rule of bigeminy until 1955.[16] In 1960, Shinji Kinoshita described the rule of multiple interectopic sinus impulses.[17] The same phenomenon was described by Schamroth and Marriott in 1961; their designation was *concealed bigeminy* or *trigeminy* caused by concealed ventricular extrasystoles from a focus that was, at least, semiprotected.[18]

ATRIAL FIBRILLATION

Robert Adams, known for his Adams-Stokes association, was probably the first to recognize atrial fibrillation and mark it in 1827 as a sign of mitral stenosis.[19] So common was rheumatic heart disease in England at the time that some 50 years later George Balfour wrote "extremely irregular action (of the heart) is almost pathognomonic of mitral stenosis."[20] (William Osler, who was gifted at refining clinical-pathologic nosology, called delirium cordis the result of multiple irregularly recurring extrasystoles. In the eighth edition [1912] of his celebrated textbook, a section titled "Fibrillation of the Heart" appeared for the first time.)

Marey, in 1863, published a pulse tracing of atrial fibrillation from a patient with mitral stenosis.[21] Because his polygraph could record no jugular pulsations in patients with atrial fibrillation, Mackenzie conceived the atria to be immobile and paralyzed, allowing the cardiac rhythm to originate in the AV node.[22] H. E. Hering in 1903

called the arrhythmia *pulsus irregularis perpetuus*.[23] In 1908, his subsequent article demonstrated the electrocardiograms of two patients with atrial fibrillation.[24] Inexplicably, he declared atrial activity to be invisible on the electrocardiogram. In 1909, Rothenberger and Winterberg first used the term *Vorhofflimmern* (fibrillation of the auricles).[25] In the same year, Thomas Lewis published a brief paper titled "Auricular Fibrillation: A Common Clinical Condition," in which he labeled the f waves.[26] He emphasized that digitalis slowed the ventricular rate "by enhancing a previously existing auriculo-ventricular heart block." In 1906, Einthoven's paper on the clinical use of the electrocardiograph contained an inscription of atrial fibrillation but no indication as to the nature or significance of irregularity.[27] Gossage and Braxton Hicks in 1913 first recognized that atrial fibrillation could occur transiently or permanently in normal hearts.[28]

Even though Engelmann, in 1894, had theorized that atrial fibrillation was caused by multiple foci in the atria, Thomas Lewis was convinced that an irregular circus movement caused atrial fibrillation.[29,30] He said he was influenced by A. G. Mayer's demonstration of a self-perpetuating contraction wave in a ring of jellyfish tissue. To clarify the issue, David Scherf in 1948 injected aconitine into the head of the sinus node to induce atrial fibrillation that could be reverted by local cooling.[31] Like Engelmann, he was convinced that high-frequency heterotopic foci were responsible for atrial fibrillation, not circus movement, a conviction he had held for 20 years.[32]

In 1951, Prinzmetal and coworkers used high-speed cinematography, later studied in slow motion, to see the fibrillating atria, which they described as being activated by "hetero-rhythmic large and small waves occurring simultaneously at rapid and irregular rates. No circus movement was found."[33]

Finally, the ventricular response to atrial fibrillation was found to be related to exit block by Söderström.[34] The computer was used by Bootsma and coworkers to analyze the R-R intervals, with the conclusion that the random nature of the ventricular rhythm is due to the "effect of randomly spaced atrial impulses of random strength reaching the A-V node from random directions."[35] The arrhythmia that was once called pathognomonic of mitral stenosis remains a physiologic mystery, despite the computer.

ATRIAL FLUTTER

In 1887, MacWilliam saw, with his naked eye, fluttering atria in a dog.[36] "The application of (faradic) current sets the auricle with a rapid flutter," he wrote. In 1905, William Ritchie first recorded flutter on the ink polygraph from a patient whose complete heart block enabled the atrial flutter to be recognized.[37] In 1909, Jolly and Ritchie used the electrocardiograph to study the same patient.[38] In 1906, Einthoven unknowingly recorded atrial flutter with 2:1 block by laying over 1.5 km of wire to connect the galvanometer in his laboratory to a patient bedded in the Academic Hospital in Leiden.[39] In 1913, Thomas Lewis enunciated the criteria for the electrocardiographic diagnosis of atrial flutter—the restless, sawtooth baseline and the inverted, regular, identical P waves in leads II and III.[40]

Prinzmetal and coworkers, in 1952, pointed out that atrial flutter was often atypical.[41] Peaked P waves in the anterior leads were not always visible, and an isoelectric interval between P waves could sometimes be seen.

In 1921, Lewis and coworkers showed that, in flutter, a circus movement circled down the right atrium and up the left atrium.[30] This was confirmed in 1947 by Cabrera and Sodi-Pollares, using the Lewis bipolar electrogram method.[42] Rytand's direct exploratory activation-mapping of a human heart exposed for surgical operation was also confirmatory.[43] Wellens,[44] however, could not find a circus movement in an exposed heart, and Prinzmetal's studies[41] showed a normal P wave axis in at least 15% of flutter, raising the question of whether there was reentry or circuits involving the right internodal tracts, but not verifying a circus movement.

Vectorcardiographic studies of P loops by the Rosen and Damato groups working in concert did not identify the mechanism of common or uncommon atrial flutter in humans.[45]

SUPRAVENTRICULAR TACHYCARDIA

Supraventricular tachycardia (SVT) afflicts the healthy; its sudden acceleration and abrupt termination nearly guarantee acute awareness by the affected individual or corroboration by an observer. Cotton described the first few instances of SVT in 1867 and 1869.[46] By 1888, Bristowe had studied nine patients with SVT, some of whom suffered from serious heart disease.[47] In 1899, Bouveret employed the term *tachycardie essentielle paroxystique* to describe this arrhythmia, and by 1900, Augustus Hoffmann, having amassed 135 cases of SVT, composed a monograph on *Die paroxysmale Tachycardie*.[48, 49]

Both Gaskell[50] and Engelmann,[10] in keeping with the myogenic theory of cardiac conduction, insisted that only the SA area could act as such a rapid pacemaker. However, because von Czermak had stopped SVT by vagal pressure in 1868 and because polyuria was deemed related to the medulla oblongata, the theory of vagal neurosis was not discarded.[51]

Polygraphic pulse tracings by Winternitz in 1886 first established that SVT consisted of a series of atrial extrasystoles.[52] Thomas Lewis demonstrated in 1909 that SVT could have its origin experimentally and clinically in either the atrium or the AV junction.[53] By 1925, in the third edition of *The Mechanism and Graphic Registration of the Heart Beat*, Lewis described all the electrocardiographic *Feinschmeckerei* of the expert.[54]

Although Vidella first described and named the posttachycardia syndrome in 1947, it was 5 years later before Mayerson and Clagett reported on it.[55, 56]

Although Lewis believed a circus movement generated atrial fibrillation and flutter, he declined to accept it as the mechanism generating SVT, mainly because of the slower rate of SVT and the inability of the small-sized atrium to accommodate a circus wave of needed speed. Both David Scherf[57] (1947) and Prinzmetal and coworkers[41] (1952) accepted the focal atrial origin of SVT.

Of all the atrial arrhythmias, SVT, particularly junctional tachycardia, gives characteristic evidence on the electrocardiogram of a rapidly activating ectopic focus. Evidence is accumulating that validates the 1928 model of Schmidt and Erlanger for reentry as a mechanism for the genesis of SVT.[58]

In 1959, Bernard Lown emphasized that paroxysmal atrial tachycardia (PAT) with block was a sign of either digitalis toxicity or was induced by hypokalemia.[59]

COMPLETE ATRIOVENTRICULAR BLOCK

A convulsive fit startles all bystanders; therefore, complete heart block is the most ancient arrhythmia to be recognized and was known at a time when the physician was served only by his five senses. When, after the seizure, a remarkable slowness of the pulse is recognized, heart block is evident even to the novice. Gaskell originated the self-explanatory term in 1883, 10 years before the conduction system was discovered.[60]

Morgagni (1761), Spens (1793), Burnett (1825), Adams (1827), Mayo (1838), Gibson (1839), Holbertson (1840), and Stokes (1846) all contributed to characterization of the Adams-Stokes syndrome. Huchard first called the syndrome Stokes-Adams disease, despite writing "noted first by Adams and then Stokes."[61] Gibson's paper, Arthur Bloomfield wrote, "is the most thorough and thoughtful of them all."[62]

In 1875, Galabin published the first graphic record of heart block, an apex cardiogram, which he thought was the result of mitral stenosis.[63] Nevertheless, he suggested that the atria and ventricles contracted independently. Chauveau, a veterinarian, described a man with heart block and found he could produce AV dissociation in the horse by stimulating the peripheral end of the cut vagus.[64]

Wilhelm His, Jr., not only described the AV conduction system in 1893, but in 1899 was the first to document a patient with heart block with syncope, presenting polygraph tracings of arterial and venous pulsations.[65,66] In 1902, Mackenzie did the same, translating Gaskell's *heart block* into *Herzblock*.

Osler could not correlate bradycardia, syncope, and the bundle of His, so he persuaded Joseph Erlanger to record the apex impulse (with Marey's cardiograph) and the radial pulse with his own recording sphygmomanometer.[67] Erlanger and Blackman also created chronic heart block with an adjustable clamp in dogs as models for Adams-Stokes attacks.[68] In three dogs, syncope was produced, not by asystole but by ventricular tachycardia. Parkinson, Papp, and Evans in 1941 found the same phenomenon in human Adams-Stokes attacks as had Robinson and Bredeck in a single case in 1917.[69,70]

Einthoven recorded the first electrocardiogram of complete heart block in 1906, and Thomas Lewis obtained one in 1910. Two years later, A. E. Cohn and Lewis published the electrocardiograms and autopsy of a patient who died of complete heart block.[71] Fibrosis of the main bundle and right bundle branch was found. This is an early and unusual verification by autopsy of an electrocardiogram. In 1905, Hay published an autopsy showing disease of the AV bundle in a patient with AV block.[72] Arrhythmias other than heart block are not subject to autopsy verification.

Complete heart block, occurring most frequently in senior citizens, had been assumed to be caused mainly by ischemic heart disease, until Yater (1935), Lev (1958), and Lenegre (1963) clarified the nonischemic cause in favor of purely mechanogenic and degenerative lesions.

VENTRICULAR TACHYCARDIA

Ventricular tachycardia (VT) was induced by Panum[73] in 1862 by injecting tallow into the coronary arteries, and Einthoven[27] recorded PVCs and ventricular bigeminy in 1906. Even so, the first electrocardiogram of VT in man was published by Thomas Lewis in 1909 as "single and successive extrasystoles."[74] The ventricular origin of the successive extrasystoles was deduced by Lewis from a simultaneous phlebogram that showed AV dissociation. In addition, although vagal stimulation slowed the atrial rate in some instances, the ventricular rate remained unaltered. Lewis' mentor, James Mackenzie, and Wenckebach had foretold that, based on studies of phlebograms and radial artery pulse-tracings, the tachycardia could originate only in the ventricle.[75,76] Case reports began to appear, including two from the United States by Palfrey and one by Willius.[77,78] The diagnosis rested on either the wide QRS or the wide QRS plus the ventricular rate exceeding that of the atria.

The first report of VT registered from a patient stricken with acute myocardial infarction was published by Robinson and Herrmann in 1921.[79] They suggested that coronary thrombosis could provoke VT, which was often fatal. Lewis had observed in 1909 that PVCs and VT were provoked by coronary artery ligation.[80] Nevertheless, he failed to appreciate that he had induced, by the same ligation, a myocardial infarction, the very malady that eventually killed him at age 64 years.

Although Gallavardin emphasized that VT caused by coronary thrombosis frequently terminated in lethal VF, he also related his experiences with "benign" VT, in which the prognosis was not unfavorable.[81,82]

The criteria for the diagnosis of VT were stated first by Robinson and Herrmann, who stressed AV dissociation and that the QRS morphology of the tachycardia resembled incidental PVCs in other electrocardiograms of the patient.[79] The importance of fusion beats was cited by Rosenberg 12 years before Dressler and Roesler emphasized that fusion signified independent atrial and ventricular contraction.[83,84]

Nevertheless, the simulation of VT by SVT remains the cloaca maxima of electrocardiology. Adding to the confusion are several stumbling blocks. First, VT, like SVT, occurs in normal hearts.[85,86] Second, the criteria for diagnosis established by Langendorf and Pick—AV dissociation plus capture beats or fusion beats—occasionally may be seen in other tachycardias.[87] In addition, there is bidirectional VT, which was first described by Schwenensen, who ascribed it to digitalis intoxication.[88] This arrhythmia has become more common because of the arrhythmogenic property of antiarrhythmic drugs. Quinidine was first convicted by Levine and Fulton as a cause of bidirectional VT in 1929.[89] However, one figure published earlier by Kerr and Bender resembles a polymorphous VT.[90] Zimdahl and Kramer dispute the ventricular origin of the bidirectional VT.[91] They demonstrated that carotid sinus stimulation obliterated the upward-directed complexes, suggesting that the inhibited focus lay above the bundle of His.

Although the term *vulnerable period* is accepted terminology, the concept is 50 years old. Louis Katz in 1928 first warned of the danger of PVCs falling on the T wave.[92] Wiggers, in 1940, repeated Lewis' experimental causation of VT by coronary artery ligation.[93] Smirk found that many patients (more than 300 by 1969) showed the R-on-T phenomenon.[94] These patients were subject to lethal VT and sudden death, which he had anticipated from animal experiments. He also described the "cardiac ballet," an arrhythmia that appeared chaotic, but actually consisted of recurrent multifocal ventricular complexes caused by asynchronous conduction and refractoriness.

VENTRICULAR FIBRILLATION

Ventricular fibrillation was first described by Erichsen[95] in 1842, induced by a faradic current by Hoffa and Ludwig[96] in 1850, and depicted vividly by MacWilliam in 1887.[36] The label *mouvement fibrillaire* was attached by Vulpian in 1874.[97]

The earliest (questioned by some) electrocardiogram of human VF was published by August Hoffmann in 1912; VF terminated the VT.[98] Because VF seemed analogous to atrial fibrillation in many ways, Lewis proffered his concept of a circus movement as the mechanism causing VF.[14] DeBoer first provoked VF in the frog ventricle by a single shock late in systole; he also favored reentry as the mechanism causing VF.[99] DeBoer's work was corroborated in 1940 when the concept and naming of the vulnerable period was firmly established by Wiggers and Wegria.[100] They induced VF by a single, localized induction and condenser shock applied during the vulnerable period of ventricular systole. In 1941, Wiggers, Wegria, and Moe found an increased duration of the vulnerable period in premature ventricular beats.[101]

The evolution of VF from VT was presented by a patient during an Adams-Stokes episode. Kerr and Bender in 1922 recorded that quinidine given to a patient with complete heart block induced VT that degenerated to VF; the electrocardiogram showing VF in their patient is the first undisputed example of human VF.[90]

ATRIOVENTRICULAR JUNCTIONAL RHYTHM

In 1903, Engelmann experimentally induced junctional rhythm in the frog heart by a ligature that isolated the sinus venosus and caused the atria and ventricles to beat simultaneously.[102] AV extrasystoles were described by Hering in 1906.[103] Lewis induced junctional rhythm in the dog's heart by cooling the sulcus terminalis.[104] He published an electrocardiogram of junctional tachycardia in humans in 1909, but gave priority to Belski. Lewis stressed the inverted P waves in leads II and III as a proof of junctional pacemaking.

PARASYSTOLE

In 1919, Kaufmann and Rothberger postulated that an ectopic focus could be protected from suppression by the normal cardiac pacemaker.[105] Subsequently, they defined parasystole to explain how certain extrasystoles and tachycardias could maintain autonomy independently of the dominant rhythm. In seven papers written over 6 years, they theorized that the ectopic center, constantly active and nearly perfectly rhythmic, was protected by a unidirectional block similar to that which is normally present in AV junctional tissue. It was considered an entrance block, to which there is added an exit block, so that the ectopic focus is protected throughout its complete cycle. They clearly described the interectopic interval, the varied coupling time, and the *Schutzblokierung* (protection).

SICK SINUS SYNDROME

Sinoatrial block was described by Mackenzie in 1902 during an epidemic of influenza.[106] At first thought to be a benign vagal phenomenon, SA block is now considered to be part of the sick sinus syndrome. In 1912, Cohn and Lewis reported an instance of Adams-Stokes attack from sudden asystole in a patient subject to paroxysmal atrial fibrillation.[107] In 1916, Samuel Levine described four patients with SA arrest following paroxysmal atrial fibrillation.[108] By 1951, Pick and coworkers instilled meaning to this phenomenon as expressed in the title of their article "Depression of Cardiac Pacemakers by Premature Impulses."[109]

However, except for Short's early (1954) and neglected article, titled "The Syndrome of Alternating Bradycardia and Tachycardia," paroxysmal atrial fibrillation, sinus bradycardia, SA arrest, SA exit block, and carotid sinus hypersensitivity were all considered unrelated nuisances.[110] When Lown in 1967 recognized that inadequate sinus node function at times appeared after cardioversion for atrial fibrillation, he coined the term *sick sinus syndrome*.[111] Both Short and Lown recognized that, because untreated atrial fibrillation was the natural cure of the sick sinus syndrome, these patients were better off without cardioversion.

In 1968, M. Irene Ferrer popularized the sick sinus syndrome.[112] However, she did not then include the bradycardia-tachycardia syndrome.

The ECG often showed intra-atrial block or a spatial orientation of the P wave different from the usual, suggesting takeover pacemaking not far from the diseased SA node. Posttachycardia bradycardia that shows delayed SA activation is also significant. Most often, however, the usual electrocardiogram was not diagnostic.

Studies using the Holter monitor, determining the SA nodal recovery time, and the induction of atrial premature depolarizations are useful for theoretic and patient-care problems, as demonstrated by Mandel and coworkers.[113]

CONCEALED CONDUCTION

After visual observation of a frog's heart, T. W. Engelmann in 1894 noted that a blocked atrial contraction was followed by prolonged AV conduction.[114] In 1905, Erlanger noted concealed conduction in his studies on complete heart block.[67] Engelmann and Erlanger postulated that the delayed conduction was caused by incomplete penetration of the junctional tissues, causing partial refractoriness. In 1925, Lewis and Master carefully studied incomplete penetration, and Ashman did the same in the turtle heart.[115,116]

The electrocardiogram was first used in the study of concealed conduction in atrial flutter with 2:1 block showing long and short cycles by Kaufmann and Rothberger in 1927.[117]

The importance of concealed conduction as the key to many arrhythmias, however, was submerged until 1948 when Richard Langendorf published "Concealed A-V Conduction: The Effect of Blocked Impulses on the Formation and Conduction of Subsequent Impulses."[118] Popularization, however, was delayed until 1956, when Katz and Pick further emphasized the mechanism and outlined its details.[119] Soon it was obvious that incomplete penetration could delay conduction, speed up conduction, cause block, slow down a pacemaker, or establish QRS aberrancy. Concealed conduction offered explanations for otherwise unexplainable electrical events in the surface electrocardiograms. In 1961, Hoffman, Cranefield, and Stuckey revealed the concealed impulse with experimental evidence that concealed conduction takes place in any part of the conduction system.[120]

Söderström pointed out in 1950 that the irregular ventricular response in atrial fibrillation is often because of concealed conduction; Moe, Abildskov, and Mendez in 1964 provided more sophisticated evidence to support this point.[34,121]

REENTRY

Reentry is not limited to the conduction tissues but can take place in any area of the heart. This concept, which is vital to the understanding of the generation of the tachyarrhythmias, was demonstrated by D. Scherf and C. Schookhoff[122] in 1926 by showing that experimental extrasystoles can return in the AV node and again activate the atria. They developed the idea that longitudinal dissociation exists in the AV node, allowing conduction up one half of the node and down the other.

Joseph Erlanger, an American physiologist and Nobel laureate, and Schmidt studied cardiac conduction in Adams-Stokes disease.[58] He published a graphic model for the reentry mechanism in which he recognized that reentry required both slowed conduction and unidirectional block. Moe and coworkers first demonstrated dual pathways in the AV node of animals in 1956.[123]

EXIT BLOCK

To explain why a parasystolic focus did not make its anticipated appearance late in diastole, in 1920, Kaufmann and Rothberger[124] and Singer and Winterberg[125] independently developed the concept of exit block. A conduction disorder involving failure of a cardiac pacemaker of any kind to propagate and depolarize adjoining myocardium, the exit block may be gradual (Wenckebach) or sudden (Mobitz).

WENCKEBACH AND MOBITZ BLOCK

The AV block that is progressively lengthened until an atrial complex is not conducted was first seen in the frog's heart by Engelmann in 1894.[114] Wenckebach, Engelmann's pupil, described this complicated arrhythmia in humans in 1899 from an insightful analysis of radial arteriograms and clearly showed that the greatest increase in conduction time occurred in the second complex of the group beats.[126] He also reported that Luciani had observed this phenomenon in the frog heart in 1872. Wenckebach called the pauses in the radial pulse *Luciani periods*. David Scherf noted that, in radial and venous pulse tracings sent by a friend to Wenckebach, dropped beats without AV hesitation were found.[127]

In a brilliant but neglected study, John Hay in 1906 published venous and arterial pulse tracings, clarified by laddergrams, that also showed normal AV conduction followed by absence of ventricular activation.[128] He believed the cause to be "depression of excitability." In 1924, Mobitz found Wenckebach periods (which he called type I) and the block described by Hay (which he called type II) in the same patient.[129] Mobitz type I was found to be a physiologic block and type II was caused by serious infra-AV nodal disease, as Wenckebach had surmised.[126]

Despite Hay's and Wenckebach's contributions, these blocks are called Mobitz I and Mobitz II.

VENTRICULAR ABERRATION

Ventricular aberration was first defined in 1925 by Thomas Lewis, whose famous book illustrates the varieties of aberration from permanent in bundle branch block, to variable in atrial fibrillation and flutter, to the single supraventricular extrasystole.[130] Lewis was acutely aware of the dilemma of deformed ventricular complexes caused by PAT that resembled VT.

However, it was 1947 before Gouaux and Ashman clarified the mechanism of aberration by relating it to the refractory period and cycle length.[131] "Aberration occurs when a short cycle follows a long one because the refractory period varies with cycle length," they wrote. Also stressed was the longer effective refractory period of the right bundle branch. Since then, the Ashman phenomenon has become an established phenomenon in arrhythmology.

Aberration was recognized clinically even before experimental verification by Moe and colleagues that the refractory period of the right bundle was longer than that of the left bundle.[132]

WOLFF-PARKINSON-WHITE SYNDROME

Because of inexplicable paroxysmal atrial fibrillation, a young athlete was referred to Paul Dudley White in 1928. The only abnormality that could be found was in the electrocardiogram, which revealed a short PR interval of only 100 milliseconds and an abnormal QRS resembling bundle branch block. Because gymnastics workouts had sometimes caused the tachycardia, the patient was asked to run up and down four flights of stairs. Unexpectedly, his electrocardiogram reverted to normal, with a PR of 160 milliseconds and a normal QRS at a heart rate of 120. After the patient rested, his electrocardiogram again became abnormal, and again reverted to normal after an injection of atropine was given. Once, when the tracing was normal, carotid sinus massage induced the abnormality of short PR and long QRS.

Dr. White unearthed six similar cases. Puzzled by these unusual electrocardiograms, he carried them with him on a tour of foreign medical centers. In Vienna, experts interpreted the abnormality as ordinary bundle branch block plus AV nodal rhythm. However, in London, Sir John Parkinson was intrigued sufficiently to search his own files and found five additional instances, which he mailed to White. The report by Wolff, Parkinson, and White in 1930 caused puzzlement, and interested electrocardiographers searched their own files.[133] In 1915, Frank Wilson had published "a case in which the vagus influenced the form of the ventricular complex of the electrocardiogram," which described the patient's "four distinct rhythms and at least three types of ventricular complexes."[134] After reading the Wolff-Parkinson-White (WPW) article, Wilson returned to his 1915 work and found that his fourth figure was a replica of the new

syndrome.[135] Similar earlier examples were found in reports by Wedd in 1921[136] and separately by Bach[137] and Hamburger[138] in 1929.

Krikler points out that the earliest publication of the electrocardiogram of a patient with WPW syndrome, undiagnosed by the authors, Cohn and Fraser, appears in the 1913–1914 volume of *Heart*.[139] The subject was a man who suffered from paroxysmal tachycardia for 57 years. He died of emphysema at age 86. An electrophysiologic study done in 1971 by Krikler demonstrated preexcitation with narrow-complex tachycardia.

The theory of an accessory conduction pathway between atria and ventricles bypassing the AV node was postulated independently by Holzmann and Scherf[140] in 1932 and by Wolferth and Wood[141] in 1933, based on Kent's anatomic discovery in animals published in 1893 and known to anatomists as the bundle of Kent.[142] The theory was confirmed in 1942 by Butterworth and Poindexter, who transmitted greatly amplified action currents from the SA node to the ventricle of a cat.[143] This electromechanical bypass of the AV node inscribed electrocardiograms resembling the WPW syndrome. By reversing the conduction pathway and sending amplified impulses from the ventricle to the atrium, bursts of tachycardia ascribable to reentry were generated. The explorations by Wilson's group of the hearts of patients with known WPW syndrome pointed to premature activation of the dorsal wall of the ventricle as a cause. Their patients' tracings showed alternating normal and anomalous conduction.[144]

Wood and coworkers[145] in 1943 and Ohnell[146] in 1944 proved the WPW syndrome by autopsy demonstration of bypass bundles. The Wood paper was based on a case of a young boy who died of tachycardia complicating his WPW syndrome. In 1967, Ferrer found sufficient studies by his own group and others to review the basic variants of preexcitation: the classic WPW syndrome, the Lown-Ganong-Levine syndrome, and the Mahaim type.[147] The Lenegre group showed multiple bypasses in certain patients, sometimes latent and sometimes active.[148]

His bundle electrophysiologic studies clarified the WPW conundrum (see Chap. 13).

TORSADE DE POINTES

If the WPW syndrome is likened to the Columbus of the arrhythmias because the original 11 cases generated thousands of investigations into the new world of bypass tracts and reentry, the atypical VT named torsade de pointes (twisting of the points) by Dessertenne in 1966 may be considered the Cinderella of the arrhythmias.[149] Dessertenne had become interested in the bizarre patterns of VF inscribed during cardiopulmonary resuscitation. An

80-year-old woman, long afflicted with complete heart block, entered his service at the Lariboisiére Hospital because of Adams-Stokes attacks that resulted in convulsions. Digitalis was discontinued. Procainamide, isoproterenol, and ephedrin were not helpful. Hydroxyzine hydrochloride, potassium, and propranolol gave only transient surcease. After ventricular asystole left the woman a neurologic cripple, her family took her home to die.

The three-channel electrocardiographic tracings showed the characteristics of torsade de points, which Dessertenne described as "a tachycardia whose frequency is 200 per minute, which displays alteration of the direction of the QRS complexes every 2 seconds, so that they successively point upwards and downwards." In another section, he writes that "the same phenomenon just described, recurring at a frequency of 200 per minute, with the difference that the amplitude of the QRS complexes now varies in a more definitely sinusoidal pattern. The first three torsades are especially interesting. Each lasts for about three seconds. . . . The complexes occurring during the transition between torsades maintain the same frequency. . . . This phenomenon of sinusoidal variation in the amplitude recalls the undulating phase of ventricular fibrillation described by Wiggers in his animal experiments."

Dessertenne suggested that "the occurrence of phasic variation in the electrical polarity of the QRS complexes during the arrhythmia could be explained by postulating two ventricular foci, one initiating QRS complexes pointing upwards, the other initiating complexes pointing downwards . . . The transition from one focus to the other generates a torsade de pointes."[150]

Even though Dessertenne's report was unique, torsade de pointes had been recognized earlier. Examples were found in works by MacWilliam[151] in 1923 and by Schwartz and associates in 1949[152] and 1954,[153] the latter work stressing the association of torsade de pointes with bradycardia and prolongation of the QT interval.

All class 1 antiarrhythmic drugs, which are therapeutic in many arrhythmias, have been found to evoke torsade de pointes in patients with normal QT intervals. Lethal torsade de pointes has even been caused by liquid-protein reducing diets.[154]

CONCLUSION

First, the many landmarks in the history of the arrhythmias show that advances have been made step by slow step. Second, it is likely that the electrocardiogram will maintain its worth, unlike the ballistocardiogram.

However, there were a few dissonant voices. P. M. Rautaharju, in a paper titled "Highways, Byways and Dead-ends in Electrocardiographic Research," declared, "There is too much information in the ECG and VCG for analysis by a human reader." Alan C. Burton concluded, "The science of electrocardiography is not purely empirical, but is based on fundamental experiments and physical laws: However, its enormous usefulness in clinical diagnosis has a basis that is almost empirical. Electrocardiography is like bird-watching, which depends not on theory, but on rules."[155]

References

1. Olmsted JMD: Claude Bernard, physiologist. New York: Schuman, 1938:25.
2. Shapiro E: Engelmann and his laddergram. Am J Cardiol 1977;39:464.
3. Cushny AR: On the action of substances of the digitalis series on the circulation in mammals. J Exp Med 1897;2:223.
4. Mobitz W: Zur Frage der atrioventrikularen Autonomie. Die Interferenz Dissoziation. Dtsch Arch klin Med 1923;141:257.
5. Wiggers CJ: Cardiac physiology of 50 years ago. Circ Res 1957;5:121.
6. Marey EJ: Des excitations électriques du coeur. In: Physiologie Experimentale. Travaux de Laboratorie de M Marey. Vol 2. Paris: Masson, 1876:63.
7. Burn JH: The relation of the autonomic nervous system to cardiac arrhythmias. Prog Cardiovasc Dis 1960;2:334.
8. Carlson AJ: Comparative physiology of the invertebrate heart. VI. The excitability of the heart during the different phases of the heart beat. Am J Physiol 1906;16:67.
9. Knoll P: Ueber die Veränderung des Herzschlages bei reflectorischer Erregnung des vasomotorischen Nervensystems. Wiener Sitzungberichte der deutschen Akademie der Wissenschafter 1872;66:195.
10. Engelmann TW: Ueber den Urspring der Herzbewegung und die physiologischen Eigenschaften der grossen Herznerven des Frosches. Arch Ges Physiol 1896–1897;65:109.
11. Wenckebach KF: Zur Analyse des unregelmässigen Pulses. Z klin Med 1900;39:293.
12. Cushny AR: On the interpretation of pulse tracings. J Exp Med 1899;4:327.
13. Kraus F, Nicolai GF: Ueber des Elektrokardiogramm unter normalen und pathologischen Verhältnissen. Berl klin Wchnschr 1908;34:1.
14. Lewis T: The mechanism and graphic registration of the heart beat, 3rd ed. London: Shaw and Sons, 1925:219.
15. Pan O: Klinische Beobachtung über ventrikuläre Extrasystolen ohne kompensatorische Pause. Dtsch Arch klin Med 1903;98:128.
16. Langendorf R, Pick A, Winternitz M: Mechanisms of intermittent bigeminy. 1 Appearance of ectopic beats dependent upon the length of the ventricular cycle, the "rule of bigeminy." Circulation 1955;11:422.
17. Satou T, Kinoshita S, Tanabe Y, et al: Impulse conductivity in the region surrounding the extrasystolic focus: Wenckebach phenomenon of the coupling intervals, and the "rule of multiples." Saishin-Igaku [Modern Medicine] 1960;15:1865 (in Japanese).

18. Schamroth L, Marriott HJL: Intermittent ventricular parasystole with observations on its relationship to extrasystolic bigeminy. Am J Cardiol 1961;7:779.

19. Adams R: Cases of diseases of heart accompanied with pathological observations. Dublin Hosp Rep 1827;4:353.

20. Balfour G: Clinical lectures on diseases of the heart and aorta. London: Churchill, 1882:256.

21. Marey EJ: Physiologie Médicale de la Circulation du Sang. Paris: Delahaye, 1863:525.

22. Mackenzie J: The inception of the rhythm of the heart by the ventricle, as the cause of continuous irregularity of the heart. BMJ 1904;1:529.

23. Hering HE: Analyse des Pulses irregularis perpetuus. Prager med Wchnschr 1903;38:377.

24. Hering HE: Das Elektrocardiogram des Pulsus irregularis perpetuus. Dtsch Arch klin Med 1908;94:205.

25. Rothenberger CJ, Winterberg H: Vorhofflimmern und Arrhythmia perpetuus. Wien klin Wchnschr 1909;22:839.

26. Lewis T: Auricular fibrillation: A common clinical condition. BMJ 1909;2:1528.

27. Einthoven W: Le Télécardiogramme. Arch Internat Physiol 1906–1907;4:132.

28. Gossage AM, Braxton Hicks JA: On auricular fibrillation. Q J Med 1913;6:435.

29. Engelmann TW: Refractäre Phase und kompensatorische Ruhe in ihrer Bedeutung für den Herzrhythmus. Arch ges Physiol 1894–1895;59:309.

30. Lewis T, Drury AN, Iliescu CC: A demonstration of circus movement on clinical fibrillation of the auricles. Heart 1921;8:361.

31. Scherf D, Romano FJ, Terranova R: Experimental studies on auricular flutter and auricular fibrillation. Am Heart J 1948; 6:241.

32. Scherf D: Versuche zur Theorie des Vorhofflatterns und Vorhofflimmerns. Z ges exp Med 1928;61:30.

33. Prinzmetal M, Oblath R, Corday E, et al: Auricular fibrillation. JAMA 1951;146:1275.

34. Söderström N: What is the reason for the ventricular arrhythmia in cases of atrial fibrillation. Am Heart J 1970; 40:212.

35. Bootsma BK, Hoelen AJ, Strackee J, et al: Analysis of R-R intervals in patients with atrial fibrillation at rest and during exercise. Circulation 1970;41:783.

36. MacWilliam JA: Fibrillar contraction of the heart. J Physiol 1887;8:296.

37. Ritchie W: Complete heart block with dissociation of the action of the auricles and ventricles. Proc R Soc Edinburgh 1905;25:1085.

38. Jolly WA, Ritchie WT: Auricular flutter and fibrillation. Heart 1910–1911;2:177.

39. Einthoven W: Le Télécardiogramme. Arch Internat Physiol 1906–1907;4:132, Fig. 32.

40. Lewis T: Observations upon a curious and not uncommon form of extreme acceleration of the auricle: "Auricular flutter." Heart 1913;4:171.

41. Prinzmetal M, Corday E, Brill C, et al: The auricular arrhythmias. Springfield, IL: Charles C Thomas, 1952:189.

42. Cabrera CE, Sodi-Pollares D: Discussion del movimento circular y prueba directa de su existencia en el flutter auricular clinico. Arch Inst Cardiol Mex 1947;17:850.

43. Rytand D: The circus movement entrapped. Circus wave hypothesis and atrial flutter. Ann Intern Med 1966;65: 125.

44. Wellens HJJ, Janse MJ, Van Dam RT, et al: Epicardial excitation of the atria in a patient with atrial flutter. Br Heart J 1971; 33:233.

45. Cohen SI, Koh D, Lau SH, et al: P loops during common and uncommon atrial flutter in man. Br Heart J 1977;39:173.

46. Cotton P: Notes and observations upon a case of unusually rapid action of the heart. BMJ 1867;1:629.

47. Bristowe JS: On recurrent palpitations of extreme rapidity in persons otherwise apparently healthy. Brain 1888;10:164.

48. Bouveret L: De la tachycardie essentielle paroxystique. Rév Méd 1889;9:753.

49. Hoffmann A: Die paroxysmale Tachycardie. Wiesbaden: Bergmann, 1900.

50. Gaskell WH: Observations on the innervation of the heart. BMJ 1882;2:572.

51. von Czermak JN: Ueber mechanische Reizung des Vagus bei Menschen. Prager Vierteljahrschrift 1868;100:30.

52. Winternitz W: Ein Beitrag zu den Motilitätsneurosen des Herzens. Berl klin Wchnschr 1883;20:93,112.

53. Lewis T: The experimental production of paroxysmal tachycardia and the effect of ligation of the coronary arteries. Heart 1909;1:98.

54. Lewis T: The mechanism and graphic registration of the heart beat. 3rd ed. London: Shaw and Sons, 1925:240–258.

55. Vidella JG: El sindrome electrocardiografico post-tachycardiaco. Rev Argent Cardiol 1947;14:30.

56. Mayerson RM, Clagett AH Jr: Transient inversion of T waves after paroxysmal tachycardia. JAMA 1952;143:193.

57. Scherf D: Studies on auricular tachycardia caused by aconitine administration. Proc Soc Exp Biol Med 1947;64:233.

58. Schmidt FO, Erlanger J: Directional differences in the conduction of the impulse through heart muscle and their possible relation to extrasystolic and fibrillary contractions. Am J Physiol 1928–1929;87:326.

59. Lown B, Marcus F, Levine HD: Digitalis and the atrial tachycardias with block. N Engl J Med 1959;260:301.

60. Gaskell WH: On the innervation of the heart, with especial reference to the heart of the tortoise. J Physiol 1883;4:43.

61. Huchard H: Maladies du Coeur et des Vaisseaux. Paris: Octave Doin, 1889:255.

62. Bloomfield AL: A bibliography of internal medicine. Chicago: University of Chicago Press, 1960:33.

63. Galabin AL: On the interpretation of cardiographic tracings and the evidence they afford as to the murmurs attendant upon mitral stenosis. Guy's Hosp Rep 1875;20:261.

64. Chauveau A: De la dissociation du rhythme auriculaire et du rhythme ventriculaire. Rév Méd 1885;5:161.

65. His W Jr: Die Tätigkeit des embryonalen Herzen und deren Bedeutung für die Lehre von der Herzbewegung beim Erwachsenen. Arbeiten aus der medizinischen Klinik zur Leipzig 1893:14–50.

66. His W Jr: Ein Fall von Adams-Stokes'scher Krankheit mit ungleichzeitigen Schlagen der Vorhöfe und Herzkammern (Herzblok). Dtsch Arch klin Med 1899;64:316.

67. Erlanger J: On the physiology of heart block in mammals, with especial reference to the causation of Stokes-Adams disease. J Exp Med 1905;7:676.

68. Erlanger J, Blackman JR: Further studies on the physiology of heart-block in mammals. Heart 1904;1:117.

69. Parkinson J, Papp C, Evans W: The electrocardiogram of the Stokes-Adams attack. Br Heart J 1941;3:171.

70. Robinson CC, Bredeck JF: Ventricular fibrillation in man with cardiac recovery. Arch Intern Med 1917;20:725.

71. Cohn AE, Lewis T: A description of a case of complete heart-block; including the postmortem examination. Heart 1912–1913;4:7.

72. Hay J: The pathology of bradycardia. BMJ 1905;2:1034.

73. Panum PL: Experimentale Beiträge zur Lehre der Emboli. Arch Pathol Anat 1862;25:308.

74. Lewis T: Single and successive extrasystoles. Lancet 1909;1:382.

75. Mackenzie J: Diseases of the heart. London: Oxford University Press, 1908:445.

76. Wenckebach KF: Beitrage zur Kenntnis der menschlichen Herztatikeit. Arch Anat Physiol 1906:297.

77. Palfrey FW: Paroxysmal tachycardia confined to the ventricles, with illustrative cases. Med Surg Rep Boston City Hospital 1913;16:182.

78. Willius FA: Paroxysmal tachycardia of ventricular origin. Boston Med Surg J 1913;178:182.

79. Robinson G, Herrmann G: Paroxysmal tachycardia of ventricular origin and its relation to coronary occlusion. Heart 1921;8:59.

80. Lewis T: The experimental production of paroxysmal tachycardia and the effect of ligation of the coronary arteries. Heart 1909;1:98.

81. Gallavardin L: Extrasystolie ventriculaire a paroxysmes tachycardiques prolonges. Arch Mal Coeur 1922;18:153.

82. Gallavardin L: Tachycardia ventriculaire terminale: complexes alternants ou multiformes; ses rapports avec une forme severe d'extra-systolie ventriculaire. Arch Mal Coeur 1926;19:153.

83. Rosenberg DH: Fusion beats. J Lab Clin Med 1940;25:919.

84. Dressler W, Roesler H: The occurrence in paroxysmal ventricular tachycardia of ventricular complexes transitional in shape to sinoauricular beats. Am Heart J 1952;44:485.

85. Wilson FN, Wishart SW, Mcloed AC, et al: A clinical type of paroxysmal tachycardia of ventricular origin in which paroxysms are induced by exertion. Am Heart J 1932;7:155.

86. Lemery R, Brugada P, Bella PD, et al: Non-ischemic ventricular tachycardia: Clinical course and long-term follow-up in patients without clinically overt heart disease. Circulation 1989;79:990.

87. Langendorf R, Pick A: Differentiation of supraventricular and ventricular tachycardias. Prog Cardiovasc Dis 1960;2:391.

88. Schwenensen C: Ventricular tachycardia as a result of the administration of digitalis. Heart 1922;9:199.

89. Levine S, Fulton MN: The effect of quinidine sulfate on ventricular tachycardia. JAMA 1929;92:1162.

90. Kerr WJ, Bender WL: Paroxysmal ventricular fibrillation with cardiac recovery in a case of auricular fibrillation and complete heart block while under quinidine sulfate therapy. Heart 1922;9:269.

91. Zimdahl WT, Kramer LI: On the mechanism of paroxysmal tachycardia with rhythmic alteration in the direction of the ventricular complexess. Am Heart J 1947;33:244.

92. Katz LN: The significance of the T wave in the electrogram and the electrocardiogram. Physiol Rev 1928;8:447.

93. Wiggers CJ, Wegria R, Pipa B: The effects of myocardial ischemia on the fibrillation threshold—the mechanism of spontaneous ventricular fibrillation following coronary occlusion. Am J Physiol 1940;131:309.

94. Smirk FH: R waves interrupting T waves. Br Heart J 1949;11:23.

95. Erichsen JE: On the influence of the coronary circulation on the action of the heart. London Med Gaz 1942;2:561.

96. Hoffa M, Ludwig C: Eine neue Versuche über Herzbewegung. Z rat Med 1850;9:107.

97. Surawicz B, Steffens T: Cardiac vulnerability in complex electrocardiography. J Cardiovasc Clin 1973;5(3):160.

98. Hoffmann A: Fibrillation of ventricles at the end of an attack of paroxysmal tachycardia in man. Heart 1912;3:213.

99. DeBoer S: Die Physiologie und Pharmakologie des Flimmerns. Ergeb Physiol 1923;21:1.

100. Wiggers CJ, Wegria R: Ventricular fibrillation due to single localized induction and condenser shocks applied during the vulnerable phase of ventricular systole. Am J Physiol 1940;128:500.

101. Wegria R, Moe GK, Wiggers CJ: Comparison of the vulnerable period and fibrillation thresholds of normal and idioventricular beats. Am J Physiol 1941;33:651.

102. Engelmann TW: Der Versuch von Stannius, seine Folgen und deren Deutung. Arch Anat Physiol (Physiol Abtheilung) 1903:505.

103. Hering HF, Rihl J: Ueber atrioventriculare Extrasystolen. Z exp Pathol Therap 1906;2:510.

104. Lewis T: Auricular fibrillation and its relationship to clinical irregularity of the heart. Heart 1909–1910;1:306.

105. Kaufmann R, Rothberger CJ: Beiträge zur Entstehungeweise extrasystolischer Aliorhythmien. Z ges exp Med 1919;7:119.

106. Mackenzie J: The cause of heart irregularity in influenza. BMJ 1902;2:1411.

107. Cohn AE, Lewis T: Auricular fibrillation and complete heart block. A description of a case of Adams-Stokes syndrome, including the post-mortem examination. Heart 1912–1913;4:15.

108. Levine S: Observations on sino-auricular heart block. Arch Intern Med 1916;17:153.

109. Pick A, Langendorf R, Katz LN: Depression of cardiac pacemakers by premature impulses. Am Heart J 1951;41:49.

110. Short DS: The syndrome of alternating bradycardia and tachycardia. Br Heart J 1954;16:208.

111. Lown B: Electrical reversion of cardiac arrhythmias. Br Heart J 1967;29:469.

112. Ferrer MI: The sick sinus syndrome in atrial disease. JAMA 1968;206:645.

113. Mandel WJ, Hawakawa H, Allen HN, et al: Assessment of sinus node function in patients with the sick sinus syndrome. Circulation 1972;46:761.

114. Engelmann TW: Beobachten und Versuche am suspendierten Herzen Pfluegers Arch 1894;56:149.

115. Lewis T, Master AM: Observations upon conduction in the mammalian heart. A-V conduction. Heart 1925;12:209.

116. Ashman K: Conductivity in compressed cardiac muscle; supernormal phase in conductivity in compressed auricular muscle in the turtle heart. Am J Physiol 1925;74:140.

117. Kaufmann R, Rothberger CJ: Der Uebergang von Kammerallorhythmien in Kammerarrhythmie in klinischen Fällen von VorhofflatterN Alternan der Reitzleitung. Z ges exp Med 1927;57:600.

118. Langendorf R: Concealed AV conduction: The effect of blocked impulses on the formation and conduction of subsequent impulses. Am Heart J 1948;35:542.

119. Katz LN, Pick A: Clinical electrocardography. 1. Arrhythmias. Philadelphia: Lea & Febiger, 1956:540.

120. Hoffman BF, Cranefield PF, Stuckey JH: Concealed conduction. Circ Res 1961;9:194.

121. Moe GK, Abildskov JA, Mendez C: An experimental study of concealed conduction. Am Heart J 1964;67:338.

122. Scherf D, Shookhoff C: Experimentelle Untersuchingen ueber die "Umkehr-Extrasystole." Wien Arch inn Med 1926; 12:50.

123. Moe GK, Preston GB, Burlington H: Physiologic evidence for a dual AV transmission system. Circ Res 1956;4:357.

124. Kaufmann R, Rothberger CJ: Beiträge zur Entstehungeweise extrasystolischer Allorhythmien. 4 Mitteilung. Z ges exp Med 1920;11:40.

125. Singer R, Winterberg H: Extrasystolen als Interferenzerscheinung. Wien Arch inn Med 1920;1:391.

126. Wenckebach KF: Zur Analyse des unregelmässigen Pulses. II Ueber den regelmässig intermitterenden Puls. Z klin Med 1899;37:475.

127. Scherf D: A cardiologist remembers. Perspect Biol Med 1968;11:615.

128. Hay J: Bradycardia and cardiac arrhythmia produced by depression of certain of the functions of the heart. Lancet 1908;1:139.

129. Mobitz W: Ueber die unvollstöndige Störung der Erregungsüberleitung zwischen Vorhof und Kammer des menschlichen Herzens. Z ges exp Med 1924;41:180.

130. Lewis T: The mechanism and graphic registration of the heart beat. 3rd ed. London: Shaw and Sons, 1925:127–133.

131. Gouaux JL, Ashman R: Auricular fibrillation with aberration simulating ventricular paroxysmal tachycardia. Am Heart J 1947;34:366.

132. Moe GK, Mendez C, Han J: Aberrant AV impulse propagation in the dog heart: A study of functional bundle branch block. Circ Res 1965;16:261.

133. Wolff L, Parkinson J, White PD: Bundle branch block with short PR interval in healthy young people prone to paroxysmal tachycardia. Am Heart J 1930;5:685.

134. Wilson FN: A case in which the vagus influenced the form of the ventricular complex of the electrocardiogram. Arch Intern Med 1915;16:1008.

135. Johnston FD, Lepeschkin E, eds: Selected Papers of Dr. Frank N. Wilson. Ann Arbor, MI: JW Edwards, 1954.

136. Wedd AM: Paroxysmal tachycardia with reference to normotropic tachycardia and the role of the intrinsic cardiac nerves. Arch Intern Med 1921;27:571.

137. Bach F: Paroxysmal tachycardia of forty-eight years duration and right bundle branch block. Proc R Soc Med 1929;22:412.

138. Hamburger WW: Bundle branch block. Four cases of intraventricular block showing interesting and unusual clinical features. Med Clin North Am 1929;13:343.

139. Krikler D: WPW syndrome: Long follow-up and an Anglo-American historical note. J Amer Coll Cardiol 1983;2:1216.

140. Holzmann M, Scherf D: Ueber Electrokardiogramme mit verkwezter Vorhof-Kammer-Distanz und positiven P-ZackeN Ztschr. F Klin Med 1932;121:404.

141. Wolferth CC, Wood FC: The mechanism of production of short PR intervals and prolonged QRS complexes in patients with presumably undamaged hearts: Hypothesis of an accessory pathway of auriculo-ventricular conduction (bundle of Kent). Am Heart J 1933;8:297.

142. Kent AFS: Researchers on structure and function of mammalian heart. J Physiol 1893;14:233.

143. Butterworth JC, Poindexter CA: Short PR interval associated with a prolonged QRS complex. A clinical and experimental study. Arch Intern Med 1942;69:437.

144. Rosenbaum FF, Hecht HH, Wilson FN, Johnston FD: The potential variations of the thorax and the esophagus in anomalous atrioventricular excitement (Wolff-Parkinson-White syndrome). Am Heart J 1945;29:281.

145. Wood FC, Wolferth CC, Geckler GD: Histological demonstration of accessory muscular connections between auricle and ventricle in a case of short PR interval and prolonged QRS complex. Am Heart J 1943;25:454.

146. Ohnell RF: Pre-excitation, a cardiac abnormality. Acta Med Scand 1944;152(suppl):74.

147. Ferrer MI: New concepts relating to the preexcitation syndrome. JAMA 1967;201:162.

148. Brechenmacher C, Laham J, Iris L, et al: Etude histologique des voies anormales de conduction dans un syndrome de Wolff Parkinson-White et dans un syndrome de Lown-Ganong-Levine. Arch Mal Coeur 1974;67:507.

149. Dessertenne F: La tachycardie ventriculaire à deux foyers opposés variables. Arch Mal Coeur 1966;59:263.

150. De Léan A: Translation of Dessertenne, F (136), distributed by Editorial Office, Ann Intern Med, Philadelphia, PA, with permission of Dr. André De Léan, Dr. Francois Dessertenne, J Ballière, Paris, France, October, 1980.

151. MacWilliam JA: Some applications of physiology to medicine. II. Ventricular fibrillation and sudden death. BMJ 1923; 2:215.

152. Schwartz SP, Orloff J, Fox C: The prefibrillatory period during established auriculoventricular dissociation, with a note on the phonocardiograms obtained at such times. Am Heart J 1949;37:21.

153. Schwartz SP, Hallinger LN: VI. Observations on the peripheral arterial pulse pressures in the course of transient ventricular fibrillation during established auriculoventricular dissociation. Am Heart J 1954;48:390.

154. Singh BN, Gaarder TD, Kanagae T, et al: Liquid protein diets and torsade de pointes. JAMA 1978;240:115–119.

155. Burton AC: Physiology and Biophysics of the Circulation. 2nd ed. Chicago: Year Book Medical Publishers, 1972:138.

Cardiac Arrhythmias, 3rd edition, edited by William J. Mandel.
J. B. Lippincott Company, Philadelphia © 1995.

2

Robert H. Anderson • Siew Yen Ho • John Wharton
Anton E. Becker

Gross Anatomy and Microscopy of the Conducting System

The morphology and microscopy described in this chapter are, for the most part, an endorsement of the initial descriptions of the conduction system by Tawara[1] and Keith and Flack[2,3] and their refinement by Monckeberg[4] and Koch.[5,6] The methodology of those early investigations (i.e., microscopic study of serial sections) is the same as that used today. Descriptions of the morphology of conduction tissue have been remarkably consistent since its discovery. Disagreements are mostly the result of interpretation of the morphologic findings in the light of electrophysiologic observations, which are rarely unequivocal.[7–10] Even though the function of a cell cannot be determined with certainty through use of microscopy, recent advances, including techniques of immunocytochemistry, are providing functional correlations.[11]

SINUS NODE

Gross Morphology

Cardiologists were aware of the site of the "ultimum moriens" before its morphologic substrate was described by Keith and Flack.[3] Wenckebach[12] suggested to Keith that

Supported in part by a grant from the British Heart Foundation.

histologic study of the site of "ultimum moriens" may prove fruitful, particularly in view of the findings of Tawara[1] and Keith and Flack[2] at the atrioventricular junction. Consequently, the sinus node was discovered and was subsequently proven to be the cardiac pacemaker by the anatomico-electrophysiologic correlations of Lewis and coworkers.[3,13] In their initial publication, Keith and Flack described the lateral position of the node in the terminal groove.[3] This finding was endorsed by Koch, who also described the variable extent of the tail of the node, which continued in the terminal groove toward the orifice of the inferior caval vein (Fig. 2-1).[5] This lateral position of the node has been substantiated by most subsequent investigators.[14,15] Hudson, however, argued that the node was related in horseshoe fashion to the junction of the superior caval vein with the crest of the right atrial appendage.[16] Our findings largely confirm the opinion of those who observed the node in lateral position (Fig. 2-2), although we found it arranged in horseshoe fashion in a minority of cases (Fig. 2-3).[17]

As Truex indicated, the precise shape of the node as seen in sections depends on the plane of section used.[14] In sections at right angles to the terminal groove, the node forms an immediately subepicardial wedge set into the junction of the wall of the superior caval vein with the terminal crest (Fig. 2-4). The wedge of tissue is usually most bulky anteriorly toward the crest of the atrial ap-

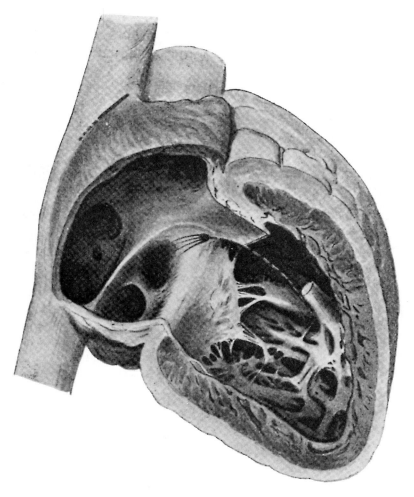

Figure 2-1. Diagram showing position of the sino-atrial node and the relation of the atrioventricular node to the triangle of Koch. (Koch W: Weitere Mitteilungen uber den Sinusknoten des Herzens. Verk Dtsch Pathol Ges 1909;13:85.

pendage and tends to taper as its tail passes posteriorly toward the inferior caval vein (see Fig. 2-2). Serial reconstructions have shown a variable extent of the nodal tissue. In infant hearts, the tail is usually extensive. An extension across the crest of the atrial appendage toward the interatrial band is rare (Fig. 2-5).

The node is usually related to a prominent nodal artery that runs toward the node in the interatrial furrow, originating from the right coronary artery in 55% of cases and from the left coronary artery in the remainder.[15] In the human heart, James has described how the artery can then run clockwise or counterclockwise around the supe-

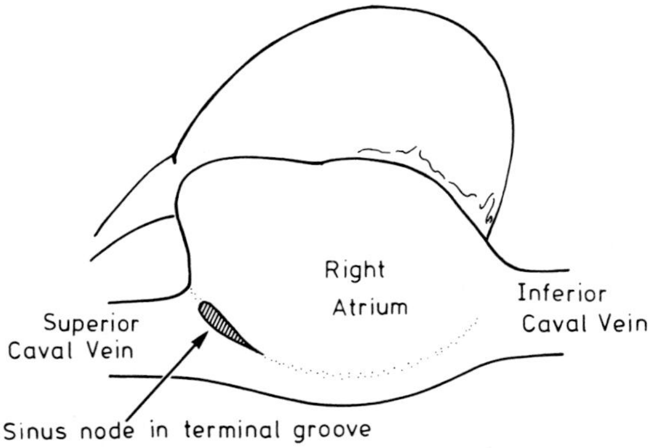

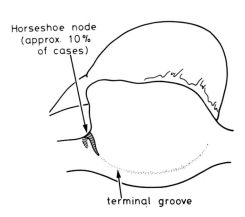

Figure 2-2. Diagram of the heart in surgical orientation showing the lateral position of the sinus node.

Figure 2-3. Horseshoe position of the sinus node.

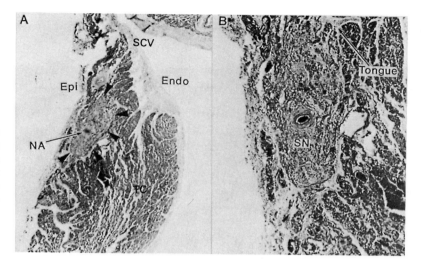

Figure 2-4. (**A**) Photomicrograph at low power showing the relation of the sinus node (SN) (*between arrows*) to the wall of the superior caval vein (SCV), the terminal crest (TC), and the epicardial (Epi) and endocardial (Endo) surfaces of the cavoatrial junction. The node is seen in a section at right angles to its long axis and the terminal groove, and is arranged around a prominent nodal artery (NA). (**B**) Enlarged view shows a tongue of transitional cells extending into the atrial musculature.

rior cavo-atrial junction.[15] Our serial reconstructions confirm and extend this observation.[17] In some cases, arteries enter the node from both sides, forming an arterial circle around the junction (Fig. 2-6A). We have also found more variation in the origin of the nodal artery, a feature noted previously by McAlpine.[18,19] Although the nodal artery arises from either the right or left coronary arteries (usually close to their origin) (Fig. 2-7), it may also arise laterally from the right artery (Fig. 2-8A) or distally from the circumflex artery (see Fig. 2-8B). These findings have major surgical significance in that they show that the precise disposition of the node and its arterial supply cannot be predicted with accuracy. The entire junction between the superior caval vein and the right atrium should be treated as a potential danger area. The anomalous routes across the atrial walls should be identified. Not only is the course of the nodal artery variable but its

relation to the nodal tissue is variable also. The artery runs completely through the nodal substance in only a proportion of cases. Otherwise, the artery ramifies within the nodal substance, runs an eccentric course through the node, or is not a prominent artery (see Fig. 2-6B). It is difficult to reconcile these findings with the contention that the sinus node and its artery function as a servomechanism.[20]

Development

Various views have been expressed concerning development of the sinus node. Some researchers contend that it is developed early; others contend that it does not become recognizable morphologically until relatively late.[21–24] Some researchers suggest that it is a derivative of the right

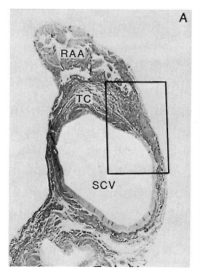
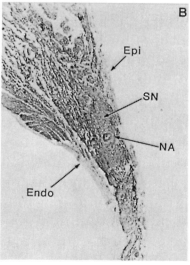

Figure 2-5. Photomicrographs at low power (**A**) and enlarged (**B**) showing the relation of the sinus node (SN) to the junction of the superior caval vein (SCV) and right atrial appendage (RAA). The node is between the terminal crest (TC) and the caval musculature. *Epi*, epicardium; *Endo*, endocardium; *NA*, nodal artery.

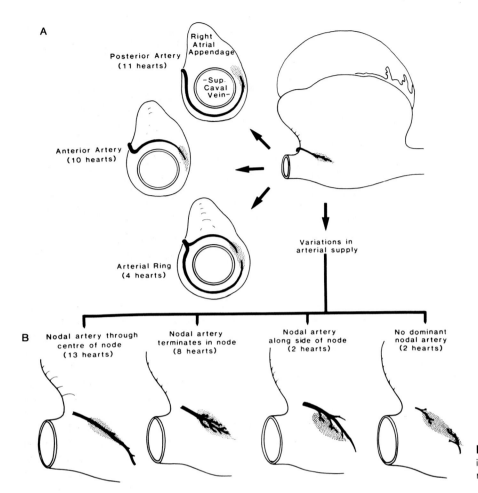

Figure 2-6. Diagram showing variability in arterial blood supply to the sinus node as reconstructed by serial section techniques.

side of a pair of specialized structures related to the sinus horns; others suggest that it is a unilateral structure related to the right sinus horn.[25–27] Our own investigation demonstrated that a histologically discrete area can be recognized at the cavo-atrial junction in the earliest embryos studied (Fig. 2-9).[28] The position of this area corresponds approximately to the position of the definitive node, being marginally more extensive in the embryo. It does not occupy the entire sinuatrial junction (Fig. 2-10). We recognized such a histological discrete structure only in relation to the superior caval vein. The area of the left sinus horn was devoid of tissue that was histologically discrete from the remainder of the atrial tissues. The size of the node relative to atrial tissues is greatest early in development. As

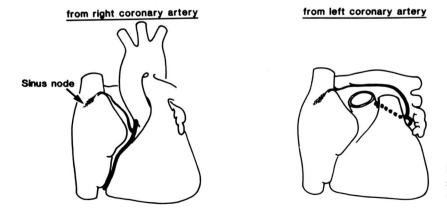

Figure 2-7. Diagram showing the origin of the sinus node artery from the proximal portion of the right or left coronary arteries.

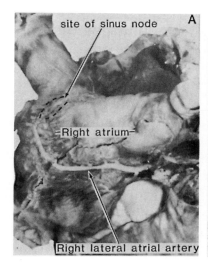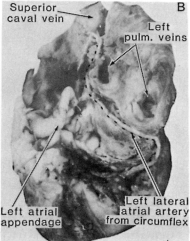

Figure 2-8. Photographs of two dissected hearts show the sinus node artery arising from a right lateral artery (**A**) and from a left lateral artery (**B**).

the heart grows, the area occupied by sinus nodal tissue decreases relative to the remainder of the atrial bulk. From the earliest stages of development, the nodal cells are set in a matrix of connective tissue. The volume of connective tissue within the node is small in the youngest embryos but becomes more evident toward term.[28]

Microscopy

The cells making up the sinus node are histologically discrete from the cells of the atrial myocardium and can be distinguished at low powers of magnification (see Figs. 2-4

and 2-5). The prominent nodal artery seen in most hearts and the fibrous tissue matrix are other good guides to nodal identification. The nodal cells are smaller than atrial myocardial cells. They are grouped together in interweaving fasciculi, the whole intermingling network of cells being set in the prominent fibrous matrix (see Fig. 2-5B). At the nodal surfaces that face the myocardium of the superior caval vein and the terminal crest, junctional zones are found between the nodal cells and the atrial myocardium. In some areas, the margin between node and atrial myocardium is discrete (see Fig. 2-5B). In other areas, tongues of nodal cells extend into the atrial myocardium, merging via short zones of transitional cells into the myocardial zones. In these interdigitating zones, the overlapping of nodal and atrial cells can be interpreted as atrial cells being present within the confines of the node.[13] These zones of interdigitation are most frequently observed on the nodal surface, which abuts against the terminal crest, but their precise distribution remains to be

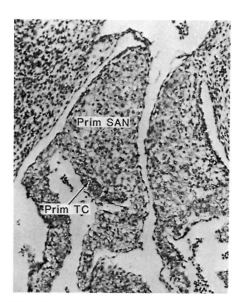

Figure 2-9. Photomicrograph of the junction of the superior caval vein and right atrium in a 15-mm human fetus. The distinction between the cells that will become the node (Prim SN) and those that will form the terminal crest (Prim TC) is already evident.

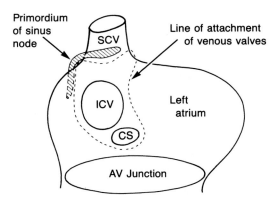

Figure 2-10. Diagram illustrating the extent of the nodal primordium shown in Figure 2-9. The primordium is related only to the junction of the right atrium with the superior caval vein (SCV). *ICV,* inferior caval vein; *CS,* coronary sinus.

quantified. Our experience has mostly been with infant and developing tissues, and we have rarely observed the large pale atrial cells sometimes described as "Purkinje" cells.[15] The function and presence of these cells in the atria is contentious, and the use of the term "Purkinje" to describe them compounds the problem. According to Truex, "It is recommended that the term 'Purkinje cell' be restricted and applied only to the specific cells of the ventricle which Purkinje described originally. The indiscriminate use of this term for large atrial cells leads not only to semantic problems but also connotes a functional pacemaker property that has never been established."

The true cellular content of the sinus node can best be established by using ultrastructural techniques in well-fixed material controlled by light microscopy. This way, the investigator can ensure that nodal material is being sampled. These criteria have thus far only been fulfilled in animal tissues. Tranum-Jensen has shown that the node of the rabbit is composed mostly of typical nodal cells.[29] These cells are irregular, roughly spindle-shaped, and sometimes branching, with thin, tapering ends. They possess poorly developed contractile apparatus and randomly distributed mitochondria. The sarcoplasmic reticulum is less well-developed than in the atrial myocardium, and a T-tubule system is lacking. However, Tranum-Jensen points out that T-tubules are not universally observed in working atrial cardiocytes, and atrial "specialized cells" cannot, therefore, be defined according to the presence or absence of T-tubules. At the margins of the rabbit node, Tranum-Jensen observed transitional cells that differed from the typical nodal cells by containing more and better-organized myofibrils and a higher content of nexus junctions. Regarding the pale cells, or "intercalated clear cells" described in the human sinus node, Tranum-Jensen suggested that the cells may be artifactual.[30]

Innervation

The mammalian sinus node is the most densely innervated region of the heart and can be distinguished from adjacent myocardium by its abundant nerve supply. Histochemical studies have indicated that the innervation comprises both presumptive cholinergic, acetylcholinesterase positive nerves and adrenergic nerves displaying catecholamine fluorescence. Ultrastructural analysis has also revealed that nodal cells are innervated by nonmyelinated varicose nerve fibers containing small clear vesicles and granular vesicles that are thought to contain acetylcholine and noradrenaline, respectively. (For reviews, see Yamauchi[31]; Canale and coworkers.[32]) The methods used in earlier studies to visualize the innervation of the conduction system were not adequate to identify the entire innervation or to differentiate between efferent and afferent subpopulations of nerves. To some extent, these limitations may be overcome by the application of immunohistochemical techniques and the use of antisera to both general neural markers and antigens considered to be selective for subtypes of nerves. The antigens include enzymes involved in neurotransmitter synthesis and several biologically active peptides that have distinct distribution patterns in autonomic and sensory nerves and which may modulate cardiac functions (see Wharton and Gulbenkian[33]).

There are extensive differences in the pattern of cardiac innervation in various species, and, while the sinus node generally receives a dense innervation, the distribution and neurochemical content of the nerves supplying it vary considerably. In the human sinus node, presumptive parasympathetic nerves appear to predominate, whereas sympathetic fiber displaying neuropeptide tyrosine and tyrosine hydroxylase immunoreactivity is prominent in perivascular networks. The extent to which the nodal innervation arises from cell bodies extrinsic or intrinsic to the heart is not clear, but local intrinsic cardiac ganglia are concentrated in tissues around the sinus node. Recent findings in the bovine heart suggest that nerves in the sinus node displaying neuropeptide tyrosine immunoreactivity are mainly of postganglionic sympathetic origin, but some may also arise from local nonsympathetic ganglion cells, which lack immunoreactivity for the catecholamine synthesizing enzymes.[34]

As in other mammals, the human heart exhibits a progressive pattern of innervation during development, with the sinus node, atrioventricular junction, and atria receiving nerves before the ventricular walls.[35] Throughout the first 7 to 24 weeks' gestation, the nerve supply to the human fetal sinus (Fig. 2-11) and atrioventricular junctional tissues is more dense than that observed in the rest of the heart. Between 7 and 10 weeks' gestation, nerves and ganglia are distributed in the adventitia surrounding the ascending aorta and pulmonary trunk and in the region of the sinus node. We have not, however, demonstrated the presence of peptide-containing nerves before 10 weeks' gestation, and, as in the adult human heart, neuropeptide tyrosine-immunoreactive nerves predominate and are concentrated in perivascular networks.[36] Somatostatin-immunoreactive nerves are also present by 10 to 12 weeks' gestation in the sinus node, atrioventricular junctional tissue and atrial myocardium may arise locally from intrinsic postganglionic cardiac neurons. Therefore, innervation of the human conduction system appears to occur at an early stage of cardiac development and is consistent with electrophysiologic findings suggesting that there is also an early functional maturation of the human conduction system.[37,38] The development of this innerva-

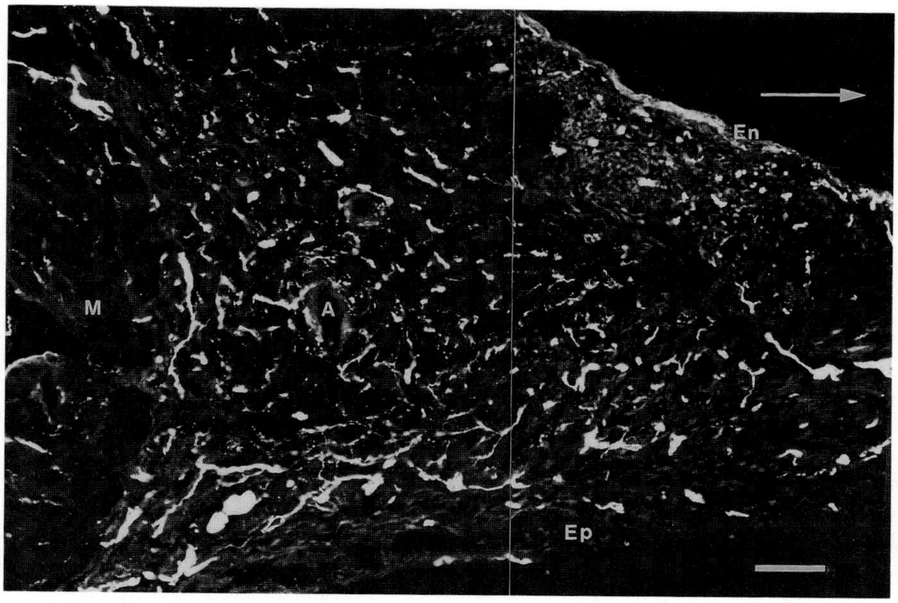

Figure 2-11. Photomicrograph of a section of a human fetal sinus node (18 weeks' gestation) showing a relatively dense innervation compared with the adjacent myocardium (M). Nerve fibers and fascicles are distributed throughout the node and surround the central artery (A). The innervation was demonstrated using an indirect immunofluorescence technique and an antiserum to the general neural marker protein gene product 9.5. *Arrow*, direction of the superior caval vein; *Ep*, epicardium; *En*, endocardium; *Bar*, 100 μm.

tion and that of the myocardium in general may be facilitated by neural cell adhesion molecules that are present on the surface of myocardial and conduction cells and that exhibit a temporal regulation that is expressed at high levels during cardiac development in both rat and man.[36,39]

INTERNODAL CONDUCTION

Controversy concerning the anatomic substrates for conduction between the sinus and atrioventricular nodes is as old as the history of the conduction system itself. Some investigators have suggested that Wenckebach described an internodal tract.[8,12] He did observe a bundle of myocardial fibers connecting the musculature of the superior caval vein to the muscle of the right atrial appendage, but he did so before the discovery of the sinus node. At the time, Wenckebach believed that this bundle of myocardial fibers might conduct the impulse from the "ultimum moriens" to the atrial myocardium and that its division might result in sinuatrial block. When Keith and Flack described the precise morphology of the sinus node, Wenckebach realized that his bundle could have no significance to sinuatrial block.[3,40]

The first real suggestion of a histologically discrete pathway between the nodes was made by Thorel.[41,42] He claimed to have traced a tract of "Purkinje" cells running along the terminal crest and connecting the nodes. This suggestion was debated at a session of the German Pathological Society in 1910.[43] The consensus of this meeting was that Thorel had not shown unequivocal evidence of a histologically discrete pathway as he claimed. In the opinions of Aschoff,[44] Monckeberg,[45] and Koch,[46] the tissue between the nodes was composed of plain atrial myocardium and did not contain histologically discrete pathways separate from this myocardium. To avoid subsequent disagreements, these observers suggested that investigators claiming to demonstrate atrial pathways should show them to be discrete in a fashion analogous to that seen in the atrioventricular conduction tissue axis. Despite this advice, authors such as Condorelli[47] and Franco[48] described atrial pathways using histologic criteria as tenuous as those of Thorel, but their suggestions were not generally accepted. The real impetus to a search for histologically specialized tracts came with the finding that not all cells in the atria had the same electrophysiologic characteristics.[49] Construing this to mean that specialized pathways had been demonstrated unequivocally using electrophysiologic techniques, James stated that the problem to be investigated was not whether pathways existed but rather where they were.[8] Based on subserial and dissection techniques, James described three "specialized pathways" connecting the nodes: anterior, middle, and posterior. James seems to have described the entire atrial septum and the terminal crest as these three specialized pathways.

The outstanding morphologic question concerning "specialized internodal pathways" is this: Does the area of the atrial septum and terminal crest contain tracts that have features distinguishing them histologically from other atrial myocardium, or is the myocardium of these areas different from the remaining atrial myocardium? In our experience, no one has suggested, based on morphologic observations, that narrow tracts exist in the atrial septum and terminal crest that are comparable with the atrioventricular bundle and bundle branches. The problem of the specialized pathways devolves simply on the criteria for specialization.

For James, the primary criterion that determined the three pathways comprised the whole atrial septum and the terminal crest was that they contained a high percentage of "Purkinje" cells, thus differentiating them from the rest of the atrial myocardium. Concerning the pathways, Truex states, "The present intensive search for anatomic evidence to substantiate the presence or absence of the much publicized atrial internodal tracts has been a tedious and time consuming task. Indeed we have looked at innumerable SAN and atrial myocardial cells in many hearts of several mammals, but alas, we have failed to delineate the widely acclaimed specific interatrial pathways. . . . It is concluded that bundles of regular atrial muscle cells are the predominant elements that provide cellular continuity between the SAN and AVN."[3] More recently, similar conclusions were reached by Lev and Bharati.[50] Chuaqui had previously voiced these opinions after an extensive review of the literature and his own stereomicroscopic investigation.[51, 52] Thus, most modern investigators, except James, substantiate the views of the early German researchers.[53]

Our own studies, mostly using fetal and infant hearts, are in keeping with the majority viewpoint. The small size of the specimens has enabled us to cut the entire right atrium, including the atrial septum and the terminal crest, in a single block of tissue. In these sections, the sinus and atrioventricular nodes are easily distinguished by their histologic characteristics. They show unequivocal evidence of histologic specialization (Fig. 2-12). The remainder of the atrial tissues (apart from the atrioventricular ring specialized tissue) shows no evidence of morphologic or histochemical specialization. As viewed through the light microscope, the atrial septum and terminal crest are composed solely of plain atrial myocardium. It was rare in our material to find large pale cells resembling so-called Purkinje cells. When present, such cells were also found in the tissues of the right atrial appendage

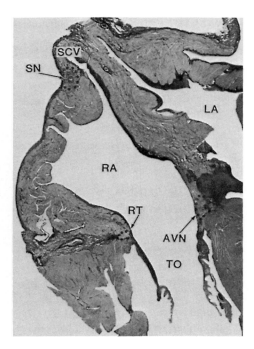

Figure 2-12. Low-power photomicrograph of a section of the right atrium (RA) cut to transect both the sinus node (SN) and atrioventricular node (AVN). Both structures can be easily recognized at low-power magnification. By using light microscopy, however, the muscle mass connecting the nodes cannot be distinguished from the remainder of the atrial myocardium. The segment of ring tissue (RT) at the lateral insertion of atrial myocardium into the tricuspid orifice (TO) can be recognized. *LA*, left atrium; *SCV*, superior caval vein.

and the left atrium. We, therefore, strongly endorse the opinions of Aschoff,[44] Monckeberg,[45] Koch,[46] Chuaqui,[51, 52] Truex,[14] and Lev and Bharati[50] that there are no histologically discrete tracts of specialized conduction tissue extending between the sinus and atrioventricular nodes. The tissue conducting the impulse is best referred to as the *internodal atrial myocardium.* Even though histologically "specialized internodal tracts" have not been identified, the possibility should not be disregarded that either there is preferential conduction of the cardiac impulse through the atrial myocardium or that cells with different electrophysiologic properties exist within the myocardium. The existence of preferential conduction is well established, but its pattern is attributed to the geometric arrangement of the muscle bundles of the right atrium (Fig. 2-13).[54-56] The behavior of given cells within the atrial myocardium may have no bearing on conduction within the atrium. The significance of this finding will only be resolved by performing marking experiments and studying the marked tissue with the electron microscope. Experiments performed so far have shown that plain atrial myocardial cells can produce both "working" and "specialized" action potentials.[57]

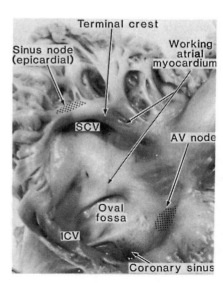

Figure 2-13. The anatomy of the right atrium is that of a bag of holes. The simple geometric arrangement of the atrial myocardium accounts fully for the preferential conduction that exists between the nodes. *AV*, atrioventricular; *ICV*, inferior caval vein; *SCV*, superior caval vein.

ATRIOVENTRICULAR ARI

The atrioventricular junctional area is the area of specialized conduction tissues forming the connection between the atrial and ventricular working myocardium.[58] It can be subdivided into various anatomic zones, namely the atrioventricular node and its transitional cell zone, the penetrating bundle, and the branching atrioventricular bundle (Fig. 2-14). Opinion varies on definition of the subdivision and extent of the zones of the specialized junctional area and whether the branching bundle should be considered part of the junctional area.[59] These differences are related to clinical correlations and can only be resolved by extensive anatomico-clinical correlations.

Gross Morphology

Koch described the gross landmarks to the site of the atrial component of the specialized junctional area.[5,6] He identified the atrioventricular node toward the apex of a triangle formed by the continuation of the eustachian valve (the

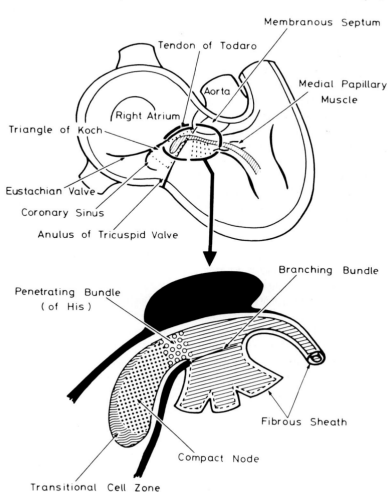

Figure 2-14. Diagram showing the gross landmarks of the atrioventricular junctional area and its cellular components and zones.

tendon of Todaro), the septal attachment of the tricuspid valve, and the orifice of the coronary sinus (see Fig. 2-1).[60] At the apex of this triangle, the tendon of Todaro inserts into the central fibrous body. Immediately posterior is the site of the penetrating atrioventricular bundle. After passing into the ventricular tissues, the axis branches on the crest of the muscular interventricular septum immediately subjacent to the interventricular component of the membranous septum. The left ventricular specialized tissues are immediately subendocardial on the septal surface of the ventricular outflow tract and cascade immediately beneath the noncoronary aortic leaflet. On the right ventricular side, the right bundle branch extends intramyocardially from the branching bundle. In the normal heart, the medial papillary muscle is an excellent guide to its position. These landmarks are valuable guides to the conduction tissues during surgery, because, in most living hearts, the triangle of Koch springs into prominence when tension is placed on the eustachian valve. In fixed hearts, it is usually possible to see the left bundle branch as it extends down the left ventricular septal surface.

Development

Knowledge of the development of the atrioventricular junctional area aids in the understanding of its subdivision and cellular architecture. Our interpretation of development is based on studies of developing hearts.[61, 62] Initially, we thought that, at the earliest stage of development, the atrial and ventricular myocardial segments were continuous all around the atrioventricular junction with a ring of histologically discrete tissue forming the muscular junction (Fig. 2-15). We argued that this atrioventricular ring was discrete from the primordium of the branching bundle, which we believed to be located on the crest of the muscular septum connecting with the subendocardial networks of both ventricles (see Fig. 2-15). We now know that the primordium of node and ventricular conduction tissues derives from a ring of specialized cells positioned between the inlet and outlet components of the ventricular segment of the heart tube, with growth of the atrioventricular and ventriculo-arterial junctions. With connection of the right atrium to the developing right ventricle and of the aorta to the left ventricle, the inlet ring transforms into a "figure of eight," enclosing the tricuspid and aortic orifices (Fig. 2-16). The only part of this ring that persists in the definitive heart is the axis of atrioventricular node and the ventricular bundle branches. The connections of the atrial myocardium to the axis occur concomitant with formation of the definitive atrial septum.

Before formation of the atrial septum, the arrangement bears no resemblance to the arrangement in the mature heart, but it is highly reminiscent of the arrange-

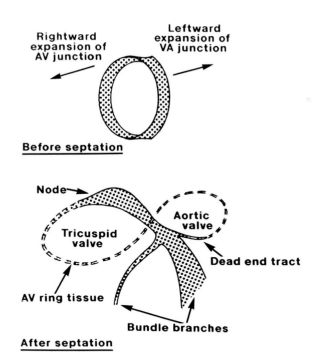

Figure 2-15. Initially, there is only one ring positioned in interventricular position in the developing heart tube (*upper panel*). It is expansion of the atrioventricular (AV) and ventriculo-arterial (VA) junctions (*lower panel*) that converts this interventricular ring to its final shape.

ment seen in hearts with atrioventricular septal defects.[63–65] At this early stage, the endocardial cushions (which help septate the atrioventricular junction) are on the endocardial aspect of the developing axis of conduction tissue. Additional tissue, the atrioventricular groove (sulcus) tissue, is present on the epicardial aspect, and extensions from this tissue surround the developing bundles (Fig. 2-17). A "sandwich" is, therefore, formed of sulcus, conduction, and cushion tissues, and persists into the definitive heart. At this stage, there is a long nonbranching bundle extending along the inlet septum, which meets with atrial tissues only at the posterior atrial wall. As the atrial septum forms, the atrial tissues are initially in contact only with the endocardial cushions, which separate the atrial myocardium from the conduction axis running on the inlet septum (Fig. 2-18A). With increasing development and growth, there is a gradual recession of the endocardial cushions, permitting the inferior rim of the atrial septum to make contact with the conduction bundle on the ventricular septum. What had originally been a long nonbranching bundle is converted into the definitive compact atrioventricular node (see Fig. 2-18B). The newly formed node is still in directly subepicardial position and is separated from the ventricular myocardium by extensions of the adipose tissue of the

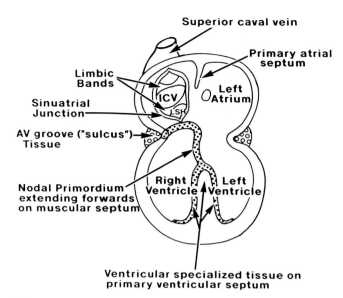

Figure 2-16. Diagram showing the location of the primordial ring of conduction tissue subsequent to expansion of the right atrioventricular junction. *IVC,* inferior caval vein.

atrioventricular groove (see Fig. 2-18C). The compact portion of the definitive node and the penetrating bundle are, therefore, derived from the same developmental source, termed the nodal–bundle axis (see Fig. 2-17). The point of division between the node and penetrating bundle depends on the degree of recession of the endocardial cushions. It is the point at which the insulating tissue of the central fibrous body (derived in part from the cushions) comes to separate the atrial myocardium from the nodal–bundle axis. Because the atrial septum grows down onto the conduction tissue axis to form the node, the definitive node is an interatrial structure.[66] The remnants of the initial ring of conduction tissue persist as the "rests" of atrioventricular ring tissue around the tricuspid orifice and the dead-end tract in the aortic root (see Fig. 2-15).

Cellular Architecture and Microscopy

The junctional area is disposed of as an axis of conduction tissue carried on the muscular interventricular septum, which then extends upward into the atrial septum. Its components are described here as it ascends from the ventricular into the atrial myocardium.

The branching bundle is arranged on the crest of the apical trabecular septum, immediately beneath the membranous septum, so that the right bundle branch is the anterior continuation of the axis. In contrast, the left bundle branch fibers cascade from the axis as a continuous fan.

Massing and James disagreed with our suggestion that the right bundle was the direct continuation of the nodal–bundle axis.[67, 68] Subsequent studies have confirmed their opinion. Thus, in neonatal hearts, a "dead-end tract" has been shown to be the direct continuation of the axis, with the tract ending blindly within the central fibrous body.[69]

We have considered the axis as the penetrating bundle proximal to the point of descent of the "first" left bundle branch fiber (Fig. 2-19). Hecht and colleagues divided this zone of the axis, in which it passes from the atrial tissues to the "first" left bundle branch fiber, into two portions, namely the penetrating bundle and the nonbranching bundle.[59] We have examined some normal hearts in which this arrangement is found. In most normal hearts, however, the nodal–bundle axis starts to branch as soon as it emerges from the central fibrous body onto the septal crest. The distinction between the penetrating bundle and the compact node is best made at the point at which the nodal–bundle axis enters the central fibrous body, thereby ceasing to make contact with the atrial myocardium (Fig. 2-20). This point depends on the formation of the central fibrous body (Fig. 2-21).

In some hearts, the "last" contact is made with the superficial overlay fibers of the right side of the atrial septum. In other hearts, it is made with the deeper left-sided septal musculature.[58] The atrial portion of the axis can be divided into the compact node and the transitional

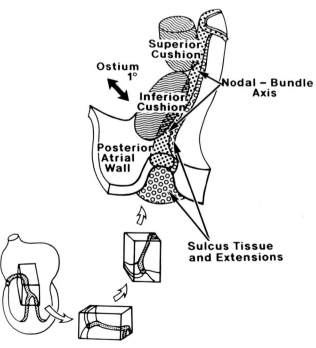

Figure 2-17. Diagram showing the mechanisms of insulation of the atrioventricular conduction axis. The insets show how the diagram is reorientated from the position shown in Figure 2-16.

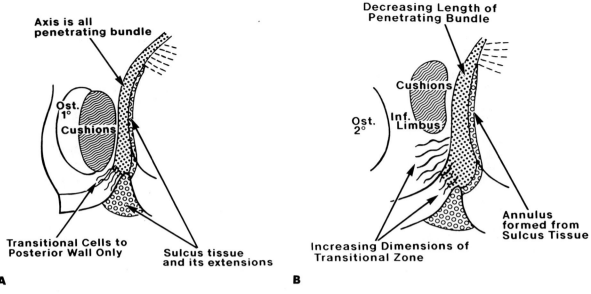

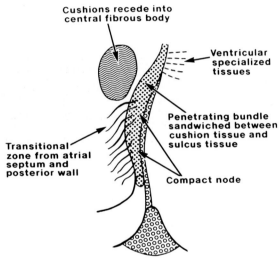

Figure 2-18. Diagram showing progressive stages in conversion of the axis of atrioventricular condition tissue, initially a penetrating bundle, into the atrioventricular node concomitant with formation of the definitive atrial septum.

cell zone. Throughout its length, the compact node retains a close relationship to the fibrous ring, which forms its baseplate (see Fig. 2-20). It can usually be traced as two extensions that continue along the baseplate, the right extension running toward the tricuspid valve and the left extension toward the mitral valve (see Fig. 2-20). This arrangement of an axis of conduction tissue penetrating the fibrous plane and bifurcating posteriorly was described and illustrated by Tawara (Fig. 2-22).[1]

The transitional cell zone is a diffuse area of atrial muscle interposed between the working myocardium and the specialized cells of the compact node. It was termed the *nodal approaches* by Hecht and coworkers.[59] In most

hearts, the transitional cells are most conspicuous posteriorly between the bifurcating extensions of the compact node (see Fig. 2-20C), but they also form a half-oval cap for the compact node itself (see Fig. 2-20B).

The working atrial myocardium approaches the node and its transitional zones from all sides. Two areas are particularly important. These are the areas identified (subsequent to ablations using surgical and radio frequency shocks) as the fast and slow pathways into the atrioventricular node. Almost certainly these pathways involve, in part, the working myocardium of the atrial approaches. The fast pathway is composed, in part, of the fibers streaming down from the anterior wall of the oval fossa and coursing

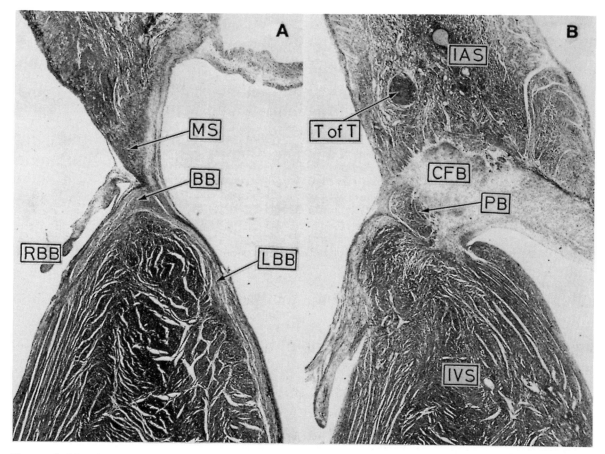

Figure 2-19. Photomicrographs through the junctional area of the heart of a child sectioned from anterior (**A**) toward posterior (**B**). In (**A**), the branching bundle (BB) is directly beneath the membranous septum (MS), which in this heart has only an atrioventricular component. The right bundle branch (RBB) is the continuation of the nodal bundle axis (see Figs. 2-16 through 2-18). The left bundle branch (LBB) fans out from the axis as a sheet of cells. In (**B**), the penetrating bundle (PB) passes through the central fibrous body (CFB). The tendon of Todaro (T of T) is already striking upward into the atrial septum (IAS). *IVS*, interventricular septum.

across the transitional cells that enclose the compact node. The slow pathway approaches the node through the musculature in the floor of the coronary sinus. By extrapolation from the locations of the lesions used to divide those pathways, it seems that they are some distance from the histologically specialized tissues of the atrioventricular node and its transitional zones, albeit that the fast pathway is much closer than the slow. The features of the pathways that give them their electrophysiologic properties have yet to be elucidated.

From the standpoint of histology, the cells of the atrial portion of the junctional area are smaller than the working atrial myocardial cells. In the transitional cell zones, the cells are long and attenuated, tending to be separated from each other by fibrous tissue strands. In the compact node, the cells are more closely packed together and are fre-

quently arranged in interconnecting fasciculi and whorls (Fig. 2-23). In many hearts, there is evidence of stratification of the compact node into deep and superficial layers, as described by Truex and Smythe.[70] The additional layer of overlying transitional cells gives the node a trilaminar appearance (Fig. 2-24). As the node becomes the penetrating bundle, there is a marginal increase in cell size, but, for the most part, the cellular architecture is comparable with that seen in the compact node.[58] It is difficult to differentiate node and penetrating bundle based on histology. For that reason, we prefer a distinction based on architecture, namely, the point at which the axis enters the fibrous body. The cells making up the branching bundle are similar in size to the ventricular myocardial cells. It is rare to observe pale or swollen cells (so-called Purkinje cells) in the specialized junctional area of infants and young children.

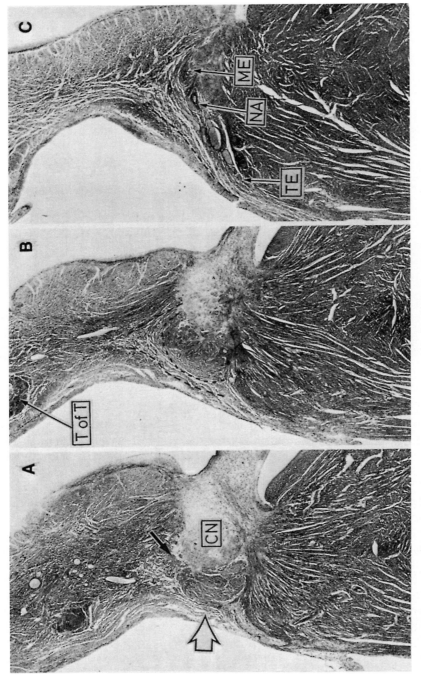

Figure 2-20. Photomicrographs continuing the series shown in Figure 2-19. (**A**) shows the junction between compact node (CN) and penetrating bundle. The axis has passed between the tricuspid anulus fibrosus and the central fibrous body, and is now the node because it is making contact with atrial transitional cells, both from the overlay area (*open arrow*) and the deep part of the septum (*closed arrow*). (**B**) shows the body of the compact node. It is set as a half-oval against the anulus fibrosus (*within dots*), with the transitional cell zone (*within dashes*) circling the compact zone. Note the tendon of Todaro passing out of the section. (**C**) shows the posterior reaches of the junctional area. The compact zone has bifurcated into extensions that pass toward the tricuspid (TE) and mitral (ME) valve attachments. The transitional cell zone surrounds these extensions (*within dashes*) and the nodal artery (NA) enters between them.

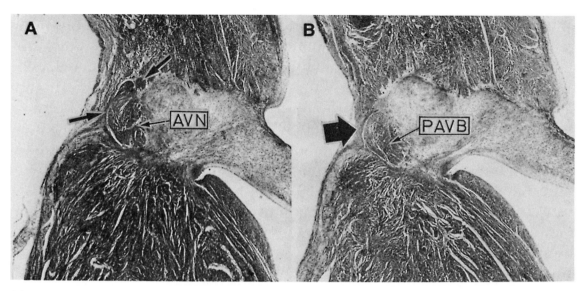

Figure 2-21. Photomicrographs showing the distinction between compact node (AVN) and penetrating bundle (PAVB) in the junctional area illustrated in Figures 2-19 and 2-20. In (**A**), the axis makes contact with atrial tissues (*between arrows*) and is, therefore, the compact node. In (**B**), the axis, identical in histologic terms, is engulfed in the central fibrous body and is prevented by fibrous tissue (*arrow*) from making contact with the atrial septum. It is, therefore, the penetrating bundle.

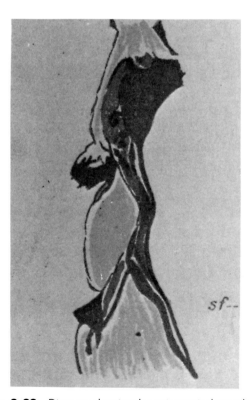

Figure 2-22. Diagram showing the atrioventricular node. In this infantile heart, the nodal–bundle axis of tissue interdigitates with the central fibrous body and has an extension that runs toward the mitral valve. This diagram can be compared with Figures 2-19 and 2-20. (Tawara S: Das Reitzleitungssystem des Saugetierherzens. Jena: Gustav Fischer, 1906.)

Electron Microscopy and Anatomico-Electrophysiologic Correlations

Most knowledge of the electrophysiology of the junctional area has come from studies of the rabbit heart. There are significant differences between the architecture of the rabbit junctional area and that of the human, so direct comparisons cannot be made. The classical studies of Paes de Carvalho[71] working in the laboratory of Hoffman[72] showed that (from an electrophysiologic standpoint) the rabbit junctional area was a trilaminar structure with AN, N, and NH zones. Some anatomic studies showed little morphologic evidence of such a nodal division.[73] In contrast, combined histologic and histochemical studies demonstrated that the rabbit junctional area was indeed a trilaminar structure. Transitional, midnodal, and lower nodal zones were identified, the latter being directly continuous with the atrioventricular bundle.[74] Subsequent anatomico-electrophysiologic correlative investigations in the rabbit using a cobalt marking technique showed that the AN potentials were produced in the transitional cell zone and the NH potentials in the anterior part of the lower nodal zone (Fig. 2-25).[75] N potentials were recorded from the small knot of middle nodal cells but were also recorded from cells in the transitional zone. The greater part of nodal delay was produced in the transitional cell area. Because the entire area of the "compact node" of the rabbit is isolated from the atrial tissues by an extensive collar derived from the central fibrous body, in terms of

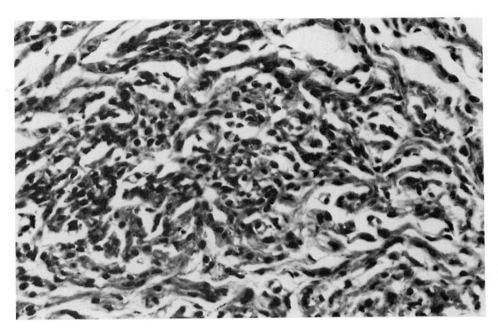

Figure 2-23. High-power photomicrograph of the cells of the compact node shown in Figures 2-19 through 2-21. The cells are small and aggregated into interweaving fasciculi.

human architecture, the whole of the rabbit "node" is considered to be the penetrating bundle.

The division of the rabbit node into morphologically discrete cellular areas has been confirmed by ultrastructural observations.[29] The cells in the different areas possess a similar ultrastructure, having few myofibrils and randomly arranged mitochondria. In this respect, the cells resemble those of the sinus node. The differences between the areas of the rabbit node are seen in the arrangement of the cells. The transitional cells are arranged individually, the upper nodal cells are aggregated in a ball, and the lower nodal cells are grouped together in cable fash-

ion.[29] Ultrastructural studies of the human node have not been performed with the precision of the study in the rabbit, largely because of the difficulty of obtaining optimal fixation.[29] Thus, the details of differences between human and animal junctional areas at the ultrastructural level remain unresolved.

Innervation

Atrioventricular junctional tissues are well innervated by both parasympathetic and sympathetic nerves. Many nerve fibers and fascicles occur amongst cells in the compact

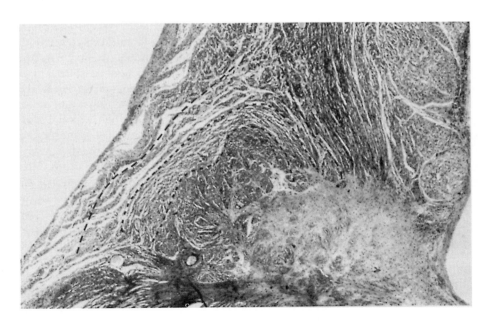

Figure 2-24. Photomicrograph of the compact node illustrated in Figures 2-19 through 2-21 showing how the compact node has two strata (*dotted lines*), with the transitional cell zone (*dashed line*) giving the atrial part of the junctional area a trilaminar appearance.

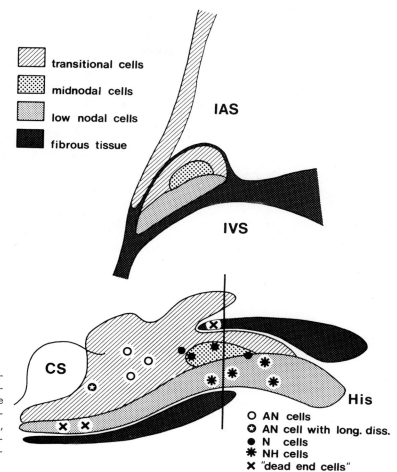

Figure 2-25. Diagram showing the correlation between action potential configuration and nodal morphology in the rabbit atrioventricular junctional area. (Janse MJ, Van Capelle FJL, Anderson RH, et al: Electrophysiology and structure of the AV node. In: Wellens HJJ, Lie KL, Janse MJ, eds. The conduction system of the heart—structure, function and clinical implications. The Hague: Martinus Nijhoff, 1976; with permission.)

node, and, in the surrounding tissue, large numbers of nerves and ganglion cells have been found. (For reviews, see Yamauchi[31]; Canale and coworkers.[32]) As with the sinus node, major species variations exist in the innervation pattern of the atrioventricular junction. For example, in the lower nodal bundle of the rabbit and atrioventricular node of the rat, there are numerous acetylcholinesterase positive and catecholamine-containing nerves.[76–79] The guinea pig atrioventricular node and ventricular conduction system contains a dense acetylcholinesterase reactive innervation as well but lacks sympathetic nerves, as demonstrated by both catecholamine fluorescence and by immunohistochemistry for tyrosine hydroxylase and neuropeptide tyrosine immunoreactivity.[80] The guinea pig atrioventricular node and bundle branches also receive a rich afferent innervation, displaying immunoreactivity for calcitonin gene-related peptide and tachykinins such as substance P, for which we have found no counterpart in other mammals, including man.[81]

There is uncertainty regarding the distribution of nerves supplying the penetrating bundle and bundle branches. As in the sinus node and atrioventricular junc-

tion, there are marked variations in the pattern of innervation of the ventricular conduction system among species. Generally, the ventricular conduction system receives fewer nerves than the nodal regions. Nerve fibers and fascicles run parallel to conduction cells in subendocardial bundle branches in man as well as in other mammals (Fig. 2-26). The sympathetic innervation may be greater than was previously thought and is of a similar density to that seen in the myocardium.[34, 82–84] Parasympathetic nerves, on the other hand, are thought to occur more frequently in association with conducting tissues than with the ventricular myocardium where they are generally sparse. Our recent studies, nonetheless, have shown that cholinesterase-containing nerves are sparse in the human atrioventricular bundle and its branches.

In addition to the distribution of nerves, the discrete anatomic relationship of receptors in the conduction system is also being examined using quantitative receptor imaging techniques on tissue sections.[85] Beta-1 and beta-2 adrenoceptors have been localized to the sinus and atrioventricular nodes of the rat and guinea pig, where the density of adrenoceptors and proportion of beta-2 recep-

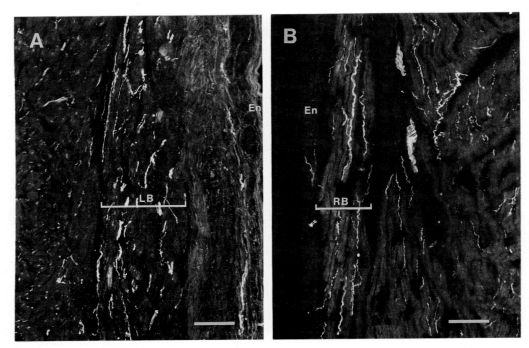

Figure 2-26. Photomicrographs of longitudinal sections of left and right bundle branches in adult human heart (**A**) and cat heart (**B**). Nerve fibers and fascicles run in the conducting tissue and underlying myocardium of the interventricular septum. The nerves display immunoreactivity for the general neural marker protein gene product 9.5 (**A**) and for neuropeptide tyrosine (**B**), which is mainly found in sympathetic nerves in the cardiovascular system. *LB*, left bundle branch; *RB*, right bundle branch; *En*, endocardium; *Bar*, 100 μm.

tors is greater than in the myocardium.[86-88] Because selective beta-2 agonists have preferential effects on heart rate, it has been suggested that beta-2 adrenoceptors may have a role in modulating heart rate. Angiotensin II also exerts positive chronotropic effects on the heart and the localization of angiotensin II binding sites in the mammalian conduction system suggests that it, too, may directly influence heart rate.[89]

Autoradiographic analysis of receptor subtypes in the conduction system should clarify their role in regulating heart rate and their possible involvement in disorders of cardiac rhythm.

SPECIALIZED ATRIOVENTRICULAR RING TISSUE

When serial sections are taken of the parietal atrioventricular junctions in many hearts, "rests" of histologically specialized tissue are found sequestrated in the atrial myocardium at its insertion to the junctions.[90] This arrangement is particularly noticeable at the anterolateral quadrant of the right atrioventricular junction. These "rests" are almost certainly the remnants of the more complete ring of spe-

cialized tissue present in fetuses, observed initially by Keith and Flack[3] and confirmed by our studies.[62] When seen in mature hearts, these areas of specialized tissue are markedly reminiscent of the structures described by Kent in 1893 and which were subsequently illustrated. We are concerned about the application of Kent's name to the accessory atrioventricular connections that unequivocally underscore the Wolff-Parkinson-White variant of preexcitation, but we do not doubt Kent's descriptions. Although we endorse Kent's illustrations, we have never observed in normal hearts these "rests" of atrioventricular ring specialized tissue effecting connections across the junction. But the structures do exist as nodes of Kent. Bundles of Kent, however, exist only in rare circumstances.

VENTRICULAR SPECIALIZED TISSUES

It has been suggested that the human left bundle branch system is bifascicular in nature.[93] Initial illustrations of the left bundle branch prepared by Tawara, however, showed the left bundle branch cascading down the septal surface in fanlike fashion from the branching bundle and ramifying into the left ventricle in some hearts in trifascicular

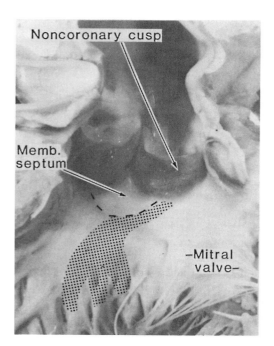

Figure 2-27. Photograph of a normal human heart illustrating the distribution of the conduction system as viewed from the left ventricle.

fashion.[1] This arrangement has been endorsed by numerous subsequent investigators including Rossi[94] and Uhley and colleagues.[95] Despite the overwhelming anatomic evidence, the concept of a bifascicular left bundle branch received enthusiastic acceptance by a clinical audience who found that it provided a basis for their electrocardiographic findings. Recent studies employing serial methods of reconstruction have shown unequivocally that the left bundle branch does not have a bifascicular structure.[67,96] Our own findings are in keeping with the majority viewpoint (Fig. 2-27). We find that the left bundle branch fibers originate as a single sheet from the branching bundle on the crest of the trabecular septum. As it descends, the sheet fans out into three broad divisions: anterior, septal, and posterior (see Fig. 2-27). On the smooth part of the septum, the left bundle branch is clearly isolated from the ventricular myocardium by a fibrous sheath (Fig. 2-28). The cells of the left bundle can be distinguished from the myocardial cells by their position and staining characteristics. Rarely in our experience with infant and child material have these cells shown "Purkinje" characteristics. When traced peripherally, the cells ramify into the ventricular myocardium. When the cells lose their aggregation and tissue sheath, it becomes

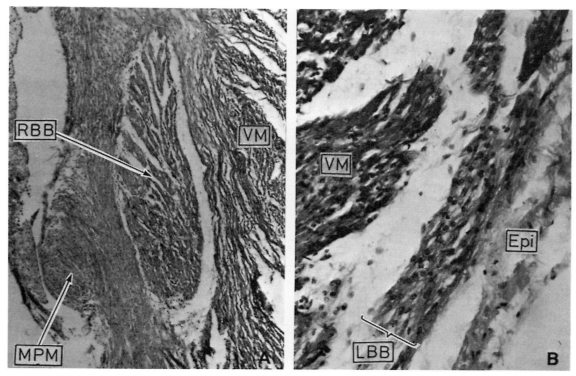

Figure 2-28. Photomicrographs showing a normal right bundle branch (RBB) (**A**) and left bundle branch (LBB) (**B**) in an infant heart. The bundles are discrete from the ventricular myocardium (VM). Their cells are in size similar to those of the myocardial cells. *MPM,* medial papillary muscle; *Epi,* epicardium.

difficult to differentiate a specialized cell from an ordinary myocardial cell.

The right bundle branch continues on from the branching bundle in the general direction of the nodal–bundle axis (see Fig. 2-14). It is a thin cordlike structure that usually runs intramyocardially. Its cells frequently cannot be distinguished on cytologic grounds from the working myocardium, but the bundle can easily be traced through serial sections because of its aggregation and fibrous sheath (see Fig. 2-28). As with the left bundle, when the right bundle branch breaks up distally, it is difficult to trace the terminal ramifications because of the cytologic similarities with myocardium.

Atrial Natriuretic Peptide and the Conduction System

Immunohistochemical techniques can be used to distinguish cells of the conduction system from myocardial cells by their content of intermediate filaments and by regional differences in the distribution of myosin heavy-chain isoforms.[97–100] The ventricular conduction system may also be delineated by the demonstration of other antigens, including the putative cardiac hormone atrial natriuretic peptide. This peptide is produced by transcription of a single gene encoding a large precursor molecule, which gives rise to

an active circulating peptide, alpha-ANP_{1-28}, that modulates the regulation of extracellular fluid volume and vasomotor tone. (For reviews, see Atlas[101]; Ballerman and Brenner[102]; Needleman and coworkers[103]; Goetz.[104]) The expression of this gene is not confined to the atria, as was originally thought, but occurs in the ventricles as well as in other extracardiac tissues. Messenger ribonucleic acid and immunoreactivity have been shown to be present in mammalian ventricular tissues and cultured cells.[105–112] Expression of the gene also exhibits developmental regulation, in that it is higher in fetal than adult tissues.[105,112–114] It has been demonstrated that immunoreactivity is present at an early stage of fetal development in the human ventricular conduction system (Fig. 2-29) as well as in atrial and ventricular myocardium.[115] Immunoreactivity has not, however, been detected in cells of the human sinus and atrioventricular nodes. A similar, differential distribution pattern has been found in the hearts of adult animals (pig, rat, guinea pig, and cat), in which immunostaining for the peptide was localized to ventricular bundle branches, atrial myocardium, and overlay and transitional cells, but was absent from cells in the compact sinus and atrioventricular nodes.[116–121] Explanted adult human hearts from transplant patients also display immunostaining of bundle branches for natriuretic peptide (see Fig. 2-29) as well as immunoreactivity for general neuroendocrine markers.[115] Regulation of gene expression in the ventricular conduc-

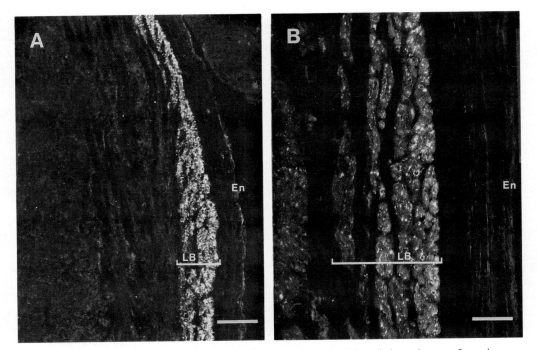

Figure 2-29. Photomicrographs of longitudinal sections through left bundle branches in a 9-week human fetus (**A**) and an explanted heart from a 21-year-old patient with cystic fibrosis (**B**). Both sections show presence of atrial natriuretic peptide (ANP) immunoreactivity in conducting cells, displaying a characteristic perinuclear localization. *Bar*, 100 μm.

tion system, therefore, appears to be distinct from that in the atrial and ventricular myocardium. The differential distribution of immunoreactivity in the ventricular conduction system seems also to be a general feature of the mammalian heart, which is consistent with the view that the ventricular conduction system is derived separately from the nodal regions.[122] Changes in cardiac rhythm effect the release of the peptide from the heart.[123-125] The conduction system may contribute to this, but the functional significance of production of the peptide in cells of the conduction system remains to be established.

ANATOMIC SUBSTRATES OF PREEXCITATION

Ventricular preexcitation happens when the ventricles are activated more rapidly than would be expected if the impulse was conducted via the normal atrioventricular junctional area.[126] Although it has been suggested that the disorder can result from a functional malformation in a normal conduction system, it is more usual to search for discrete anatomic "short circuits" of the junctional area as its cause.[127] To understand the site and morphology of such substrates, the disposition of the normal junctional specialized tissues and the morphology of the atrioventricular junctional insulating mechanism must be understood.

Atrioventricular Fibrous Rings

In the normal heart, the atrioventricular bundle is believed to be the only muscular structure connecting the atrial and ventricular myocardial tissues, although, as James has indicated, studies comparable to those carried out in hearts with ventricular preexcitation are lacking in normal hearts.[128] In any search for accessory muscular atrioventricular connections in hearts with preexcitation, the entire atrioventricular junction must be studied. As Lev has commented, such studies are exceedingly time-consuming.[129] To provide some information on this topic and on the structure of the fibrous rings themselves, we have conducted subserial sectioning of the atrioventricular muscular junctions in human hearts (Fig. 2-30). These studies do not provide the precision demanded in hearts with preexcitation.[128] Nevertheless, we believe the studies provide important information regarding the anatomic substrates for this malformation. In the subserial sections, we never observed any atrioventricular muscular connections outside the specialized junctional area. We did observe that the fibrous ring of the mitral valve was a solid, well-formed collagenous structure which, at all points, separated the atrial and ventricular myocardial tissues and

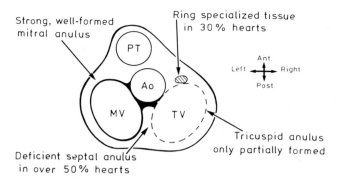

Figure 2-30. Results obtained from the study of the anulus fibrosus in normal hearts. *Ao,* aorta; *MV,* mitral valve; *PT,* pulmonary trunk; *TV,* tricuspid valve.

supported the mitral valve leaflets. In contrast, the ring of the tricuspid valve was variably formed, even in individual hearts. At some points in each of the hearts studied, segments of collagenous tissue separated atrial and ventricular myocardial segments. At other points in the same hearts, the junction was turned in and the collagenous ring supported only the tricuspid leaflets, with the atrial and ventricular muscular tissues being separated only by the adipose tissue of the atrioventricular groove. A similar variability was found in the region of the septum. In most of the hearts studied, only the adipose atrioventricular groove tissue separated the posterior reaches of the compact atrioventricular node and the base of the atrial septum from the ventricular septum. Furthermore, when viewed from within the right atrium, the compact node appears as an anterior structure close to the central fibrous body.[130] The node, nonetheless, is also a directly subepicardial structure (Figs. 2-31 and 2-32). The tissue plane of the posterior atrioventricular groove extends beneath the coronary sinus toward the central fibrous body. The artery to the atrioventricular node runs through the plane (see Fig. 2-32). Rests of histologically specialized tissue are found adjacent to the tricuspid valve fibrous ring (see Fig. 2-30). These are the remnants of the atrioventricular ring specialized tissue initially illustrated by Kent.[91,92]

Anatomic Substrates for Preexcitation

The function of the specialized atrioventricular junctional area is to produce delay. In animal hearts, most of the delay occurs in the transitional cell zones of the area.[75] Some delay is also produced in the atrioventricular bundle and bundle branches because these structures are isolated from the septal myocardium and the normal impulse must traverse their length before activating the ventricular myocardium. Consequently, there are several possibilities whereby anatomic connections could "short-circuit" all or

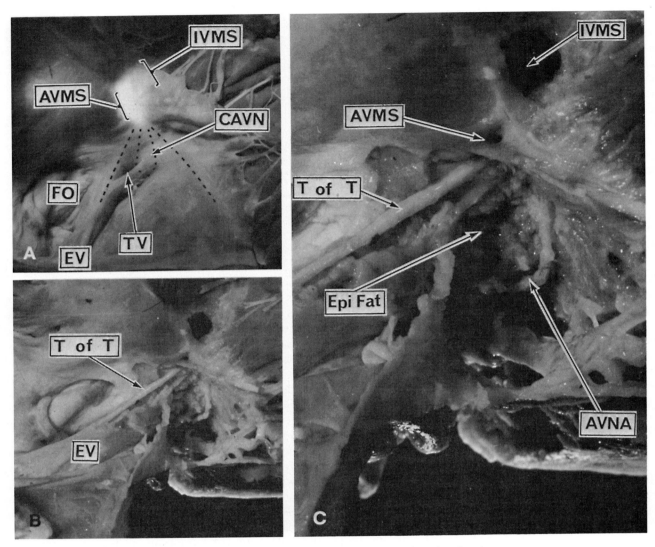

Figure 2-31. Dissection illustrating the position of the atrioventricular node and its directly subepicardial position. *AVMS,* atrioventricular membranous septum; *AVNA,* atrioventricular nodal artery; *CAVN,* compact atrioventricular node; *EpiFat,* epicardial fat; *EV,* eustachian valve; *FO,* oval foramen; *IVMS,* intraventricular membranous septum; *T of T,* tendon of Todaro; *TV,* tricuspid valve.

part of this normal delay. The morphology of these connections has been described by several investigators, notably by Lev.[129]

The use of eponyms to describe various connections confuses the correlation of anatomic and clinical studies. For example, accessory atrioventricular connections existing outside the specialized junctional area are widely termed "bundles of Kent," yet the connections thus described bear no resemblance to the structures observed by Kent himself, which are the remnants of the atrioventricular ring specialized tissue.[91,92] According to Sherf and James, because there is no resemblance between these structures and the actual connections, "bundles of Kent" is an inappropriate eponym.[131] This point is conceded by

those who use it in the interests of brevity.[132] The propriety of the eponym has been debated by ourselves[133] and Sealy.[134] The structures illustrated by Kent do not resemble the accessory atrioventricular connections, which, in almost all cases, are the substrates of preexcitation.

The fibers initially described by Mahaim do short-circuit the specialized junctional area.[135] They are found in normal hearts and can be divided into groups that arise from the node and others that arise from the fascicular portion of the conduction axis. These fibers must be distinguished from other fibers in the parietal atrioventricular junction producing so-called Mahaim physiology.

Further confusion exists with regard to the nodal bypass fibers described by James as being present in the

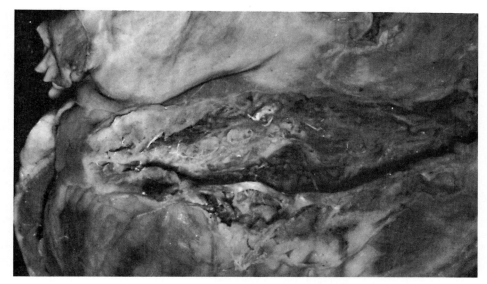

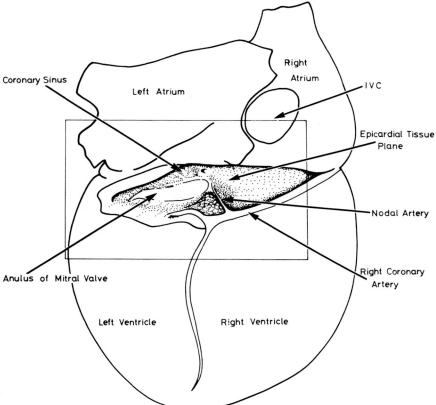

Coronary Sinus

Left Atrium

Right Atrium

IVC

Epicardial Tissue Plane

Nodal Artery

Right Coronary Artery

Anulus of Mitral Valve

Left Ventricle

Right Ventricle

Figure 2-32. Dissection of a normal human heart showing the tissue plane beneath the coronary sinus, which extends from the posterior atrioventricular sulcus to the region of the atrioventricular node and the central fibrous body.

normal heart.[7] These tracts do not resemble the fiber tract described by Brechenmacher in hearts with short PR-normal QRS syndrome, yet such syndromes are frequently explained based on so-called James fibers.[136]

We suggested that eponyms be avoided in the nomenclature of preexcitation and that descriptive terms be used instead.[137] The possibilities for a short-circuit of the junc-tional area, therefore, can be considered in terms of accessory atrioventricular connections, accessory nodo-ventricular connections, accessory fasciculoventricular connections, accessory atriofascicular connections, and intranodal bypass tracts (Fig. 2-33). For the historical background of the various eponyms, refer to the review by Burchell.[138]

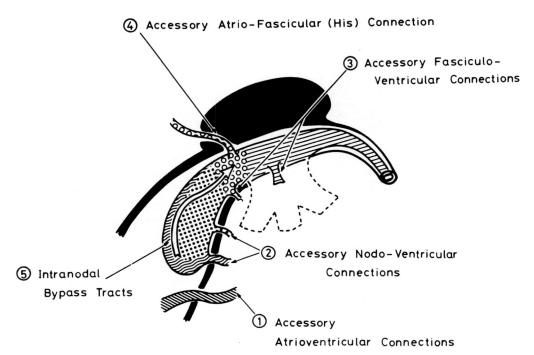

④ Accessory Atrio-Fascicular (His) Connection

③ Accessory Fasciculo-Ventricular Connections

② Accessory Nodo-Ventricular Connections

⑤ Intranodal Bypass Tracts

① Accessory Atrioventricular Connections

Figure 2-33. Diagram showing the theoretic ways in which accessory anatomic connections could "short-circuit" the delay-producing area of the specialized atrioventricular junctional area. This figure can be compared with Figure 2-14.

Accessory Atrioventricular Connections

Accessory atrioventricular connections are pathways that connect the atrial and ventricular myocardial tissues outside the specialized junctional area. Except when the pathways originate in the segments of specialized atrioventricular ring tissue originally described by Kent,[91,92] it is incorrect to refer to these pathways as "Kent bundles." The first accessory atrioventricular pathway to be demonstrated histologically was that studied by Wood and coworkers,[139] but the most exemplary demonstration was that given by Ohnell[140] (Fig. 2-34). Nearly all left-sided pathways studied subsequently are similar to this pathway (Fig. 2-35). Subsequent histologic studies, together with recent electrophysiologic mapping studies such as those of Gallagher and colleagues, have demonstrated unequivocally that these pathways are the anatomic substrates for the classical Wolff-Parkinson-White variety of preexcitation.[141] It has also been demonstrated that the pathways can be successfully divided at surgery, either by standard surgical techniques or by cryothermy.[142] Surgical procedures, however, are being replaced because accessory connections can be destroyed with equal facility using radio frequency current delivered through catheters.[143]

Regardless of how the accessory connections are destroyed, their architecture and relations to the fibrous rings should be understood. The pathways can exist at any point around the atrioventricular junctions where the

atrial tissues are adjacent to ventricular myocardium. In this respect, at least one pathway has been demonstrated extending across the area of fibrous continuity between the mitral and aortic valves.[144] Considered together, the accessory connections can be divided into left-sided, right-sided, or septal pathways. The lateral pathways do not pass

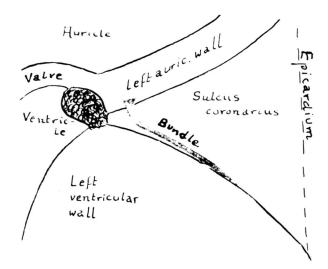

Figure 2-34. Thesis diagram demonstrating the epicardial course of a left-sided accessory atrioventricular connection. (Ohnell RF: Preexcitation, a cardiac abnormality. Acta Med Scand 1944; 152 (Suppl):1.

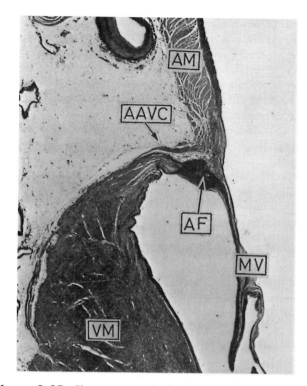

Figure 2-35. Photomicrograph of a left-sided accessory atrio-ventricular (AAVC) connection from a patient with preexcitation. The epicardial course is shown relative to the anulus fibrosus (AF) of the mitral valve (MV). *AM,* atrial myocardium; *VM,* ventricular myocardium.

through gaps in the fibrous ring. In most cases, left-sided pathways skirt a well-formed fibrous ring on its epicardial aspect (see Figs. 2-34 and 2-35). They traverse the fat of the epicardial groove and are closely adherent to the fibrous ring. Cuts used by the surgeons who intend to divide these pathways probably divide the atrial wall above the connection rather than extirpating the pathway itself (Fig. 2-36). It is almost always necessary to dissect the epicardial aspect of the groove to avulse the pathway. When delivering radio frequency energy, the pathway can be ablated from either the atrial or ventricular aspect. The position of right-sided pathways is complicated by the absence of a well-formed tricuspid fibrous ring. Thus, the pathways can pass directly through the adipose tissue, dividing atrial and ventricular musculatures. However, the pathways may also directly traverse the subendocardial tissues, particularly when accompanying an Ebstein's malformation, a frequent association of right-sided preexcitation (Fig. 2-37). Theoretically, septal pathways can cross the septal ring at any point from the tricuspid to the mitral side of the septum. The only septal pathway we have identified, however, crossed the ring at the point of origin of the tricuspid valve.[145] Septal pathways are the hardest to divide. The convention of dividing the "septum" into anterior, mid, and posterior septal components has no anatomic foundation.[146] The "posterior septum" is the floor of the coronary sinus (see Fig. 2-32); the "anterior septum" is the supraventricular crest and, as such, is part of the right parietal atrioventricular junction.

Most connections identified histologically have been tiny threads of working myocardium (see Fig. 2-35). In our experience,[145] they have been thicker at their atrial origin and have ramified like the roots of a tree at their ventricu-

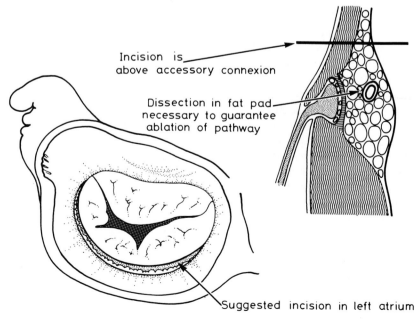

Incision is above accessory connexion

Dissection in fat pad necessary to guarantee ablation of pathway

Suggested incision in left atrium

Figure 2-36. Diagram showing the likely site of a surgical incision to divide an accessory pathway. It is unlikely to divide the actual connection.

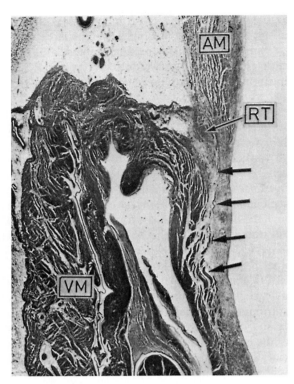

Figure 2-37. Photomicrograph of a right-sided accessory connection (*arrows*) from a patient with preexcitation. The connection is directly subendocardial. This pathway originates from a segment of specialized atrioventricular ring tissue (RT) and can be compared with Figure 2-36. *AM*, atrial myocardium; *VM*, ventricular myocardium.

lar insertion. One of the pathways we studied had its atrial origin in a segment of atrioventricular specialized tissue (see Fig. 2-37). This connection could be considered a Kent bundle. The bundle was composed of specialized conduction tissue, a finding described by other investigators. It seems probable that these connections, originating in segments of ring tissue, can produce "Mahaim" physiology.[147–149] The bundle originating from the node of Kent probably joins the right bundle branch. The fibers have, therefore, been renamed "atriofascicular fibers" and should not be confused with atrio-Hisian tract.[150] Multiple connections have been identified histologically by several investigators and this finding has also been reported on the basis of clinical studies.[139, 145, 151, 152]

The precise structure and morphology of nodoventricular and fasciculoventricular connections (see Fig. 2-33) and their relation to ventricular preexcitation remain to be elucidated. During development, the septal fibrous ring is perforated by numerous strands of specialized tissue which pass between the nodal–bundle axis and the crest of the muscular septum. Despite this ana-

tomic continuity, electrophysiologic studies have shown that conduction occurred as though the nodal–bundle axis was totally isolated from the ventricular septal myocardium as in the definitive heart.[37] The septal fibrous plane is much better developed at birth, but, in most hearts, it is still possible to trace archipelagos of conduction tissue that pass through the central fibrous body in such a position that the compact node and penetrating bundle are in anatomic continuity with the ventricular tissues (Fig. 2-38). The subsequent fate of these tenuous connections has not, to the best of our knowledge, been studied in a systematic manner in the hearts of children and young adults. Nonetheless, in our experience, it is frequent to find direct nodoventricular and fasciculoventricular connections in the hearts of "normal" children and young adults (Fig. 2-39). Systematic studies should be performed to establish the "normal" complement of these connections. A relationship between their presence and preexcitation has been strongly suggested in two cases by correlative anatomico-clinical studies.[153, 154] Even so, the type of preexcitation produced (so-called Mahaim physiology) has been shown to be mediated more frequently by specialized muscular connections originating in the nodes of Kent.[147, 148] Accessory atriofascicular connections connecting the atrial myocardium directly to the penetrating bundle (atrio-Hisian tract) produce preexcitation with a normal QRS complex, that is, the Lown-Ganong-Levine syndrome. Such preexcitation is also explained based on the "James" fiber, but an anatomic distinction must be made between a "James" fiber and an atrio-Hisian accessory connection (Fig. 2-40). The fibers described by James are a finding in normal hearts.[7] He described them as a gathering together of fibers from the eustachian ridge, which passed forward to insert into the junction of the atrioventricular node and bundle. In contrast, atrio-Hisian connections are fibers that insert directly through the fibrous tissue collar to enter the penetrating atrioventricular bundle. The latter fibers were identified by Brechenmacher in hearts from patients known to have exhibited preexcitation of the short PR-normal QRS variety.[136] The key to distinction of an atrio-Hisian connection is that it must enter the nodal–bundle axis after the axis has entered the central fibrous body and becomes the penetrating atrioventricular bundle. The atrio-Hisian connection should be distinguished from the specialized muscular connections originating in the nodes of Kent, because the latter structures are sometimes described as atriofascicular tracts.[150] The fibers described by James are best considered as intranodal bypass tracts.[7] They are confined entirely to the atrial component of the specialized junctional area. Because they are found in normal hearts, it is difficult to implicate them as a source of preexcitation. It is likely that any evidence would be circumstantial, such as the

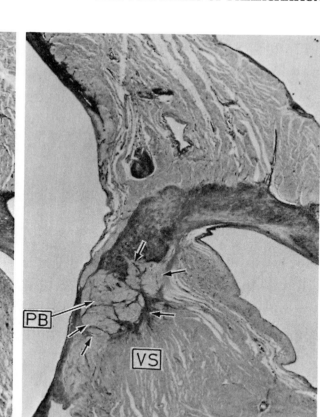

Figure 2-38. Photomicrograph of a junctional area from a neonate showing the archipelagos of conduction tissue (*arrows*), which pass through the anulus fibrosus and connect the compact node (CN) and penetrating bundle (PB) to the crest of the ventricular septum (VS).

finding of short PR–normal QRS preexcitation in patients without accessory atriofascicular connections. There are numerous possibilities for bypass within the atrial component of the specialized junctional area (Fig. 2-41). There is considerable variation in the normal heart in the architecture of the "last" atrial fiber to make contact with the nodal–bundle axis before it becomes the penetrating bundle.[58] In most hearts, this fiber is an atrial overlay transitional fiber. In other hearts, the fiber originates deep from the left atrial aspect of the septum.

Further variation exists with regard to the morphology of the compact node and its posterior extension. In some hearts, the major axis is toward the mitral valve and the left side of the septum. In other hearts, the tricuspid extension of the compact node is dominant. Within the node itself, the stratification of the normal node gives multiple possibilities for bypass pathways. These variations and the problem of the substrates for normal PR–short QRS preexcitation will only be elucidated

after extensive studies of "normal" hearts compared with hearts known to have exhibited this form of preexcitation.

The possible candidates for pathways as intranodal bypass tracts must also be considered as substrates for dual nodal pathways and longitudinal dissociation. In anatomico-electrophysiologic studies performed in the specialized junctional area of the rabbit, an area of longitudinal dissociation was positively identified within the transitional cell zone of the atrioventricular node.[75] In this area, the transitional cells were attenuated and separated by strands of connective tissue. Similar cell arrangements are found in the posterior transitional area of the human node. Surprisingly, the grosser alternative pathways studied in the rabbit node, such as the anterior atrial overlay fibers and the extensive posterior bundle-like prolongation of the lower nodal cells, both proved to be electrophysiologic "dead-end pathways" when examined by anterograde and retrograde stimulation.[75]

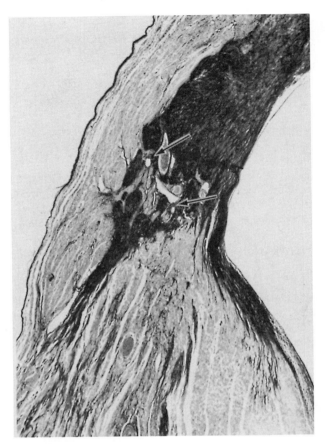

Figure 2-39. Photomicrograph of a normal adult junctional area showing persistent archipelagos (*arrows*), which penetrate the anulus fibrosus when traced in serial sections to form a nodoventricular connection.

CONDUCTION TISSUES AND SUDDEN INFANT DEATH SYNDROME

That fatal arrhythmias may be responsible for some of the cases of sudden infant death is both feasible and of preventive significance.[155] Histologic studies of the conduction system of infants who have died suddenly, however, have helped little in alleviating the problem, and the contention that surrounds the topic may have a deleterious effect.[156] Some observers have considered that changes in archipelagos of conduction tissue that extend into the central fibrous body of infant hearts (see Fig. 2-38) may play a role in the production of sudden death.[155–158] Others question these interpretations, either because they were unable to find the described changes or because they found similar changes in the conduction systems of infants dying from known causes.[159–161] Lesions in these archipelagos were first implicated as a possible substrate for sudden infant death by James.[155] He described a process of "orderly resorptive degeneration of portions of the undivided His bundle and A-V node" in all hearts he studied, both from infants who died suddenly and from those dying from known causes. While denying the presence of inflammatory changes, massive necrosis, or hemorrhage, James nonetheless described "a slowly destructive process in which neighbouring fibroblasts were replacing necrotic fibers of the His bundle or A-V node." He further stated that "macrophages were present adjacent to the small foci of necrosis, acting as scavenger cells" and that "those pockets of tissue were in various stages of degeneration and resorption, some with relatively little necrosis and others in which nearly all the fibers had been destroyed and were being removed by macrophages and replaced by fibroblastic invasion." Subsequent observers were unable to confirm these interpretations,[159–161] because they were unable to identify any necrosis or macrophage aggregation. James, in a subsequent editorial,[156] suggested that these negative reports were adopting a "straw-man approach," because he had intended to indicate that "resorptive degeneration" was a normal developmental process. The argument centers on whether there is evidence of focal cell death in the infant junctional area, and, if it is present, whether it represents a pathologic process. James described such focal necrosis but evidently did not consider it pathologic.[155, 156] Others have not observed any

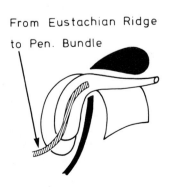

a)"James Fiber"

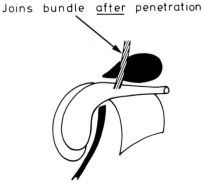

Joins bundle <u>after</u> penetration

b) Atrio-fascicular Fiber

Figure 2-40. Diagram showing the anatomic difference between a "James" fiber and an atriofascicular accessory connection such as described by Brechenmacher.[7, 136]

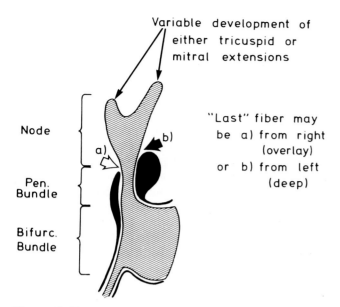

Variable development of either tricuspid or mitral extensions

Node

Pen. Bundle

Bifurc. Bundle

a)

b)

"Last" fiber may be a) from right (overlay) or b) from left (deep)

Figure 2-41. Diagram showing possibilities for bypass tracts provided by variations in a normal specialized junctional area.

evidence of the reported focal necrosis, considering that the appearance of the archipelagos of conduction tissue in the central fibrous body was consistent with normal development of the junctional area.[159–161]

It must also be considered whether there is evidence to link this process of normal development (or focal necrosis) to arrhythmias. James argued that cell death may cause release of intracellular potassium and produce local tissue acidosis, which may affect function in adjacent surviving tissue.[155] Alternatively, he opined that the degenerating tissue in the archipelagos may become hyperexcitable and give rise to ectopic beats or ectopic rhythm. He also directed attention to the studies of Preston and coworkers which demonstrated "immaturity" of the junctional area in three different species of young mammals.[162] James further reasoned that the shaggy, large atrioventricular bundle of the fetus was electrophysiologically unsafe and that orderly conduction is better performed by the thin, smooth bundle of the adult.

Electrophysiologic studies in the human fetal heart have subsequently demonstrated that the conduction patterns are mature before midterm, even though the specialized tissue at this stage is in extensive anatomic continuity throughout its length with the ventricular myocardium.[37] Histologic studies in hearts of infants dying suddenly have demonstrated the archipelagos of conduction tissue extending into the central fibrous body observed by James and others.[155, 157–161] In keeping with other investigators, we have not observed the changes, normal or abnormal, described as "resorptive degeneration."[159, 161] In a series of control hearts compared with

hearts from infants dying suddenly, we found similar changes in both series.[163] Having antemortem evidence of conduction disorders would be ideal before suggesting that changes occurring as a normal developmental process may be substrates for sudden death.

Yet, arrhythmias may cause some sudden deaths in infancy. Hearts from two infants who died suddenly and who were known to have a gross abnormality in the conduction system were studied. In the first, an accessory connection was observed in the region of the compact node.[160] In the other, there was stenosis of the penetrating bundle, a lesion suggested to be a cause of sudden death in some canine species.[164, 165] But, there was no evidence that these anatomic substrates were the mechanisms of arrhythmia.[161] To discover if these are the substrates for some cases of sudden infant death, the conduction systems from infants dying suddenly who have had prior electrocardiographic investigation must be studied. We endorse the observation of James who said it would be regrettable if the interpretations offered by Lie and coworkers discouraged others from investigating the functional aspect of the conduction system in infancy.[155, 161]

AGING EFFECTS IN THE CONDUCTION TISSUES

The process of aging and its effect on the histologic appearances of the conduction tissues have been much neglected. Apart from the studies of Lev[166] and Erickson[167] and the investigations on the sinus node and internodal atrial myocardium by Davies and Pomerance,[168] we are unaware of any systematic research on this important topic. As the body ages, there is a general increase in the amount of fibrous tissue present in the conduction tissues. Whether this increase in fibrosis is caused by increased deposition of fibrous tissue or by a decrease in the amount of conduction tissues relative to the heart remains to be established. The fetal penetrating bundle has been shown to be a vast structure compared with its adult counterpart.[21, 155] This is equally true of the atrial component of the junctional area and the sinus node. Our studies of fetal tissues show that all these structures are laid down within a matrix of connective tissue, particularly the sinus node (see Fig. 2-4), although James[169] indicated that the fetal sinus node was lacking in fibrous tissue. Our studies show rather that the content of nodal tissue per unit area of node decreases with increasing age.[28] The excessive fibrosis reported in aged nodes may be a continuation of this process because few nodal cells persist in these nodes. Our observations suggest a similar progression in the atrioventricular junctional area, notably on the archipelagos of conduction tissue in the central fibrous body of fetal and infant hearts.[58] In his editorial, James asks what happens to the archipelagos if they are not removed by the "resorptive degeneration."[156] The islands become less evident with increasing growth of the heart, but they continue to protrude into the fibrous body. We have found some of these remnants in the majority of adult and adolescent hearts studied.[170]

CONDUCTION TISSUES IN CONGENITAL HEART DISEASE

The disposition of the conduction tissues (both the atrial conduction tissues and the atrioventricular bundle) must be known by any surgeon intending to correct congenital cardiac malformations. This section reviews the conduction tissue architecture in the more important anomalies.

Sinus Node and Internodal Atrial Myocardium

When performing surgery, damage must be avoided not only to the sinus node but also to its nutrient artery. These structures are at risk during incisions into the right atrium as well as during the placement of atrial cannulas. The entire junction of the superior caval vein with the right atrium should be considered a danger area. The area of maximal danger is the part of the terminal groove between the crest of the atrial appendage and the orifice of the inferior caval vein (see Fig. 2-2). The sinus node is directly subepicardial in this position and particularly susceptible to any form of trauma.

The sinus node is likely to be in most danger during operations for complete transposition, which redirect the systemic and pulmonary venous returns (Mustard and Senning procedures). Much has been written concerning the role of the "specialized internodal tracts" in the genesis of postoperative arrhythmias in this condition.[171] Histologic studies are conflicting in this respect. One investiga-

tion suggested damage to the tracts as the cause.[172] Another pointed to the high incidence of sinus node trauma in patients dying after repair.[173] Other studies have not demonstrated the narrow tracts of specialized cells presumed by some to exist in the atrial septum and walls.[10, 58, 171] After removal of the atrial septum, the impulse passes either in front of the hole thus created or behind it in the remainder of the atrial myocardium. This premise was borne out by the mapping studies carried out at Great Ormond Street Hospital, London.[174] Therefore, incisions across the major muscle bundles such as the terminal crest should be avoided in the repair procedure. Even if the crest is cut (as was the policy of Lincoln at the Royal Brompton Hospital, London), postoperative arrhythmias can be prevented if the areas of the sinus and atrioventricular nodes are avoided and if the abnormal rhythms that existed before the operation are accounted for.[175, 176]

Now that the operation of choice for repair of complete transposition is the arterial switch procedure, these discussions are moot. However, the surgeon should still avoid damage to the artery supplying the sinus node, particularly when transferring the coronary arteries to the new aortic root. One condition that must be considered when planning an atrial incision is that of juxtaposition of the atrial appendages. This anomaly (a frequent accompaniment of tricuspid atresia and occasionally encountered with transposed great arteries) alters the position of the sinus node. Our results show that the node is unrelated to the juxtaposed right atrial appendage.[177] Instead, it remains within the displaced terminal groove, either at the orifice of the superior caval vein or near the atrioventricular groove (Fig. 2-42). The node is smaller than anticipated for normal hearts.[177]

Atrioventricular Conduction Tissues

Formation of the normal node and bundle demands contributions from both the atrial and ventricular tissues. The ventricular component is formed in relation to the muscular interventricular septum. To produce a normal atrioven-

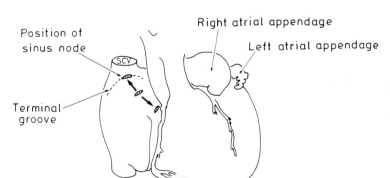

Figure 2-42. Diagram showing the position of the sinus node in five cases studied with juxtaposition of the atrial appendages. *SCV,* superior caval vein.

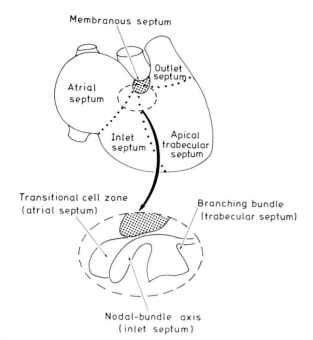

Figure 2-43. Diagram showing how the alignment of the atrial septum, inlet septum, and trabecular septum is necessary for formation of a normal atrioventricular junctional area.

tricular conduction mechanism, there must be normal formation and alignment of the atrial septum and the muscular septum (Fig. 2-43). If this alignment does not occur, an anomalous node can be derived from the ring of conduction tissue that surrounded the right side of the atrioventricular junction during development (see Fig. 2-30). These considerations underscore the disposition of the atrioventricular conduction mechanism in those hearts with normally aligned septal structures as opposed to those with either septal malalignment or absence of the ventricular inlet septum.

Hearts With Normally Aligned Septal Structures

Hearts with "isolated" ventricular septal defects, Fallot's tetralogy, atrioventricular septal defects, and abnormal ventriculo-arterial connections associated with concordant atrioventricular connections all are considered hearts with normally aligned septal structures. Although there are minor differences in each subgroup, they all have the landmark of the penetrating atrioventricular bundle at the apex of the triangle of Koch, as in the normal heart (see Fig. 2-14). In hearts with atrioventricular septal defects, this nodal triangle (not the triangle of Koch) is displaced posteriorly by the defect (Fig. 2-44).[65]

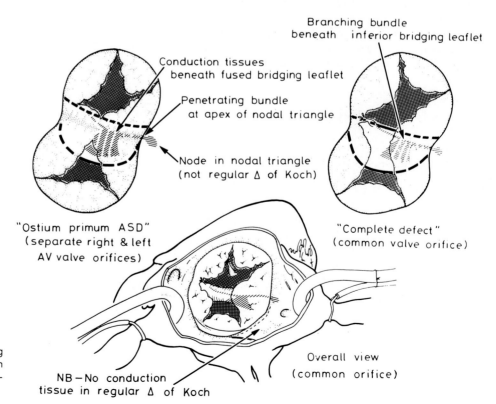

Figure 2-44. Diagrams showing the position of the conducting tissues in hearts with atrioventricular septal defects.

In hearts with ventricular septal defects (Fig. 2-45), the disposition of the atrioventricular bundle depends on the type of defect.[178] Most defects result from absence of the crest of the muscular ventricular septum in the environs of the membranous septum (so-called membranous defects, but better referred to as perimembranous defects). In these defects, all of which have the central fibrous body in their posteroinferior rims and roof, the ventricular conducting tissues are related to the crest of the septum. The atrioventricular bundle penetrates through the fibrous tissue, which is the area of greatest danger. In some hearts, the branching bundle sits directly on the septal crest, but, in most, the bundle may be to the left side as in tetralogy of Fallot.[179–182] When defects are in the muscular part of the inlet septum, the bundle bears a significantly different relation.[178] The defect is within the muscular inlet septum and is, thus, below and behind the penetrating and branching atrioventricular bundles. Therefore, the superoanterior and anterior quadrants are those parts of the defect "at risk" (see Fig. 2-45). Such muscular inlet defects can be distinguished from perimembranous inlet defects because of their complete muscular rim. Muscular defects of the outlet septum are remote from the ventricular conducting tissues (see Fig. 2-45). Muscular defects in the apical trabecular septum can be related to the peripheral bundle branches.[181]

In tetralogy of Fallot, the conducting tissue is disposed in a similar fashion to perimembranous defects, and, in most cases, the branching bundle is to the left side of the septal crest.[183] The septal crest is, therefore, devoid of conducting tissues, with the major danger area being the posteroinferior angle where the penetrating bundle passes through the central fibrous body.[184] In a few cases

of tetralogy of Fallot, the branching bundle can be positioned directly on the septal crest (Fig. 2-46).[180, 184] In these cases, which cannot be distinguished on gross anatomic observations, it is dangerous to place sutures directly into the septal crest during repair as advocated by Starr and coworkers.[185] When the defect in tetralogy has a muscular posteroinferior rim (such as occurs with muscular outlet ventricular septal defects), the ventricular conduction tissues are remote from the defect rim.

The ventricular component of an atrioventricular septal defect can be considered as a large perimembranous inlet defect extending to the crux of the heart (see Fig. 2-44). The disposition of conduction tissue is similar in the varieties with either separate valve orifices or a common valve.[63–65] The nodal triangle is displaced posteroinferiorly by the septal defect and is not the usual triangle of Koch. The penetrating bundle is found at its apex. Because of the septal deficiency, the atrioventricular node is hypoplastic. The posterior displacement contributes both to the longer nonbranching bundle seen in these hearts and the posteriorly situated left bundle branch, which runs down from the branching bundle positioned along the full length of the crest of the inlet septum. In the anomaly with separate right and left valvar orifices (i.e., ostium primum atrial septal defect), the penetrating and branching bundles are directly inferior to the conjoined bridging leaflets.

In hearts with abnormal ventriculo-arterial connections but concordant atrioventricular connections, the variability of conduction tissue disposition depends on the type of ventricular septal defect (e.g., perimembranous or with a muscular posteroinferior rim). These anomalies include complete transposition, double outlet

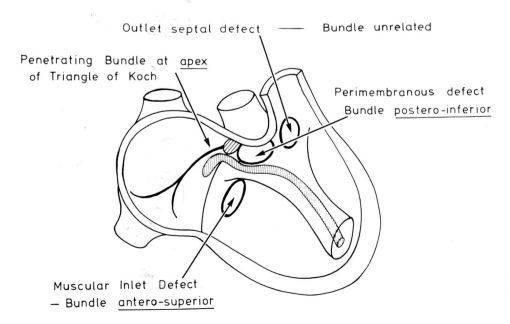

Outlet septal defect —— Bundle unrelated

Penetrating Bundle at apex of Triangle of Koch

Perimembranous defect
Bundle postero-inferior

Muscular Inlet Defect
— Bundle antero-superior

Figure 2-45. Diagram illustrating the relation of the ventricular conducting tissues to different types of ventricular septal defects.

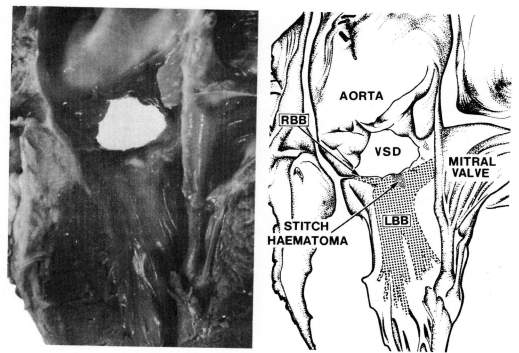

Figure 2-46. Photograph and drawing illustrating the left aspect of a heart with tetralogy of Fallot. The conducting tissues (RBB, LBB) are directly astride the crest of the defect (VSD). In this case, stitches placed directly into the septal crest (stitch hematoma) resulted in traumatic heart block. (Anderson RH, Monroe JL, Ho SY, Smith A, Deverall PB. Les voies de conduction auriculo-ventriculaires dans le tetralogy of Fallot. Coeur 1977;8:793.)

right ventricle with subaortic or subpulmonary defect, and common arterial trunk.[186–188] The septal crest of the muscular septum is usually devoid of conducting tissues, but there are exceptions.[189]

Hearts With Malaligned Septal Structures

The defect typifying hearts with malaligned septal structures is congenitally corrected transposition, which is the combination of discordant atrioventricular and ventriculoarterial connections.[190] When this anomaly exists in individuals with normally arranged atria, there is a vital derangement in disposition of the conduction tissues. Because of septal malalignment, the apex of tue triangle of Koch is out of line with the inlet component of the muscular septum. The regular atrioventricular node at the apex of the triangle of Koch cannot make contact with the ventricular conduction tissues on the trabecular septum.[191, 192] Instead, an anterior atrioventricular node communicates via a long nonbranching bundle with ventricular conduction tissues. In the presence of a ventricular septal defect, the bundle passes lateral to the pulmonary outflow tract (Fig. 2-47).[193] Some researchers have suggested that the bundle passes between the pulmonary

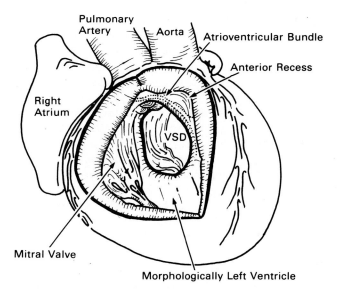

Figure 2-47. Diagram showing the position of conducting tissues in congenitally corrected transposition in hearts with usual atrial arrangement. (Becker AE, Anderson RH: Anatomy of conditions with atrioventricular discordance. In: Anderson RH, Shinebourne EA, eds. Paediatric cardiology, 1977. Edinburgh: Churchill Livingstone, 1978; with permission.)

valve and the defect.[194] Anatomic considerations suggest that this apparent difference is related to perspective and interpretation rather than variable disposition of the bundle.[195]

When there is mirror-image arrangement of the atria in congenitally corrected transposition, all the cases studied have had posterior atrioventricular nodes and penetrating bundles.[196–198] This is probably related to the better alignment of septal structures seen in these hearts. Even so, anterior connections may exist in any heart with atrioventricular discordance, or there may be an entire sling of ventricular conduction tissue connected to both anterior and regular nodes. Such a sling was first observed by Monckeberg[199] and has since been identified by us[200] as well as Bharati and Lev.[201]

Hearts With Univentricular Atrioventricular Connections

The conduction tissues have a grossly abnormal disposition in most hearts with univentricular atrioventricular connections. The most common example is the heart with double inlet left ventricle. The feature of these hearts is lack of a septum extending to the crux, which disables the regular node from making contact with the ventricular conduction tissues, and an anterior node assumes this role.[202, 203] In the variety with left-sided rudimentary right ventricle, the disposition of the ventricular conduction tissues is similar to that seen in congenitally corrected transposition with usually arranged atria (Fig. 2-48 and see Fig. 2-47). In double inlet left ventricle with a right-sided rudimentary right ventricle, any surgery to the dominant ventricle might involve a left-sided incision. If approached this way, the bundle is seen to pass beneath the defect, despite originating from an anterior node (Fig. 2-49). If the surgeon approaches any heart with double inlet left ventricle through the rudimentary right ventricle, the conduction tissue is always distant and lies on the left ventricular side beneath the crest of the ventricular septal defect (Fig. 2-50). The identifying feature of the abnormal disposition of the conducting tissues is the presence or absence of a septum running to the crux. In double inlet to a solitary and indeterminate ventricle, there is no such septum. An anterior or anterolateral node is, therefore, present.[204, 205] In contrast, in double inlet right ventricle with left-sided rudimentary left ventricle, or in hearts with huge ventricular septal defects, a septum or septal remnant does extend to the crux, and a regular connecting node is found in these anomalies.[205, 206] Ventricular surgery in classical tricuspid atresia is likely to be confined to the rudimentary right ventricle. The conduction tissues are related to the septum exactly as in double inlet left ventricle (see Fig. 2-50). In all these hearts with univentricular

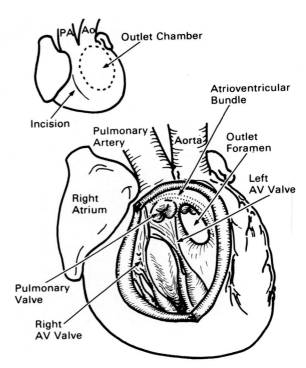

Figure 2-48. Diagram showing the position of the conducting tissues in double inlet left ventricle with left-sided rudimentary right ventricle. (Anderson RH, Wilkinson JL, Becker AE: The conducting tissues in the univentricular heart. In: Van Mierop LHS, Oppenheimer-Decker A, Bruins CHLCh,, eds. Embryology and teratology of the heart and great arteries. The Hague: Leiden University Press, 1978.)

atrioventricular connection to a dominant left ventricle, if it is necessary to enlarge the ventricular septal defect, it is always the margin of the apical trabecular septum closest to the left border of the heart that can most safely be excised.

CONGENITAL HEART BLOCK

Lev has divided congenitally complete heart block into two basic varieties, one of which occurs in a congenitally malformed heart and the other in an otherwise normal heart.[207]

Congenital heart block associated with a cardiac malformation is most frequently seen with congenitally corrected transposition and atrioventricular septal defects having separate right and left orifices (i.e., ostium primum atrial septal defect). Although it may be complete at birth, it is more usual for the arrhythmia to be progressive, starting with first degree block and leading to complete block. Histologic studies suggest that the progression may be related to increasing fibrosis of the atrioventricular

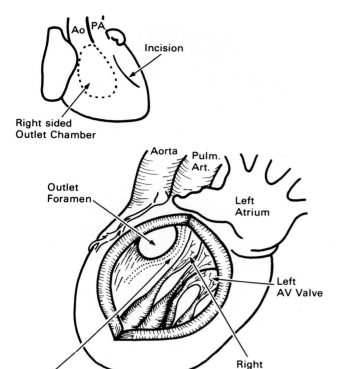

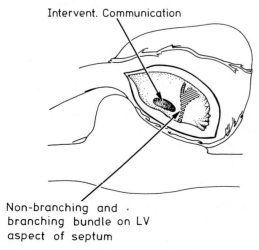

Figure 2-49. Diagram showing the position of the conducting tissues in double inlet left ventricle with right-sided rudimentary right ventricle. (Anderson RH, Wilkinson JL, Becker AE: The conducting tissues in the univentricular heart. In: Van Mierop LHS, Oppenheimer-Decker A, Bruins CHLCh, eds. Embryology and teratology of the heart and great arteries. The Hague: Leiden University Press, 1978; with permission.

Figure 2-50. Diagram showing the relation of the conducting tissues to the outlet foramen when viewed from the rudimentary right ventricle in a heart with any form of univentricular atrioventricular connection to a dominant left ventricle.

bundle, which is situated in a mobile part of the heart compared to the normal heart.[192] The degree of fibrosis of the ventricular conduction tissues may also be related to the known vulnerability to the mildest trauma, with the block being known to occur during induction of anesthesia or at an initial thoracotomy.[208]

Congenitally complete heart block occurring in an otherwise normal heart can also be divided into various forms depending on the histology of the junctional area.[209,210] Three types are described. In the first type, discontinuity is found between the atrial tissues and a hypoplastic nodal–bundle axis.[209] In the second type, the atrioventricular node is normally formed but is discontinuous from the ventricular specialized tissues (Fig. 2-51).[210] The third and rarest type exists when the bundle branches are discontinuous from the branching bundle.[211] A recent study pointed to a strong correlation between isolated congenitally complete heart block and anti-RO (SS-A) antibody in maternal serum.[212] Histologic studies of seven hearts from children whose maternal serum was anti-RO positive shared absence of the atrioventricular node.[213] In its place were fibrous and adipose tissues.

ACQUIRED DISEASES OF THE CONDUCTION SYSTEM

Many disease processes that affect the heart can involve the normally situated conduction tissues. Any disease affecting the endocardium, myocardium, or pericardium may produce functional and anatomic abnormalities in the conduction tissues. (For review, see Davies and co-workers.[214]) The most important acquired diseases are coronary arterial disease and the effect of aging processes on the ventricular conduction system.

Coronary Arterial Disease and Conduction Abnormalities

Acute myocardial infarction may become complicated either by bundle branch block or atrioventricular dissociation. The prognostic significance of these findings depends on the localization of the primary infarct. In patients with anteroseptal infarction, the development of bundle branch block carries a grave prognosis, contrasting with the relatively benign course in those with posteroinferior wall infarction. The pathologic substrate of the arrhythmias is a matter of dispute, in part because the conduction tissues are more resistant to ischemia than the working myocardium, making the interpretation of histologic findings more difficult.[215–220] Bundle branch block in the setting of an acute myocardial infarction is rarely attributed to overt bundle branch necrosis.[218–220] Still, ischemic changes,

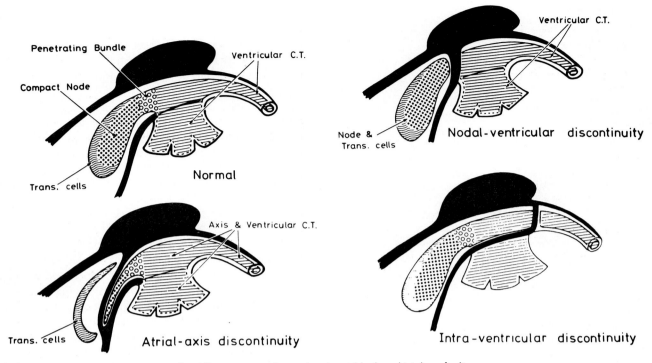

Figure 2-51. Diagram showing the differentiations of complete heart block on histology findings.

such as edema and inflammatory cell infiltration present in the direct vicinity of the bundle branches or within the conduction fibers, are found in the majority of cases with electrocardiographic changes. The development of bundle branch block is related to the extent of the infarction rather than actual necrosis of conduction fibers. If the patient survives, regression of electrocardiographic changes might be expected. It is common in posteroinferior wall infarction to find atrioventricular dissociation in the early phase, which is nearly always reversible. The underlying pathology is similar to that described for anteroseptal infarctions.[221]

The frequency of chronic conduction disturbances directly resulting from myocardial infarction has not been determined. It is widely accepted that the usual case of atrioventricular dissociation or bundle branch block in the elderly patient is not directly related to coronary artery disease.

area. The precise nature of these changes is not fully understood. The degenerative changes may affect the penetrating and nonbranching segments of the bundle in their position on the crest of the ventricular septum. Abnormalities at these sites are claimed to be the substrates of so-called Lev's disease.[222,223] Similar changes affecting the more distal portions of the bundle branches, often found with patchy distribution, most likely underlie so-called Lenegre's disease.[224,225] Whether these disease processes form the extreme ends of a spectrum of pathology of the ventricular conduction tissues or whether they are discrete entities with their own pathogenesis is not determined.[226] Progression of the pathologic changes found in these disease entities, whatever their cause, may result in complete heart block. This so-called idiopathic complete heart block is the most common reason for pacemaker insertion in the elderly.[227]

Aging Processes in the Ventricular Conduction Tissues

In general, increasing age is accompanied by increasing fibrosis of the ventricular conduction tissues as well as a fall-off in the number of conduction fibers present per unit

Acknowledgments

We are greatly indebted to our colleagues and collaborators who have been involved in many of the investigations abstracted in this review, notably, Wout Lamers, M.D., Antoon Moorman, Ph.D., and Audrey Smith, Ph.D. Mrs. Christine Anderson helped considerably in compiling the manuscript.

References

1. Tawara S: Das Reizleitungssystem des Saugetierherzens. Jena: Gustav Fischer, 1906.
2. Keith A, Flack M: The auriculo-ventricular bundle of the human heart. Lancet 1906;2:359.
3. Keith A, Flack M: The form and nature of the muscular connections between the primary divisions of the vertebrate heart. J Anatomy Physiology 1907;41:172.
4. Monckeberg JG: Das spezifische Muskelsystem in menschlichen Herzen. Ergebnisse allgmeiner Pathologie Anatomie 1921;19:328.
5. Koch W: Weiter Mitteilungen uber den Sinusknoten der Herzens. Verhandlungen der Deutschen Pathologische Anatomie 1909;13:85.
6. Koch W: Der funktionelle Bau des menschlichen Herzens. Berlin: Urban v. Schwarzenburg, 1922:92.
7. James TN: Morphology of the human atrioventricular node, with remarks pertinent to its electrophysiology. Am Heart J 1961;62:756.
8. James TN: The connecting pathways between the sinus node and the A-V node and between the right and the left atrium in the human heart. Am Heart J 1963;66:498.
9. Racker DK: Transmission and reentrant activity in the sinoventricular conducting system and in the circumferential lamina of the tricuspid valve. J Cardiovascular Electrophysiology 1993;4:513.
10. Janse MJ, Anderson RH: Specialized internodal atrial pathways—Fact or fiction. Eur J Cardiol 1974;2:117.
11. Oosthoek PW, Viragh S, Lamers WH, Moorman AFM: Immunohistochemical delineation of the conduction system. II. The atrioventricular node and Purkinje fibers. Circ Res 1993;73:482.
12. Wenckebach KF: Beitrage zur Kenntis der menschlichen Herztatigkeit. Archiv Anat u Physiol 1906;2:297.
13. Lewis T, Oppenheimer BS, Oppenheimer A: Site of origin of the mammalian heart beat: The pacemaker in the dog. Heart 1910;2:147.
14. Truex RC: The sinuatrial node and its connections with the atrial tissues. In: Wellens HJJ, Lie KI, Janse MJ, eds. The conduction system of the heart: Structure, function and clinical implications. Leiden: HE Stenfert Kroese BV, 1976:209.
15. James TN: Anatomy of the human sinus node. Anat Rec 1961;141:109.
16. Hudson REB: Surgical pathology of the conducting system of the heart. Br Heart J 1967;29:646.
17. Anderson KR, Ho SY, Anderson RH: The location and vascular supply of the sinus node in the human heart. Br Heart J 1979;41:28.
18. Busquet J, Fontan F, Anderson RH, Ho SY, Davies MJ: The surgical significance of the atrial branches of the coronary arteries. Int J Cardiol 1984;6:223.
19. McAlpine WA: Heart and Coronary Arteries. An Anatomical Atlas for Clinical Diagnosis, Radiological Investigation and Surgical Treatment. New York: Springer-Verlag, 1975:154.
20. James TN: The sinus node as a servomechanism. Circ Res 1973;32:307.
21. Walls EW: The development of the specialized conducting tissue of the human heart. J Anat 1947;81:93.
22. Sanabria T: Recherches sur la differenciation du tissu nodal et connecteur du coeur des mammiferes. Arch Biol, Leige 1936;47:1.
23. Shaner RF: The development of the atrioventricular node, bundle of His and sinoatrial node in the calf with a description of a third embryonic nodelike structure. Anat Rec 1929;44:85.
24. Robb JS, Kaylor CT, Turman WG: A study of specialized heart tissue at various stages of development of the human fetal heart. Am J Med 1948;5:324.
25. Patten BM: Development of the sinoventricular conduction system. Univ Mich Med Bull 1956;22:1.
26. Heinzberger CFM: The development of the sinoatrial node in the mouse. Acta Morphol Neerl Scand 1974;12:317.
27. Van Mierop LHS, Gessner IH: The morphologic development of the sinoatrial node in the mouse. Am J Cardiol 1970;25:204.
28. Anderson RH, Ho SY, Becker AE, Gosling JA: The development of the sinoatrial node. In: Bonke FIM, ed. The Sinus Node. Structure, Function and Clinical Relevance. Hague: Martinus Nijhoff, 1978:166.
29. Tranum-Jensen J: The fine structure of the atrial and atrioventricular (AV) junctional specialized tissues of the rabbit heart. In: Wellens HJJ, Lie KI, Janse MJ, eds. Conduction system of the heart: Structure, function and clinical implications. Leiden: HE Stenfert Kroese BV, 1976:55.
30. James TN, Sherf L, Fine G, Morales AR: Comparative ultrastructure of the sinus node in man and dog. Circulation 1966;34:139.
31. Yamauchi A: Ultrastructure of the innervation of the mammalian heart. In: Challice CE, Viragh S, eds. Ultrastructure of the Mammalian Heart. New York: Academic Press, 1973:127.
32. Canale ED, Campbell GR, Smolich JJ, Campbell JH: Cardiac Muscle. Berlin: Springer Verlag, 1986.
33. Wharton J, Gulbenkian S: Peptides in the mammalian cardiovascular system. Experientia 1987;43:821.
34. Forsgren S: Neuropeptide Y-like immunoreactivity in relation to the distribution of sympathetic nerve fibers in the heart conduction system. J Mol Cell Cardiol 1989;21:279.
35. Lipp JAM, Rudolph AM: Sympathetic nerve development in the rat and guinea-pig heart. Biol Neonate 1972;21:76.
36. Wharton J, Anderson RH, Espejo R, Smith A, Penketh R, Polak JM: Development of peptide-containing neural and endocrine elements in the human heart. (Abstract) Br Heart J 1989;61:112.
37. Janse MJ, Anderson RH, Van Capelle FJL, Durrer D: A combined electrophysiological and anatomical study of the human fetal heart. Am Heart J 1976;91:556.
38. Fine C, Sutton MGStJ, Cartier MS, Doubilet PM: Variation in heart rate in the normal fetus during and after cardiogenesis. (Abstract) Circ Res 1988;78:II-397.
39. Wharton J, Gordon L, Walsh FS, Flanigan TP, Moore SE, Polak JM: Neural cell adhesion molecule (N-CAM) expression during cardiac development in the rat. Brain Res 1989;483:170.
40. Lewis T: The mechanism and graphic registration of the heart beat. London: Shaw and Sons, 1920:1.

41. Thorel C: Verlaufige Mitteilung uber eine besondere Muskelverbindung zwischen der Cava Superior und dem Hisschen Bundel. Munch Med Woch 1909;56:2159.

42. Thorel C: Uber den Aufbau des Sinusknotens und seine Verbindung mit der Cava superior und den Wenckbachschen bundel. Munch Med Wochenschr 1910;57:186.

43. German Pathological Society: Bericht uber die Verhandlungen der XIV Tagung der Deutschen pathologischen Gesellschaft in Erlangen vom 4–6 April 1910. Z all Path u Path Anat 1910;21:433.

44. Aschoff L: Referat uber die Herzstorungen in ihren Beziehungen zu den Spezifischen Muskelsystem des Herzens. Verh Dtsch Pathol Ges 1910;14:3.

45. Monckeberg JG: Beitrage zur normalen und pathologischen Anatomie des Herzens. Verh Dtsch Pathol Ges 1910;14:64.

46. Koch W: Discussion in The German Pathological Society. Bericht uber die Verhandlungen der XIV Tagung der Deutschen pathologischen Gesellschaft in Erlangen vom 4–6 April 1910. Z all Path u Path Anat 1910;21:433.

47. Condorelli L: Uber die Bahnen der Reizleitung vom Keithr-Flackschen Knoten zu den Vorhofen. Z Ges exp Med 1929;68:493.

48. Franco PM: Recherches sur les faisceaux de connexion auriculaires dans les conditions normales et pathologues. Arch Mal Coeur 1951;44:287.

49. Paes de Carvalho A: Cellular electrophysiology of the atrial specialized tissues. In: Paes de Carvalho A, Mello WC, Hoffman BF, eds. Specialized tissues of the heart. Amsterdam: Elsevier, 1961:115.

50. Lev M, Bharati S: Lesions of the conduction system and their functional significance. In: Sommers SC, ed. Pathology Annual, 1974. New York: Appleton-Century-Crofts, 1974:157.

51. Chuaqui B: Uber die Ausbreitungsbundel des Sinusknoten. Eine kritische analyse der wichtigsten Arbeiten. Virchows Arch (Pathol Anat) 1972;355:179.

52. Chuaqui B: Lupenpraparatorische Darstellung der Ausbreitungszuge des Sinusknotens. (Stereomicroscopic demonstration of the extensions of the sinus node). Virchows Arch Path Anat 1972;356:141.

53. James TN: Sir Thomas Lewis redivivus: From pebbles in a quiet pond to autonomic storms. Br Heart J 1984;52:1.

54. Spach MS, Lieberman M, Scott JG, Barr RC, Johnson EA, Kootsey JM: Excitation sequences of the atrial septum and AV node in isolated hearts of the dog and the rabbit. Circ Res 1971;29:156.

55. Spach MS, King TD, Barr RC, Boaz DE, Morrow MN, Herman-Giddens S: Electrical potential distribution surrounding the atria during depolarization and repolarization in the dog. Circ Res 1969;24:857.

56. Spach MS, Kootsey JM: The nature of electrical propagation in cardiac muscle. Am J Physiol 1983;244:H-3.

57. Tranum-Jensen J, Janse MJ: Fine structural identification of individual cells subjected to microelectrode recording in perfused cardiac preparations. J Mol Cell Cardiol 1982;14:233.

58. Becker AE, Anderson RH: Morphology of the human atrioventricular junctional area. In: Wellens HJJ, Lie KI, Janse MJ,

eds. The conduction system of the heart: Structure, function and clinical implications. Leiden: HE Stenfert Kroese BV, 1976:263.

59. Hecht HH, Kossmann CE, Childers RW, et al: Atrioventricular and intraventricular conduction—revised nomenclature and concepts. Am J Cardiol 1973;31:232.

60. Todaro F: Novelle richerche sopra la struttura muscolare delle orecchiette del coure umano e sopra la valvola d'Eustachio. Sperimentale 1865;16:217.

61. Anderson RH, Taylor IM: Development of atrioventricular specialized tissue in the human heart. Br Heart J 1972;34:1205.

62. Lamers WH, Wessels A, Verbeek FJ, et al: New findings concerning ventricular septation in the human heart. Implications for maldevelopment. Circulation 1992;86:1194.

63. Lev M: The architecture of the conduction system in congenital heart disease. I. Common atrioventricular orifice. Arch Pathol 1958;65:174.

64. Feldt RH, DuShane JW, Titus JL: The atrioventricular conduction system in persistent common atrioventricular canal defect: correlations with electrocardiogram. Circulation 1970;42:437.

65. Thiene G, Wenink ACG, Frescura C, et al: The surgical anatomy of the conduction tissues in atrioventricular defects. J Thorac Cardiovasc Surg 1981;82:928.

66. Scherf D, Cohen J: The atrioventricular node and selected cardiac arrhythmias. New York: Grune and Stratton, 1964.

67. Massing GK, James TN: Anatomical configuration of the His bundle and bundle branches in the human heart. Circulation 1976;53:609.

68. Davies MJ: The conduction system of the heart. London: Butterworths, 1971.

69. Kurasawa H, Becker AE. Dead-end tract of the conduction axis. Int J Cardiol 1985;7:13.

70. Truex RC, Smythe MQ: Reconstruction of the human atrioventricular node. Anat Rec 1967;158:11.

71. Paes de Carvalho A, De Mello WG, Hoffman BF: Electrophysiological evidence for specialised fiber types in rabbit atrium. Am J Physiol 1959;196:483.

72. Hoffman BF, Cranefield PF: Electrophysiology of the heart. New York: McGraw-Hill, 1960:48.

73. James TN: Anatomy of the cardiac conduction system in the rabbit. Circ Res 1967;20:638.

74. Anderson RH: Histologic and histochemical evidence concerning the presence of morphologically distinct cellular zones within the rabbit atrioventricular node. Anat Rec 1972;173:7.

75. Anderson RH, Janse MJ, Van Capelle FJL, Billette J, Becker AE, Durrer D: A combined morphological and electrophysiological study of the atrioventricular node of the rabbit heart. Circ Res 1974;35:909.

76. Anderson RH: Histologic and histochemical evidence concerning the presence of morphologically distinct cellular zones within the rabbit atrioventricular node. Anat Rec 1972;173:7.

77. Anderson RH: The disposition and innervation of atrioventricular ring specialized tissue in rats and rabbits. J Anat 1972;113:197.

78. Bojsen-Moller F, Tranum-Jensen J: Rabbit heart nodal tissue,

sinuatrial ring bundle and atrioventricular connexions identified as a neuromuscular system. J Anat 1972;112:367.

79. Finlay M, Anderson RH: The development of cholinesterase activity in the rat heart. J Anat 1974;117:239.

80. Anderson RH: The disposition, morphology and innervation of cardiac specialized tissues in the guinea pig. J Anat 1972; 111:453.

81. Wharton J, Polak JM, McGregor GP, Bishop AE, Bloom SR: The distribution of substance P-like immunoreactive nerves in the guinea-pig heart. Neurosci 1981;56:2193.

82. Forsgren S: The distribution of sympathetic nerve fibres in the AV node and AV bundle of the bovine heart. Histochem J 1986;18:625.

83. Forsgren S: Marked sympathetic innervation in the regions of the bundle branches shown by catecholamine histofluorescence. J Mol Cell Cardiol 1987;19:555.

84. Forsgren S: The distribution of terminal sympathetic nerve fibers in bundle branches and false tendons of bovine heart. Anat Embryol 1988;177:437.

85. Summers RJ, Molenaar P, Stephenson JA: Autoradiographic localization of receptors in the cardiovascular system. Trends Pharmacol Sci 1987;8:272.

86. Molenaar P, Canale E, Summers RJ: Autoradiographic localization of beta-1 and beta-2 adrenoreceptors in guinea pig atrium and regions of the conducting system. J Pharmacol Exp Ther 1987;241:1048.

87. Saito K, Kurihara M, Cruciani R, Potter WZ, Saavedra JM: Characterization of B1- and B2-adrenoreceptor subtypes in the rat atrioventricular node by quantitative autoradiography. Circ Res 1988;62:173.

88. Saito K, Torda T, Potter WZ, Saavedra JM: Characterization of B1-B2-adrenoreceptor subtypes in the rat sinoatrial node and stellate ganglia by quantitative autoradiography. Neurosci Lett 1989;96:35.

89. Saito K, Gutkind JS, Saavedra JM: Angiotensin II binding sites in the conduction system of rat hearts. Am J Physiol 1987; 253:H-1618.

90. Anderson RH, Davies MJ, Becker AE: Atrioventricular ring specialized tissue in the normal heart. Eur J Cardiol 1974; 2:219.

91. Kent AFS: Researchers on the structure and function of the mammalian heart. J Physiol 1893;14:233.

92. Kent AFS: The right lateral auriculo-ventricular junction of the heart. J Physiol 1914;48:22.

93. Rosenbaum MB, Elizari MV, Lazzari JO: The hemiblocks. In: Tampa Tracings. Oldsmar, FL: 1970.

94. Rossi L: Histopathology of the conducting system. G Ital Cardiol 1972;2:484.

95. Uhley HN: The quadrifascicular nature of the peripheral conduction system. In: Dreifus LS, Liboff W, eds. Cardiac arrhythmias. New York: Grune & Stratton, 1973:339.

96. Demoulin JC, Kulbertus HE: Histopathological examination of concept of left hemiblock. Br Heart J 1972;34:807.

97. Eriksson A, Thornell L-E, Stigbrand T: Skeletin immunoreactivity in heart Purkinje fibers from several species. J Histochem Cytochem 1979;27:1604.

98. Kuro-o M, Tsuchimochi H, Ueda S, Takaku F, Yazaki Y: Distribution of cardiac myosin isozymes in human conduction system. J Clin Invest 1986;77:340.

99. Bouvagnet P, Neveu S, Montoya M, Leger JJ: Developmental changes in the human cardiac isomyosin distribution: An immunohistochemical study using monoclonal antibodies. Circ Res 1987;61:329.

100. Gorza L, Thornell L-E, Schiaffino S: Nodal myosin distribution in the bovine heart during prenatal development: An immunohistochemical study. Circ Res 1988;62:1182.

101. Atlas SA: Atrial natriuretic factor: A new hormone of cardiac origin. Recent Prog Horm Res 1986;42:207.

102. Ballerman BJ, Brenner BM: Role of atrial peptides in body fluid homeostasis. Circ Res 1986;58:619.

103. Needleman P, Adams SP, Cole BR, et al: Atriopeptins as cardiac hormones. Hypertension 1986;7:469.

104. Goetz KL: Physiology and pathophysiology of atrial peptides. Am J Physiol 1988;254:E-1.

105. Block KD, Seidman JG, Naftilan JD, Fallon JT, Seidman CE: Neonatal atria and ventricles secrete atrial natriuretic factor via tissue-specific secretory pathways. Cells 1986;47:695.

106. Gardner DG, Gertz BJ, Hane S: Thyroid hormone increases rat atrial natriuretic peptide messenger ribonucleic acid accumulation in vivo and vitro. Mol Endocrinol 1987;1:260.

107. Nemer M, Lavigne J-P, Drouin J, Thibault G, Gannon M, Antakly T: Expression of atrial natriuretic factor gene in heart ventricular tissue. Peptides 1987;7:1147.

108. Hamid Q, Wharton J, Terenghi G, et al: Localisation of atrial natriuretic peptide mRNA and immunoreactivity in the heart and human atrial appendage. Proc Natl Acad Sci U S A 1987;84:105.

109. Hassal CJS, Wharton J, Gulbenkian S, et al: Ventricular and atrial myocytes of newborn rats synthesise and secrete atrial natriuretic peptide in culture: Light and electron-microscopical localisation and chromotographic examination of stored and secreted molecular forms. Cell Tissue Res 1988;- 251:161.

110. Cantin M, Ding J, Thibault G, et al: Immunoreactive atrial natriuretic factor is present in both atria and ventricles. Mol Cell Endocrinol 1987;52:105.

111. Claycomb WC: Atrial-natriuretic-factor mRNA is developmentally regulated in heart ventricles and actively expressed in cultures of ventricular cardiac muscle cells of rat and human. Biochem J 1988;255:617.

112. Mercadier JJ, Zongazo MA, Wisnewsky C, et al: Atrial natriuretic factor messenger ribonucleic acid and peptides in the human heart during ontogenic development. Biochem Biophys Res Commun 1989;159:777.

113. Wei Y, Rodi CP, Day ML, et al: Developmental changes in the rat atriopeptide hormonal system. J Clin Invest 1987;79:1325.

114. Kikuchi K, Nakao K, Hayashi K, et al: Ontogeny of atrial natriuretic polypeptide in the human heart. Acta Endocrinol 1987;115:211.

115. Wharton J, Anderson RH, Springhall D, et al: Localisation of atrial natriuretic peptide immunoreactivity in the ventricular myocardium and conduction system of the human fetal heart. Br Heart J 1988;60:267.

116. Back J, Stumpf WE, Ando E, Nokihara K, Forsmann WG: Immunocytochemical evidence for CDD/ANP-like peptides in strands of myoendocrine cells associated with the ventricular conduction system of the rat heart. Anat Embryol 1986;175:223.

117. Scott JN, Jennes L: Distribution of atrial natriuretic factor in fetal rat atria and ventricles. Cell Tissue Res 1987;248:479.

118. Toshimori H, Toshimori K, Oura C, Matsuo H: Immunohistochemical study of atrial natriuretic polypeptides in the embryonic, fetal and neonatal rat heart. Cell Tissue Res 1987; 248:627.

119. Toshimori H, Toshimori K, Oura C, Matsuo H: Immunohistochemistry and immunocytochemistry of atrial natriuretic polypeptide in porcine heart. Histochemistry 1987;86:595.

120. Toshimori H, Toshimori K, Oura C, Matsuo H, Matsukura S: Immunohistochemical identification of Purkinje fibers and transitional cells in a terminal portion of the impulse-conducting system of porcine heart. Cell Tissue Res 1988; 253:47.

121. Toshimori H, Toshimori K, Oura C, Matsuo H, Matsukura S: The distribution of atrial natriuretic polypeptide (ANP)-containing cells in the adult rat heart. Anat Embryol 1988; 177:477.

122. Wenink ACG: Embryology of the heart. In: Anderson RH, Macartney FJ, Shinebourne EA, Tynan M, eds. Paediatric cardiology. Vol 1. Edinburgh: Churchill Livingstone, 1987:83.

123. Tikkanen I, Fyhrquist F, Metsarine K, Leidenius R: Plasma atrial natriuretic peptide in cardiac disease and during infusion in healthy volunteers. Lancet 1985;2:66.

124. Roy D, Pillard F, Cassidy D, et al: Atrial natriuretic factor during atrial fibrillation and supraventricular tachycardia. J Am Coll Cardiol 1987;9:509.

125. Anderson JV, Gibbs JS, Woodruff PIW, Creco C, Rowland E, Bloom SR: The plasma atrial natriuretic peptide response to treatment of acute cardiac failure, spontaneous supra-ventricular tachycardia and induced re-entrant tachycardia in man. J Hypertens 1986;4:2.

126. Durrer D, Schuilenberg RM, Wellens HJJ. Preexcitation revisited. Am J Cardiol 1970;25:690.

127. Sherf L, James TN: A new electrocardiographic concept: Synchronized sino-ventricular conduction. Dis Chest 1969; 55:127.

128. James TN: Heuristic thoughts on the Wolff-Parkinson-White syndrome. In: Schlant RC, Hurst JW, eds. Advances in electrophysiology. New York: Grune & Stratton, 1972:269.

129. Lev M. The pre-excitation syndrome: Anatomic considerations of anomalous A-V pathways. In: Dreifus LS, Koff WS, eds. Mechanisms and therapy of cardiac arrhythmias. New York: Grune & Stratton, 1966:665.

130. Anderson RH, Becker AE: Anatomy of conducting tissues revisited. Br Heart J 1978;40(suppl):2.

131. Sherf L, James TN: Wolff-Parkinson-White syndrome. Circulation 1971;43:456.

132. Durrer D, Wellens HJ: The Wolff-Parkinson-White syndrome. Eur J Cardiol 1974;1:347.

133. Anderson RH, Becker AE: Stanley Kent and accessory atrioventricular connexions. J Thorac Cardiovasc Surg 1981; 81:649.

134. Sealy WC: Reply to: Accessory atrioventricular connections. J Thorac Cardiovasc Surg 1979;78:311.

135. Mahaim I: Kent's fiber in the A-V paraspecific conduction through the upper connection of the bundle of His-Tawara. Am Heart J 1947;33:651.

136. Brechenmacher C: Atrio-His bundle tracts. Br Heart J 1975; 37:853.

137. Anderson RH, Becker AE, Brechenmacher C, Davies MJ, Rossi L: Ventricular preexcitation. A proposed nomenclature for its substrates. Eur J Cardiol 1975;3:27.

138. Burchell HB: Ventricular pre-excitation historical overview. In: Benditt DG, Benson DW, eds. Cardiac preexcitation syndromes. The Hague: Martinus Nijhoff Publishing, 1986:3.

139. Wood FC, Wolferth CG, Geckeler GD: Histologic demonstration of accessory muscular connections between auricle and ventricle in a case of short P-R interval and prolonged QRS complex. Am Heart J 1943;25:454.

140. Ohnell RF: Preexcitation, a cardiac abnormality. Acta Med Scand 1944;152:1.

141. Gallagher J, Svenson R, Sealy WC, Wallace A: The Wolff-Parkinson-White syndrome and the pre-excitation dysrhythmias. Med Clin North Am 1976;60:101.

142. Sealy WC, Wallace AG, Ramming KP, Gallagher JJ, Svenson RH: An improved operation for the definitive treatment of the Wolff-Parkinson-White syndrome. Ann Thorac Surg 1974;17:107.

143. Warin J-F, Haissaguerre M, D'Ivernois C, Le Metayer P, Monserrat P: Catheter ablation of accessory pathways: Technique and results in 248 patients. PACE 1989;13:1609.

144. Gotlieb AI, Chan M, Palmer WH, Huang S-N: Ventricular preexcitation syndrome. Accessory left atrioventricular connection and rhabdomyomatous myocardial fibers. Arch Pathol Lab Med 1977;101:486.

145. Becker AE, Anderson RH, Durrer D, Wellens HJJ: The anatomical substrates of Wolff-Parkinson-White syndrome: A clinico-pathologic correlation in seven patients. Circulation 1978;57:870.

146. Sealy WC, Gallagher JJ: The surgical approach to the septal area of the heart based on experience with 45 patients with Kent bundles. J Thorac Cardiovasc Surg 1980;79:542.

147. Gillette PC, Garson A Jr, Cooley DA, McNamara DG: Prolonged and decremental antegrade conduction properties in right anterior accessory connections: Wide QRS antidromic tachycardia of left bundle branch block pattern without Wolff-Parkinson-White configuration in sinus rhythm. Am Heart J 1982;103:66.

148. Klein GJ, Guiraudon GM, Kerr CR, et al: "Nodoventricular" accessory pathway: Evidence for a distinct accessory atrioventricular pathway with atrioventricular node-like properties. J Am Coll Cardiol 1988;11:1035.

149. Guiraudon CM, Guiraudon GM, Klein GJ: "Nodal ventricular" Mahaim pathway: Histologic evidence for an accessory atrioventricular pathway with an AV node-like morphology. Circulation 1988;78:II-40.

150. Leitch J, Klein GJ, Yee R, Murdock C: New concepts on nodoventricular accessory pathways. J Cardiovasc Electrophysiol 1990;1:220.

151. Dreifus LS, Wellens HJ, Watanabe Y, Kimbiris D, Truex R: Sinus bradycardia and atrial fibrillation associated with the Wolff-Parkinson-White syndrome. Am J Cardiol 1976;38:149.

152. Denes P, Amat-y-Leon F, Wyndham C, Wu D, Levitsky S, Rosen K: Electrophysiological demonstration of bilateral anomalous pathways in a patient with Wolff-Parkinson-

White syndrome (Type B pre-excitation). Am J Cardiol 1976;37:93.

153. Lev M, Fox SM, Bharati S, Greenfield JC, Rosen KM, Pick A: Mahaim and James fibers as a basis for a unique variety of ventricular pre-excitation. Am J Cardiol 1975;36:880.

154. Gmeiner R, Ng CK, Hammer I, Becker AE: Tachycardia caused by an accessory nodoventricular tract: A clinico-pathologic correlation. Eur Heart J 1984;5:233.

155. James TN: Sudden death in babies: New observations in the heart. Am J Cardiol 1968;22:479.

156. James TN: Sudden death of babies. Circulation 1976;53:1.

157. Anderson WR, Edland JF, Schenk EA: Conducting system changes in the sudden infant death syndrome. (Abstract) Am J Pathol 1970;59:35a.

158. Ferris JAJ: Hypoxic changes in conducting tissue of the heart in sudden death in infancy syndrome. BMJ 1973;2:23.

159. Valdes-Dapena MA, Greene M, Basavarand N, Catherman C, Truex RC: The myocardial conduction system in sudden death in infancy. N Engl J Med 1973;289:1179.

160. Anderson RH, Bouton J, Burrow CT, Smith A: Sudden death in infancy: A study of the cardiac specialized tissue. BMJ 1974;2:135.

161. Lie JT, Rosenberg HS, Erickson EE: Histopathology of the conduction system in the sudden infant death syndrome. Circulation 1976;53:3.

162. Preston JB, McFadden S, Moe GK: Atrioventricular transmission in young mammals. Am J Physiol 1959;197:236.

163. Ho SY, Anderson RH: Conduction tissue and SIDS. Ann N Y Acad Sci 1988;533:176.

164. Southall DP, Vulliamy DG, Davies MJ, Anderson RH, Shinebourne EA, Johnson AM. A new look at the neonatal electro-cardiogram. BMJ 1976;2:615.

165. James TN, Robertson BT, Waldo AL, Branch CE: De subitaneis mortibus. XV. Hereditary stenosis of His bundle in pug dogs. Circulation 1975;52:1152.

166. Lev M. Ageing changes in the human sinoatrial node. J Gerontol 1954;9:1.

167. Erickson EE, Lev M: Ageing changes in the human AV node, bundle and bundle branches. J Gerontol 1952;7:1.

168. Davies MJ, Pomerance A: Quantitative study of ageing changes in the human sinoatrial node and internodal tracts. Br Heart J 1972;34:150.

169. James TN: The sinus node. Am J Cardiol 1977;40:965.

170. Davies MJ, Anderson RH, Becker AE: The conduction system of the heart. London: Butterworths, 1983:306.

171. Angelini P, Sandiford FM: Functional correction of transposition of the great arteries: A new approach to avoid post-operative arrhythmias. J Thorac Cardiovasc Surg 1973;66:87.

172. Isaacson R, Titus JL, Merideth J, Feldt RH, McGoon DC: Apparent interruption of atrial conduction pathways after surgical repair of transposition of the great arteries. Am J Cardiol 1972;30:533.

173. El-Said G, Rosenberg HS, Mullins CE, Hallman GL, Colley DA, McNamara DG: Dysrhythmias after Mustard's operation for transposition of the great arteries. Am J Cardiol 1972;39:526.

174. Wittig JH, De Leval MR, Stark J: Intraoperative mapping of

atrial activation before, during and after Mustard's operation. J Thorac Cardiovasc Surg 1977;73:1.

175. Ullal RR, Anderson RH, Lincoln C: Mustard's operation modified to avoid dysrhythmias and pulmonary and systemic venous obstruction. J Thorac Cardiovasc Surg 1979;78:431.

176. Southall DP, Keeton BR, Leanage R, et al: Cardiac rhythm and conduction before and after Mustard's operation for complete transposition of the great arteries. Br Heart J 1980;43:21.

177. Ho SY, Monro JL, Anderson RH: The disposition of the sinus node in left-sided juxtaposition of the atrial appendage. Br Heart J 1979;41:129.

178. Truex RC, Bishof JK: Conduction system in human hearts with interventricular septal defects. J Thorac Surg 1958;35:421.

179. Lev M: The architecture of the conduction system in congenital heart disease. III. Ventricular septal defect. Arch Pathol 1960;70:529.

180. Titus JL, Daugherty GW, Edwards JE: Anatomy of the atrioventricular conduction system in ventricular septal defect. Circulation 1963;28:72.

181. Latham RA, Anderson RH: Anatomical variations in atrioventricular conduction system with reference to ventricular septal defects. Br Heart J 1972;34:185.

182. Milo S, Ho SY, Wilkinson JL, Anderson RH: The surgical anatomy and atrioventricular conduction tissues of hearts with isolated ventricular septal defects. J Thorac Cardiovasc Surg 1980;79:244.

183. Lev M: The architecture of the conduction system in congenital heart disease II. Tetralogy of Fallot. Arch Pathol 1959;67:572.

184. Anderson RH, Monro JL, Ho SY, Smith A, Deverall PB: Les voies de conduction auriculo-ventriculaires dans le tetralogie de Fallot. Coeur 1977;8:793.

185. Starr A, Bonchek LI, Sunderland CO: Total correction of tetralogy of Fallot in infancy. J Thorac Cardiovasc Surg 1973;65:45.

186. Bharati S, Lev M: The conduction system in simple, regular (d-), complete transposition with ventricular septal defect. J Thorac Cardiovasc Surg 1976;72:194.

187. Bharati S, Lev M: The conduction system in double outlet right ventricle with sub-pulmonic ventricular septal defect and related hearts (The Taussig-Bing Group). Circulation 1976;54:459.

188. Thiene G, Bortolotti V, Gallucci V, Terrible V, Pellegrino PA: Anatomical study of truncus arteriosus communis with embryological and surgical considerations. Br Heart J 1976;38:II-1109.

189. Lincoln C, Anderson RH, Shinebourne EA, English TAH, Wilkinson JL: Double outlet right ventricle with l-malposition of the aorta. Br Heart J 1975;37:453.

190. Allwork SP, Bentall HH, Becker AE, et al: Congenitally corrected transposition of the great arteries: Morphologic study of 32 cases. Am J Cardiol 1976;38:910.

191. Anderson RH, Arnold R, Wilkinson JL: The conducting system in congenitally corrected transposition. Lancet 1973;1:1286.

192. Anderson RH, Becker AE, Arnold R, Wilkinson JL: The con-

ducting tissues in congenitally corrected transposition. Circulation 1974;50:911.

193. De Leval M, Bastos P, Stark J, Taylor JFN, Macartney FJ, Anderson RH: Surgical technique to reduce the risks of heart block following closure of ventricular septal defect in atrioventricular discordance. J Thorac Cardiovasc Surg 1979;78:515.

194. Kupersmith J, Krongrad E, Gersony WM, Bowman FO: Electrophysiologic identification of the specialized conduction system in corrected transposition of the great arteries. Circulation 1974;50:795.

195. Anderson RH, Danielson GK, Maloney JD, Becker AE: Atrioventricular bundle in corrected transposition. Ann Thor Surg 1978;26:95.

196. Dick M, Van Praagh R, Rudd M, Folkerth T, Castaneda AR: Electrophysiological delineation of the specialised atrioventricular conduction system in two patients with corrected transposition of the great arteries with situs inversus (I,D,D). Circulation 1977;55:896.

197. Thiene G, Nava A, Rossi L: The conduction system in corrected transposition with situs inversus. Eur J Cardiol 1977; 6:57.

198. Wilkinson JL, Smith A, Lincoln C, Anderson RH: The conducting tissues in congenitally corrected transposition with situs inversus. Br Heart J 1978;40:41.

199. Monckeberg JG: Zur Entwicklungsgeschichte des Atrioventrikularsystems. Ver deutsch Path Ges 1913;16:228.

200. Symons JC, Shinebourne EA, Joseph MC, Lincoln C, Ho Y, Anderson RH: Criss-cross heart with congenitally corrected transposition: Report of a case with d-transposed aorta and ventricular preexcitation. Eur J Cardiol 1977;5:493.

201. Bharati S, Lev M: The course of the conduction system in dextrocardia. Circulation 1978;50:163.

202. Anderson RH, Arnold R, Thaper MK, Jones RS, Hamilton DI: Cardiac specialized tissues in hearts with an apparently single ventricular chamber (Double inlet left ventricle). Am J Cardiol 1974;33:95.

203. Bharati S, Lev M: The course of the conduction system in single ventricle with inverted (L) loop and inverted (L) transposition. Circulation 1975;51:723.

204. Wilkinson JL, Anderson RH, Arnold R, Hamilton DI, Smith A: The conducting tissues in primitive ventricular hearts without an outlet chamber. Circulation 1976;53:930.

205. Anderson RH, Wilkinson JL, Becker AE: Conducting tissues in the univentricular heart. In: Van Mierop LHS, Oppenheimer-Dekker A, Bruins CLD Ch, eds. Embryology and teratology of the heart and the great arteries (Boerhaave Course 13). The Hague: Leiden University Press, 1978: 62.

206. Wilkinson JL, Macartney FJ, Keeton BR, Tynan MJ, Hunter S, Anderson RH: Morphology and conducting tissue in univentricular hearts of right ventricular type. Herz 1979;4:151.

207. Lev M: Pathogenesis of congenital atrioventricular block. Prog Cardiovasc Dis 1972;15:145.

208. El Sayed H, Cleland WP, Bentall HH, Melrose DG, Bishop MB, Morgan J: Corrected transposition of the great arterial

trunks: Surgical treatment of the associated defects. J Thorac Cardiovasc Surg 1962;44:443.

209. Lev M, Silverman J, Fitzmaurice FM, Paul MH, Cassels DE, Miller RA: Lack of connection between the atria and the more peripheral conduction system in congenital atrioventricular block. Am J Cardiol 27:481, 1971.

210. Lev M, Cuadros H, Paul MH: Interruption of the atrioventricular bundle with congenital atrioventricular block. Circulation 1971;43:703.

211. Husson GS, Blackman MS, Rogers MC, Bharati S, Lev M: Familial congenital bundle branch system disease. Am J Cardiol 1973;32:365.

212. Scott JS, Maddison PJ, Taylor PV, Esscher E, Scott O, Skinner RD: Connective tissue disease, antibodies to ribonucleoprotein, and congenital heart block. N Engl J Med 1983;4:209.

213. Ho SY, Esscher E, Anderson RH, Michaelsson M: Anatomy of congenital complete heart block and relation to maternal anti-Ro bodies. Am J Cardiol 1986;58:291.

214. Davies MJ, Anderson RH, Becker AE: The conduction system of the heart. London: Butterworths, 1983.

215. Blondeau M, Maurice P, Reverdy V, Lenegre J: Troubles de rhythme de la conduction auriculo-ventriculaire dans l'infarctus du myocarde recent. Considerations anatomiques. Arch Mal Coeur Vaiss 1967;60:1733.

216. Blondeau M, Rizzon P, Lenegre J: Les troubles de la conduction auriculo-ventriculaire dans l'infarctus myocardiaque recent. Il etude anatomique. Arch Mal Coeur Vaiss 1961;53:1104.

217. Sutton R, Davies M: The conduction system in acute myocardial infarction complicated by complete heart block. Circulation 1968;8:987.

218. Hunt D, Lie JT, Vohra J, Sloman G: Histopathology of heart block complicating acute myocardial infarction. Correlation with the His bundle electrogram. Circulation 1973;48:1252.

219. Hackel DG, Estes EH Jr: Pathologic features of atrioventricular and intraventricular conduction disturbances in acute myocardial infarction. Circulation 1971;43:977.

220. Hackel DB, Wagner G, Ratliff NB, Cies AB, Estes EH Jr: Anatomic studies of the cardiac conducting system in acute myocardial infarction. Am Heart J 1972;83:77.

221. Becker AE, Lie KI, Anderson RH: Bundle branch block in the setting of acute anteroseptal myocardial infarction: A clinico-pathologic investigation. Br Heart J 1978;40:773.

222. Lev M: The pathology of complete atrioventricular block. Prog Cardiovasc Dis 1964;6:317.

223. Lev M. Anatomic basis for atrioventricular block. Am J Med 1964;37:742.

224. Lenegre J: Etiology and pathology of bilateral bundle branch block in relation to complete heart block. Prog Cardiovasc Dis 1964;6:409.

225. Lenegre J: Bilateral bundle branch block. Cardiology (Basel) 1966;46:261.

226. Davies M: Pathology of the conducting tissue of the heart. London: Butterworths, 1971:92.

227. Davies M: Pathology of the conducting tissues of the heart. London: Butterworths, 1971:67.

Cardiac Arrhythmias, 3rd edition, edited by William J. Mandel.
J. B. Lippincott Company, Philadelphia © 1995.

3

David C. Gadsby • Hrayr S. Karagueuzian • Andrew L. Wit

Normal and Abnormal Electrical Activity in Cardiac Cells

In general, an arrhythmia is any abnormality in the rate, regularity, or site of origin of the cardiac impulse or disturbance in the conduction of that impulse, such that the normal sequence of activation of atria and ventricles is altered.[1] Arrhythmias may thus be said to result from abnormalities of impulse initiation, impulse conduction, or both.[2] Such abnormalities may result from quite small changes in the mechanisms underlying the generation of the normal transmembrane action potential. They may also be caused by more substantial changes, resulting in electrical activity with characteristics unlike those found in normal cardiac cells.

As discussed throughout this book, cardiac arrhythmias and conduction disturbances have many pathologic causes. However, all arrhythmias and conduction abnormalities result from critical alterations in the electrical activity of myocardial cells. This chapter outlines the mechanisms underlying normal activity of cardiac cells and shows how this activity may be changed by disease to cause arrhythmias. More detailed treatment of specific types of arrhythmias, for example, supraventricular tachycardia, ventricular fibrillation, and ischemic arrhythmias, are discussed elsewhere in this book.

RESTING AND ACTION POTENTIAL OF NORMAL ATRIAL, VENTRICULAR, AND PURKINJE FIBERS

The normal, regular beating of the heart is accompanied by cyclic changes in the membrane potential of cardiac cells. The use of intracellular microelectrodes has allowed these membrane potential changes to be measured directly; the changes vary in amplitude and time course as the impulse travels through the heart.[3] The microelectrode technique involves the insertion of a fine glass needle into a cell, so that the membrane potential, that is, the potential difference between the cell interior and the extracellular fluid, may be recorded directly and continuously. A micromanipulator is used to advance the microelectrode until its tip (usually less than 0.1 μm in diameter) pierces the cell membrane. At the moment the microelectrode tip passes from the outside to the inside of the cell, it records a negative potential difference with respect to a reference electrode placed in the extracellular fluid (Fig. 3-1). Microelectrode studies are usually made on isolated bundles of cardiac fibers mounted in a tissue bath and superfused with warmed, oxygenated solutions.

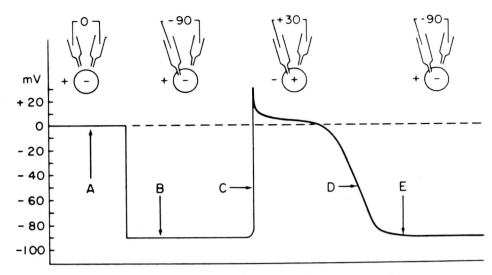

Figure 3-1. The resting and action potential of a cardiac cell. The upper row of diagrams shows a cell (*the circle*) and two microelectrodes. In *A*, both electrodes are in the extracellular space, and there is no potential difference between them. *B* shows the tip of one microelectrode inside the cell; the potential difference between the inside and outside of the cell, the resting potential (-90 mV) is now recorded. *C* shows the upstroke of the action potential, which occurs when the cell is excited. At the peak of the upstroke, the inside of this cell is 30 mV positive with respect to the outside. *D* represents the final phase of repolarization, which returns membrane potential to its resting level, shown at *E*. (Cranefield PF: The conduction of the cardiac impulse. Mt Kisco NY. Futura, 1975; with permission.)

Action potentials may be initiated in such preparations by the application of brief current pulses through electrodes placed on the fiber surface (see Fig. 3-1). In the absence of stimulated action potentials, however, the interior of most cardiac cells (except those of the sinus and atrioventricular node, which are discussed separately) remains 80 to 90 mV negative with respect to the extracellular space.[3] This transmembrane potential during electrical quiescence is referred to as the *resting potential.*

As with many other excitable cells, the resting potential of cardiac cells is largely determined by the concentration gradient for potassium ions across the cell membrane, whereas the rapid potential change during impulse initiation depends on the concentration gradient for sodium ions.[4-6] These concentration gradients run in opposite directions. The intracellular potassium concentration, $[K^+]_i$, is approximately 30 times greater than the extracellular concentration, $[K^+]_o$. In Purkinje fibers, for example, $[K^+]_i$ and $[K^+]_o$ are typically 140 to 150 mM and 4 to 5 mM, respectively.[7] The intracellular sodium concentration, $[Na^+]_i$, is much smaller than the extracellular concentration, $[Na^+]_o$; $[Na^+]_i$ and $[Na^+]_o$ are usually about 10 mM and 150 mM, respectively, in Purkinje fibers.[8] During each action potential, a small amount of sodium enters the cell and a small amount of potassium is lost from the cell. Normal electrical activity depends on the existence of the steep concentration gradients for Na^+ and K^+, and the

long-term maintenance of these gradients depends on an active transport mechanism called the sodium pump. This mechanism, which has been studied extensively, is a Mg^{++}-ATPase (adenosine triphosphatase) that is located within the cell membrane and that uses the energy stored as ATP (adenosine triphosphate) to pump sodium ions out of the cell and potassium ions into the cell. These ion movements must expend energy, because they are both normally uphill, that is, against the respective electrochemical potential gradients. The pumped ion movements, however, are probably not equal in the two directions, because more than one Na^+ is pumped out for each K^+ that is pumped in.[9] Thus, the sodium pump generates a net outward movement of positive charge, or a net outward current across the cell membrane. This pump current is usually small, but it may make a significant contribution to membrane potential changes under certain conditions.

Resting Potential

As discussed, the level of the resting potential is predominantly determined by the potassium ion concentration gradient. This is because, at rest, the cell membrane is relatively permeable to potassium ions but relatively impermeable to other ions such as sodium, calcium, or chloride ions. Because of the concentration gradient, potassium ions tend to diffuse out of the cell across the membrane. Electroneutrality cannot be maintained by an outward movement of cellular anions, because these are mainly large polyvalent ions (often associated with cell proteins) to which the cell membrane is impermeable.[10] The outward movement of the positively charged potassium ions, therefore, causes a net negative charge to build up inside the cell (Fig. 3-2). If the cell membrane was permeable only to potassium ions, then these would continue to diffuse from the cell until the cell interior became sufficiently negative that electrostatic attraction would oppose further net outward potassium movement. In this case, the inwardly directed electrical force exactly counters the outwardly directed force, because the concentration gradient and net movement of potassium ions cease. The algebraic sum of these two forces, called the electrochemical potential gradient, is then zero. The intracellular potential at which the net passive flux of potassium ions is zero is called the equilibrium potential for potassium ions, E_K, and its value is given by the Nernst equation[3-5]:

$$E_K = \frac{RT}{F} \ln \frac{[K^+]_o}{[K^+]_i}$$

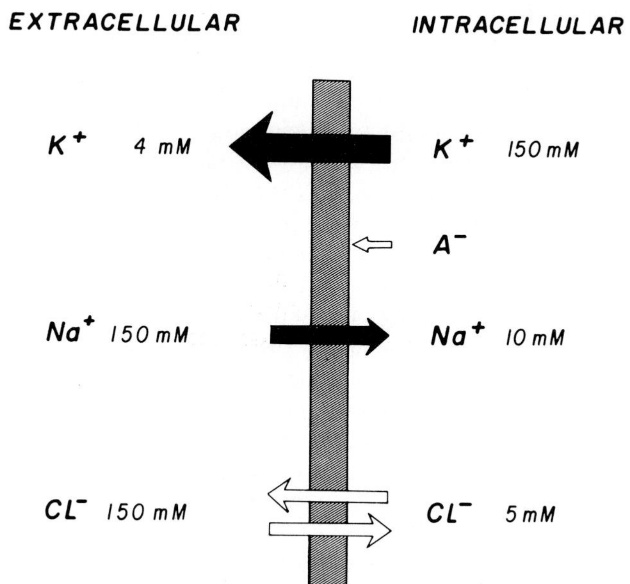

EXTRACELLULAR   **INTRACELLULAR**

Figure 3-2. Distribution of ions contributing to the resting potential. Typical concentrations of ions inside and outside the cell are shown. At rest, the membrane is highly permeable to K^+ but impermeable to large anions (A^-), and the permeability to Na^+ is low. The permeability to Cl^- is also relatively low, and the distribution of Cl^- is most probably determined by the average value of the membrane potential.

where R is the gas constant, T is the absolute temperature, F is Faraday's constant, and $[K^+]_o$ and $[K^+]_i$ are the extracellular and intracellular concentrations of potassium ions, respectively. (The ratio of the ion activities should be used in place of the concentration ratio, but these two ratios are approximately the same when the internal and external activity coefficients for K^+ are similar.) For example, the value of E_K for a Purkinje fiber at 36°C for which $[K^+]_o$ is 4 mM and $[K^+]_i$ is 150 mM would be:

$$E_K = \frac{RT}{F} \ln \frac{4}{150} = 26.6 \ln \frac{4}{150}$$

$$= 61.4 \log \frac{4}{150} = -96.6 \text{ mV}$$

The Nernst equation shows that E_K changes by 61.4 mV after a 10-fold change in either $[K^+]_o$ or $[K^+]_i$. If the cell membrane was exclusively permeable to K^+, then the cell would behave just like a potassium electrode, and its intracellular potential would change with variations in $[K^+]_o$ and $[K^+]_i$ just as predicted by the Nernst equation. The membrane potentials of resting Purkinje fibers and atrial and ventricular myocardial fibers are well approximated by the Nernst relation when $[K^+]_o$ is higher than approximately 10 mM. At lower values of $[K^+]_o$, however, the resting potentials of these cells are less negative than the potassium equilibrium potential, and this discrepancy increases as $[K^+]_o$ is lowered.[5, 11] For instance, the resting potential of Purkinje fibers exposed to a solution containing 4 mM K^+ is a few millivolts less negative than the estimated value of E_K. The reason for this is because the cell membrane is not exclusively permeable to K^+, but has a relatively low permeability to Na^+. Because both the electrical gradient and the concentration gradient favor the inward movement of Na^+, a small inward depolarizing current of sodium ions flows across the cell membrane. The depolarization caused by this Na^+ current is negligibly small when $[K^+]_o$ is high and the membrane K^+ conductance, therefore, is also high, but it becomes significant when $[K^+]_o$ is low, because membrane K^+ currents also become small under these conditions.

This depolarizing influence of Na^+ is most easily discussed in terms of the Goldman[12] and Hodgkin and Katz[13] "constant field" equation for the resting potential, V_r, of a cell permeable to both K^+ and Na^+:

$$V_r = \frac{RT}{F} \ln \frac{[K^+]_o + (P_{Na}/P_K)[Na^+]_o}{[K^+]_i + (P_{Na}/P_K)[Na^+]_i}$$

$$V_r = \frac{RT}{F} \ln \frac{[K^+]_o + 0.01 [Na^+]_o}{[K^+]_i}$$

$$V_r = \frac{RT}{F} \ln \frac{[K^+]_o + 1.5}{[K^+]_i}$$

This equation shows that the resting potential, V_r, approximates the K^+ equilibrium potential, E_K, only when $[K^+]_o$ is much greater than 1.5 mM; at low $[K^+]_o$ values, the second term in the numerator makes an important contribution. For example, at a $[K^+]_o$ of 1.5 mM, V_r is less negative than E_K by 61.4 log (3/1.5) = 61.4 log 2, or approximately 18 mV. So far, only the relative permeability of the membrane to potassium and sodium ions has been discussed; the absolute magnitude of these permeability coefficients has not been considered. As the Goldman and Hodgkin and Katz equation shows, the resting potential is sensitive to the ratio of the permeabilities of the ions involved but not to the permeability values themselves. For example, even if the Na^+ permeability is substantial, the resting potential is determined predominantly by the K^+ concentration gradient as long as the membrane retains a much higher permeability to K^+ than to Na^+. The membrane channels through which K ions move to generate the K^+ currents that determine the resting membrane potential are called inward rectifier K^+ channels. K^+ currents flowing in these channels depend on the size and direction of the electrochemical driving force on K^+, that is, the difference between the membrane potential, V_m, and the K^+ equilibrium potential, E_K, or $V_m - E_K$. The channels are called inward rectifiers because they allow passage of large inward K^+ currents when $V_m - E_k$ is large and negative, but they allow only very small outward K^+ currents when the driving force is large and positive.[10,11,15]

Changes in the resting potential level may be a primary cause of arrhythmias and conduction disturbances, and such changes might come about under pathologic conditions. For example, cardiac disease might result in alterations in the level of intracellular or extracellular K^+ concentration, or both, thereby causing a change in the resting membrane potential. Alternatively, the characteristics of the cell membrane might change in such a way that the relative permeability of the membrane to Na^+ or other ions (such as Ca^{++}) is increased, also resulting in a change in the level of resting potential.

Depolarization Phases of the Cardiac Action Potential

The electrical impulse that travels through the heart to initiate each heartbeat is called the action potential; it is a propagated wave of transient depolarization during which the intracellular potential of each cell, in turn, briefly becomes positive, then returns to its initial negative level. The potential changes during the normal cardiac action potential have a characteristic time course that is subdivided into the following phases[3]: phase 0 is the initial, rapid membrane depolarization; phase 1 consists of rapid but limited repolarization; phase 2 is the "plateau" or prolonged depolarization characteristic of the action potential of cardiac cells; phase 3 is the final rapid repolarization; and phase 4 is the period of diastole.

The intracellular potential becomes positive during the action potential because the excited membrane temporarily becomes more permeable to Na^+ than to K^+, so the membrane potential transiently approaches the equilibrium potential for sodium ions, E_{Na}. E_{Na} can be estimated by use of the Nernst relation, and for extracellular and intracellular Na^+ concentrations of 150 mM and 10 mM, respectively, it amounts to:

$$E_{Na} = \frac{RT}{F} \ln \frac{[Na^+]_o}{[Na^+]_i} = 26.6 \ln \frac{150}{10}$$
$$= 61.4 \log \frac{150}{10} = +72.2 \text{ mV}$$

The increased Na^+ permeability is not maintained, however, so the membrane potential does not reach E_{Na} but returns toward its resting level during termination of the action potential.

Permeability changes, which cause the depolarization phase of the action potential, result from the opening and closing of special membrane channels, or pores, through which sodium ions can easily pass. It is believed that "gates" control the opening and closing of individual channels and exist in at least three conformations—closed, open, and inactivated. One gate, corresponding to the activation variable "m" in the Hodgkin-Huxley analysis of sodium currents in the membrane of squid giant axons, moves rapidly to open the channel when the membrane is suddenly depolarized by a stimulus.[15] The other gate, corresponding to the inactivation variable "h" in the Hodgkin-Huxley analysis, moves more slowly on depolarization; its function is to close the channel (Fig. 3-3). Both the steady-state distribution of the gates within the channel population and the speed with which they move into and out of position depend on the level of the membrane potential. Hence, the adjectives time- and voltage-dependent describe membrane Na^+ conductance.

If step depolarization to a positive potential level is suddenly applied to the resting membrane (in a voltage clamp experiment, for example), the activation gates move rapidly to open the sodium channels, then the inactivation gates slowly close them (see Fig. 3-3). "Slowly" means that inactivation takes several milliseconds, whereas activation occurs in a fraction of a millisecond. The gates remain in these positions until the membrane potential is changed again, and, to return all the gates to their resting positions, the membrane must be fully repolarized to large negative potential levels. If the membrane is repolarized to only small negative potential levels, some of the inactivation gates remain closed and the maximum number of sodium channels available to be

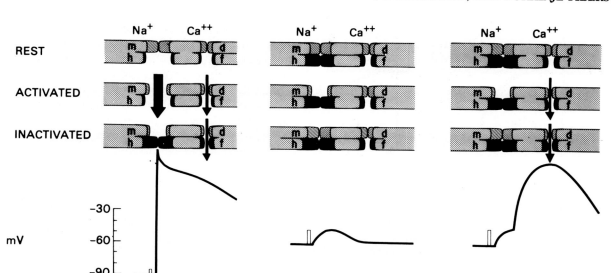

Figure 3-3. Schematic representation of membrane channels for inward current at the resting potential and during activation and inactivation. The left panel illustrates the sequence of events in a fiber with a normal resting potential of −90 mV. The inactivation gates of the Na$^+$ channel (h) and the slow Ca^{++}/Na$^+$ channel (f) are both open at rest. During activation (when the cell is excited), the m gates of the Na$^+$ channel open and the resulting inward current of Na ions depolarizes the cell, giving rise to the upstroke of the action potential depicted below. The h gates then close the channel, thereby inactivating the Na$^+$ conductance. During the upstroke of the action potential, the membrane potential exceeds the more positive threshold potential of the slow channel; the activation (d) gates of this channel then open, and Ca^{++} and Na$^+$ flow into the cell, giving rise to the plateau phase of the action potential. The f gates, which inactivate the Ca^{++}/Na$^+$ channel, close much more slowly than the h gates, which inactivate the Na$^+$ channel. The middle panel shows the behavior of the channels when the resting potential is reduced to below −60 mV. The majority of the inactivation gates of the Na$^+$ channel remain closed as long as the membrane remains depolarized; when the cell is stimulated, the resulting inward Na$^+$ current is too small to cause an action potential. The inactivation (f) gates of the slow channel, however, are not closed, and, as shown in the right panel, excitation of the cell sufficient to open the slow channel, permitting the flow of slow inward current, may cause a slow response action potential to occur. (Wit AL, Bigger JT: Possible electrophysiological mechanisms for lethal arrhythmias accompanying myocardial ischemia and infarction. Circulation 1975; 52:III-96(suppl): with permission.)

opened by subsequent depolarization is reduced.[15] (The electrical behavior of cardiac cells in which some Na$^+$ channels remain inactivated is discussed in subsequent paragraphs.) The full membrane repolarization at the end of a normal action potential ensures that the sodium channel gates are reset, ready for the next action potential.

The rapid depolarization at the beginning of the action potential is caused by a large inward current of sodium ions flowing into the cell, down their electrochemical potential gradient, through the opened sodium channels.[6,16] However, first the sodium channels must be opened effectively, which requires that a sufficiently large area of membrane be depolarized rapidly enough to a level called the *threshold potential* (Fig. 3-4). This can be achieved experimentally by applying current to the membrane from an outside source through either an extracellular or an intracellular stimulating electrode. Usually, the local circuit currents flowing across the membrane just in front of a propagating action potential serve this same

purpose. At the threshold potential, enough sodium channels are opened to give rise to an inward sodium current of sufficient magnitude to cause further membrane depolarization; this, in turn, causes a greater number of channels to open, resulting in more inward current, so that the depolarization becomes self-regenerative. The speed of this regenerative depolarization (or "upstroke" of the action potential) depends on the intensity of the inward sodium current, which itself depends on factors such as the size of the Na$^+$ electrochemical potential gradient and the fraction of available (or noninactivated) sodium channels. In Purkinje fibers, the maximum rate of depolarization during the action potential, referred to as dV/dt$_{max}$ or $\dot{V}_{max}$, reaches about 500 V/sec. If this rate was maintained throughout the entire upstroke from −90 mV to +30 mV, the 120 mV excursion would take about 0.25 millisecond. The maximum rate of depolarization of fibers in ventricular muscle is about 200 V/sec; in atrial muscle, it is between 100 and 200 V/sec.[3] (The depolarization phase of the

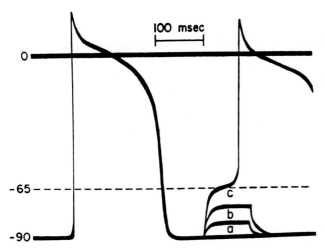

Figure 3-4. The threshold potential for excitation of a cardiac cell. The action potential shown at the left arises from a resting potential of −90 mV; this occurs when the fiber is excited by a propagating impulse or by any suprathreshold stimulus that rapidly lowers the membrane potential to below the threshold level of −65 mV. At the right, the effects of two subthreshold stimuli and a third threshold stimulus are shown. The subthreshold stimuli (a and b) do not lower the membrane potential to the threshold level, and, therefore, an action potential is not elicited. The threshold stimulus (c) reduces the membrane potential just to the threshold level from which an action potential then arises. (Hoffman BF, Cranefield PF: Electrophysiology of the heart. New York: McGraw-Hill, 1960.)

action potentials in sinus and atrioventricular [AV] nodal cells is different and is discussed separately.)

Action potentials with such rapid rates of rise are often called *fast responses*, and they propagate rapidly through the heart.[17] In cells with similar membrane capacitance and axial resistance properties, the speed of action potential propagation is largely determined by the magnitude of the inward current flowing during the upstroke of the action potential, which also determines $\dot{V}_{max}$. This is because the local circuit currents that flow through the cells just ahead of the action potentials are larger during faster upstrokes, thus bringing the membrane potential of those cells to the threshold level sooner than can smaller currents (see Fig. 3-4). These local currents also flow across the membrane just behind an advancing action potential, but they are unable to excite this membrane because it is refractory.

The prolonged refractory period following excitation of cardiac cells results from the long duration of the action potential and the voltage dependence of the gating of the Na^+ channels. After the upstroke of the action potential, there is a period of a hundred to several hundred milliseconds during which there is no regenerative electrical response to a second stimulus (Fig. 3-5). This is called the *absolute refractory period*, and it usually covers the plateau (phase 2) of the action potential. As described, the

sodium channels become inactivated and remain closed during such a maintained depolarization. During the repolarization phase of the action potential (phase 3), a progressive removal of inactivation occurs so that a progressively increasing fraction of the sodium channels becomes available again for subsequent activation. Consequently, it is possible to induce only small inward sodium currents by applying a stimulus at the beginning of repolarization, but these currents increase as action potential repolarization proceeds. Inward Na^+ currents elicited when some Na^+ channels remain inactivated can cause regenerative depolarization and thus give rise to action potentials. However, the rate and extent of the depolarization and, hence, the conduction velocity of these action potentials are all greatly reduced (see Fig. 3-5) and only return to normal values after full repolarization.[18, 19] The time during which a second stimulus can elicit these "graded" action potentials is called the *relative refractory period*. The voltage dependence of the removal of inactivation was studied by Weidmann, who found that the rate of rise of an action potential and the potential level at which that action potential was elicited were related by an S-shaped curve, which is also known as the *membrane responsiveness curve*.

The small rate of rise of action potentials initiated during the relative refractory period causes them to propagate slowly, and such action potentials may form the basis of conduction abnormalities such as conduction delay, decrement, and block and may even cause reentrant excitation. These phenomena are discussed in subsequent paragraphs.

In normal cardiac cells, the inward sodium current responsible for the fast upstroke of the action potential is followed by a second inward current that is smaller and slower than the sodium current and that is probably carried mainly by calcium ions.[20, 21] This current is generally referred to as *slow inward current*, although it is slow only in comparison to the fast sodium current. Other important current changes, such as those occurring during repolarization, are probably slower still. The slow inward current flows through a channel, called the *slow channel*, which exhibits time- and voltage-dependent conductance characteristics (see Fig. 3-3).[22] The threshold for activation of this conductance (i.e., for the activation gates [d] to begin opening) is thought to be around −30 to −40 mV compared with −60 to −70 mV for the sodium conductance.[21] The regenerative depolarization caused by the fast Na^+ current normally activates the slow inward current conductance, and current flows in both channels during the latter part of the action potential upstroke. The Ca^{++} current is much smaller than the peak fast Na^+ current, however, so it contributes little to the action potential until the fast Na^+ current becomes largely inactivated, that is, after the initial rapid upstroke. Because the slow inward

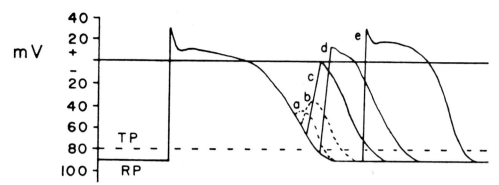

Figure 3-5. Diagrammatic representation of a normal action potential and of responses elicited by stimuli applied at various stages of repolarization. The amplitude and upstroke velocity of the responses elicited during repolarization and are related to the level of the membrane potential from which they arise. The earliest responses (*a* and *b*) arise from such low levels of membrane potential that they are too small to propagate (graded or local responses). Response *c* represents the earliest propagated action potential, but it propagates slowly because of its low upstroke velocity and low amplitude. Response *d* is elicited just before complete repolarization, and its rate of rise and amplitude are greater than those of *c* because it arises from a higher membrane potential; however, it still propagates more slowly than normal. Response *e* is elicited after complete repolarization and, therefore, has a normal rate of depolarization and amplitude and so propagates rapidly. (Singer DH, Ten Eick RE: Pharmacology of cardiac arrhythmias. Progr Cardiovasc Dis 1969;11:488; with permission.)

current inactivates only slowly, it contributes mainly to the plateau of the action potential. Thus, the plateau is shifted in a depolarizing direction when the electrochemical potential gradient for Ca^{++} is enhanced by raising the external Ca^{++} concentration, $[Ca^{++}]_o$, and lowering $[Ca^{++}]_o$ produces a shift in the opposite direction.[23,24] In some cases, however, a contribution of the Ca^{++} current to the rising phase of the action potential can be observed. For example, the upstrokes of action potentials in fibers of the frog ventricle sometimes show an inflection near 0 mV, at which point the initial rapid depolarization gives way to a slower depolarization that continues to the peak of the action potential overshoot. Both the rate of the slower depolarization and the extent of the overshoot have been shown to increase as $[Ca^{++}]_o$ is raised.[24,25]

In addition to the different dependence characteristics of these two conductances on membrane potential and time, they are pharmacologically distinct. Thus, current through the fast Na^+ channel is reduced by tetrodotoxin (TTX), whereas the slow Ca^{++} current is unaffected by TTX but is enhanced by catecholamines and reduced by manganese ions and by the drugs verapamil and D600.[21,26–29] It seems likely, at least in the frog heart, that much of the calcium needed to activate the contractile proteins during each heartbeat enters the cell during the action potential through the slow inward current channel. In mammalian cardiac cells, an additional source of Ca^{++} is available in the stores of the sarcoplasmic reticulum. Two types of slow calcium current, T current and L current, have been described in sinoatrial node cells, atrial cells, ventricular muscle cells, and in Purkinje fibers.[30–35] These

currents are also known by other names. For example, the T current is also called fast current, or SD, for slow deactivation, or type I, and the L current is known as slow current, or FD for fast deactivation, or type II.[30–35] These two currents differ in terms of kinetics of activation and inactivation, voltage dependence of activation and inactivation, sensitivity to various pharmacologic agents, and conductance properties at the single channel level.[30–35] Figure 3-6 shows two types of calcium channels in a single canine Purkinje cell, the T current, the current component seen at more negative holding voltages (i.e., −70 mV) and L current for the current component remaining at less negative holding voltages (i.e., −30 mV). The apparent reversal potential for the L current is about +75 mV, as determined by extrapolating the ascending limb of the peak current-voltage relation recorded at a holding potential of −30 mV to the point where it intercepted the voltage axis (see Fig. 3-6). The apparent reversal potential for the T current, as determined by the intersection of the difference current with the voltage axis, is +37 mV (see Fig. 3-6). The modulation of T and L type calcium currents by catecholamines occur via different adrenoreceptors.[35]

Repolarization Phases of the Cardiac Action Potential

Action potentials recorded in Purkinje fibers and in some ventricular muscle fibers show a brief, rapid phase of repolarization (phase 1) immediately following the action

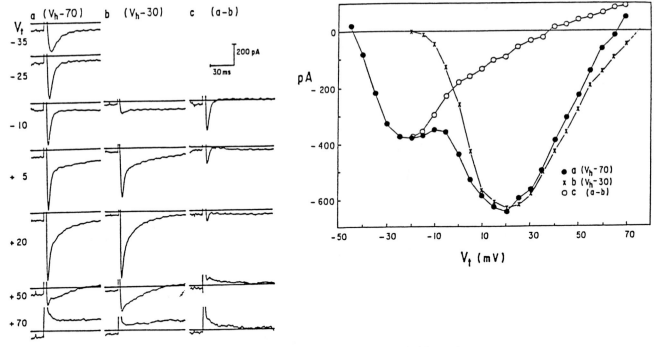

Figure 3-6. Tracing and graph showing Ca^{2+} channel currents recorded at two holding voltages (V_hs) in a canine Purkinje cell. The currents were recorded under conditions that suppressed Na^+ and K^+ currents, with the bath solution containing 5 mM Ca^{2+} at 36° C. Depolarizaion pulses to different voltages (V_ts) for 300 msec were applied at an interval of 7 seconds. *Left panel:* Selected original current tracings at a V_h of −70 mV (column a), −30 mV (column b), and the difference current (column c). V_t is marked on the left. The horizontal lines denote the zero current level. *Right panel:* Peak current-voltage relations at the two levels of V_h and of the difference current. The current recorded at the V_h of −30 mV was extrapolated to cross the voltage axis at +75 mV (*dashed line*). (From Tseng GN, Boyden PA: Multiple types of Ca 2+ currents in single canine Purkinje cells. Circ Res 1989; 65:1735.)

potential upstroke (see Fig. 3-1). This phase temporarily returns the membrane potential to near 0 mV, from which level the plateau phase of the action potential arises, and a well-defined notch is sometimes seen between these two phases. The rapid repolarization has been shown (in Purkinje fibers) to result from a transient surge of outward current.[36] This outward current is activated by the depolarization to positive potential levels during the upstroke of the action potential and is then inactivated both by a time-dependent process and by the resulting repolarization. Although it was originally thought that this outward current was carried largely by chloride ions, it seems more likely that it is carried largely by potassium ions and that only a small component is carried by chloride ions.[37] Two components of transient outward current have been identified in ventricular muscle cells and in Purkinje fibers.[38–41] These two currents differ in terms of their kinetics of activation and inactivation, voltage dependence, sensitivity to intracellular calcium ion concentration, and pharmacologic probes, namely 4-aminopyridine.[38–41] Transient outward current is more pronounced in the epicardium

than in the endocardium, causing a characteristic spike and dome morphology in epicardial action potential.[42] It is suggested that the more prominent transient outward current in the epicardium is largely because of the 4-aminopyridine sensitive component of the transient outward current.[42] Figure 3-7 shows a composite of 6–9 sweeps of the oscilloscope. The first response in each panel is the last of a train of 10 basic beats; subsequent beats represent the response to premature stimuli applied progressively later in the cycle. In the epicardium, the amplitudes of the phase 0, 1, and 2 of premature beats elicited early in diastole were greater than those of the basic beats. These changes were attended by the disappearance of their spike and dome morphology so that the action potential morphology of early premature beats in the epicardium resemble those of the endocardium. Similar changes were observed in the basic responses when the stimulation rate was accelerated. In the example shown in Figure 3-7, the spike and dome configuration of epicardium was greatly attenuated when the stimulation rate was changed from a basic cycle length of 2000 msec to

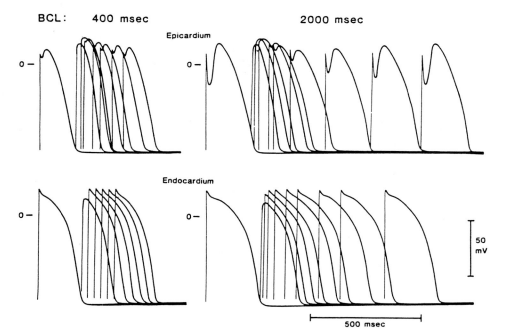

Figure 3-7. Restitution of action potential parameters in epicardium (*top panels*) and endocardium (papillary muscle) (*bottom panels*). BCL = 2,000 msec. Time dependence of the spike and dome morphology in epicardium becomes more evident at slower basic stimulation rates. Note also the biphasic restitution of total amplitude in epicardium and absence of this phenomenon in endocardium. (From Litovsky SH, Antzelevitch C: Transient outward current prominent in canine ventricular epicardium and not in endocardium. Circ Res 1988; 62:116.)

400 msec. The morphology of the endocardial action potential was clearly less rate-dependent; aside from the changes in action potential duration, the restitution of scan revealed only slight changes in other parameters.[42] The prominent presence of transient outward current in epicardium, but not endocardium, appears to contribute to the differences in the time and rate dependence of action potential duration and refractoriness in these two cell types.[43] The presence of a prominent spike and dome in the epicardium but not in the endocardium may produce a voltage gradient during ventricular activation that should manifest in the electrocardiogram as a low amplitude, late delta wave, or what is commonly referred to as a J wave (Osborne wave). Although J wave is often not present in the standard electrocardiogram, signal-averaged electrocardiography often manifests a deflection at the end of the QRS that may be representative of J wave.[43] These contentions are supported in that conditions that exacerbate the magnitude of spike and dome, such as hypercalcemia and hypothermia, also give rise to J wave.[43-45]

During the plateau phase of the action potential, which may last for hundreds of milliseconds, the rate of membrane repolarization is very low, because the net outward membrane current is small: the inward currents that remain as a result of incomplete inactivation of Na^+ and Ca^{++} channels are approximately balanced by outwardly directed membrane currents.[36,46] At least one of these currents is likely to be a potassium current flowing through a gated, time- and voltage-dependent conductance. Activation of this conductance takes place only slowly at plateau levels of membrane potential. Other

small contributions to outward (repolarizing) membrane current at this potential level are expected to be made by inward movements of chloride ions and by the activity of the Na–K exchange pump, which generates a net outward current of Na^+.[47] As the net membrane current (i.e., the algebraic sum of all outward and inward current components) at the plateau potential becomes more outward, the membrane potential shifts more rapidly in a negative direction and the final rapid phase of action potential repolarization takes place. This final repolarization, like the initial fast depolarization, is regenerative, but unlike the upstroke, it probably involves conductance changes that are predominantly voltage dependent and not time dependent; its time course, therefore, reflects the time taken for the outward current to charge the membrane capacitance.[48]

Spontaneous Diastolic Depolarization and Automaticity

The membrane potential of normal working atrial and ventricular muscle cells remains steady at its resting level throughout diastole (see Fig. 3-1). If these cells are not excited by a propagating impulse, then the resting potential is maintained. In other cardiac fibers, such as specialized atrial fibers or Purkinje fibers of the ventricular conducting system, the membrane potential is not steady during diastole, rather it declines. If such a fiber is not excited by propagating impulses before the membrane potential reaches threshold level, a spontaneous action potential may arise in that cell (Fig. 3-8). The decline of membrane potential during diastole is called *spontaneous, diastolic*, or *phase 4 depolarization*. By initiating action potentials, this mechanism forms the basis of automaticity. Automaticity is a normal property of cells in the sinus node, in the muscle of the mitral and tricuspid valves, in some parts of the atrium, in the distal part of the AV node, and in the His–Purkinje system. In the normal heart, the rate of impulse initiation due to automaticity of cells in the sinus node is sufficiently high that these propagated impulses excite other potentially automatic cells before they spontaneously depolarize to threshold potential. In this way, the potential automaticity of other cells is normally suppressed, although it may be revealed under a number of physiologic and pathologic conditions.

Spontaneous diastolic depolarization results from a gradual shift in the balance between inward and outward components of membrane current in favor of net inward

(depolarizing) currents. This pacemaker current shows both time- and voltage-dependent gating properties when investigated with the voltage clamp technique in Purkinje fibers and in nodal pacemakers.[14,48–51] Initial studies of the potential levels at which these pacemaker current changes reversed their direction strongly suggested that an outward pacemaker current, carried by K^+, gradually declined and so allowed inwardly directed background current to depolarize the cell membrane.[14,48,49] More recent experiments, however, are interpreted as suggesting that the normal pacemaker current is an inward current, carried predominantly by Na^+, that gradually increases with time, thereby causing the gradual diastolic depolarization.[50,51] When the depolarization reaches threshold potential, an impulse is initiated and the pacemaker conductance is then switched off by the depolarization, only to be reactivated after repolarization of the action potential. The pacemaker rate is determined by the time taken for di-

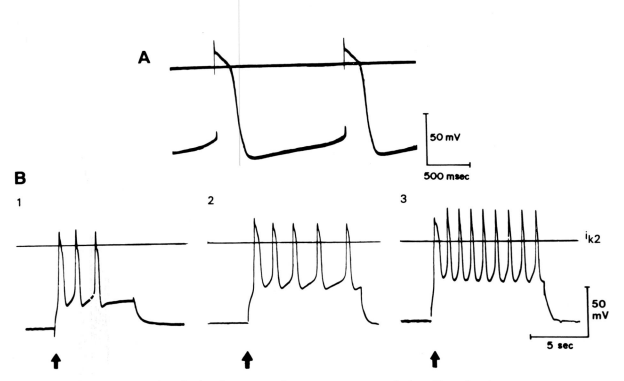

Figure 3-8. Spontaneous diastolic depolarization and automaticity in canine Purkinje fibers. Panel (**A**) shows automatic firing of a Purkinje fiber with a maximum diastolic potential of −85 mV. The diastolic depolarization results from the decay of the pacemaker current. Panel (**B**) shows the automaticity that can occur when membrane potential is decreased. This record was obtained from a Purkinje fiber superfused with a Na^+-free solution, but similar activity is seen in a normal, Na^+-containing Tyrode's solution. In *B1*, when the fiber is depolarized (*at the arrow*) from a resting potential of −60 mV to −45 mV by injecting a long-lasting current pulse through a microelectrode, three nondriven action potentials occur. In *B2*, a larger amplitude current pulse reduces the membrane potential to −40 mV, resulting in sustained rhythmic activity. In *B3*, a still larger current pulse reduces the membrane potential to −30 mV, and sustained rhythmic activity then occurs at a higher rate. Such rhythmic activity occurring at membrane potentials less negative then −60 mV probably depends on different pacemaker currents than the rhythmic activity shown in (**A**). (Wit AL, Friedman PF: Basis for ventricular arrhythmias accompanying myocardial infarction. Arch Intern Med 1975;135:459; with permission.)

astolic depolarization to carry the membrane potential to threshold, so that changes in either the threshold potential or the rate of diastolic depolarization, such as that caused by epinephrine in Purkinje fibers, can alter the rate of automaticity. Spontaneous phase 4 depolarization and automatic impulse initiation are also observed in partially depolarized (approximately -50 mV of resting membrane potential) and dilated human atrial fibers.[52] Abnormal atrial pacemaking is promoted by chamber dilatation (stretch) and strongly modulated by intracellular calcium ion concentration involving the sarcoplasmic reticulum.[52] Because sarcoplasmic reticular-dependent current is inhibited by low sodium media,[52] low sodium perfusate are expected to terminate such activity. Figure 3-9 illustrates the effects of sodium-poor superfusate on spontaneous automaticity in an atrial fiber isolated from a dilated right human atrium.[52]

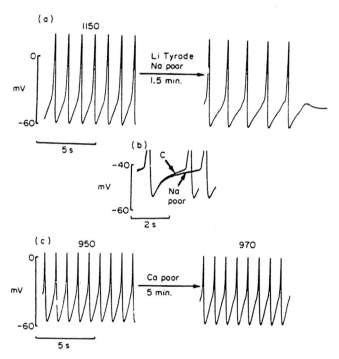

Figure 3-9. (**A**) Effects of a reduction in the extracellular Na concentration (Na$_o$ = 24 mm) in an automatic fiber, isolated from diolated human right atrium. Spontaneous firing ceased within 1.5 mins after the superfusion had been switched to the low Na medium. (**B**) Superimposed expanded traces of the lower part of the slow responses showing diastolic configurations in control Tyrode (**C**) and after 1 min in the low Na Li-substitute medium in a different fiber. In (**A**) and (**B**), Cs 2 mm was appplied 10 mins before and throughout the experiments. (**C**) Low Ca medium (Ca$_o$ = 0.5 mm) failed to suppress abnormal pace-making within the first 5 mins of action. In (**A**) and (**C**), numbers above traces indicate spontaneous basic cycle length in ms. (From Escande D, Coraboeuf E, Planche C: Abnormal pacemaking is modulated by sarcoplasmic reticulum in partially-depolarized myocardium from dilated right atria in humans. J Mol Cell Cardiol 1987; 19:231.)

Delayed Afterdepolarizations and Triggered Sustained Rhythmic Activity

In addition to automaticity, there is another mechanism by which impulses may be rhythmically initiated in normal cardiac cells. The mechanism of impulse initiation depends on delayed afterdepolarizations (DAD), and the resulting nondriven rhythmic impulses are called *triggered action potentials*.[21,47] As described, automatic activity is characterized by the spontaneous initiation of each impulse. Thus, if an automatic fiber is not excited by a propagated impulse, it does not remain quiescent but undergoes spontaneous diastolic depolarization until an action potential is initiated. This accords with the use of the adjective "automatic," which is defined as "having the power of self-motion." In contrast, if a triggerable fiber is not excited by a propagated impulse, it remains quiescent. Because a triggered impulse is one that results from and arises after another impulse, triggered activity cannot occur until the fiber is excited at least once by a propagating impulse. Triggered activity is a form of rhythmic activity in which each impulse arises as a result of the preceding impulse, except the first triggering action potential, which must be driven.

Triggered impulses arise from delayed afterdepolarizations that are large enough to bring the membrane potential to threshold. Delayed afterdepolarizations are transient depolarizations that occur after termination of an action potential but that arise as a result of that action potential. Delayed afterdepolarizations have been recorded in atrial fibers of the mitral valve and in fibers of the coronary sinus and atrial pectinate muscles of normal hearts.[53–55] As shown in Figure 3-10, delayed afterdepolarizations are often preceded by an afterhyperpolarization. After the action potential, the membrane potential transiently becomes more negative than it was just before the

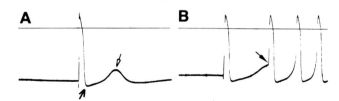

Figure 3-10. Afterdepolarizations and triggered activity in an atrial fiber in the canine coronary sinus. In (**A**), the fiber is stimulated once and a single action potential is elicited; that action potential is followed by an afterhyperpolarization (*solid arrow*) and then a delayed afterdepolarization (*open arrow*). (**B**) shows recordings from a different cell; the first action potential (*at left*) is elicited by a stimulus, but the delayed afterdepolarization (*black arrow*) that follows it reaches threshold potential and gives rise to a nondriven action potential. This first nondriven action potential is then followed by more nondriven action potentials; the nondriven impulses are triggered impulses, constituting "triggered activity."

action potential. After the decay of this afterhyperpolarization, the membrane potential transiently becomes more positive than it was just before the action potential. The transient nature of this afterdepolarization distinguishes it from normal spontaneous diastolic (pacemaker) depolarization, during which the membrane potential declines monotonically until the next action potential occurs.

Delayed afterdepolarizations may be subthreshold, but under certain conditions, they may exceed threshold potential; when this occurs a nondriven action potential arises from the afterdepolarization. In the atrial fibers cited above, catecholamines increase the amplitude of afterdepolarizations, causing them to reach threshold potential.[53, 54] The amplitude of subthreshold afterdepolarizations is also highly sensitive to the rate at which action potentials are elicited.[47, 55] An increase in drive rate is accompanied by an increase in the amplitude of afterdepolarizations (Fig. 3-11), and, conversely, a reduction in the rate of stimulation leads to a decline in afterdepolarization amplitude. In addition, when a premature action potential is elicited during stimulation at a regular rate, the afterdepolarization following the premature action potential is larger than that following the regular action potential. Furthermore, the amplitude of that premature

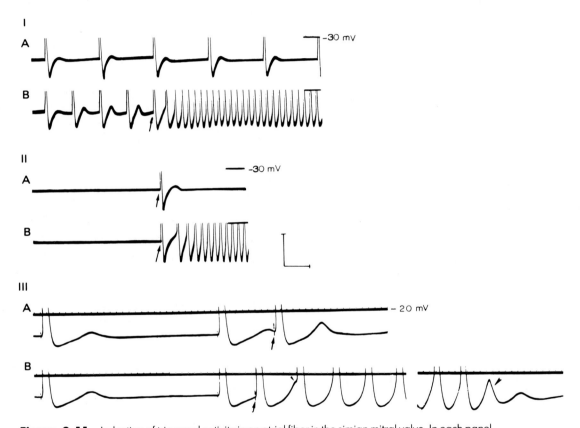

Figure 3-11. Induction of triggered activity in an atrial fiber in the simian mitral valve. In each panel, only the lower parts of the action potentials are shown. Horizontal lines in panels *I* and *II* are drawn at −30 mV; the top trace in *III* is at −20 mV. Panels *IA* and *IB* show triggered activity initiated as a result of decreasing the basic stimulus cycle length. In *IA*, stimulus cycle length was 3400 milliseconds, and a subthreshold delayed afterdepolarization follows each action potential. At the start of *IB*, the stimulus cycle length was reduced to 1750 milliseconds and a progressive increase is seen in the amplitude of the afterdepolarization that follows each of the first four driven action potentials. The last driven action potential (*arrow*) is followed by a nondriven action potential and then by sustained rhythmic activity at a rate higher than the drive rate. Panels *IIA* and *IIB* show triggering caused by a single driven impulse. In *IIA*, after a period of quiescence, a single stimulated action potential (*arrow*) is followed by a subthreshold afterdepolarization. In *IIB*, under slightly different conditions, a single stimulated action potential (*arrow*) is followed by a sustained rhythmic activity. Panels *IIIA* and *IIIB* show how triggered activity may be induced by premature stimulation. In *IIIA*, when the premature impulse (*arrow*) was elicited during the repolarization phase of the afterdepolarization, the amplitude of the subsequent afterdepolarization was increased. In *IIIB*, the premature impulse (*arrowhead*) was followed by an afterdepolarization that just reached threshold (*arrow*) and initiated a train of triggered impulses. (Wit AL, Cranefield PF: Triggered activity in cardiac muscle fibers of the simian mitral valve. Circ Res 1975;38:85; with permission.)

afterdepolarization increases as the premature action potential is elicited earlier during the basic cycle. At a sufficiently high rate of regular stimulation or after a sufficiently early premature stimulus, afterdepolarizations may reach threshold and initiate nondriven action potentials. The first nondriven impulse arises after an interval shorter than the basic cycle length because the afterdepolarization from which it arises occurs soon after repolarization of the preceding action potential. Therefore, that nondriven impulse gives rise to another afterdepolarization that also reaches threshold, causing a second nondriven impulse (see Fig. 3-11). The latter impulse gives rise to the afterdepolarization that initiates a third nondriven impulse and so on for the duration of the triggered activity. The triggered activity may eventually terminate spontaneously. When it does, the last nondriven impulse is usually followed by one or more subthreshold afterdepolarizations.

The ionic basis of the currents underlying the appearance of afterdepolarizations and the mechanism by which afterdepolarization amplitude is altered by changes in stimulus cycle length are not known. The amplitude of afterdepolarizations can be reduced by drugs that are known to reduce current flowing through the slow inward (Na^+/Ca^{++}) channel. These drugs can also prevent the appearance of triggered activity.[47,53,54] It is believed, however, that the slow inward current is not involved directly in the initiation of afterdepolarizations, but that calcium ions entering the cell through this and possibly other routes give rise in some other way to the delayed inward current that causes afterdepolarizations.[56]

A causative role of increased intracellular calcium ion concentration and the genesis of DAD with subsequent triggering is suggested during intoxication with cardiotonic steroids both in Purkinje fibers[57,58] and in ventricular muscle cells.[59,60] Figure 3-12 schematically illustrates events leading to cellular calcium overload. It is believed that during digitalis intoxication, increased resting contractile tension and DADs are induced by calcium overload secondary to inhibition of Na–K pump.[57–60] Further support for an important role for the Na–K pump is provided

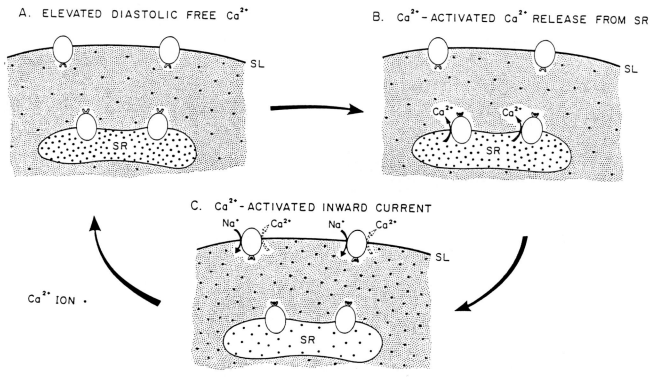

Figure 3-12. Mechanism of abnormal electrical and mechanical activity in calcium-overloaded cells. When the diastolic level of free calcium becomes elevated (**A**), calcium ions interact with sites on the surface of the sarcoplasmic reticulum (SR), causing release of the sequestered store (**B**). In **C**, the resulting further elevation of free calcium causes an inward sodium current across the sarcolemma (SL), which may be coupled to extrusion of calcium ions from the cell. Subsequent uptake of calcium by the sarcoplasmic reticulum terminates the abnormal inward current, allowing the cycle to repeat. This chain of events mediates oscillatory afterpotentials, aftercontractions, and abnormal automaticity in calcium overloaded cells, and can produce fibrillation when the calcium overload becomes severe. The inward and outward currents in **C** resemble one another because the stoichiometry is not specified. (From Clusin TW, Bristow MR, Karagueuzian HS, Katzung BG, Schroeder JS: Do calcium-dependent ion currents mediate ischemic ventricular fibrillation. Am J Cardiol 1982; 49:606.)

in triggerable atrial fibers.[61] The initial rapid rates of triggered activity is associated with increased $[K]_o$ and depolarization, while later slowing is and termination are accompanied with low $[K]_o$ and hyperpolarization. Figure 3-13 illustrates a hyperpolarization of maximum diastolic potential and depletion of extracellular potassium ions after the termination of the triggered activity. The decline of $[K]_o$ and slowing of rate are known responses to enhanced Na–K pump activation, as is the post triggering depletion of extracellular K.[61] Thus, it appears that the duration of tachycardia caused by triggered activity may depend in part on the ability of cardiac tissue to activate an electrogenic membrane pump and clear accumulated K from the extracellular space.[61] As pump activity modulates DAD through calcium overload, it was found that agents that directly interfere with intracellular calcium concentration (such as caffeine) through effects on the sarcoplasmic reticulum also exert important modulatory roles on the DAD and subsequent triggering.[62] Furthermore, it was found that diabetic myocardial cells, unlike normal myocardial cells, are very susceptible to development of myoplasmic calcium overload and DADs.[63] It is entirely possible that during ischemia DADs develop secondary to myoplasmic calcium overload.[64, 65] In addition to calcium overload, an increase in the action potential duration can also facilitate the induction of DAD and subsequent triggering both in atrial (Fig. 3-14)[66] and in digitalis intoxicated ventricular muscle cells (Fig. 3-15).[59] When action potential duration was shortened in canine coronar

sinus fibers,[66] by passing hyperpolarizing current pulses, the amplitude of the DAD was decreased (see Fig. 3-14), however when depolarizing current pulses where passed, so as to increase repolarization time, DAD amplitude was increased (see Fig. 3-14). Similar results are also obtained when action potential dureation is prolonged in digitalis intoxicated ventricular muscle cells (see Fig. 3-15). The effects of increasing the degree of applied depolarizing pulses. The greater the degree of the depolarization, (more positive) the higher is the amplitude of the DAD (see Fig. 3-15). Agents that release endogeneous catecholamines, can increase intracellular calcium ion concentration, and thus may enhance DAD amplitude and initiate triggering.[59] Figure 3-16 illustrates the augmenting effects of amantadine, and tyramine (agents that release endogenous catecholamines),[59] on DAD amplitude.

RESTING AND ACTION POTENTIALS OF NORMAL SINUS AND ATRIOVENTRICULAR NODE CELLS

The electrical activity of cells in the sinus and AV nodes is different from that of cells in the ventricular specialized conducting system and in the working myocardium of the atria and ventricles, which has been discussed. Because of their unusual electrophysiologic characteristics, nodal cells are often involved in the initiation and maintenance of arrhythmias. Because of the important differences be-

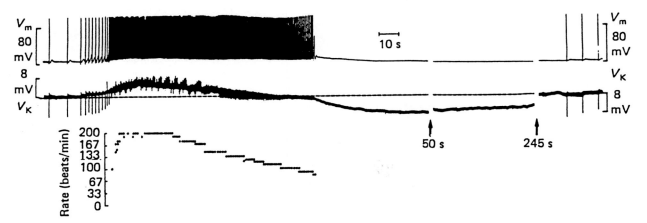

Figure 3-13. An episode of triggering was induced by a train of 10 rapid stimulated beats following two slower control beats. The top panel shows intracellular membrane potential recordings (top of 80 mV vertical calibration bracket indicates zero potential). The middle trace is the output of a potassium sensitive electrode (V_k). The 8 mV vertical calibration bracket indicates a $[K^+]_o$ increase of 2.25 mM (4 mV indicates 1.0 mM increase in $[K^+]_o$). For V_k changes negative to bath levels (i.e. K^+ depletions), the changes in $[K^+]_o$ indicated by an 8 or 4 mV deflexion are respectively −1.6 and 0.9 mM. The two breaks in the record following the triggered are indicated with arrows. The durations of the omitted records in seconds are indicated under the arrows. The bottom vertical axis indicates the instantaneous rate of triggering calculated during the entire triggering run in beats per minute. The rate was derived directly from the inverse of the interval between beats. Some duplicate points were omitted for clarity. The adrenaline concentration in the bath was 1 μg/mL. (Henning B, Kline RP, Siegal MS, Wit AL: Triggered activity in atrial fibers of canine coronary sinus: Role of extracellular potassium accumulation and depletion. J Physiol (Lond) 1987; 383:191.)

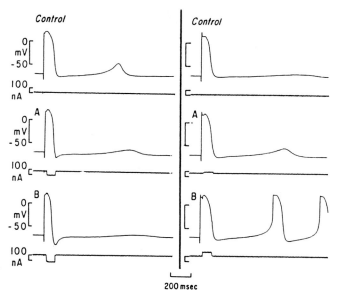

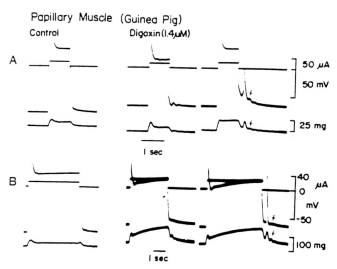

Figure 3-14. Effects of accelerating (*left panels*) and prolonging (*right panels*) the time course of action potential repolarization on delayed afterdepolarizations (DAD). The bottom traces show the amount of current passed through the intracellular microelectrode (hyperpolarizing current shown by downward deflection). Norepinephrine concentration in the superfusate was 1×10^{-8} M. Records from two different preparations are shown. In the left panels, the control action potential duration to the 0-mV level (APD$_o$) is 88 msec; DAD amplitude to 28 mV. In panel A, APD$_o$ is decreased to 75 msec, and DAD amplitude to 13 mV; in panel B, APD$_o$ is decreased to 60 msec, and DAD amplitude to 5 mV. In the right panels, the control APD$_o$ is 63 msec, while DAD amplitude is 4 mV. In panel A, APD$_o$ is increased to 75 msec, and DAD amplitude to 23 mV, in panel B, APD$_o$ is increased to 88 msec and triggered activity occurs. (From Henning B, Wit AL: The time course of action potential repolarization affects delayed afterdepolarization amplitude in atrial fibers of the canine coronary sinus. Circ Res 1984; 55:110.)

Figure 3-15. Electrical and mechanical responses of a normal papillary muscle to long current clamps. Photographs of oscilloscope records. The top trace shows the rectangular current steps applied across the sucrose gap. The middle trace shows the transmembrane potential which is deflected in the high positive range by these pulses. the bottom trace is the contractile tension. As shown in the upper row of panels, the smaller current pulse (*middle panel*) applied during digoxin exposure resulted in a distinct OAP and a very small aftercontraction. A slightly larger current pulse evoked a larger OAP which reached threshold. The extrasystole evoked a secondary OAP and aftercontraction (*arrows, top right panel*). The lower row of panels (**B**) shows the effect of current pulse duration. The control pulse of 4.4 sec evoked no measurable OAP or aftercontraction (*left panel*). After digoxin was begun, even a shorter pulse of 3.2 sec resulted in a clear aftercontraction, although the OAP was not marked. However, a longer pulse of 4.8 sec (*right panel*) was followed by a large OAP which reached threshold. The resulting action potential generated a secondary OAP and aftercontraction (*arrows*). Single impalement. (Karagueuzian HS, Katsung BG: Relative inotropic and arrhythmic effects of five cardiac steroids in ventricular myocardium. Oscillatory after potentials and the role of endogenous catecholamines. J Pharmacol Exp Ther 1981; 218:348.)

tween nodal and other cardiac cells, the normal electrical characteristics of the nodes are discussed separately.

Resting Potential

Cells of the sinus node are usually continuously active and rarely at rest, so the term *resting potential* should not be used. However, the maximum diastolic potential (the most negative level of the membrane potential immediately following action potential repolarization) is easily measured and is much less negative (by about 20 mV) than the maximum diastolic potential of Purkinje fibers or atrial or ventricular fibers (Fig. 3-17). The maximum diastolic potential of AV nodal cells is similar to that of sinus nodal cells. The measured levels of intracellular K$^+$ concentration (and thus the level of E$_K$) in sinus nodal cells appear to be similar to those of cardiac cells with much higher resting potentials.[67] It is likely, therefore, that the lower membrane potential of sinus and AV nodal cells results

from a higher ratio of the Na$^+$ to the K$^+$ permeability coefficient (P$_{Na}$/P$_K$) of the membrane of these cells in comparison with that of atrial, ventricular, and Purkinje cells. It is not yet clear how much the larger ratio P$_{Na}$/P$_K$ of nodal cells reflects a lower P$_K$, as opposed to a higher P$_{Na}$, than exists in the other cardiac cells. Further experiments should indicate, however, whether nodal cells have an unusually high resting permeability to Na$^+$ or an unusually low permeability to K$^+$.

Sinus node refractoriness may play an important regulatory role in the rate of pacemaker activity or during retrograde activation by atrial impulses. A method of measuring sinoatrial refractory period by premature stimulation has been described in isolated sinoatrial tissue preparations.[68] This technique was also used to measure human sinoatrial refractoriness.[69] In a series of 12 patients with sick sinus syndrome, characterized by severe bradycardia and sinus arrests, the sinus nodal refractory period was

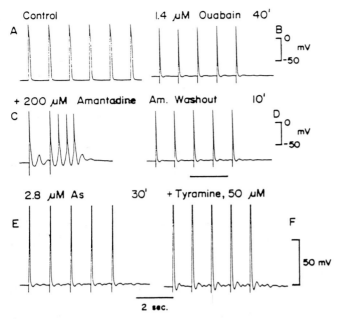

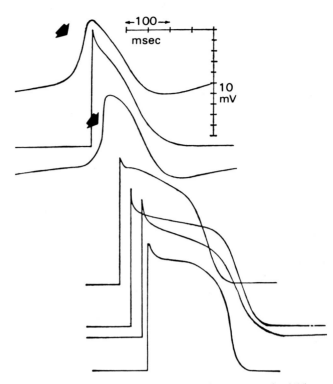

Figure 3-16. Effects of catecholamine-releasing agents. Panels A, control action potentials. Panel B, effect of 40-min exposure to ouabain (1.4 μM). OAPs are small because of the slow (1 Hz) drive rate. Panel C, effects 8 min after addition of AM to the ouabain superfusate. OAP amplitude is markedly increased and triggering of several automatic impulses shown. Panel D shows the result of removing AM from the ouabain superfusate. A single cell impalement was maintained throughout the entire period. Panels E and F, effects of tyramine on acetylstrophanthidin (As)-induced OAPs. The effect of 2.8 μM AS superfusion for 30 min is shown in panel E. Action potential overshoots were offscale in this recording. Addition of tyramine (panel F) resulted in a 4-fold increase in OAP amplitude. (Karagueuzian HS, Katsung BG: Relative inotropic and arrhythmic effects of five cardiac steroids in ventricular myocardium. Oscillatory after potentials and the role of endogenous catecholamines. J Pharmacol Exp Ther 1981; 218:348.)

Figure 3-17. Comparison of sinus and atrioventricular (AV) nodal action potentials (*arrows*) with action potentials of working myocardium and Purkinje fibers. Drawings of action potentials are recorded from the following sites, starting at the top: sinoatrial node, atrium, AV node, bundle of His, Purkinje fiber in a false tendon, terminal Purkinje fiber, and ventricular muscle fiber. Note that the upstroke velocity and amplitude of sinus and AV nodal action potentials are both smaller than those of the action potentials of the other cells. (Hoffman BF, Cranefield PF: Electrophysiology of the heart. New York: McGraw-Hill, 1960.)

significantly increased compared to patients with normal sinus node function (from a mean of 325 ± 39 milliseconds to 522 ± 20 milliseconds).[69] Because of their low resting membrane potential, AV nodal cells are characterized by their properties of slow impulse conduction velocity and by their ability to undergo rate-induced dynamic variations in their functional refractory period.[70] These dynamic changes in the AV nodal functional refractory period were suggested to result from complex interaction between facilitation and fatigue phenomena.[70, 71] The slowly developing, rate-induced prolongation in the AV nodal conduction time is termed *fatigue*.[70, 71]

Depolarization and Repolarization Phases of the Nodal Action Potential

Sinus and AV nodal cells exhibit a much lower rate of phase 0 depolarization (1 to 20 V/sec) than normal Purkinje or working myocardial cells (see Fig. 3-17). The

amplitude of the action potentials is also quite small (60 to 80 mV), and, in some fibers, the peak of the action potential might not exceed 0 mV.[3] The slower upstroke and the lower amplitude of the action potential of nodal cells both reflect the much smaller inward current underlying the phase 0 depolarization of these cells in comparison with that of other cardiac cells. Evidence strongly suggests that this smaller inward current of sinus and AV nodal cells flows not through the fast Na^+ channel but through the slow inward channel and is carried by calcium and sodium ions.[72-74] Such action potentials with upstrokes dependent on slow inward current are often called *slow responses* to distinguish them from the more usual *fast response* action potentials in which the upstroke depends on the fast Na^+ current.[21] Because of the small net inward current and the slow phase 0 depolarization, the slow response action potentials conduct only slowly (0.01 to 0.1 m/sec) through the nodes. It is this slow conduction that, under certain conditions, can cause arrhythmias to arise in the nodes. As described, the slow inward current channel has different time- and voltage-dependent properties than the fast sodium channel. The slow inward current turns on and also turns off, or inactivates, much more slowly than the fast sodium current. After the upstroke of the nodal action potential, therefore, the slow inward current inactivates only slowly and contributes to the membrane depolarization throughout the action potential plateau. Activation of a time- and voltage-dependent outward K^+ current coupled with inactivation of the slow inward current probably causes repolarization of nodal cells as described for termination of the action potential of other cardiac fibers.

The slow inward channel conductance is also much slower to reactivate after membrane repolarization than the fast Na^+ channel conductance.[21,22] In contrast to the other cardiac cells, nodal cells do not respond to premature stimuli applied during the terminal repolarization phase by giving action potentials. Sufficient inactivation of the slow inward conductance may persist even after full repolarization for the cells still to be absolutely refractory to applied stimuli.[75] Reactivation then occurs gradually throughout diastole; premature impulses elicited soon after full repolarization have slower upstrokes and lower amplitudes than normal and conduct more slowly. Premature impulses initiated later in diastole have correspondingly faster upstrokes and higher amplitudes and, therefore, conduct more rapidly.[76] This behavior reflects the long time course for reactivation of the slow channel. The resulting long refractory period of the nodes and the markedly slowed conduction through them of premature impulses can be an important factor in the initiation of some arrhythmias.

Automaticity

Sinus node cells are usually automatic, each action potential apparently being initiated as a result of spontaneous diastolic depolarization, and AV nodal cells can also fire automatically, especially when disconnected from surrounding atrial myocardium.[77] It, therefore, appears that electrotonic interaction between atrium and node suppresses automaticity through atrio-nodal connections. Automaticity of sinus node cells might not be caused by the same pacemaker current as described for Purkinje fibers. The gating variable of the membrane conductance responsible for normal Purkinje fiber automaticity changes only between membrane potential levels of -90 and -60 mV.[14] Such conductance changes seem unlikely to provide an explanation of spontaneous diastolic depolarization of sinus node cells, because the maximum diastolic potential in these cells is usually less negative than -60 mV. However, evidence suggests that the pacemaker current in the sinus node is at least partly carried by K^+, and the decay of this outward current against a steady background inward current results in gradual membrane depolarization.[51] In addition, it appears that an inward current that can be activated by hyperpolarization (called i_f) plays an important role.[51,78] i_f is carried primarily by sodium ions and is blocked by cesium ions.[79] In addition to the inward i_f current, two additional time-dependent membrane currents also contribute to pacemaker depolarization of sinus node cells.[78-80] The first is decay of potassium current (i_K); the second is a slow inward calcium current.[30,78-80] Computer simulation studies indicate that the slow calcium current contributes only to the last third of the pacemaker depolarization and the action potential upstroke.[80] Variations in the amount of activation of the inward current (i_f) can modulate the rate of the sinoatrial pacemaker.[50,51,78-80]

Two modes of sinus nodal pacemaker synchronization have been proposed. In one scheme, a cell or small group of cells acts as the dominant pacemaker, and all other intrinsically active pacemakers in the node having slower rates would be driven by the dominant pacemaker to fire at its faster intrinsic frequency. A second scheme suggests that synchronization of sinus pacemaker activity may be a more democratic process, whereby the individual cells, each beating at slightly different intrinsic rates, mutually interact through electrical coupling to achieve a "consensus" as to when to fire.[81] Experimental and computer simulation studies suggest that the process of sinus nodal synchronization occurs by this latter phenomenon of mutual entrainment.[81,82]

EFFECTS OF CARDIAC DISEASE ON THE RESTING AND ACTION POTENTIAL OF CARDIAC FIBERS

Cardiac arrhythmias and conduction disturbances can occur as a result of alterations in the electrical properties of cardiac fibers due to disease, and recent investigations have been aimed at characterizing some of these changes. Microelectrodes have been used to record electrical activity of cells in pieces of myocardium isolated from diseased human and experimental animal hearts. Results from such studies can often be correlated with other data obtained in studies on normal myocardial tissue exposed to an altered extracellular environment in order to mimic conditions existing during certain cardiac diseases.

Resting Potential

It appears that many diseases that affect the heart, causing arrhythmias, tend to depolarize the membrane of cardiac cells. Membrane potentials have been recorded in atrial cells from hearts with rheumatic and congenital disease and with cardiomyopathy and from cells in both ventricular muscle and ventricular conducting fibers in areas of ischemia and infarction.[83-88] In each instance, resting membrane potentials were found to be less negative than those of cells from similar regions of normal hearts (Fig. 3-18).

The reasons for the decline in resting potential in each of these cases are not completely understood, but several factors might contribute. These are best considered in terms of the Goldman and Hodgkin and Katz equation that approximates the resting potentials of Purkinje fibers exposed to a wide range of extracellular K+ concentrations:

$$V_r = \frac{RT}{F} \ln \frac{[K^+]_o + (P_{Na}/P_K)[Na^+]_o}{[K^+]_i + (P_{Na}/P_K)[Na^+]_i}$$

If typical values for the ion concentrations and permeability ratio in this equation are approximately $[K^+]_o = 4$ mM; $[K^+]_i = 150$ mM; $[Na^+]_o = 150$ mM; $[Na^+]_i = 10$ mM; and $P_{Na}/P_K = 1/100$, then, in the absence of large temperature changes, there are four ways in which the resting potential, V_r, can readily be made less negative: (1) increase the extracellular K+ concentration, $[K^+]_o$; (2) decrease the intracellular K+ concentration, $[K^+]_i$; (3) increase membrane Na+ permeability, P_{Na}, which in-

creases the P_{Na}/P_K ratio, or (4) decrease membrane K+ permeability, P_K, which also increases the P_{Na}/P_K ratio. Any of these changes causes the resting potential to decline, but more than one of them might occur in diseased cells. For example, any pathologic condition that results in impaired activity of the sodium pump is expected to lead to depolarization of the affected cells, probably as a result of both an increase in $[K^+]_o$ and a decrease in $[K^+]_i$. The normal loss of cellular K+ and gain of Na+ that accompanies electrical activity (and that occurs, to a smaller extent, even at rest) is, therefore, not easily reversed, as it usually is, by the sodium pump. In other words, there is a continuous net loss of K+ from the cells (the cellular K+ effectively being replaced by Na+), and $[K^+]_i$ gradually declines. Because diffusion of ions from the extracellular spaces is somewhat restricted and slow, the potassium ions lost by the cells tend to accumulate in these spaces, causing $[K^+]_o$ to rise. As noted, both the fall in $[K^+]_i$ and the rise in $[K^+]_o$ may contribute to the decline in resting membrane potential.

Just as changes in both $[K^+]_o$ and $[K^+]_i$ may simultaneously contribute to a fall in resting potential, it is likely that complementary changes in both P_{Na} and P_K combine

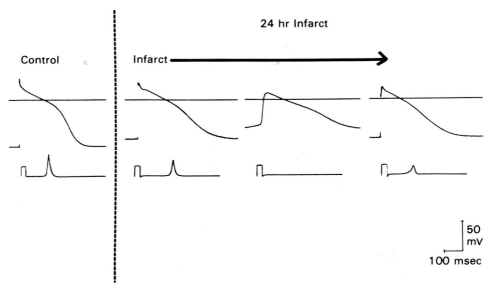

Figure 3-18. Changes in the action potentials recorded from Purkinje fibers as a result of infarction in the canine heart. The bottom trace in each panel (recorded with a faster sweep) shows the differentiated upstroke of the action potential preceded by a differentiated calibration signal with a 200-V/sec slope of depolarization; the differentiated calibration pulse appears as a square wave. The control panel (*left*) shows the action potential recorded from a Purkinje fiber in a noninfarcted region; it has a normal maximum diastolic, or resting, potential and a rapid upstroke. The right panel shows action potentials recorded from three different Purkinje fibers on the endocardial surface of the infarct. Note that maximum diastolic potential, action potential amplitude, and upstroke velocity (V_{max}) were all diminished in the infarct as compared to the control region. Depression of the resting potential and action potential in the middle infarct panel is particularly severe. (Friedman PL, Stewart JR, Fenoglio JJ Jr, Wit AL: Survival of subendocardial Purkinje fibers after extensive infarction in dogs: In vitro and in vivo correlations. Circ Res 1973;33:597 with permission.)

to cause membrane depolarization in the following way. If a certain pathologic condition was associated with an increase in the "leakiness" of cell membranes to Na ions (or, P_{Na} is increased), then the ratio P_{Na}/P_K would be increased and the resting potential would be reduced. Because this depolarization might occur in the absence of any significant change in $[K^+]_o$ or $[K^+]_i$, the K^+ equilibrium potential would remain unchanged. However, the outward driving force on K^+, given by $(V_m - E_K)$, would be greater than normal, and, as a result of inward rectification, the K^+ conductance and, therefore, the K^+ permeability coefficient, P_K, would be smaller than normal. The steady membrane depolarization under these conditions would be associated with an enhanced ratio, P_{Na}/P_K, but both an increase in P_{Na} and a decrease in P_K contribute to this change.

On the other hand, if some cardiac disease led specifically to a reduction in P_K (as a result of alterations in the chemical composition of the membrane due to abnormal protein or lipid metabolism, for example), the ratio P_{Na}/P_K would still increase and depolarization would occur, while P_{Na} remained unchanged. Such a specific decline in P_K has not yet been demonstrated in diseased cardiac cells, although a similar effect may be artificially produced in isolated tissue preparations by including millimolar concentrations of cesium ions in the bathing solution.[89] A large, maintained increase in the leakiness of cell membranes to Na^+ might eventually lead to changes in the cation distributions across the membrane if the sodium pump could not keep pace with the resulting increased fluxes of Na^+ and K^+. An initial depolarization would occur in response to the relative increase in sodium permeability, but then a more gradual, secondary depolarization might occur, reflecting a fall in intracellular K^+ concentration. This is because K^+ would leave the cells as Na^+ entered in order to preserve electroneutrality. Although chloride ion permeability is generally thought to be small in cardiac cells, some chloride ions may be expected to enter the cells along with Na^+, together with some water; the cells would swell slightly, leading to a corresponding further fall in $[K^+]_i$. Because the rate of sodium pump activity is predominantly determined by the level of $[Na^+]_i$, pump activity would be increased in these leaky cells with raised $[Na^+]_i$. If the passive movements of Na^+ and K^+ were large, however, or if pump activity was impaired, substantial changes in the levels of $[Na^+]_i$ and $[K^+]_i$ would still occur despite this pump activation by internal Na^+.

Dresdner and coworkers evaluated the ionic basis of partial depolarization of myocardial infarct surviving subendocardial Purkinje cells using ion-sensitive microelectrodes.[90,91] The researchers, using pH-, Na^+-, and K^+-sensitive microelectrodes, suggested that intracellular acidification did not appear to be the cause of partial depolarization, and that only a portion of the maximum diastolic potential changes could be accounted for by a reduction of the potassium equilibrium potential.[90,91] Other mechanisms, such as alteration of membrane Na–K pump activity or membrane conductances of ions, were suggested as additional likely mechanisms.[90]

Phase 0 Depolarization

Under most pathologic conditions investigated, the upstroke of the action potential (phase 0) of Purkinje fibers or atrial or ventricular myocardial cells is slowed and reduced in amplitude.[83–88,92] These changes are probably largely caused by the reduced membrane potentials of the diseased cells, although similar changes could also arise as a result of specific disease-related alterations in the underlying conductance mechanisms in the absence of any resting potential changes. There is little detailed information about the specific primary effects of diseases on the conductance mechanisms underlying the inward current that causes the action potential upstroke.

As discussed, the fast Na^+ conductance inactivates during prolonged membrane depolarization (after the upstroke of the action potential) and full membrane repolarization to large negative potential levels (e.g., the repolarization of the action potential) is necessary to remove this inactivation completely. Incomplete membrane repolarization leads to only partial removal of inactivation in the steady state. Thus, following complete activation of the Na^+ conductance, a steady hyperpolarization to about -100 mV suffices to remove inactivation fully, leaving all Na^+ channels available for reactivation by a subsequent depolarizing stimulus, whereas steady repolarization to between -60 and -70 mV would leave about 50% of the sodium channels inactivated and, therefore, unavailable for reactivation by a depolarizing stimulus. At a potential level of -50 mV, most of the sodium channels remain inactivated and so are unavailable for immediate reactivation (see Fig. 3-3).

Thus, in cardiac cells depolarized as a result of disease, only a fraction of the total population of fast Na^+ channels may be available to carry inward current. In this case, the magnitude of the net inward current during phase 0 of the action potential would be reduced, and, consequently, both the speed and amplitude of the upstroke would be diminished (see Fig. 3-10). Such action potentials, with upstrokes dependent on inward current flowing through partially inactivated Na^+ conductance, are sometimes referred to as *depressed fast responses* to distinguish them from *slow responses*, which also have slow upstrokes but which depend on inward current flowing in different, pharmacologically distinct, membrane channels.[17,21] Because of their slow upstrokes and diminished amplitudes the conduction velocity of depressed fast responses is much reduced. For example, the conduction velocity of Purkinje fiber action potentials may be reduced from 2 to 4 m/sec to less than 0.5 m/sec because of steady state Na$^+$ channel inactivation resulting from membrane depolarization. Further depolarization and inactivation of the Na$^+$ channel may render the fiber inexcitable so that it may become a site of conduction block. However, although the fast Na$^+$ conductance may be completely inactivated near -50 mV, the slow inward conductance (Na$^+$/Ca^{++} channel) is still available for activation below this potential.[21,22] Under these conditions, therefore, a strong depolarizing stimulus can still elicit a slow inward current. Whether this normally weak, slow inward current gives rise to the regenerative depolarization characteristic of a propagated slow response action potential depends on the relative magnitude of the membrane K$^+$ conductance. As discussed for resting potential, membrane depolarization caused by a small increase in Na$^+$ permeability, for instance, is expected to result in a reduction in K$^+$ conductance because of the presence of inward-going rectification. Under these conditions, the slow inward current may suffice to initiate a slow response action potential (see Fig. 3-3). On the other hand, membrane depolarization resulting from an increase in [K$^+$]$_o$ is associated with an increase in K$^+$ conductance, so that, in this case, the same weak, slow inward current may give rise to only a negligibly small depolarization. However, if the slow inward current is enhanced, as in the presence of catecholamines, slow response action potentials can also be elicited when [K$^+$]$_o$ is elevated.[93] Because of its slow upstroke, the conduction velocity of slow response action potentials is low. The conduction velocity of Purkinje fiber action potentials may thus be reduced to less than 0.1 m/sec as a result of severe membrane depolarization.[21]

When phase 0 depolarization is slowed to a critical degree, unidirectional conduction block may occur.[1] In bundles of atrial, ventricular, or Purkinje fibers, stimulated at either end to elicit normal action potentials, the impulse conducts at almost equal velocities in either direction along the bundle. As the upstroke velocity and amplitude of the action potential decrease, conduction velocity is slowed in both directions. At a critical degree of depression of the action potential upstroke velocity, conduction may fail in one direction but proceed slowly in the other direction (Fig. 3-19). The critical degree of depression varies in different regions of the heart and depends partly on the geometry of the cardiac syncytium. Further depression of the action potential upstroke and amplitude usually results in conduction block in both directions. Slow conduction or unidirectional conduction block can occur in bundles of fibers showing either depressed fast response or slow response action potentials.

Because it is unlikely that there will be a uniform reduction in membrane potential in diseased areas of the heart, it seems reasonable to expect varying degrees of

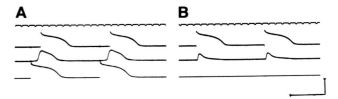

Figure 3-19. Unidirectional conduction block in a bundle of canine Purkinje fibers. The top line shows time marks at 100-msec intervals. The three traces beneath show action potentials recorded from three different cells along the length of a Purkinje fiber bundle. The action potentials on the upper trace were recorded from the near end of the bundle, those on the middle trace were recorded from the center, and those on the bottom trace were recorded from the far end of the bundle. The cells in the center segment of the bundle were depolarized by perfusion with high (K$^+$)$_o$ solution, and the action potentials recorded there have slow upstrokes and low amplitudes. Panel (**A**) shows records obtained by stimulating the bundle at the far end. The impulse was first recorded in the cell at the far end of the bundle (*bottom trace*), and then it conducted through the center segment (*middle trace*) to finally excite the cells at the near end of the bundle (*top trace*). Panel (**B**) shows records obtained when the near end of the bundle was stimulated. The cell monitored by the top trace was excited, because this was near the region of stimulation, but conduction block occurred in the depressed area (*middle trace*), so the far end of the bundle (*bottom trace*) was not activated. (Cranefield PF, Wit AL, Hoffman BF: The genesis of cardiac arrhythmias. Circulation 1973;47:190; with permission.)

Na$^+$ channel inactivation in these areas, ranging from little inactivation (impulses conducted rapidly in the form of fast response action potentials), through moderate inactivation (impulses conducted relatively slowly as depressed fast responses), to full inactivation (impulses, if any, conducted very slowly as slow response action potentials).

Repolarization and Refractoriness

As described for normal action potentials, the relative refractory period of normal Purkinje or atrial or ventricular myocardial cells (with maximum diastolic potentials near -90 mV) lasts until action potential repolarization is complete. Premature action potentials elicited during this period have reduced rates of rise and reduced amplitudes because of persisting, partial inactivation of the Na$^+$ conductance. This inactivation is removed within a few milliseconds after repolarization to about -90 mV, then action potential upstrokes regain their normal speed and amplitude. However, the rate of removal of Na$^+$ current inactivation (and, therefore, the rate of recovery of the maximum rate of depolarization) depends strongly on the steady level of membrane potential: recovery occurs rapidly (within 20 milliseconds) at -90 mV but takes longer (more than 100 milliseconds) at -60 mV.[94] In cardiac cells depolarized by disease, therefore, recovery of the action potential upstroke may be prolonged. Because the upstrokes of action potentials in these cells are already slowed as a result of the steady membrane depolarization, premature action potentials elicited during the prolonged relative refractory period have even slower upstrokes and correspondingly lower conduction velocities. If the cells are so depolarized that the Na^+ conductance remains fully inactivated and only slow response action potentials can be initiated, then the relative refractory period still extends into diastole because removal of inactivation of the slow inward current also occurs very slowly. In this case, the absolute refractory period may last until action potential repolarization is complete, and full recovery of the upstroke of a premature impulse may not be achieved for hundreds of milliseconds after that time. The greatly slowed conduction of premature impulses in cardiac fibers with low membrane potentials can lead to reentry, and the premature impulses that cause reentry in these fibers may arise long after complete repolarization.

Large alterations in the refractory periods can also be brought about by changes in action potential duration in cells with large negative resting potentials, because, in this case, removal of inactivation is complete soon after action potential repolarization. A shortening of the action potential in these cells, such as that resulting from an increase in stimulation rate, is therefore accompanied by a corresponding shortening of the effective and relative refractory periods.[3] In cells with very low resting potentials, on the other hand, removal of inactivation may occur so slowly that the relative refractory period is practically independent of action potential duration.

The following are examples of changes in action potential duration caused by cardiac disease. The action potential of ventricular muscle cells shortens soon after the onset of ischemia, before the resting potential declines significantly.[87,95,96] The effective and relative refractory periods of such ischemic cells are decreased accordingly. In areas that are chronically ischemic, action potential duration of ventricular muscle and Purkinje fibers may be markedly prolonged, and, therefore, the relative and effective refractory periods of these cells are increased.[85,86,97] Vagal stimulation causes atrial action potential duration and refractory periods to decrease.[98] Such changes in action potential duration and refractoriness can markedly alter conduction properties and thereby cause arrhythmias.

Abnormal Automaticity and Triggered Activity

As discussed, automaticity is a normal property of certain types of cardiac fibers. Working atrial and ventricular myocardial cells do not normally develop spontaneous diastolic depolarization and do not initiate spontaneous impulses. However, when the membrane potential of atrial or ventricular fibers is experimentally reduced to less than approximately -60 mV, "spontaneous" diastolic depolarization and automatic impulse initiation may occur in these cells.[99-101] The spontaneously occurring action potentials are slow responses. The decrease in membrane potential that may lead to this abnormal automaticity, however, might also be caused by disease (Fig. 3-20). Automaticity may occur also in Purkinje fibers when the membrane is depolarized to less than -60 mV (see Fig. 3-8).[102] As discussed, for propagated action potentials to occur at these low membrane potentials in atrial, ventricular, or Purkinje fibers, membrane K^+ conductance must be low. In cells depolarized by an increase in $[K^+]_o$, such automaticity is usually not seen because the membrane K^+ conductance is also increased under these conditions. Canine subepicardial ventricular muscle cells that survive in 24-hour transmural infarcts have been found to be capable of generating abnormal automaticity and triggered activity in the same manner as surviving subendocardial Purkinje fibers.[103]

The ionic currents underlying the automaticity at low membrane potentials have not yet been elucidated, but it is unlikely that the pacemaker current described for normal Purkinje fibers is involved, because the gating variable for this channel does not change at membrane potentials less negative than approximately -60 mV.

Delayed afterdepolarizations may follow the action potentials of working atrial fibers and of Purkinje fibers when the membrane potentials are reduced by cardiac disease.[84,104,105] The amplitude of these afterdepolarizations increases when the dominant rhythm becomes faster or after a premature impulse, and triggered activity may occur in such cells if the afterdepolarizations reach threshold potential. The mechanism by which afterdepolarizations arise in diseased cardiac cells is not yet clear but is probably related to an increase in intracellular Ca.

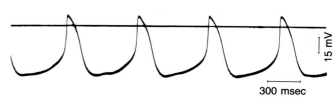

Figure 3-20. Abnormal automaticity recorded from a left atrial fiber in an isolated preparation obtained from a failed canine heart. The left atrium was markedly dilated, and resting potentials of the atrial cells were generally very low. The automaticity in this cell may have been initiated as a result of the fall in resting membrane potential.

GENESIS OF CARDIAC ARRHYTHMIAS

This section describes how the site of origin of the dominant pacemaker may shift from the sinus node to an ectopic site, thereby causing ectopic beats and tachycardia. This change in the locus of impulse initiation is often a consequence of the alterations in electrical activity of cardiac cells that accompany disease. Although arrhythmias may also occur in clinically normal hearts, these arrhythmias might be initiated by similar alterations in cellular electrophysiology that occur in only a limited region of the heart and may, therefore, be too small to be detected by clinical examination.

Arrhythmias Caused by Reentry

In the heart driven by the sinus rhythm, the conducting impulse dies out after sequential activation of the atria and ventricles because it is surrounded by refractory tissue that it has recently excited. The heart then must await a new impulse arising in the sinus node for subsequent activation. The phenomenon of reentry occurs when the propagating impulse does not die out after complete activation of the heart but persists to reexcite the heart after the end of the refractory period.[106] For this to happen, the impulse must remain somewhere in the heart while the recently excited cardiac fibers regain excitability so that the impulse can reenter and reactivate them.

The effective refractory period of cardiac fibers is long, ranging from 150 milliseconds in the atrium to about 300 to 500 milliseconds in the ventricular specialized conducting system.[3] An impulse destined to reenter or reexcite the heart must survive for at least this amount of time if it is to outlast the refractory period. However, it cannot remain stationary while waiting out the refractory period but must continue to travel over a pathway that is functionally isolated from the rest of the heart. Such a conduction pathway must provide a return route to the regions previously excited and must be sufficiently long to permit propagation of the impulse during the entire refractory period. The cardiac impulse normally conducts at a velocity of 0.5 to 5 m/second in cardiac fibers other than those in the sinus and atrioventricular nodes. If the impulse traveled at these speeds for the duration of the refractory period, it would have to travel in a pathway between 7.5 cm and 2.5 m long. Cranefield and Hoffman have stated "that so long a path, however circuitous, could exist in functional isolation from the rest of the heart has never seemed likely."[107]

Travel at a normal velocity is not the only way in which the impulse, destined to reenter, might persist during the refractory period: a reduction of the conduction velocity obviates the need for such a long conduction pathway. For example, if conduction is slowed to 0.02 m/second, the impulse would travel only 6 mm during a refractory period of 300 milliseconds.[107] As discussed in the previous section, cardiac disease can give rise to such slow impulse conduction, and pathways of this length are readily available in the heart.

Alterations in the duration of the refractory period also may facilitate reentry. For example, a shortening of the effective refractory period, which usually occurs when repolarization of the action potential is accelerated, reduces the time during which the impulse must conduct through the functionally isolated pathway while awaiting the recovery of excitability of the rest of the heart.

Reentry Caused by Slow Conduction and Unidirectional Conduction Block in Cardiac Fibers With Low Resting Potentials and Low Upstroke Velocities

The occurrence of reentry depends on the presence of slow conduction and unidirectional conduction block. The basic principles that enable reentry to occur are illustrated in Figure 3-21, which is a modified form of a figure published by Mines in 1914.[106] His data were obtained from isolated rings of cardiac tissue. Similar studies that also contributed to the modern concepts on reentrant excitation were performed by Mayer in rings of jellyfish subumbrella tissue.[108] Figure 3-21 shows that if a ring of excitable tissue is stimulated at one point, two waves of excitation start at this point and progress in opposite directions around the ring, with only one excitation of the ring occurring, because the waves collide and die out. However, by temporarily applying pressure near the site of stimulation, an excitation wave can be induced to progress in only one direction around the ring. The area of com-

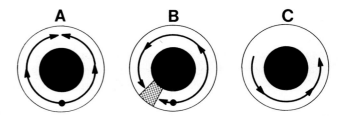

Figure 3-21. Schematic representation of reentry in a ring of excitable tissue as described by Mayer and by Mines. In (**A**), the ring was stimulated in the area indicated by the black dot, and impulses propagated away from the point of stimulation, in both directions, and collided; no reentry occurred. In (**B**), the cross-hatched area was compressed while the ring was stimulated, again at the black dot. The impulse propagated around the ring in only one direction, having been blocked in the other direction by the area of compression; immediately after stimulation the compression was relieved. In (**C**), the unidirectionally circulating impulse returns to its point of origin, then continues around the loop.

pression prevents the conduction of a wave in the other direction. The wave conducting in one direction returns to its point of origin (by which time pressure is no longer being applied to the ring) and then conducts around the ring again. The impulse is able to conduct around the ring an indefinite number of times because each time it returns to its point of origin, that part of the ring has recovered excitability.[106, 108]

Reentry can occur in a similar manner in loops composed of bundles of cardiac fibers, whether they be atrial, ventricular, or Purkinje fibers. For example, the anatomy of the ventricular specialized conducting system provides conduction pathways that are functionally suitable for reentry. Bundles of interconnecting Purkinje fibers are surrounded by connective tissue that separates them from the ventricular myocardium. In peripheral regions of the conducting system, such Purkinje fiber bundles often arborize into many branches. Where these branches make contact with ventricular muscle, anatomic loops composed of the Purkinje fiber bundles and the muscle are often formed (Fig. 3-22). Loops composed entirely of Purkinje fiber bundles are also known to exist in the peripheral ventricular conducting system.

Purkinje fibers normally have fast response action potentials that conduct rapidly at a velocity of 1 to 4 m/second. Under normal circumstances, the rapidly conducting impulse of sinus origin invades all Purkinje fiber bundles of a distal loop and conducts into ventricular muscle, where impulses collide and die out because they are surrounded by refractory tissue (Fig. 3-23). For reentry to occur in the distal ventricular specialized conducting system, conduction must be slowed and a strategically located region of unidirectional block must be present. Slow conduction may occur when the loop of fibers is in a diseased region of the heart. In this case, both the rate of phase 0 depolarization and the overshoot of the action potential of the Purkinje fibers in the loop may be reduced, possibly because of a decrease in resting potential. Depression of the resting potential and action potential upstroke is rarely uniform in regions of disease, and, in areas where the action potential is severely depressed, unidirectional block may occur.

The mechanism by which slowed conduction and unidirectional block can result in reentry is illustrated in the left panel of Figure 3-22.[109, 110] In the distal loop, composed of Purkinje fiber bundles and ventricular muscle, an area of unidirectional conduction block is located near the origin of branch B; an impulse cannot conduct through this area in the antegrade direction but it can in the retrograde direction. Slow conduction is assumed to occur in the rest of the loop. An impulse of sinus origin conducting into the loop through the main Purkinje fiber bundle blocks near the origin of branch B can enter only branch A, through which it conducts slowly into the ventricular muscle. This impulse can then invade branch B at its myocardial end. This branch had not been excited initially because of the unidirectional block at its origin, and so the impulse can conduct in the retrograde direction in branch B, through the region of unidirectional block, and then reexcite the main bundle from which it entered the loop (see Fig. 3-22).

The reentering impulse will block if it returns to the main bundle while the fibers in that region are still effectively refractory (see Fig. 3-23). It is necessary, then, for slowly conducting action potentials around the loop. The region of unidirectional conduction block prevents one part of the loop from being invaded by the antegrade impulse and so provides a return excitable pathway for the reentering impulse.

When the reentrant impulse returns to the main bundle, it may travel throughout the conducting system to reactivate the ventricles, causing a premature ventricular beat. It may also reinvade the bundle of Purkinje fibers through which it originally excited the ventricular muscle (see Fig. 3-22, branch A) and once again propagate back through the reentrant pathway. This may result in a continuous circling of the impulse around the loop or "circus movement," much like the circling of the impulse around the ring of tissue observed by Mines and Mayer. In the loop just described, however, the continuous circling would result in repetitive excitation of the ventricles.

If, during normal activation of the heart, conduction in the loop of Purkinje fibers and ventricular muscle is not slowed sufficiently to permit reentry, or if there is not a strategically located site of unidirectional block, reentry might still be induced by premature activation. The basic impulse may spread through the Purkinje bundles and ventricular muscle in any of the ways indicated in Figure 3-23. If these Purkinje fibers are then reactivated prematurely, before they have completely recovered excitability, the premature impulse may be expected to conduct even more slowly than the basic impulse. Premature activation may also result in unidirectional block because of the low safety margin for conduction in partially refractory tissue. Premature activation may then lead to reentry as shown in Figure 3-22.

Although the peripheral Purkinje system has been used as an example in describing the mechanism for reentry in a loop caused by depressed conduction, reentry may occur by a similar mechanism in other regions of the heart. For example, rheumatic heart disease in the atrium or infarction of the ventricle can leave discrete areas of inexcitable tissue in addition to depressing the resting potential and action potential upstroke.[84, 87] Conduction around these areas may then be circular, as described for the peripheral Purkinje system and as shown in Figure 3-22.

Gross anatomic loops are not a prerequisite for the

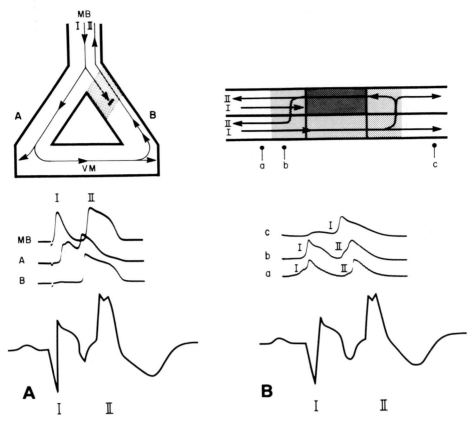

Figure 3-22. Possible mechanisms for reentry resulting from slow conduction and unidirectional conduction block. (**A**) shows a main bundle of Purkinje fibers (MB), which divides into two branches (A and B) before terminating on ventricular muscle (VM). A severely depressed area in which unidirectional conductional block occurs in the antegrade direction is located in branch B (*shaded area*). Conduction is slow throughout the rest of the loop because the Purkinje fibers have low resting potentials; consequently, their action potentials have slow upstrokes. The arrows indicate the sequence of activation of the loop by the conducting impulse. Arrow *I* represents an impulse of sinus origin entering the loop; arrow *II* is the reentering impulse leaving the loop. Action potentials recorded from MB and branches A and B are shown below, together with an example of how the electrocardiogram might appear. Action potential *I* in the MB trace was recorded as the impulse entered the loop. The action potentials in A and B were recorded as the impulse conducted around the loop. Action potential *II* in the MB trace occurred when the impulse reexcited the main bundle. Impulse *I* would cause ventricular depolarization I on the electrocardiogram and impulse II would cause a ventricular extrasystole (ventricular depolarization II). Panel (**B**) shows, at the top, how reentry can occur even in a single bundle of muscle or Purkinje fibers. The diagram depicts two adjacent fibers in a bundle; the entire shaded area is depressed, but depression in the darker area of the upper fiber is so severe that unidirectional conduction block occurs. The arrows indicate the sequence of activation in the bundle; arrows labeled *I* show the impulse entering the bundle; arrows labeled *II* show the reentrant impulse returning to reexcite the left end of the bundle. Action potentials recorded from sites a, b, and c in the lower fiber are shown below. Action potentials *I* were recorded as the impulse conducted from left to right, and action potentials *II* were recorded as the impulse returned to its origin. The bottom trace shows how such events would appear on the electrocardiogram. (Wit AL, Bigger JT: Possible electrophysiological mechanisms for lethal arrhythmias accompanying myocardial ischemia and infarction. Circulation 1975; 52:III-96(suppl):51–52; with permission.)

I

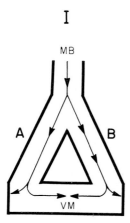

II

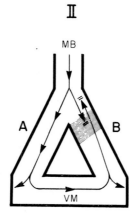

III

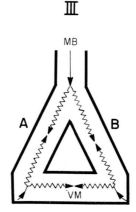

Figure 3-23. Schematic representation of a bundle of Purkinje fibers (MB) in the distal ventricular conducting system, which divides into two branches (*A* and *B*) before making contact with ventricular muscle (VM) to form a loop. Panel *I* shows the sequence of activation under normal conditions; the impulse of sinus origin invades the main bundle (MB) leading to the loop and conducts through both branches *A* and *B* into ventricular muscle, where the impulses collide and die out. Panel *II* shows the sequence of activation in the presence of an area of unidirectional conduction block (*shaded area*); conduction is blocked in the antegrade direction (from B to VM) but not in the retrograde direction (from VM to B). Conduction velocity is normal in the rest of the loop, because this is not depressed, and, therefore, the impulse conducts rapidly around the loop, returning to the main bundle (MB) before it has recovered excitability and is then blocked in this refractory tissue. Panel *III* indicates a possible sequence of activation when conduction is slowed throughout the loop, but no region of unidirectional conduction block is present. Thus, the impulse conducts slowly from the main bundle through both branches. However, the ventricular muscle is first activated by impulses conducting rapidly from other regions where conduction is not depressed. Again, there is no excitable return pathway through which reentry can take place. (Wit AL, Rosen MR, Hoffman BF: Electrophysiology and pharmacology of cardiac arrhythmias. II. Relationship of normal and abnormal electrical activity of cardiac fibers to the genesis of arrhythmias. Am Heart J 1974;88:664; with permission.)

occurrence of reentry. Reentry caused by slow conduction and unidirectional block can also occur in unbranched bundles of muscle fibers, and the same general principles apply as discussed for reentry in discrete loops of tissue.[109–111] A mechanism for reentry in an unbranched bundle of Purkinje or muscle fibers, called reflection, is shown in Figure 3-22B. In these structures, individual fibers are arranged predominantly in parallel with lateral connections in some regions. An example of nonuniform reduction of membrane potential as a result of disease in such an unbranched structure is shown in the top part of the diagram. Cells in the midregion of the upper fiber are assumed to have lower resting potentials than those in the lower fiber, so that unidirectional conduction block occurs in the upper fiber and slow conduction occurs in the lower one. An impulse propagating through this unbranched bundle is, therefore, blocked near the midregion of the upper fiber but conducts slowly along the lower fiber. Once past the midregion, the impulse may then travel laterally into the upper fiber and conduct in both antegrade and retrograde directions (see Fig. 3-22). In this way, the impulse can reenter and reexcite the unbranched structure in the retrograde direction, thereby reexciting other parts of the heart.

Another mechanism that may cause reflection is one in which, because of depressed transmembrane potentials, slow conduction does not occur along the entire bundle as illustrated in Figure 3-22B.[112] Instead, there is delayed activation of part of the bundle, resulting from electrotonic excitation of a region distal to an inexcitable segment. The inexcitable segment may be caused by a depressed resting potential and subsequent inactivation of the Na channels. (For details, see Antzelevitch and coworkers.[112])

Reentry Caused by Dispersion of Refractoriness

Reentry can also occur in the absence of disease-induced steady-state reduction in resting membrane potential and depression of phase 0 depolarization. However, the two essential conditions for the occurrence of reentry are slow conduction and unidirectional conduction block. Both these conditions may be met in healthy cardiac fibers when premature impulses are elicited within the relative refractory period, particularly if the refractory periods of adjacent groups of cardiac fibers differ markedly. The differences in refractory periods of adjacent groups of fibers can also be accentuated by cardiac disease. The following are examples of reentry caused by such dispersion of refractoriness.

The refractory periods of cells in the normal AV node vary considerably. Cells at the atrial end of the node (AN region) appear to comprise at least two populations, each with a different refractory period (Fig. 3-24).[113] Under certain conditions, this difference in refractoriness of cells in the upper nodal region may lead to the formation of a

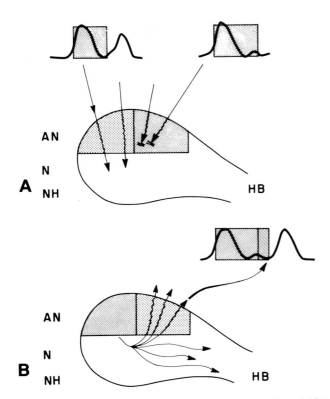

Figure 3-24. Reentry of an atrial impulse in the AV node. Both (**A**) and (**B**) show diagrammatic representations of the AV node with the upper (AN), middle (N), and lower (NH) node indicated; HB indicates the His bundle. In (**A**), action potentials recorded from two regions of the upper node are illustrated at the top. The action potential at the left has a shorter refractory period than that shown at the right, as indicated by the shaded area. Therefore, when a premature atrial impulse enters the AV node (*arrows*), it may be able to propagate through the part of the upper node with the shorter refractory period but blocks in the region with the longer refractory period. This is also depicted in the action potential recordings at the top. Panel (**B**) shows a possible continuation of these events. The propagating impulse (*arrows*) can return to excite the area of the node in which antegrade conduction block had occurred and thereby reenter the atrium; action potentials recorded from the return nodal pathway are shown above. The impulse can also conduct into the His bundle (Wit AL, Rosen MR, Hoffman BF: Electrophysiology and pharmacology of cardiac arrhythmias. II. Relationship of normal and abnormal electrical activity of cardiac fibers to the genesis of arrhythmias. Am Heart J 1974;88:799; with permission.)

functional reentrant pathway.[113] Normally, the sinus impulse reaches the AV node long after both groups of cells recover excitability and so conducts through all these fibers to the His bundle. Similarly, a premature atrial impulse occurring late enough in the basic cycle length usually propagates through all the fibers in the AV node. However, the disparity in refractoriness of upper nodal fibers becomes significant in determining conduction patterns of frequent irregular impulses or early premature impulses. Early premature atrial impulses conducting into the node may encounter a region of unidirectional block where the refractory periods of the cells are the longest but may still conduct slowly through upper nodal fibers, which have somewhat shorter effective refractory periods (see Fig. 3-24). If conduction of the early premature impulses through these fibers is slow enough, the impulse may enter the region of unidirectional block in a retrograde direction after fibers in this region have recovered excitability and then return to reexcite the atrium as a reentrant impulse or return extrasystole (see Fig. 3-24). The "antegrade" conduction pathway, with the shorter refractory period, has been called the *alpha pathway* by Mendez and Moe, whereas the "retrograde" pathway, with the longer refractory period, has been called the *beta pathway*.[113] Because the lower region of the AV node is not part of the reentrant pathway, a premature atrial impulse can reenter whether or not that impulse is also conducted in an antegrade direction to activate the His bundle and the ventricles.[113]

The mechanisms described for single reentry of atrial impulses in the AV node can also result in continuous reentry. If an impulse reenters the atrium when the nodal fibers it previously excited in the antegrade pathway have recovered excitability, then the impulse can once again enter the AV node and conduct around the circuit.[114-116] This can become a repetitive process, the atrium being activated each time the impulse conducts around the reentrant loop. This is one of the possible mechanisms for supraventricular tachycardia and is discussed further in Chapter 10.

Differences in refractoriness of adjacent groups of cells can also cause reentry in atrial, ventricular, or Purkinje fibers with normal electrophysiologic characteristics, although pathologic changes that tend to accentuate local differences in refractoriness facilitate reentry.[117-123] As in the example of reentry in the AV node, a premature impulse is necessary for reentry to occur. Reentry in the atrium resulting from the leading circle mechanism is described in Chapter 6.[118] Figure 3-25 illustrates reentry resulting from dispersion of refractoriness in the Purkinje system surviving in a region of myocardial infarction. The action potential duration of these fibers is prolonged, as are the relative and effective refractory periods compared to Purkinje fibers in surrounding noninfarcted regions. In

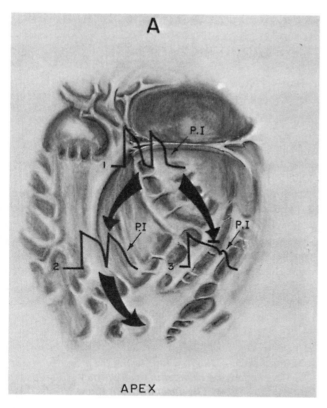
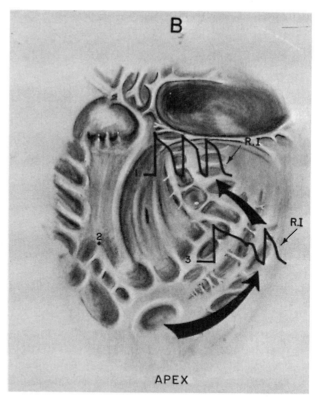

Figure 3-25. Mechanism for reentry resulting from dispersion of refractoriness in the subendocardial Purkinje fiber network over an area of extensive myocardial infarction. Both (**A**) and (**B**) show the endocardial surface of the left ventricular anterior papillary muscle (*to the left*) and the anterior interventricular septum (*to the right*). The light area in each diagram is the infarcted region, which is covered by a blanket of surviving Purkinje fibers.[53] Purkinje fibers in different regions have action potentials with markedly different durations and refractory periods. Action potentials recorded from a subendocardial Purkinje fiber at the border of the infarcted region and normal tissue (*site 1*) and from subendocardial Purkinje fibers with prolonged repolarization phases (*sites 2* and *3*) surviving in the infarct are shown in the diagrams.[53] In (**A**), a premature impulse (P.I.) occurs at *site 1* at the infarct border and conducts into the infarcted regions (curved arrows), where action potentials are prolonged; the action potential at *site 3* is longer than that at *site 2* in the infarct. Consequently, the premature impulse can excite cells at *site 2* but conduction blocks at *site 3*. Panel (**B**) shows the continuation of these events. The premature impulse, after conducting through *site 2*, activates the cells at *site 3* as a reentering impulse (R.I.), then proceeds to its site of origin, *site 1*, which it also reexcites as an R.I. (Wit AL, Rosen MR, Hoffman BF: Electrophysiology and pharmacology of cardiac arrhythmias. II. Relationship of normal and abnormal electrical activity of cardiac fibers to the genesis of arrhythmias. Am Heart J 1974; 88:799; with permission.)

addition, the action potential duration of adjacent fibers in the infarct is not homogeneous; action potential duration and refractoriness are prolonged more in some fibers than in others. Marked differences in the effective refractory periods of cells in adjacent regions result in an early premature impulse being blocked in the region with the longest effective refractory period, yet conducting slowly through relatively refractory regions with a shorter effective refractory period (see Fig. 3-25 A). While the impulse conducts slowly through the excitable tissue, the region of block recovers excitability so that the premature impulse eventually excites these regions and returns to its site of origin as a reentrant impulse. Reentry caused by this mechanism can also be repetitive and give rise to tachycardias.

The premature impulses that are responsible for the stated types of reentry can arise in several ways. These impulses may arise spontaneously in the sinus node, for example, or in an ectopic pacemaker, or they may be elicited by electrical stimulation of the heart.

Slow Conduction and Reentrant Excitation Caused by the Anisotropic Structure of Cardiac Muscle

Cardiac muscle is anisotropic, that is, its anatomic and biophysical properties vary according to the direction in the cardiac syncytium in which they are measured.[124] These anisotropic properties might sometimes cause reentry by affecting conduction of the cardiac impulse.[125, 126] Impulse conduction velocity in a direction that is perpendicular to the long axis of orientation of atrial or ventricular fibers is much slower than parallel to the long axis. Very slow conduction occurs even though resting potentials and action potential upstrokes are normal. The slow conduction is caused by an effective axial resistivity (resistance to current flow in the direction of propagation), which is much higher in the direction perpendicular to fiber orientation than parallel to fiber orientation.[124–126] This higher axial resistivity results in part from fewer and shorter intercalated disks connecting myocardial fibers in a side-to-side direction than in the end-to-end direction. The slow conduction provides one of the components necessary for reentry to occur and may be one of the factors enabling reentry to occur in normal atrial or ventricular muscle. The role of ventricular anisotropy in the genesis of reentry in a setting of chronic myocardial infarction was studied by Dillon and coworkers using epicardial isochronal activation maps.[127] During induced tachycardia when the lines of apparent conduction block were functional (i.e., block occurred only during tachycardia and not during sinus rhythm or ventricular pacing), those lines were oriented parallel to the long axis of epicardial muscle bundles. Excitation across the lines of block (transverse) occurred slowly because of anisotropic tissue properties.[127] It was concluded from these studies that parallel orientation of the muscle bundles in the epicardial border zone with nonuniform interstitial tissue fibrosis are an important cause of ventricular tachycardia because activation transverse to myocardial fibers is sufficiently slow to permit reentry.[127] The combined presence of repolarization inhomogeneities and anisotropy further facilitates the occurrence of reentry.[128]

The demonstration of dynamic variations of action potential properties and conduction patterns on a beat-to-beat basis has suggested that such irregular properties could promote electrophysiologic heterogeneity that may lead to reentry.[129, 130] The induction of such dynamic variations in action potential duration and action potential amplitude, both in ventricular muscle cells and in Purkinje fibers isolated from quinidine-induced arrhythmic ventricles, supports such a contention.[131]

ARRHYTHMIAS CAUSED BY AUTOMATICITY AND TRIGGERED ACTIVITY

Sinus Node Domination of Subsidiary Pacemakers

Cells in many regions of the normal heart are capable of spontaneous impulse initiation. These regions include the sinus node, atrial specialized fibers, coronary sinus, AV junction and valves, and the ventricular specialized conducting system. In the diseased heart, however, impulse initiation can occur almost anywhere, even in working atrial and ventricular muscle. The cell (or small group of cells) that becomes the pacemaker of the heart is the cell that first depolarizes to threshold and initiates an impulse, provided that the impulse conducts throughout the heart and excites other potential pacemakers before they can spontaneously depolarize to threshold. The site of impulse initiation is known as the *dominant pacemaker*. Other regions that are capable of pacemaking but are driven by the dominant pacemaker are called *subsidiary* or *latent pacemakers*.

The intrinsic rate at which a pacemaker cell initiates impulses is determined by the interplay of three factors: (1) the level of the maximum diastolic potential, (2) the level of the threshold potential, and (3) the steepness of phase 4 depolarization. A change in any one of these factors alters the time taken for phase 4 depolarization to carry the membrane potential from the maximum diastolic level to the threshold level (Fig. 3-26) and, therefore, alters the rate of impulse initiation. For example, if maximum diastolic potential increases (becomes more negative), spontaneous depolarization to threshold potential takes longer and the rate of impulse initiation falls (see Fig. 3-26). Conversely, a decrease in maximum diastolic potential increases the rate of impulse initiation. Similarly, changes in threshold potential level or changes in the slope of phase 4 depolarization alter the rate of impulse initiation. In the normal heart, cells in the sinus node are the quickest to depolarize to threshold, so the intrinsic rate of the sinus node is faster than that of other cells. Therefore, the sinus node is usually the dominant pacemaker.

If sinus node activity is suddenly stopped, impulse initiation by some subsidiary pacemaker does not occur immediately but usually follows a long period of quiescence. The initial rate of impulse initiation by the subsidiary pacemaker is then slow and only gradually accelerates to a steady rate, which is still lower than the original sinus rate.[132] The quiescent period that follows abolition of the sinus rhythm reflects the wearing off of an inhibitory influence exerted on subsidiary pacemakers by the dominant pacemaker. This type of inhibition ensures that the

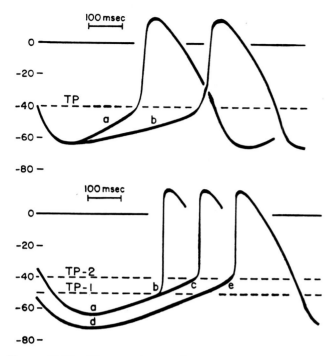

Figure 3-26. Diagram showing the principal mechanisms underlying changes in the frequency of discharge of a pacemaker fiber. The upper diagram shows a reduction in rate caused by a decrease in the slope of diastolic, or pacemaker, depolarization, from *a* to *b*, and thus an increase in the time required for the membrane potential to decline to the threshold potential level (TP). The lower diagram shows the reduction in rate associated with a shift in the level of the threshold potential from TP-1 to TP-2 and a corresponding increase in cycle length (*b* to *c*); also illustrated is a further reduction in rate due to an increase in the maximum diastolic potential level. (Hoffman BF, Cranefield PF: Electrophysiology of the heart. New York: McGraw-Hill, 1960; with permission.)

sinus node usually functions as the only pacemaker in the normal heart and is called *overdrive suppression.*

Overdrive suppression results from driving a pacemaker cell faster than its intrinsic spontaneous rate and is mediated by enhanced activity of the Na–K exchange pump. Because sodium ions enter the cell during each action potential, the higher the rate of stimulation, the greater is the amount of Na$^+$ entering the cell over a given time. The rate of activity of the sodium pump is largely determined by the level of intracellular sodium concentration, so that pump activity is enhanced during high rates of stimulation.[133] As discussed, the Na–K exchange pump usually moves more Na$^+$ outward than K$^+$ inward, thereby effectively generating a net outward (hyperpolarizing) current of Na$^+$. When subsidiary pacemaker cells are driven faster than their intrinsic rate, this hyperpolarizing pump current further suppresses spontaneous impulse initiation in these cells. After cessation of activity by the

dominant pacemaker, this suppression of subsidiary pacemakers is responsible for the period of quiescence that lasts until the intracellular Na$^+$ concentration; hence, the pump current becomes small enough to allow subsidiary pacemaking cells to depolarize to threshold and initiate the next impulse. It seems likely that the dominant pacemaker subordinates other potential pacemakers by the mechanism of overdrive suppression, whether pacemaking in these other cells depends on normal automaticity or on triggered activity, because the amplitude of the afterdepolarizations from which triggered impulses arise is also expected to be reduced by enhanced pump current. However, there is an important distinction between the effects of the dominant sinus pacemaker on abnormal automaticity (automaticity at low membrane potentials) and normal automaticity. Unlike normal automaticity, abnormal automaticity may not be overdrive suppressed.[134] Therefore, if sinus node activity is suddenly stopped, impulse initiation by subsidiary pacemakers with abnormal automaticity might occur immediately.

Mechanisms for a Shift in the Pacemaker

A shift in the site of impulse initiation (the pacemaker) to a region other than the sinus can result either from failure of the sinus impulse to activate the heart or from enhancement of impulse initiation in a subsidiary pacemaker. The rate of impulse initiation by the sinus node may be slowed, or impulse initiation may be inhibited altogether by either the autonomic nervous system or by sinus node disease.[135, 136] A decrease in sympathetic activity or an increase in vagal (parasympathetic) activity suppresses sinus node automaticity; sinus node disease may lead to degeneration of sinus node cells. Alternatively, impulse conduction from the sinus node to the atrium might be impaired in some way. Under any of these conditions, there may be escape of a subsidiary pacemaker. Removal of overdrive suppression resulting from a decrease in, or abolition of, sinus rate enables spontaneous diastolic depolarization in a latent pacemaker to proceed to threshold and initiate impulses. Such escape rhythms normally arise in the AV junction (AV node or His bundle) because cells in this region have faster intrinsic rates than other ectopic sites. Sometimes, however, pathologic processes that suppress impulse initiation in the sinus node also suppress it in the AV junction, and the site of ectopic impulse initiation usually resides at some other site in the atria or ventricular conducting system.[136] The mechanism for spontaneous diastolic depolarization underlying the ectopic rhythm may be the normal pacemaker current that occurs at high levels of membrane potential in normal Purkinje fibers, or it may be a pacemaker current occurring at lower levels of membrane potential in the AV valves or AV node.

Many factors can enhance subsidiary pacemaker activity and cause impulse initiation to shift to ectopic sites, even when sinus node function is normal. For example, norepinephrine released from sympathetic nerves increases the slope of spontaneous diastolic depolarization of most ectopic pacemaker cells, enabling the membrane potential to reach threshold level in these cells before they are activated by an impulse conducting from the sinus node.[137] The norepinephrine may be released locally at discrete ectopic sites, thereby causing a shift of the pacemaker.[138,139] This effect of the catecholamine may result from its known action on the normal pacemaker current in Purkinje fibers or an action on pacemaker currents occurring at lower levels of membrane potential.[140] Norepinephrine is also known to increase the amplitude of delayed afterdepolarizations in mitral valve and coronary sinus fibers, and if the afterdepolarizations reach threshold, then triggered activity might be initiated at a higher rate than the sinus rate.[53,54] Cardiac disease can also lead to subsidiary pacemaker activity; thus, a reduction in membrane potential can result in automatic activity in atrial, ventricular, and Purkinje fibers. This type of spontaneous activity often occurs at higher rates than the sinus rate; hence, impulse initiation may shift to a diseased area of the heart. As discussed, the automaticity caused by a reduction in membrane potential is probably not suppressed by overdrive from the sinus node.

References

1. Cranefield PF, Wit AL, Hoffman BF: The genesis of cardiac arrhythmias. Circulation 1973;47:190.
2. Hoffman BF, Cranefield PF: Physiologic basis of cardiac arrhythmias. Am J Med 1964;37:670.
3. Hoffman BF, Cranefield PF: Electrophysiology of the heart. New York: McGraw-Hill, 1960.
4. Hodgkin AL: Ionic movements and electrical activity in giant nerve fibers. Proc R Soc Lond (Biol) 1957;148:1.
5. Weidmann S: Elektrophysiologie der herzmuskelfaser. Bern: Medizinischer Verlag Hans Huber, 1956.
6. Draper MH, Weidmann S: Cardiac resting and action potentials recorded with an intracellular electrode. J Physiol 1951;115:74.
7. Miura DS, Hoffman BF, Rosen MR: The effect of extracellular potassium on the intracellular potassium ion activity and transmembrane potentials of beating canine cardiac Purkinje fibers. J Gen Physiol 1977;69:463.
8. Ellis D: The effects of external cations and ouabain on the intracellular sodium activity of sheep heart Purkinje fibers. J Physiol (Lond) 1977;273:211.
9. Thomas RC: Electrogenic sodium pump in nerve and muscle cells. Physiol Rev 1972;52:563.
10. Adrian RH: Potassium chloride movement and the membrane potential of frog muscle. J Physiol 1960;151:154.
11. Gadsby DC, Cranefield PF: Two levels of resting potential in cardiac Purkinje fibers. J Gen Physiol 1977;70:725.
12. Goldman DE: Potential, impedance and rectification in membranes. J Gen Physiol 1943;27:27.
13. Hodgkin AL, Katz B: The effect of sodium ions on the electrical activity of the giant axon of the squid. J Physiol 1949;108:37.
14. Noble D, Tsien RW: The kinetics and rectifier properties of the slow potassium current in cardiac Purkinje fibers. J Physiol (Lond) 1968;195:185.
15. Hodgkin AL, Huxley AF: A quantitative description of membrane currents and its application to conduction and excitation in nerve. J Physiol 1952;117:500.
16. Dudel J: Excitation process in heart cells. In: De Mello WC, ed. Electrical phenomena in the heart. New York: Academic Press, 1972.
17. Wit AL, Rosen MR, Hoffman BF: Electrophysiology and pharmacology of cardiac arrhythmias. II. Relation of normal and abnormal electrical activity of cardiac fibers to the genesis of arrhythmias. Am Heart J 1974;88:515.
18. Weidmann S: The effect of the cardiac membrane potential on the rapid availability of the sodium carrying system. J Physiol (Lond) 1955a;127:213.
19. Van Dam RT, Moore EN, Hoffman BF: Initiation and conduction of impulses in partially depolarized cardiac fibers. Am J Physiol 1963;204:1133.
20. Reuter H: The dependence of slow inward current in Purkinje fibers on the extracellular calcium concentration. J Physiol (Lond) 1967;192:479.
21. Cranefield PF: The conduction of the cardiac impulse. Mt Kisco, NY: Futura, 1975.
22. Reuter H: Divalent cations as charge carriers in excitable membranes. In: Butler JAV, Noble D, eds. Progress in biophysics and molecular biology 26. New York: Pergamon Press, 1973:3.
23. Kass RS, Tsien RW: Control of action potential duration by calcium ions in Purkinje fibers. J Gen Physiol 1976;67:599.
24. Niedergerke R, Orkand RK: The dual effect of calcium on the action potential of the frog's heart. J Physiol (Lond) 1966;184:291.
25. Niedergerke R, Orkand RK: The dependence of the action potential of the frog's heart on the external and intracellular sodium concentration. J Physiol (Lond) 1966;184:312.
26. Kao CY: Tetrodotoxin, saxitoxin and their significance in the study of excitation phenomena. Pharmacol Rev 1966;18:998.
27. Vassort G, Rougier O, Garnier D, et al: Effects of adrenaline on membrane inward currents during the cardiac action potential. Pflugers Arch 1969;309:70.
28. Hagiwara S, Nakajima S: Differences in Na and Ca spikes as examined by application of tetrodotoxin, procaine and manganese ions. J Gen Physiol 1966;49:793.
29. Kolhardt M, Bauer B, Krause H, Fleckenstein A: Differentiation of the transmembrane Na and Ca channels in mammalian cardiac fibers by the use of specific inhibitors. Pflugers Arch 1972;335:309.
30. Hagiwara N, Irisawa H, Kameyama M: Contribution of two types of calcium currents to the pacemaker potential of rabbit sinoatrial node cells. J Physiol (Lond) 1988;395:233.
31. Bean B: Two kinds of calcium channels in canine atrial cells. J Gen Physiol 1985;87:161.
32. McCleskey EW, Fox AP, Feldman D, Tsien RW: Different types of calcium channels. J Exp Biol 1986;1124:177.

33. Nilius B, Hess P, Lansman JB, Tsien RW: A novel type of cardiac calcium channel in ventricular cells. Nature 1985; 316:443.

34. Mitra R, Morad M: Two types of calcium channels in guinea pig ventricular myocytes. Proc Natl Acad Sci U S A 1986; 83:5340.

35. Tseng GN, Boyden PA: Multiple types of Ca 2 + currents in single canine Purkinje cells. Circ Res 1989;65:1735.

36. Trautwein W: Membrane currents in cardiac muscle fibers. Physiol Rev 1973;53:793.

37. Kenyon JL, Gibbons WR: Effects of low-chloride solutions on action potentials of sheep cardiac Purkinje fibers. J Gen Physiol 1977;70:635.

38. Hiraoka M, Kawano S: Calcium-sensitive and insensitive transient outward current in rabbit ventricular myocytes. J Physiol (Lond) 1989;410:187.

39. Tsen GN, Robinson RB, Hoffman BF: Passive properties and membrane currents of canine ventricular myocytes. J Gen Physiol 1987;90:671.

40. Coraboeuf E, Carmeliet E: Existence of two transient outward currents in sheep cardiac Purkinje fibers. Pflugers Arch 1982;392:352.

41. Siegelbaum SA, Tsien RW: Calcium-activated transient outward current in calf cardiac Purkinje fibers. J Physiol (Lond) 1980;299:485.

42. Litovsky SH, Antzelevitch C: Transient outward current prominent in canine ventricular epicardium and not in endocardium. Circ Res 1988;62:116.

43. Litovsky SH, Antzelevitch C: Rate dependence of action potential duration and refractoriness in canine ventricular endocardium differs from that of epicardium: Role of transient outward current. J Am Coll Cardiol 1989;14:1053.

44. West T, Frederickson E, Amory D: Single fiber recording of the ventricular response to induced hypothermia in the anesthetized dog: Correlation with multicellular parameters. Circ Res 1959;7:880.

45. Sridharan MR, Horan LG: Electrocardiographic J wave of hypercalcemia. Am J Cardiol 1984;54:672.

46. Noble D, Tsien RW: Outward membrane currents activated in the plateau range of potentials in cardiac Purkinje fibers. J Physiol (Lond) 1969a;200:205.

47. Cranefield PF: Action potentials, afterpotentials and arrhythmias. Circ Res 1977;41:415.

48. Vassalle M: Analysis of cardiac pacemaker potential using a "voltage clamp" technique. Am J Physiol 1966;210:1335.

49. Vassalle M: Cardiac pacemaker potentials at different extracellular and intracellular K concentrations. Am J Physiol 1965;208:770.

50. DiFrancesco D: A new interpretation of the pace-maker current in Purkinje fibers. J Physiol (Lond) 1981;314:359.

51. DiFrancesco D, Ojeda C: Properties of the current i_f in the sino-atrial node of the rabbit compared with those of the current i_{K2} in Purkinje fibres. J Physiol (Lond) 1980; 308:353.

52. Escande D, Coraboeuf E, Planche C: Abnormal pacemaking is modulated by sarcoplasmic reticulum in partially-depolarized myocardium from dilated right atria in humans. J Mol Cell Cardiol 1987;19:231.

53. Wit AL, Cranefield PF: Triggered activity in cardiac muscle fibers of the simian mitral valve. Circ Res 1976;38:85.

54. Wit AL, Cranefield PF: Triggered and automatic activity in the canine coronary sinus. Circ Res 1977;41:435.

55. Saito T, Otoguro M, Matsubara T: Electrophysiological studies on the mechanism of electrically induced sustained rhythmic activity in the rabbit right atrium. Circ Res 1978; 42:199.

56. Weingart R, Kass RS, Tsien RW: Role of calcium and sodium ions in the transient inward current induced by strophanthidin in cardiac Purkinje fibers. Biophys J 1977;17:3A.

57. Kass RS, Lederer WJ, Tsien TW, et al: Role of cation ion in transient inward currents and after contractions induced by strophanthidin in cardiac Purkinje fibers. J Physiol (Lond) 1978;281:187.

58. Kass RS, Tsien WJ, Weingart R: Ionic basis of transient current induced by strophanthidin in cardiac Purkinje fibers. J Physiol (Lond) 1978;281:209.

59. Karagueuzian HS, Katzung BG: Relative inotropic and arrhythmic effects of five cardiac steroids in ventricular myocardium. Oscillatory after potentials and the role of endogenous catecholamines. J Pharmacol Exp Ther 1981;218:348.

60. Karagueuzian HS, Katzung BG: Voltage-clamp studies of transient inward current and mechanical oscillations induced by ouabain in ferret papillary muscle. J Physiol (Lond) 1982;327:255.

61. Henning B, Kline RP, Siegal MS, Wit AL: Triggered activity in atrial fibers of canine coronary sinus: Role of extracellular potassium accumulation and depletion. J Physiol (Lond) 1987;383:191.

62. Aronson R, Cranefield PF, Wit AL: The effects of caffeine and ryanodine on the electrical activity of the canine coronary sinus. J Physiol (Lond) 1985;368:593.

63. Nordin C, Gilat E, Aronson RS: Delayed afterdepolarization and triggered activity in ventricular muscle from rats with streptozocin-induced diabetes. Circ Res 1985;57:28.

64. Clusin TW, Bristow MR, Karagueuzian HS, Katzung BG, Schroeder JS: Do calcium-dependent ionic currents mediate ischemic ventricular fibrillation. Am J Cardiol 1982;49:606.

65. Ferrier GR, Moffat MP, Lukas A, et al: Possible mechanisms of ventricular arrhythmias elicited by ischemia followed by reperfusion: Studies on isolated canine ventricular tissues. Circ Res 1985;56:184.

66. Henning B, Wit AL: The time course of action potential repolarization affects delayed afterdepolarization amplitude in atrial fibers of the canine coronary sinus. Circ Res 1984;55:110.

67. Grant AO, Strauss HC: Intracellular potassium activity in rabbit sinoatrial node. Evaluation during spontaneous activity and arrest. Circ Res 1982;51:271.

68. Kerr CR, Prystowsky EN, Browning DJ, Strauss HC: Characterization of refractoriness in the sinus node of the rabbit. Circ Res 1980;47:742.

69. Kerr CR, Strauss HC: The measurement of sinus node refractoriness in man. Circulation 1983;68:1231.

70. Billette J, Metayer R: Origin, domain, and dynamics of rate-induced variations of functional refractory period in rabbit atrioventricular node. Circ Res 1989;65:164.

71. Billette J, Metayer R, St-Vincent M: Selective functional characteristics of rate-induced fatigue in rabbit atrioventricular node. Circ Res 1988;62:790.

72. Paes de Carvalho A, Hoffman BF, de Paula Carvalho M: Two components of the cardiac action potential. I. Voltage time course and the effect of acetylcholine on atrial and nodal cells of the rabbit heart. J Gen Physiol 1969;54:607.

73. Zipes DP, Mendez C: Action of manganese ions and tetrodotoxin on atrioventricular nodal transmembrane potentials in isolated rabbit hearts. Circ Res 1973;32:447.

74. Wit AL, Cranefield PF: Effect of verapamil on the sinoatrial and atrioventricular nodes of the rabbit and the mechanism by which it arrests reentrant atrioventricular nodal tachycardia. Circ Res 1974;35:413.

75. Merideth J, Mendez C, Mueller WJ, Moe GK: Electrical excitability of atrioventricular nodal cells. Circ Res 1968;23:69.

76. Mendez C, Moe GK: Some characteristics of transmembrane potentials of AV nodal cells during propagation of premature beats. Circ Res 1966;19:993.

77. Kokubun S, Nishimura M, Noma A, Irisawa A: The spontaneous action potential of rabbit atrioventricular nodal cells. Jpn J Physiol 1980;30:529.

78. Brown HF: Electrophysiology of the sino-atrial node. Physiol Rev 1982;62:505.

79. Maylie J, Morad M: Ionic currents responsible for the generation of pace-maker current in the rabbit sino-atrial node. J Physiol (Lond) 1984;355:215.

80. Brown HF, Kimura J, Noble D, Noble SJ, Taupignon A: The ionic currents underlying pacemaker activity in rabbit sino-atrial node: Experimental results and computer simulation. Proc R Soc Lond 1984;B222:329.

81. Jalife J: Mutual entrainment and electrical coupling as mechanisms for synchronous firing of rabbit sino-atrial pace-maker cells. J Physiol (Lond) 1984;356:221.

82. Michaels DC, Matyas EP, Jose J: Mechanisms of sinoatrial pacemaker synchronization: A new hypothesis. Circ Res 1987;61:704.

83. Hordof AJ, Edie R, Malm JR, et al: Electrophysiologic properties and response to pharmacologic agents of fibers from diseased human atria. Circulation 1976;54:774.

84. Boyden PA, Tilley LP, Albala A, et al: Mechanisms for atrial arrhythmias associated with cardiomyopathy: A study of feline hearts with primary myocardial disease. Circulation 1984;69:1036.

85. Friedman PL, Stewart JR, Fenoglio JJ Jr, Wit AL: Survival of subendocardial Purkinje fibers after extensive myocardial infarction in dogs: In vitro and in vivo correlations. Circ Res 1973;33:597.

86. Lazzara R, El-Sherif N, Scherlag BJ: Early and late effects of coronary artery occlusion on canine Purkinje fibers. Circ Res 1974;35:391.

87. Downar E, Janse MJ, Durrer D: The effect of acute coronary artery occlusion on subepicardial transmembrane potentials in the intact porcine heart. Circulation 1977;56:217.

88. Lazzara R, El-Sherif N, Befeler B, Scherlag BJ: Lidocaine action on depressed cardiac cells. Circulation 1975;52:II-85.

89. Isenberg G: Cardiac Purkinje fibers: Cesium as a tool to block inward rectifying potassium currents. Pflugers Arch 1976;365:99.

90. Dresdner KP, Kline RP, Wit AL: Intracellular K^+ activity, intracellular Na^+ activity and maximum diastolic potential of canine subendocardial Purkinje cells from one day old infarct. Circ Res 1987;60:122.

91. Dresdner KP, Kline RP, Wit AL: Intracellular pH of canine subendocardial Purkinje cells surviving in 1-day old myocardial infarcts. Circ Res 1989;65:554.

92. Lazzara R, El-Sherif N, Scherlag BJ: Disorders of cellular electrophysiology produced by ischemia of the canine His bundle. Circ Res 1975;36:444.

93. Carmeliet E, Vereecke J: Adrenaline and the plateau phase of the cardiac action potential. Importance of Ca^{++}, Na^+, and K^+ conductance. Pflugers Arch 1969;313:300.

94. Gettes LS, Reuter H: Slow recovery from inactivation of inward currents in mammalian myocardial fibers. J Physiol (Lond) 1974;240:703.

95. MacLeod DP, Prasad K: Influence of glucose on the transmembrane action potential of papillary muscle. J Gen Physiol 1969;53:792.

96. Han J: Ventricular ectopic activity in myocardial infarction. In: Han J, ed. Cardiac arrhythmias. A symposium edited by J. Han. Springfield, IL: Charles C Thomas, 1972:171.

97. Lazzara R, El-Sherif N, Scherlag BJ: Electrophysiological properties of canine Purkinje cells in one-day-old myocardial infarction. Circ Res 1973;33:722.

98. Alessi R, Nusynowitz M, Abildskov JA, Moe GK: Nonuniform distribution of vagal effects on the atrial refractory period. Am J Physiol 1968;194:406.

99. Katzung B: Effects of extracellular calcium and sodium on depolarization-induced automaticity in guinea pig papillary muscle. Circ Res 1975;37:118.

100. Brown HF, Noble SJ: Membrane currents underlying delayed rectification and pacemaker activity in frog atrial muscle. J Physiol (Lond) 1969;204:717.

101. Imanishi S, Surawicz B: Automatic activity in depolarized guinea pig ventricular myocardium: Characteristics and mechanisms. Circ Res 1976;39:751.

102. Imanishi S: Calcium-sensitive discharges in canine Purkinje fibers. Jpn J Physiol 1971;21:443.

103. Dangman KH, Dresdner KP, Zaim S: Automatic and triggered impulse initiation in canine subepicardial ventricular muscle cells from border zone of 24-hour transmural infarcts. New mechanism for malignant cardiac arrhythmias. Circulation 1988;78:1020.

104. Mary-Rabine L, Hordof AJ, Daniels P Jr, et al: Mechanisms for impulse initiation in isolated human atrial fibers. Circ Res 1980;47:267.

105. El-Sherif N, Gough WB, Zeiler RH, Mehra R: Triggered ventricular rhythms in 1-day-old myocardial infarction in the dog. Circ Res 1983;52:566.

106. Mines GR: On circulating excitations in heart muscle and their possible relations to tachycardia and fibrillation. Transactions of the Royal Society of Canada (Ser 3 Sec 4) 1914;8:43.

107. Cranefield PF, Hoffman BF: Reentry: Slow conduction, summation and inhibition. Circulation 1971;44:309.

108. Mayer AG: Rhythmical pulsation in scyphomedusae II. Papers from the Tortugar Laboratory of the Carnegie Institute of Washington 1:113. Carnegie Institution of Washington Publication No. 102, part VII, 1908.

109. Schmitt FO, Erlanger J: Directional differences in the conduction of the impulse through heart muscle and their possible relation to extrasystolic and fibrillary contractions. Am J Physiol 1928.

110. Wit AL, Cranefield PF, Hoffman BF: Slow conduction and reentry in the ventricular conducting system. II. Single and sustained circus movement in networks of canine and bovine Purkinje fibers. Circ Res 1972;30:11.

111. Wit AL, Hoffman BF, Cranefield PF: Slow conduction and reentry in the ventricular conducting system. I. Return extrasystole in canine Purkinje fibers. Circ Res 1972;30:1.

112. Antzelevitch C, Jalife J, Moe GK: Characteristics of reflection as a mechanism of reentrant arrhythmias and its relationship to parasystole. Circulation 1980;61:182.

113. Mendez C, Moe GK: Demonstration of a dual A-V nodal conduction system in the isolated rabbit heart. Circ Res 1966;29:378.

114. Wit AL, Goldreyer BN, Damato AN: An in vitro model of paroxysmal supraventricular tachycardia. Circulation 1971;43:862.

115. Janse MJ, van Capelle FJL, Freud GE, Durrer D: Circus movement within the AV node. Circ Res 1971;28:403.

116. Coumel P: Mechanism of supraventricular tachycardia. In: Narula OS, ed. His bundle electrocardiography and clinical electrophysiology. Philadelphia: FA Davis, 1975.

117. Moe GK: On the multiple wavelet hypothesis of atrial fibrillation. Arch Int Pharmacodyn 1962;140:183.

118. Allessie MA, Bonke FIM, Schopman FJG: Circus movement in rabbit atrial muscle as a mechanism of tachycardia. III. The "leading circle" concept: A new model of circus movement in cardiac tissue without the involvement of an anatomical obstacle. Circ Res 1977;41:9.

119. Moe GK: Evidence for reentry as a mechanism for cardiac arrhythmias. Rev Physiol Biochem Pharmacol 1975;72:56.

120. Kuo CS, Munakata K, Reddy P, Surawicz B: Characteristics and possible mechanism of ventricular arrhythmias dependent on the dispersion of action potential durations. Circulation 1983;67;1356.

121. Sasyniuk BI, Mendez C: A mechanism for reentry in canine ventricular tissue. Circ Res 1973;28:3.

122. Myerburg RJ, Stewart JW, Hoffman BF: Electrophysiological properties of the canine peripheral AV conducting system. Circ Res 1970;26:361.

123. Friedman PL, Stewart JR, Wit AL: Spontaneous and induced cardiac arrhythmias in subendocardial Purkinje fibers surviving extensive myocardial infarction in dogs. Circ Res 1973;22:612.

124. Clerc L: Directional differences of impulse spread in trabecular muscle from mammalian heart. J Physiol (Lond) 1976;255:335.

125. Spach M, Miller WT, Geselowitz DB, et al: The discontinuous nature of propagation in normal canine cardiac muscle: Evidence for recurrent discontinuities of intracellular resistance that affect the membrane currents. Circ Res 1981;48:39.

126. Spach M, Miller WT, Dolber PC, et al: The functional role of structural complexities in the propagation of depolarization in the atrium of the dog: Cardiac conduction disturbances due to discontinuities of effective axial resistivity. Circ Res 1982;50:175.

127. Dillon SM, Allessie MA, Urcell PC, Wit AL: Influence of anisotropic tissue structure on reentrant circuits in the epicardial border zone of subacute infarcts. Circ Res 1988;63:182.

128. Spach MS, Dolber PC, Heidlage JF: Interaction of inhomogeneities of repolarization with anisotropic propagation in dog atria. A mechanism for both preventing and initiating reentry. Circ Res 1989;65:1612.

129. Chialvo DR, Jalife J: Non-linear dynamics of cardiac excitation and impulse propagation. Nature 1987;330:749.

130. Chialvo DR, Michaels D, Jalife J: Supernormal excitability as a mechanism of chaotic dynamics of activation in cardiac Purkinje fibers. Circ Res 1990;66:525.

131. Karagueuzian HS, Khan SS, Hong K, Kobayash Y, Denton T, Mandel WJ, Diamond GA: Action potential alternans and irregular dynamics in quinidine-intoxicated ventricular muscle cells. Implications for ventricular proarrhythmia. Circulation 1993;87:1661.

132. Vassalle M: The relationship among cardiac pacemakers: Overdrive suppression. Circ Res 1977;41:269.

133. Vassalle M: Electrogenic suppression of automaticity in sheep and dog Purkinje fibers. Circ Res 1970;27:361.

134. Dangman KH, Hoffman BF: Studies on overdrive stimulation of canine cardiac Purkinje fibers: Maximum diastolic potential as a determinant of the response. J Am Coll Cardiol 1983;2:1183.

135. Trautwein W, Kuffler SW, Edwards C: Changes in membrane characteristics of heart muscle during inhibition. J Gen Physiol 1956;40:135.

136. Ferrer MI: The sick sinus syndrome. Mt Kisco, NY: Futura, 1974.

137. Wit AL, Hoffman BF, Rosen MR: Electrophysiology and pharmacology of cardiac arrhythmias. IX. Cardiac electrophysiologic effects of beta adrenergic receptor stimulation and blockade. Am Heart J 1975;90:521.

138. Armour JA, Hageman GR, Randall WC: Arrhythmias induced by local cardiac nerve stimulation. Am J Physiol 1972;223:1068.

139. Geesbreght JM, Randall WC: Area localization of shifting cardiac pacemakers during sympathetic stimulation. Am J Physiol 1971;220:1522.

140. Tsien RW: Effect of epinephrine on the pacemaker potassium current of cardiac Purkinje fibers. J Gen Physiol 1974;64:293.

Cardiac Arrhythmias, 3rd edition, edited by William J. Mandel.
J. B. Lippincott Company, Philadelphia © 1995.

4

Borys Surawicz

The Interrelationship of Electrolyte Abnormalities and Arrhythmias

The electrical activity in the excitable tissues is accompanied by changes in membrane permeability and transmembrane fluxes of ions. For background material on these phenomena, refer to Hoffman and Cranefield,[1] Noble,[2] and Chapter 3 of this book. The following discussion of the electrophysiologic theory is limited to the phenomena that are directly related to the clinical observations described in this chapter. Therefore, the experimental background is confined to the ranges of electrolyte concentrations that may be encountered in clinical practice. A large portion of text is devoted to discussion of potassium, because this ion has a more prominent role in arrhythmias than other ions.

Supported in part by the Herman C. Krannert Fund, by grants HL-06308 and HL-07182 from the National Heart, Lung, and Blood Institute of the National Institutes of Health, U.S. Public Health Service, the American Heart Association, Indiana Affiliate, Inc., by the Attorney General of Indiana Public Health Trust, and by the Roudebush Veterans Administration Medical Center, Indianapolis.

HYPERKALEMIA

Electrophysiologic Mechanism

1. Resting membrane potential (RMP), or maximal diastolic potential (MDP),* decreases (i.e., becomes less negative) with increasing extracellular potassium concentration. Within the range of plasma potassium concentrations encountered in vivo, intracellular potassium concentration stays within narrow limits and, therefore, is not expected to play a major role in the determination of RMP or MDP.[3] Depolarization caused by increased extracellular potassium concentration brings the membrane potential to an approximate value expected from the Nernst equation for a membrane freely permeable to K^+. This means that, at plasma potassium concentrations higher than normal, the membrane acts like a potassium electrode. The value of RMP in the ventricular myocardium is approximately -84 mV at $(K)_o = 5.4$ mM/L,

* Refers to myocardial fibers of the atria or the ventricles, and to the Purkinje fibers.

-67 mV at $(K)_o = 10.0$ mM/L, and -60 mV at $(K)_o = 16.2$ mM/L. At less negative levels of RMP, the fibers are usually no longer excitable, at least in response to stimuli of ordinary strength.

2. Repolarization becomes more rapid because increased $(K)_o$ increases membrane permeability to potassium and shortens the duration of the action potential. In the ventricular myocardial fibers, this shortening is predominantly because of a more rapid slope of phase 3.

3. Diastolic depolarization in Purkinje fibers is attributed to increasing membrane permeability to Na^+, and perhaps to decreasing membrane permeability to K^+. Hyperkalemia, which increases membrane permeability to potassium, decreases the slope of phase 4 (diastolic depolarization), thereby decreasing or suppressing automaticity.

4. Threshold potential decreases (becomes less negative) with increasing depolarization (less negative RMP or MDP). However, hyperkalemia usually causes a greater shift of the RMP in the depolarizing direction than the shift of the threshold potential. This may cause a decrease in the "distance" (difference) between the RMP and the threshold potential. Therefore, an increase in $(K)_o$ does not always decrease conduction velocity or the rate of the pacemaker fibers. Rather, moderate increase in $(K)_o$ may improve conduction without changing the rate of pacemaker.

5. Biphasic effect of increased $(K)_o$ on conduction and excitability results from the dependence of conduction and excitability on both the absolute level of RMP and the difference between RMP and threshold potential. When $(K)_o$ increases gradually, the conduction becomes at first more rapid and the excitability threshold decreases because of the decreased difference between RMP and threshold potential. Afterward, the conduction becomes slower and the threshold of excitability increases because of the absolute decrease in the level of RMP.[4] Increase in $(K)_o$ may have the same biphasic effect on the rate of firing of the Purkinje fibers, that is, first an increase, then a decrease and arrest.

6. Differences in sensitivity to potassium among different types of cardiac fibers are prominent.[5] Thus, the depression of excitability and conduction in atrial myocardial fibers takes place at lower $(K)_o$ than in other types of myocardial fibers. In isolated preparations, the sinus node and the His bundle are more "resistant" to the increased $(K)_o$ than the ventricular myocardium, which is more "resistant" to high potassium concentration than the atrial myocardium. The phenomenon has been demonstrated in a patient with a dual chamber pacemaker in whom hyper-

kalemia suppressed the atrial pacing while the ventricular pacing was maintained.[6]

7. "Injury currents" may result from differences in potassium concentration in different parts of myocardium. In one study, every site in the ischemic region of an isolated perfused pig heart showed a linear relationship between local extracellular potassium concentration and the intensity of local current of injury manifested by QT segment depression.[7]

8. Increased potassium concentration tends to decrease the dispersion of refractoriness because it shortens action potential duration at all heart rates and decreases the rate-dependent differences in action potential duration in both ventricular muscle and Purkinje fibers. It also decreases the difference between the duration of action potentials in Purkinje and ventricular fibers at all heart rates.[8] The decrease in dispersion of refractoriness in the myocardium caused by these factors affects predominantly the nonpremature complexes. However, a marked shortening of the action potential in the early premature complexes can contribute to an increase in dispersion.

9. Moderate hyperkalemia abolishes supernormal conduction and excitability. This effect has been observed both in vitro and in vivo in the Purkinje fibers and bundle branches.[9] A similar phenomenon in the ventricular myocardium can suppress the dip in the excitability curve.[10]

10. The negative inotropic effect of hyperkalemia, which may play an indirect role in the genesis of arrhythmias, appears to be more pronounced in the failing heart than in the normal heart.[11] In animal experiments, the depression of contractility by potassium is associated with myocardial K^+ uptake and is related to the rate of $(K)_o$ rise rather than to the absolute $(K)_o$ value.[12]

Electrocardiographic Manifestations

When the plasma potassium concentration exceeds approximately 5.5 mEq/L, the electrocardiogram (ECG) shows the T waves as tall and peaked; when the plasma potassium concentration exceeds 6.5 mEq/L, QRS changes are usually present. The diagnosis of hyperkalemia cannot be based solely on T wave changes.

A correct ECG diagnosis of hyperkalemia can usually be made when plasma potassium concentrations exceed 6.7 mEq/L.[13] The uniformly wide QRS complex caused by hyperkalemia differs from the ECG pattern of bundle branch block or preexcitation because widening affects both the initial and the terminal portions of the QRS complex. The wide S wave in the left precordial leads helps to differentiate a pattern of hyperkalemia from a typical left bundle branch block and the wide initial portion from a right bundle branch block. In vitro, the high–K-induced delay of transmission across the Purkinje ventricular junction has been associated with uniformly slowed conduction resulting from depolarization.[14] However, in patients with hyperkalemia, the wide QRS complex may resemble the typical pattern of left bundle branch block. The QRS axis sometimes shifts superiorly and sometimes inferiorly. This suggests a nonuniform delay of conduction in the major divisions of left bundle branch. Slow intraventricular conduction is associated with a prolonged HV interval; this prolonged interval parallels the increase in QRS duration.[15] QRS duration increases progressively with an increasing plasma potassium concentration, and there is a rough correlation between the duration of the QRS complex and plasma potassium concentration.

The pattern of advanced hyperkalemia is similar to that recorded in dying hearts. Sometimes, in patients with advanced hyperkalemia, the ST segment deviates appreciably from the baseline and simulates the "acute injury" pattern, which resembles the pattern of acute myocardial ischemia. Such ST deviation disappears rapidly when the pattern of hyperkalemia regresses during treatment with hemodialysis.[16] The injury current responsible for the ST segment deviation is probably caused by nonhomogeneous depolarization in different portions of the myocardium. Deviation of the ST segment or a monophasic pattern can be readily produced by topical application of potassium on the ventricular surface or an intracoronary potassium chloride (KCl) injection.[12]

When the plasma potassium concentration exceeds 7.0 mEq/L, the P wave amplitude usually decreases and the duration of the P wave increases because of the slower conduction in the atria. The PR interval is frequently prolonged, but most of the prolongation is caused by an increase in P wave duration. When the plasma potassium concentration exceeds 8.8 mEq/L, the P wave frequently becomes invisible. In the presence of a wide QRS complex, a low or absent P wave helps to differentiate the pattern of hyperkalemia from intraventricular conduction disturbance of other origin. A regular rhythm in the absence of P waves has been attributed to sinoventricular conduction in the presence of sinoatrial block. This concept is supported by experiments in dogs. Even when the P wave disappeared during hyperkalemia, the electrical activity was recorded from the sinoatrial node, atrionodal tracts, and crista terminals, and each QRS complex was preceded by a His bundle electrogram.[17,18] A regular rhythm in the absence of P waves can be caused by a displacement of the pacemaker into the atrioventricular (AV) junction or the Purkinje fibers, but precise localization of the pacemaker in patients with absent P waves is

usually not possible. When the plasma potassium concentration exceeds about 10 mEq/L, the ventricular rhythm may become irregular because of the simultaneous activity of several escape pacemakers in the depressed myocardium. The combination of an irregular rhythm and an absent P wave may simulate atrial fibrillation.

An increase in the plasma potassium concentration above 12 to 14 mEq/L causes ventricular asystole or ventricular fibrillation. Ventricular fibrillation may be preceded by an acceleration of the ventricular rate.[19] Ventricular fibrillation probably results from reentry, which is facilitated by the slow intraventricular conduction and the short duration of the ventricular action potential. Experiments in dogs have shown that advanced intraventricular conduction disturbances may be associated with a change or even a reversal of the activation sequence (i.e., the epicardial excitation occurring before the endocardial excitation).[15]

The ECG pattern of hyperkalemia can be made more normal by increasing the concentration of plasma calcium and sodium and more abnormal by decreasing the concentration of plasma calcium and possibly sodium.[20]

To understand ECG changes produced by hyperkalemia, these changes may be correlated with concomitant changes in the atrial and ventricular transmembrane action potential (Fig. 4-1), which is based on experimental work in isolated perfused rabbit hearts. Except for the difference in the QRS and the QT durations, the normal ECG and various electrolyte imbalance patterns in the rabbit are almost identical with those in humans.[21] Figure 4-1 shows that the duration of action potential in the atrial fibers is shorter than in the ventricular fibers. It is assumed that the sum of all depolarizations and repolarization of the atrial fibers is responsible for the origin of the P wave and the Ta wave, and the sum of the ventricular fibers is responsible for the origin of the QRS complex, ST segment, and the T wave. Phase 0 lasts only a few milliseconds, but the time required to depolarize all fibers is represented by the duration of the QRS complex. The duration of phase 2 corresponds approximately to the duration of the ST segment, and the duration of phase 3 corresponds to the duration of the T wave. The end of the T wave corresponds approximately to the termination of ventricular action potentials on the ventricular surface. The slope of phase 3 is usually similar to the slope of the terminal portion of the T wave. The end of the T wave coincides approximately with the end of the ventricular ejection, and the U wave is usually inscribed during relaxation. Figure 4-1B shows the effect on repolarization, which is responsible for the narrow and peaked T wave, when the potassium concentration is increased to 6.0 mEq/L. At this concentration, the effects of slight lowering of RMP are still not evident. Figure 4-1C through E demonstrates that a progressive increase in potassium concentration produces a

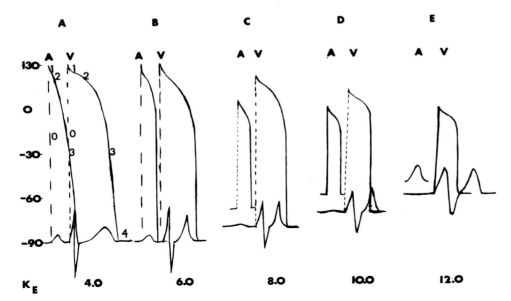

Figure 4-1. Diagram of an atrial (A) and ventricular (V) action potential superimposed on the electrocardiogram. The numbers on the left designate the transmembrane potential in millivolts (mV), and the numbers at the bottom designate extracellular K concentration $(K)_E$ in milliequivalents per liter (mEq/L). (Surawicz B: Relation between electrocardiogram and electrolytes. Am Heart J 1967;73:814.)

progressive decrease in RMP, which decreases the upstroke velocity of the action potential. This, in turn, slows the intra-atrial and intraventricular conduction, thereby increasing the duration of the P wave and the QRS complex, respectively.[22] At the potassium concentration of 12.0 mEq/L, ventricular depolarization is slow, portions of the ventricular myocardium undergo repolarization before depolarization is completed, and the end of the QRS complex may be difficult to impossible to determine (see Fig. 4-1E). Figure 4-1C and D shows that the depolarization of the atrial fibers is more pronounced than that of the ventricular fiber. In Figure 4-1C, the P wave is wide and of low amplitude, and, in Figure 4-1D, the P wave is barely discernible. In Figure 4-1E, the P wave is absent because the low amplitude impulse does not reach the threshold and does not produce a propagated response.[23] The disappearance of the P wave while ventricular complex is still well defined indicates that excitability of the atrial fibers is abolished at a lower potassium concentration than is the excitability of the ventricular fibers. Figure 4-2 shows gradual regression of hyperkalemia pattern during treatment. Note the absence of P waves when K = 8.6 mEq/L, the decreasing QRS duration, and the typical pointed narrow T waves. From top to bottom are leads I, II, III, V_1, V_5, and V_6.

Antiarrhythmic Effects of Potassium

Patients with moderate hyperkalemia (i.e., potassium concentrations from 5.5. to 7.5 mEq/L) rarely have ectopic beats. Disturbances of AV conduction are also uncommon at this stage of hyperkalemia. The antiarrhythmic effects of

increased potassium concentration may be due to one of the following mechanisms: (1) depression of automaticity of ectopic pacemakers caused by slowed diastolic depolarization, (2) termination of reentry caused by improved conduction (i.e., dissipation of unidirectional block), (3) termination of reentry caused by impaired conduction (i.e., change from a unidirectional to a bidirectional block), (4) decreased dispersion of refractoriness within the myocardium and between Purkinje fibers and ventricular myocardium, and (5) abolition of supernormal conduction and excitability. Depression of automaticity of ectopic pacemakers is probably of greatest clinical interest, at least after a slight to moderate increase in plasma potassium concentration.

The effect of potassium administration on cardiac rhythm and conduction depends on the integrity of the myocardium, the initial plasma potassium concentration, the amount of administered potassium, and the rate of change of the plasma potassium concentration. In Bettinger and coworkers' study, intravenous administration of potassium suppressed supraventricular and ventricular ectopic beats, except for atrial fibrillation and flutter, in about 80% of patients; the incidence of suppression was not influenced by the presence or absence of heart disease and treatment with digitalis.[24] The margin between the therapeutic and the toxic dose of potassium was narrow, and the antiarrhythmic effect usually occurred when the plasma potassium concentration increased by 0.5 to 1.0 mEq/L to a level of 5.0 to 6.5 mEq/L.[24] Such an increase of plasma potassium concentration usually had no effect on sinus rate.

The therapeutic effect of potassium administration is usually transient, and therapy must be monitored by a

M.R. 75F. Rx. of hyperkalemia

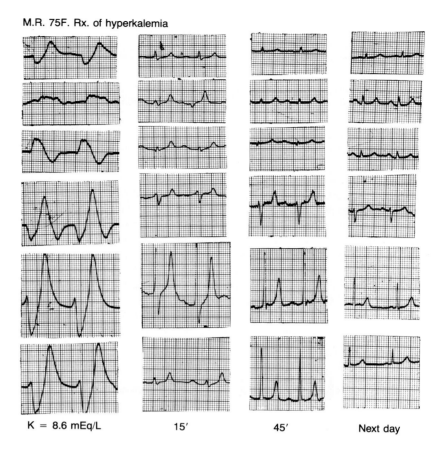

Figure 4-2. Regression of hyperkalemia pattern during treatment.

K = 8.6 mEq/L   15'   45'   Next day

physician who is familiar with the effect of potassium on the ECG. Observations of the T and P waves are helpful, because peaking of the T wave or a marked decrease of P wave amplitude usually precedes the appearance of serious effects of increased potassium concentration on the QRS duration and AV conduction. However, in certain patients with impaired AV conduction, administration of potassium at a safe rate produces a high degree AV block before the T wave configuration is appreciably altered.[24] This is more likely to occur in patients treated with digitalis because of the synergistic action of potassium and digitalis on the AV conduction.[25]

Administration of potassium salts with glucose at a slow rate may precipitate serious arrhythmias in patients with hypokalemia, severe potassium depletion, or digitalis toxicity.[26] In these patients, potassium is apparently avidly taken up by the cells, and, when it is administered slowly, plasma potassium concentration decreases, which may precipitate ectopic complexes and ventricular tachycardia or fibrillation.[26]

The effect of potassium on arrhythmias is nonspecific. Potassium is equally effective in abolishing ectopic complexes in patients with low and normal plasma potassium concentrations and of digitalis treatment. However, po-

tassium is most frequently used for the treatment of ectopic complexes and AV conduction disturbances precipitated by hypokalemia and for the treatment of ectopic supraventricular tachycardias with 1:1 or 2:1 conduction and ventricular tachycardia induced by digitalis. The tachycardias are frequently precipitated by hypokalemia and possibly by potassium depletion without hypokalemia. In these patients, correction of hypokalemia and potassium deficiency restores more normal digitalis tolerance and prevents the recurrence of life-threatening arrhythmias. When the ectopic rhythms and complexes are not caused by hypokalemia or digitalis toxicity, the duration of the nonspecific antiarrhythmic potassium effect may be short and the arrhythmias may recur as soon as the treatment is discontinued and potassium concentration returns to control value. Even in patients without hypokalemia or digitalis toxicity, the use of potassium may sometimes be desirable because it causes no hypotensive effect. Potassium is effective in the treatment of ectopic complexes and rapid ectopic rhythms after open-heart operations. Even when these patients have no hypokalemia before operation, hypokalemia may appear because of hemodilution, use of glucose, and large potassium losses in the urine. Because many candidates for open-heart operations receive digitalis, the incidence of postoperative arrhythmias is high. These arrhythmias can often be effectively suppressed by single or repeated administration of 2 to 5 mEq of potassium intravenously within 20 to 60 minutes. The antiarrhythmic effect of potassium usually occurs in the absence of significant change in sinus rate, probably because the sinoatrial (SA) node is less sensitive to potassium than are the Purkinje fibers.[27]

Administration of potassium may occasionally terminate an ectopic supraventricular or ventricular tachycardia abruptly, but more often the rate of the ectopic rhythms decreases gradually (Fig. 4-3).[28] Atrial flutter and fibrillation usually do not revert to sinus rhythm after potassium administration, probably because the doses used in the therapy of arrhythmias do not achieve the appropriate potassium concentrations. Clinical and laboratory observations suggest that the defibrillation of the atria can be expected when the plasma potassium concentration exceeds 7.0 mEq/L. Spontaneous atrial defibrillation in patients with chronic fibrillation has been reported in patients with severe hyperkalemia.[5,24] The defibrillatory

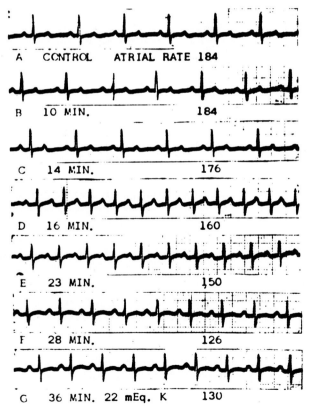

Figure 4-3. Effect of intravenous KCl administration on the rate of an ectopic atrial pacemaker. Note the gradual decrease of atrial rate. In strips A, B, and C, the atrioventricular conduction is 2:1; in the remaining strips, it is 1:1. (Surawicz B: Antiarrhythmic properties of potassium salts. In: Brest AN, Moreover JH, eds. Cardiovascular drug therapy. New York: Grune & Stratton, 1964.)

effect of potassium in the ventricles has been known since the beginning of this century. In an emergency situation, when a defibrillator is not available, the ventricles can be defibrillated using concentrated potassium solution intravenously.[5]

Effects of Potassium on the Sinoatrial Node and the Atrioventricular Node

The SA node and the AV node require separate consideration because the automaticity, conduction, and refractoriness in these tissues depend considerably on the membrane current carried predominantly by calcium current. This dependence on calcium current may be, in part, responsible for the apparent decreased sensitivity of these fibers to hyperkalemia.[29] During regional perfusion of the SA node ion in the dog, the electrical activity of the SA node persisted when the $(K)_o$ concentration increased to 21.6 mM/L but was suppressed at lower $(K)_o$ concentration when sympathetic influences were eliminated or calcium concentration was decreased.[29]

High potassium concentration depresses the conduction in the AV node less than in the Purkinje fibers and in the ventricles. Moderate hyperkalemia (i.e., increase of plasma K concentration to 5.0 to 6.5 mEq) may shorten the PR interval or even abolish second or third degree AV block, probably because optimal AV conduction occurs at potassium concentrations that are near or slightly above the upper limits of normal potassium concentration.[22]

Biphasic Effects of Potassium on Excitability and Intraventricular Conduction

In dogs, the ventricular threshold of excitability decreases when the plasma potassium concentration is moderately elevated, but increases sharply when plasma potassium concentration exceeds about 7 to 9 mEq/L.[8] In humans, gradual increase in the plasma potassium concentration failed to reproduce the expected initial decrease in the excitability threshold, which increased when the plasma potassium concentration exceeded about 7 mEq/L (Fig. 4-4).[30] However, certain clinical observations suggest that a slight increase in potassium concentration may increase the excitability threshold. Thus, occasionally, a normal response to pacemaker stimulation could be restored by the administration of potassium, possibly because the excitability threshold is lowered.[31] The lowest excitability threshold and the most rapid intraventricular conduction in humans occur probably when the plasma potassium concentration is close to 6.0 mEq/L. Both lower and higher potassium concentrations are expected to slow the con-

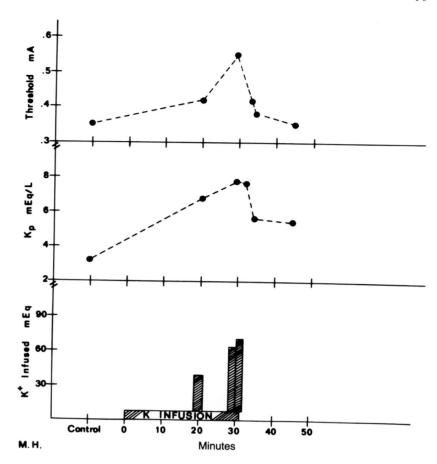

Figure 4-4. Changes in diastolic threshold and plasma potassium concentration (K_p) during the infusion of KCl. (Gettes LS, Shabetai R, Down TA, Surawicz B: Effect of changes in potassium and calcium concentrations on diastolic threshold and strength-interval relationship of the human heart. Ann NY Acad Sci 1969;167:693.)

duction and increase the excitability threshold. Therefore, within normal ranges of $(K)_o$, potassium administration may increase the intraventricular conduction velocity.[23,32] During rapid administration of potassium intravenously, the duration of the QRS interval first decreases, then increases.[32] An initial decrease in QRS duration was also observed during intracoronary infusions of potassium salts.[12]

Arrhythmogenic Effects of High $(K)_o$

Lethal hyperkalemia in humans is predominantly due to uremia and occasionally to an accidental error in the amount of potassium administered intravenously (e.g., therapy with massive doses of potassium salts of penicillin). Also, large doses of orally administered potassium can be lethal in certain patients with low cardiac output or impaired renal function.

Effects of intravenously administered potassium depend on the rate of administration rather than on an absolute amount of administered potassium. Large amounts of potassium can be administered at a slow rate, which allows the potassium to be excreted through the kidneys or transferred into the cells. However, at rapid rates of administration, even small amounts of potassium can be lethal. Thus, in a dog, rapid intravenous administration of 2 to 4 mEq of KCl produced ventricular fibrillation.[19] Figure 4-5 shows that such ventricular fibrillation may be initiated by a single ectopic complex and that it may not be preceded by any of the usual manifestations of potassium toxicity such as wide QRS complex, prolonged PR interval, or bradycardia. Similar effects, but after smaller doses of administered potassium, occur during administration of potassium salts directly into coronary arteries. In dogs, ventricular fibrillation occurred when potassium was administered at a rate of 1.6 μEq/kg/sec into the left anterior descending artery, or at a rate of 0.8 μEq/kg/sec into the right coronary artery.[12] The total amount of potassium that caused ventricular fibrillation in these experiments was within the range of approximately 0.25 to 0.5 mEq. Electrophysiologic studies in dogs have shown that ventricular fibrillation induced by regional hyperkalemia is preceded by the appearance of injury current, increased duration of the vulnerable period, and reversal of the normal endocardial to epicardial sequence of excitation.[12,15] The latter observation suggested that the origin of the ventricular ectopic activity was within the myocardium rather than the conducting system.[15]

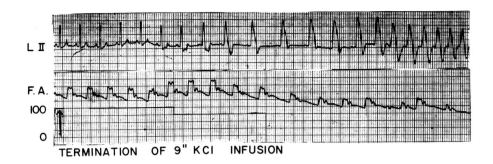

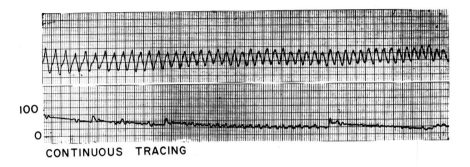

Figure 4-5. Lead II (L II) and femoral artery (F. A.) pressures of a dog after an infusion of 2.5 mEq of KCl into the pulmonary artery within 9 seconds. The arrow indicates termination of infusion. (Surawicz B, Pellegrino E, eds: Sudden cardiac death. New York: Grune & Stratton, 1964.)

Role of Increased Potassium Concentration in Myocardial Ischemia

Animal experiments have suggested that sudden death after myocardial infarction may be caused by ventricular fibrillation induced by liberation of potassium from the ischemic myocardium.[33] Harris and coworkers have demonstrated that the onset of arrhythmias in dogs with coronary occlusion coincided with an increase in potassium concentration in a coronary vein draining the infarcted area.[33] In humans, loss of potassium during myocardial ischemia can be induced by pacing. Studies of Weiss and coworkers in rabbit myocardium showed that the potassium loss during the first 30 to 45 minutes of total ischemia could not be explained by the impairment of sodium–potassium adenosine triphosphatase (ATPase) activity ("pump"). Therefore, the more likely cause of transient ischemic injury and potassium loss is an increased cell membrane permeability. Recent studies have shown that increased potassium efflux during myocardial ischemia was associated with acidosis, which prompted passive electrodiffusion of potassium accompanying the efflux of lactate and phosphate.[34,35] Also, increased potassium conductance contributes to loss of intracellular potassium, presumably through the recently discovered adenosine triphosphate (ATP)-dependent potassium channels.[36]

The development of the K^+-sensitive electrode enabled several groups of investigators to directly measure potassium concentration changes in the interstitial fluid in the area of acute myocardial ischemia.[37,38] These studies have demonstrated close correlation between the rise in extracellular potassium concentration and the development of current of injury, shortening of refractory period, slowing of conduction, ventricular fibrillation (Fig. 4-6), and depression of contractility immediately after coronary ligation in dogs and pigs.[37,38] These observations strongly support the "potassium theory" of ventricular arrhythmias during acute myocardial ischemia but do not exclude the role of acidosis and other factors.

Effects Peculiar to Nonsteady State During Rapid Changes of Potassium Concentration

Rapid changes in extracellular potassium concentration can produce electrophysiologic effects that differ from those occurring at the corresponding $(K)_o$ concentrations during steady state. An example of such phenomenon is the "paradoxical" Zwaardemaker-Libbrecht effect, which consists of a transient arrest of pacemaker fibers, shortening of action potential duration, and hyperpolarization after change from low to normal or high extracellular potassium concentration. This phenomenon was studied in perfused rabbit hearts, isolated Purkinje fibers, and anesthetized potassium-depleted dogs and was attributed to sudden increase in potassium permeability and increased activity of the sodium pump.[8,21,23,32,39] The clinical significance of the Zwaardemaker-Libbrecht effect is prob-

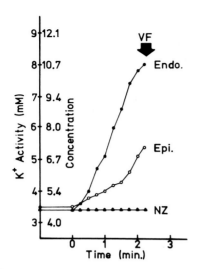

Figure 4-6. Changes in subendocardial (Endo) and subepicardial (Epi) extracellular K$^+$ activity (a_{K^+}) recorded in the center of the ischemic zone by two double-barrel K$^+$ electrodes fused together with their tips positioned 8 mm apart. *NZ,* nonischemic zone; *VF,* ventricular fibrillation.

ably limited to an occasional episode of bradycardia or AV block during administration of potassium at a rapid rate in patients with severe hypokalemia and potassium depletion.[13]

Other examples of the "paradoxical" effect of potassium during the nonsteady state are the decrease in QRS duration observed during the rapid administration of potassium in dogs and the negative inotropic effect of potassium dependent on the rate of potassium administration rather than on the absolute value of extracellular potassium concentration.[12,32]

HYPOKALEMIA

Electrophysiologic Mechanisms

Resting membrane potential or MDP* of cardiac fibers increases (i.e., becomes more negative) with decreasing extracellular potassium concentration. However, this increase (i.e., the hyperpolarization) is not as large as might be expected from the calculation based on the Nernst equation for a membrane freely permeable to K$^+$. The hyperpolarization can be demonstrated in all types of cardiac fibers, but its time course is different in myocardial and pacemaker (e.g., Purkinje) fibers.[8,39] In the nonpacemaker fibers, perfusion with low potassium solution (i.e.,

---

* Refers to myocardial fibers of the atria or the ventricles, and to the Purkinje fibers.

0.54 mM/L) produces long-lasting hyperpolarization, but in the Purkinje fibers the hyperpolarization is brief and transient, and is rapidly succeeded by progressive depolarization caused by marked increase in the slope of diastolic depolarization. Thereafter, spontaneous automatic activity appears, during which MDP becomes progressively less negative until the fiber becomes nonexcitable.

Repolarization

With decreasing (K)$_o$ concentration, repolarization becomes slower and AP duration increases.[22] The duration of phase 2 first increases, and subsequently shortens. As the slope of phase 2 becomes steeper, the slope of phase 3 becomes slower, causing a prolonged "tail" of the AP. Furthermore, the repolarization slope changes progressively from convex to concave. The lengthened AP duration is caused by reduction of both the delayed rectifying (i_K) and inward rectifying (i_{K1}) K currents.

When repolarization is prolonged, there is a longer interval during which the difference between the diastolic potential and the threshold potential is small. This means that the period of increased excitability is prolonged and the appearance of ectopic complexes is facilitated.[21,22] Hypokalemia prolongs the "tail" of the AP in the conducting system more than in the ventricles, so that the period of incomplete repolarization is longer in the Purkinje fibers than in the ventricular fibers.

Diastolic Depolarization

Hypokalemia increases diastolic depolarization in the Purkinje fibers and, therefore, promotes automatic activity and early afterdepolarizations in quiescent Purkinje fibers.[8,27,40] When such fibers are depolarized from a level of membrane potential that is less negative than the maximal diastolic potential, the upstroke velocity of the action potential and the conduction velocity decrease. Increased automaticity of Purkinje fibers may cause ventricular ectopic complexes and rhythms. Automaticity can appear even in ventricular myocardial (nonpacemaker) fibers when the repolarization of these fibers becomes slow, and the threshold potential is reached before the repolarization is completed.[22] This type of automaticity may be triggered by repetitive stimulation.[41]

Other Effects

Gettes and Surawicz have shown that hypokalemia increases the difference between the action potential duration of the Purkinje and ventricular fibers.[8] Initially, prolonged duration of the action potential was associated with prolonged refractoriness, but the subsequent shortening of phase 2 and the slow rate of phase 3 repolarization allowed the fiber to reach the threshold potential earlier than in the presence of normal potassium concentration, resulting in a shortened refractory period.[8] Clinical observations also suggest that hypokalemia shortens the effective refractory period because atrial and ventricular premature complexes in patients with hypokalemia frequently appear after a short coupling interval (Fig. 4-7).

Hypokalemia frequently slows conduction because the depolarization begins in incompletely repolarized fibers, and probably also because there is an increased difference between the resting membrane potential and the threshold potential.[22]

Electrocardiograms

Electrocardiogram changes caused by hypokalemia may be correlated with concomitant changes in the ventricular action potential (Fig. 4-8.) Progressive changes in repolarization are reflected in the ECG as progressive depression of the ST segment, a decrease in the T wave amplitude, and an increase in the U wave amplitude in the standard limb and precordial leads. As long as the T wave and the U wave

are separated by a notch, the duration of the QT interval is unchanged. In more advanced stages of hypokalemia, the T wave and U wave are fused, and an accurate measurement of the QT interval is not possible.[13] Because the duration of mechanical systole does not change in hypokalemia, the pattern of hypokalemia is seen as a gradual shift of the major repolarization wave from systole into diastole. In Figure 4-8A, the amplitude of the repolarization wave is inscribed during diastole (U). In Figure 4-8B, both waves are of equal amplitude, whereas in Figure 4-8C and D, the amplitude of the repolarization wave inscribed during diastole is greater than that inscribed during systole. The latter two types of ECG pattern of hypokalemia are most frequently encountered when the plasma concentration is less than 2.7 mEq/L.[13, 42]

When hypokalemia is advanced, the amplitude and duration of the QRS interval are increased. The QRS complex is widened diffusely, but, in adults, seldom by more than 0.02 second. In children, the QRS widening may be more pronounced. The increased duration of the QRS is the result of widening without change in the shape of the QRS complex, which suggests that this is caused by slower intraventricular conduction without changes in the sequence of depolarization. As discussed, the slowing of intraventricular conduction in hypokalemia may be

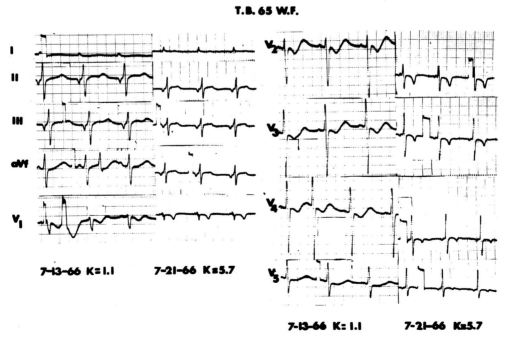

T.B. 65 W.F.

7-13-66 K= 1.1   7-21-66 K=5.7

7-13-66 K= 1.1   7-21-66 K=5.7

Figure 4-7. Electrocardiogram of a 65-year-old woman with chronic pyelonephritis and vomiting before and after treatment with potassium salts. Note the typical pattern of hypokalemia on July 13, 1966, and the short coupling interval of the ventricular ectopic beats in leads aVF and V. Plasma potassium concentration is in mEq/L. (Surawicz B: Relation between electrocardiogram and electrolytes. Am Heart J 1967; 73:814.)

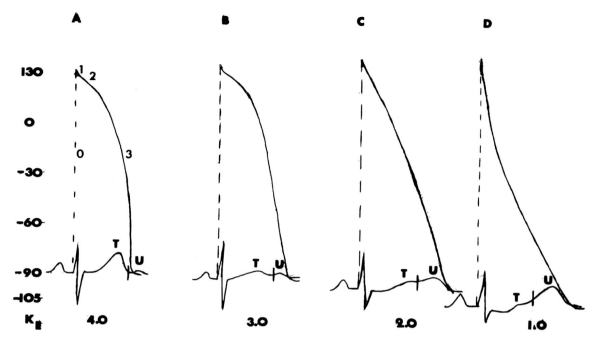

Figure 4-8. Diagram of the ventricular action potential superimposed on the electrocardiogram for extracellular potassium (K_E) at 4.0, 3.0, 2.0, and 1.0 mEq/L. The numbers on the left designate the transmembrane potential in millivolts. (Surawicz B: Relation between electrocardiogram and electrolytes. Am Heart J 1967;73:814.

caused by hyperpolarization of ventricular fibers or by a slower propagation in the incompletely repolarized Purkinje and ventricular fibers.

The amplitude and duration of the P wave in hypokalemia is usually increased, and frequently the PR interval is slightly or moderately prolonged.

Arrhythmogenic Effects

Hypokalemia precipitates ectopic complexes and rhythms caused by increased automaticity and facilitation of reentry. Reentry can be caused by slow conduction during the prolonged relative refractory period, increased dispersion of refractoriness, and decreased threshold of excitability.[8] The low–K-induced facilitation of arrhythmias in the atria has been attributed to both abnormal impulse formation and decreased wavelength of propagation resulting from shortening of effective refractory period and slight increase in conduction velocity.[43]

Another arrhythmogenic effect of low $(K)_o$ is similar to that of digitalis toxicity in that it is caused by the block of Na–K pump. This results in increased intracellular calcium concentration, transient inward current, delayed afterdepolarizations, and aftercontractions.[44] These effects are attenuated by lowering extracellular calcium concentration.

In humans, hypokalemia promotes the appearance of supraventricular and ventricular ectopic complexes. In one study of 81 patients not treated with digitalis and who had a plasma potassium concentration 3.2 mEq/L or less, ventricular ectopic complexes occurred in 28%, supraventricular ectopic complexes in 22%, and AV conduction disturbances in 12%.[42] Ectopic complexes occurred three times and AV conduction two times more frequently than in the control hospital population.[42]

Arrhythmias appearing in patients with severe hypokalemia are of the same type as in patients with digitalis toxicity, that is, nonparoxysmal atrial tachycardia with block (Fig. 4-9) and various types of AV dissociation. These arrhythmias are attributed to a combination of increased automaticity of ectopic pacemakers and at least some degree of AV conduction disturbance. Like digitalis, hypokalemia increases sensitivity to vagal stimulation. Potassium depletion achieved by diet and administration of diuretics increases the incidence of both spontaneous and induced ventricular fibrillation in dogs with myocardial infarction and acute myocardial ischemia.[45,46]

Perfusion of isolated hearts with potassium-deficient solutions produces ventricular fibrillation.[21] This may be caused by a combination of increased ventricular automaticity, slow conduction, short effective refractory period, and prolonged relative refractory period. In patients with severe hypokalemia, serious ventricular tachyarrhythmias (e.g., ventricular tachycardia, torsade de pointe, ventricu-

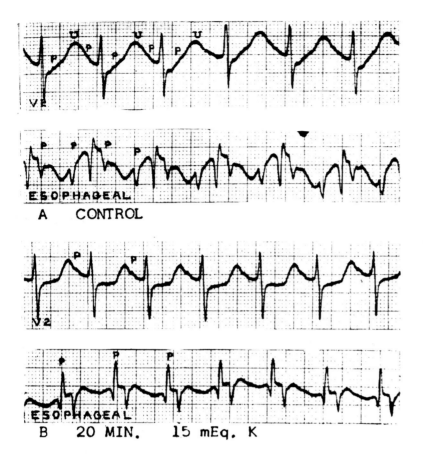

A   CONTROL

B   20 MIN.   15 mEq. K

Figure 4-9. Electrocardiogram of a 34-year-old woman with vomiting and plasma potassium concentration of 1.0 mEq/L. The upper strip shows hypokalemia pattern and indistinct P waves in lead V₂. The P waves and the 2:1 atrioventricular block are clearly seen in the esophageal lead. Following intravenous administration of 15 mEq of potassium (lower two strips), ectopic atrial tachycardia and 2:1 block are no longer present (Bettinger JC, Surawicz B, Bryfogle JW, Anderson BN, Bellet S: The effect of intravenous administration of potassium chloride on ectopic rhythms, ectopic beats and disturbances in AV conduction. Am J Med 1956;21:521.)

lar fibrillation) have been reported in the absence of heart disease or digitalis therapy (Fig. 4-10).[26, 42, 47–49] Hypokalemia is frequently present in patients with acute myocardial infarction or after resuscitation from out-of-hospital ventricular fibrillation, possibly due to previous treatment with thiazide-diuretics or administration of sodium bicarbonate during resuscitation (Fig. 4-11).[48, 50–52] In addition, hypokalemia may be precipitated by intense sympathetic stimulation, which shifts potassium into the skeletal muscle and the liver, an effect attributed to beta₂-receptor stimulation by the circulating epinephrine (Fig. 4-12).[53, 54] However, the arrhythmogenic effect of adrenaline may result not only from the hypokalemic effect of beta-adrenergic stimulation but also from an increase in extracellular calcium mediated by alpha₁-adrenergic stimulation.[55]

Presence of hypokalemia in patients with acute myocardial infarction increases the incidence of serious ventricular arrhythmias.[50, 51] Also, some investigators maintain that treatment with diuretics increases the risk of ventricular arrhythmias but others find such risk to be overstated.[56–60] For prevention of hypokalemia in patients with acute myocardial infarction, administration of nonselective beta-adrenergic blockers appears to be preferable to treatment with selective beta₁-adrenergic blockers.[61–63]

Modification of Potassium Effects by Other Electrolytes

In patients with hyperkalemia, calcium concentration may be the important factor that determines the severity of AV and intraventricular conduction disturbance and the vulnerability to ventricular fibrillation. Hypocalcemia frequently accompanies hyperkalemia in patients with renal insufficiency. It may be expected to aggravate the AV and intraventricular conduction disturbances and facilitate the appearance of ventricular fibrillation.

In some patients with renal insufficiency and hyperkalemia, hypercalcemia may also be present because of secondary hyperparathyroidism or overzealous therapy with calcium. Hypercalcemia may be expected to counteract the effect of hyperkalemia on the AV and intraventricular conduction disturbances and to prevent ventricular fibrillation.

Arrhythmias have been frequently reported during dialysis in both patients treated and patients not treated with digitalis. However, the effect of dialysis on the relationship between arrhythmias and electrolyte disturbances is difficult to evaluate because the dialysis aims at correcting several electrolyte disorders simultaneously.

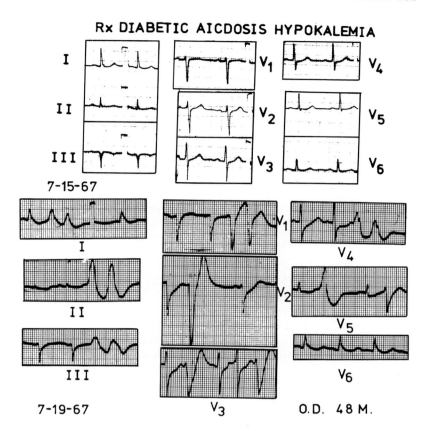

Rx DIABETIC AICDOSIS HYPOKALEMIA

Figure 4-10. Electrocardiographic pattern of hypokalemia with ventricular ectopic beats during treatment of diabetic ketoacidosis (7-15-67). (Surawicz B, Mangiardi ML: Electrocardiogram in endocrine and metabolic disorders. In: Rios J, ed. Clinical electrocardiographic correlations. Cardiovascular Clinics 8/3. Philadelphia: FA Davis, 1977.)

Abnormal sodium and magnesium concentrations may also modify the ECG pattern of hyperkalemia. Hypernatremia may counteract and hyponatremia may augment the effects of increased potassium concentration on AV and intraventricular conduction disturbances. Hypermagnesemia could also augment the effect of hyperkalemia on conduction disturbances. In one study, arrhythmias were as common in hypokalemic patients with hypocalcemia as they were in those without hypocalcemia.[42] Similarly, the incidence of arrhythmias was the same in hypokalemic patients with and without acidosis.[42]

CALCIUM

Electrophysiologic Mechanisms

Only extremely high or low concentrations of calcium produce electrophysiologic abnormalities of clinical importance. Within the range of concentrations compatible with life, calcium has relatively little effect on the resting membrane potential. Low calcium prolongs and high calcium shortens the phase 2 of the action potential, the total action potential duration, and the duration of the effective refractory period.[64] The effects appear to be secondary to changes in potassium currents, partly due to changes in the intracellular calcium concentration and partly to the changes in the plateau amplitude of the action potential.[65] The changes also depend on the heart rate and magnesium concentration.[64, 66] Low calcium depresses contractility, lowers the excitability threshold, and slightly decreases the rate of diastolic depolarization in Purkinje

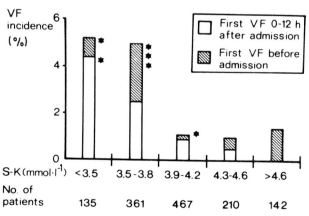

Figure 4-11. Relation between serum potassium concentration and incidence of ventricular fibrillation (VF) in patients with acute myocardial infarction before and after hospital admission. (Hulting J: In-hospital ventricular fibrillation and its relation to serum potassium. Acta Med Scand 1981;645:109.)

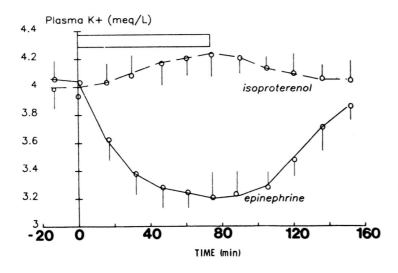

Figure 4-12. Differences between the effect of epinephrine and isoproterenol infusion on plasma potassium concentration. The values determined both during and after infusion were significantly different (P < 0.01). (Brown MJ, Brown DC, Murphy MB: Hypokalemia from beta$_2$-receptor stimulation by circulating epinephrine. N Engl J Med 1983;309:1414.)

fibers. High calcium has a positive inotropic effect, increases the excitability threshold, and slightly increases the rate of diastolic depolarization in the Purkinje fibers. Calcium plays an important role in the conduction of impulses dependent on the flow of ions through the calcium channel.

Effects on Electrocardiogram and Cardiac Arrhythmias

In patients with hypercalcemia, the ST segment is short or absent, and the duration of the QTc interval is decreased.[13] Experimental hypercalcemia increases the duration of the PR interval and QRS complex, and produces ectopic complexes and ventricular fibrillation. In one study in dogs, hypercalcemia decreased the sinus rate and prolonged the AH interval during atrial pacing, but these effects occurred when plasma calcium concentrations reached levels of 10.5 and 9.6 mEq/L, respectively.[67] In patients with severe hypercalcemia, QRS and PR intervals are frequently prolonged, and second or third degree AV block is occasionally present.[68] However, the incidence of these events is low. Thus, in a series of 20 patients with primary hyperparathyroidism, high degree AV block was not observed before operation.[69]

There is no firm evidence that the incidence of ectopic beats in patients with hypercalcemia is increased. However, it has been postulated that sudden death of patients during hyperparathyroid crisis and other conditions associated with severe hypercalcemia may be caused by ventricular fibrillation.[68] In one case, the sudden postoperative death of a patient with a plasma calcium concentration of 18 mEq/L was attributed to arrhythmia.

In patients with hypocalcemia, the ST segment and the QTc interval are prolonged. The duration of the ST segment is inversely related to plasma calcium concentration.[13] Prolongation of the QTc interval is associated with increased duration of the ventricular refractory period. This effect, in the absence of concomitant increase in dispersion of refractoriness or changes in conduction, may produce an antiarrhythmic action. In one study, moderate hypocalcemia induced by administration of Na$_2$-EDTA suppressed supraventricular and ventricular ectopic complexes in about 50% of patients.[70] Ectopic complexes suppressed by hypocalcemia reappeared after calcium administration.[70]

After successful surgical treatment of 20 patients with hyperparathyroidism, serum calcium decreased and QT interval lengthened, but there was no difference in the incidence of supraventricular and ventricular arrhythmias.[69]

SODIUM

High sodium concentration increases and low sodium concentration decreases the upstroke velocity of the action potential. Increased sodium concentration counteracts many effects of hyperkalemia by increasing the rate of depolarization. High sodium prolongs the duration of the action potential, but the clinical significance of this is uncertain.

The effect of high or low sodium on the ECG, cardiac rhythm, and conduction are probably negligible within limits of plasma sodium concentration compatible with life. However, in patients with intraventricular conduction disturbances caused by hyperkalemia, hypernatremia shortens and hyponatremia prolongs the duration of the QRS complex.

MAGNESIUM

Biologic Role

Magnesium is essential to normal growth and development. The magnesium complex with adenosine triphosphate (Mg-ATP) is the substrate for the enzymatic reaction that underlies the sliding filament mechanism of contraction and relaxation. Magnesium ion is transported in and out of the cells at a much slower rate than the rates of potassium, sodium, and chlorine. The very slow rate of magnesium exchange is independent of the frequency of contractions and the external work done by the heart.[71]

Electrophysiologic Effects

Magnesium concentrations within the range encountered in clinical situations have no important effect on the AP at normal potassium and calcium concentrations.[64] In isolated rabbit hearts, perfusion with magnesium-deficient fluids for up to 22 minutes produced no changes in left intraventricular pressure, shape and duration of ventricular AP, heart rate, PR interval, or shape and duration of the atrial and ventricular complex in the ECG. When magnesium was omitted, however, from a calcium-free solution, the duration of ST segment, QT interval, and ventricular monophasic AP increased. Similar, less pronounced changes were observed during perfusion with one sixteenth of normal calcium and one fourth to one sixteenth normal magnesium concentration.[66] These experiments showed that, in the presence of extremely low extracellular calcium concentration, magnesium exerts an effect on the current or currents that modulate the plateau duration of the ventricular AP. The current is probably not the slow inward calcium current because the calcium channel is not measurably permeable to magnesium.[72]

Electrocardiogram

Hypomagnesemia and hypermagnesemia do not produce specific ECG patterns in animals and humans. In dogs depleted of magnesium by means of dialysis, reduction of extracellular magnesium concentration to less than half normal concentration failed to produce any ECG changes.[73] Personal experience suggests that neither hypermagnesemia nor hypomagnesemia has a detectable effect on the QT interval in humans. In children with tetany, lack of QT prolongation favors deficiency of magnesium rather than deficiency of calcium.

Systemic Effects of Magnesium Deficiency

Prolonged hypomagnesemia may be associated with hypocalcemia but has no effect on the levels of serum sodium, chloride, or potassium. However, magnesium deficiency causes depletion of muscle potassium.[73] This depletion persists despite treatments with large of potassium, which suggests that magnesium deficiency influences the ability of cells to maintain an appropriate potassium gradient. This finding, believed to affect the magnesium-depleted patients, is the basis of the hypothesis that intracellular potassium depletion predisposes to cardiac arrhythmias that defy correction in the absence of magnesium.[73] However, none of the studies in animals with chronic magnesium depletion reported occurrence of cardiac arrhythmias or sudden death from arrhythmias.[73] Admittedly, none of the animals were monitored for the purpose of arrhythmia detection.

Role of Magnesium in Cardiac Arrhythmias

The evidence that hypomagnesemia is responsible for cardiac arrhythmias is limited to case reports. In some of these, the causes of the arrhythmias were suspected because of either QT prolongation or presence of hypokalemia on admission.[73]

In patients who had suffered myocardial infarction, there was no correlation between hypomagnesemia and ventricular arrhythmias or late potentials.[74]

In patients with congestive heart failure, magnesium supplementation reduced the frequency of asymptomatic arrhythmias.[75] Magnesium sulfate solution administered intravenously has been used empirically for several decades to suppress a variety of supraventricular and ventricular arrhythmias both in the absence and in the presence of digitalis therapy.[76–81] Several investigators have reported the efficacy of magnesium sulfate in the treatment of torsade de pointes and have considered magnesium as the treatment of choice of this arrhythmia, particularly when other methods have failed.[82–85] The precise mechanism of magnesium effect on these and other arrhythmias remains to be elucidated. Magnesium blocks the calcium channel and exerts modulating effects on several potassium currents.[86,87] It is plausible that the antiarrhythmic effect of magnesium is caused by improved conduction in depolarized myocardium. In vitro, high magnesium concentration restores excitability in myocardium depolarized by high extracellular potassium concentration and shifts the relation between membrane potential and velocity of depolarization in the depolarizing direction.[88, 89] The resulting conduction improvement may suppress arrhythmias generated by various mechanisms, for example, after depolarizations, abnormal automaticity, and reentry.

Hypermagnesemia depresses AV and intraventricular conduction. In animal experiments, the depression of intraventricular conduction occurs when magnesium concentration reaches 3 to 5 mM, that is, close to concentrations that may cause respiratory arrest.[66]

In humans, infusion of magnesium salt solutions lengthens sinus node recovery time, AV conduction time, and QRS duration during ventricular pacing.[90] These actions can influence cardiac arrhythmias and conduction disturbances.

Lithium

Lithium readily enters cardiac cells and replaces potassium. Sinus bradycardia, sinus node dysfunction, and minor T wave abnormalities have been reported in patients treated with lithium for manic-depressive disorder.[91]

pH

Acidosis and alkalosis are usually associated with altered concentration of potassium and ionized calcium. Whether the modifications of extracellular pH cause specific ECG changes is difficult to determine.

INTERACTION OF ELECTROLYTES WITH DIGITALIS AND ANTIARRHYTHMIC DRUGS

The action of all cardioactive and antiarrhythmic drugs produces various changes in membrane permeability to ions and is influenced by altered intracellular and extracellular ionic concentrations. Some of the important clinical interactions are discussed here.

Digitalis

Increased extracellular potassium concentration inhibits glycoside binding to (Na^+, K^+) ATPase, decreases the inotropic effect of digitalis, and suppresses digitalis-induced ectopic rhythms.[92-94] Accordingly, hyperkalemic animals and humans can tolerate large doses of digitalis without developing ectopic activity.[95] Conversely, hypokalemia increases glycoside binding to (Na^+, K^+) ATPase, decreases rate of digoxin elimination, and potentiates

toxic effects of digitalis.[96] However, at plasma potassium concentrations encountered in patients with hypokalemia, the inhibition of the sodium pump would be small.[97] Recent study in isolated guinea pig myocytes attributed late afterdepolarizations (a presumed substrate of digitalis-induced arrhythmias) to the combined effects of low–K-induced decrease in outward potassium current and digitalis-induced increase in transient inward current.[97] In hypokalemic animals, ectopic complexes and rhythms may appear after administration of unusually small doses of glycosides. In patients treated with digitalis, arrhythmias may be precipitated by carbohydrate administration, removal of potassium by dialysis, and, most frequently, by treatment with diuretic drugs.[98] Combination of hyperkalemia and digitalis causes serious AV conduction disturbances only in patients with preexisting first degree AV block.[99] In patients without preexisting AV block, the rate of the escape pacemaker is either normal or rapid. Figure 4-13 shows an ECG of a patient with atrial fibrillation and renal insufficiency treated with a maintenance dose of 0.5 mg digoxin daily. In this patient, the rhythm and the rate are the same when plasma potassium concentration is 8.4, 6.7, and 4.4 mEq/L.

Hypokalemia may augment the digitalis-induced depression of AV conduction. The most characteristic arrhythmias are nonparoxysmal supraventricular tachycardia with block and AV junctional tachycardia either during sinus rhythm (AV dissociation) or during atrial fibrillation. These types of arrhythmia are caused by a combination of increased ectopic pacemaker activity and depression at the AV conduction. Both hypokalemia and digitalis shorten the effective refractory period of the ventricles and the coupling interval of the ventricular ectopic complexes. Slow propagation of the early premature ectopic impulses may result in reentry and cause ventricular fibrillation (Fig. 4-14). The synergistic effect of hypokalemia and digitalis on automaticity of ectopic pacemakers and AV conduction explains the low digitalis tolerance of patients with hypokalemia. In these patients, nonparoxysmal atrial tachycardia with block or AV dissociation with AV junctional tachycardia may appear after the administration of 0.75 to 2.0 mg of digoxin.

Digitalis and hypercalcemia have similar effects on the automaticity of ectopic pacemakers. At the same time, both increase the threshold of excitability and shorten the effective refractory period in the ventricles. Recent studies also show that increased calcium concentration increases the transient diastolic depolarization induced by glycosides. Although observations in vitro suggest that hypercalcemia may be expected to increase ectopic activity in patients treated with digitalis, there is no convincing clinical or experimental support of this hypothesis. The clinical examples of an alleged synergism between hypercalcemia and digitalis are 40 to 50 years old; more recent informa-

T. B. 53 W.M.
cont. mainten. digoxin 0.5 mg. daily

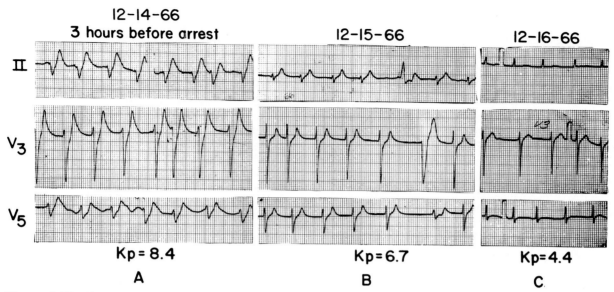

Figure 4-13. Electrocardiogram of a 53-year-old patient with atrial fibrillation treated with a maintenance dose of 0.5 mg digoxin daily. Note pattern of hyperkalemia 3 hours before "cardiac arrest" (**A**) and after treatment with sodium lactate, glucose, and insulin (**B** and **C**). Ventricular rate is about 95 per minute in all three tracings. (Surawicz B: Arrhythmias and electrolyte disturbances. Bull N Y Acad Med 1967;43:1160.)

Figure 4-14. Electrocardiogram of a 26-year-old patient with rheumatic heart disease treated with a maintenance dose of 0.25 mg digoxin daily. On August 25, 1964, ventricular fibrillation begins after a ventricular premature beat with a short coupling interval. On the next day, the electrocardiographic pattern of hypokalemia and regular rhythm is attributed to an ectopic escape pacemaker. (Davidson S, Surawicz B: Ectopic beats and atrioventricular conduction disturbances in patients with hypopotassemia. Arch Intern Med 1967; 120:280.)

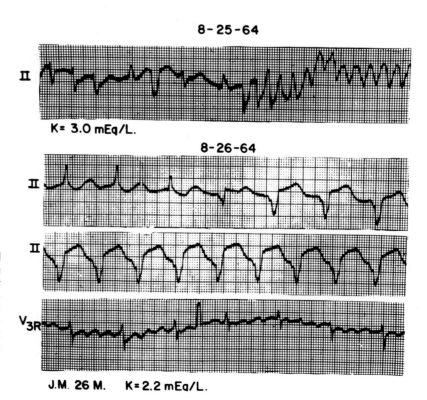

tion on this subject is lacking.[70] In animals treated with digitalis and calcium, hypercalcemia produced ectopic rhythms only when the animals received more than 95% of the toxic dose of ouabain, whereas animals that received 90% of the toxic glycoside dose had no arrhythmia when their plasma calcium concentration was 46.2 mg per 100 mL. This confirmed an earlier study in dogs which failed to show important synergistic or additive effects of calcium and digitalis on cardiac rhythm and conduction.

Hypocalcemia induced by administration of Na$_2$-EDTA or citrate salts is believed to suppress ectopic complexes induced by digitalis. However, personal experience suggests that Na$_2$-EDTA is equally effective in suppressing ectopic complexes and rhythms both in patients receiving and those not receiving digitalis.[70] Hypomagnesemia decreases the dose of digitalis required to induce ectopic rhythms in both animals and humans.[100, 101]

Antiarrhythmic Drugs

In animal experiments, hyperkalemia and quinidine exert synergistic effects on the rate of rise of cardiac action potential and conduction velocity. Therefore, hyperkalemia augments quinidine toxicity. Hypokalemia augmented the toxic effects of quinidine on conduction in isolated rabbit hearts and anesthetized dogs, presumably because of the greater prolongation of repolarization by low potassium and quinidine together than by either alone.[22] This, in turn, increased the duration of the relative refractory period during which slow conduction is caused by impulse propagation in incompletely repolarized fibers. Quinidine administration can produce hypokalemia that may possibly contribute to quinidine toxicity. Also, quinine, which causes the same electrophysiologic effects as quinidine, can induce serious ventricular arrhythmias associated with drug-induced hypokalemia.

Other antiarrhythmic drugs that increase the action potential duration have similar interactions with potassium, particularly in the presence of hypokalemia when the drug-induced prolongation of QT appears to facilitate the occurrence of ventricular arrhythmias, especially torsade de pointes.[102–104] Class I antiarrhythmic drugs exaggerate the slowing of conduction induced by hyperkalemia, and the effect of these drugs on conduction is influenced by potassium concentration. For instance, therapeutic concentrations of lidocaine have little effect on rate of depolarization when extracellular potassium concentration is less than 4.5 mM, but they may be expected to cause a decrease in the rate of depolarization when potassium concentration is elevated in depolarized, infarcted myocardium.[105–107]

Toxic effects of quinidine on AV and intraventricular conduction in dogs are reversed by administration of sodium lactate or sodium chloride. This effect of sodium is not specific for quinidine because it is also present when conduction is depressed by potassium and certain drugs. Administration of calcium aggravates conduction disturbances produced by quinidine.

References

1. Hoffman BF, Cranefield PF: Electrophysiology of the heart. New York: McGraw-Hill, 1960.
2. Noble D: The initiation of the heartbeat. Oxford: Clarendon Press, 1975.
3. Fozzard HA, Sheu SS: The resting potential in heart muscle. Adv Myocardiol 1982;3:125.
4. Dominguez G, Fozzard HA: Influence of extracellular K$^+$ concentration on cable properties and excitability of sheep cardiac Purkinje fibers. Circ Res 1970;26:565.
5. Surawicz B: Role of electrolytes in etiology and management of cardiac arrhythmias. Prog Cardiovasc Dis 1966;8:364.
6. Barold S, Falkoff MD, Ong LS, Heinle RA: Hyperkalemia-induced failure of atrial capture during dual-chamber cardiac pacing. J Am Coll Cardiol 1987;10:467.
7. Coronel R, Fiolet JW, Francien JG, et al: Distribution of extracellular potassium and its relation to electrophysiologic changes during acute myocardial ischemia in the isolated perfused porcine heart. Circulation 1988;77:1125.
8. Gettes L, Surawicz B: Effects of low and high concentrations of potassium on the simultaneously recorded Purkinje and ventricular action potentials of the perfused pig moderator band. Circ Res 1968;23:717.
9. Spear JF, Moore EN: Effect of potassium on supernormal conduction in the bundle branch Purkinje system of the dog. Am J Cardiol 1977;40:923.
10. Lyons CJ, Burgess MJ, Abildskov JA: Effects of acute hyperkalemia on cardiac excitability. Am Heart J 1977;94:755.
11. Kaseno K, Sugimoto T, Hirasaisa K, Nohara T, Uraoki T, Takerichi J: The effects of hyperpotassemia on cardiac performance. Cardiovasc Res 1975;9:212.
12. Logic JR, Krotkiewski A, Koppius A, Surawicz B: Negative inotropic effects of K$^+$: Its modification by Ca^{++} and acetylstrophanthidin in dogs. Am J Physiol 1968;215:14.
13. Surawicz B: Relation between electrocardiogram and electrolytes. Am Heart J 1967;73:814.
14. Tan RC, Ramza BM, Joyner RW: Modulation of the Purkinje-ventricular muscle junctional conduction by elevated potassium and hypoxia. Circulation 1989;79:1100.
15. Ettinger PO, Regan TJ, Oldewurtel HA: Hyperkalemia, cardiac conduction and the electrocardiogram: A review. Am Heart J 1974;88:360.
16. Levine HD, Wanzer SH, Merrill JP: Dialyzable currents of injury in potassium intoxication resembling acute myocardial infarction or pericarditis. Circulation 1956;13:29.
17. Hariman RJ, Chen Chia M: Effects of hyperkalemia on sinus nodal function in dog: Sino-ventricular conduction. Cardiovasc Res 1983;17:509.
18. Racker DK: Sinoventricular transmission in 10 mM K$^+$ by canine atrioventricular nodal inputs. Circulation 1991; 83:1738.

19. Surawicz B: Methods of production of ventricular fibrillation. In: Surawicz B, Pellegrino E, eds. Sudden cardiac death. New York: Grune & Stratton, 1964:64.

20. Garcia-Palmieri MR: Reversal of hyperkalemic cardiotoxicity with hypertonic saline. Am Heart J 1962;64:483.

21. Surawicz B, Lepeschkin E, Herrlich HC, Hoffman BF: Effect of potassium and calcium deficiency on the monophasic action potential, electrocardiogram and contractility of isolated rabbit hearts. Am J Physiol 1959;196:1302.

22. Gettes LS, Surawicz B, Shiue JC: Effect of high K, low K, and quinidine on QRS duration and ventricular action potential. Am J Physiol 1962;203:1135.

23. Surawicz B, Gettes LS: Two mechanisms of cardiac arrest produced by potassium. Circ Res 1963;12:415.

24. Bettinger JC, Surawicz B, Bryfogle JW, Anderson BN, Bellet S: The effect of intravenous administration of potassium chloride on ectopic rhythms, ectopic beats and disturbances in A-V conduction. Am J Med 1956;21:521.

25. Fisch C, Martz BL, Priebe FH: Enhancement of potassium induced atrioventricular block by doses of digitalis drugs. J Clin Invest 1960;39:1885.

26. Kunin AS, Surawicz B, Sims EAH: Decrease in serum potassium concentration and appearance of cardiac arrhythmias during infusion of potassium with glucose in potassium-depleted patients. N Engl J Med 1962;266:228.

27. Vassalle M: Cardiac pacemaker potentials at different extra- and intracellular K concentrations. Am J Physiol 1965;208:770.

28. Surawicz B: Arrhythmias and electrolyte disturbances. Bull N Y Acad Med 1967;43:1160.

29. Vassalle M, Greineder JK, Stuckey JH: Role of the sympathetic nervous system in the sinus node resistance to high potassium. Circ Res 1973;32:348.

30. Gettes LS, Shabetai R, Downs TA, Surawicz B: Effect of changes in potassium and calcium concentrations on diastolic threshold and strength-interval relationship of the human heart. Ann N Y Acad Sci 1969;167:693.

31. Walker WJ, Elkins JT, Wood LW: Effects of potassium in restoring myocardial response to a subthreshold cardiac pacemaker. N Engl J Med 1964;271:597.

32. Surawicz B, Chlebus H, Mazzoleni A: Hemodynamic and electrocardiographic effects of hyperpotassemia. Differences in response to slow and rapid increases in concentration of plasma K. Am Heart J 1967;73:647.

33. Harris AS, Bisteni A, Russell RA, Brigham JC, Firestone JE: Excitatory factors in ventricular tachycardia resulting from myocardial ischemia: Potassium a major excitant. Science 1954;119:797.

34. Kleber AG, Riegger CB, Janse MJ: Extracellular K^+ and H^+ shifts in early ischemia: Mechanisms and relation to impulse propagation. J Mol Cell Cardiol 1987;19:35.

35. Weiss JN, Lamp ST, Shine KI: Cellular K^+ loss and anion efflux during myocardial ischemia and metabolic inhibition. Am J Physiol 1989;256:1165.

36. Noma A: ATP regulated K^+ channels in cardiac muscle. Nature 1983;305:147.

37. Hill JL, Gettes LS: Effect of coronary artery occlusion on local myocardial extracellular K^+ activity in swine. Circulation 1980;61:768.

38. Franz C, Box L, Hirche H, Schramm MP: Extracellular K^+ activity and ventricular fibrillation during myocardial ischemia in pigs. Pflugers Arch 1978;373(suppl):R17.

39. Ito S, Surawicz B: Transient "paradoxical" effects of increasing extracellular K^+ concentration on transmembrane potential in canine cardiac Purkinje fibers. Circ Res 1977;41:799.

40. Christe G: Effects of low (K^+) on the electrical activity of human cardiac ventricular and Purkinje cells. Cardiovasc Res 1982;17:243.

41. Hiraoka M, Kawano S: Triggered tachycardia of guinea pig papillary muscle in the low K^+ solution. In: Ueda H, Murao S, Yamada K, Harumi K, Mashima S, Hiraoka M, eds. Recent advances in electrocardiology. Jap Heart J 1982;23:69.

42. Davidson S, Surawicz B: Ectopic beats and atrioventricular conduction disturbances in patients with hypopotassemia. Arch Intern Med 1967;120:280.

43. Lammers WJ, Allessie MA, Bonke FM: Reentrant and focal arrhythmias in low potassium in isolated rabbit atrium. Am J Physiol (Heart Circ Physiol 24) 1988;255:H1359.

44. Eisner DA, Lederer WJ: Inotropic and arrhythmogenic effects of potassium-depleted solutions on mammalian cardiac muscle. J Physiol 1979;294:255.

45. Garan H, McGovern BA, Canzanello VJ, et al: The effect of potassium ion depletion on postinfarction canine cardiac arrhythmias. Circulation 1988;77:696.

46. Hohnloser SH, Verrier RL, Lown B, Raeder EA: Effect of hypokalemia on susceptibility to ventricular fibrillation in the normal and ischemic canine heart. Am Heart J 1986;112:32.

47. Surawicz B, Braun AH, Crum WB, Wagner S, Bellet S, Kemp RL: Quantitative analysis of the electrocardiographic pattern of hypopotassemia. Circulation 1957;16:750.

48. Redleaf PD, Lerner IJ: Thiazide-induced hypokalemia with associated major ventricular arrhythmia. JAMA 1968;206:1302.

49. Salvador M, Thomas C, Mazeng M, Conte J, Meriel P, Lesbre P: Troubles du rhythme directment induits ou favorises par les depletions potassiques. Arch Mal Coeur Vaiss 1970;63:230.

50. Beck OA, Hochrein H: Initial serum potassium level in relation to cardiac arrhythmias in acute myocardial infarction. Z Kardiol 1977;66:187.

51. Hulting J: In-hospital ventricular fibrillation and its relation to serum potassium. Acta Med Scand 1981;647(suppl):109.

52. Thompson RG, Cobb LA: Hypokalemia after resuscitation from out-of-hospital ventricular fibrillation. JAMA 1982;248:2860.

53. Vick RL, Todd EP, Luedke DW: Epinephrine-induced hypokalemia: Relation to liver and skeletal muscle. J Pharmacol Exp Ther 1972;181:139.

54. Brown MJ, Brown DC, Murphy MB: Hypokalemia from beta$_2$-receptor stimulation by circulating epinephrine. N Engl J Med 1983;309:1414.

55. Takamura T, Sugiyama S, Ozawa T: Effects of bunazosin and propranolol on ventricular arrhythmias in dogs with hypokalemia. J Electrocardiol 1987;20:147.

56. Holland OB, Kuhnert L, Pollard J, Padia M, Anderson RJ, Blomqvist G: Ventricular ectopic activity with diuretic therapy. Am J Hypertens 1988;1:380.

57. Stewart DE, Ikram H, Espiner EA, Nicholls MG: Arrhyth-

mogenic potential of diuretic induced hypokalemia in patients with mild hypertension and ischemic heart disease. Br Heart J 1985;54:290.

58. Hirsch IA, Tomlinson DL, Slogoff S, Keats AS: The overstated risk of preoperative hypokalemia. Anesth Analg 1988;67:131.

59. Papademetriou V, Burris JF, Notargiacomo A, Fletcher RD, Freis ED: Thiazide therapy is not a cause of arrhythmias in patients with systemic hypertension. Arch Intern Med 1988;148:1272.

60. Madias JE, Madias NE, Gavras HP: Nonarrhythmogenicity of diuretic-induced hypokalemia. Arch Intern Med 1984; 144:2171.

61. Vincent HH, Boomsma F, Man in't Veld AJ, Derkx FHM, Wenting GJ, Schalekamp MADH: Effects of selective and nonselective beta-agonists on plasma potassium and norepinephrine. J Cardiovasc Pharmacol 1984;6:107.

62. Johansson BW: Effect of beta blockade on ventricular fibrillation and ventricular tachycardia-induced circulatory arrest in acute myocardial infarction. Am J Cardiol 1986;57:34.

63. Simpson E, Rodger JC, Raj SM, Wong C, Wilkie L, Robertson C: Pre-treatment with beta blockers and the frequency of hypokalaemia in patient with acute chest pain. Br Heart J 1987;58:499.

64. Hoffman BF, Suckling EE: Effect of several cations on transmembrane potentials of cardiac muscle. Am J Physiol 1956; 186:317.

65. Munakata K, Dominic JA, Surawicz B: Variable effects of isoproterenol on action potential duration in guinea pig papillary muscle: Differences between nonsteady and steady state—role of extracellular calcium concentration. J Pharmacol Exp Ther 1982;221:806.

66. Surawicz B, Lepeschkin E, Herrlich HC: Low and high magnesium concentrations at various calcium levels. Effect on the monophasic action potential, electrocardiogram and contractility of isolated rabbit hearts. Circ Res 1961;9:811.

67. Hariman J, Mangiardi LM, McAllister RG, Surawicz B, Shabetai R, Kishida K: Reversal of the cardiovascular effects of verapamil by calcium and sodium: Differences between the electrophysiological and the hemodynamic response. Circulation 1979;59:797.

68. Voss DM, Drake EH: Cardiac manifestations of hyperparathyroidism, with presentation of a previously unreported arrhythmia. Am Heart J 1967;73:235.

69. Rosenquist N, Norderstrom J, Andersson M, Edhag OK: Cardiac conduction in patients with hypercalcemia due to primary hyperparathyroidism. Clin Endocrinol 1992;37:1129.

70. Surawicz B: Use of the chelating agent, EDTA, in digitalis intoxication and cardiac arrhythmias. Prog Cardiovasc Dis 1959;2:432.

71. Polimeni PI, Page E. Magnesium in heart muscle. Circ Res 1973;33:367.

72. Hess P, Lansman JB, Tsien RW. Calcium channel selectivity for divalent and monovalent cations: Voltage and concentration dependence of single channel current in ventricular heart cells. J Gen Physiol 1986;88:293.

73. Surawicz B: Is hypomagnesemia or magnesium deficiency arrhythmogenic? J Am Coll Cardiol 1989;14:1093.

74. Pohl W, Mory P, Nurnberg M, Bayer P, Steinbach K: Serum magnesium, serum potassium and arrhythmia profile in patients with acute myocardial infarct. Wien Klin Wochenschr 1993;105:163.

75. Bashir Y, Sneddon JF, Staunton A, et al: Effect of long-term oral magnesium chloride replacement in congestive heart failure secondary to coronary artery disease. Am J Cardiol 1993;72:1156.

76. Boyd LJ, Scherf D: Magnesium sulphate in paroxysmal tachycardia. Am J Med Sci 1943;206:43.

77. Szekely P, Wynne NA: The effects of magnesium on cardiac arrhythmias caused by digitalis. Clin Sci 1951;10:241.

78. Iseri LT, Fairshter RD, Hardemann JL, Brodsky MA: Magnesium and potassium therapy in multifocal atrial tachycardia. Am Heart J 1985;110:789.

79. Wesley RC Jr, Haines DE, Lerman BB, DiMarco JP, Crampton RS: Effect of intravenous magnesium sulfate on supraventricular tachycardia. Am J Cardiol 1989;63:1129.

80. Allen BJ, Brodsky MA, Capparelli EV, Luckett CR, Iseri LT: Magnesium sulfate therapy for sustained monomorphic ventricular tachycardia. Am J Cardiol 1989;64:1202.

81. Gottlieb SS, Fisher ML, Pressel MD, Patten RD, Weinberg M, Greenberg N: Effects of intravenous magnesium sulfate on arrhythmias in patients with congestive heart failure. Am Heart J 1993;125:1645.

82. Tzivoni D, Keren A, Cohen AM, et al: Magnesium therapy for torsades de pointes. Am J Cardiol 1984;528:53.

83. Artigou JY, Lemonnier MP, Devys J, et al: Treatment of torsade de pointes by intravenous magnesium. Arch Mal Coeur Vaiss 1986;7:1094.

84. Perticone F, Adinolfi L, Bonaduce D: Efficacy of magnesium sulfate in the treatment of torsade de pointes. Am Heart J 1986;112:847.

85. Tzivoni D, Banai S, Schuger C, et al: Treatment of torsade de pointes with magnesium sulfate. Circulation 1988;77:392.

86. Lansman JB, Hess P, Tsien RW. Blockade of current through single calcium channels by Cd^{2+}, Mg^{2+}, and Ca^{2+}. J Gen Physiol 1986;88:321.

87. Horie M, Irisawa H: Rectification of muscarinic K+ current by magnesium ion in guinea pig atrial cells. Am J Physiol 1987;253:H210.

88. Spaeh F, Fleckenstein A: Evidence of a new preferentially Mg-carrying transport system besides the fast Na and slow Ca channels in the excited myocardial sarcolemma membrane. J Mol Cell Cardiol 1979;11:1109.

89. Kiyosue T, Arita M. Magnesium restores high K-induced inactivation of the fast Na channel in guinea pig ventricular muscle. Pflugers Arch 1982;395:78.

90. DiCarlo LA Jr, Morady F, de Buitleir M, Krol RB, Schurig L, Annesley TM: Effects of magnesium sulfate on cardiac conduction and refractoriness in humans. J Am Coll Cardiol 1986;7:1356.

91. Wellens HJJ, Manger Cats V, Dueren DR: Symptomatic sinus node abnormalities following lithium carbonate therapy. Am J Med 1975;59:285.

92. Lown B, Levine HD: Atrial arrhythmias, digitalis and potassium. New York: Lansberger, 1958.

93. Vassalle M, Greenspan K: Effects of potassium on ouabain-induced arrhythmias. Am J Cardiol 1963;12:692.

94. Fisch C, Knoebel SB, Feigenbaum H, Greenspan K: Potassium and the monophasic action potential, ECG, conduction and arrhythmias. Prog Cardiovasc Dis 1966;8:387.

95. Williams JF, Klocke FJ, Braunwald E: Studies on digitalis XIII. A comparison of the effects of potassium on the inotropic and arrhythmic producing actions of ouabain. J Clin Invest 1966;45:346.

96. Steiness E: Diuretics, digitalis, and arrhythmias. Acta Med Scand 1981;647(suppl):75.

97. Aronson R, Nordin C: Arrhythmogenic interaction between low potassium and ouabain in isolated guinea-pig ventricular myocytes. J Physiol (Lond) 1988;400:113.

98. Lown B, Levine SA: Current concepts in digitalis therapy. N Engl J Med 1954;25:771.

99. Weizenberg A, Class RN, Surawicz B: Effects of hyperkalemia on the electrocardiogram of patients receiving digitalis. Am J Cardiol 1985;55:968.

100. Sellers RH, Cangrario J, Kim KE, Mendelssohn D, Rust AN, Swartz C: Digitalis toxicity and hypomagnesemia. Am Heart J 1970;79:57.

101. Beller GA, Hood WD Jr, Smith TW, Abelmann WH, Wacker WEL: Correlation of serum magnesium levels and cardiac digitalis intoxication. Am J Cardiol 1974;33:225.

102. Winslow E, Campbell JK, Marshall RJ: Comparative electrophysiological effects of disopyramide and bepridil on rabbit atrial, papillary, and Purkinje tissue: Modification by reduced extracellular potassium. J Cardiovasc Pharmacol 1986;8:1208.

103. McKibbin JK, Pocock WA, Barlow JB, Millar RN, Obel IW: Sotalol, hypokalemia, syncope, and torsade de pointes. Br Heart J 1984;51:157.

104. Santinelli V, Chiariello M, Santinelli C, Condorelli M: Ventricular tachyarrhythmias complicating amiodarone therapy in the presence of hypokalemia. Am J Cardiol 1984;53:1462.

105. Surawicz B: Pharmacologic treatment of cardiac arrhythmias: 25 years of progress. J Am Coll Cardiol 1983;1:365.

106. Singh BN, Vaughan Williams EM: Effect of altering potassium concentration on the action of lidocaine and diphenylhydantoin on rabbit atrial and ventricular muscle. Circ Res 1971;29:286.

107. Saito S, Chen CM, Buchanan J Jr, Gettes LS, Lynch MR: Steady state and time-dependent slowing of conduction in canine hearts. Effects of potassium and lidocaine. Circ Res 1978;42:246.

Cardiac Arrhythmias, 3rd edition, edited by William J. Mandel.
J. B. Lippincott Company, Philadelphia © 1995.

5

Hrayr S. Karagueuzian • William J. Mandel

Antiarrhythmic Drugs: Mode of Action, Pharmacokinetic Properties, and Therapeutic Uses

Cardiac arrhythmias are thought to be caused by abnormalities of cellular electrophysiologic properties of cardiac cells in a given region of the heart.[1,2] The use of antiarrhythmic drugs for the management and prevention of these arrhythmias is based on (1) the cellular electrophysiologic mechanisms leading to the genesis of arrhythmias, (2) the cellular electropharmacologic properties of antiarrhythmic drugs on cardiac cells at the presumed arrhythmogenic site of origin, and (3) the pharmacokinetic properties of antiarrhythmic drugs. These criteria are not complete, and antiarrhythmic drug therapy is largely empirical. However, in the last decade, there have been significant advances in clarifying arrhythmia mechanisms, electropharmacology, and drug assays in biologic samples. The differential electropharmacologic properties of antiarrhythmic drugs on normal versus diseased myocardium and the profound influence exerted by extracellular ions (e.g., H^+ and K^+) on the action of antiarrhythmic drugs have guided arrhythmia management and prevention. Programmed electrical stimulation of the heart to induce arrhythmias for on-line evaluation of antiarrhythmic drug efficacy has provided a new way of selecting effective drug therapy. In this chapter, the cellular electrophysiologic mechanisms of antiarrhythmic drugs

are discussed in relation to the cellular mechanisms of cardiac arrhythmias. The clinical pharmacokinetic profile of various drugs and their clinical applications are also examined.

ELECTROPHYSIOLOGIC BASIS FOR CARDIAC ELECTRICAL ACTIVITY

A review of the normal cellular mechanisms responsible for cardiac electrical activity (see Chap. 3) aids in the understanding of the cellular mechanisms responsible for the genesis of cardiac arrhythmias. Much of the information has been obtained using the microelectrode technique to record the transmembrane potential of cardiac fibers and by studying the nature and properties of transmembrane flow of ionic current using voltage-clamp studies, ion replacements, and pharmacologic manipulations.

Cardiac fibers maintain a transmembrane resting potential because of the dominant permeability of the membrane to potassium ions (K). If the permeability of K ions is much higher than the permeability of other ions, then, according to the Nernst equation, the resting membrane potential (Er) would equal the equilibrium potential for K ions (Ek). However, Er usually approaches but does not equal Ek because of the presence of residual background ionic currents carried by other ions such as sodium and calcium.[3]

Action potentials are inscribed because of sequential changes in the conductance (permeability) of transmembrane ionic currents. Ions move across the membrane in a direction and rate determined by concentration and voltage gradients. Inward currents correspond to a net entry of positive charges, that is, of cations into the cell; outward currents correspond to a net positive charge leaving the cell. Ionic currents responsible for the generation of action potentials are not the same for all cardiac fibers. Atrial, ventricular, and Purkinje fibers maintain a relatively high Er (close to Ek) and have many similarities in their processes of depolarization and repolarization. The cells of the sinoatrial node and of certain parts of the AV node maintain a much lower Er (less negative, that is, approximately − 50 mV), and their excitatory (depolarizing) currents differ from those of atrial and ventricular fibers. These electrophysiologic differences have profound pharmacologic implications, as discussed later in this chapter.

In the absence of excitation, atrial and ventricular fibers not engaged in pacemaker activity sustain a steady resting potential (phase 4). During excitation (depolarizing pulses), a transmembrane action potential is inscribed. Rapid depolarization (phase 0) carries the membrane potential from − 90 to + 40 mV. Phase 0 is generated whenever the resting potential is rapidly reduced to the threshold potential. This occurs because threshold depolarization increases conductance (activates) the fast sodium channel (GNa). Inward depolarizing (excitatory) sodium current carries the membrane potential toward the sodium equilibrium potential (ENa). Before equilibrium is attained, GNa decreases again, thus inactivating the fast sodium channel. Both activation and inactivation depend on membrane potential.[3] Repolarization does not immediately follow depolarization as it does in nerve and muscle. A plateau (phase 2) region precedes the rapid repolarization (phase 3). Depolarization activates another depolarizing channel, called the secondary, or slow inward current (Isi). This channel permits calcium and probably some sodium to enter the cell (inward current) and keep membrane potential at a fairly constant depolarized state during phase 2 (plateau). Toward the end of phase 2, Isi decreases because of inactivation, causing a decrease in inward current. Then, another conductance (IX1) is fully activated (the delayed rectifier), which permits rapid outward current carried by K$^+$ to repolarize the cell (phase 3) and shifts membrane potential back to the resting state. When this occurs, the depolarizing conductance, GNa and Isi, are restored and become available again for reactivation. In sinoatrial and AV nodal cells, the fast inward current is absent because the normally present low resting potential inactivates the fast sodium channels. In these cells, the excitatory inward current depends solely on Isi.[1-3]

Automaticity

Automaticity is the ability of specialized cardiac cells to develop action potentials in the absence of external stimuli. At the end of repolarization (phase 3), the transmembrane potential spontaneously decreases slowly (spontaneous phase 4 depolarization) until threshold potential is attained. A nondriven (spontaneous) action potential is initiated. The pacemaker current responsible for spontaneous depolarization and automatic impulse initiation is brought about by decay of a time-dependent outward potassium current (that differs in various tissues), which, in the presence of an inward background depolarizing current (carried mainly by sodium and calcium ions), brings about a spontaneous phase 4 depolarization.[4] The inward background current has a conditioning role in spontaneous diastolic depolarization because, in the absence of inward background current, the potential would nearly equal EK, whereas a decrease in time-dependent potassium conductance alone would fail to depolarize the cell. In normal Purkinje fibers, the pacemaker current seems to arise from deactivation of a potassium current that is activated at + 20 mV and deactivated at − 50 mV. Pacemaker activity can also occur in myocardial fibers when long depolarizing pulses are applied, a mechanism known as depolarization-induced automaticity (DIA) or automaticity caused by early afterdepolarization.[5] DIA is perhaps caused by the deactivation of the IX1 current. The range of activation is − 30 to + 20 mV, and deactivation occurs at − 90 mV. In Purkinje fibers depolarized to − 60 mV or less, and manifesting pacemaker activity (abnormal automaticity), the pacemaker current seems to be brought about by a decay of the slow outward current.[4]

Triggered Automaticity

Triggered automatic impulses are a direct result of prior electrical activity. One or more impulses initiate (trigger) one impulse or sustained rhythmic activity.[5,6] After full repolarization, the triggerable fiber (e.g., atrial, ventricular, mitral valve, Purkinje fiber) develops one or more spontaneous small depolarizations (pacemaker activity). These postrepolarization potentials, called transient depolarizations or delayed afterdepolarizations (DAD), are oscillatory afterpotentials that can reach threshold potential and initiate one or more triggered automatic impulses.[5-7] The pacemaker current responsible for triggered automaticity, known as TI, is activated in the range of − 20 to + 40 mV and does not follow the characteristic Hodgkin-Huxley kinetics described for other ionic currents. The reversal potential of this current is −5 to −8 mV.[7,8] The TI emerges by various procedures that elevate intracellular calcium ions. The current seems to be carried by sodium and perhaps by calcium ions in both Purkinje and ventricular muscle cells.[7,8]

Cellular Mechanisms of Cardiac Arrhythmias and Effects of Antiarrhythmic Drugs

Cardiac arrhythmias result from abnormalities of impulse initiation, impulse conduction, or both.[9]

Normal Automatic Mechanisms and Effects of Antiarrhythmic Drugs

Arrhythmias caused by normal automatic mechanisms (enhanced normal automaticity) may arise if impulse initiation in the sinus node is too slow or too fast or if the automaticity of latent pacemakers (atrial, junctional, or ventricular) increases and is faster than the sinus rate. These abnormalities in automatic rates can lead to single or multiple premature impulses or to sustained ectopic rhythms (tachycardia). Quinidine, procainamide, lidocaine, diphenylhydantoin (DPH), disopyramide, aprindine, mexiletine, tocainide, propafenone, and cibenzoline (class I) and beta-blocker (class II) antiarrhythmic agents depress enhanced normal automaticity by depressing the spontaneous phase 4 depolarization of Purkinje fibers in a concentration-dependent manner.[10,11]

Abnormal Automatic Mechanisms and Effects of Antiarrhythmic Drugs

Arrhythmias resulting from abnormal (spontaneous) automaticity (i.e., Er approximately −60 mV) are resistant to "therapeutic" concentrations of all the above mentioned antiarrhythmic agents but are suppressed promptly by verapamil, a calcium channel blocker. Similar electropharmacologic profiles are applicable to arrhythmias caused by triggered automatic mechanism and by DIA. Verapamil, a secondary inward (slow) channel blocking agent (class IV agent), promptly suppresses both these arrhythmogenic mechanisms.[5–8]

Arrhythmias Caused by Abnormal Conduction (Reentry) and Effects of Antiarrhythmic Drugs

Both unidirectional conduction block and slow conduction are prerequisites for reentrant excitation. In the Wolff-Parkinson-White (WPW) syndrome, an anomalous accessory pathway exists between the atrium and the ventricle. If in such a heart there is unidirectional conduction block in either the normal or the abnormal atrioventricular (AV) pathway, reentrant excitation of both ventricle and atria may result from continuous and circulatory propagation of the wave of excitation. For example, if anterograde conduction block exists in the abnormal pathway, the impulse propagates from atria to ventricles over the normal AV nodal route, then, if permitted by atrial refractoriness, the impulse returns from the ventricles to the atria over the abnormal pathway. It may then propagate again to the ventricles over the normal pathway.[9] In such a setting, prolongation of the refractory period of either anterograde or retrograde direction with, for example, amiodarone (i.e., a class III agent) could be useful.

Unidirectional block and slow conduction are highly likely to occur in any part of the heart, causing atrial, junctional, or ventricular reentrant rhythms. Theoretically, all antiarrhythmic drugs at appropriate myocardial concentrations can change the refractoriness or conduction properties of affected cells, with two possible outcomes. One, the balance between conduction and refractoriness that is necessary to perpetuate reentry may be altered and reentrant activity promptly terminated.[12] Two, drug-induced changes in conduction and refractoriness may facilitate reentrant excitation.[12,13] There are many examples of drug-induced aggravation of arrhythmias.[14–16] It is impossible to predict whether an antiarrhythmic drug will successfully terminate a reentrant arrhythmia because (1) the cellular electrophysiologic basis for reentry in the intact human heart or in an animal model is unknown and (2) it is not known how a given drug will interact with affected (diseased) myocardial cells engaged in the genesis of reentrant excitation because normal and diseased cells respond differently to a given antiarrhythmic agent.[17]

Arrhythmias Caused by Simultaneous Abnormalities of Impulse Formation and Impulse Conduction: Effects of Antiarrhythmic Drugs

Under a number of conditions, both impulse formation and impulse conduction may be abnormal.[9,18] Because phase 4 depolarization (normal, abnormal, or oscillatory afterpotentials) shifts membrane potential toward zero, there is partial inactivation of the fast inward depolarizing channel with attendant slowing of conduction, thus favoring reentry. A drug that stabilizes phase 4 is likely to improve conduction velocity, a property that may terminate reentrant excitation. Other coexisting abnormalities of conduction and automaticity are provided by parasystolic foci and are discussed in Chapter 11.

Nonlinear Dynamics and Cardiac Arrhythmias: Effects of Antiarrhythmic Drugs

The complex and irregular rate-dependent variability in impulse conduction and excitability follows a well described pattern that can be accurately predicted by mathematical theory.[19,20] Such temporal variability in action potential parameters at a given myocardial site is an additional input to the overall spatial variability of action potential parameters (electrophysiologic heterogeneity) that, so far, assumed only the presence of fixed variability over space. Temporal and spatial variabilities increase the degree of electrophysiologic heterogeneity and decrease the electrical stability of the myocardium by promoting sustained reentrant premature excitation.[21] The pattern of beat to beat variability of cardiac electrical responses resembles many other physical systems (nonlinear) that are dynamically well characterized. Therefore, cardiac electrical dynamics may be studied using established methods of analysis used in various nonlinear dynamical systems.[22] The benefits from taking such an approach for potential drug-induced proarrhythmia recognition are promising. The nonlinear dynamic activity of cardiac excitation, conduction, and refractoriness has been demonstrated in disparate experimental settings and in various cardiac tissues: in isolated myocardial cells, either beating spontaneously or under voltage-clamped conditions, in closed-chest

anesthetized dogs, and in AV conduction in humans.[23–26] Furthermore, various ionic mechanisms controlling the inscription of cardiac action potentials are governed by nonlinear differential equations.[3,27] The importance of these findings and their potential usefulness in arrhythmia prediction and control by pharmacologic agents is as follows: a major mechanism of reentrant premature excitation has been shown to be promoted by nonhomogeneous dispersion of action potential duration and conduction patterns within a critical tissue matrix.[28–30] The larger the dispersion, the greater is the ease of induction of reentrant excitation in a given tissue volume.[28–30] An important determinant of action potential duration is the recovery time, that is, the diastolic interval available before activation.[31–34] The longer the recovery time, the longer is the action potential duration, until a plateau is reached. Then, further prolonging of the diastolic interval has no important effect on the action potential duration. Such a relationship, that is, recovery time versus action potential duration, is known as electrical restitution curve, or action potential duration restitution curve.[31–34] The nonlinear nature of such a curve is the prominent characteristic of the action potential duration restitution curve (Fig. 5-1). The greater the nonlinearity (i.e., the steeper the initial slope of the curve, which typically occurs at short diastolic intervals), the wider is the dispersion of action potential duration for a given recovery time.[20–22,31–34] As the degree of action potential dispersion is critically involved in the

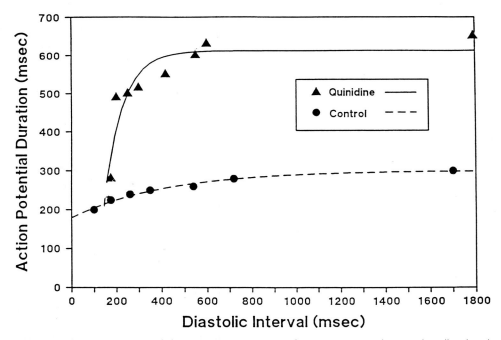

Figure 5-1. Action potential duration restitution curve of a canine ventricular muscle cell isolated from a dog with quinidine-induced ventricular fibrillation (*solid line*) and from a normal untreated dog (*dashed line*). Note the steeper slope at short diastolic intervals.

induction of reentrant premature excitation, it is apparent that the slope of action potential duration restitution curve offers a quantitative measure of the cardiac tissue in question to display dispersion of repolarization, in the face of subtle changes in the recovery time (i.e., diastolic interval).[28-30] This indicates that an increase in the slope (nonlinearity) of action potential restitution curve will be associated with enhanced propensity for reentrant arrhythmias caused by dispersion of action potential duration.[21,28-30] The pharmacologic implications of such an arrhythmic potential are immense. For a drug to effectively prevent the initiation of reentrant cardiac arrhythmias caused by dispersion of repolarization, the drug must decrease the slope of action potential restitution curve so that the dispersion of repolarization process for a given recovery interval is minimized, thus preventing reentry. Conversely, if a drug increases the slope of action potential restitution curve, the drug is expected to encourage (aggravate) the arrhythmia. Data indicate that many ventricular tachycardias, especially with healed myocardial infarction, are caused by circus movement reentry and that antiarrhythmic drugs can aggravate such tachycardias in a substantial number of patients.[14-16,35,36] The increased slope of the action potential duration restitution curve offers an explanation for such an aggravation and provides a theoretically sound hypothesis that can be tested in humans with relative ease by recording monophasic action potentials with contact or pressure electrode.[37,38] However, minimal data are available on the effects of antiarrhythmic drugs on action potential duration restitution curves and these are mostly on normal cardiac fibers.[39,40] The effects of antiarrhythmic drugs on abnormal and diseased tissue, which appears to manifest an altered restitution curve, are virtually unknown.[41] Ventricular fibrillation, ventricular tachycardia, and wide QRS slow ventricular "agonal" rhythms in dogs, induced by incremental intravenous toxic doses of quinidine, have been shown to manifest a significantly increased slope of action potential duration restitution curve for both Purkinje and ventricular muscle cells (Fig. 5-1).[21,42,43] These data strongly suggest that an increased slope of action potential duration restitution curve may be one important mechanism of quinidine-induced ventricular tachyarrhythmias.[21,42,43] Alternatively, increased slope of action potential duration restitution curve may indicate increased electrical instability and enhanced susceptibility for inducible tachycardias. Kobayashi and coworkers have shown that the slope of the action potential duration restitution curve of the second premature stimulus has a significantly steeper slope compared to a single premature stimulus both in isolated tissue studies and in the intact in situ ventricles, thus suggesting the increased incidence of inducible ventricular tachycardias during double premature stimulation.[44,45] It has been demonstrated in patients with ventricular disease and complicat-

ing ventricular tachycardia that the slope of the monophasic action potential duration (MAPD) restitution curve is steeper compared to that in patients without inducible arrhythmias.[46] In addition, Gang and coworkers showed that the ventricular fibrillation threshold was significantly lower when the test was made after double premature stimuli were applied.[47] Computer simulation studies corroborate these experimental and clinical findings by showing that increasing the steepness of the action potential duration restitution causes the induction of double counterclockwise nonstationary spiral waves (i.e., reentrant wavefront of activation) in a two-dimensional matrix made of 16,000 excitable elements.[48,49] The use of nonlinear dynamical system theory is expected to provide greater understanding of arrhythmia mechanisms and suppression.[50] In addition to quantitating dispersion of repolarization, use of dynamic methods to evaluate excitation and conduction offers important indices for cardiac electrical instability that can be evaluated both in vitro and in vivo.

Classification of Antiarrhythmic Drugs

Antiarrhythmic drugs are classified into four types (types I to IV) based on observations made on normal cells and reflects the effects of an agent.[51] In type I, the agent (e.g., quinidine) depresses fast sodium current. In type II, the agent (e.g., propranolol) blocks beta adrenergic receptors. In type III, the agent (e.g., amiodarone) prolongs action potential duration without appreciable blockade of fast sodium current. In type IV, the agent (e.g., verapamil) blocks secondary inward current (i.e., slow inward current) carried mainly by calcium and some sodium ions. Type I is subclassified by the Harrison modification of the Vaughan Williams classification into types IA (quinidine, procainamide, disopyramide, cibenzoline), IB (lidocaine, tocainide, mexiletine, moricizine), and IC (encainide, flecainide, lorcainide, propafenone, indecainide) (Table 5-1).[52] Type IA prolongs action potential duration, whereas type IB shortens it, and type IC has no appreciable effect on action potential duration.[52] Supporters say the classifications "provide valuable conceptual framework for the understanding of the clinical electrophysiologic properties of antiarrhythmic drugs"[53] and that they "enable the more rational and effective use of antiarrhythmics drugs."[52] Critics say (1) such classification is flawed because it is based on electrophysiologic effects exerted by an arbitrary concentration of the drug, generally on normal Purkinje fibers, often not even on arrhythmic preparations; (2) the effects of antiarrhythmic drugs depend on tissue type, species, the degree of acute or chronic ischemia or damage, heart rate, membrane potential, ionic composition and other modulating factors; (3) many drugs have actions that belong to multiple categories or exert indirect effects such as altering hemodynamics, myocardial metabolism, or autonomic

TABLE 5-1. Harrison Modification of Class I Agents

Class	Actions	Agents
1A	Widens QRS and slows conduction at high concentrations Prolongs QT interval and lengthens duration of action potential Lengthens refractory periods	Quinidine Procainamide Disopyramide Cibenzoline
1B	Limited effect on QRS and conduction Shortens repolarization and QT Elevates fibrillation thresholds	Lidocaine Tocainide Mexiletine Ethmozine
1C	Widens QRS and slows conduction at low concentrations Little effect on repolarization and duration of action potential Small changes in refractoriness	Encainide Lorcainide Flecainide Propafenone Indecainide

transmission; (4) some drugs have active metabolites that exert effects different from the parent compound; and (5) not all drugs in the same class have identical effects, whereas some drugs in different classes have similar actions.[54] For example, the effect of lidocaine on the fast sodium current is strongly voltage- and rate-dependent.[55] Based on the critical considerations, it is more appropriate to address antiarrhythmic "class action" rather than antiarrhythmic "drug class." Even Vaughan Williams, who originally proposed the classification of antiarrhythmic drugs, seems to advocate such a claim.[56] It is our opinion that such classification is useful only as a conversational shorthand and its value in recommending a prescription for a given clinical setting is highly questionable.

Dissatisfaction with the existing classification of antiarrhythmic drugs led a group of investigators in a meeting held in Sicily to consider a different approach for the classification of antiarrhythmic drugs. This new approach is based on a variety of factors, including drug actions on the various arrhythmogenic mechanisms at clinical, cellular, and molecular levels.[57] Called the "Sicilian Gambit," the new approach is somewhat tutorial, designed to provide background information in the field of antiarrhythmic drug development and antiarrhythmic drug testing.

Antiarrhythmic Drugs and Proarrhythmia

The widespread use of antiarrhythmic drugs has made it increasingly evident that antiarrhythmic drugs can worsen the "arrhythmic condition."[58–65] Such a toxic potential of antiarrhythmic drugs is recognized when arrhythmias are exposed in the cardiac catheterization lab with programmed electrical stimulation that allows on-line determination of the patient's arrhythmic response before and after the adminis-

tration of a drug. Terms that describe such a toxic effect of antiarrhythmic drugs include *arrhythmia aggravation, worsening, exacerbation,* or *facilitation* of the arrhythmia, or *proarrhythmic* or *arrhythmogenic.* The term *proarrhythmia* is used here. The criteria used to define proarrythmia are arbitrary, because their mechanisms are unknown, and there is no way to predict with certainty their occurrences. This problem arises because proarrhythmia occurs in patients who have blood levels within accepted therapeutic range, and the electrocardiogram intervals do not show gross or significant abnormalities compared with patients who are on similar drug regimens and who do not manifest proarrhythmia.[58, 60, 64] Furthermore, in a study involving a large number of patients (n = 506) undergoing 1268 drug trials, it was suggested that the age, gender, cardiac diagnosis, location of prior myocardial infarction, and New York Heart Association functional class for heart failure were not related to the occurrence of drug-induced proarrhythmias.[64] The general consensus is that proarrhythmia is defined as (1) the development of spontaneous ventricular tachycardia or ventricular fibrillation associated with the administration of the drug that subsides after the elimination of the drug from the body, (2) reduction in the number of premature stimuli needed for the induction of ventricular tachycardia, (3) the induction of monomorphic sustained ventricular tachycardia when only nonsustained ventricular tachycardia could be induced before the administration of the drug, (4) ventricular tachycardia requiring cardioversion that, before administration of the drug, could either be terminated spontaneously or by ventricular burst pacing, and (5) induction of ventricular tachycardia after drug administration that could not be induced during control, predrug state.[58–60, 64] The incidence of proarrhythmia with antiarrhythmic drug therapy reportedly varies between 6% and 28%.[58–65] The incidence seems to be related to the type of drug used and the definition adopted to describe the phenomenon of worsening of the patient's arrhythmic condition.[58–65]

From Cardiac Arrhythmia Pilot Study to Cardiac Arrhythmia Suppression Trial

The Cardiac Arrhythmia Suppression Trial (CAST), a multicenter, randomized, placebo-controlled study, was designed to test whether the suppression of asymptomatic or mildly symptomatic ventricular arrhythmias after myocardial infarction would reduce the rate of death from arrhythmia.[66] In an earlier multicenter study, the Cardiac Arrhythmia Pilot Study (CAPS), it was established that adequate suppression of arrhythmias could be attained with encainide, flecainide, and moricizine in patients with myocardial infarction.[67, 68] In the CAST study during an average of 10 months' follow-up, the patients assigned to the active drug therapy had a higher rate of death from arrhythmia than the patients on placebo therapy.[66] Administration of encainide and flecainide accounted for the excess rate of deaths from arrhythmia and nonfatal cardiac arrest, that is, 33 of 730 patients taking encainide or flecainide (4.5%), 9 of 725 patients taking placebo (1.2%), with a relative risk of 3.6 (95% confidence interval, 1.7 to 8.5). Patients on active drugs also accounted for the higher total mortality, that is, 56 of 730 patients taking active drugs (7.7%) as opposed to 22 of 725 patients in the placebo group (3%), with a relative risk of 2.5 (95% confidence interval, 1.6 to 4.5). These results were sufficiently compelling to discontinue the portion of the trial involving encainide and flecainide.[66] The mechanism of drug-induced increased incidence of death in this trial, however, remains undefined. It was recommended that "neither encainide nor flecainide should be used in the treatment of patients with asymptomatic or minimally symptomatic ventricular arrhythmias, after myocardial infarction, even though these drugs may be effective initially in suppressing ventricular arrhythmias." In addition, it is not known from the CAST study if this recommendation applies to other patients who might be candidates for antiarrhythmic drug therapy.

The second CAST trial (CAST-II) tested the effectiveness of moricizine to reduce mortality by suppressing asymptomatic or mildly symptomatic ventricular premature depolarizations after myocardial infarction.[69] As with flecainide and encainide, moricizine was found to be not only ineffective but also harmful. Seventeen of 665 patients died or had cardiac arrest in the moricizine group compared with three deaths out of 660 patients with no treatment or placebo. The trial was terminated because it was considered highly unlikely that a survival benefit from moricizine would be observed if the trial were completed.[69] The rationale for selecting flecainide, encainide, and moricizine for the CAST trials are explained in a recent article by Green and coworkers.[70] The mechanisms of increased deaths in the treatment groups (ventricular tachycardia and ventricular fibrillation) are discussed in an article by Echt and coworkers.[71] In an evaluation of the effects of the drugs used in the two CAST trials and on the timing of arrhythmic death, Peters and coworkers reported that the onset of the arrhythmic death displayed a bimodal variation, with significant peaks in midmorning and late afternoon/early evening; more than half of the symptomatic events were accompanied by angina-like symptoms.[72]

Basic Pharmacokinetic Principles and Antiarrhythmic Drug Efficacy

The ability of an antiarrhythmic drug to reliably suppress or even exaggerate an arrhythmia is often related to drug plasma concentration. Changes in plasma drug concentration reflect myocardial drug concentration at the receptor site or near the site of action in the myocardium. The next section, Time Course of Plasma Drug Concentration, discusses the general principles that govern the time course of plasma drug concentration and defines how various factors modify the time versus blood concentration profile. A general knowledge of the pharmacokinetic principles and the pharmacokinetic properties of antiarrhythmic drugs provides a good base for therapy. After therapy is initiated, however, subsequent doses and the establishment of long-term drug therapy must be adjusted strictly in relation to the patient's clinical outcome. Because of the narrow therapeutic ratio of minimum effective plasma concentration to toxic plasma concentration, a working knowledge of basic pharmacokinetic principles is needed to effectively manage and control patients with cardiac arrhythmias. Skillful dose adjustment is necessary to prevent undesirable side effects. Subtherapeutic concentrations may be ineffective in preventing recurrences of potentially life-threatening arrhythmias, and toxic doses may be lethal. Furthermore, as the patient's clinical status changes during the protracted antiarrhythmic drug therapy, the initial dosage regimen must be constantly reevaluated.

Time Course of Plasma Drug Concentration

Rapid Intravenous Injection

When a drug is rapidly injected intravenously (bolus injection), it undergoes many physiologic processes (e.g., metabolism, distribution, elimination), all of which act together to reduce the plasma drug concentration until the plasma becomes free of the drug. Plasma decay of the drug is often exponential, and experience shows that simple mathematic transformation, that is, a plot of log plasma concentration ($\ln Cp$) versus time, results in a straight line (monoexponential) (Fig. 5-2). A monoexponential decay is expressed as follows:

$$cp = Cp_0 \, e - Ket$$

or

$$\ln Cp = \ln Cp0 - Ket$$

where Cp is plasma drug concentration at time t, Ke is the elimination rate constant (time -1), and Cp_0 is plasma drug concentration at time zero, obtained by extrapolating the line relating $\ln Cp$ versus time to time zero. If the time course of a drug is linear ($\ln Cp$ versus time), then the drug behaves according to a one-compartment model (first-order plot). Usually, all antiarrhythmic drugs show a plasma decay consistent with a two-compartment model,

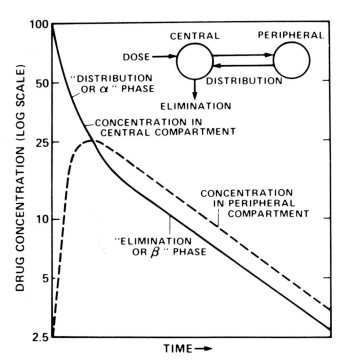

Figure 5-2. Drug concentrations at various times following a bolus dose, when the body has the characteristics of a one-compartment model. *Inset* shows the same information with concentration plotted on a logarithmic scale. (Harrison DC, Meffin PJ, Winkle RA: Clinical pharmacokinetics of antiarrhythmic drugs. Prog Cardiovasc Dis 1977;20:217.

with the initial, rapid phase of decline corresponding to the rapid distribution of the drug in the body (central compartment) and the slower compartment corresponding to drug elimination and distribution to a more slowly accessible (peripheral) compartment (Fig. 5-3). Most antiarrhythmic drugs are eliminated from the body by renal excretion and by hepatic biotransformation, an elimination that proceeds as a first-order process.[73,74] The linear first-order plot offers many useful pharmacokinetic drug properties.

Half-life

The half-life ($t^{1/2}$) of a drug is defined as the time required for any given plasma concentration to decrease to half, that is, in the first equation, ln Cp/ln Cp0 becomes $^{1/2}$:

$$\ln \frac{1}{2} = 0.693 = Ket$$

Contrary to a first-order process, a zero-order process does not have a constant half-life. A zero-order process continues at a constant rate independent of the fraction of the process already completed. The following formula describes a zero-order process:

$$t^{1/2} = 0.5 \times Cp/Ko$$

In such a case, there is no definitive half-life for that particular drug, because the zero-order rate constant (Ko) in the denominator represents a constant value, so the larger the initial concentration (Cp), the longer the apparent half-life is. Therefore, such drugs appear to have half-lives that increase with increased dose. Such a phenomenon is called *dose-dependent pharmacokinetics*. Although commonly referred to as nonlinear kinetics, this is a misnomer because the plot is linear on ordinary graph paper. The concept refers to dose-dependent kinetics. As the drug dose increases, the kinetic data may change from those of apparent first order (state of no metabolic [enzyme] saturation) to apparent zero order (state of metabolic [enzyme] saturation). Thus, plasma levels of such drugs may not be a linear function of the dose, and their kinetics are termed nonlinear. Of the conventional antiarrhythmic drugs, DPH is one drug that manifests this pharmacokinetic behavior.

Volume of Distribution

The volume of distribution or, more properly termed, the apparent volume of distribution (Vd), is determined by dividing the concentration of the drug at time zero (see extrapolation above) to the total amount of the drug administered intravenously (M). The phrase volume of distribution, which is often confusing, defines a hypothetical volume into which the total amount of the administered drug must be diluted to result in a plasma concentration at time zero:

$$Vd = M/Cp_0$$

where M is the amount of drug administered (in grams) and Cp_0 is plasma drug concentration at time zero (in grams/liter). Note that Vd has the unit of volume, liters in this example, and is best considered as a factor that will convert plasma concentration (Cp) to total amount in the body at any desired time (i.e., amount in the body = Cp × Vd).

Continuous Intravenous Infusion

When a drug is continuously infused, the plasma level increases until a constant or steady-state plasma level is achieved. During the steady state (i.e., the period during which the plasma level of the drug is maintained at a constant), the rate of drug infusion (input) is equal to the rate of elimination (output):

$$(a) \quad Ki = Cpss \times Cl$$

where Ki is the rate of infusion of the drug (e.g., in milligrams per minute), Cpss is plasma drug concentration at steady state, and Cl is total body clearance of the

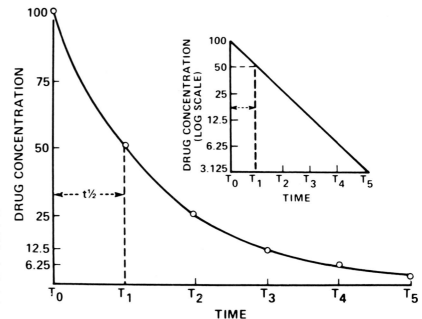

Figure 5-3. Conceptual representation of a two-compartment model showing reversible distribution between a rapidly equilibrating peripheral compartment. Also shown are the concentrations of drug at various times in both the central and peripheral compartments after an intravenous bolus into the central compartment. (Harrison DC, Meffin PJ, and Winkle RA: Clinical pharmacokinetics of antiarrhythmic drugs. Prog Cardiovasc Dis 1977;20:217.

drug (e.g., in milliliters per minute). This equation can be rewritten using the parameter of Vd:

$$(b) \quad Cl = Ke \times Vd$$

where Ke is the apparent first-order elimination rate constant (time − 1) and Vd is the apparent volume of distribution. Substituting equation (a) for clearance in equation (b) yields:

$$(c) \quad Ki = Cpss \times Ke \times Vd$$

For the one-compartment model of plasma drug decay (linear semi-logarithmic plot), Ke = 0.693/t½, equation (c) becomes

$$(d) \quad Ki = Cpss \times 0.693 \times VD/t½$$

Consequently, if the clearance (Cl) or the volume of vdistribution (Vd) and the half-life (t½) are known or if the elimination rate constant (Ke) is known, then equations (a) and (d) can be used to calculate the required intravenous infusion rate to achieve any desired steady-state plasma level of a drug. If 90% of the plasma steady state is acceptable as a reasonable estimate of the desired therapeutic concentration, then 3.3 half-lives are required for onset of drug action. Therefore, for a drug with a half-life of 2 hours, 6.6 hours are needed to achieve 90% of the desired steady-state plasma drug concentration. Therefore, slow continuous intravenous infusion does not lead to a rapid therapeutic effect (arrhythmia suppression), which may be crucial, especially in the setting of intensive

coronary care unit where rapid suppression of the arrhythmia, for example with lidocaine, is urgently needed. This problem can be overcome by an initial rapid administration of a single dose (i.e., a loading dose) to "fill" the apparent volume of distribution. A loading dose is a rapid intravenous injection of a calculated amount of a drug to provide a plasma steady-state amount in the body. This amount can be calculated from the equation Vd = M/Cp by substituting the desired steady-state plasma concentration (Cpss) for the value of Cp.

When steady-state plasma drug concentration is attained by multiple intermittent intravenous doses (D) of a drug, clearance (Cl) and dose (D) become the principal determinants of the average plasma drug concentration (Cav) of the area under the plasma concentration versus time curve (AUC) (Fig. 5-4):

$$AUC = D/Cl$$

Furthermore, the average plasma drug concentration (Cav) can be equated to D and Cl:

$$Cav = Cl \cdot t$$

where t is the time interval between intravenous doses.

Oral Drug Administration

When a drug is administered orally or by a route requiring absorption (e.g., buccal, intramuscular, subcutaneous, topical), the time course of the plasma drug concentration

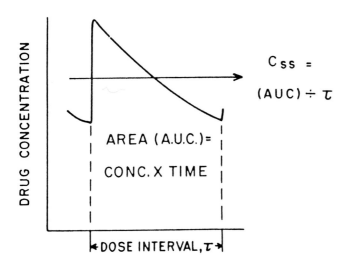

Figure 5-4. Steady-state concentrations (Css) and the area under the concentration/time profile (AUC). AUC = concentration × time.

initially increases (input > output), then the concentration reaches a maximum (input = output) and finally decays (output > input). The terminal portion of the blood level curve becomes linear (semilogarithmic plot), and when absorption is sufficiently fast, the slope of this curve represents the rate constant for elimination; therefore, the half-life of the drug can be calculated from the equation $t^{1/2} = 0.693/Ke$. However, if absorption of the drug is sufficiently slow, the terminal slope of such a plot does not represent Ke, because absorption still occurs while part of the drug is being eliminated. Therefore, the true half-life of a given drug should be regarded as the one determined by rapid intravenous administration, showing linear kinetics that exclusively reflect elimination. When the observed half-life of a drug after oral administration is longer than that reported by rapid intravenous administration, a slow rate of absorption is presumed to be present. Measurement should reflect the parent drug and not that of a parent compound and a metabolite combination.

Bioavailability

When drugs require an absorption site, absorption becomes complete (100%) when (1) the drug molecules are fully available at the absorption site and (2) the drug molecules are completely absorbed into the systemic circulation without loss. However, this is often not possible, and the labeled dose on the pharmaceutical form should be differentiated from the bioavailable dose to the systemic circulation. The labeled dose (e.g., the amount per tablet) is the actual chemical content of the dose form, and the bioavailable dose is the amount of the drug that actually enters the bloodstream on administration. The bio-

available fraction, F, is the fraction of the labeled dose that is absorbed and enters the bloodstream (systemic circulation). For example, if 200 mg of a drug was absorbed from a tablet containing 250 mg, the bioavailable fraction F is 200/250 = 0.8.

In intravenous dosing, F = 1 because all the drug is delivered directly to the bloodstream. The amount of a drug that reaches the bloodstream after oral administration can be determined by rearranging the equation AUC = D/Cl, by replacing D with F × D, where D is the bioavailable dose and F = 1 because of intravenous administration:

$$AUC = F \times Dose/Cl, \text{ or } F = AUC \times CL/Dose$$

This equation states that the fraction of the drug absorbed may be calculated from a knowledge of the AUC following the oral dose, along with the clearance for that drug and the size of the dose administered. Furthermore, F can be calculated as the fraction of a drug absorbed orally:

$$F = AUC\infty \text{ (oral)}/AUC\infty \text{ (IV)} \times Dose \text{ (IV)}/Dose \text{ (oral)}$$

∞AUC is the area under the curve from time equals zero to time equals infinity. Some of the antiarrhythmic drugs in which bioavailability problems have been of clinical significance include DPH, procainamide, and quinidine. Food intake may modulate bioavailability of antiarrhythmic drugs. Specifically, when tocainide or mexiletine are taken on an empty stomach, side effects appear, possibly reflecting more rapid absorption. However, if either agent is taken with a meal, absorption is slowed, but its amount is unaltered.[75,76] Therefore, the same amount of drug is bioavailable, but the rapid rise in plasma seen when the drugs are taken on an empty stomach is minimized when the drugs are ingested with meals. Meals also raise plasma lipoprotein levels, at least transiently, which may displace drugs from their protein binding sites. This becomes particularly important for drugs that are highly protein bound, such as propranolol and propafenone.[75]

Intestinal and First-Pass Metabolism

First-pass metabolism is so termed because an absorbed drug, after oral administration, undergoes metabolism or degradation, usually by the liver, before reaching the systemic circulation. This can result in reduced blood levels of the the parent drug. For example, the area under the blood level–time curve for lidocaine is significantly greater when the drug is infused into a peripheral vein of a dog than when an equal amount is infused into the portal vein. Introducing the drug directly into the portal vein may be analogous to the pathway after oral administration. Thus, the area under the curve is reduced because the drug is exposed to the liver before it is sampled to determine bioavailability. Furthermore, an intravenous dose is simultaneously distributed to all parts of the body including the liver. Drugs initially distributed to other organs may be temporarily protected from metabolism by the liver. Other mechanisms by which drugs can be metabolized before reaching the systemic circulation may exist. Unless the actual mechanism for metabolism is clearly identified (i.e., first-pass metabolism), it is more appropriate to refer to such metabolic loss of drug as presystemic metabolism. The presystemic, or first-pass elimination, occurs with lidocaine and propranolol (i.e., high hepatic clearance); therefore, alterations of hepatic blood flow have a major impact on the clearances of these drugs. Because first-pass drug metabolism may be subject to saturation (zero-order), it is possible to observe a nonlinear dependency for the AUC as a function of the oral dose. As the drug-metabolizing enzyme becomes saturated with increasing oral doses of the drug, more drug enters the bloodstream in intact (unmetabolized) form and raises the blood levels abruptly (positive deviation form linearity), a phenomenon previously discussed as nonlinear kinetics or dose-dependent kinetics.

Absorption and Diseased States

Physiologic and pathologic differences between patients or in a given patient at different times can affect gastrointestinal absorption of drugs. In general, most antiarrhythmic drugs are well absorbed from the small intestine, and absorption from the stomach is relatively insignificant. As a result, any factor that delays the rate of gastric emptying potentially reduces the rate of absorption of orally administered drugs and prevents attainment of peak plasma concentration in the blood, resulting in failure of arrhythmia suppression. Furthermore, the patient's physiologic state, including the level of physical activity, the presence or absence of food components forming poorly absorbable complexes with antiarrhythmic drug molecules, and the disease state can affect gastrointestinal motility and may alter the bioavailability of antiarrhythmic agents.

GENETICS, DISEASED STATES, AND KINETIC DISPOSITION OF ANTIARRHYTHMIC DRUGS

The genetic composition of the patient can exert profound influence on the metabolism of the drug, thus modifying the disposition kinetics of the drug. Evidence for such effects for individual antiarrhythmic drugs is presented here whenever data are available. Genetic influences on

the pharmacokinetics of certain antiarrhythmic drugs, including procainamide, propafenone, and encainide, have been reported. Other modulators of antiarrhythmic drug disposition include altered protein binding during various disease conditions and the newly recognized stereospecific or stereoselective properties of antiarrhythmic drugs. For example, myocardial infarction causes alpha-1-acid glycoprotein plasma levels to rise, which, in turn, can bind to antiarrhythmic drugs and alter their disposition kinetics and actions.[77] This indicates the importance of monitoring free plasma drug levels (protein unbound) rather than the total plasma drug concentration. The potential pharmacokinetic and pharmacodynamic consequences of stereoselectivity of antiarrhythmic drugs are discussed under drug headings for quinidine, disopyramide, verapamil, and propafenone.

The following paragraphs are a discussion of the mode of action, pharmacokinetic properties, clinical use, and toxic side effects of standard and new investigational antiarrhythmic agents.

Standard Agents

Quinidine

MODE OF ACTION. Microelectrode studies on isolated superfused cardiac preparations have shown that quinidine (Fig. 5-5), at concentrations considered clinically effective, decreases the slope of spontaneous phase 4 depolarization in Purkinje fibers, which arise from a resting potential of -90 to -70 mV, thus decreasing the rate of automatic impulse initiation.[78] In cardiac fibers manifesting abnormal or triggered automatic mechanisms, quinidine has no significant effect.[78-81] The drug causes a concentration and rate-dependent decrease in the maximum rate of depolarization ($\dot{V}_{max}$) and in the overshoot potential of canine Purkinje fibers, ventricular muscle cells, and human atrial tissue.[78,82-86] Moderate lengthening of action potential duration (at 90% repolarization) and effective refractory period occurs in Purkinje fibers, whereas the plateau phase of the action potential becomes shortened. In ventricular muscle cells, quinidine prolongs the duration at all phases of the action potential.[78,82,83,85] No significant change in resting membrane potential occurs in either fiber type with "therapeutic concentration" of quinidine.[78,81,82,84,85] The depression of conduction in the direction parallel to fiber orientation (axis) is more important than in the direction transverse to fiber orientation.[87] A rate-dependent decrease in conduction velocity in the canine Purkinje–ventricular muscle junction also occurs with quinidine.[88] The increase in the effective refractory period (ERP) caused by quinidine is greater than the increase in the action potential duration (APD) (i.e., ratio of ERP to APD is greater than 1), an effect that indicates delay in the

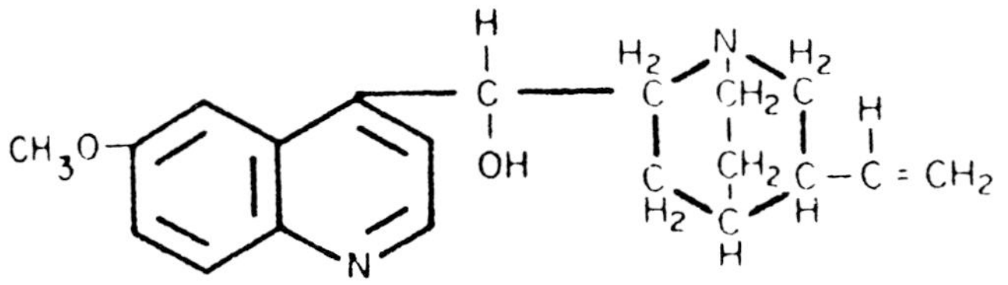

Figure 5-5. Quinidine.

reactivation kinetics of the fast sodium channel.[82] Quinidine decreases excitability of atrial and ventricular fibers (i.e., a higher stimulus intensity is needed to elicit a propagated action potential), an effect that appears to be rate-dependent, at least in canine ventricular endocardium in vivo.[83,89] However, studies on isolated sheep Purkinje fibers indicate that therapeutically relevant concentrations (4 µg/mL) of quinidine actually increase cardiac excitability as manifested by a decrease in the current required to attain threshold despite a depression of the fast sodium current and conduction velocity.[90] This indicates that the interaction of quinidine with the passive properties (i.e., input membrane resistance, space and time constants, all significantly increased with quinidine) of Purkinje fibers has major influence on the excitability. During quinidine washout, both passive properties and excitability were observed to remain altered while active properties, such as resting potential, $\dot{V}_{max}$, action potential duration, and overshoot, returned to normal.[90] Recent voltage-clamp studies on enzymatically isolated canine myocytes have shown that quinidine reduces steady-state outward current (iK1), the slow inward current (isi), and both the sodium (tetrodotoxin sensitive) and calcium (tetrodotoxin insensitive) window currents.[91] A block of time-dependent outward current was also observed in isolated guinea pig ventricular myocytes exposed to quinidine.[92] A reduction of the transient outward current by quinidine was also observed in rabbit atrial tissue, an effect that contributes to the overall lengthening of the action potential duration.[93] This multitude of actions on transmembrane ionic current flows during the plateau phase of action potential perhaps explains the differing effects of quinidine on action potential duration in Purkinje and ventricular muscle fibers.[78,82-85] Quinidine in vitro preparations were found to cause greater slowing of conduction velocity in the longitudinal to myocardial fiber orientation than transverse to it, a finding that may be caused by lesser availability of sodium current ("safety factor") in the longitudinal direction.[94]

Using monophasic action potential recordings in humans, it has been shown that quinidine has a frequency-dependent effect on the ventricular action potential and QRS duration.[95] At slower rates, quinidine had a significant effect on the action potential duration, repolarization, and voltage-dependent refractory period. As the heart rate was increased, the effect of quinidine on these variables diminished, but its effect on the time-dependent refractory period became more pronounced. In contrast to the effect of quinidine on the action potential duration, the drug prolonged the QRS duration in a use-dependent manner.[95,96] Furthermore, the observed quinidine-induced increase in QT duration as cycle length is prolonged is consistent with a reverse use-dependent effect of quinidine on ventricular repolarization.[97]

In addition to the use-dependent block of the sodium channel, greater binding of quinidine to the cardiac sodium channel and, thus, greater depression of $\dot{V}_{max}$ occur in partially depolarized cardiac muscle and Purkinje fibers.[17,82-85] These findings suggest that quinidine might selectively slow conduction in partially depolarized "sick" myocardial cells engaged in a reentrant circuit, thus terminating reentrant arrhythmias.[17,82] In an in vitro model of reflected reentry, quinidine terminated the reentry when the initial conditions of conduction were highly impaired; no such effect could be observed when the initial conditions were moderately severe.[98] These observations support the hypothesis of selective depression of "sick" myocardial cells.[17] Furthermore, membrane-depressant effects (decrease in $\dot{V}_{max}$) and prolongation of effective refractory period by quinidine are potentiated by an elevated extracellular potassium concentration.[99]

Dreifus and coworkers found that a return to normal values of $\dot{V}_{max}$ and action potential amplitude occurred in the presence of lowered potassium ion concentration.[99] Potentiation of the electrophysiologic effects of quinidine were also seen during combination therapy with mexiletine.[100] Combinations of quinidine and mexiletine, at concentrations which alone had little effect, produced antiarrhythmic activity that was greater than that seen with high concentrations of either quinidine or mexiletine.[100] Because effects of tetrodotoxin mimic effects of mexiletine, it was suggested that the combination therapy involved enhanced sodium channel blockade, in accordance with the modulated receptor hypothesis of the cardiac sodium channel.[17,82,101]

The direct depressant effects of quinidine are masked by its indirect vagolytic and antiadrenergic effects on the heart and vasculature.[102,103] The vagolytic action of the drug may increase heart rate, whereas its antiadrenergic property tends to reduce it. Therefore, quinidine administration in unanesthetized humans causes either no change or a slight acceleration in the sinus rate.[104] When excessive sympathetic activity is present, such as during thyrotoxicosis or general anesthesia, quinidine almost invariably produces bradycardia. Intravenous administration of quinidine can cause hypotension. It was suggested that quinidine can cause vasodilation by its direct action, an effect that is associated with baroreflex-mediated increase in sympathetic nerve activity.[105]

The interaction between the direct and indirect (autonomic) effects of quinidine has great clinical significance. Josephson and coworkers found that quinidine prolonged His–Purkinje and intraventricular conduction time in humans.[106] In addition, the refractory period of the atria and the His–Purkinje system was prolonged, whereas the effective period of the AV node was consistently shortened. Furthermore, quinidine consistently slowed conduction and increased refractoriness in the accessory pathways in various preexcitation syndromes, a property found effective in reducing the ventricular rate in patients with the WPW syndrome complicated by atrial flutter or fibrillation.[107,108] Heissenbuttel and Bigger have attempted to correlate the electrophysiologic effects of quinidine to its plasma concentration in humans.[109] They found increased QRS duration with increased quinidine plasma concentration (r = 0.56, $p > 0.0001$). The correlation of the QTc interval with plasma quinidine level was, however, not as high as that of the QRS (r = 0.28, $p < 0.01$). More consistent prolongation of the QTc interval was found with toxic plasma concentrations of quinidine. It has been suggested that a nonhomogenous prolongation of refractoriness by quinidine (i.e., temporal and spatial dispersion of excitability) favors the development of ventricular fibrillation or atypical ventricular tachycardia known as torsades de pointes.[110] A recent report indicates that torsades de pointes may be initiated by the mechanism of early afterdepolarizations and subsequent triggering of automaticity.[111] This contention gains credence by the in vitro observations made on isolated Purkinje fibers. These fibers manifest early afterdepolarizations and triggered automatic activity under conditions of hypokalemia and bradycardia during superfusion with low concentrations of quinidine.[85,112,113] These arrhythmias are thought to be the basis of quinidine syncope in many patients.[114] In some patients, torsades de pointes has been observed with quinidine plasma levels considered well below those usually considered toxic, a requirement (i.e., low concentrations of quinidine 1 to 2μg/mL) for the induction of early afterdepolarization and triggered activity in isolated Purkinje fibers.[85,112,113,115,116]

METABOLISM AND PHARMACOKINETICS. Quinidine is usually administered orally, occasionally intrasmuscularly, and infrequently intravenously.[104] In humans, quinidine is metabolized (up to 85%) in the liver to two hydroxylated metabolites with potential antiarrhythmic activity both in experimental arrhythmia models and in humans.[117,118] These metabolites and the remainder (15% to 20%) of unchanged quinidine are excreted in the urine. The amount of unchanged quinidine recovered in the urine varies inversely with urine pH. In alkaline urine, quinidine excretion is decreased. These findings are based on specific quinidine assay methods.[119] Plasma clearance of quinidine averages 4.7 mL/kg/min (range, 1.5 to 7.1 mL/kg/min), with a half-life of 6.3 hours (range, 3.6 to 8.2 hours). The low clearance of the drug in relation to liver blood flow indicates poor hepatic extraction and explains the high percentage of bioavailability of the drug (76%). The intravenous route is generally not recommended because a large single dose can cause profound circulatory depression. However, very slow infusion rates of quinidine have been found to be safe in a number of patients.[104,120]

In humans, quinidine is well absorbed orally, mainly in the small intestine. Gastric acidity does not influence quinidine bioavailability; however, gastrointestinal motility and the presence of food in the gut can influence its rate of absorption.[121] Quinidine can be detected in serum within 15 minutes of an oral dose; its onset of action begins within 30 minutes, and peak effects are attained in 1 to 3 hours. Several different oral quinidine salt preparations are prescribed. Quinidine sulfate is rapidly absorbed (peak levels at about 1 to 2 hours), with 60% to 100% of the salt being available for systemic circulation. In contrast, quinidine gluconate is more slowly absorbed, with peak blood levels attained about 4 hours after administration. This salt is less available, and absorption is more erratic (40% to 90%) than with the sulfate salt.[122] The slower absorption rate of gluconate salt allows less frequent administration of quinidine than the sulfate salt (8 to 12 hours as opposed to 4 to 6 hours). The slower absorption process, however, results in lower peak plasma levels of quinidine. The principle of prolonging absorption, with no concomitant change in elimination half-life, is used commercially to increase the duration of action of quinidine in slow-release preparations of sulfate, gluconate, and polygalacturonate. These various salts of quinidine contain different amounts of quinidine base. For example, the sulfate contains 83% of the base, the gluconate, 62%, and the polygalacturonate, 60%.[73] About 80% of plasma quinidine is bound to albumin. Although the bound fraction of quinidine does not diffuse out of the vascular compartment, quinidine is still extensively and rapidly distributed to various body tissues.

Ueda and coworkers studied the time course of quinidine plasma concentration after intravenous injection and described its disposition by a two-compartment model system.[119] A rapid phase of distribution (i.e., central compartment [alpha phase]) is followed by slower plasma decline (distribution to the peripheral compartment [beta phase]). The volume of the central compartment was 0.9 ± 0.11 L/kg, and the steady-state volume of distribution was 3.03 ± 0.25 L/kg. The initial rapid phase of distribution half-life ($t^{1/2}$ alpha) was 7.2 ± 0.7 minutes, and the apparent elimination half-life ($t^{1/2}$ beta) was 6.3 ± 0.47 hours. After an intravenous injection $t^{1/2}$ alpha was similar to $t^{1/2}$ beta obtained after both oral and intramuscular injections. Concentrations of 1.5 to 6 μg/mL are generally considered therapeutic, and levels of 7 μg/mL and more are associated with an increased incidence of toxicity.

Effects of Renal, Hepatic, and Cardiac Failure on Quinidine Pharmacokinetics.

Kessler and coworkers analyzed the kinetics of quinidine in patients with renal failure by determining quinidine levels using two different assay methods.[123] They concluded that quinidine doses should not be reduced in patients with renal failure, a recommendation consistent with the minor role played by the kidney in eliminating quinidine. No data are available on the effects of liver disease on the kinetics of quinidine. In patients with congestive heart failure, however, the volume of distribution of quinidine and its absorption rate appear to be reduced, with no change in the elimination half-life.[123] These effects should tend to increase plasma quinidine levels. The clinical significance of such an increase remains unknown, especially because there are large variations in quinidine plasma levels among patients.

DRUG INTERACTIONS WITH QUINIDINE. Quinidine has been shown to potentiate the muscle-relaxing effects of certain neuromuscular junction blocking agents and of aminoglycoside antibiotics such as gentamicin, kanamycin, and streptomycin.[124, 125] Because urine pH can influence quinidine elimination (in alkaline urine, excretion is decreased), coadministration of drugs that acidify (e.g., acetazolamide, ascorbic acid) or alkalinize (e.g., sodium bicarbonate) the urine are expected to alter the clearance of quinidine. Displacement of quinidine from protein-binding sites with drugs increases the likelihood of toxicity (cinchonism).[126] Koch-Weser observed a potentiation of the anticoagulant effect of warfarin with quinidine, possibly caused by displacement of warfarin from its protein-binding sites.[127] Finally, when quinidine is given to patients taking digoxin, the serum digoxin concentration increases.[128–130] In patients receiving constant glycoside maintenance doses, the addition of quinidine to digoxin therapy resulted in a mean 2.5 times increase in digoxin plasma levels (from 0.98 ± 0.37 to 2.47 ± 0.7 ng/mL).[128] Although the clinical significance of an increased digoxin level is not clear, patients receiving quinidine and digoxin simultaneously should be closely monitored for a possible reduction in digoxin dose to prevent digitalis-induced toxic arrhythmias.[128] A 30% to 40% reduction of digoxin has been suggested.[128] Heparin administration was found to displace protein-bound quinidine from 0.3 ± 0.1 to 0.6 ± 0.1 μg/mL in 10 patients, an effect that may have therapeutic implications.[131]

THERAPEUTIC ACTION, DOSE, AND SIDE EFFECTS. Quinidine, the oldest primary antiarrhythmic drug in clinical use, was first described by Wenckebach in 1918.[102] As early as 1749, however, French physician Jean-Baptiste de Senac of Paris used quinidine successfully in the management of patients with a rhythm disorder that he referred to as rebellious palpitation (most likely atrial fibrillation) (Fig. 5-6). He described the usefulness of quinidine as follows:[36, 132, 133]

"Of all the stomachic remedies the one whose effects have appeared to be the most constant and the most prompt in many cases is quinidine mixed with a little rhubarb. Long and rebellious palpitation have ceded to this febrifuge seconded with a light purgative."

This important observation was overlooked for more than two centuries. Even Wenckebach and Frey, who were responsible for the modern use of quinidine, were unaware of de Senac's early findings.[102]

Quinidine is used to treat a wide variety of arrhythmias of atrial, junctional, and ventricular origin; it is thus classified as a "broad-spectrum" antiarrhythmic drug. Used alone or in combination with beta blockers or digoxin, it is valuable in terminating atrial flutter and fibrillation. In patients with AV nodal reentrant supraventricular tachycardia, quinidine alone may not be effective because it does not slow AV nodal conduction. However, it may be successfully used in patients with premature atrial or ventricular depolarizations, which may be responsible for initiating the tachycardia. However, quinidine is frequently effective in atrial tachycardia, with or without WPW syndrome.[107, 108] Before initiating quinidine therapy in

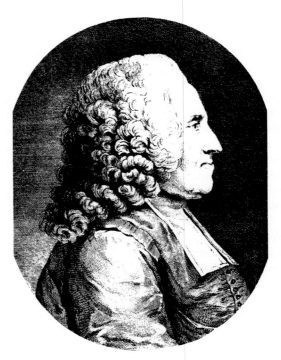

Figure 5-6. Jean-Baptiste de Senac, a French physician, first recorded the efficacy of quinidine in the management of "rebellious palpitation" in 1749. (From Willius FA, Keys TE. Classics of Cardiology. Vol 1. New York: Dover Publications, Inc., 1983:158.)

patients with atrial arrhythmias with a rapid ventricular response (i.e., atrial fibrillation, atrial flutter), either digoxin or a beta blocker should be administered to prevent sudden acceleration of the ventricular rate. This may occur because quinidine exerts vagolytic action on the AV node while progressively slowing the atrial rate of depolarization (decrease in atrial rate). This can facilitate AV transmission by removing concealed AV conduction, which allows more atrial impulses to propagate successfully through the AV node, thereby increasing the ventricular rate. Prophylactic digitalis therapy to prolong AV refractoriness prevents sudden acceleration of ventricular rate. Although quinidine is effective in suppressing most types of ventricular arrhythmias, either alone or in combination with beta blockers, tocainide, or mexiletine, it is usually not effective in controlling digitalis-induced arrhythmias.[85, 100, 134–136] It has been suggested that the efficacy of quinidine against inducible ventricular tachycardias may be related to the ability of quinidine to prolong ventricular refractoriness.[137] In this setting, lidocaine and DPH are effective.

Quinidine has potentially proarrhythmic effects, perhaps by increasing the action potential duration restitution curve, inducing prolongation of the QTc interval, and causing early afterdepolarizations, that is, torsades de pointes.[21, 111–113] Elevation of plasma epinephrine levels within reported physiologic levels may antagonize the antiarrhythmic efficacy of quinidine.[138, 139, 140] In this context, in some patients in whom quinidine prevented inducible sustained ventricular tachycardia, it was found that tachycardia was inducible again during epinephrine infusion. It has also been reported that quinidine can convert nonsustained to sustained ventricular tachycardia.[141] Alternatively, the proarrhythmic effect of quinidine may be caused by its ability to induce chaotic cellular dynamics.[21, 42]

A number of methods have been suggested for rapidly achieving and maintaining therapeutic plasma levels of quinidine. For example, quinidine sulfate has often been given orally in 200- to 400-mg doses every 2 hours, followed by maintenance therapy of up to 3.0 g/d. The bihourly dose regimen is particularly useful in the chemical conversion of atrial fibrillation. An initial loading dose, which is twice the maintenance dose, has also been recommended for rapid attainment of a plateau plasma concentration. In this way, a single oral dose of 600 mg is administered safely.[142] If rapid attainment of therapeutic plasma levels is not essential, the maintenance dose of the drug (200 to 400 mg every 6 hours) may be commenced and a steady-state plasma concentration achieved after at least five eliminating half-lives have been exceeded (32 to 38 hours). Adjustment in dose should be dictated by patient response, serum levels, and toxic manifestations. The doses of quinidine gluconate and quinidine polygalacturo-

nate are larger than that of sulfate. A 324-mg tablet of the gluconate is equivalent to 240 mg of quinidine sulfate, and a 275-mg tablet of the polygalacturonate is equivalent to 200 mg of quinidine sulfate. When quinidine is given intravenously, 6 to 10 mg/kg of the gluconate should be administered slowly (i.e., 30 to 50 mg/min) with careful and continuous monitoring of the patient's clinical status, blood pressure, and electrocardiogram.[143] Quinidine is potentially very toxic, and its kinetics are highly variable, making plasma level monitoring highly desirable.

Quinidine toxicity (i.e., cinchonism) is characterized by various symptoms ranging from tinnitus, temporary deafness, headache, and blurred vision to diplopia, photophobia, vertigo, confusion, delirium, and, in severe cases, psychosis. Anorexia, nausea, vomiting, diarrhea, and abdominal colic occur frequently (i.e., in 20% of patients taking oral quinidine). These gastrointestinal disturbances, probably caused by local irritation, have been reported to be less severe when the polygalacturonate or a slow-release formulation of the sulfate was used.[144] Hypersensitivity reaction to quinidine is not common, but drug fever, urticaria, maculopapular rash, and exfoliative dermatitis have all been reported. Of the other allergic manifestations, anaphylactic reactions are rare, although a variety of hematologic effects have developed during protracted oral quinidine therapy, of which, thrombocytopenia is the best known.

Electrocardiographic monitoring of patients receiving maintenance quinidine therapy can detect early signs of toxicity by identifying characteristic widening of the QRS and the QTc intervals, with the QRS widening occurring at a lower concentration of the drug.[109] In advanced toxicity, the P wave becomes widened and deformed, and the sinus rate slows, eventually leading to intra-atrial conduction block and atrial arrest. Simultaneous intraventricular conduction abnormalities lead to ventricular tachycardia and fibrillation (quinidine syncope and sudden death).[114] Quinidine syncope appears to be related to the emergence of torsades de pointes.

In a study evaluating the mortality rate by meta-analysis, quinidine was found to be associated with significantly higher mortality (12 out of 502) when compared to flecainide (1 of 141), mexiletine (2 out of 246), propafenone (0 out of 53), and tocainide (1 out of 53).[145]

Procainamide

MODE OF ACTION. The cellular electrophysiologic properties of procainamide (Fig. 5-7) in isolated cardiac preparations, in both intact animals and humans, are similar to those of quinidine. Microelectrode studies have shown that the drug prolongs action potential duration and refractory period, decreases the rate of automatic impulse initiation and the rate of rise of phase zero ($\dot{V}_{max}$) in a

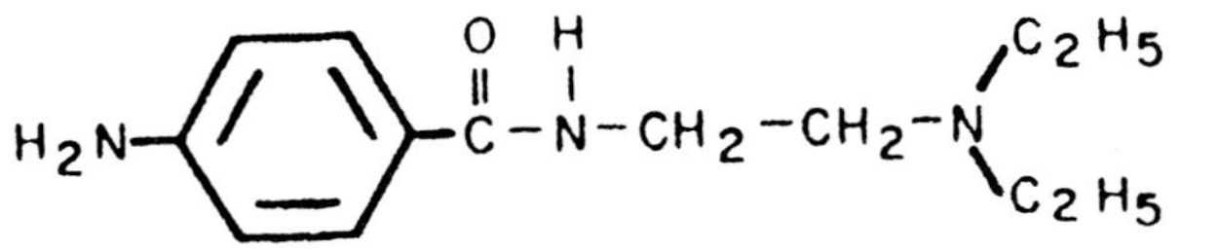

Figure 5-7. Procainamide.

rate-dependent manner, and slows conduction velocity.[17, 102, 146, 147] Procainamide-induced use-dependent block of the sodium channel seen in isolated tissues appeared to closely resemble the rate-dependent changes in conduction velocity that were observed in intact anesthetized dogs.[148] Slowed conduction induced by procainamide is greater in the direction longitudinal to myocardial fiber orientation than in the direction transverse to it, a phenomenon that could be ascribed to directional differences in effective membrane capacitance and axial resistivity.[94, 149] Furthermore, $\dot{V}_{max}$ is higher in the transverse direction than in the longitudinal direction despite slower conduction in the former.[94] This may be the reason, in part, for the greater slowing effects of the drugs (quinidine, procainamide, and lidocaine) on the longitudinal rather than on the transverse direction to myocardial fiber orientation.[94, 149] Arnsdorf and Bigger have shown that, in isolated Purkinje fibers, therapeutic concentrations of procainamide shifted threshold potential to a less negative value and shifted the non-normalized strength duration curve upward and to the right, indicating decreased excitability and increased refractoriness.[150] The decrease in excitability induced by procainamide, however, was not uniform. Rather, it depended on the relative contribution of procainamide-induced changes in both passive and active membrane properties.[150] Furthermore, the authors suggested that these findings may explain the conflicting results of cardiac excitability both in clinical and experimental studies, an effect that may also explain the proarrhythmic potential of procainamide in some patients. Procainamide shifts the strength interval curve of the right ventricular endocardium in humans upward and to the right as it does in isolated cardiac tissue preparations.[151]

It has recently been suggested that procainamide has a preferential effect on the reentry loop in patients with sustained monomorphic ventricular tachycardia, presumably by acting on diseased myocardial fibers, a suggestion consistent with the modulated receptor hypothesis of selective inhibition of sodium current in partially depolarized cells.[17, 152, 153] Procainamide-induced slowing of conduction can delay retrograde conduction in the depressed segment of a reentry loop, an effect that could convert unidirectional conduction block to bidirectional block. Once this occurs, a reentrant premature depolarization is terminated. Similar suggestions of preferential depression of area of abnormal conduction by procainamide were also made in a canine model of chronic (2 to 74

months) infarction.[154] Giardina and Bigger studied the effects of intravenous procainamide in patients with frequent premature ventricular depolarizations.[155] As plasma procainamide concentration was increased (2 to 7 μg/mL), the coupling interval of the premature complexes progressively increased until the premature beat was suppressed. The pharmacodynamic consequences of procainamide in humans were also evaluated by Morady and coworkers who showed that procainamide-induced changes in ventricular refractoriness and QRS duration in humans parallel changes in the plasma procainamide concentration and that relatively high infusion rates (8 mg/min) of the drug that causes higher plasma procainamide concentration did not cause additional increase in either refractoriness or QRS duration.[156] Rate-dependent increase in QRS duration has also observed with procainamide.[157] Consistent with these pharmacodynamic properties of procainamide, various clinical electrophysiologic studies have shown that procainamide prolonged refractory periods in the atrium, ventricle, and His–Purkinje system and slowed conduction in the His–Purkinje system as indicated by a 10% to 30% prolongation of the HV interval.[158] Gang and coworkers have shown that procainamide causes a rate-dependent prolongation of HV interval in humans.[159] In this study, the HV interval was measured during atrial pacing.[159] Similarly, procainamide causes a rate-dependent increase of intraventricular electrogram duration in humans, an effect that appears to be more accentuated in chronically infarcted tissue than in normal ventricular myocardium, an observation consistent with the modulated receptor hypothesis of sodium channels (i.e., selective depression of partially depolarized cells).[17, 160] These authors also reported, however, that during sinus rhythm, the prolonging effects of procainamide on indices of conduction in normal and abnormal myocardium were similar.[385]

The cardiac electrophysiologic effects of procainamide, along with its effects on heart rate and AV conduction, are variable because of the vagolytic actions of procainamide on the heart.[102] Vagal inhibition induced by procainamide offsets its direct myocardial depressant actions.

METABOLISM AND PHARMACOKINETICS. Absorption of oral procainamide is rapid and virtually complete. Koch-Weser and Klein studied the gastrointestinal absorption of the hydrochloride salt of procainamide in fasting healthy subjects.[162] After 15 to 20 minutes, first-order absorption kinetics were seen with a $t^{1/2}$ of absorption of 20 to 30 minutes. In healthy subjects, peak plasma levels are reached in 1 hour. Using titrated procainamide, Graffner and coworkers found that the AUC, after a single oral dose, was 75% of that observed after intravenous injection of the same dose.[163] The researchers estimated that the first-pass, or presystemic, elimination was approximately 15%. The extent of oral procainamide absorption in patients, however, is more variable. In patients with severe heart failure or myocardial infarction, intestinal absorption of procainamide is usually delayed and produces lower peak plasma levels.[164] An initial intravenous administration of procainamide in such patients was suggested as being more effective. Absorption of procainamide from sustained-release preparations is slower, which could lead to less fluctuation in plasma procainamide levels.[165] Absorption after intramuscular injection is fast and complete; peak levels are reached within 20 to 30 minutes.[166] However, intramuscular injections are painful and may raise plasma creatine phosphokinase. In patients with low cardiac output, peak plasma levels may be delayed.

Procainamide is metabolized in the liver through the action of polymorphic enzyme N-acetyltransferase, with conversion of the parent product to N-acetylprocainamide (NAPA). Dreyfuss and coworkers were the first to discover NAPA in the urine of rhesus monkeys and, later, in the pooled urine of four humans.[167] The rate and extent of procainamide acetylation depends on the genetically determined "acetylator phenotype."[167–172] Renal clearance is the major route of elimination of procainamide, with approximately 40% to 54% of the administered dose appearing in the urine. The 24-hour urinary excretion of NAPA under steady-state conditions varies between 6% and 25% of the administered dose. Between 2% and 10% of the administered dose is hydrolyzed to para-aminobenzoic acid.

The electrophysiologic and antiarrhythmic properties of NAPA are similar to those of procainamide.[146, 173] In addition, like procainamide, NAPA has vagolytic activity.[174] In a canine study, NAPA was found to decrease defibrillation energy requirements, whereas procainamide, at similar mean plasma concentrations (12 μg/mL), had no effect on defibrillation energy requirements.[175] NAPA, in contrast to its parent compound, is almost entirely eliminated by the kidney, necessitating extreme caution and careful titration of procainamide in patients with renal failure; constant monitoring of blood levels is necessary.[169, 176] The half-life of elimination of NAPA in patients with normal renal function is about twice that of procainamide (6 to 8 hours for NAPA); its apparent volume of distribution is 1.38 L/kg, and it appears to be well tolerated to levels as high as 40 μg/mL. Urinary excretion of both procainamide and NAPA correlates well with creatine clearance. Gibson and coworkers found the half-life (t^{1}/$_{2}$ beta) of procainamide to increase 11.3 to 16 hours in patients with renal failure.[169] Urinary pH can influence the elimination of procainamide. Renal clearance of procainamide increases with decreasing urine pH (aciduria) and decreases with increasing urine pH (alkaluria). This can be explained by the phenomenon of ion trapping. As the free base, procainamide enters the urine from the plasma by passive diffusion, it becomes charged (protonated) in acid urine. This charged form cannot reenter the plasma (ion trapping) and is eliminated in the urine.

THERAPEUTIC ACTION, DOSE, AND SIDE EFFECTS. Procainamide is effective in preventing and suppressing both ventricular and supraventricular arrhythmias. It is of particular value in patients with life-threatening ventricular arrhythmias who fail to respond to lidocaine.[177] Kuchar and coworkers showed that noninducibility of ventricular tachycardia with intravenous procainamide predicted long-term successful response to various oral antiarrhythmic drug therapies.[178] Interian and coworkers reported a study that sharply contrasts an earlier report on the value of acute intravenous procainamide for predicting long-term oral procainamide therapy.[179] The authors found that, in patients with inducible ventricular arrhythmia during predrug control study, the response to intravenous procainamide did not predict the arrhythmic outcome of subsequent oral administration of procainamide in doses that yielded similar or slightly higher plasma concentrations. The authors questioned the value of administering intravenous procainamide during serial electrophysiologic testing.[179] Similarly, a significant correlation between percent increases in rate-dependent QRS duration after procainamide administration and lengthening of ventricular tachycardia cycle was also reported, a finding that was attributed to rate-dependent changes in conduction caused by procainamide.[180] Morady and coworkers determined that there was an optimal plasma procainamide concentration range within which inducible sustained ventricular tachycardia could be suppressed and that additional procainamide administration (total of 22.5 mg/kg intravenously) causing undue elevation of plasma procainamide levels made the tachycardia reinducible.[157] The authors suggested that, during long-term therapy with procainamide, monitoring of its plasma concentration are important to remain within the effective plasma concentration range. Procainamide therapy is also effective in patients with the WPW syndrome; however, this effect does not seem to be uniform.[107, 108, 177, 181] Intravenous procainamide produces somewhat less cardiovascular depression than quinidine, although its negative inotropic effects are not negligible. Giardina and coworkers found that 100 mg of the drug can be safely given intravenously every 5 minutes to a total of 1 g.[182] During intravenous administration of procainamide, however, both blood pressure and electrocardiogram should be monitored continuously and the rate of drug administration should not exceed 50 mg/min.[162] The average patient requires 50 mg/kg/day of oral procainamide to achieve and maintain an acceptable therapeutic plasma level of 4 to 8 μg/mL.[162, 165] In some patients, plasma levels of 10 to 15 μg/mL are needed to suppress life-threatening arrhythmias. The intramuscular route offers little advantage over the oral route in most instances. It may be necessary to adjust the dose of procainamide to take into account plasma NAPA concentrations, because this metabolite has antiarrhythmic efficacy and a longer half-life especially in patients with renal failure. The patient who is a fast or slow "acetylator" may be unmasked by monitoring plasma levels of both compounds.

The limitations of procainamide therapy are largely caused by potentially troublesome side effects, which often occur after prolonged use of (high doses of) the drug. Toxic cardiac effects of procainamide, manifested by progressive lengthening of the QTc interval and QRS duration, are, in general, similar to those of quinidine and appear with a plasma concentration over 12 μg/mL. However, sudden death or recurrent syncope caused by ventricular tachycardia or ventricular fibrillation is less common than with quinidine use. During chronic oral administration, gastrointestinal side effects, especially with high doses, include anorexia, nausea, vomiting, and diarrhea. Hematologic complications such as leukopenia and agranulocytosis have been reported; these generally occur in the first 3 months of therapy and necessitate serial white blood cell count determinations.[182] A syndrome resembling systemic lupus erythematosus may appear in as many as 40% of patients chronically treated with procainamide.[183] The initial symptoms may appear as early as 2 weeks after the start of therapy or as late as several years later and include fever, rash, myalgia, arthralgia, arthritis, pericarditis, pleuritis, hepatosplenomegaly, and, occasionally, pericardial tamponade. This syndrome is associated with high antinuclear titers and is more likely to occur in patients who are slow acetylators of procainamide.[184] These drug-induced symptoms disappear when procainamide is discontinued. If they persist, corticosteroid therapy may help eliminate them.

Procainamide was found to exert less hemodynamic deterioration in patients with congestive heart failure than either encainide or tocainide.[185]

Disopyramide

MODE OF ACTION. Disopyramide (Norpace) has been approved for general clinical use since 1977. The cellular electrophysiologic properties of disopyramide are similar to those of quinidine and procainamide (Fig. 5-8). Disopyramide, in isolated Purkinje fibers, increases action potential duration and refractory periods with a concomitant decrease in action potential amplitude and maximum rate of rise of phase zero ($\dot{V}_{max}$) and conduction velocity; it does not affect resting membrane potential (Fig. 5-9).[33] The block of $\dot{V}_{max}$ by disopyramide does not dissipate with increasing diastolic intervals (up to seconds), suggesting that this block, unlike quinidine and procainamide, is

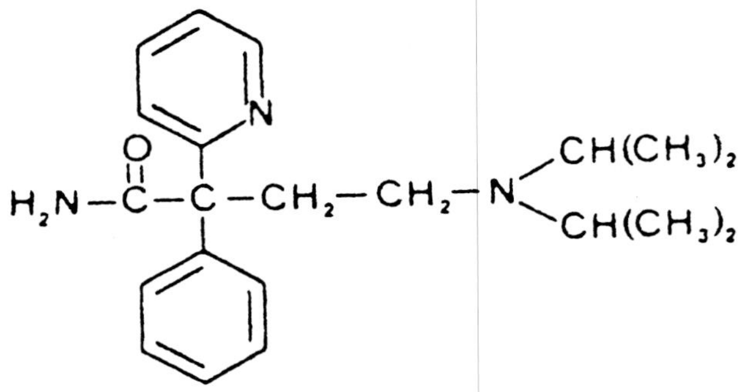

Figure 5-8. Disopyramide.

tonic and not use-dependent.[33] Disopyramide did not change the kinetics of action potential duration restitution.[33] The electropharmacologic effects of disopyramide are influenced by its stereochemical properties. The racemic disopyramide and (+)-disopyramide prolong action potential duration measured at 95% repolarization in canine Purkinje fibers, whereas the (−)-disopyramide shortens the action potential duration in a time and concentration-dependent manner.[186] These directionally opposite effects of disopyramide indicate that the stereochemical configuration of disopyramide determines its effect on repolarization of cardiac Purkinje fibers.[186] The clinical significance of these observations with respect to arrhythmia suppression is undefined.

Disopyramide has no appreciable effect on slow-response action potentials but suppresses the slope of spontaneous diastolic depolarization in Purkinje fibers with high resting membrane potentials.[187] Lowering the extracellular potassium concentration tends to reverse the membrane-depressant effects of the drug.[99] In addition, disopyramide has important anticholinergic (atropine-like) properties that often offset its direct membrane-depressant effects on the myocardium.[103] For example, its depressant effect on AV conduction is nullified or even reversed so that the PR interval may be little altered or even shortened.[188] Pretreatment with atropine (0.02 mg/kg) allows more uniform inducement of the depressant effects of disopyramide, namely, prolonged AH interval and functional refractory period of the AV node, prolonged sinus nodal recovery time, and slowed heart rate.[189] Using microelectrode technique on isolated rabbit sinoatrial preparations, Katoh and coworkers have shown that disopyramide depresses sinus nodal automaticity at upper therapeutic and toxic levels during cholinergic blockade; its acceleratory action on the sinus node appears at a much lower concentration and only during cholinergic stimulation.[190] These results indicate that earlier reports of the variable effects of disopyramide on conduction and sinus rate could have been caused by its inhibitory effects on vagal tone. However, in high doses, direct depressant

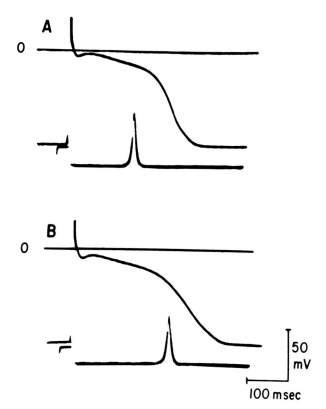

Figure 5-9. Effect of disopyramide, 10^{-5} M, on Purkinje fiber action potential (cycle length = 500 msec; T = 37° C). In (**A**) and (**B**), the top trace is a reference, zero potential; the middle trace is an action potential recorded using an intracellular glass microelectrode; and the bottom trace is the electronically differentiated upstroke of a sawtooth wave, with a rate of rise of 200 V/sec followed by the differentiated phase 0 upstroke of the action potential, V_{max}. (**A**) is a control. (**B**) shows effects of disopyramide, 10^{-3} M. Note the decrease in action potential amplitude and V_{max} and the prolongation of the voltage-time course of repolarization. (Danilo P, Rosen MR: Cardiac effects of disopyramide. Am Heart J 1976;92:532.)

effects predominate, including widening of the QRS and QT intervals and slowing of the sinus rate.

METABOLISM AND PHARMACOKINETICS. The metabolism and pharmacokinetic disposition of disopyramide have not been completely determined, particularly in various disease states.[191] Ward and Kingham reported that postinfarction patients achieved about a twofold lower concentration of disopyramide after oral administration of 100 mg than did healthy subjects who attained a peak level of about 3 μg/mL.[192] Orally administered disopyramide phosphate is well absorbed, albeit relatively slowly, with a bioavailability of approximately 90%.[193,194] Peak serum concentrations generally occur 2 to 3 hours after administration and may be maintained for several hours, because the terminal half-life (t½ beta) of disopyramide is 5 to 6 hours in healthy persons.[192–195] Total disopyramide clearance is ap-

proximately 1.5 mL/min/kg, and its apparent volume of distribution is 0.8 L/kg. Serum binding of disopyramide decreases with increasing serum concentration; at therapeutic concentration (range, 2 to 6 μg/mL), about 30% to 50% of the drug in the serum is free.[194–196] In this concentration range, the free fraction varies relatively little, and no important clinical consequences related to the protein binding of disopyramide have been reported. Because the clearance of the drug depends on its free levels and because the level of free drug increases as the concentration of disopyramide increases (protein unbinding), disopyramide displays nonlinear pharmacokinetics with respect to total drug concentration.[191,197] For this reason, there is less than proportional increase in total drug concentration as the dose is increased. With multiple doses, however, the free concentration does not increase linearly with dose. The major metabolite of disopyramide, the N-dealkylated form, has some antiarrhythmic efficacy (about 50% of the parent drug); it is formed in the liver and excreted in the urine.

THERAPEUTIC ACTION, DOSE, AND SIDE EFFECTS. Disopyramide is effective in suppressing premature depolarizations and tachycardias of both supraventricular and ventricular origin.[197–199] Its ability to prolong conduction time and refractory period of the accessory pathway in patients with the WPW syndrome may also be useful in the management of arrhythmias associated with the preexcitation syndrome.[200] In patients with supraventricular arrhythmias, disopyramide has been used to prevent recurrences of atrial fibrillation after direct current conversion to sinus rhythm. Disopyramide was also found to terminate paroxysmal supraventricular tachycardia, atrial flutter, and atrial fibrillation of recent onset.[197] However, the atropine-like actions of disopyramide make the drug of limited value in the management of patients with paroxysmal atrial tachycardia resulting from AV nodal reentry. Moreover, facilitation of AV conduction in susceptible patients may increase the ventricular response rate in atrial flutter and fibrillation.

In a large multicenter study, disopyramide was found to suppress ventricular arrhythmias effectively.[201] Furthermore, in a double-blind comparative study with quinidine, disopyramide was found to have similar efficacy in suppressing ventricular premature depolarizations, with an overall decrease of about 88% with disopyramide and 93% with quinidine.[94] The incidence of side effects, however, was higher with quinidine. Disopyramide has potential proarrhythmic effects [???]. Recent studies have also indicated that disopyramide may be of value in the prophylaxis of ventricular arrhythmias in patients with recent myocardial infarction.[203,204] Rangno and coworkers showed that, in postinfarction patients, the drug had a somewhat reduced clearance and prolonged half-life of about 12 hours, presumably because of impaired renal function.[205] The authors suggested that a suitable intravenous regimen would be 2 mg/kg over 15 minutes, then 2 mg/kg over the next 45 minutes, followed by a maintenance infusion of 0.4 mg/kg/h. Such a regimen would yield a plasma level of about 4 μg/mL in patients with an average clearance level of 57 mL/min. These doses should be reduced in patients who show greater reductions in creatine clearance.

In most patients, plasma levels of disopyramide within a 2- to 4-μg/mL range can be achieved with daily divided doses of 400 to 1200 mg. If rapid attainment of therapeutic levels is desired, a loading dose of the drug (200 to 300 mg) can be given, followed by maintenance doses every half-life (5 to 6 hours). Recently, a sustained-release preparation (Norpace) has become available, allowing a 12-hour dosage schedule. Intravenous disopyramide (2 mg/kg) exerts mild negative inotropic action on the heart, an effect less apparent after oral administration. Although disopyramide is well tolerated after oral administration, 10% to 40% of patients reported side effects caused by the anticholinergic activity of the drug. Side effects included dry mouth, urinary hesitancy, constipation, blurred vision, and dry eyes, nose, and throat.[202] Although the drug is similar to quinidine, disopyramide-induced syncope (ventricular tachycardia and ventricular fibrillation) or marked QTc prolongation has not been reported with usual maintenance doses of disopyramide.

Observations in patients with recent myocardial infarction have suggested that the drug exerts more profound negative inotropic effects in this patient group.[206] The exact cause of this effect in the setting of acute myocardial infarction is unclear.

Lidocaine

MODE OF ACTION. Microelectrode studies on isolated cardiac tissue preparations have shown that lidocaine (Fig. 5-10) invariably shortens action potential duration and refractoriness but delays the reactivation process of excitability.[33,82,102,207–209] Maximum rate of rise of phase zero ($\dot{V}_{max}$) is decreased in a concentration-dependent and use-dependent manner, with a depression of membrane responsiveness.[17,33,82,209,210] The development of sodium channel block and recovery from it appear to depend on temperature.[211] These effects are more pronounced in the presence of 4- to 5.4-mM extracellular potassium concentration and are negligible or nonexistent when extracellular potassium concentration is lowered to 2.7 mM.[208,212,213] The decrease in the action potential duration, $\dot{V}_{max}$, and contractile force have been suggested to be caused by a reduction in intracellular sodium ion concentration.[209] Voltage-clamp studies on isolated rabbit myocytes, using single channel analysis, have shown that lidocaine blocks

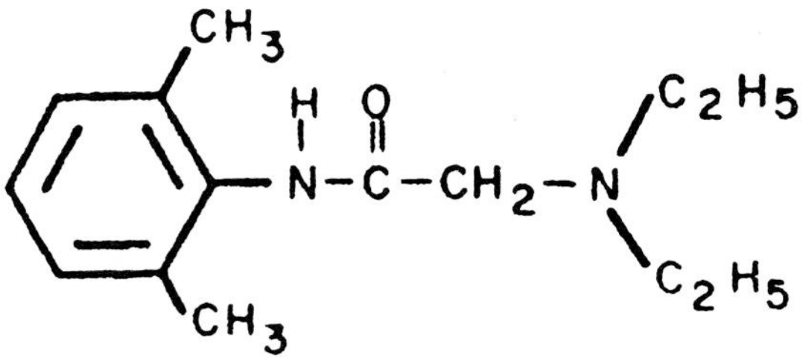

Figure 5-10. Lidocaine.

the sodium channel.[214] This block occurs as a result of binding of lidocaine to a specific receptor site, presumably in the cardiac sodium channel, that is also common to quinidine, and which can competitively be displaced by lidocaine's metabolite, glycilxylidide.[101,215] According to the modulated receptor hypothesis, lidocaine blocks the sodium channel in the inactive state (channel closed).[17,216] Because atrial action potential duration is relatively short, the degree of lidocaine block of sodium channel is, therefore, limited; the duration for which atrial fibers spend in the closed state is short.[216] This property of lidocaine may explain, in part, the relative inefficacy of lidocaine against atrial arrhythmias caused by reentry.

These membrane-depressant effects, when present, are expected to slow conduction velocity and could theoretically convert areas of unidirectional conduction block into bidirectional block, thus terminating reentrant arrhythmias.[13,99] However, study of normal atrial tissue has shown that lidocaine has no effect on the wavelength of the atrial impulse (wavelength = refractory period × conduction velocity), thus explaining, in part, the lack of antiarrhythmic efficacy of lidocaine against reentrant atrial tachycardias.[12] For a drug to be effective against reentrant arrhythmias, it must prolong the wavelength.[12] Whether lidocaine increases the wavelength of the ventricular impulse remains undefined. In canine Purkinje fibers, Elharrar has shown that lidocaine, unlike disopyramide, slows the kinetics of action potential duration restitution (prolongation) (i.e., a decrease in the time constant of the fast decaying exponential component of the restitution curve), the mechanism of which may be caused by slowing of the deactivation kinetics of the delayed rectifier current (iX1).[33]

Lidocaine seems to exert a preferentially greater membrane-depressant effect on ischemic and hypoxic myocardial cells than on normal cardiac fibers.[82] Isolated tissue studies with microelectrodes have shown a greater degree of depression of $\dot{V}_{max}$ and conduction velocity as well as slower recovery from the process of inactivation with lidocaine in acidic and hypoxic media.[217,218] Lidocaine at therapeutic concentrations can abolish tetrodotoxin-sensitive depressed fast responses in depolarized tissues that still depend on the sodium channel.[219,220]

Lamenna and coworkers have shown that lidocaine

impairs conduction through potassium-depolarized isolated Purkinje fibers, an effect the authors suggest is caused by suppression of a background sodium current.[221] This may impart significant antiarrhythmic properties to lidocaine in a setting of ischemic arrhythmias.[13,99] The degree of shortening of action potential duration and refractoriness of Purkinje fibers by lidocaine is related to the location of the Purkinje fiber cell, because the most pronounced effect is seen at a site close to where the free running strands insert into the ventricular myocardium. Furthermore, lidocaine causes the greatest changes in action potential duration and refractoriness in normal Purkinje fibers, where the parameters are very long.[208] Lidocaine suppresses spontaneous diastolic depolarization and automatic impulse initiation at membrane potentials between -90 and -70 mV. This occurs at lidocaine concentrations that do not affect sinus node automaticity.[222] Lidocaine was also found to decrease the amplitude of ouabain-induced delayed afterdepolarization in Purkinje fibers; however, such an effect was not seen in ventricular fibers.[223,224] In long mammalian Purkinje fibers superfused with lidocaine containing 4 mM of potassium, Arnsdorf and Bigger found that lidocaine shifted the normalized strength-duration curve toward higher current levels to elicit an action potential without altering the resting membrane or threshold potential.[207,225] These effects differ from those of procainamide in that lidocaine does not shift membrane threshold potential to less negative values; rather, it increases threshold current primarily by increasing subthreshold membrane conductance. More recently, Karagueuzian and coworkers have shown that lidocaine had no effect on the strength-interval curve of the right ventricular endocardium in intact dogs.[226,227]

METABOLISM AND PHARMACOKINETICS. Lidocaine is primarily eliminated by metabolism in the liver, which efficiently removes the drug from the circulation. As a result of this high hepatic extraction, the clearance of lidocaine approaches hepatic blood flow.[73,228] Furthermore, lidocaine clearance and lidocaine plasma concentration are greatly influenced by alteration in liver blood flow and liver disease.[75,228] A number of lidocaine metabolites have been identified. Two such metabolites with some pharmacologic action that have undergone clinical experimental investigations are monoethylglycine xylidide (MEGX), which has some antiarrhythmic efficacy, and glycine xylidide (GX), which potentiates the convulsant action of both lidocaine and MEGX and which can displace lidocaine from its binding sites.[229,215] Lidocaine is not recommended to be administered orally because of high presystemic (hepatic) elimination of approximately 80% of the dose.[73] When doses four to five times higher are administered to achieve therapeutic plasma levels similar to procainamide, considerable toxic side effects occur. In addition, gastric irritation becomes a major clinical problem. Attempts have been made to develop congeners of lidocaine that are less efficiently extracted by the liver so that they could be orally effective. Tocainide and mexiletine seem useful in this regard.

Disposition of lidocaine may be explained based on the linear two-compartment model. In healthy persons, the $t\frac{1}{2}$ alpha of the rapid phase of distribution is about 8 minutes, and the $t\frac{1}{2}$ beta of elimination from the peripheral compartment is about 100 minutes. The volume of the central compartment is approximately 0.44 L/kg, and the volume of distribution steady state is 1.1 L/kg, with a total body clearance averaging 10 mL/min/kg.[73,74] Little (<3%) lidocaine is excreted unchanged in the urine. Thus, renal function impairment has no significant effect on lidocaine pharmacokinetics. However, in patients with heart failure, lidocaine clearance is reduced to about 60% because of reduced liver blood flow.[73-75] Consequently, approximately 60% reduction in the maintenance dose of lidocaine should be contemplated in these patients to avoid toxic side effects. Similar considerations should also apply in patients with liver disease and reduced hepatic blood flow.[73,74]

THERAPEUTIC ACTION, DOSE, AND SIDE EFFECTS. Lidocaine is effective against ventricular arrhythmias of diverse clinical causes (e.g., surgery, ischemic heart disease, digitalis toxicity). It is considered the drug of choice for the emergency intravenous therapy of patients with ventricular arrhythmias because it is relatively devoid of toxic side effects and because antiarrhythmic plasma concentration can be rapidly achieved by intravenous titration.[73,230] Intravenous prophylactic lidocaine given for 48 hours after the onset of symptoms indicating acute myocardial infarction was found to be of value in preventing primary ventricular fibrillation.[231-234] Lidocaine with a mean plasma concentration of 8.2 μg/mL was found to double the energy required for defibrillation in experimental canine studies.[175] The clinical significance of these findings in otherwise nondiseased normal canine ventricular myocardium remains undefined. In rare cases, lidocaine may aggravate arrhythmias and may even be lethal.[235,236] The mechanism of these paradoxic effects (proarrhythmia) of lidocaine require further investigation.[237] Lidocaine is relatively ineffective in the management of patients with supraventricular arrhythmias.[230,238,239] However, lidocaine may be useful against supraventricular tachyarrhythmias in patients with WPW syndrome, in whom atrial impulses conducting antegradely over an AV bypass tract may be slowed.[240] Lidocaine is also effective against ventricular tachycardia that occurs 1 day after either left or right coronary artery occlusion in the dog.[226,241] The mechanism of these tachycardias are thought to be caused by an automatic mechanism.[226,241]

The therapeutic range of plasma lidocaine levels is 1.6 to 5 μg/mL.[73] As discussed, the infusion rate at steady state is equal to the desired steady-state plasma concentration multiplied by the clearance. For example, if a 3-μg/mL steady-state plasma lidocaine level is desired, with a clearance of 10 mL/kg/min, the infusion rate of lidocaine should be 30 μg/kg/min. If, in patients with heart failure, the clearance is reduced by 50%, the infusion rate becomes 15 μg/kg/min. Discontinuing lidocaine 5 half-lives (90 minutes per half-life) before electrophysiologic testing could not ensure lack of electrophysiologic effects of either the parent drug or its metabolite.[242] Therefore, more than 5.5 half-lives were necessary to wash out the effects of lidocaine and its metabolites.

In patients with normal weight and cardiac output, approximately 175 mg of lidocaine should be given in the first 10 to 15 minutes. This dose is given as a single intravenous injection over 5 to 10 minutes or as a series of small injections several minutes apart.[243] If arrhythmias recur during this initial phase, a small (25 to 50 mg) bolus injection should be given while a constant infusion of 2 to 4 mg/min, initiated after the loading dose, is continued. When breakthrough arrhythmias occur after steady-state conditions have been attained, a further small bolus and a temporary increase in infusion rate become necessary.

Lidocaine is considered relatively safe and free from adverse hemodynamic side effects. The most commonly reported adverse effects are related to central nervous system toxicity and include dizziness, paresthesias, confusion, delirium, stupor, seizure, and coma. The drug normally has minimal depressant effects on the cardiac conducting system.[240] Larger doses, however, may produce heart block because of a preexisting abnormally long His–Purkinje conduction time.[244] Life-threatening increases in ventricular rates have been reported after lidocaine administration in patients with atrial tachyarrhythmia and rapid ventricular response.[236] However, clinically significant adverse hemodynamic effects rarely occur. When propranolol is administered with lidocaine, clearance is decreased and plasma level of lidocaine increases because propranolol decreases hepatic blood flow.[73, 245]

Diphenylhydantoin

Because it is devoid of potent inherent antiarrhythmic effects and is associated with a wide range of toxic side effects, DPH (Fig. 5-11), formerly known as phenytoin, has a limited role in the management of patients with cardiac arrhythmias.

MODE OF ACTION. Microelectrode studies have shown that DPH depresses the slope of both spontaneous phase 4 depolarization and the amplitude of ouabain-induced af-

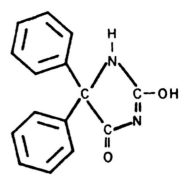

Figure 5-11. Diphenylhydantoin.

terdepolarizations in Purkinje fibers, effects that slow the rate of automatic impulse initiation that may eventually suppress ectopic automatic foci.[246–248] Like lidocaine, DPH depresses the maximum rate of phase zero depolarization in a use- and concentration-dependent manner.[249] These effects appear to depend on extracellular potassium concentration.[250] With a low potassium level (3 mM), the membrane-depressant effect of DPH is minimal. The drug markedly shortens action potential duration and delays reactivation kinetics of the fast sodium inward current, as do other antiarrhythmic drugs.[82, 102] This effect leads to delay in the recovery of excitability.

Some of the antiarrhythmic properties of DPH may be mediated through its central nervous system depressant actions.[11, 102] Because AV nodal cells are highly innervated, DPH-induced effects on the AV transmission may be partly attributed to the initial state of autonomic tone and the nature and extent of interaction of DPH with sympathetic or parasympathetic components of the autonomic nervous system.

METABOLISM AND PHARMACOKINETICS. Diphenylhydantoin is eliminated almost entirely by metabolism by way of hepatic microsomal enzyme systems, which convert DPH to 5-phenylhydantoin by parahydroxylation.[251] The elimination of DPH is an example of zero-order kinetics (nonlinear); that is, the metabolism (elimination) becomes a saturated process over the therapeutic range of plasma concentration (10 to 20 μg/mL). Once the process of elimination becomes saturated, the clearance of DPH progressively reduces and its half-life is prolonged as dose increases.[251–253] Most patients can metabolize at least 10 mg/kg/d; however, this may change with disease states and administration of other drugs.[254] Bishydroxycoumarin, chloramphenicol, isoniazid, chlorpromazine, prochlorperazine, chlordiazepoxide, and diazepam inhibit DPH metabolism by competing for hepatic enzymes, whereas carbamazepine and phenobarbital stimulate DPH metabolism, mostly through microsomal enzyme induction.[73] The dose at which metabolism becomes saturated varies widely among patients, and, at best, the clinician can approximate average pharmacokinetic values. Therefore, continuous plasma monitoring of DPH levels is highly desirable. An average half-life value of 22 hours can be used as a guide.[73] Thus, 3 to 5 half-lives (3 to 4 days) are required to reach a steady state.

In healthy subjects, 90% of DPH is protein bound, mostly to albumin, but this percentage can be altered by various disease states.[255] Decreased binding was seen in patients with renal failure, hypoalbuminemia, the nephrotic syndrome, and hyperbilirubinemia as well as in those receiving phenylbutazone and salicylic acid. In these patients, therefore, the concentration of free DPH tends to increase, causing toxic side effects. However, as greater free-to-bound DPH ratios become available, greater metabolism of DPH is expected, if microsomal enzymes are not yet saturated. Similar total DPH plasma concentrations may be associated with variable free, unbound plasma DPH levels. Therefore, total DPH plasma levels should not be used for accurate monitoring; free DPH levels should be considered instead. Finally, DPH metabolism can be altered significantly by a genetically determined defect in parahydroxylation.[256] Such patients are expected to maintain higher DPH levels for a given dose, with an attendant decrease in clearance and prolonged half-life.

THERAPEUTIC ACTION, DOSE, AND SIDE EFFECTS. The use of DPH as an antiarrhythmic agent is usually limited to the management of patients with atrial and ventricular arrhythmias caused by digitalis toxicity.[257,258] Ventricular arrhythmias associated with other disease processes respond much less frequently to DPH.[257,259–261] Some success has been noted in the management of patients with ventricular arrhythmias associated with general anesthesia, cardiac surgery, and direct current cardioversion of atrial tachyarrhythmias.[238] DPH is not considered effective in the management of atrial arrhythmias not caused by digitalis toxicity. DPH is generally given orally, 750 to 1000 mg in divided doses for loading, followed by 300 to 400 mg daily. If given intravenously, small doses (30 to 50 mg/min) are injected to avoid hypotension, until toxicity develops (nystagmus) or 1000 mg is reached.[261] For oral maintenance, appropriate allowances should be made for other drugs being given and for the state of the patient's hepatic function.

Intravenous DPH can cause severe hypotension, especially in the elderly. This effect is dose related and occurs with rapid intravenous loading. It is, however, transient, rarely lasting more than 20 minutes. The most common manifestations of DPH toxicity relate to central nervous system effects, including nystagmus, dizziness, ataxia, stupor, and coma. Adverse electrophysiologic effects are rare. DPH may cause sinus node depression and bradycardia,

increased ventricular response to atrial flutter or fibrillation (facilitation of AV conduction), or even AV block.[248]

A number of unusual syndromes with unknown cause may also develop in patients receiving chronic oral DPH therapy. Gingival hyperplasia may develop in as many as 40% of patients. Other complications include systemic lupus erythematosus, pseudolymphoma, osteomalacia, peripheral neuropathy, megaloblastic anemia, and a variety of dermatologic disorders including pigmentation and hirsutism. The development of lymphadenopathy is often diagnostically confusing but disappears when DPH is withdrawn.

Propranolol

MODE OF ACTION. The antiarrhythmic properties of propranolol (Fig. 5-12) are brought about by beta-adrenergic receptor blocking properties, which occur at low plasma levels (25 to 500 ng/mL), and by direct "membrane-depressant" actions, which occur at higher plasma levels.

On isolated cardiac tissue preparations, microelectrode studies have shown that beta-blocking concentrations of propranolol have little or no effect on transmembrane potential properties. However, such beta-blocking concentrations effectively decrease the slope of spontaneous phase 4 depolarization and the rate of automatic impulse initiation in both sinus and ectopic pacemakers, especially when automaticity is promoted by catecholamines or ouabain.[262] Therefore, arrhythmias caused by enhanced automaticity with sympathetic hyperactivity are likely to respond to beta-adrenergic blockade. At higher concentrations, propranolol, like lidocaine, exerts membrane-depressant effects by depressing fast sodium inward current on Purkinje fibers (i.e., there is a decrease in membrane responsiveness).[262] Although propranolol possesses stereospecific beta-adrenergic properties, racemic propranolol and the optical stereoisomers are equally potent in decreasing the maximum rate of depolarization and action potential amplitude of human and canine cardiac fibers.[263] Both ventricular action potential duration and refractoriness are shortened, although the former is

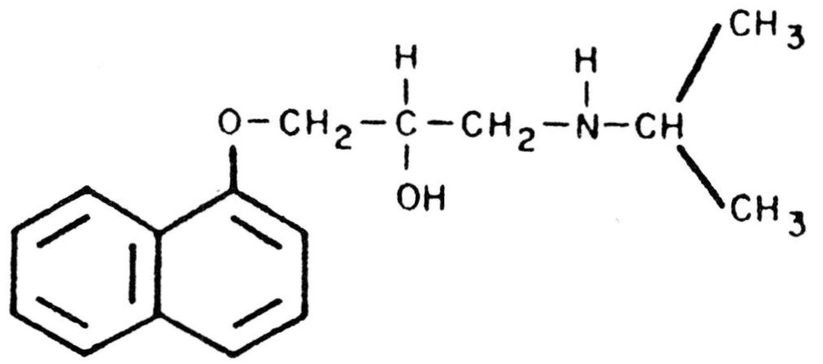

Figure 5-12. Propranolol.

shortened more than the latter. This effect is similar to that of lidocaine, because propranolol delays the reactivation kinetics of the fast sodium current, thereby delaying recovery of excitability.[82, 102, 262] Beta-blocking effects of propranolol are expected to increase AV nodal refractoriness and slow conduction velocity (i.e., remove the sympathetic facilitation effect). Both of these effects are of great value in suppressing reentrant supraventricular tachycardia using the AV node as part of the reentry circuit. This action of propranolol on the AV node can also be of value in decreasing ventricular response rate during atrial tachycardias, particularly when used in combination with digitalis.[99, 238, 262]

METABOLISM AND PHARMACOKINETICS. Propranolol is eliminated almost entirely by hepatic metabolism. Bioavailability of a single oral dose of propranolol is very low because of presystemic elimination caused by a high hepatic extraction ratio. Large variations in peak plasma levels (up to 20-fold) occur in patients given the same oral dose of propranolol.[73] These variabilities may be partly related to the level of hepatic blood flow, the ability of hepatic microsomal enzyme to metabolize propranolol, and the dose. At low propranolol concentrations, virtually all of the drug is removed by the liver. The major metabolite of propranolol is 4-hydroxypropranolol. Its role in arrhythmia suppression is not defined. During chronic oral therapy, the hepatic extraction ratio of propranolol falls to almost 65% as hepatic microsomal sites become saturated. Plasma propranolol levels under these conditions become a function of the administered dose. The clearance of propranolol, like lidocaine, is limited by hepatic blood flow. The half-life of elimination of propranolol is between 2 and 5 hours (3.2 hours after a single oral dose and 4.6 hours after chronic therapy). The clearance of propranolol is approximately 1 L/min, and its apparent volume of distribution is 3 L/kg. About 90% of the drug is bound to protein. Patient variations in plasma propranolol levels reflect variations in hepatic blood flow.[73, 262, 264]

Although pharmacokinetic interaction with other drugs has not been described in clinical reports, drugs that stimulate microsomal enzymes, such as phenobarbital, probably decrease the half-life of propranolol; drugs that inhibit these enzymes, such as chlorpromazine, tend to increase its half-life and plasma level, causing toxic side effects.

THERAPEUTIC ACTION, DOSE, AND SIDE EFFECTS. The ability of propranolol to slow conduction and increase refractoriness in the AV node makes it useful in the management and prevention of paroxysmal supraventricular tachycardia. However, for supraventricular tachycardias, especially those that occur after cardiac surgery, the ultra-short beta blocker esmolol, which is easily titrated, is preferred over

propranolol.[265] When prophylaxis is considered, propranolol combined with digitalis is particularly useful. Arrhythmias that are largely caused by excess sympathetic nervous activity, such as exercise-induced arrhythmias and those associated with pheochromocytoma, thyrotoxicosis, and anesthesization with cyclopropane or halothane, can be suppressed with propranolol.[266, 267] Patients with resistant arrhythmias after myocardial infarction may respond well to propranolol. Propranolol and other beta blockers may reduce the incidence of sudden cardiac death in survivors of myocardial infarction.[268–270] Propranolol is the drug of choice in the treatment of arrhythmias associated with prolonged QT interval.[262] Similarly, propranolol is helpful in treating patients with arrhythmias associated with mitral valve prolapse.[271, 272] It has been suggested that combination therapy with beta blockers and class I antiarrhythmic agents is safe and effective in the management of patients whose ventricular arrhythmias are refractory to therapeutic doses of class I drugs alone.[135]

Propranolol may be administered orally or intravenously. An average plasma level of 50 ng/mL is expected when 160 mg/d of propranolol is given orally, but the range in plasma levels is so wide that this figure is only an approximation.[272] Individual titration of the dosing schedule is therefore necessary. Reduction of resting heart rate to 50 to 55 beats per minute after propranolol administration may reflect achievement of adequate sympathetic blockade. If arrhythmias fail to respond to propranolol, daily doses of up to 640 mg should be considered, unless side effects limit this regimen.

When intravenous propranolol is indicated, doses of 0.1 to 0.15 mg/kg can be administered slowly at a rate not exceeding 1 mg/min. McAllister proposed a single dose of 11.4 mg (1 mg/min) followed by an infusion at a rate of 0.055 mg/min.[273] This regimen causes a steady-state plasma propranolol level of 38 ng/mL after 30 minutes. Continuous hemodynamic and electrocardiographic monitoring during intravenous propranolol infusion is necessary, especially in patients with cardiac decompensation.

The most common side effects of propranolol include worsening of asthmatic attacks, congestive heart failure, and depression of sinus node function and AV nodal conduction. Among insulin-dependent diabetics, propranolol may increase the risk of hypoglycemia. Impaired sexual activity (impotence) and easy fatigability occur with chronic propranolol therapy. Symptoms probably related to sympathetic supersensitivity have been observed after abrupt withdrawal from chronic (i.e., 12 weeks') propranolol therapy.[274, 275] Diarrhea may also occur. Sympathetic supersensitivity to the chronotropic effect of isoproterenol has been demonstrated among patients with essential hypertension who are abruptly withdrawn from propranolol therapy. Therefore, gradual reduction of propranolol doses should be considered to avoid withdrawal

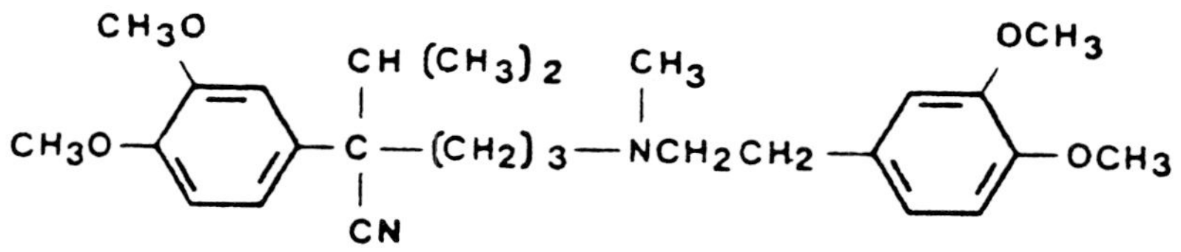

Figure 5-13. Verapamil.

symptoms, which may include unstable angina, myocardial infarction, and even sudden death. Even gradual withdrawal has, at times, been associated with failure.[276]

Verapamil

MODE OF ACTION. In 1982, verapamil (Fig. 5-13), a slow channel blocking agent, became available for clinical use in the United States, mainly for the management of patients with supraventricular tachyarrhythmias.

Microelectrode studies in isolated cardiac tissue have shown that the electrophysiologic effects of verapamil differ from those of other antiarrhythmic agents. At concentrations considered therapeutic, verapamil exerts little or no effect on normal Purkinje fibers except for minor acceleration of phase 2 repolarization and a slight depression of the plateau (Fig. 5-14).[277] In depressed fibers (resting potential less negative than -60 mV) and sinus nodal fibers, verapamil suppresses the excitatory depolarizing current, which is mainly carried by calcium and sodium ions.[277–279] In depressed fibers (atrial or ventricular) manifesting spontaneous automatic activity or delayed afterdepolarization with the potential for triggered automatic activity, verapamil can terminate such ectopic automatic foci (Fig. 5-15). Therefore, it seems that verapamil could terminate reentrant arrhythmias by further reducing the slow conduction in one limb of a reentry circuit as well as terminating arrhythmias caused by abnormal automatic activity. Because these arrhythmic mechanisms are generated by the secondary, or slow inward, current to initiate and maintain cardiac arrhythmias, verapamil, which suppresses this current, can eliminate these arrhythmic mechanisms. Although verapamil can suppress triggered automaticity in both Purkinje and ventricular muscle fibers, its role in the management of patients with ventricular tachycardia is still controversial.[223, 224] Verapamil exerts stereospecific effects on both the fast sodium current and the slow inward current.[280, 281] The $(+)$-stereoisomer exerts potent inhibitory effects on the fast inward current, whereas the $(-)$-isomer has little effect on the fast current, yet it produces a marked reduction in the magnitude of the slow inward current.[280, 281] The different effects of the stereoisomers of verapamil on these two depolarizing currents suggest that each isomer binds to different specific membrane "receptor" sites to alter transmembrane flow of

sodium and calcium currents. Results obtained in humans are in line with these experimental observations. The $(-)$-isomer of verapamil is 8 to 10 times more potent than the $(+)$-isomer in prolonging the PR interval.[282] The $(-)$-isomer of verapamil is more potent in prolonging the AV nodal conduction time because AV nodal cells rely mainly on the slow inward current for impulse transmission.[282]

METABOLISM AND PHARMACOKINETICS. Verapamil is eliminated largely by metabolism in the liver; only 5% is found in urine in the unchanged form. The major metabolite with pharmacologic activity has been identified as N-demethyl verapamil, or norverapamil.[282, 283] The large hepatic capacity to metabolize verapamil is consistent with

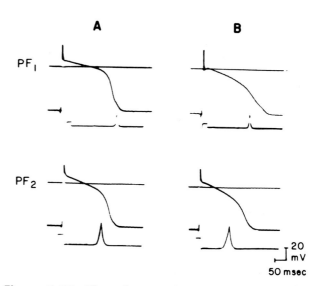

Figure 5-14. Effects of verapamil on normal canine cardiac Purkinje fibers. (**A**) is the action potential, and (**B**) shows a 200-V/sec calibration followed by electronic differentiation of the maximum rate of rise of phase 0 (V_{max}). (**A**) is a control record of two Purkinje fiber potentials: PF_1 and PF_2. (**B**) shows the same action potentials 30 minutes after onset of superfusion with verapamil, 1 mg/L. Note that this concentration of verapamil has no effect on action potential amplitude or V_{max} or on resting membrane potential. However, the voltage at which the plateau originates is decreased and the slope of phase 2 repolarization is increased by verapamil. These changes are consistent with the block of a slow inward current such as that of calcium ion. (Rosen MR, Wit AL, Hoffman BF: Electrophysiology and pharmacology of cardiac arrhythmias. VI. Cardiac effects of verapamil. Am Heart J 1975;89:665.)

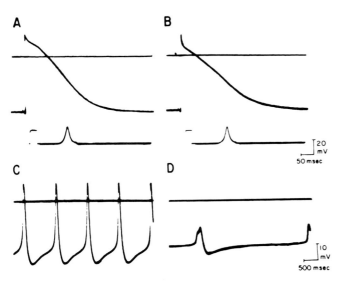

Figure 5-15. Effects of verapamil on specialized conducting fibers from normal and diseased human atria. (**A**) and (**B**) are from a segment of normal human atrium stimulated at a cycle length of 800 msec. (**A**) is a control. In (**B**), after 30 minutes of superfusion with verapamil, 1 mg/L, resting membrane potential, action potential amplitude, and $\dot{V}_{max}$ are unchanged. However, the voltage at which the plateau originates is decreased and the slope of phase 2 is increased. (**C**) and (**D**) were recorded from an isolated sample of diseased human atrium. (**C**) is a control record of the spontaneous rhythm occurring in this tissue. In (**D**), following 7 minutes of superfusion with verapamil, 1 mg/L, the maximum diastolic potential, the slope of phase 4, and the spontaneous rate have decreased, and action potential amplitude is markedly diminished. Within 1 minute, the preparation became quiescent. Both samples were obtained from human right atria as part of the routine procedure for cardiac bypass. (Rosen MR, Wit AL, Hoffman BF: Electrophysiology and pharmacology of cardiac arrhythmias. VI. Cardiac effects of verapamil. Am Heart J 1975;89:665.)

its relatively low bioavailability (35%), which is largely due to presystemic (first-pass) hepatic elimination (metabolism).[283] Systemic and oral clearance of (−)-verapamil is substantially higher than that of (+)-verapamil. The bioavailability of (−)-verapamil (50%) is 2.5 times higher than that of of the (+)-verapamil (20%).[282] The positive to negative isomer ratio of plasma verapamil after intravenous administration is approximately 2, whereas, after oral administration, the positive to negative ratio is 5; therefore, there is a lack of strong negative dromotropic effect of oral verapamil on the AV transmission compared to that of intravenous verapamil.[282] Therapeutically, the effective plasma verapamil concentration is within 0.1 to 0.3 μg/mL.[283–285] The half-life of the drug is related to dose. In one report, after a single oral dose of verapamil, mean half-life was 6 hours (range, 2 to 15 hours), but this figure increased to 12 hours (range, 9 to 25 hours) 10 to 12 weeks after daily oral maintenance therapy with verapamil.[283–285] Similar prolongation of the half-life was seen with nor-

verapamil when the half-life increased from 10 to 16 hours.[284, 285] Although the mechanism of such slowing of elimination is not clear, reduced hepatic flow and subsequent reduced clearance of verapamil might be responsible. These findings are crucial for a rational and effective design of a maintenance dose of verapamil or less frequent administration of the drug becomes mandatory to avoid or minimize toxic side effects. Like the stereospecific actions of verapamil isomers on the AV nodal conduction, oral verapamil was found to be ineffective in preventing spontaneously occurring paroxysmal supraventricular tachycardia in patients in whom intravenous verapamil had previously suppressed tachycardia induced by programmed electrical stimulation.[286] McAllister and Kirsten have shown that double to triple plasma verapamil concentrations were needed after oral verapamil administration to prolong the PR interval as much as an intravenous bolus injection.[287] Similar results were obtained by Reiter and coworkers who found that plasma verapamil concentration corresponding to a 10% prolongation of the PR interval was 36 ng/mL after intravenous bolus, 132 ng/mL after an oral dose, and 85 ng/mL after steady intravenous infusion.[288] Maximum PR prolongation in this study, however, was comparable for the three methods of administration. Similar observations were made by Eichelbaum.[282]

The clearance of verapamil is 13 mL/min/kg, and its steady-state volume of distribution is 4.3 L/kg.[283] Woodcock and coworkers have demonstrated a reduction in the elimination of single doses of verapamil in patients with liver disease or compromised left ventricular function, which could be caused by differences in hepatic flow and subsequent hepatic clearance of verapamil.[289] Approximately 90% of verapamil is bound to plasma protein.

THERAPEUTIC ACTION, DOSE, AND SIDE EFFECTS. The antiarrhythmic properties of verapamil are caused mainly by its ability to suppress slow-response action potentials, which are initiated by the secondary or slow inward current and carried by calcium and sodium ions. Abnormal automaticity and triggered automatic activity, mechanisms that depend on the slow inward current, are also suppressed by verapamil.

Intravenous verapamil is highly effective in treating patients with paroxysmal supraventricular tachycardias and may be the drug of choice in reverting acute episodes of supraventricular tachycardia to normal sinus rhythm.[286, 290–294] Furthermore, intravenous verapamil has a fast onset of action (usually less than 1 minute). Successful and prompt conversion of this arrhythmia has been reported to be 80% to 100% after intravenous administration.[292] Conversion of atrial fibrillation to normal sinus rhythm with verapamil is uncommon; however, verapamil can slow the ventricular rate during atrial flutter and fibrillation by slowing conduction velocity and increasing AV nodal refractoriness. Verapamil has minimal effect on anterograde and retrograde conduction and on refractoriness in the anomalous pathway in patients with WPW syndrome. Therefore, verapamil is unlikely to be of value in the management of WPW syndrome when it is complicated by atrial flutter or fibrillation, and, in some instances, verapamil may be associated with a paradoxic increase in the ventricular rate. Ventricular arrhythmias frequently fail to respond to verapamil, but a good response to verapamil was observed in patients with ventricular arrhythmias during anesthetization with halothane.[295, 296] Overall, the role of verapamil in the management of patients with ventricular arrhythmias has not been established. For the conversion of atrial arrhythmias, the most commonly used dosage is a single bolus intravenous injection of 5 to 10 mg over 1 to 2 minutes. Although not customary, continuous intravenous infusion can also be instituted after a bolus. An infusion rate of 5 to 10 mg/h can be used, with adjustment dependent on clinical response. An oral regimen of verapamil is generally 80 to 120 mg every 6 to 8 hours. Rarely, higher doses are used. With chronic oral therapy, subsequent adjustments may be necessary because clearance of the drug decreases with time.[284, 285]

Verapamil is generally well tolerated. Side effects are not common, and they are mainly limited to the cardiovascular system. Verapamil may cause mild congestive heart failure because it depresses myocardial contractility and, thus, should not be used in the presence of frank heart failure. Nevertheless, through its peripheral vasodilation effects, verapamil may increase cardiac output in some patients. Verapamil causes sinus bradycardia and depresses AV nodal conduction (i.e., PR prolongation); therefore, it is contraindicated in patients with sick sinus syndrome.[297] Intravenous verapamil has rarely been associated with severe hypotension, severe bradycardia, or, in some instances, asystole. Continuous monitoring in these settings is necessary. Unlike beta blockers, verapamil does not increase airway resistance and, therefore, can be given to patients with bronchial asthma. Constipation, headache, gastrointestinal upset, vertigo, dizziness, and nervousness are uncommon but have been reported to occur with oral verapamil.

Amiodarone

Amiodarone has been approved by the Food and Drug Administration (FDA) and is marketed under the brand name of Cordarone for the management of ventricular arrhythmias.

MODE OF ACTION. Amiodarone (Fig. 5-16) differs from all other antiarrhythmic drugs by its very slow onset of action, requiring weeks to months before full antiarrhythmic efficacy is manifest. No explanation is available for such pecu-

Figure 5-16. Amiodarone.

liar behavior. Microelectrode studies on isolated cardiac preparations obtained from rabbits and dogs receiving daily doses of amiodarone for up to 6 weeks have shown considerable prolongation of action potential duration of atrial, ventricular muscle, and Purkinje fibers, with no significant alteration in other transmembrane potential properties.[298, 299] Amiodarone reduces the maximum rate of depolarization of action potential upstroke ($\dot{V}_{max}$) both in guinea pig ventricular muscle cells and in canine Purkinje fibers and ventricular muscle.[300, 301] The block of sodium current was found to be frequency- and voltage-dependent, and the block occurred with the binding of amiodarone with the sodium channel in its inactivated state.[300, 301] Similarly, amiodarone was shown to cause use-dependent block of secondary slow inward current, which is carried by calcium and sodium ions, in "slow response" canine Purkinje fibers.[302] Microelectrode studies have also shown that amiodarone slows sinus node automaticity by actions that slow sinus rate, that is, depression of phase 4 depolarization and prolongation of action potential duration.[303] Ohta and coworkers have shown that amiodarone reduces the amplitude of DAD and reduces subsequent triggered automaticity in isolated rabbit ventricular myocardium, effects that were more pronounced during chronic therapy than acute (superfusion) therapy.[304] Similar antiautomatic actions of amiodarone were also reported in canine Purkinje fibers and in guinea pig ventricular muscle cells.[300, 305] Radioligand binding studies have shown that amiodarone, like class I antiarrhythmic drugs, binds to the inactivated sodium channel, thus possibly accounting for the drug's class I action on the sodium current.[306]

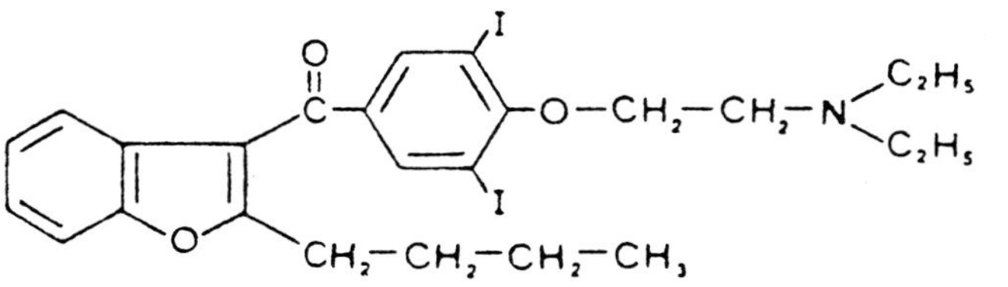

In intact dogs, amiodarone, 10 mg/kg administered intravenously, had maximum electrophysiologic effects in 5 to 10 minutes. The sinus rate was slowed by 36%, and atrial and ventricular monophasic action potentials and refractory periods were prolonged, as was AV node conduction time.[307] However, during oral amiodarone therapy in dogs, the onset of electrophysiologic actions took between 2 and 9 days depending on the site of action in the heart.[308] Effects on the atria were faster than effects on the ventricle (prolongation of the refractory period).[308] Similarly, after the cessation of amiodarone therapy, effects lasted longer on the ventricular myocardium than on the atria, with effects on the AV node being intermediate.[308] It has been suggested that delay in the maximum (steady state) effects of amiodarone is caused partly by the accumulation of the active metabolite desethylamiodarone, which has potent electrophysiologic, biochemical, and antiarrhythmic effects.[309–311]

In unanesthetized dogs with complete heart block and idioventricular escape rhythm, intravenous amiodarone was ineffective.[312] Such ventricular rhythm could be caused by enhanced normal automatic mechanisms that have different ionic mechanisms than DADs and by depolarization-induced automaticity. These mechanisms are suppressed by amiodarone.[300, 304, 305]

In dogs with coronary artery occlusion, Patterson and coworkers demonstrated that both short-term intravenous amiodarone and long-term (24 days) oral amiodarone therapy significantly reduced the incidence of ventricular fibrillation.[313] Long-term oral amiodarone therapy, however, was more effective against ventricular fibrillation and caused greater prolongation of the effective refractory period and the QT segment of the right ventricle.[313] Amiodarone was also effective against reperfusion ventricular fibrillation.[311]

METABOLISM AND PHARMACOKINETICS. Amiodarone is a unique antiarrhythmic agent in both its pharmacokinetic and pharmacologic properties. High-pressure liquid chromatographic assay techniques have only recently provided data on the pharmacokinetic and metabolic properties of amiodarone.[314–316] The full spectrum of the disposition kinetics of the drug, however, remains poorly understood.

The salient pharmacologic feature of amiodarone (i.e., delay in onset of antiarrhythmic action) has been attributed to slow accumulation of the drug and its major metabolite, desethylamiodarone, in the myocardium and to extensive uptake by adipose tissue, causing slow attainment of steady-state plasma drug concentration.[309, 314–316] In four patients (explanted human hearts) who underwent cardiac transplantation, significant interindividual variations in myocardial concentrations of amiodarone and desethylamiodarone were observed, with plasma concentrations being poorly correlated with myocardial amiodarone and desethylamiodarone concentrations.[317] The slow development of metabolic alterations in thyroid hormone activity may have an antiarrhythmic implication in the efficacy of long-term amiodarone therapy.[310, 318, 319, 320] Long-term oral amiodarone therapy increases plasma concentrations of reverse triiodothyronine (T3) and thyroxine (T4), changes that parallel the onset and magnitude of QT prolongation and suppression of ventricular premature depolarizations.[318] Finally, desethylamiodarone, a major metabolite of amiodarone that accumulates with long-term amiodarone therapy, and a possible antagonism of the sympathetic nervous system by both amiodarone and

its major metabolite may influence the ability of this drug to suppress arrhythmias. The full spectrum of pharmacologic activity of amiodarone remains unresolved.

Oral absorption of amiodarone is relatively slow, and peak serum concentration after an oral dose of 800 mg is reached after 5.2 hours, with a half-life of absorption of 1.62 hours.[314] The maximum serum concentration after a single oral dose of 800 mg is reported to be 1.7 μg/mL (range, 0.6 to 3.2 μg/mL).[314] The plasma half-life of amiodarone after a single oral dose is 4.62 hours. Oral bioavailability of amiodarone (Cordarone) is 35%.[316] The half-life of amiodarone after a single intravenous dose (5 mg/kg) is similar to that after a single oral dose. However, with chronic oral therapy, the half-life of amiodarone is considerably prolonged, up to 30 days. The mechanism of this prolongation is unknown but could reflect amiodarone tissue distribution (slow process) and perhaps formation of metabolites that slow clearance of the parent drug.[315] Neither amiodarone nor its pharmacologically active metabolite, desethylamiodarone, is found in the urine for 24 hours after a single oral dose.[314–316] Animal studies have also failed to show amiodarone in feces after intravenous administration.[314] It appears that amiodarone has a strong affinity to concentrate in various tissues, resulting in a huge apparent volume of distribution (5000 L).[321] The preliminary studies of Haffajee and coworkers have shown that amiodarone can concentrate to values up to 385 times that of plasma amiodarone concentration in the fatty mesenteric tissue and up to 36 times in the heart.[314]

In the dog, mean right ventricular amiodarone concentration after long-term oral administration (28 days) was 13 μg/g, representing a sevenfold uptake; concentration was 54 μg/g for desethylamiodarone, representing a 20-fold uptake.[178] How amiodarone becomes so concentrated in various tissues is unknown. One important electrophysiologic consequence of such a concentrating ability in myocardial tissue is the lack of any apparent correlation between plasma amiodarone levels and antiarrhythmic efficacy. Many patients who responded to amiodarone had plasma amiodarone levels lower than those of patients who did not respond.[314] This may reflect lower myocardial uptake of amiodarone in patients who did not respond, assuming that amiodarone has the necessary antiarrhythmic properties. These considerations need further research and experimental verification. Wellens and coworkers have shown that oral and intravenous amiodarone have different electrophysiologic effects.[322] Oral amiodarone prolonged the HV interval and the effective refractory period of the atrium and ventricle, whereas intravenous amiodarone had no effect on these parameters. Despite these differences in electrophysiologic responses, intravenous amiodarone predicted outcome with oral amiodarone in preventing inducible tachycardia.[314] If similar observations are made on a larger patient population, then additional electrophysiologic mechanisms by which amiodarone suppresses tachycardia (other than prolongation of refractory period) should be invoked on the heart.[323]

THERAPEUTIC ACTION, DOSE, AND SIDE EFFECTS. The ability of amiodarone to prolong refractoriness of almost all cardiac tissues makes it useful in the clinical management of patients with supraventricular and ventricular arrhythmias as well as arrhythmias associated with the WPW syndrome.[314,323–329] Amiodarone is often effective in the management of these arrhythmias when conventional antiarrhythmics fail to correct the rhythm disorder. Amiodarone does not exert frequency-dependent effects on ventricular repolarization, and its absence of reverse frequency-dependent effects on repolarization, along with its time-dependent effects on refractoriness, were considered to account for the high efficacy of the drug against ventricular tachyarrhythmias.[330] Epinephrine was found to only partially reverse the antiarrhythmic efficacy of amiodarone, an effect that may be caused by the beta-adrenergic antagonism of amiodarone.[140,331] Epinephrine had greater potential to reverse the antiarrhythmic efficacy of quinidine.[140] A therapeutic role for amiodarone in the management of atrial fibrillation has been emphasized.[332,333] The full antiarrhythmic efficacy of oral amiodarone does not manifest for days, sometimes weeks.[320,334,335] Although high oral amiodarone dose and intravenous amiodarone administration have been found to be effective in both adults and children, it has been suggested that an adequate response after short-term therapy does not guarantee a similar response after long-term treatment, and an inadequate response after short-term therapy does not always predict a similar response after long-term therapy.[336–339] The considerable prolongation of its half-life of elimination seems to be the result of its accumulation in various body tissues. Such "body stores" may, in part, be the reason for the persistence of amiodarone's antiarrhythmic and electrophysiologic effects for at least several weeks after therapy is stopped.[308]

Intravenous amiodarone, 5 mg/kg, may be administered at a rate of 30 to 50 mg/min in a central line. Most commonly, the drug is given orally, usually with a loading dose of 800 to 1800 mg/d during the first week, followed by a daily maintenance dose of 200 to 800 mg/d. Amiodarone seems to be well tolerated by most patients; however, with its increased use, several unwanted side effects have been recognized.[340] The incidence of side effects varies between 17% and 30%.[341,342] In animal models, however, it was reported that cardiac performance could be preserved during amiodarone therapy while recovering from surgery, and that long-term amiodarone therapy in younger patients had no effect on growth.[343,344] Exercise-induced QRS prolongation, consistent with the drug's ability to cause use-dependent sodium channel block, has been observed in patients on amiodarone therapy.[345] Among the side effects that complicate amiodarone therapy is pulmonary fibrosis.[346,347] No reliable test can predict the likelihood of this complication. The frequency (approximately 5%), however, can be reduced by lowering the maintenance dose. A recent multicenter study showed pulmonary toxicity to occur in as many as 45% of patients over a 4-year period with a daily maintenance dose of 500 mg of amiodarone. The most consistent complication of amiodarone therapy is corneal microdeposits (lipofuscin), which appear as yellow-brown granular pigmentation in the cornea that may cause photophobia.[340] These symptoms disappear within weeks or months after amiodarone is discontinued. Amiodarone may also cause thyroid dysfunction, and patients may manifest either hypothyroidism or hyperthyroidism.[340] In long-term amiodarone therapy (generally more than 1 year), the skin may occasionally turn bluish or slate-gray. This discoloration generally begins nasally, then spreads to encompass the entire face. It may not clear completely for months to years after discontinuation of the drug. Approximately 5% of patients must discontinue amiodarone therapy because of more serious, even life-threatening, side effects, but it has been suggested that the benefits of amiodarone therapy often outweigh the side effects.[348,349] Side effects include refractory heart failure, pulmonary fibrosis, central nervous system side effects (e.g., tremor, ataxia, paresthesias, headache, nightmares), sinus arrest, aplastic anemia, and exacerbation of ventricular tachycardia. Testicular dysfunction may also result from prolonged amiodarone therapy.[350]

Amiodarone interacts with several drugs with important clinical implications; chief among these interactions is potentiation of the anticoagulant effect of warfarin.[351] Although increases in prothrombin time vary, the maintenance dose of warfarin should be reduced by one third to one half in patients receiving amiodarone.[351] Torsades de pointes has been observed when quinidine, propafenone, or mexiletine is given with amiodarone.[352] Adding amiodarone to maintenance digoxin therapy causes a progressive increase (up to 70%) in serum digoxin concentration, with the emergence of symptoms compatible with digoxin toxicity.[352] Combination of amiodarone and a class 1 agent seldom results in noninducibility of sustained ventricular tachycardia in patients, although greater reduction in tachycardia cycle length and perhaps greater tolerance to the tachycardia may result from such a combination.[353] Finally, amiodarone may interact with beta blockers and certain calcium channel antagonists (verapamil and diltiazem) to cause severe sinus bradycardia and even sinus arrest, especially in patients with sick sinus syndrome.[352] Oral amiodarone but not intravenous amiodarone was found to elevate the ventricular defibrillation threshold.[354,355]

Mexiletine

Mexiletine (Fig. 5-17), a structural analog of lidocaine, shares many of its electrophysiologic effects on the transmembrane potential of cardiac fibers. Mexiletine differs from lidocaine in that it is effective orally and is not eliminated by first-pass hepatic metabolism.

MODE OF ACTION. Microelectrode studies on isolated Purkinje fibers have shown that mexiletine decreases the maximum rate of phase-zero depolarization and membrane responsiveness and shortens the effective refractory period more than it shortens action potential duration.[87,100,356–360] Mexiletine causes frequency and myocardial fiber orientation-dependent prolongation of conduction time in normal canine epicardium.[87] The degree of conduction slowing is greater in orientation for which predrug conduction is faster, an observation consistent with the known effects of myocardial anisotropy on conduction (i.e., faster conduction parallel to fiber orientation).[87]

Mexiletine suppresses normal, abnormal, and triggered automatic mechanisms in Purkinje fibers at concentrations that have little or no effect on sinus node automaticity.[358] In isolated guinea pig hearts, mexiletine was

effective against reperfusion arrhythmias after a period of ischemia and hypoxia.[359] Furthermore, in isolated Purkinje fibers, mexiletine decreased the amplitude of delayed afterdepolarizations and triggered automaticity induced by either barium or strophanthidin.[358,359] Mexiletine does not appear to have any effect on the slow response action potentials; however, on partially depolarized Purkinje fibers manifesting spontaneous automatic activity (abnormal automaticity), mexiletine, at concentrations of 0.4 to 2.0 µg/mL, depressed phase 4 depolarization and reduced the rate of automatic impulse initiation.[358,361] Furthermore, when partially depolarized Purkinje fibers were electrically driven, the application of mexiletine rendered the maximum diastolic potential more negative, with a concomitant decrease of pacemaker slope and an increase in the $\dot{V}_{max}$ of the phase-zero action potential.[358] In Purkinje fibers with normal resting potential, mexiletine decreases the rate of automatic impulse initiation by shifting the threshold potential to less negative values.[358] In vivo daily administration of mexiletine in rats induced upregulation of sodium ion channels (i.e., increased the number of sodium channels) 3 days after drug therapy.[362]

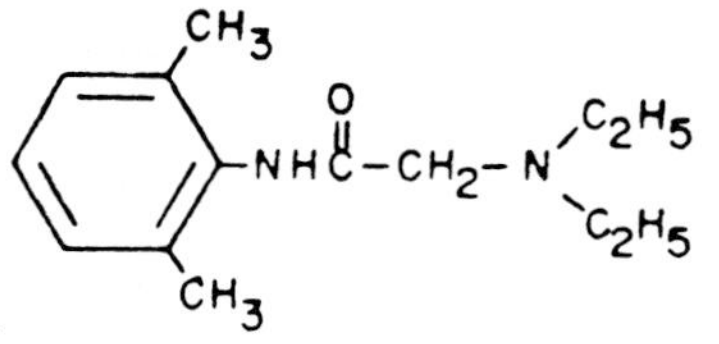

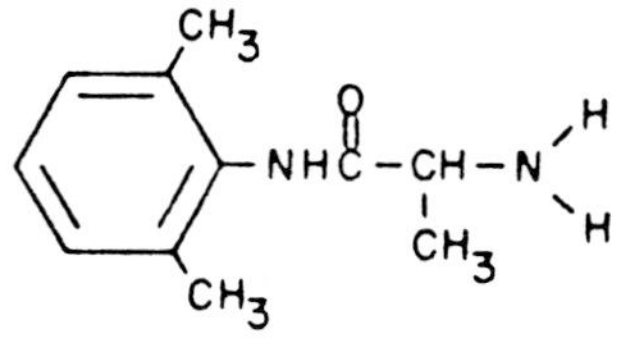

In humans, mexiletine increases the functional refractory period of the AV node and the relative and effective refractory periods of the His–Purkinje system and prolongs the HV interval. These findings are not always uniform, however. Differences may reflect differences between patients or between therapeutic regimens. Harper and Olsson found that mexiletine had no effect on the duration of endocardial right ventricular monophasic action potentials in humans, nor did it alter the effective refractory period of this site when the ventricles were regularly driven at cycle lengths of 500 to 600 milliseconds.[363] However, mexiletine did prolong the MAPD of early premature ventricular beats.[363] The authors concluded that this property of the drug may be related to its antiarrhythmic activity. Furthermore, they showed that mexiletine abolished the supernormal conduction phase, which occurs immediately after repolarization, presumably as a result of phase 4 depolarization in the cells of the specialized conducting system.[363] The antiarrhythmic significance of such an effect is undefined.

METABOLISM AND PHARMACOKINETICS. Mexiletine is rapidly and well absorbed after oral administration in healthy volunteers.[364] However, absorption is incomplete and delayed in patients with myocardial infarction and in patients receiving narcotic analgesics that retard gastric emptying. Mexiletine is eliminated largely by liver metabolism, with only less than 10% excreted by the kidneys unchanged. Renal clearance of mexiletine decreases as urinary pH increases.[364] The half-life of elimination is approximately 12 hours, and therapeutic plasma concentrations (1 to 2

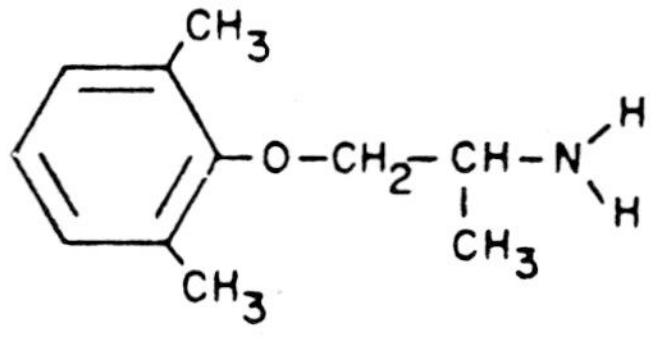

Figure 5-17. (**A**) Lidocaine. (**B**) Tocainide. (**C**) Mexiletine.

μg/mL) can be maintained with 200- to 300-mg oral doses every 6 to 8 hours. The half-life of mexiletine increases in patients with myocardial infarction, and careful monitoring for dose readjustment is needed. About 70% of the drug is protein bound.[364]

THERAPEUTIC ACTION, DOSE, AND SIDE EFFECTS. Mexiletine can be given orally, 100 to 400 mg every 6 to 8 hours. For urgent therapy, the intravenous route may be considered, with 200 to 250 mg over 5 minutes followed by an infusion of 60 to 90 mg/h. Mexiletine is effective in suppressing ventricular arrhythmias, and its relatively long half-life is beneficial for patient compliance.[365–367] Its definite role in controlling ventricular arrhythmias remains undefined. Mexiletine is found to have greater antiarrhythmic potential when used in combination with quinidine.[366] According to the modulated receptor hypothesis, combinations of drugs having different kinetics of binding (block) and unbinding (recovery from block) to sodium channels could provide enhanced diastolic binding to sodium channels that could not be attained by either alone.[216] Mexiletine–quinidine combinations provide such effective diastolic block of sodium channels and decrease excitability by decreasing $\dot{V}_{max}$.[216] Such an effect provides more effective suppression of arrhythmias in selected patient populations.[366]

In a double-blind, placebo-controlled trial involving 630 patients with documented myocardial infarction, the International Mexiletine and Placebo Antiarrhythmic Coronary Trial (IMPACT) reported that mexiletine therapy was not associated with reduced mortality rate (7.6% in mexiletine group versus 4.8% in the placebo group, difference not significant).[368] Similar to encainide and flecainide studies (CAST), although mexiletine suppressed ventricular premature complexes and arrhythmias in patients after myocardial infarction, these effects, however, did not result in reduced mortality rate. The addition of mexiletine to propafenone increases the efficacy against sustained ventricular tachycardia in some patients.[369]

Most side effects are seen during the initial period of therapy and disappear during maintenance therapy; most are of central nervous system origin. They include tremor, nystagmus, dizziness, dysarthria, paresthesias, ataxia, and confusion.[368] Gastrointestinal side effects are common and include nausea, vomiting, and dyspepsia.[368] Thrombocytopenia and positive antinuclear antibody occur rarely but have been reported. Side effects are more likely to occur at mexiletine plasma concentrations over 1.5 to 2 μg/mL, which is close to the therapeutic level. Cardiovascular effects of mexiletine are infrequent and include hypotension, bradycardia, and exacerbation of arrhythmias. Mexiletine may aggravate congestive heart failure in patients with reduced left ventricular ejection fraction or a history of congestive heart failure; however, the incidence

rate is relatively low and unpredictable.[370] The drug is generally well tolerated. Mexiletine was found to be associated with a lesser mortality rate than quinidine.[145]

Tocainide

MODE OF ACTION. Tocainide (Tonocard), a lidocaine analog, has many electrophysiologic similarities to mexiletine (see Fig. 5-17). It also resembles mexiletine in that it is active orally and does not undergo presystemic elimination by first-pass hepatic degradation.

Microelectrode studies have shown that tocainide has similar electrophysiologic effects to those of lidocaine on resting and action potential, namely a reduction in the $\dot{V}_{max}$ and shortening of action potential duration.[84,371,372] Its effects on $\dot{V}_{max}$ are potassium dependent. At normal extracellular potassium concentration (3 to 5 mM), tocainide slightly reduces $\dot{V}_{max}$. However, at elevated potassium concentration, at which $\dot{V}_{max}$ is already depressed, tocainide has a much greater depressant effect.[371,372] A microelectrode study on isolated Purkinje fibers has shown that tocainide depresses $\dot{V}_{max}$ in a voltage- and use-dependent manner.[84] The rate constant for onset of block for sodium current is faster with tocainide than with quinidine (0.9 versus 5.6 pulses).[84]

Tocainide increases the amount of current necessary to evoke an action potential by intracellular current injection in a concentration-dependent manner, an indication of decreased excitability.[371] Tocainide decreases the amplitude and plateau phase of the action potential in a concentration-dependent manner, thereby decreasing time to 50% and 95% repolarization, respectively.[84,371] However, tocainide had no effect on total duration of action potential, maximal action potential amplitude, or resting membrane potential in Purkinje fibers.[84,371] Although the drug had no consistent effect on the effective refractory period of Purkinje fibers, the ratio of effective refractory period to action potential duration was consistently increased in a concentration-dependent manner after tocainide superfusion.[371,373] One study showed that tocainide has no effect on action potential duration of surviving canine subendocardial Purkinje fibers 1 day after left anterior descending coronary artery occlusion, while shortening both 50% and 90% repolarization of adjoining normal Purkinje fibers.[373] This study suggested that decreased disparity in repolarization induced by tocainide may have antiarrhythmic relevance.[373]

Tocainide completely suppresses ventricular tachycardia induced by ouabain intoxication in dogs, with an average plasma level of 18 μg/mL. Similarly, tocainide suppresses the 24-hour ventricular arrhythmias induced by coronary artery occlusion in the dog, with an average plasma level of 42 μg/mL (range, 28 to 67 μg/mL).[371] Although the 24-hour postcoronary artery occlusion ventricular arrhythmias were suppressed by tocainide, tachycardia induced by electrical stimulation during the chronic phase were less responsive to tocainide therapy.[374] With lower plasma levels of tocainide (mean, 18 μg/mL), these ischemic ventricular arrhythmias were suppressed by about 50%. Tocainide increased the ventricular fibrillation threshold, with a maximum increase of about 150% achieved with a plasma tocainide concentration of 48 μg/mL.[371]

METABOLISM AND PHARMACOKINETICS. Tocainide is rapidly and predictably well absorbed by the oral route and has a high systemic bioavailability.[375,376] Plasma tocainide levels are highly predictable after an oral dose. The drug undergoes hepatic degradation (40–60%); the remainder is eliminated by the kidney unchanged. The half-life of elimination of tocainide is 12 hours (range, 10 to 17 hours), and it is 50% bound to plasma protein. Tocainide clearance is 2.2 mL/min/kg, and its steady-state volume of distribution is 1.6 L/kg. Renal elimination of tocainide is reduced with an increase in urinary pH.[375,376]

THERAPEUTIC ACTION, DOSE, AND SIDE EFFECTS. Clinical studies have shown that tocainide can decrease the frequency of ventricular premature depolarizations and has variable effects on ventricular tachycardias.[377,378] The precise role of tocainide and the clinical setting in which it may eventually be used remain undefined. In one study involving 54 patients with drug-resistant sustained ventricular tachycardia, tocainide was of limited use because it was effective in only 13% of the patients (i.e., seven of 54 patients).[379] As for the control of premature ventricular depolarizations, tocainide was found to exert similar effects as lidocaine.[380] Tocainide apparently exerts its antiarrhythmic efficacy at plasma concentrations above 6 μg/mL, if at all. The oral regimen for tocainide is usually 400 to 600 mg every 8 hours. Tocainide is generally well tolerated. Side effects include central nervous system disorders such as tremor, headache, sweating, altered hearing, dizziness, nervousness, hot flashes, paresthesias, blurred vision of diplopia, anxiety, and light-headedness. Gastrointestinal complaints are more common and include anorexia, vomiting, nausea, abdominal pain, and constipation.[378] In patients with myocardial infarction and taking beta blockers, tocainide was found to slightly and transiently depress left ventricular function.[381] Although tocainide may cause greater hemodynamic compromise than procainamide, mortality in the first few days after myocardial infarction may be reduced with tocainide therapy in a canine model of infarction.[382,383]

Flecainide

MODE OF ACTION. Flecainide (Fig. 5-18) (Tambocor) has been approved by the FDA for the management of life-threatening ventricular arrhythmias.[384]

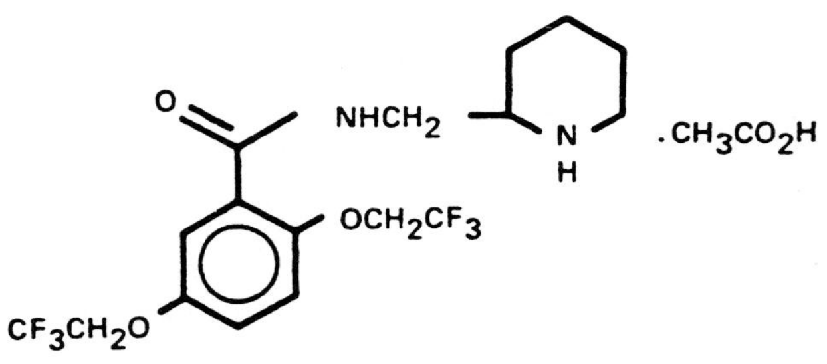

Figure 5-18. Flecainide acetate.

Microelectrode studies on isolated tissue preparations have shown that flecainide decreases $\dot{V}_{max}$ of the upstroke of canine Purkinje and ventricular muscle cells in a concentration-dependent manner.[385] The decrease in the $\dot{V}_{max}$ of ventricular action potential is voltage- and time-dependent.[386] The rate-dependent block of sodium current may be responsible for the observed rate-dependent conduction slowing (i.e., QRS widening seen in humans).[96] Ventricular muscle action potential duration was increased and Purkinje fiber duration decreased. Furthermore, flecainide depressed Purkinje fiber automaticity by elevating threshold potential.[387] These effects were considered relevant for the antiarrhythmic actions of the drug. In human atrial tissue, flecainide increased the action potential duration and the atrial refractoriness more at faster than at slower pacing rates.[86] In open-chest anesthetized dogs, flecainide prolonged epicardial refractoriness more in the infarct zone than in the normal zone.[388] In this study, flecainide had no efficacy against inducible sustained ventricular tachycardia; rather, the drug had the potential to aggravate arrhythmias in this canine model.[388]

METABOLISM AND PHARMACOKINETICS. In anesthetized open-chest canine preparations, intravenous flecainide infusion, 0.1 to 0.25 mg/kg/min, with plasma levels of 0.5 to 6.5 μg/mL, caused a concentration-dependent prolongation in atrial effective refractory periods and AV nodal functional and relative refractory periods.[384,385] At a lower flecainide concentration (0.7 μg/mL), the drug significantly reduced ventricular rate during atrial fibrillation and appeared to increase the ventricular fibrillation threshold.[387] In a canine study, flecainide infusion, with mean plasma levels of 0.6 μg/mL, increased the level of energy needed for defibrillation by 75%.[389] Pretreatment with flecainide (2 mg/kg intravenously) appeared to reduce the incidence of ventricular fibrillation in open-chest swine preparations during the first 30 minutes of partial ischemia caused by 75% reduction in flow in the left anterior descending coronary artery.[390] However, flecainide had no effect on the incidence of ventricular fibrillation after complete occlusion of this artery.[390] Furthermore, flecainide depressed myocardial contractility (LV dP/dt max), caused hypotension, and increased QRS duration in a concentration-dependent manner.[384,390] Similar antiarrhythmic and electrophysiologic effects were also seen in humans. Prolonged PR and QT intervals and QRS widening were seen after flecainide administration.[391–395] Furthermore, flecainide appeared to be effective in suppressing premature ventricular complexes of various causes.[66,391–394]

THERAPEUTIC ACTION, DOSE, AND SIDE EFFECTS. In most patients, an oral regimen of 200 mg twice daily has been shown to be effective; a few patients require 300 mg twice daily. The half-life of flecainide is between 13 and 16 hours in normal subjects and approximately 20 hours in patients with heart disease.[396] The average effective flecainide plasma concentrations is 650 ng/mL (range, 200 to 1000 ng/mL), which can be achieved with the above oral dosing schedule.[396] Flecainide was found to be effective against atrial fibrillation that failed to respond to either quinidine or propafenone.[397,398] A single oral dose of flecainide was also found to be effective against paroxysmal supraventricular tachycardia in children and young adults.[399] In a preliminary report, intravenous flecainide (2 mg/kg over 5 minutes) was found to be effective in patients with the WPW syndrome because it increased both anterograde and retrograde effective refractory periods of the accessory pathway.[384,400] Oral flecainide was found to be effective in a young patient population manifesting a broad range of atrial and ventricular tachyarrhythmias.[401] Intravenous flecainide (2 gm/kg) and oral flecainide were found to effectively suppress premature ventricular complexes.[66,402] Although flecainide was found to effectively suppress ventricular ectopy in a multicenter trial (CAST) involving 730 patients with myocardial infarction, follow-up studies have shown that the mortality rate in patients treated with flecainide was significantly higher than in the placebo group.[66] The mechanism of increased mortality rate with flecainide remains undefined. In another study involving 1330 patients with sustained ventricular tachycardia and with a mean follow-up period of 292 days, the safety of flecainide increased when "slow incremental approach to dosing" was practiced, especially in high risk patients with structural heart disease.[403] The long-term benefit of flecainide in patients with myocardial infarction seems of questionable value, because of increased mortality rate, and because of potential proarrhythmic effects of the drug.[64–66,395,396,403] In one study, exercise exacerbated flecainide-induced conduction slowing (QRS widening), consistent with flecainde's use-dependent block of the sodium channel.[386,395] Other side effects of flecainide include dizziness, blurred vision, headache, and nausea.[384,391–394,396] Some patients experience abnormal taste sensations, flushing, tinnitus, sleepiness, and paresthesias.[391] A search of world literature on the use of flecainide in children found the drug to be relatively safe and effective against supraventricular tachyarrhythmias.[404]

Encainide

MODE OF ACTION. Encainide (Fig. 5-19) (ENKAID) has been approved by the FDA for the management of life-threatening ventricular arrhythmias.

Encainide (4-methoxy-2'[2-(1 methyl-2-piperidyl)ethyl] benzanilide hydrochloride) seems to be an effective and potent antiarrhythmic agent when administered either orally or intravenously.[405] Isolated tissue studies with microelectrodes have shown that encainide, like flecainide, decreases the $\dot{V}_{max}$ of the action potential of Purkinje fibers in a rate-dependent manner and shortens action potential duration of Purkinje but not ventricular muscle fibers.[406,407] Encainide also suppresses normal Purkinje fiber automaticity but has no effect on abnormal automaticity initiated in partially depolarized Purkinje fibers and induced by high extracellular potassium or depolarizing current injections.[406] Thus, the drug appears not to affect slow-response action potentials. Furthermore, encainide decreases excitability (increased current threshold) by shifting threshold voltage to less negative values.[408] A metabolite of encainide, O-demethylencanide, has more potent cellular electrophysiologic effects than the parent drugs in in vitro studies and a higher antiarrhythmic activity in a rat model of arrhythmia induced by aconitine.[406,409] In anesthetized open-chest dogs, encainide prolonged the refractory period and the duration of the MAPD in both atrial and right ventricular endocardial tissues, with a more pronounced increase in the atrium.[410] Furthermore, in this study, encainide also caused an increase in the AH, HV, QRS, and QTc intervals.

METABOLISM AND PHARMACOKINETICS. The metabolism of encainide appears to be polymorphically distributed similarly to the genetically determined oxidative biotransformation of debrisoquine.[411] Poor metabolizers of debri-

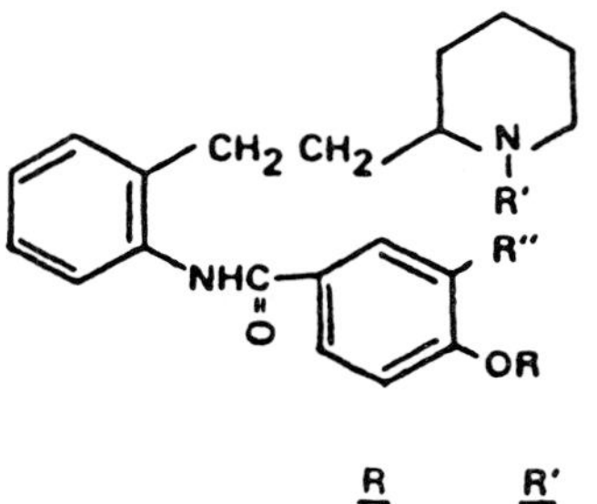

	R	R'	R''
ENCAINIDE	$-CH_3$	$-CH_3$	$-H$
ODE	$-H$	$-CH_3$	$-H$
MODE	$-H$	$-CH_3$	$-OCH_3$
NDE	$-CH_3$	$-H$	$-H$

Figure 5-19. Encainide.

soquine are also poor metabolizers of encainide. O-demethylencainide, a major metabolite, abolishes spontaneously occurring ventricular arrhythmias in dogs 48 hours after a 2-hour left anterior descending coronary artery occlusion followed by reperfusion.[412] However, O-demethylencainide appears to facilitate initiation of ventricular fibrillation by brief right ventricular pacing at 200 beats per minute, which could not be defibrillated in the majority of dogs studied.[412] The experimental studies of the electrophysiologic, antiarrhythmic, and proarrhythmic properties of encainide and of O-demethylencainide seem to corroborate well with the clinical findings. Encainide prolongs AH, HV, and QRS intervals in humans.[396, 413, 414] Prolongation of the QT interval, however, was noted only during long-term therapy, possibly because of the accumulation of the active metabolite.[415]

Oral absorption of encainide is highly variable. Bioavailability ranges between 7.4% and 82% (mean, 42%).[416] Such variability may be due to presystemic elimination.[405] The half-life after intravenous dosing was 3.3 ± 1.68 hours (range, 2 to 6.9 hours), and it tended to be shorter after oral dosing, averaging 2.4 hours (range, 1.5 to 3.7 hours).[416] Clearance also varied widely, ranging from 210 to 1790 mL/min (average, 1157 mL/min). The time to peak plasma concentration after oral dosing was 1.5 to 3 hours (average, 1.6 hours).[396, 416] The major route of elimination of encainide is hepatic metabolism, which should be considered when long-term oral encainide therapy is contemplated because the metabolites have important antiarrhythmic efficacy.[396, 415, 417, 418]

THERAPEUTIC ACTION, DOSE, AND SIDE EFFECTS. Encainide is somewhat effective against frequent and complex premature ventricular depolarizations and arrhythmias associated with the WPW syndrome.[66, 416, 419, 420] Encainide is also effective against AV nodal reentrant tachycardia by depressing conduction in the retrograde limb of the reentrant cicuit.[421] Encainide appears to be more effective and better tolerated than quinidine in patients with premature ventricular complexes.[422] Minimal antiarrhythmic plasma concentration after intravenous dosing is higher than after oral dosing (39 versus 14 ng/mL), suggesting the presence of an active metabolite after oral dosing.[416, 423] Note that in a patient who did not respond to encainide, no O-demethylencainide was found in the plasma. Subsequent studies have shown 6% to 10% of patients cannot metabolize encainide.[415] It is neither clear if patients who do not respond cannot metabolize encainide nor whether such deficiency in metabolism causes arrhythmias in the WPW syndrome.[420] Dose schedule should carefully be reevaluated in each patient based on the ability of the drug to suppress arrhythmias or QRS widening. Rate-dependent increases in the QRS duration caused by encainide may be used as a "marker" for evaluating drug effect;

alternatively, changes in the QRS duration may be used as a means for recognizing subgroups of patients with different phenotypic patterns of encainide metabolism.[424] Daily oral doses of encainide are between 75 to 300 mg, given in divided doses every 4 to 6 hours. Peak plasma level after an intravenous dose of 75 mg is 996 ng/mL; after an oral dose, it is 241 ng/mL.[416]

The most troublesome side effect of encainide therapy is aggravation of ventricular arrhythmias, including induction of ventricular fibrillation.[65, 416, 422, 425, 426] A common type of arrhythmia induced by encainide seems to be polymorphic ventricular tachycardia, resulting in cardiac arrest.[426] Such arrhythmia aggravation appears to differ from other quinidine-like drug-induced arrhythmias in that encainide-induced rhythm disorders were not associated with marked QT prolongation and usually did not self-terminate.[426] The risk of encainide-induced ventricular tachyarrhythmias was 11% in 90 patients receiving the drug for recurrent sustained ventricular tachycardia or ventricular fibrillation and was 2.2% in 47 patients receiving the drug for chronic complex premature ventricular depolarizations.[422] Similar results were seen in a large patient population (506 patients) receiving encainide.[65] Rhythm aggravation occurs 17 to 48 hours after the start of chronic oral maintenance dosing with encainide.[426] Patients with a history of recurrent sustained ventricular tachycardia and ventricular fibrillation should receive encainide therapy only in the hospital under close surveillance and with continuous electrocardiographic monitoring. The effect of encainide as well as flecainide on mortality rate in patients with myocardial infarction was evaluated in the CAST study.[66] Even though premature ventricular depolarizations were effectively suppressed in patients on encainide therapy, those patients had a significantly higher mortality rate than patients on placebo therapy.[66] The mechanism of encainide-induced increased mortality rate is undefined.

New Agents

Aprindine

Aprindine (Fig. 5-20), developed in Belgium, has important local anesthetic effects. It is still an investigational agent in the United States.

MODE OF ACTION. On isolated canine Purkinje fibers and atrial and ventricular muscle fibers, aprindine shortens action potential duration and, to a lesser extent, effective refractory period.[427–430] The ratio of effective refractory period shortening to action potential duration shortening is greater than 1.[427–429] The effects of the drug on Purkinje fibers occur at lower concentrations than on atrial and ventricular fibers. Aprindine depresses maximum rate of

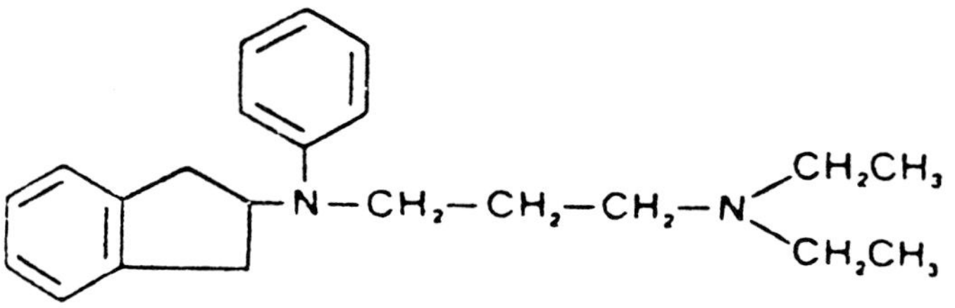

Figure 5-20. Aprindine.

rise of phase zero of the action potential in a frequency-dependent manner; greater depression occurs at a faster rate of drive.[427–430] Membrane responsiveness is shifted to the right with aprindine superfusion in a concentration-dependent manner. Aprindine also decreases the slope of spontaneous phase 4 depolarization of Purkinje fibers with high resting membrane potential (normal enhanced automaticity), thereby decreasing the rate of automatic impulse initiation and eventually arresting automaticity.[427–430] In anesthetized dogs, aprindine injected into the sinus node artery slows sinus discharge rate; when injected into the AV nodal artery, aprindine prolongs the conduction time and the functional refractory period of the AV node.[431] These nodal effects are independent of indirect autonomic nervous system influences. Furthermore, aprindine prolongs both atrial and ventricular effective refractory periods.[431]

Aprindine suppresses transient depolarization and subsequent triggered automatic activity induced by ouabain in Purkinje fibers.[430] However, it does not have any effect on transmembrane potential properties of "slow-response" Purkinje fibers induced with a 22-mM potassium superfusion in the presence of isoproterenol.[430] Aprindine (2.8 mg/kg) administered intravenously completely eliminated accelerated idioventricular rhythm induced by ouabain in all 14 dogs studied, an effect not seen with other antiarrhythmic agents, and it significantly reduced the frequency of premature ventricular depolarization 24 hours after permanent coronary artery occlusion in dogs.[432, 433] The precise cellular ionic mechanisms by which aprindine suppresses digitalis arrhythmias are unknown. The reduction in the amplitude of delayed after-depolarizations and suppression of subsequent triggered automatic activity may be one operative mechanism.

METABOLISM AND PHARMACOKINETICS. Aprindine is active orally and has a high systemic bioavailability, with a rapid rate of oral absorption. Pharmacokinetic parameters of aprindine are not defined. In healthy volunteers, clearance of aprindine was 2.55 mL/min/kg, and its half-life of elimination was 30 hours, with a steady-state volume of distribution of 3.6 L/kg. Less than 1% of the dose is excreted unchanged in the urine. Therapeutic plasma levels (1 to 2 μg/mL) of aprindine overlap with toxic side effects (i.e.,

there is a low toxic-to-therapeutic ratio). As much as 95% of the drug is protein bound.[434, 435]

THERAPEUTIC ACTION, DOSE, AND SIDE EFFECTS. Aprindine appears to be very effective against both supraventricular and ventricular arrhythmias of various causes.[434] It has been used orally in a loading dose of 200 to 300 mg, followed by a maintenance dose of 150 mg/d. This dosage regimen achieved mean plasma aprindine levels of 1.7 μg/mL. In a mean follow-up period of 23 months involving 64 patients with high risk of sudden death, oral aprindine therapy with mean blood levels higher than 1.5 μg/mL was associated with greater protection against sudden death and recurrences of symptomatic ventricular tachycardias than patients having lower aprindine levels (65% and 35%, respectively).[436] The ability of aprindine to slow conduction through the AV node and to increase atrial refractoriness makes aprindine potentially useful in the management of patients with the WPW syndrome.[434, 437] Electrophysiologic studies in such patients have demonstrated that aprindine increased refractoriness of the accessory pathway in both the anterograde and retrograde directions in most patients.[434, 437] In 143 high-risk patients with acute myocardial infarction, the prophylactic antiarrhythmic value of aprindine was evaluated in a double-blind, placebo-controlled study.[438] No significant difference was found between the two groups with respect to overall 1-year mortality, even though mortality in the aprindine arm was delayed (86 days versus 21 days).[438] In this study, it was suggested that aprindine may be effective in the short term, before more aggressive intervention (surgery) is sought.[438]

The potential usefulness of aprindine is limited by its narrow toxic-to-therapeutic ratio, which is particularly evident during the initial loading period. To decrease the incidence of side effects, therapy should be initiated without an initial loading dose, if possible. The central nervous system is the major site of toxic side effects, the most common being tremor. With high plasma levels (1.5 to 2.5 μg/mL) dizziness, intention tremor ataxia, nervousness, hallucinations, diplopia, memory impairment, or seizures may also occur. These neurologic disorders are minimal or absent with aprindine plasma levels of less than 1 μg/mL.[434, 435] Gastrointestinal side effects, which are less common, include nausea and occasional diarrhea. Agranulocytosis has been reported to occur in 5% of patients and is manifest idiosyncratically.

Sotalol

Sotalol (Fig. 5-21) is a beta-adrenergic blocking agent that differs from propranolol in that it prolongs considerably both the action potential duration and the effective refractory period without affecting the fast sodium inward current.

MODE OF ACTION. Microelectrode studies on isolated tissue preparations have shown that sotalol considerably prolongs action potential duration and effective refractory period, more so in Purkinje fibers than in ventricular muscle.[439,440] Sotalol, however, had no appreciable effect on other transmembrane potential properties, namely, resting membrane potential, action potential amplitude, and maximum rate of rise of phase zero action potential.[439–441] In atrial tissue, sotalol was found to increase atrial refractory period without affecting conduction velocity, thus increasing the wavelength of excitation (i.e., the product of refractory period and conduction velocity).[12] In this study, shorter wavelengths were associated with increased incidence of reentrant repetitive activity; it was suggested, therefore, that the mechanism of the antiarrhythmic activity against reentrant atrial premature excitation may be caused by the lengthening effect of sotalol on the excitation wavelength.[12,442] Whether similar effects are seen in the ventricular myocardium is unknown. Sotalol manifests reverse use-dependent effect on the ventricular MAPD in humans.[443] The reverse use-dependent effect of sotalol means that its prolonging effect of the MAPD is diminished at faster pacing rates. For example, sotalol caused a 6% increase in the MAPD at a 300-millisecond pacing cycle length and a 13% reduction at a 600-millisecond cycle length of stimulation.[443]

Sotalol antagonizes, in a concentration-dependent manner, isoproterenol-induced sinus acceleration.[444] In partially depolarized Purkinje fibers, sotalol terminated abnormal automatic mechanisms, suppressing spontaneous phase 4 depolarization.[104] In intact dogs with induced AV block, sotalol (2 mg/kg intravenously) slowed the rate of idioventricular rhythm and the idioventricular escape interval.[439] Sotalol was also found to prevent or slow the rate of induced reentrant ventricular tachycardia in 11 of 19 dogs with coronary artery occlusion.[445] This effect of sotalol was found to be superior to that of metoprolol, which led Cobbe and coworkers to suggest that its greater efficacy might be caused by its ability to prolong both action potential duration and effective refractory period.[445]

The acute electrophysiologic effects of sotalol have also been studied in humans.[446–448] These studies have shown, as predicted by animal studies, that sotalol significantly increases the refractory period of ventricular myocardium. An increase in the atrial–His conduction time, effective refractory period of the AV node, and AV nodal functional refractory period was also observed. Later studies by Nathan and coworkers found that sotalol prolongs the effective refractory period of both atrial and ventricular tissue.[449] It thus appears that sotalol prolongs refractoriness uniformly in all cardiac tissues. Prolonging the refractory period without concomitant slowing of conduction velocity increases the wavelength and prevents recurrence of reentrant tachyarrhythmias.[450,451] Sotalol, alone or in combination, was effective against "drug-refractory" ventricular tachycardia.[452–454] Acute intravenous sotalol was effective against paroxysmal supraventricular tachycardia.[455]

METABOLISM AND PHARMACOKINETICS. Schnelle and coworkers found that after an intravenous dose of sotalol in healthy subjects, its elimination half-life was 6 to 8 hours.[456] The drug was excreted mainly by glomerular filtration, and metabolites were not found.[456]

Plasma concentration of sotalol was measured after oral administration of increasing doses to healthy subjects.[457] Plasma levels 2 hours after oral doses of 400 and 800 mg showed a fourfold variation among subjects. This may be caused by differences in presystemic elimination (perhaps first-pass hepatic metabolism), causing variations in systemic bioavailability. Peak plasma levels of sotalol after oral administration are reached within 2 to 3 hours. Plasma time course of sotalol decays in a biexponential manner; the apparent half-life of the terminal phase (t¹/₂ beta, the elimination phase) is approximately 13 hours. Beta-blocking effects of sotalol, determined by attenuation of the chronotropic effects of isoproterenol, is seen at 0.8 μg/mL, whereas 6.9 μg/mL are needed to cause half-maximal increases in either atrial or ventricular refractoriness.[444]

The half-life of sotalol is considerably prolonged in patients with renal failure because the drug appears to be eliminated mainly by glomerular filtration.[458] Tjandramaga and coworkers reported that the half-life of sotalol was 2 hours in patients with renal failure. Considerable prolongation of half-life in anuric patients was also reported in another study.[458,459]

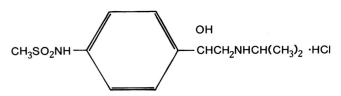

Figure 5-21. Sotalol.

THERAPEUTIC ACTION, DOSE, AND SIDE EFFECTS. Sotalol is effective against supraventricular and ventricular arrhythmias and arrhythmias associated with the WPW syndrome.[460–464] Sotalol suppresses premature ventricular depolarizations with daily oral doses of 160 to 960 mg.[460] Mean daily oral doses of 400 mg (beta-blocking dosage) in humans is associated with a mean plasma level of 1.4 μg/mL; the so-called class II action (i.e., prolonging the refractory period) occurs with mean oral daily dose of 920 mg, giving plasma levels of 3 μg/mL.[463] Side effects of sotalol include exacerbation of congestive heart failure and proarrhythmia.[461,462,465] The proarrhythmic effect of sotalol is most likely to occur in instances of renal failure, hypokalemia, bradycardia, and high concentration of the drug and when there are preexisting long QT intervals.[461] Torsades de pointes resulting from sotalol therapy may be obviated by drug withdrawal, isoproterenol therapy, and ventricular pacing.[466] Correction of electrolyte imbalance may also be useful. During sotalol therapy, administration of drugs that prolong the QT interval is contraindicated.

Propafenone

Propafenone (Fig. 5-22) (RHYTHMOL), newly released for clinical use, has been used with varied success in the management of patients with supraventricular and ventricular arrhythmias and arrhythmias associated with the WPW syndrome.[467,468]

MODE OF ACTION. Microelectrode studies on isolated cardiac tissues have shown that propafenone decreases the maximum rate of depolarization of phase zero of the action potential without changing the resting membrane potential of atrial and ventricular muscle and Purkinje fibers.[469–471] The decrease in $\dot{V}_{max}$ induced by propafenone is use-dependent.[472]

Propafenone shortens action potential duration more than it shortens the effective refractory period, making the ratio of decrease in effective refractory period to action potential shortening greater than 1.[469,471] Propafenone also decreases the slope of spontaneous phase 4 depolarization in Purkinje fibers with relatively high resting membrane potential (-7 mV), causing a decrease in the rate of automatic impulse initiation.[473] The antiautomatic concen-

trations of propafenone on Purkinje fibers have no appreciable effect on sinus node automaticity.[473] Thus, it appears that propafenone has no, or a mild, blocking effect on the sinus node pacemaker current. However, similar concentrations of propafenone caused severe sinus slowing during cholinergic blockade with atropine, indicating that propafenone exerts vagolytic action on the sinus node and offsets its depressant effects.[473] On ventricular and atrial tissue, propafenone prolonged action potential duration and elevated diastolic excitability threshold.[469,471,474] In Purkinje fibers with barium-induced automaticity at low levels of membrane potentials (approximately -50 mV), only the metabolite of propafenone (5-OH propafenone) was effective in slowing the automatic activity; the parent compound and the other metabolite (NDPP) were relatively ineffective.[475] In studies involving dogs with coronary artery occlusion, propafenone suppressed ventricular arrhythmias promptly during the 24-hour post-occlusion arrhythmic period, an effect that was found to be superior to that of lidocaine.[226,475] The two major metabolites of propafenone were found to be more potent than the parent compound against the 24-hour post-occlusion arrhythmias.[475] Electrophysiologic studies in humans have shown that propafenone slows both AV nodal (AH interval), and intra-atrial conduction and prolongs QRS duration and QT interval.[476–478] Both atrial and ventricular effective refractory periods are prolonged.[476,478]

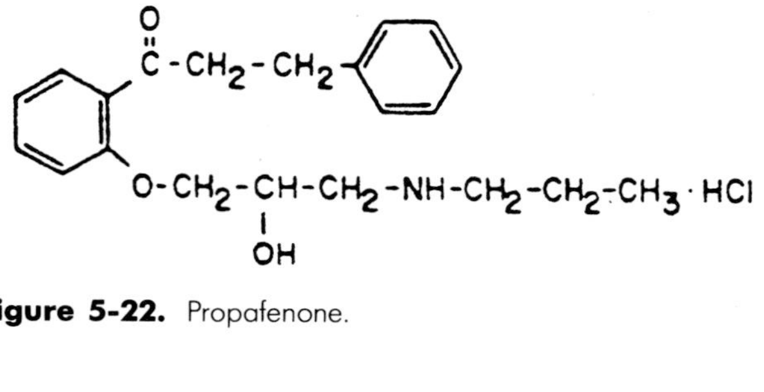

METABOLISM AND PHARMACOKINETICS. Propafenone is metabolized into two major metabolites, 5-OH propafenone and N-depropylpropafenone (NDPP).[479–481] Propafenone seems to be well absorbed orally, but considerable patient variation exists in its half-life of elimination.[476,479,482] Keller and coworkers found peak plasma propafenone levels of about 2.4 μg/mL after an oral dose of 900 mg, with a mean half-life of 3.6 hours.[483] Later studies by Connolly and coworkers showed large patient variability in elimination half-life (range, 2.4 to 11.8 hours).[482] These authors dismissed liver disease, age, heart failure, and the presence of concomitant medication as factors that could interfere with elimination of propafenone, suggesting instead that patient differences in metabolism cause the differences seen in the elimination half-life. Furthermore, in this study, great variability was found in the steady-state mean propafenone concentration in different patients receiving the same dose of propafenone. Although some of these variabilities can be explained by differences in elimination half-life, no strong correlation between half-life and steady-state concentration could be found, indicating the involvement of other factors. One such possible factor, the role of which is still ill-defined, is systemic bioavailability and presystemic elimination (first-pass metabolism). A nonlinear relationship between dose and steady-state concentration was seen; that is, a large increase in plasma

Figure 5-22. Propafenone.

propafenone level followed a small increase in propafenone dose.[482] The mechanism of such plasma elevation of propafenone concentration is unknown but could be caused by saturation of the first-pass metabolic process. Recent studies have shown that the patient's ability to hydroxylate propafenone by the P-450 cytochrome system greatly varies between patients, depending on the patient's genetic composition.[480] Thus, some patients are poor metabolizers and others are fast or extensive metabolizers, which may, in part, be the reason for the various plasma propafenone levels.[480] Because the 5-OH metabolite has antiarrhythmic effects that may be more important than the parent compound, differences in the therapeutic outcome between poor and extensive metabolizers of propafenone are of potential clinical significance.[480] The clinical impact of different stereospecific dispositions of propafenone in poor and extensive metabolizers remains undefined.[484] Propafenone is administered as a racemic mixture of (+)-S- and (−)-R-enantiomers. It is suggested that the beta-blocking activity of propafenone is related to the (+)-S-enantiomer of propafenone.[485] The lower beta-blocking activity of the (−)-R-enantiomer, without significant difference in sodium channel blockade, suggests that administration of this enantiomer rather than the racemic mixture may be advantageous in patients intolerant of beta blockade.[485]

Both propafenone and its major metabolite are extensively distributed in the body. In one experimental study on rabbits, the average myocardial propafenone concentration was 114 times that of the perfusate.[486, 487] During steady-state therapy, saliva propafenone concentrations in healthy volunteers were about 25% that of the plasma.[488] Food intake was found to increase propafenone bioavailability, causing faster and greater peak plasma propafenone concentrations.[489] Cimetidine administration had little or no clinical consequence on the pharmacokinetics or pharmacodynamics of propafenone.[490] However, concomitant administration of propafenone and warfarin leads to an enhanced anticoagulant effect that may require a reduction in the warfarin dose.[491, 492]

THERAPEUTIC ACTION, DOSE, AND SIDE EFFECTS. Propafenone is reported to be effective against premature ventricular depolarizations, paroxysmal supraventricular tachycardia, and arrhythmias associated with the WPW syndrome.[483, 477, 493–504] The drug is not as effective against inducible sustained ventricular tachycardia and is comparable to other antiarrhythmic drugs.[476, 493, 478] Thus, determination of its efficacy and role against inducible ventricular tachycardia awaits further studies involving a larger patient population with a variety of underlying heart diseases. Propafenone has been found to be somewhat effective against ventricular arrhythmias as judged by exercise testing, because 70% of patients responded to propafe-

none therapy.[474] Intravenous injections of propafenone, 1 to 2 mg/kg followed by 0.3 to 0.5 mg/min constant infusion, achieved impressive results in patients with torsades de pointes. Torsades de pointes ceased even during bolus injections.[505] The mild beta-blocking effect of propafenone seen in experimental studies was found to be of no clinical significance.[470, 506, 507]

Propafenone is usually given orally, 150 mg to 300 mg every 8 hours.[479] A therapeutic window of propafenone has not yet been established, but the drug appears to exert its antiarrhythmic efficacy in the plasma level range of 0.5 to 1.8 μg/mL.[479, 482] Side effects include potential block of AV transmission, requiring caution in the use of propafenone in patients with preexisting AV conduction abnormalities.[482] However, in patients with impaired left ventricular function, propafenone was found to be well tolerated, although other studies suggested otherwise.[474, 508] We recommend caution when administering propafenone to patients with impaired left ventricular function. The combination of propafenone and mexiletine is effective in suppressing the induction of ventricular tachycardia in some patients refractory to procainamide and propafenone alone.[369] In those patients in whom ventricular tachycardia could still be induced, the rate was slower and hemodynamically tolerated during the combination therapy.[369] Propafenone may also aggravate ventricular arrhythmias.[65, 493, 502] In one study, propafenone, like other antiarrhythmic drugs with class I action, was found to provide adequate protection against acute ischemic inducible ventricular tachycardias.[509] Neurologic disorders are not uncommon and may include weakness and disorientation, dry mouth, metallic taste, and sometimes nausea, not often necessitating discontinuation of the drug.[476, 479, 502] In one study, caution in the use of propafenone was suggested in asthmatics because it decreased the dose of methacholine required to reduce the forced expiratory volume.[510] More studies are needed to clarify the clinical significance of this observation. In a 2-year-old child, inadvertent ingestion of 1.8 g of propafenone induced seizures and severe conduction abnormalities in which intravenous phenytoin administration caused cardiopulmonary collapse, necessitating aggressive cardiopulmonary life support.[511]

Bretylium

Bretylium (Fig. 5-23) is used in the United States for the treatment of recurrent life-threatening ventricular arrhythmias (i.e., ventricular fibrillation), such as those seen in postmyocardial infarction patients. It is marketed under the brand name of Bretylol.

MODE OF ACTION. The antiarrhythmic mechanisms of bretylium are not fully understood. It has been suggested that

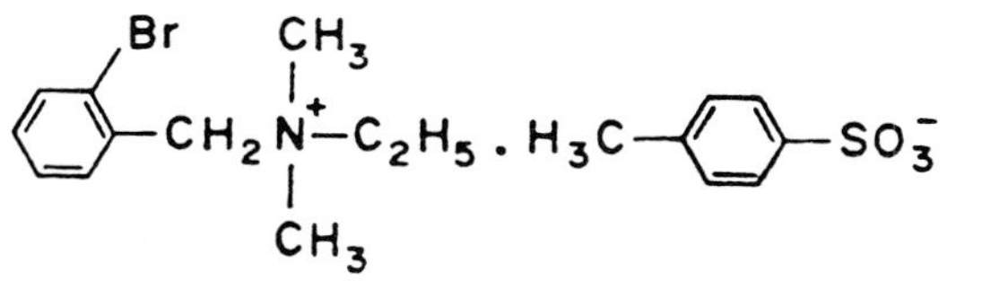

Figure 5-23. Bretylium tosylate.

arrhythmia suppression may result from the ability of bretylium to interact with the sympathetic nervous system, from its direct effects on the transmembrane potentials of cardiac fibers, or by a combination of these mechanisms. In vitro studies on isolated papillary muscle preparations have shown that bretylium, at clinically relevant concentrations, causes a concentration-dependent increase in the force of contraction.[512] Pretreating animals with reserpine (to produce catecholamine depletion) or a beta blocker (e.g., propranolol) prevents this positive inotropic effect, suggesting that bretylium has indirect inotropic action mediated through myocardial catecholamine release.[512, 513] Although other studies ascribe a direct effect to increased force of contraction, the primary action of bretylium on myocardial force of contraction results from the release of catecholamines from the adrenergic nerve endings.[513, 514] However, prolonged administration of bretylium produces peripheral vasodilation, probably caused by adrenergic blockade.[515–517]

Microelectrode studies on isolated cardiac fibers have shown that bretylium, in concentrations up to 20 μg/mL, has no effect on resting membrane potential, upstroke velocity, or action potential amplitude, both in Purkinje and ventricular myocardial fibers.[518, 519] However, the drug may transiently increase resting potential (make it more negative) and upstroke velocity, with an attendant increase in conduction velocity. These effects may be caused by release of norepinephrine from sympathetic nerve endings.[513, 518] At concentrations above 20 μg/mL, bretylium exerts a direct membrane-depressant effect, decreasing upstroke velocity and action potential amplitude and slowing conduction velocity.[513] Bretylium markedly prolongs the duration of action potential and effective refractory period of both ventricular and Purkinje fibers.[513, 518–520] It is postulated that such remarkable prolongation of action potential duration and refractory period, without concomitant changes in other action potential properties, may terminate reentrant arrhythmias during acute myocardial infarction.[17] In this respect, it has been argued that bretylium has an action that is "antifibrillatory."[17] Furthermore, bretylium-induced prolongation of action potential duration is greater in regions of the heart where action potentials are shortest.[513, 518, 519] Cardinal and Sasyniuk have shown that bretylium prolonged action potential duration of subendocardial Purkinje fibers in the normal zone more than in ischemic Purkinje fibers in the infarcted zone, where the action potential duration was already considerably prolonged (due to ischemia) before bretylium superfusion.[521] Such a differential effect on action potential duration and, presumably, on refractoriness decreases the disparity in the repolarization process, thereby decreasing the likelihood of reentrant premature excitation.

The antiarrhythmic effects of bretylium may be delayed after parenteral administration, sometimes for more than 1 hour. Animal studies have shown that myocardial bretylium concentrations, after intravenous injection (6 mg/kg over 1 minute), rise slowly and reach a peak 1.5 to 6 hours after injection.[522] At 12 hours after injection, the ratio of myocardial to serum drug concentration reaches 7.[522] It could be postulated that the delay required for the development of full antiarrhythmic efficacy is caused by the slowly rising myocardial bretylium concentration. The antifibrillatory effect of bretylium was demonstrated by Wenger and coworkers.[523] In a canine model of ischemic ventricular fibrillation caused by transient occlusion, bretylium decreased the incidence of ventricular fibrillation during subsequent coronary artery reperfusion.[523] Bretylium is one of the few antiarrhythmic drugs that significantly reduces the incidence of ventricular fibrillation in dogs after release of an acute coronary artery occlusion. Most of the commonly used antiarrhythmic drugs, including amiodarone, are ineffective against reperfusion-induced ventricular fibrillation in the canine model.[524] It is, perhaps, for this unique action that bretylium was characterized as an antifibrillatory drug.

METABOLISM AND PHARMACOKINETICS. Bretylium can be administered by oral, intramuscular, or intravenous route, although the oral route is least preferred because bretylium has a poor and erratic pattern of absorption.[435] Similar considerations apply for the intramuscular route. The pharmacokinetic disposition of bretylium is not yet fully described. The drug is not metabolized significantly and is largely eliminated by the kidney.[75] Bretylium maintenance doses should be reduced in patients with renal failure.[75]

THERAPEUTIC ACTION, DOSE, AND SIDE EFFECTS. The major clinical use of bretylium is the emergency treatment of life-threatening, drug-resistant ventricular tachycardia and ventricular fibrillation.[513, 522–526] Bretylium tosylate has also been used orally in the management of patients with ventricular tachycardia, with 200 to 400 mg given every 8 hours. Although orthostatic hypotension may develop in the initial stages of oral drug administration, tolerance usually develops without loss of antiarrhythmic efficacy. Much of the reported clinical experience is, however, with parenterally administered bretylium. A suitable dosage regimen is a loading dose of 600 to 900 mg (5 to 10 mg/kg) intramuscularly with incremental doses of 200 mg every 1 to 2 hours, until the arrhythmia is controlled or approximately 2 g of drug has been given. The recommended maintenance dosage is 5 mg/kg every 6 to 8 hours. During intravenous infusion, bretylium should be diluted in 50 to 100 mL of 5% dextrose in water, and the loading dose (5 to 10 mg/kg) should be administered slowly over 15 to 30 minutes. This regimen may be followed by a constant infusion of 1 to 10 mg/min. The initial release of catecholamines induced by bretylium results in increased heart rate and blood pressure.[527] Bretylium has been used with variable success against torsades de pointes.[528]

The most common adverse effect is hypotension, usually postural.[206] Nausea and vomiting have occasionally been reported. Parotid enlargement commonly develops after 2 to 4 months of oral bretylium therapy. The consequences of bretylium-induced beta-adrenergic blockade, which usually follows an initial activation, include exacerbation of AV conduction slowing, congestive heart failure, and asthmatic attacks. Caution must be exercised when catecholamine administration is sought to counteract the effects of bretylium because there may be supersensitivity reactions caused by blockade by adrenergic nerve endings of norepinephrine uptake. Arrhythmias may be aggravated and heart failure exacerbated.[527] It has been suggested that bretylium not be used in combination with other antiarrhythmic drugs, because complete nullification of either drug may result from combination therapy.[99]

Moricizine

Ethmozine (Fig. 5-24) is the trade name of moricizine, a phenothiazine derivative (10-[morpholinopropionyl]-phenothiazine-2-carbamic acid), which has been used clinically in the fomer Soviet Union for the management of patients with atrial and ventricular arrhythmias associated with a variety of heart diseases.[529, 530] Its clinical use in the United States began in the late 1970s, and increasing data are becoming available on its clinical usefulness, efficacy, and indications.[59, 60, 63, 66, 68, 531–533]

MODE OF ACTION. Microelectrode studies on isolated Purkinje fibers have shown that moricizine decreases the $\dot{V}_{max}$ of phase zero and the amplitude of the action potential, with a concomitant shortening of action potential dura-

Figure 5-24. Ethmozin.

tion.[531, 534] These effects are concentration-dependent. Voltage-clamp studies on isolated frog atrial muscle preparations have shown that moricizine decreases the fast inward sodium current by decreasing the maximum conductance of sodium (GNa), without affecting the kinetics of sodium channel activation, inactivation, and reactivation.[529] Such an effect, if also present in mammalian cardiac fibers, differs from that of other antiarrhythmic agents, which almost always delay the reactivation kinetics of the fast sodium inward current. Moricizine does not seem to affect slow-response action potentials, because, in the results of open-chest anesthetized canine studies, moricizine did not change spontaneous sinus node cycle length or AV conduction time when selectively injected into the sinus node artery and the posterior septal artery, respectively.[535] Although the drug decreases Purkinje fiber action potential duration, intact canine studies have shown that moricizine, following intravenous administration (4 mg/kg), increases both the right and left ventricular muscle cell refractory period and diastolic excitability threshold.[535] Moricizine appears to be effective against spontaneously occurring ventricular arrhythmias 24 hours after coronary artery occlusion in dogs as well as against ventricular arrhythmias induced by epinephrine 2 to 5 days after coronary artery occlusion.[534]

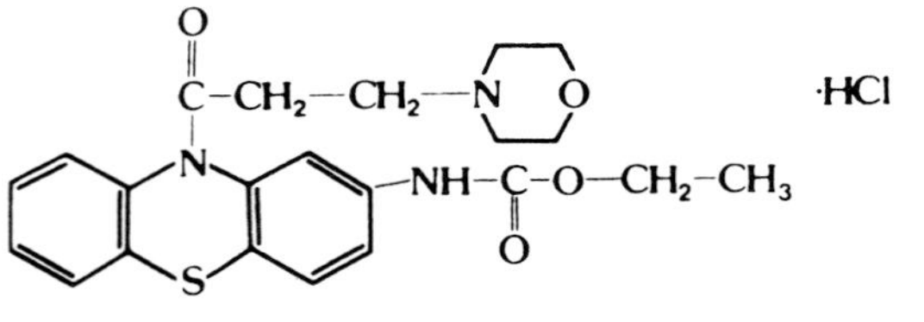

METABOLISM AND PHARMACOKINETICS. Little information has been published on the pharmacokinetics of moricizine in humans. The drug appears to be well absorbed when given orally, and only small amounts of the agent (0.25%) appear unchanged in the urine and feces, suggesting extensive metabolism.[529, 531, 532] Peak plasma levels of moricizine after an oral dose are reached in 1 to 3 hours.[536] The elimination half-life of moricizine in five healthy volunteers after an oral dose of 500 mg was 4 hours, with a range of 2.1 to 5.1 hours.[531, 536] However, the half-life is longer in patients with arrhythmia, reaching up to 6.7 hours.[537] Therefore, the drug has been prescribed every 8 hours with trough plasma levels averaging 114 ng/mL.[537] According to one study, therapeutic efficacy is maintained using twice daily dosing.[538] Plasma levels of moricizine associated with significant antiarrhythmic effects were 244 to 1300 ng/mL. Atrial premature depolarizations appeared to be suppressed with lower moricizine plasma levels than ventricular premature depolarizations.[531, 532]

THERAPEUTIC ACTION, DOSE, AND SIDE EFFECTS. Moricizine is well tolerated by patients receiving up to 600 mg daily. The drug has almost no adverse effects.[531, 535] Good control of premature ventricular complexes was achieved with a 600-mg total daily oral dose of moricizine (200 mg three times daily), which was found to be more effective than oral disopyramide in controlling complex ventricular arrhythmias.[59] Moricizine was found ineffective against inducible sustained ventricular tachycardia in humans.[539] As with encainide and flecainide, moricizine was also associated with increased death rate in the CAST study.[69, 70] The study of the long-term effects of moricizine in suppressing ventricular premature depolarizations in patients with myocardial infarction is ongoing.[66] The incidence of proarrhythmic effects with moricizine, both during Holter monitoring (noninvasive) and electrical stimulation (invasive) studies, was less than 10%.[63] Similarly, moricizine has relatively low potential to aggravate congestive heart failure.[370] Furthermore, moricizine was associated with minimal extracardiac side effects.[533] The near absence of toxic side effects makes moricizine an attractive alternative antiarrhythmic agent; however, its value and effectiveness in the control of life-threatening ventricular arrhythmias are unknown.

Lorcainide

MODE OF ACTION. Carmeliet and Zaman evaluated the effects of lorcainide (Fig. 5-25) on the transmembrane potential characteristics of isolated tissue preparations with microelectrodes.[540, 541] The drug decreased the $\dot{V}_{max}$ of the action potential of Purkinje fibers and prolonged the effective refractory periods of both Purkinje and ventricular muscle fibers. The depression of $\dot{V}_{max}$ in isolated guinea pig muscle is use-dependent.[386] Slow-response action potentials are unaffected by lorcainide concentrations of up to 5 μg/mL.[541] Lorcainide decreases conduction velocity and automaticity in isolated normal Purkinje fibers and causes a concentration-dependent prolongation in the HV interval in both basic and premature impulses in intact guinea pig hearts.[541, 542] Experimental ventricular arrhythmias caused by left anterior descending coronary artery occlusion during the 24-hour arrhythmic phase, as well as arrhythmias caused by ouabain toxicity, respond well to lorcainide.[542]

Electrophysiologic studies in humans have shown that lorcainide consistently prolongs the HV interval in a dose-dependent manner and, thus, is contraindicated in patients with preexisting intraventricular conduction abnormalities.[542] Lorcainide has a variable effect on the AV nodal effective and functional refractory periods and the effective refractory period of the right ventricle. Most studies, however, found prolonged PR, QRS, and QT intervals.[542] Furthermore, lorcainide prolonged both anterograde and retrograde conduction times and effective refractory periods of the accessory pathway in patients with WPW syndrome; therefore, it can be useful in such a patient population.[543] Lorcainide is classified as having class 1C action.

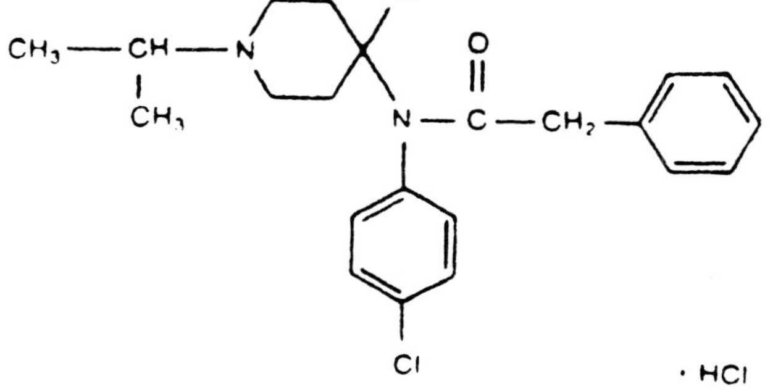

METABOLISM AND PHARMACOKINETICS. Lorcainide is rapidly distributed to well-perfused tissues, with early decline in plasma lorcainide concentrations, necessitating a three-compartment model system to describe the kinetics adequately, at least in patients with ventricular arrhythmias.[544] The volume of distribution of lorcainide at steady state is 6.3 L/kg, and its terminal half-life is 7.8 hours.[544] Clearance of lorcainide is high and approximates normal blood flow.[542, 544] The drug is 83% bound to protein, with significantly lower binding in patients with congestive heart failure.[542] Oral bioavailability of lorcainide increases with higher and long-term oral doses and ranges from 2% to 4% after a single oral dose of 100 mg to 100% after 200 mg of long-term oral administration.[543, 545–547] This occurs because of presystemic elimination of lorcainide, primarily caused by first-pass metabolism.[545] Only 2% of lorcainide is excreted unchanged in the urine. The elimination half-life of lorcainide averages from 8 to 13 hours.[544, 546, 548] Its elimination half-life may, however, reach 26.8 hours after 1 week of oral lorcainide administration in patients with ventricular arrhythmias.[544]

The major metabolite of lorcainide is norlorcainide, which has potent antiarrhythmic efficacy.[542] Norlorcainide gradually accumulates in serum because it has a longer half-life (26 hours) than the parent compound.[544, 546] At steady state, norlorcainide levels are about twice the level of lorcainide.[396] Plasma concentration of lorcainide associated with effective suppression of ventricular arrhythmias seems to be variable but usually ranges between 150 and 400 ng/mL, a concentration range usually achieved with 100 mg twice or three times daily.[542, 546, 549] The complete elimination of lorcainide by hepatic metabolism indicates that hepatic function and hepatic blood flow could influence the disposition kinetics of this drug. Klots and co-workers have shown that the half-life of lorcainide increases from 7.7 to 12.5 hours in patients with alcoholic cirrhosis.[550] Furthermore, in patients with congestive heart failure, the half-life increased from 7.7 to 15.6 hours, with a concomitant decrease in clearance from 1000 to 385 mL/min, probably caused by a decrease in hepatic blood flow.[550, 551]

Figure 5-25. Lorcainide.

THERAPEUTIC ACTION, DOSE, AND SIDE EFFECTS. Lorcainide appears to suppress ventricular premature depolarizations and to prevent induction of sustained ventricular tachycardia by programmed electrical stimulation (in up to 70% of patients).[178, 552–557] Intravenous lorcainide was found to be as effective as lidocaine against symptomatic ventricular tachyarrhythmias, but 30% of patients responded to only one of the two agents.[558] The agent also appears to be effective in patients with the preexcitation syndrome but is relatively ineffective against atrial arrhythmias.[542, 543, 559] Typical doses are 1 to 2 mg/kg intravenously and 100 to 200 mg orally twice daily.[396] The most common side effect, occurring at the start of therapy, is sleep disturbance, characterized by frequent awakening, hot flashes, and vivid dreams.[542, 552, 554] It appears, however, that patients do not complain of fatigue during the day.[552] Although the severity of the sleep disturbances diminishes with chronic therapy, most patients who develop this side effect continue to have symptoms after 1 year of therapy and often require chronic treatment with benzodiazepines for sleep.[560] Other side effects include central nervous system toxicity, metallic taste, gastrointestinal distress, headache, nausea, excessive perspiration, and mild potential to aggravate congestive heart failure and arrhythmias.[59, 370, 517, 542, 552, 561] Long-term efficacy and adverse effects of this agent remain to be seen.

Ajmaline

Ajmaline (Fig. 5-26), a tertiary indoline alkaloid, was first isolated from the root of *Rauwolfia serpentina*, an Indian plant, by Siddiqui and Siddiqui in 1932.[562] Unlike the reserpine-like alkaloids, the ajmaline-like alkaloids isolated from the plant do not seem to affect adrenergic nerve terminals. Microelectrode studies on isolated cardiac tissues have shown that ajmaline (1 μg/mL) has no effect on resting membrane potential but decreases $\dot{V}_{max}$, action potential amplitude, and overshoot of canine atrial, Purkinje, and ventricular muscle fibers.[563] Furthermore, ajmaline shortens Purkinje fiber action potential but prolongs both atrial and ventricular muscle action potential duration.[563] Similar findings were observed by Dreifus and coworkers on partially depolarized (resting membrane potential approximately − 60 mV) ventricular muscle fibers when superfused with 3 μg/mL of 17-monochloroacetyl ajmaline hydrochloride.[99] Ajmaline decreases excitability of both canine atrial and ventricular tissue.[563] Ajmaline also decreases the slope of phase 4 depolarization and slows linear conduction velocity in isolated strands of canine Purkinje fibers.[564]

Ajmaline is effective against digitalis-induced ventricular arrhythmias in dogs.[563, 565] However, this drug is most effective against aconitine-induced atrial tachyarrhyth-

Figure 5-26. Ajmaline.

mias.[563] Electrophysiologic studies in both anesthetized and conscious dogs demonstrated a significant depression of intraventricular conduction with QRS widening but without significant prolongation of the AH interval.[566] In addition, ajmaline was effective against ventricular arrhythmias that occur 24 hours after left anterior descending coronary artery occlusion in the dog.[566] Early clinical studies indicate that ajmaline can be of some value in the management of paroxysmal supraventricular tachycardia.[563, 567] Bojorges and coworkers have shown that 1 mg/kg of ajmaline given over 5 minutes suppressed these arrhythmias in 30 of 36 patients.[563] In a later study, intravenous administration of ajmaline (50 mg) was found to be effective in 10 patients with paroxysmal supraventricular tachycardia mediated by dual AV nodal pathways.[567] Furthermore, ajmaline was found to be relatively ineffective against arrhythmias of ventricular origin.[563] Wellens and coworkers found that ajmaline caused complete antegrade block in the accessory pathway in 32 of 59 patients with WPW syndrome.[568] Furthermore, failure of ajmaline to produce completed anterograde block appeared to be related to a shorter (less than 270 milliseconds) refractory period of this pathway.

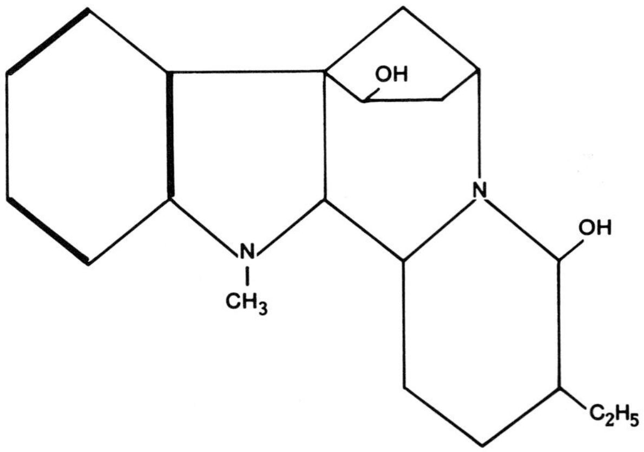

The role of ajmaline in the long-term management of arrhythmias of various causes and the role, if any, of its metabolites remain undefined. The drug does not seem to be associated with serious side effects.[568] Mild side effects include flushing, nausea, and blinking of eyes. However, severe toxicity can cause worsening of congestive heart failure, shock, sinoatrial block, and even ventricular tachycardia and ventricular fibrillation.[567, 568] The drug should be used with caution in patients with conduction disturbances of the AV node and the His–Purkinje system. Hypotension may develop during intravenous administration; therefore, it is imperative to infuse the drug slowly, 1 mg/kg over 3 to 5 minutes.[563, 568]

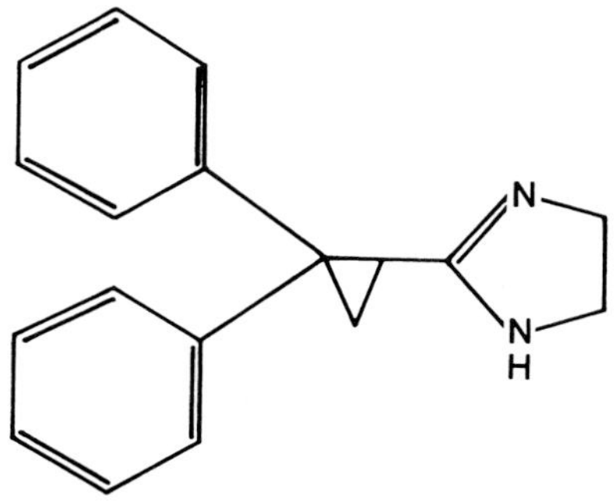

Figure 5-27. Cibenzoline.

Cibenzoline

MODE OF ACTION.   Cibenzoline (Fig. 5-27), an antiarrhythmic drug of imidazoline derivation (2-[2,-diphenyl-cyclopropyl]), is not related chemically to any other known antiarrhythmic drug. The succinate salt is used. Preliminary clinical trials indicate the potential usefulness of this agent to suppress ventricular premature depolarizations and arrhythmias associated with the WPW syndrome.[569, 570]

Microelectrode studies on isolated cardiac tissue have shown that cibenzoline prolongs the action potential duration of atrial and ventricular muscle cells while shortening action potential duration in Purkinje fibers.[571–573] Furthermore, cibenzoline appears to prevent action potential shortening during hypoxia.[572] Cibenzoline decreases V_{max} in atrial and ventricular tissues and slows conduction velocity in isolated ventricular preparations.[571–573] The drug does not interfere with sinus nodal automaticity but causes a concentration-dependent prolongation of sinus node cell action potential duration, which tends to decrease the rate of sinus firing.[571, 572] Cibenzoline decreases the slope of phase 4 depolarization in normal Purkinje fibers, causing a decrease in the rate of automatic impulse initiation.[571] However, such an effect was not observed in Dangman's studies; instead, cibenzoline depressed automaticity in normal Purkinje fibers induced by isoproterenol by a mechanism independent of beta-adrenergic receptor blockade.[573] Cibenzoline was found to depress abnormal automatic mechanism (resting potential, −60 to 40 mV) in Purkinje fibers induced by barium ions.[573]

In clinical studies, cibenzoline increased the PR, HV, and QTC intervals, with QRS widening following oral or intravenous administration.[574–577]

METABOLISM AND PHARMACOKINETICS.   Both the oral and intravenous forms of cibenzoline have been studied. The half-life of elimination of cibenzoline in healthy subjects varies between 3.5 to 10.5 hours.[578, 579] The elimination half-life of cibenzoline is prolonged in patients with heart disease to reach between 7.6 to 22.3 hours.[580] Twice daily dosing appears adequate based on the characteristics of cibenzoline disposition kinetics. The half-life increases with age and declining kidney function.[579, 580] Approximately 60% of the drug is excreted unchanged in the urine.[581, 582] Clearance of cibenzoline correlates well with creatinine clearance, with an average rate of 495 mL/min.[583] Approximately 60% of cibenzoline is protein bound.[584] Bioavailability of oral cibenzoline is reported to be 92%.[581] Peak plasma cibenzoline level after an oral dose is reached within 2.5 hours, and effective plasma cibenzoline concentrations appear to be 215 to 400 ng/mL.[582, 585] No information is yet available on the metabolic fate of cibenzoline.

THERAPEUTIC ACTION, DOSE, AND SIDE EFFECTS.   Cibenzoline is effective in suppressing or decreasing the frequency of premature ventricular depolarizations of various causes.[569, 574, 577, 586] In patients in whom ventricular tachycardia was induced by electrical stimulation, cibenzoline prevented tachycardia induction in 40% to 58% (total of 17 patients in two studies).[574, 575] In another report, cibenzoline eliminated nonsustained ventricular tachycardia in 16 of 26 patients.[587] Cibenzoline appears to be ineffective in patients with sustained ventricular tachycardia or ventricular fibrillation.[588] In two studies, cibenzoline was found to be effective in terminating supraventricular tachycardia with and without the involvement of accessory pathways.[570, 589] Intravenous doses range between 1 and 3 mg/kg and oral doses between 130 and 380 mg/kg.[65, 396] The drug appears to be well tolerated. Side effects include congestive heart failure that may require discontinuation of therapy, bundle branch block, and syncope.[577, 590] In 10% to 20% of patients on cibenzoline therapy, arrhythmia aggravation occurs.[60, 65] Epigastric burning, blurred vision, nausea, and vomiting have also been reported.[577, 588, 590]

Imipramine

Imipramine (Fig. 5-28) is a tricyclic antidepressant drug that also has cardiac antiarrhythmic effects. The early description of the cardiac effects of the tricyclic antidepres-

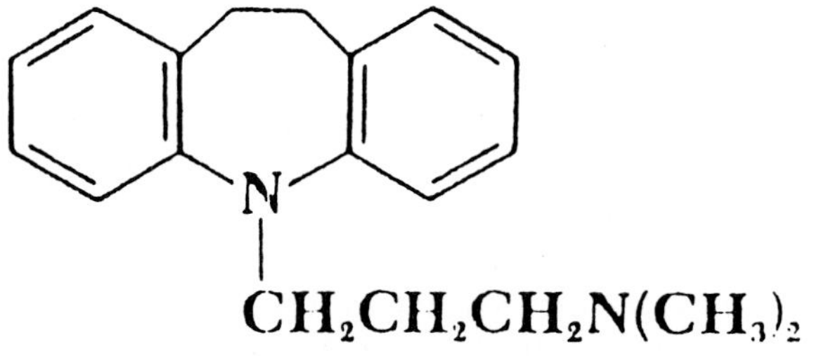

$$CH_2CH_2CH_2N(CH_3)_2$$

Figure 5-28. Imipramine.

Amiloride

Guanidinium

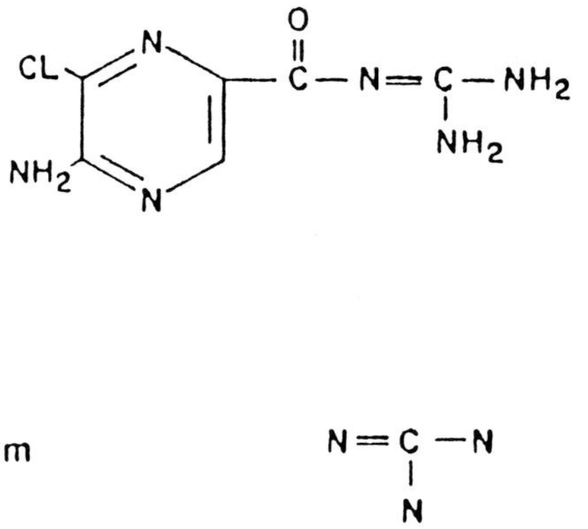

Figure 5-29. Amiloride and guanidinium.

sants came as reports of cardiac side effects associated with both therapeutic and toxic doses. Imipramine is marketed as an antidepressant, and its use as an antiarrhythmic agent has not yet been approved by the FDA.

Microelectrode studies on Purkinje fibers have shown that imipramine decreases $\dot{V}_{max}$ of action potential upstroke, shortens action potential duration, and slows conduction velocity (i.e., quinidine-like effect).[591,592] Imipramine also exerts potent autonomic influences in that it blocks norepinephrine uptake by adrenergic nerve endings and has strong anticholinergic activity.[593,594] These direct and indirect actions of imipramine affect the cardiac electrophysiologic and vascular hemodynamic functions in an important manner. Clinical studies have shown that imipramine increases HV interval and QRS duration, and QT interval also becomes prolonged with toxic doses of imipramine.[595,596]

METABOLISM AND PHARMACOKINETICS. Imipramine undergoes significant first-pass hepatic metabolism by N-demethylation to give two active metabolites, desipramine and nortriptyline.[597] As a result of this high first-pass hepatic extraction, the steady-state volume of distribution of imipramine is large, reaching approximately 1100 L, or about 15 L/kg.[598] Imipramine is 85% protein bound, and its elimination half-life in the young is 16 hours, which is prolonged to 30 hours in the elderly.[598] The bioavailability of imipramine is approximately 50%.[598]

THERAPEUTIC ACTION, DOSE, AND SIDE EFFECTS. Imipramine was used in the CAPS trial in patients with myocardial infarction and frequent premature ventricular depolarizations.[68] Imipramine was found to be less effective than either encainide or flecainide in suppressing ventricular ectopy evaluated in 102 patients (52% versus 80%).[68] Similarly, in patients with inducible ventricular tachycardia, imipramine prevented inducibility of the tachycardia in only 2 of 12 patients studied.[595] Imipramine has serious side effects, including proarrhythmia, orthostatic hypotension, and depression of ventricular function.[68,595] Daily oral doses of imipramine are 100 to 380 mg with therapeutic plasma levels ranging between 100 and 300 ng/mL.[68,599]

Amiloride

Amiloride is a widely used potassium-sparing diuretic agent, marketed under the trade name of Midamor. Structurally, amiloride is a guanidinium (Fig. 5-29) and is related to bethanidine and meobentine (Fig. 5-30).

Microelectrode studies on isolated canine Purkinje fibers showed that prolonged exposure to amiloride caused progressive time and concentration-dependent prolongation of action potential duration without affecting $\dot{V}_{max}$ of the action potential upstrokes.[600] The time constant

Bethanidine

Meobentine

Amiloride

Guanidinium

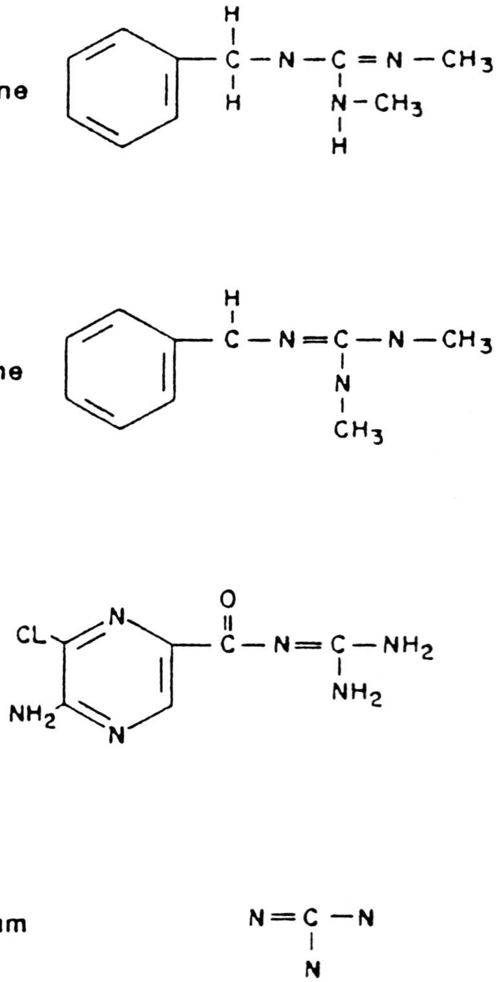

Figure 5-30. Drugs with guanidinium-related chemical structures.

of action potential prolongation was 1.8 hours.[600] At a relatively long cycle length of stimulation (>2000 milliseconds), early afterdepolarizations were induced that could be suppressed by tetrodotoxin and nisoldipine.[600] In dogs with experimental myocardial infarction and inducible ventricular tachycardia, prolonged loading and maintenance intravenous infusion of amiloride prevented tachycardia inducibility in 6 of 12 dogs.[601] In this study, it was found that the dogs that responded had significantly smaller infarct size than those that did not respond.[601] In another study, the efficacy of amiloride was tested in 35 patients with inducible sustained ventricular tachycardia that was refractory to an antiarrhythmic drug therapy (average of 3.6 drugs tested).[602] Twelve of 35 patients responded to oral amiloride therapy, 10 and 20 mg/d on a twice-daily regimen.[602] The patients who responded had significantly higher plasma amiloride levels than those who did not (52 ng/mL and 30 ng/mL, respectively).[602] Amiloride was also found to be effective against ventricular premature depolarizations in 8 of 15 patients studied.[602]

Although these preliminary results indicate the antiarrhythmic potential of amiloride both in experimental and clinical settings of ischemic heart disease, its long-term efficacy and its role in arrhythmia suppression are unclear.

Adenosine

Adenosine (Fig. 5-31) is an endogenous, naturally occurring compound found in the human body. It is composed of adenine, a nitrogenous base of purine class bonded to D-ribose, a pentose. The hydroxyl group attached to C5 on the adenine ring can form an ester bond with one, two, or three molecules of phosphate. When this occurs, the resultant compounds are adenosine monophosphate (AMP), adenosine diphosphate (ADP), and adenosine triphosphate (ATP), respectively. Adenosine itself is formed in the body by two major mechanisms. The first is by the dephosphorylation of AMP to adenosine and phosphate. The second pathway is by the breakdown of S-adenosyl homocysteine to adenosine and homocysteine.[603] Adenosine was approved by the FDA for intravenous use in patients with supraventricular tachycardia.

Adenosine acts through extracellular adenosine receptors and causes transient slowing or block of AV nodal conduction.[603] In a multicenter study involving 359 patients, adenosine in graded doses of up to 12 mg (bolus) rapidly and effectively terminated acute episodes of paroxysmal supraventricular tachycardia in which the AV node was an integral part of the reentry circuit.[604] The overall efficacy of adenosine is similar to that of verapamil, but its onset of action is more rapid, and its adverse effects are minor but brief.[604] After cardiac transplantation, the denervated atria and ventricles demonstrate increased sensitivity to adenosine, a phenomenon that appears to be consistent with adenosine receptor supersensitivity in denervated human heart.[605] In contrast to atrial tissue, adenosine has no direct effect in ventricular myocardium. However, both inotropic and electrophysiologic effects of adenosine on ventricular myocardium can be demonstrated during stimulation of the adenyl cyclase-cAMP system with catecholamines.[606]

Future Directions

None of the available antiarrhythmic drugs, whether they are standard, conventional, or investigational, are ideal in terms of efficacy and safety. A substantial number of patients still do not respond to "therapeutic" doses of all the antiarrhythmic drugs discussed here.[607] In such "drug-refractory" patients, other therapeutic modalities, such as catheter ablation, antitachycardia devices (e.g., implantable defibrillators), and cardiac surgery, are sought.

The search for new agents that are site-specific and have high toxic to therapeutic ratios is essential. New ways of drug delivery for antiarrhythmic drugs have been investigated. We found that coronary venous retroinfusion of procainamide was superior to the systemic intravenous route against spontaneous and inducible sustained ventricular tachycardia in a canine model of complete and permanent coronary artery occlusion.[608] Although the drug could not reach the site of the arrhythmia with sufficient concentration by systemic injection (coronary obstruction), the delivery of the same agent through the vein draining the occluded bed achieved superior antiar-

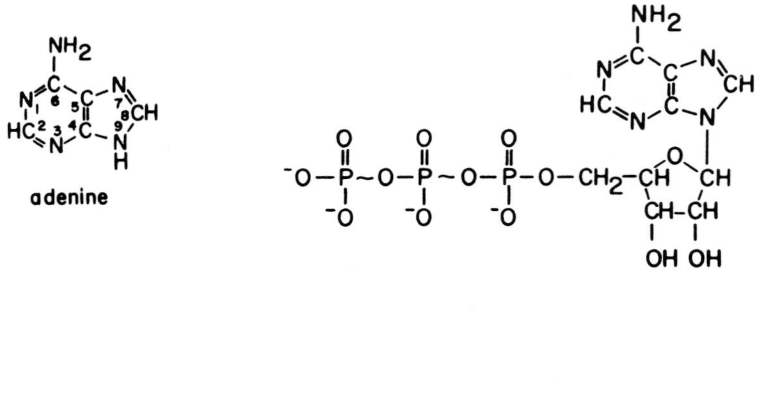

Figure 5-31. Adenine (adenosine triphosphate).

rhythmic efficacy.[608] Future work should address the possibility of "tagging" an antiarrhythmic drug with a ligand that will deliver the drug exclusively to specific diseased myocardial sites where arrhythmias are thought to originate. Such targeted delivery of drugs would eliminate the toxic side effects of those drugs.

The complex and unusual features of amiodarone may contain important clues for potential drug developers. It may be possible to identify beneficial and toxic properties of amiodarone more accurately to separate these two actions and create a safe amiodarone-like drug.[607]

References

1. Wit AL, Rosen MR, Hoffman BF: Electrophysiology and pharmacology of cardiac arrhythmias. II. Relationship of normal and abnormal electrical activity of cardiac fibers to the genesis of arrhythmias. B. Reentry sec 1. Am Heart J 1974; 88:664.

2. Wit AL, Rosen MR, Hoffman BF: Electrophysiology and pharmacology of cardiac arrhythmias. II. Relationship of normal and abnormal electrical activity of cardiac fibers to the genesis of arrhythmias. B. Reentry sec 2. Am Heart J 1974; 88:798.

3. Coraboeuf E: Ionic basis of electrical activity in cardiac tissues. Am J Physiol 1978;234:H101.

4. Vassalle M: Electrogenesis of the plateau and pacemaker potential. Annu Rev Physiol 1977;41:425.

5. Cranefield PF: Action potentials and arrhythmias. Circ Res 1977;41:415.

6. Wit AL, Cranfield PF: Triggered and automatic activity in the canine coronary sinus. Circ Res 1977;41:435.

7. Tsien RW, Kass RS, Weingart R: Cellular and subcellular mechanisms of cardiac pacemaker oscillations. J Exp Biol 1979;81:205.

8. Karagueuzian HS, Katzung BG: Voltage-clamp studies of transient inward current and mechanical oscillations induced by ouabain in ferret papillary muscle. J Physiol (Lond) 1982;327:255.

9. Hoffman BF, Rosen MR: Cellular mechanisms of cardiac arrhythmias. Circ Res 1981;49:1.

10. Vaughan Williams EM: Classification of antiarrhythmic drugs. J Pharmacol Exp Ther 1975;1:115.

11. Singh BN, Hauswirth O: Comparative mechanisms of action of antiarrhythmic drugs. Am Heart J 1974;87:367.

12. Rensma PL, Allessie MA, Lammers WJEP, Bonke FIM, Schalij M: Length of excitation wave and susceptibility to reentrant arrhythmias in normal conscious dogs. Circ Res 1988;62:395.

13. Rosen MR: Effects of pharmacological agents on mechanisms responsible for re-entry. In: Kulbertus HE, ed. Reentrant arrhythmias. Mechanisms and treatment. Baltimore: University Park Press, 1976:283.

14. Podrid PJ, Lampert S, Graboys TB, Blatt CM, Lown B: Aggravation of arrhythmia by antiarrhythmic drugs—incidence and predictors. Am J Cardiol 1987;59:38E.

15. Rae AP, Kay HR, Horowitz LN, Spielman SR, Greenspan AM: Proarrhythmic effects of antiarrhythmic drugs in patients with malignant ventricular arrhythmias evaluated by electrophysiologic testing. J Am Coll Cardiol 1988;12:131.

16. Stanton MS, Prystowsky EN, Fineberg NS, et al: Arrhythmogenic effects of antiarrhythmic drugs: A study of 506 patients treated for ventricular tachycardia or fibrillation. J Am Coll Cardiol 1989;14:209.

17. Katzung BG: New concepts of antiarrhythmic drug action. Prog Cardiol 1987;15:5.

18. Antzelevitch C, Bernstein MJ, Feldman HN, Moe GK: Parasystole reentry and tachycardia: A canine preparation of cardiac arrhythmia occurring across inexcitable segment of tissue. Circulation 1983;68:1101.

19. Chialvo DR, Jalife J: Non-linear dynamics of cardiac excitation and impulse propagation. Nature 1987;330:749.

20. Chialvo DR, Jalife J: On the nonlinear equilibrium of the heart, locking behavior and chaos in Purkinje fibers. In: Zipes DP, Jalife J, eds. Cardiac electrophysiology, from cell to bedside. Philadelphia: WB Saunders, 1990:201.

21. Karagueuzian HS, Khan SS, Mandel WJ, Diamond AG: Nonlinear dynamic analysis of temporally heterogenous action potential characteristics. PACE, 1990;13:2113.

22. Glass L, Mckay MC: From clocks to chaos. The rhythms of life. Princeton, NJ: Princeton University Press, 1988.

23. Guevara MR, Shrier A, Glass L: Phase-locked rhythms in periodically stimulated heart cell aggregates. Am J Physiol 1988;254:H1.

24. Delmar M, Glass L, Michaels DC, Jalife J: Ionic basis and analytical solution of the Wenckebach phenomenon in guinea pig ventricular myocytes. Circ Res 1989;65:775.

25. Ritzenberg AL, Adam DR, Cohen RJ: Period multipling: Evidence for nonlinear behaviour in the canine heart. Nature 1984;307:159.

26. Shrier A, Dubarsky H, Rosengarten M, Guevara MR, Nattel S, Glass L: Prediction of complex atrioventricular conduction rhythms in humans with use of the atrioventricular nodal recovery curve. Circulation 1987;76:1196.

27. Beeler GW, Reuter H: Reconstruction of the action potential of ventricular myocardial fibers. J Physiol (Lond) 1977;268:177.

28. Kuo CH, Reddy CP, Munakata K, Surawicz B: Arrhythmias dependent predominantly on dispersion of repolarization. In: Zipes D, Jalife J, ed. Cardiac electrophysiology and arrhythmias. New York: Grune & Stratton, 1985:277.

29. Gough WB, Mehra R, Restivo M, Zeiler RH, El-Sherif N: Reentrant ventricular arrhythmias in the late myocardial infarction period in the dog. 13. Correlation of activation and refractory maps. Circ Res 1985;57:432.

30. Spach M, Dolber PC, Heidage FJ: Interaction of inhomogeneities of repolarization with anisotropic propagation in dog atria. Circ Res 1989;65:1612.

31. Boyett MR, Jewell BR: A study of the factors responsible for rate-dependent shortening of the action potential in mammalian ventricular muscle. J Physiol (Lond) 1978;285:359.

32. Elharrar V, Surawicz B: Cycle length effect on restitution of action potential duration in dog cardiac fibers. Am J Physiol 1983;244:H782.

33. Elharrar V: Recovery from use-dependent block of Vmax and restitution of action potential duration in canine cardiac Purkinje fibers. J Pharmacol Exp Ther 1988;246:235.

34. Saitoh H, Bailey JC, Surawicz B: Alternans of action potential duration after abrupt shortening of cycle length: Differences between dog Purkinje and ventricular muscle fibers. Circ Res 1988;62:1027.

35. De Bakke JMT, Van Capelle FJL, Janse MJ, et al: Reentry as cause of ventricular tachycardia in patients with chronic ischemic heart disease: Electrophysiologic and anatomic correlation. Circulation 1988;77:589.

36. Gorget C: Du quinquina a l'hydroquinidine. ALFRED HOUDE', Perennite des Alcaloides. Paris: Laboratoires Houde', 1985:167.

37. Franz MR, Schaefer J, Schottler M, Seed WA, Noble MIM: Electrical and mechanical restitution of the human heart at different rates of stimulation. Circ Res 1983;53:815.

38. Franz MR, Swerdlow CD, Liem LB, Schaefer J: Cycle length dependence of human action potential duration in vivo. Effects of cardiology extrastimuli, sudden sustained rate acceleration and deceleration, and different steady-state frequencies. J Clin Invest 1988;82:972.

39. Elharrar V, Atarashi H, Surawicz B: Cycle length-dependent action potential duration in canine cardiac Purkinje fibers. Am J Physiol 1984;247:936.

40. Varro A, Elharrar V, Surawicz B: Effect of antiarrhythmic drugs on the premature action potential duration in canine cardiac Purkinje fibers. J Pharmacol Exp Ther 1985;233:304.

41. Boyden PA, Albala A, Dresdner KP Jr: Electrophysiology and ultrastructure of canine subendocardial Purkinje cells isolated from control and 24-hour infarcted hearts. Circ Res 1989;65:955.

42. Karagueuzian HS, Kobayashi Y, Khan SS, et al: Action potential alternans and irregular dynamics during quinidine intoxication in ventricular muscle cells. Implications to proarrhythmias. Circulation 1993;87:1661.

43. Karagueuzian HS, Kogan BY, Khan SS, et al: Induction of cellular chaos during quinidine toxicity. The predictive power on nonlinear dynamical analysis for drug-induced proarrhythmias. A hypothesis. J Electrocardiol 1992;24 (suppl):91.

44. Kobayashi Y, Peters W, Khan SS, Mandel WJ, Karagueuzian HS: Cellular mechanisms of differential action potential duration in canine ventricular muscle cells during single vs double premature stimuli. Circulation 1992;86:955.

45. Kobayashi Y, Gotoh M, Mandel WJ, Karagueuzian HS: Increased tempo-spatial dispersion of repolarization during double premature stimulation in the intact ventricle. PACE 1992;15:II2194.

46. Morgan JM, Cunningham D, Rowland E: Dispersion of monophasic action potential duration: Demonstrable in humans after premature ventricular stimulation but not in the steady-state. J Am Coll Cardiol 1992;19:1244.

47. Gang ES, Peter T, Karagueuzian HS, Mandel WJ, Meesmann M: A decline in the ventricular fibrillation threshold following successive premature ventricular extrastimuli: A possible explanation for the induction of fibrillation during programmed stimulation with multiple extrastimuli. Cardiovasc Res 1987;21:790.

48. Kogan BY, Karplus WJ, Billett BS, Pang AT, Karagueuzian HS, Khan SS: The simplified FitzHugh-Nagumo model with ac-tion potential restitution: Effects on 2-D wave propagation. PHYSICA-D 1991;50:327.

49. Kogan BY, Karplus WJ, Billett BS, et al: The role of diastolic outward current deactivation kinetics on the induction of spiral waves. PACE 1991;14:1688.

50. Denton TA, Diamond GA, Khan SS, Karagueuzian HS: Fascinating rhythms: A primer on chaos theory and its application to cardiology. Am Heart J 1990;120:1419.

51. Vaughan Williams EM: Classification of anti-arrhythmic drugs. In: Sandoe E, Flensted-Jensen E, Olsen KH, eds. Symposium on cardiac arrhythmias. Sodertalje, Sweden: AB Astra, 1980:449.

52. Harrison DC: Antiarrhythmic drug classification: New science and practical applications. Am J Cardiol 1985;56:185.

53. Cobbe SM: Clinical usefulness of the Vaughan Williams classification system. Eur Heart J 1987;8:65.

54. Zipes DP: A consideration of antiarrhythmic therapy. Circulation 1985;72:949.

55. Hondeghem LM: Antiarrhythmic agents: Modulated receptor applications. Circulation 1987;75:514.

56. Vaughan Williams EM: A classification of antiarrhythmic actions reassessed after a decade of new drugs. J Clin Pharmacol 1984;24:129.

57. The Task Force of the Working Group on Arrhythmias of the European Society of Cardiology. The "Sicilian Gambit." A new approach for the classification of antiarrhythmic drugs based on their actions on arrhythmogenic mechanisms. Eur Heart J 1991;12:1112.

58. Velbeit V, Podrid P, Lown B, Cohen BH, Graboys TB: Aggravation of ventricular arrhythmias by antiarrhythmic drugs. Circulation 1982;65:886.

59. Podrid PJ: Aggravation of ventricular arrhythmias. A drug-induced complication. Drugs 1985;29(suppl 4):33.

60. Torres V, Flowers D, Somberg JC: The arrhythmogenicity of antiarrhythmic drugs. Am Heart J 1985;109:1090.

61. Bigger JT Jr, Sahar DI: Clinical types of proarrhythmic response to antiarrhythmic drugs. Am J Cardiol 1987;59:2E.

62. Zipes DP: Proarrhythmic effects of antiarrhythmic drugs. Am J Cardiol 1987;59:26E.

63. Creamer JE, Nathan AW, Camm AJ: The proarrhythmic effects of antiarrhythmic drugs. Am Heart J 1987;114:397.

64. Rae AP, Kay HR, Horowitz LN, Spielman SR, Greenspan AM: Proarrhythmic effects of antiarrhythmic drugs in patients with malignant ventricular arrhythmias evaluated by electrophysiologic testing. J Am Coll Cardiol 1988;12:131.

65. Stanton MS, Prystowsky EN, Fineberg NS, Miles WM, Zipes DP, Heger JJ: Arrhythmogenic effects of antiarrhythmic drugs: A study of 506 patients treated for ventricular tachycardia of fibrillation. J Am Coll Cardiol 1989;14:209.

66. The Cardiac Arrhythmias Suppression Trial (CAST) Investigators: Preliminary report: Effect of encainide and flecainide on mortality in a randomized trial of arrhythmias suppression after myocardial infarction. N Engl J Med 1989;321:406.

67. The Cardiac Arrhythmia Pilot Study (CAPS) Investigators: The Cardiac Arrhythmias Pilot Study. Am J Cardiol 1986;57:91.

68. The Cardiac Arrhythmia Pilot Study (CAPS) Investigators: Effects of encainide, flecainide, imipramine and moricizine

on ventricular arrhythmias during the year after acute myocardial infarction: The CAPS. Am J Cardiol 1988;61:501.

69. The Cardiac Arrhythmias Suppression Trial (CAST) II Investigators. Effects of the antiarrhythmic agent moricizine on survival after myocardial infarction. New Engl J Med 1992; 327:227.

70. Green LH, Roden DM, Katz RJ: The Cardiac Arrhythmia Suppression Trial: The first CAST . . . then CAST-II. J Am Coll Cardiol 1992;19:894.

71. Echt DS, Liebson PR, Mitchell LB, et al: Mortality and morbidity in patients receiving encainide and flecainide or placebo. The Cardiac Arrhythmias Suppression Trial. N Engl J Med 1991;324:781.

72. Peters RW, Mitchell LB, Brooks MM, et al: Circadian pattern of arrhythmic death in patients receiving encainide, flecainide, or moricizine in the Cardiac Arrhythmias Suppression Trial (CAST). J Am Coll Cardiol 1994;23:283.

73. Woosley RL, Shand DG: Pharmacokinetics of antiarrhythmic drugs. Am J Cardiol 1978;41:986.

74. Harrison DC, Meffin PJ, Winkle RA: Clinical pharmacokinetics of antiarrhythmic drugs. Prog Cardiovasc Dis 1977; 20:217.

75. Roden D: New concepts in antiarrhythmic drug pharmacokinetics. Prog Cardiol 1987;15:19.

76. Lalka D, et al: Kinetics of the oral antiarrhythmic lidocaine congener, tocainide. Clin Pharmacol Ther 1976;19:757.

77. Kessler KM, Kissane B, Cassidy J, et al: Dynamic variability of binding of antiarrhythmic drugs during the evolution of acute myocardial infarction. Circulation 1984;70:472.

78. Hoffman BF, Rosen MR, Wit AL: Electrophysiology and pharmacology of cardiac arrhythmias. VII. Cardiac effects of quinidine and procainamide. Am Heart J 1975;90:117.

79. Hong K, Karagueuzian HS, Mandel WJ: Comparative electrophysiologic, antiarrhythmic and proarrhythmic effects of quinidine and dihydroquinidine. In vivo and in vitro studies. Journal of Electrophysiology 1989;3:393.

80. Davidenko JM, Cohen L, Goodrow R, Antzeletvich C: Quinidine-induced action potential prolongation, early afterdepolarizations, and triggered activity in canine Purkinje fibers. Effects of stimulation rate, potassium ad magnesium. Circulation 1989;79:674.

81. Takanaka C, Singh BN: Barium-induced nondriven action potentials as a model triggered poentials from early afterdepolarizations: Significance of slow channel activity and different effects of quinidine and amiodarone. J Am Coll Cardiol 1990;15:213.

82. Hondeghem L, Katzung BG: Test of a model of antiarrhythmic drug action. Effects of quinidine and lidocaine on myocardial conduction. Circulation 1980;61:1217.

83. Weld FM, Coromilas J, Rottman JN, Bigger JT Jr: Mechanisms of quinidine-induced depression of maximum upstroke velocity in ovine cardiac Purkinje fibers. Circ Res 1982; 50:369.

84. Valois M, Sasyniuk BI: Modification of the frequency- and voltage-dependent effects of quinidine when administered in combination with tocainide in canine Purkinje fibers. Circulation 1987;76:427.

85. Hong K, Karagueuzian HS, Mandel WJ: Comparative electrophysiologic, antiarrhythmic, and proarrhythmic effects of

quinidine and dihydroquinidine: In vivo and in vitro studies. Journal of Electrophysiology 1989;3:393.

86. Wang Z, Pelletier LC, Talajic M, Nattel S: Effects of flecainide and quinidine on human atrial action potentials. Role of rate-dependence and comparison with guinea pig, rabbit, and dog tissues. Circulation 1990;82:274.

87. Bajaj AK, Kopelman HA, Wikswo JP, Cassidy F, Woosley RL, Roden DM: Frequency- and orientation-dependent effects of mexiletine and quinidine on conduction in the intact dog heart. Circulation 1987;75:1065.

88. Veenstra RD, Johner RW, Rawling DA: Purkinje and ventricular activation sequences of canine papillary muscle. Circ Res 1984;54:500.

89. Franz MR, Costard AC: Frequency-dependent effects of quinidine on the relationship between action potential duration and refractoriness in the canine heart in situ. Circulation 1988;77:1177.

90. Arnsdorf MF, Sawicki GJ: Effects of quinidine sulfate on the balance among active and passive cellular properties that comprise the electrophysiologic matrix and determine excitability in sheep Purkinje fibers. Circ Res 1987;61:244.

91. Salata JJ, Wasserstrom A: Effects of quinidine on action potentials and ionic currents in isolated canine ventricular myocytes. Circ Res 1988;62:324.

92. Balser JR, Bennett PB, Hondeghem LM, Roden DM: Suppression of time-dependent outward current in guinea pig ventricular myocytes. Actions of quinidine and amiodarone. Circ Res 1991;69:519.

93. Imaizumi Y, Giles WR: Quinidine-induced inhibition of transient outward current in cardiac muscle. Am J Physiol 1987; 253:H704.

94. Spach MS, Dolber PC, Heidlage JF, Kootsey JM, Johnson EA: Propagation depolarization and canine cardiac muscle: Apparent directional differences in membrane capacitance. A simplified model for selective directional effects of modifying the sodium conductance on Vmax, t foot, and propagation safety factor. Circ Res 1987;60:209.

95. Nademanee K, Stevenson WG, Weiss JN: Frequency-dependent effects of quinidine on the ventricular action potential and QRS duration in humans. Circulation 1990;81:790.

96. Ranger S, Talajic M, Lemery R, Roy D, Villemaire C, Nattel S: Kinetics of use-dependent ventricular conduction slowing by antiarrhythmic drugs in humans. Circulation 1991;83:1987.

97. Cappato R, Alboni P, Codeca L, Guardigli G, Toselli T, Antonioli GE: Direct and autonomically mediated effects of oral quinidine on RR/QR relation after abrupt increase in heart rate. J Am Coll Cardiol 1993;22:99.

98. Sheng X, Antzelevitch C: Mechanisms underlying the antiarrhythmic and arrhythmogenic actions of quinidine in a Purkinje fiber-ischemic gap preparation of reflected reentry. Circulation 1986;73:1342.

99. Dreifus LS, Watanabe Y, Dreifus HN, Azevedo ID: The effect of antiarrhythmic agents on impulse formation and impulse conduction. In: Wellens HJJ, Lie KI, Janse MJ, eds. The conduction system of the heart. Philadelphia: Lea & Febiger, 1976:182.

100. Duff HJ, Cannon NJ, Sheldon RS: Mexiletine–quinidine in isolated hearts: An interaction involving the sodium channel. Cardiovasc Res 1989;23:584.

101. Clarkson CW, Hondeghem LM: Evidence for a specific receptor site for lidocaine, quinidine, and bupivacaine associated with cardiac sodium channels in guinea pig ventricular myocardium. Circ Res 1985;56:496.

102. Hoffman BF, Bigger JT Jr: Antiarrhythmic drugs. In: Dipalma JR, ed. Drill's pharmacology in medicine. New York: McGraw-Hill, 1971:824.

103. Mirro MJ, Manalan AS, Bailey JC, Watanabe AM: Anticholinergic effects of disopyramide and quinidine on guinea pig myocardium. Mediation by direct muscarinic receptor blockade. Circ Res 1980;47:855.

104. Ochs HR, Grube E, Greenblatt DJ, et al: Intravenous quinidine: Pharmacokinetic properties and effects on left ventricular performance in humans. Am Heart J 1980;99:468.

105. Mariano DJ, Schomer SJ, Rea RF: Effects of quinidine on vascular resistance and sympathetic nerve activity in humans. J Am Coll Cardiol 1992;20:1411.

106. Josephson ME, Seides SE, Battsford WP, et al: The electrophysiological effects of intramuscular quinidine on the atrioventricular conducting system in man. Am Heart J 1974; 87:55.

107. Seller TD, Campbell RWF, Bashore TM, Gallagher JG: Effects of procainamide and quinidine sulfate in the Wolff-Parkinson-White syndrome. Circulation 1977;55:15.

108. Wellens HJ, Durrer D: Effect of procainamide, quinidine, and ajmaline in the Wolff-Parkinson-White syndrome. Circulation 1974;50:116.

109. Heissenbuttel RH, Bigger JT Jr: The effect of oral quinidine on intraventricular conduction in man: Correlation of plasma quinidine with changes in QRS duration. Am Heart J 1970;80:453.

110. Krikler DM, Curry PVL: Torsades de pointes, an atypical ventricular tachycardia. Br Heart J 1976;38:117.

111. El-Sherif N, Bekheit SS, Henkin R: Quinidine-induced long QTU interval and torsade de pointes: Role of bradycardia-dependent early after depolarizations. J Am Coll Cardiol 1989;14:252.

112. Roden DM, Hoffman BF: Action potential prolongation and induction of abnormal automaticity by low quinidine concentrations in canine Purkinje fibers. Circ Res 1985;56:857.

113. Davidenko JM, Cohen L, Goodrow R, Antzelevitch C: Quinidine-induced action potential prolongation, early afterdepolarizations, and triggered activity in canine Purkinje fibers. Circulation 1989;79:674.

114. Selzer A, Wray HW: Quinidine syncope: Paroxysmal ventricular fibrillation occurring during treatment of chronic atrial fibrillation. Circulation 1964;30:17.

115. Karen A, Tzivoni D, Gavish D, et al: Etiology, warning signs and therapy of torsades de pointes. A study of 10 patients. Circulation 1981;64:1164.

116. Jenger HR, Hagemaijer F: Quinidine syncope: Torsades de pointes with low quinidine plasma concentrations. Eur J Cardiol 1976;4:447.

117. Lecocq B, Jaillon P, Lecocq V, et al: Clinical pharmacology of hydroxy-3(S)-dihydroquinidine in healthy volunteers following oral administration. J Cardiovasc Pharmacol 1988; 12:445.

118. Vozeh S, Oti-Amoako K, Uematsu T, Follath F: Antiarrhythmic activity of two quinidine metabolites in experimental

119. Ueda CT, Hirschfeld DS, Scheinman MM, et al: Disposition kinetics of quinidine. Clin Pharmacol Ther 1976;19:30.

120. Hirschfeld DS, Veda CT, Rowland M, et al: Clinical and electrophysiological effects of intravenous quinidine in man. (Abstract) Circulation 1974;50(suppl III):230.

121. Khorsandian R, Chaplan RF, Feinberg JF, Bellet S: Plasma quinidine content levels following single oral doses of quinidine polygalacturonate. Am J Med Sci 1963;245:311.

122. Greenblatt DJ, Pfeifer HJ, Ochs HR, et al: Pharmacokinetics of quinidine in humans after intravenous intramuscular and oral administration. J Pharmacol Exp Ther 1977; 202:365.

123. Kessler KM, Lowenthal DT, Warner H, et al: Quinidine elimination in patients with congestive heart failure or poor renal function. N Engl J Med 1974;290:706.

124. Miller RD, Way WL, Katzung BG: The potentiation of neuromuscular blocking agents by quinidine. Anesthesiology 1972;28:1036.

125. Aviado DM, Salem H: Drug action, reaction and interaction. I. Quinidine for cardiac arrhythmia. J Clin Pharmacol 1975; 15:447.

126. Blout RE: Management of chloroquinine resistant falciparum mala. Arch Intern Med 1967;119:557.

127. Koch-Weser J: Quinidine induced hypoprothrombinemia hemorrhage in patients on chronic warfarin therapy. Ann Intern Med 1968;68:511.

128. Doering W: Quinidine–digoxin interaction. Pharmacokinetics, underlying mechanism, and clinical implication. N Engl J Med 1979;301:400.

129. Bigger JT Jr: The quinidine–digoxin interaction. What do we know about it? N Engl J Med 1979;301:779.

130. Hirsh PD, Weiner HJ, North RL: Further insights into digoxin–quinidine interaction. Lack of correlation between serum digoxin concentration and inotropic state of the heart. Am J Cardiol 1980;46:863.

131. Kessler KM, Wozniak PM, Mcauliffe D, et al: The clinical implications of changing unbound quinidine levels. Am Heart J 1989;118:63.

132. de Senac JB: Traite de la structure du coeur, de son action et de ses maladies. Paris J Vincent 1749;2:504.

133. Willius FA, Keys TE: A remarkably early reference to the use of cinchona in cardiac arrhythmias. Staff meetings of the Mayo Clinic May 13, 1942:294.

134. Karagueuzian HS, Liu ZY, Yao F, Fishbein MC, Mandel WJ: Reperfusion ventricular fibrillation: Its suppression by high dose metaprolol–quinidine combination and its relation to occlusion arrhythmias. (Submitted).

135. Deedwania PC, Olukotun AY, Kupersmith J, Jenkins P, Golden P: Beta blockers in combination with class 1 antiarrhythmic agents. Am J Cardiol 1987;60:21D.

136. Karagueuzian HS, Liu ZY, Yao F, Fishbein MC, Mandel WJ: Suppression of reperfusion ventricular fibrillation by metaprolol–quinidine combination. (Abstract) Revue Europeene de Technologie Biomedicale 1990;12:81.

137. Kus T, Costi P, Dubuc M, Shenasa M: Prolongation of ventricular refractoriness by class Ia antiarrhythmic drugs in the

reperfusion arrhythmia: Relative potency and pharmacodynamic interaction with the parent drug. J Pharmacol Exp Ther 1987;243:297.

prevention of ventricular tachycardia induction. Am Heart J 1990;120:855.

138. Morady F, Kou WH, Kadish AH, et al: Antagonism of quinidine's electrophysiologic effects by epinephrine in patients with ventricular tachycardia. J Am Coll Cardiol 1988;12:388.

139. Jazayeri MR, VanWyhe G, Avitall B, McKinnie J, Tchou P, Akhtar M: Isoproterenol reversal of antiarrhythmic effects in patients with inducible sustained ventricular tachyarrhythmias. J Am Coll Cardiol 1989;14:705.

140. Calkins H, Sousa J, El-Atassi R, Schmalts S, Kadish A, Morady F: Reversal of antiarrhythmic drug effects by epinephrine: Quinidine versus amiodarone. J Am Coll Cardiol 1992;19:347.

141. Rinkenerger RL, Prystowsky EN, Jackman WM, et al: Drug conversion of nonsustained ventricular tachycardia to sustained ventricular tachycardia during serial electrophysiologic studies: Identification of drugs that exacerbate tachycardia and potential mechanisms. Am Heart J 1982;103:179.

142. Gaughan CE, Lown B, Lanigan J, et al: Acute oral testing for determining antiarrhythmic drug efficacy. I. Quinidine. Am J Cardiol 1976;38:677.

143. Hirschfeld DS, Veda CT, Rowland M, et al: Clinical and electrophysiological effects of intravenous quinidine in man. Br Heart J 1977;37:309.

144. Torok E, Bajkay G, Guylas A, Maklary E: Comparative study of a long acting quinidine preparation and quinidine sulfate in chronic atrial fibrillation. Pharmacol Clin 1970;2:90.

145. Morganroth J, Goin JE: Quinidine-related mortality in the short–to–medium-term treatment of ventricular arrhythmias. A meta-analysis. Circulation 1991;84:1977.

146. Bagwell EE, Walle T, Drayer DE, et al: Correlation of the electrophysiological and antiarrhythmic properties of the N-acetyl metabolite of procainamide with plasma and tissue drug concentrations in the dog. J Pharmacol Exp Ther 1976;197:38.

147. Rosen MR, Gelband H, Hoffman BF: Canine electrocardiographic and cardiac electrophysiologic changes induced by procainamide. Circulation 1972;46:528.

148. Villemaire C, Savad P, Talajic M, Nattel S: A quantitative analysis of use-dependent ventricular conduction slowing by procainamide in anesthetized dogs. Circulation 1992;85:2255.

149. Kadish AH, Spear JF, Levine JH, Moore EN: The effects of procainamide on conduction in anisotropic canine ventricular myocardium. Circulation 1986;74:612.

150. Arnsdorf MF, Bigger JT: The effect of procainamide on components of excitability in long mammalian cardiac Purkinje fibers. Circ Res 1976;38:115.

151. Camardo JS, Greenspan AM, Horowitz LN, et al: Strength-interval relation in the human ventricle: Effect of procainamide. Am J Cardiol 1980;45:856.

152. Kay GN, Epstein AE, Plumb VJ: Preferential effect of procainamide on the reentrant circuit of ventricular tachycardia. J Am Coll Cardiol 1989;14:382.

153. Schmitt C, Kadish AH, Balke WC, et al: Cycle length-dependent effects on normal and abnormal intraventricular electrograms: Effect of procainamide. J Am Coll Cardiol 1988;12:395.

154. De Langen CDJ, Hanich RF, Michelson EL, et al: Differential

effects of procainamide, lidocaine and acetylstrophanthidin on body surface potentials and epicardial conduction in dogs with chronic myocardial infarction. J Am Coll Cardiol 1988;11:403.

155. Giardina EC, Bigger JT: Procainamide against reentrant ventricular arrhythmias. Lengthening R-V intervals of coupled ventricular premature depolarization as an insight into the mechanism of action procainamide. Circulation 1973;48:959.

156. Morady F, Kou WH, Schmaltz S, et al: Pharmacodynamics of intravenous procainamide as used during acute electropharmacologic testing. Am J Cardiol 1988;61:93.

157. Morady F, DiCarlo LA, De Buttler M, et al: Effects of incremental doses of procainamide on ventricular refractoriness, intraventricular conduction, and induction of ventricular tachycardia. Circulation 1986;74:1355.

158. Josephson ME, Caracta AR, Ricciutti MA, et al: Electrophysiologic properties of procainamide in man. Am J Cardiol 1974;33:596.

159. Gang ES, Peter T, Oseran D, Mandel WJ: Rate-dependent effects of procainamide on His–Purkinje conduction in man. Am J Cardiol 1985;55:525.

160. Schmitt C, Kadish AH, Balke WC, et al: Cycle length-dependent effects on normal and abnormal intraventricular electrograms: Effects of procainamide. J Am Coll Cardiol 1988;12:395.

161. Schmitt CG, Kadish AH, Marchlinski FE: Effects of lidocaine and procainamide on normal and abnormal intraventricular electrograms during sinus rhythm. Circulation 1988;77:1030.

162. Koch-Weser J, Klein SW: Procainamide dosage schedules, plasma concentrations and clinical effects. JAMA 1971;215:1454.

163. Graffner C, Johnsson G, Sjogren J: Pharmacokinetics of procainamide intravenously and orally as conventional slow-release tablets. Clin Pharmacol Ther 1975;17:414.

164. Shaw TRD, Kumana DR, Royds RD, et al: Use of plasma level in evaluation of procainamide dosage. Br Heart J 1974;36:265.

165. Giardina EGV, Fenster PE, Bigger JT Jr, et al: Efficacy, plasma concentrations and adverse effects of a new sustained release procainamide preparation. Am J Cardiol 1980;46:855.

166. Koch-Weser J: Pharmacokinetics of procainamide in man. Ann N Y Acad Sci 1971;179:370.

167. Dreyfuss J, Bigger JT Jr, Cohen AI, Schreiber EC: Metabolism of procainamide in rhesus monkey and man. Clin Pharmacol Ther 1972;13:366.

168. Strong JM, Dutcher JS, Lee WK, et al: Pharmacokinetics in man of the N-acetylated metabolite of procainamide. J Pharmacokinet Biopharm 1975;3:223.

169. Gibson TP, Matusik E, Matusik J, et al: Acetylation of procainamide in man and its relationship to isonicotinic acid hydrazide acetylation phenotype. Clin Pharmacol Ther 1975;17:395.

170. Gibson RP, Matuski EJ, Briggs WA: N-acetylprocainamide levels in patients with end-stage renal failure. Clin Pharmacol Ther 1976;19:206.

171. Giardina EGV, Dreyfuss J, Bigger JT Jr, et al: Metabolism of procainamide in normal and cardiac subjects. Clin Pharmacol Ther 1976;17:339.

172. Reidenberg MM, Drayer DE, Levy M, et al: Polymorphic

acetylation of procainamide in man. Clin Pharmacol Ther 1975;17:722.

173. Wenger TL, Masterton CE, Abou-Donia MB, et al: Relationship between regional myocardial procainamide concentration and regional myocardial blood flow during ischemia in the dog. Circ Res 1978;42:846.

174. Reynolds RD, Gorczynski RJ: Comparison of autonomic effects of procainamide and N-acetylprocainamide in the dog. J Pharmacol Exp Ther 1980;212:579.

175. Echt DS, Black JN, Barbey JT, Coxe DR, Cato E: Evaluation of antiarrhythmic drugs on defibrillation requirement in dogs. Sodium channel block and action potential prolongation. Circulation 1989;79:1106.

176. Elson J, Strong JM, Lee WK, et al: Antiarrhythmic potency of N-acetylprocainamide. Clin Pharmacol Ther 1975;17:137.

177. Bigger JT Jr, Heissenbuttel RH: The use of procainamide and lidocaine in the treatment of cardiac arrhythmias. Prog Cardiovasc Dis 1969;11:515.

178. Kuchar DL, Rottman J, Berger E: Prediction of successful sustained ventricular tachyarrhythmias by serial drug testing from data derived at the initial electrophysiologic study. J Am Coll Cardiol 1988;12:982.

179. Interian A Jr, Zaman L, Velez-Robinson E, Kozlovskis P, Castellanos A, Myerburg RJ: Paired comparison of efficacy of intravenous and oral procainamide in patients with inducible sustained ventricular tachyarrhythmias. J Am Coll Cardiol 1991;17:1581.

180. Marchlinski FE, Buxton AE, Josephson ME, Schmitt C: Predicting ventricular tachycardia cycle length after procainamide by assessing cycle length-dependent changes in paced QRS duration. Circulation 1989;79:39.

181. Mandel WJ, Laks MM, Obayshi K, et al: The Wolff-Parkinson-White syndrome. Pharmacologic effects of procaine amide. Am Heart J 1975;90:744.

182. Giardina EGV, Heissenbuttel RH, Bigger JT Jr: Intermittent intravenous procainamide to treat ventricular arrhythmias. Ann Intern Med 1973;78:183.

183. Blomgren SE, Condemi JJ, Vaughan JH: Procainamide-induced lupus erythematosus. Clinical and laboratory observations. Am J Med 1972;52:338.

184. Woosley RL, Drayer DE, Reidenburg MM, et al: Effect of acetylator on the rate at which procainamide induces antinuclear antibodies and the lupus syndrome. N Engl J Med 1978;298:1157.

185. Gottlieb SS, Kukin ML, Medina N, Yushak M, Packer M: Comparative hemodynamic effects of procainamide, tocainide, and encainide in severe chronic heart failure. Circulation 1990;81:860.

186. Ehring GR, Hondeghem LM: Rate rhythm and voltage dependent effects of phenytoin: A test of a model of the mechanism of action of antiarrhythmic drugs. Proc West Pharmacol Soc 1978;21:63.

187. Danilo P, Hordof AJ, Rosen MR: Effects of disopyramide on electrophysiologic properties of canine cardiac Purkinje fibers. J Pharmacol Ther 1977;201:701.

188. Josephson ME, Caracta AR, Lau SR, et al: Electrophysiological evaluation of disopyramide in man. Am Heart J 1973;86:771.

189. Birkhead JS, Vaughan Williams EM: Dual effect of disopyramide on atrial and atrioventricular conduction and refractory periods. Br Heart J 1977;39:657.

190. Katoh T, Karagueuzian HS, Jordan J, Mandel WJ: The cellular electrophysiologic mechanism of the dual actions of disopyramide on rabbit sinus node function. Circulation 1982; 6:1216.

191. Hinderling PH, Garrett ET: Pharmacokinetics of the antiarrhythmic disopyramide in healthy humans. J Pharmacokinet Biopharm 1976;4:199.

192. Ward JW, Kingham CR: The pharmacokinetics of disopyramide following myocardial infarction with special reference to oral and intravenous dose regimen. J Intern Med Res 1976;4(suppl 1):49.

193. Bryson SM, Whiting B, Lawrence JR: Disopyramide serum and pharmacologic effect kinetics applied to the assessment of bioavailability. Br J Clin Pharmacol 1978;6:409.

194. Dubetz DK, Brown NN, Hooper WD, et al: Disopyramide pharmacokinetics and bioavailability. Br J Clin Pharmacol 1976;6:279.

195. Hinderling PH, Garrett ER: Pharmacokinetics of the antiarrhythmic disopyramide in healthy humans. J Pharmacokinet Biopharm 1976;4:199.

196. Cunningham JL, Shen DD, Shudo L, et al: The effects of urine pH and plasma protein binding on the renal clearance of disopyramide. Clin Pharmacokinet 1977;2:373.

197. Koch-Weser J: Disopyramide. N Engl J Med 1979;300:957.

198. Hartel G, Louhua A, Konttinen A: Disopyramide in the prevention of recurrence of atrial fibrillation after electroconversion. Clin Pharmacol Ther 1974;15:551.

199. Vismara LA, Vera Z, Miller RR, et al: Efficacy of disopyramide phosphate in the treatment of refractory ventricular tachycardia. Am J Cardiol 1977;39:1027.

200. Spurrell RAJ, Thorburn CW, Camm J, et al: Effects of disopyramide on electrophysiological properties of specialized conduction system in man and on accessory atrioventricular pathway in Wolff-Parkinson-White syndrome. Br Heart J 1975;37:861.

201. Investigational brochure: Norpace (disopyramide phosphate) an antiarrhythmic drug. Searle Laboratories, May 1977.

202. Heel RC, Brogden RN, Speight TM, Avery GS: Disopyramide: A review of its pharmacological properties and therapeutic use in treating cardiac arrhythmias. Drugs 1978;15:331.

203. Jennings G, Model DG, Jones MBS, et al: Oral disopyramide in prophylaxis of arrhythmias following myocardial infarction. Lancet 1976;1:51.

204. Zainal N, Carmichael DJS, Griffiths JW, et al: Oral dysopyramide for the prevention of arrhythmias in patients with acute myocardial infarction admitted to open wards. Lancet 1977;2:887.

205. Rangno RE, Warnica W, Ogilvie RL, et al: Correlation of disopyramide pharmacokinetics with efficacy in ventricular tachyarrhythmias. J Intern Med Res 1976;4(suppl):54.

206. Block PJ, Winkle RA: Hemodynamic effects of antiarrhythmic drugs. Am J Cardiol 1983;52:146.

207. Arnsdorf MF, Bigger JT Jr: The effect of lidocaine on membrane conductance in mammalian Purkinje fibers. J Clin Invest 1972;51:2252.

208. Bigger JT Jr, Mandel WJ: Effect of lidocaine on conduction in canine Purkinje fibers and at the ventricular muscle Purkinje fiber junction. J Pharmacol Exp Ther 1970;174:487.

209. Sheu SS, Lederer WJ: Lidocaine's negative inotropic and

antiarrhythmic actions. Dependence on shortening of action potential duration and reduction on intracellular sodium activity. Circ Res 1985;57:578.

210. Clarkson CW, Follmer CH, Tne Eick RE, Honeghem LM, Yeh JZ: Evidence for two components of sodium channel block by lidocaine in isolated cardiac myocytes. Circ Res 1988; 63:869.

211. Maklieski JC, Falleroni MJ: Temperature dependence of sodium current block by lidocaine in cardiac Purkinje cells. Am J Physiol 1991;260:H681.

212. Singh BN, Vaughan Williams EM: Effect of altering potassium concentration on the action of lidocaine and diphenylhydantoin on rabbit and ventricular muscle. Circ Res 1971; 29:286.

213. Rosen MR, Merker C, Pippenger CE: The effects of lidocaine on the canine ECG and electrophysiological properties of Purkinje fibers. Am Heart J 1976;91:191.

214. Grant AO, Dietz MA, Gilliam R III, Starmer CF: Blockade of sodium channels by lidocaine. Single channel analysis. Circ Res 1989;65:1247.

215. Bennett PB, Woosley RL, Hondeghem LM: Competition between lidocaine and one of its metabolites, glycylxylidide, for cardiac sodium channels. Circulation 1988;78:692.

216. Hondeghem LM: Antiarrhythmic agents: Modulated receptor applications. Circulation 1987;75:514.

217. Kimura S, Nakaya H, Kanno M: Effects of verapamil and lidocaine on changes in action potential characteristics and conduction time induced by combined hypoxia, hyperkalemia and acidosis in canine ventricular myocardium. J Cardiovasc Pharmacol 1982;4:658.

218. Grant AO, Strauss LJ, Wallace AG, Strauss HC: The influence of pH on the electrophysiological effects of lidocaine in guinea pig ventricular myocardium. Circ Res 1980;47:542.

219. Brennan FJ, Cranefield PF, Wit AL: Effects of lidocaine on slow response and depressed fast response action potentials of canine Purkinje fibers. J Pharmacol Exp Ther 1978; 204:312.

220. El-Sherif N, Sherlag BJ, Lazzara R, Hope RR: Reentrant ventricular arrhythmias in the late myocardial infarction period. Mechanism of action of lidocaine. Circulation 1977;56:395.

221. Lamenna V, Antzelevitch C, Moe GK: Effects of lidocaine on conduction through depolarized canine false tendons and on a model of reflected reentry. J Pharmacol Exp Ther 1982;221:353.

222. Mandel WJ, Bigger JT Jr: Electrophysiologic effects of lidocaine on isolated canine rabbit atrial tissue. J Pharmacol Exp Ther 1973;185:438.

223. Rosen MR, Danilo P Jr: Effects of tetrodotoxin, lidocaine, verapamil, and AHR-2666 on ouabain induced delayed after depolarizations in canine Purkinje fibers. Circ Res 1980; 46:117.

224. Karagueuzian HS, Katzung BG: Relative inotropic and arrhythmogenic effects of five cardiac steroids in ventricular myocardium: Oscillatory after potentials and the role of endogenous catecholamines. J Pharmacol Exp Ther 1981; 218:348.

225. Arnsdorf MF, Bigger JT Jr: The effect of lidocaine on components of excitability in long mammalian cardiac Purkinje fibers. J Pharmacol Exp Ther 1975;195:206.

226. Karagueuzian HS, Fujimoto T, Katoh T, et al: Suppression of ventricular arrhythmias by propafenone, a new antiarrhythmic agent, during acute myocardial infarction in the conscious dog. A comparative study with lidocaine. Circulation 1982;66:1190.

227. Karagueuzian HS, Katoh T, McCullen A, et al: Electrophysiologic and hemodynamic effects of propafenone, a new antiarrhythmic agent, on the anesthetized closed-chest dog: Comparative study with lidocaine. Am Heart J 1984;107:418.

228. Stenson RE, Constantino RT, Harrison DC: Interrelationships of hepatic blood flow, cardiac output, and blood levels of lidocaine in man. Circulation 1971;43:205.

229. Blumer J, Strong JM, Atkinson AJ: The convulsant potency of lidocaine and its N-dealkylated metabolites. J Pharmacol Exp Ther 1973;186:31.

230. Rosen MR, Hoffman BF, Wit AL: Electrophysiology and pharmacology of cardiac arrhythmias. V. Cardiac antiarrhythmic effects of lidocaine. Am Heart J 1975;89:526.

231. Noreman JW, Rogers JF: Lidocaine prophylaxis for acute myocardial infarction. Medicine 1978;57:501.

232. Lie KL, Wellens HJ, Van Capelle FJ, et al: Lidocaine in the prevention of primary ventricular fibrillation. N Engl J Med 1974;291:1324.

233. Harrison DC: Should lidocaine be administered routinely to all patients after acute myocardial infarction. Circulation 1978;58:581.

234. Antman E, Berlin JA: Declining incidence of ventricular fibrillation in myocardial infarction. Implications for the prophylactic use of lidocaine. Circulation 1992;86:764.

235. Burket MW, Fraker TD, Temesy-Armos PN: Polymorphous ventricular tachycardia provoked by lidocaine. Am J Cardiol 1985;55:592.

236. Marriott HJL, Bieza CF: Alarming ventricular acceleration after lidocaine administration. Chest 1972;61:682.

237. Anderson KP, Walker R, Lux RL, et al: Conduction velocity depression and drug-induced ventricular tachyarrhythmias. Effects of lidocaine in the intact canine heart. Circulation 1990;81:1024.

238. Nattel A, Zipes DP: Clinical pharmacology of old and new antiarrythmic drugs. In: Castellanos A, ed. Cardiac arrhythmias, mechanisms and management. Philadelphia: FA Davis, 1980:221.

239. Kabela E: The effects of lidocaine on potassium efflux from various tissues of the heart. J Pharmacol Exp Ther 1973; 184:611.

240. Rosen KM, Barwolf C, Ehsani A, Rahimtoola S: Effects of lidocaine and propranolol on the normal and abnormal pathways in patients with preexcitation. Am J Cardiol 1972; 30:801.

241. Karagueuzian HS, Sugi K, Ohta M, Mandel WJ, Peter T, McCullen A: The efficacy of lidocaine and verapamil alone and in combination on spontaneously occurring automatic ventricular tachycardia in conscious dogs one day after right coronary artery occlusion. Am Heart J 1986;111:438.

242. Estes NAM, Manolis AS, Greenblatt DJ, Garan H, Ruskin JN: Therapeutic serum lidocaine and metabolite concentrations in patients undergoing electrophysiologic study after discontinuation of intravenous lidocaine infusion. Am Heart J 1989;117:1060.

243. Harrison DC, Alderman EL: The pharmacology and clinical use of lidocaine as an antiarrhythmic drug. Modern Treatment Monograph No. 9. Hagerstown, MD: Harper & Row, 1972.

244. Gupta PK, Lichstein E, Chadda KD: Lidocaine-induced heart block in patients with bundle branch block. Am J Cardiol 1974;33:487.

245. Feely J, Wade D, McAllister CB, et al: Effect of hypertension on liver blood flow and lidocaine disposition. N Engl J Med 1982;307:866.

246. Strauss HC, Bigger JT Jr, Basset AL, Hoffman BF: Actions of diphenylhydantoin on the electrical properties of isolated rabbit and canine atria. Circ Res 1968;23:463.

247. Rosen MR, Danilo P, Alonso MB, Pippenger CE: Effect of therapeutic concentrations of diphenylhydantoin on transmembrane potentials of normal and depressed Purkinje fibers. J Pharmacol Exp Ther 1976;197:594.

248. Wit AL, Rosen MR, Hoffman BF: Electrophysiology and pharmacology of cardiac arrhythmias. VIII. Cardiac effects of diphenylhydantoin. Am Heart J 1975;90:397.

249. Mirro MJ, Watanabe AM, Bailey JC: Electrophysiological effects of the optical isomers of disopyramide and quinidine in the dog. Dependence on stereochemistry. Circ Res 1981; 48:867.

250. Singh BN, Vaughan Williams EM: Explanation for the discrepancy in reported cardiac electrophysiological actions of diphenylhydantoin and lidocaine. Br J Pharmacol 1971;41:385.

251. Butler TC: The metabolic conversion of 4, 5-diphenylhydantoin to 5-(p-hydroxphenyl) 5 phenylhydantoin. J Pharmacol Exp Ther 1957;119:1.

252. Glazko AJ, Chang T, Baukema J, et al: Metabolic disposition of diphenylhydantoin in normal human subjects following intravenous administration. Clin Pharmacol Ther 1969;10:498.

253. Houghsen GW, Richens A: Rate of elimination of tracer doses of phenytoin at different steady-state serum phenytoin concentrations in epileptic patients. Br J Clin Pharmacol 1974;1:155.

254. Kutt H: Biochemical and genetic factors regulating dilantin metabolism in man. Ann N Y Acad Sci 1971;179:704.

255. Lunde PKM, Rane A, Yaffe SL, et al: Plasma protein binding of diphenylhydantoin in man: Interaction with other drugs and the effect of temperature and plasma dilution. Clin Pharmacol Ther 1970;11:846.

256. Kutt H, Wolk M, Scherman R, et al: Insufficient parahydroxylation as a cause of diphenylhydantoin toxicity. Neurology 1964;14:542.

257. Bigger JT, Strauss HC: Digitalis toxicity: Drug interactions promoting toxicity and the management of toxicity. Seminars in Drug Treat 1972;2:147.

258. Salerno DM: Review: Antiarrhythmic drugs: 1987. Part II. Class IA and class IB antiarrhythmic drugs. A review of their pharmacokinetics, electrophysiology, efficacy, and toxicity. Journal of Electrophysiology 1987;1:300.

259. Mercer EN, Osborne JA: The current status of diphenylhydantoin in heart disease. Ann Intern Med 1967;67:1084.

260. Stone N, Klein MD, Lown B: Diphenylhydantoin in the prevention of recurring ventricular tachycardia. Circulation 1971;43:420.

261. Bigger JT, Schmidt DH, Kult H: Relationship between plasma level of diphenylhydantoin sodium and its cardiac antiarrhythmic effects. Circulation 1968;38:363.

262. Wit AL, Hoffman BF, Rosen MR: Electrophysiology and pharmacology of cardiac arrhythmias. IX. Cardiac electrophysiologic effects of beta adrenergic receptor stimulation and blockade. Am Heart J 1975;90:665.

263. Coltrat DJ, Meldrum SJ: The effect of racemic propranolol, dextropropranolol and racemic practolol on the human and canine transmembrane action potential. Arch Int Pharmacodyn Ther 1971;192:188.

264. Shand DG, Nuckolls EM, Oates JA: Plasma propranolol in adults. Clin Pharmacol Ther 1970;11:112.

265. Ko W-J, Chu S-H: A new regimen for esmolol to treat supraventricular tachyarrhythmia in Chinese patients. J Am Coll Cardiol 1994;23:302.

266. Davis LD, Temte JV, Murphy QR: Epinephrine-cyclopropane effects on Purkinje fibers. Anesthesiology 1969;36:369.

267. Nixon JV, Pennington W, Ritter W, et al: Efficacy of propranolol in the control of exercise-induced or augmented ventricular ectopic activity. Circulation 1978;57:115.

268. Lemberg L, Castellanos A, Arcebal AG: The use of propranolol in arrhythmias complicating acute myocardial infarction. Am Heart J 1970;80:479.

269. Multicentre International Study: Improvement in prognosis of myocardial infarction by long-term beta adrenoreceptor blockade using practolol. BMJ 1975;3:735.

270. Singh BN: B-adrenoreceptor blocking drugs and acute myocardial infarction. Drugs 1978;15:218.

271. Barlow JR, Bosman CK, Pocock WA, et al: Late systolic murmurs and non-ejection ("mid-late") systolic clicks. Br Heart J 1968;30:203.

272. Nies AS, Shand DG: Clinical pharmacology of propranolol. Circulation 1975;52:6.

273. McAllister RG: Intravenous propranolol administration: A method for rapidly achieving and sustaining desired plasma levels. Clin Pharmacol Ther 1976;20:517.

274. Mizgala HF, Counsell J: Acute coronary syndromes following abrupt cessation of oral propranolol therapy. Can Med Assoc J 1976;114:1123.

275. Nattel S, Shanks J, Rangno RE: Propranolol withdrawal. Ann Intern Med 1978;89:288.

276. Nattel A, Rangno RE: Failure of gradual withdrawal of propranolol to prevent beta adrenergic supersensitivity. Circulation 1978;57,58(suppl III):103.

277. Cranefield PF, Aronson RS, Wit AL: Effect of verapamil on the normal action potential and on a calcium-dependent slow response of canine cardiac Purkinje fibers. Circ Res 1974; 34:204.

278. Wit AL, Cranefield PF: Effect of verapamil on the sinoatrial and atrioventricular nodes of the rabbit and the mechanism by which it arrests reentrant atrioventricular nodal tachycardia. Circ Res 1974;35:413.

279. Zipes DP, Fischer JC: Effects of agents which inhibit the slow channel on sinus node automaticity and atrioventricular conduction in the dog. Circ Res 1974;34:184.

280. Bayer R, Kalusche D, Kaufman R, Mannold R: Inotropic and electrophysiologic actions of verapamil and D600 in mammalian myocardium. III. Effects of the optical isomers on

transmembrane action potentials, Naunyn Schmiedebergs Arch Pharmacol 1975;290:81.

281. Ehara T, Kaufman R: The voltage-and time-dependent effects of (−) verapamil on the slow inward current in ventricular myocardium. J Pharmacol Exp Ther 1978;207:49.

282. Eichelbaum M: Pharmacokinetic and pharmacodynamic consequences of stereoselective drug metabolism in man. Biochem Pharmacol 1988;37:93.

283. Kates RE, Keefe DLD, Schwatz J, et al: Verapamil disposition: Kinetics in chronic atrial fibrillation. J Clin Pharmacol Ther 1981;30:44.

284. Schwartz JB, Keefe DL, Kirsten E, et al: Prolongation of verapamil elimination kinetics during chronic oral administration. Am Heart J 1982;104:198.

285. Shand DG, Hammil SC, Aanosen L, Pritchett ELC: Reduced verapamil clearance during long term oral administration. Clin Pharmacol Ther 1981;30:701.

286. Rikenberger RL, Prystowsky EN, Heger JJ, et al: Effects of intravenous and chronic oral verapamil administration in patients with supraventricular tachyarrhythmias. Circulation 1980;62:996.

287. McAllister RG, Kirsten EB: The pharmacology of verapamil IV kinetic and dynamic effects after single intravenous and oral doses. Clin Pharmacol Ther 1982;31:418.

288. Reiter MJ, Shand DG, Pritchett ELC: Comparison of intravenous and oral verapamil dosing. Clin Pharmacol Ther 1982;32:711.

289. Woodcock BG, Reitbrock L, Vohringer HF, Reitbrock N: Verapamil disposition in liver disease and intensive care patients. Kinetics, clearance and apparent blood flow relationships. Clin Pharmacol Ther 1981;29:27.

290. Klein GJ, Gulamhusein S, Prystowsky EN, et al.: Comparison of the electrophysiologic effects of intravenous and oral verapamil in patients with paroxysmal supraventricular tachycardia. Am J Cardiol 1982;49:117.

291. Mauriston DR, Winnifold MD, Walker WS, et al: Oral verapamil for paroxysmal supraventricular tachycardia. A long term, double blind randomized trial. Ann Intern Med 1982; 96:409.

292. Singh BN, Ellrodt G, Peter CT: Verapamil: A review of its pharmacologic properties and therapeutic use. Drugs 1978; 15:169.

293. Belhassen B, Glick A, Laniado S: Comparative clinical and electrophysiologic effects of adenosine triphosphate and verapamil on paroxysmal reciprocating junctional tachycardia. Circulation 1988;77:795.

294. Barnett JC, Touchon RC: Short-term control of supraventricular tachycardia with verapamil infusion and calcium pretreatment. Chest 1990;97:1106.

295. Wellens HJJ, Bar FW, Lie KI, et al: Effect of procainamide, propranolol and verapamil on mechanism of tachycardia in patients with chronic recurrent ventricular tachycardia. Am J Cardiol 1977;40:579.

296. Brichard G, Zimmerman PE: Verapamil in cardiac dysrhythmias during anesthesia. Br J Anaesth 1970;41:1005.

297. Karagueuzian HS, Mandel WJ: The effects of drugs on sinus node function. In: Masoni A, Alboni P, eds. Cardiac electrophysiology today. New York: Academic Press, 1982:123.

298. Singh BN, Vaughan Williams EM: The effects of amiodarone, a new antianginal drug, on cardiac muscle. Br J Pharmacol 1970;39:657.

299. Rosenbaum MB, Chiale PA, Halpern MS, et al: Clinical efficacy of amiodarone as an antiarrhythmic agent. Am J Cardiol 1966;38:934.

300. Mason JW, Hondeghem LM, Katzung BG: Block of inactivated sodium channels and of depolarization-induced automaticity in guinea pig papillary muscle by amiodarone. Circ Res 1984;55:277.

301. Yabek SM, Kato R, Singh BN: Acute effects of amiodarone of the electrophysiological properties of isolated neonatal and adult cardiac fibers. J Am Coll Cardiol 1985;5:1109.

302. Nattel S, Talajic M, Quantz M, DeRoode M: Frequency-dependent effects of amiodarone on atrioventricular nodal function and slow-channel action potentials: Evidence for calcium channel-blocking activity. Circulation 1987;76: 442.

303. Gooupil N, Lenfant J: The effects of amiodarone on sinus node activity of the rabbit heart. Eur J Pharmacol 1976;39:23.

304. Ohta M, Karagueuzian HS, McCullen A, et al: Chronic and acute effect of amiodarone on delayed after depolarization and triggered automaticity in rabbit ventricular myocardium. Am Heart J 1987;113:289.

305. Takanaka C, Singh BN: Barium-induced nondriven action potentials as a model of triggered potentials from early afterdepolarizations: Significance of slow channel activity and differing effects of quinidine and amiodarone. J Am Coll Cardiol 1990;15:213.

306. Sheldon RS, Hill RJ, Cannon NJ, Duff HJ: Amiodarone: Biochemical evidence for binding to a receptor for class I drugs associated with the rat cardiac sodium channel. Circ Res 1989;65:477.

307. Cabasson J, Puch P, Mellet JD, et al: Analyse des effects electrophysiologigues de l'amiodarone par l'enregistrement silmutane' des potentiels d'action monophasiques et da faisceau de His. Arch Mal Coeur 1976;7:691.

308. Tuna IC, Qi A, Gornick C, Bolman RM, Benditt DG: Kinetics of electrophysiologic changes during oral loading of amiodarone and after withdrawal of amiodarone in the unsedated dog. Circulation 1985;72:1380.

309. Talajic M, DeRoode MR, Nattel S: Comparative electrophysiologic effects of intravenous amiodarone and desethylamiodarone in dogs: Evidence for clinically relevant activity of the metabolite. Circulation 1987;75:265.

310. Venkatesh N, Padbury JF, Singh BN: Effects of amiodarone and desethylamiodarone on rabbit myocardial B-adrenoceptors and serum thyroid hormones—absence of relationship to serum and myocardial drug concentrations. J Cardiovasc Pharmacol 1986;8:989.

311. Riva E, Hearse DJ: Anti-arrhythmic effects of amiodarone and desethylamiodarone on malignant ventricular arrhythmias arising as a consequence of ischaemia and reperfusion in the anaesthetised rat. Cardiovasc Res 1989;23:331.

312. Boucher M, Duchene-Marullaz P: Comparative effects of amiodarone perhexilline and bepridil on the cardiac rhythms of the unanesthetized dog in chronic heart block. Arch Int Pharmacodyn Ther 1978;233:65.

313. Patterson E, Eller BT, Abrams GD, et al: Ventricular fibrillation in a conscious canine preparation of sudden coronary

death—prevention by short and long term amiodarone administration. Circulation 1983;68:857.

314. Haffajee CT, Love JC, Canada AT, et al: Clinical pharmacokinetics and efficacy of amiodarone for refractory tachyarrhythmias. Circulation 1983;67:1347.

315. Siddoway LA, McAllister CB, Wilkinson GR, et al: Amiodarone dosing: A proposal based on its pharmacokinetics. Am Heart J 1983;106:951.

316. Zipes DP, Prystowsky EN, Heger JJ: Amiodarone: Electrophysiologic actions, pharmacokinetics and clinical effects. J Am Coll Cardiol 1984;3:1059.

317. Giardina EGV, Schneider MS, Barr ML: Myocardial amiodarone and desethylamiodarone concentrations in patients undergoing cardiac transplantations. J Am Coll Cardiol 1990;16:943.

318. Nademanee K, Singh BN, Hendrickson JA, et al: Pharmacokinetics significance of serum reverse T3 levels during amiodarone treatment: A potential method for monitoring chronic drug therapy. Circulation 1982;66:202.

319. Venkatesh N, Somani P, Bersohn M, Phair R, Kato R, Singh BN: Electropharmacology of amiodarone: Absence of relationship to serum, myocardial, and cardiac sarcolemmal membrane drug concentrations. Am Heart J 1986;112:916.

320. Mitchell LB, Wyse G, Gillis AM, Duff HJ: Electropharmacology of amiodarone therapy initiation. Time course of onset of electrophysiologic and antiarrhythmic effects. Circulation 1989;80:34.

321. Holt DW, Tucker GT, Jackson PR, Storey GCA: Amiodarone pharmacokinetics. Am Heart J 1983;106:840.

322. Wellens HJJ, Brugada P, Abdollah H, Dassen WR: A comparison of the electrophysiologic effects of intravenous and oral amiodarone in the same patients. Circulation 1984;69:120.

323. Hamer AW, Finnerman WB, Peter T, Mandel WJ: Disparity between the clinical and electrophysiologic effects of amiodarone in the treatment of recurrent ventricular tachycardias. Am Heart J 1981;102:992.

324. Feld GK, Nadamanee K, Weiss J, et al: Electrophysiologic basis for the suppression by amiodarone of orthodromic supraventricular tachycardia complicating pre-excitation syndromes. J Am Coll Cardiol 1984;3:1298.

325. Nademanee K, Handrickson J, Cannom DS, et al: Control of refractory life-threatening ventricular tachyarrhythmias by amiodarone. Am Heart J 1981;101:759.

326. Heger JJ, Prystowsky EN, Zipes DP: Clinical efficacy of amiodarone in the treatment of recurrent ventricular tachycardia and ventricular fibrillation. Am Heart J 1983;106:887.

327. Graboys TB, Podrid PJ, Lown B: Efficacy of amiodarone for refractory supraventricular tachyarrythmias. Am Heart J 1983;106:870.

328. Wellens HJJ, Brugada P, Abdollah H: Effect of amiodarone in paroxysmal supraventricular tachycardia with and without WPW syndrome. Am Heart J 1983;106:876.

329. Hamer AWF, Mandel WJ, Zaher CA, et al: The electrophysiological basis for the use of amiodarone for treatment of cardiac arrhythmias. PACE 1983;6:784.

330. Sager PT, Uppal P, Follmer C, Antimisiaris M, Pruitt C, Singh BN: Frequency-dependent electrophsyiologic effects of amiodarone in humans. Circulation 1993;88:1063.

331. Kadish AH, Chen R-F, Achmaltz S, Morady F: Magnitude and time course of beta-adrenergic antagonism during oral amiodarone therapy. J Am Coll Cardiol 1990;16:1240.

332. Zehender M, Hohnloser S, Muller B, Meinertz T, Just H: Effects of amiodarone versus quinidine and verapamil in patients with chronic atrial fibrillation: Results of a comparative study and a 2-year follow-up. J Am Coll Cardiol 1992; 19:1054.

333. Mostow ND, Vrobel TR, Noon D, Rakita L: Rapid control of refractory atrial tachyarrhythmias with high-dose oral amiodarone. Am Heart J 1990;120:1356.

334. Zhu J, Haines DE, Lerman BB, DiMarco JP: Predictors of efficacy of amiodarone and characteristics of recurrence of arrhythmia in patients with sustained ventricular tachycardia and coronary artery disease. Circulation 1987;76:802.

335. Greenspon AJ, Volosin KJ, Greenberg RM, Jeferies L, Rotmensch HH: Amiodarone therapy: Role of early and late electrophysiologic studies. J Am Coll Cardiol 1988;11:117.

336. Evans SJL, Myers M, Zaher C, et al: High dose oral amiodarone loading: Electrophysiologic effects and clinical tolerance. J Am Coll Cardiol 1992;19:169.

337. Nalos PC, Ismail Y, Pappas JM, Nyitray W, DonMichel TA: Intravenous amiodarone for short-term treatment of refractory ventricular tachycardia or fibrillation. Am Heart J 1991; 122:1629.

338. Perry JC, Knilans TK, Marlow D, Denfield SW, Fenrich AL, Friedman RA: Intravenous amiodarone for life-threatening tachyarrhythmias in children and young adults. J Am Coll Cardiol 1993;22:95.

339. Rosenheck S, Sousa J, Calkins H, et al: Comparison of the results of electrophysiologic testing after short-term and long-term treatment with amiodarone in patients with ventricular tachycardia. Am Heart J 1991;121:1693.

340. Harris L, McKenna WJ, Roland E, et al: Amiodarone: Side effects of long term therapy. Circulation 1983;67:45.

341. Myers M, Peter T, Weiss D, et al. Benefit and risks of long-term amiodarone therapy for sustained ventricular tachycardia: Minimum of three-year follow-up in 145 patients. Am Heart J 1990;119:8.

342. Ceremuzynsky L, Klecar E, Krzeminska-Pakula M, et al: Effect of amiodarone on mortality after myocardial infarction: A double-blind, placebo-controlled pilot study. J Am Coll Cardiol 1992;20:1056.

343. Bjorn-Hansen L, Pederson EM, Keld D, Paulsen PK: Reduced cardiac reserve in amiodarone-treated pigs after cardiopulmonary bypass cardioplegic arrest. J Am coll Cardiol 1992;20:236.

344. Guccione P, Paul T, Garson A Jr: Long-term follow-up of amiodarone therapy in the young: Continued efficacy, unimpaired growth, moderate side effects. J Am Coll Cardiol 1990;15:1118.

345. Cascio WE, Woelfel A, Knisley SB, Buchanan JW, Foster JR, Gettes LS: Use dependence of amiodarone during the sinus tachycardia of exercise in coronary artery disease. Am J Cardiol 1988;61:1042.

346. Rakita L, Sobol SM, Mostow N, Vrobel T: Amiodarone pulmonary toxicity. Am Heart J 1983;106:906.

347. Dusman RE, Stanton MS, Miles WM, et al: Clinical features of amiodarone-induced pulmonary toxicity. Circulation 1990; 82:51.

348. Wilson JS, Podrid PJ: Side effects of amiodarone. Am Heart J 1991;121:158.

349. Weinberg BA, Miles WM, Klein LS, et al: Five-year follow-up of 589 patients treated with amiodarone. Am Heart J 1993; 125:109.

350. Dobs AS, Sarma PS, Guarnieri T, Griffith L: Testicular dysfunction with amiodarone use. J Am Coll Cardiol 1991; 18:1328.

351. Hamer A, Peter T, Mandel WJ, et al: The potentiation of warfarin anticoagulation by amiodarone and anticoagulant treatment. Circulation 1982;65:1025.

352. Marcus FI: Drug interactions with amiodarone. Am Heart J 1983;106:924.

353. Toivonen L, Kadish A, Morady F: A prospective comparison of class 1A, B, and C antiarrhythmic agents in combination with amiodarone in patients with inducible sustained ventricular tachycardia. Circulation 1991;84:101.

354. Frame LH: The effect of chronic oral and acute intravenous amiodarine administration on ventricular defibrillation threshold using implanted electrodes in dogs. PACE 1989; 12:339.

355. Jung W, Manz M, Pizzulli L, Pfeiffer D, Luderitz B: Effects of chronic amiodarone therapy on defibrillation threshold. Am J Cardiol 1992;70:1023.

356. Singh BN, Vaughan Williams EM: Investigations of the mode of action of a new antidysrhythmic drug (KO 1173). Br J Pharmacol 1972;44:1.

357. Yamaguchi I, Singh BN, Mandel WJ: Electrophysiological actions of mexiletine on isolated rabbit atrial and canine ventricular muscle and Purkinje fiber. Cardiovasc Res 1979; 13:288.

358. Weld FM, Bigger JT, Swister D, et al: Electrophysiological effects of mexiletine (KO 1173) on ovine cardiac Purkinje fibers. J Pharmacol Exp Ther 1979;210:222.

359. Amerini S, Carbonin P, Cerbai E, et al: Electrophysiological mechanisms for the antiarrhythmic action of mexiletine on digitalis, reperfusion, and reoxy-generation-induced arrhythmias. Br J Pharmacol 1985;86:805.

360. Arita M, Masayosi G, Nagamoto Y, Saikawa T: Electrophysiological actions of mexiletine (KO 1173) on canine Purkinje fibers and ventricular muscle. Br J Pharmacol 1979; 67:143.

361. Carmeliet E: Mechanisms of arrhythmias and of antiarrhythmic activity with special reference to mexiletine. Acta Cardiol 1980;25(suppl):5.

362. Taouris M, Sheldon RS, Duff HJ: Upregulation of the rat cardiac sodium channel by in vivo treatment with a class 1 antiarrhythmic drug. J Clin Invest 1991;88:375.

363. Harper RW, Olsson B: Effect of mexiletine on conduction of premature ventricular beats in man: A study using monophasic action potential recordings from the right ventricle. Cardiovasc Res 1979;13:311.

364. Prescott LF, Pottage A, Clements JA: Absorption, distribution and elimination of mexiletine. Postgrad Med J 1977;53(suppl I):50.

365. Hegger JJ, Nattel S, Rinkenberger RL, Zipes DP: Mexiletine therapy in 15 patients with drug resistant ventricular tachycardia. Am J Cardiol 1980;45:627.

366. Duff HJ, Roden D, Prim RK, et al: Mexiletine in the treatment of resistant ventricular arrhythmias: Enhancement of efficacy and reduction of dose related side effects by combination with quinidine. Circulation 1983;67:1124.

367. Podrid PJ, Lown B: Mexiletine for ventricular arrhythmias. Am J Cardiol 1981;47:895.

368. Impact Research Group: International Mexiletine and Placebo Antiarrhythmic Coronary Trial: I. Report on arrhythmia and other findings. J Am Coll Cardiol 1984;4:1148.

369. Yeung-Lai-Wah JA, Murdock CJ, Boone J, Kerr CR: Propafenone–mexiletine combination for the treatment of sustained ventricular tachycardia. J Am Coll Cardiol 1992;20:547.

370. Ravid S, Podrid PJ, Lampert S, Lown B: Congestive heart failure induced by six of the newer antiarrhythmic drugs. J Am Coll Cardiol 1988;14:1326.

371. Moore EM, Spear JF, Horowitz LN, et al: Electrophysiologic properties of a new antiarrhythmic drug tocainide. Am J Cardiol 1978;41:703.

372. Oshita S, Sada H, Kojima M, Ban T: Effects of tocainide and lidocaine on the transmembrane action potentials as related to external potassium and calcium concentrations in guinea pig papillary muscles. Arch Pharmacol 1980;314:62.

373. Dersham GH, Han J, Cameron JS, O'Connel DP: Effects of tocainide on Purkinje fibers from normal and infarcted ventricular tissues. J Electrocardiol 1986;19:355.

374. Wallace AA, Stupienski RF, Heaney LA, Gehret JR, Lynch JJ Jr: Antiarrhythmic actions of tocainide in canine models of previous myocardial infarction. Am Heart J 1991;121:1413.

375. Winkle RA, Meffin PJ, Fitzgerald JW, et al: Clinical efficacy and pharmacokinetics of a new orally effective antiarrhythmic—tocainide. Circulation 1976;54:884.

376. Lalks D, Meyer MB, Duce BR, et al: Kinetics of oral antiarrhythmic lidocaine congener—tocainide. Clin Pharmacol Ther 1976;19:767.

377. Lewinter MM, Engler RL, Karliner JS: Tocainide therapy of ventricular arrhythmias: Assessment with ambulatory electrocardiographic monitoring and treadmill exercise. Am J Cardiol 1980;45:1045.

378. Pottage A: Clinical profiles of newer class I antiarrhythmic agents—tocainide, mexiletine, encainide, flecainide, and lorcainide. Am J Cardiol 1983;52:24C.

379. Adhar GC, Swerdlow CD, Lance BL, Clay D, Bardy GH, Greene HL: Tocainide for drug-resistant sustained ventricular tachyarrhythmias. J Am Coll Cardiol 1988;11:124.

380. Mohiuddin SM, Hilleman DE, Mooses AN, Esterbrooks D, Sdetch MH, Stengel LA, Butler ML: Double-blind randomized comparison of intravenous tocainide versus lidocaine in the treatment of chronic ventricular arrhythmias. Am Heart J 1987;114:296.

381. Renard MB, Bernard RM, Ewalenko MB, Englert M: Hemodynamic effects of concurrent administration of metoprolol and tocainide in acute myocardial infarction. J Cardiovasc Pharmacol 1983;5:116.

382. Gottlieb SS, Kukin ML, Median N, Yushak M, Packer M: Comparative hemodynamic effects of procainamide, tocainide, and encainide in severe chronic heart failure. Circulation 1990;81:860.

383. Vanoli E, Hull SS, Stith RD, Adamson PB, Foreman RD, Schwartz PJ: Tocainide and mortality after myocardial infarctions: A prospective study in conscious dogs.

384. Holmes B, Heel RC: Flecainide: A preliminary review of its pharmacodynamic properties and therapeutic efficacy. Drugs 1985;29:1.

385. Ikeda N, Singh BN, Davis LD, Hauswirth O: Effects of flecainide on the electrophysiological properties of isolated canine and rabbit myocardial fibers. J Am Coll Cardiol 1985; 5:303.

386. Campbell TJ, Vaughan Williams EMV: Voltage- and time-dependent depression of maximum rate of depolarisation of guinea-pig ventricular action potentials by two new antiarrhythmic drugs, flecainide and lorcainide. Cardiovasc Res 1983;17:251.

387. Hodess AB, Follansbee WP, Spear JF, Moore EW: Electrophysiological effects of a new antiarrhythmic agent, flecainide, on the intact canine heart. J Cardiovasc Pharmacol 1979;1:427.

388. Sakai T, Ogawa S, Hosokawa M, Miyazaki T, Sakurai K, Nakamura Y: Electrophysiologic effects of flecainide in a canine 7 day old myocardial infarction model. Cardiovasc Res 1989;23:177.

389. Hernandez R, Mann DE, Breckinridge S, Williams GR, Reiter MJ: Effects of flecainide on defibrillation thresholds in the anesthetized dog. J Am Coll Cardiol 1989;14:777.

390. Verdouw PD, Deckers JW, Connad GJ: Antiarrhythmic and hemodynamic actions of flecainide acetate (R818) in the ischemic porcine heart. J Cardiovasc Pharmacol 1979;1:473.

391. Anderson JL, Stewart JR, Perry BA, et al: Oral flecainide acetate for the treatment of ventricular arrhythmias. N Engl J Med 1981;305:473.

392. Duff HJ, Roden DM, Maffucci RJ, et al: Suppression of resistant ventricular arrhythmias by twice daily dosing with flecainide. Am J Cardiol 1981;48:1133.

393. Hodges M, Haugland M, Granrud G: Suppression of ventricular ectopic depolarizations by flecainide acetate, a new antiarrhythmic agent. Circulation 1982;65:879.

394. The Flecainide–Quinidine Research Group: Flecainide versus quinidine for treatment of chronic ventricular arrhythmias. A multicenter clinical trial. Circulation 1983; 67:1117.

395. Ranger S, Talajic M, Lemery R, Roy D, Nattel S: Amplification of flecainide-induced ventricular conduction slowing by exercise. Circulation 1989;79:1000.

396. Salerno DM: Part III: Class IC antiarrhythmic drugs. A review of their pharmacokinetics, electrophysiology, efficacy, and toxicity. Journal of Electrophysiology 1987;1:435.

397. Leclerq JF, Chouty F, Denjoy I, Coumel P, Slama R: Flecainide in quinidine-resistant atrial fibrillation. Am J Cardiol 1992;70:62A.

398. Suttorp MJ, Kingma H, Jessurun ER, Lie-A-Huen L, van Hemel NM: The value of class IC antiarrhythmic drugs for acute conversion of paroxysmal atrial fibrillation or flutter to sinus rhythm. J Am Coll Cardiol 1990;16:1722.

399. Musto B, Cavallaro C, Musto A, D'onfrio A, Belli A, De Vincentis L: Flecainide single oral dose for management of paroxysmal supraventricular tachycardia in children and young adults. Am Heart J 1992;124:110.

400. Hellestrand KJ, Nathan AW, Bexton RS, Camm AJ: Effect of flecainide on anomalous pathways and reentrant junctional tachycardia. (Abstract) Circulation 1982;66(suppl II):273.

401. Perry JC, McQuinn RL, Smith RT, Gothing C, Fredell P, Garson A: Flecainide acetate for resistant arrhythmias in the young: Efficacy and pharmacokinetics. J Am Coll Cardiol 1989;14:185.

402. Abitbol H, Califano JE, Abate C, et al: Use of flecainide acetate in the treatment of premature ventricular contractions. Am Heart J 1983;105:227.

403. Morganroth J, Anderson JL, Gentzkow GD: Classification by type of ventricular arrhythmia predicts frequency of adverse cardiac events from flecainide. J Am Coll Cardiol 1986;8:607.

404. Perry JC, Garson A: Flecainide acetate for treatment of tachyarrhythmias in children: Review of world literature on efficacy safety and dosing. Am Heart J 1992;124:1614.

405. Pottage A: Clinical profiles of newer class 1 antiarrhythmic agents. Tocainide, mexiletine, encainide, flecainide, and lorcainide. Am J Cardiol 1983;52:24C.

406. Elharrar V, Zipes DP: Effects on encainide and metabolites (MJ 14030 and MJ 9444) on canine cardiac Purkinje and ventricular fibers. J Pharmacol Exp Ther 1982;220:440.

407. Gibson JK, Somani P, Bassett AL: Electrophysiologic effects of encainide (MJ9067) on canine Purkinje fibers. Eur J Pharmacol 1978l;52:161.

408. Schmidt G, Sawicki GJ, Arnsdorf MF: Effects of encainide on components of excitability in cardiac Purkinje fibers. (Abstract) Circulation 1981;64(suppl IV):1037.

409. Roden DM, Duff HJ, Altenberg D, Woosley RL: Antiarrhythmic activity of the o-demethyl metabolite of encainide. J Pharmacol Ther 1982;221:552.

410. Samuelsson RG, Harrison DC: Electrophysiologic evaluation of encainide with use of monophasic action potential recording. Am J Cardiol 1981;48:871.

411. Roden WDM, Wolfenden HT, Woosley RL, Wood AJJ, Wilkinson GR: Influence of genetic polymorphism on the metabolism and disposition of encainide in man. J Pharmacol Exp Ther 1983;228:605.

412. Dawson AK, Duff HJ, Woosley RL: Paradoxical response to o-demethyl encainide in a canine infarction model. (Abstract) Circulation 1981;64:(suppl IV):1039.

413. Jackman WM, Zipes DP, Naccarelli GV, et al: Electrophysiology of oral encainide. Am J Cardiol 1982;49:1270.

414. Sami M, Mason JW, Peters F, Harrison DC: Clinical electrophysiologic effects of encainide, a newly developed antiarrhythmic agent. Am J Cardiol 1979;44:526.

415. Woosley RL, Roden DM: Importance of metabolites in antiarrhythmic therapy. Am J Cardiol 1983;52:3c.

416. Winkle RA, Peters F, Kates RE, et al: Clinical pharmacology and antiarrhythmic efficacy of encainide in patients with chronic ventricular arrhythmias. Circulation 1981;64:290.

417. Kates RE, Harrison DC, Winkle RA: Metabolite accumulation during long-term oral encainide administration. Clin Pharmacol Ther 1982;31:427.

418. Carey EL, Duff HJ, Roden DM: Encainide and its metabolites: Comparative effects in man on ventricular arrhythmias and electrocardiography intervals. J Clin Invest 1984;73:539.

419. Roden DM, Reele SB, Higgins SB, et al: Total suppression of ventricular arrhythmias by encainide. N Engl J Med 1980; 302:877.

420. Prystowsky EN, Klein GJ, Rinkenberger RL, et al: Clinical efficacy and electrophysiologic effects of encainide in pa-

tients with Wolff-Parkinson-White syndrome. Circulation 1984;69:278.

421. Chimienti M, Bergolis ML, Moizi M, Salerno JA: Electrophysiologic and clinical effects of oral encainide in paroxysmal atrioventricular node reentrant tachycardia. J Am Coll Cardiol 1989;14:992.

422. Sami M, Harrison DC, Kramer H, et al: Antiarrhythmic efficacy of encainide and quinidine: Validation of a model for drug assessment. Am J Cardiol 1982;48:147.

423. Duff HJ, Dawson AK, Roden DM: Electrophysiologic actions of o-demethyl encainide: An active metabolite. Circulation 1983;68:385.

424. Karalis DG, Nydegger C, Porter RS, et al: Effects of encainide and metabolizer phenotype on ventricular conduction during exercise. Am J Cardiol 1990;66;1393.

425. Posen R, Lombardi E, Podrid P, Lown B: Aggravation of induced arrhythmias with antiarrhythmic drugs during electrophysiological testing. (Abstract) Am J Cardiol 1983;1: 709.

426. Winkle RA, Mason JW, Griffin JC, Ross D: Malignant ventricular tachyarrhythmias associated with the use of encainide. Am Heart J 1981;102:857.

427. Carmeliet E, Verdonck F: Effects of aprindine and lidocaine on transmembrane potentials and radioactive K efflux in different cardiac tissues. Acta Cardiol 1974;18:73.

428. Verdonck F, Vereecke J, Vleugels A: Electrophysiological effects of aprindine on isolated heart preparations. Eur J Pharmacol 1974;26:338.

429. Steinberg MI, Greenspan K: Intracellular electrophysiological alternations in canine conducting tissue induced by aprindine and lidocaine. Cardiovasc Res 1976;10:236.

430. Elharrar V, Bailey JC, Lathrop DA, Zipes DP: Effects of aprindine on slow channel action potentials and transient depolarizations in canine Purkinje fibers. J Pharmacol Exp Ther 1978;205:410.

431. Elharrar V, Foster PR, Zipes DP: Effects of aprindine HCL on cardiac tissue. J Pharmacol Exp Ther 1975;195:201.

432. Foster PR, King RM, Dehnicoll A, Zipes DP: Suppression of ouabain-induced ventricular rhythms with aprindine HCL: A comparison with other antiarrhythmic agents. Circulation 1976;53:315.

433. Zipes DP, Elharrar V, Gilmour RF Jr, et al: Studies with aprindine. Am Heart J 1980;100:1055.

434. Reid PR, Greene HL, Varphese PJ: Suppression of refractory arrhythmias by aprindine in patients with the WPW syndrome. Br Heart J 1977;39:1353.

435. Ronfeld RA: Comparative pharmacokinetics of new antiarrhythmic drugs. Am Heart J 1980;100:978.

436. Vlay SC, Kallman CH, Reid PR: The utility of aprindine blood levels in the management of ventricular arrhythmias. J Am Coll Cardiol 1985;5:738.

437. Zipes DP, Guam WE, Foster PR, et al: Aprindine treatment of supraventricular tachycardia, with particular application to Wolff-Parkinson-White syndrome. Am J Cardiol 1977;40:586.

438. Gottlien SH, Achuff SC, Mellits ED, et al: Prophylactic antiarrhythmic therapy of high-risk survivors of myocardial infarction: Lower mortality at 1 month but not at 1 year. Circulation 1987;75:792.

439. Strauss HC, Bigger JT Jr, Hoffman BF: Electrophysiological

and beta-receptor blocking effects of MJ1999 on dog and rabbit tissue. Circ Res 1970;26:661.

440. Singh BN, Vaughan Williams EM: A third class of antiarrhythmic action. Effect on atrial and ventricular intracellular potentials, and other pharmacological actions on cardiac muscle of MJ 1999 and AH-3474. Br J Pharmacol 1970;39:675.

441. Yabek SM, Kato R, Ikeda N, Singh BN: Cellular electrophysiologic responses of isolated neonatal and adult cardiac fibers to d-sotalol. J Am Coll Cardiol 1988;11:1094.

442. Feld GK, Venkatesh N, Singh BN: Pharmacologic conversion and suppression of experimental canine atrial flutter: Differing effects of d-sotalol, quinidine, and lidocaine and significance of changes in refractoriness and conduction. Circulation 1986;74:197.

443. Schmitt C, Brachmann J, Karch M, et al: Reverse use-dependent effects of sotalol demonstrated by recording monophasic action potentials of the right ventricle. Am J Cardiol 1991;68:1183.

444. Nattel S, Elituv RF, Matthews C, Nayebpour M, Talajic M: Concentration dependence of class III and beta-adrenergic blocking effects of sotalol in anesthetized dogs. J Am Coll Cardiol 1989;13:1190.

445. Cobbe SM, Hoffman E, Ritzenhoff A, et al: Action of sotalol on potential reentrant pathways and ventricular tachyarrhythmias in conscious dogs in the late postmyocardial infarction phase. Circulation 1983;68:865.

446. Edvardson N, Hirsch I, Emanuelsson H, et al: Sotalol induced delayed ventricular repolarization in man. Eur Heart J 1980;1:335.

447. Echt DS, Berte LE, Clusin WT, et al: Prolongation of the human cardiac monophasic action potential by sotalol. Am J Cardiol 1982;50:1082.

448. Bennett DH: Acute prolongation of myocardial refractoriness by sotalol. Br Heart J 1982;47:521.

449. Nathan AW, Hellestrand KI, Bexton RS, et al: Electrophysiological effects of sotalol—just another beta blocker? Br Heart J 1982;47:515.

450. Funck-Brentano C, Kibleur Y, LeCoz F, Poirier JM, Mallet A, Jaillon P: Rate dependence of sotalol-induced prolongation of ventricular repolarization during exercise in humans. Circulation 1991;83:536.

451. Kus T, Aurora C, Nadeau R, Dubuc M, Kaltenbrunner W, Shenasa M: Efficacy and electrophysiologic effects of oral sotalol in patients with sustained ventricular tachycardia caused by coronary disease. Am Heart J 1992;123:82.

452. Ruder MA, Ellis T, Lebsack C, Mead RH, Smith NA, Winkle RA: Clinical experience with sotalol in patients with drug-refractory ventricular arrhythmias. J Am Coll Cardiol 1989;13:145.

453. Hohnloser SH, Zabel M, Krause T, Just H: Short- and long-term antiarrhythmic and hemodynamic effects of d,l-sotalol in patients with symptomatic ventricular arrhythmias. Am Heart J 1992;123:1220.

454. Dorian P, Newman D, Berman N, Hardy J, Mitchell J: Sotalol and type 1A drugs in combination prevent recurrence of sustained ventricular tachycardia. J Am Coll Cardiol 1993; 22:106.

455. Jordaens L, Gorgels A, Stroobandt R, Temmerman J: For the Sotalol Versus Placebo Multicenter Study Group. Am J Cardiol 1991;68:35.

456. Schnelle K, Klein G, Schinz A: Studies on the pharmacokinetics and pharmacodynamics of the beta-adrenergic blocking agent sotalol in normal man. J Clin Pharmacol 1979;19:516.

457. Investigator's Brochure MJ 1999, Sotalol, Evansville, IN: Bristol-Myers Company, March 31, 1983, Rev June 24, 1983.

458. Tjandramaga S, Thoma T, Verbeeck R, Venbeselt R, et al: The effect of end-stage renal failure and haemodialysis on the elimination kinetics of sotalol. Br J Clin Pharmacol 1976; 3:259.

459. Berglund G, Descamps R, Thomis S: Pharmacokinetics of sotalol after chronic administration to patients with renal insufficiency. Eur J Clin Pharmacol 1980;18:321.

460. Salerno DM: Part IV: Class II, class III, and class IV antiarrhythmic drugs, comparative efficacy of drugs, and effect of drugs on mortality—a review of their pharmacokinetics, efficacy, and toxicity. J Electrophysiol 1988;2:55.

461. Singh BN, Nademanee K: Sotalol: A beta blocker with unique antiarrhythmic properties. Am Heart J 1987;114:120.

462. Golzalez R, Scheinman MM, Herre JM, Griffin JC, Sauve MJ, Sharkey H: Usefulness of sotalol for drug-refractory malignant ventricular arrhythmias. J Am Coll Cardiol 1988; 12:1568.

463. Mithcell BL, Wyse G, Duff HJ: Electropharmacology of sotalol in patients with Wolff-Parkinson-White syndrome. Circulation 1987;76:810.

464. Kunze KP, Schluter M, Kuck HK: Sotalol in patients with Wolff-Parkinson-White syndrome. Circulation 1987;75:1050.

465. Mahmarian JJ, Verani MS, Hohmann T, et al: The hemodynamic effects of sotalol and quinidine: Analysis by use of rest and exercise gated radionuclide angiography. Circulation 1987;76:324.

466. Totterman KJ, Turto H, Pellinen T: Overdrive pacing as treatment of sotalol-induced ventricular tachyarrhythmias (torsades des pointes). Acta Med Scand 1982;668:28.

467. Funck-Brentano C, Kroemer HK, Roden DM: Propafenone. N Engl J Med 1990;322:518.

468. Shen EN: Propafenone: A promising new antiarrhythmic agent. Chest 1990;98:434.

469. Karagueuzian HS, Katoh T, Sugi K, et al: Electrophysiologic effects of propafenone, a new antiarrhythmic drug, on isolated cardiac tissue. Circulation 1982;66(suppl II):378.

470. Ledda F, Mantella L, Manzini S, et al: Electrophysiologic effects of propafenone in isolated cardiac preparations. J Cardiovasc Pharmacol 1981;3:1162.

471. Dukes ID, Vaughan Williams EMV: The multiple modes of action of propafenone. Eur Heart J 1984;5:115.

472. Kohlhardt M, Seifert C: Tonic and phasic I Na blockade by antiarrhythmics. Different properties of drug binding to fast sodium channels as judged from Vmax studies with propafenone and derivatives in mammalian ventricular myocardium. Pflugers Arch 1983;396:199.

473. Katoh T, Karagueuzian HS, Sugi K, Ohta M, Mandel WJ, Peter T: Effects of propafenone on sinus nodal and ventricular automaticity: In vitro and in vivo correlation. Am Heart J 1987;113:941.

474. Podrid PJ, Lown B: Propafenone: A new agent for ventricular arrhythmias. J Am Coll Cardiol 1984;4:117.

475. Malfatto G, Zaza A, Forster M, Sodowick B, Danilo P Jr, Rosen M: Electrophysiologic, inotropic and antiarrhythmic effects of propafenone, 5-hydroxypropafenone and N-depropyl-propafenone. J Pharmacol Exp Ther 1988;246:419.

476. Connolly SJ, Katz RE, Lebsack CS, et al: Clinical efficacy and electrophysiology of oral propafenone for ventricular tachycardia. Am J Cardiol 1983;52:1208.

477. Hammill SC, McLaran CJ, Wood DL, et al: Double-blind study of intravenous propafenone for paroxysmal supraventricular reentrant tachycardia. J Am Coll Cardiol 1987;9:1364.

478. Chilson DA, Heger JJ, Zipes DP, Browne KF, Prystowsky EN: Electrophysiologic effects and clinical efficacy of oral propafenone therapy in patients with ventricular tachycardia. J Am Coll Cardiol 1985;5:1407.

479. Harron WG, Brogden RN: Propafenone: A review of its pharmacodynamic and pharmacokinetic properties, and therapeutic use in the treatment of arrhythmias. Drugs 1987;34:617.

480. Siddoway LA, Thompson KA, McAllister B, et al: Polymorphism of propafenone metabolism and disposition in man: Clinical and pharmacokinetic consequences. Circulation 1987;75:785.

481. Kates RE, Yee YG, Winkle RA: Metabolic cumulation during chronic propafenone dosing in arrhythmia. Clin Pharmacol Ther 1985;37:610.

482. Connolly SJ, Katz RE, Lebsack CS, et al: Clinical pharmacology of propafenone. Circulation 1983;68:589.

483. Keller K, Meyer-Estorg G, Beck OA, Hochrein H: Correlation between serum concentration and pharmacological effect on the atrioventricular conduction time of the antiarrhythmic drug propafenone. Eur J Clin Pharmacol 1978;13:17.

485. Kroemer HK, Funck-Breantano C, Silberstein DJ, et al: Stereoselective disposition and pharmacologic activity of propafenone enantiomers. Circulation 1989;79:1068.

486. Latini R, Marchi S, Riva E, et al: Distribution of propafenone and its active metabolite, 5-hydroxypropafenone, in human tissues. Am Heart J 1987;113:843.

487. Gillis AM, Kates RE: Myocardial uptake kinetics and pharmacodynamics of propafenone in the isolated perfused rabbit heart. J Pharmacol Exp Ther 1986;237:708.

488. Mason WD, Lanman RC, Kirsten EB: Plasma and saliva propafenone concentrations at steady state. J Pharm Sci 1987; 76:437.

489. Axelon JE, Chan GLY, Kirsten EB, et al: Food increases the bioavailability of propafenone. Br J Clin Pharmacol 1987; 23:735.

490. Pitchett ELC, Smith WM, Kirsten EB: Pharmacokinetic and pharmacodynamic interactions of propafenone and cimetidine. J Clin Pharmacol 1988;28:619.

491. Kates RE, Yee YG, Kirsten EB: Interaction between warfarin and propafenone in healthy volunteer subjects. Clin Pharmacol Ther 1987;42:305.

492. Stohler JL, Kowe PR, Marinchak RA, Friehling TD: Drug interaction with propafenone. Journal of Electrophysiology 1987;1:568.

493. Shen EN, Sung RJ, Morady F, et al: Electrophysiologic and hemodynamic effects of intravenous propafenone in patients with recurrent ventricular tachycardia. J Am Coll Cardiol 1984;3:1291.

494. Klein RC, Huang SK, Marcus FI, et al: Enhanced antiarrhythmic efficacy of propafenone when used in combina-

tion with procainamide or quinidine. Am Heart J 1987; 114:551.

495. Dinh H, Murphy ML, Baker BJ, et al: Efficacy of propafenone compared with quinidine in chronic ventricular arrhythmias. Am J Cardiol 1985;55:1520.

496. Naccarella F, Bracchetti D, Palmieri M, et al: Comparison of propafenone and disopyramide for treatment of chronic ventricular arrhythmias: Placebo-controlled, double-blind, randomized crossover study. Am Heart J 1985;109:833.

497. Nacarella F, Bracchetti D, Palmieri M, et al: Propafenone for refractory ventricular arrhythmias: Correlation with drug plasma levels during long-term treatment. Am J Cardiol 1984;54:1008.

498. Hammil SC, Sorenson PB, Wood DL, et al: Propafenone for the treatment of refractory complex ventricular ectopic activity. Mayo Clin Proc 1986;61:98.

499. Hernandez M, Reder RF, Marinchak RA, Rials SJ, Kowey PR: Propafenone for malignant ventricular arrhythmias: An analysis of the literature. Am Heart J 1991;121:1178.

500. Pritchett EL, McCarthy EA, Wilkinson WE: Propafenone treatment of symptomatic paroxysmal supraventricular tachycardia. Ann Intern Med 1991;114:539.

501. Gentili C, Giordano F, Alois A, Massa E, Bianconi L: Efficacy of intravenous propafenone in acute atrial fibrillation complicating open-heart surgery. Am Heart J 1992;123:1225.

502. Karagueuzian HS, Mandel WJ, Peter T: Propafenone. In: Scriabine A, ed. New drugs annual: Cardiovascular drugs. Vol 3. New York: Raven Press, 1985:285.

503. Rudolph W, Petri H, Kafka W, et al: Effects of propafenone on the accessory pathway (AP) in patients with WPW syndrome. (Abstract) Am J Cardiol 1979;43:430.

504. Ludmer PL, Mcgwan NE, Antman EM, Friedman PL: Efficacy of propafenone in Wolff-Parkinson-White syndrome: Electrophysiologic findings and long-term follow-up. J Am Coll Cardiol 1987;9:1357.

505. Zilcher H, Glogar D, Kaindl R: Torsades de pointes: Occurrence in myocardial ischemia as a separate entity. Multiform ventricular tachycardia or not? Eur Heart J 1980;1:63.

506. Alboni P, Pirani R, Paparella N, et al: A method for evaluating different modes of action of an antiarrhythmic drug in man. The effects of propafenone on sinus nodal function. Int J Cardiol 1985;7:255.

507. Cheriex EC, Krijne R, Heymerikas J, Wellens HJJ: Lack of clinically significant beta-blocking effect of propafenone. Eur Heart J 1987;8:53.

508. Brodsky MA, Allen BJ: Ventricular tachycardia in patients with impaired left ventricular function: The role of propafenone. Clin Prog Electrophysiol Pacing 1986;4:546.

509. Hanaki Y, Sugiyama S, Hieda N, et al: Cardioprotective effects of various class 1 antiarrhythmic drugs in canine hearts. J Am Coll Cardiol 1989;14:219.

510. Hill MR, Gotz VP, Herman E, et al: Evaluation of the asthmogenicity of propafenone, a new antiarrhythmic drug. Chest 1986;90;698.

511. McHugh T, Perina DG: Propafenone ingestion. Ann Emerg Med 1987;16:437.

512. Hammermeister KE, Boerth RC, Warbase JR: The comparative inotropic effects of six clinically used antiarrhythmic agents. Am Heart J 1972;84:643.

513. Heissenbuttel RH, Bigger JT: Bretylium tosylate: A newly available antiarrhythmic drug for ventricular arrhythmia. Ann Intern Med 1979;91:229.

514. Markis JE, Koch-Weser J: Characteristics and mechanism of the positive inotropic action of bretylium tosylate: Combined norepinephrine release and direct effect. Circulation 1971;43(suppl II):183.

515. Chatterjee K, Mandel WJ, Vyden JK, et al: Cardiovascular effects of bretylium tosylate in acute myocardial infarction. JAMA 1973;223:757.

516. Taylor SH, Saxton C, Davies PS, Stoker JB: Bretylium tosylate in prevention of cardiac arrhythmias after myocardial infarction. Br Heart J 1970;23:326.

517. Block PJ, Winkle RA: Hemodynamic effects of antiarrhythmic drugs. Am J Cardiol 1983;52:14C.

518. Bigger JR, Jaffe C: The effect of bretylium tosylate on the electrophysiological properties of ventricular muscle and Purkinje fibers. Am J Cardiol 1971;27:82.

519. Wit AL, Steiner C, Damato AN: Electrophysiologic effects of bretylium tosylate on single fibers of the canine specialized conducting system and ventricle. J Pharmacol Exp Ther 1970;173:344.

520. Kowey PR, Friehling TD, O'Connor KM, et al: The effects of bretylium and clofilium on dispersion of refractoriness and vulnerability to ventricular fibrillation in the ischemic feline heart. Am Heart J 1985;110:363.

521. Cardinal R, Sasyniuk BI: Electrophysiological effects of bretylium tosylate on subendocardial Purkinje fibers from infarcted canine hearts. J Pharmacol Exp Ther 1978;204:159.

522. Anderson JC, Patterson E, Conlon M, et al: Kinetics of antifibrillatory effects of bretylium: Correlation with myocardial drug concentration. Am J Cardiol 1980;46:583.

523. Wenger TC, Lederman S, Starmer FC, et al: A method for quantitating antifibrillatory effects of drugs after coronary reperfusion in dogs: Improved outcome with bretylium. Circulation 1984;69:142.

524. Naito M, Michelson EL, Kmetz JJ, et al: Failure of antiarrhythmic drug to prevent experimental reperfusion ventricular fibrillation. Circulation 1981;63:70.

525. Bernstein JG, Koch-Weser J: Effectiveness of bretylium tosylate against refractory ventricular arrhythmias. Circulation 1972;45:1024.

526. Bacaner MD: Quantitative comparison of bretylium with other antifibrillatory drugs. Am J Cardiol 1968;21:504.

527. Wilson JR: Use of antiarrhythmic drugs in patients with heart failure: Clinical efficacy, hemodynamic results, and relation to survival. Circulation 1987;75(suppl IV):64.

528. Stratman HG, Kennedy HL: Torsades de pointes associated with drugs and toxins: Recognition and management. Am Heart J 1987;113:1470.

529. Zipes DP, Troup PJ: New antiarrhythmic agents. Amiodarone, aprindine, disopyramide, ethmozin, mexiletine, tocainide, verapamil. Am J Cardiol 1978;41:1005.

530. Clyne CA, Estes NAM, Wang PJ: Moricizine. N Engl J Med 1992;327:255.

531. Morganroth J, Pearlman AS, Dunkman WB: Ethmozin: A new antiarrhythmic agent developed in the USSR. Efficacy and tolerance. Am Heart J 1979;98:621.

532. Podrid PJ, Lyakishev A, Lown B, Mazur N: Ethmozin: A new antiarrhythmic drug for suppressing ventricular premature complexes. Circulation 1980;61:450.

533. Pratt CM, English LJ, Yepsen SC, et al: Double-blind placebo control crossover trial of ethmozin and dispyramide in the suppression of complex ventricular arrhythmias. (Abstract) Circulation 1983;(suppl III)68:1659.

534. Denilo PJ, Lanfan WB, Rosen MR, Hoffman BF: Effects of the phenothiazine analog, EN-313, on ventricular arrhythmias in the dog. Eur J Pharmacol 1977;45:127.

535. Ruffy R, Rozenshtraukh S, Elharrar V, Zipes DP: Electrophysiological effects of ethmozin on canine myocardium. Cardiovasc Res 1979;13:354.

536. Whitney CC, Weinstein SH, Gaylord JC: High performance liquid chromatography determination of Ethmozine in plasma. J Pharm Sci 1981;70:462.

537. Salerno DM, Sharky PJ, Granurd G, et al: Efficacy, safety, and pharmacokinetics of high dose Ethmozine during short and long-term therapy. Circulation 1984;70(suppl II):440.

538. Morganroth J: Safety and efficacy of a twice-daily dosing regimen of moricizine (Ethmozine). Am Heart J 1985;110:1188.

539. Damle R, Levine J, Matos J, et al: Efficacy and risks of moricizine in inducible sustained ventricular tachycardia. Ann Intern Med 1992;116:375.

540. Carmeliet E, Jansen PAJ, Marsboom R, et al: Antiarrhythmic electrophysiologic and hemodynamic effect of lorcainide. Arch Int Pharmacodyn Ther 1978;231:104.

541. Carmeliet E, Zaman MY: Comparative effects of lignocaine and lorcainide on conduction in the Langendorff-perfused guinea pig heart. J Cardiovasc Pharmacol 1979;13:439.

542. Eriksson CE, Brogden RN: Lorcainide, a preliminary review of its pharmacodynamic properties and therapeutic efficacy. Drugs 1984;27:279.

543. Kasper W, Treese N, Meinertz T, et al: Electrophysiologic effects of lorcainide on the accessory pathway in the Wolff-Parkinson-White syndrome. Am J Cardiol 1983;51:1618.

544. Kates RE, Keefe DL, Winkle RA: Lorcainide disposition kinetics in arrhythmia patients. Clin Pharmacol Ther 1983;33:28.

545. Jahnchen E, Bechtold H, Kasper W, et al: Lorcainide. I. Saturable presystemic elimination. Clin Pharmacol Ther 1979;26:187.

546. Keefe DL: Pharmacology of lorcainide. Am J Cardiol 1984;54:18B.

547. Amery WK, Heykants J, Bruyneel K, et al: Bioavailability and saturation of the presystemic metabolism of oral lorcainide therapy initiated in three different dose regimens. Eur J Clin Pharmacol 1983;24:517.

548. Somani P: Pharmacokinetics of lorcainide, a new antiarrhythmic drug, in patients with cardiac rhythm disorder. Am J Cardiol 1981;48:157.

549. Meinertz T, Kasper W, Kersting F, et al: Lorcainide. II. Plasma concentration-effect relationship. Clin Pharmacol Ther 1979;26:196.

550. Klots U, Fischer C, Muller-Scydlitz P, et al: Alterations in the disposition of differently cleared drugs in patients with cirrhosis. Clin Pharmacol Ther 1979;26:221.

551. Klotz U: Disposition and antiarrhythmic effects of lorcainide. Int J Clin Pharmacol Biopharm 1979;17:152.

552. Keefe DL, Peters F, Winkle RA: Randomized double-blind placebo controlled crossover trial documenting oral lorcainide efficacy in suppression of symptomatic ventricular tachyarrhythmias. Am Heart J 1982;103:511.

553. Schmidt G, Klein G, Wirtzfeld C: Acute effects of antiarrhythmic drugs on stable ventricular premature beats. Controlled comparison of lorcainide and lidocaine. Eur J Clin Pharmacol 1985;27:633.

554. Saksena S, Rothbart ST, Capello G, et al: Clinical and electrophysiological effects of chronic lorcainide therapy in refractory ventricular tachycardia. J Am Coll Cardiol 1983;2:538.

555. Somberg JC, Butler B, Flowers D, et al: Comparison of noninvasive arrhythmia induction technique with electrophysiologic studies and evaluation of lorcainide in patients with symptomatic ventricular tachycardia. Am J Cardiol 1984;54:49B.

556. Somberg JC, Butler B, Flowers D, et al: Evaluation of lorcainide in patients with symptomatic ventricular tachycardia. Am J Cardiol 1984;54:43B.

557. Somberg JC, Butler B, Torres V, et al: Lorcainide therapy for high-risk patient post-myocardial infarction. Am J Cardiol 1984;54:37B.

558. Hohnloser SH, Podrid PJ, Lown B: Intravenous lorcainide for symptomatic ventricular tachyarrhythmias: Comparison with lidocaine and oral lorcainide. Am Heart J 1989;115:824.

559. Manz M, Steinbeck G, Luderitz B: Electrophysiological effects of lorcainide in sino-atrial disease and in Wolff-Parkinson-White syndrome. Eur Heart J 1982;3:56.

560. Mead RH, Keefe DL, Kates RE, et al: Chronic lorcainide therapy for symptomatic premature ventricular complexes: Efficacy, pharmacokinetics and evidence for norlorcainide antiarrhythmic effect. Am J Cardiol 1985;55:72.

561. Vlay SC, Mallis GI: Intravenous and oral lorcainide: Assessment of central nervous system toxicity and antiarrhythmic efficacy. Am Heart J 1986;111:452.

562. Siddiqui S, Siddiqui RH: The alkaloids of Rauwolfia serpentina. J Indian Chem Soc 1932;9:539.

563. Bojorges R, Pastelin G, Sanchez-Perez A, et al: The effects of ajmaline in experimental and clinical arrhythmias and their relation to some electrophysiological parameters of the heart. J Exp Pharmacol Ther 1975;193:183.

564. Obayashi K, Mandel WJ: Electrophysiological effects of ajmaline in isolated cardiac tissue. Cardiovasc Res 1976;10:20.

565. Bazika V, Lang TW, Pappelbaum S, Corday E: Ajmaline, a Rauwolfia alkaloid for the treatment of digitalis arrhythmias. Am J Cardiol 1966;17:227.

566. Obayashi K, Hagasawa K, Mandel WJ, et al: Cardiovascular effects of ajmaline. Am Heart J 1976;92:487.

567. Sethi KK, Jaishankar S, Gupta MP: Salutary effects of intravenous ajmaline in patients with paroxysmal supraventricular tachycardia by dual atrioventricular nodal pathways: Blockade of the retrograde fast pathway. Circulation 1984;70:876.

568. Wellens HJJ, Bar FW, Gorgel AP, Vanagt EJ: Use of ajmaline in patients with the Wolff-Parkinson-White syndrome to disclose short refractory period of the accessory pathway. Am J Cardiol 1980;45:130.

569. Herpin D, Gaudeau B, Amid A, et al: Etude de l'activite et de la tolerance d'un nouvel anti-arythmique la cibenzoline (Cipralan) administre par voie orale. Acta Cardiol 1981;36:131.

570. Thebaut JF, Archard F, deLangenhagen B: Etude electrophysiologique chez l'homme d'un nouvel antiarythmic, la

cibenzoline, dans de syndrome de Wolff-Parkinson-White. L'Inform Cardiol 1980;4:393.

571. Ohta M, Sugi K, McCullen A, et al: Electrophysiologic effects of cibenzoline, a new antiarrhythmic drug on isolated cardiac tissue. (Abstract) Circulation 1983;68(suppl III):220.

572. Millar JS, Vaughan Williams EM: Effects on rabbit nodal atrial ventricular and Purkinje cell potentials of a new antiarrhythmic drug, cibenzoline, which protects against action potential shortening in hypoxia. Br J Pharmacol 1982;75: 469.

573. Dangman KH: Cardiac effects of cibenzoline. J Cardiovasc Pharmacol 1984;6:300.

574. Browne KF, Hegger JJ, Zipes DP, et al: Clinical and electrophysiologic effects of cibenzoline in patients with ventricular arrhythmias. (Abstract) J Am Coll Cardiol 1983;1:699.

575. Miura DS, Karen G, Siegel L, et al: Effect of cibenzoline in suppressing ventricular tachycardia induced by programmed electrical stimulation. (Abstract) J Am Coll Cardiol 1983;1: 699.

576. Miura DS, Dangman KH: New therapy focus: Cibenzoline. Cardiovasc Res 1986;7:55.

577. Klein RC, Horowitz LD, Rushforth N: Efficacy and safety of oral cibenzoline for ventricular arrhythmia. Am J Cardiol 1986;57:592.

578. Khool KC, Szuna AJ, Colburn WA, et al: Single-dose pharmacokinetics and dose proportionality of oral cibenzoline. J Clin Pharmacol 1984;24:283.

579. Massarella JW, Khoo KC, Szuna AJ, et al: Pharmacokinetics of cibenzoline after single and repetitive dosing in healthy volunteers. J Clin Pharmacol 1986;26:125.

580. Brazzell RK, Colburn WA, Aogaichi K, et al: Pharmacokinetics of oral cibenzoline in arrhythmia patients. Clin Pharmacokinet 1985;10:178.

581. Canal M, Flouvat B, Tremblay D, et al: Pharmacokinetics in man of a new antiarrhythmic drug, cibenzoline. Eur J Pharmacol 1983;24:509.

582. Brazzell RK, Rees MMC, Khoo KC, et al: Age and cibenzoline disposition. Clin Pharmacol Ther 1984;36:613.

583. Canal M, Flouvat B, Tremblay D, Disfour A: Pharmacokinetics in man of a new antiarrhythmic drug: Cibenzoline. Eur J Clin Pharmacol 1983;24:509.

584. Brown KF, Prystowsky EN, Zipes DP, et al: Clinical efficacy and electrophysiologic effects of cibenzoline therapy in patients with ventricular arrhythmias. J Am Coll Cardiol 1984;3:857.

585. Cibenzoline (RO 22-7796) Investigational Brochure: Nutley, NJ: Hoffman-LaRoche, Inc, 1982.

586. Brazzell RK, Aogaichi K, Meger JJ Jr, et al: Cibenzoline plasma concentration and antiarrhythmic effect. Clin Pharmacol Ther 1984;35:307.

587. Browne KF, Prystowky EN, Zipes DP, et al: Clinical efficacy and electrophysiologic effects of cibenzoline therapy in patients with ventricular arrhythmias. J Am Coll Cardiol 1984;3:857.

588. Miura DS, Keren G, Torres V, et al: Antiarrhythmic effects of cibenzoline. Am Heart J 1985;109:827.

589. Waleffe A, Dufour A, Aymard MF, et al: Electrophysiologic effects, antiarrhythmic activity and pharmacokinetics of cibenzoline studied with programmed stimulation of the heart in patients with supraventricular reentrant tachycardia. Eur Heart J 1985;6:253.

590. Kostis JB, Krieger S, Moreyra AA, et al: Cibenzoline for the treatment of ventricular arrhythmias: A double-blind placebo-controlled study. J Am Coll Cardiol 1985;4:372.

591. Rawling D, Fozzard HA: Electrophysiological effects of imipramine on cardiac Purkinje fibers. Am J Cardiol 1978; 41:387.

592. Weld FM, Bigger JT, Swistel D, Bordulk J: Effects of imipramine hydrochloride on electrophysiological properties of sheep cardiac Purkinje fibers. Am J Cardiol 1978;41:386.

593. Williams RD, Sherter C: Cardiac complication of tricyclic anti-depressant therapy. Ann Intern Med 1971;74:395.

594. Raisfeld IH: Appraisal and reappraisal of cardiac therapy. Am Heart J 1972;83:129.

595. Connolly SJ, Mitchell BL, Swerdlow CD, et al: Clinical efficacy and electrophysiology of imipramine for ventricular tachycardia. Am J Cardiol 1984;53:516.

596. Neimann JT, Bessen HA, Rothstein RJ, Laks MM: Electrocardiographic criteria for tricyclic antidepressant cardiotoxicity. Am J Cardiol 1986;57:1154.

597. Gram LF, Christiansen J: First-pass metabolism of imipramine in man. Clin Pharmacol Ther 1975;17:555.

598. Abernathy DR, Greenblatt DJ, Shader RI: Imipramine and desipramine disposition in the elderly. 1985;232:183.

599. Giardina EGV, Johnson LL, Vita J, et al: Effect of imipramine and nortriptyline on left ventricular function and blood pressure in patients treated for arrhythmias. Am Heart J 1985;109:992.

600. Marchese AC, Hill JA, Xie PD Jr, Strauss HC: Electrophysiologic effects of amiloride in canine Purkinje fibers: Evidence for a delayed effect on repolarization. J Pharmacol Exp Ther 1985;232:485.

601. Duff HJ, Lester WM, Rahmberg M: Amiloride. Antiarrhythmic and electrophysiologic activity in the dog. Circulation 1988; 78:1469.

602. Duff HJ, Mitchell B, Kavanagh KM, et al: Amiloride. Antiarrhythmic and electrophysiologic actions in patients with inducible sustained ventricular tachycardia. Circulation 1989;79:1257.

603. Bellardinelli L, Linden J, Berne R: The cardiac effects of adenosine. Prog Cardiovasc Dis 1989;32:73.

604. DiMarco JP, Miles W, Akhtar M, the Adenosine for PSVT Study Group: Ann Intern Med 1990;113:104.

605. Ellenbogen KA, Thames MD, DiMarco JP, Sheehan H, Lerman BB: Electrophysiological effects of adenosine in the transplanted human heart. Evidence of supersensitivity. Circulation 1990;81:821.

606. Bellardinelli L, Wu S-N, Visentin S: Adenosine regulation of cardiac electrical activity. In: Zipes DP, Jalife J, eds. Cardiac electrophysiology, from cell to bedside. Philadelphia: WB Saunders, 1990:284.

607. Surawicz B: Ventricular arrhythmias: Why is it so difficult to find a pharmacologic cure? J Am Coll Cardiol 1989;14:1401.

608. Karagueuzian HS, Ohta M, Drury JK, et al: Coronary venous retroinfusion of procainamide: A new approach for the management of spontaneous and inducible sustained ventricular tachycardia during myocardial infarction. J Am Coll Cardiol 1986;7:551.

Cardiac Arrhythmias, 3rd edition, edited by William J. Mandel.
J. B. Lippincott Company, Philadelphia © 1995.

6

Jeffrey S. Goodman • C. Thomas Peter

Proarrhythmia: Primum Non Nocere

It is well documented that antiarrhythmic agents may produce or aggravate arrhythmias. Proarrhythmia may be loosely defined as any arrhythmia or conduction disturbance that is pharmacologically induced. Although it is sometimes difficult to distinguish definitively between the patient's underlying arrhythmia and a detrimental drug effect, there are ample data to support the important role that proarrhythmia plays. These iatrogenically induced rhythms may be ventricular tachyarrhythmias, supraventricular tachyarrhythmias, or bradyarrhythmias. As shown in Table 6-1, proarrhythmia may take several forms, including the worsening of the underlying arrhythmia, the induction of a new arrhythmia, or rendering a previously well-tolerated rhythm hemodynamically unstable. Although most of the culprit drugs are specifically those agents given in an attempt to suppress cardiac arrhythmias, nonantiarrhythmic drugs may also be implicated.

The first documented report of proarrhythmia appeared in 1785, when William Withering described bradycardia among the manifestations of foxglove toxicity in his book, *An Account of the Foxglove and Some of its Medical Uses With Practical Remarks on Dropsy and Other Diseases*.[1] In 1922, 4 years after its clinical introduction, separate publications by Kerr and Bender and Drury and coworkers reported cases of ventricular fibrillation in pa-

tients receiving therapy with quinidine sulfate.[2,3] The clinical significance of proarrhythmia was reemphasized in 1964 when Selzer and Wray reported the incidence of ventricular fibrillation in patients receiving quinidine for atrial fibrillation.[4] It was not until the release of the Cardiac Arrhythmia Suppression Trial (CAST) results in 1988 (showing a threefold increase in mortality in treated patients, as compared with untreated patients) that it became widely known that antiarrhythmic agents were responsible for fatal ventricular arrhythmias in a significant percentage of patients.[5] Although historically the emphasis has been on drug-induced tachyarrhythmias, clinicians must realize that the spectrum of proarrhythmia is indeed wide and varied (see Table 6-1).

DRUG-INDUCED BRADYARRHYTHMIAS

Induction or exacerbation of sinoatrial or atrioventricular (AV) node block has been clearly documented in patients treated with antiarrhythmic agents.[6-10] As with most proarrhythmic effects, patients with underlying heart disease are at greatest risk. Patients having baseline conduction disturbances have a higher incidence of drug-induced

TABLE 6-1. Manifestations of Proarrhythmia

I. Drug-induced bradyarrhythmias
  A. Exacerbation or induction of sinus node dysfunction
    1. Decreased sinus node automaticity, resulting in sinus bradycardia or sinus arrest
    2. Sinus node/sinoatrial exit block
    3. Exacerbation of sinus node dysfunction in patients with sick sinus syndrome
  B. Exacerbation or induction of atrioventricular (AV) block
    1. AV node
    2. His-Purkinje system
II. Drug-induced tachyarrhythmias
  A. Exacerbation or induction of supraventricular arrhythmias
    1. Increased frequency/duration of paroxysmal atrial fibrillation or flutter
    2. Acceleration or ventricular response due to enhanced AV node conduction
    3. Acceleration of ventricular response in atrial flutter due to decreased flutter cycle length and resultant 1:1 AV node conduction
    4. Atrial tachycardia with AV block
    5. Acceleration of ventricular rate in patients with Wolff-Parkinson-White syndrome and atrial fibrillation
    6. Nonparoxysmal AV junction tachycardia
    7. Aberrant conduction
  B. Exacerbation or induction of ventricular arrhythmias
    1. Increased frequency of underlying ventricular tachycardia
    2. Induction of ventricular tachycardia or tachycardias of different or multiform morphology or morphologies
    3. Rate acceleration of underlying ventricular tachycardia
    4. Increased frequency of baseline ventricular ectopy (premature ventricular complexes [PVCs], nonsustained ventricular tachycardia)
    5. Induction of ventricular ectopy (PVCs, nonsustained ventricular tachycardia) of new or multiform morphology or morphologies
    6. Induction of incessant ventricular tachycardia
    7. Torsades de pointes (QT-interval prolongation) with polymorphic ventricular tachycardia
    8. Induction of bidirectional ventricular tachycardia
    9. Induction of ventricular fibrillation/sudden cardiac death
    10. Change in response to programmed electric stimulation
      a. Easier induction of VT
      b. Conversion of previously nonsustained to sustained ventricular tachycardia
      c. Conversion of previously hemodynamically stable to unstable ventricular tachycardia or ventricular fibrillation, requiring cardioversion
      d. Rate acceleration of induced ventricular tachycardia
      e. A combination of any of the above

bradyarrhythmias when compared with patients with no clinically evident conduction disease.[10]

Sinus node dysfunction may take the form of decreased automaticity, which may range from sinus bradycardia to sinus arrest and sinus node or sinoatrial exit block. β-Adrenergic blockers (class II agents), digitalis, and class I agents are the most commonly associated antiarrhythmic agents, although amiodarone and calcium channel blockers are also reported.[6-9] Although sinus node dysfunction as a proarrhythmic manifestation is more frequent with drug levels above the therapeutic range, it may even be seen with therapeutic plasma levels. Patients with underlying sinus node disease, such as the sick sinus syndrome, seem to be at highest risk for advanced sinus bradycardia and sinus arrest, especially when they convert from atrial fibrillation to sinus rhythm in the presence of class I antiarrhythmic agents.[8] In addition to a direct depressant effect on sinus node function, sinoatrial exit block may occur, especially with the use of class I antiarrhythmics such as quinidine.[11]

Patients who have underlying sinus node disease benefit from careful rhythm monitoring during the initiation of drug therapy. Although patients with underlying conduction disturbances are at greatest risk, significant sinus node depression can occur in those patients with apparently normal sinus node function. It is possible that there are patients with clinically undetected baseline sinus node dysfunction who may be at higher risk for drug-induced bradycardia.

Drug-induced AV block may be due to effects on the AV node or His-Purkinje system, resulting in prolongations in AH or less commonly in HV intervals, as detected in the electrophysiology laboratory. Patients with baseline PR interval prolongation or evidence of advanced AV block are a higher risk than those with normal AV conduction.[12,13] β-Adrenergic blockers, calcium channel blockers, class III agents, and digitalis have all been shown to aggravate or induce AV nodal conduction block with normal or supratherapeutic plasma levels (Fig. 6-1).[14-17] This block may range in severity from PR interval prolongation to complete heart block and the development of an idioventricular rhythm.[13]

Class I antiarrhythmic agents are particularly notorious for their depressant effects on AV nodal conduction and have been shown to cause delay or block in the His-Purkinje system with a resultant increase in the HV interval or the HV-interval prolongation.[10] This is most commonly seen with class IC agents but class IA and to a lesser extent class IB agents have induced infra- or intra-Hisian block. Disopyramide has been shown to increase the HV interval by 18% to 25% and may cause hemiblock or even complete heart block.[12,18,19] Procainamide and quinidine have also been shown to significantly increase the HV interval, with procainamide's effects on AV nodal conduction becoming more pronounced at higher drug levels.[20-22] Conduction systems with underlying disease are at greatest risk but advanced block has also been seen in patients with normal baseline conduction who have class I drug overdose.[13] Treatment of drug-induced bradycardia is primarily by removal of the offending agent. The use of atropine or temporary transvenous pacing (although rarely required) is indicated if bradycardia is persistent or hemodynamically intolerated. In patients with renal failure, dialysis may be necessary to remove dialyzable antiar-

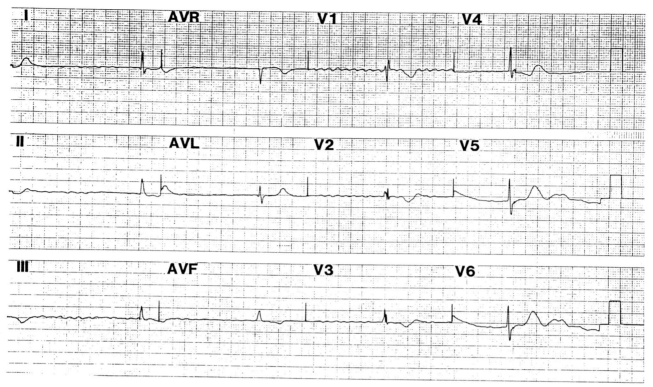

Figure 6-1. Twelve-lead electrocardiogram of a 69-year-old man with chronic atrial fibrillation who presented with congestive heart failure and weakness. Electrocardiogram demonstrates atrial fibrillation with heart block and a ventricular escape rhythm of 30. Note prominent U waves in the lateral precordial leads, which may be secondary to hypokalemia. Serum digoxin level was 3.4 ng/mL and serum potassium level was 3.4 mEq/L. This patient required temporary transvenous pacing because of hemodynamic compromise but did well with discontinuation of digitalis and potassium repletion.

rhythmic agents or their active metabolites. In some cases of drug overdose (e.g., beta blockade, digitalis), agents that are directed at binding, inactivating, or minimizing drug effects may be given if clinically indicated. The use of digoxin-specific antibodies is discussed in the section on drug-induced supraventricular tachyarrhythmias.

In cases of hemodynamically significant conduction block due to therapy with β-adrenergic blockade, intravenous glucagon may be given. Glucagon may produce a positive chronotropic and inotropic effect, which may overcome the influence of beta blockade even in patients unresponsive to isoproterenol.[23] Glucagon is given as an initial bolus of 50 to 150 μg/kg intravenously over 1 minute, followed by a continuous infusion of 1 to 5 mg/hour.[24]

DRUG-INDUCED SUPRAVENTRICULAR TACHYARRHYMIAS

As shown in Table 6-1, drug-induced or -exacerbated supraventricular arrhythmias may take many forms. In pa-

tients with underlying paroxysmal atrial fibrillation, atrial flutter or ectopic atrial tachycardia proarrhythmic drug effect may dramatically increase the frequency or duration of arrhythmia. Digitalis and the class IV agents diltiazem and verapamil have been implicated.[25–27] Previously, paroxysmal supraventricular arrhythmias may be rendered incessant with class I agents—particularly class IC agents.[28] A possible mechanism for this phenomenon is the drug's effect of slowing of atrial conduction without significant effects on atrial refractoriness, hence improving conditions for sustained reentry. In patients with Wolff-Parkinson-White syndrome another possible mechanism is drug-induced anterograde block in the bypass tract in addition to slowing of AV nodal conduction, creating the milieu for incessant reentry.

Class I agents—particularly quinidine, disopyramide, flecainide, and propafenone—have been demonstrated to enhance AV nodal conduction, leading to an accelerated ventricular response in patients with atrial fibrillation or flutter.[28–30] These advanced rates may be associated with aberrant ventricular conduction or hemodynamic compromise. The development of aberrantly conducted complexes may be significant when differentiation from ventricular tachycardia (VT) becomes difficult.[31] Another interesting phenomenon occurs in patients who have atrial flutter. Antiarrhythmic drug therapy may slow the flutter cycle length and may enhance AV nodal conduction to the point at which 1:1 conduction of atrial flutter may occur.[32]

In patients with atrial fibrillation and Wolff-Parkinson-White syndrome, use of digitalis, beta blockade, or the intravenous forms of diltiazem, or verapamil may be associated with an enhanced ventricular response (Fig. 6-2) that may degenerate into ventricular fibrillation.[33–35]

Two supraventricular tachyarrhythmias are almost pathognomonic of digitalis intoxication: atrial tachycardia with AV block (Fig. 6-3) and nonparoxysmal junctional tachycardia.[36] In digitalis-induced atrial tachycardia with block, the atrial rate is often slow and the nonparoxysmal junctional tachycardia is often associated with AV dissociation. Studies suggest that digitalis toxicity–induced accelerated idioventricular rhythm may be due to delayed afterdepolarizations (DADs).[37,38] Delayed afterdepolarizations are oscillations of transmembrane activity that are seen after complete repolarization of the cardiac action potential (Fig. 6-4). Delayed afterdepolarizations that reach threshold may generate spontaneous triggered activity and are seen in conditions of increased intracellular calcium, such as digoxin-induced sodium–potassium pump inhibition or an increase in catecholamines.[39]

Delayed afterdepolarization triggered activity may clinically manifest as an accelerated junctional rhythm or ventricular tachyarrhythmias.[40] As opposed to early afterdepolarizations, DADs tend to increase with increasing heart rates; thus, the risk of DAD-induced triggered arrhythmias increases as heart rate accelerates (Fig. 6-5).[37]

Most digitalis-induced supraventricular arrhythmias are associated with above normal plasma levels of digoxin but several other factors may predispose patients to digoxin proarrhythmia, even with therapeutic digoxin levels.[41] These include electrolyte disturbances such as hypokalemia, hypercalcemia, hyponatremia, and hypomagnesemia. In a study of 21 consecutive patients having digoxin toxicity, hypomagnesemia was identified as being the most common electrolyte abnormality associated with the development of digoxin toxicity.[42] Other coexistent conditions include increased adrenergic stimulation, thyroid disease, acid–base imbalance, renal dysfunction, respiratory disease, and drug–drug interactions. Some of the most common drug interaction are those that increase plasma levels of digoxin and include verapamil, amiodarone, propafenone, quinidine, spironolactone, anesthetics, and various sympathomimetics.[42,43]

Treatment of drug-induced supraventricular arrhythmias requires the immediate removal of the offending agent. Concomitant exacerbating factors such as electrolyte imbalances and drug–drug interactions should be corrected.

In addition to the above-mentioned measures, several other actions may be taken in the treatment of hemodynamically unstable digitalis toxicity–associated rhythms. Magnesium sulfate may be given as a 2- to 4-g intravenous bolus, and intravenous phenytoin (dilantin) or lidocaine has been used in the treatment of rapid supraventricular or new-onset ventricular arrhythmias.

In 1967, digoxin-specific antibodies were first produced and tested in assays of human serum; in 1971, they were successfully tested in animal studies of digoxin toxicity.[44,45,46] The first reported use of digoxin-binding antibodies in humans was in 1976 in a case of life-threatening digoxin toxicity.[47]

The United States Food and Drug Administration–released product Digibind is a 50,000d ovine-produced IgG–Fab antibody fragment made to a human albumin-digoxin complex. Each Fab fragment is a third the molecular size of IgG and binds one molecule of digoxin. The smaller size of the antibody enables it to distribute and work rapidly. When given intravenously, these fragments bind membrane-bound digoxin and the combination is excreted renally. Because of its cost, use of Digibind should be restricted to several specific situations (Table 6-2).

Digibind is packaged in 40-mg vials and is given in doses according to total body digoxin burden or empirically if steady-state drug concentrations are unknown. Each vial of lyophilized powder neutralizes 0.6 mg of digoxin, which is the usual total body digoxin burden in patients with therapeutic digoxin levels. The total body digoxin load can be calculated by the following formula:

$$\frac{\text{serum digoxin level [ng/mL]} \times 6 \text{ L/kg} \times \text{body wt [kg]}}{1000}$$

The number of vials of Digibind that are necessary is then calculated as the total body digoxin load divided by 0.6 mg/vial. As is often the case, steady-state digoxin levels may not be reliable; in these situations, 5 to 10 vials of Digibind may be empirically given. Digibind is given as an intravenous infusion over 30 minutes but may be given in bolus form if cardiac arrest is imminent. Digibind rapidly binds free digoxin and displaces membrane-bound digoxin. Paradoxically, this displacement results in even higher plasma digoxin levels (up to 30 times the pre-Digibind level) but it is critical for the clinician to realize that this represents inactive digoxin. Marked clinical improvement, including reversal of hyperkalemia, is usually seen within 30 minutes of administration, with complete reversal of cardiac toxicity within 3 to 4 hours. It is important to realize that in addition to the toxic effects, the therapeutic benefits of digoxin therapy are also abolished. It is important to monitor patients for signs of worsening congestive heart failure or atrial fibrillation with rapid AV nodal conduction. Most of the digoxin-bound Digibind is

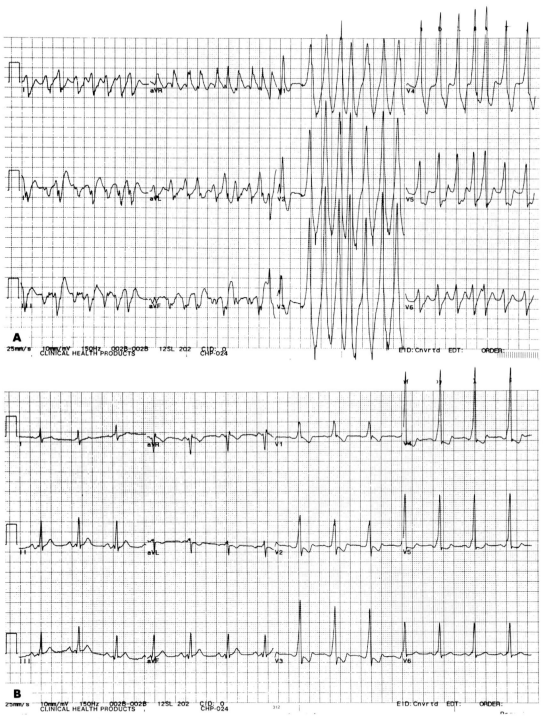

Figure 6-2. (**A**) Twelve-lead electrocardiogram (ECG) of a 24-year-old man who presented to the emergency room complaining of palpitations and was found to be in a atrial fibrillation with occasional wide complex beats. He was given 5 mg of intravenous verapamil, after which the ECG in A was obtained. The ECG demonstrates atrial fibrillation with a rapid ventricular response as fast as 300 beats per minute, with wide complexes of varying degrees. The patient became hemodynamically unstable, requiring synchronized cardioversion, after which the ECG in B was obtained. (**B**) Electrocardiogram demonstrates sinus rhythm with the Wolff-Parkinson-White syndrome and an anterolateral accessory bypass tract, which was successfully ablated with radiofrequency energy.

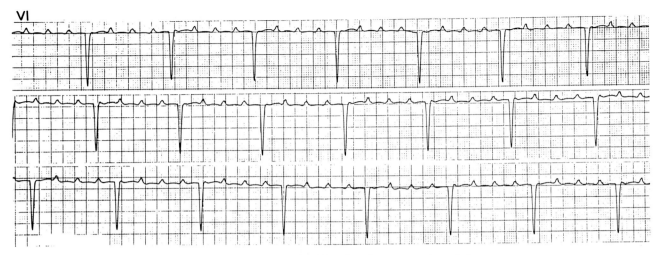

Figure 6-3. Continuous-lead V₁ rhythm strip from a 72-year-old female with congestive heart failure who presented with complaints of neck pulsations. Rhythm strip demonstrates atrial tachycardia with a ventricular response of 40. Serum digoxin level was 4.2 ng/mL, with a serum potassium of 5.2 mEq/L. Patient was hemodynamically stable and was treated conservatively, including withdraw of digoxin. Seventy-two hours later, the serum digoxin level was 0.7 ng/mL and electrocardiogram demonstrated sinus rhythm. Later that day, the patient suffered acute exacerbation of congestive heart failure and eventually required reinstitution of digitalis therapy at lower doses.

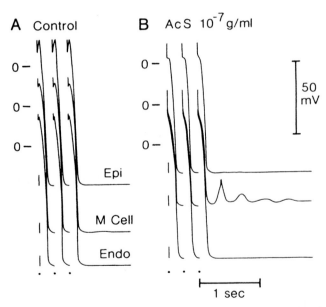

Figure 6-4. Transmembrane recordings from epicardial (*Epi*), endocardial (*Endo*), and M cell preparations of canine cardiac tissue. Shown are the last three beats of a train of 10 beats paced at a cycle length of 250 milliseconds. (**A**) The control, and (**B**) tissue exposed to a digitalis analog (acetylstrophanthidin [AcS]). AcS elicits oscillations of transmembrane potential that occur after repolarization. These oscillations are prominent delayed afterdepolarizations that are only recorded in M cells and not in the endocardial or epicardial layers. (Reprinted with permission from Antzelevitch C, Sicouri S: Clinical relevance of cardiac arrhythmias generated by afterdepolarizations: role of M cells in the generation of U waves, triggered activity and torsade de pointes. J Am Coll Cardiol 1994:23:259)

excreted renally within 24 hours, although this may be longer in patients with renal insufficiency. A small percentage of patients may demonstrate recrudescence of digoxin toxicity in 24 hours, and a second dose of Digibind may be given if clinically indicated.[48] More than 50% of digoxin-toxic patients have a complete response and another third demonstrate a partial response. Less than 1% of patients have an allergic reaction to Digibind, and there are no known contraindications to therapy.[48]

DRUG-INDUCED VENTRICULAR TACHYARRHYTHMIAS

The most serious form of proarrhythmia is the induction or exacerbation of ventricular tachyarrhythmias. Published studies indicate that the use of antiarrhythmic agents is associated with ventricular tachyarrhythmias in up to 31% of all treated patients.[49] These effects can range from an asymptomatic increase in spontaneous ventricular ectopy to ventricular fibrillation and sudden cardiac death. The danger of drug-induced sudden cardiac death is highly significant, with the CAST study demonstrating a relative risk as high as 3.6 in patients receiving antiarrhythmic drug therapy as compared to patients not receiving drug treatment.[50]

Concomitant risk factors for proarrhythmia are shown in Table 6-3. Some of these include coexistent cardiac ischemia, left ventricular dysfunction, and electrolyte imbalance.

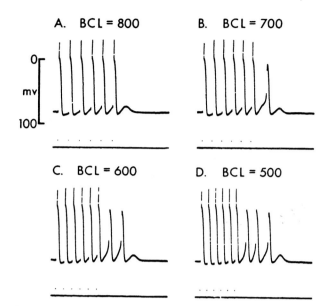

Figure 6-5. Rate-dependence of delayed afterdepolarizations (DAD) in a canine digitalis-toxic model. As paced cycle length decreases, the amplitude of DADs increase, as does DAD-induced triggered activity. (Reprinted with permission from Antzelevitch C, Sicouri S: Clinical relevance of cardiac arrhythmias generated by afterdepolarizations: role of M cells in the generation of U waves, triggered activity and torsade de pointes. J Am Coll Cardiol 1994:23:259)

Increased frequency of VT can be seen in up to 15% of patients treated with antiarrhythmic drugs.[49] This may be defined as an increase in the frequency or duration of VT episodes or an increase in the rate of VT. Ventricular tachycardia cycle length may decrease 10% to 25%, rendering a previously well-tolerated VT hemodynamically unstable. All class I and class III drugs have been associated an increased frequency of spontaneous episodes of VT. Generally, class IC agents such as encainide and fle-

TABLE 6-2. Indications for the Use of Digoxin Antibody for Digoxin Toxicity

Hemodynamically significant arrhythmias
 Ventricular fibrillation, asystole, ventricular tachycardia, complete heart block, symptomatic second-degree heart block, intolerant supraventricular tachyarrhythmia
Potassium level ≥5.5 mEq/L in adults or ≥6.0 mEq/L in children
Serum digoxin level >6.0 ng/mL in adults or >5.0 ng/mL in children and with signs or symptoms[43] of digitalis toxicity
Consumption of >10 mg digoxin in adults or >0.1 mg/kg in children[43]

*Visual changes, nausea/vomiting, weakness/fatigue, abdominal pain, lightheadedness, headache, diarrhea

(Modified from Smith TW, Austman EM, Friedman PL, et al: Digitalis glycosides: mechanisms and manifestations of toxicity. Prog Cardiovasc Dis 1984;27:21.)

TABLE 6-3. Concomitant Risk Factors for Developing Drug-Induced Ventricular Tachyarrhythmias

Depressed left ventricular ejection fraction (<35%)
Congestive heart failure
Concomitant myocardial ischemia
Use of diuretics
Use of digitalis
Age
Male gender
History of myocardial infarction
Malignant ventricular arrhythmia at presentation
Electrolyte imbalance
Prolonged QTc interval
Coexistent liver or renal disease
High plasma concentrations of class IC agents
Previous history of proarrhythmia

cainide demonstrate the highest incidence, followed by the class IA agents quinidine, disopyramide, and procainamide, and finally class III drugs.

As with most forms of proarrhythmia, it may be difficult to differentiate changes in the spontaneous nature of the underlying disease with specific drug effects. Patients at greatest risk are shown in Table 6-3 and are particularly those in whom the baseline frequency of spontaneous VT is greatest. If a patient treated with antiarrhythmic agents experiences a worsening of the baseline arrhythmia, it is important to assess several factors before attributing this to proarrhythmia. Some of these include drug levels, active ischemia, and electrolyte imbalance. Assessment of drug levels is critical in differentiating whether the increased VT frequency is due to drug inefficacy, inadequate serum levels, or drug levels in excess of the therapeutic range. If levels are therapeutic or higher, it is imperative to remove the offending drug. Hemodynamically compromised patients may require pressor support, and frequent bursts of VT may require cardioversion or temporizing treatment with intravenous antiarrhythmic agents such as lidocaine. When stable, the search for efficacious pharmacologic or nonpharmacologic arrhythmia suppression may be sought.

A less serious form of ventricular proarrhythmia is a marked increase in baseline premature ventricular complexes (PVCs) or short bursts of nonsustained VT. This increase is considered significant when there is either a fourfold increase in hourly PVCs or a tenfold increase in the mean hourly frequency of couplets or bursts of nonsustained VT.[51] Previously asymptomatic patients may become symptomatic with this increase in spontaneous ectopy. Although this type of proarrhythmic response has not been conclusively proved to be a harbinger of sustained VT, it may serve as a warning that therapy with a particular drug may not be efficacious or prudent. Class IC agents, followed by class IA and, to a lesser extent, class III, are the most prevalent offenders, and discontinuation of therapy is indicated. In the post-CAST era, antiarrhythmic drug therapy for patients with asymptomatic nonsustained VT or PVCs is generally contraindicated.

Another manifestation of proarrhythmia is the induction of sustained or nonsustained VT of one or more new morphologies.[51] This is separate from polymorphous VT, torsades de pointes, and bidirectional VT. Offending agents and treatment are similar to those described above.

A serious complication of antiarrhythmic drug use is the development of incessant VT. The VT may be of the spontaneous VT morphology but more frequently, it takes a sinusoidal form, with a relatively slow rate (Fig. 6-6). This form is primarily associated with the use of class IC antiarrhythmic agents.[52, 53] Incessant VT is defined as continuous VT that is not terminated by electric cardioversion or overdrive pacing or VT that recurs immediately after termination. Incessant VT temporally occurs near the time of drug initiation or dosage increase and is more common in patients with depressed ejection fraction and a history of sustained VT. In a study of 506 patients treated pharmacologically for recurrent VT or ventricular fibrillation, incessant VT was found in 66% of the 35 documented proarrhythmic events.[54] Encainide-induced incessant VT was the most common, followed by that induced by amiodarone and propafenone.[55] The other class IC agents flecainide and moricizine are also documented offenders.[56, 57]

Incessant VT is a form of proarrhythmia that is associated with a significant morbidity and mortality. Patients often develop hemodynamic compromise that sometimes progresses to cariogenic shock and even death. After drug discontinuation, supportive care in the form of pressors and intraaortic balloon counterpulsation may be necessary until drug washout is achieved. The use of emergent intravenous antiarrhythmic agents, including amiodarone, has occasionally proved effective in patients with class IC–induced incessant VT.

First described in 1966 by Dessertenne, torsades de pointes is a polymorphic VT that is associated with a prolonged QT interval.[58] The typical corrected QT or QTc interval (calculated by Bazett's formula, QTc = QT/RR interval) is frequently greater than 600 milliseconds. The tachycardia rate is usually 200 to 300 beats per minute, and the tachycardia is such that rapid changes in QRS morphology wind around an isoelectric baseline, resembling

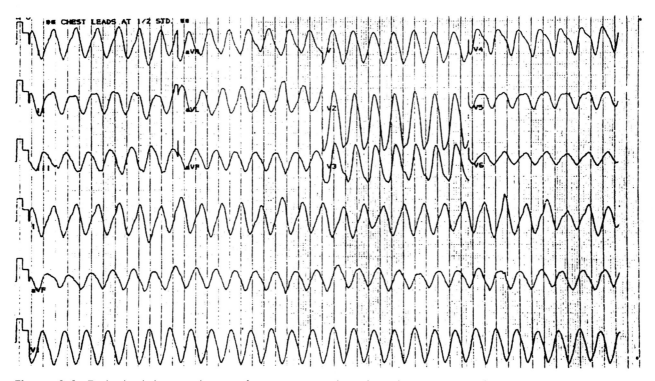

Figure 6-6. Twelve-lead electrocardiogram of incessant ventricular tachycardia in a patient with depressed ejection fraction and encainide toxicity. Note the sinusoidal pattern and relatively slow rate (160 beats/min) of the tachycardia, which is typical of class IC toxicity. (Reprinted with permission from Herre JM, Titus C, Oeff M, et al: Inefficacy and proarrhythmic effects of flecainide and encainide for sustained ventricular tachycardia and ventricular fibrillation. Ann Intern Med 1990;113:671)

a "twisting of the points" (Fig. 6-7). Torsade de pointes is often associated with a sine wave type of appearance and in the past has been confused with ventricular fibrillation (Fig. 6-8). Episodes are usually highly symptomatic and self-limiting but may degenerate into true ventricular fibrillation.

Electrophysiologically, a prolonged QT or QTU interval is presumed to represent a dispersion of refractoriness in the ventricle, which is considered to be due to early afterdepolarizations (EADs). Early afterdepolarizations are oscillations of transmembrane potential that occur during repolarization of the cardiac action potential (Fig. 6-9). Early afterdepolarizations can be documented in vitro with transmembrane recordings or in vitro with the use of monophasic action potential (MAP) recordings made in the electrophysiology laboratory. In humans, EADs have been documented in Purkinje fibers and in cardiac M cells, which are found in the deep subepicardial to mid-myocardial regions.[39] M cells are a subgroup of ventricular cells that, similar to Purkinje cells, have the ability to prolong their action potential duration at decreased stimulation rates and, similar to endocardial or epicardial muscle cells, do not demonstrate phase 4 activity (Fig. 6-10). Early afterdepolarizations occur during phase 2 or 3 of the cardiac action potential (see Fig. 6-9) and when sufficiently large to depolarize the cell membrane to its threshold may induce spontaneous action potentials, referred to as triggered responses (see Fig. 6-10). These triggered responses can lead to tachyarrhythmias, including polymorphous VT (see Fig. 6-7).[40] One possible mechanism for the genesis of the twisting points of torsades is that dispersion of refractoriness between M cells and the ventricular myocardium may create a column of functional refractoriness in the mid-myocardium. Early afterdepolarization-induced triggered activity may create an excitation wavefront that travels along the border zone and enters the M-cell region once it is no longer refractory. The wavefront would then exit the refractory M-cell region and reenter the recovered border zone. Repetition of this type of activity may produce the type of polymorphous VT seen in torsades de pointes. Unlike delayed afterdepolarizations, EADs and their associated triggered activity increase with decreasing stimulation rates (see Fig. 6-10). As shown in Table 6-4, EADs are known to be associated with a wide variety of drugs as well as certain pathologic conditions.

Correlation has been made of MAP-documented EADs with QTU prolongation seen on the surface electrocardiogram (Fig. 6-11).[59] Specifically, the U wave may correspond to prolongation of the M cell action potential by drugs or any of the other conditions seen in Table 6-3. Occasionally, EADs in the form of U waves may be directly visualized on the surface electrocardiogram (Fig. 6-12). Because EADs are most prominent with slow heart rates, it is not surprising that the associated triggered electric activity is accentuated after a long RR interval. As shown in Figure 6-7, tachycardia is typically initiated by a pattern in which a pause (long RR interval) is followed by a PVC (i.e., a long–short sequence). The PVC after the pause has a markedly prolonged repolarization phase (manifest by marked QT prolongation) and creates a milieu for R and T initiated tachycardia due to triggered activity.

Another electrocardiographic precursor of torsades de pointes is TU or U wave alternans (Fig. 6-13). Described as early as 1913 by Mines and later in 1931 by Padilla and Cossio, TU alternans occurs when a significant beat-to-beat change in TU axis is seen and is often more pronounced at shorter cycle lengths (Fig. 6-14).[60,61] TU alternans has been described in patients with congenital QT interval prolongation, hypokalemia, hypomagnesemia, and hypocalcemia. Although seen, it is less common in patients with acquired QT interval prolongation. If it occurs, TU alternans is seen immediately preceding the initiation of torsades de pointes (see Fig. 6-14).

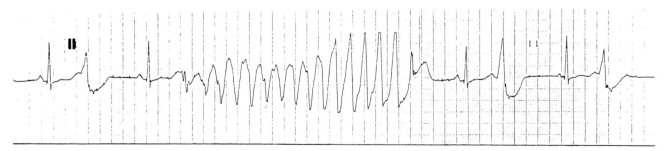

Figure 6-7. Continuous rhythm strip of a short run of torsades de pointes. Note the polymorphic morphology of the tachycardia with rapidly changing axis, characteristic of the "twisting of the points." This episode of ventricular tachycardia is self-limiting and is initiated with a premature ventricular complex followed by a pause and a capture beat, characteristic of the "long–short" sequence. This is a 58-year-old patient with a previous infarction, recently started on quinidine sulfate for paroxysmal atrial fibrillation. Patient did well with discontinuation of class IA therapy.

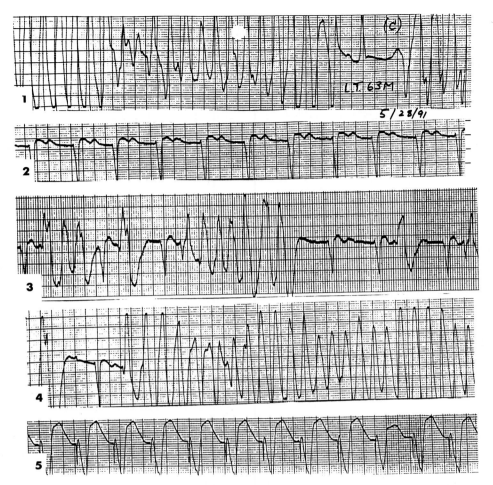

Figure 6-8. Multiple noncontinuous rhythm strips in a 63-year-old man with ischemic cardiomyopathy treated with procainamide for asymptomatic nonsustained ventricular tachycardia. Strips 1, 3, and 4 demonstrate runs of non-sustained torsades de pointes with plasma levels of procainamide and NAPA within the therapeutic range. Initiation of tachycardia is preceded by long–short sequences, and the tachycardia demonstrates sudden changes in axis, consistent with twisting of the points. Strip 4 demonstrates the sine wave appearance of torsades de pointes that may be mistaken for ventricular fibrillation. Note that in strip 2, prominent U waves are present, resulting in marked QTU-interval prolongation. Because of multiple symptomatic episodes, a temporary transvenous pacemaker was placed; with overdrive ventricular pacing at a rate of 95 (Strip 5), the patient did well and had no further episodes. Pacing was discontinued after 2 days and the patient was discharged on no antiarrhythmic medications.

Although the mechanisms for TU alternans has not been conclusively elucidated, several possibilities exist. One potential explanation is alternate 2:1 propagation of EADs.[62] A second theory suggests that TU alternans may occur because of differences in ionic membrane recovery currents.

The role of QT interval dispersion in the development of torsades de pointes has been described. QT dispersion refers to the difference between the maximum measured QT and the minimum measured QT on the same 12-lead electrocardiogram. For the purposes of QT dispersion, the QT interval is measured manually from the onset of the QRS complex to the terminal point of the T wave. When a U wave is present, the terminal portion of the visible T wave is extrapolated to the TP baseline to identify the point of T wave offset.[63] Some investigators examine all 12 leads, whereas others use only the six precordial leads.

In most reported studies, QT dispersion normally averages 50 ± 15 milliseconds. In patients having torsades de pointes, QT dispersion is often doubled, measuring as high as 100 ± 40 milliseconds from a 12-lead electrocardiogram nearest the episode.[63, 64]

It is interesting to note that QT dispersion may be independent of total QT or QTU interval prolongation as a

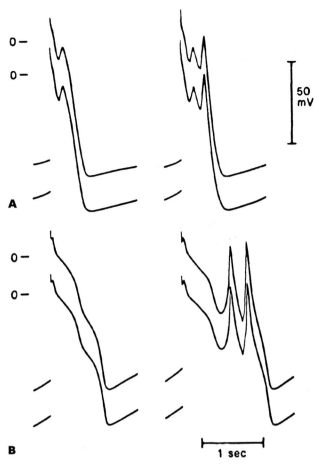

Figure 6-9. Early afterdepolarizations (EAD) occurring during phase 2 (left panel **A**) and phase 3 (left panel, **B**) of the cardiac action potential. These transmembrane recordings were made in canine Purkinje cells exposed to quinidine. The right panels demonstrate EAD-induced triggered activity during both phase 2 (**A**) and phase 3 (**B**). (Reprinted with permission from Antzelevitch C, Sicouri S: Clinical relevance of cardiac arrhythmias generated by afterdepolarizations: role of M cells in the generation of U waves, triggered activity and torsade de pointes. J Am Coll Cardiol 1994:23:259)

risk factor in antiarrhythmic medication–associated torsades de pointes. Studies show that amiodarone demonstrates less QT dispersion when compared with class IA agents, even though absolute QT or QTU interval prolongation may be similar.[63] This finding is corroborated further by the clinical observation that the incidence of amiodarone-induced torsades de pointes is less than that associated with administration of class IA agents.

Acquired QT prolongation is most common with class IA antiarrhythmics and was likely responsible for the findings of Selzer and Wray's 1964 publication of quinidine-induced ventricular fibrillation. Several other antiarrhythmic agents can cause QT prolongation and resultant

torsades de pointes, including procainamide, disopyramide, amiodarone, and sotalol.[65–68] As shown in Table 6-5, multiple nonantiarrhythmic agents also cause torsades de pointes, including pentamidine, terfenadine, erythromycin, and tricyclic antidepressants.[69]

Other causes of QT prolongation can be seen in Table 6-6 and include a congenital form, hypokalemia, hypomagnesemia, low-protein fad diets, severe bradycardia, and CNS disease. A combination of antiarrhythmic-induced QT prolongation with electrolyte imbalance (particularly hypokalemia) creates an even more dangerous milieu for the development of torsades de pointes. Similarly, patients with the congenital form of long QT syndrome (isolated to specific chromosomal patterns), those with bradycardia-induced QT prolongation, and those with acquired QT syndrome due to nonantiarrhythmic agents are especially susceptible to torsades de pointes with concomitant antiarrhythmic agent use.[70] It should be noted that although less common, there is a form of polymorphous VT that is not associated with a prolonged QT interval.[71]

Treatment of torsades de pointes first involves discontinuation of the causative agent. The need for further treatment must be individualized, depending on each patient's presentation. Correction of any electrolyte imbalance is critical. Empiric intravenous magnesium sulfate given in doses as high as 4 to 8 g intravenously over 1 hour, followed by a continuous infusion of 1 to 2 g/hour has proved effective. Patients should be monitored for hypotensive responses during high-dose magnesium loading, and some patients experience an uncomfortable flushing feeling with rapid infusions. In patients with recurrent episodes of torsades de pointes, treatment aimed at reducing heterogenous repolarization or reducing EADs may be used while waiting for drug washout to occur. Because EADs and their associated triggered activity are more pronounced at slower heart rates, rate-dependent sup-

TABLE 6-4. Drugs and Conditions Associated With Early Afterdepolarizations

CONDITIONS	DRUGS
Hypokalemia	Quinidine
Hypocalcemia	Procainamide
Acidosis	N-acetyl procainamide
Hypoxia	Disopyramide
Hypoxemia	Sotalol
Bradycardia	Bretylium
	Amiloride
	Erythromycin
	Catecholamines
	Cesium
	Veratridine

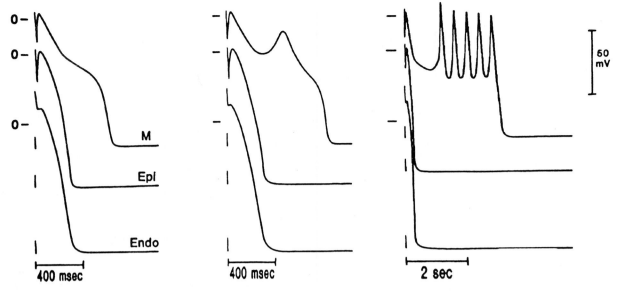

Figure 6-10. Demonstration of reverse rate-dependence of early afterdepolarizations (EADs) and their triggered activity, recorded in endocardial (*Endo*), epicardial (*Epi*), and M cells of canine heart tissue exposed to quinidine and hypokalemia. As the paced cycle length increases (**A** 3500 milliseconds, **B** 5000 milliseconds; **C** 20 seconds), the amplitude of EADs and EAD-induced triggered activity increases in the M-cell layer. Early afterdepolarizations are not recorded in endocardial and epicardial cell layers. (Reprinted with permission from Antzelevitch C, Sicouri S: Clinical relevance of cardiac arrhythmias generated by afterdepolarizations: role of M cells in the generation of U waves, triggered activity and torsade de pointes. J Am Coll Cardiol 1994:23:259)

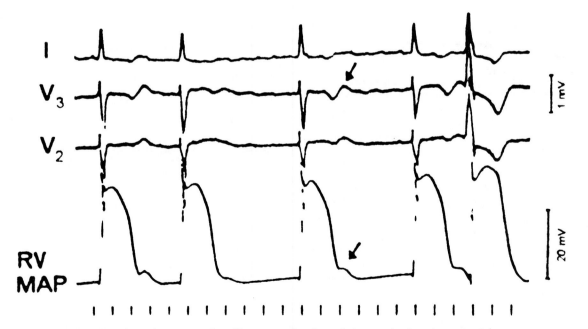

Figure 6-11. Correlation between surface U waves and endocardial monophasic action potential (*MAP*) recordings. Three-lead surface electrocardiogram and simultaneous endocardial MAP recordings from the posteroseptal region of the right ventricle in a patient treated with quinidine sulfate. Patient experienced runs of torsades de pointes. Note the increased prominence of the surface U wave and synchronous MAP-recorded early afterdepolarization after a longer RR interval.

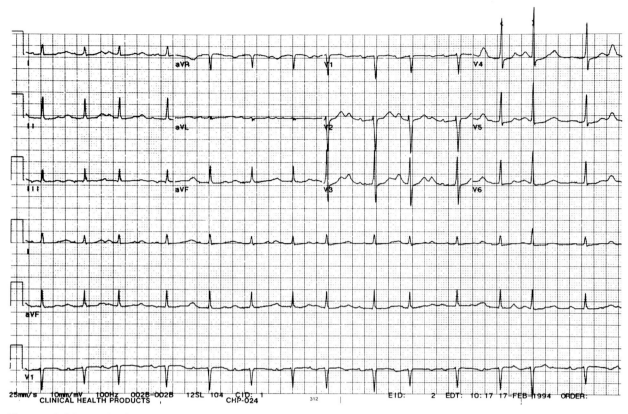

Figure 6-12. Twelve-lead electrocardiogram of a 72-year-old female treated with sotalol, 80 mg bid, for paroxysmal atrial fibrillation. Prominent U waves are noted, especially in the anterior precordial leads after the T wave and before the P wave. The patient suffered long runs of torsades de pointes, requiring multiple cardioversions, and suffered irreversible neurologic deficits.

TABLE 6-5. Drugs Associated With the Development of Torsades de Pointes

ANTIARRHYTHMIC AGENTS
- Quinidine
- Procainamide
- N-acetyl procainamide
- Disopyramide
- Amiodarone
- Sotalol
- Flecainide
- Encainide
- Proparfenone

ANTIMICROBIC AGENTS
- Erythromycin
- Trimethoprim-sulfamethoxazole
- Pentamidine
- Amantadine
- Chloroquine
- Ketaconazole
- Itraconazole
- Halofantrine

ANTIHISTAMINES
- Terfenadine
- Astemizole

ANTIDEPRESSANTS
- Amoxapine
- Maprotiline
- Trazadone
- MAO inhibitors
- Haloperidol
- Droperidol
- Promethazine
- Thioridizine
- Sulpiride

VASODILATORS
- Prenylamine
- Lidoflazin
- Bepridil
- Lidoflazine
- Perhexaline

CORTICOSTEROIDS

INOTROPIC AGENTS
- Amrinone
- Milrinone
- Dobutamine

HYPERLIPIDEMIC AGENTS
- Probucol

MISCELLANEOUS
- Furosemide
- Vasopressin
- Ketanserin
- Liquid protein diets
- Organophosphates
- Chloral hydrate
- Adenosine
- Indapamine
- Terodiline
- Papaverine
- Arsenic
- Cocaine
- Chlopromazine

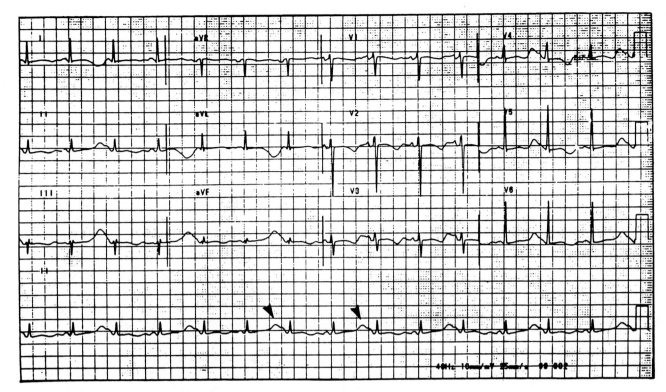

Figure 6-13. Twelve-lead electrocardiogram of a 23-year-old HIV-positive female with marked hypokalemia and hypomagnesemia (potassium, 2.3 mEq/L; magnesium, 0.7 mEq/L) admitted with dizzy spells. Electrocardiogram demonstrates marked TU alternans and QTU prolongation (>600 milliseconds). *Arrows* demonstrate the alterations in the TU wave with every other beat, consistent with TU alternans. Patient had documented runs of torsades de pointes and was treated with electrolyte repletion and temporary transvenous pacing but eventually succumbed to recurrent cardiac arrest and could not be resuscitated. (Reprinted with permission from Habbab MA, El-Sherif N: TU Alternans, long QTU, and torsade de pointes: clinical and experimental observations. Pacing Clin Electrophysiol 1992;15:916)

pression of these phenomenon may be achieved with the use of atrial or ventricular pacing at a rate exceeding the underlying rhythm (see Fig. 6-8) or by the use of intravenous isoproterenol. Dialysis is sometimes necessary in patients with renal failure. Occasionally, defibrillation may be necessary for prolonged hemodynamically significant episodes or if degeneration into true ventricular fibrillation results.

Bidirectional VT is a unique manifestation of proarrhythmia (Fig. 6-15). Typically seen in digitalis toxicity, bidirectional VT displays two families of QRS complexes with different axes alternating on a beat-to-beat basis at a rate of 150 to 200 beats per minute.[72] Although typical for digitalis toxicity, cases independent of digoxin (including a familial form) are reported.[73] Treatment with intravenous lidocaine or phenytoin is often effective in acute tachycardia conversion. Electrolyte imbalances must be

corrected; if digitalis toxicity is present, binding-antibody administration should be considered.

Induction of ventricular fibrillation or sudden cardiac death is the ultimate example of proarrhythmia. The pathophysiology relates to progression of VT or polymorphous VT to ventricular fibrillation or the spontaneous generation of ventricular fibrillation and resultant sudden cardiac death. The additional role that the concomitant factors listed in Table 6-3 play cannot be overemphasized.

The frequency of proarrhythmic-induced ventricular fibrillation became apparent when the CAST trial documented an incidence of 4.5% arrhythmic deaths and nonfatal cardiac arrests in patients treated with flecainide or encainide, compared with 1.2% in those treated with placebo. In this group of 2300 patients treated for asymptomatic or mildly symptomatic ventricular ectopy (6 or more PVCs/hour), the relative risk of arrhythmic death for

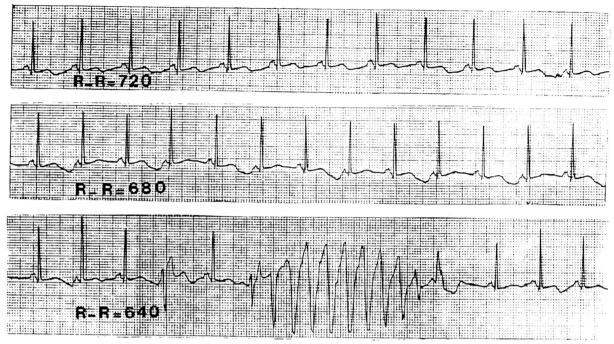

Figure 6-14. Rhythm strips from same patient as in Figure 6-13. Note how TU alternans becomes more apparent with decreasing RR intervals. Short run of torsades de pointes occurs at a critical cycle length (640 milliseconds) and is initiated with a "long–short" sequence. (Reprinted with permission from Habbab MA, El-Sherif N: TU Alternans, long QTU, and torsade de pointes: clinical and experimental observations. Pacing Clin Electrophysiol 1992;15:916)

patients receiving drug therapy was 3.6, as compared with placebo. These striking results are even more impressive when one realizes that these were relatively asymptomatic patients with an average ejection fraction of 40%. Other studies found that with antiarrhythmic drug therapy in patients with depressed left ventricular ejection fractions, the relative risk of an arrhythmic death may be as high as 5.8, compared with a similar population not on medication.[74]

PROARRHYTHMIA AS EVALUATED WITH PROGRAMMED ELECTRICAL STIMULATION

Several studies have addressed proarrhythmic responses during electrophysiologic testing; the overall incidence of antiarrhythmic agent–mediated changes with programmed electrical stimulation (PES) ranges from 5% to 32%.[75,76] These changes in response to PES may take several forms. The two most common forms of PES-documented proarrhythmia are conversion of a previously nonsustained VT to sustained VT and easier induction of sustained VT.[75]

Conversion of a previously induced nonsustained VT to a sustained VT in patients treated with antiarrhythmic medications may be seen in up to 28% of patients.[75] The VT cycle length is often longer (up to 65 milliseconds) and a more aggressive stimulation protocol may be needed. Most class I and III agents have been implicated.

Easier induction of sustained VT on antiarrhythmic therapy is frequently seen. Although this definition of proarrhythmia is more controversial than others, a 19% to 38% incidence has been described.[77] Investigators have defined less aggressive stimulation as requiring at least one less extrastimuli at PES to induce the underlying sustained VT. Once again, class I and III agents and combination drug therapy have been demonstrated.

Conversion of a previously well-tolerated VT to hemodynamically unstable VT or ventricular fibrillation is a serious proarrhythmic complication seen in the electrophysiology lab. This has been seen in up to 13% of patients and by definition requires direct current cardioversion. The mechanism by which a previously stable VT becomes hemodynamically unstable may be either VT rate acceleration or a negative inotropic effect of the antiarrhythmic medication, rendering the baseline VT less tolerable. Pro-

TABLE 6-6. Etiology of Long-QT Syndromes

CONGENITAL CAUSES

Romano-Ward syndrome
  Autosomal dominant

Jervell and Lange-Nielsen syndrome
  Autosomal recessive
  Associated with neural deafness

ACQUIRED CAUSES

Drugs (see Table 6-4)

Bradyarrhythmias

Electrolyte disturbances
  Hypokalemia
  Hypomagnesemia
  Hypocalcemia

Liquid protein diets

Central nervous system disease

Hypothyroidism

Mitral valve prolapse

Myocarditis

arrhythmic rate acceleration of VT may also develop without hemodynamic deterioration, and multiple proarrhythmic events may be seen in up to 21% of patients.[78]

MECHANISMS OF PROARRHYTHMIA

The mechanisms by which antiarrhythmic agents promote arrhythmia are most likely similar to those mechanisms that induce spontaneous arrhythmias. The two major general categories of proarrhythmic arrhythmogenesis are conduction block leading to reentry and abnormal impulse initiation, such as those which manifest by early or late afterdepolarizations.

Antiarrhythmic medications may induce bidirectional conduction block and therefore terminate a reentrant circuit, ending the tachyarrhythmia for which they were prescribed. When there are areas of myocardium in which conduction is delayed (e.g., in the presence of ischemia or

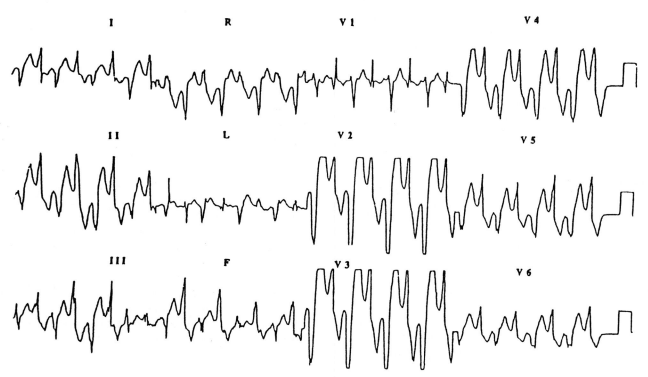

Figure 6-15. Twelve-lead electrocardiogram of bidirectional ventricular tachycardia in this 26-year-old female with a familial form of sudden cardiac death due to bidirectional ventricular tachycardia. Note the beat-to-beat alteration in axis from −600 to −800 in the beats with left bundle branch block to +1200 in the beats with right bundle branch block morphology. (Reprinted with permission from Cohen TJ, Lien LB, Hancock EW: Association of bidirectional ventricular tachycardia with familial sudden death syndrome. Am J Cardiol 1989;64:1078)

infarction), medications may have differential effects on conduction. In some areas of myocardium, drugs may create bidirectional block; yet at other sites, unidirectional block may be created, setting up the milieu for reentry.[76] Different drug concentrations at different sites within the heart may also create differential conduction block, leading to reentry also.[79]

The combination of concomitant physiologic derangements with antiarrhythmic drugs increases the risk of proarrhythmia.[80] Hill and Gettes, Kagiyama and co-workers, Ireda and associates and others have demonstrated that hyperkalemia and acidosis associated with myocardial ischemia can markedly increase the risk of antiarrhythmic-mediated proarrhythmia by further delaying conduction.[81–83]

Inappropriate drug dosing may result in the development of proarrhythmia. One example is the erroneous extrapolation of therapeutic drug dosing in normal healthy volunteers to ill patients with arrhythmias.[79] This may have been the cause of the high frequency of proarrhythmia that occurred when disopyramide was first released. Proarrythmia may also be due to decreased drug clearance because of hepatic disease, renal disease, genetic factors, and the presence of active drug metabolites.

Factors that increase or decrease drug clearance once steady state has been achieved may also be significant. This includes drugs that may increase or decrease hepatic metabolism (e.g., cimetidine, alcohol, rifampin, and the barbiturates), resulting in increased antiarrhythmic drug levels. Drug–drug interactions may occur with the use of multiple antiarrhythmic agents. This includes quinidine-induced increases in digoxin levels and the amiodarone induced increases in the levels of procainamide, N-acetyl procainamide and aprinidine.

CONCLUSIONS

Close monitoring of patients who are receiving antiarrhythmic drug therapy can help to minimize the risks and morbidity of proarrhythmia. It is essential to be aware of the warning signs of proarrhythmic manifestations. A regularization of rhythm in patients with chronic atrial fibrillation may represent a manifestation of digitalis toxicity. Initiation of drug therapy under telemetric monitoring may allow early detection of post-PVC TU-wave accentuation. Serial 12-lead electrocardiograms and periodic 24-hour Holter-monitor recordings may be helpful in monitoring patients for QTU-interval prolongation, increased QT-interval dispersion, or TU alternans. Changes in concomitant drug therapy (including diuretic use and initiation of therapy with agents that may interact with antiarrhythmic drug therapy) should be accompanied by even more vigilant patient supervision.

Our knowledge of the mechanisms and natural history of cardiac dysarrhythmias has progressed significantly since the time of Withering but in many ways, antiarrhythmic drug treatment has not. We have learned that all of the clinically available drugs used to suppress arrhythmias have the potential to either worsen the baseline arrhythmia or create new ones. It is crucial for the contemporary clinician to be certain of the indications for antiarrhythmic drug therapy and to have a heightened awareness of the warning signs of and the risk factors for potential proarrhythmic consequences to uphold the dictum primum non nocere.

References

1. Withering W: An account of the foxglove and some of its medical uses with practical remarks on dropsy and other diseases. In: Willis FA, Keys TED (adduce). Classics of cardiology. New York: Henry Shuman, 1941:231.
2. Kerr WJ, Bender WL: Paroxysmal ventricular fibrillation with cardiac recovery in a case of auricular fibrillation and complete heart-block while under quinidine sulphate therapy. Heart 1922;9:269.
3. Drury AN, Horsfall WN, Munly WC: Observations related to the action of quinidine upon the dog's heart; the refractory period of, and conduction in, ventricular muscle. Heart 1922;9:365.
4. Selzer A, Wray HW: Quinidine syncope; paroxysmal ventricular fibrillation occurring during treatment of chronic atrial arrhythmias. Circulation 1964;30:17.
5. Preliminary report: effect of encainide and flecainide on mortality in a randomized trial of arrhythmia suppression after myocardial infarction. N Engl J Med 321:406.
6. Talley JD, Wathen MS, Jurst JW: Hyperthyroid-induced atrial flutter-fibrillation with profound sinoatrial nodal pauses due to small doses of digoxin, verapamil, and propanolol. Clin Cardiol 1989;12:45.
7. Margolis JR, Strauss JC, Miller HC, Gilbert M, Wallace AG: Digitalis and the sick sinus syndrome. Clinical and electrophysiologic documentation of a severe toxic effect on sinus node function. Circulation 1975;52:162.
8. LaBarre A, Strauss JC, Scheinman MM, Evans GT, Bashore T, Teideman JS: Electrophysiologic effects of disopyramide phosphate on sinus node function in patients with sinus node dysfunction. Circulation 1979;59:226.
9. Touboul P, Atallah G, Gressard A, Kirkorian G: Effects of amiodarone on sinus node function in man. Br Heart J 1979;42:5.
10. Falk RH: Proarrhythmia in patients treated for atrial fibrillation or flutter. Ann Intern Med 1992;117:141.
11. Brayzel J, Angeles J: Sino-atrial block in man provoked by quinidine. J Electrocardiol 1972;5:289.
12. Bergfeldt L, Rosenqvist M, Vallin H, Edhag O: Disopyramide induced second and third degree atrioventricular block in patients with bifascicular block: an acute stress test to predict atrioventricular block progression. Br Heart J 1985;53:328.

13. Intermittent atrioventricular block: procainamide adminis-tration as a provocative test. Aust NZ J Med 1978;8:594.

14. Antonaccio MJ, ed: Cardiovascular pharmacology. New York: Raven Press, 1990:444.

15. de-Langen CD, Meijboom EJ, Kingma JH: Heart rate depend-ent atrioventricular nodal conduction and the effects of calcium channel blocking drugs: comparison of verpamil and nifedipine. J Cardiovasc Pharmacol 1984;6:267.

16. Fogoros RN, Anderson KP, Winkle RA, Swerdlow CD, Mason JW: Amiodarone: clinical efficacy and toxicity in 96 patients with recurrent drug-refractory arrhythmias. Circulation 1983;68:88.

17. Bigger JT Jr: Digitalis toxicity. J Clin Pharmacol 1985;25:514.

18. Morady F, Scheinman MM, Desai J: Disopyramide. Ann In-tern Med 1982;96:337.

19. Timins BI, Gutman JA, Haft JI: Disopyramide-induced heart block. Chest 1981;79:477.

20. Scheinman MM, Weiss AN, Shafton E, Benowitz N, Rowland M: Electrophysiologic effects of procainamide in patients with intra-ventricular conduction delay. Circulation 1974; 49:522.

21. Josephson ME, Caracta AR, Ricciutti MA, Lau SH, Damato AN: Electrophysiologic properties of procainamide in man. Am J Cardiol 1974;33:596.

22. Wyse DG, McAnulty JH, Rahimtoola SH: Influence of plasma drug level and the presence of conduction disease on the electrophysiologic effects of procainamide. Am J Cardiol 1979;43:619.

23. Kosinski EJ, Malindzak GS: Glucagon and isoproterenol in reversing propranolol toxicity. Arch Intern Med 1973; 132:683.

24. Ward DE, Jones B: Glucagon and beta-blocker toxicity. Br Med J 1976;2:151.

25. Rawles JM, Metcalfe MJ, Jennings K: Time of occurrence, duration, and ventricular rate for paroxysmal atrial fibrilla-tion: the effect of digoxin. Br Heart J 1990;63:225.

26. Shenassa M, Kus T, Fromer M, LeBlanc RA, Dubuc M, Nadeau R: Effect of intravenous and oral calcium antagonists (diltiazem and verapamil) on sustenance of atrial fibrilla-tion. Am J Cardiol 1988;62:403.

27. Kasanuki H, Ohnishi S: Verapamil increasing inducibility and persistence of atrial fibrillation. Circulation 1986;74:II. Abstract.

28. Feld GK, Chen PS, Nicod P, Fleck RP, Meyer D: Possible atrial proarrhythmic effects of class IC antiarrhythmic agents. Am J Cardiol 1990;66:378.

29. Robertson CE, Miller HC: Extreme tachycardia complicating the use of disopyraminde in atrial flutter. Br Heart J 1980; 44:602.

30. Falk RH, Leavitt JI: Digoxin for atrial fibrillation: a drug whose time has gone? Ann Intern Med 1991;114:573.

31. Greer GS, Wilkinson WE, McCarthy EA, Pritchett EL: Random and nonrandom behavior of symptomatic paroxysmal atrial fibrillation. Am J Cardiol 1989;64:339.

32. Cheng TO: Atrial flutter during quinidine therapy of atrial fibrillation. Am Heart J 1956;52:273.

33. Sellers TD Jr, Bashore TM, Gallagher JJ: Digitalis in the pre-excitation syndrome. Analysis during atrial fibrillation. Cir-culation 1977;56:260.

34. Morady F, DiCarlo LA Jr, Baerman JM, De Buitleir M: Effect of propanolol on ventricular rate during atrial fibrillation in the Wolff-Parkinson-White syndrome. Am Heart J 1980; 10:492.

35. Bulamhusein S, Ko P, Klein GJ: Ventricular fibrillation fol-lowing verapamil in the Wolff-Parkinson-White syndrome. Am Heart J 1983;106:145.

36. Kastor JA, Yurchak P: Recogniton of digitalis intoxication in the presence of atrail fibrillation. Ann Intern Med 1967; 67:1045.

37. Rosen MR, Gelband J, Merker C, Hoffman BF: Mechanisms of digitalis-toxicity—effects of ouabain on phase four of canine Purkinje fiber transmembrane potentials. Circulation 19; 47:681.

38. Rosen MR: Delayed afterdepolarizations induced by dig-italis. Cardiac electrophysiology: a text book. Mt. Kisco, NY: Futura Publishing, 1990:2.

39. Antzelevitch C, Sicouri S: Clinical relevance of cardiac ar-rhythmias generated by afterdepolarizations: role of M cells in the generation of U waves, triggered activity and torsade de pointes. J Am Coll Cardiol 1994:23:259.

40. Wit AL, Rosen MR: Afterdepolarizations and triggered activ-ity. In: Fozzard HA, Haber E, Jenning RB, et al, eds. The heart and cardiovascular system. New York: Raven Press, 1986: 1449.

41. Bellar GA, Smith TW, Abelmann WH, et al: Digitalis intoxica-tion: a prospective clinical study with serum level correla-tions. N Engl J Med 1971;284:989.

42. Young IS, Goh EM, McKillop UH, Stanford CF, Nicholls DP, Trimble ER: Magnesium status and digoxin toxicity. Br J Clin Pharmacol 1991;32:717.

43. Smith TW, Anstman EM, Friedman PL, et al: Digitalis gly-cosides: mechanisms and manifestations of toxicity. Prog Cardiovasc Dis 1084;27:21.

44. Butler VP Jr, Chen JP: Digoxin-specific antibodies. Proc Natl Acad Sci USA 1967;57:71.

45. Schmidt DH, Butler VP Jr: Immunological protection against digoxin toxicity. J Clin Invest 1971;50:866.

46. Schmidt DH, Butler VP Jr: Reversal of digoxin toxicity with specific antibodies. J Clin Invest 1971;50:1738.

47. Smith TW, Haber E, Yeatman L, Butler VP Jr: Reversal of advanced digoxin intoxication with Fab fragments of di-goxin-specific antibodies. N Engl J Med 1976;294:797.

48. Hickey AR, Wenger TL, Carpenter VP, et al: Digoxin immune Fab therapy in the management of digitalis intoxication: safety and efficacy results of an observational surveillance study. J Am Coll Cardiol 1991;17:590.

49. Herre JM, Titus C, Oeff M, et al: Inefficacy and proarrhythmic effects of flecainide and encainide for sustained ventricular tachycardia and ventricular fibrillation. Ann Intern Med 1990;113:671.

50. Echt DS, Leibson PR, Mitchell LB, et al: Mortality and mor-bidity in patients receiving encainide, flecainide or placebo: the Cardiac Arrhythmia Suppression Trial. N Engl J Med 1991;324:781.

51. Velbit V, Podrid P, Lown B, Cohen BH, Grayboys TB: Aggrava-tion and provocation of ventricular arrhythmias by antiar-rhythmic drugs. Circulation 1982;65:886.

52. Winkle RA, Mason JW, Griffin JC, Ross D: Malignant ventricu-

lar tachyarrhythmias associated with the use of encainide. Am Heart J 1981;102:857.

53. Morganroth J, Horowitz LN: Flecainide: its proarrhythmic effects and expected changes on the surface electrocardiogram. Am J Cardiol 1984;58:89B.

54. Stanton MS, Prystowsky EN, Finegerg NS, Miles WM, Zipes DP, Heger JJ: Arrhythmogenic effects of antiarrhythmic drugs: a study of 506 patients treated for ventricular tachycardia or fibrillation. J Am Coll Cardiol 1989;14:209.

55. Stavens CS, McGovern B, Garan H, Ruskin JM: Aggravation of electrically provoked ventricular tachycardia during treatment with propafenone. Am Heart J 1985;110:24.

56. Tschaidse O, Graboys TB, Lown B, Lampert S, Ravid S: The prevalence of proarrhythmic events during moricizine therapy and their relationship to ventricular function. Am Heart J 1992;124:912.

57. Ruskin JN, McGovern B, Garan H, DiMarco JP, Kely E: Antiarrhythmic drugs: a possible cause of out-of-hospital cardiac arrest. N Engl J Med 1983;309:1302.

58. Dessertenne F: La Tachycardie ventriculaire a deux foyers opposes variable. Arch Mal Coeur 1966;59:263.

59. Hoffman BF, Cranefield PF: Electrocardiology of the heart. New York: McGraw-Hill 1960:202.

60. Mines GR: On functional analysis by the action of electrolytes. J Physiol 1913;46:188.

61. Padilla T, Cossio P: Alternacia electrica ventricular. La Semana Medica 1931;24:15.

62. Habbab MA, El-Sherif N: TU Alternans, long QTU, and torsade de pointes: clinical and experimental observations. Pacing Clin Electrophysiol 1992;15:916.

63. Hii JTY, Wyse DG, Gillis AM, Duff HJ, Solylo MA, Mitchell LB: Precordial QT interval dispersion as a marker of torsade de pointes: disparate effects of class IA antiarrhythmic drugs and amiodarone. Circulation 1992;86:1376.

64. Barr CS, Naas A, Freeman M, Lang CC, Struthers AD: QT dispersion and sudden unexpected death in chronic heart failure. Lancet 1994;343:327.

65. Schechter JA, Caine R, Friehling T, Kowney PR, Engel TR: Effect of procainamide on dispersion of ventricular refractoriness. Am J Cardiol 1983;52:279.

66. Wald RW, Waxman MB, Colman JM: Torsade de pointes ventricular tachycardia: a complication of disopyramide shared with quinidine. J Electrocardiol 1981;14:301.

67. Mitchell LB, Wyse DG, Gillis AM, Duff HJ: Electropharmacology of amiodarone therapy initiation: time courses of onset of electrophysiologic and antiarrhythmic effects. Circulation 1989;80:34.

68. El-Sherif N: Early afterdepolarizations and arrhythmogenesis: experimental and clinical aspects. Arch Mal Coeur 1991;84:227.

69. Martyn R, Somberg JC, Kerin NZ: Proarrhythmia of nonantiarrhythmic drugs. Am Heart J 1993;126:201.

70. Keating M, Atkinson D, Dunn C, Timothy K, Vincent GM, Leppert M: Linkage of a cardiac arrhythmia, the long QT syndrome, and the Harvey ras-1 gene. Science 1991;252:704.

71. Sclarovsky S, Strasberg B, Lewin RF, Agmon J: Polymorphous ventricular tachycardia: clinical features and treatment. Am J Cardiol 1979;44:339.

72. Rosenbaum MB, Elizari MV, Lazzari JO: The mechanism of bidirectional tachycardia. Am Heart J 1969;78:4.

73. Cohen TJ, Lien LB, Hancock EW: Association of bidirectional ventricular tachycardia with familial sudden death syndrome. Am J Cardiol 1989;64:1078.

74. Flaker GC, Blackshear JL, McBride R, Kronmal RA, Halperin JL, Hart RG: Antiarrhythmic drug therapy and cardiac mortality in atrial fibrillation. J Am Coll Cardiol 1992;20:527.

75. Rae AP, Kay HR, Horowitz LN, Spielman SR, Greenspan AM: Proarrhythmic effects of antiarrhythmic drugs in patients with mailignant ventricular arrhythmias evaluated by electrophysiologic testing. J Am Coll Cardiol 1988;12:131.

76. Rosen MR, Wit AL: Arrhythmogenic actions of antiarrhythmic drugs. Am J Cardiol 1987;59:10E.

77. Sager PT, Perlmutter RA, Rosenfeld LE, Batsford WP: Antiarrhythmic drug exacerbation of ventricular tachycardia inducibility during electrophysiologic study. Am Heart J 1992;123:926.

78. Bigger JT Jr, Shahar DI: Clinical types of proarrhythmic response to antiarrhythmic drugs. Am J Cardiol 1987;59:2E.

79. Woosley RL, Roden DM: Pharmacologic causes of arrhythmogenic actions of antiarrhythmic drugs. Am J Cardiol 1987;59:19E.

80. Podrid PJ, Lampert S, Grayboys TB, Blatt CM, Lown B: Aggravation of arrhythmia by antiarrhythmic drugs: incidence and predictors. Am J Cardiol 1987;59:38E.

81. Hill JL, Gettes LS: Effect of acute coronary occlusion on local myocardial extracellular K^+ activity in swine. Circulation 1980;61:768.

82. Kagiyama Y, Hill JL, Gettes LS: Interaction of acidosis and increased extracellular potassium on action potential characteristics and conduction in guinea pig ventricular muscle. Circ Res 1981;51:614.

83. Ireda N, Singh BN, Davis LD, Hauswirth O: Effects of flecainide on the electrophysiologic properties of isolated canine and rabbit myocardial fibers. J Am Coll Cardiol 1985;5:303.

Cardiac Arrhythmias, 3rd edition, edited by William J. Mandel.
J. B. Lippincott Company, Philadelphia © 1995.

7

Thomas F. Ross • William J. Mandel

Invasive Cardiac Electrophysiologic Testing

INDICATIONS

Invasive electrophysiologic study of the heart has been available for clinical use since the late 1960s, when the procedure for reproducible recording of His-bundle electrograms was described. The technique has since been expanded to include the use of multiple intracardiac recording electrodes with programmed electric stimulation. It is being used as a diagnostic, therapeutic, and prognostic tool in a variety of clinical situations. Despite this, controversy still exists about its clinical use. Clinical use is an important issue because what began as a sophisticated research tool in select universities is available in many local medical centers.

Given the financial constraints in contemporary medicine, the clinical use of such a technique must include consideration not only of the risk–benefit ratio but also of cost-effectiveness. Establishing an electrophysiology laboratory may be quite expensive.[1] The procedures are time-consuming and can present major scheduling problems if performed in a laboratory that also does standard cardiac catheterizations. Catheter insertion times range from 30 to 60 minutes, and programmed stimulation adds an additional 120 to 210 minutes. In-depth analysis of tracings may require 2 to 5 additional hours. Several personnel are needed to perform each study; two technicians and two physicians are present in our laboratory. The cost to the patient is considerable. The basic laboratory charge is compounded by additional fees for more lengthy procedures requiring extra catheters, drugs, and equipment as well as the cost of hospitalization and the physician's fee. The use of such a costly and time-consuming procedure must therefore be carefully reviewed. Interventional procedures, being more complex and time-consuming, add considerably to the cost.

Electrophysiologic studies are a basic research tool to investigate mechanisms of arrhythmias and conduction disorders. Extrapolation of these findings to prospective clinical situations has resulted in considerable controversy and confusion.[2–5] Contemporary and future clinical use of electrophysiologic studies involves four areas: diagnostic testing, therapeutic uses (medical and surgical therapy), interventional (ablation), and prognosis.

DIAGNOSTIC USES

The necessity for electrophysiologic testing in diagnosing arrhythmias and conduction disorders depends not only on the nature of the rhythm disturbance but also on its clinical consequences. A patient with asymptomatic arrhythmia may warrant no therapy or simply an empiric trial of medication rather than a costly invasive evaluation of etiology. Conversely, a person with recurrent syncope may benefit considerably from invasive investigation of possible arrhythmic causes and appropriately tailored therapy. A variety of neurologic, cardiac, pulmonary, and constitutional symptoms can be caused by rhythm disturbances. Poor cardiac reserve, secondary to associated cardiovascular and pulmonary disorders, can worsen any clinical manifestation. Supraventricular tachycardia in a young, otherwise healthy person may produce few or no symptoms. The same arrhythmia in a person with coronary artery disease can precipitate angina, infarction, or congestive heart failure.

Before invasive diagnostic studies are initiated, a careful review of the results of noninvasive electrophysiologic tests is needed. These range from static resting 12-lead electrocardiograms to dynamic studies such as ambulatory Holter monitoring or exercise stress tests. Additional noninvasive tests may be forthcoming. Delayed low-amplitude signals after the end of the QRS complex on the surface electrocardiogram are a marker for ventricular tachycardia in certain subsets of patients.[6] In many cases, these studies obviate the need for further costly diagnostic testing.

Bradyarrhythmias

Sick sinus syndrome is the term applied to disorders of sinus node function that result in clinical bradyarrhythmias. These are generally considered in three groups: (1) sinus bradycardia (less than 60 beats/minute); (2) sinus arrest with junctional or ventricular escape rhythms; and (3) bradycardia–tachycardia syndrome. Most patients with these disorders are easily diagnosed by standard electrocardiograms or ambulatory monitoring.

Asymptomatic patients require no treatment, and invasive diagnostic studies add little to their management.[7] If symptoms clearly related to sinus node dysfunction are present, a pacemaker is required. In this setting, electrophysiologic studies can provide information on the presence or absence of associated conduction defects that may influence the type of pacemaker (atrial, ventricular, or dual chamber) used. More than 50% of patients with sinus bradycardia or symptomatic sinus node disease have associated AV conduction abnormalities.[8, 9]

Many patients present with symptoms such as syncope or fatigue and have undergone noninvasive studies that reveal no abnormalities or mild sinus bradycardia. Sinus bradycardia occurs in young and elderly persons without apparent cardiac abnormalities.[10, 11] It may also result from autonomic dysfunction with excessive vagal tone rather than from intrinsic sinus node abnormality.[12] In these settings, electrophysiologic studies help to establish the presence of sinus node dysfunction and examine the relation between symptoms and the rhythm disturbance. An approach to the use of invasive testing in patients with bradyarrhythmias is summarized in Table 7-1.

Conduction Disorders

Major goals in evaluating patients with AV conduction disorders include determining the site of block, establishing the relation between the conduction abnormality and symptoms, and evaluating the likelihood of progression to high grades of AV block with attendant morbidity and mortality. Given this information, appropriate decisions regarding pacemaker therapy can be made. In most situations, this is accomplished without invasive electrophysiologic investigation (Table 7-2).

Although lesions throughout the conduction system may cause first-degree AV block, the most common site of

TABLE 7-1. Indications for Electrophysiologic Studies: Bradyarrhythmias

	Indication for Electrophysiologic Study	
Surface ECG	**Symptoms**	**No Symptoms**
Sinus bradycardia	Possible	No
Sick sinus syndrome	Pacemaker (No electrophysiologic study)*	No

*Electrophysiologic study may be indicated to diagnose associated conduction abnormalities or aid in choice of pacemaker.

TABLE 7-2. Indications for Electrophysiologic Studies: Atrioventricular Conduction Abnormalities

Surface ECG	Site of Block*	Indication for Electrophysiologic Study	
		Symptoms	No Symptoms
First-Degree AV	AVN >> HPS	Rare	No
Second-Degree AV			
Type I—normal QRS	AVN >>>> HPS	Pacemaker (no EPS)†	No
Type I—wide QRS	AVN > HPS	Pacemaker (no EPS)†	Yes
Type II—normal QRS	HPS > AVN	Pacemaker (no EPS)†	Yes
Type II—wide QRS	HPS >>>> AVN	Pacemaker (no EPS)†	Yes‡
2:1 normal QRS	HPS = AVN	Pacemaker (no EPS)†	Yes
2:1 wide QRS	HPS >> AVN	Pacemaker (no EPS)†	Yes‡
Complete heart block			
Normal QRS	HPS = AVN	Pacemaker (no EPS)†	Yes
Wide QRS	HPS >> AVN	Pacemaker (no EPS)†	Yes‡

†Electrophysiologic study may be indicated to aid in choice of pacemaker.
‡Pacemaker without electrophysiologic study is also an option.
AVN, atrioventricular node; EPS, electrophysiologic study; HPS, His Purkinje system.
*(From Zipes DP: Second degree atrioventricular block. Clrculation 1979;60:465.

delay is the AV node. The rate of progression to high-grade block in asymptomatic persons is extremely low, and evaluation or therapy is not needed. Symptomatic persons with first-degree AV block warrant electrophysiologic studies only if the symptoms are recurring or disabling (e.g., syncope) or if they occur in the setting of other arrhythmias and conduction disorders that warrant such studies in their own right.

Chronic second-degree heart block, localized to the AV node, has a benign prognosis in persons without organic heart disease. In the setting of cardiac pathology, however, the prognosis is poor, with 27% of patients requiring pacemakers for symptoms and 47% mortality over 3½ years.[15] Lesions within the bundle of His that result in second-degree AV block usually occur in the setting of organic heart disease and result in congestive heart failure, fatigue, dizziness, or syncope.[16,17] In studies, 86% of persons required pacemakers for symptoms, with 36% mortality over 20 months. Too few asymptomatic persons with second-degree intra-Hisian block have been followed-up to draw conclusions regarding the need for pacemaker therapy. Second-degree AV block due to infra-Hisian lesions usually requires pacemaker therapy for symptoms; such patients have a high rate of progression to complete heart block and excessive mortality.[18] Asymptomatic persons with infra-Hisian second-degree block are at high risk for syncope and sudden death and are candidates for prophylactic pacemakers.[19]

As described above, the site of block, presence of underlying heart disease, and presence or absence of symptoms are key factors in the morbidity and mortality associated with second-degree heart block. The site of block can usually be inferred from surface electrocardiograms in conjunction with provocative maneuvers such as carotid sinus massage and the administration of atropine.[20,21] Symptomatic persons usually require pacemakers unless a reversible etiology is found. In this setting, invasive studies are not needed. If the site of block is uncertain from surface electrocardiograms in asymptomatic persons, an electrophysiologic study can be of value to identify high-risk subgroups (patients with intra-Hisian or infra-Hisian block). Table 7-2 summarizes the indications for invasive electrophysiologic testing in patients with second-degree AV block, based on their surface electrocardiograms and presence or absence of symptoms.

An additional setting in which electrophysiologic testing is of diagnostic value is in persons with second-degree heart block and junctional premature beats. Pseudo-AV block has been reported to occur in patients with frequent, nonpropagated, junctional extrasystoles due to their concealed conduction within the AV node.[22] His-bundle studies are required to document this phenomenon.

As with other types of AV conduction disorders, the lesions producing complete heart block can occur at any level of the conduction system. In 70% to 80% of patients, this is within or below the bundle of His.[23] This is usually accompanied by an unstable wide QRS escape rhythm and bradycardia-related symptoms. In these and other forms of symptomatic complete heart block, pacemaker therapy is required and electrophysiologic studies are not needed.

Invasive studies may be used in this setting, however, to determine the optimal pacing mode (ventricular or AV synchronous). Asymptomatic persons with complete heart block are more likely to have lesions involving the AV node or within the His bundle. For these patients, electrophysiologic studies are useful to delineate the site of block and assess the stability of escape pacemakers.[24] This permits a rational approach to the use of prophylactic pacemakers.

The long-term mortality of patients with asymptomatic intraventricular conduction abnormalities (right bundle branch block, left bundle branch block, left anterior fascicular block, left posterior fascicular block) is reported as high as 50% in those with newly acquired left bundle branch block yet is no higher than matched controls in persons with right bundle branch block.[25, 26] These discrepancies are most likely explained by differences in the population studied. Morbidity and mortality in these groups reflect the severity of underlying cardiac pathology, with few people progressing to high-grade block. Prospective studies of patients with chronic bundle branch block reveal progression to complete heart block at only 1% to 2% per year. Sudden death was observed in 3% to 5% per year but most of these were due to tachyarrhythmias and myocardial infarction rather than to bradyarrhythmias.[27, 28]

Because prophylactic pacing may benefit some of these persons, attempts have been made to identify high-risk groups. Analysis of surface electrocardiograms and categorization of patients with a combination of conduction defects (such as bifascicular and trifascicular block) does not improve diagnostic sensitivity and specificity. Several prospective studies used invasive electrophysiologic studies to categorize persons based on their HV interval.[27–29] Although different populations were examined, 31% to 63% had a normal HV interval (less than or equal to 55 milliseconds) and 37% to 69% had a prolonged HV interval. The average annual rate of progression to high-grade block was 0.15% to 1.3% in the former group and 1.2% to 2.4% in the latter. The sensitivity of a prolonged HV interval in these studies was similar at 80% but the specificity varied from 32% to 64%, with a positive predictive value of only 5% to 7%. One study suggests that the longer the abnormal HV interval, the higher the risk; an HV interval of greater than or equal to 70 milliseconds was associated with 4% annual progression and an HV interval greater than or equal to 100 milliseconds with 8% annual progression. Few patients had such prolonged conduction times—37% and 5%, respectively. Incremental atrial pacing has been performed to enhance the sensitivity and specificity of electrophysiologic studies by stressing the conduction system to reveal occult abnormalities. In patients with intact AV nodal conduction, those who developed infranodal block during pacing pro-

gressed to second- or third-degree AV block at a rate of 14% per year. Only 3% of all patients studied had this finding but pacing predicted 60% of all episodes of high-grade block.[30] Using this approach, diagnostic sensitivity is 60%, specificity is 98%, and positive predictive value is 43%.

The poor predictive value of such electrophysiologic testing in asymptomatic persons reflects the slow progression of conduction system disease. Also, serial electrophysiologic studies show that AV nodal and infranodal conduction disease progress independently. As many as 50% of cases of high-grade heart block, which develop in persons with bifascicular block, occur in the AV node rather than in the infranodal tissues.[31, 32]

Neurologic and cardiac symptoms in patients with intraventricular conduction disturbances may be a manifestation of intermittent high-grade block. Evaluation of such patients should include a complete neurologic and medical workup, with extended ambulatory electrocardiographic monitoring. Electrophysiologic testing may provide additional diagnostic information. Through this technique, heart block was thought to be the cause of transient neurologic symptoms in 17% to 47% of persons with bifascicular block.[33–35] Patients with prolonged HV intervals (more than 60 milliseconds in one study and 80 or more milliseconds in another study) or infra-Hisian block during incremental atrial pacing appear to benefit most from permanent pacing.

Despite these findings, several points should be emphasized: (1) arrhythmias other than high-grade block are the cause of symptoms in more than 50% of patients with bifascicular block; (2) progression to complete AV block can occur despite a normal HV interval, presumably due to AV nodal block; and (3) long-term mortality may not be improved by prophylactic pacing. Table 7-3 summarizes the use of electrophysiologic testing in patients with bundle branch and fascicular blocks.

TABLE 7-3. Indications for Electrophysiologic Studies: Intraventricular Conduction Abnormalities

Surface ECG		Indication for Electrophysiologic Study	
		Symptoms	No Symptoms
RBBB LAFB LPFB LBBB		Rare	No
RBBB + LAFB RBBB + LPFB	Bifascicular Block	Possible	No

LAFB, left anterior fascicular block; LBBB, left bundle branch block; LPFB, left posterior fascicular block; RBBB, right bundle branch block.

Conduction abnormalities are reported in 15% of patients with acute myocardial infarction. Although morbidity and mortality in this group are primarily due to associated pump failure, an increased incidence of progression to high-grade AV block also exists. There is considerable controversy about the selection of patients with conduction abnormalities for temporary and permanent pacemakers. Contemporary approaches use infarct location and surface electrocardiogram categorization of conduction abnormalities.[36] Several studies have investigated the use of His-bundle recordings to further identify high-risk subgroups. Lie and colleagues found that an HV interval of more than 60 milliseconds predicted a high rate of progression to complete AV block and death in patients with bundle branch block complicating anteroseptal infarction.[37] Subsequent investigators, however, have failed to demonstrate the prognostic value of a prolonged HV interval in the postinfarct patient.[38,39]

Tachyarrhythmias

Diagnostic electrophysiologic studies are performed in persons with tachyarrhythmias for two major purposes: (1) to guide therapy of documented arrhythmias by determining underlying electrophysiologic mechanisms, and (2) to evaluate the etiology of wide QRS complex tachycardias.

Supraventricular Tachycardia

Examination of the surface electrocardiograms during supraventricular tachycardia may provide clues to underlying electrophysiologic mechanisms.[40] This information is often adequate as a basis for empiric drug therapy in patients with infrequent episodes or minimal symptoms. Several groups of patients, however, warrant more invasive diagnostic testing. Persons in whom the occurrence of tachycardia results in disabling or life-threatening symptoms such as hypotension, syncope, or pulmonary edema require rapid diagnosis of the type of tachycardia and appropriate effective drug therapy. Similarly, patients with recurrent supraventricular tachycardias refractory to conventional antiarrhythmic therapy need electrophysiologic testing as a basis for other therapeutic options, among them investigational drugs, antitachycardia pacemakers, and ablation.

Another group that may benefit from electrophysiologic therapy is patients with ventricular preexcitation. Paroxysmal supraventricular tachycardia in these persons can usually be approached as described above, with invasive studies limited to patients with severe symptoms or refractory arrhythmias. Despite the presence of ventricular preexcitation on the surface electrocardiogram, symptoms in these patients may be due to arrhythmias other

than those using the accessory pathway. Electrophysiologic testing may be the only method to diagnose such problems.[41] Atrial fibrillation occurs in 20% of patients with Wolff-Parkinson-White syndrome. If the anterograde refractory period of the bypass tract is short, conduction can result in a rapid ventricular response. In addition to severe symptoms, this rhythm can degenerate into ventricular fibrillation.[42] Electrophysiologic studies are necessary in this setting to guide the type of intervention.[43]

Controversy exists on the management of asymptomatic persons with evidence of ventricular preexcitation on their resting electrocardiogram. Although most such persons have a good prognosis, atrial fibrillation with rapid ventricular responses and ventricular fibrillation are reported.[42] The induction of anterograde block in the accessory pathway with normalization of the QRS complex during exercise or after the administration of procainamide has been used to identify persons thought to be at low risk.[44,45] Whether electrophysiologic testing should be performed in persons who do not respond to such provocative maneuvers remains to be determined.

Wide QRS Complex Tachycardias

Differentiation between a supraventricular rhythm with aberrant conduction and a ventricular rhythm in patients with wide QRS complex tachycardias has important therapeutic implications. Traditional approaches use clinical and electrocardiographic findings.[46] In many cases, however, these criteria are inadequate to make such a distinction. Electrophysiologic testing can provide valuable information in this setting. The rationale for such testing is based on the finding that most supraventricular and ventricular tachycardias are reentrant arrhythmias and as such can be reproducibly initiated and terminated by atrial or ventricular stimulation.[47,48] Findings that differentiate supraventricular tachycardia from ventricular tachycardia include (1) the temporal relation between the atrial, His-bundle, and ventricular depolarizations; (2) the atrial activation sequence; (3) the mode of initiation of tachycardia; and (4) the response of the arrhythmia to atrial and ventricular stimuli.

Sudden Cardiac Death and Ventricular Tachyarrhythmias

The use of electrophysiologic testing in the management of survivors of sudden cardiac death is controversial. Prognosis after survival of cardiac arrest appears to be poor, with reported mortalities of 24% to 30% at 1 year, 34% to 40% at 2 years, and 51% to 60% at 4 years follow-up.[49,50] The cause of death is usually a recurrence of the original arrhythmia. There is considerable variability in the rhythm first recorded in this setting.[51-56] Bradyarrhythmias or asystole occur in 0% to 31%, ventricular tachycardia in 0% to 38%, and ventricular fibrillation in 58% to 87% of patients. This range is partly explained by different patient populations. Also, the first recorded rhythm may not be identical to that which initiated the event. The degeneration of ventricular tachycardia into ventricular fibrillation or asystole is reported.[57,58]

Empiric antiarrhythmic therapy has had no major impact on these statistics. Sudden death occurred in 50% of patients treated empirically with either quinidine or procainamide.[59] Improved survival is reported, however, when persons with documented tachyarrhythmias are treated with drugs chosen for their ability to suppress certain forms of complex ventricular ectopy during both extended ambulatory monitoring and exercise stress testing.[60] Criticism of this technique is based on the poor relation between such ectopy and ventricular tachyarrhythmias and the prolonged hospitalization necessary to choose an appropriate drug regimen.[61] Improved survival is also reported with empiric therapy using amiodarone.[62] In this study, the recurrence of sudden death was only 7% after 12 months. Empiric use of drugs is limited by a lack of parameters with which to judge therapeutic efficacy. Sustained ventricular tachyarrhythmias are infrequent random events. To use the arrhythmia itself as an end point may require many months and failure may be fatal. These are major limitations given data that suggest that any single drug is effective in only a third of patients and may worsen the arrhythmia in 16%.[63,64]

Electrophysiologic testing has been used as an adjunct to the diagnosis and therapy of persons who have undergone sudden death and recurrent ventricular tachyarrhythmias. The purpose is to induce reproducibly the patient's ventricular arrhythmia and judge therapeutic efficacy by the inability to induce the same arrhythmia after appropriate therapy. The rationale for this approach is based on two points: (1) electrophysiologic study is a diagnostic test with suitable sensitivity and specificity, and (2) based on test results, medical or surgical therapy is superior to conventional empiric drug therapy. Determination of sensitivity and specificity has been hampered by different stimulation protocols used by various investigators, including (1) stimulus intensity (current amplitude and pulse width); (2) rates of pacing; (3) number of extrastimuli (one to four); (4) number of sites stimulated (right ventricle and left ventricle); (5) stimulation during provocative drug infusions (isoproterenol); and (6) definition of a positive response (sustained ventricular tachycardia versus nonsustained ventricular tachycardia versus repetitive ventricular response). In addition, patients with different arrhythmias (ventricular tachycardia versus ventricular fibrillation) and drug histories have been compared.

Tables 7-4 through 7-6 list the sensitivity, specificity, and predictive values of a variety of stimulation protocols.

The more aggressive the induction (e.g., multiple ventricular sites with an isoproterenol infusion and multiple extrastimuli), the greater the sensitivity but the lower the specificity. Our procedure includes burst ventricular pacing and insertion of one to three extrastimuli during ventricular pacing at multiple-paced cycle lengths and multiple locations within the right ventricle. In patients with documented sustained ventricular tachycardia, the sensitivity and specificity of this protocol are about 85%. If ventricular fibrillation is the underlying rhythm, the sensitivity is decreased by 10% to 25%.

Table 7-7 describes the rate of recurrence of sudden death or arrhythmia in patients whose therapy was guided by electropharmacologic testing. Early reports suggested that the inability to induce a tachyarrhythmia was a good prognostic sign. Newer reports, however, describe a 35% recurrence at 18 months, similar to that of conventional therapy. Patients with inducible tachycardias that are suppressible with drugs or surgery have a lower recurrence (0% to 33% at 14 to 22 months) than do those patients whose arrhythmias are not suppressible (9% to 91%).

Electrophysiologic testing in the diagnosis and treatment of patients with sudden death and ventricular tachyarrhythmias has several limitations and uncertainties. The ideal stimulation protocol has yet to be determined. There is debate about the definition of a positive response. Is nonsustained (less than 30 seconds) polymorphic ventricular tachycardia an abnormal response with the aggressive stimulation protocols? Electropharmacologic testing may not predict the clinical response of certain drugs, such as amiodarone. What is the role of invasive testing in patients with nonsustained ventricular tachycardia and torsades de pointes? Despite these limitations, electrophysiologic testing appears superior to conventional empiric antiarrhythmic therapy. It identifies persons at high risk for recurrence and permits a more rational approach to drug therapy. In patients requiring cardiac electrosurgery or implantable antitachycardia devices, it is essential.

Evaluation of Symptoms

Despite extensive cardiac and neurologic evaluation (including ambulatory Holter monitoring), the etiology of transient neurologic and cardiovascular symptoms is often unclear.[79] In this setting, electrophysiologic testing may reveal the presence of arrhythmias or conduction abnormalities. Perhaps the most widely investigated symptom is syncope.[33,80–82] Prospective studies of unexplained syncope demonstrate possible electrophysiologic causes in 12% to 68% of patients. Factors that explain this variation include (1) different populations with respect to prevalence of underlying heart disease, (2) variable stimulation protocols, and (3) different definitions of significant elec-

TABLE 7-4. Diagnostic Value of Electrophysiologic Studies in Patients With Ventricular Tachyarrhythmias

Study (Reference)	Sensitivity (%)	Specificity (%)	Positive Predictive Value (%)	Negative Predictive Value (%)
Underlying Arrhythmia: Sudden Death (Ventricular Tachycardia + Ventricular Fibrillation)				
Ruskin[53]	81			
Myerburg[52]	29			
Josephson[54]	60			
Ruskin[65]	75			
Mason[73]	89			
Morady[55]	76			
Benditt[66]	88			
Roy[74]	61			
Underlying Arrhythmia: Ventricular Tachycardia				
Ruskin[53]	100			
Myerburg[52]	83			
Josephson[54]	85			
Vandepol[67]	84	99	96	97
Fisher[71]	85	95	94	87
Naccarelli[68]	51	—	—	—
Livelli[69]	65	98	97	75
Morady[148]	83	—	—	—
Benditt[66]	100	—	—	—
Mann[70]	83	88	85	87
Underlying Arrhythmia: Ventricular Fibrillation				
Ruskin[53]	74			
Myerburg[52]	0			
Josephson[54]	43			
Kehoe[72]	64			
Morady[55]	77			
Benditt[66]	86			

TABLE 7-5. Diagnostic Value of the Number of Ventricular Extrastimuli in Electrophysiologic Studies in Patients With Ventricular Tachyarrhythmias

Study (Reference)	Arrhythmia	Number of Extrastimuli	Sensitivity (%)	Specificity (%)	Positive Predictive Value (%)	Negative Predictive Value (%)
Morady[55]	Ventricular tachycardia + ventricular fibrillation	1	2	—	—	—
		2	26	—	—	—
		3	67	—	—	—
Benditt[66]	Ventricular tachycardia + ventricular fibrillation	1	6	—	—	—
		2	44	—	—	—
		3	79	—	—	—
Fisher[71]	Ventricular tachycardia	1	15	100	100	56
		2	42	98	98	49
		3	82	86	94	65
Mann[70]	Ventricular tachycardia	1	17	99	90	60
		2	45	96	89	69
		3	68	90	84	78
		4	83	88	85	87
Brugada[75]	None	4	—	60	—	—

TABLE 7-6. Stimulation Protocols Used in Electrophysiologic Studies in Patients With Ventricular Tachyarrhythmias

| Study (Reference) | Patients (n) | Maximum Extrastimuli (n) | Sites Stimulated | | | Burst Pacing | Definition of Minimum Positive Response |
			Right Ventricle (Multiple)	Left Ventricle	Isoproterenol		
Ruskin[53]	31	2	N	N	Y	Y	Three repetitive beats
Myerburg[52]	17	1	Y	N	N	Y	Sustained ventricular tachycardia
Josephson[54]	50	2	N	Y	N	Y	Nonsustained ventricular tachycardia
Vandepol[67]	529	2	Y	Y	N	Y	Three repetitive beats
Fisher[71]	203	3	?	?	?	?	?
Ruskin[65]	82	?	?	?	?	?	Three repetitive beats
Naccarelli[68]	83	2	Y	Y	N	Y	Nonsustained ventricular tachycardia
Livelli[69]	100	2	Y	N	N	Y	Three repetitive beats
Kehoe[72]	44	?	?	?	?	?	Sustained ventricular tachycardia
Mason[73]	186	3	?	?	?	?	Nonsustained ventricular tachycardia
Morady[55]	42	3	N	Y	Y	Y	Six repetitive beats
Benditt[66]	34	3	N	N	N	Y	Six repetitive beats
Roy[74]	119	3	Y	Y	Y	Y	Sustained ventricular tachycardia(>30 sec)
Mann[70]	121	4	Y	N	N	Y	Six repetitive beats

Y, Yes; N, No.

trophysiologic abnormalities and arrhythmias. Electrophysiologic testing has its highest diagnostic yield in patients with syncope and clinical evidence of organic heart disease. The importance of identifying the cause of syncope is emphasized by a study that demonstrates a 24% incidence of sudden death in patients with a cardiovascular etiology, as compared with 4% in patients with a noncardiovascular cause.[79] In addition, if drug or pacemaker therapy is directed by the result of such testing, syncope rarely recurs. The evaluation of other possible arrhythmic-related symptoms such as palpitations or dizziness should include electrophysiologic testing only if noninvasive investigation has been unrevealing and symptoms are recurrent and disabling.

Electropharmacologic Testing

Antiarrhythmic drugs have different effects on the various electrophysiologic parameters of the heart (Table 7-8). Attempts have been made to use such effects on cardiac conduction, refractoriness, and automaticity to enhance the diagnostic sensitivity and specificity of electrophysiologic testing. The use of procainamide and ajmaline to screen asymptomatic persons with Wolff-Parkinson-White syndrome is one such example.[45] The normalization of the QRS complex after administration of these agents suggests a long anterograde refractory period in the bypass tract. This correlates well with a slow ventricular response to spontaneous or induced atrial fibrillation and suggests a good prognosis in these patients.

Procainamide has been used in patients with bundle branch block during electrophysiologic testing in an attempt to provoke infra-Hisian block and thus identify persons at high risk for spontaneous AV block.[83, 84] The results of these studies suggest only a limited role for this agent. Electrophysiologic testing may be of value to screen patients with sinus node dysfunction or conduction abnormalities before beginning antiarrhythmic therapy that may exacerbate these disorders. Measurements of electrophysiologic parameters after administration of drugs may identify patients at high risk to encounter worsening of bradyarrhythmias or conduction abnormalities during chronic use.[85] Studies have not been performed, however, to compare the benefit of electrophysiologic testing with drug administration with cautious empiric therapy with ambulatory monitoring.

TABLE 7-7. Rate of Recurrence of Sudden Death or Ventricular Tachyarrhythmias Based on Therapy Guided by Electrophysiologic Testing

| Study (Reference) | Patients (n) | Months of Follow-up | Inducible Arrhythmia | | | | Noninducible Arrhythmia |
| | | | Suppressed by RX | | Nonsuppressed by RX | | |
			(%) Frequency	(%) Recurrence	(%) Frequency	(%) Recurrence	(%) Recurrence
Ruskin[53]	31	15	76	0	24	50	0
Mason[76]	51	18	67	32	33	89	—
Kehoe[72]	44	14	64	0	36	78	0
Ruskin[65]	61	18	77	5	23	16	0
Horowitz[77]	111	18	59	6	41	91	—
Morady[55]	45	22	26	33	74	9*	0
Schoenfeld[78]	72	16	—	—	—	—	11
Benditt[66]	34	18	62	5	15	40	38
Roy[74]	119	18	60	15	40	19*	32

*Some patients were tested with amiodarone.
RX, drug therapy.

THERAPEUTIC USES

Medical Therapy

Much of the rationale for using electropharmacologic testing in the treatment of tachyarrhythmias has been previously discussed. Major limitations in conventional empiric drug therapy include (1) the random nature of spontaneous tachycardias, (2) the lack of noninvasive parameters with which to guide therapeutic efficacy, (3) major morbidity and mortality associated with tachyarrhythmias, and (4) inadequate knowledge of the electrophysiologic mechanism of many arrhythmias. The clinical use of electropharmacologic testing is based on its ability to induce the patient's underlying tachycardia. This provides a reliable tool with which to judge drug efficacy rapidly. The ability of a drug to prevent the induction of a tachycardia correlates to long-term efficacy in patients with a ventricular tachyarrhythmia. Similar findings using electropharmacologic therapy are reported in patients with paroxysmal supraventricular tachycardia.[86,87]

Pacemaker Use

The decision to insert a permanent pacemaker for symptomatic bradyarrhythmias and conduction disorders can usually be made without invasive testing. Although many patients continue to receive single-chamber models, a wide array of dual-chamber pacemakers have been introduced. This has occurred as evidence supporting the physiologic benefit of maintaining AV synchrony has been forthcoming.[88] Hemodynamic assessment during ventricular or AV synchronous pacing provides a method to evaluate patients in whom the decision between implanting single- and dual-chamber models is difficult to make. Patients with existing VVI pacemakers who experience fatigue, exercise intolerance, symptomatic worsening of underlying cardiac disorders, and pacemaker syndrome may also be evaluated to assess the potential benefit of conversion to a dual-chamber system. Table 7-9 shows the results of such a study in a man with AV block and exercise intolerance. Ventricular pacing would have resulted in only modest increments in cardiac output, with the additional burden of mitral regurgitation. Synchronized AV pacing, however, increased cardiac output without significant mitral regurgitation.

Pacing techniques learned in the electrophysiology laboratory have been expanded and are applied in the treatment of patients with tachycardias.[89,90] Underdrive pacing, overdrive pacing, and the insertion of one or more extrastimuli have been used to terminate a wide array of reentrant tachyarrhythmias in the acute-care setting.

Successful termination of atrial flutter by rapid atrial pacing has been reported in 75% of cases.[91] Rapid ventricular pacing and ventricular extrastimuli can terminate ventricular tachyarrhythmias in up to 79% of cases.[92] Under investigation are a wide variety of permanently implanted pacemakers with programmable features to terminate tachyarrhythmias.[93] Early models required patient activation but technologic advances permit automatic sensing of the tachycardia and initiation of a preprogrammed termination sequence. These pacemakers are restricted to patients who are not candidates for or do not improve with conventional therapeutic approaches. In addition, extensive preimplant electrophysiologic testing is required to determine suitability for this mode of ther-

TABLE 7-8. Electrophysiologic Effects of Drugs

Class	Drug	QRS	QTc	Sinus Node			Atrium		AV Node			His-Purkinje		Ventricle	Accessory Pathway
				SCL	SNRT	SACT	A-ERP	Threshold	AH	AV-ERP	AV-FRP	HV	HP-ERP	V-ERP	ERP
I	Quinidine	+	+	0–	V	0+	+	+	V+	V	0	0+	0+	+	+
	Procainamide	+	+	0–	0+	0+	+	+	0+	0	0	0+	0+	+	+
	Disopyramide	+	+	0–	V	V	+	+	V+	V–	0	0+	0+	+	V
	Lidocaine	0	0–	0	0	0	0	0–	0–	0	0	0	–	0–	V
	Diphenylhydantoin	0	0–	–	0	0+	0	0–	0–	0–	0–	0	–	–	V
	Aprindine	+	0+	0–	0–		+	–	+	+	+	+	+	+	+
	Mexiletine	0	0	0+		0	0	0	0+	0+	0+	0+	0+	0	+
	Tocainide	0	0–	0+	0–		0–		0+	0–	0	0	0–	0–	+
	Encainide	+	0+				0+	0	0+	0+	0+	+	+	0+	+
	Flecainide	0+	0				0		0+	0	0	+		+	+
	Ajmaline			+			+	0+	0+	H	+	+	+	+	0
II	Propranolol	0	0–	+	+	+	0	–	0+	0+	+	0	0–	0–	0
III	Bretylium	0	0+	0+	0	0	0–	0	0	V	+	0	–	–	
	Amiodarone	0	+	+	0	0	+	–	+	+	+	0+	+	+	+
IV	Verapamil	0	0	0+	0+	0	0	–	+	+	+	0	0	0	V
Other	Digoxin	0	–	0–	–	–	0–	–	+	–	+0–	0	0	–	0–
	Atropine			–	–		0–	+	–	–	–	0	0	0	0–
	Isoproterenol			–	–		0–	+	–	–	–	0	0	0–	–

+, increase; –, decrease; 0, no significant change; V, variable (reports of increases, decreases, and no significant change).

TABLE 7-9. Hemodynamic Effects of Ventricular and Atrioventricular Sequential Pacing

Pacing Rate	Pacing Mode	PA (mm)	PCW (mm)	CI (L/min/m)	SVI (L/min/m)	Comments
50		25/12	11	2.3	46	Baseline 2:1 AV block
70	Ventricular	28/15	15	2.69	38	6-mm ventricular waves
90	Ventricular	30/16	17	3.08	34	10-mm ventricular waves
110	Ventricular	34/18	19	2.74	25	16-mm ventricular waves
70	AV sequential	25/12	12	3.23	46	
90	AV sequential	26/13	12	3.72	41	4-mm ventricular waves
110	AV sequential	28/14	13	4.07	37	6-mm ventricular waves

AV, atrioventricular; CI, cardiac index; PA, pulmonary artery; PCW, pulmonary capillary wedge, SVR, systemic vascular resistance.

apy and the most effective pacing termination sequence for the tachycardia. Another use of electric stimulation in the treatment of patients with tachycardias is the development of implantable automatic defibrillators. Reports suggest a 52% decrease in mortality in patients using this device.[94]

Surgical Therapy

Despite the use of conventional or investigational antiarrhythmic drugs and implantable antitachycardia pacemakers, some patients continue to have disabling or life-threatening tachycardias. Electrophysiologic-guided surgical techniques have been developed to aid these persons.

Atrioventricular electrical connections include the normal AV node–His-Purkinje system and accessory pathways. These connections may be a vital link in the reentrant pathway of a supraventricular arrhythmia (e.g., orthodromic reciprocating tachycardia) or they may act as passive conduits for rapid atrial impulses (e.g., in atrial flutter). Mechanical disruption of these connections either terminates the arrhythmia in the former or blocks conduction to the ventricle in the latter. If additional AV connections are not present, the ventricular rate subsequently depends on a junctional or ventricular escape focus or an implanted pacemaker. Intraoperative electrophysiologic studies are required to map the location of these pathways. Endocardial mapping with cryosurgical ablation of the AV node–His bundle produced AV block in 17 of 22 patients with disabling supraventricular tachycardia.[95] Epicardial mapping has been used to locate accessory AV pathways. Surgical excision based on mapping was successful in ablating 80% of pathways in a report of patients with the Wolff-Parkinson-White syndrome.[96] Surgical mortality in both these studies was 0%.

Sustained ventricular tachyarrhythmias usually occur in the setting of severe coronary artery disease, often with prior infarction and aneurysm formation. Coronary artery revascularization and aneurysmectomy have been used to treat recurrent ventricular tachycardia in these patients. Early reports suggested short-term survivals as high as 87% with these techniques.[97] Later studies question these statistics and report arrhythmia recurrence rates of 50%.[97,98] Electrophysiologic studies have been performed, both preoperatively and postoperatively, on patients undergoing coronary revascularization for ventricular tachyarrhythmias; 40% had either spontaneously occurring or inducible ventricular tachycardia postoperatively.[99]

Using endocardial or epicardial mapping, electrophysiologic techniques can localize early sites of ventricular activation during ventricular tachycardia. These areas are usually on the endocardial border zone of a myocardial scar and when excised by a variety of surgical techniques, terminate the tachycardia and prevent its reinduction. With these procedures, the recurrence of tachyarrhythmias is reported to be less than 30%.[98–100] These encouraging results suggest that electrophysiologically guided surgery is superior to conventional revascularization and aneurysmectomy in the treatment of patients with intractable ventricular tachyarrhythmias. Similar techniques have also been successfully used in patients with tachycardias unrelated to ischemic heart disease.[101]

Catheter Ablation

Despite the low mortality reported with surgical ablation of the AV node and accessory AV pathways, alternative techniques have been sought to avoid the cost and potential morbidity of an open-chest procedure. One such technique is catheter ablation. In this technique, a conventional pacing catheter is positioned through endocardial electrophysiologic mapping adjacent to the structure of interest. Initially, a synchronized direct current shock was delivered. Several groups reported successful ablation of the AV node–His-Purkinje region in patients with refractory supraventricular tachycardia.[102,103] Similar success was reported in patients with accessory AV pathways, junctional ectopic arrhythmias, and focal ventricular tachycardias.[104–106] Interventional electrophysiology has expanded logarithmically especially since the introduction of radiofrequency energy. Use of transesophageal ultrasound has aided in placement of catheters in specific locations for selected ablations.[107]

PROGNOSIS

Attempts have been made to use the data obtained during invasive electrophysiologic studies as markers for subsequent morbidity and mortality. This was initially done in patients with conduction disorders to identify those at high risk for complete heart block. As previously discussed, the tests have inadequate specificity in most such patients. Attempts to enhance the specificity by provocative drug administration in conjunction with electrophysiologic testing have also met with limited success in patients with conduction abnormalities and sinus node disorders.[83–85]

Numerous studies support the prognostic value of electrophysiologic testing in survivors of sudden cardiac death.[53,55,65,72,76–78] Noninducibility of ventricular tachyarrhythmias predicts a low rate of recurrence over subsequent months. Similarly, the inability to medically or surgically suppress an induced tachycardia is associated with recurrence rates as high as 90%. Two studies question these findings.[66,74] Major limitations in comparing the results of these studies are the use of markedly different stimulation protocols and different definitions of a positive response. Using regression analysis, Swerdlow and associates demonstrated that response to therapy during electrophysiologic study was an independent predictor of survival in patients with ventricular tachyarrhythmias.[108]

Electrophysiologic testing has been used in survivors of myocardial infarction to predict groups at high risk for sudden death.[109–111] Although such testing appears to have prognostic value, less invasive and less costly techniques such as determination of left ventricular ejection fraction appear to be equally or more valuable. Other areas in which investigation of the clinical use of electrophysiologic testing is in progress include patients with stable coronary artery disease and nonsustained ventricular tachycardia.[112,113]

METHODOLOGY

Early electrophysiologic studies consisted of recording intracavitary electric activity during spontaneous rhythms with conventional pacemaker electrodes. Contemporary methodology uses electrodes in several intracardiac positions for simultaneous pacing and recording. An array of electrophysiologic parameters are then measured during both spontaneous and paced rhythms. With programmed stimulation, a variety of arrhythmias can be induced and their electrical substrate defined through mapping techniques. Modalities for the treatment and prophylaxis of patients with such arrhythmias can also be evaluated. Each electrophysiologic study must be tailored to the individual patient to minimize time, cost, and morbidity. To provide such services, an investigator must be fully trained in all aspects of electrophysiology and have available a well-equipped catheterization laboratory.

Equipment

A fully equipped catheterization laboratory is a prerequisite. It must be adapted for electrophysiologic testing through the addition of special catheters, amplifiers, recording devices, and stimulators. Intracavitary electric activity is best recorded from platinum ring electrodes incorporated into woven Dacron catheters. This form of construction allows good torque control yet sufficient pliability exists to bend and loop the catheter within the vascular system for accurate positioning. The choice of catheter size is generally based on vessel size. 6-French catheters are routinely used in adults. Smaller sizes have better pliability but less torque control. Large catheters often have more electrodes or are lumenal; these have greater torque control but are stiffer and may increase the risk of vascular perforation. Intracardiac electric activity is usually recorded in a bipolar fashion to evaluate local events. This requires at least two ring electrodes per catheter. Commercially available catheters have two (bipolar), three (tripolar), four (quadrapolar), six (hexapolar), or even 10 (decapolar) electrodes positioned 0.5, 1.0, or 2.5 cm apart. Closely positioned electrodes permit electric activity to be recorded from small areas of endocardium. Accurate mapping studies require interelectrode distances of 1 cm or less.

Selection of an electrode catheter is based on its use in the individual patient. Bipolar catheters with an interelectrode distance of 1 cm are used for intracavitary recordings. If simultaneous pacing (two electrodes) and recording (two electrodes) is desired, a quadripolar catheter is necessary. His-bundle potentials can usually be recorded from a bipolar catheter. Continuous His-bundle recording is sometimes not possible, however, because of an unstable catheter position. In that case, a tripolar or quadripolar catheter may allow a more stable position, with a His potential recorded from one of the possible combinations of electrodes. Uniquely designed catheters are used in some clinical situations. For coronary sinus studies, we use a preshaped 7-French lumenal hexapolar

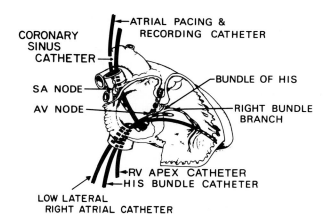

Figure 7-1. Diagnostic representation of catheter placement for electrophysiologic investigations. Two catheters (atrial pacing, coronary sinus) are shown as they would be introduced from an arm, interval jugular, or subclavian entry site. They also may be introduced from the femoral venous route. The coronary sinus catheter should have multiple poles (see Fig. 7-2). The low atrial catheter may be of the mapping type (see Fig. 7-3). The atrial pacing catheter, when inserted from the femoral route, is usually positioned in the right atrial appendage. The His-bundle catheter may also have four poles to allow recording of low atrial or right ventricular inflow electrograms.

or secapolar catheter. Preshaping the catheter facilitates its introduction into the coronary sinus (Figs. 7-1 and 7-2).

Once positioned, electrode catheters are connected to appropriate amplifiers and recorders. Connecting cables should be shielded to minimize extraneous electric noise. Sources of such 60-cycle interference include fluoroscopy equipment, overhead lights, and recording devices themselves. Cables must be kept as short as possible to reduce waveform distortion, whereas leakage currents are minimized to prevent induction of undesired arrhythmias. Before being permanently recorded, intracavitary

electric signals are amplified and filtered. Atrial and ventricular electrograms have an amplitude greater than 1 mV. His-bundle potentials are smaller, and adequate visualization requires a sensitivity of 0.1 to 0.2 mV. Intracavitary electrograms are recorded primarily to time local cardiac electric events. This requires reproduction of the local depolarizing wavefront, a medium-frequency event. Examination of waveform morphology is less important. Conventional surface electrocardiographic records require an accurate reproduction of waveform morphology. ST segments and repolarization phenomena such as T waves are low-frequency events; thus, diagnostic electrocardiogram amplifiers use a 0.5- to 100-Hz frequency response. To eliminate these repolarization phenomena and other low-frequency events, respiration, body movement, tremor, and special electrical interference filters have been incorporated into intracardiac–His-bundle amplifiers. Extremely high frequencies are also excluded. Most commercial amplifiers use a frequency response of 40 to 500 Hz.

After the electric signal has been amplified and filtered, it is visualized on an oscilloscope and recorded on hard copy. This permanent record can be made during the initial study or later if signals have been stored on a tape or disk recorder. Various available devices use ink jet, ultraviolet light, heat, or photographic techniques to produce a permanent record. Computer-based electrophysiologic recording devices have been used. These systems have significant storage capabilities using optical discs. Furthermore, they are able to display in excess of 16 channels of data, which are designed to function even during radiofrequency ablation. Although considerable differences in cost and ease of use exist, all devices must be capable of frequency responses greater than 500 Hz at paper speeds of 100 to 200 mm per second. High speeds are necessary to

Figure 7-2. Still frame from angiographic film during contrast injection from °A coronary sinus catheter. This 7-French catheter has three bipolar electrode pairs to record distal, mid- and proximal coronary sinus electrograms. The coronary sinus and its atrium are easily identified. The catheter was introduced from a left medial antecubital vein through a cutdown. Additional catheters, inserted by the femoral route, are positioned in the high right atrium (*HRA*), His bundle (*His*), and right ventricular apex (*RVa*) regions.

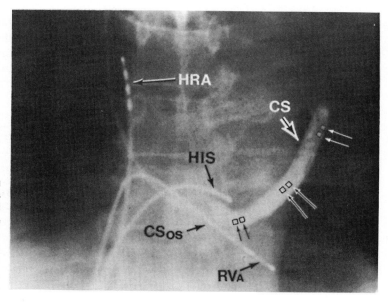

permit accurate measurement of closely timed electric events with a resolution of 5 to 10 milliseconds. The recording system must have multiple channels to permit simultaneous visualization of surface and intracardiac electric events. Ideally, three surface leads—I, aV_F, and V_1—should be used for accurate analysis of P-wave or QRS morphology. Most electrophysiologic studies require two or three intracardiac channels but additional channels may be needed in some clinical situations. One to two channels should also be available for hemodynamic measurements. If not already integrated into the system, a channel should be available to provide time markers. In complex studies, a marker channel to identify electric stimuli is also useful.

The system described above is adequate to evaluate electric events present during spontaneous rhythms. The introduction of programmed-stimulation techniques has expanded the use of these systems. Conventional external pacing devices permit simple incremental pacing, which is sufficient to evaluate sinus node recovery time (SNRT) and AV Wenckebach threshold. Sophisticated electrophysiologic testing, including the induction and termination of arrhythmias, requires a more versatile stimulator. Several models are available. Important features include (1) incremental pacing from less than 60 beats per minute to more than 500 beats per minute, (2) multiple channels for dual-chamber pacing, (3) a variable constant current source to regulate current output at different pacing thresholds, (4) at least three programmable extrastimuli, and (5) the ability to sense intracardiac electrocardiograms and synchronize stimulation to these events. In addition to shielding connecting cables, all equipment must be well grounded and inspected for leakage currents. These should be less than 10 μA to minimize accidental induction of potentially lethal cardiac arrhythmias. A defibrillator, which can be synchronized off intracardiac or surface leads, is also needed.

Catheterization Technique

Patients are prepared for electrophysiologic testing just as for conventional diagnostic cardiac catheterization. Food and liquids are withheld for 6 hours before study. Essential medications can be continued but drugs with antiarrhythmic properties should be stopped for at least five half-lives. In some situations, it may be clinically important to continue antiarrhythmic agents. An example would be a patient being tested for ventricular arrhythmias who is taking therapeutic doses of digoxin to control the ventricular response in atrial fibrillation. In this situation, digoxin should be continued to prevent an acceleration in ventricular rate but its electrophysiologic effects should be carefully considered. Diazepam or medazolam can be used if a sedative is required because they have no major

direct electrophysiologic effects.[114] These and similar agents may have indirect electrophysiologic effects, however, because they affect the central nervous system. Lidocaine is used for local anesthesia during catheter insertion. It is preferable to use a 1% solution and limit the total dose to less than 2.5 mg/kg (0.25 mL/kg of 1% solution or 17.5 mL for a 70-kg person). Larger subcutaneous doses result in therapeutic blood concentrations of lidocaine.[115]

Most electrode catheters are positioned in the right heart and thus require access to the venous system. The modified percutaneous Seldinger technique is preferred because of the ease and speed of access, simplicity of catheter exchange and removal, and ability to reuse the vein for subsequent studies. Occasionally, it may be difficult to cannulate the femoral or internal jugular veins; the use of Valsalva's maneuver on ultrasound-assisted cannulation may be useful.[116,117] A large vein, as in the femoral area, accommodates two or more 6-French catheters. Direct venous exposure through a cutdown is occasionally used in the upper extremities when a percutaneous procedure is not possible or a special large catheter must be introduced into a small vein. Venous access can be obtained from the femoral, antecubital, subclavian, and internal jugular veins. The femoral veins are most commonly used. Upper extremity veins are of value when additional catheters are needed or the femoral veins cannot be safely cannulated. Use of antecubital veins may facilitate catheterization of the coronary sinus and are often used when a catheter is left in position on completion of the study. Subclavian and jugular veins have been used but may lead to a higher incidence of complications, particularly pneumothorax.[118] Catheters are ultimately positioned in their appropriate intracardiac locations through fluoroscopic visualization. This can be confirmed by recording intracavitary electrograms, using lumenal catheters, examining pressure waveforms, and injecting contrast. The choice of catheter location and technical features for accurately positioning each catheter are described below and in Table 7-10. Although the risk of thromboembolic complications is low, 2500 to 5000 U of heparin is routinely administered in procedures lasting longer than 2 hours or when a catheter is introduced into the arterial circulation.

Catheter Placement

Right Atrium

Electrode catheters can be positioned in the right atrium from a variety of access sites, although stable recording and pacing may be difficult to maintain because of poor endocardial contact. The atrial appendage provides a stable catheter position and is easily approached from the femoral vein. J-tipped temporary pacing catheters facilitate

TABLE 7-10. Common Electrode Catheter Locations in Electrophysiologic Studies

Location	Type of Study	
	Recording	*Pacing*
Right atrium	Sinus node SVT Mapping	Sinus node SVT AV conduction
Left atrium	SVT Mapping	SVT
His-bundle catheter	AV conduction VA conduction SVT VT	Confirm catheter position
Right ventricle	SVT VT Mapping	SVT VT VA conduction
Left ventricle	VT Mapping	VT
Coronary sinus	As per left atrium and left ventricle	As per left atrium and left ventricle

SVT, supraventricular tachycardias (includes evaluation of bypass tracts); VT, ventricular tachyarrhythmias; AV conduction, antero-grade conduction through the AV node–His-Purkinje system; VA conduction, retrograde conduction through the AV node–His-Purkinje system.

entry into the appendage from upper extremity veins.[119] Patients who have undergone open heart surgery with cardiopulmonary bypass have had their atrial appendages ligated. A remnant stump is often present, which may allow a stable catheter position. Another commonly used location is the high posterolateral wall near the origin of the superior vena cava. This location also facilitates direct recordings of sinus node activity.[120] Accurate positioning of catheters is important when atrial mapping is performed. In addition to the high right atrium and atrial appendage, other commonly used right atrium sites include the low right atrium at the junction of the inferior vena cava, the os of the coronary sinus, and the AV junction near the tricuspid valve (see Figs. 7-1 and 7-2).[121] The latter is best recorded in conjunction with His-bundle studies. (Mapping of the tricuspid ring is facilitated with the use of a catheter with a steerable tip, Fig. 7-3.) Common clinical uses for right atrial catheters are listed in Table 7-10.

Left Atrium

Direct placement of an electrode catheter in the left atrium is rarely required. Most atrial electrical studies can be performed from the right atrium. Additional sites are needed, however, in evaluating patients with supraventricular tachyarrhythmias and accessory AV connections. Although the left atrium can be entered directly through a patent foramen ovale or transseptal puncture or retrogradely across the mitral valve, indirect approaches are preferred. Catheters positioned in the coronary sinus, main pulmonary artery, and esophagus have been used for left atrial recording and pacing. The coronary sinus location allows catheter stability with both recording and pacing capabilities. The main pulmonary artery is useful

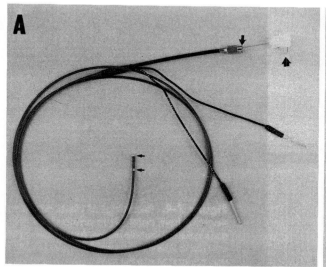
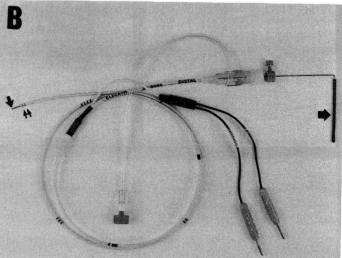

Figure 7-3. Two types of mapping catheters for use in recording bipolar electrograms from multiple sites. The tips of these catheters can be manipulated with the use of a stiff guide wire, which is inserted and positioned according to the position of its distal "handle." The catheter in **A** has no lumen, whereas the catheter in **B** has both a lumen and a side arm for flushing. These catheters are most useful for mapping the tricuspid ring in patients with Wolff-Parkinson-White syndrome but they are also useful for mapping the right atrium and possibly the left ventricle.

for recording electric signals when other techniques are not possible but left atrial pacing from this site is not practical. Esophageal leads have been used for both recording and pacing. Reports suggest that the electrogram recorded from this position reflects paraseptal atrial depolarization rather than true left atrial activation.

His-Bundle Electrograms

His-bundle recordings are used in most electrophysiologic studies. They are necessary to evaluate anterograde and retrograde AV conduction, supraventricular arrhythmias, and the etiology of wide QRS tachycardias. During ventricular tachycardia studies, they are used to confirm a ventricular origin. His-bundle pacing has been used to confirm proper catheter position but has limited clinical value. The His-bundle recording is best obtained from a bipolar catheter inserted through a femoral vein. It is advanced into the right ventricle and then withdrawn using clockwise torque, with final positioning near the septal leaflet of the tricuspid valve (see Fig. 7-1). The endocardial electrogram is recorded during catheter positioning. With the catheter in the right ventricle, a large ventricular electrogram with little or no atrial activity is recorded. As the catheter is withdrawn, the ventricular

electrogram becomes smaller as the atrial signal increases. His-bundle activity is a biphasic or triphasic signal located between the atrial and ventricular electrograms. The ideal His-bundle recording is that recorded with the largest atrial potential, representing proximal His-bundle activity in the membranous atrial septum (Fig. 7-4). This is often found with about equal atrial and ventricular electrograms. It is extremely important to scan the entire His-bundle area (see Fig. 7-4). The normal His-bundle potential has a duration of 15 to 20 milliseconds, with an HV interval of 35 to 55 milliseconds. Intra-Hisian abnormalities with a split or widened His potential may be missed unless the entire area is adequately explored and recorded.[124] An HV interval of less than 30 milliseconds may reflect recording of a right bundle branch potential rather than true His-bundle activity. If a stable His-bundle recording is not achieved despite repeated attempts at positioning, a tripolar or quadrapolar catheter can be used. This catheter is positioned in a similar fashion, with recordings made between various pairs of electrodes. Using this technique, an adequate His bundle can be recorded in more than 90% of patients. Procedures for obtaining His-bundle studies using upper extremity or retrograde arterial approaches are described but are technically more difficult and rarely necessary.

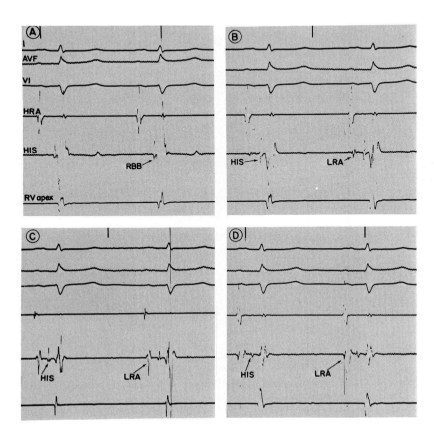

Figure 7-4. Recordings of His-bundle electrograms from distal (**A**) to proximal (**D**) positions in the His-bundle region. As the His-bundle catheter is slowly withdrawn from inside the right ventricular cavity to the right atrium, one can see the following: (**A**) a right bundle potential—note the short RBB–QRS interval; (**B**) a large His bundle and small atrial potential; (**C**) a larger atrial but still prominent His-bundle potential (ideal position to record most reproducible AH, HV intervals); and (**D**) a large atrial and small His-bundle potential (catheter too far in atrium).

Right Ventricle

Electrode catheters are positioned in the right ventricle to evaluate retrograde ventriculoatrial conduction, supraventricular tachycardia, and ventricular tachycardia. The right ventricular apex is the most widely used position and can easily be approached from both upper and lower extremity veins (see Fig. 7-1). Additional sites, such as the inflow and outflow tracts, may be needed for pacing and mapping in the investigation of ventricular tachycardia.

Left Ventricle

Left ventricular pacing may be required to initiate ventricular tachyarrhythmias if they cannot be induced by conventional right ventricle pacing. Detailed mapping of these arrhythmias also requires access to the left ventricle. Left ventricle pacing and electrogram recording may rarely be needed in evaluating patients with supraventricular tachycardia. Retrograde arterial catheterization is the most widely used technique and allows access to multiple left ventricular sites, including aneurysms.

Coronary Sinus

The coronary sinus is a venous structure that lies in the posterior AV groove. An electrode catheter in this location allows indirect electrogram recording and pacing of both the left atrium and ventricle, which is useful for many clinical situations in which electrophysiologic evaluation of these chambers is needed. Coronary sinus pacing and recording is used to locate accessory AV connections in patients with supraventricular arrhythmias. Direct left atrium catheters are rarely needed if stable coronary sinus pacing and recording is achieved. The coronary sinus is also adjacent to the posterobasal portion of the left ventricle, and ventricular pacing can be achieved in 50% to 75% of patients. If stable left ventricular pacing cannot be achieved or if detailed ventricular mapping is required, retrograde arterial catheterization is necessary.

Because of the anatomic arrangement of the os of the coronary sinus, it is best cannulated with a catheter inserted from the left arm or by the right internal jugular vein. We use a preshaped 7-French hexapolar or decapolar lumenal catheter (see Figs. 7-1 and 7-2). Continuous recording of a pressure waveform from a catheter tip during insertion facilitates its placement. Inadvertent advancement of the catheter into the right ventricle rather than the coronary sinus is immediately recognized by a change from a venous to a ventricular waveform. Proper catheter position can be confirmed by several methods. Fluoroscopic location is of value but may be misleading if the coronary sinus is short or the catheter cannot be fully advanced. A lumenal catheter permits analysis of the pressure waveform recorded at the distal tip and the injection of contrast media to opacify the coronary sinus. Further confirmation is provided by recording left atrial and left ventricular electrograms or by the appearance of a left atrial or left ventricular rhythm during coronary sinus pacing. Localization of the os of the coronary sinus and definition of anomalies of the coronary sinus have become more important with interventional electrophysiologic techniques. Several studies have helped the clinician clarify these issues.[125, 126]

Complications

Despite the use of multiple intracardiac catheters and lengthy studies, the incidence of complications in electrophysiologic studies is similar to conventional diagnostic catheterizations (Table 7-11).[118, 127] The use of multiple catheters increases the risk of significant bleeding. Careful attention to venous and arterial access sites immediately after catheter removal and minimal patient movement for several hours lower the risk of hemorrhage. A low rate of phlebitis and thromboembolic phenomena can be achieved by careful catheterization technique by experienced physicians. Systemic heparin is used for procedures lasting longer than 2 hours or when a catheter is introduced into the arterial circulation. Infection is minimized by proper sterile technique. Antibiotics are not routinely used. In a subclavian or internal jugular approach, care must be taken to avoid pneumothorax.

Arrhythmias are often initiated during electrophysiologic testing and can occur in patients without known clinical arrhythmias. These are usually self-terminating or nonsustained atrial or ventricular tachyarrhythmias. Hemodynamic stability is determined by the rate of the tachycardia, its duration, and the patient's underlying cardiovascular status. Hemodynamically unstable rhythms must be quickly terminated with programmed stimulation techniques or if this is unsuccessful, electric cardioversion. The success rate of cardioversion approaches 100% be-

TABLE 7-11. Complications From Electrophysiologic Studies

Complication	Percentage of Patients
Hemorrhage	< 1
Phlebitis/thromboembolism	0.2–2.2
Infection	0.6–1.7
Arrhythmias	
Requiring cardioverion	17
Unsuccessful cardioversion	0
Myocardial infarction or CVA	0
Mortality	0

cause of the controlled setting and termination of arrhythmias before irreversible metabolic derangements arise. A significant advance in cardioversion and defibrillation has occurred with the use of adhesive electrode patches connected directly to the defibrillator (Fig. 7-5). Extreme caution must be exercised, however, in testing patients with unstable clinical conditions. Electrophysiologic studies should be deferred in such patients until they have been stabilized, especially those with severe left ventricular dysfunction. If patients are chosen carefully and the above precautions are taken, the mortality from electrophysiologic testing, even in patients with malignant ventricular arrhythmias, should approach 0%.

Conduction Intervals and Refractory Periods

Electric activity is conducted through the heart through a series of specialized tissues with different electrophysiologic characteristics. Measurable parameters have been devised to assess these characteristics and distinguish normal from pathologic conditions. The two most commonly used are conduction intervals and refractory periods. The former refers to the time taken for a single spontaneous or paced electric impulse to traverse one or more portions of the cardiac conduction system. The latter assesses the ability of a tissue to conduct two sequential electric impulses.

Conduction Intervals

A conduction interval is merely a measurement of the time it takes for electric activity to spread through the portion of the heart under study. Surface electrocardiograms have crudely examined atrial, AV, and ventricular conduction through P, PR, and QRS interval durations. The use of multiple electrodes and recordings made at high paper speeds (100 or more mm/second) permits accurate measurement of a variety of intracardiac conduction times. The most commonly used intervals are:

PA—measurement of intraatrial conduction; the interval from onset of the P wave on surface leads to onset of low atrial activity in the His-bundle recording

AH—measurement of low atrial and AV node conduction; the interval from onset of low atrial activity to onset of His potential; both are measured in the His-bundle recording

His potential—measurement of conduction through the His bundle; the interval from onset to conclusion of the His potential in the His-bundle recording

HV—measurement of His-Purkinje conduction; the interval from onset of His potential in the His-bundle recording to the earliest onset of ventricular activation in any intracardiac or surface leads

Reported normal values are listed in Table 7-12. The variation noted reflects different populations, number of persons studied, catheter positions, criteria for measurements, and statistical methods used. Our normal range reflects the techniques and measurements described above, as applied to 243 patients between 1981 and 1983. This represents 85% of all electrophysiologic studies performed during that period. Fifty-three patients were excluded because they were taking medications that might have affected electrophysiologic parameters; thus, 190 patients were available for comparison. To define the normal population for each parameter, patients with a clinical or

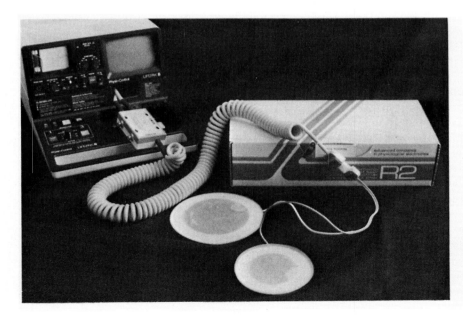

Figure 7-5. A commercially available defibrillator pad system, which allows a "hands-off" operation in the case of rapid application of direct-current transthoracic shock or shocks.

TABLE 7-12. Normal Conduction Intervals

Study (Reference)	PA	AH	His	HV
Castellanos[128]	20–50	50–120		25–55
Gallagher[129]	24–45	60–140	10–15	30–55
Josephson[130]		60–125	10–25	35–55
Narula[131]	25–60	50–120	25	35–45
Rosen[132]	9–45	54–130		31–45
Ross and Mandel	20–45	60–125		35–55

electrophysiologic diagnosis that might significantly affect the measured variable were excluded. As an example, all patients referred for testing for AV block would be excluded from the determination of the normal range of AH and HV intervals. For each group, the 10th through 90th percentile of measured values was used as the normal range.

Determination of these intervals requires a His-bundle catheter and one or more surface leads (see Figs. 7-1, 7-4, and Fig. 7-6). Abnormal autonomic tone or cardiac drugs (see Table 7-8) may markedly alter these intervals. Although measurements are usually made in spontaneous sinus rhythm, their response to incremental pacing can be of clinical value. As with other cardiac structures, a stress applied to the conduction system (e.g., pacing) may unmask otherwise occult disorders. An abrupt increase in the HV interval during slow atrial pacing can indicate His-Purkinje system dysfunction. Quantitative analysis of the effect of pacing is limited for several reasons. Pacing from different sites can result in varying intervals because of altered atrial activation and entry into the conduction system. Rapid pacing may cause catheter artifact and movement, making accurate measurements difficult. Finally, faster heart rates can produce hemodynamic changes that alter autonomic tone and thus indirectly influence conduction intervals.

Refractory Periods

Refractory periods evaluate the capacity of tissues to conduct two sequential impulses. The second impulse is a paced beat; the first can be spontaneous or paced. Refractory periods do not directly measure conduction time. This difference is illustrated in Figure 7-7, which describes a portion of the conduction system, with the AV node used as an example. Electric activity is recorded from electrodes positioned near the input and output of this system. For the AV node, both input (low atrial electrogram) and output (His-bundle potential) are measured from the same electrode. For other tissues, separate electrodes may

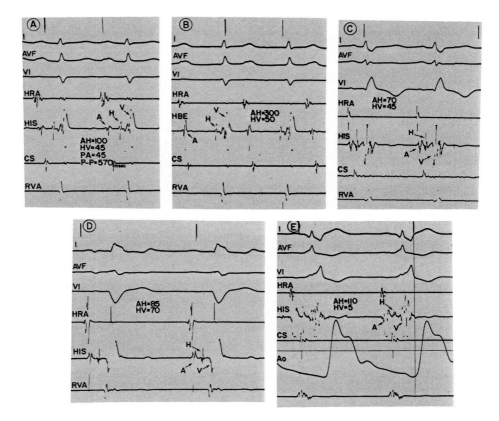

Figure 7-6. Recordings of three surface electrocardiogram leads (*I*, *aV$_F$*, *V$_1$*) and electrogram recordings from the high right atrium (*HRA*). His-bundle region (*His*), coronary sinus (*CS*), and right ventricular apex (*RVA*). AH and HV intervals are listed for all panels. (**A**) AH, HV, and PA intervals are all normal. (**B**) There is a marked prolongation of the AH interval. (**C**) In a patient with RBBB, the AH and HV intervals are also normal. (**D**) In a patient with LBBB, however, the HV is prolonged (70 milliseconds). (**E**) Data from a patient with ventricular preexcitation (Wolff-Parkinson-White syndrome). Note the normal AH interval but the very short HV (QRS) interval of only 5 milliseconds.

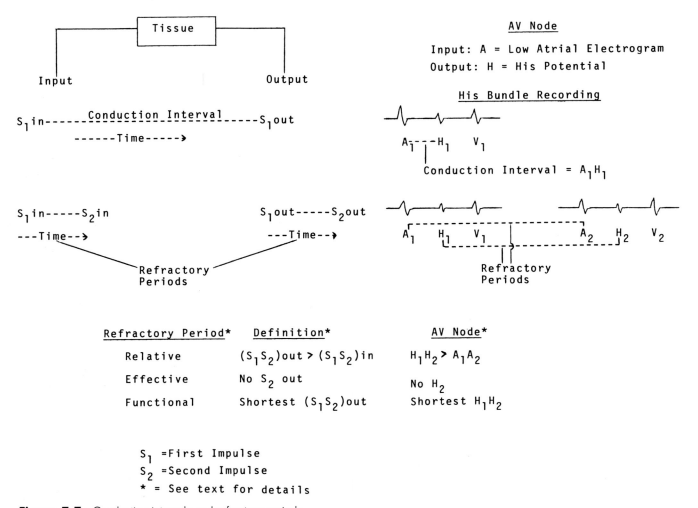

Figure 7-7. Conduction intervals and refractory periods.

be needed. The conduction interval is the absolute time taken for a single impulse (S_1) to travel through the tissue—in the case of the AV node, the AH interval (A_1H_1).

Refractory periods analyze the difference in conduction between two consecutive impulses, S_1 (spontaneous or paced) and S_2 (paced). They describe not absolute conduction time but the delay between impulses as they exit a tissue, compared with the delay at their input. The more closely coupled the two impulses, the more likely that the second will encounter refractoriness and delay during its conduction. Refractoriness results in a longer S_1S_2 interval measured at output than that measured at input. For the AV node, the exit delay (H_1H_2) is compared with the input coupling interval (A_1A_2). If refractoriness is absent, there is no difference in conduction between the two impulses, and A_1A_2 equals H_1H_2. This is usually observed at relatively long coupling intervals between S_1 and S_2. As the second impulse becomes more premature, it encounters refractoriness and consequently takes longer

to conduct through the AV node. Thus, H_1H_2 becomes longer than A_1A_2 or put in another way, the AH conduction interval of S_2 becomes longer than that of S_1. The longest coupling interval (A_1A_2) at which this occurs is the relative refractory period of the tissue. This can be illustrated by a graph of the coupling interval at the input versus the output (see Fig. 7-7). The coupling interval measured at the output of the AV node (H_1H_2) is influenced by the degree of prematurity (shortening H_1H_2 because A_1A_2 is less) and the amount of refractoriness encountered (lengthening H_1H_2 because of delayed conduction with increasing A_2H_2). As shown in Figure 7-8, with more premature impulses, the H_1H_2 interval continues to decrease but more slowly because of increasing refractoriness. A point is often reached at which the increment in conduction delay is greater than the decrement in prematurity, and the H_1H_2 interval actually becomes longer than it was for less premature impulses. This represents the ascending limb of the refractory-period curve. Eventually, a point

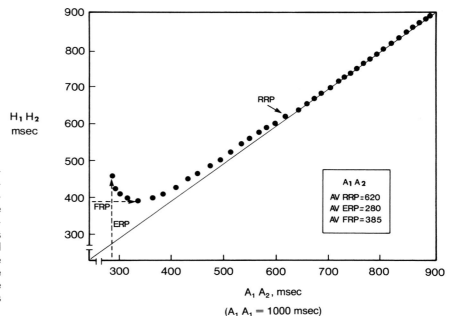

Figure 7-8. Graph of test-stimulus intervals (A_1A_2) on the horizontal axis versus response intervals (H_1H_2) obtained from the His-bundle recordings to determine the AV node refractory periods. The relative refractory period (*RRP*) of the AV node begins when there is deviation off the line of identity. The functional refractory period of the AV node (*FRP*) is the shortest H_1H_2 interval observed. The effective refractory period of the AV node (*ERP*) is the shortest A_1A_2 interval that conducts to the His bundle.

comes at which complete refractoriness exists. The second impulse is then blocked within the AV node and no output (H_2) is recorded. The effective refractory period (ERP) is the longest coupling interval (A_1A_2) at which there is *no* conduction. Examination of the curve shows that there is a minimum output interval (H_1H_2) over the entire range of conducted premature impulses; this represents the functional refractory period (FRP).

Refractory periods have been determined for a variety of tissues in both an anterograde and retrograde direction. The input and output signals necessary to access these are listed in Table 7-13. Table 7-14 shows reported normal ranges for commonly measured refractory periods. In addition to different absolute refractory periods, various cardiac tissues demonstrate different refractory-period curves. The AV node often has a prominent ascending curve, and its FRP is significantly greater than its ERP. Atrial and ventricular refractory period curves usually lie close to the line of identity, with their FRP often being only 10 to 30 milliseconds greater than their ERP.

Note that the FRP and ERP are defined as coupling intervals measured at the input of the system, at which point critical conduction changes occur, whereas the FRP is defined as an interval measured at the output. Thus, to characterize fully the refractory periods of a tissue, one must be able to measure electrical events on each side. This can be difficult in many situations. AV node refractory periods are measured based on differences between A_1A_2 and H_1H_2 but this requires no limitation in atrial refractoriness during the insertion of premature stimuli. If the atrial FRP is greater than the AV node ERP, the latter can never be

accurately determined because refractoriness in the atrium limits the degree of prematurity of input into the AV node; this occurs in 36% of patients. It is often difficult to assess retrograde conduction in the His-Purkinje system because of the inability to record a retrograde His-bundle potential in many cases. Refractoriness can be influenced by many factors. Drugs and changes in autonomic tone can have considerable impact on measured values (see Table 7-8). In addition, the basic heart rate at which a refractory period is measured also has an impact. Refractory periods

TABLE 7-13. Measurements Necessary to Determine Refractory Periods

Structure	Input	Output
ANTEROGRADE CONDUCTION		
Atrium	S_1S_2	A_1A_2
AV node	A_1A_2	H_1H_2
H-P system	H_1H_2	V_1V_2
Entire conduction system	S_1S_2	V_1V_2
RETROGRADE CONDUCTION		
Ventricle	S_1S_2	V_1V_2
H-P system	V_1V_2	H_1H_2*
AV node	H_1H_2*	A_1A_2
Entire conduction system	S_1S_2	A_1A_2

* Retrograde His potential.

S, stimulus artifact; A, atrial electrogram; H, His-bundle potential; V, ventricular electrogram; 1, first impulse; 2, second impulse; AV, atrioventricular; H-P, His-Purkinje.

TABLE 7-14. Normal Refractory Periods

Study (Reference)	ERP Atrium	FRP Atrium	ERP AVN	FRP AVN	ERP HPS	ERP V
Akhtar[133]	230–330		280–430	320–680	340–430	190–290
Denes[134]	150–360	190–390	250–365	350–495		
Josephson[130]	170–300		230–425	330–525	330–450	170–290
Schuilenburg[135]			230–390	330–500		
Ross and Mandel	200–300	235–340	260–430*	355–550		205–270

* AV node ERP limited by atrial FRP in 36% of patients.
AVN, atrioventricular node; *ERP*, effective refravtory period; *FRP*, functional refractory period; *HPS*, His-Purkinje system; *V*, ventricle.

of the atrium, His-Purkinje system, and ventricle shorten with faster heart rates, whereas those of the AV node lengthen.

Principles of Arrhythmia Induction and Termination

Research supports the concept that several electrophysiologic mechanisms can cause arrhythmias, including enhanced automaticity, delayed afterpotentials, triggered automaticity, and reentry.[136] The latter is thought to be responsible for more than 90% of supraventricular and ventricular tachyarrhythmias. Contemporary electrophysiologic techniques are most suitable for initiating and terminating triggered and reentrant arrhythmias. Automatic arrhythmias are diagnosed by their inability to be initiated or terminated by electrophysiologic techniques and by the characteristic common to most automatic foci, overdrive suppression. Reentrant arrhythmias are initiated and terminated by incremental pacing and extrastimulus techniques. Under pathologic conditions, tissues or portions thereof may exhibit variable refractoriness. In this setting, these electrophysiologic techniques alter conduction and cause unidirectional block, which is critical to the initiation of reentrant events.

Figure 7-9 illustrates these principles in more detail.

An area of the conduction system is illustrated that has two limbs with different refractoriness. These limbs join proximally and distally and have the capacity for anterograde and retrograde conduction, as do most cardiac tissues. Conduction times through each pathway are listed when appropriate. Dispersion of refractoriness is illustrated by the longer anterograde ERP of pathway B. As shown in Figure 7-9B, if two sequential impulses are introduced with a coupling interval of 450 milliseconds, both are conducted in a normal anterograde fashion through each limb. Conduction is intact, although conduction times may vary through each portion. In Figure 7-9C, two impulses are introduced, with a coupling interval of 400 milliseconds. This is close to the ERP of Figure 7-9A; thus, conduction may slow but remains intact. Anterograde conduction through pathway B is blocked, however, because the coupling interval is shorter than the ERP of that path. Because of slowed conduction through pathway A, as the impulse reaches its distal connection with pathway B, it finds the latter no longer refractory and capable of conducting in a retrograde direction. The transit time around the reentrant circuit is 400 milliseconds, which allows time for pathway A to recover from its refractoriness and conduct another anterograde cycle. The resulting tachycardia will have a cycle length of 400 milliseconds, equivalent to a rate of 150 beats per minute. The arrhythmia can be terminated by the introduction of one or more critically timed

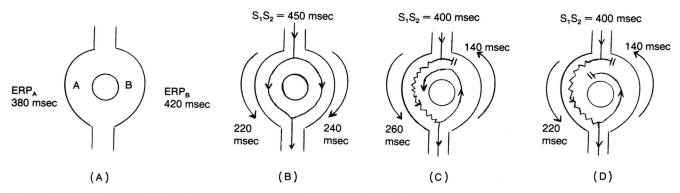

Figure 7-9. Schematic of AV node activity in a patient with dual AV nodal pathways.

impulses into the circuit, which induce additional unidirectional or bidirectional blocks and stop the reentrant wavefront.

This example uses a single extrastimulus to initiate the arrhythmia. In some cases, the critical degree of refractoriness cannot be reached and a second or third extrastimulus is needed. Multiple extrastimuli allow refractoriness to be "peeled back." Refractory periods vary with different physiologic conditions, including the rate at which a tissue is being paced and the coupling interval of previously introduced extrastimuli. Using Figure 7-9D as an example, let us examine the effect of inserting a single extrastimulus, S_2, with a coupling interval of 400 milliseconds but without the marked delay in conduction through pathway A. Assume that this conduction time is only 220 milliseconds. Unidirectional anterograde block will still occur in pathway B. If retrograde conduction occurs through pathway B, the transit time of the reentrant cycle would be 360 milliseconds rather than the 400 milliseconds noted in Figure 7-9C. Such a rapid circuit time would result in anterograde block in pathway A after the first circuit because its anterograde refractory period is only 380 milliseconds. A second or third extrastimulus is used to peel back this refractory period. The first extrastimulus (S_2) is introduced just beyond its ERP—in this case, at about 390 milliseconds—permitting conduction. A second extrastimulus (S_3) is then introduced, with progressively closer and closer coupling intervals. Using this procedure, the ERP of S_3 will be less than S_2 and so on if a third extrastimulus (S_4) is introduced.

The use of multiple extrastimuli to peel back refractoriness in pathway A may also alter the refractory period in pathway B. Initiation of reentrant arrhythmias requires a critical interplay of refractory periods, delayed conduction, and unidirectional block. By shortening refractory periods with multiple extrastimuli, dispersion in refractoriness will more likely be uncovered, thus fostering the critical electrical milieu for reentry. Incremental pacing serves the same purpose by introducing multiple impulses until a critical degree of conduction delay and unidirectional block occurs. Pacing at faster rates allows refractoriness to be peeled back in a fashion similar to the introduction of multiple extrastimuli. Given this understanding of the principles underlying conduction intervals, refractory periods, and the initiation of arrhythmias, the techniques of incremental pacing and insertion of extrastimuli can be applied to the conduction system in a systematic fashion.

Measurements in Spontaneous Rhythm

Before initiating pacing, the clinician must measure various conduction intervals during normal sinus rhythm.

These include the PA, AH, His-potential, HV, QRS, and QT intervals (see Fig. 7-6). These measurements are compared with reported normal values and interpreted in light of the surface electrocardiogram. In most patients with arrhythmias and conduction disorders, the abnormality is rarely present in the resting state and must be unmasked by pacing techniques. In some situations, however, the arrhythmia may occur spontaneously. The analysis of conduction intervals and the order of atrial and ventricular activation during these spontaneous events is extremely valuable, particularly if the arrhythmia cannot be initiated by standard electrophysiologic techniques.

Atrial Pacing Studies

Incremental pacing and the insertion of extrastimuli in the right atrium are used to assess sinus node, AV node, and atrial function in addition to initiating and terminating tachyarrhythmias.

Sinus Node Function

A detailed analysis of techniques used to assess sinus node function is provided elsewhere in this text. The most commonly used procedure is overdrive suppression to determine SNRT.[137] Pacing in the high right atrium is initiated and maintained for more than 30 seconds and then abruptly terminated. The interval from the last paced complex to the onset of the first sinus beat, as measured from high right atrium electrogram, is the SNRT (Fig. 7-10). This interval is often corrected for the underlying sinus rate by subtracting the sinus cycle length ($SNRT_c$). This maneuver is performed over a wide range of paced rates, and the maximum SNRT is defined as the longest recovery time recorded. The normal range for maximum $SNRT_c$ in our laboratory is 180 to 500 milliseconds. We commonly measure this parameter at the following rates: 100, 110, 120, 130, 150, and 170 beats per minute. The SNRT lengthens as the paced rate is increased up to heart rates of 120 to 150, after which it frequently shortens. The cause of this paradoxical shortening at high paced rates is unknown but contributing factors include changes in autonomic tone, neurotransmitter levels, hemodynamics, or variable entrance block of paced beats into the sinus node. In addition to the SNRT, cycle lengths of the subsequent 8 to 10 beats after termination of overdrive pacing are examined. During this period, the cycle length gradually returns to that of the underlying sinus rate. Prolonged secondary pauses may indicate sinus node dysfunction despite a normal SNRT.

Another widely measured parameter is sinoatrial conduction time (SACT). This is an estimate of conduction time in to and out of the sinus node. Three techniques are

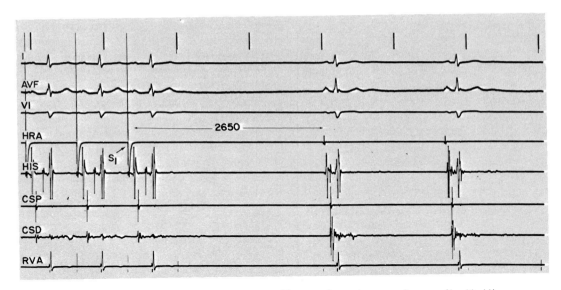

Figure 7-10. Abnormal sinus node recovery time. Three surface electrocardiogram (*I*, *aV_F*, *V_1*) recordings and electrogram recordings from the high right atrium (*HRA*); His-bundle region (*His*): proximal (*CSP*) and distal (*CSD*) coronary sinus; and the right ventricular apex (*RVA*) are displayed. The first three complexes are obtained during atrial pacing, which is discontinued abruptly after the third QRS (S_1). The first complex seen after termination of pacing occurs 2650 milliseconds later.

in clinical use. The first involves an analysis of the response of the sinus node to premature atrial extrastimuli.[138] After eight to ten sinus beats (A_1), a premature atrial extrastimulus (A_2) is introduced. The return interval (A_2A_3) is compared with the coupling interval of the premature impulse (A_1A_2), where A_1 represents the last sinus beat, A_2 the premature atrial extrastimulus, and A_3 the first sinus return beat. Measurements are made from a high right atrial electrode catheter, and impulses are introduced throughout diastole at 10- to 20-millisecond decrements. To facilitate analysis, these cycle lengths are normalized by dividing by the spontaneous sinus cycle length (A_1A_1). Figure 7-11 is a graph of the normalized premature cycle ($A_1A_2 \div A_1A_1$) plotted against the normalized return cycle ($A_2A_3 \div A_1A_1$). Figure 7-12 illustrates various zones encountered as the atrial extrastimulus is scanned through diastole. In late diastole, there is a period of compensation when premature atrial impulses are followed by a full compensatory pause:

$$A_1A_2 + A_2A_3 = 2(A_1A_1).$$

Through mid-diastole, a plateau is noticed in Figure 7-11. This represents a reset zone, in which the premature extrastimulus has reset the sinus node pacemaker without changing its underlying cycle length; A_1A_3 is less than two times A_1A_1. Because sinus node automaticity is unchanged, in the return cycle $A_2A_3 = A_1A_1 + SACT$, the latter being the conduction time in to and out of the sinus node to the

recording electrode. During early diastole, premature atrial extrastimuli may result in interpolation, so that A_2A_3 is less than A_1A_1, or in reentry, so that $A_1A_2 + A_2A_3$ is less than A_1A_1.

Sinoatrial conduction time is an estimate of perinodal conduction time. Using the premature atrial extrastimulus technique, the total conduction time in to and out of the sinus node is measured. A wide range of normal values has been reported; 100 to 250 milliseconds represents the normal values, as determined by our laboratory. Variables that may influence this measurement include location of the high right atrium pacing and recording electrode, atrial conduction abnormalities, sinus arrhythmia, and the possibility that the premature atrial impulse may suppress the sinus node and alter its automaticity.

An alternative approach to measuring SACT has been developed by Narula and colleagues.[139] In this technique, the atrium is paced for eight beats, 10 beats per minute faster than the underlying sinus rate. The interval from the last paced beat to the first return sinus beat, recorded in the high right atrium, is measured. The SACT is this interval minus the mean sinus cycle length. This is analogous to measurement of SNRT but pacing at this rate is thought not to suppress sinus node automaticity. This method is easier and faster than the atrial extrastimulus technique and also overcomes the limitations of sinus arrhythmia. The newest technique developed to measure SACT uses direct recording of sinoatrial electric activity.[140] An electrode catheter is positioned in the high right atrium in proximity to the

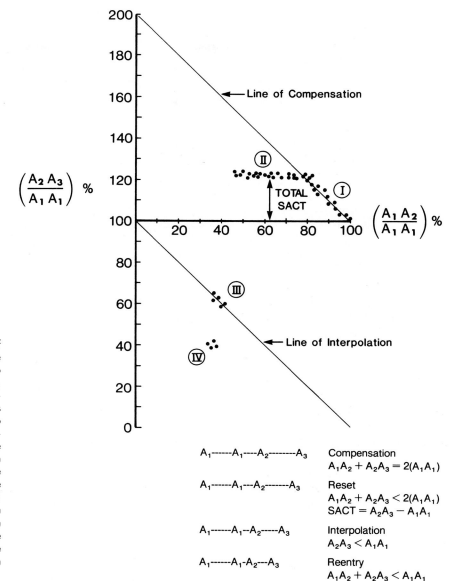

Figure 7-11. Method of determination of sinoatrial conduction time (*SACT*) using the Strauss technique. The ventrical axis is the ratio of the A_2A_3 interval (return cycle) to the A_1A_1 interval (sinus cycle length), expressed in percentage from 0% to 200%. The horizontal axis is the ratio of the A_1A_2 interval (test interval) to the A_1A_1 interval (sinus cycle length), expressed in percentage from 0% to 100%. The diagonal lines identify a line of compensation and a line of interpolation. Four zones are identified: (*I*) zone of compensation, (*II*) zone of reset, (*III*) zone of interpolation, and (*IV*) zone of reentry. The total SACT is measured in the zone of reset (*II*) at the area identified with the line with two *arrowheads*. A_1A_1, sinus cycle length; A_1A_2, coupling interval of premature atrial extrastimulus; A_2A_3, cycle length of return sinus impulse.

sinus node. High amplification (50 to 100 mV/cm) and low-pass filters (0.1 to 20 Hz) are employed to record slow diastolic electric activity of the sinus node. Sinoatrial conduction time is the interval from the beginning of the upstroke of the sinus node electrogram to the onset of atrial activity in that lead. Although each of these techniques purports to measure SACT, given their marked procedural differences, it is unlikely that they examine identical electric events. This partly explains the poor correlation between methods in certain clinical situations.[141]

Abnormalities in SNRT and SACT may reflect variations in autonomic tone rather than true sinus node dysfunction. This effect can be eliminated through autonomic blockade with atropine, 0.04 mg/kg intravenously, and propranolol, 0.2 mg/kg intravenously. The resultant spontaneous sinus rate is defined as the intrinsic heart rate (IHR). The measured value is compared with normal values predicted by the linear regression formula:[142]

$$IHR_p = 118.1 - (0.57 \times age).$$

The 95% confidence limit is plus or minus 14% for people younger than 45 years of age and plus or minus 18% for people older than 45 years of age. An abnormal SNRT or SACT with a normal IHR suggests abnormal autonomic activity, whereas an abnormal IHR indicates intrinsic sinus node dysfunction. To assess sinus node function, we measure maximum $SNRT_c$ and one or more measure-

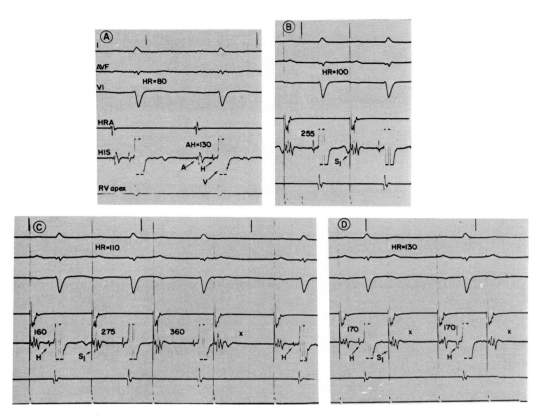

Figure 7-12. Atrioventricular node Wenckebach phenomenon. Three surface electrocardiogram leads (*I, aV_F, V_1*) and intracardiac electrograms recorded from the high right atrium (*HRA*), His-bundle region (*His*), and right ventricular apex (*RV apex*) are shown. (**A**; sinus rhythm) The AH interval is prolonged (130 milliseconds); atrial pacing is then performed (*S_1*) and at a heart rate of 100/min (**B**), the AH interval is markedly prolonged (255 milliseconds). (**C**) As the pacing rate was increased to 110/min, 4:3 node Wenckebach phenomenon occurs; there is no His-bundle spike or QRS after the fourth paced P wave. Progressive AH-interval prolongation occurred (160, 275, and 360 milliseconds) before the blocked P wave. (**D**) As the paced rate is increased further (130/min), 2:1 AV conduction occurs, with block occurring at the AV node; no His spike is seen after the nonconducted P wave.

ments of SACT in all patients undergoing electrophysiologic testing. If there are significant abnormalities in these results or if the patient is being tested primarily for sinus node dysfunction, autonomic blockade with termination of IHR is performed.

AV Node–His-Purkinje Function

The same electrophysiologic techniques, incremental atrial pacing and the insertion of premature atrial extrastimuli, are used to assess sinus node and AV node function. During incremental atrial pacing, AH interval prolongation occurs, with faster rates due to encroachment on the relative refractory period of the AV node. At a critical rate, long-cycle AV node–Wenckebach phenomenon occurs (see Fig. 7-12). This is confirmed by incremental lengthening of the AH interval, with the dropped ventricular complex showing paced atrial activity but no

His-bundle activity. The rate at which the AV node–Wenckebach cycle occurs varies because of differing refractory periods and autonomic nervous system activity. The normal range in our laboratory is 120 to 200 beats per minute. Although the usual response to incremental atrial pacing is block within the AV node, infra-Hisian block may occur in some healthy persons. If the AV node is capable of conducting at high rates, the refractory periods of the normal His-Purkinje system can be encroached on. Infra-Hisian or bundle branch block occurring at rates of less than 160 to 170 beats per minute usually represents a pathologic process. The extrastimulus technique is used to determine anterograde AV node refractory periods and if applicable, bundle branch and His-Purkinje system refractory periods. In our laboratory, these are routinely measured during pacing at 100 to 110 beats per minute. Frequent spontaneous extrasystoles or other arrhythmias may necessitate a faster basic drive rate. A change in cycle length, however, can affect the measured refractory periods, although this is usually not clinically significant.[143]

In some persons, analysis of the AV node refractory curve reveals a break in the curve, with a marked increase in conduction time (A_2H_2 or H_1H_2) with progressively premature extrastimuli. This discontinuous response reflects the presence of dual AV node pathways (Fig. 7-13). The faster conducting pathway masks the slower pathway at long coupling intervals but has a longer ERP. When the refractory period has been reached, more premature impulses unmask the slow pathway, with a sudden increase

in the A_2H_2 interval. This abnormality is present in about 75% of patients with clinical AV node reentrant tachycardia but it is also seen in persons without a history of clinical arrhythmias.

Atrial Function

Techniques similar to those described above are used to evaluate atrial function. The clinical significance of such findings is not as well understood as for the AV node and His-Purkinje system. The PA interval is used to measure

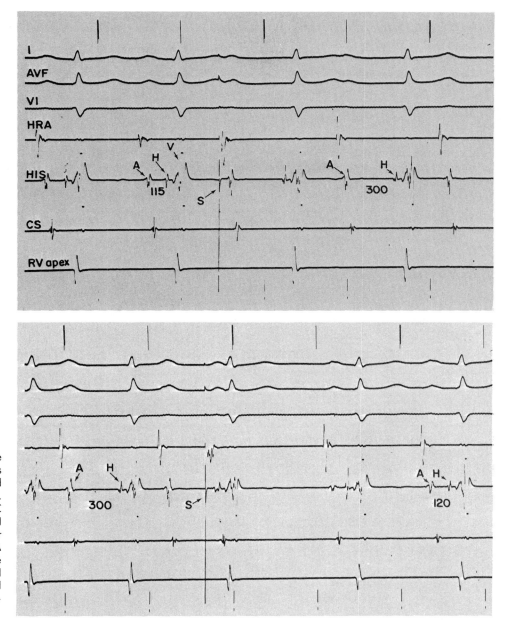

Figure 7-13. Dual AV node pathways. (**A**) Two sinus complexes precede an electrically stimulated atrial premature complex (APC; S). The AH intervals before the APC were 115 milliseconds but the AH interval in the sinus complex after the APC is 300 milliseconds. (**B**) A second APC is induced, and the previously prolonged AH interval (300 milliseconds) is now followed by sinus complexes with an AH interval of 120 milliseconds.

intraatrial conduction but has many limitations. It represents the conduction interval from the onset of P-wave activity on the surface electrocardiogram to the onset of low right atrial activity in the His-bundle electrogram. As such, it is a crude index of right atrial activation. In many cases, endocardial atrial activity, as measured by other atrial electrograms, often precedes the onset of surface P-wave activity. A more extensive analysis of atrial conduction requires mapping techniques.

With stimulation currents of two to three times diastolic threshold, incremental atrial pacing should result in 1:1 capture to rates higher than 250 beats per minute. Loss of capture before this point is usually due to unstable catheter position and can be corrected by increasing current intensity or repositioning the pacing catheter. Atrial pacing at rates higher than 250 beats per minute may induce atrial fibrillation or flutter in normal persons (Fig. 7-14). These arrhythmias usually terminate spontaneously in a few seconds or minutes. Atrial refractory periods are measured with the extrastimulus technique. Caution must be used during atrial pacing in persons with a clinical history of atrial fibrillation and flutter. Rapid atrial pacing (greater than 200 beats/minute) or the insertion of premature atrial extrastimuli close to the atrial ERP may induce sustained atrial fibrillation or flutter. This may preclude further analysis of sinus node, atrial, and AV node function unless the arrhythmia can be terminated. Electric cardioversion may be required to terminate atrial fibrillation in this setting.

Gap Phenomenon

The conduction system is organized as an electric circuit with specialized tissues connected in series, AV node and His-Purkinje system, or parallel bundle branches. As such,

the electrophysiologic parameters of one area may influence those of another. An example of this is the inability to determine AV node ERP in 36% of persons because of atrial refractoriness. Another example is the gap phenomenon (Fig. 7-15). This is a situation in which progressively more premature impulses result in paradoxical improvement in conduction. This is most commonly seen during measurement of AV node and His-Purkinje refractory periods using the extrastimulus technique. In some situations, the ERP of the His-Purkinje system or bundle branches is reached while the AV node is still capable of conduction. At this point, either infra-Hisian or bundle branch block occurs. As progressively more premature impulses are delivered, the infra-Hisian or bundle branch block is noted to resolve, an apparent paradox. This is explained by the gap phenomenon. Premature extrastimuli are being introduced into the high right atrium and must traverse the atrium and AV node before reaching the input to the His-Purkinje system. These impulses are thus subject to conduction delays at several sites. In the example noted above, more premature atrial impulses can encounter the ascending limb of the AV node refractory period curve, producing marked AV node delay and allowing the His-Purkinje system to recover from refractoriness. Although the extrastimulus is more premature (A_1A_2 is shorter), the input to the His-Purkinje system (H_1H_2) or bundle branches is actually longer because of the delay in AV node conduction. This same phenomenon can be encountered elsewhere in the conduction system and is one explanation for accelerated conduction.

Supraventricular Arrhythmias

The principles underlying initiation and termination of reentrant arrhythmias have been discussed. In most pa-

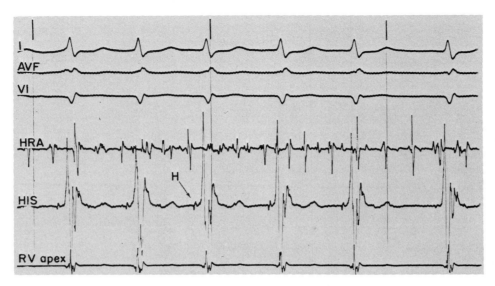

Figure 7-14. Atrial fibrillation. Three surface electrocardiogram (ECG) leads (*I, aV_F, V_1*) are recorded with intracardiac leads from the high right atrium (*HRA*), His bundle (*His*), and right ventricular apex (*RV apex*). Note the irregular RR intervals on the surface ECG leads. The HRA recording shows a rapid, irregular pattern of atrial discharge. The His recording is obtained with the catheter introduced further into the ventricle to lower atrial depolarization amplitude. Note the readily identifiable His-bundle deflection with each QRS.

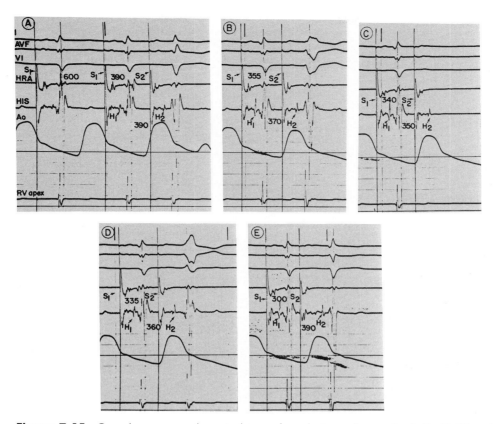

Figure 7-15. Gap phenomenon, shown in three surface electrocardiogram leads (*I*, *aV$_F$*, *V$_1$*) and intracardiac electrograms recorded from the high right atrium (*HRA*), His bundle (*His*), and right ventricular apex (*RV apex*). An intraarterial pulse tracing is also shown (A$_0$). (**A**) The last two of a train of eight basic drives (S$_1$) are shown and a test pulse (S$_2$) is then delivered. The basic drive cycle length is 600 milliseconds (100/min). The S$_1$S$_2$ test interval is 390 milliseconds, and the H$_1$H$_2$ response interval is also 390 milliseconds. The resultant QRS interval demonstrates slight aberration, and the H$_2$V$_2$ intervals are prolonged. (**B** to **E**) Further sequences during the stimulation run as the S$_1$S$_2$ interval is shortened. (**B**) The test interval was shortened to 355 milliseconds. The H$_1$H$_2$ interval is greater than the S$_1$S$_2$ interval, and the QRS interval is grossly aberrant. (**C**) The test interval was shortened to 340 milliseconds, the H$_1$H$_2$ interval was 350 milliseconds but block occurred below the His. (**D**) The test interval was reduced to 335 milliseconds and conduction resumed with an aberrant QRS interval similar to that in *B* but with a longer HV interval. (**E**) The test interval was shortened to 300 milliseconds. Conduction persisted but aberration was lessened significantly because the S$_2$H$_2$ interval was markedly prolonged (390 milliseconds).

tients with a clinical history of supraventricular tachycardia, the techniques used to assess sinus, atrial, and AV node function are sufficient. These include incremental atrial pacing to a rate of 200 to 250 beats per minute and scanning diastole by 10- to 20-milliseconds decrements with premature atrial extrastimuli. In some situations, more rapid pacing rates or multiple extrastimuli are needed. Certain supraventricular tachyarrhythmias require critical alterations in autonomic tone for initiation. Intravenous atropine, 0.5 to 2 mg, or isoproterenol sufficient to produce a resting sinus rate of 110 to 120 beats per minute can be used in conjunction with pacing techniques if the latter alone fails to initiate the tachycardia. Occasionally, these agents may be administered together to enhance further

tachycardia inducibility. These aggressive techniques are capable of inducing transient atrial arrhythmias in some healthy persons, however. Arrhythmias are terminated by similar techniques—bursts (10 to 20 beats) of more rapid atrial pacing or the introduction of progressively more premature extrastimuli. Hemodynamically unstable arrhythmias require immediate termination with synchronized cardioversion.

These techniques are used to initiate a variety of supraventricular tachycardias, including atrial fibrillation, atrial flutter, sinus node reentry, atrial reentry, AV node reentry, and tachycardias, using accessory AV connections with orthodromic or antidromic conduction (Figs. 7-16 and 7-17). These are easily distinguished by their rate,

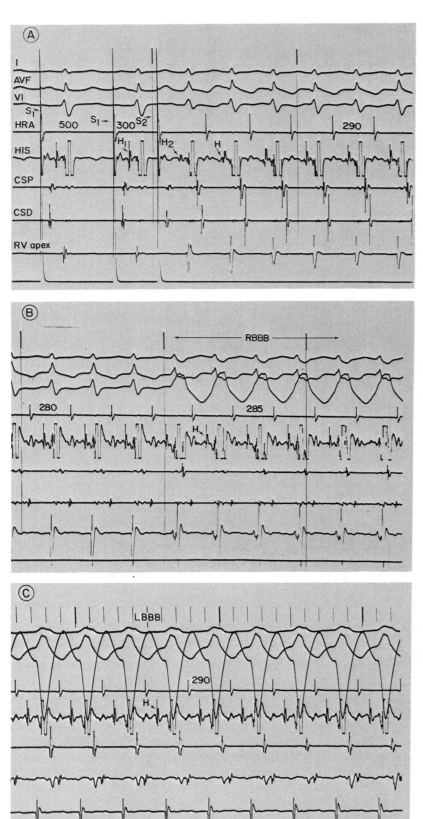

Figure 7-16. Supraventricular tachycardia. (**A**) Three surface electrocardiogram leads (*I, aV_F, V_1*) are recorded, along with intracardiac electrograms from the high right atrium (*HRA*); His bundle (*His*); the proximal (*CSP*) and distal (*CSD*) coronary sinuses; and the right ventricular apex (*RV apex*). The basic drive (S_1S_1) is 500 milliseconds (120/min). An atrial premature complex is initiated with a test interval (S_1S_2) of 300 milliseconds. Supraventricular tachycardia occurs, with a cycle length of 290 milliseconds. Review of the activation sequence identifies that the proximal coronary sinus electrogram precedes all other atrial electrograms, indicating a left paraseptal bypass tract operating in the retrograde direction. (**B**) Spontaneous right bundle branch block occurs, with no significant change in tachycardia cycle length or HA or AH intervals. (**C**) Spontaneous left bundle branch block occurs and again, no significant change in the tachycardia cycle length is observed.

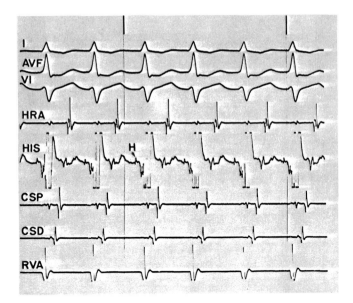

Figure 7-17. Supraventricular tachycardia. The format is similar to that of Figure 7-16. Recordings obtained in a patient with a left lateral bypass tract are shown. Note that in contrast to Figure 7-16, the *distal* coronary sinus electrogram occurs first, with atrial activation proceeding in a stepwise fashion from proximal coronary sinus (*CSP*), atrial septum (*His*) to high right atrium (*HRA*).

P-wave and atrial endocardial electrogram morphology, and atrial activation sequence (Table 7-15).

In some cases, however, more sophisticated electrophysiologic techniques are needed to define the underlying abnormality. These are beyond the scope of this discussion but include analysis of response of the tachycardia to bundle branch block, atrial or ventricular pacing, and premature atrial or ventricular extrastimuli. In rare patients, atrial pacing studies may induce ventricular tachycardia. This occurs in patients capable of 1:1 AV conduction at rapid pacing rates. The effect is probably similar to direct ventricular pacing techniques used to induce ventricular tachyarrhythmias. Ventricular tachycardia must therefore be included in the differential diagnoses of wide QRS tachycardias induced during atrial stimulation (see Table 7-15).

Ventricular Pacing Studies

Ventricular pacing is typically performed using an impulse 2 milliseconds in duration with a current intensity equal to twice the diastolic pacing threshold. The techniques employed in the ventricle are similar to those used in the atrium; namely, incremental pacing, usually from the right ventricular apex, and the introduction of one or more premature ventricular extrastimuli. Such techniques are used to evaluate ventricular electrophysiologic character-

istics, retrograde VA conduction, supraventricular tachycardia, and ventricular tachyarrhythmias.

Ventricular Function and VA Conduction

Incremental pacing from the right ventricular apex should result in 1:1 capture up to rates of 200 beats per minute. Faster rates may result in variable ventricular capture. Ventricular refractory periods are derived by scanning diastole with single ventricular extrastimuli. This is usually performed during ventricular pacing at 100 to 120 beats per minute for eight beats. This allows sufficient time for the influence of the pacing rate to stabilize. As with atrial muscle, the refractory period curve usually lies close to the line of identity, with minimal conduction delay and a short ascending limb.

Retrograde VA conduction is present in about 50% of healthy persons. Conduction can be evaluated in a manner analogous to anterograde AV conduction. With incremental ventricular pacing, there is gradual prolongation in retrograde conduction through the His-Purkinje system and AV node (Fig. 7-18). This is documented by an increase in the VA conduction interval. The VA interval is measured as the time between onset of ventricular activity, usually measured by the right ventricular apex electrogram, and onset of earliest retrograde atrial activity, usually measured in the His-bundle recording. Retrograde VA block occurs at a critical rate, usually with Wenckebach periodicity. The level of retrograde block (His-Purkinje versus AV node) is difficult to determine because a retrograde His potential is visualized in only 10% of persons. With intact VA conduction, we have found retrograde conduction to be better than anterograde conduction in 27% of persons, the same in 20%, and worse in 53%. Retrograde VA refractory periods are determined with the extrastimulus technique. As with incremental ventricular pacing, the level of block may be difficult to determine because of an inability to visualize a retrograde His potential. Indirect methods suggest the site of block is the AV node in 90% of patients.[144] Retrograde VA gap phenomena may be seen during the insertion of premature ventricular extrastimuli. This usually occurs when the ERP of the AV node is reached, resulting in retrograde VA block. More premature ventricular extrastimuli paradoxically restore VA conduction by inducing delay in the His-Purkinje system sufficient to allow recovery of AV node conduction.

It is important to examine the sequence of retrograde atrial activation during ventricular pacing. In normal persons, the earliest activity should appear in the low atrial septum, best visualized from the atrial electrogram in the His-bundle recording. Early electric activity in other portions of the atrium suggests the presence of an accessory AV connection. The order of retrograde atrial activation during ventricular pacing should be compared with

TABLE 7-15. Common Arrhythmias Induced by Programmed Stimulation

Arrhythmia	Atrial Rate beats/min	P-Wave Morphology	Atrial Electrogram	P-Wave and QRS Relation	Atrial Activation Sequence	His Potential	Dual AV Node Pathways (%)	Effect of BBB on Cycle Lengths	Atrial Participation Required	Atrial Activation Sequence During V Pacing	AV Node H-P System Required	Atrial Advancement by PVC
Sinus node reentry	80–150	Similar to sinus	Discrete	P > QRS	Similar to sinus	Yes	<10	None	Yes	Retrograde	No	No
Atrial reentry	150–200	Variable	Discrete	P > QRS	Variable	Yes	<10	None	Yes	Retrograde	No	No
AV node reentry	150–250	Variable	Discrete	Variable	Retrograde	Yes	>75	None	No	Retrograde	Yes	No
Reentry with bypass tracts Orthodromic	150–250	Variable	Discrete	QRS > P	Variable	Yes	<10	↑ If BBB ipsilateral to bypass tract	Yes (in part)	Same as in SVT	Yes	Yes
Antidromic	150–250	Variable	Discrete	P > QRS	Retrograde	Rare (retrograde)	<10	—	Yes (in part)	Variable	Yes	Yes
Atrial fibrillation	400–650	Absent	Fibrillatory waves	—	Disorganized	Yes	<10	None	Yes	—	No	No
Atrial flutter	230–450	Flutter waves	Discrete	Variable	Variable	Yes	<10	None	Yes	—	No	No
Ventricular tachycardia	AV dissociation	→Sinus	Discrete	Variable	Sinus	No	<10	—	No	Sinus	No	No
	Retrograde VA conduction	→Variable	Discrete	QRS > P	Retrograde	No	<10	—	No	Retrograde	No	Variable

V, ventricular; BBB, bundle branch block; PVC, premature ventricular complexes; H-P, His-Purkinje; AV, atrioventricular; SVT, supraventricular tachycardia.

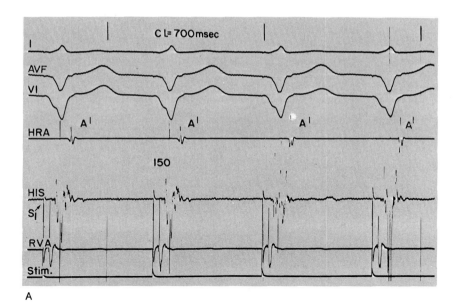

Figure 7-18. VA Wenckebach. (**A**) The ventricle is being paced at a cycle length of 700 milliseconds (85 beats/min). One-to-one VA conduction is present, with a VA interval of 150 milliseconds. *Stim.* represents a display of the stimulus artifact only. The remainder of A is similar to previous figures. (**B**) The ventricular cycle length has been shortened to 500 milliseconds (120 beats/min). Note the 4:3 retrograde Wenckebach period, with progressive VA delay (150, 325, and 400 milliseconds) until VA block occurs.

atrial activation during supraventricular tachycardia to understand better the mechanism of the arrhythmia (see Table 7-15).

Supraventricular Arrhythmias

Incremental pacing and the extrastimulus technique are used to evaluate supraventricular tachycardias. If the ventricle is part of the reentrant circuit, these techniques may directly initiate and terminate the arrhythmia. Ventricular pacing can initiate supraventricular tachycardia, even when the ventricle does not participate in the arrhythmia. If retrograde conduction is intact, ventricular impulses can reach critical portions of the tachycardia circuit such as the atrium or AV node. The response of an arrhythmia to burst ventricular pacing and premature ventricular extrastimuli is also of diagnostic value (see Table 7-15).

Ventricular Arrhythmias

Ventricular pacing is most widely used during electrophysiologic studies to evaluate patients with sudden death and recurrent ventricular tachycardia. The sensitivity, specificity, and predictive value of numerous ventricular pacing protocols has been discussed. Our protocol includes incremental ventricular pacing from 100 to 250 beats per minute for bursts of 5 to 10 seconds at twice diastolic threshold from the right ventricular apex. This is followed by pacing for eight beats at 100 to 120 beats per minute, with the sequential insertion of single, double, and triple ventricular extrastimuli carried down to the point of refractoriness (Fig. 7-19). If this fails to induce sustained ventricular tachycardia, the extrastimulus technique is repeated, initially with a higher basic drive rate of 150 beats per minute and subsequently with a high pacing rate and increased current strength (five times diastolic threshold).

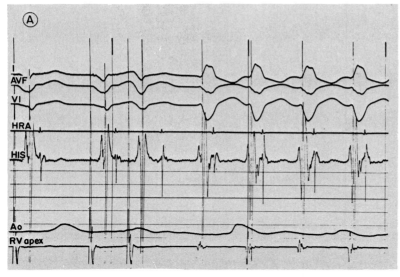

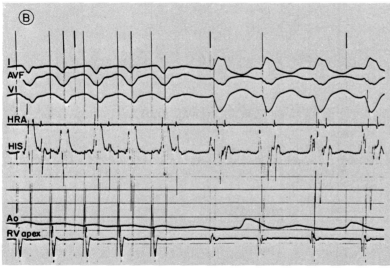

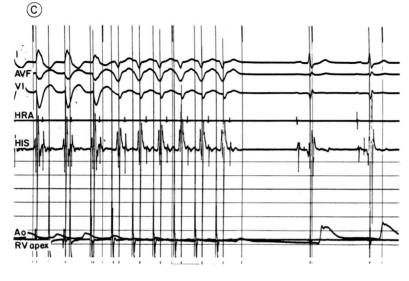

Figure 7-19. Ventricular tachycardia. (**A**) The first two complexes are the last two ventricular paced complexes in an eight-beat train (S_1S_1 = 550 milliseconds; 110 beats/min). The third complex is induced ventricular premature complex with an S_1S_2 test interval of 275 milliseconds. Ventricular tachycardia then occurs with a cycle length of 365 milliseconds (167 beats/min). (**B**) The first five complexes are the result of right ventricular overdrive at a cycle length of 250 milliseconds (240 beats/min). Pacing is discontinued and ventricular tachycardia is then observed, with a morphology and cycle length similar to A. (**C**) Ventricular overdrive is performed at a cycle length of 300 milliseconds (200 beats/min) for six complexes. After overdrive is terminated, sinus rhythm is restored.

These changes peel back ventricular refractoriness and facilitate initiation of tachyarrhythmias. If this is unsuccessful, the latter pacing sequence is repeated in at least one other location within the right ventricle, usually the outflow tract. These techniques have a sensitivity and specificity of about 85% to 90%. Occasionally, a long–short stimulation sequence is used, which may be especially helpful in patients with potential repolarization abnormalities. In certain clinical situations, additional stimulation is performed during an isoproterenol infusion or from the left ventricle. The latter procedures are not routinely used (despite an increase in sensitivity) for several reasons: (1) their use may decrease specificity and increase morbidity, (2) most patients with ventricular arrhythmias have underlying coronary artery disease, and (3) an isoproterenol infusion may worsen angina or myocardial infarction. These techniques also limit the ease of serial drug testing. Evaluation of proper pharmacologic therapy requires serial stimulation, using the same procedures as those required to initiate the arrhythmia in the drug-free state. A right ventricular pacing catheter can be safely left in place for 7 to 10 days, with serial studies performed at bedside. If left ventricular stimulation is required, multiple left ventricular catheterizations may be necessary. Serial antiarrhythmic drug studies during an isoproterenol infusion may be difficult to interpret because of drug interactions.

The ability to quickly and safely terminate sustained ventricular arrhythmias is critical. The hemodynamic response to such arrhythmias depends on their rate and the severity of underlying cardiac disorders. Left ventricular function is a critical factor. Most patients with good left ventricular function tolerate tachycardias with rates up to 200 beats per minute without hemodynamic deterioration. Ventricular mapping studies and response to drug infusions can be examined in clinically stable patients. Hemodynamic compromise, either initially or after several minutes, requires prompt intervention. The electrophysiologic mechanisms underlying the termination of reentrant arrhythmias with pacing techniques have been discussed. Programmed stimulation techniques are successful in terminating ventricular tachycardia in up to 80% of patients. The remainder require cardioversion.[92] The insertion of one to three extrastimuli results in termination in 27% to 63% of attempts. Burst pacing is successful in 76% of trials. Acceleration of the tachycardia occurs in 20%. The rate of the tachycardia is critical to successful termination by pacing techniques. Programmed extrastimuli are successful in only 15% when the tachycardia is faster than 200 beats per minute. Burst ventricular pacing is successful in 49% at similar tachycardia rates. Other techniques, such as ultrarapid stimulation or rapid pacing plus extrastimuli, are reported to terminate ventricular

tachycardia.[145,146] These methods, however, require further investigation.

When a hemodynamically unstable rhythm causes loss of consciousness, direct-current cardioversion is immediately performed, with 200 watt-second used initially, followed by higher energies if additional countershocks are necessary. If the rhythm is hemodynamically stable, burst ventricular pacing for 10 to 15 beats is attempted at a rate 10 to 20 beats per minute faster than the tachycardia. If this is unsuccessful or acceleration occurs and the patient remains clinically stable, faster overdrive rates or premature extrastimuli are used.

Coronary Sinus Pacing Studies

The coronary sinus provides an additional site for electrogram recording and pacing in evaluating supraventricular and ventricular arrhythmias. Because of its location, it allows indirect electric access to the left atrium and ventricle. The pacing techniques used are identical to those described elsewhere; namely, incremental pacing and insertion of one or more extrastimuli. Greater current intensity may be needed to achieve stable left atrial or left ventricular pacing from the coronary sinus than with direct electric contact against the endocardium.

Coronary sinus studies are important in patients with supraventricular tachycardia using accessory AV connections because many of these tracts are left sided. If anterograde conduction is present (Wolff-Parkinson-White syndrome), the location of the bypass tract can be located by comparing the stimulus-to-delta–wave interval and degree of ventricular preexcitation at different paced sites with similar rates. Proximity of the pacing site to the origin of the accessory tract shortens the stimulus-to-delta–wave interval and increases the degree of preexcitation. The tract is likely to be in the left free wall when this occurs during distal coronary sinus pacing. A paraseptal tract should be suspected when maximal preexcitation occurs with proximal coronary sinus or low atrial septum pacing. Coronary sinus stimulation can initiate supraventricular tachycardia. Critical tachycardia zones may be encountered because of proximity to bypass tracts and altered atrial activation or conduction.

Indirect left ventricular stimulation through coronary sinus pacing can be used to initiate and terminate ventricular tachycardias that were unprovokable from right ventricular sites. Direct left ventricle stimulation has been reported necessary for induction in 11% of patients with recurrent ventricular tachycardia.[147] Indirect left ventricle pacing may decrease morbidity associated with retrograde left ventricle catheterization. Left ventricular stimulation is also reported to enhance the evaluation of drug efficacy in patients with ventricular arrhythmias.[148] Because such testing takes place over several days, a coronary sinus catheter can be left in place for repeated use rather than performing multiple retrograde left ventricle catheterizations.

Drug Testing

Drugs are used in conjunction with electrophysiologic studies to enhance the sensitivity and specificity of diagnostic testing and to treat a variety of arrhythmias. Atropine and propranolol are used to produce autonomic blockade in the evaluation of patients for sick sinus syndrome. Similar agents may facilitate the initiation of tachyarrhythmias in cases wherein standard programmed stimulation techniques have been unsuccessful. Because of their electrophysiologic effects, atropine (0.01 to 0.04 mg/kg) and isoproterenol (0.5 to 5.0 μg/minute) enhance the initiation of a variety of supraventricular arrhythmias. Isoproterenol in comparable doses is used to facilitate the initiation of ventricular tachycardia.

Antiarrhythmic agents can be tested for their ability to terminate or prevent the initiation of tachyarrhythmias. Most electropharmacologic testing is performed for the latter purpose. Once it has been demonstrated that programmed stimulation can reproducibly initiate a tachyarrhythmia, a series of drugs is administered and repeat stimulation studies are performed. Dose is adjusted to achieve therapeutic serum levels. The drug that best prevents the induction of the same tachycardia is subsequently used for long-term therapy. During the initial electrophysiologic study, pharmacologic testing is usually performed with an intravenous preparation. If this is successful, the patient is given an oral form and repeat testing is performed in several days. If the initial drug is unsuccessful, another type of agent is then tested. It is important to allow a suitable length of time (five or more drug half-lives) for steady-state levels to be achieved.

The choice of drugs is dictated by the nature of the arrhythmia, side effects, left ventricular function, and any potential drug–drug or drug–disease interactions. For supraventricular tachycardia, we test the effectiveness of a class I agent (quinidine, procainamide, or disopyramide) alone and in combination with a different class of drug (propranolol, digoxin, or verapamil). If these are unsuccessful, an experimental agent may be considered.

Considerable controversy exists regarding the choice of drugs to treat ventricular tachyarrhythmias. During the initial electrophysiologic study, an intravenous preparation of a type I agent is usually tested, such as procainamide (15 mg/kg) or quinidine (10 mg/kg). If the arrhythmia is noninducible, repeat testing is performed after a steady-state level has been achieved on an oral regimen. It has been suggested that a negative response to a class I agent predicts a poor response to other conventional drugs and that further therapy should involve experimental agents, surgery, or an implantable cardioverter defibrillator.[63] Any single agent has an efficacy less than 33%.[55,63,73] Given the low rate of initial response, however, the testing of multiple drugs improves the overall response rate by 25% to 30%. The testing of combinations of drugs does not improve therapeutic efficacy.[149,150] Our approach is to test a minimum of two conventional antiarrhythmic drugs before using investigational agents. Experimental drugs are tested in a similar fashion, with the exception of amiodarone. There is a poor correlation between the results of electropharmacologic testing and clinical response with this agent.[151]

Mapping Studies

Mapping studies are performed to localize electrophysiologic areas for surgical or catheter ablation. Preliminary mapping is done in the catheterization laboratory, with more detailed studies at the time of surgery. In the evaluation of supraventricular tachycardia, mapping is most often performed to localize accessory AV connections. If the pathway shows evidence of anterograde conduction (Wolff-Parkinson-White syndrome), it can be localized by two methods: (1) evaluation of the stimulus-to-delta–wave interval and degree of preexcitation during atrial pacing at different sites, and (2) ventricular mapping during atrial pacing. The former is used to locate the bypass tract in the catheterization laboratory; the latter technique is used at surgery. Ventricular mapping can be performed in the catheterization laboratory but requires positioning catheters at multiple points around the AV valve rings in both the right and left ventricles. This is technically difficult because of supporting valvular structures. Intraoperative studies are performed with epicardial rather than endocardial mapping because of the location of most accessory AV connections. A hand-held mapping electrode is moved around the valve rings along the ventricular aspect of the AV groove during atrial pacing. The timing of the ventricular electrogram is compared with that of right and left ventricle reference epicardial electrograms and multiple surface leads. The site of earliest ventricular activity identifies the bypass tract. Mapping must be performed when there is manifest preexcitation on the surface electrocardiogram. If pacing is performed at a rate that results in anterograde block in the bypass tract, conduction to the ventricle is solely through the AV node. Computer-assisted mapping has enhanced the accuracy and markedly increased the speed of epicardial mapping studies.

If retrograde conduction is present, atrial mapping is performed during ventricular pacing. In the catheteriza-

TABLE 7-16. Electrophysiologic Pacing Protocols

SINUS NODE STUDIES

Catheters
1. HRA (pacing and recording)

Procedures
1. Incremental atrial pacing (to rates greater than 150 beats/min)
2. Atrial extrastimulus technique (single)
3. Autonomic blockade (atropine and propranolol)

CONDUCTION SYSTEM STUDIES

Catheters
1. HRA (pacing)
2. HBE (recording)
3. RV (pacing)

Procedures
1. Baseline conduction intervals
2. Anterograde conduction
   A. Incremental atrial pacing (to development of AV block)
   B. Atrial extra stimulus technique (single)
3. Retrograde conduction
   A. Incremental ventricular pacing (to development of VA block)
   B. Ventricular extra stimulus technique (single)
4. Atropine (repeat 1, 2, and 3)

SUPRAVENTRICULAR TACHYCARDIA

Catheters
1. HRA (pacing and recording)
2. HBE (recording)
3. RV (pacing and recording)
4. CS (pacing and recording)

Procedures
1. Baseline conduction intervals
2. Atrial pacing (possible multiple sites)
   A. Incremental pacing (to rates greater than 200 beats/min)
   B. Extrastimulus technique (single; possible double and triple)
3. Coronary sinus pacing (possible multiple sites)
   A. Incremental pacing (to rates greater than 200 beats/min)
   B. Extrastimulus technique (single; possible double and triple)
4. Ventricular pacing
   A. Incremental pacing (to rates greater than 200 beats/min)
   B. Extrastimulus technique (single; possible double and triple)
5. During tachycardia (repeat 1, 2, 3, and 4)
6. Drug studies

VENTRICULAR TACHYCARDIA

Catheters
1. RV (pacing and recording)
2. HBE (recording)
3. CS or LV (possible; pacing and recording)

Procedures
1. Baseline conduction intervals
2. RV pacing
   A. From apex at two times diastolic threshold
      i. Incremental pacing (to 250 beats/min)
      ii. Extrastimulus technique (single, double, and triple; paced rate of 110 and 150 beats/min)
   B. From apex at five times diastolic threshold
      i. Extrastimulus technique (single, double, and triple; paced rate of 150 beats/min)
   C. From outflow tract at five times diastolic threshold
      i. Extrastimulus technique (single, double, and triple; paced rate of 150 beats/min)
3. LV (direct or from CS)
   A. Two times diastolic threshold
      i. Extrastimulus technique (single, double, and triple; paced rate of 150 beats/min)
4. Isoproterenol (repeat 2B, 2C, and 3)
5. During tachycardia (hemodynamically stable)
   A. Mapping of LV and RV
   B. Termination
      i. Burst overdrive pacing
      ii. Extrastimulus technique (single, double, and triple)
6. Drug studies

AV, atrioventricular; CS, coronary sinus; HBE, His-bundle electrogram; HRA, high right atrium; LV, left ventricle; RV right ventricle; VA, ventriculo-atrial.

tion laboratory, the right atrium is mapped through a standard electrode catheter and the left atrium is indirectly mapped through a coronary sinus catheter. The sequence and timing of retrograde atrial activation is compared with reference atrial electrograms from the high right atrium and low septal atrium, the latter from the His-bundle electrogram recording. It is important to confirm that retrograde atrial activation is indeed through an accessory AV connection rather than the normal His-Purkinje–AV node pathway. In the latter, the earliest site of retrograde atrial activity will appear in the His-bundle recording. Paraseptal bypass tracts may be difficult to distinguish from normal retrograde conduction. Intraoperative retrograde mapping is performed in a similar fashion during ventricular pacing, except that the atrial epicardial surface around the AV groove rather than the endocardial surface is mapped.

Studies suggest that electrophysiologically guided resection of myocardial scar markedly decreases the recurrence of ventricular tachyarrhythmias.[98–100] These areas are usually on the endocardial border zone of a myocardial scar, often a ventricular aneurysm. Preliminary mapping can be performed in the catheterization laboratory in some patients, with more detailed mapping at surgery.[152,153]

Only those patients with hemodynamically stable tachycardias can be mapped in the catheterization laboratory; 30% to 50% have tachycardias that are too rapid. Administration of an antiarrhythmic drug may sufficiently slow the tachycardias to permit mapping yet not alter the site of origin. The timing and morphology of ventricular electrograms from a mapping catheter are compared with those of multiple surface leads and a reference endocardial catheter, usually at the right ventricular apex. The earliest recorded presystolic ventricular electrogram, whether discrete or fragmented, locates the site of the tachycardia. In some patients, holodiastolic fragmented activity is recorded. This is thought to represent electric activity within the reentrant circuit. All catheter positions are confirmed by fluoroscopy in multiple planes. In patients whose ventricular tachycardia has multiple morphologies, an attempt should be made to map each form.

More detailed mapping is performed in the operating room on full cardiopulmonary bypass at a temperature of 37° to 38°C. Endocardial mapping is performed with a ring or hand-held electrode, with an interelectrode distance of 1 to 2 mm, through a ventriculotomy through an area of myocardial scar. If an aneurysm is present, it is first resected, and mapping is started at the border zone. The tachycardia is induced through a previously paced right ventricle pacing catheter, and mapping is performed under direct vision in a radial fashion around the ventriculotomy in successive circles 1 cm apart. Ventricular electrograms are compared with the right and left ventricle reference electrograms, recorded from plunge electrodes

inserted at the time of surgery; multiple surface leads are also recorded. Similar criteria are used for locating the site of origin as in the catheterization laboratory. Areas of origin are subsequently resected, and an attempt is made to reinduce the tachycardia. If inducible, mapping and resection are repeated.

Several limitations exist with these techniques. Programmed stimulation is successful in initiating ventricular tachycardia during surgery in only 80% of patients, despite preoperative induction in the catheterization laboratory. Limiting factors include cardiac temperature, presence of antiarrhythmic drugs, electrolyte imbalance, and anesthetic agents. Temperature is an important variable. Ventricular tachycardia can rarely be induced when the patient is hypothermic. Intraoperative studies should thus be performed with a cardiac temperature of 37° to 38°C. All antiarrhythmic drugs should be stopped at least four to five half-lives before surgery. Mapping requires a stable sustained monomorphic arrhythmia. Nonsustained ventricular tachycardia can be mapped if the morphology is constant but requires repeated induction. Rapid polymorphic tachycardias can rarely be accurately mapped. Because of these limitations, an attempt has been made to perform intraoperative mapping during normal sinus rhythm.[154] With this technique, endocardial areas showing fragmented electric activity are resected. Further investigation is needed to confirm this approach.

CONCLUSION

Invasive electrophysiologic testing is a valuable diagnostic and therapeutic tool. A variety of pacing and recording techniques are available to examine the cardiac electric system. Each study must be tailored to the individual patient's clinical needs. Table 7-16 summarizes our approach to the evaluation of the more common electrophysiologic disorders. These are often combined to assess multiple areas of the electric system with the same technique (e.g., evaluation of sinus and AV node function and initiation of supraventricular tachycardia with atrial pacing studies). In the hands of an experienced electrophysiologist, these techniques can be applied with minimal morbidity and facilitate the diagnosis and therapy of complex clinical situations.

References

1. Ross DL, Farre J, Bar FW, et al: Comprehensive clinical electrophysiologic studies in the investigation of documented tachycardias; time, staff, problems and costs. Circulation 1980;61:1010.

2. Dreifus LS: Clinical judgement is sufficient for the management of conduction defects. Cardiovasc Clin 1977;8:195.

3. Wu D, Rosen KM: Clinical judgment is not sufficient for the management of conduction defects. (Indications for diagnostic electrophysiologic studies.) Cardiovasc Clin 1977; 8:203.

4. Weiner I: Current applications of clinical electrophysiologic study in the diagnosis and treatment of cardiac arrhythmias. Am J Cardiol 1982;49:1287.

5. Scheinman MM, Morady F: Invasive cardiac electrophysiologic testing: The current state of the art. Circulation 1983;67:1169.

6. Simson MB: Use of signals in the terminal QRS complex to identify patients with ventricular tachycardia after myocardial infarction. Circulation 1981;64:235.

7. Shaw DB, Holman RR, Gowers JI: Survival in sinoatrial disorder. Br Med J 1980;1:139.

8. Narula OS: Atrioventricular conduction defects in patients with sinus bradycardia. Circulation 1974;44:1096.

9. Rosen KM, Loeb HS, Sinno MZ, et al: Cardiac conduction in patients with symptomatic sinus node disease. Circulation 1971;43:836.

10. Brodsky M, Wu D, Denes P, et al: Arrhythmias documented by 24-hour continuous electrocardiographic monitoring in 50 male medical students without apparent heart disease. Am J Cardiol 1977;39:390.

11. Agruss NS, Rosin EY, Adolph RJ, Fowler NO: Significance of chronic sinus bradycardia in elderly people. Circulation 1972;46:924.

12. Thormann J, Schwarz F, Ensslen R, Sesto M: Vagal tone, significance of electrophysiologic findings and clinical course in symptomatic sinus node dysfunction. Am Heart J 1978;95:725.

13. Gann D, Tolentino A, Samet P: Electrophysiologic evaluation of elderly patients with sinus bradycardia. Ann Intern Med 1979;90:24.

14. Reiffel JA, Bigger JT, Cramer M, Reid DS: Ability of Holter electrocardiographic recording and atrial stimulation to detect sinus nodal dysfunction in symptomatic and asymptomatic patients with sinus bradycardia. Am J Cardiol 1977; 40:189.

15. Strasberg B, Amat-Y-Leon F, Dhingra RC, et al: Natural history of chronic second degree atrioventricular nodal block. Circulation 1981;63:1043.

16. Amat-Y-Leon F, Dhingra R, Denes P, et al: The clinical spectrum of chronic HIS bundle block. Chest 1976;70:747.

17. Gupta PK, Lichstein E, Chadda KD: Chronic HIS bundle block: Clinical, electrocardiographic, electrophysiological and follow-up studies on 16 patients. Br Heart J 1976;38:1343.

18. Ranganathan N, Dhurandes R, Phillips JH, Wigle ED: HIS bundle electrogram in bundle-branch block. Circulation 1972;45:282.

19. Dhingra RC, Denes P, Wu D, et al: The significance of second degree atrioventricular block and bundle branch block: observations regarding site and type of block. Circulation 1974;49:638.

20. Zipes DP: Second degree atrioventricular block. Circulation 1979;60:465.

21. Mangiardi LM, Bonamini R, Conte M, et al: Bedside evaluation of atrioventricular block with narrow QRS complexes: usefulness of carotid sinus massage and atropine administration. Am J Cardiol 1982;49:1136.

22. Rosen KM, Rahimtoola SH, Gunnar RM: Pseudo AV block secondary to premature non-propagated HIS bundle depolarizations: documentation by HIS bundle electrocardiography. Circulation 1970;42:367.

23. Narula OS, Scherlag BJ, Javier RP, et al: Analysis of the AV conduction defect in complete heart block utilizing HIS bundle electrograms. Circulation 1970;41:437.

24. Narula OS, Narula JT: Junctional pacemakers in man: response to overdrive suppression with and without parasympathetic blockade. Circulation 1978;57:880.

25. Schneider JF, Thomas HE, Sorlie P, et al: Comparative features of newly acquired left and right bundle branch block in the general population: the Framingham study. Am J Cardiol 1981;47:931.

26. Fleg JL, Das DH, Lakatta EG: Right bundle branch block: long term prognosis in apparently healthy men. J Am Coll Cardiol 1983;1:887.

27. McAnulty JH, Rahimtoola SH, Murphy E, et al: Natural history of "high risk" bundle branch block. N Engl J Med 1982;307: 137.

28. Scheinman MM, Peters RW, Sauve MJ, et al: Value of the H-Q interval in patients with bundle branch block and the role of prophylactic permanent pacing. Am J Cardiol 1982;50:1316.

29. Rosen KM, Dhingra RC, Wyndham CR: Significance of H-V interval in 515 patients with chronic bifascicular block. Am J Cardiol 45:405 1980. Abstract.

30. Dhingra RC, Wyndham C, Baurnfeind R, et al: Significance of block distal to the HIS bundle induced by atrial pacing in patients with chronic bifascicular block. Circulation 1979; 60:1455.

31. Dhingra RC, Wyndham C, Amat-Y-Leon F, et al: Incidence and site of atrioventricular block in patients with chronic bifascicular block. Circulation 1979;59:238.

32. Peters RW, Scheinman MM, Dhingra R, et al: Serial electrophysiologic studies in patients with chronic bundle branch block. Circulation 1982;65:1480.

33. Dhingra RC, Denes P, Wu D, et al: Syncope in patients with chronic bifascicular block: significance, causative mechanisms, and clinical implications. Ann Intern Med 1974;81: 302.

34. Scheinman M, Weiss A, Kunkel F: His bundle recordings in patients with bundle branch block and transient neurologic symptoms. Circulation 1973;48:322.

35. Altschuler H, Fisher JD, Furman S: Significance of isolated H-V interval prolongation in symptomatic patients without documented heart block. Am Heart J 1979;97:19.

36. DeGuzman M, Rahimtoola SH: What is the role of pacemakers in patients with coronary artery disease and conduction abnormalities. Cardiovasc Clin 1983;13:191.

37. Lie KI, Wellens HJ, Schuilenberg RM, et al: Factors influencing prognosis of bundle branch block complicating acute antero-septal infarction. Circulation 1974;50:935.

38. Harper R, Hunt D, Vohra J, et al: His bundle electrogram in patients with acute myocardial infarction complicated by atrioventricular or intraventricular conduction disturbances. Br Heart J 1974;37:705.

39. Gould L, Reddy CV, Kim SG, Oh KC: His bundle electrogram in patients with acute myocardial infarction. Pacing Clin Electrophysiol 1979;2:428.

40. Wu D, Denes P, Amat-Y-Leon F, et al: Clinical, electrocardiographic and electrophysiologic observations in patients with paroxysmal supraventricular tachycardia. Am J Cardiol 1978;41:1045.

41. Lloyd EA, Hauer RN, Zipes DP, et al: Syncope and ventricular tachycardia in patients with ventricular pre-excitation. Am J Cardiol 1983;52:79.

42. Klein GJ, Bashare TM, Sellers TD, et al: Ventricular fibrillation in the Wolff-Parkinson-White syndrome. N Engl J Med 1979;301:1080.

43. Morady F, Sledge C, Shen E, et al: Electrophysiologic testing in the management of patients with the Wolff-Parkinson-White syndrome and atrial fibrillation. Am J Cardiol 1983; 51:1623.

44. Strasberg B, Ashley WW, Wyndham CR, et al: Treadmill exercise testing in the Wolff-Parkinson-White syndrome. Am J Cardiol 1980;45:742.

45. Wellens HJ, Braat S, Brugada P, et al: Use of procainamide in patients with the Wolff-Parkinson-White syndrome to disclose a short refractory period of the accessory pathway. Am J Cardiol 1982;50:1087.

46. Wellens HJ, Bar FW, Lie KI: The value of the electrocardiogram in the differential diagnosis of a tachycardia with a widened QRS complex. Am J Med 1978;64:27.

47. Josephson ME: Paroxysmal supraventricular tachycardia: an electrophysiologic approach. Am J Cardiol 1978;41:1123.

48. Kastor JA, Horowitz LN, Harken AH, Josephson ME: Clinical electrophysiology of ventricular tachycardia. N Engl J Med 1981;304:1004.

49. Cobb LA, Baum RS, Alvarez H, Schaffer WA: Resuscitation from out-of-hospital ventricular fibrillation: 4 years of follow-up. Circulation 1975;III(Suppl 52):223.

50. Eisenberg MS, Hallstrom A, Bergner L: Long term survival after out-of-hospital cardiac arrest. N Engl J Med 1982;22:1340.

51. Iseri LT, Humphrey SB, Siner EJ: Prehospital bradyasystolic cardiac arrest. Ann Intern Med 1978;88:741.

52. Myerburg RJ, Conde CA, Sung RJ, et al: Clinical, electrophysiologic and hemodynamic profile of patients resusciated from prehospital cardiac arrest. Am J Med 1980;68:568.

53. Ruskin JN, DiMarco JP Garan H: Out-of-hospital cardiac arrest: electrophysiologic observations and selection of long term antiarrhythmic therapy. N Engl J Med 1980;303:607.

54. Josephson ME, Horowitz LN, Spielman SR, Greenspan AM: Electrophysiologic and hemodynamic studies in patients resuscitated from cardiac arrest. Am J Cardiol 1980;46:948.

55. Morady F, Scheinman MM, Hess DS, et al: Electrophysiologic testing in the management of survivors of out-of-hospital cardiac arrest. Am J Cardiol 1983;51:85.

56. Longstreth WT, Inui TS, Cobb L, Copass MK: Neurologic recovery after out-of-hospital cardiac arrest. Ann Intern Med 1983;98:588.

57. Panidis IP, Morganroth J: Sudden death in hospitalized patients: cardiac rhythm disturbances detected by ambulatory electrocardiographic monitoring. J Am Coll Cardiol 1983; 2:798.

58. Pratt CM, Francis MJ, Luck JC, et al: Analysis of ambulatory electrocardiograms in 15 patients during spontaneous ventricular fibrillation with special reference to preceding arrhythmic events. J Am Coll Cardiol 1983;2:789.

59. Myerburg RJ, Conde C, Sheps DS, et al: Antiarrhythmic drug therapy in survivors of prehospital cardiac arrest: comparison of effects on chronic ventricular arrhythmias and recurrent cardiac arrest. Circulation 1979;59:855.

60. Graboys TB, Lown B, Podrid PJ, DeSilva R: Longterm survival of patients with malignant ventricular arrhythmia treated with antiarrhythmic drugs. Am J Cardiol 1982;50:437.

61. Winkle R: Measuring antiarrhythmic drug efficacy by suppression of asymptomatic ventricular arrhythmias. Ann Intern Med 1979;91:480.

62. Peter T, Hamer A, Weiss D, Mandel W: Sudden death survivors: experience with long-term empiric therapy with amiodarone. Circulation 1981;64(Suppl IV):36. Abstract.

63. Waxman HL, Buxton AE, Sadowski LM, Josephson ME: The response to procainamide during electrophysiologic study for sustained ventricular tachyarrhythmias predicts the response to other medications. Circulation 1983;67:30.

64. Velebit V, Podrid P, Lown B, et al: Aggravation and provocation of ventricular arrhythmias by antiarrhythmic drugs. Circulation 1982;65:886.

65. Ruskin JN, Garan H, Dimarco JP, Kelly E: Electrophysiologic testing in survivors of prehospital cardiac arrest. Am J Cardiol 1982;49:958. Abstract.

66. Benditt DG, Benson DW, Klein GJ, et al: Prevention of recurrent sudden cardiac arrest: role of provocative electropharmacologic testing. J Am Coll Cardiol 1983;2:418.

67. Vandepol CJ, Farshidi A, Spielman SR, et al: Incidence and clinical significance of induced ventricular tachycardia. Am J Cardiol 1980;45:725.

68. Naccarelli GV, Prystowksy EN, Jackman WM, et al: Role of electrophysiologic testing in managing patients who have ventricular tachycardia unrelated to coronary artery disease. Am J Cardiol 1982;50:165.

69. Livelli FD, Bigger JT, Reiffel JA, et al: Response to programmed ventricular stimulation: Sensitivity, specificity, and relation to heart disease. Am J Cardiol 1982;50:452.

70. Mann DE, Luch JC, Griffin JC, et al: Induction of clinical ventricular tachycardia using programmed stimulation: value of third and fourth extrastimuli. Am J Cardiol 1983; 52:501.

71. Fisher JD: Role of electrophysiologic testing in the diagnosis and treatment of patients with known and suspected bradycardias and tachycardias. Prog Cardiovasc Dis 1981;24:25.

72. Kehoe RF, Moran JM, Zheutin T, Lesch M: Electrophysiological study to direct therapy in survivors of pre-hospital ventricular fibrillation. Am J Cardiol 1982;49:928. Abstract.

73. Mason JW, Swerdlow CD, Winkle RA, et al: Programmed ventricular stimulation in predicting vulnerability to ventricular arrhythmias and their response to antiarrhythmic therapy. Am Heart J 1982;103:633.

74. Roy D, Waxman HL, Kienzle MG, et al: Clinical characteristics and long-term follow-up in 119 survivors of cardiac arrest: relation to inducibility at electrophysiologic testing. Am J Cardiol 1983;52:969.

75. Brugada P, Adbollah H, Heddle B, Wellens HJ: Results of a ventricular stimulation protocol using a maximum of 4 pre-

mature stimuli in patients without documented or suspected ventricular arrhythmias. Am J Cardiol 1983;52:1214.

76. Mason JW, Winkle RA: Accuracy of the ventricular tachycardia-induction study for predicting long-term efficacy and inefficacy of antiarrhythmic drugs. N Engl J Med 1980; 303:1073.

77. Horowitz LN, Spielman SR, Greenspan AM, Josephson ME: Role of programmed stimulation in assessing vulnerability to ventricular arrhythmias. Am Heart J 1982;103:604.

78. Schoenfeld MH, McGovern B, Garan H, et al: Long-term follow-up of patients with ventricular tachycardia or fibrillation with no inducible arrhythmia during programmed cardiac stimulation. J Am Coll Cardiol 1983;1:606. Abstract.

79. Kapoor WN, Karpf M, Wieand S, et al: A prospective evaluation and follow-up of patients with syncope. N Engl J Med 1983;309:197.

80. DiMarco JP, Garan H, Harthorne JW, Ruskin JN: Intracardiac electrophysiologic techniques in recurrent syncope of unknown cause. Ann Intern Med 1981;95:542.

81. Gulamhusein S, Nacarelli GV, Ko PT, et al: Value and limitations of clinical electrophysiologic study in assessment of patients with unexplained syncope. Am J Med 1982;73:700.

82. Hess DS, Morady F, Scheinman MM: Electrophysiologic testing in the evaluation of patients with syncope of undetermined origin. Am J Cardiol 1982;50:1309.

83. Tonkin AM, Heddle WF, Tornos P: Intermittent atrioventricular block: procainamide administration as a provocative test. Aust NZ J Med 1978;8:594.

84. Zaher C, Hamer A, Peter T, Mandel W: The use of intravenous procainamide to evaluate the potential etiology of syncope in patients with bundle branch block. Pacing Clin Electrophysiol 1983;6:A-104.

85. LaBarre A, Strauss HC, Scheinman MM, et al: Electrophysiologic effects of disopyramide phosphate on sinus node function in patients with sinus node dysfunction. Circulation 1979;59:226.

86. Wu D, Amat-Y-Leon F, Simpson RJ, et al: Electrophysiological studies with multiple drugs in patients with atrioventricular re-entrant tachycardias utilizing an extranodal pathway. Circulation 1977;56:727.

87. Bauernfiend RA, Wyndham CR, Dhingra RC, et al: Serial electrophysiologic testing of multiple drugs in patients with atrioventricular nodal re-entrant paroxysmal tachycardia. Circulation 1980;62:1341.

88. Kruse I, Arnman K, Conradson TB, Rydén L: A comparison of the acute and long-term hemodynamic effects of ventricular inhibited and atrial synchronous ventricular inhibited pacing. Circulation 1982;65:846.

89. Weiner I: Pacing techniques in the treatment of tachycardias. Ann Intern Med 1980;93:326.

90. Kowey PR, Engel TR: Overdrive pacing for ventricular tachyarrhythmias: a reassessment. Ann Intern Med 1983;99:651.

91. Wells JL, MacLean WA, James TN, Waldo AL: Characterization of atrial flutter: studies in man after open heart surgery using fixed atrial electrodes. Circulation 1979;60:665.

92. Roy D, Waxman HL, Buxton AE, et al: Termination of ventricular tachycardia: Role of tachycardia cycle length. Am J Cardiol 1982;50:1346.

93. Fisher JD, Kim SG, Furman S, Matos J: Role of implantable pacemakers in control of recurrent ventricular tachycardia. Am J Cardiol 1982;49:194.

94. Mirowski M, Reid PR, Winkle RA, et al: Mortality in patients with implanted automatic defibrillators. Ann Intern Med 1983;98:585.

95. Klein GJ, Sealy WC, Pritchett EL, et al: Cryosurgical ablation of the atrioventricular node—His bundle: Long term follow-up and properties of the junctional pacemaker. Circulation 1980;61:8.

96. Holmes DR, Osborn MJ, Gersh B, et al: The Wolff-Parkinson-White syndrome: a surgical approach. Mayo Clin Proc 1982; 57:345.

97. Mason JW, Stinson EB, Winkle RA, et al: Relative efficacy of blind left ventricular aneurysm resection for the treatment of recurrent ventricular tachycardia. Am J Cardiol 1982; 49:241.

98. Mason JW, Stinson EB, Winkle RA, et al: Surgery for ventricular tachycardia: efficacy of left ventricular aneurysm resection compared with operation guided by electrical activation mapping. Circulation 1982;65:1148.

99. Garan H, Ruskin JN, DiMarco JP, et al: Electrophysiologic studies before and after myocardial revascularization in patients with life-threatening ventricular arrhythmias. Am J Cardiol 1983;51:519.

100. Josephson ME, Harken AH, Horowitz LN: Long-term results of endocardial resection for sustained ventricular tachycardia in coronary disease patients. Am Heart J 1982;104:51.

101. Fontaine G, Guirandon G, Frank R, et al: Surgical management of ventricular tachycardia unrelated to myocardial ischemia or infarction. Am J Cardiol 1982;49:397.

102. Gallagher JJ, Svenson RH, Kasell JH, et al: Catheter technique for closed-chest ablation of the atrioventricular conduction system. N Engl J Med 1982;306:194.

103. Wood DL, Hammill SC, Holmes DR, et al: Catheter ablation of the atrioventricular conduction system in patients with supraventricular tachycardia. Mayo Clin Proc 1983;58:791.

104. Weber H, Schmitz L: Catheter technique for closed-chest ablation of an accessory atrioventricular pathway. N Engl J Med 1983;308:653.

105. Gillette PC, Garson A, Porter CJ: Junctional automatic ectopic tachycardia: new proposed treatment by transcatheter His bundle ablation. Am Heart J 1983;106:619.

106. Hartler GO: Electrode catheter ablation of refractory focal ventricular tachycardia. J Am Coll Cardiol 1983;2:1107.

107. Saxon LA, Stevenson WG, Fonarow GC, et al: Transesophageal echocardiography during radiofrequency catheter ablation of ventricular tachycardia. Am J Cardiol 1993;72:658.

108. Swerdlow CD, Winkle RA, Mason JW: Determinants of survival in patients with ventricular tachyarrhythmias. N Engl J Med 1983;308:1436.

109. Hamer A, Vohra J, Hunt D, Sloman G: Prediction of sudden death by electrophysiologic studies in high risk patients surviving acute myocardial infarction. Am J Cardiol 1982; 50:223.

110. Richards DA, Cody DV, Denniss AR, et al: Ventricular electrical instability: a predictor of death after myocardial infarction. Am J Cardiol 1983;51:75.

111. Marchlinski FE, Buxton AE, Waxman HL, Josephson ME: Indentifying patients at risk of sudden death after myocar-

dial infarction: value of the response to programmed stimulation, degree of ventricular ectopic activity and severity of left ventricular dysfunction. Am J Cardiol 1983;52:1190.

112. Kowey PR, Folland ED, Parisi AF, Lown B: Programmed electrical stimulation of the heart in coronary artery disease. Am J Cardiol 1983;51:531.

113. Buxton AE, Waxman HL, Marchlinski FE, Josephson ME: Electrophysiologic studies in nonsustained ventricular tachycardia: relation to underlying heart disease. Am J Cardiol 1983;52:985.

114. Ruskin JN, Caracta AR, Batsford WP, et al: Electrophysiologic effects of diazepam in man. Clin Res 1974;22:302A.

115. Nattel S, Rinkenberger RL, Lehrman LL, Zipes DP: Therapeutic blood lidocaine concentrations after local anesthesia for cardiac electrophysiologic studies. N Engl J Med 1979;301: 418.

116. Bombardini T, Picano E, Magagnini E: Reduced time for femoral venipuncture by simple bedside application of valsalva maneuver (the poor cardiologist's smart needle). Am J Cardiol 1994;73:1023.

117. Denys BG, Uretsky BF, Reddy PS: Untrasound-assisted cannulation of the internal jugular vein. Circulation 1993;87: 1557.

118. Dimarco JP, Garan H, Ruskin JN: Complications in patients undergoing cardiac electrophysiologic procedures. Ann Intern Med 1982;97:490.

119. Littleford PO, Curry RC, Schwartz KM, Pepine CJ: Clinical evaluation of a new temporary atrial pacing catheter: results in 100 patients. Am Heart J 1984;107:237.

120. Reiffel JA, Gang E, Gliklich J, et al: The human sinus node electrogram: a transvenous catheter technique and a comparison of directly measured and indirectly estimated sinoatrial conduction time in adults. Circulation 1980;62:1324.

121. Josephson ME, Scharf DL, Kastor JA, Kitchen JG: Atrial endocardial activation in man. Am J Cardiol 1977;39:972.

122. Breithardt G, Seipel L: Recording of left atrial potentials from pulmonary artery in man. Br Heart J 1980;43:689.

123. Prystowsky EN, Pritchett EL, Gallagher JJ: Origin of the atrial electrogram recorded from the esophagus. Circulation 1980;61:1017.

124. Guimond C, Puech P: Intra-His bundle blocks (102 cases). Eur J Cardiol 1976;4:481.

125. Davis LM, Byth K, Lau KC, Uther JB, Richards DAB, Ross DL: Accuracy of various methods of localization of the orifice of the coronary sinus at electrophysiologic study. Am J Cardiol 1992;70:343.

126. Chiang CE, Chen SA, Yang CR, et al: Major coronary sinus abnormalities: identification of occurrence and significance in radiofrequency ablation of supraventricular tachycardia. Am Heart J 1994;127:1279.

127. Josephson ME, Seides SF: Clinical cardiac electrophysiology; techniques and interpretations. Philadelphia: Lea & Febiger, 1979:18.

128. Castellanos A, Castillo C, Agha A: Contribution of His bundle recording to the understanding of clinical arrhythmias. Am J Cardiol 1971;28:499.

129. Gallagher JJ, Damato AN: Techniques of recording His bundle activity in man. In: Grossman W, ed. Cardiac catheterization and angiography. Philadelphia: Lea & Febiger, 1980:283.

130. Josephson ME, Seides SF: Clinical cardiac electrophysiology: techniques and interpretations. Philadelphia: Lea & Febiger, 1979:23.

131. Narula OS, Scherlag BJ, Samet P, Javier RP: Atrioventricular block: localization and classification by His bundle recordings. Am J Med 1971;50:146.

132. Rosen KM: Evaluation of cardiac conduction in the cardiac catheterization laboratory. Am J Cardiol 1972;30:701.

133. Akhtar M, Damato AN, Batsford WP, et al: A comparative analysis of antegrade and retrograde conduction patterns in man. Circulation 1975;52:766.

134. Denes P, Wu D, Dhingra R, et al: The effects of cycle length on cardiac refractory periods in man. Circulation 1974; 49:32.

135. Schuilenberg RM, Durrer D: Conduction disturbances within the His bundle. Circulation 1972;45:612.

136. Hoffman BF, Rosen MR: Cellular mechanisms for cardiac arrhythmias. Circ Res 1981;49:1.

137. Mandel WJ, Hayakawa H, Danzig R, Marcus HS: Evaluation of sinoatrial node function in man by overdrive suppression. Circulation 1971;44:59.

138. Strauss HC, Saroff AL, Bigger JT, Giardina EG: Premature atrial stimulation as a key to the understanding of sinoatrial conduction in man. Circulation 1973;47:86.

139. Narula OS, Shanto N, Vasquez M, et al: A new method for measurement of sinoatrial conduction time in man. Circulation 1978;58:706.

140. Hariman RJ, Krongrad E, Boxer RA, et al: Method for recording electrical activity of the sinoatrial node and automatic atrial foci during cardiac catheterization in human subjects. Am J Cardiol 1980;45:775.

141. Juillard A, Guillerm F, Chuong HV, et al: Sinus node electrogram recording in 59 patients: comparison with simultaneous estimation of sinoatrial conduction using premature atrial stimulation. Br Heart J 1983;50:75.

142. Jose AD, Collison D: The normal range and determinants of the intrinsic heart rate in man. Cardiovasc Res 19704:160 1970.

143. Denes P, Wu D, Dhingra R, et al: The effects of cycle length on cardiac refractory periods in man. Circulation 1974;49:32.

144. Josephson ME, Seides SF: Clinical cardiac electrophysiology: techniques and interpretations. Philadelphia: Lea & Febiger, 1979:39.

145. Fisher JD, Ostrow E, Kim SG, Matos JA: Ultrarapid single-capture train stimulation for termination of ventricular tachycardia. Am J Cardiol 1983;51:1334.

146. Gardner MJ, Waxman HL, Buxton AE, et al: Termination of ventricular tachycardia: evaluation of a new pacing method. Am J Cardiol 1982;50:1338.

147. Robertson JF, Cain ME, Horowitz LN, et al: Anatomic and electrophysiologic correlates of ventricular tachycardia requiring left ventricular stimulation. Am J Cardiol 1981;48: 263.

148. Morady F, Hess D, Scheinman MM: Electrophysiologic drug testing in patients with malignant ventricular arrhythmias: importance of stimulation at more than one ventricular site. Am J Cardiol 1982;50:1055.

149. Ross DL, Sze DY, Keffe DL, et al: Antiarrhythmic drug combinations in the treatment of ventricular tachycardia. Circulation 1982;66:1205.

150. Duffy CE, Swiryn S, Bauernfeind RA, et al: Inducible sus-

tained ventricular tachycardia refractory to individual class I drugs: effect of adding a second class I drug. Am Heart J 1983;106:450.

151. Hammer AW, Finerman WB, Peter T, Mandel WJ: Disparity between the clinical and electrophysiologic effects of amiodarone in the treatment of recurrent ventricular tachyarrhythmias. Am Heart J 1981;102:992.

152. Josephson ME, Horowitz LN, Farshidi A, et al: Recurrent sustained ventricular tachycardia. II. Endocardial mapping. Circulation 1978;57:440.

153. Josephson ME, Horowitz LN, Spielman SR, et al: Comparison of endocardial catheter mapping with intraoperative mapping of ventricular tachycardia. Circulation 1980;61:395.

154. Weiner I, Mindich B, Pitchon R: Fragmented endocardial electrical activity in patients with ventricular tachycardia: a new guide to surgical therapy. Am Heart J 1984;107:86.

Cardiac Arrhythmias, 3rd edition, edited by William J. Mandel.
J. B. Lippincott Company, Philadelphia © 1995.

8

Paul C. Gillette • David S. Buckles • Christopher L. Case
Derek A. Fyfe • Ashby B. Taylor • Henry B. Wiles • Vicki L. Zeigler

The Use of Electrophysiologic Testing in Pediatric Patients

Cardiac dysrhythmias, which have been considered rare in children, are now recognized frequently, probably because of three factors: (1) increased awareness, (2) improved detection techniques, and (3) a true increase in incidence secondary to successful cardiac surgical procedures.

The tools with which clinicians may detect and treat these dysrhythmias have improved manyfold. Noninvasive techniques, such as ambulatory, transtelephonic, and exercise electrocardiography, and inpatient telemetric monitoring have been useful.[1] Fetal echocardiography has also increased detection. Invasive electrophysiologic testing, however, has been the most important tool, both in studying the mechanisms of dysrhythmias and in their day-to-day management.[2] The techniques of electrophysiologic testing are similar for children and adults, but equipment, techniques, and indications differ. This chapter highlights these differences and gives an overall picture of pediatric electrophysiologic studies (EPS).

TECHNIQUES

Electrophysiologic studies are carried out by the percutaneous sheath technique.[3] Slightly longer sheaths can be used for the left femoral vein to ease the transition into the inferior vena cava. Most catheters are introduced into the femoral veins. The same percutaneous sheath technique is used to introduce a catheter into the coronary sinus by way of the brachial vein (Fig. 8-1).[4] Subclavian, internal jugular, and axillary venipuncture have also been used but may carry a greater risk and are usually reserved for patients in whom the more distal veins are not usable. Anticoagulation is used only in patients with right to left shunts or when catheters are positioned in the left atrium or ventricle. Antibiotic prophylaxis is not used. In patients undergoing radio frequency catheter ablation, 150 U/kg of heparin are given. Activated clotting times are measured in the electrophysiology laboratory and are maintained for approximately 320 seconds. At the end of the procedure, the heparin is not reversed but is allowed to wear off slowly. Antibiotic prophylaxis, Ancef, 12.5 mg/hg kg, is given for catheter ablation cases. Xylocaine 0.5% is injected subcutaneously at each puncture site in the smallest amount possible to produce analgesia. Serum xylocaine concentrations are measured 1 hour after injection to ensure proper amounts are administered.[5]

Sedation is necessary for pediatric EPS. Each sedative affects the patient's electrophysiology.[6] We usually use meperidine and promethazine for premedication and ketamine for additional sedation. Ketamine is short acting and does not depress respiration. Versed may be used in addi-

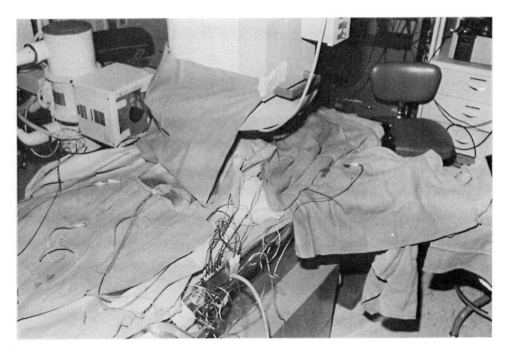

Figure 8-1. View from the left leg of a pediatric patient undergoing a four-catheter electrophysiology study. Two electrode catheters have been introduced into the right femoral vein, one in the left femoral vein and one in the left brachial vein. A plastic cannula is in the left femoral artery. The catheters are attached into junction boxes. Posterior, anterior, and lateral x-ray equipment is also demonstrated.

tion in very small doses. In patients younger than 1 year of age, general anesthesia is necessary for catheter ablation or pacemaker implantation.

A 12- to 24-channel oscilloscopic recorder should be used. Instant developing paper or paper that is developed later by photographic techniques are both adequate. Electrical isolation and elimination of 60-Hz and radio frequency interference are critical. A tape or disc recorder to back up the physiological recorder is necessary. We use a 24-channel system that digitizes the electrograms at the patient's bedside and passes them to the recorder by fiber optics, thus minimizing interference. The data can be stored intermittently on paper and continuously on optical disc. The data can be viewed continuously on one screen and "frozen" on a separate screen. Electronic calipers allow instantaneous measurements. The data can be reanalyzed at a separate workstation. Several other semiautomatic systems are available. Stimulation and automated measurement are carried out by a custom software system.[7] Several commercial stimulation systems are available.

A second, more simple stimulator is kept as a backup and to use for portable studies (Fig. 8-2). Two defibrillators are in the laboratory. In high-risk cases, radiolucent patches are prepositioned for rapid defibrillation or transcutaneous pacing.

CATHETERS

The catheters used for pediatric EPS differ in French size and electrode spacing. We use numbers 4, 5, 6, and 7 French catheters with 1- to 5-mm electrode spacing. For mapping, we use six French catheters with up to 12 electrodes spaced at 2, 5, 2, 5, and 2, 5 mm, or at 2, 2 mm (Fig. 8-3). We record between the 2 mm spacings in a bipolar fashion. Because the catheters do not have lumens, we use two sidearm sheaths that are one French size greater than their catheters for fluid, drug, and sedation infusion. A small plastic arterial cannula is used in each patient for blood pressure monitoring and arterial blood sampling.

In general, long sheaths that reach the heart are used only when transseptal puncture is used to reach the left atrium. In this case, the sheath is the same size as the catheter (usually number 7 French). Continuous flushing is not used. Each time the catheter is withdrawn, careful flushing is performed by the physician. Each such patient is fully heparinized.

Transseptal puncture is performed under biplane fluoroscopy with continuous pressure monitoring. The coronary sinus catheter is positioned first and outlines the posterior wall of the heart in the lateral projection. If it is positioned through the superior vena cava (SVC), the SVC part of the catheter delineates the position of the aorta in the lateral projection in normal hearts.

In the posterior–anterior projection, the J of the coronary sinus catheter delineates the lower border of the safe puncture zone. The other electrode catheters are usually withdrawn because they get in the way of the puncture. A catheter is not routinely placed in the aortic root. Puncture is otherwise performed by standard techniques. Heparinization is not used until the long sheath is documented to be in the left atrium, that is, red blood is withdrawn and there is a clear pressure waveform. On occasion, we have performed transseptal puncture after

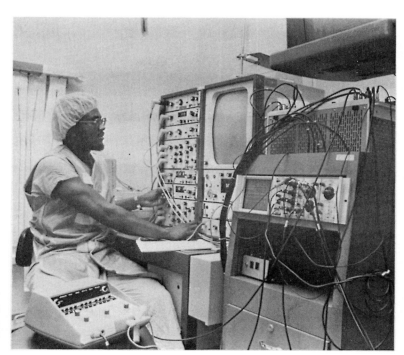

Figure 8-2. Demonstration of recording equipment for pediatric electrophysiology study. Data are recorded on paper from an oscillographic recorder, on magnetic tape, and on a storage oscilloscope. The simple stimulator is in the foreground.

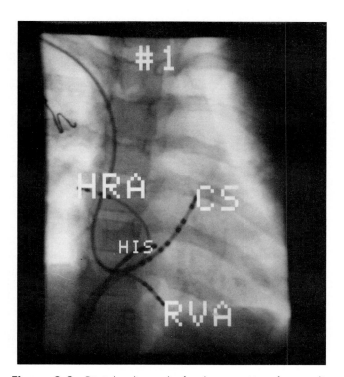

Figure 8-3. Digital radiograph of catheter positions for a pediatric electrophysiology study of supraventricular tachycardia. Four catheters have been introduced, three from the femoral veins positioned at the high right atrium, the His bundle area, and the right ventricular apex. The fourth catheter was introduced from the right brachial vein and is positioned into the coronary sinus.

heparinization when a left-sided pathway is found late. We have used standard transseptal sheaths, although a variety of shapes and lengths are available.

Standard, commercially available junction boxes are used to connect the patient to a standard physiologic recorder. A recording is made of each maneuver, and a compact disc (CD) read-only memory (ROM) is used to record any transient event. Biplane fluoroscopy is used to position the catheters, and biplane digital images are used to document catheter positions for later comparisons to EPS recordings. Certain catheter positions can be marked with a felt-tip pen on the fluoroscopy screen for later use.

Angiographic delineation of the coronary sinus, either directly or by left coronary artery angiography, is useful when the coronary sinus is difficult to enter or when it is necessary to enter the posterior descending vein.

Full resuscitation equipment is available and is tested frequently. A pulse oximeter is monitored continuously.

Electrophysiologic studies are frequently carried out during hemodynamic catheterization and angiography. Pressures and oxygen saturation are frequently recorded before EPS, but angiography is always deferred because of its possible effect on the patient's physiology.

AUTOMATION

We have designed an automated system to carry out each of our stimulation and measurement protocols.[8-10] Patient information is entered, and the initial protocol is selected (e.g., sinus node recovery time). The initial stimulation cycle length and decrement cycle length are selected, and the protocol in automaticity is carried out and measured. The recorder and a storage oscilloscope are automatically controlled. The results are immediately presented in tabular and graphic form. Tachycardia or bradycardia are automatically detected, and treatment options are presented to the operator.

Each new protocol is begun by the operator. The measured points on electrograms that were selected by the system are shown to the operator for confirmation for interactive changes with movable cursors (Fig. 8-4). Measurements are made of the same points that were hand measured (Fig. 8-5). At the end of the procedure, a report is prepared and added to the patient's chart. Each report is stored in a data base and indexed to an overall clinical data base for retrieval.

This system has greatly shortened the time required for our studies and has improved their reproducibility.

INDICATIONS

An EPS should be performed when any information that is clinically needed cannot be obtained by noninvasive means or when a therapeutic procedure is needed. Patients with recurrent supraventricular tachycardia are the most frequently studied in our laboratory.[11] The mechanisms of supraventricular tachycardia are more varied in pediatric patients. Wolff-Parkinson-White (WPW) syndrome makes up 44% of all cases; atrial automatic focus, 10%; and junctional automatic focus, 4%.[12] Atrioventricular (AV) nodal reentry makes up only 30% of our supraventricular tachycardia cases. Determination of the mechanism not only directs drug therapy but often clarifies the choice of pacemaker and surgical or catheter ablative procedures.

Ventricular tachycardia makes up only 20% of pediatric tachycardias seen in the pediatric electrophysiology laboratory.[13] Five situations account for most cases of ventricular tachycardia: (1) infants with tumors, (2) adolescents who have undergone surgery for congenital heart disease, (3) patients with arrhythmogenic right ventricular dysplasia, (4) patients with mild to severe cardiomyopathy, and (5) patients with subacute myocarditis.[14–16] Angiography is usually performed in all of these studies, except in patients with supraventricular tachycardia if two-dimensional and Doppler echocardiograms are normal.

In our experience, almost half of biopsy studies of the right ventricle are abnormal in outpatients with ventricular dysrhythmias. Most have findings undistinguishable from chronic dilated cardiomyopathy. Ten percent, however, have findings of subacute myocarditis, and about half

of these respond fully to treatment with corticosteroids and do not require antiarrhythmic treatment. Subsequent biopsies are normal.

Recently, catheter ablation has become possible for ventricular tachycardia. The best candidates are those with structurally normal hearts and right ventricular outflow tract ventricular tachycardia. Patients with left ventricular and posterior fascicular ventricular tachycardia have had successful results as well. Patients with arrhythmogenic right ventricular dysplasia and postoperative ventricular tachycardia have also had success, although long-term follow-up reports are not yet available.

In each tachycardia study, a thorough evaluation of sinus node, atrial, AV nodal, and His–Purkinje function is performed first. Tachycardia induction protocols are similar to those in adults. We induce only two premature ventricular contractions (PVCs) in patients who have never had documented ventricular tachycardia. In those with previously documented tachycardia, we use as many as three PVCs and carefully compare induced ventricular tachycardia to clinical ventricular tachycardia.

Drugs such as atropine and isoproterenol may be necessary to induce tachycardia. A tachycardia study, either supraventricular or ventricular, cannot be considered negative until isoproterenol infusion is performed. In addition, each patient with antegrade conduction over an accessory pathway must have isoproterenol infusion to test the properties of the pathway. Other drugs such as digoxin and propranolol may be given to predict clinical efficacy.[17] Repeat drug studies are done by reinducing catheters on another day.

Mapping is done with up to 21 channels using closely spaced bipolar and sometimes unipolar electrograms displayed on the storage oscilloscope and paper recorder (Figs. 8-6 and 8-7).

Functional and anatomic properties of the arrhythmogenic focus or reentrant circuit are considered together with the patient's previous clinical course and any other heart disease.[18–20] During the procedure, the best treatment (e.g., medication, pacing, catheter ablation, surgery) is tentatively identified. If pacing or ablation is chosen and parental permission has been obtained, treatment may be done at that time. If pharmacologic therapy is chosen, a drug may be given intravenously and arrhythmia induction again attempted.

SYNCOPE

Patients with syncope that is not caused by an autonomic or neurologic cause require a complete evaluation, including testing of their sinus nodes and conduction systems and inducibility of supraventricular or ventricular tachy-

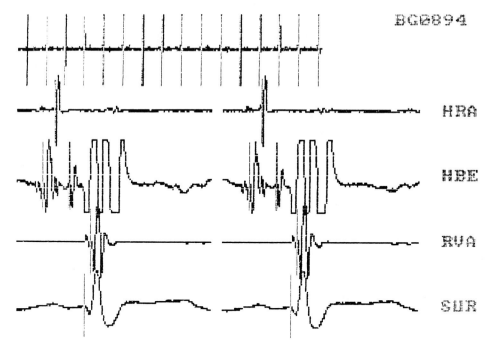

Figure 8-4. Print of a computer screen measuring resting intervals during a pediatric electrophysiology study. The case number is displayed in the upper right-hand corner. The high right atrial electrograms used to measure the resting cycle length are displayed at slow sweep speed on top. Two beats are presented as measured from high right atrium (HRA), His bundle electrogram (HBE), right ventricular apex (RVA), and surface electrocardiogram. Cursors can be seen at the beginning of the high right atrial depolarization, lower right atrial depolarization, His bundle depolarization, right ventricular apex, and surface electrocardiogram. These cursors are placed by the computer software and confirmed by the operator. The operator can move the cursors if the necessary. A low right atrial rhythm is demonstrated.

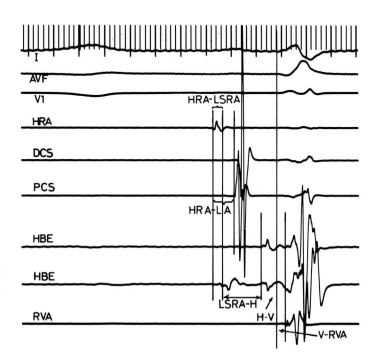

Figure 8-5. Demonstration of hand measurement of intracardiac electrophysiology intervals from the high right atrium to the low septal right atrium (HRA-LSRA), from the high right atrium to the left atrium (HRA-LA), AV node conduction time (LSRA-H), His Purkinje conduction time (H-V), and right bundle branch conduction time (V-RVA). Also displayed are surface leads I, aVF, and V1. *DCS*, distal coronary sinus; *PCS*, proximal coronary sinus, *HBE*, His bundle electrogram; *RVA*, right ventricular apex.

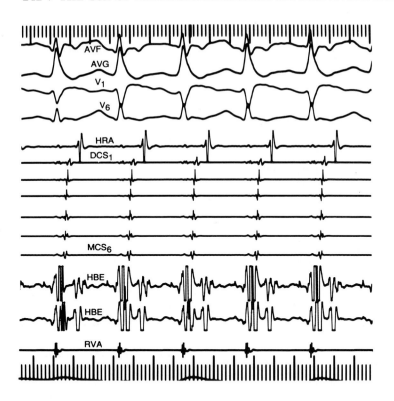

Figure 8-6. Electrocardiographic mapping of a posterior septal accessory connection. Shown are surface leads I, aVF, V₁, and V₆, together with intracardiac recording of the high right atrium (HRA), distal coronary sinus (DCS) to midcoronary sinus (MCS), His bundle (HBE), and right ventricular apex (RVA). The patient is in supraventricular tachycardia with a normal, narrow QRS complex. Earliest activation is at the sixth pair of coronary sinus electrodes, which are in the proximal coronary sinus near the os of the coronary sinus. Both high right atrium and low septal right atrium are activated later. His bundle electrogram precedes each QRS complex.

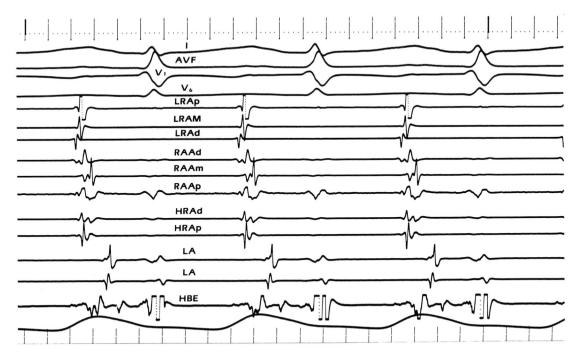

Figure 8-7. Demonstration of electrocardiographic mapping of an atrial automatic focus tachycardia. Shown are simultaneously recorded surface leads I, aVF, V₁, and 2V₆, together with low right atrium (LRA)—proximal, mid, and distal; right atrial appendage (RAP)—distal, mid, and proximal; high right atrium (HRA)—distal and proximal; left atrium (LA); and His bundle electrogram (HBE), along with femoral artery pressure. The low right atrial distal electrogram is the earliest for this atrial automatic focus tachycardia. Comparison of this tracing with a digitally recorded radiograph of the catheter allows pinpoint measurement of the tachycardia focus.

dysrhythmias. Even if one possible cause for syncope is found, evaluation should be completed. Once the study is completed, the treatment of choice can be identified.

POSTOPERATIVE MANAGEMENT

Patients who have had certain major open-heart repairs of congenital cardiac defects should undergo postoperative EPS.[21–23] These repairs include those for tetralogy of Fallot, truncus arteriosus, endocardial cushion defect, ventricular septal defect with pulmonary hypertension, and Mustard, Senning, and Fontan repairs. Each of these defects carries the significant possibility of sudden death within 5 years postoperatively.

These deaths are felt to be due to abnormalities of impulse initiation or conduction or tachydysrhythmias. It is likely that more than one factor plays a role in a single patient. For example, sinus bradycardia coupled with prolonged intra-atrial conduction may predispose patients who have undergone atrial repairs to atrial flutter or fibrillation.

Because the exact mode of death in these patients is speculative, a complete evaluation should be performed in each. Data can be obtained to determine a normal versus an abnormal response in the postoperative situation (Fig. 8-8). Although most patients who require treatment are symptomatic, some asymptomatic patients probably should be treated. The induction of a sustained monomorphic ventricular tachycardia by two or fewer

PVCs in a patient after repair of tetralogy of Fallot is such a situation. The induction of sustained atrial flutter in a patient who has undergone a Mustard procedure is another. In almost 15 years of follow-up study, we have found that a mildly prolonged HV interval (≤ 90 milliseconds) is a benign finding. A corrected sinus node recovery time greater than 150% of normal is frequently found and does not seem to be of adverse prognostic significance. Other benign findings include splitting of the His bundle potential, presence of block below the His bundle, and presence of single ventricular reentrant beats using the conduction system.

WOLFF-PARKINSON-WHITE SYNDROME

Patients with the WPW syndrome, even those without tachycardia or symptoms, should be considered for study. In some patients, the first symptom is sudden death, which may be more frequent in pediatric patients. Patients who are resuscitated from sudden death and who are found to have the WPW syndrome almost always have short antegrade refractory periods of their accessory connections. Because accessory pathways with the shortest refractory periods are the least sensitive to medication and because patient compliance is known to be poor, we recommend catheter ablation of these pathways.

Radio frequency catheter ablation is increasingly being used in pediatric patients. Each mechanism of tachycardia may be treated with a high degree of success. The

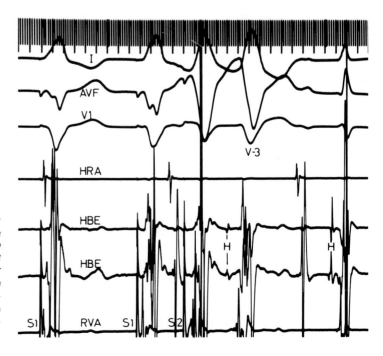

Figure 8-8. Demonstration of a reentry beat during ventricular pacing with premature ventricular stimulation. The S₂ beat given at the right ventricular apex (RVA) has failed to conduct retrogradely over the right bundle branch; instead it has passed through the septum, conducted retrogradely over the left bundle branch anterogradely over the right bundle branch, and caused a reentrant beat with the same morphology as the pace beat and with the His bundle potential in between the two ventricular beats. This is a normal phenomenon. *HRA*, high right atrium; *HBE*, His bundle electrogram.

WPW syndrome or concealed WPW with left-sided pathways AV node reentry and automatic atrial and His bundle foci are also successfully treated. Complications, although rare, do occur. In our first 250 cases, there were no deaths or strokes. Two patients developed AV block long enough to receive pacemakers, although in both, normal AV conduction resumed. Two patients had cardiac perforation with tamponade. One required surgery, and one did not. One patient developed intractable ventricular fibrillation before the EPS began, but was successfully rescued with percutaneous cardiopulmonary bypass with no apparent sequelae. Our success rate during those first 250 cases, which included many postoperative cases and ventricular tachycardia cases, was 90%. For left-sided WPW cases, the success rate approached 100%. Careful follow-up with Holter monitoring and exercise testing has revealed only one patient with apparent dysrhythmia from the procedure; the case was a failed right-sided WPW with more than 50 lesions. We have made exclusively atrial lesions. Recently, we have incorporated the use of a closed-loop temperature control device with an omnidirectional steerable catheter. This device has significantly reduced fluoroscopy time and impedance rises.

CONCLUSION

Electrophysiologic testing is now an integral part of the practice of pediatric cardiology, as it is for adult cardiology. It has allowed clinicians to care for the increasing number of patients with dysrhythmias. Together with noninvasive testing, electrophysiologic testing allows clinicians to determine which patients require treatment and which do not. Surgical and catheter treatment allows physicians to "cure" some patients without lifelong treatment. The use of pacemakers, including antitachycardia pacemakers, may be lifesaving for some patients and may simplify treatment for others.

References

1. Hesslein PS: Noninvasive diagnosis of dysrhythmias. In: Gillette PC, Garson A Jr, eds. Pediatric cardiac dysrhythmias. New York: Grune & Stratton, 1981.
2. Gillette PC, Garson A Jr: Intracardiac electrophysiologic studies: Use in determining the site and mechanism of dysrhythmias. New York: Grune & Stratton, 1981.
3. Gillette PC, Reitman JJ, Gutgesell HP, et al: Intracardiac electrography in children and young adults. Am Heart J 1975;89:36.
4. Gillette PC, Garson A Jr: Pediatric cardiac dysrhythmias. New York: Grune & Stratton, 1981:77.
5. Buckles CS, Gillette PC, Buckles DS: Subcutaneous lidocaine affects inducibility in programmed electrophysiologic testing of children. J Cardiovasc Electrophysiol 1991;2:103.
6. Clapp S, Driscoll DJ, Mitrani I, Lewis RM, Gillette PC: Comparative effects of age and sedation on sinus node automaticity and atrioventricular conduction. Dev Pharmacol Ther 1981;2:180.
7. Buckles DS, Gillette PC: A remotely controlled, programmable stimulator for clinical cardiac electrophysiology testing. IEEE Proceedings of the EMBS, 1991.
8. Zinner A, Gillette PC, Combs W: Totally automated electrophysiologic testing of sinus node function. Am Heart J 1984; 108:1024.
9. Gillette PC, Garson A, Zinner A, Kugler JD: Continuous computer automated measurement of electrophysiologic data during cardiac catheterization. Comput Cardiol 1981.
10. Gillette PC, Garson A, Zinner A, et al: Automated online measurement of electrophysiologic intervals during cardiac catheterization. PACE 1980;3:456.
11. Garson A Jr: Supraventricular tachycardia. In: Gillette PC, Garson A Jr, eds. Pediatric cardiac dysrhythmias. New York: Grune & Stratton, 1981.
12. Gillette PC: The preexcitation syndromes. In: Gillette PC, Garson A Jr, eds. Pediatric cardiac dysrhythmias. New York: Grune & Stratton, 1981.
13. Garson A Jr: Ventricular dysrhythmias. In: Gillette PC, Garson A Jr, eds. Pediatric cardiac dysrhythmias. New York: Grune & Stratton, 1981.
14. Garson A Jr, Gillette PC, Titus JL, et al: Surgical treatment of ventricular tachycardia in infants: Infant ventricular tachycardia surgery. N Engl J Med 1984;310:1443.
15. Garson A Jr, Kugler JD, Gillette PC, et al: Control of last postoperative ventricular arrhythmias with phenytoin in young patients. Am J Cardiol 1980;46:290.
16. Dungan WT, Garson A Jr, Gillette PC: Arrhythmogenic right ventricular dysplasia: A cause of ventricular tachycardia in children with apparently normal hearts. Am Heart J 1981; 102:745.
17. Jedeikin R, Gillette PC, Garson A Jr, et al: Effect of ouabain on the antegrade effective refractory period of accessory atrioventricular connection in children. J Am Coll Cardiol 1983; 1:869.
18. Gillette PC, Garson A Jr, Porter CJ, et al: Junctional automatic ectopic tachycardia: New proposed treatment by transcatheter His bundle ablation. Am Heart J 1983;106:619.
19. Silka MJ, Gillette PC, Carson A Jr, Zinner A: Transvenous catheter ablation of a right atrial automatic ectopic tachycardia. J Am Coll Cardiol 1985;5:999.
20. Gillette PC, Wampler DG, Garson A Jr, et al: Treatment of atrial automatic tachycardia by ablation procedures. J Am Coll Cardiol 1985;6:405.
21. Garson A Jr, Porter CJ, Gillette PC, McNamara DG: Induction of ventricular tachycardia during electrophysiology study after repair of tetralogy of Fallot. J Am Coll Cardiol 1983; 1:1493.
22. Gillette PC, El-Said GM, Sivarajan N, et al: Electrophysiologic abnormalities after Mustard's operation for transposition of the great arteries. Br Heart J 1974;36:186.
23. El-Said GM, Gillette PC, Cooley DA, et al: Protection of the sinus node in Mustard's operation. Circulation 1976;53:788.

Cardiac Arrhythmias, 3rd edition, edited by William J. Mandel.
J. B. Lippincott Company, Philadelphia © 1995.

9

Jay L. Jordan • William J. Mandel

Disorders of Sinus Function

The sinus node is a highly organized cluster of specialized cells located at the junction between the superior vena cava and right atrium.[1] Crescent shaped, it varies in length from 9 to 15 mm and has a central body (5 mm wide and 1.5 to 2 mm thick) and tapering ends. Its anatomic, microscopic, and ultrastructural features are described in Chapter 2. An important ultrastructural characteristic of the sinus node is a sarcolemma composed of a trilaminar unit plasma membrane surrounded by an external glycoprotein coat. The glycoprotein coat may concentrate and bind cations to its surface, thereby, in part, determining the local ionic environment of the sinus node independent of the actual concentration of cations in the surrounding media.[2-8] This property of the glycoprotein coat could confound the interpretation of voltage-clamp studies designed to identify the ionic currents involved in sinoatrial electrogenesis.

A perinodal zone of unique cell type surrounds the sinus node of the rabbit. These perinodal fibers have electrophysiologic characteristics distinct from the sinus node and normal atrial tissue and may represent a buffer zone through which electrical activity must pass. Although an anatomically distinct perinodal zone and specialized pathways of conduction between the sinus node and atrium have not been demonstrated in humans, there is considerable indirect evidence supporting their functional existence. Because some investigators have failed to trace discrete or continuous anatomic tracts of Purkinje-like cells between the sinus and atrioventricular (AV) nodes, it has been suggested that the spatial orientation of atrial myocardial fibers facilitates preferential routes of conduction.

The vascular supply to the mammalian sinus node region comes from a central artery that does not appear to terminate in the sinus node. A rich supply of collateral vessels, densest centrally and sparser peripherally, is a constant feature. Although some animals, particularly the dog, occasionally have more than one sinus node artery or have a single vessel with multiple origins, humans do not. A single sinus node artery originates from the proximal 2 to 3 cm of the right coronary artery in 55% of humans and from the proximal 1 cm of the left circumflex artery in 45%.

SINOATRIAL NODE ELECTROGENESIS

Spontaneous phase 4 depolarization is the electrophysiologic characteristic that distinguishes pacemaker cells from other cells. The sinus node emerges as the dominant cardiac pacemaker because of two basic electrophysiologic properties of the sinus node pacemaker cells: (1) the low level of the resting or maximum diastolic membrane potential (-60 mV) and (2) the rapid rate of rise of phase 4 diastolic depolarization. Only recently has a technique been developed to perform voltage-clamp experiments in the sinus node, enabling characterization of the ionic events that give rise to spontaneous diastolic depolarization.[9] Extensive microelectrode studies show the following changes in membrane properties, either singly or in combination, as possible mechanisms responsible for phase 4 depolarization: (1) decreased outward permeability to potassium, (2) increased inward permeability to sodium, (3) reduced sodium pump activity, and (4) increased inward permeability to calcium.

Although the most accepted explanation for the initiation of spontaneous pacemaker depolarization is that there is a voltage greater than the time-dependent decay in outward potassium (ik) current, several facts mitigate against applying this theory to the sinus node. First, the potential range over which phase 4 depolarization occurs in sinus node cells is in a voltage range in which the pacemaker current is fully activated in pacemaker cells that are dependent on decay of outward potassium current (i.e., Purkinje fibers).[10-12] Second, the slope of phase 4 depolarization in sinus node cells is relatively resistant to the depressant effect of an increase in external potassium concentration when compared to Purkinje fibers.[13]

Evidence suggests that the passive sodium current plays a minimal role in initiating the sinus node impulse. Specifically, changes in the extracellular concentration of sodium have little effect on the slope of phase 4 depolarization.[14] Likewise, active sodium transport appears to contribute little to generating the sinus node impulse: neither tetrodotoxin nor lithium substitution, both of which make the electrogenic sodium pump inoperative, significantly affects the slope of phase 4 depolarization.[15-17]

Our understanding of the mechanisms of the generation of the sinus node impulse has recently been expanded by recognizing the importance of the slow (isi) channel.[18,19] Both sodium and calcium have been implicated as the ionic elements participating in a slow inward current that follows closely behind an initial fast inward current in both the sinus and AV nodes. Although the threshold of activation for the slow current (-30 to -40 mV) is positive to the voltage range over which pacemaking largely occurs, microelectrode studies suggest that the slow current may play a significant role in generating the sinus node impulse. Specifically, slow channel inhibitors such as D-600, Mg^{++}, and verapamil depress sinus node phase 4 depolarization.[20-24] It has been suggested that sluggish inactivation occurs of the slow current that had been activated during the plateau of the previous action potential, thus accounting for its persistence at the level of the sinus node maximum diastolic membrane potential.[25]

Explanations of the extreme complexity of the relationship between the various ions participating in the generation of slow diastolic depolarization in the sinus node pacemaker cell must contend with recent observations regarding the role of anion currents. An inward chloride ionic current seems to participate in slow diastolic depolarization in the sinus node. Via the if channel, a hyperpolarizing-activated current is carried by Na^+, K^+, and Cl^- ions and is activated during the diastolic phase of the sinus node action potential and blocked by alinidine and cesium ion.[26-42] Anion permeability of the sinus node is much greater than that of Purkinje cells. Substitution of extracellular anions that are more permeant than chloride (e.g., bromide) results in faster rates of spontaneous diastolic depolarization of the isolated sinus node cell. Substitution of anions that are less permeant than chloride (e.g., methyl sulfate) results in slower rates of spontaneous diastolic depolarization. That being said, it should be emphasized that it is unclear how chloride contributes to phase 4 depolarization. Furthermore, it is likely that chloride contributes only a part of the current responsible for slow diastolic depolarization in the sinus node cell, possibly in the latter half of phase 4 diastolic depolarization.[43] Specifically, although sinus rate is slowed significantly by the blocking agents cesium and alinidine, pacemaker activity cannot be completely abolished, suggesting that the current is not necessary to sustain sinus node automaticity.

Phase 4 depolarization is probably composed of two components in the sinus node and in subsidiary atrial pacemakers.[44-46] The second, later component appears to involve the participation of a very slow intracellular calcium current, separate from the transmembrane slow isi current, that moves across membranes of the sarcoplasmic reticulum. Ryanodine interferes with calcium-release channels in the sarcoplasmic reticulum and significantly reduces the slope of the latter portion of phase 4. Norepinephrine raises intracellular calcium and increases sinus rate by increasing the slope of the latter third of phase 4, an effect mediated predominantly through beta-1 adrenoreceptors. Despite combined inhibition of the if current and the intracellular calcium current, pacemaker activity persists, suggesting that neither current is the primary pacemaker current in the sinus node.

Voltage-clamp studies have shown that cells in different parts of the sinus node have different electrophysiologic characteristics with participation of different ions, making it difficult to identify precise ionic currents involved in generating diastolic depolarization. The "dominant pacemaker site" probably lies in the center of the node where a group of approximately 5000 cells (p cells) with identical synchronous activity show maximum diastolic potentials of about -50 mV and have short times halfway between maximum diastolic potential and peak action potential. For technical reasons, most voltage-clamp studies have been performed in the periphery of the sinus node near the crista terminalis where the most negative maximum diastolic potential is between −70 and −75 mV. Central cells appear to be slow channel dependent, whereas peripheral cells are less dependent on the slow channel.

B-cells, found between the caval border of the crista terminalis and the primary pacemaker cells, rest at maximum diastolic potentials of approximately −60 mV and demonstrate diastolic depolarization activated at very negative potentials ranging between −60 and −35 mV.[47] Because diastolic depolarization is reduced by cesium ion and because the rate of rise of the ascending phase of the action potential is strongly depressed by tetrodotoxin, it is concluded that the pacemaker mechanism in these B-cells arises mostly as a result of the onset of the if current.

As important as discovery of the primary ionic pacemaker current is to understanding sinoatrial electrogenesis, identification and characterization of background currents are also important. The background currents impact, alter, and modulate the behavior of the primary pacemaker current. Experimental manipulations of these background currents and the channels through which they move can have profound effects on the primary pacemaker current and the channel through which it migrates. These secondary effects can make it impossible to determine if any specific manipulation has not affected the primary current itself. This may be confusing when determining which ionic elements play a role in sinoatrial electrogenesis. Specifically, voltage-clamp studies can characterize individual ionic currents, but the interaction between them in vivo is more difficult to study. The interaction of any given background current with the primary

current depends on time and voltage characteristics, which are constantly changing in response to intrinsic and extrinsic influences on the sinus node. Under certain circumstances, such as with various diseases of the sinus node, the background currents may even assume dominance over the primary pacemaker current. Furthermore, Becker and coworkers[48] have recently discovered gap junctions in the sinus node, prompting Michaels and coworkers[49] and, more recently, Anumonwo and colleagues[50] to consider the possibility of cell-to-cell interaction via electrical coupling and mutual entrainment with possible resultant synchronization of pacemaker activity in the whole sinus node rather than the possibility of a single dominant cell assuming the pacemaker role.

The rate of spontaneous depolarization of a pacemaker cell is determined by the level of maximum diastolic potential, the rate or slope of phase 4 depolarization, the level of the threshold potential, the rate of rise and amplitude of phase 0, and duration of the action potential (Fig. 9-1). Thus, slowing of the rate of spontaneous sinus node discharge may be due to an increased maximum diastolic potential, a reduced slope of diastolic depolarization, a threshold potential less negative than normal, a reduced slope and amplitude of phase 0, or a prolonged duration of the action potential.

As with phase 4 depolarization, the determinants of the other characteristics of the sinus node action potential are voltage- or time-dependent fluctuations in membrane permeability to various ions. Phase 0 appears to depend on both the activation of a fast sodium channel and a second slow channel, the dominant current being determined by the level of the takeoff potential.[29–32] Mainte-

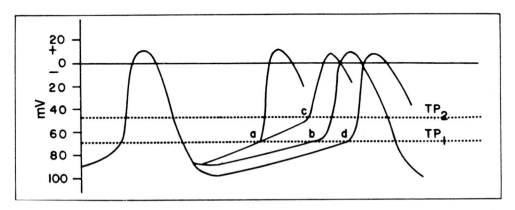

Figure 9-1. A typical sinus node action potential is seen on this graph. An indication of action potential voltage in millivolts is shown on the vertical axis. Points *a* and *b* identify different frequencies of sinus node depolarization dependent on the slope of phase 4 depolarization. In action potentials *b* and *d*, with equal slopes of phase 4 depolarization, maximum diastolic potential in *b* is greater (more negative than in *d*); therefore, the rate of discharge of the sinus node pacemaker in *d* is slower than in *b*. Another feature that alters the rate of discharge of the sinus node is the threshold potential. At points *a*, *b*, and *d*, the threshold potential is approximately −70 mV; at point *c*, the threshold potential is approximately −48 mV. This upward shift in the threshold potential (i.e., to less negative) results in a slowing in the rate of discharge when points *a* and *c* are compared.

nance of the resting membrane potential probably depends on the electrogenic sodium pump and changes in potassium flux, although the precise mechanisms involved are unclear.[17,33-35] The duration of the action potential probably depends on characteristics of slow channel currents as well as potassium conductance.

An apparent slowing of sinus node automaticity, which is electrocardiographically indistinguishable from abnormalities of sinus node pacemaker function, may result from slowing of conduction through the sinoatrial junction. Depression of sinoatrial conduction by verapamil in isolated rabbit sinus node preparations suggests that the slow channel plays a significant role in determining the conduction properties of the perinodal zone.[36]

EXTRINSIC FACTORS MODIFYING THE INTRINSIC ELECTROPHYSIOLOGIC CHARACTERISTICS OF THE SINUS NODE

Role of the Autonomic Nervous System

The mechanisms of initiating spontaneous phase 4 depolarization and the determinants of the rate of spontaneous depolarization are intrinsic properties of the pacemaker cell. Similarly, sinoatrial conduction time (SACT) is a function of the intrinsic electrophysiologic properties of the sinoatrial junction. However, the characteristics of these intrinsic properties can be modified by parasympathetic and sympathetic influences.

Vagal stimulation or acetylcholine slows the sinus rate and intranodal conduction velocity, lengthens the effective and relative refractory periods of the sinus node, causes pacemaker shift, and affects the electrotonic interaction with the sinus node which in turn may influence synchronization of the sinoatrial nodal fibers.[37,38] Corresponding changes in the sinus node action potential include increased negativity of the maximum diastolic potential and reduced slope of phase 4 diastolic depolarization.[39,40] Evidence suggests that these effects are mediated, in part, by increased conductance of potassium.[41-47] However, DiFrancesco has suggested that the if current may play a fundamental role in the underlying negative chronotropic action of acetylcholine.[51] Parasympathetic stimulation causes a marked slowing and inhibition of the if current. Parasympathetic effects on sodium conductance are minimal, whereas effects on the slow channel, even independent of an increased maximum diastolic potential, are probably substantial.[17,47,48] As an aside, but of significant importance, SACT is prolonged by parasympathetic stimuli.[49]

In contrast, sympathetic stimulation or catecholamine infusion increases the spontaneous sinus node discharge rate, primarily because the rate of phase 4 depolarization is increased.[37,52] This change in phase 4 slope presumably relates to a decrease in time-dependent potassium conductance.[53] However, sympathetic stimulation also increases calcium conductance at all levels of maximum diastolic potential, probably through a nonspecific effect on adenyl cyclase induction, and increases the probability that if channels will open on hyperpolarization.[39,41,54,55] SACT is shortened by sympathetic stimulation.

It has been proposed that the sinoatrial region contains both beta-1 and beta-2 adrenergic receptors. Moreover, it has been suggested that either beta-1 or beta-2 receptors in the sinus node may predominate under different circumstances. Friedman and coworkers concluded that sinoatrial beta-2 receptors are stimulated by circulating catecholamines to a greater extent than beta-1 adrenergic receptors.[56] This conclusion was based on the finding that doses of the nonselective beta antagonist propranolol that lowered resting sinus rate equivalent to doses of the selective beta-1 antagonist atenolol, produced progressively greater antagonism of heart rate in dogs during exercise as workload was increased than did atenolol.

During simultaneous stimulation of the sympathetic and parasympathetic systems, deceleration of sinus rate to cholinergic stimulation predominates over the acceleratory effects of sympathetic stimulation. In an elegant series of experiments, MacKary and coworkers determined that when acetylcholine is added to a sinus node preparation, either alone or in combination with epinephrine, pacemaker shift occurs from the superior part of the sinus node to the inferior part.[57] Pacemaker cells in the inferior portion demonstrate deceleration because of the acetylcholine, which is enhanced in the presence of epinephrine. Thus, functional inhomogeneity of the sinus node seems to be a reason, in part, for the predominance of the effect of cholinergic stimulation over that of sympathetic stimulation.

Role of the Endocrine System

Although less extensively investigated than the interaction between intrinsic sinus node function and the autonomic nervous system, humoral factors also modify the electrophysiologic characteristics of the sinus node. This modification appears to be independent of any interaction with the autonomic nervous system. For example, sinus node cells isolated from the hearts of thyrotoxic rabbits have an increased rate of diastolic depolarization and a decreased action potential duration. In contrast, sinus node cells isolated from hypothyroid rabbits have a decreased rate of diastolic depolarization and an increased action potential duration.[58]

Role of the Sinus Node Artery

The sinus node artery is larger than expected considering the extent of the area that it supplies. This disproportionately large size is considered by James to be of physiologic importance.[59, 60] Based on predictable responses of the sinus rate to stretch and on the special arrangement of the sinus node cells around the sinus node artery, James suggests that the distention and collapse of this vessel play an important role in regulating sinus rate.[61, 62] Collapse of the artery increases the tension on pacemaker cells because the cells and artery are attached through collagen to both the nodal cells and the arterial wall. Thus, collapse of the artery increases sinus rate. Distention of the artery has the opposite effect, leading to relaxation of the nodal cells and slowing of the heart rate. The precise intrinsic electrophysiologic properties of the sinus node that are modified by stretch and, therefore, by sinus node artery perfusion pressure have not been clearly defined.

Other Extrinsic Factors

Hypothermia depresses sinus automaticity by increasing the negativity of the maximum diastolic membrane potential, an effect mediated through inhibition of the sodium pump and resulting in accumulation of intracellular sodium. Hypothermia also reverses the acceleratory effect of increased extracellular calcium concentration and, therefore, may retard conductance through the slow channel.[63, 64] Moreover, hypothermia causes pacemaker shifts and, usually, a consequent shortening of SACT, as demonstrated recently in microelectrode and extracellular recordings in isolated rabbit hearts.[65] Conversely, hyperthermia in the isolated preparation and fever in humans increase sinus rate.[63] Drugs that interfere with oxidative metabolism (e.g., cyanide, phenobarbital) depress intrinsic sinus node automaticity, whereas aspirin enhances automaticity.

SINUS NODE DYSFUNCTION

The *sick sinus syndrome* is a term coined by Lown[66] and popularized by Ferrer[67] to refer to a constellation of signs, symptoms, and electrocardiographic criteria defining sinus node dysfunction in a clinical setting. The syndrome is characterized by syncope or other manifestations of cerebral dysfunction in association with sinus bradycardia, sinus arrest, sinoatrial block, alternating bradyarrhythmias and tachyarrhythmias, or carotid hypersensitivity. However, clinical signs and symptoms result from failure of escape pacemaker function, not from sinus node malfunc-

tion per se. Thus, the sick sinus syndrome may represent a generalized disorder of the conduction system of the heart, with sinus node dysfunction being only one aspect.

Incidence

The incidence of sinus node dysfunction in the general population is unknown. Limited information suggests that, in cardiac patients, the incidence of sinus node dysfunction is approximately 3 in 5000.[68] Between 6.3% and 24% of all patients with permanent pacemakers followed in pacemaker clinics worldwide have evidence of sinus node disease.[69-74] With increasing clinical awareness of the sick sinus syndrome and more liberal criteria for pacemaker insertion in general, abnormalities of sinus node function may have been the primary indication for permanent pacing in as many as 50% of permanently paced patients in recent years. Men and women appear to be equally affected by disturbances of sinus node function.[75] There seems to be a bimodal distribution of incidence of sinus node dysfunction among age groups, with peaks occurring in the third and fourth decades of life and again in the seventh (Fig. 9-2). Most patients in the older age group have coexisting hypertensive heart disease or coronary artery disease, although many exceptions have been cited.[75-77]

Etiology

Many etiologic factors have been implicated in the development of abnormalities of sinus node function.[78-81] The most frequent anatomic findings in patients with sick sinus are coronary atherosclerosis, atrial amyloidosis, and diffuse fibrosis. Although sinus node dysfunction is characteristically thought of as a disease of the aged, the precise anatomic concomitants of the aging process responsible for sinus node dysfunction in the elderly have not been elucidated. Anatomic studies have demonstrated that the fibrous stroma gradually increases with age and that there is a corresponding decrease in the number of nodal cells.[82] The syndrome has also been described in association with other infiltrative disorders, collagen vascular disease, infectious processes (e.g., diphtheria, rheumatic fever, viral myocarditis), as a familial pattern, and in pericardial disease. Drug-induced abnormalities of sinus node function have been recognized with increasing frequency.

Perhaps the most common form of the sick sinus syndrome is the idiopathic variety. However, the recent discovery of antibodies to the human sinus node in the sick sinus syndrome may clarify the cause in many patients previously categorized as idiopathic. In a group of sick sinus patients with bradycardia and with carotid sinus

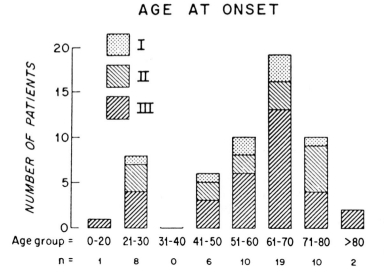

Figure 9-2. This figure demonstrates the age of onset of sinus node dysfunction in a group of sinus node dysfunction patients. Note the bimodal distribution of the patient population, with the majority being older than 50 years of age. However, a small subgroup of patients are younger than age 30 years. (Rubenstein JJ et al.: Clinical spectrum of the sick sinus syndrome. Circulation 1972;46:5; with permission.)

syndrome, two subtypes of anti–sinus-node antibodies have been characterized by Maisch and coworkers[83]: forms both absorbable and nonabsorbable with ventricular myocardium. A 10-fold increased risk of sick sinus syndrome could be calculated in patients with antibodies as compared to age-matched normals. Patients with sick sinus syndrome and prior myocarditis or rheumatic fever had a three-fold increased incidence of antibodies. Anti–sinus-node antibodies were found to be highly specific and moderately sensitive for sinus node disorders. However, the investigators caution that, although anti–sinus-node antibodies are present in sick sinus syndrome, it cannot be concluded that they are pathogenic.

Special consideration should be given to sinus node dysfunction in the setting of acute myocardial infarction. Sinus bradycardia is a common clinical manifestation of acute inferior and lateral myocardial infarction, and even sinus arrest occasionally has been reported.[84–86] Whether these manifestations of sinus node dysfunction are the consequence of ischemia to the sinus node per se or reflect local autonomic neural effects or edematous changes in surrounding tissue is speculative.[87,88] A recent report by Bashour and coworkers describing restoration of normal sinus node function after right coronary angioplasty in a 77-year-old woman seems to confirm the importance of the former mechanism.[89] Although most patients demonstrate only transient depression of sinus node function during the acute stage of the infarct, a few develop evidence of permanent sinus node dysfunction. No long-term follow-up study of a large population of these patients has been reported to allow a statement on the incidence of permanent sinus node dysfunction following an acute myocardial infarction. Experimental occlusion of the sinus node artery in dogs has resulted in

varying degrees of sinus node dysfunction, ranging from profound slowing to no response.[90,91] The variability in response has been attributed to differences in extent of collaterals and the occasional multiplicity of sinus node arteries in canine hearts.[92,93]

Electrocardiographic Manifestations of Sinus Node Dysfunction

Regular sinus rhythm is the normal rhythm of the heart. The normal rate of impulse formation by the sinus node in the adult is conventionally accepted as 60 to 100 beats per minute. Sinus rhythm has a frontal plane P vector oriented to the left and inferior, generally between $+30°$ and $+60°$ (Fig. 9-3). A regular sinus rhythm with a rate over 100 defines sinus tachycardia. Sinus tachycardia rarely exceeds 160 beats per minute in the adult; however, in the young adult, the normal sinus node is probably capable of discharging at rates over 180 beats per minute under the influence of maximum physiologic or pharmacologic stimulation. The maximum rate at which the sinoatrial junction is normally able to conduct sinus impulses is unknown. A regular sinus rhythm with a rate less than 60 beats per minute defines sinus bradycardia, perhaps the most common electrocardiographic manifestation of sinus node dysfunction.

Sinus Arrhythmia

In sinus arrhythmia, the pacemaker is the sinus node but the rhythm is irregular. Until recently, the definition of sinus arrhythmia was not standardized; some authorities

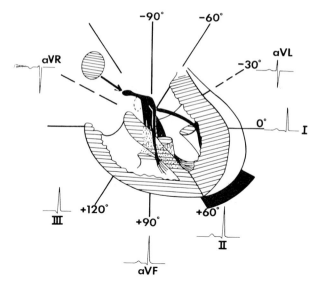

Figure 9-3. Diagram showing normal P wave activation. The normal P wave vector is between +30° and +60° in the frontal plane, leading to an isoelectric P wave in lead III and a negative P wave in lead aVR.

considered sinus arrhythmia to be present when the difference between the shortest P-P interval and the longest P-P interval was at least 120 milliseconds.[94,95] Other criteria defining sinus arrhythmia included variations in sinus cycle length of 10% or more.[96] However, Persson and Solders have reported their effort to establish more rigid and standardized normal values for maximal change in sinus cycle length and range of variation of sinus cycle length for different age groups during a 1-minute continuous electrocardiogram (Table 9-1).[97] In normals, both mean maximum changes in sinus cycle length and mean range of variation of sinus cycle length decreased with age.

Under control of the parasympathetic nervous system, sinus rate varies normally with the phases of respiration, increasing with inspiration and slowing with expiration. In the past it had been assumed that sinus arrhythmia bearing no relationship to respiration probably had little clinical significance; rarely is this rhythm a forerunner of atrial dysrhythmias. However, studying patients more than 40 years of age, Bergfelt and coworkers have suggested that an excessive range of variation of sinus cycle length and an excessive maximal change of sinus cycle length between any two consecutive cycles (measured during a 1-minute continuous rhythm strip) can distinguish patients with severe sinus node dysfunction from healthy subjects (see Table 9-1).[98] Also, the presence of nonrespiratory sinus arrhythmia should raise the suspicion of sinus parasystole, a rare and difficult arrhythmia to diagnose.[99]

Variations in ventricular rate are often accompanied by parallel variations in sinus rate. This arrhythmia is termed *ventriculophasic arrhythmia* and may relate to variations in coronary flow, carotid flow, or alterations in autonomic tone (Fig. 9-4).

It is not possible to distinguish irregularity of sinus impulse formation from variable conduction velocities through the sinoatrial junction on the surface electrocardiogram.

Sinus Arrest

Alternatively designated *sinus pause* or *atrial standstill*, sinus arrest denotes a cessation of sinus node impulse formation. Criteria for minimum duration of a pause that would qualify it as an arrest of sinus activity have not been established. Characteristically, the pause is not an exact multiple of the normal P-P interval.

Typically, the period of sinus arrest in patients with sick sinus is terminated by a sinus beat (Fig. 9-5). Escape pacemakers often fail to assume dominance of the cardiac rhythm despite markedly prolonged durations of sinus

TABLE 9-1. One-Minute ECG Recordings

Variation range of sinus cycle length (SCL) (msec) standardized by dividing by mean SCL* (msec) in healthy individuals at rest during quiet breathing

Age (y)	no.	$\overline{X}$	SD	$\overline{X}; \pm 2$ SD	
20–29	23	29.2	8.7	12–46	
30–39	16	29.0	6.6	16–42	
40–49	15	21.3	7.6	6–36	Reference limits
50–59	12	14.2	4.5	5–23	
60–69	9	13.0	2.9	7–19	
70†	—	—	—		

Maximal changes in sinus cycle length between any two consecutive sinus cycles (max ΔSCL) (msec) in healthy individuals at rest during quiet breathing

Age (y)	no.	$\overline{X}$	SD	$\overline{X} + 2$ SD	
20–29	20	114	65	245	
30–39	14	82	47	175	
40–49	12	69	41	150	Reference limits
50–59	9	32	13	60	
60–69	9	29	13	55	
70†	—	—	—	55	

Linear correlation to age strata: $r = -0.91$, $P < 0.001$.

*Standardization (%): $\dfrac{\text{maximal SCL} - \text{minimal SCL}}{\text{mean SCL}} \times 100$.

†The same reference limits as for ages 60 to 69 were used.

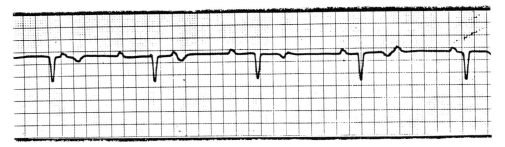

Figure 9-4. This rhythm strip was obtained from a patient with advanced atrioventricular block and a junctional escape pacemaker. When the P-P interval encompassing a QRS is plotted against the P-P interval in cycles without a QRS, the cycle encompassing the QRS has a shorter P-P interval. This is characteristic of ventriculophasic sinus arrhythmia.

arrest. When subsidiary pacemakers are capable of escaping, the pause may be terminated by either AV junctional (see Fig. 9-5) or ventricular automatic foci.

Sinoatrial Exit Block

Sinoatrial exit block is that which denotes failure of the sinus node impulse to conduct normally to the atrium. The site of block may be within the sinus node itself or within the sinoatrial junction. Furthermore, spontaneous sinus node impulse formation may be normal or abnormal.

First degree sinoatrial block describes an abnormal prolongation of the SACT. In this situation, each spontaneously generated nodal impulse does arrive at the atrium, albeit the arrival is delayed. First degree sinoatrial block cannot be recognized on the surface electrocardiogram.

Its recognition by the technique of programmed premature atrial stimulation is described later in this chapter.

Second degree sinoatrial block is characterized by periodic failure of the sinus node impulse to conduct to the atrium, which is manifested as periodic absence of a P wave on the surface electrocardiogram. Sinoatrial Wenckebach periodicity results from progressive delay of sinoatrial conduction in the face of regular sinus node pacemaker activity.[100] Electrocardiographically, this phenomenon is manifested as a progressive shortening of the P-P interval preceding the dropped P wave (Fig. 9-6).

Advanced second degree sinoatrial block occurs when there is a regular interruption of anterograde sinoatrial conduction not preceded by progressive prolongation of sinoatrial conduction. Absence of a P wave on the surface electrocardiogram associated with second degree sinoatrial block can be distinguished from that observed

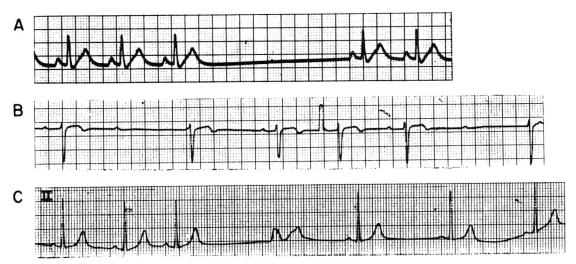

Figure 9-5. (**A**) An episode of sinus arrest occurs in which the P-P cycle of the long pause is not a multiple of basic sinus cycle length. There is no escape complex present. (**B**), During an episode of atrioventricular block, probably of the Wenckebach type, junctional escape complexes are noted. (**C**), During a sinus arrhythmia, a ventricular escape complex is noted.

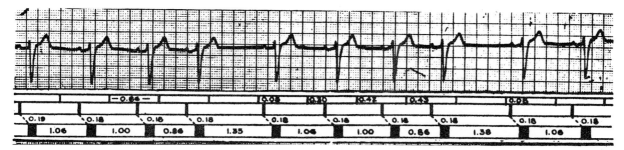

Figure 9-6. This electrocardiogram rhythm strip demonstrates repetitive group beating with fixed PR relationships but abbreviated R-R relationships followed by a pause. The laddergram below the tracing identifies that sinoatrial (SA) Wenckebach phenomenon occurs due to progressive delay at the SA junction. (Greenwood RJ, Finkelstein D, Monheit R: Sinoatrial heart block with Wenckebach phenomenon. Am J Cardiol 1961;8:141.)

with sinus arrest; characteristically, the pause between P waves in the former circumstance is an exact multiple of the normal P-P interval (Fig. 9-7).

Third degree or complete sinoatrial block cannot be distinguished from prolonged sinus arrest on the surface electrocardiogram. P waves are absent in both circumstances. Regardless of the cause, advanced sinoatrial block or profound sinoatrial arrest is always associated with significant clinical symptoms.

Bradycardia-Tachycardia Syndrome

A frequent electrocardiographic manifestation of sinus node dysfunction is a pattern of slow sinus or subsidiary rhythms alternating with tachyarrhythmia, which is typically supraventricular in origin (Fig. 9-8). In keeping with the high incidence of atrial disease in patients with sick sinus syndrome, atrial fibrillation is probably the supraventricular tachycardia most frequently observed in this setting. However, atrial flutter, accelerated AV junctional rhythms, and reentrant AV junctional tachycardias are also observed. Ventricular tachycardia is less frequently encountered, even though slow supraventricular rhythms could theoretically predispose to ventricular dysrhythmias.[101, 102]

Abrupt spontaneous termination of a tachycardia episode is often accompanied by exaggerated suppression of sinus and subsidiary pacemaker activity in patients with sick sinus syndrome. Electrocardiogram abnormalities and central nervous system symptoms may become manifest only during this posttachycardia period; sinus node dysfunction is otherwise occult in many patients with sick sinus syndrome.

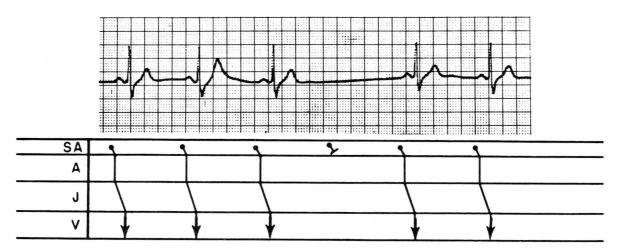

Figure 9-7. This rhythm strip and its accompanying laddergram identify the cause of the pause seen on the rhythm strip. The P-P interval encompassing the pause is twice the normal sinus cycle length, identifying that paroxysmal second degree sinoatrial (SA) block occurs with delay at the SA junction.

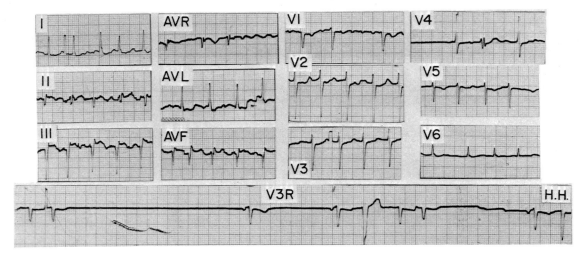

Figure 9-8. This standard electrocardiogram was obtained from a patient with a history of palpitations and dizziness. The 12-lead electrocardiogram identifies the presence of atrial fibrillation with a moderately rapid ventricular rate. During the rhythm strip (V_{3R}), atrial fibrillation terminates spontaneously with a pronounced pause followed by a sinus escape complex. This tracing is typical for episodes of bradycardia-tachycardia.

Sinus Node Reentry

A supraventricular tachyarrhythmia unique to patients with sick sinus is sinus node reentry tachycardia. Although evidence suggests that sinus node reentry is a genuine phenomenon, some investigators doubt that the sinus node itself is involved in a tachycardia circuit.[103–109] Nonetheless, to qualify as a sinus node reentrant tachycardia, a supraventricular rhythm must meet certain criteria. It is usually initiated by premature atrial depolarizations occurring early in diastole, P waves during the tachyarrhythmia must have the same shape as P waves during normal sinus rhythm, the rate of the tachyarrhythmia is characteristically, but not invariably, slow (100 to 120 beats per minute), and the duration of the arrhythmia is often brief (several beats) (Fig. 9-9).[110,111]

Gomes and coworkers found that, of 65 consecutive patients with paroxysmal supraventricular tachycardia, 11 (16.9%) demonstrated sustained sinus node reentrant tachycardia.[112] This arrhythmia could be induced reproducibly during atrial pacing or by premature atrial stimulation over a wide echo zone. The tachycardia could be terminated by carotid sinus massage, atrial pacing, and premature atrial stimulation. In different patients, cycle lengths of 250 to 590 milliseconds were observed with wide fluctuations of 20 to 180 milliseconds in individual patients. The tachycardia was responsive to ouabain, verapamil, and amiodarone administration, but resistant to beta blockers. The investigators concluded that sinus node reentrant tachycardia is not as benign as previously believed and that many patients with this arrhythmia have evidence of organic heart disease.

The mechanism of sinus node reentry is further discussed under Premature Atrial Stimulation (see below).

MECHANISMS OF SINUS NODE DYSFUNCTION IN THE SICK SINUS SYNDROME

Evaluation of sinus node function must take into account that its normal function depends on a delicately balanced interaction between intact intrinsic electrophysiologic properties of pacemaker automaticity and sinoatrial conduction and factors extrinsic to the sinoatrial region. Thus, not only must the integrity of intrinsic electrophysiologic determinants of sinoatrial function be tested, but the integrity of the autonomic nervous system, the endocrine system, and the sinus node blood supply must also be evaluated. These extrinsic elements exert profound modifying influences on intrinsic electrophysiologic mechanisms of the sinus node and perinodal structures; dysfunction at any one of these sites may become clinically manifest as the sick sinus syndrome. Furthermore, each component of this complex network of factors, upon which normal sinus function depends, may be intact, but the interaction between them may be abnormal. Possible disturbances of reflex feedback mechanisms should, therefore, be considered and explored.

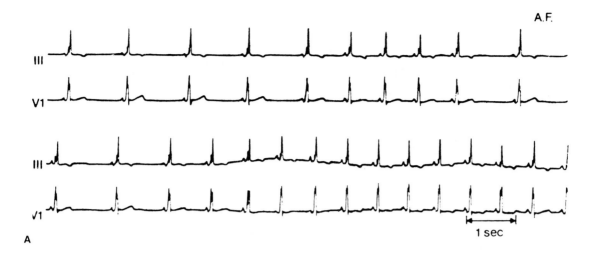

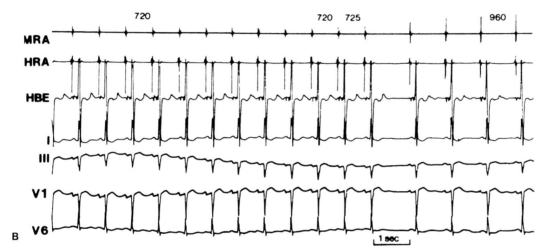

Figure 9-9. (**A**) In the upper panel, sinus rhythm is interrupted by a short burst of accelerated sinus rate. In the lower panel, there is a more sustained episode of sinus rhythm. (**B**) In a different patient, termination of an episode of "sinus" tachycardia is seen, with the prompt restoration of sinus rhythm at a rate of approximately 65 per minute. Note the lack of change in P-wave morphology in the various surface electrocardiographic leads during the burst of more rapid "sinus" rhythm. Both (**A**) and (**B**) are typical of paroxysmal sinus node reentry. (Curry PVL, Krinkler DM: Paroxysmal reciprocating sinus tachycardia. In: Kulbertus HE, ed. Re-entrant arrhythmias: Mechanisms and treatment. Baltimore: University Park Press, 1976:39.)

CLINICAL EVALUATION OF SINUS NODE FUNCTION

The sick sinus syndrome must be included in the differential diagnosis of the patient giving a clinical history of palpitations, vague neurologic complaints of intermittent dizziness and light headedness, or alarming symptoms related to hypotension and reduced cardiac output (e.g., syncope). However, the intermittency of symptoms and electrocardiographic features so characteristic of the syndrome may frustrate efforts to document a cause-and-effect relationship between clinical presentation and electrophysiologic events. Sophisticated electrophysiologic studies should be reserved for those patients in whom the diagnosis of sinus node dysfunction is in question. Furthermore, the diagnostic situation in which the studies are performed should be optimized to enhance the probability that symptoms and electrocardiographic abnormalities occur at that time.

Electrocardiogram Monitoring

Resting Electrocardiogram: Analysis of Sinus Cycle Variation

Studying patients older than 40 years of age, Bergfelt and coworkers analyzed 1-minute resting rhythm strips in 18 normal, healthy patients and in 30 patients with severe sinus node dysfunction and found that the two groups were distinguished by sinus cycle variation.[98] Two parameters were studied: the maximum change in sinus cycle length (max SCL) and the range of variation of sinus cycle length. The range of variation was defined by the difference between the maximal and minimal sinus cycle lengths. Max SCL was standardized by either dividing by the mean sinus cycle length or by the total range of variation. The range of variation of sinus cycle length was standardized by dividing by the mean sinus cycle length.

Normal max SCL and normal ranges of variation of sinus cycle length were established for different age groups. Both mean variation range and mean maximum changes of sinus cycle length decreased with age in normals and in sick sinus patients (see Table 9-1). Although both parameters distinguished sick sinus patients from healthy patients, the sensitivity was higher for increased max SCL (78%) than for increased range of variation (63%). However, the specificity was lower for increased max SCL than for increased range of variation (94%). The predictive values of a positive test were 88% and 95%, respectively, for the two measures. In the presence of both an increased max SCL and an increased standardized range of sinus cycle length, the specificity as well as the predictive value was 100%. However, only 63% of the sick sinus patients had this combination. Even though the investigators cautioned that the results of this study might not apply to patients with less severe sinus node dysfunction, the observations do represent a major advance in the analysis of the resting electrocardiogram in terms of diagnosing sick sinus syndrome in patients older than 40 years.

Exercise Testing

Exercise testing assesses the ability of the sinus node to accelerate in response to internal physiologic chronotropic stimuli. Although a patient may have no evidence of sinus node dysfunction on the resting electrocardiogram, abnormal sinus node responses to stress may be uncovered by treadmill testing, especially in sick sinus patients with abnormal beta-2 adrenergic receptors. Established norms for sinus node rate response for standard stress testing protocols for age and sex are available.[113, 114]

Although some investigators have found that mean oxygen consumption at maximum stress was significantly lower for patients with sick sinus compared with predicted maximum oxygen consumption for controls, recent reports indicate that maximum oxygen consumption may not differ between the two groups.[112] Thus, for any given oxygen consumption, patients with sick sinus and no myocardial disease have slower heart rate responses than healthy patients.

Exercise testing potentially allows distinction between patients with sick sinus and other groups of patients with slow resting or exercise heart rates.[113] For example, age-matched "healthy" patients with autonomic chronotropic incompetence secondary to myocardial disease have lower oxygen consumption for any given heart rate during exercise because of the inability to increase cardiac output by increasing stroke volume. These patients usually cannot reach as high a peak oxygen consumption as patients with sick sinus with normal myocardial function.[113, 114]

In contrast to patients with sick sinus, otherwise normal individuals with sinus node dysfunction, primarily as a consequence of heightened vagal tone, are expected to have normal heart rate responses to exercise.[115] Specifically, exercise is vagolytic, which eliminates parasympathetic influences on sinus node function in all groups of patients; therefore, there is no effect on the maximum heart rate achieved during exercise and atropine administration.

Patients with sick sinus can be distinguished from physically well-trained persons during exercise, although both groups seem to have similar heart rates at similar levels of oxygen consumption. However, the physically well-conditioned individual can ultimately achieve a greater peak oxygen uptake and, therefore, a greater maximum heart rate response.

Thus, exercise testing appears useful for distinguishing patients with sick sinus from other groups of individuals with slow heart rates. However, the sensitivity of the method is not perfect. Some patients with sick sinus demonstrate normal heart rate responses to exercise, theoretically relating to relatively normal sinus node beta-2 adrenergic receptors and normal adrenomedullary epinephrine production. On the other hand, in sick sinus patients with abnormal heart rate responses to exercise, abnormalities of beta-2 adrenergic receptors on the sinus node may be pathogenic. Alternatively, some of these patients may have a deficiency in production of adrenomedullary epinephrine. Unfortunately, studies measuring serum and urine epinephrine levels before and after exercise in age-matched normals and in both groups of sick sinus patients are lacking. Pre- and post-propranolol and atenolol heart rate responses to exercise in sick sinus patients with normal post-exercise epinephrine levels might prove or disprove the theory that some sick sinus patients with abnormal heart rate responses to exercise have abnormalities of sinus node beta-2 adrenergic receptors.

Finally, there is the rare phenomenon of exercise-induced sinus node deceleration. Miller and coworkers reported that only two of eight patients studied angiographically who had sinus node slowing during exercise had significant disease of the right coronary artery proximal to the origin of the sinus node artery.[116] The authors concluded that exercise-induced sinus slowing is not a valid marker for exercise-induced sinoatrial node ischemia.

Holter Monitoring

Ambulatory monitoring with a Holter device may be a more useful physiologic technique than exercise testing for assessing sinus node function, if performed during normal daily activities.[117] The intermittent occurrence of both bradyarrhythmias and tachyarrhythmias in patients with the sick sinus syndrome frequently is missed on a routine resting electrocardiogram. Furthermore, ambulatory monitoring can be virtually diagnostic of many cases of the sick sinus syndrome if the simultaneous occurrence of symptoms and sinus dysrhythmia is documented. Patients can carry a device to be used only when symptoms occur, transmitting an electrocardiogram to a central station by telephone or recording the electrocardiogram on a portable recorder. "Intelligent recorders" are being developed to record the electrocardiogram only when abnormalities of rate or rhythm occur.

Testing the Sinus Node–Autonomic Nervous System Axis

Tests of Sinus Node Responsiveness to Autonomic Activity

The signs, symptoms, and electrocardiogram features of the sick sinus syndrome may be secondary to sinus node overresponsiveness or underresponsiveness to autonomic activity. Arguss and coworkers[115] have demonstrated that slowing of the sinus rate with age may be, in part, secondary to inappropriate parasympathetic tone in many elderly individuals. Other investigators have shown that, in some patients, sinoatrial block may be mediated by abnormal autonomic tone.[118, 119] Furthermore, it has been demonstrated that sinus arrhythmia is often produced primarily by periodic alterations in parasympathetic efferent cardiac activity.[120] Finally, patients with myocardial dysfunction have been shown to have profound abnormalities of parasympathetic and sympathetic control of heart rate.[94, 95, 121, 122]

The importance of the autonomic nervous system to intrinsic sinus node function has led some investigators to recommend that heart rate response to sympathomimetic (isoproterenol), sympatholytic (propranolol), vagotonic (bethanechol or edrophonium), and vagolytic (atropine) drugs be employed routinely in the clinical evaluation of patients with the sick sinus syndrome.[123] However, no standardized or systematic protocols have been described for administration of these agents to evaluate heart rate response. Furthermore, before abnormalities of heart rate response to these agents can be quantified, dose-response curves in healthy subjects must be described for comparison. In general, patients with intrinsic sinus node dysfunction may be expected to exhibit all, some, or various combinations of the following abnormal responses: (1) a blunted heart rate acceleration for age with isoproterenol administration, suggesting sinus node unresponsiveness to appropriate beta-adrenergic stimulation, (2) a blunted acceleration response to atropine for age, suggesting that sinus node dysfunction is a result of oversensitivity to parasympathetic tone, (3) an exaggerated response to atropine, indicating that oversensitivity to parasympathetic tone or increased parasympathetic tone are etiologic factors, and (4) an exaggerated slowing response to bethanechol or edrophonium, indicating oversensitivity to parasympathetic stimulation.

Testing the Integrity of the Autonomic Nervous System

When the possibility that the sinus node responds inappropriately to changes in the autonomic environment after the above pharmacologic tests are excluded, it is then necessary to verify that the autonomic nervous system is itself intact. A characteristic clinical presentation of patients with the sick sinus syndrome may result from primary dysfunction of the autonomic nervous system. To test this possibility, autonomic activity should be provoked mechanically or pharmacologically. Carotid massage, the Valsalva maneuver, or phenylephrine-induced hypertension should normally produce slowing of the heart rate by reflex responses of the autonomic nervous system.[94, 95, 97, 122, 123] In contrast, lowering the blood pressure by titrated nitroprusside infusion normally results in a reflex increase in heart rate.[94, 95, 124–126] Heart rate changes induced by rapid positional changes should also be studied. Regretably, blood pressure—heart rate response curves are not available for healthy subjects.

With the combined results of studies designed to test the integrity of sinus node response to direct autonomic stimulation and inhibition and studies testing the integrity of the autonomic nervous system, the status of autonomic regulation of sinus node function can be completely characterized. Dighton has suggested that patients with symptomatic sinus bradycardia are more likely to have an abnormal sinus rate response to autonomic stimulation and inhibition than asymptomatic patients.[127]

The integrity of the autonomic nervous system is relative. The autonomic nervous system normally changes with age, and what may be considered an intact autonomic nervous system in one age group may not apply to a different age group. That is, the autonomic nervous system normally ages to accommodate the aging intrinsic electrophysiologic properties of the sinus node, thereby maintaining the interdependent systems in harmony and equilibrium. Therefore, abnormalities of the autonomic nervous system should be defined as disturbances that alter the equilibrium and harmony with intrinsic sinoatrial properties of automaticity and conduction. Therefore, what is normal for the age of the patient being tested should be considered when defining and testing the integrity of the autonomic nervous system.

Reporting on the relationship between aging and the autonomic nervous system, Pfeifer and coworkers found evidence of an age-related increase in cardiovascular sympathetic nervous activity and an age-related reduction in parasympathetic nervous activity.[128] The investigators concluded that the findings were consistent with the hypothesis that there is a sympathetic and parasympathetic nervous system compensation of cardiovascular function in response to an age-related decrease in baroreceptor sensitivity. DeMarneefe and coworkers, finding similar age-related changes in the autonomic nervous system in relation to sinus node function, postulated that these findings could reflect a compensation in response to age-related deterioration of intrinsic sinus node function.[129]

Intrinsic Heart Rate Determination

The intrinsic heart rate (IHR) is defined as the rate of spontaneous sinus node depolarization independent of the effects of the autonomic nervous system. The significance of the IHR is that its value theoretically depends only on intrinsic electrophysiologic mechanisms of sinus node automaticity. Complete autonomic blockade can be achieved with a modification of the protocol of Jose.[130–136] Propranolol, 0.2 mg/kg, is administered intravenously at a rate of 1 mg per minute to obtain a dose-response curve of heart rate response to beta blockade. Ten minutes later, atropine sulfate, 0.04 mg/kg, is administered intravenously over 2 minutes. The resultant sinus rate is the observed IHR (IHRo). The dose of propranolol used abolishes the positive beta-adrenergic effects of large doses of isoproterenol for approximately 20 minutes. After atropine is administered, the IHR remains stable for approximately 30 minutes.[130] Therefore, within the physiologic range, functional autonomic blockade appears to be complete.

With the technique of IHR determination, patients with sick sinus syndrome with intrinsic sinus node dysfunction can be distinguished from patients with disturbed autonomic regulation of sinus node function. Because the observed IHR theoretically depends only on

intrinsic electrophysiologic properties of sinus node automaticity, an abnormal IHRo reflects an abnormality of one or more of these intrinsic properties. In contrast, when the heart rate is normal after autonomic blockade, disturbed autonomic regulation is most likely the underlying mechanism responsible for the manifestations of sinus node dysfunction.

Intrinsic heart rate decreases with age in a linear fashion in normal subjects as well as in patients with sick sinus syndrome. The normal deterioration of sinus node function with age must be distinguished from pathologic abnormalities of sinus node function defining the sick sinus syndrome.

Normal values for IHR can be determined using the linear regression equation derived by Jose, which relates predicted IHR (IHRp) to age:[130]

$$IHRp = 118.1 - (0.57 \times age)$$

For individuals younger than 45 years, the 95% confidence limit of IHRp is $\pm 14\%$; for individuals older than 45 years, the 95% confidence limit of IHRp is $\pm 18\%$. An IHRo falling within two standard deviations (SD) of the predicted IHR is indicative of normal sinus node function. Conversely, an IHRo falling below and outside the 95% confidence limit of IHRp is compatible with abnormal intrinsic sinus node function.

A comparative measure of intrinsic sinus node function has also been derived.[131] The ratio of IHRo to its lowest normal point (i.e., IHRp − 2 SD) represents a quantitative measure of the integrity of intrinsic sinus node function. By this method, a ratio of 1 or greater indicates normal sinus node function.

Autonomic influences on intrinsic electrophysiologic properties of the sinus node vary from moment to moment depending on internal and external stimuli and inhibitors. Moreover, autonomic influences can either mask or exaggerate abnormalities of intrinsic electrophysiologic properties, contributing to the evanescent quality of electrocardiographic features of the sick sinus syndrome. On the other hand, the IHR has been shown to be stable on repeated determinations over extended periods.

The magnitude and direction of autonomic tone at any point can be semiquantitated in humans by using the technique of IHR determination. The percentage of a person's resting heart rate (RHR) attributable to negative or positive autonomic chronotropic influences on intrinsic electrophysiologic mechanisms of sinus node automaticity can be determined by the following formula[131]:

$$(RHR/IHR - 1.00) \times 100$$

If RHR is less than IHR, the resultant value is negative,

indicating that net negative autonomic chronotropy is present. When RHR is greater than IHR, net positive autonomic chronotropy is present and the value is positive.

Atrial Overdrive

Mechanisms and Determinants of Sinus Node Suppression

In 1884, Gaskell reported that termination of rapid cardiac rhythms in the turtle heart resulted in a delay of return of spontaneous pacemaker activity.[132] Subsequent clinical reports emphasized this phenomenon in ventricular pacemakers.[133–135] Using these clinical observations, Lange systematically studied overdrive suppression of the sinus node in the laboratory.[136] With the use of transvenous pacing catheters, overdrive suppression evolved into a means of evaluating sinus node function in humans.[137]

"Suppression" of sinus node pacemaker automaticity by intra-atrial overdrive pacing has been considered useful in unmasking occult sinus node dysfunction in many patients with the sick sinus syndrome.[137–139] Recent observations suggest that this phenomenon may provide a key to understanding fundamental electrophysiologic properties of pacemaker automaticity itself.

Transient arrest of spontaneous sinus node activity follows cessation of overdrive atrial pacing as an apparent physiologic event. In general, patients with sinus node dysfunction demonstrate longer periods of sinus arrest than do healthy subjects (Fig. 9-10). The mechanisms by which overdrive pacing suppresses pacemaker automaticity have been the subject of speculation. Two general hypotheses have received serious consideration in the clinical and experimental laboratory: (1) suppression is mediated by the release of autonomic neurotransmitters and (2) overdrive pacing directly disrupts intrinsic mechanisms of pacemaker automaticity.[136, 140, 141]

Atrial overdrive pacing results in a release of autonomic neurotransmitters from storage sites within myocardial tissue and nerve endings.[40, 142] If there is a net release of a negative chronotropic neurotransmitter, presumably acetylcholine, suppression of sinus node automaticity may be mediated by this neurohumoral agent. Vagal stimulation or acetylcholine administration prolongs sinus node recovery.[13]

That catecholamine release also plays a role in postoverdrive electrophysiologic events is suggested by the observation that the often-seen postoverdrive acceleration of sinus rate can be abolished by reserpine or propranolol pretreatment.[141] Moreover, isoproterenol infusion results in a predictable shortening of the sinus node recovery time.[13]

Clinical and experimental observations suggest that release of autonomic neurotransmitters is not the only mechanism by which overdrive atrial pacing suppresses sinus node pacemaker automaticity. Because the sinus node recovery time is longer than the spontaneous sinus cycle length, even after complete autonomic blockade, overdrive pacing may directly disrupt intrinsic electrophysiologic determinants of sinus node automaticity.[136] Some patients with sick sinus syndrome exhibit longer corrected sinus node recovery times (SNRTCs) than healthy subjects after autonomic blockade, suggesting that overdrive pacing may actually exaggerate abnormalities of these intrinsic properties.[136] Some individuals have net release of a positive chronotropic neurotransmitter in the face of overdrive suppression, suggesting that a direct effect on intrinsic electrophysiologic properties may be the primary mechanism of suppression.[136]

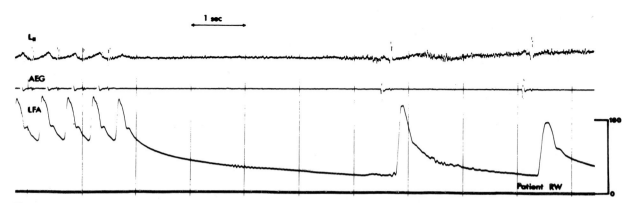

Figure 9-10. A typical example of marked suppression of sinus function following overdrive pacing. The tracings are, from the top down, lead II electrocardiogram, a high right atrial electrocardiogram, and left femoral artery blood pressure. Right atrial overdrive pacing at a rate of 130 per minute was abruptly turned off, resulting in a pause of approximately 5 seconds that was terminated by a sinus complex.

Recent observations in the microelectrode laboratory on the relationship between rate of overdrive pacing and sinus node recovery time have significantly advanced the understanding of the mechanisms and determinants of sinus node recovery time.[143,144]

1. Using small sinus node preparations and pacing at a closer proximity to the pacemaker cell (<5 mm) minimizes acetylcholine release and unmasks the direct disruptive effects of overdrive pacing on pacemaker automaticity. These effects on the sinus pacemaker action potential are directly proportional to the rate of penetration of paced beats and are not reversed by atropine.

2. The extent of sinus node pacemaker suppression is directly related to the number of paced beats that penetrate the sinus node per unit of time. Paced beats that fail to penetrate the sinus node do not suppress pacemaker automaticity to the same extent as do paced beats penetrating the sinus pacemaker.

3. Activation of the electrogenic sodium pump is eliminated as a mechanism of pacemaker suppression in the sinus node because overdrive pacing has been observed to directly hypopolarize the sinus node pacemaker cell.

4. Sinus node recovery time cannot be interpreted only in terms of overdrive suppression of sinus node automaticity but is the result of a complex interaction between conduction and impulse formation in the sinoatrial region. The faster the rate of overdrive pacing, the slower is retrograde sinoatrial conduction because of progressive impingement on the relative refractory period of the perinodal zone. The faster the rate of overdrive pacing, the slower is antegrade sinoatrial conduction because of decreased amplitude of the sinus node pacemaker action potential.

5. The mechanism by which overdrive pacing reduces the amplitude of the pacemaker action potential may be prevention of completion of phase 3 when pacing rates are rapid.

Abnormalities of only one potential intrinsic mechanism of sinus node automaticity have been studied with the object of uncovering the mechanism of suppression by overdrive pacing. When isolated rabbit sinus node preparations are perfused with the slow channel inhibitor verapamil, 1×10^{-7}M, the SNRTC is prolonged.[145] This finding is reproducible even when the influence of released autonomic neurotransmitters is blocked with atropine and propranolol added to the perfusate.[146] Therefore, some patients with sick sinus syndrome demonstrating abnormal prolongation of the sinus node recovery time may have intrinsic slow channel abnormalities. An exaggeration of Na^+, K^+, intracellular calcium, and anion current abnormalities by atrial pacing has not been investigated.

Another mechanism that has been considered as a possible cause of overdrive suppression is the transient induction of ischemia of the sinus node by rapid atrial pacing. Against this hypothesis is the clinical finding that sinus node recovery time is not prolonged in patients with chronic or acute ischemia of the sinoatrial node.[147–149] The possibility that pH changes induced by rapid pacing may contribute to ionic current alterations and, therefore, to abnormal pacemaker suppression has not been specifically investigated. However, sinus node automaticity is influenced by acid-base imbalances.[150]

Methods, Characteristics, and Clinical Application of Sinus Node Recovery Time

Intracardiac pacing is performed in the cardiac catheterization laboratory with patients in the fasting state. All cardiac drugs and medications known to interfere with sinus node or autonomic neural function should be withdrawn for at least 48 hours or two half-lives before the study. Mild sedation is achieved with Seconal, 100 mg orally, given 30 minutes before the procedure. After local anesthesia is achieved, a quadripolar pacing catheter is positioned at the high right atrium. Multiple electrocardiographic leads as well as an intra-atrial electrogram are monitored on a photographic oscillographic recorder. Atrial pacing is performed at a milliamperage two times the diastolic threshold. An initial intra-atrial pacing rate of approximately 20 beats per minute faster than the patient's RHR is chosen, with increments of 20 beats per minute in succeeding pacing trials, up to a rate of 170 beats per minute. Pacing is continued for 30, 60, and 180 seconds at each pacing rate, then is abruptly terminated; 60 seconds is allowed to elapse between each pacing trial. The SNRT is measured in milliseconds as the time elapsing from the last paced P wave to the first spontaneous depolarization on the intra-atrial electrogram. The shape of the P wave confirms that the complex ending the sinus pause is indeed sinoatrial in origin.

To control for differences in spontaneous sinus rate between patients and for the influence that it would have on the apparent time it would take the sinus node to recover its automaticity, the sinus node recovery time (SNRT) may be corrected for the spontaneous sinus cycle length (SCL); thus, SNRTC = SNRT − SCL. Benditt and associates expressed sinus node recovery time as a ratio of sinus cycle length.[151] Accordingly, SNRT/SCL ≤ 1.61 was used as the normal value for patients with sinus cycle lengths less than 800 milliseconds. For patients with sinus cycle lengths greater than 800 milliseconds, SNRT/SCL ≤ 1.83 was considered normal.

Reported sinus node recovery time values for normal subjects include 1400 milliseconds, 1040 ± 56 milliseconds (M ± SEM), and 958 ± 149 milliseconds.[112,152,153]

Reported normal SNRTC values range from <450 milliseconds to <525 milliseconds.[138,154]

In humans and animals, SNRT increases slightlty as the pacing rate increases. However, at rapid rates (>130 beats per minute), sinus node recovery time decreases somewhat.[112] In patients with sick sinus syndrome, maximum sinus node recovery time (SNRT$_{max}$) often occurs at rates slower than the pacing rate at which SNRT$_{max}$ occurs in normal subjects.[155,156] It has been suggested that the pacing cycle length at which the longest postpacing pause occurs (peak paced cycle length, or PCL$_p$) be considered when interpreting the meaning of any particular sinus node recovery time value. Reiffel and coworkers found that PCL$_p$ was equal to or less than 600 milliseconds in normal subjects and tended to be prolonged in patients with sick sinus syndrome.[157] The authors explained that a prolonged PCL$_p$ is a manifestation of disturbed atriosinus conduction during pacing and a prolonged perinodal refractory period.[161b] Furthermore, they suggested that rate-dependent retrograde sinoatrial block during atrial pacing could result in spuriously short sinus node recovery time values in patients with sick sinus because of failure of each paced beat to reach and depolarize sinus node pacemaker cells.[161b] Therefore, a patient with a normal sinus node recovery time but a long PCL$_p$ may actually have a disorder of sinus node pacemaker function that escapes detection through overdrive atrial pacing if an abnormally prolonged PCL$_p$ is not recognized. In microelectrode studies,

Kerr and colleagues have confirmed that the PCL$_p$ is determined by the refractory period of the perinodal zone and the occurrence of retrograde sinoatrial block.[208]

In contrast to the sinus node pacemaker, subsidiary pacemakers demonstrate significant proportional increases in recovery time with increasing pacing rates (Fig. 9-11).[158] Of more importance clinically, subsidiary pacemakers have more sustained periods of suppression than the sinus node following overdrive, that is, an average of eight beats in the sinus node versus 66 to 100 beats in the AV node of the dog.[159]

Most normal subjects demonstrate little correlation between duration of pacing and sinus node recovery time (Fig. 9-12).[158] The correlation in patients with sick sinus is variable. Subsidiary pacemakers generally show a positive correlation between pacing duration and recovery time (see Fig. 9-11); this finding may reflect different mechanisms mediating overdrive suppression in different pacemaker sites.[158]

The proximity of the pacing catheter to the intrinsic pacemaker being studied appears to be an important determinant of the magnitude of that pacemaker's overdrive suppression. Ventricular pacing results in less depression of AV junctional pacemakers than does atrial pacing and even less suppression of the sinus node.[136] On the other hand, suppression of Purkinje fiber automaticity is best achieved by ventricular pacing.[13] Within the atrium, it has been demonstrated in experimental preparations that a

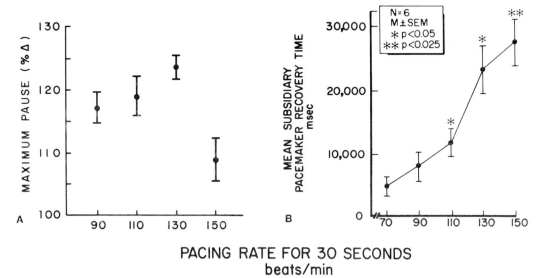

PACING RATE FOR 30 SECONDS
beats/min

Figure 9-11. The influence of pacing rate on sinus node recovery time. The horizontal axis indicates the pacing rate used for 30 seconds of overdrive. The vertical axis demonstrates the maximum sinus node recovery time in milliseconds. (**A**) Using data obtained from normal patients, a peak in sinus node recovery time is observed at a rate of 130 per minute. (**B**) In contrast, data obtained from animal investigations show that, in subsidiary pacemakers (i.e., junctional escape pacemakers), overdrive suppression is more pronounced and has a linear relationship with the frequency of overdrive used.

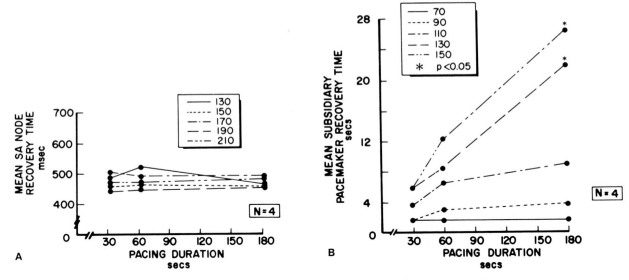

Figure 9-12. Influence of various durations of overdrive pacing on the sinus node recovery time. In both (**A**) and (**B**), the horizontal axis indicates the duration of pacing in seconds; the vertical axis in (**A**) indicates the recovery time of the sinus node pacemaker, and in (**B**), the subsidiary pacemaker recovery time. Note the lack of influence of pacing duration on sinus node recovery time in normal patients. In patients with subsidiary pacemakers, there appears to be significant influence on recovery times dependent on the duration of pacing. This is especially evident at the faster overdrive pacing rates.

premature impulse results in a longer return cycle if delivered in the region of the coronary sinus or crista terminalis than in the intra-atrial septum.[159] In the clinical laboratory, atrial pacing is performed in the high right atrium. Variations in pacing amperage cause no significant change in sinus node recovery time or SNRTC.[112]

In normal subjects, the uncorrected sinus node recovery time prolongs in a linear fashion with longer resting sinus cycle lengths. However, at abnormally slow heart rates, the recovery time generally becomes disproportionately prolonged.[112]

Neely and coworkers have reported on the relative determinants of recovery times in the sinus node and AV nodal pacemakers with regard to features of overdrive pacing in anesthetized dogs.[159] For the sinus node, pre-pacing cycle length was the most important factor in 73%, site of pacing in 3.5%, pacing rate in 2%, and interaction between the site of pacing and pacing rate in 1%. For slow AV junctional pacemakers, the duration of pacing was the most important factor in 40%, interaction between duration and rate of pacing in 27%, and prepacing cycle length in 9%.

The sinus node recovery time in children and in elderly normal subjects is not significantly different from mean values found in the general population.[160, 161] The pacing rate at which there is a sudden decrease in sinus node recovery time seems to be slower in the elderly,

suggesting that sinoatrial entrance block occurs at a slower rate.[155] This phenomenon may represent differential aging of the perinodal zone.

Generally, patients with sick sinus with documented sinus arrest of marked duration (5 seconds or longer) and central nervous system symptoms have relatively longer SNRTCs than asymptomatic patients with sinus arrest of lesser magnitude. However, dramatic exceptions to this rule demonstrate that there is probably no direct linear relationship between magnitude of sinus bradycardia or sinus arrest and the duration of SNRTC in patients with sick sinus syndrome.

Patients with congestive heart failure, independent of its cause, have diminished sinus rate responses to variations in autonomic tone as well as significantly slower IHRs.[94, 95, 121, 122, 161] Jose suggested that, in congestive heart failure, the same biochemical abnormality exists in both myocardial and pacemaker cells.[161] However, the relationship between sinus node recovery time and the presence of heart failure has not been specifically investigated.

Atherosclerotic disease of the sinus node artery is not associated with abnormalities of sinus node recovery time.[162] In addition, mild to moderate hypertension in the absence of cardiomegaly or heart failure does not influence sinus node response to overdrive pacing.[131]

Despite the theoretic potential for marked variations in autonomic tone, sinus node recovery time and SNRTC have been shown to be remarkably reproducible whether pacing is performed on consecutive days or at intervals of many months.[138, 155]

In some instances, SACT appears to be a clinically more sensitive indicator of electrophysiologic abnormalities of the sinoatrial region than sinus node recovery time (e.g., in the setting of atherosclerotic involvement of the sinus node artery).[155] Even patients with gross manifestations of the sick sinus syndrome may have an abnormal SACT in association with a normal sinus node recovery time.[139, 163, 164] The comparative insensitivity of sinus node recovery time may be a consequence of sinoatrial entrance block in the diseased perinodal zone and inconsistent penetration of the sinus node.[128] The occasional finding of a paradoxical effect of atropine on sinus node recovery time (i.e., increased prolongation) may thus be accounted for based on improved retrograde conduction of paced beats into the sinoatrial node.[165, 166]

Observations of abnormal calcium current in isolated tissue preparations suggest that a disparity of sinus node recovery time and SACT may be artifactual. In these preparations, sinus node recovery time and SACT abnormalities invariably parallel one another.[146, 167] The relative magnitude of abnormalities of sinus node recovery time and SACT may depend on the mechanisms of sinoatrial dysfunction that are operative in any patient with sick sinus syndrome, because the calcium current is equally important to both automaticity and sinoatrial conduction.

Limited information suggests that sick sinus patients with abnormalities of AV nodal or intraventicular conduction may have a greater incidence of abnormal sinus node recovery time than patients without distal conduction abnormalities.[152]

Intrinsic Sinus Node Recovery Time

The value of the sinus node recovery time as a diagnostic tool in the sick sinus syndrome has been questioned. Not all patients with sick sinus demonstrate abnormal prolongation of the sinus node recovery time.[168] However, to expect the sinus node recovery time to be prolonged in all patients with sick sinus syndrome presupposes that the technique of intra-atrial overdrive pacing tests an underlying pathophysiologic mechanism that is common to all cases. Based on our knowledge of the large number of potential determinants of sinus node automaticity and overdrive suppression, it is unlikely that sick sinus syndrome is a homogeneous entity in terms of pathophysiologic mechanisms.

Normal sinus node function depends on a complex and delicately balanced interaction among intrinsic sinus node electrophysiologic properties, sinoatrial conduction properties, and factors extrinsic to the sinoatrial region.

Among the extrinsic factors capable of exerting modifying influences on intrinsic sinus node function, the role of the autonomic nervous system is perhaps the most important. However, persons differ in extent and direction of net autonomic tone and perhaps also in end-organ sensitivity to similar levels of autonomic tone. Individuals may also differ in the relative and absolute amounts of epinephrine and acetylcholine released during intra-atrial pacing. Because abnormalities of different intrinsic electrophysiologic properties of sinus node automaticity may be differentially influenced directly by overdrive pacing and because pacing takes place at different levels of autonomic activity, all patients with sick sinus syndrome do not demonstrate abnormal prolongation of the sinus node recovery time. Chadda and coworkers have suggested that the finding of an abnormal SNRTC should be evaluated in terms of the role that autonomic tone plays in its value before concluding that sinus node dysfunction per se caused the abnormality.[169]

Based on observations that many patients with sick sinus have blunted sinus rate acceleration to the administration of atropine and that atropine shortens the sinus node recovery time in normal subjects, this drug has been employed to distinguish patients with sick sinus with intrinsic sinus node disease from those with abnormally exaggerated parasympathetic influences.[170] The effects of atropine on the sinus node recovery time vary in patients with sick sinus, shortening it in some, having no effect in others, and paradoxically prolonging it in a few.[165, 166, 171] These different results may represent differences in residual parasympathetic tone, which must be considered before comparing the effect of parasympathetic blockade on sinus node recovery time in different persons. Differences in resting sympathetic tone, which is unopposed after atropine is administered, also must be considered. All attempts to determine absolute normal values for sinus node recovery time in the postatropine state may be thwarted because of the problems encountered in quantifying sympathetic and residual parasympathetic tone.

The problems associated with determining normal values for postpropranolol sinus node recovery time are similar to those discussed for atropine. Standards for completeness of sympathetic blockade must be established. Differences in unopposed parasympathetic tone must be considered.

Most of the disadvantages of separate atropine and propranolol administration can be overcome by the simultaneous administration of these drugs and determination of IHR at the time of atrial overdrive pacing. With the doses of atropine and propranolol employed with IHRo determination, sinus node recovery time can be automatically adjusted for the role that autonomic influences might play in its value to yield a measure of intrinsic sinus node recovery time. Alternatively, control sinus node recovery time can be adjusted mathematically for the role of autonomic influences.[131] In the past, we proposed that this could be achieved according to the following formula:

$$\text{Intrinsic SNRTC} = \text{SNRTC} + \text{SNRTC} \times (\text{RHR/IHR} - 1.00)$$

In our unit, observed IHRs have been determined in 17 patients with symptomatic sinus bradycardia; 10 patients had normal IHRo. Six of these patients had normal control SNRTC (>450 milliseconds), and four had abnormal control SNRTC. Seven patients had abnormal IHRo, and all seven patients had abnormal control SNRTC. When overdrive pacing was performed after autonomic blockade, all 10 patients with normal IHRo had normal intrinsic SNRTC, whereas all seven patients with abnormal IHRo continued to demonstrate abnormal SNRTCs (Fig. 9-13). We concluded that (1) sick sinus syndrome is not a homogeneous entity in terms of pathophysiologic mechanisms, (2) patients with sick sinus who demonstrate normal sinus node recovery times corrected for the magnitude and direction of autonomic chronotropy consistently have normal IHRs and, therefore, abnormalities of autonomic regulation of sinus node function, and (3) patients with sick

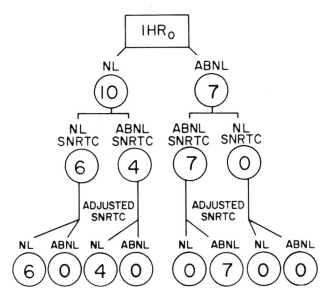

Figure 9-13. Use of the intrinsic heart rate to separate normal and abnormal sinus node recovery times based on intrinsic or extrinsic sinus node dysfunction. The flow diagram demonstrates that patients with normal intrinsic heart rates who have abnormal sinus node recovery times corrected for basic sinus cycle length will have corrected normal values if there SNRTC is adjusted for the degree of positive or negative chronotropic activity. The latter is based on differences between the observed intrinsic heart rate and the basal heart rate. *NL*, normal; *ABNL*, abnormal; *IHRo*, observed intrinsic heart rate; *SNRTC*, corrected sinus node recovery time.

sinus who demonstrate abnormal intrinsic sinus node recovery times consistently have abnormal IHRs and, therefore, abnormalities of intrinsic sinus node function.

Most authorities agree that, with refinement, the technique of pharmacologic autonomic blockade has potential for improving the sensitivity and specificity of the sinus node recovery time as well as for clarifying mechanisms of sinus node dysfunction in patients with sick sinus syndrome. Refinements in the technique are necessary because subsequent investigators have demonstrated occasional exceptions to our results. Furthermore, recent studies have brought forth new observations that force us to modify some basic assumptions.

First, Kang and coworkers have found that neither SNRTC nor intrinsic SNRTC correlates with IHR in a linear fashion.[172] Sinus node recovery time is not a function of sinus node automaticity alone, but is also a function of sinoatrial conduction. Some investigators have even proposed that sinoatrial conduction is the major determinant of sinus node recovery time. Even so, the original interpretation of our results unwittingly minimized the fact that paced beats entering the sinus node and sinus beats exiting the sinus node must pass through the sinoatrial junction and that electrophysiologic properties of the sinoatrial junction may influence sinus node recovery time as much as does sinus node automaticity.

Second, it has been found that intrinsic sinus node recovery time, derived in the setting of autonomic blockade, often does not correlate well with the value for adjusted sinus node recovery time derived from the above formula.[173] Again, sinus node recovery time is determined both by properties of sinus node automaticity and by properties of sinoatrial conduction. Because IHR depends solely on sinus node automaticity, the ratio RHR/IHR cannot be properly applied to sinus node recovery time because it does not include sinoatrial conduction. This omission becomes more significant because sinoatrial conduction and sinus node automaticity are often affected differently by similar levels of autonomic tone. Kuga and coworkers have proposed a more appropriate formula for adjusting for the role that autonomic influences might play in the value of sinus node recovery time[174]:

$$\text{Intrinsic SNRTC} = \text{SNRTC} + \text{SNRTC} \\ \times (\text{SNRTC/INTRINSIC HEART RATE} - 1.00)$$

Third, SNRTC does not correlate with age, but intrinsic SNRTC does increase proportionally with age in a linear fashion similar to IHR.[129] This revelation has led to perhaps the most significant refinement in the application of the technique of autonomic blockade to the assessment of sinus node function. Specifically, comparison of sinus node recovery time between different groups is flawed unless the groups are matched for age. Similarly, intrinsic sinus node recovery time for any individual has meaning only if its value is compared to a mean normal value or to a predicted normal value for age.

Recently, Alboni and coworkers reported a mean normal value for intrinsic SNRTC in 20 subjects who were chosen from a general population of normal persons to be 169 ± 39 milliseconds or 247 milliseconds (M + 2 SD).[175] More importantly, De Marneefe and coworkers have reported age-related normal intrinsic SNRTC values.[129] Mean intrinsic SNRTC was 98 ± 42 milliseconds in eight normal patients younger than 40 years, 323 ± 85 milliseconds in eight normal patients aged 40 to 60 years, and 338 ± 76 milliseconds in 14 normal patients older than 60 years. Thus, the upper limits of normal (M + 2 SD) for these age groups were 182 milliseconds, 497 milliseconds, and 490 milliseconds, respectively. Larger numbers of patients in each group will be required to establish truer normal values. However, these data represent a major advance in understanding sinus node recovery time and applying it to the study of sinus node dysfunction.

Because the autonomic nervous system compensates for age-related deterioration of intrinsic sinoatrial properties, SNRTC does not correlate with age. That is, younger persons have greater parasympathetic tone and less sympathetic tone than elderly persons. Intrinsic SNRTC does increase with age as shown by pharmacologic elimination of the autonomic nervous system, which unmasks the age-related deterioration of intrinsic sinoatrial function. The construction of a linear regression equation relating intrinsic SNRTC to age in normals has not been reported. Therefore, there is no mechanism for predicting exact intrinsic sinus node recovery time.

Fourth, not only does intrinsic sinus node recovery time increase with age in normals, it is also linearly proportional to age in sick sinus patients.[174] It must be proven that differences in sinus node recovery time between any two patients is truly based on the presence of sinus node dysfunction and not merely on difference in age. In our study, we determined whether an intrinsic SNRTC value was normal by comparing it to a mean value that was derived from a healthy general population of all ages. We now believe that these measures are not truly comparable.

Exceptions to our findings include the occasional patient with normal IHR showing abnormal SNRTC after, but not before, autonomic blockade. Sethi and coworkers theorized that this exception meant that intrinsic SNRTC is a more sensitive measure of depressed intrinsic sinus node automaticity than IHR.[176] However, a more likely explanation is that this exception emphasizes the fact that, unlike IHR, sinus node recovery time is not a function of sinus node automaticity alone. The consequences of atrial overdrive pacing also depend on properties of sinoatrial conduction. Thus, when the effects of cholinergic blockade outweigh the effects of beta-adrenergic blockade in

the sinoatrial junction, the net effect is facilitation of retrograde sinoatrial conduction and more consistent penetration into the sinus node by the paced beats. This differential effect of autonomic blockade on the sinus node and sinoatrial junction cannot be anticipated based solely on IHR.

The rare patient with an abnormal IHR and a normal SNRTC both before and after autonomic blockade has been described. In the absence of abnormal retrograde sinoatrial conduction preventing consistent penetration of paced beats into the sinus node, no adequate explanation has been offered to account for this phenomenon.

Finally, the rare patient with an abnormal IHRo but a normal SNRTC before and after autonomic blockade has been described. Kang and coworkers had no explanation for this finding, although it may relate to the fact that normal SNRTC values were determined in the preautonomic blockade state.[172] Intrinsic SNRTC can only be declared normal if it is found to be less than or equal to a normal postautonomic blockade value determined in a group of age-matched normal subjects.

Mason has reported results of overdrive atrial pacing in denervated transplanted human hearts.[171] Sinus rate was significantly faster in denervated donor hearts than in remnant atrial and control subsets. No significant difference was found between donor SNRTC (300 ± 117 milliseconds) and recipient SNRTC (291 ± 171 milliseconds) or control SNRTC (273 ± 171 milliseconds). These values compare favorably with SNRTC after pharmacologic blockade in patients with normal IHRs (287 ± 114 milliseconds).[177] The most dramatic finding was that $SNRT_{max}$ resulted from shorter overdrive cycle lengths in the donor hearts (359 ± 46 milliseconds) than in recipient hearts (491 ± 111 milliseconds) ($P < 0.005$) or in control hearts (499 ± 82 milliseconds) ($P < 0.005$). This latter finding suggests that the sinoatrial junction is particularly sensitive to negative dromotropic effects of resting autonomic tone. Thus, elimination of resting autonomic tone resulted in shortening the retrograde sinoatrial refractory period, allowing more rapidly delivered paced beats to conduct into the sinus node.

After autonomic blockade is achieved, the acute administration of ouabain, 0.1 mg/kg intravenously, may rarely produce marked prolongation of the sinus node recovery time. This phenomenon has only been observed in patients with sick sinus with abnormal IHRs. The mechanism of action is not certain; however, this finding may further improve the sensitivity of SNRTC.

There does not appear to be a correlation between the duration of overdrive pacing and the magnitude of SNRTC in patients with normal IHRs.[178] However, preliminary observations suggest that patients with abnormal IHRs may show progressively longer recovery times with longer durations of pacing.[178] Recognizing this phenomenon as an abnormal response to overdrive pacing could increase the sensitivity of the technique.

In the healthy subject, the sinus cycles following the first recovery sinus beat are either shorter (secondary acceleration) or initially longer than the basic sinus cycle with gradual but progressive return to the basic sinus cycle length. In some patients with sick sinus, the P-P interval immediately following cessation of pacing is not the longest, or even abnormally prolonged, but is followed by longer P-P intervals (Fig. 9-14). This secondary suppression may persist for 10 to 20 beats or more. Instances of secondary suppression have been reported in patients with sick sinus but less frequently in healthy subjects. Desai and colleagues have reported that, in the pre-autonomic blockade state, the incidence of secondary pauses was significantly higher in patients with abnormal IHRs than in those with normal IHRs (five of eight versus two of 13) ($P < 0.05$).[177] Furthermore, after autonomic blockade, secondary pauses in patients with abnormal IHRs persisted or increased, whereas secondary pauses in patients with normal IHRs tended to disappear. Similarly, Mason reported that secondary pauses seen in 78% of recipient atria and in 45% of control atria were virtually absent in denervated donor hearts (6%).[171] These observations suggest that careful examination of the phenomenon of secondary pauses, especially after autonomic block, increases the sensitivity and specificity of overdrive atrial pacing in the diagnosis of the patient with sick sinus syndrome.

Recently, Prinsze and Bouman investigated the mechanism of the intrinsic sinus node recovery time.[180] In isolated rabbit sinus node preparations to which atropine and propranolol were added, overdrive pacing resulted in decreased action potential duration, amplitude, maximum diastolic potential, and diastolic depolarization rate in primary pacemaker fibers. Action potential duration, amplitude, and diastolic potential returned to control value during the first cycle after overdrive pacing. Only diastolic depolarization remained depressed during many consecutive cycles. In primary pacemaker fibers, diastolic depolarization appeared to be depressed throughout diastole. In latent pacemaker fibers, diastolic depolarization was depressed only in the second part of diastole.

Based on the finding that depression of anterograde and retrograde conduction recovers more quickly than depression of phase 4 diastolic depolarization after overdrive pacing in the setting of pharmacologic autonomic blockade, Prinsze and Bouman suggest an indirect method for determining, at least qualitatively, the relative importance of the contribution of the two components of recovery time, that is, conduction and automaticity. The authors suggest that prolongation of each subsequent recovery beat compared to the recovery time of the first return beat might be useful.

Premature Atrial Stimulation

Analysis of sinus node responses to premature atrial depolarizations has revealed important electrophysiologic features of normal and abnormal sinus node function and sinoatrial conduction.[177,181-183] With methods similar to

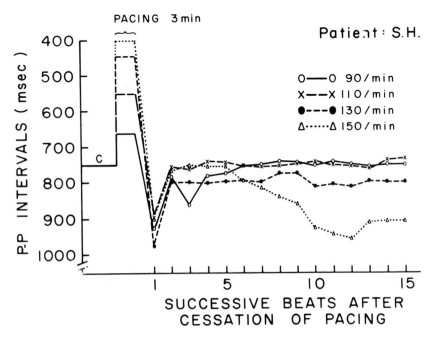

Figure 9-14. The influence of overdrive pacing at different rates on the sinus cycle length after termination of pacing. After overdrive pacing at rates of 90, 110, and 130 beats per minute, sinus cycle length promptly returns to control values. However, after overdrive pacing at a rate of 150 beats per minute, initial overdrive suppression is followed, after approximately 10 beats, by additional suppression (i.e., secondary suppression).

those described in the section on sinus node recovery times, premature atrial stimuli are introduced in late diastole during spontaneous sinus rhythm after every eighth beat at progressively decreasing coupling intervals (in 10-millisecond increments). In this fashion, the sinus cycle length is scanned until atrial capture is lost.

Four types of sinus node responses to atrial premature depolarizations (APDs), depending on the timing of the APD in the sinus cycle (A_1–A_1) and whether the APD retrogradely penetrates the sinus node, have been identified: (1) compensation resulting from a late diastolic extra stimulus that fails to depolarize the sinus node because of collision with the normal sinus depolarization; (2) reset, produced by premature depolarization of the sinus node by the extra stimulus resulting in A_2–A_3 interval of shorter duration than a compensatory pause; (3) interpolation, produced by failure of the extra stimulus to enter the sinus node, but not barring conduction to the atrium of the next sinus impulse; and (4) reentry resulting from reflection of the premature complex, producing an early "sinus" depolarization (Fig. 9-15).

Identification of a perinodal zone of tissue in the right atrium of the rabbit by Strauss and Bigger has contributed significantly to the understanding of the above events.[184] The perinodal cells have electrophysiologic characteristics distinct from atrial muscle and sinus node cells and may represent a potential conduction barrier.

The fibers of the sinoatrial node and perinodal zone share some electrophysiologic properties with AV junctional tissue. Specifically, the depolarization velocity of the action potential of an APD progressively slows as the extrasystole is delivered earlier in diastole, exhibiting decremental conduction.[184] Moreover, an APD may be completely blocked in the retrograde direction within the perinodal zone or within the sinoatrial node if it encounters these tissues in the absolute refractory period of excitability.[128,181–183]

The compensatory pause seen when APDs are introduced late in the sinus cycle may be caused by the electrophysiologic properties of the perinodal zone because the APD does not penetrate or disturb the sinus node and the subsequent sinus beat occurs on time. If the perinodal zone is abnormal, as might be the case in patients with the sick sinus syndrome, the zone of compensation may be expected to occupy a greater percentage of the sinus cycle than in patients with normal perinodal tissue. Thus, even earlier APDs would encounter the existing sinus beat in the perinodal zone. These events form the electrophysiologic basis of first degree sinoatrial block, a manifestation of the sick sinus syndrome (Fig. 9-16).[186,187]

During a portion of the zone of sinus node reset, the postextrasystolic pause (A_2–A_3) lengthens progressively as the premature beat is elicited earlier in the midportion of the atrial cycle. Three mechanisms of this lengthening have been proposed: (1) a progressive slowing of the conduction velocity of the premature impulse, (2) a temporary depression of rhythmicity of sinus node pacemaker cells, and (3) intrasinoatrial nodal pacemaker shifts.[15,177,182,183,188] In patients with abnormalities of sinoatrial conduction, the zone of reset theoretically occupies less of the sinus cycle than in healthy subjects.[163]

Early APDs encounter a perinodal zone that remains effectively refractory in the wake of the preceding sinus impulse, are blocked from entering the sinus node, and fail to reset it. The next spontaneous impulse occurs on schedule, traverses a perinodal zone that has recovered from refractoriness, enters the atrium on schedule, and results in interpolation of the APD. The zone of interpolation has been examined in detail in the microelectrode laboratory.[189] Progressively earlier premature beats are blocked at progressively greater distances from the node. Therefore, the sinoatrial junction provides a progressive gradation of refractoriness rather than a discrete barrier. Furthermore, APDs occurring later in the zone of interpolation may actually penetrate the sinus node. However, their amplitude is so low that they cannot reset the node. Rather, these earlier APDs appear to reduce the maximum diastolic potential, impose a phase delay in attaining maximum diastolic potential, and perturb the terminal part of phase 3 or the early part of phase 4 of the transmembrane action potential, or both. The appearance of the spontaneous recovery beat is delayed, resulting in incomplete interpolation.

Very early APDs may find a portion of the perinodal zone and sinus node recovered sufficiently from the previous spontaneous sinus beat to enter these tissues. However, retrograde conduction would be markedly slowed, allowing other portions of the sinus node and perinodal zone to recover excitability. Such an electrophysiologic circumstance would allow for sinus node reentry. Theoretically, abnormalities of the sinoatrial region should increase the probability of sinus node reentry and the occurrence of atrial arrhythmias.[103,104,190,191] These events may be the underlying electrophysiologic basis for the observed increased frequency of occurrence of supraventricular tachyarrhythmias in patients with the sick sinus syndrome.

In summary, patients with sick sinus with electrophysiologic abnormalities of the sinoatrial junction might be expected to demonstrate the following responses to premature atrial stimulation: (1) a prolonged zone of compensation, (2) a shortened zone of sinus node reset, (3) a prolonged zone of interpolation, and (4) a prolonged zone of sinus node reentry (see Fig. 9-16).

A fifth type of sinus node response to APD has been described: a second compensatory pause following very early APDs (Fig. 9-17).[192] Collision between early APDs and the next sinus beat cannot be merely a consequence of

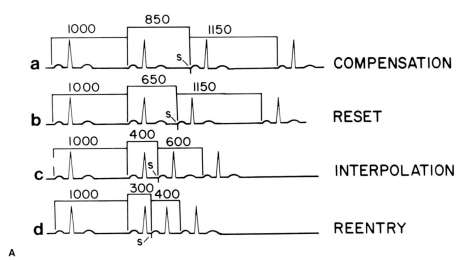

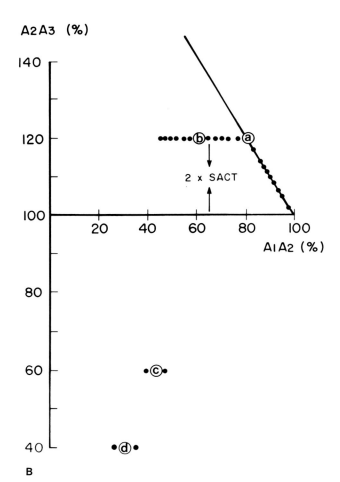

Figure 9-15. (**A**) Various types of sinus node response to atrial extra stimuli—compensation, reset, interpolation, and reentry. Compensation implies that the atrial premature depolarization did not depolarize the sinus node, leading to the development of a compensatory pause. Atrial premature complexes that occur earlier in the sinus cycle lead to the premature depolarization of the sinus node with subsequent reset (i.e., a less than compensatory pause). On rare occasions, an atrial premature depolarization can be interpolated and not disturb the manifest sinus cycle length. On very rare occasions, an atrial premature depolarization that occurs early in the diastole can lead to delayed entrance into the sinus node region, followed by sinus node reentry. (**B**) The horizontal axis identifies the test coupling interval (i.e., the A_1A_2 interval expressed as a percentage of the basic sinus cycle, A_1A_{-1} interval). The vertical axis identifies the return cycle length (i.e., the A_2A_3 interval, again expressed as a percentage of basic sinus cycle length). Points a, b, c, and d refer to compensation, reset, interpolation, and reentry. The oblique line at the upper right identifies the line of compensation.

fortuitous timing, as in the case with late APDs. The marked prematurity of early APDs should allow more than sufficient time for retrograde sinoatrial conduction before the next sinus discharge. Thus, conduction of these APDs must be significantly slowed in the sinoatrial junction. In short, early APDs followed by a compensatory sinus pause

have encountered the relative refractory period of the sinoatrial junction, where decremental conduction becomes electrocardiographically manifest.

In 1962, Langendorf and coworkers deduced some of the functional characteristics of conduction between the sinoatrial node and the atrium from an analysis of the

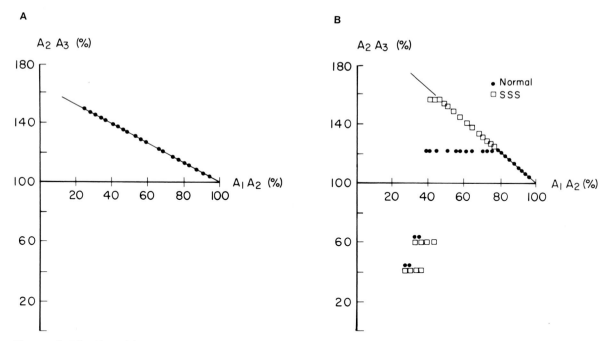

Figure 9-16. Plots of the A_1A_2/A_2A_3 relationships that might be expected in normal patients and in patients with sinus node dysfunction. (**A**), All points fall on the line of identity, indicating inability of even early atrial premature depolarizations to enter the sinus node and reset it. This is an example of first degree sinoatrial block. (**B**) Patients with sinus node dysfunction may be expected to have prolongation of the compensatory zone, a decrease in the reset zone, and increase in the interpolation and reentry zone.

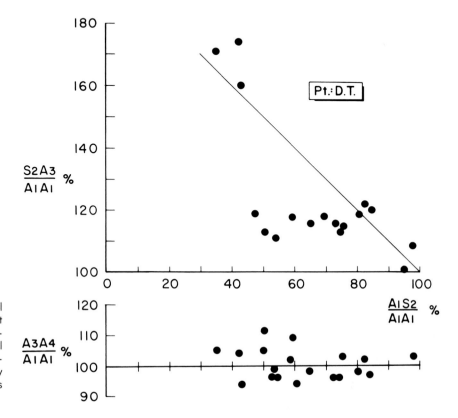

Figure 9-17. Plot of the A_1S_2 test interval versus the S_2A_3 response intervals. The plot at the lower portion of the panel identifies subsequent A_3A_4 intervals plotted against control A_1A_1. In the upper portion of this graph, a compensatory zone and a reset zone are followed by a second zone of compensation, which occurs with very early atrial premature complexes.

surface electrocardiogram in a patient with atrial parasystole.[193] Based on their clinical observations and on the experimental observations of Bonke and coworkers,[181] Strauss and coworkers[183] described how to assess SACT using programmed atrial stimulation. The calculation of SACT assumes that the difference between the mean return cycle length (A_2–A_3) in the zone of sinus node reset and the spontaneous cycle length (A_1–A_1) is equal to the time required for the APD to retrogradely conduct through the perinodal zone plus the time required for the reset sinus impulse to traverse the perinodal zone anterogradely and enter the atrium (Fig. 9-18). An abnormally prolonged SACT is compatible with first degree sinoatrial block, a characteristic of some patients with the sick sinus syndrome.[139, 184, 194–196, 196a]

However, this method requires certain assumptions: (1) all APDs resulting in a postextrasystolic pause that is less than compensatory must reset the sinus node, (2) APDs must not depress sinus node automaticity, an event that would cause an overestimation of SACT, (3) anterograde and retrograde conduction must be equally influenced by an APD, (4) SACT must be independent of variations in spontaneous sinus rate, a phenomenon common to many patients with sinus node dysfunction, and (5) the velocity of retrograde sinoatrial conduction must be independent of the site of atrial stimulation.

In isolated tissue, Miller and Strauss demonstrated that the transition between compensatory and less than compensatory postextrasystolic pauses included APDs that did not penetrate and reset the sinus node.[197] Shortening of the sinus node return cycle in these cases was due to a shortening of the sinus node action potential by elec-

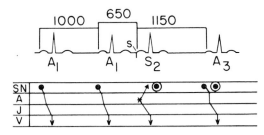

Figure 9-18. Diagrammatic explanation of the method of calculating sinoatrial conduction time (SACT). The electrocardiographic strip identifies the events seen before and after an atrial premature complex. In the laddergram, the asterisk identifies the atrial premature depolarization that prematurely excites the sinus node (arrowhead), the double circles identify where the anticipated sinus node depolarization should normally have been, and the solid circle identifies the reset sinus node discharge point. In the lowest portion of the diagram. SACT is calculated by subtracting the basal A_1A_1 interval (1000 msec) from the observed recovery time S_2A_3 interval (1150 msec). The total SACT, that is, the anterograde and retrograde conduction times, is 150 msec; the unidirectional conduction time, as expressed in the formula is 75 msec.

tronic interaction between sinus node and adjacent cells during repolarization. This artifactual shortening of the return cycle resulted in underestimation of the actual SACT. Furthermore, APDs delivered in the middle of the sinus cycle in animal hearts may depress sinus node automaticity and cause pacemaker shifts.[177] However, differences of opinion exist concerning the magnitude of the influence of depressed pacemaker automaticity on estimated SACT in humans.[198]

Miller and Strauss noted that measured anterograde and retrograde conduction times are not equal, retrograde conduction usually being faster than anterograde conduction.[197] In addition, SACT appears to vary as a function of the spontaneous sinus cycle length. At slower heart rates, estimated SACT is shorter than at faster heart rates.[199, 200]

Finally, Yamaguchi and Mandel have demonstrated that the speed of retrograde conduction of an APD depends on the site of atrial stimulation (see Table 9-1).[196a] This observation may relate to the existence of specialized functional pathways of conduction between the sinus node and the atrium.[201]

Despite these inherent problems, the method of Strauss and coworkers has proved a valuable addition to the diagnostic modalities available for evaluating sinus node dysfunction.[183] Differentiation between abnormalities of sinus node generator function and impulse conduction is now possible.

Reported ranges of normal values for calculated SACT in patients without apparent sinus node dysfunction include 56 ± 22 milliseconds; 70 ± 30 milliseconds; 84.5 ± 26 milliseconds; 92 ± 60 milliseconds; 82 ± 19.2 milliseconds; and 88 ± 7 milliseconds.[155, 163, 164, 188, 198, 202] However, many of these patients had evidence of organic heart disease, some with abnormalities of the distal conduction system, many with ischemic heart disease, and others with valvular abnormalities. Jordan and coworkers reported that patients with atherosclerotic involvement of the sinus node artery and no clinical or electrocardiographic evidence of sinus node dysfunction have significantly longer (although "normal") SACT values than do patients with coronary artery disease without such lesions.[162] Similar differences in SACT may eventually be found in patients without apparent sinus node dysfunction, depending on other underlying pathologic processes. Sinoatrial disease progression to overt clinical and electrocardiographic manifestations may be a dynamic but gradual process.

Furthermore, as sinus node recovery time may be influenced by differences in autonomic tone, so may SACT be modified by changes in autonomic activity. Bonke and coworkers[177] and Klein and coworkers[182] could demonstrate no effect of atropine on sinoatrial conduction. Miller and Strauss found that shortening of the sinus node action potential by APDs was not affected by atropine or propranolol.[197] However, in 17 normal human subjects, Dhingra and coworkers reported a significant shortening of calculated SACT after administration of 1 to 2 mg of atropine (from 103 ± 5.7 milliseconds to 58 ± 3.9 milliseconds) as well as a shortening of the zone of compensation.[203]

That SACT is shortened in humans by the administration of atropine, independent of any change in heart rate, is suggested by the observation that the return cycle following an APD shortened more than did the sinus cycle length.[203] In keeping with a hypothesis that atropine facilitates perinodal conduction, this drug has been shown to eliminate interpolation and echo responses in some persons.[203] Techniques for lengthening the perinodal refractory period, such as pacing the atrium at a rate faster than the sinus rate, have increased the number of normal subjects with zones of interpolation and reentry.[202]

The effect of atropine on SACT in patients with sinus node dysfunction varies. Some patients with sick sinus have marked shortening of SACT after receiving atropine; others have only minimal shortening.[203, 204] Dhingra and coworkers found that mean preatropine and postatropine SACTs in 21 patients with sick sinus did not differ significantly than previously reported mean postatropine SACTs in 17 patients without evidence of sinus node dysfunction.[203, 205] Sick sinus patients who show significant shortening of SACT after atropine administration may have lower levels of resting parasympathetic activity and, therefore, less residual parasympathetic tone after similar doses of atropine. Alternatively, these patients may have greater resting sympathetic activity than patients failing to demonstrate SACT shortening. Finally, these patients may have no abnormalities of intrinsic electrophysiologic properties of sinoatrial conduction, their sinus node dysfunction being primarily a manifestation of abnormal autonomic control of sinoatrial conduction.

Dhingra and coworkers did not find an overall shortening of the zone of compensation following atropine administration or a lengthening of the zone of sinus reset in patients with sick sinus.[205] Similarly, interpolation and echo responses were unaffected by atropine in these patients.

Strauss and coworkers found that propranolol, 1 mg/kg, significantly lengthened SACT in patients with sick sinus.[206] However, effects on sinus node automaticity may have contributed to this finding.

As a group, in the control state, patients with sick sinus and abnormal IHRs have significantly longer SACT than patients with sick sinus and normal IHRs. Also, patients with sick sinus and normal IHRs have significantly greater decreases in SACT than patients with abnormal IHRs after autonomic blockade. However, individual patients do not neatly separate in terms of normal and abnormal SACT based on normal versus abnormal IHRs, either in the control state or after complete pharmacologic autonomic

blockade. That is, many patients with sick sinus and normal IHRs have abnormal SACT; many patients with sick sinus and abnormal IHRs have normal SACT. Thus, autonomic blockade appears to be a better discriminator of intrinsic sinus node pacemaker dysfunction than of intrinsic sinoatrial conduction abnormalities. However, to assess sinoatrial conduction based on sinus node automaticity (i.e., IHR) may not be appropriate. To declare intrinsic sinoatrial conduction abnormal, comparison between known or predicted normal intrinsic SACT values would be more appropriate. Specifically, similar levels of autonomic tone do not influence heart rate and sinoatrial conduction to a similar degree. Thus, rather than adjusting SACT for the role that autonomic tone plays in its value by the ratio RHR/IHRo, a more accurate formula, suggested by Kuga and coworkers, might be[174]:

Adjusted SACT = SACT + SACT
$$\times \ (\text{SACT/Intrinsic SACT} - 1.00)$$

Although SACT does not correlate with age, intrinsic SACT does increase in a linear fashion with age (similar to IHR and intrinsic SNRTC) in normals and in patients with sick sinus syndrome.[129] Therefore, because age is a major determinant of the value of intrinsic SACT, patients may be found to have SACT values that track with IHR, if intrinsic SACT (rather than control SACT) is studied and if sick sinus patients are compared only to normal patients who are matched for age.

Few studies have attempted to establish normal values for intrinsic SACT. Alboni and coworkers reported a mean intrinsic SACT value in 20 normal patients to be 154 ± 30 milliseconds (i.e., upper limits of normal, 214 milliseconds).[149] More importantly, DeMarneefe and coworkers have reported normal intrinsic SACT values for different age groups in 30 healthy patients.[129] Mean intrinsic SACT was 81 ± 18 milliseconds in eight patients older than 40 years, 128 ± 26 milliseconds in eight patients aged 40 to 60 years, and 179 ± 78 milliseconds in 14 patients older than 60 years. Thus, upper limits of normal (M + 2 SD) in these age groups are 127 milliseconds, 180 milliseconds, and 335 milliseconds, respectively. Although these values may be valid, various age groups of larger numbers of patients may have to be studied to establish truer norms for intrinsic SACT. The construction of a linear regression equation relating intrinsic SACT to age in normals has not been reported; therefore, there is no mechanism for predicting intrinsic SACT.

The incidence of abnormal prolongation of calculated SACT in 418 patients without evidence of sinus node dysfunction was found to be 2% by Dhingra and coworkers.[195] However, these investigators used an SACT of 152 milliseconds as their criterion for abnormal, a figure considerably greater than other investigators have used. Therefore, their number of false-positive results may be spuriously low. This high cut-off value for normal subjects may also explain the low incidence of abnormal SACT found in patients suspected of having sinus node dysfunction (29% of 52 patients). Breithardt and coworkers reported that 45% of 41 patients with various manifestations of sinus dysfunction had prolonged SACT when 120 milliseconds was used as the upper limit of normal.[196] Using a normal value of 215 milliseconds for total anterograde plus retrograde conduction, Strauss and coworkers reported that 38% of 16 patients with sinus node dysfunction demonstrated an abnormally long total SACT.[139]

Breithardt and coworkers attempted to correlate prolongation of SACT and sinus node recovery time with specific electrocardiographic abnormalities in patients with sick sinus.[196] Patients with asymptomatic sinus bradycardia did not have significantly longer SNRTC or SACT values than control subjects, whereas patients with symptoms did. Patients with the bradycardia-tachycardia syndrome, episodic sinoatrial block, or both demonstrated significantly longer sinus node recovery time values than control subjects, although SACT in the bradycardia-tachycardia group did not differ from that of the control patients. Sinus node recovery time was found to be a somewhat more sensitive measure than SACT, showing fewer false-negative results in patients with sinus node dysfunc-

tion (Fig. 9-19). Nonetheless, SACT determination proved to be a better method of distinguishing patients with sick sinus from healthy subjects than had previously been reported.[138]

Continuous Pacing Method for Determining Sinoatrial Conduction Time

Limitations of the atrial premature stimulus technique for determining the SACT have been reviewed. To circumvent sinus node suppression, pacemaker shift, and other variables, Narula and coworkers described a new method for determining SACT using overdrive atrial pacing.[207] The atrium is paced 10 beats per minute faster than the basic sinus rate for eight beats. The interval in milliseconds from the last paced beat to the first return sinus beat on the intra-atrial electrogram is taken as the total time of retrograde and anterograde sinoatrial conduction (Fig. 9-20). Clinically, at this pacing rate, the sinus node pacemaker does not appear to be suppressed and there is no suggestion of pacemaker shift when postreturn cycles (A_3–A_4, A_4–A_5, and so on) are examined. The measure appears to be reproducible. The advantages of the methods are that complex equipment (i.e., programmed stimulator) and

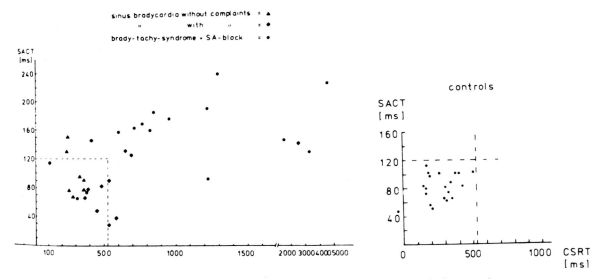

Figure 9-19. In this figure, the corrected sinus node recovery time (CSRT) is plotted on the horizontal axis and the sinoatrial conduction time (SACT) is plotted on the vertical axis. In the right-hand graph, data on control patients without clinical evidence of sinus node dysfunction are plotted. In all patients, CSRT and SACT fall within the normal zone. The left-hand graph shows data for patients with sinus bradycardia but no significant complaints (*triangles*), sinus bradycardia with cardiovascular complaints (*diamonds*), and data for patients with bradycardia-tachycardia syndrome with sinoatrial block (*circles*). The most abnormal data points for both sinoatrial conduction and sinus node recovery times occur with patients with bradycardia-tachycardia syndrome with sinoatrial block. Most patients with sinus bradycardia but no central nervous system symptoms fall within the normal zone. (Breithardt G, Seipel L, Loogan F: Sinus node recovery time and calculated sinoatrial conduction time in normal subjects and patients with sinus node dysfunction. Circulation 1977;56:43; with permission.)

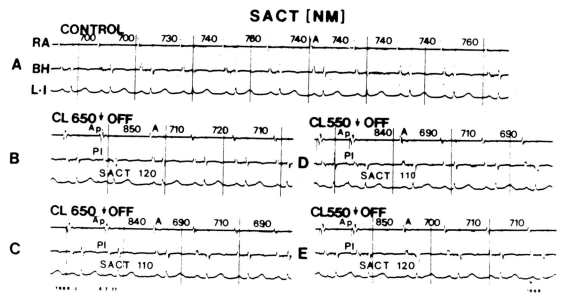

Figure 9-20. This figure shows a different method of calculating the sinoatrial conduction time. Recordings are shown in the control state and after overdrive pacing, at cycle lengths of 650 and 550. Note the similarity of sinoatrial conduction times measured after the last paced beats to the onset of the next spontaneous sinus complex. (Narula OS, Narashimhan S, Vaszuez M et al: A new method for measurement of sinoatrial conduction time. Circulation 1978;58:706; with permission.)

laborious calculations required for SACT determination with the premature atrial stimulation technique are unnecessary.

The validity of SACT as estimated by the constant atrial pacing technique has been examined in the micro-electrode laboratory (Table 9-2).[172] Many of the same difficulties encountered in the premature atrial stimulus technique exist in the constant atrial pacing method. Shortening of sinus node action potential, depression of automacity, and shifts in the primary pacemaker contributed to errors in both techniques. Estimation of SACT by the constant atrial pacing method was further complicated by failure of sinus node capture, especially at slow pacing rates (≤ 5 beats per minute faster than the basic sinus rate). Total SACT 5, 10, and 15 beats per minute faster than the RHR were 76 ± 10, 86 ± 10, and 96 ± 10 milliseconds; correlation coefficients with measured SACT were 0.7, 0.54, and 0.4, respectively. Estimates of SACT by constant atrial stimulation compared well with estimates by premature atrial stimulation. The mean $\pm$ SEM were similar for both techniques. SACTs overestimated by constant pacing tended to be overestimated by premature atrial stimulation. The correlation coefficient for the two methods was 0.85. When the two estimates were compared with measured SACTs, the determinations were not significantly different from each other ($P \geq 0.9$), and both were subject to a mean error of approximately 30%. Pretreatment with atropine and propranolol did not prevent shortening of

the sinus node action potential duration. The antegrade conduction time preceding the train of paced beats was 30 milliseconds and 10 milliseconds for the first return sinus beat, possibly reflecting a shift in the pacemaker site toward the crista terminalis and leading to an underestimation of SACT; antegrade conduction time usually returned to its prepacing value in five to 10 cycles.

Clinically, Kang and coworkers found that the two methods correlated very well ($r = 0.80$) during control and after autonomic blockade ($r = 0.85$).[173] In addition, the directional changes in SACT after autonomic blockade were always similar. For each method, eight of 12 patients with sick sinus demonstrated shortening of SACT and four of 12 demonstrated lengthening of SACT after autonomic blockade. The investigators suggested that prolongation of SACT after autonomic blockade is an abnormal response in patients in whom sinus node suppression cannot be demonstrated by examining postpacing or post-extra stimulus cycle lengths. They proposed that an increase in SACT may be related to intrinsic abnormalities of sinoatrial conduction previously masked by sympathetic activity.

Breithardt and Seipel reported a poor correlation between SACTs by the constant atrial stimulation method and the premature atrial stimulation method ($r = 0.45$).[207a] The investigators suggested that the poor correlation resulted from greater depression of sinus node automaticity by the premature atrial stimulus technique. However, Grant and coworkers believe that the disparity was more

TABLE 9-2. Sinoatrial Conduction Times and Transition Points During Crista Terminalis, Coronary Sinus, and Atrial Septal Stimulation

	Crista Terminalis	Coronary Sinus	Atrial Septum
Retrograde conduction time (msec)	19.7 ± 1.1	18.6 ± 1.6	15.7 ± 1.0 ‡
Anterograde conduction time (msec)	32.5 ± 2.6 ΔΔΔ	33.5 ± 2.6 ΔΔΔ	34.7 ± 2.8 ΔΔΔ*
Total measured conduction time (msec)	52.2 ± 3.3	52.1 ± 4.1	50.4 ± 3.0
Estimated conduction time (msec)	57.8 ± 6.3	66.4 ± 10.7	43.6 ± 4.8 †
Transition point (%)	83.6 ± 1.2	83.0 ± 11.9	88.7 ± 0.9 ‡

Key: mean ± SEM; N = 18; * = significantly different from crista terminalis stimulation; Δ = significantly different from retrograde conduction time. (SEM, standard error of the mean)

Δ* $P < 0.05$

ΔΔ† $P < 0.01$

ΔΔΔ† $P < 0.005$

likely related to failure of penetration and reset of the sinus node during pacing at slow pacing rates, an effect that disappeared when pacing rates were increased by as little as 3 beats per minute.[207b]

SINOATRIAL REFRACTORINESS

Goldreyer and Damato postulated the phenomenon of sinoatrial entrance block to explain why a critically coupled APD becomes interpolated and suggested that entrance block is a manifestation of sinoatrial refractoriness.[161a] The property of sinoatrial refractoriness has been studied and confirmed in the microelectrode laboratory by Kerr and coworkers. More recently, Kerr and Strauss have attempted to explore the difference in sinoatrial refractoriness in patients with and without sick sinus syndrome.[208] These investigators found that, in a group of normal subjects of all ages, the sinus node refractory period was between 250 and 380 milliseconds, whereas the sinus node refractory period in patients of all ages with sick sinus syndrome was between 500 and 550 milliseconds. Atropine shortens the sinoatrial refractory period in normals but the effect in sick sinus patients is variable. In a more recent study during an atrial pacing cycle length of 660 milliseconds, Kerr[209] observed that sinoatrial refrac-

tory period in 12 normal subjects shortened after the administration of atropine and propranolol from a mean value of 360 ± 40 milliseconds to 320 ± 40 milliseconds ($P = 0.05$), suggesting that the upper limits of normal for intrinsic sinoatrial refractory period is 360 milliseconds. Age-related normal intrinsic refractory periods have not yet been determined. Two recent studies have confirmed the theoretically expected result that intrinsic sinus node effective refractory period prolongs as pacing cycle length decreases.[209, 210]

Sinus Node Extracellular Potential Recordings

Developments in electrophysiologic techniques have permitted the recording of the sinus node action potential from the endocardial and epicardial surfaces of the intact heart.[175, 176, 211, 212] With unipolar recordings through Ag-AgCI electrodes (0.5 mm in diameter), covered to the tip with polyethylene, directly coupled to a preamplifier and positioned 0.2 to 0.5 mm above the sinus node, identification of pacemaker action potentials from the epicardial surface has been substantiated by simultaneous transmembrane recordings in isolated rabbit hearts.[175] A similar technique that obtains both unipolar and bipolar recordings has permitted extracellular action potentials to be recorded from the epicardial surface in humans during open-heart surgery (Fig. 9-21).[176] Hariman and coworkers found that SACTs were 32.4 ± 2.8 milliseconds at sinus cycle lengths 587.6 ± 35.6 milliseconds for the bipolar method and 38.2 ± 3.2 milliseconds at sinus cycle lengths of 712.2 ± 50.7 milliseconds for the unipolar method.[213]

Finally, a transvenous catheter technique has been developed to record endocardial surface sinoatrial pacemaker potentials in the intact canine heart and, more recently, in humans.[211, 214–216] Gomes and coworkers have reported that when the catheter was looped in the right atrium and advanced to the junction of the superior vena cava and right atrium so that the distal poles of the catheter were in direct contact with the right atrial endocardium underlying the area of the sinoatrial node, stable sinoatrial electrograms could be obtained in 18 of 21 (86%) patients.[217] The method was reported to be superior to the technique of Reiffel and colleagues, in which the catheter tip was only in close proximity to the right atrial endocardium.[215] The former technique minimized baseline drift of the sinoatrial electrogram. Patients with sick sinus syndrome consistently had longer directly measured SACT (1.35 ± 30 milliseconds) than did patients without sick sinus syndrome (87 ± 12 milliseconds), measurements in agreement with those found by Reiffel and coworkers. The discrepancy between SACT recorded from the endocardial surface and SACT recorded from the epicardial surface

HUMAN SAN ELECTROGRAMS

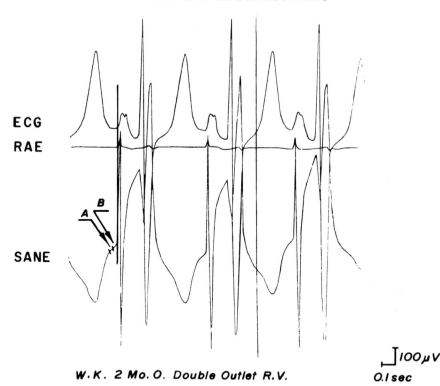

ECG
RAE

SANE

Figure 9-21. Extracellular recordings obtained from human sinus node at the time of open heart surgery. From top to bottom are surface electrocardiogram (ECG), right atrial electrogram (RAE), and a sinoatrial node electrogram (SANE). Note the appearance of pre–P-wave electrical activity in the sinoatrial node electrogram. (Courtesy of Roger Hariman, MD.)

W.K. 2 Mo. 0. Double Outlet R.V.

$\rfloor 100 \mu V$

0.1 sec

by Hariman and colleagues[213] was not explained, although Haberl and coworkers[218] suggest that Hariman may have underestimated true SACT because of failure to center the electrode over the primary pacemaker. These investigators demonstrated that even a small distance away from the primary pacemaker results in an underestimation of true SACT as determined by simultaneous intracellular recordings. These investigators warn that the positioning of the extracellular electrode cannot be precisely controlled in humans; therefore, absolute findings of SACT in milliseconds, derived from the technique, should be interpreted with caution and may be shorter than true SACT.

There was good correlation between direct and indirect SACTs estimated by Narula's pacing method (r = 0.843, N = 28) and by the premature stimulation method (r = 0.778, N = 18). The direct method, $SACT_d$, appears superior to the indirect methods, $SATC_i$, for measuring SACT in patients in whom no zone of reset can be obtained and in patients in whom frequent atrial premature complexes are present.

Based on their findings that $SACT_i$ often overestimates $SACT_d$, Reiffel and coworkers have suggested that when $SACT_i$ is normal, $SACT_d$ is normal; however, if $SACT_i$ is prolonged, $SACT_d$ may be normal.[215] On the other hand, Gomes and coworkers found that $SACT_i$ often underestimates $SACT_d$.[217] The discrepancy between these results

needs further explanation, but it may relate to differences in methodology.

Although these techniques await further confirmation and wider application, such developments are major advances in electrophysiologic methodology. The surface electrocardiogram and intracavitary recordings often grossly misrepresent underlying electrophysiologic events in the sinus node and sinoatrial junction in the setting of overdrive pacing and premature atrial stimulation. Applying these new methods of recording surface electrical potentials from the sinoatrial region in humans may provide new insights into the mechanisms of function and dysfunction in the human sinus node.

The most controversial application of sinoatrial electrogram recordings in humans comes from a report by Asseman and colleagues.[219] These investigators studied eight patients with sick sinus whose sinus node recovery time was greater than 1500 milliseconds. In six patients, sinus node electrograms, appearing at a rate similar to the basic sinus rate, persisted during the postpacing pause. The authors concluded that the pause following cessation of atrial overdrive is often caused by overdrive-induced sinoatrial block rather than by sinus node pacemaker suppression in patients with sick sinus. This conclusion directly conflicts with findings in microelectrode studies that clearly demonstrate suppression of sinus node pacemaker activity by atrial overdrive pacing in both the normal sinus node and in the sinus node made abnormal by the addition of verapamil to the isolated tissue preparation.[146, 220] Moreover, microelectrode studies that do confirm alteration in sinoatrial conduction following overdrive pacing (as a consequence of decreased sinus pacemaker action potential amplitude) also show slowing of pacemaker rate.[221, 222] Asseman and coworkers reported that overdrive pacing resulted in no sinus rate suppression, despite obvious changes in action potential characteristics. Despite these inconsistencies, the findings of Asseman's group are provocative, especially because there is a complex interaction between conduction and impulse formation that determines sinus node recovery time.

More in keeping with microelectrode findings is a report of Gomes and coworkers in which direct sinus node recordings in humans revealed that $SNRT_i$ reflects both sinus node automaticity and sinoatrial conduction.[223] In all 16 patients, overdrive atrial pacing appeared to result in marked prolongation of $SACT_d$ for the first postpacing beat, which was longer in patients with sick sinus than in healthy subjects. However, only one patient demonstrated actual sinoatrial block. Postpacing $SACT_d$ prolongation persisted for 3.6 ± 0.96 beats. Sinus node suppression was seen in 56% of total patients, that is, in 44% of normal patients and in 71% of patients with sick sinus syndrome. Sinus node acceleration was noted in 26% of patients, and no appreciable change in sinus node automaticity was observed in 19%. Insensitive to the contribution of increased SACT to sinus node recovery after overdrive pacing, $SNRT_i$ consistently overestimated $SNRT_d$, although $SNRT_d$ was significantly longer in patients with sick sinus.

To what extent sinoatrial block, either entrance or exit, influences sinus node recovery time probably depends on many variables including the level of parasympathetic tone present, the presence of drugs that either enhance or suppress sinoatrial conduction, differential aging of the sinoatrial junction and the sinus node, and the differential effects that disease has on the sinoatrial junction and the sinus node, which is, in part, determined by the fact that the two regions of the sinoatrial area depend on different ionic currents, possibly with different susceptibilities to disease.

Spontaneous pacemaker cell shifts and postoverdrive pacemaker shifts have been recorded in humans by sinus node extracellular potential recordings.[224] These shifts occur more often in sick sinus patients than in normals. When the primary pacemaker cell shifts to subsidiary pacemaker cells within the sinus node, sinus rate slows and there are changes in the characteristics of the new pacemaker action potential, including the resting membrane potential and the slope of phase 4 diastolic depolar-

ization. In the sick sinus syndrome, these subsidiary intranodal pacemakers may regularly assume dominance over the "sick" primary pacemaker. Furthermore, the intrinsic determinants of subsidiary pacemakers (e.g., the if or ik current) may be more susceptible to the effects of overdrive than the primary pacemaker, as is suggested by exaggerated suppression by overdrive of pacemakers outside the sinoatrial area (e.g., AV nodal and Purkinje fiber pacemakers).[225-228]

Direct sinoatrial electrogram recordings have exposed the importance of the role of alterations in sinoatrial conduction in other bradycardic situations previously ascribed to depression of sinus node automaticity alone. Using this recording technique, Gang and coworkers have shown that sinoatrial block is an important component of the asystolic pause that occurs in patients with the cardioinhibitory form of the hypersensitive carotid sinus syndrome (Fig. 9-22).[229] This finding is predictable because the baroreceptor reflex is mediated by enhanced parasympathetic tone and the sinoatrial junction is particularly sensitive to vagal stimulation compared to the sinus node.

Carotid sinus hypersensitivity may be manifested in two ways, apparently independent of each other.[230, 231] The cardioinhibitory type is expressed as an apparent slowing of the heart rate with mechanical stimulation of the carotid sinus and is inhibited by atropine. The less common vasodepressor type is accompanied by vasodilation and hypotension and is often inhibited by epinephrine. The cardioinhibitory type appears to be mediated by the parasympathetic nervous system and is most commonly found in elderly men with coronary atherosclerosis and hypertensive heart disease.[232-234] The precise mechanism of the cardioinhibitory type is not known, although four possibilities have been proposed: (1) a high level of resting vagal tone, (2) excessive release of acetylcholine, (3) inadequate cholinesterase activity, and (4) hyperresponsiveness to acetylcholine. If the latter mechanism is the predominant one, carotid hypersensitivity is properly part of the sick sinus syndrome. However, the findings of Marley and coworkers that normals and sick sinus patients have similar sinus node bradycardia responses to phenylephrine—induced hypertension suggested to the investigators that sick sinus patients have normal responses to reflex vagal stimulation.[235a]

Most patients with carotid hypersensitivity have normal sinus node recovery time and SACT.[231, 235-237]

Reiffel and coworkers have employed sinus node extracellular potential recordings to demonstrate the existence of two controversial electrical events in the sinoatrial region: sinoatrial reentry and concealed conduction.[238] Evidence for sinus node echoes includes fixed coupling between the sinus node deflections and the preceding retrograde

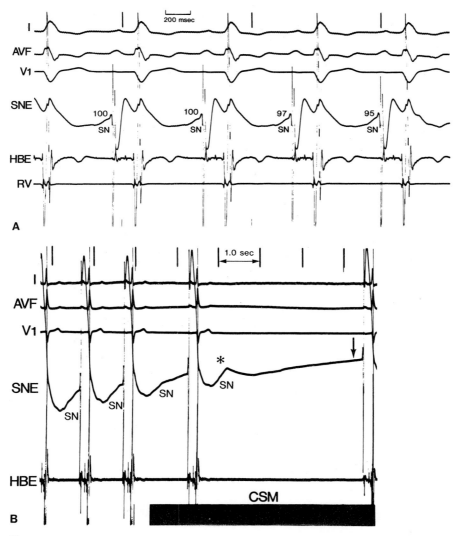

Figure 9-22. (**A**) The sinus node electrogram. Surface electrocardiogram leads I, aVF, and V₁ are displayed along with intracavitary electrocardiograms from the region of the sinus node, His bundle, and right ventricle. Sinus node potentials are the positive-going, low-frequency deflections preceding each atrial depolarization. The directly measured sinoatrial conduction times are labeled above each sinus node deflection. SNE, sinus node; *HBE*, His bundle; *RV*, right ventricle; SN, sinus node potentials. (**B**) Carotid sinus massage in a patient with the hypersensitive carotid sinus syndrome. Surface and intracardiac electrocardiograms are labeled as in (**A**). The onset of carotid sinus massage is followed by profound prolongation in the sinus node deflection, signifying probable prolongation in the sinoatrial conduction time. Sinoatrial block is then illustrated, because a sinus node impulse is shown to occur without subsequent atrial depolarization (*asterisk*). Sinus node quiescence is then recorded until the inscription of the next atrial impulse, which is not preceded by a sinus node potential (*arrow*). The absence of a sinus node potential suggests a shifting of the primary pacemaker focus out of the sinus node or to another region without the sinus node. *CSM*, cardiac sinus massage.

sinus node depolarization, retrograde conduction delay from an atrial premature depolarization into the sinus node preceding the echo, prolongation of the sinus cycle length following the atrial echo, and similar coupling intervals to those seen in sinus node echoes studied by indirect techniques. Evidence for concealed sinoatrial conduction included antegrade conduction delay in the cycle following an interpolated premature depolarization that could not be seen on the body surface electrocardiogram.

HUMAN SINUS NODE ANTIBODY DETECTION

Maisch and coworkers have determined that a 10-fold increase in incidence of sick sinus syndrome could be calculated in patients with anti–sinus-node antibodies as compared with age-matched controls.[83] Patients with sick sinus syndrome and prior myocarditis or rheumatic fever had a three-fold incidence of that antibody. Anti–sinus-node antibodies were found to be highly specific for sinus node disorders; their sensitivity was less and was probably dependent on their cause.

Determination of anti–sinus-node antibody titers is not yet routinely performed in all cases of suspected sick sinus syndrome. Such determinations may revolutionize methods of establishing the diagnosis of sick sinus syndrome, especially when considered in the context of electrophysiologic test results. Serial titers of anti–sinus-node antibodies may even provide information about the natural history of the sick sinus syndrome and predict the course of sinus node dysfunction in any patient, guiding therapeutic decisions regarding timing of pacemaker implantation and the use of other therapeutic modalities. Additionally, the magnitude of abnormalities of electrophysiologic test results may correlate with the magnitude of anti–sinus-node antibodies. Finally, if anti–sinus-node antibodies are not only markers of the disease but also important to the pathophysiology of some cases, new therapeutic approaches may be developed, including the use of anti-inflammatory and immunosuppressive agents.

EFFECTS OF DRUGS ON NORMAL AND ABNORMAL SINUS NODE FUNCTION

Sinus node response to any particular pharmacologic agent varies and may even appear to be almost idiosyncratic. In any given person, a specific drug may have negligible, profound stimulatory, or marked inhibitory effects on sinus node automaticity or sinoatrial conduction. Furthermore, the electrophysiologic effects of many antiarrhythmic agents, as observed in isolated tissue preparations, often do not correspond to the clinical response witnessed in humans. The effect of a drug on sinus node function may differ significantly when it is given as an acute single intravenous dose or as chronic oral administration. These apparent inconsistencies can be explained when several facts are considered: (1) the effects of a drug on sinus node function may be mediated by indirect (interaction with the autonomic and central nervous systems) as well as direct mechanisms of action, (2) the sinus node response to a specific cardiac drug may differ in the setting of abnormal intrinsic sinoatrial function than when no intrinsic sinus node abnormalities are present, (3) in sinoatrial dysfunction, the clinical response to a pharmacologic agent may be determined by the specific electrophysiologic property that is abnormal as well as the magnitude of the abnormality, (4) drugs may have differential effects on properties of sinus node automaticity and sinoatrial conduction, and (5) the electrophysiologic assumptions on which the technique of premature atrial stimulation are based may be invalid in the sinus node, and sinoatrial junction may be made abnormal by cardioactive drugs.

Even if the electrophysiologic mode of action of all antiarrhythmic drugs was understood and even if the primary electrophysiologic mechanisms of electrogenesis were certain, it is unlikely that the effect on sinus node function by any antiarrhythmic drug would be entirely predictable. Specifically, background currents in the sinus node interact with and modulate the properties and behavior of the primary ionic channel. Although not all antiarrhythmic drugs affect the primary channel directly, a particular agent may affect a background current that impacts on the primary channel in a major way, a minor way, or not at all.

Finally, intranodal subsidiary pacemakers may often assume dominance over the "sick" primary pacemaker in the sick sinus patient. These subsidiary pacemakers probably have different intrinsic ionic determinants of automaticity (e.g., if current or ik current) than does the primary pacemaker, leading to susceptibility to certain drugs that otherwise would not be anticipated to affect sinus node function based on their known electrophysiologic action.

Established Antiarrhythmic Agents

Digitalis

Digitalis preparations slow sinus rate by slowing the rate of rise of phase 4 of the sinus node action potential. Changes in action potential amplitude and threshold potential have also been reported.[239] Most studies indicate that an interaction with the autonomic nervous system is probably the primary mechanism of action of digitalis on sinus node function.[240–244] However, negative chronotropic responses have also been demonstrated in denervated human hearts and in humans after complete pharmacologic blockade.[245] Gomes and coworkers found that ouabain, 0.01 mg/kg administered intravenously after pharmacologic autonomic blockade, significantly lengthened sinus node recovery time in patients with normal and abnormal IHRs.[246] On the other hand, ouabain had no significant effect on SACT as determined by the continuous pacing method after autonomic blockade. Reports have described a positive chronotropic response to digitalis preparations in animals that may have been due to release of endogenous catecholamines or an increase in preganglionic sympathetic tone.[247–249]

In healthy subjects, digitalis generally has little effect on sinus rate, sinus node recovery time, or sinoatrial conduction. However, Dhingra and coworkers reported that digitalis shortened sinus node recovery time, and several clinical studies have indicated that digitalis lengthened estimated SACT.[208, 250, 251] This latter finding might suggest that shortening of sinus node recovery time is artifactual, because fewer paced beats are expected to penetrate the sinus node in the presence of digitalis. However, microelectrode studies in isolated rabbit atria demonstrate that ouabain produces almost no change in refractoriness of perinodal fibers in the retrograde direction (Fig. 9-23) (Yamaguchi I, Jordan JL, Mandel WJ: Antiarrhythmic drug effects on sinus node function during early premature stimulation, personal communication.) Furthermore, the premature atrial stimulus technique overestimates SACT in the presence of ouabain because depression of sinus node automaticity is depressed by the APD (Fig. 9-24) (Yamaguchi, personal communication).

In examining the effect of digitalis on sinoatrial function, Harriman and Hoffman, using sinoatrial electrogram recordings in instrumented dogs, found that ouabain caused beat-to-beat variation in sinus cycles, abnormalities of sinoatrial conduction, and pacemaker shifts.[251a] The effects could be abolished by atropine. Ouabain-induced failure of sinoatrial conduction appeared to result by one of two mechanisms. First, failure of sinoatrial conduction can occur if the amplitude of the sinus pacemaker potential is reduced so that it is unable to excite the surrounding tissue. Second, sinoatrial conduction can fail if the effects of ouabain are more intense on the fibers of the sinoatrial junction than on the sinus node pacemaker, resulting in sinoatrial block. Both mechanisms of failure of sinoatrial conduction have also been described in response to vagal stimulation. Because acetylcholine reduced SACT but not pacemaker action potential amplitude, the authors suggested that the effects of ouabain result from different densities of vagal fibers in different areas of the sinoatrial region rather than from differing sensitivities of pacemaker cells and perinodal cells to the drug.

Numerous investigators have cautioned against administering digitalis to patients with sick sinus syndrome.[210, 252, 253] However, adverse effects on sinus node function in patients with this syndrome vary, and exaggerated responses cannot be predicted in any given patient.[252, 253]

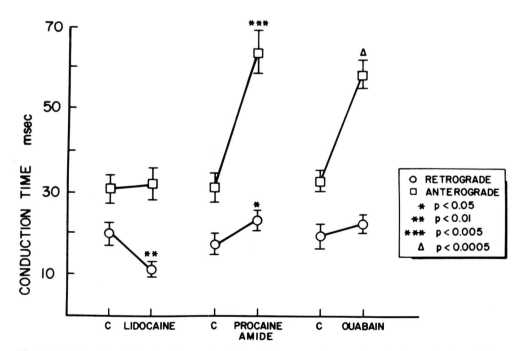

CRISTA TERMINALIS STIMULATION

Figure 9-23. The effect of various antiarrhythmic drugs on anterograde and retrograde sinoatrial conduction time in isolated cardiac tissue. With lidocaine, retrograde conduction time is significantly shortened, whereas with procainamide and ouabain, retrograde and, to a greater extent, anterograde conduction times are significantly prolonged.

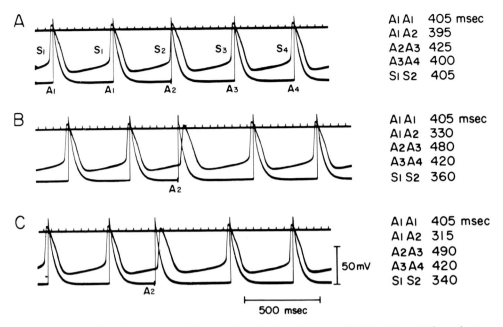

AI AI	405 msec
AI A2	395
A2A3	425
A3A4	400
SI S2	405

AI AI	405 msec
AI A2	330
A2A3	480
A3A4	420
SI S2	360

AI AI	405 msec
AI A2	315
A2A3	490
A3A4	420
SI S2	340

50 mV

500 msec

Figure 9-24. Plots showing the influence of ouabain on features of indirect sinoatrial conduction time measurements and the influence of premature atrial depolarizations on sinus node cycle lengths and the indirect measurement of sinoatrial conduction. (**A**), Very late diastolic atrial premature complexes (A_2) do not influence (capture) the sinus node. (**B**), An earlier A_1A_2 interval of 330 msec results in sinus node capture, but the test and return cycles are compensatory. (**C**) At an even earlier A_1A_2 interval, the test and return cycles are in the zone of reset. With ouabain, the sinus node could be prematurely discharged and reset at a time when the atrial electrograms indicate compensatory response (i.e., noncapture). These atrial records result in an apparent upward shift in the point of transition and would, therefore, lead to false prolongation of the indirectly measured sinoatrial conduction time.

Quinidine

In humans, the usual effect of quinidine is acceleration of sinus rate, believed to be mediated by an interaction with the autonomic nervous system.[254,255] Infrequent negative chronotropic effects on sinus node function do not appear to be related to beta-adrenergic blocking properties of the drug.[256] Mason and coworkers administered quinidine gluconate intravenously to cardiac allograft recipients (mean plasma level 4.3 μg/liter) 8 to 20 months after transplantation.[257] The sinus cycle length increased in all transplanted hearts but decreased in the innervated atrial remnant. The investigators concluded that direct membrane effects of quinidine slow the rate of depolarization of the sinus node whereas enhancement of sinus node in humans is neurally mediated. In persons without sinus node disease, quinidine-induced abnormalities of sinoatrial dysfunction are probably clinically rare.[258–260] No information is available on the incidence of adverse effects of quinidine in patients with sick sinus.

Procainamide

Consistent with microelectrode observations that procainamide has no significant effect on the characteristics of the spontaneous sinus node action potential, clinical reports of its adverse effects on sinus node function are infrequent.[239] Procainamide does prolong SACT in isolated tissue preparations, primarily by prolonging anterograde conduction (see Fig. 9-23).[239]

Clinically, Josephson and coworkers observed an increase in sinus rate (mean 7%) in response to intravenous procainamide administration.[260a] Although not extensively investigated, enhanced automaticity of the sinus pacemaker has been attributed to a vagolytic effect of procainamide. Reflex sympathetic discharge, because of negative ionotropic actions and vasodilatory effect of procainamide, may also play a role in accelerating heart rate. Goldberg and coworkers reported that procainamide tended to prolong SNRTC by enhancing sinoatrial conduction in patients with sinus node dysfunction.[261] In contrast, procainamide shortened SNRTC in patients without sinus node dysfunction.

Disopyramide

Disopyramide usually (but not invariably) shortens sinus cycle length in healthy persons, presumably by a vagolytic effect.[262] Negative ionotropic effects with reflex sympathetic discharge may also play a role in sinus rate acceleration.[263] In isolated sinoatrial preparations, disopyramide has little effect on sinus node recovery time or sinoatrial conduction regardless of the magnitude of cholinergic tone.[264]

There appears to be a difference between the effect of disopyramide on normal and abnormal sinus node function. Disopyramide shortens sinus node recovery time in healthy persons but significantly prolongs recovery time in patients with sick sinus.[262, 265] LaBarre and coworkers reported that disopyramide slowed the sinus rate in some patients with sick sinus and shortened the estimated SACT in patients with sinus pauses, sinoatrial block, and secondary pauses after overdrive pacing.[265a]

Lidocaine

Contrary to microelectrode studies in isolated tissue, which demonstrate lidocaine to have little effect on characteristics of the sinus node action potential, Dhingra and coworkers reported that administration of this drug resulted in a significant decrease in the sinus cycle length in patients with normal and abnormal sinus node function. Positive chronotropic effects of lidocaine on the sinus node in humans may be secondary to the vagolytic properties of the drug.[265b]

Dhingra and coworkers reported that lidocaine shortened the mean maximal sinus node recovery time in humans, an effect presumably not artifactual, because lidocaine actually shortens the retrograde absolute refractory period of perinodal fibers and thus would not be expected to block penetration of paced beats into the sinus node.[265c] (Yamaguchi I, Jordan JL, Mandel WJ: Antiarrythmic drug effects on sinus node function during early premature stimulation, unpublished.) Estimated SACTs were significantly prolonged in patients with sick sinus but were unchanged in patients with normal sinus node function. In contrast, Yamaguchi and coworkers found that measured SACT was significantly shortened in isolated rabbit tissue after lidocaine superfusion (see Fig. 9-23).[239]

Lidocaine has been implicated in the precipitation of exaggeration of abnormalities of sinoatrial function in a number of clinical reports.[266] However, adverse effects of lidocaine on sinus node function cannot be reliably predicted.

Mexiletine

Mexiletine is structurally related to lidocaine and has many class IB antidysrhythmic actions. Yamaguchi and coworkers reported that, in isolated sinus node tissue, mexiletine slowed the sinus rate only in concentrations exceeding the equivalent of therapeutic plasma levels in humans.[267] In contrast, mexiletine prolonged SACT at concentrations below the equivalent of toxic plasma levels.

In animals and humans, mexiletine can cause sinus bradycardia.[268, 269] However, a slight acceleration in heart rate and decrease in sinus node recovery time have also been observed in some patients. Roos and coworkers reported that three of five patients demonstrating prolongation of sinus node recovery time after mexiletine administration had sick sinus syndrome, and in only one patient with sinus node dysfunction did recovery time decrease.[268] These investigators cautioned against using mexiletine in patients with dysfunction of impulse formation.

Tocainide

Tocainide is also structurally related to lidocaine, having class IB effects on the monophasic action potential. Although no reports suggest adverse effects on sinus node function, reported experiences with lidocaine and mexiletine warrant caution with the use of tocainide in patients with sick sinus syndrome.

Encainide

Encainide is a class IC antiarrhythmic agent with electrophysiologic properties similar to those of quinidine, except that it does not significantly alter action potential duration. In anesthetized dogs, Samuelsson and Harrison reported a significant reduction in heart rate with intravenous administration of encainide, 2.7 mg/kg.[270] Maximal increase in basic cycle length was reached within 15 to 30 minutes. These results were not confirmed by Sami and coworkers.[271] Furthermore, these investigators found no significant effect of encainide on sinus node recovery time. In humans, neither intravenous nor oral encainide has been shown to significantly affect heart rate or sinus node recovery time.[272]

Flecainide

Flecainide is an antiarrhythmic drug with a predominantly class IC mode of action. In doses of 1 mg/kg given intravenously, Seipel and coworkers found that it had no significant effect on sinus node function in patients with normal sinus node function.[273] However, at 2 mg/kg, sinus node recovery time increased 37% in these patients, although no effect was observed on spontaneous sinus rate. Vik-Mo and coworkers reported a statistically significant increase in corrected sinus node recovery time in patients with sinus node dysfunction when 1.5 mg/kg of flecainide was administered intravenously.[274] Sinus cycle length and SACT were not significantly changed. The investigators advised caution in using flecainide in patients with sinus node dysfunction.

Lorcainide

Lorcainide, another antiarrhythmic agent with class IC electrophysiologic properties, was shown in clinical electrophysiologic studies to prolong sinus node recovery time, particularly in patients with sinus node dysfunction.[275,276]

Diphenylhydantoin

Direct membrane effects, interaction with the autonomic nervous system, and central system effects could all contribute to the electrophysiologic effects of diphenylhydantoin (DPH).[277-279] In humans, heart rate response to DPH may vary. A cardioacceleratory effect may be secondary to an anticholinergic action; in the denervated dog heart, DPH slows the sinus rate.[277] Strauss and coworkers could find no significant effect of DPH on the sinus node action potential in isolated tissue preparations; however, the sinus node that had been depressed by stretch, mechanical trauma, or toxic concentrations of acetylcholine, propranolol, or potassium became markedly more susceptible to toxic concentrations of DPH.[280] Sinoatrial block, however, was not a manifestation of DPH-induced sinoatrial dysfunction in these experimentally depressed preparations.

Examples of sinus node dysfunction in the setting of intravenous DPH administration are well documented but may not be solely the effect of the drug. The solvent for DPH contains propylene glycol, a substance that has been shown to cause marked sinus bradycardia.[281]

Slow Channel Inhibitors

Verapamil

Verapamil is a slow channel blocking agent. It has not been established whether it blocks only calcium conductance or the sodium component of the slow channel as well. Verapamil has been demonstrated to affect all aspects of the sinus node action potential, with the possible exception of the maximum diastolic membrane potential. Wit and Cranefield reported that verapamil produced linear dose-related decreases in sinus rate.[282] The negative chronotropic effect of verapamil does not appear to be mediated by interaction with the autonomic nervous system.[283,284] Sinus node recovery time is prolonged after verapamil administration, as is SACT (in the anterograde direction only).[285-287]

In humans and intact animals, variable effects on heart rate have been demonstrated after intravenous verapamil administration. Most commonly, an increase in sinus rate is observed in the clinical settings after administration of the drug, presumably the result of a reflex autonomic response to hypotension.[288] Verapamil is contraindicated in patients with sick sinus syndrome.

Nifedipine

The effects of nifedipine on sinoatrial node transmembrane potentials are identical to the effects of verapamil, although these depressant effects require a much higher concentration of nifedipine.[289] More intense peripheral vasodilatory effects probably result in greater reflex sympathetic activity than is seen with verapamil, usually offsetting the negative chronotropic effects of nifedipine. Nonetheless, nifedipine should be used with caution in patients with sick sinus syndrome.

Diltiazem

Direct negative chronotropic effects of diltiazem are less than verapamil but greater than nifedipine.[290] Extreme caution is advised when using this drug in the setting of sinus node dysfunction.

Newer Antiarrhythmic Agents

Amiodarone

The mechanism of antiarrhythmic action of amiodarone is unknown. The drug appears to have major antimetabolic activity, significantly reducing myocardial oxygen consumption and increasing the ratio of ATP and creatine phosphate to ADP, creatine, and inorganic phosphate.[291]

Amiodarone, 1.5×10^{-5}M, slows spontaneous sinus rate activity. The most significant changes in the sinus node action potential include a depression of phase 4 diastolic depolarization and prolongation of the action potential duration.[292] The negative chronotropic action of amiodarone is enhanced under conditions of low calcium concentration. Autonomic blockade has little or no effect on the negative chronotropic action of amiodarone.[293]

Ajmaline

Ajmaline is a derivative of *Rauwolfia serpentina* and might be expected to depress sinus node function on the basis of catecholamine depletion as well as through direct membrane effects. Obayashi and Mandel observed no significant effect of ajmaline on sinus node automaticity in isolated sinus node preparations at concentrations less than 1×10^{-4}M/L.[294] In contrast, ajmaline prolonged anterograde sinoatrial conduction. In the intact dog heart, ajmaline slowed sinus rate only at high doses (8 mg/kg); at lower doses (4 mg/kg) an increase in heart rate was observed, perhaps due to a local (atrial) release of catecholamines.[295]

Aprindine

Aprindine hydrochloride has local anesthetic properties and may also possess significant slow channel blocking properties.[296] Direct membrane effects of the drug cause a dose-dependent slowing of sinus rate.[297] In humans, sinus rate is probably little affected by aprindine; reflex sympathetic activity in response to negative inotropic effects may offset direct membrane-depressant effects.[297]

Propafenone

Propafenone is a new antiarrhythmic agent with complex mechanisms of action, including (1) inhibition of fast sodium current, (2) lidocaine-like effects on transmembrane action potentials at low concentrations, (3) beta-sympatholytic actions, and (4) a weakly inhibitory effect on slow calcium inward current at high concentrations.[298, 299] In a dose-dependent fashion, propafenone reduces action potential amplitude, the maximum diastolic potential, and the rate of phase 4 depolarization while prolonging action potential duration.[300] In voltage-clamp studies. Satoh and Hashimoto concluded that the negative chronotropic effects of propafenone are predominantly mediated by decreases in the outward ik current in the sinus node.[300]

Sotalol

Sotalol is a unique antiarrhythmic agent with both classic beta-adrenergic blocking properties and class III antiarrhythmic effects on the human monophasic action potential.[301] Sotalol slows sinus rate and may precipitate significant exaggeration of sinus node dysfunction in patients with sick sinus syndrome.

Ethmozin

Ethmozin is the first phenothiazine derivative with primarily cardiac antiarrhythmic properties. Its exact modes of action are not known, although voltage-clamp studies in frog atrial muscle suggest that, at least, ethmozin depresses rapid inward current.[302] Roffy and coworkers perfused ethmozin directly into the sinus node artery of dogs and found no significant effect on heart rate.[303] The drug has mild, transient vasolytic effects.

Ethacizin

Ethacizin is the diethylamine analog of ethmozin. In contrast to ethmozin, after injection into the sinus node artery, this agent has significant negative chronotropic effects on the sinus node, which appear to be the result of a direct membrane effect.[304] Significant atropine-like action attenuates much of the negative chronotropic effects. For this reason, the drug has been considered to have a low incidence of clinically important consequences of its negative chronotropic and negative dromotropic actions. However, the drug has not been tested in patients with sick sinus

syndrome and until further data are available, the drug should be used with great caution in this group of patients.

Cibenzoline

Cibenzoline is a new antiarrhythmic agent of imidazole derivation unrelated to any other known antiarrhythmic drug. This agent does not interfere with sinus node diastolic depolarization and, therefore, does not alter sinus node automaticity per se. However, the drug causes a concentration-dependent prolongation of the sinus node action potential duration, which tends to decrease the rate of sinus node discharge.

Adenosine Triphosphate

Adenosine triphosphate (ATP) has potent inhibitory effects on AV nodal conduction and has become the parenteral drug of choice for rapid termination of reentrant supraventricular tachycardia.[305, 306] In normal subjects, ATP produces a dose-dependent prolongation of spontaneous sinus cycle length. Patients with sick sinus syndrome have been reported to have more exaggerated responses to ATP.

Sharma and Klein found a negative correlation between control sinus cycle length and the dose required to produce a maximal prolongation of cycle length.[307] This negative correlation may result because low resting parasympathetic tone may shorten sinus cycle length but increase the dose of ATP required. Consistent with this theory, West and Belardinelli found that ATP and acetylcholine produce hyperpolarization in the rabbit sinus node cell by similar mechanisms.[308] In contrast to the negative correlation between control SCL and the dose of ATP required to produce a maximal prolongation of sinus cycle length, there was a positive correlation between the AV nodal functional refractory period and the AH interval with a 2-mg dose. The authors suggested that ATP potentially has different mechanisms of action on sinus node automaticity and AV conduction, a theory supported by the fact that negative chronotropic actions of the drug are not mediated by interaction with the sympathetic nervous system, whereas negative dromotropic effects of the drug, in part, are so mediated. Secondary effects on ik current have been suggested.[309, 310]

Alinidine

Alinidine, a newly created compound chemically related to clonidine, specifically reduces sinus rate.[311] Miller and Vaughn Williams have proposed that this compound may represent a fifth class of antiarrhythmic drug.[28] These investigators have published the results of microelectrode studies on isolated sinus node preparations that strongly suggest that the mechanism by which alinidine decreased the slope of slow diastolic depolarization and increased action potential duration was by restricting inward current through anion-selective channels. Potential antiarrhythmic uses for this drug have not been explored. Because alinidine reduces heart rate without affecting blood pressure, myocardial contractility, or AV conduction, the drug may have important use as an antianginal agent.

Alinidine has not been studied in the setting of complete autonomic blockade. Its effects on sinus node recovery time, SACT, and heart rate response to exercise have not been examined.

MANAGEMENT OF PATIENTS WITH SICK SINUS SYNDROME

The indications for permanent pacing in patients with sick sinus syndrome must be clearly defined.[312-317] The benefits to be realistically expected from pacemaker insertion must be understood by the clinician so that sound judgment, based on well-controlled clinical trials, may prevail. Thus, the natural history, complications, morbidity, and mortality of the sick sinus syndrome must be elucidated. Furthermore, electrophysiologic and clinical predictors of the potential for complications must be developed and refined to improve decisions concerning the timing of pacemaker insertion.

Not only is the sick sinus syndrome a heterogeneous entity in underlying pathophysiologic mechanism, but it also occurs in a heterogeneous population having associated cardiovascular diseases. Patients with sick sinus with ischemic heart disease, congestive heart failure, or primary cerebrovascular disease form a higher risk population for sudden death than patients without these associated risk factors.[317-320] Therefore, clinical data concerning the benefits of permanent pacing in terms of reduction in mortality and morbidity should be assessed independently in patients with and without other cardiovascular diseases. In addition, patients with the bradycardia-tachycardia syndrome present therapeutic challenges not encountered in patients with sinus bradycardia, sinus arrest, or sinoatrial block alone.

If central nervous system symptoms have been shown to be unequivocally associated with episodes of sinus node dysfunction and failure of subsidiary pacemakers to escape, artificial pacing has been consistently successful in eliminating cerebral symptoms.[312,317-319] When an adequate cardiac output does not depend on atrial contribution, ventricular pacing has been as successful as atrial or AV sequential pacing in eliminating dizziness or syncope. With severe heart failure, subtle symptoms of fatigue and failing mental acuity may be as much a consequence of diminished stroke volume as an inappropriately slow heart rate. Only prepacing and postpacing hemodynamic studies at a variety of rates will support an assumption that a faster heart rate increases cerebral perfusion by increasing cardiac output. In patients with myocardial dysfunction, cardiac performance must be assessed in the basal state as well as with atrial and ventricular pacing.

Improvement in symptoms of congestive heart failure, with and without the addition of digitalis, has been reported after pacemaker implantation in some patients with the sick sinus syndrome.[314,317] In patients with ventriculoatrial conduction, however, VVI pacing can worsen congestive heart failure. Stewart and coworkers reported that dual-chamber pacing enhanced ventricular filling by restoring atrial transport function and increased cardiac output by as much as 30% compared to VVI pacing with 1:1 ventriculoatrial conduction.[321] Furthermore, Rediker and coworkers have suggested that hemodynamic improvement with dual-chamber pacing may remain stable, whereas the hemodynamic benefits of ventricular pacing tend to dissipate over time.[322] In an additional group of patients without overt congestive heart failure, patients were noted to achieve improved exercise tolerance after pacemaker insertion, which may be applicable to even more sick sinus patients with the introduction of rate-responsive pacemakers.[318]

Because the sick sinus syndrome is probably a diffuse disease of the AV conduction system, His bundle recordings should be performed when atrial pacing is considered. Frequently, abnormalities of AV nodal and distal pathways of conduction coexist with sinus node dysfunction. If atrial contribution to diastolic ventricular filling is necessary for adequate ventricular performance, sequential AV pacing should be considered in these patients. Although technical problems and malfunctions appear to be more common with these pacemakers, the clinical situation may allow no alternative.

In general, pharmacologic approaches to the management of sinus bradycardia have been disappointing.[313,323,324] However, notable exceptions have been reported, with symptom-free states lasting for 5 years or longer. Atropine-like drugs and sublingual beta-adrenergic drugs have obvious disadvantages. These include short durations of action, intolerable side effects, irregular and unreliable absorption, and the need for unfaltering patient compliance to a demanding dose schedule. Moreover, these drugs have been shown to worsen or precipitate atrial and ventricular tachyarrhythmias.

Bradyarrhythmias are less well tolerated by patients with significant cerebrovascular disease. In these patients, even short episodes of moderately slow heart rates can be catastrophic. Moreover, a stable sinus bradycardia may have variable central nervous system consequences depending on the relative distribution of blood flow during periods of stress or exercise; blood flow may be diverted to the periphery, "stealing" flow from the cerebral circulation in the absence of compensatory cardioacceleration. Thus, in patients with significant cerebral vascular disease, symptoms may occur even in the absence of gross changes in cardiac rhythm. In addition, cerebral atherosclerosis is a progressive disease, and some patients may have recurrences of central nervous system symptoms after a considerable period of being asymptomatic following artificial pacing. In most series, failure of pacing to improve dizziness or syncopal episodes has been attributed to coexistent severe cerebral vascular disease.[318]

The therapeutic approach to the patient with the bradycardia-tachycardia syndrome is complex and must be individualized. In the absence of central nervous system symptoms, the bradycardia may be observed closely while antiarrhythmic agents alone are tried in progressive incremental doses. When the tachyarrhythmias are supraventricular, digitalis has been the mainstay of therapy. However, the effect of digitalis on sinus node function in these patients varies, and caution is warranted. Therapy is best started in the hospital while the patient is electrocardiographically monitored. Propranolol and verapamil, documented to be highly effective in supraventricular arrhythmias, probably carry a higher risk of suppressing sinus node function than do digitalis preparations, and the combination of the two drugs is contraindicated in patients with sinus node disease without permanent pacing.

Some investigators have suggested that artificial pacing may not only allow higher doses of antiarrhythmic drugs to be given but also that many patients may have better results with lower doses that failed to control the tachyarrhythmias before pacemaker application.[312, 314, 315] Certain electrophysiologic principles suggest that a beneficial synergism between atrial or coronary sinus pacing and antiarrhythmic drugs could exist; however, more extensive and well-controlled studies are necessary. The potential for distal conduction system problems occurring secondary to the use of antiarrhythmic agents alone might be anticipated from the results of His bundle recordings.[317, 325, 327]

Considerable controversy exists regarding the efficacy of pacing alone for controlling the occurrence of supraventricular tachyarrhythmias in patients with sick sinus syndrome.[325, 327] Rubinstein and others have been unable to limit the frequency of episodes or entirely suppress them without adding antiarrhythmic agents.[312, 321] Others, however, have met with better success with atrial or coronary sinus pacing alone, and more recently with dual chamber pacemakers.[313, 328–331] Ohe and coworkers recently reported on the efficacy of atrial pacing as it relates to cycle length and reduction of the fragmented atrial activity zone.[347]

Some investigators have reported successful prophylaxis with ventricular pacing when retrograde AV conduction is present.[332] At the other extreme, refractoriness to antiarrhythmic agents has continued in a few patients despite permanent pacing.[319] The relative refractoriness to pharmacologic therapy of supraventricular tachyarrhythmias in the bradycardia-tachycardia syndrome compared to other settings has not been specifically investigated. A realistic approach to the control of supraventricular arrhythmias is to (1) initiate drug therapy if central nervous system symptomatology permits, (2) proceed with atrial or coronary sinus pacing alone if drugs fail or precipitate symptomatic sinus node dysfunction, and (3) combine antiarrhythmic agents with pacing if pacing alone is ineffectual.

Despite a potential electrophysiologic predisposition for ventricular arrhythmias to occur in the presence of slow heart rates, arrhythmias in patients with the sick sinus syndrome are more often supraventricular.[333–335] When ventricular ectopy or malignant ventricular rhythms do occur, atrial or ventricular pacing may not invariably abolish them without the assistance of antiarrhythmic drugs. However, pacing may facilitate pharmacologic management by shortening the Purkinje fiber refractory period, increasing the threshold for ventricular fibrillation, and minimizing asynchronous recovery of excitability in the ventricles.[333–336]

PROGNOSIS IN PATIENTS WITH SICK SINUS SYNDROME

From the standpoint of mortality and morbidity, the sick sinus syndrome is a discouraging disease entity to treat. The 5-year mortality in these patients is high and does not appear to be significantly influenced by artificial pacing. Skagen and coworkers[318] followed 50 patients with sinoatrial block treated with permanent pacing for 1 to 14 years. They reported survival after 1, 2, 5, and 8 years to be 94%, 85%, 64%, and 48%, respectively. These figures indicate an excess yearly mortality in the first 5 years of 4% to 5% compared with a control population of the same age and sex. Mortality was significantly influenced by the coexistence of cardiovascular and valvular heart disease (Fig. 9-25). Chokshi and coworkers reported 1- and 4-year survival rates in 52 permanently paced patients with sick sinus of 85% and 47%, respectively.[318] Krishnaswami and coworkers followed 17 patients with sinus bradycardia or sinus arrest in a pacemaker clinic for a mean duration of 19.4 months and reported a 30% mortality.[319] In 16 patients with alternating bradycardia-tachycardia, these investigators reported a 36% mortality over 16.3 months, half the deaths being secondary to massive cerebral infarction. In a follow-up study of 90 patients for a mean of 23 months after pacemaker implantation, Hartel and

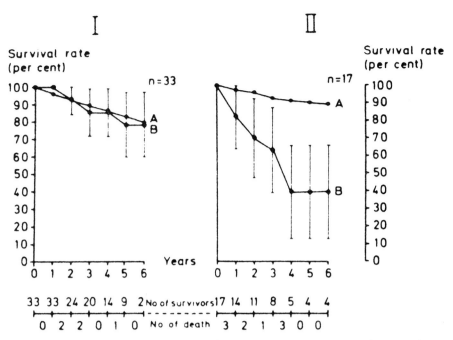

Figure 9-25. Graphs illustrating survival curves in two groups, one without significant cardiac disease (*I*) and one with significant cardiac disease (*II*). All patients had significant sinus node dysfunction and were treated with permanent cardiac pacing. In each graph, age-matched controls are illustrated by the line marked *A*, and the index patients are illustrated by the line marked *B*. Survival rates are shown for group *I* and group *II* patients. Note the significant deviation from the expected survival in group *II* patients without significant underlying disease. (Skagen K, Hansen JF: The long-term prognosis for patients with sinoatrial block treated with permanent pacemaker. Acta Med Scand 1975;199:13.)

Talvensaari reported an annual mortality of 11%.[316] As a group, the patients who died did not differ significantly from the survivors with regard to type of sinus dysfunction, occurrence of tachyarrhythmias, or distal conduction abnormalities.

Hauser and coworkers followed 301 patients with ventricular pacemakers; survival rates at 1, 3, and 5 years were 94%, 79%, and 69%, respectively, in patients with bradycardias alone versus 86%, 73%, and 63% in patients with the bradycardia-tachycardia syndrome.[348] The differences in survival rates were not significant. Simon and coworkers reported similar results in 71 patients, although patients with sick sinus and congestive heart failure had significantly lower survivals of 69%, 50%, and 41%.[349]

In all series, death in patients with this syndrome with permanent pacing most frequently results from complications of associated cardiovascular or cerebrovascular disease and not from complications of sinus node and subsidiary pacemaker dysfunction. However, the incidence of embolic events involving the lungs, brain, and peripheral arterial tree remains high in patients with permanent pacing and the sick sinus syndrome. The frequency of embolic events suggests that the instances of alternating bradyarrhythmias and tachyarrhythmias are more common than appreciated from random electrophysiologic evaluation. Although more extensive use of Holter monitoring to detect cases of inadequate pharmacologic prophylaxis of tachyarrhythmias may reduce the incidence of embolization somewhat, the paroxysmal nature of these arrhythmias would allow many episodes to escape detection. Thus, it has been proposed that all patients exhibiting the bradycardia-tachycardia syndrome be fully anticoagulated. While the benefit–risk argument of chronic anticoagulation has not been entirely resolved, the issue of anticoagulation in these patients is less controversial than it has been in the past. Prevention of life-threatening embolization appears to be the only area in which the physician can potentially favorably influence the high rate of mortality and morbidity in the permanently paced patient with sick sinus syndrome. However, not all cerebral vascular accidents in these patients are secondary to embolic events. Elderly patients with atherosclerotic cerebral vascular disease may have transient ischemic attacks or frank cerebral infarction if a tachyarrhythmia is associated with a fall in cardiac output. This group of patients does not benefit from anticoagulant therapy and must be distinguished from patients with cerebral embolization.

On a more positive note, a study by Sutton and Kenny involved 177 patients over 2½ years and found that the incidence of atrial fibrillation in patients with ventricular pacing was significantly higher than in patients with atrial demand pacing (22.3% versus 3.9%).[350] Furthermore, this reduction in atrial fibrillation was accompanied by a decreased incidence of systemic embolization (13% versus 1.6%).

Reports comparing survival with dual-chamber pacing versus ventricular pacing are encouraging. Alpert and coworkers reported survival rates in 79 patients for VVI pacing at 1, 3, and 5 years to be, respectively, 89%, 82%, and 74% for DDI and 94%, 86%, and 78% for DDD pacing.[351] In patients with congestive heart failure, survival rates with VVI pacing were 78%, 69%, and 87%. Survival rates for DDI and DDD pacing were significantly better at 90%, 83%, and 75% ($P > 0.03$).

Even more encouraging is the report by Rosenquist and coworkers on a 4-year follow-up of 168 patients.[352] These investigators found the incidence of atrial fibrillation to be higher in the VVI paced group (47%) than in the AAI paced group ($P > 0.005$). The incidence of congestive heart failure was greater in the VVI group (37%) than in the AAI group (15%) ($P > 0.005$). Furthermore, mortality was higher in the VVI group (23%) than in the AAI group (8%) ($P > 0.005$).

Finally, the issue of prophylactic permanent pacing in the asymptomatic patient with sick sinus syndrome must be addressed. At present, the natural history of the disease is unknown; furthermore, clinical risk factors for the development of symptoms have not been defined, and no electrophysiologic measure of sinus node function has been demonstrated to have reliable predictive value. Therefore, common practice has been to withhold pacemaker therapy in the asymptomatic patient. However, if more reports of the sort published by Rosenqvist begin appearing in the literature, the philosophy regarding pacemaker therapy in the asymptomatic patient may change.

References

1. James TN: Anatomy of the human sinus node. Anat Rec 1961;141:109.
2. Truex RC, Smythe MQ, Taylor MJ: Reconstruction of the human sinoatrial node. Anat Rec 1967;159:371.
3. James TN, Scherf L, Fine G: Comparative ultrastructure of the sinus node in man and dog. Circulation 1966;34:139.
4. Howse ND, Ferrnas VJ, Hibbs RG: A comparative histochemical and electron microscopic study of the surface coatings of cardiac muscle cells. J Mol Cell Cardiol 1970;1:57.
5. Kawamura K, James TN: Comparative ultrastructure of cellular junctions in working myocardium and the conduction system under normal and pathologic conditions. J Mol Cell Cardiol 1971;3:31.
6. DeMello WC: Membrane lipids and cardiac electrogenesis. In: DeMello WC, ed. Electrical phenomena in the heart. New York: Academic Press, 1972:89.
7. Langer GA, Frank JS: Lanthanum in heart cell cultures. Effect on localization. J Cell Biol 1972;54:441.
8. Tranum-Jensen J: The fine structure of the atrial and atrioventricular (AV) junctional specialized tissue of the rabbit heart. In: Wellen HJJ, Lie KI, Janse MJ, eds. The conduction system of the heart. Structure, function and clinical implications. Leiden: Stenfert Kraese BV, 1976:55.
9. Noma A, Irisawa H: Membrane currents in the rabbit sinoatrial node cell as studied by the double microelectrode method. Pflugers Arch 1976;364:45.
10. Noble D: The initiation of the heartbeat. Oxford: Clarendon, 1975.
11. Brown HF, Clark A, Noble SJ: Identification of the pacemaker current in frog atrium. J Physiol 1976;258:52.
12. Brown HF, Clark A, Noble SJ: Analysis of pacemaker repolarization currents in frog atrial muscle. J Physiol 1976;258:547.
13. Brooks C McC, Lu H-H: The sinoatrial pacemaker of the heart. Springfield, IL: Charles C Thomas, 1972:109.
14. Hoffman BF, Cranefield P: Electrophysiology of the heart. New York: McGraw-Hill, 1960.
15. West TCL: Effects of chronotropic influences on subthreshold oscillations in the sinoatrial node. In: Pae de Carvalho A, DeMello WC, Hoffman BF, eds. Specialized tissues of the heart. New York: Elsevier, 1961.
16. Yamagishi S, Sano T: Effect of tetrodotoxin on the pacemaker action potential of the sinus node. Prac Jpn Acad 1966;42:1194.
17. Toda N, West TC: Interaction of K, Na, and vagal stimulation in the SA node of the rabbit. Am J Physiol 1967;212:426.
18. Rougier O, et al: Existence and role of slow inward current during the frog atrial action potential. Pflugers Arch 1969;308:91.
19. Reuter H: Divalent cations as charge carriers in excitable membranes. Prog Biophys 1973;26:1.
20. Kohlhardt M, Bauer B, Krause H: Differentiation of the transmembrane Na and Ca channels in mammalian cardiac fibers by the use of specific inhibitors. Pflugers Arch 1972;335:309.
21. Wit AL, Cranefield P: Effect of verapamil on the sinoatrial and atrioventricular nodes of the rabbit and the mechanism by which it arrests reentrant atrioventricular nodal tachycardia. Circ Res 1974;35:413.
22. Zipes DP, Fischer JC: Effects of agents which inhibit the slow channel on sinus node automaticity and atrioventricular conduction in the dog. Circ Res 1974;34:184.
23. Haastert HP, Fleckenstein A: Ca-dependence of supraventricular pacemaker activity and its responsiveness to Ca-antagonistic compounds (verapamil, D-600, nifedipine). Arch Pharmacol 1975;287(suppl i):R39.
24. Kolhardt M, Figulla H-R, Tripathi O: The slow membrane channel as the predominant mediator of the excitation process of the sinoatrial pacemaker cell. Basic Res Cardiol 1976;71:17.
25. Strauss HC, Prystowsky EN, Scheinman MM: Sinoatrial and atrial electrogenesis. Prog Cardiovasc Dis 1977;19:385.
26. DeMello WC: Role of chloride ions in cardiac and pacemaker potentials. Am J Physiol 1963;295:567.

27. Seyama I: Characteristics of the anion channel in the sinoatrial node cell of the rabbit. J Physiol 1979;294:447.

28. Miller JS, Vaughn Williams EM: Pacemaker selectivity: Influence on rabbit atria of ionic environment and of alinidine, a possible anion antagonist. Cardiovasc Res 1981;15:335.

29. Yanagihera K, Irisawa H: Inward current activated during hyperpolarization in the rabbit SA-node cell. Pflugers Arch 1980;385:11.

30. DiFrancesco D, Ojeda C: Properties of the current i-f in the sinoatrial node of the rabbit compared with those of the current ik2 in Purkinje fibers. J Physiol (Lond) 1980;308:353.

31. Brown HF, DiFrancesco D: Voltage clamp investigations of membrane currents underlying pacemaker activity in rabbit sino-atrial node. J Physiol 1980;308:331.

32. Brown H, DiFrancesco D: Voltage-clamp investigations of membrane currents underlying pacemaker activity in rabbit sino-atrial node. J Physiol (Lond) 1980;308:331.

33. Yanagihera K, Noma A, Irisawa H: Reconstruction of sinoatrial node pacemaker potential based on the voltage clamp experiments. Jpn J Physiol 1980;30:841.

34. Irisawa H, Noma A: Pacemaker mechanisms of rabbit sinoatrial node cells. In: Bowman LN, Jongma HJ, eds. Cardiac rate and rhythm. The Hague: Martinus Nijhoff, 1982:33.

35. Noma A, Morad M: Does the "pacemaker current" generate the diastolic depolarization in the rabbit SA-node cells. Pflugers Arch 1983;397:190.

36. Brown HF, Kimura J, Noble D: The ionic currents underlying pacemaker activity in rabbit sino-atrial node: Experimental results and computer simulation. Proc R Soc Lond (Biol) 1984;222:305.

37. Maylie J, Morad M: Ionic currents responsible for the generation of pacemaker current in the rabbit sino-atrial node. J Physiol (Lond) 1984;355:215.

38. Duivenvoordan JJ, Bouman LN, Opthof T, Bukauskas FF, Jongsma HJ. Effect of transmural vagal stimulation on electrotonic spread in the rabbit sinoatrial node. Cardiovasc Res 1992;26:678.

39. DiFrancesco D: The cardiac hyperpolarizing-activated current if. Origins and development. Biophys Molec Biol 1985;46:163.

40. DiFrancesco D, Ferroni A, Massanti M, et al: Properties of the hyperpolarizing-activated current (if) in cells isolated from the rabbit sino-atrial node. J Physiol (Lond) 1986;377:61.

41. DiFrancesco D: Characterization of single pacemaker channels in cardiac sinoatrial node cells. Nature 1986;324:470.

42. Brown H, DiFrancesco D, Kimura J: Cesium: A useful tool for investigating sino-atrial (S-A) node pacemaking. J Physiol 1989;317:549.

43. Gilsa R, VanGinnekeu ACG: Voltage clamp analysis of the if current in isolated cells from the rabbit sino-atrial node. J Gen Physiol (in press).

44. Brown HF, Kimura J, Noble D, et al: The slow inward current isi in the rabbit sinoatrial node investigated by voltage clamp and computer simulation. Proc R Soc Lond (Biol) 1984;B222:305.

45. Noble D: The surprising heart: A review of recent progress in cardiac electrophysiology. J Physiol (Lond) 1984;353:1.

46. Rubenstein DS, Lipsius SL: Mechanisms of automaticity in subsidiary pacemakers from cat right atrium. Circ Res 1989;64(4):648.

47. Kreitner D: Electrophysiological study of the two main pacemaker mechanisms in the rabbit sinus node. Cardiovas Res 1985;19:(5):304.

48. Becker WK, MacKaary AJC, Masson P, et al: Functional and morphological organization of the rabbit sinus node. Circ Res 1980;46:11.

49. Michaels DC, Matyas EP, Jalike J: Mechanisms of sinoatrial pacemaker synchronization. A new hypothesis. Circ Res 1987;61:704.

50. Anumonwo JMB, Wang H-Z, Trabke-Jaulk E, et al: Gap junctional channels in adult mammalian sinus node cells: Immunolocalization and electrophysiology. Circ Res 1992;71:229.

51. DiFrancesco D, Tromba C: Acetylcholine inhibiting activation of the cardiac pacemaker current if. J Physiol 1987;410:39.

52. Kassebaum DG: Membrane effects of epinephrine in the heart. In: Krays O, Kovarikova A, eds. Second international pharmacologic meeting. Vol 5. Pharmacology of cardiac function. Oxford: Pergamon Press, 1964:95.

53. Tsien RWL: Effects of epinephrine on the pacemaker potassium current of cardiac Purkinje fibers. J Gen Physiol 1974;64:293.

54. Vassort G, Rougier O, Garmer D: Effects of adrenaline on membrane inward currents during the cardiac action potential. Pflugers Arch 1969;309:70.

55. Watanabe AM, Besch HR: Cyclic adenosine monophosphate modulation of slow calcium influx channels in guinea pig hearts. Circ Res 1974;35:316.

56. Friedman DB, Musch TI, Williams RS, et al: Beta adrenergic blockade with propanolol and atenolol in the exercising dog: Evidence for beta2 adrenoreceptors in the sinoatrial node. Cardiovasc Res 1987;21:124.

57. MacKary AJC, Hof TO, Bkekerwk SA, et al: Interaction of adrenaline and acetylcholine on cardiac pacemaker function. Functional inhomogeneity of the rabbit sinus node. J Pharmacol Exp Therap 1980;214:417.

58. Johnson PN, Freeberg AS, Marshall JM: Action of thyroid hormone on the transmembrane potentials from sinoatrial node cells and atrial muscle in isolated atria of rabbits. Cardiology 1973;58:273.

59. James TN, Nadeau RA: Sinus bradycardia during injections directly into the sinus node artery. Am J Physiol 1963;204:9.

60. James TN: Pulse and impulse formation in the sinus node. Henry Ford Hosp Med J 1967;15:275.

61. Brooks C McC, et al: Effects of localized stretch of the sinoatrial node region of the dog heart. Am J Physiol 1966;211:1197.

62. Lange G, et al: Effect of stretch of the isolated cat sinoatrial node. Am J Physiol 1966;211:1192.

63. Bouman LN, Van der Westen HM: Pacemaker shift in the sinoatrial node induced by a change of temperature. Pflugers Arch 1970;318:262.

64. Bouman LN, et al: Pacemaker shifts in the sinus node: Effects of vagal stimulation, temperature and reduction of extracellular calcium. In: Bonke FIM, ed. The sinus node: Structure, function and clinical relevance. The Hague: Martinus Nijhoff, 1978:245.

65. LeHeuzey J-Y, Guize L, Valty J, et al: Intracellular and extracellular recordings of sinus node activity: Comparison with

estimated sinoatrial conduction times during pacemaker shifts in rabbit heart. Cardiovasc Res 1986;20:81.

66. Lown B: In: Dreifus L, Likoff W, Moyer J, eds. Fourteenth Hahnemann Symposium on Mechanisms and Therapy of Cardiac Arrhythmias. New York: Grune & Stratton, 1966:185.

67. Ferrer MI: Sick sinus syndrome in atrial disease. JAMA 1968; 206:645.

68. Kulbertus HE, De Leval-Turren F, Demoulin JC: Sinoatrial disease: A report on 13 cases. J Electrocardiol 1973;6:303.

69. Rasmussen K: Chronic sinoatrial heart block. Am Heart J 1971;81:38.

70. Conde C, et al: Effectiveness of pacemaker treatment in the bradycardia-tachycardia syndrome. Am J Cardiol 1973; 32:209.

71. Sigurd B, et al: Adams-Stokes syndrome caused by sinoatrial block. Br Heart J 1973;35:1002.

72. Radford DJ, Julian DG: Sick sinus syndrome: Experience of a cardiac pacemaker clinic. BMJ 1974;3:155.

73. Sowton E, Hendrix G, Roy P: Ten-year survey of treatment with implanted cardiac pacemaker. BMJ 1974;3:155.

74. Hartel G, Talvensaari T: Treatment of sinoatrial syndrome with permanent cardiac pacing in 90 patients. Acta Med Scand 1975;198:341.

75. Rubenstein JJ, et al: Clinical spectrum of the sick sinus syndrome. Circulation 1972;46:5.

76. Wan SH, Lee GS, Ton CS: The sick sinus syndrome. A study of 15 cases. Br Heart J 1972;34:942.

77. Moss AJ, Davis RJ: Brady-tachy syndrome. Prog Cardiovasc Dis 1974;16:439.

78. Fraser GR, Froggatt P, James TN: Congenital deafness associated with electrocardiographic abnormalities, fainting attacks and sudden death: A recessive syndrome. Q J Med 1964;33:361.

79. Metzger AL, Goldberg AN, Hunter RL: Sick sinus node syndrome as the presenting manifestation of reticulum cell sarcoma. Chest 1971;60:602.

80. Kaplin BM, et al: Tachycardia-bradycardia syndrome (so-called "sick sinus syndrome"). Pathology, mechanisms and treatment. Am J Cardiol 1973;31:497.

81. Jordan JL, Yamaguchi I, Mandel WJ: Characteristics of sinoatrial conduction in patients with coronary artery disease. Circulation 1977;55:569.

82. Davies MJ, Pomerance A: Quantitative study of aging changes in the human sinoatrial node and internodal tract. Br Heart J 1972;34:150.

83. Maisch B, Loite O, Schneider J: Antibodies to human sinus node in sick sinus syndrome. PACE 1986;9:1101.

84. Haden RF, et al: The significance of sinus bradycardia in acute myocardial infarction. Dis Chest 1963;44:168.

85. Adgey AJJ, et al: Incidence, significance and management of early bradyarrhythmia complicating acute myocardial infarction. Lancet 1968;2:1097.

86. Rokseth R, Hattle L: Sinus arrest in acute myocardial infarction. Br Heart J 1971;33:639.

87. Thomas M, Goodgate D: Effect of atropine on bradycardia and hypotension in acute myocardial infarction. Br Heart J 1966;28:409.

88. Brown AM: Excitation of afferent cardiac sympathetic nerve fibers during myocardial ischemia. J Physiol 1967;190:35.

89. Bashaor TT, Chen F, Feeney J. Ischemic sinus node hiberna-tion: Resolution following angioplasty. Am Heart J 1991; 122:1156.

90. James TN, Reemtsma K: The response of sinus node function to ligation of the sinus node artery. Henry Ford Hosp Med Bull 1960;8:129.

91. Billette J, et al: Sinus slowing produced by experimental ischemia of the sinus node in dogs. Am J Cardiol 1973; 31:331.

92. Meck WJ, Keenan M, Theisen HJ: Auricular blood supply in the dog. I. General auricular supply with special reference to sino-auricular node. Am Heart J 1929;4:591.

93. Halpern MH: Arterial supply to the nodal tissue in the dog heart. Circulation 1954;9:547.

94. Eckberg DL, Drabinsky M, Braunwald E: Defective cardiac parasympathetic control in patients with heart disease. N Engl J Med 1971;285:877.

95. Goldstein RE, et al: Impairment of autonomically mediated heart rate control in patients with cardiac dysfunction. Circ Res 1975;36:571.

96. Friedman HH: Diagnostic electrocardiography and vector-cardiography. New York: McGraw-Hill, 1977:432.

97. Persson A, Solders G: R-R variations, a test of autonomic dysfunction. Acta Neurol Scand 1983;67:285.

98. Bergfelt BL, Ednag KO, Solders GE, et al: Analysis of sinus cycle variation: A new method for evaluation of suspected sinus node dysfunction. Am Heart J 1987;114:321.

99. Satullo G, Oreto G, Luzza F, Consolo A, Donato A: Sinus parasystole. Am Heart J 1991;121:1507.

100. LeHeuzey J-Y, Caron J, Guize L, et al: Wenckebach periods in sinoatrial block: Experimental and clinical evidence. PACE 1991;14:1032.

101. Han J, et al: Incidence of ectopic beats as a function of basic rate in the ventricle. Am Heart J 1966;72:632.

102. Han J, et al: Temporal dispersion of recovery of excitability in atrium and ventricle as a function of heart rate. Am Heart J 1966;71:481.

103. Han J, Malozzi AM, Moe GK: Sinoatrial reciprocation in the isolated rabbit heart. Circ Res 1968;22:355.

104. Paulay KL, Varghese JP, Damato AN: Sinus node reentry. An in vivo demonstration in the dog. Circ Res 1973b;32:455.

105. Narula OS: Sinus node reentry. A mechanism for supraventricular tachycardia. Circulation 1974;50:1114.

106. Weisfogel GM, et al: Sinus node reentrant tachycardia in man. Am Heart J 1975;90:295.

107. Breithardt G, Seipel L: Sequence of atrial activation in patients with atrial echo beats. In: Bonke FIM, ed. The sinus node: Structure, function and clinical relevance. The Hague: Martinus Nijhoff, 1978:389.

108. Allessie MA, Bonke FIM: Re-entry within the sinoatrial node as demonstrated by multiple microelectrode recordings in the isolated rabbit heart. In: Bonke FIM, ed. The sinus node: Structure, function and clinical relevance. The Hague: Martinus Nijhoff, 1978:409.

109. Damato AN: Clinical evidence for sinus node reentry. In: Bonke FIM, ed: The sinus node: Structure, function and clinical relevance. The Hague: Martinus Nijhoff, 1978:379.

110. Curry PVL, Callowhill E, Krikler DM: Paroxysmal re-entry sinus tachycardia. Br Heart J 1976;38:311.

111. Curry PVL, Krikler DM: Paroxysmal reciprocating sinus tachycardia. In: Kulbertus H, ed. Re-entrant arrhythmias.

Mechanisms and treatment. Baltimore: University Park Press, 1977:39.

112. Scheinman MM, et al: The sick sinus and ailing atrium. West J Med 1974;121:473.

112a. Gomes JA, Hariman RJ, Kang PS: Sustained symptomatic sinus node reentrant tachycardia: Incidence, clinical significance, electrophysiologic observations and the effects of antiarrhythmic agents. J Am Coll Card 1985;5:45.

113. Holden W, McAnulty JW, Rahimotoola SN: Characterization of heart rate response to exercise in the sick sinus syndrome. Br Heart J 1978;40:923.

114. Ellestad MH: Stress testing: Principles and practice. Philadelphia: FA Davis, 1975:38.

115. Arguss NS, et al: Significance of chronic sinus bradycardia in elderly people. Circulation 1972;46:924.

116. Miller TD, Gibbons RJ, Squires RW, Allison TG, Gau GT. Sinus node deceleration during exercise as a marker of significant narrowing of the right coronary artery. Am J Cardiol 1993;71:371.

117. Crook BRM, et al: Tape monitoring of the electrocardiogram in ambulant patients with sinoatrial disease. Br Heart J 1973;35:1009.

118. Brasil A: Autonomic sinoatrial block. A new disturbance of the heart mechanism. Arq Bras Cardiol 1955;8:159.

119. Dighton DH: Sinoatrial block: Autonomic influences and clinical assessment. Br Heart J 1975;37:321.

120. Hamlin RL, Smith CR, Smeler DL: Sinus arrhythmia in the dog. Am J Physiol 1966;210:321.

121. Covell JW, Chidsey CP, Braunwald E: Reduction of the cardiac responses to postganglionic sympathetic nerve stimulation in patients with cardiac decompensation. Circ Res 1966;19:51.

122. Beiser GD, et al: Impaired heart rate response to sympathetic nerve stimulation in patients with cardiac decompensation. Circulation 1968;38:VI-40.

123. Mandel WJ, Laks MM, Obayashi K: Sinus node function: Evaluation in patients with and without sinus node disease. Arch Intern Med 1975;135:388.

124. Robinson BF, et al: Control of heart rate by the autonomic nervous system. Circ Res 1966;19:400.

125. Deuleeschhouwer GC, Heymen E: In: Kezdi P, ed. Baroreceptors and hypertension. New York: Pergamon Press, 1967:187.

126. Thomas MD, Kontos HA: Mechanisms of baroreceptor-induced changes in heart rate. Am J Physiol 1970;218:251.

127. Dighton DH: Sinus bradycardia autonomic influences and clinical assessment. Br Heart J 1974;36:791.

128. Pfeifer MA, Weinberg CR, Cook D: Differential changes of autonomic nervous system function in man. Am J Med 1983;75:249.

129. DeMarneefe M, Jacobs P, Haardt R: Variations of normal sinus node function in relation to age: Role of autonomic influence. Surg Heart J 1986;7:662.

130. Jose AD, Collison D: The normal range and determinants of the intrinsic heart rate in man. Cardiovasc Res 1970;4:160.

131. Jordan JL, Yamaguchi I, Mandel WJ: Studies on the mechanism of sinus node dysfunction in the sick sinus syndrome. Circulation 1978;57:217.

132. Gaskell WH: On the innervation of the heart with especial reference to the heart of the tortoise. J Physiol 1884;4:43.

133. Cohn AE, Lewis T: Auricular fibrillation and complete heart block: A description of a case of Adams-Stokes syndrome including the post-mortem examination. Heart 1912;4:15.

134. Parkinson J, Papp C, Evans W: The electrocardiogram of the Stokes-Adams attack. Br Heart J 1941;3:171.

135. Pick A, Langendorf R, Katz LN: Depression of cardiac pacemakers by premature impulses. Am Heart J 1951;41:49.

136. Lange G: Action of driving stimuli from intrinsic and extrinsic sources on in situ cardiac pacemaker tissues. Circ Res 1965;17:449.

137. Mandel WJ, et al: Assessment of sinus node function in patients with sick sinus syndrome. Circulation 1972;43:761.

138. Narula OS, Samet P, Javier RP: Significance of the sinus node recovery time. Circulation 1972;45:140.

139. Strauss HC, et al: Electrophysiologic evaluation of sinus node function in patients with sinus node dysfunction. Circulation 1976;53:763.

140. Vincenzi FF, West TC: Release of autonomic mediators in cardiac tissue by direct subthreshold electrical stimulation. J Pharmacol Exp Ther 1963;141:185.

141. Lu H-H, Lange G, Brooks C McC: Factors controlling pacemaker action in cells of the sinoatrial node. Circ Res 1965;17:461.

142. Furchgott RF, DeGubareff T, Grossman A: Release of autonomic mediators in cardiac tissue by subthreshold stimulation. Science 1959;129:328.

143. Kodama I, Goto J, Anso S, et al: Effects of rapid stimulation on the transmembrane action potentials of rabbit sinus node pacemaker cells. Circ Res 1980;46:90.

144. Steinbeck G, Haberl R, Luderitz B: Effects of atrial pacing on atrio-sinus conduction and overdrive suppression in the isolated rabbit sinus node. Circ Res 1981;46:859.

145. Konsai T: Electrophysiologic consideration of sick sinus syndrome. Jpn Circ J 1976;40:194.

146. Jordan JL, et al: Studies on the mechanism of suppression of sinus node pacemaker automaticity by atrial overdrive pacing. Clin Res 1978;26:241A.

147. Engel TR, et al: Appraisal of sinus node artery disease. Circulation 1975;52:286.

148. Singer D, Parameswaran R, Goldberg H: Sinus and AV nodal dysfunction following myocardial infarction. J Electrocardiol 1975;8:281.

149. Alboni P, Baggioni GF, Scart-o' S, et al: Role of sinus node artery disease in sick sinus syndrome in inferior wall myocardial infarction. Am J Cardiol 1991;67:1180.

150. Mandel WJ, Yamaguchi I: The effects of changes in extracellular pH on sinoatrial conduction. Am J Cardiol 1977;39:265.

151. Benditt DC, Strauss HC, Scheinman MM, et al: Analysis of secondary pauses following termination of rapid atrial pacing in man. Circulation 1976;54:436.

152. Rosen RM, et al: Cardiac conduction in patients with symptomatic sinus node disease. Circulation 1971;43:836.

153. Engel TR, Schaal SF: Digitalis in the sick sinus syndrome: The effects of digitalis on sinoatrial automaticity and atrioventricular conduction. Circulation 1973;48:1201.

154. Jordan JL, Yamaguchi I, Mandel WJ: The sick sinus syndrome: Pathophysiology, significance and treatment. Cardiol Dig 1977;12:11.

155. Kulbertus HE, deLeval-Rutten F, Casters L: Sinus node recovery time in elderly. Br Heart J 1975;37:420.

156. Scheinman MM, Strauss HC, Abbott JA: Electrophysiologic testing for patients with sinus node dysfunction. J Electrocardiol 1979;12:211.

157. Reiffel JA, Gang E, Bigger JT Jr, et al: Sinus node recovery time related to paced cycle length in normal and patients with sinoatrial dysfunction. Am Heart J 1982;104:746.

158. Jordan J, et al: Comparative effects of overdrive on sinus and subsidiary pacemaker function. Am Heart J 1977;93:367.

159. Neely BH, Urthaler F, Hageman GR: Differences in determinants of overdrive suppression between sinus rhythm and slow atrio-ventricular junctional rhythm. Circ Res 1985; 57(1):182.

160. Yabek SM, Jarmakani JM, Roberts NK: Sinus node function in children. Factors influencing its evaluation. Circulation 1976;53:28.

161. Jose AD, Taylor RR: Autonomic blockade by propranolol and atropine to study myocardial function in man. J Clin Invest 1969;48:2019.

161a. Goldreyer BN, Damato AN: Sinoatrial node entrance block. Circulation 1971;44:789.

162. Jordan JL, Yamaguchi E, Mandel WJ: Characteristics of sinoatrial conduction in patients with coronary artery disease. Circulation 1977;55:569.

163. Massini G, Dianda R, Grazina A: Analysis of sino-atrial conduction in man using premature atrial stimulation. Cardiovasc Res 1975;9:498.

164. Steinbeck G, Luderitz G: Comparative study of sino-atrial conduction time and sinus node recovery time. Br Heart J 1975;37:956.

165. Bashour T, et al: An unusual effect of atropine on overdrive suppression. Circulation 1973;48:911.

166. Reiffel JP, Bigger JT Jr, Giardina EGV: "Paradoxical" prolongation of sinus nodal recovery time after atropine in the sick sinus syndrome. Am J Cardiol 1975;36:98.

167. Jordan JL, et al: The effects of verapamil on sinoatrial conduction in isolated tissue. Clin Res 1978;26:279A.

168. Gupta PK, et al: Appraisal of sinus nodal recovery time in patients with sick sinus syndrome. Am J Cardiol 1974; 34:265.

169. Chadda KD, et al: Corrected sinus node recovery: Experimental, physiological and pathologic determinants. Circulation 1975;51:797.

170. Okimoto T, et al: Sinus node recovery time and abnormal post-pacing phase in the aged patients with sick sinus syndrome. Jpn Heart J 1976;17:290.

171. Mason JW: Overdrive suppression in the transplanted heart: Effect of the autonomic nervous system on human sinus node recovery. Circulation 1980;62:688.

172. Kang PS, Gomes JAC, El-Sherif N: Differential effects of functional autonomic blockade on the variables of sinus nodal automaticity in sick sinus syndrome. Am J Cardiol 1982;49:273.

173. Kang P, Gomes J, Kelen G, et al: Role of autonomic regulatory mechanisms in sinoatrial conduction and sinus node automaticity in sick sinus syndrome. Circulation 1981; 64:832.

174. Kuga K, Yamaguchi I, Sugishita Y: Assessment by autonomic blockade of age-related changes of the sinus node function and autonomic regulation in sick sinus syndrome. Am J Cardiol 1988;61:361.

175. Alboni P, Macarne C, Pedroni P: Electrophysiology of normal sinus node with and without autonomic blockade. Circulation 1982;65:1236.

176. Sethi KK, Jaishankar S, Balachander J: Sinus node function after autonomic blockade in normals and in sick sinus syndrome. Int Cardiol 1984;5:707.

177. Bonke FIM, Bouman LN, VanRisn HE: Change of cardiac rhythm in the rabbit after an atrial premature beat. Circ Res 1969;24:533.

178. Jordan JL, Mandel WJ: Comparative effects of duration of atrial overdrive pacing in patients with and without intrinsic sinus node dysfunction. In preparation.

179. Desai JM, Scheinman MM, Strauss HC, et al: Electrophysiologic effects of combined autonomic blockade in patients with sinus node disease. Circulation 1981;63:953.

180. Prinsze FJ, Bouman LN. The cellular basis of intrinsic sinus node recovery time. Cardiovasc Res 1991;25:546.

181. Bonke FIM, Bouman LN, Schopman FJG: Effect of an early atrial premature beat on activity of the sinoatrial rhythm in the rabbit. Circ Res 1971;24:704.

182. Klein HO, Singer DH, Hoffman BF: Effects of atrial premature systoles on sinus rhythm in the rabbit. Circ Res 1973; 32:480.

183. Strauss NC, et al: Premature atrial stimulation as a key to the understanding of sinoatrial conduction in man. Presentation of data and critical review of the literature. Circulation 1973;47:86.

184. Strauss NC, Bigger JT Jr: Electrophysiological properties of rabbit sinoatrial perinodal fibers. Circ Res 1972;31:490.

185. Pasmooij JH, Bonke FIM: Influence of stimulus frequency on the depolarization of the action: Comparison between atrium and SA node. (Abstract) Pflugers Arch 1970;318:263.

186. Rasmussen K: Chronic sinoatrial heart block. Am Heart J 1971;81:38.

187. Scherf D: The mechanisms of sinoatrial block. Am J Cardiol 1969;23:769.

188. Engel TR, Bond RC, Schaal SF: First degree sinoatrial heart block: Sinoatrial block in the sick sinus syndrome. Am Heart J 1976;91:303.

189. Kerr CR, Prystowsky ER, Browning DJ, Strauss HC: Characterization or refractoriness in the sinus node of the rabbit. Circulation 1980;47:742.

190. Childers RW, et al: Sinus node echoes. Am J Cardiol 1973; 31:220.

191. Paritsky Z, Obayashi K, Mandel WJ: Atrial tachycardia secondary to sinoatrial node reentry. Chest 1974;66:526.

192. Tzivoni D, Jordan JL, Barrett P, et al: Two zones of full compensation: An unexpected finding related to alterations in conduction at the sinoatrial junction. Clin Res 1978;26:241.

193. Langendorf R, et al: Atrial parasystole with interpolation: Observations on prolonged sinoatrial conduction. Am Heart J 1962;63:649.

194. Scheinman MM, et al: Sinoatrial function and atrial refractoriness in patients with sick sinus syndrome. Circulation 1973;48:IV-215.

195. Dhingra RC, et al: Clinical significance of prolonged sinoatrial conduction time. Circulation 1977;55:8.

196. Breithardt G, Seipel L, Loogen F: Sinus node recovery time

and calculated sinoatrial conduction time in normal subjects and patients with sinus node dysfunction. Circulation 1977;56:43.

196a. Yamaguchi I, Mandel WJ: Alterations in measured and estimated sinus node conduction times: Effects of site stimulation and drug infusion. Arch Ven Cardiol 1976;3:78.

197. Miller HC, Strauss HC: Measurement of sinoatrial conduction time by premature atrial stimulation in the rabbit. Circ Res 1974;35:935.

198. Breithardt G, Seipel L: The effect of premature atrial depolarization on sinus node automaticity in man. Circulation 1976;53:920.

199. Denes P, Wu D, Dhingra R: The effects of cycle length on cardiac refractory periods in man. Circulation 1974;49:32.

200. Reiffel JA, Bigger JT Jr, Konstam MA: The relationship between sinoatrial conduction time and sinus cycle length during spontaneous sinus arrhythmia in adults. Circulation 1974;50:924.

201. Sanot T, Yamagishi S: Spread of excitation from the sinus node. Circ Res 1965;16:423.

202. Dhingra RC, et al: Sinus nodal responses to atrial extrastimuli in patients without apparent sinus node disease. Am J Cardiol 1975;36:445.

203. Dhingra RC, et al: Electrophysiologic effects of atropine on human sinus node and atrium. Am J Cardiol 1976;38:429.

204. Breithardt G, et al: The effect of atropine on calculated sinoatrial conduction time in man. Eur J Cardiol 1976;4:49.

205. Dhingra RC, et al: Electrophysiologic effects of atropine on sinus node and atrium in patients with sinus node dysfunction. Am J Cardiol 1976;38:848.

206. Strauss HC, et al: Electrophysiologic effects of propranolol on sinus node function in patients with sinus node dysfunction. Circulation 1976;54:452.

207. Narula OS, Narashimhan S, Vasquez M, et al: A new method for measurement of sinoatrial conduction time. Circulation 1978;58:706.

207a. Breithardt G, Seipel L: Comparative study of two methods of estimating sinoatrial conduction time in man. Am J Cardiol 1978;42:965.

207b. Grant AO, Kirkorian G, Benditt DG, Strauss HC: The estimation of sinoatrial conduction time in rabbit hearts by the constant atrial pacing technique. Circulation 1979;60:597.

208. Kerr CR, Strauss HC: The measurement of sinus node refractoriness in man. Circulation 1983;68:1231.

209. Kerr CR: Effects of pacing cycle length and autonomic blockade on sinus node refractoriness. Am J Cardiol 1988;62:1192.

210. Omori I, Inove D, Shirayama T, et al: Effect of paced cycle length on sinus node effective refractory period before and after autonomic blockade in patients with sick sinus syndrome. European Heart Journal 1989;10:409.

211. Cramer M, Hariman RJ, Boxer RA, et al: Catheter recording of sinoatrial node potentials in the in situ canine heart. Am J Cardiol 1978;41:374.

212. Cramer M, Seigal M, Hoffman BF: Electrogram of the canine sinus node. Circulation 1976;54:II-156.

213. Hariman RJ, Krongrad E, Bexer RA, et al: Methods for recording electrograms of the sinoatrial node during cardiac surgery in man. Circulation 1980;61:1024.

214. Castillo-Fesnoy A, Thebaut JF, Achard F, DeLangenhagen B: Identification du potentiel sinusal chez l'homme. Arch Mol Coeur 1977;72:948.

215. Reiffel JA, Gang E, Glicklich J, et al: The human sinus node electrogram: A transvenous catheter technique and a comparison of directly measured and indirectly estimated sinoatrial conduction time in adults. Circulation 1980;62:1324.

216. Hariman RJ, Krongrad E, Beyer RA, et al: Method for recording electrical activity of the sinoatrial node and automatic atrial foci during cardiac catheterization in human subjects. Am J Cardiol 1980;45:775.

217. Gomes JAC, Kang PS, El-Sherif N: The sinus node electrogram in patients with and without sick sinus syndrome. Techniques and correlation between directly measured and indirectly estimated sinoatrial conduction time. Circulation 1982;66:864.

218. Haberl R, Steinbeck G, Luderitz B: Comparison between intracellular and extra-cellular direct current recordings of sinus node activity for evaluation of sinoatrial conduction time. Circulation 1984;70(4):760.

219. Asseman P, Berzun B, Desry DR, et al: Persistent sinus nodal electrograms during abnormally prolonged post pacing atrial pauses in sick sinus syndrome in humans: Sinoatrial block vs. overdrive suppression. Circulation 1983;68:33.

220. Koniski T: Electrophysiological consideration of sick sinus syndrome. Jpn Circ J 1976;40:194.

221. Kodama I, Goto J, Ando S, et al: Effects of rapid atrial stimulation on the transmembrane potentials of rabbit sinus node pacemaker cell. Circ Res 1980;46:90.

222. Steinbeck G, Naberi R, Luderitz B: Effects of atrial pacing on atriosinus conduction and overdrive suppression in the isolated rabbit sinus node. Circ Res 1980;46:859.

223. Gomes JA, Hariman BI, Chowdry IA: New application of direct sinus node recordings in man: Assessment of sinus node recovery time. Circulation 1984;70:663.

224. Gomes JA, Winters SL: The origins of the sinus node pacemaker complex in man: Demonstration of dominant and subsidiary foci. JACC 1987;9(1):45.

225. Noma A, Irisawa H: Electrogenic sodium pump in the sinoatrial node. Pflugers Arch 1974;352:177.

226. Vasalle M: Cardiac automaticity. In: Vasalle M, ed. Cardiac physiology for the clinician. New York: Academic Press, 1976:27.

227. Vasalle M: The relationship among cardiac pacemakers. Circ Res 1977;41:269.

228. Sperelakis N: Origin of the cardiac resting potential. In: Riebierne, ed. Handbook of physiology, the heart. Washington, DC: American Physiological Society, 1979:187.

229. Gang ES, Oseran DS, Mandel WJ, Peter T: Sinus node electrogram in patients with the hypersensitive carotid sinus syndrome. J Am Coll Cardiol 1985;5:1484.

230. Weiss S, Baker JP: The cardotid sinus reflex in health and disease; its role in the causation of fainting and convulsions. Medicine 1933;12:297.

231. Walter PF, Crawley IS, Derney ER: Carotid hypersensitivity and syncope. Am J Cardiol 1978;42:396.

232. Thomas JE: Hyperactive carotid sinus reflex and carotid sinus syncope. Mayo Clin Proc 1969;44:127.

233. Nathanson MH: Hyperactive cardioinhibitory carotid sinus reflex. Arch Intern Med 1946;77:491.

234. Sigler LH: The cardioinhibitory carotid sinus reflex. Am J Cardiol 1963;12:175.

235. Hartzler GO, Maloney JD: Cardioinhibitory carotid sinus hypersensitivity. Arch Intern Med 1977;137:727.

235a. Marley CA, Dehn KB, Perrin EJ, et al: Baroreflex sensitivity measured by the phenylephrine pressor test in patients with carotid sinus and sick sinus syndromes. Cardiovasc Res 1984;18:752.

236. Davies AB, Stephens MR, Davies AG: Carotid sinus hypersensitivity in patients presenting with syncope. Br Heart J 1979;42:583.

237. Probst P, Muhlberger V, Lederbauer M, et al: Electrophysiologic findings in carotid sinus massage. PACE 1983;6:689.

238. Reiffel JA, Bigger JT, Ferrick K, et al: Sinus node echoes concealed conduction: Additional sinus node phenomena confirmed in man direct sinus node electrocardiography. J Electrophysiology 1985;18(3):259.

239. Yamaguchi I, Jordan JL, Mandel WJ: The effect of anti-arrhythmic drugs on estimated and measured sinoatrial conduction. In preparation.

240. Perry WLM, Reiihert H: The action of cardiac glycosides on autonomic ganglia. Br J Pharmacol 1954;9:324.

241. Mendez C, Aceves J, Mendez R: Inhibition of adrenergic cardiac acceleration by cardiac glycosides. J Pharmacol Exp Ther 1961;81:191.

242. Nadeau RA, James TN: Antagonistic effects on the sinus node of acetylstrophanthidin and adrenergic stimulation. Circ Res 1963;13:388.

243. Ten Eick RE, Hoffman BF: Chronotropic effect of cardiac glyscosides in dogs, cats and rabbits. Circ Res 1967;25:305.

244. Ten Eick RE, Hoffman BF: The effect of digitalis on the excitability of autonomic nerves. J Pharmacol Exp Ther 1969;109:95.

245. Goodman DJ, et al: Sinus node function in the denervated human heart: Effect of digitalis. Br Heart J 1975;37:618.

246. Gomes JAC, Kang PS, El-Sherif N: Effects of digitalis on the human sick sinus node after pharmacologic autonomic blockade. Am J Cardiol 1981;48:783.

247. Hashimoto K, Kimura T, Kubota K: Study of the therapeutic and toxic effects of ouabain by simultaneous observations on the excised and blood-perfused sinoatrial node and papillary muscle preparations and in the heart of dogs. J Pharmacol Exp Ther 1973;186:463.

248. Dick HLH, McCawley EL, Fisher WA: Reserpine-digitalis toxicity. Arch Intern Med 1962;109:503.

249. Gillis RA: Cardiac sympathetic nerve activity: Changes induced by ouabain and propranolol. Science 1969;166:508.

250. Dhingra RC, et al: The electrophysiological effects of ouabain on sinus node and atrium in man. J Clin Invest 1975;56:555.

251. Bond RC, Engel TR, Schaal SF: The effect of digitalis on sinoatrial conduction in man. Circulation 1973;48(suppl IV):147.

251a. Hariman RJ, Hoffman BF: Effects of ouabain in vagal stimulation on sinus nodal function in conscious dogs. Circ Res 1982;51:760.

252. Scherlag BJ, Abelleira JL, Narula OS: The differential effects of ouabain on sinus, AV nodal, His bundle and idioventricular arrhythmias. Am Heart J 1971;81:227.

253. Engel TR, Schaal SF: Digitalis in the sick sinus syndrome: The effects of digitalis on sinoatrial automaticity and atrioventricular conduction. Circulation 1973;48:1201.

254. Wallace AG, et al: Electrophysiological effects of quinidine. Circ Res 1966;19:960.

255. Hoffman BF, Rosen MR, Wit AL: Electrophysiology and pharmacology of cardiac arrhythmias. VIII. Cardiac effects of quinidine and procainamide. Am Heart J 1975;89:804.

256. Chiba S: Absence of blocking effect of quinidine on response to norepinephrine in the isolated dog atrium. Jpn Heart J 1976;17:506.

257. Mason JW, et al: The electrophysiological effects of quinidine in the transplanted human heart. J Clin Invest 1977;59:481.

258. Josephson ME, et al: The electrophysiological effects of intramuscular quinidine on the atrioventricular conducting system in man. Am Heart J 1974;87:55.

259. Cohen IS, Jick H, Cohen SI: Adverse reactions to quinidine in hospitalized patients: Findings based on data from the Boston Collaborative Drug Surveillance Program. Prog Cardiovasc Dis 1977;20:151.

260. Hirschfield DS, et al: Clinical and electrophysiological effects of intravenous quinidine in man. Br Heart J 1977;39:309.

260a. Josephson ME, et al.: Electrophysiological properties of procainamide in man. Am J Cardiol 1974;33:596.

261. Goldberg D, Reiffel JA, Davis JC, et al: Electrophysiologic effects of procainamide on sinus function in patients with and without sinus node disease. Am Heart J 1982;103:75.

262. Befeler B, et al: Electrophysiologic effects of the antiarrhythmic agent disopyramide phosphate. Am J Cardiol 1975;35:282.

263. Marrot PK, et al: A study of acute electrophysiological and cardiovascular action of disopyramide in man. Eur J Cardiol 1976;413:303.

264. Katoh T, Karagueuzian HS, Jordan JL, Mandel WJ: The cellular electrophysiologic mechanism of the dual actions of disopyramide on rabbit sinus node function. Circulation 1982;66:1216.

265. Seipel L, Breithardt G: Sinus recovery time after disopyramide phosphate. Am J Cardiol 1976;37:118.

265a. LaBarre AB, et al.: Electrophysiological effects of disopyramide phosphate on sinus node function in patients with sinus node dysfunction. Circulation 1979;59:226.

265b. Lieberman NA, et al.: The effects of lidocaine on the electrical and mechanical activity of the heart. Am J Cardiol 1968;22:375.

265c. Dhigra RC, et al.: Electrophysiologic effects of lidocaine on sinus node and atrium in patients with and without sinoatrial dysfunction. Circulation 1978;57:448.

266. Parameswaran R, et al: Sinus bradycardia due to lidocaine. Clinical electrophysiologic correlations. J Electrocardiol 1974;7:75.

267. Yamaguchi I, Singh BN, Mandel WJ: Electrophysiological actions of mexiletine on isolated rabbit atria and canine ventricular muscle and Purkinje fibers. Cardiovasc Res 1979;13:288.

268. Roos JC, Paalman ACA, Dunning AG: Electrophysiological effects of mexiletine in man. Br Heart J 1976;38:1262.

269. Campbell RWF, et al: Mexiletine (KO1173) in the management of ventricular dysrhythmias. Lancet 1973;2:204.

270. Samuelsson RG, Harrison DC: Electrophysiologic evaluation of encainide with use of monophasic action potential recording. Am J Cardiol 1981;48:871.

271. Sami M, Mason JW, Al JC, Harrison DC: Canine electrophysiology of encainide, a new antiarrhythmic drug. Am J Cardiol 1979;43:1149.

272. Jackman WM, Zipes DP, Nacarelli GV, et al: Electrophysiology of oral encainide. Am J Cardiol 1982;49:1270.

273. Seipel L, Abendroth RR, Breithardt G: Electrophysiological effects of flecainide (R818) in man. (Abstract) Circulation 1980;62(suppl):III-153.

274. Vik-Mo H, Ohm OJ, Lund-Johansen P: Electrophysiological effects of flecainide acetate in patients with sinus nodal dysfunction. Am J Cardiol 1982;50:1090.

275. Bar F, Farre J, Ross D, et al: Electrophysiological effects of lorcainide, a new antiarrhythmic drug. Observations in patients with and without pre-excitation. Br Heart J 1981; 45:292.

276. Manz M, Steinbeck G, Ludentz B: Action of lorcainide (RT 15889) on sinoatrial node function and intracardiac conduction. Herz Kreislauf 1979;11:192.

277. Rosati RA, et al: Influence of diphenylhydantoin on electrophysiological properties of the canine heart. Circ Res 1967; 21:757.

278. Wit AL, Rosen MR, Hoffman BF: Electrophysiology and pharmacology of cardiac arrhythmias. VIII. Cardiac effects of diphenylhydantoin. Am Heart J 1975;90:397.

279. Mercer EN, Osborne JA: Current status of diphenylhydantoin in heart disease. Ann Intern Med 1967;67:1084.

280. Strauss HC, Bigger JT Jr, Bassett AL: Actions of diphenylhydantoin on the electrical properties of isolated rabbit and canine atria. Circ Res 1968;23:463.

281. Louis S, Kutt H, McDowell F: Cardiocirculatory changes caused by intravenous dilantin and its solvents. Am Heart J 1967;74:523.

282. Wit AL, Cranefield P: Effects of verapamil on the sinoatrial and atrioventricular nodes of the rabbit and the mechanism by which it arrests atrioventricular nodal tachycardia. Circ Res 1974;35:413.

283. Singh BN, Vaughan-Williams EM: A fourth class of antidysrhythmic action? Effect of verapamil on ouabain toxicity and on atrial and ventricular intracellular potentials and on other features of cardiac function. Cardiovasc Res 1972; 6:109.

284. Zipes DP, Fischer JC: Effects of agents which inhibit the slow channel on sinus node automaticity and atrioventricular conduction in the dog. Circ Res 1984;34:184.

285. Konishi T: Electrophysiological consideration of sick sinus syndrome. Jpn Circ J 1976;40:194.

286. Jordan JL, Yamaguchi I, Mandel WJ: Studies on the mechanism of suppression of sinus node automaticity by atrial overdrive pacing. Clin Res 1978;26:241.

287. Jordan JL, Yamaguchi I, Mandel WJ: The effects of verapamil on sinoatrial conduction in isolated tissue. Clin Res 1978; 26:241.

288. Singh BN, Roche AHG: Effects of intravenous verapamil on hemodynamics in patients with heart disease. Am Heart J (in press).

289. Ning W, Wit AL: Comparison of the direct effects of nifedipine and verapamil on the electrical activity of the sinoatrial and atrioventricular nodes of the rabbit heart. Am Heart J 1983;106:345.

290. Henry PD: Comparative pharmacology of calcium antagonists: Nifedipine, verapamil and diltiazem. Am J Cardiol 1980;46:1047.

291. Broekhysen J, Deltour G, Ghislain M: Some biochemical effects of amiodarone. Arzneimittelforschung Forsch 1969;19:1850.

292. Goupil N, Lenfant J: The effects of amiodarone on the sinus node activity of the rabbit heart. Eur J Pharmacol 1976;39:23.

293. Gloor HO, Urthaler F, James TN: Acute effects of amiodarone upon the canine sinus node and atrioventricular junctional region. J Clin Invest 1983;71:1457.

294. Obayashi R, Mandel WJ: Electrophysiological effects of ajmaline in isolated cardiac tissue. Cardiovasc Res 1976; 10:20.

295. Obayashi K, Nagasawa K, Mandel WJ, et al: Cardiovascular effects of ajmaline. Am Heart J 1976;92:487.

296. Reiser J, Freeman AR, Greenspan K: Aprindine—a calcium mediated antidysrhythmic. Fed Proc 1974;33:476.

297. Elharrour V, Foster PR, Zipes DP: Effects of aprindine HCL on cardiac tissue. J Pharmacol Exp Ther 1975;195:201.

298. Ledda E, Mantelli L, Manzini S, et al: Electrophysiological and antiarrhythmic properties of propafenone in isolated cardiac preparations. J Cardiovasc Pharmacol 1981;3:1162.

299. Kohlhardt M: Der Einflus von propafenon auf den transmembranaien Na$^+$ und Ca$^+$ strom der Warmbliiter myokard fasermembran. In: Hechrein H, Hapke HJ, Beck OA, eds. Fortshritte in der Pharmako Therapie von Herzrhythmusstorungen. Stuttgart: Fischer, 1977:38.

300. Satoh H, Hashimoto K: Effect of propafenone on the membrane currents of rabbit sinoatrial node cells. Eur J Pharmacol 1984;99:185.

301. Echt DS, Berte LE, Clusin WT, et al: Prolongation of the human monophasic action potential by sotalol. Am J Cardiol 1982;51:1082.

302. Rosenshtraukh LV, Yurgavichyus IA, Undrovinas AI, et al: Effects of Ethmozine on the contractile force, transmembrane action potential, and sodium current in frog auriculat muscle. First US–USSR Symposium of Sudden Death. Yalta, USSR, Oct. 3–5, 1977.

303. Roffy R, Rosenshtraukh LV, Elharrar V, Zipes DP: Electrophysiological effects of ethmozin on canine myocardium. Cardiovasc Res 1979;13:354.

304. Urthaler F, Rosenshtraukh LV, Hageman GR, et al: Differential modulation of autonomic activity by Ethmozin and Ethacizin (analog of Ethmozin) on the canine sinus node and atrioventricular junction. J Am Coll Cardiol 1986;8:86A.

305. Belhassev B, Pelleg A, Shoshani D, et al: Electrophysiologic effects of Adenosine-5-triphosphate on atrioventricular reentrant tachycardia. Circulation 1983;68:827.

306. Belardinnelli L, Shryock J, West AG, et al: Effects of adenosine and adenine nucleotides on atrioventricular node of the isolated guinea pig heart. Circulation 1984;70:1083.

307. Sharma AD, Klein GJ: Comparative quantitative electrophysiologic effects of adenosine triphosphate on the sinus node and atrioventricular node. Am J Cardiol 1988;61(4):330.

308. West GA, Belardinelli L: Correlation of sinus slowing and hyperpolarization caused by adenosine in sinus node. Pfluger Arch 1985;403(1):75.

309. Opt Hef T, Duivenviofden JJ, VanGinneken ACG, et al: Electrophysiological effects of alinidine (ST 567) on sinoatrial node fibers in the rabbit heart. Cardiovasc Res 1986;20:727.

310. VanGinneken ACG, Bouman LN, Jongsma NJ: Alinidine as a model of the mode of action of specific bradycardic agents on SA node activity. Eur Heart J 1985;(suppl L):25.

311. Kobinger W, Lillier C, Pichler L: N-allyl derivative of clonidine, a substance with specific bradycardia action at a cardiac site. Arch Pharmacol 1979;306:255.

312. Conde C, Leppo J, Lipski J, et al: Effectiveness of pacemaker treatment in the bradycardia-tachycardia syndrome. Am J Cardiol 1973;32:209.

313. Sigurd B, Jensen G, Melbom J, et al: Adams-Stokes syndrome caused by sinoatrial block. Br Heart J 1973;35:1002.

314. Rokseth R, Hatle L: Prospective study on the occurrence and management of chronic sinoatrial disease, with follow-up. Br Heart J 1974;36:582.

315. Radford DJ, Julian DG: Sick sinus syndrome: Experience of a cardiac pacemaker clinic. Br Med J 1974;3:504.

316. Sowton E, Hendrix G, Roy P: Ten-year survey of treatment with implanted cardiac pacemaker. Br Med J 1974;3:155.

317. Hartel G, Talvensaari T: Treatment of sinoatrial syndrome with permanent cardiac pacing in 90 patients. Acta Med Scand 1975;198:341.

318. Chokshi DS, Mascarenhas E, Sanet P, et al: Treatment of sinoatrial rhythm disturbances with permanent cardiac pacing. Am J Cardiol 1973;32:215.

319. Skagen K, Hansen JF: The long-term prognosis for patients with sinoatrial block treated with permanent pacemaker. Acta Med Scand 1975;199:13.

320. Krishnaswami K, Geraci AR: Permanent pacing in disorders of sinus node function. Am Heart J 1975;89:579.

321. Stewart WJ, DiCola VL, Hawthorne JW: Doppler ultrasound measurement of cardiac output in patients with physiologic pacemakers: Effects of left ventricular function and retrograde ventriculo-atrial conduction. Am J Cardiol 1984;54:308.

322. Rediker DE, Eagle KA, Homma S, et al.: Clinical and hemodynamic comparison of VVI versus DDD pacing in patients with DDD pacemakers. Am J Cardiol 1988;61:323.

323. Rubenstein JJ, et al: Clinical spectrum of the sick sinus syndrome. Circulation 1972;46:5.

324. Wan SH, Lee GS, Toh CCS: The sick sinus syndrome. A study of 15 cases. Br Heart J 1972;34:942.

325. Rosen K, Loeb H, Sinno MZ: Cardiac conduction in patients with symptomatic sinus node disease. Circulation 1971;43:836.

326. Narula O: Atrioventricular conduction defects in patients with sinus bradycardia. Analysis by His bundle recordings. Circulation 1971;44:1096.

327. Lasmas GA, Estres NM III, Schneller S, Flaker GC. Does dual chamber or atrial pacing prevent atrial fibrillation? The need for a randomized controlled trial. PACE 1992;15:1109.

328. Zipes DP, Wallace RG, Sealy WC, et al: Artificial atrial and ventricular pacing in the treatment of arrhythmias. Ann Intern Med 1969;70:885.

329. Hayes DL, Neubauer SA. Incidence of atrial fibrillation after DDD pacing. PACE 1990;13:501.

330. Nurnberg M, Frehmner K, Podzeck A, Steinbach K. Is VVI pacing more dangerous than AV sequential pacing in patients with sick sinus syndrome. PACE 1991;14:674.

331. Zanini R, Facchinetti A, Gallo G, Cazzamalli L, Binandi L, Dei Cas L. Morbidity and mortality of patients with sinus node disease: Comparative effects of atrial and ventricular pacing. PACE 1990;13:2076.

332. Chen TO: Transvenous ventricular pacing in the treatment of paroxysmal atrial tachyarrhythmias alternating with sinus bradycardia and standstill. Am J Cardiol 1968;22:874.

333. Zoll PM, Linenthal DJ, Zarsky LRN: Ventricular fibrillation. Treatment and prevention by external cardiac currents. N Engl J Med 1960;262:105.

334. Han J, Millet D, Chizzonitti B, et al: Temporal dispersion of recovery of excitability in atrium and ventricle as a function of heart rate. Am Heart J 1966;71:481.

335. Han J, De Traglia J, Millet D, et al: Incidence of ectopic beats as a function of basic rate in the ventricle. Am Heart J 1966;72:632.

336. Sandoe E, Flensted-Jensen E: Adams-Stokes seizures in patients with attacks of both tachy and bradycardia, a therapeutic challenge. Acta Med Scand 1969;186:111.

344. Lillie C, Kobinger W: Actions of alinidine and AK-A 39 on the rate and contractility of guinea pig atria during B-adrenoreceptor stimulation. J Cardiovasc Pharmacol 1983;5:1048.

346. Kruc I, Ryden L: A comparison of physical work capacity and systolic time intervals with ventricular inhibited and atrial synchronous ventricular inhibited pacing. Br Heart J 1981;46:129.

347. Ohe T, Shimemura K, Inagaki M: The effects of cycle length on fragmented atrial activity zone in patients with sick sinus syndrome. J Electrocardiog 1987;20(5):364.

348. Hauser RG, Jones JJ, Moss K, et al: Survival after permanent pacemaker implantation. In: Proceedings of the 7th World Symposium on Cardiac Pacing, Vienna. Darmstadt: Steinkopft Verlag, 1983:483.

349. Simon AB, Janz N: Symptomatic bradyarrhythmias in the adult: Natural history following ventricular pacemaker implantation. PACE 1982;5:372.

350. Sutton R, Kenny RA: The natural history of sick sinus syndrome. PACE 1986;9:1110.

351. Alpert MA, Curtis JJ, Sanfelippo JF, et al: Comparative survival following permanent ventricular and dual-chamber pacing for patients with chronic symptomatic sinus node dysfunction with and without congestive heart failure. Am Heart J 1987;113(4):958.

352. Rosenqvist M, Brandt S, Schuller H: Long term pacing in sinus node disease: Effects of stimulation mode of cardiovascular morbidity and mortality. Am Heart J 1988;116:16.

Cardiac Arrhythmias, 3rd edition, edited by William J. Mandel.
J. B. Lippincott Company, Philadelphia © 1995.

10

Maurits A. Allessie • Felix I. M. Bonke

Atrial Arrhythmias: Basic Concepts

Several problems are inherent in writing about the concepts of atrial premature beats and tachyarrhythmias. The main difficulty is that despite the extensive and excellent research done in this field, the underlying mechanisms of most human arrhythmias have still not been determined. Therefore, we cannot describe in this chapter the mechanism of each of the different atrial arrhythmias as a circumscribed well-defined scientific fact. We are forced to present the various theoretic mechanisms for tachyarrhythmias as they are found in experimental studies.

Nevertheless, by comparing experimental data obtained from animal studies with clinical observations, we will try to indicate which of the possible mechanisms seems most likely to be responsible for each of the different arrhythmias encountered in humans.

CLASSIFICATION OF ATRIAL ARRHYTHMIAS

Another difficulty caused by the lack of knowledge concerning the underlying mechanisms of atrial arrhythmias is that the clinical classification of supraventricular tachyarrhythmias in tachycardia, flutter, and fibrillation is primarily arbitrary; the most important criterion used for this classification is the rate of the arrhythmias. Figure 10-1 shows the different rate scales several authors use to classify atrial tachyarrhythmias. As seems inevitable in medicine when some arbitrary criterion is used, opinions diverge widely on the rate at which a tachycardia should be called *flutter* or when flutter changes into *fibrillation*. Actually, no sharp division exists between the different arrhythmias. As indicated by some authors, there is overlap in rate between tachycardia and flutter and an area of "no man's land" between flutter and fibrillation. Terms such as *impure flutter*, *flutter-fibrillation*, and *coarse fibrillation* are used to describe the intermediate form between flutter and fibrillation.

The close interrelation between different atrial arrhythmias is further illustrated by the observation that one arrhythmia may change into another. The transition from atrial flutter into fibrillation or vice versa is well known, occurring either spontaneously or during the administration of digitalis or quinidine. All this clarifies that the present classification of atrial arrhythmias does not necessarily mean that each has a different fundamental mechanism. In addition, tachyarrhythmias of about the same rate and of similar clinical appearance may be based on completely different mechanisms. Because of this, another

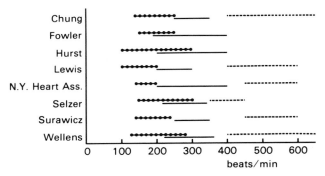

Figure 10-1. Classification of supraventricular tachyarrhythmia in tachycardia, flutter, and fibrillation, according to the rate of the arrhythmia. A wide variability exists in the criteria used by several authors. There is overlap between the definition of tachycardia and flutter, whereas an undefined area exists between flutter and fibrillation. (●—●—●—●, tachycardia; ———, flutter; - - - - -, fibrillation) (Data from Chung EK: Principles of cardiac arrhythmias. Baltimore: Waverly Press, 1977; Fowler N: Cardiac diagnosis. Hagerstown, MD: Harper & Row, 1968; Hurst J: The heart. New York: McGraw-Hill, 1974; Lewis T: The mechanism and graphic registration of the heart beat. London: Shaw & sons, 1925; New York Heart Association: nomenclature and criteria for diagnosis of diseases of the heart and great vessels, 7th ed., 1973; Selsen A: Principles of clinical cardiology. Philadelphia: WB Saunders, 1975; Surawicz B, et al: Standardization of terminology and interpretation. Am J Cardiol 1978;41:130; Wellens HJJ: Electrical stimulation of the heart in the study and treatment of tachycardias. Leiden: Stenfert Kroese, 1971)

classification based on the underlying mechanisms would be far preferable. Such classification cannot be made, however, until the various mechanisms underlying atrial arrhythmias are better understood and clinical criteria and diagnostic tests are developed to differentiate the various mechanisms of arrhythmias operative in humans.

Atrial Premature Complexes

A premature atrial complex is an early depolarization that may originate anywhere in the atria outside the sinus node. The propagation of the impulse in the atria from an atrial ectopic focus is usually different from that of the sinus impulse, so that the shape of the resultant P wave is more or less different from the P wave of sinus origin. Depending on the degree of prematurity and whether the pacemaker in the sinus node is reset, an atrial premature complex may be interpolated, followed by a full compensatory pause or followed by an interval that is only somewhat longer than a normal sinus interval. Furthermore, it may also trigger a bout of rapid repetitive atrial activity.

Atrial Tachycardia

As do atrial premature complexes, atrial tachycardia may originate from anywhere in the atria. There is a rapid and regular succession of P waves of different form, compared with the P wave of sinus origin, and an isoelectric segment exists between P waves. Atrial tachycardia frequently occurs in paroxysms but on rare occasions, it may become chronic. It usually has a rate between 140 and 200 beats per minute, generally with each atrial impulse conducted to the ventricle (1:1 response).

Atrial Flutter

Atrial flutter is characterized by a rapid, highly regular rhythm of the atria (200 to 350 beats/minute). Because of the refractory period in the atrioventricular (AV) junctional tissue, the ventricular response is usually at half this rate because a 2:1 or greater AV block almost always exists. Atrial activity is represented in the electrocardiogram by regular biphasic oscillations (F waves) of uniform shape. There is no intervening isoelectric segment between the F waves, and the atrial oscillations have a continuous sawtooth type of appearance. Atrial flutter has been classified into two different types.[1] Type I, similar to classic or common atrial flutter, has an atrial rate between 240 and 340 beats per minute and can be entrained by rapid pacing. Type II flutter, with an atrial rate between 340 and 430 beats per minute, cannot be reset or entrained by programmed electric stimulation. Atrial flutter may (1) occur in paroxysms, with spontaneous termination; (2) be a continuous chronic process if not treated; or (3) change into atrial fibrillation. Generally, flutter is less stable than fibrillation.

Atrial Fibrillation

During atrial fibrillation, atrial activity is chaotic and uncoordinated. On the electrocardiogram, the completely irregular atrial activation is recorded in the form of small waves that constantly vary in amplitude and configuration. It is usually impossible to count accurately the number of atrial responses from the ordinary electrocardiogram but it has been estimated to vary between 400 and 650 "beats" per minute. Not uncommonly, fibrillation is so fine and activation of the atria so fragmented that it becomes difficult to distinguish any atrial activity on the electrocardiogram. Local electrograms, however, recorded directly from the surface of the atria under these circumstances, still show well-defined (although irregular) electric activity.[2] The ventricular rhythm during atrial fibrillation is completely irregular. Atrial fibrillation may occur in a paroxysmal form or it may become chronic. Generally, paroxysms of atrial fibrillation must be considered to be a precursor of permanent atrial fibrillation.

POSSIBLE MECHANISMS OF ATRIAL TACHYARRHYTHMIAS

Two groups of fundamentally different mechanisms may be responsible for producing tachyarrhythmias. Group I contains those mechanisms that are based on some form of abnormal impulse formation. Group II is based on a disorder of impulse conduction, leading to circulating excitation or reentry. Figure 10-2 summarizes the different types of abnormal impulse formation and the two types of circus movement that have been recognized in experimental studies.

Abnormal Impulse Formation

Abnormal impulse formation may be defined as the generation of impulses by fibers other than the dominant pacemaker fibers in the center of the sinus node, regardless of whether the abnormal impulse is generated spontaneously or induced by foregoing normal or abnormal

activities. According to this definition, abnormal impulse formation is the same as ectopic impulse formation.

It is also possible to use a definition based more on the mechanism underlying impulse formation. Normal impulse formation is the occurrence of a spontaneous depolarization before the onset of an action potential, the so-called diastolic depolarization. If depolarization occurs either during repolarization or under special conditions directly after repolarization, the term "abnormal impulse formation" may be used.

Under normal conditions, the fibers in the atrium that show spontaneous depolarization (diastolic depolarization) are located in the sinus node, the region of the AV node, and perhaps around the orifices of the pulmonary veins in the left atrium (these fibers are present in the rabbit but perhaps not in all other species). Furthermore, there are fibers in the vicinity of the coronary sinus (at least in the dog) and in the leaflets of the AV valves that have a relatively low resting potential and develop spontaneous depolarization under certain conditions.

Finally, Hashimoto and Moe describe fibers in the canine right atrium close to the crista terminalis that have some characteristics of Purkinje fibers (i.e., spontaneous depolarization).[3] It is not known whether these fibers are also present in other species.

The spontaneous depolarization in the fibers in the center of the sinus node is normally the fastest and therefore, this depolarization brings these fibers to a discharge

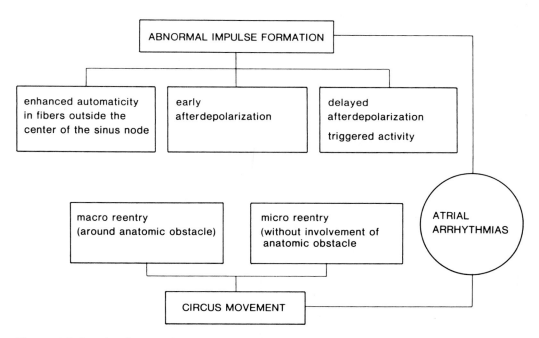

Figure 10-2. Classification of atrial tachyarrhythmias on the basis of their possible underlying mechanisms.

before others. Thus, under normal conditions, automaticity of the dominant pacemaker in the center of the sinus node suppresses the subsidiary pacemakers in the atria.

Enhanced Automaticity in Fibers Outside the Center of the Sinus Node

A certain agent can perhaps differentially enhance the spontaneous depolarization in a subsidiary pacemaker without affecting the sinus node or by influencing it only to a lesser extent. For example, when extracellular potassium concentration is reduced, diastolic depolarization (phase 4 depolarization) may be enhanced in subsidiary pacemaker fibers, whereas fibers within the center of the sinus node remain relatively insensitive. Similarly, although catecholamines enhance diastolic depolarization in both the dominant and subsidiary pacemakers, this effect could be more pronounced on subsidiary pacemakers than on sinus node fibers. Vagal influences may also preferentially suppress the dominant pacemaker to such an extent that subsidiary pacemakers generate either one or a series of spontaneous discharges.

If the normal function of the pacemaker of the sinus node is severely depressed by whatever cause or if the impulse from the pacemaker does not reach the atrium (sinoatrial block), automaticity in subsidiary pacemaker fibers may generate an impulse or even take over pacemaker function. In an isolated preparation of the coronary sinus region of the canine atrium, Wit and Cranefield were able to induce automaticity by adding catecholamines to the tissue bath and increase the rate to a range similar to the sinus rate in an isolated canine right atrium preparation (Fig. 10-3).[4]

Early Afterdepolarizations

Depolarization may also occur during repolarization or before repolarization is completed. It is incorrect to call this a phase 4 depolarization because the depolarization starts from a low level of membrane potential (e.g., -30 mV). Cranefield uses the term "early afterdepolarization" (EAD).[5] If such an afterdepolarization is strong enough, it may lead to an action potential with a low amplitude.

Normally, the net ionic current through the cell membrane during repolarization is directed outward. If the outward current is depressed or if the background inward current is enhanced, the net current may become inward; this means that a depolarization of the membrane occurs and such a depolarization may excite the fiber again. Such decrease of outward (repolarizing) current may occur if the membrane conductance for potassium ions is reduced (e.g., as is the case if the extracellular potassium concentration is markedly reduced). An increase of background inward current may result from hypoxia, injury, or some drugs.[6] An example of the latter is the demonstration by Scherf that focal application of aconitine to the surface of the canine atrium produced a tachycardia with a rate of 200 to 300 beats per minute, originating at the site where aconitine was applied.[7] Although this drug has no significance for practical use, it illustrates well the phenomenon of EAD. Matsuda and coworkers showed that in isolated dog ventricular myocardium, focal application of aconitine prolonged the repolarization and subsequently the occurrence of "spontaneous" or "nondriven" action potentials.[8] This has also been demonstrated by Schmidt; Figure 10-4 is taken from his publication.[9] Peper and Trautwein were able to demonstrate that aconitine inhibits or postpones the inactivation of the sodium influx system, so that the background inward current is strongly increased during repolarization.[10] If the membrane potential of a group of fibers is brought artificially (e.g., through depolarizing current) to a level between -40 and -10 mV, spontaneous action potentials may occur. This is illustrated in Figure 10-5, taken from the work of Lenfant and coworkers, using atrial trabecula of the frog.[11] In principle, the same phenomena were demonstrated in ventricular muscle of the guinea pig.[12, 13] The same phenomenon may be present in diseased human atrial tissue; if these fibers are put in a tissue bath, they become depolarized and spontaneously active.[14]

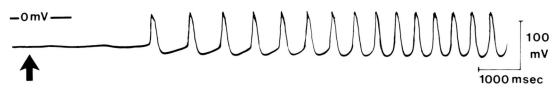

Figure 10-3. Spontaneous impulse initiation in atrial fibers outside the coronary sinus ostium (dog). Norepinephrine, 10^{-6} g/mL, was added to the tissue bath at the moment indicated by the arrow (*left*). Small oscillations in membrane potential then occurred and led to the first spontaneous impulse; the slope of the diastolic depolarization increased with each subsequent spontaneous impulse, by which the rate of the focal discharge increased. (Wit AL, Cranefield PF: Triggered and automatic activity in the canine coronary sinus. Circ Res 1977;41:435. By permission of the American Heart Association.)

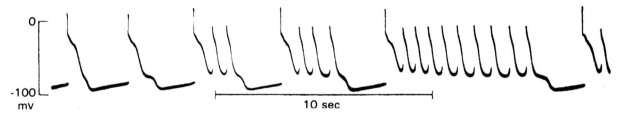

Figure 10-4. Isolated Purkinje fibers of the dog, showing spontaneous activity. Aconitine is added to the tissue bath in a low concentration (10^{-6}–10^{-8} g/mL). This slows the repolarization, and the third action potential is followed by two spontaneous, nondriven impulses. The fourth and fifth action potentials are followed by a series of these impulses. (Schmidt RF: Versuche mit Aconitin zum Problem der spontanen Erregungsbildung im Herzen. Pflugers Arch 1960;271:526.)

Delayed Afterdepolarizations

An afterdepolarization may also occur after the fiber is repolarized completely or almost completely. If the amplitude of such an afterdepolarization is large enough, a single or a series of nondriven action potentials may arise. Afterdepolarizations of this type have been recorded in experimental studies in which cardiac tissue was exposed to toxic concentrations of cardiac glycosides; this is true not only in Purkinje and ventricular fibers but also in specialized atrial fibers and diseased human atrial tissue.[3,15,16] Conversely, Saito and coworkers described that in isolated rabbit right atrium preparations, it was possible under special conditions (no spontaneous activity, K_o = 2.6 mmol, and the temperature of the superfusate at 32°C) to induce by regular drive, delayed afterpotentials, and by

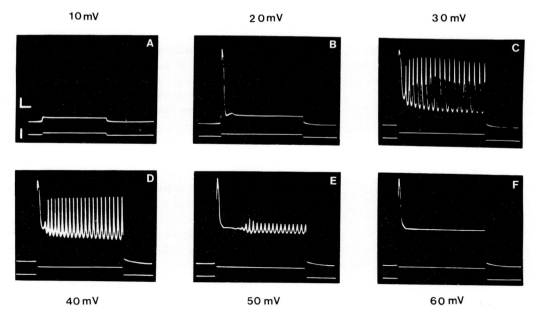

Figure 10-5. The effect of depolarizing current on frog atrial trabecula. The upper trace in panel represents the membrane potential; the lower trace, the amount of current that is given to the preparation. (**A**) The current causes a depolarization of 10 mV, whereas a depolarization of 20 mV (**B**) causes a single action potential followed by an oscillation. More current causes a stronger depolarization (30 mV in **C** and 40 mV in **D**), and sustained rhythmic activity follows the first-induced action potential. If the membrane is depolarized with 50 mV (**E**), only small oscillations are present, whereas in the case of a depolarization with 60 mV (**F**), a stable membrane potential is reached after the action potential.

In the first panel (**A**), calibrations are given, namely, 20 mV and 1 second for the first trace and 5 × 10^{-7} A for the current trace (*second trace*). Measurements were made with a double-sucrose-gap technique. (Lenfant J, Mironneau J, Akar JR: Activité répétitive de la fibre sino-auriculaire de grenouille: analyse des courants membranaires responsables de l'automatisme cardiaque. J Physiol (Paris) 1972;64:5.)

an extra stimulus, sustained rhythmic activity.[17] This is illustrated in Figure 10-6. Saito mentioned that some of the spontaneously active preparations became quiescent when the external potassium concentration was raised from 2.6 to 5.2 mmol. It is unclear whether this phenomenon is important under normal conditions and in the human heart.

Furthermore, these delayed afterdepolarizations (DAD) also occur in canine, simian, and human valvular fibers; in the canine coronary sinus; and in diseased human atrium.[4,18-21] In all these cases, the afterdepolarizations only occur in relation to a preceding action potential and never develop spontaneously. Therefore, the term "triggered activity" is used when an afterdepolarization is strong enough to initiate a nondriven action potential (Fig. 10-7).[4] Wit and Cranefield demonstrated that triggered sustained tachycardias are characterized by a progressive decrease of the cycle length (the rate increases; warming-up phenomenon) during the first 10 to 20 beats.[4] The sustained activity always subsides spontaneously after some seconds to minutes. Preceding termination, the rate slows down and the last nondriven action potential is followed by one or more subthreshold afterdepolarizations. In a few seconds, the membrane potential then

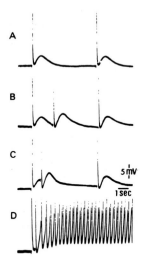

Figure 10-6. In isolated right atrium of the rabbit, it is sometimes possible to find fibers showing afterpotentials. In this experiment, the preparation was electrically stimulated every 6 seconds. Only the foot of the action potential is shown in this recording (note the calibration). (**A**) The control recording, where an extra stimulus was given in the other records; (**B**) With a coupling of 2 seconds; (**C**) of 1 second; and (**D**) of 500 milliseconds. In **D**, the extra response is followed by a series of nondriven impulses. (Saito T, Otoguro M, and Matsubara T: Electrophysiological studies on the mechanism of electrically induced sustained rhythmic activity in the rabbit right atrium. Circ Res 1978;42:199. By permission of the American Heart Association.)

increases to the level attained just before triggering (Fig. 10-8).

The mechanism for DAD is still unclear. Calcium probably plays an important role because the amplitude of afterdeplarizations is increased by catecholamines and by an increase of extracellular calcium. In contrast, the amplitude is lowered by calcium entry blockers (e.g., verapamil). Sodium is also important because the amplitude of the afterdepolarizations is reduced by lowering the extracellular sodium concentration, by TTX (tetrodotoxin), and by class I antiarrhythmic drugs. It seems that during the delayed afterdepolarization, the transient inward (depolarizing) current is carried by sodium ions, whereas the membrane conductance is modulated by the intracellular calcium concentration.[22] Such a contention gains support from the experiments using low doses of caffeine, an agent that enhances calcium release from intracellular stores (i.e., the sarcoplasmic reticulum and causes elevation of intracellular calcium ion concentration).[23] The presence of caffeine caused both DAD to move earlier in the cycle and larger amplitudes, so that triggered activity could more easily be induced and lasted longer than in the absence of caffeine.[23] During the triggered activity, there is an initial acceleration (warming up) of the rate that is associated with depolarization of the maximum diastolic membrane potential, followed by slowing of the rate and termination accompanied by membrane hyperpolarization. It was found that the initial increase in the rate during triggered activity was accompanied by an initial increase in $[K^+]_o$ and depolarization, and the later slowing of the rate and membrane hyperpolarization was accompanied by a decline in $[K^+]_o$. It is proposed that enhanced Na^+/K^+ pump activity could be responsible for the decline in $[K]_o$ and slowing of the rate and could posttrigger depletion of extracellular K^+.[24] The amplitude of the DAD was found to increase with the superfusion of lysophosphatidylcholine at concentrations comparable to those present in ischemic myocardium[25]. These lysophosphatidylcholine-induced DADs persisted even in the presence of hyperkalemia ($[K^+]_o$ 7 mmol) and acidosis.[3]

Early Afterdepolarizations

Arrhythmias may also result by the mechanism of EAD. Although the precise mechanism or mechanisms of EAD in atrial fibers remain undefined, a number of studies on ventricular tissue suggest that EAD induction requires first a conditioning phase, characterized by prolongation of the action potential duration that is controlled by the sum of membrane currents present at the plateau voltage range of the action potential (i.e., inward depolarizing current and outward repolarizing current).[26] It has been shown that a calcium channel current agonist (BAY K 8644) can induce both lengthening of action potential plateau and recovery

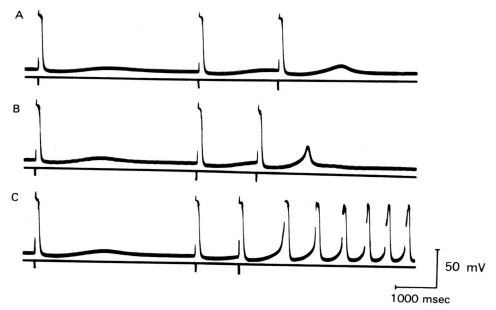

Figure 10-7. Recording from a canine coronary sinus fiber while norepinephrine (10^{-6} g/mL) was in the tissue bath. Each panel shows the last two impulses of a series of 10 driven beats, with an interval of 4000 milliseconds after which a premature pulse was induced at progressively shorter coupling intervals (**A**) 2000 milliseconds, (**B**) 1400 milliseconds; and (**C**) 1000 milliseconds. In **B**, the premature action potential is followed by an afterdepolarization of about 30 mV, whereas in **C**, sustained rhythmic activity is triggered by the afterdepolarization following the premature action potential. (Wit AL, Cranefield PF: Triggered and automatic activity in the canine coronary sinus. Circ Res 1977;41:435. By permission of the American Heart Association)

from inactivation and reactivation of the L-type calcium current that leads to EAD formation and repetitive activity.[27] It has been suggested by Kimura and associates that cocaine-induced blocking of the delayed outward current (IK) could be responsible for the induction of EADs and triggered activity.[28] These authors, however, suggest that

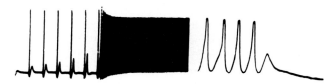

Figure 10-8. Recording from a canine coronary sinus fiber stimulated with an interval of 4000 milliseconds. The afterdepolarizations progressively increase in amplitude until rapid sustained rhythmic activity is triggered. During this rapid rhythm, the membrane potential and the amplitude of the action potentials are decreased. At the right, the end of the rapid rhythm is shown while the paper speed of the recorder is 10 times faster than at the left. The last action potential is followed by an afterdepolarization and the membrane potential then returns to the level present before triggering. The interval at the end of the period of rapid rhythm is about 440 milliseconds in this case. The amplitude of the action potential shown at the left is about 90 mV. Norepinephrine (10^{-6}g/mL) was added to the superfusing fluid. (Wit AL, Cranefield PF: Triggered and automatic activity in the canine coronary sinus. Circ Res 1977;41:435. By permission of the American Heart Association)

the lengthening of the action potential duration at the plateau voltage range by blocking IK may result in recovery from inactivation and reactivation of the calcium current. This was suggested by cocaine-induced EADs and triggered activity being enhanced by isoproterenol and suppressed by verapamil.[28] Sympathetic stimulation, α-adrenoceptor stimulation, and acidosis all reliably augment EAD amplitude and facilitate the induction of triggered activity.[29–31] Whether these factors also augment EAD amplitude and triggering in atrial tissue to cause atrial tachyarrhythmias remain to be seen.

In Figure 10-9, the three different types of abnormal impulse formation (enhanced automaticity, EAD, and DAD-triggered activity) are summarized schematically.

CIRCUS MOVEMENT

General Considerations

The concept of the electric impulse being entrapped in a circus movement somewhere in the heart dates from the end of the 19th century. As an alternative to the earlier proposed possibility of enhanced automaticity, in an article about fibrillar contraction of the heart, McWilliam wrote:

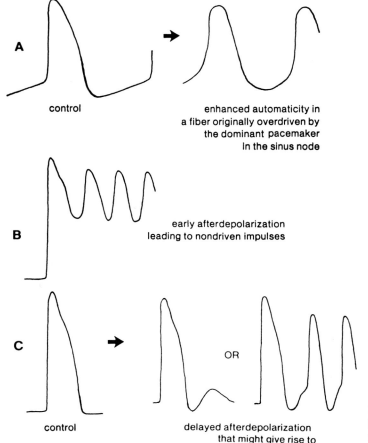

control

enhanced automaticity in
a fiber originally overdriven by
the dominant pacemaker
in the sinus node

early afterdepolarization
leading to nondriven impulses

OR

control

delayed afterdepolarization
that might give rise to
nondriven impulses

Figure 10-9. (**A**) Enhanced automaticity (diastolic depolarization). (**B**) Early afterdepolarization, leading to nondriven impulses. (**C**) Delayed afterdepolarization that may give rise to nondriven impulses.

For apart from the possibility of rapid spontaneous discharges of energy by the muscular fibers, there seems to be another probable cause of continued and rapid movement. The peristaltic contraction travelling along such a structure as that of the ventricular wall must reach adjacent muscle bundles at different points of time, and because these bundles are connected with one another by anastomosing branches the contraction would naturally be propagated from one contracting fiber to another over which the contraction wave had already passed. Hence if the fibers are sufficiently excitable and ready to respond to contraction waves reaching them there would evidently be a more or less rapid series of contractions in each muscular bundle in consequence of the successive contraction waves reaching that bundle from different directions along its fibers of anastomosis with other bundles.[32]

It is an interesting detail that the first observations about circulating excitation were not of the heart but on an animal bearing close resemblance to the heart: the jellyfish. In 1906, Mayer, studying the nature of rhythmic pulsation of the jellyfish, found that a strip of paralyzed subumbrella tissue of the jellyfish *Scyphomedusa* cut in the shape of a ring or closed circuit pulsates rhythmically again if a contraction wave is initiated in the circuit.[33] The rate of this rhythm, based on a continuous circus movement of the impulse around the ring, was about three to four times as rapid as the normal rhythm of the Medusa, originating from its marginal sense organs. The analogy with atrial flutter and sinus rhythm is indeed striking.

It seems questionable whether Mayer himself was aware of the importance of his observations with respect to cardiac arrhythmias. Although he repeated his experiments on ring-shaped strips of turtle ventricle, in which he found the same phenomena as in the rings of the jellyfish, he emphasized:

It is remarkable that these isolated circuit waves, moving constantly in one direction through a circuit, are not met with in nature. Indeed, the heart, or pulsating Medusa, contains within itself the means to prevent any single pulsation wave from coursing constantly in one direction through the tissues. . . . Such a circuit cannot take possession of the vertebrate heart.[33]

Two contemporary physiologists immediately understood the fundamental significance of Mayer's observations in respect to cardiac arrhythmias. Independent of each other, Mines and Garrey extended Mayer's studies on rings cut from atria, ventricles, or both.[34-36] These studies resulted in a concept of circulating excitation that has survived 65 years of extensive research on the electrophysiology of the heart. Since then, this early model of Mines as a basis for tachyarrhythmias has not lost its validity. It still gives a good and complete description of the properties of a rhythm based on the circulation of an excitation wave in a relatively large anatomically defined circuit. Investigations have discovered, however, that in contrast to this classic model of circus movement, many tachyarrhythmias seem to arise from circus movement in a small circuit, without involving a gross anatomic obstacle. The behavior of this type of circus movement differs from circus movement around a large anatomically determined circuit. Instead of being determined by the length of the circuit, this circus movement is completely governed by the functional electrophysiologic properties of the tissue composing the circuit. Circus movement tachycardias within the AV and sinoatrial (SA) nodes are probably the best known examples of such microreentry but sustained microreentry is also possible in ordinary working myocardium.[37-41] These investigations have led to the description of a second model of circus movement that—in contrast to the classic anatomic model—is based solely on the functional electrophysiologic properties of cardiac muscle.[42] We first describe these two fundamental models of circulating excitation in the heart, emphasizing the similarities and differences between macroreentry and microreentry.

For a better appreciation of the importance of the active cellular mechanism or mechanisms and the passive electric properties of atrial tissue in the induction of these two different types of reentrant excitation (rotor formation), an overview of the newest findings in atrial electrophysiology is in order. This allows a better appreciation of the cellular and ionic mechanism or mechanisms of impulse initiation (excitation) and impulse propagation.

Atrial Gap Junctions

The rapid propagation and synchronization of action potentials in cardiac tissue is insured by specialized ionic channels that link adjacent cells by a specialized structure known as gap junctions. In the adult atrial tissue, unlike in ventricular gap junctions, the transjunctional conductance is dependent of transjunctional voltage.[43] This finding is especially true in weakly coupled atrial cells. It is suggested that transjunctional ionic currents result from the all-or-none gating of a population of gap junction channels and that such voltage-dependence gating of gap junction channels provides a rapid control mechanism of cell-to-cell interaction, especially in poorly coupled cells, and determines impulse initiation and impulse propagation.[43]

Sodium Current

Using the whole-cell voltage-clamp technique, it is reported that isolated human atrial myocytes manifest the same kinetics of activation of the fast inward sodium current and recovery from inactivation as do other mammalian cardiac cells.[44,45] Similarly, atrial fast sodium channel currents also manifest the phenomenon of use-dependent block when exposed to antiarrhythmic drugs.[46] The determinants of steady-state availability of the fast sodium current in isolated human myocytes did not differ in cells from patients with different disease states and different ages.[44] Furthermore, myocytes from patients in sinus rhythm and atrial fibrillation also did not differ in this regard.[44] More studies are clearly needed to substantiate the role of fast sodium current in the induction of reentry rotors that lead to atrial fibrillation.

Calcium Current

Two different calcium currents have been demonstrated in cardiac and noncardiac tissues.[47] One current results from the activation of low-threshold, rapidly inactivating T-type channels and the other from the activation of the classic high-threshold, slowly inactivating L-type calcium channels.[47] Only the L-type calcium channel is sensitive to organic calcium antagonists (i.e., nifedipine, diltiazem, nicarpidine) and they are usually referred to as dihydropyridine-sensitive channels. Relatively little is known about the slow inward current in human atrial myocytes.[48] The T-type calcium channel was never observed in human atrial myocytes and it is reported that chronic therapy with organic calcium antagonists results in down-regulation of the L-type calcium channel.[49] This indicates that a depression of calcium current persists long after removal of the blocking agent. The L-type current density in the atrial myocytes isolated from nontreated patients was 19 $\mu A/cm^2$, compared with 5 $\mu A/cm^2$ in the treated cells.[49] Threshold of activation and reversal potential of the L-type calcium current was similar in the treated and the nontreated groups.[49] The mechanism of L-type calcium channel down-regulation with chronic antagonist therapy remains undefined.[49]

Repolarizing Outward Currents

It has been suggested that repolarization in human atrial tissue is mainly governed by time- and voltage-dependent transient outward currents and that the inwardly rectifying background potassium current (IK1) and the delayed rectifier potassium current (IK) play a more minor role.[50,51] Measurements of action potential shape changes and phasic tension as a function of stimulus frequency indicate that in human atrium, the transient outward current can produce pronounced changes in both early repolarization of the action potential and force generation.[51] Complete block of this current by quinidine in rabbit atrium suggests that if quinidine's antiarrhythmic actions involve regulation of atrial action potential plateau and duration, the transient outward current may be an important factor in the genesis and control of some types of reentrant atrial tachyarrhythmias, with or without the presence of an anatomic obstacle.[52] Action potential shapes of adult human atrial fibers differ from young human atrial fibers.[53] Adult fibers have an initial notch, followed by a low-level prolonged plateau, whereas atrial fibers in the younger population are more triangular and manifest a short plateau approaching zero potential.[53] Using various pharmacologic ionic probes (4-aminopyridine, caffeine), it is suggested that an age-related increase in transient outward current can explain the differences in action potential plateau shape between the younger and the adult population.[53] Differences in action potential duration between epicaridal and endocardial atrial fibers were observed in mammalian atrium.[54] It was suggested that shorter epicardial action potential duration may be caused by the more prominent transient outward current in the epicardium, compared with the endocardium.[54] Whether similar regional (epicardium versus endocardium) differences also exist in humans remains undefined.

Circus Movement in an Anatomically Defined Pathway

Figure 10-10 shows the original diagrams drawn by Mines to illustrate the conditions required for initiation of circulating excitation in an anatomically defined circuit. It also shows the electrophysiologic situation during a sustained circus movement of the impulse. Shown in this figure is a series of images of the electrophysiologic state of a ring of cardiac muscle; the impulse is assumed to travel exclusively in a clockwise direction. The part of the circuit in the absolute refractory period is indicated by black, whereas the phase of the relative refractory period is represented by dots. The white area in the ring represents the fibers that have completely restored their excitability after the foregoing excitation.

Two prerequisites must be fulfilled to capture the impulse in a continuous circus movement around a ring: (1) the conduction of the impulse must be blocked in one direction around the ring while it continues to propagate in the other direction, and (2) the conduction time of the impulse around the circuit must be long enough to enable each part of the ring to restore its excitability sufficiently to respond to the next impulse.

The first condition of local conduction block can arise under many circumstances—the common cause being some kind of spatial inhomogeneity in the ability to propagate an excitation wave. The second condition is emphasized in Figure 10-10.

Figure 10-10A depicts a situation that arises if the rate of propagation is rapid when compared with the length of the circuitous pathway, the duration of the refractory period, or both. If the conduction velocity is too rapid, the circuit too small, or the refractory period too long, the impulse returns to its point of origin at a moment when the fibers have not yet recovered their excitability. Consequently, after one circuit around the ring, the excitation dies out and sustained circus movement is prevented. If the dimensions of the circuit are large, conduction velocity is low, or the refractory period is short, the region where the excitation started restores its excitability before the impulse returns to this point of the ring; consequently, the impulse reenters the ring for a second time (see Fig. 10-10B). Once started in this way, the impulse may continue to circulate for many revolutions, resulting in a sustained regular rhythm, the rate of which is determined by the conduction time of the activation wave around the circuit.

Figure 10-11 summarizes the properties of such sustained circus movement in a large anatomic circuit. The main characteristics are as follows:

1. The length of the circuit is fixed, being determined by the perimeter of the anatomic structure that forms the inexcitable center of the circuit.

2. The rate of the tachycardia is given by the following equation:

$$\text{Rate of tachycardia (beats/second)} = \frac{\text{conduction velocity}}{\text{length of circuit}}$$

because,

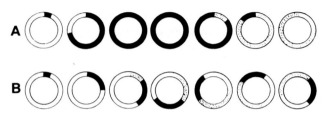

Figure 10-10. Original diagrams drawn by Mines to illustrate the conditions under which circulating excitation can occur. The absolute refractory period is indicated in black, whereas the condition of depressed excitability that exists during the relative refractory period is represented by dots. (Mines GR: On dynamic equilibrium in the heart. J Physiol 1913;46:349)

CIRCUS MOVEMENT AROUND ANATOMIC OBSTACLE (MINES 1913)

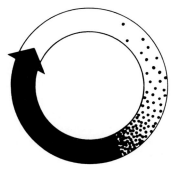

1. Length of circuit is fixed
   (given by perimeter of obstacle)

2. Rate of reentrant rhythm is
   proportional to $\dfrac{\text{conduction velocity}}{\text{length of circuit}}$

3. There is a gap of full excitability
   in the circuit (white part of the circuit)

4. Shortening of the refractory period
   does not affect the rate of the circus movement

Figure 10-11. Properties of circus movement in a gross anatomic circuit.

$$\text{rate} = \frac{1}{\text{revolution time}}$$

and,

$$\text{revolution time} = \frac{\text{length of circuit}}{\text{conduction velocity}}.$$

Thus, the rate is governed by two parameters: the length of the circuit and the average conduction velocity of the circulating impulse. If the circuit is small or the conduction velocity is high, the resulting rhythm is fast. Conversely, if the circuit is large or the impulse conducts slowly in all or part of the circuit, the rate of the arrhythmia is slow.

3. There exists an excitable gap in the circuit (see Figs. 10-10 and 10-11, white area). If the length of the circuit is longer than the wavelength of the circulating excitation wave, the fibers ahead of the circulating depolarization front have completely restored their excitability. This means that a stimulus (approaching depolarization wave) of diastolic threshold may already interfere with this circus movement rhythm. This is significant for the behavior of this type of circus movement when confronted with wavefronts of other origin, either occurring spontaneously or induced by electric stimulation.

4. This type of circus movement is insensitive to changes in duration of the effective refractory period in parts of the ring. A shortened refractory period further enlarges the gap of full excitability, whereas a prolonged refractory period will narrows the excitable gap without affecting the actual rate of the tachycardia. Only after marked prolongation of the refractory period is the excitable gap closed and the circulating activation wave encounters fibers that are still in their relative refractory state. This eventually leads to either a slowing of conduction of the circulating wavefront and a concomitant slowing of the tachycardia or termination of the arrhythmia.

Frame and associates developed in vivo and in vitro canine models of atrial reentry that involved a central anatomic obstacle.[55-58] The mechanism of the induced tachycardia was thought to be due to circus movement reentry, based on the (1) ability to induce and terminate it by premature impulses or by overdrive, (2) ability to reset the tachycardia by single premature stimuli, (3) pattern of entrainment during overdrive stimulation, and (4) ability to terminate the tachycardia by interrupting the conducting pathway. The window of reset, determined by the range of coupling intervals of premature impulses capable of entering and resetting the tachycardia (excitable gap), ranged about 70 milliseconds. It appeared that the excitable gap could recover only partially, as evidenced by the observation that, even when stimulated late, premature impulses that entered the circuit conducted slowly. No depressed segments could be identified in the reentry circuit.[55] Termination of these types of induced atrial tachycardias in the canine model was associated with undamped oscillations of action potential duration, refractoriness, and conduction velocities. The slope of the action potential duration restitution curve (also known as electric restitution) of the atrial fibers comprising the reentry circuit may identify whether the atrial reentry will be stable or unstable. Stable tachycardias exhibited damped oscillations when challenged with a premature stimulus, whereas unstable tachycardias were associated with undamped oscillation, which often led to termination. Because both conduction velocity and action potential duration contribute to the termination of reentry, the characteristics of the interval–conduction time relation and the action potential duration–diastolic interval relation (electric restitution curve) should provide some insight whether tachycardia will be stable or unstable (i.e., terminate). It was suggested that when the slope of the interval-dependent changes in conduction time is less than -1, the cycle length oscillates, with progressively increasing alternation of long and short cycles until a sufficiently short cycle causes block. This would terminate the reentry tachycardia.[57] Similarly, the value of the slope of the action potential duration restitution curve influences the magnitude of the oscillation and therefore the stability of the tachycardia. When the slope was larger than 0.96 and larger oscillation occurred, the tachycardia terminates. When the slope was less than 0.66, however, oscillation was damped or did not occur and the tachycardia was stable.[57] It must be noted that these arguments are based on a reentry mechanism that involves a central anatomic obstacle with a partially excitable gap. It is unknown whether similar arguments of oscillation versus atrial reentrant tachycardia stability (relative to restitution of conduction time and action potential duration) also apply to reentry without a central anatomic obstacle (the leading circle concept).

CIRCUS MOVEMENT WITHOUT THE INVOLVEMENT OF AN ANATOMIC OBSTACLE

Over the years, little attention has been given to circus movement without the involvement of an anatomically preformed pathway. The question of whether an anatomic obstacle is involved has important consequences for the properties of a circus movement tachycardia, however.

Lewis was one of the few who realized that the behavior of circulating waves in the intact heart probably would be more complicated than in artificial narrow rings of muscle. In his famous monograph, *The Mechanism and Graphic Registration of the Heart Beat*, he spent an entire chapter on this subject.[59] He proposed some early theoretic considerations about the properties of circulating excitation in a simple narrow ring, compared with circus movement in a sheet of muscle. Because these early ideas seem to be have been ignored by many later investigators and because Lewis predicted a kind of circus movement similar to that described in this chapter, the relevant passage is given below.

After having described the properties of circus movement in a narrow ring, Lewis continues:

> We have been dealing, in speaking of circus movement, with a simple and narrow ring of muscle of fixed circumference; such does not exist in the auricle. It is true that there are natural rings of tissue around the mouths of the great vessels and around the auriculoventricular orifices, but each of these is more correctly viewed as a circular hole in a flat sheet of muscle. Thus, there is a ring adjoining the orifice; there are also outer rings,

greater in circumference, at distances more removed from the orifice. These outer rings provide optional paths for the wave and introduce a new possibility, namely, change in the length of circuit travelled. Suppose that the responsive gap in a ring of tissue immediately surrounding a natural auricular orifice is represented by Figure 310A* (Fig. 10-12), and supposing that for some reason the refractory period becomes longer, the gap will close (Fig. 310B). This closure will not end the circus movement if there are longer paths open to the wave; it can still circulate and will circulate, on such a new path if the conditions are there suitable (Fig. 310B). When a wave circulates around an orifice in a sheet of muscle the size of the gap will be greater if we pass from inner to outer circles of muscle, as is shown in Figure 310C. At any given instant the gap is represented by a wedge of tissue, its point (x) lying toward the center and its base (y-z) lying peripherally.

The conditions existing in the circle of muscle in which the gap is shortest—the circle that includes the point of this wedge in the diagram—are those that determine the rate of beating of the muscle sheet as a whole. That is, the rate of beating is not controlled by the length of path if sufficient optional paths are available because the length of path is determined by the remaining factors. It is probable that the rate of conduction in these circumstances does not influence the rate of beating because a change in conduction would at once be balanced by an appropriate change in the length of path. It is impossible to visualize the precise paths followed by and available to a circulating wave in the auricle but it would seem from these considerations that when a circus movement is established and *when shorter or longer paths become available, the length of the refractory period is in sole control of the rate of beating.*

Later studies demonstrate that the central aperture, still present in the above-cited theoretic considerations, is not essential for the initiation and continuation of circus movement.[41, 42, 60–64] Sustained tachyarrhythmia can be electrically induced in isolated small segments of ordinary atrial muscle. The mechanism of this tachyarrhythmia was extensively studied, leading to the description of a second type of circus movement, the leading circle concept, which is completely determined by the electrophysiologic properties of cardiac tissue.[41, 42, 64]

In Figures 10-13 and 10-14, the phenomenon of circus movement in the absence of an anatomic obstacle is depicted. In isolated pieces of the left atrium of the rabbit (15 × 20 mm), paroxysms of a rapid regular rhythm (rate between 400 and 800 beats/minute) were produced by the

---

* Figure numbers given in Lewis's quote refer to illustrations in Lewis's book and not to illustrations in this text, except Figure 9-12.

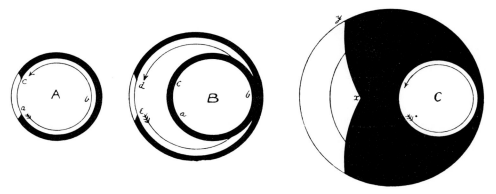

Figure 10-12. Original diagrams drawn by Lewis to illustrate the difference in behavior between circus movement in a narrow ring of cardiac tissue and in a sheet of cardiac muscle. (Lewis T: The mechanism and graphic registration of the heart beat. London: Shaw & Sons, 1925)

induction of a single premature beat. The spread of the excitation wave in the sheet of atrial myocardium was mapped accurately, during both initiation and perpetuation of atrial flutter.

In Figure 10-13, an activation map is given that was reconstructed from more than 100 intracellular recordings during a single period of sustained tachycardia. The map clearly shows a circus movement of the depolariza-tion wave in a clockwise direction, with a revolution time of 105 milliseconds (rate, 550 beats/minute). The dimensions of the circuit are remarkably small. In this case, the diameter can be estimated to be about 0.6 cm. Hence, the total length of the circular pathway is no more than 2 cm.

Figure 10-14 shows the intracellular recordings of seven fibers located on a straight line through the center of the circuit. The most peripheral fibers lying along the

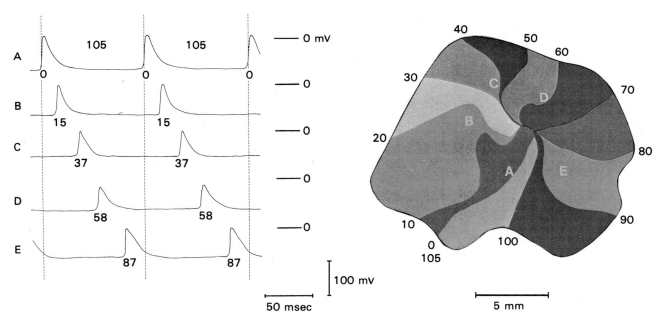

Figure 10-13. Map of the spread of activation in a piece of isolated left atrial muscle of the rabbit during sustained flutter. The map was constructed from time measurements of the intracellular recordings of 94 different fibers. The impulse was rotating in a clockwise direction, with a revolution time of 105 milliseconds. At the left, the transmembrane potentials of 5 fibers (**A** to **E**) are shown that lie along the circular pathway. The activation times are given in milliseconds together with the action potentials and the isochronic lines of the map. (Allessie MA, Bonke FIM, Schopman FJG: Circus movement in rabbit atrial muscle as a mechanism of tachycardia. III. The "leading circle" concept: a new model of circus movement in cardiac tissue without the involvement of an anatomic obstacle. Circ Res 1977;41:9. By permission of the American Heart Association)

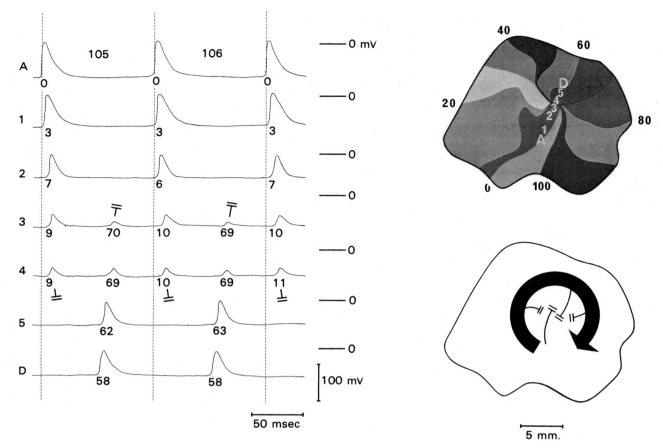

Figure 10-14. Same experiment as in Figure 10-13. The transmembrane potentials of seven fibers (A, D, and 1 to 5) located on a straight line through the center of the circus movement are shown. Fibers A and D are the same as in Figure 10-13. This figure demonstrates that the central area is activated by centripetal wavelets. Note that the fibers in the central point of the circuit (fibers 3 and 4) show double responses of subnormal amplitude. Both responses are unable to propagate beyond the center, thus preventing the impulse from short-circuiting. Below the map, the activation pattern is given schematically, showing the "leading circuit," with the converging wavelets in the center. Block is indicated by double bars. (Allessie MA, Bonke FIM, Schopman FJG: Circus movement in rabbit atrial muscle as a mechanism of tachycardia. III. The "leading circle" concept: a new model of circus movement in cardiac tissue without the involvement of an anatomic obstacle. Circ Res 1977;41:9. By permission of the American Heart Association)

circuit (see Fig. 10-14A and D) are the same as in Figure 10-13. The fibers in the center are marked by numerals (see Fig. 10-14, 1 to 5). As can be read from the time measurements of these fibers, the central area of the circuit is activated in a centripetal direction. From fiber A (see Fig. 10-14), the impulse excites fibers 1, 2, 3, and 4, in that order. When penetrating deeper into the center of the vortex, the centripetal wavelets lose more and more of their "stimulating efficacy" until they are unable to excite the tissue ahead. Going from fiber 1 to 4 (Fig. 10-14), amplitude, rate of rise, and duration of the responses are all gradually decreasing, finally resulting in complete extinction of the impulse somewhere between fibers 4 and

5. Essentially the same sequence of events takes place at the opposite side of the circuit, where half a revolution time later, the circulating impulse penetrates the center again, traveling from fiber D to fibers 5, 4, and 3 (see Fig. 10-14). Again, the centripetal wavelet is conducted with decrement, resulting in extinction of the impulse between fibers 3 and 2.

As a result of this course of events, the center of the vortex is continuously invaded by multiple centripetal wavelets that collide in the center of the circuit. In this way, the circulating impulse is prevented from short-circuiting, whereas the area of converging wavelets serves as a functional "obstacle" for the impulse to turn around. In the diagram beneath the map in Figure 10-14, the sequence of excitation is summarized schematically. It can be described as a "leading" circulating wavefront that activates both the periphery and the center of this circle. It is this leading circuit that determines the rate of beating of the rest of the heart. With more than one circuit available (and a sheet of muscle can be regarded as being composed of numerous circles of different diameter), the circuit with the shortest revolution time takes the lead. The situation is highly analogous to the competition between pacemakers, wherein the fibers with the most rapid rate of diastolic depolarization act as the dominant pacemaker; all the other optional pacemakers with a slower intrinsic rate of discharge are under the control of the fastest rhythm.

Usually, the circuit with the smallest diameter also exhibits the shortest revolution time. In the smallest possible circuit, the stimulating efficacy of the circulating wavefront is just enough to excite the tissue ahead, which is still in its relative refractory phase. In other words, on the leading circuit, the head of the circulating wave is continuously biting its own tail of refractoriness.

Because of this tight fit, the length of the leading circuit is defined by and equal to the "wavelength" of the impulse (i.e., the product of conduction velocity and refractory period). In the center of the leading circuit, dimensions are too small for sustained circus movement. Within this area, a circulating impulse would encounter tissue in which excitability had not yet recovered sufficiently, and the conduction velocity of the impulse would be secondarily depressed below some minimal value, at which successful impulse propagation would no longer be possible.

The properties of circus movement without the involvement of an anatomic obstacle are summarized in Figure 10-15. The main characteristics are:

1. The dimensions of the leading circuit are not fixed but are variable, with the length of the circuit being equal to the wave length of the impulse. Because the wavelength is given by the product of conduction velocity and functional refractory period, a change in either of these electrophysiologic parameters results in a shift of the leading circle to another circuit of different dimensions. Again, this situation is highly analogous to the competition between pacemaker fibers. A shift in the pacemaker occurs if the electrophysiologic properties of pacemaker fibers (e.g., phase 4 depolarization) are changed by maneuvers such as stimulation of the vagal nerves.[65] Thus, a shortening of the functional refractory period or a slowing of conduction velocity in the myocardium results in a narrowing of the leading circuit. In contrast, when the refractory period is long or the conduction velocity is fast, the minimal dimensions for a sustained circus movement are large.

2. By definition, there is no gap of full excitability within the circuit. This implies that a stimulus or depolarization of greater than diastolic threshold is required to influence this type of circus movement.

3. The rate of this reentrant rhythm is inversely related to the refractory period. A shortening of the functional refractory period enables the impulse to circulate in a smaller circuit with a shorter revolution time, accelerating the circus rhythm. Conversely, a prolonged refractory period forces the impulse to find a larger circular pathway, resulting in deceleration of the tachycardia. If a larger circuit is not available, the circus movement suddenly terminates.

Note that in contrast to circus movement around an obstacle, the rate of the functionally determined circus movement does *not* depend directly on conduction velocity because a change in conduction velocity is immediately neutralized by a change in length of the circuitous pathway. If a change in conduction velocity is caused by a change in the stimulating efficacy of the impulse, however, an indirect effect on the rate of circus rhythm may be

CIRCUS MOVEMENT WITHOUT ANATOMIC OBSTACLE (Leading circle model)

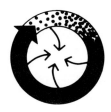

1. Length of circuit is variable (determined by electrophysiologic properties)

2. There is no gap of full excitability

3. The rate of the circus movement is proportional to $\dfrac{1}{\text{refractory period}}$

Figure 10-15. Properties of circus movement without an anatomic obstacle being involved.

expected. This can be understood by realizing that a decrease of the stimulating efficacy of the depolarization wave not only depresses conduction velocity but also prolongs the functional refractory period.

Significance of Refractory Period, Conduction Velocity, and Wavelength in the Induction of Atrial Reentry

To study the relative importance of various electrophysiologic properties of the atrium in relation to atrial fibrillation, we developed a chronically instrumented conscious dog model in which refractory periods, conduction velocity, and wavelength could be measured and directly correlated with the inducibility of arrhythmias.[66] Figure 10-16 shows a set of double-row electrodes designed for measurement of the wavelength in the bundle of Bachmann and the free wall of the right and left atria. The lower part of the figure shows superimposed unipolar electrograms recorded from the neighboring electrodes along the bundle of Bachmann. The principle of the wavelength measurement consists of the simultaneous determination of conduction velocity and refractory period.[67] The wavelength is defined as the product of conduction velocity and refractory period. If the corresponding electrodes of the double row are activated simultaneously, the impulse propagates parallel to the long axis of he electrode and the measured conduction times can be used to calculate the actual conduction velocity. To measure the refractory period, the atrium is driven at a basic rate. After every 15th beat, a premature stimulus is given at progressively shorter intervals in steps of 2 to 5 milliseconds. The shortest possible A_1 to A_2 interval that results in a response (measured at the recording electrode closest to the stimulus site) is taken as the functional refractory period. By applying a second premature stimulus, the refractory period of the first premature impulse can be measured from the shortest A_2 to A_3 interval. The wavelength of the basic rhythm is calculated by multiplying the conduction velocity during A_1 with the A_1 to A_2 interval. The wavelength of the premature beat is the product of conduction velocity of the A_2 impulse and the A_2 to A_3 interval. Figure 10-17 shows the different types of arrhythmias that were induced by premature stimulations with varying degrees of prematurity. Premature stimuli with long coupling intervals (Fig. 10-17A) only elicited single premature responses (A_2), after which sinus rhythm resumed. Moderately premature stimuli (Fig 10-17B) were followed by short series of rapid repetitive responses (RRR). Early premature stimuli (Fig. 10-17C) result in longer or shorter paroxysm of atrial flutter. Premature stimuli given immediately after the end of the refractory period frequently induced atrial fibrillation (Fig. 10-17D).

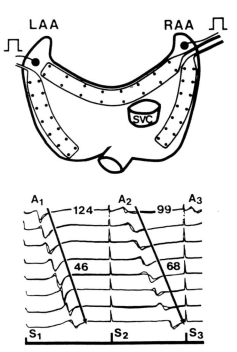

Figure 10-16. (*Upper panel*) Schematic representation of chronically implanted double-row electrodes for the measurement of wavelength. The long electrode is positioned on Bachmann's bundle, extending from the right to the left atrial appendage (*RAA* and *LAA*). The other electrodes are attached to the free wall of the right or left atrium parallel to the atrioventricular ring. Two pairs of stimulating electrodes (*black dots*) are sutured to the atrial appendages (SVC, superior vena cava). (*Lower panel*) Superimposed unipolar electrograms recorded from neighboring electrodes of the double-row electrodes (interelectrode distance, 8 mm). The signals recorded at each pair of electrodes are simultaneous, indicating that the impulse is propagating parallel to the long axis of the electrode. Conduction under the electrode was uniform, as can be seen from the constant conduction time between pairs of electrodes. Total conduction time for the basic impulse (A_1) was 46 milliseconds and for the premature impulse (A_2) 68 milliseconds. The shortest A_1–A_2 interval was 124 milliseconds. The wavelength of the basic impulse thus can be calculated to be 56 mm/46 milliseconds × 124 milliseconds = 15.0 cm. The wavelength of the premature impulse was 8.2 cm. (Reproduced with permission from Rensma PL, Allessie MA, Lammers WJEP, Bonke FIM, Schalij MJ: Length of excitation and susceptibility to reentrant atrial arrhythmias in normal conscious dogs. Circ Res 1988;62:395)

Comparison with the left panel shows that the observed atrial response to progressively shorter coupled premature stimuli coincided with a progressive decrease in refractory period, conduction velocity, and wavelength. To determine how these different parameters affected the induction of arrhythmias, the electrophysiologic properties of the atrial tissue were changed with a variety of drugs. The values of the refractory period, conduction velocity, and wavelength of the premature impulse were correlated with the induction of atrial arrhythmias. Figure 10-18 shows cumulative histograms of the induction of

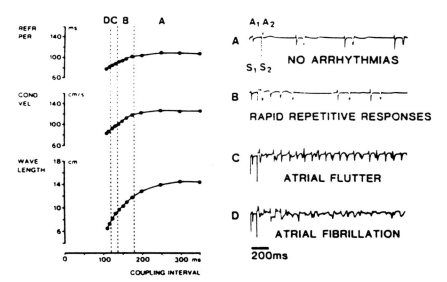

Figure 10-17. Atrial arrhythmias induced by single premature stimulus (S₂). The left panel shows the relation between the coupling interval and refractory period, conduction velocity, and wavelength of premature impulses. The prematurity zones in the left panel correspond to the tracings in the right panels. Premature stimuli with a long coupling interval (*zone A*) elicited only single premature responses (A₂). Moderately premature stimuli (*B*) were followed by a short run of rapid repetitive responses. Still earlier extrasystoles (*zone C*) resulted in a paroxysm of atrial flutter. Premature stimuli given immediately after the refractory period (*zone D*) induced episodes of atrial fibrillation. (Reproduced with permission from Rensma PL, Allessie MA, Lammers WJEP, Bonke FIM, Schalij MJ: Length of excitation and susceptibility to reentrant atrial arrhythmias in normal conscious dogs. Circ Res 1988; 62:395)

arrhythmias under a variety of drug-induced electrophysiologic changes of the atrial tissue. Although a relatively higher incidence of atrial fibrillation was observed with shorter refractory periods (*upper panel*), prolongation of the refractory period per se did not prevent the induction of arrhythmias. Atrial fibrillation, flutter, and RRR were inducible at a wide range of refractory period values and at certain refractory period, any type of atrial response to the test stimulus could be expected. Furthermore, the predictive power of conduction velocity for induction of arrhythmias was also low (*middle panel*). At most values of conduction velocity, any of the four types of responses could be found. The histograms correlating induction of atrial arrhythmias to the wavelength (*lower panel*) showed a different pattern. Although the different arrhythmias were still not completely separated by the wavelength into four individual subpopulations, the degree of overlap of the subgroups was far less, compared with the histograms of refractory period and conduction velocity. When the wavelength was long, no arrhythmias were induced. When the wavelength became progressively shorter, RRR, then flutter, and finally atrial fibrillation was observed. By linear discriminant analysis, optimal cutoff points between the four subpopulations were calculated. The critical wavelength for the induction of the

various types of reentrant arrhythmias are indicated by arrows. For induction of RRR, a critical wavelength of shorter than 12.3 cm was computed; for atrial flutter, the critical wavelength was below 9.7 cm; and for atrial fibrillation, the wavelength was shorter than 7.8 cm. The overall correct prediction of the several types of arrhythmias by the corresponding value of the wavelength was 75%, compared with 48% and 38% for refractory period and conduction velocity, respectively.[66] The concept of critical wavelength for reentrant arrhythmias suggests that it might be useful to describe the antiarrhythmic properties of cardiac drugs in terms of changes in the wavelength.

Role of Wavelength in Reentrant Arrhythmias

For the perpetuation of the reentrant rhythm, the wavelength is crucial. Interventions that prolong the wavelength increase the minimal size of intramyocardial circuits. If an excitable gap is present in the reentrant loop, prolongation of the wavelength first reduces and finally closes the excitable gap, leading to instability and a high chance of block of the circulating impulse. In the case where multiple wavelets are present, a prolongation of the wavelength results in an increase in the average circuit

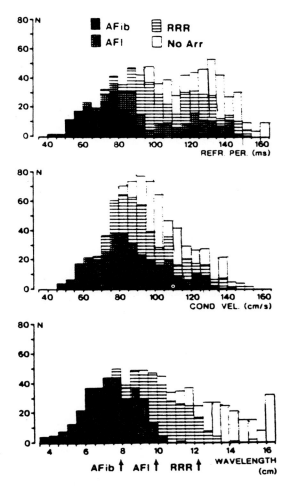

Figure 10-18. Histograms (n = 750) correlating the occurrence of arrhythmias (short series of rapid repetitive responses [*RRR*], atrial flutter [*AFl*], and atrial fibrillation [*AFib*], with the refractory period, conduction velocity, and wavelength of the provoking premature beats. The values of refracting period (RP), conduction velocity (CV), and wavelength were varied by administration of various drugs. Each bar represents the total number of observations at the various values of RP, CV, and wavelength. The different shadings indicate the different types of responses. The optimal cutoff points of the wavelength, as computed by discriminant analysis and predicting the induction of the type of arrhythmia, are indicated by *vertical arrows* (predictive power, 75%). RRR was induced at a wavelength shorter than 12.3 cm. Atrial flutter occurred below a wavelength of 9.7 cm, whereas fibrillation was initiated when the length of the excitation wave became shorter than 7.8 cm. (Reproduced with permission from Rensma PL, Allessie MA, Lammers WJEP, Bonke FIM, Schalij MJ: Length of excitation and susceptibility to reentrant atrial arrhythmias in normal conscious dogs. Circ Res 1988;62:395)

size. Because the finite atrial tissue size cannot accommodate so many circuits, the total of the wandering impulses diminishes and the likelihood of fusion and dying out of the wavelets increases. As a consequence, prolongation of the wavelength during fibrillation may lead to spontaneous termination of the arrhythmia.[68] In contrast, inter-

ventions that shorten the wavelength might stabilize the reentrant process by creating or enlarging an excitable gap or might lead to degeneration into multiple smaller circuits. Electrically induced rapid atrial rhythms during acetylcholine perfusion was mapped, using an isolated canine atrial epicardium.[69] Multiple reentrant circuits were identified in the absence of a central anatomic obstacle. The number of circuits and wavelets increased in a concentration-dependent manner (acetylcholine). Unexpectedly, this trend did not continue when the rapid rhythm became sustained. Instead, reentry tended to stabilize to a small, single, relatively stable reentrant circuit. This suggests that below a critical level of refractory period (less than 95 milliseconds), atrial reentrant circuits without an anatomic obstacle can become stable and dominate activation.[69] This unexpected finding (the presence of single, stable rotor during sustained tachyarrhythmias fibrillation) is contrary to the long-held Moe's multiple-wavelets hypothesis of atrial fibrillation.[92–94] In this study, multiple simultaneous circuits were unstable but usually one of the circuits would dominate and extinguish the others. This could be related to tissue distribution of refractory period. In Moe's simulation model of atrial fibrillation, the refractory periods were randomly distributed, whereas studies of distribution in the normal intact dog suggest an underlying pattern or gradient of inhomogeneity.[70–72] A discrete pattern of refractory period inhomogeneity would produce fewer potential reentry sites.[69]

Excitable Gap in Functional and Anatomic Reentry

The presence of tissue anisotropy modifies the characteristics of both functional (leading circle model) and anatomic types of reentry. The geometry of cardiac fibers is such that the fibers are arranged and oriented parallel to each other. This creates myocardial tissue anisotropy because conduction parallel to the long axis of the fibers is faster than conduction transverse to it; this is explained by differences in cell coupling in different directions.[73,74] In the case of reentry with an anatomic obstacle, anisotropy causes slow conduction in the segment of the circuit in which propagation occurs transverse to the fiber orientation. This creates a large excitable gap or allows rotor formation (circulating excitation) to occur in a smaller tissue volume.[75] An excitable gap is not only present in anatomic reentry but also in functional models. The excitable gap in functional anisotropic circuits (rotors) may occur as a result of three possible mechanisms:

1. Microanatomic barrier at the pivoting points: the presence of microanatomic obstacles at both pivoting

points of the circuit may enlarge the central functionally determined line of block of the circuit. It also stabilizes the position of the reentrant loop at a fixed location in the myocardium. Small conduction barriers may exist as a result of interposition of collagenous septa, causing electric separation of adjacent atrial fibers, as occurs during aging and myocardial hypertrophy.[76]

2. Block at the pivoting point because of high electrotonic load: the stimulating efficacy of a propagating action potential is influenced by sudden changes in the axial current load.[77] A sudden increase of current load occurs when an abrupt change in the direction of impulse propagation occurs. This may occur during circulation of a wavefront during reentry, leading to conduction slowing (decremental conduction) or even block, despite the cells being fully excitable. For example, at the pivoting points of anisotropic reentry, the slowly conducting transverse wavefront encounters a sudden increase of axial current load (low resistance) when the longitudinal limb of the circuit has to be excited. It is possible that because of mismatch between the generated excitatory current and the high axial electrotonic load at the pivoting points, the impulse may fail to immediately activate the longitudinal limb of the circuit. It is only after a certain delay (during which a larger part of the wavefront has rotated around the pivoting point) that the impulse succeeds in making a 180° turn. Such a temporary halt of the impulse at the pivoting points may create an excitable gap because it results in functional lengthening of the central line of conduction block and consequently of the cycle length of the tachycardia.

3. Electrotonic prolongation of the action potential at the pivoting points: spatial differences of action potential duration may also contribute to the creation of excitable gap. Because the sequence of activation affects the duration of action potential, it is possible that such changes at the pivoting points of a reentry circuit may modify the excitable gap.[71]

Experimental Atrial Flutter and Fibrillation: Initial Results of High-Resolution Activation Mapping

Figures 10-19 and 10-20 show activation maps of atrial fibrillation in isolated normal canine hearts, induced by programmed electric stimulation. The activation maps were constructed based on local electrograms recorded with a right and left multiple endocardial electrode, containing 960 leads (spatial resolution, 2 to 3 mm).[78]

Figure 10-19 depicts the excitation of the right atrium during atrial fibrillation and Figure 10-20 shows that of the left atrium. Each series of activation maps covers a time window of about half a second. Although the right and left atria were mapped consecutively and cannot be directly time-aligned, it seems justified to consider the two different episodes as part of the same process. In Figure 10-19A of the right atrium, which begins at an arbitrary moment during sustained atrial fibrillation, we encounter three independent wavelets. One wavelet (*shortest arrow*) is traveling down the septum and is extinguished at time 30 at the AV junction. The other two waves originally propagated in opposite directions, with the middle wave traveling along the medial wall of the atrium in a posterior direction (downward in the map) and the right wave traveling upward to the tip of the appendage. At time 20, the two waves collide, resulting in a sudden narrowing of the middle wave. The right wave, finding its way to the appendage suddenly blocked, changes its direction of propagation by 180° and continues its course as a narrow wavelet in the lateral wall until at time 80, it dies out at the AV ring. In Figure 10-19B, the large activation wave at the end of Figure 10-19A is split into smaller wavelets. One wavelet (Figure 10-19B, *lower arrow*) encounters an area in the posterior wall of the right atrium, which obviously has not yet restored its excitability, resulting in a 180° clockwise turn. At time 170, this turning wavelet is extinguished at the atrial border. A second wave (Figure 10-19B, *counterclockwise arrow*) enters the lateral wall of the appendage and makes a full 360° turn in the anterior part of the lateral wall. As can be seen from Figure 10-19C, this wavelet creates a closed local circuit that continues for another revolution, although the size and location of the circuit change (compare *counterclockwise arrows* in Fig. 10-19B and C). Figure 10-19C shows two other interesting phenomena. First, at time 180, a new impulse appears at the site indicated by the asterisk. The origin of this impulse cannot be explained from the propagation of wavelets in the right atrium and most probably is the continuation of a wavelet in the left atrium. The second noteworthy phenomenon is the event indicated by the four small arrows. We can see here what can happen if two narrow wavelets collide. Instead of mutual extinction, we see something that we term the "clash-and-go" phenomenon. The two narrow impulses approaching each other collide and after the collision, diverge again in opposite directions, with a 90° change in direction. The phenomena in Figure 10-19C lead to the presence of three clearly separated and narrow wavelets in Figure 10-19D. That on the right is an offspring of the circuit around the appendage, which has ceased to exist. The other two are the result of the clash-and-go phenomenon. After the right wavelet has died out at time 260 at the AV ring in Figure 10-19E, only two wavefronts are left. At time 290, these two remaining wavelets are simultaneously extinguished by the coincidental combi-

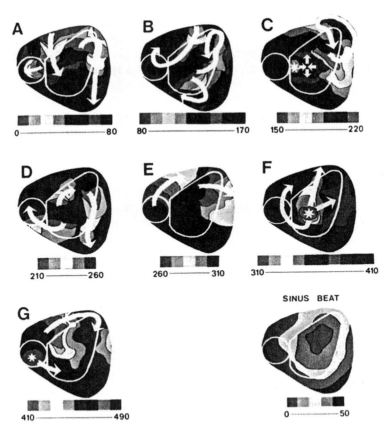

Figure 10-19. A series of consecutive activation maps covering the spread of excitation in the right atrium during 400–500 milliseconds of stable atrial fibrillation. The propagation of impulses is visualized by color-coded isochrones of 10 milliseconds; the general direction of wavelets is indicated by *white arrows*. *Asterisks* indicate sites of origin of "new" impulses, which must be regarded as offspring from impulses wandering through the left atrium. The time window covered by the maps is given with the color scale below each map. For comparison, at the lower right corner, the activation during sinus rhythm is given. See text for detailed description. (Reproduced with permission from Allessie MA, Rensma PL, Lammers WJEP, Kirchhof CJHJ: The role of refractoriness, conduction velocity, and wavelength in initiation of atrial fibrillation in normal conscious dogs. In: Attuel P, Coumel P, Janse MJ, eds. The atrium in health and disease. Mt. Kisco, NY: Futura Publishing, 1989:27)

nation of reaching the AV ring and conduction block at refractory tissue. This sudden disappearance of multiple wandering wavelets in the right atrium did *not* result in termination of atrial fibrillation. About 20 milliseconds after the right atrium had become electrically silent, a new impulse penetrated the right atrium from the left (Fig. 10-19*F*, asterisk). The activation map in Figure 10-19*F* further illustrates that the impulse entering the right atrium at time 310 is immediately broken into three separate depolarization waves. Obviously, the short time that the right atrium was electrically silent was not long enough to bring the fibers to the same phase of excitability. The new impulse therefore encounters islands of refractoriness, and the process of fragmented multiple wandering wavelets is restarted.

Figure 10-20 shows the fibrillatory process in the left atrium. Generally, the left atrium exhibits the same pattern of excitation as described for the right atrium. During sustained fibrillation, each atrium contained an average of about three wandering wavelets. Also, in the left atrium, frequent entries of "new" impulses from the right atrium were seen (Fig. 10-20*C,D*, and *E*, asterisks). Again, the ever-changing pathways of the multiple reentering wavelets become evident.

RELATION OF THE DIFFERENT BASIC MECHANISMS TO CLINICAL ARRHYTHMIAS

Atrial Premature Depolarizations

Many textbooks state that atrial premature beats can occur in persons of all ages and in the absence of heart disease. Emotional stress, fatigue, or excessive use of alcohol, tobacco, or coffee may be associated with a higher incidence of premature complexes, atrial as well as ventricular. Furthermore, premature complexes are "normal" in ischemia of the myocardium and are often seen after the use of cardiac drugs such as digitalis, quinidine, and procainamide, in which case they may indicate a toxic reaction to these drugs. The incidence of atrial premature contractions and other atrial arrhythmias is greater in distention of the atrium. Furthermore, atrial premature complexes that occur at rest often disappear during exercise. All the above should be kept in mind during the discussion of the possible underlying mechanisms of atrial premature beats.

The normal impulse formation in the sinus node is strongly influenced by the autonomic nervous system.

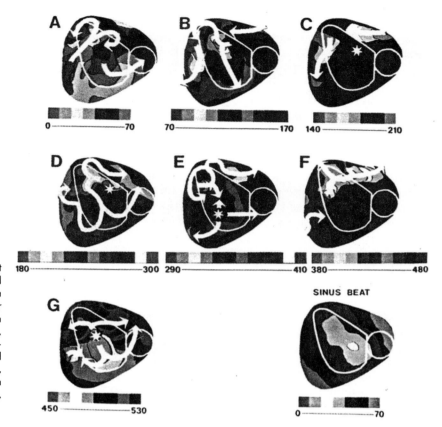

Figure 10-20. Excitation maps of the left atrium during the same episode of sustained atrial fibrillation as in Figure 10-19. The recordings from right and left atria were taken immediately after each other in time. (Reproduced with permission from Allessie MA, Rensma PL, Lammers WJEP, Kirchhof CJHJ: The role of refractoriness, conduction velocity, and wavelength in initiation of atrial fibrillation in normal conscious dogs. In: Attuel P, Coumel P, Janse MJ, eds. The atrium in health and disease. Mt. Kisco, NY: Futura Publishing, 1989:27)

Although vagal and sympathetic nerves influence the atrial myocardium and the AV node, it is not clear whether these structures are always influenced to the same degree as the sinus node. Therefore, the automaticity in one of the subsidiary pacemakers might be fast enough to produce an impulse that activates the rest of the atrium, especially if the sinus node is under vagal influence. This hypothesis agrees with the observation that during exercise and thus with less vagal influence, atrial premature complexes often disappear. The second possible mechanism of abnormal impulse formation—the occurrence of an EAD—is unlikely to be the cause of atrial premature depolarizations because it demands unusual circumstances. If such circumstances are present, a series of impulses rather than a single premature complex can be expected.

A premature atrial complex can also be induced or triggered. The studies of Wit and Cranefield show sustained triggered activity but it is also possible to trigger only a singular impulse with the appropriate concentration of catecholamines.[4, 19]

Most textbooks mention a reentrant mechanism as the primary cause for atrial premature complexes. If the impulse coming from the sinus node is blocked somewhere in the atrium (the first prerequisite for reentry)

and the area of block is relatively large, the area of block may be activated retrogradely; from this region, the atrium may be reentered, creating an atrial premature beat. This may occur more easily if the impulse is conducted slowly; therefore, if the impulse on its way through the AV node is blocked in one part of the node, conduction may proceed through the rest of the node and because of slow conduction in this tissue may retrogradely excite the area of block and reenter the atrium. In the literature, this is often referred to as "return extrasystole" or "AV nodal echo beat."

If one atrial premature beat exists, this impulse can set the stage for another reentry—either in the atrium or through the AV node or the sinus node. Therefore, a premature impulse coming from the atrium may invade part of the sinus node while the entrance to other parts of the sinus node is blocked. The impulse can then find a way through the slowly conducting tissue of the sinus node and find an exit to the atrium, which has meanwhile restored its excitability. The impulse then reenters the atrium. The existence of such a sinus echo has been demonstrated by Allessie and Bonke.[40] The same is possible in the AV node, as was demonstrated experimentally by Moe and coworkers, Mendez and Moe, and clinically by Schuilenburg and Durrer.[37,79,80] Generally, a reentrant mechanism is well-reconciled with a fixed coupling interval of atrial premature beats.

Atrial Tachycardia

If impulse generation in the dominant pacemaker in the sinus node is enhanced (e.g., because of a high sympathetic activity), sinus tachycardia occurs. If the impulse formation outside the sinus node is enhanced, atrial or nodal tachycardia is present. This is demonstrated in Figure 10-3. The rate of such atrial tachycardias increases if catecholamines are administered, whereas it slows or is even interrupted by acetylcholine or vagal stimulation (carotid sinus massage).

Sustained rhythmic activity may be induced or triggered by a relatively rapid sinus nodal or atrial rhythm as well as by a premature atrial beat. Triggering only occurs if catecholamines are present and therefore depends on the equilibrium of the autonomic nervous system. Furthermore, the rate of such a tachycardia diminishes or the tachycardia may even stop with the administration of acetylcholine and also by a drug such as verapamil. Also, triggered rhythmic activity not only can be started but also can be stopped by a single premature complex.

From a theoretic point of view, the third possible cause of abnormal impulse formation, the occurrence of EAD, may induce a rapid-firing atrial focus. Under normal conditions, however, this is unlikely. Theoretically, tachycardias based on this mechanism are stopped by the administration of acetylcholine (or vagal stimulation) because it increases membrane conductance for potassium and therefore repolarizes the fibers. Thus, acetylcholine does not enable the clinician to distinguish among tachycardias.

The underlying mechanism for supraventricular tachycardia may also be a circus movement of the impulse. If the circus movement is purely within the atrial myocardium, however, the length of such a pathway should be between 20 and 26 cm, assuming a mean conduction velocity of the impulse in the atrium during tachycardia of about 60 cm per second (normally during sinus rhythm, this is between 60 and 100 cm/second) and a rate of the tachycardia between 140 and 180 beats per minute. These long circuits are unlikely in the atrium. Conversely, if part of the circuit has properties of slow conduction, the circuit may be considerably smaller, making circus movement as a cause of atrial tachycardia more probable. Slow conduction is present if the sinus node or the AV node is part of the circuit. In these cases, the terminology "sinus nodal reentrant tachycardia" or "AV junctional tachycardia" is used. Both kinds of tachycardia can frequently be slowed or even converted to sinus rhythm by carotid sinus massage. This agrees with the observation that acetylcholine slows down or even blocks conduction in the SA or AV node.

Tachycardia based on a circus movement can be started or terminated by a single premature beat. Because this is the case for "triggered" sustained rhythmicity also, it is not a good method to distinguish between these two mechanisms.

Therefore, if a patient has (paroxysmal) supraventricular tachycardia, enhanced automaticity, triggered activity, and circus movement must be considered, it may be difficult to distinguish among these possible mechanisms.

Atrial Flutter

Atrial flutter has never been satisfactorily defined. Lewis emphasized that a high degree of regularity in both beat-to-beat interval and configuration of the atrial complexes in the electrocardiogram is the most prominent characteristic of atrial flutter.[59] Realizing that the boundaries between atrial tachycardia and atrial flutter are not sharp and that the rates of the two arrhythmias may overlap, atrial flutter can be defined as any regular atrial rhythm faster than 200 beats per minute. This is a wide definition, and subdivision of atrial flutter into different types is helpful. Based on the polarity of the flutter waves, Lewis distinguished a "common" form of atrial flutter (with F waves inverted in leads II, III, and aV_F and upright in lead a V_R) and an "uncommon" form (with F waves upright in leads II, III, and aV_F and inverted in lead aV_R).[59] No differences in rate have been found between these two types of flutter.[81] Because of the similarity between the F waves during uncommon flutter and P waves during subsequent sinus rhythm, it has been suggested that uncommon flutter arises from the high right atrium. Many examples of clinical atrial flutter can be found, however, with F waves somewhere intermediate between the two extreme forms representing common and uncommon flutter.

Wells and colleagues distinguished two different types of atrial flutter, primarily based on differences in atrial rate.[1] They divided 27 patients who developed atrial flutter after open-heart surgery into two groups. Group I consisted of 18 patients with classic (common) atrial flutter, with an atrial rate ranging from 240 to 338 beats per minute. In group II (nine patients), the atrial rates ranged from 340 to 433 beats per minute. Both types of flutter were characterized by a strikingly constant beat-to-beat interval, morphology, polarity, and amplitude of the atrial electrograms. The authors separated atrial flutter into two categories because they observed that rapid atrial pacing from the high right atrium always influenced type I flutter but never influenced type II flutter.[2] Conversion of atrial flutter by rapid pacing or reset of the flutter cycle with a properly timed single stimulus strongly points to the existence of a reentry circuit with an excitable gap.[82-84] Thus, the slower examples of atrial flutter (type I) should be based on circus movement, including an appreciable excitable gap. In contrast, failure to interrupt type II flutter by overdrive pacing suggests that the excitable gap is either small or absent, resulting in effective shielding of the circuit from interference with oncoming activation waves.

There is considerable experimental evidence that circus movement around an anatomic obstacle can cause atrial flutter. This concept was first introduced by Lewis and coworkers based on multiple recordings during long-lasting periods of atrial flutter induced by weak faradic stimulation of the auricle.[85] Figure 10-21 shows the spread of the excitation process during such a period of atrial flutter. A large part of the pathway taken by the activation waves could be identified by this method. During one cycle of the flutter (beat-to-beat interval, 0.16 second), the wave travels from the inferior cava up along the crista terminalis and to the right auricular appendage. It then turns around the orifice of the superior cava and passes along the interatrial band to the left atrium; a little later, a new wave appears behind the inferior cava and the same sequence of activation is repeated. As Lewis emphasized, "It remains to ascertain if this new wave is a continuation of the old one; if so, then a circus movement is proved."

Unfortunately, direct measurements along the left side of the entrances of the caval veins were not obtained but based on indirect evidence, Lewis decided that, "there remains little doubt that we are dealing with a wave mov-

ing around the cavae, the movement being continuous and completes once during each auricular cycle."

Later studies draw the same conclusion.[86-89] The studies of Kimura and coworkers supplied complementary data on the spread of excitation at the left side of the venae cavae, where Lewis was unable to take records.[87] Figure 10-22 is the complete map of the pathway of the excitation wave during flutter. The results confirm Lewis's conclusions. The involvement of artificial or pathologic obstacles in atrial flutter was emphasized by Rosenblueth and Garcia Ramos and later by Kimura and coworkers.[86, 87] These authors found that crushing the conducting bridge between the two venae cavae, which converted the two orifices into a single obstacle, markedly facilitated the induction of flutter by rapid stimulation. Further enlargement of the obstacle decreased the rate of flutter. When the

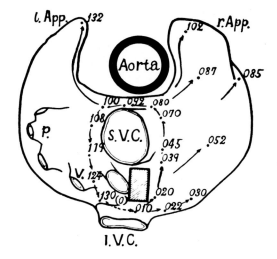

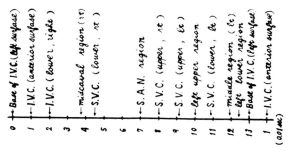

Figure 10-22. Recordings taken during atrial flutter induced by rapid stimulation of the left appendage. To facilitate the induction of atrial flutter, the conducting bridge between the two venae cavae was crushed. In this study, the left side of the caval veins was also mapped. It is demonstrated that the impulse turns around the superior vena cava and a right pulmonary vein. The revolution time is 0.13 second. A chart is given below the map, showing the time relation of the different recording sites during one cycle of the flutter. (Kimura E, Kato K, Murao S, et al: Experimental studies on the mechanism of the auricular flutter. Tohoku J Exp Med 1954;60:197)

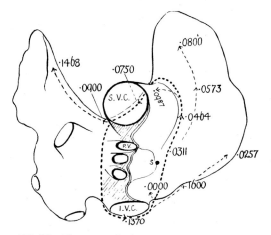

Figure 10-21. The spread of excitation in the atria of a dog, measured by Lewis and coworkers, during a period of electrically induced atrial flutter. Local activation times are expressed as parts of a second, and the *broken lines* and *arrows* indicate the course taken by the excitation wave. Note that recordings were not obtained at the left side of the entrances of the caval veins. *S* marks the point that was originally stimulated to induce flutter. (Lewis T, Feil, HS, Stroud WD: Observations upon flutter and fibrillation. II. Nature of auricular flutter. Heart 1920;7:191)

lesion was extended to the auriculoventricular groove (i.e., as soon as the obstacle was no longer entirely surrounded by conducting tissue), the flutter suddenly terminated and could no longer be reinitiated. More anatomically defined circuits exist in the atria, however. A list of the possible anatomic circuits in the human atria, together with the estimated length of the pathways, is given below.

1. Circuit around the orifices of all atrial veins (superior vena cava [SVC], inferior vena cava [IVC], left and right pulmonary veins) — 26 cm
2. Around SVC, IVC, and right pulmonary veins — 23 cm
3. Around IVC and right pulmonary veins — 20 cm
4. Around SVC and right pulmonary veins — 18 cm
5. Around SVC and IVC — 18 cm
6. Around right and left pulmonary veins — 17 cm
7. Around SVC and upper right pulmonary veins — 16 cm
8. Around IVC and lower right pulmonary veins — 16 cm
9. Around right pulmonary veins — 12 cm
10. Around left pulmonary veins — 12 cm
11. Around tricuspid orifice — 12 cm
12. Around mitral orifice — 12 cm
13. Around SVC — 9 cm
14. Around IVC — 9 cm
15. Around one pulmonary vein — 3 cm to 6 cm[90]

In this list, pathways course around a combination of cardiac veins. Such long loops do not exist in a normal heart because the intact muscle bands between the orifices of the veins short-circuit these loops.

When the atria are diseased (e.g., by coronary artery disease or mitral stenosis) and the conduction properties in parts of the atrial myocardium are lost, large circuits may result, either by a loss of excitability in the muscle bands between two or more veins or by the presence of hypoplastic or fibrotic areas lying as an island in the myocardium or in close opposition to one of the natural openings in the atria.

Figure 10-23 shows a graph relating the length of a given circuit to the rate of the related reentrant rhythm, as calculated for different conduction velocities. From this graph, it can be seen that at the normal conduction velocity in the atrium of 70 cm per second, to get a tachyarrhythmia that is classified as atrial flutter, the length of the circuit must be between 12 and 20 cm. Such long pathways are not available in the normal heart. In contrast, when the conduction velocity of the impulse in the atrial myocardium is decreased to 40 cm per second (as an example),

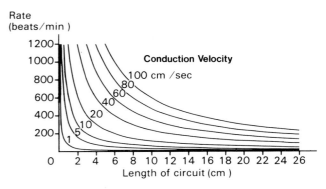

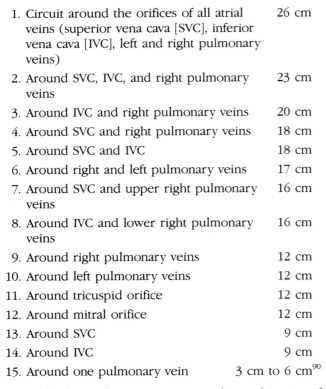

Figure 10-23. Graph relating the rate of circus movement to the length of the circuitous pathway at different conduction velocities of the impulse.

an obstacle with a perimeter of only 9 cm may be adequate to serve as a center for circus movement, with a rate of 300 beats per minute.

The activation during acetylcholine-induced rapid atrial flutter has been mapped in the isolated canine heart.[91] Figure 10-24 has been taken from this study. In all cases, atrial flutter was based on continuous circus movement of the impulse in the atrial myocardium. The localization and dimensions of the circuit differed from case to case, however. In most cases, a gross anatomic obstacle was not involved in this type of atrial flutter.

Atrial Fibrillation

The most likely mechanism underlying fibrillation of the atria is the presence of multiple circus movements of the leading circle type. According to this theory, in "coarse" fibrillation, the number of circuits is small and circuit dimensions are relatively large, whereas in "fine" fibrillation, numerous circuits of small dimension may exist. Conditions that facilitate the induction of atrial fibrillation, such as vagal stimulation, rapid pacing, distention of the atria, ischemia, and the presence of conduction disturbances, all cause shortening of the refractory period, lowering of conduction velocity, or both and thus a shortening of the dimension of a leading circuit. If there exists a single circus movement as a cause of atrial flutter, shortening of the minimum dimension of that circuit (e.g., by vagal stimulation) creates a situation in which there is room for more than one circuit. As soon as a second or third circuit is established, flutter converts into fibrillation. As the conditions that favored the initiation of multiple small circuits wane, the small circuits may die out, one after the other, and fibrillation may convert to flutter again if a single circus movement remains; if not, fibrillation is terminated completely and sinus rhythm resumes. Because of the complexity of this situation, no one has been able to

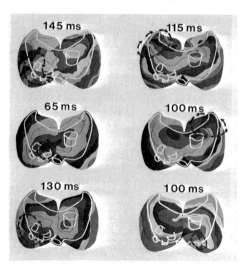

Figure 10-24. Atrial excitation maps of six different cases of rapid atrial flutter. In all cases, atrial flutter was based on intraatrial reentry. There was marked variation in both the rate of the flutter and the localization of the circuit responsible for the arrhythmia. In the upper left panel the circuit (cycle length, 145 milliseconds) was found in the inferolateral wall of the left atrium. In the *upper right panel*, the impulse circulated around the left atrial appendage with a revolution time of 115 milliseconds. The extremely rapid flutter shown in the middle left panel (cycle length, 65 milliseconds) was based on a circuit in the posterior wall of the left atrium. The episodes of the other three cases of atrial flutter were caused by an intraatrial circuit located around the right atrial appendage (*middle right panel*), in the free wall of the left atrium (*lower left panel*), and in the posterior right atrium (*lower right panel*), respectively. Estimated circuit size varied between 5 and 10 cm. Each shade of gray represents an isochrone of 10 milliseconds. (Allessie MA, Lammers WJEP, Bonke FIM, Hollen J: Intra-atrial reentry as a mechanism for atrial flutter induced by acetylcholine and rapid pacing in the dog. Circulation 1985;70:123. By permission of the American Heart Association)

analyze the activation of the atria during fibrillation. In a computer simulation, however, Moe and coworkers succeeded in producing fibrillation in a mathematic two-dimensional area or in a closed surface without holes.[92–94] In this model, multiple circulating wavefronts were shown to occur during fibrillation: "reentry occurred over numerous loops of varying size and position, wandering over the excitable surface like eddies in a turbulent pool."[93]

If fibrillation is caused by the presence of multiple circulating wavelets, its persistence is a matter of statistical probability. Circus movement without the involvement of an anatomic obstacle is not a stable phenomenon; as a rule, spontaneous termination occurs after a shorter or longer period.[41] If many circuits exist, however, it is unlikely that they will stop at the same time. The crucial factor for induction and termination of fibrillation is the *dimension of the heart relative to the dimension of the smallest possible circuit in the myocardium.* If the heart is large or the

dimension of a functionally determined circuit is small, many circuits can exist in the heart and the statistical chance for spontaneous termination of fibrillation is low. In contrast, if the heart is small or the dimension of the "leading circuit" is large, the heart can accommodate only a few circuits; in this situation, the probability of conversion of fibrillation to sinus rhythm is great. According to this concept, interventions that either decrease the dimension of the heart (diminishing of the atrial distention) or increase the dimension of a functionally determined circuit (drugs that increase refractory period or conduction velocity or both) decrease the chance for induction of fibrillation and increase the probability of its spontaneous termination.

INTRAATRIAL REENTRY AS A BASIS FOR ATRIAL FLUTTER AND FIBRILLATION

We postulate that all cases of clinical atrial flutter and fibrillation are based on a reentrant mechanism because any positive proof for a different mechanism is lacking. The evidence in favor of a focus of some form of rapid automaticity is based on experiments performed with aconitine or in the case of triggered activity, the rate of abnormal impulse generation is too slow to explain atrial flutter or fibrillation. There is no doubt that topical application of aconitine produces rapid abnormal automaticity in the atrium, precipitating atrial flutter or fibrillation.[7] This, however, cannot be regarded as evidence that a similar mechanism is operative in clinical flutter. Triggered activity has been elicited in several parts of the heart under a variety of circumstances.[3–6, 18–20] The rate of this abnormal rhythm is usually about 140 beats per minute and rarely exceeds 200 beats per minute. Another argument that speaks against triggered activity as a mechanism for atrial flutter or fibrillation is the observation that DAD and sustained triggered activity are inhibited by acetylcholine, whereas in human atrial flutter or fibrillation, the rate of the F waves either remains unchanged or is accelerated by vagal stimulation.[4, 95–96] Furthermore, study of the electrophysiologic properties of pieces of diseased atrium taken from patients exhibiting atrial arrhythmias failed to demonstrate the presence of rapid automaticity in diseased atrial myocardium.[14, 21]

In considering circus movement in the atria as cause for atrial flutter and fibrillation, many possibilities exist. At one end there is circus movement around a large anatomic obstacle; at the other is the possibility of a small functional intramyocardial circuit without an excitable gap, originally identified in isolated pieces of rabbit myocardium and later confirmed in the canine heart.[41, 42, 64, 91] Between these two extremes, a wide variety of intermediate types of reentry of various sizes and with different excitable gaps may exist. The presence of diseased atrial tissue with abnormal electrophysiologic properties may further add to the complexity of intraatrial circus movement in patients.

Figure 10-25 diagrams various types of intraatrial circus movement. Figure 10-25A shows the earliest model of circus movement, introduced by Mines in 1913.[34] It is the simplest model of reentry, in which the impulse continuously encircles a large anatomic obstacle. Implicit to

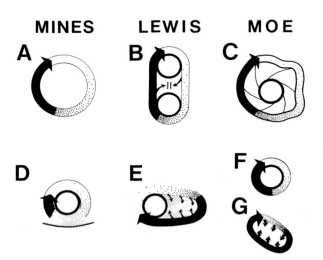

Figure 10-25. Schematic representation of various possible types of circus movement in the atria. The *black arrow* represents the crest of a circulating depolarization wave, with the area that is in the absolute refractory phase in its wake. The *dotted area* indicates the tail of relative refractory tissue. (**A**) Circus movement around a gross anatomic obstacle as introduced by Mines[34] is given. Essential characteristics of this model are the presence of an excitable gap (*white part* of the circuit) and the fact that the size and location of the reentrant pathway are anatomically determined. (**B**) Circus movement around the orifices of two (or more) veins, as suggested by Lewis[59] to be responsible for atrial flutter, is given. The main difference with the model in **A** is the presence of a bridge of conductive tissue between the two obstacles through which shortcut of the circuit can take place. (**C**) The model of circus movement, as recently introduced by Moe and colleagues,[97] in which the impulse is thought to circulate in a loop composed of atrial bundles exhibiting a faster conduction velocity than the atrial tissue within the loop. The types of circus movement diagrammed in **D** and **E** are based on a combination of an anatomic obstacle and an adjacent area of diseased atrium exhibiting depressed conduction (*hatched area*). (**F**) Circus movement around a relatively small obstacle has become possible because of alterations in the refractory period and the conduction velocity, resulting in a shortening of the wavelength of the impulse. (**G**) Circus movement without the involvement of an anatomic obstacle.[42, 91] This kind of intraatrial reentry is completely determined by the electrophysiologic properties of the myocardium. The impulse is circulating around a functional arc of conduction block. The rate of the resulting arrhythmia is the highest of all models of circus movement summarized in this figure. Its dimension is the smallest, however, with the length of the circular pathway being equal to the length of the excitation wave. (Allessie MA, et al: Circulation 1985;70:123. By permission of the American Heart Association.)

this model is the existence of an excitable gap (*white* part of the circuit) between the crest of the excitation wave and its tail of refractoriness (*dotted area*). The presence of such an excitable gap explains the high degree of regularity and stability of this kind of rhythm. Since the studies of Rosenblueth and Garcia Ramos, there is little doubt that by creating a large obstacle in the atria, atrial flutter based on this mechanism can be produced.[86] The problem, however, is that in patients suffering from atrial flutter, such large anatomic obstacles have never actually been demonstrated.

In Figure 10-25B, circus movement around two obstacles (e.g., the venae cavae), as popularized by Lewis, is given schematically.[59] A functional arc of conduction block is assumed in the isthmus between the two obstacles. As long as the excitable gap remains *shorter* than the circumference of the *smallest* of the two obstacles, short-circuit of the circulating impulse through the interobstacle band is prevented and the flutter rate is determined by the revolution time of the impulse around both obstacles. The behavior of this type of reentry is identical to the model given in Figure 10-25A, with one exception. As soon as the excitable gap gets larger than the perimeter of the smallest obstacle, the impulse can shortcut the circuit. This may result in sudden termination of flutter (an event that occurred so frequently in Lewis's experiments that it almost invariably prevented complete mapping of the excitation of the atria) or when the impulse continues to circulate around the larger obstacle may cause the flutter to accelerate abruptly. If other parts of the atria cannot follow the higher rate, degeneration into atrial fibrillation occurs.

In another attempt to overcome the problem that natural obstacles in the atria do not seem to be large enough to allow sustained circus movement, Moe and collaborators modified the early model of Mines by incorporating differences in conduction velocity in the atrium.[97] In Moe's model (Fig. 10-25C), the role of rapidly conducting muscle bundles (e.g., the internodal bands and the bundle of Bachmann) is emphasized. The idea is that the internodal pathways that form closed loops may serve as preferential circuits, through which flutter waves may circulate. The greater conduction velocity in these muscle bundles would abandon the necessity for a large physical obstacle. For instance, by assuming that the conduction velocity in a loop of internodal bands is twice as rapid as in normal myocardium, the *effective* perimeter of any natural opening present within that loop is doubled.

In Figure 10-25D and E, we propose some additional variants of intraatrial circus movement that may be responsible for common atrial flutter in humans. They are based on a *combination* of a physical obstacle and an adjacent area of diseased tissue. In Figure 10-25D, an area of depressed conduction is assumed in the inferior atrium between an internal obstacle (e.g., a pulmonary vein or the IVC) and the AV ring. Assume that the circumference of the internal obstacle is 9 cm and let the shortest possible cycle length of a sustained atrial rhythm be 140 milliseconds at a conduction velocity of 70 cm per second. If the obstacle is completely surrounded by healthy tissue, circus movement around the obstacle is impossible because the impulse would complete a full cycle within 130 milliseconds, 10 milliseconds less than the atrial fibers need to restore their excitability. If a third of the loop in the isthmus between the internal obstacle and the anulus fibrosis consists of depressed atrial tissue with a conduction velocity of 30 cm per second, it would take the impulse 190 milliseconds to travel around the orifice. Not only would the rate of such reentrant rhythm be within the range of common atrial flutter but it would most likely be stable and long-lasting because in the healthy segment of the circuit, an excitable gap of 50 milliseconds exists.

In Figure 10-25E, a functional arc of conduction block extends to an internal anatomic obstacle. The revolution time in such a circular pathway may be long enough to create an excitable gap in the normal atrial myocardium. Only at the free end of the arc of conduction block is there a tight fit between the crest of the circulating depolarization wave and its tail of refractoriness. This functionally determined turning point is the only unstable part of the circuit. During subsequent cycles, the impulse may pivot at slightly different points, resulting in minor variations in size and cycle length of the circuit. The localization of the circuit is fixed, however, and the resulting flutter may last for a long period.

Another way to facilitate intraatrial reentry is shortening of the wavelength of the impulse. The wavelength is defined as the distance traveled by the impulse during the time equal to the functional refractory period. If this occurs, the size of natural openings in the atria may suffice as central anatomic obstacles for stable circus movement (Fig. 10-25F). Conditions that shorten the excitation wave also favor circus movement without involving any physical obstacle. Relatively small arcs of functional conduction block that may arise during atrial premature beats or rapid pacing may then be sufficiently large to permit rapid self-sustained reentry (Fig. 10-25G).

When the different types of circus movement are compared with the different atrial tachyarrhythmias, the following concepts are evident.

Intraatrial reentry without the involvement of an anatomic obstacle (Fig. 10-25G) generates the fastest possible atrial rhythm. If only one circuit is present and the rest of the atria can follow the high rate in a 1:1 way, rapid atrial flutter results. The episodes of acetylcholine-induced atrial flutter analyzed in the present studies were based on this type of reentry. Most of the rapid atrial flutters found after cardiac surgery are probably based on this mechanism.[1] In our experiments, rapid atrial flutter was not a stable arrhythmia. Because of the absence of a clear excitable gap, the chances for conduction block of the circulating impulse, leading to sudden termination of flutter, are high. Another reason this rhythm was not stable for prolonged periods is that because of the extremely high rate, degeneration into atrial fibrillation may easily occur.

The same type of intraatrial circus movement (around a functional arc of conduction block) is the basic element underlying atrial fibrillation. Atrial fibrillation may result from two different mechanisms. One possibility is that a *single* intramyocardial circuit is operative, in which the circulation rate is so high that it causes conduction disturbances in other parts of the atria. This kind of fibrillation is more adequately described as *rapid flutter with fibrillatory conduction*. The other type of atrial fibrillation (true fibrillation) is based on the presence of multiple wandering wavelets.[92]

We do not believe that reentry without an anatomic obstacle is responsible for the slower type of atrial flutter. Not only would the rate of this type of reentry be higher than the rate of common atrial flutter but the absence of an appreciable excitable gap excludes such rhythm persisting for weeks, months, or even years. Evidence shows that an excitable gap of about 15% to 25% of the flutter cycle exists in human atrial flutter.[81-84] The crucial point to be elucidated regarding mechanism of classic atrial flutter is which electrophysiologic or structural abnormalities create the appropriate conditions for an excitable gap. Catheter mapping and programmed electric stimulation during atrial flutter point to an area of slow conduction located somewhere in the inferior atrium. Puech noted an isthmus of slow conduction in the inferior right atrium in the vicinity of the coronary sinus: "la partie occulte de la depolarisation auriculaire droite correspond au front d'onde d'excitation qui occupe le bas fond de l'oreillette entre la partie externe et basse de la paroi anterieure et la septum interauriculaire."[81] Using programmed electric stimulation, Inoue and colleagues and Disertori and colleagues reported that the degree of reset of the flutter cycle by the application of a single premature stimulus depended on both the site of stimulation and the site of recording.[83, 84] Together with the studies of Leier and associates and Cosio and associates, who showed that clinical atrial flutter is associated with depressed atrial conduction, these observations make us believe that common atrial flutter can best be understood by a special interplay at some strategic areas (see Fig. 10-25D and E).[98, 99]

References

1. Wells JL, Maclean WAH, James TN, Waldo AL: Characterization of atrial flutter. Studies in man after open heart surgery using fixed atrial electrodes. Circulation 1979;60:665.
2. Waldo AL, Maclean WAH, Karp RB, et al: Entrainment and

interruption of atrial flutter with atrial pacing. Studies in man following open heart surgery. Circulation 1977;56:737.

3. Hashimoto K, Moe GK: Transient depolarizations induced by acetylstrophantidin in specialized tissue of dog atrium and ventricle. Circ Res 1973;32:618.

4. Wit AL, Cranefield PF: Triggered and automatic activity in the canine coronary sinus. Circ Res 1977;41:435.

5. Cranefield PF: The conduction of the cardiac impulse. New York: Futura, 1975.

6. Cranefield PF: Action potentials, afterpotentials and arrhythmias. Circ Res 1977;41:415.

7. Scherf D: Studies on auricular tachycardia caused by aconitine administration. Proc Soc Exp Biol Med 1947;64:233.

8. Matsuda K, Hoshi T, Kameyama S: Effects of aconinitine on the cardiac membrane potential of the dog. Jpn J Physiol 1959;9:419.

9. Schmidt RF: Versuch mit Aconitin zum Problem der spontanen Erregungsbildung im Herzen. Pflugers Arch 1960; 271:526.

10. Peper K, Trautwein W: The effect of aconitine on the membrane current in cardiac muscle. Pflugers Arch 1967;296: 328.

11. Lenfant J, Mironneau J, Aka JK: Activitē rēpētitive de la fibre sino-auriculaire de grenouille: analyse des courants membranaire responsables de l'automatisme cardiaque. J Physiol (Paris) 1972;64:5.

12. Imanishi S, Surawicz B: Automatic activity in depolarized guinea pig ventricular myocardium. Characteristics and mechanisms. Circ Res 1976;39:751.

13. Katzung BG: Effects of extracellular calcium and sodium on depolarization-induced automaticity in guinea pig papillary muscle. Circ Res 1975;37:118.

14. Hordof AJ, Edie R, Malm J, et al: Electrophysiologic properties and response to pharmacologic agents of fibers from diseased human atria. Circulation 1976;54:774.

15. Rosen MR, Reder RF: Does triggered activity have a role in the genesis of cardiac arrhythmias? Ann Intern Med 1981; 94:794.

16. Hordof AJ, Spotnitz A, Mary-Rabine L, et al: The cellular electrophysiologic effects of digitalis on human atrial fibers. Circulation 1978;57:223.

17. Saito T, Otoguro M, Matsubara T: Electrophysiological studies on the mechanisms of electrically induced sustained rhythmic activity in the rabbit right atrium. Circ Res 1978; 42:199.

18. Wit AL, Fenoglio JJ, Wagner BM, Bassett AL: Electrophysiological properties of cardiac muscle in the anterior mitral valve leaflet and the adjacent atrium in the dog: possible implications for the genesis of atrial dysrhythmias. Circ Res 1973; 32:731.

19. Wit AL, Cranefield PF: Triggered activity in cardiac muscle fibers of the simian mitral valve. Circ Res 1976;38:85.

20. Wit AL, Fenoglio JJ, Hordof AJ, Reemtsma K: Ultrastructure and transmembrane potentials of cardiac muscle in the human anterior mitral valve leaflet. Circulation 1979;59: 1284.

21. Mary-Rabine L, Hordof AJ, Danilo P, et al: Mechanisms for impulse initiation in isolated human atrial fibers. Circ Res 1980;47:267.

22. Hoffman BF, Rosen MR: Cellular mechanisms for cardiac arrhythmias. Circ Res 1981;49:1.

23. Aronson RS, Cranefield PF, Wit AL: The effects of caffeine and ryanodine on the electrical activity of the canine coronary sinus. J Physiol (Lond) 1985;368:593.

24. Henning B, Kline RP, Siegal MS, Wit AL: Triggered activity in atrial fibers of canine coronary sinus: role of extracellular potassium accumulation and depletion. J Physiol (Lond) 1987;383:191.

25. Pogwizd SM, Onufer JR, Kramer JB, Sobel BE, Corr PB: Induction of delayed afterdepolarizations and triggered activity in canine Purkinje fibers by lysophosphoglycerides. Circ Res 1986;59:416.

26. January CT, Riddle JM: early afterdepolarizations: mechanism of induction and block. A role for L-type Ca^{2+} current. Circ Res 1989;64:977.

27. January CT, Riddle JM, Salata JJ: A model for early afterdepolarizations: induction with the Ca^{2+} channel agonist BAY K 8644. Circ Res 1988;62:563.

28. Kimura S, Bassett AL, Xi H, Myerberg RJ: Early afterdepolarizations and triggered activity induced by cocaine. Possible mechanism of cocaine arrhythmogenesis. Circulation 1992; 85:2227.

29. Ben-David J, Zipes DP: Differential response to right and left ansa subclaviae stimulation of eraly afterdepolarizations and ventricular tachycardia induced by cesium. Circulation 1988;78:1241.

30. Ben-David J, Zipes DP: Alpha-adrenoceptor stimulation and blockade modulates cesium-induced early afterdepolarizations and ventricular tachycardia in dogs. Circulation 1990; 82:225.

31. Rozanski GJ, Witt RC: Early afterdepolarizations and triggered activity in rabbit cardiac Purkinje fibers recovering from ischemic-like conditions. Role of acidosis. Circulation 1991;83:1352.

32. McWilliam JA: Fibrillar contraction of the heart. J Physiol 1887;8:296.

33. Mayer AG: Rhythmical pulsation in scyphomedusae. Washington, DC: Carnegie Institution, 1906. Publication 47.

34. Mines GR: On dynamic equilibrium in the heart. J Physiol 1913;46:349.

35. Mines GR: On circulating excitations in heart muscles and their possible relation to tachycardia and fibrillation. Trans R Soc Canad 1914;IV:43.

36. Garrey WE: The nature of fibrillary contraction of the heart. Its relation to tissue mass and form. Am J Physiol 1914;33:397.

37. Moe GK, Preston JB, Burlington H: Physiologic evidence for a dual AV transmission system. Circ Res 1956;4:357.

38. Janse MJ, Van Capelle FJL, Freud GE, Durrer D: Circus movement within the AV node as a basis for supraventricular tachycardia as shown by multiple microelectrode recordings in the isolated rabbit heart. Circ Res 1971;28:403.

39. Han J, Malozzi AM, Moe GK: Sinoatrial reciprocation in the isolated rabbit heart. Circ Res 1968;44:355.

40. Allessie MA, Bonke FIM: Direct demonstration of sinus node reentry in the rabbit heart. Circ Res 1979;44:557.

41. Allessie MA, Bonke FIM, Schopman FJG: Circus movement in rabbit atrial muscle as a mechanism of tachycardia. Circ Res 1973;33:54.

42. Allessie MA, Bonke FIM, Schopman FJG: Circus movement in rabbit atrial muscle as a mechanism of tachycardia. III. The "leading circle" concept: a new model of circus movement in cardiac tissue without the involvement of an anatomic obstacle. Circ Res 1977;41:9.

43. Lal R, Arnsdorf MF: Voltage-dependent gating and single-channel conductance of adult mammalian atrial gap junctions. Circ Res 1992;71:737.

44. Sakakibara Y, Wasserstorm JA, Furukawa T, et al: Characterization of sodium current in single human atrial myocytes. Circ Res 1992;71:536.

45. Fozzard HA, January CT, Makieski JC: New studies of the excitatory sodium currents in heart muscle. Circ Res 1985; 56:475.

46. Barber MJ, Starmer CF, Grant TO: Blockade of cardiac sodium channels by amitriptyline and diphenylhydantoin. Evidence for two use-dependent binding sites. Circ Res 1991; 69:677.

47. Bean BP: Classes of calcium channels in vertebrate cells. Annu Rev Physiol 1989;51:367.

48. Escande D, Coulombe A, Faivre J-F, Coraboeuf E: Characteristics of the time-dependent slow inward current in adult human atrial single myocytes. J Mol Cell Cardiol 1986; 18:547.

49. Le Grand B, Hatem S, Deroubaix D, Couetil JP, Coraboeuf E: Calcium current depression in isolated human atrial myocytes after cessation of chronic treatment with calcium antagonist. Circ Res 1991;69:292.

50. Escande D, Coulombe A, Faivre J-F, Deroubaix E, Coraboeuf E: Two types of transient outward current in adult human atrial myocytes. Am J Physiol 1987;252:H142.

51. Shibata EF, Refsum DH, Aldrette V, Giles W: Contribution of fast transient outward current to repolarization in human atrium. Am J Physiol 1989;257:H1773.

52. Imaizumi Y, Giles WR: Quinidine-induced inhibition of transient outward current in cardiac muscle. Am J Physiol 1987; 253:H704.

53. Escande D, Loisance D, Planche C, Coraboeuf E: Age-related changes in action potential plateau and shape in isolated human atrial fibers. Am J Physiol 1985;249:H843.

54. Wang Z, Fermini B, Nattel S: Repolarization differences between guinea pig atrial endocardium and epicardium: evidence for a role of Ito. Am J Physiol 1991;260:H1501.

55. Frame LH, Page RL, Hoffman BF: Atrial reentry around an anatomical barrier with a partially refractory excitable gap. A canine model of atrial flutter. Circ Res 1986;48:495.

56. Frame LH, Page RL, Boyden PA, Fenoglio JJ Jr, Hoffman BF: Circus movement in the canine atrium around the tricuspid ring during experimental atrial flutter and during reentry in vitro. Circulation 1987;76:1155.

57. Frame LH, Simson MB: Oscillations of conduction, action potential duration, and refractoriness. A mechanism for spontaneous termination of reentrant tachycardia. Circulation 1988;78:1277.

58. Frame LH, Rhee EK: Spontaneous termination of reentry after abrupt one cycle or short nonsustained runs. Role of oscillations and excess dispersion of refractoriness. Circ Res 1991;68:493.

59. Lewis T: The mechanism and graphic registration of the heart beat. London: Shaw & Sons, 1925.

60. Dawes GS, Vane JR: Repetitive discharges from the isolated atria. J Physiol 1951;112:28P.

61. Dawes GS: Experimental cardiac arrhythmias and quinidine-like drugs. Pharmacol Rev 1952;4:43.

62. West TC, Cox AR: Single fiber recording during the production and control of flutter in the isolated atrium of the rabbit. J Pharmacol Exp Ther 1960;130:303.

63. West TC, Landa JF: Minimal mass required for induction of a sustained arrhythmia in isolated atrial segments. Am J Physiol 1962;202:232.

64. Allessie MA, Bonke FIM, Schopman FJG: Circus movement in rabbit atrial muscle as a mechanism of tachycardia. II. The role of nonuniform recovery of excitability in the occurrence of unidirectional block as studied with multiple microelectrodes. Circ Res 1976;39:168.

65. Bouman LN, Gerlings ED, Biersteker PA, Bonke FIM: Pacemakershift in the sinoatrial node during vagal stimulation. Pflugers Arch 1968;302:255.

66. Rensma PL, Allessie MA, Lammers WJEP, Bonke FIM, Schalij MJ: Length of excitation and susceptibility to reentrant atrial arrhythmias in normal conscious dogs. Circ Res 1988;62:395.

67. Smeets JLRM, Allessie MA, Lammers WJEP, Bonke FIM, Hollen J: The wavelength o of the cardiac impulse and reentrant arrhythmias in isolated rabbit atrium. The role of heart rate, autonomic transmitters, temperature, and potassium. Circ Res 1986;58:96.

68. Allessie MA, Rensma PL, Brugada J, Smeets JLRM, Penn O, Kirchhof CJHJ: Pathophysiology of atrial fibrillation. In: Zipes DP, Jalife J, eds. Cardiac electrophysiology. From cell to bedside. Philadelphia: WB Saunders, 1990:548.

69. Schuessler RB, Grayson TM, Bromberg BI, Cox JL, Boineau JP: Cholinergically mediated tachyarrhythmisa induced by a single extrastimulus in the isolated canine right atrium. Circ Res 1992;71:1254.

70. Spach MS, Dolber PC, Heidlage JF: Interaction of inhomogeneities of repolarization with anisotropic propagation in dog atria. A mechanism for both preventing and initiating reentry. Circ Res 1989;65:1612.

71. Spach SM, Dolber PC, Anderson PAW: Multiple regional differences in cellular properties that regulate repolarization and contraction in right atrium of adult and newborn dogs. Circ Res 1989;65:1594.

72. Sato S, Yamauchi S, Schuessler RB, Boineau JP, Matsunaga Y, Cox JL: The effect of augmented atrial hypothermia on atrial refractory period, conduction, and atrial flutter/fibrillation in the canine heart. J Thorac Cardiovasc Surg 1992;104:297.

73. Clerc L: Directional differences in impulse spread in trabecular muscle from mammalian heart. J Physiol (Lond) 1976;255:335.

74. Spach MS, Miller WT, Dolber PC, Kootsey M, Sommer JR, Mosher CE: The functional role of structural complexities in the propagation of depolarization in the atrium of the dog. Cardiac conduction disturbances due to discontinuities of effective axial resistivity. Circ Res 1982;50:175.

75. Allessie MA, Schalij MJ, Kirchhof CJHJ, Boersma L, Huyberts M, Hollen J: Electrophysiology of spiral waves in two dimensions: the role of anisotropy. Ann NY Acad Sci 1990;591:247.

76. Spach MS, Dolber PC, Heidlage JF: Influence of the passive anisotropic properties on directional differences in propagation following modification of sodium conductance in human atrial muscle. A model of reentry based on anisotropic discontinuous propagation. Circ Res 1988;62:811.

77. Spach MS, Dolber PC, Heidlage JF, Kootsey JM, Johnson EA: Propagating depolarization inanisotropic human and canine cardiac muscle: apparent directional differences in membrane capacitance. A simplified model for selective directional effects of modifying the sodium conductance on V_{max}, tau_{foot}, and propagation safety factor. Circ Res 1987;60:206.

78. Allessie MA, Rensma PL, Lammers WJEP, Kirchhoh CJHJ: The role of refractoriness, conduction velocity, and wavelength in initiation of atrial fibrillation in normal conscious dogs. In: Attuel P, Coumel P, Janse MJ, eds. The atrium in health and disease. Mt. Kisco, NY: Futura Publishing, 1989:27.

79. Mendez C, Moe GK: Demonstration of a dual AV nodal conduction system in isolated rabbit heart. Circ Res 1966;19:378.

80. Schuilenburg RM, Durrer D: Atrial echo beats in the human heart elicited by induced atrial premature beats. Circulation 1968;37:680.

81. Puech P, Latour H, Grolleau R: Le flutter et ses limites. Arch Mal Coeur 1970;61:116.

82. Watson RM, Josephson ME: Atrial flutter. I. Electrophysiologic substrates and modes of initiation and termination. Am J Cardiol 1980;45:732.

83. Inoue H, Matsuo H, Takayanagi K, Murao S: Clinical and experimental studies of the effects of atrial extrastimulation and rapid pacing on atrial flutter cycle. Am J Cardiol 1981;48:623.

84. Disertori M, Inama G, Vergara G, et al: Evidence of a reentry circuit in the common type of atrial flutter in man. Circulation 1983;67:434.

85. Lewis T, Feil HS, Stroud WD: Observations upon flutter and fibrillation. II. Nature of auricular flutter. Heart 1920;7:191.

86. Rosenblueth A, Garcia Ramos J: Studies on flutter and fibrillation. II. The influence of artificial obstacles on experimental auricular flutter. Am Heart J 1947;33:677.

87. Kimura E, Kato K, Murao S, et al: Experimental studies on the mechanism of the auricular flutter. Tohoku J Exp Med 1954;60:197.

88. Lanari A, Lambertini A, Ravin A: Mechanism of experimental atrial flutter. Circ Res 1956;4:282.

89. Hayden WG, Hurley EJ, Rytand DA: The mechanism of canine atrial flutter. Circ Res 1967;20:496.

90. McAlpine WA: Heart and coronary arteries. Berlin: Springer-Verlag, 1975.

91. Allessie MA, Lammers WJEP, Bonke FIM, Hollen J: Intra-atrial reentry as a mechanism for atrial flutter induced by acetylcholine and rapid pacing in the dog. Circulation 1985;70:123.

92. Moe GK: On the multiple wavelet hypothesis of atrial fibrillation. Arch Int Pharmacodyn Ther 1962;140:183.

93. Moe GK, Rheinboldt WC, Abildskov JA: A computer model of atrial fibrillation. Am Heart J 1964;67:200.

94. Moe GK: In: Stacy RW, Waxman BD, eds. Computers in Biomedical Research. Vol 2. New York: Academic Press, 1965.

95. Lewis T, Drury AN, Bulger HA: Flutter and fibrillation; the effects of vagal stimulation. Heart 1921;8:141.

96. Wilson FN: Report of a case of auricular flutter in which vagus stimulation was followed by an increase in the rate of the circus rhythm. Heart 1924;11:61.

97. Moe GK, Pastelin G, Mendez R: Circus movement excitation of the atria. In: Little RC, ed. Physiology of atrial pacemakers and conductive tissues. New York: Futura Publishing, 1980:207.

98. Leier CV, Meacham JA, Schaal SF: Prolonged atrial conduction. A major predisposing factor for the development of atrial flutter. Circulation 1978;57:213.

99. Cosio FG, Palacios J, Vidal J, et al: Electrophysiologic studies in atrial fibrillation. Slow conduction of premature impulses: a possible manifestation of the background for reentry. Am J Cardiol 1983;51:122.

Cardiac Arrhythmias, 3rd edition, edited by William J. Mandel.
J. B. Lippincott Company, Philadelphia © 1995.

11

Hossein Shenasa • Paul V.L. Curry • Mohammad Shenasa

Atrial Arrhythmias: Clinical Concepts and Advances in Mechanism and Management[*]

About 60% of all cardiac arrhythmias encountered clinically either arise in or involve the atria.[1] The spectrum of such atrial arrhythmias includes, at one extreme, single atrial extrasystoles of dubious significance and at the other, chronic irreversible atrial fibrillation (Table 11-1). Between these two extremes are atrial tachycardias of varying rate and regularity, such as paroxysmal sinus node tachycardia, atrial tachycardia, "chaotic" or multifocal atrial tachycardia, and atrial flutter. There are also disorders of intraatrial and interatrial conduction. Despite such diversity, atrial arrhythmias have much in common, especially regarding their etiology and management.

PATHOPHYSIOLOGY

The many pathologic and functional conditions that can affect the atria, thereby causing atrial arrhythmias, are summarized in Table 11-2. Most such pathologic processes affect not only working atrial myocardium but also the

sinus and sometimes the atrioventricular (AV) nodes that are also situated within the atria.[2] When this occurs, it does not necessarily produce arrhythmias that fairly represent the degree of involvement of each site; indeed, many atrial tachyarrhythmias can arise with sinus node disease alone and in the absence of overt atrial myocardial involvement. Frequently, atrial arrhythmias arise as part of the sick sinus syndrome or the atrial bradycardia–tachycardia syndrome (Fig. 11-1) before the bradycardia component has developed.[3,4] Hudson, in 1965, suggested that damage to the SA node was a necessary precursor to the occurrence of atrial arrhythmias.[5] Direct damage to atrial muscle, atrial dilation, and occlusion of the sinus node artery were also thought to be predominant factors responsible for atrial arrhythmias.[6-8]

Davies and Pomerance undertook pathologic studies of 100 hearts from patients coming to autopsy who had atrial fibrillation.[9] Examining specifically both the SA node and atrial tissue, they found that patients with either recent or rare atrial fibrillation had atrial dilation but essentially preserved sinus node and atrial myocardium. In contrast, patients with long-term atrial tachyarrhythmias such as atrial fibrillation showed combinations of SA node artery stenosis and muscle loss within the SA node or main

[*]Dedicated to the memory of Edgar Sawton.

TABLE 11-1. Types of Atrial Arrhythmias

Atrial extrasystoles, echo beats, and parasystole
Sinoatrial nodal reentrant tachycardia
Atrial tachycardia
Atrial flutter
Atrial fibrillation
First-, second-, and third-degree intraatrial block
Atrial standstill

TABLE 11-2. Disorders Affecting Sinus Node, Atrium, and Atrioventricular Node

General Type of Disorder	Specific Disorder or Cause
ACUTE	
Vascular	
Inflammatory	Acute myocardial infarction
	Viral myocarditis
	Rheumatic carditis
	Collagen disease
	Bacterial carditis
Trauma	
Surgery	
Distention	Raised atrial pressure
Distortion	From within or externally
Tumor	Infiltration (including leukemia)
Radiation	
Toxic carditis	
Drugs	(e.g., digoxin)
Endocrine and metabolic disorder	(e.g., acute electrolyte imbalance)
Bronchopulmonary disease (acute)	
Bradycardia with hyper-vagotonia	
CHRONIC	
Rheumatic heart disease	
Cardiomyopathy	(Primary or secondary)
Coronary artery disease	
Idiopathic atrial fibrosis	(Sclerodegenerative)
Infiltrations	(e.g., slow neoplasia, amyloid, hemochromatosis)
Collagen disease	
Chronic infections	(e.g., tuberculosis, carditis, sarcoid, Chagas' disease)
Congenital	(e.g., atrial septal defect, SA node development)
Chronic dilation or hyper-trophy	(e.g., mitral valve disease, hypertension)
Bronchopulmonary disease (chronic)	e.g., thyroid disease
Endocrine	

intraatrial bundles in addition to dilation. The underlying pathologic conditions found most commonly in this group were chronic rheumatic valvular disease, ischemic heart disease, hypertension, and cor pulmonale. Occasionally in some aged patients, atrial fibrillation had occurred in association with loss of muscle fibers and increased fibrosis within the SA node, for which there was no clear underlying pathologic cause and no atrial involvement. Sims reported similar findings.[10]

The precise form of atrial arrhythmia is often independent of the nature of the causative atrial disease and may relate more to the extent and location of the disease process within the atria and to prevailing autonomic tone. Certain arrhythmias, however, are more common with acute atrial disturbance. It is known that atrial fibrillation can even occur in the absence of both atrial and sinus node disease, possibly as a result of sudden changes in autonomic tone.[11] Pharmacologic interventions can have the same effect.[9, 12–15] Atrial arrhythmias may "escape" during transient bradycardia or may be precipitated by either physical or emotional stress (Fig. 11-2).[16]

Other conditions within the chest but remote from the heart can precipitate atrial arrhythmias (e.g., pleurisy or trauma, chest infection), possibly through reflex mechanisms. Neuromuscular disorders such as myotonia dystrophica and metabolic disorders such as thyroid over- or underactivity, diabetes, uremia, and pheochromocytoma can cause atrial arrhythmias.[16] Paroxysmal or acute atrial arrhythmias may also be precipitated by toxic states, hypoxia, alcohol, nicotine, caffeine, digitalis, adrenergic stimulants, and exercise.

Sometimes atrial arrhythmias are caused by other tachycardias that either directly (Wolff-Parkinson-White syndrome or AV nodal reentrant tachycardia) involve the atria or secondarily affect atrial electrophysiologic behavior (e.g., rapid ventricular tachycardia). Atrial arrhythmias can even be precipitated by permanent endocardial pacing leads as they course through or impinge on the right atrium. It has also been postulated that certain rapid atrial arrhythmias may arise as a result of conduction of premature ventricular impulses retrogradely up functional bypasses of the AV node, which then arrive in the atria during their vulnerable period, precipitating the fibrillation process.

Arrhythmias can arise anywhere within the atria, even within the sinus node.[17] Furthermore, most of atrial tachycardias originate in the right atrium, and about 10% arise from the left atrium.[19] Atrial arrhythmias can either involve both atria or be isolated to one part of either the left or right atrium while another atrial rhythm prevails elsewhere; however, the simultaneous occurrence of dissimilar atrial rhythms has been requestioned.[20, 21] Concomitant supraventricular tachycardias have been reported in patients with SA nodal reentrant tachycardia and in patients with atrial tachycardia (Fig. 11-3).[22]

The abnormal electrophysiologic mechanisms underlying such arrhythmias include enhanced focal automat-

I.R. 591193

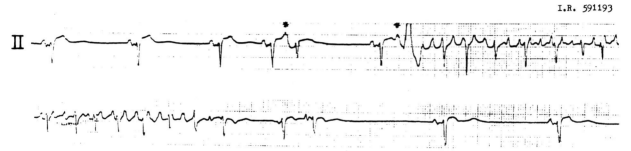

Figure 11-1. Atypical atrial flutter arising in association with sinoatrial disease in a form of brady-cardia-tachycardia syndrome. Some of the atrial extrasystoles appear to rise from a site in the atrium in common with that for the tachycardia.

icity, triggered activity, and reentry (Fig. 11-4). In the latter case, circus movement can occur either within a closed anatomic circuit, perhaps formed by divisive structures such as caval orifices and foramina within the atria, or by the leading-circle mechanism without necessarily involving fixed anatomic features.[23] Abnormalities of intraatrial conduction can also occur either alone or in association with atrial tachyarrhythmias.[24] Generally, such abnormal electrophysiologic mechanisms arise as a result of atrial disease. This is in marked contrast to the occurrence of reentrant tachycardias at the AV junction in patients who most often have otherwise normal hearts.

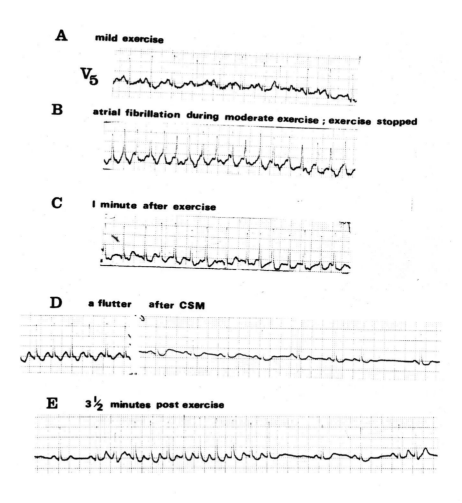

Figure 11-2. Paroxysmal atrial fibrillation and flutter provoked by exercise. *CSM*, carotid sinus massage.

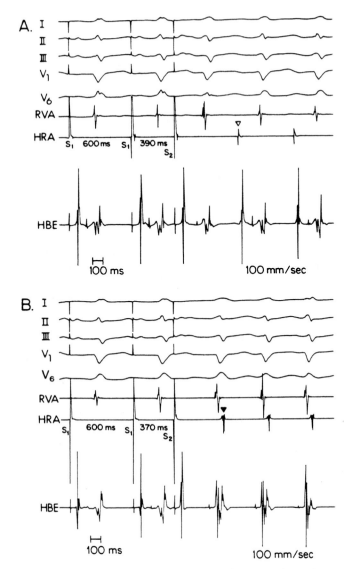

Figure 11-3. (**A**) Surface and intracardiac recordings during atrial programmed stimulation at the drive cycle (S_1) length of 600 milliseconds, with the introduction of an atrial extrastimulus (S_2) at a coupling interval of 390 milliseconds. Sinoatrial node reentrant tachycardia (▽) was induced. (**B**) The introduction of S_2 at a slightly shorter coupling interval (370 milliseconds) initiated atrioventricular node reentrant tachycardia (▼). (From Sanders WE, et al: Sinoatrial node reentrant tachycardia ablation. J Am Coll Cardiol 1994; 23(4):926)

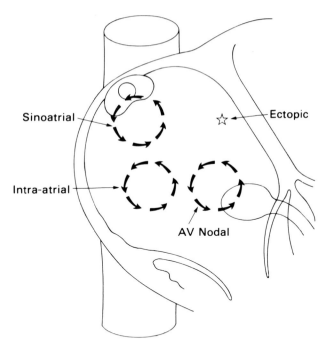

Figure 11-4. Sites and mechanisms of atrial tachyarrhythmias. Proximity to nodal tissue confers increasing sensitivity to alterations in autonomic nervous tone.

ATRIAL EXTRASYSTOLES, ECHOES, AND PARASYSTOLE

Neither the incidence nor the significance of these arrhythmias is fully known. Undoubtedly they occur in otherwise normal individuals, whether adults or children.[25,26] Atrial parasystole is relatively infrequent.[27–29] We have

found a 10% incidence of minor atrial arrhythmias in normal subjects, compared with a 30% incidence in patients with complete heart block and an 88% incidence in patients with the sick sinus syndrome.[30]

Mostly, the occurrence of atrial arrhythmias goes unnoticed, although long compensatory or reset pauses may be detected by the patient as transient dizziness with a characteristic precordial discomfort and a stronger post-ectopic impulse, especially in hypertensive patients. The effects of exercise, emotion, sudden deep breathing, and vagal tone on such arrhythmias are individual. Responses are inconsistent even in the same patient on differing occasions.[29,31,32] Most often, "atrial transport" is retained and unpleasant cannon-wave reflexes avoided.[33]

The electrocardiographic features of such arrhythmias are well known. The P-wave configuration of the premature atrial beat, when examined in all 12 conventional surface electrocardiogram (ECG) leads, portrays its approximate site of origin.[34] Atrial parasystole is suspected if there is a constant short interectopic P-wave interval and there are atrial fusion beats. The clinical value of this diagnostic achievement, however, is less clear unless it is associated in a particular case with recurrent atrial tachycardia, flutter, or fibrillation due to the atrial R-on-T phenomenon. Rarely, such foci require ablation because of this phenomenon.

Similarly, atrial echo beats may reflect a latent predisposition to reentrant or junctional tachycardia; sinus node, atrial, and junctional echoes are commonly elicited during intracardiac extrastimulation tests.[35]

WANDERING ATRIAL PACEMAKER

Typically, the atrial rate during this arrhythmia is about 100 beats per minute or less, and P-P intervals vary at random (Fig. 11-5).[35] The P wave may be hidden if it occurs simultaneously with a junctional beat during a relative bradycardia phase. The ventricular response is usually 1:1, with the exception of concealed premature impulses that arise at a time when the AV node is refractory.[36]

Investigation, if indicated for such minor atrial arrhythmias, is with 24-hour continuous ECG recording and perhaps with monitored stress testing. The occurrence of echoes and extrasystoles during clinical electrophysiologic studies is standard, especially during the functional refractory periods of the different regions comprising the atrium (Fig. 11-6).

Because most patients with such arrhythmias are unaware of their occurrence, treatment is rarely required. The nature and frequency of such arrhythmias should be noted for serial assessment, however. Occasionally, their occurrence heralds thyroid overactivity before it is otherwise clinically overt.

SINOATRIAL NODAL REENTRANT TACHYCARDIA

Paroxysmal SA nodal reentrant tachycardia is a relatively new clinical arrhythmia, at least regarding its recognition (Fig. 11-7).[17] More than 30 years ago, Barker and coworkers postulated that one form of paroxysmal supra-ventricular tachycardia might be due to sustained impulse reentry within the region of the SA node, a concept reiterated by Wallace and Daggett.[37,38] During clinical intracardiac studies, the underlying electrophysiologic mechanism behaves as if it were reentrant; that is, such tachycardias can be both initiated and terminated reproducibly and over a critical zone during atrial diastole by a single triggered atrial extrastimulus (see Fig. 11-3), although triggered activity cannot be excluded. Support for the reentrant hypothesis came from the work of Han and associates and from that of Allessie and Bonke.[39,40] Knowledge of the precise mechanism, however, is of little consequence to therapy in this particular instance.

The frequency of SA nodal reentrant tachycardia has grown rapidly since its recognition. Most early examples were seen incidentally during intracardiac studies but 43 cases have been diagnosed electrocardiographically on suspicion of their occurrence.[46] Continuous 24-hour ECG monitoring is especially applicable to the diagnosis and assessment of this arrhythmia. With the emergence of radiofrequency catheter ablation for elimination of supraventricular tachycardias, the frequency of SA nodal reentrant tachycardias has been reexamined.[22] The frequency of 3.2% among patients referred for evaluation of paroxysmal supraventricular tachycardias is consistent with that observed by Josephson (3%) and Wellens (1.8%) in the preablation era.[22,41,42]

Patients with SA nodal reentrant tachycardia are typically older than those having other forms of supraventricular tachycardia and often present during or after the fifth decade of life.[22]

Structural heart disease is not present in most patients with SA nodal reentrant tachycardia and its occurrence in normal subjects is well described.[22,43–46] Some of these patients may have other features of SA disease. In some patients, the only additional finding is a substrate for another supraventricular tachycardia such as ventricular pre-excitation syndrome or the presence of dual AV nodal

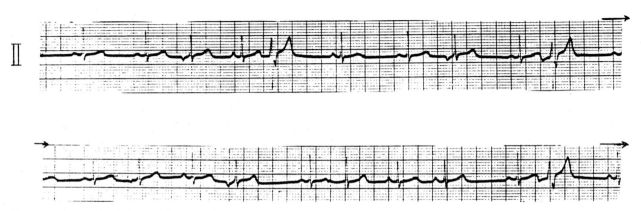

Figure 11-5. Wandering atrial pacemaker.

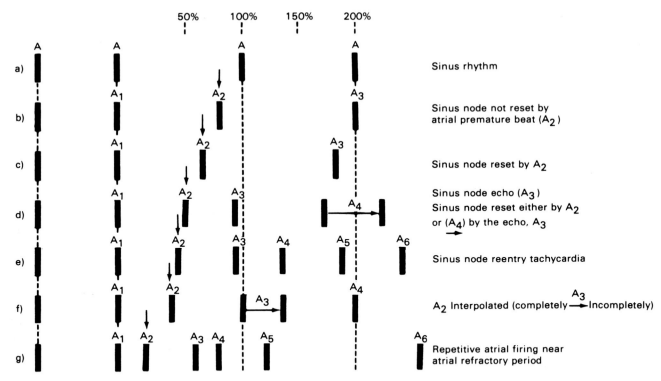

Figure 11-6. Diagram of responses seen variably with programmed atrial extrastimulation (nonsinus reset; sinus node reset, sinus node or atrial echoes and tachycardias; atrial repetitive firing or local reentry, sometimes leading to atrial flutter or fibrillation as the extra stimulus is given more prematurely).

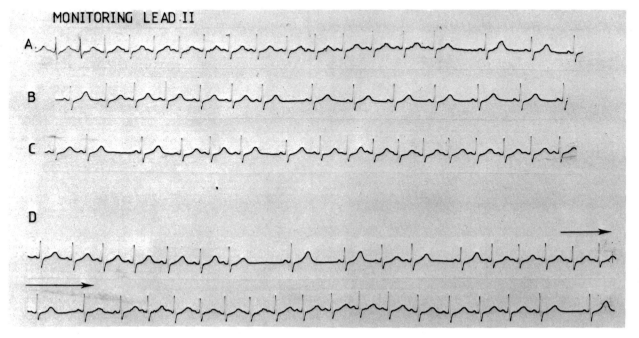

Figure 11-7. Repetitive paroxysmal sinus node reentrant tachycardia. Note P waves during sinus rhythms (slower rate) are similar to those of the tachycardia. The lower two panels (**D**) are continuous.

pathway and AV nodal reentrant tachycardia.[22, 46, 47] Sinus node echo responses have been reported as occurring in up to 11% of patients without SA node disease.[48]

Heart rates during paroxysmal SA nodal reentrant tachycardia are slower than those in most other forms of supraventricular tachycardia, usually between 80 and 150 beats per minute, although faster rates have been reported.[44–46] When heart rates during tachycardia are below 90 beats per minute, this is a relative tachycardia with sudden onset and sudden offset, occurring in patients with sinus bradycardia. Symptoms are usually mild, and most attacks probably pass unnoticed except when the rate in tachycardia is above 120 beats per minute. Most attacks are short-lived, usually lasting for no more than 10 to 20 beats (Fig. 11-8) but they are repetitive, being characteristically sensitive to changes in autonomic tone, including even those changes associated with normal breathing. This last feature occasionally makes distinction from sinus arrhythmia almost impossible (Fig. 11-9). More persistent attacks last for some minutes but rarely longer.

It would be interesting to know how often patients with this arrhythmia are mistakenly diagnosed as suffering from anxiety. Reassurance and tranquilizers have little effect on the occurrence of attacks; however, close questioning reveals that their tachycardias are truly paroxysmal. Although most attacks are only a mild nuisance (once recognized and their significance explained), others can cause angina, breathlessness, and syncope, especially in those with associated heart disease and the sick sinus syndrome. The similarity to normal sinus rhythm extends to hemodynamic considerations such as appropriate atrial systole and transport but the rate is inappropriate.

Electrocardiographic Features

The electrocardiographic features of this tachycardia are well described and consist of the sudden onset and termination of the tachycardia, the appearances of which suggest a paroxysmal and regular sinus tachycardia. Although P-wave morphology in the tachycardia may be indistinguishable from that in basic sinus rhythm in all 12 leads of the conventional ECG, more often the P waves are similar but not identical. The sequence of atrial activation, however, remains one of high to low and right to left, even for nonidentical P waves, suggesting an origin for the arrhythmia in the region of sinus node in the high right atrium. Mostly, attacks arise without antecedent premature spontaneous extrasystoles—a distinction from most other such apparently reentrant supraventricular tachycardias, although their initiation by prior sinus node acceleration is similar to the mechanism of initiation that is sometimes seen with paroxysmal reentry AV tachycardias that have a wide initiation zone.[49]

As a rule, attacks slow before terminating spontaneously, again without prompting by spontaneously occurring premature extrasystolic activity (Fig. 11-10). Termination can be encouraged by carotid sinus massage or similar vagotonic maneuvers to which this arrhythmia is supremely sensitive (Fig. 11-11). In our experience, carotid sinus massage during sustained SA reentrant tachycardia slowed the tachycardia in all and terminated it in all but one case.[22] The paroxysm may terminate with cycle-length alteration—a feature that suggests an underlying reentrant mechanism (Fig. 11-12).[50] The post-termination pause resembles that seen after moderate overdrive atrial

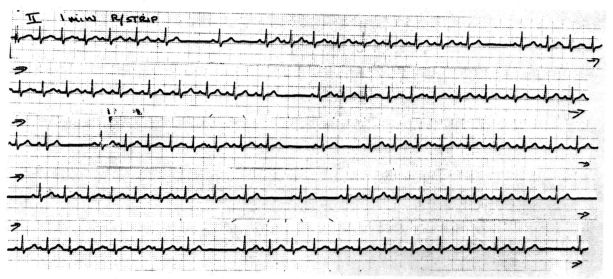

Figure 11-8. Repetitive paroxysmal sinus node reentrant tachycardia. Atrial rate-related functional prolongation of the PR interval is seen, a feature that distinguishes this arrhythmia from sinus tachycardia where PR may be shortened by increased adrenergic tone.

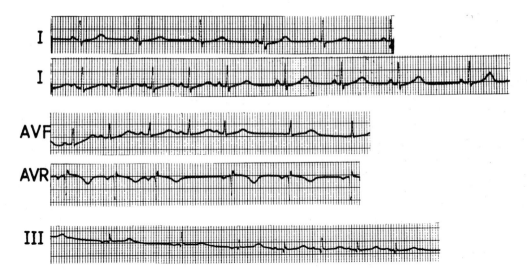

Figure 11-9. In these electrocardiogram strips, paroxysmal sinus node reentrant tachycardia can be distinguished from sinus arrhythmia by the minor alteration in P-wave morphology and the slight lengthening of the PR interval.

pacing, as performed in studies of sinus node recovery, confirming the conflicts within the region of the SA node. Preliminary reports indicate that rapid intravenous administration of adenosine during sustained SA reentrant tachycardia may terminate the tachycardia in most cases (Fig. 11-13).[51,52]

Perhaps the most important electrocardiographic sign that distinguishes this arrhythmia from appropriate and physiologic sinus tachycardia is prolongation of the PR interval in accordance with inherent functional properties of delay within the AV node when this is traversed by impulses other than those of natural sinus rhythm. The

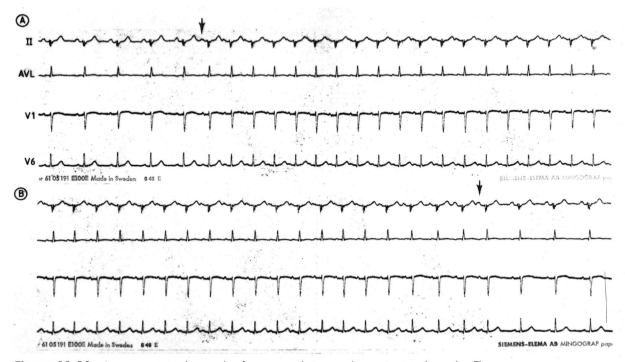

Figure 11-10. A more sustained example of paroxysmal sinus node reentrant tachycardia. The *arrows* show the spontaneous onset and termination. Interestingly, the minor aberration in P-wave morphology in the tachycardia recovers just before the tachycardia stops, so that the last two P waves are identical to those of the ensuing normal sinus rhythm.

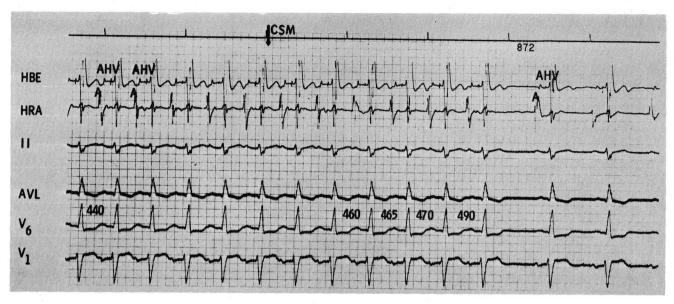

Figure 11-11. Carotid sinus massage (*CSM*) slows and then stops an attack of paroxysmal sinus node reentrant tachycardia. *HBE*, His-bundle electrogram; *HRA*, high right atrial electrogram.

degree of prolongation is mild but so is the stress imposed on the AV node by this relatively slow atrial tachycardia. Figure 11-8 shows this phenomenon most clearly as each new tachycardia arises. In contrast, autonomically mediated sinus tachycardia shows little change or even shortening of the PR interval. Rarely, variable AV conduction occurs at the onset of such tachycardias, with some impulses failing to traverse the AV node (Fig. 11-14). Both functional patterns of disturbed AV conduction are passive phenomena and exclude participation of the AV node in the mechanism of the arrhythmia.

Intracardiac Studies

Characteristically, attacks can be both initiated and terminated reproducibly with programmed extrastimulation (Figs. 11-15 and 11-16; see Fig. 11-14). Termination by this method, however, requires that the tachycardia is sufficiently sustained before application, a feature that is not always forthcoming, although small amounts of atropine are persuasive.[46] Such extrastimuli are most effective when introduced near the sinus node except when delivered with antecedent paced rhythm, in which case they

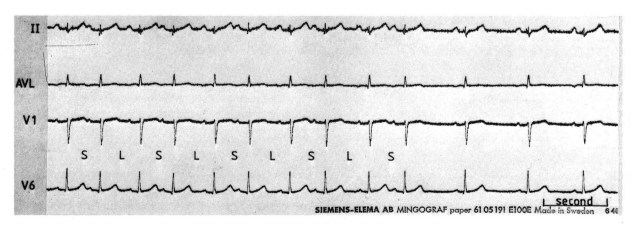

Figure 11-12. Termination of paroxysmal sinus node reentrant tachycardia, with alternately long (*L*) short (*S*) cycle lengths.

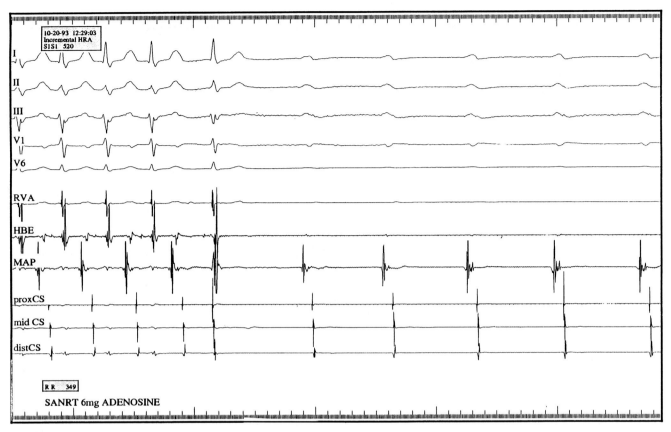

Figure 11-13. Administration of 6 mg intravenous adenosine during a sinoatrial nodal reentrant tachycardia. Prolongation of tachycardia cycle length before its termination and transient high-degree atrioventricular block is present. Sequence of atrial activation during tachycardia is similar to that of sinus rhythm. *I, II, III, V₁, V₆,* surface-lead electrocardiogram; *RVA,* right ventricular apex; *HBE,* His-bundle electrogram; *MAP,* mapping catheter recording; *proxCS, mid-CS,* and *distCS,* coronary sinus.

are equally effective from any site, as long as effective prematurity is maintained in transit to the SA node. Initiation by ventricular extrastimulation has been observed (Fig. 11-17).

Simultaneous multipoint atrial mapping confirms the direction of atrial activation during paroxysmal sinus node reentrant tachycardia as being similar to that of natural sinus rhythm. Minor alterations in the configuration of the high right atrial electrograms and of the initial P wave vector are to be expected because the pattern of atrial activation within the immediate vicinity of the SA node must be affected if the circuit partially includes extranodal atrial myocardium. Intrasinus node aberration and a shifting sinus node pacemaker would have similar effects, however (see Fig. 11-16).[49, 53] Incremental atrial pacing also initiates the tachycardia, whereas overdrive pacing may suppress or terminate it. Spontaneous termination is never long awaited (Fig. 11-18). Direct recording of the sinus node electrogram during sinus rhythm and sinus node reentry may further elucidate the mechanisms and

electrophysiologic characteristics of this arrhythmia.[54] Early, fractionated, and prolonged atrial electric activation times during the tachycardia are found to be the characteristics of a promising radiofrequency catheter ablation site (Fig. 11-19).[22]

Management

Only symptomatic attacks require treatment, which is best achieved with beta-blocking drugs (Fig. 11-20); but these can only be used in the absence of other features of sinus node disease. Both digoxin and verapamil have also been effective. Only rarely is this arrhythmia relatively more responsive to the quinidine-like antiarrhythmic drugs. Permanent pacing to either overdrive or interrupt attacks has so far not been required, although pacemaker implantation might conceivably be needed if antiarrhythmic drugs became necessary for the control of attacks in a patient with associated SA node disease at risk of sinus

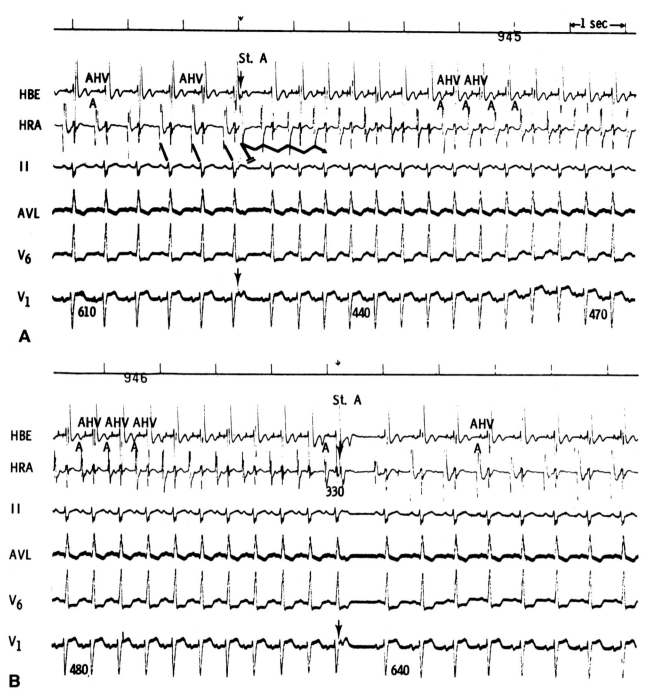

Figure 11-14. Initiation and termination of paroxysmal sinus node reentrant tachycardia by programmed atrial extrastimulation. Note that the initiating atrial extrastimulus fails to traverse the atrioventricular node, thereby excluding this structure from participation in the atrial tachycardia mechanism. (*St. A*, induced premature atrial extra beat)

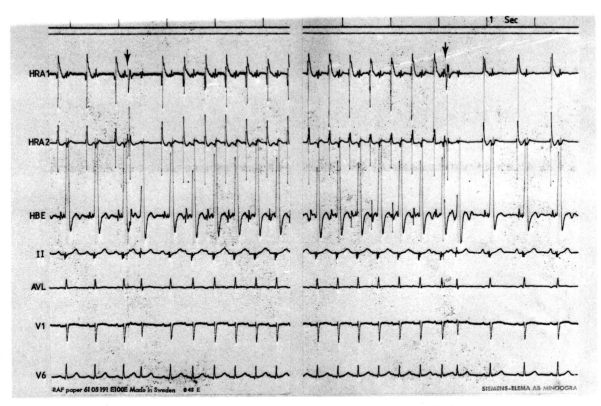

Figure 11-15. Initiation and termination of paroxysmal sinus node reentrant tachycardia by programmed extrastimulation.

arrest. Propafenone, a class IC agent, has also been useful in the management of this arrhythmia. Flecainide, although reported to be effective in the management of a variety of atrial arrhythmias but considering its proarrhythmic effect even in the absence of left ventricular dysfunction, should be used cautiously. Although resistant cases are rare, sotalol and amiodarone has been found effective. Again, one should be aware of the possible association with sinus node dysfunction.

Although occasionally in mildly symptomatic cases, reassurance through accurate diagnosis is all the treatment the patient requires of the physician, in drug refractory cases, the option of radiofrequency catheter ablation of this tachycardia must be considered. In our experience, up to 80% of patients with SA nodal reentrant tachycardia have other forms of supraventricular tachycardia—most commonly, AV nodal reentrant tachycardia.[22] In these conditions, radiofrequency catheter ablation of all tachycardias in the same session should be considered.

Most of these arrhythmias require medical therapy; however, because of the side effects and lifelong treatment required for these tachycardias and the safety and efficacy of radiofrequency catheter ablation, this technique is increasingly popular for curative treatment.[22] Characteristics of successful ablation sites during this tachycardia are similar to those of atrial tachycardia and include early, fractionated, and prolonged endocardial atrial activation regarding the timing of the surface P wave (see Fig. 11-19). Of interest, in our series, none of the patients who underwent radiofrequency ablation of SA nodal reentrant tachycardia required pacemaker implantation.[22]

Inappropriate Sinus Tachycardia

Previously, the term inappropriate sinus tachycardia has been applied to any sinus tachycardia occurring in the absence of a physiologic explanation such as exercise, fever, and catecholamine release due to anxiety or panic attack. This broad definition includes what is called SA nodal reentrant tachycardia and nonphysiologic sinus tachycardia. The latter is commonly called inappropriate sinus tachycardia with the following characteristics: (1) P-wave morphology and axis during tachycardia similar to that of sinus rhythm, (2) lack of initiation or termination of tachycardia by a critically timed atrial premature stimulus, and (3) initiation of tachycardia with β-adrenergic stimulation such as isoproterenol or aminophylline and a blunted response to administration of atropine, indicating low vagal tone.

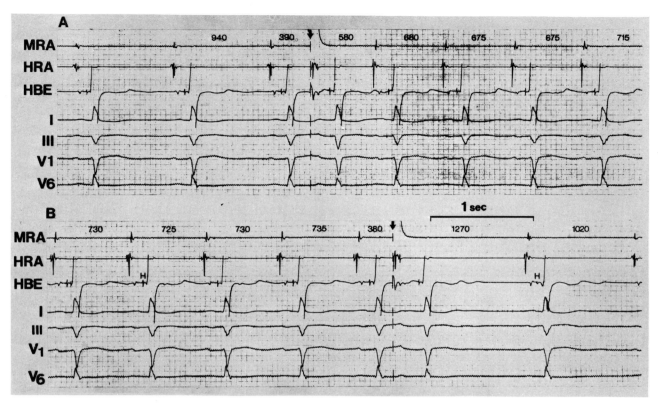

Figure 11-16. The sequence of atrial activation in the initiated attack of paroxysmal sinus node reentrant tachycardia is identical to that in normal sinus beats seen before (first three beats, *upper panel*) and after (last two atrial beats, *lower panel*) the tachycardia. The heart rate in tachycardia is only about 85 beats per minute. Sinus node recovery is affected by the preceding tachycardia—not a feature of normal sinus rhythm. Note the subtle change in configuration of the high right atrial electrogram (*HRA*) at the onset of tachycardia. *HBE*, His bundle electrogram; *MRA*, mid-right atrial electrogram.

Management of inappropriate sinus tachycardia is difficult. These patients often fail multiple medications, including β-adrenergic blockers, calcium channel blockers, and class I antiarrhythmics. Cardiovascular fitness and physical conditioning may improve their symptoms by increasing resting vagal tone. The preliminary results of radiofrequency catheter ablation and modification of sinus node in five patients with inappropriate sinus tachycardia indicate that it may be a promising therapy of last resort, although three patients required permanent pacemaker.[55]

ATRIAL TACHYCARDIA

Terminology

Several terms (e.g., ectopic atrial tachycardia, focal atrial tachycardia, primary atrial tachycardia, interatrial reentrant tachycardia, SA nodal reentrant tachycardia, and auto-matic atrial tachycardia) have been used for atrial tachycardia, depending on its underlying mechanism. The term "atrial tachycardia" may actually be applied to all these tachycardias, regardless of underlying mechanism.

Mechanism

Reentry is thought to be the most common mechanism for atrial tachycardias. Less often, the underlying mechanism is presumed to be enhanced automaticity or triggered activity. As reported by Brugada and Wellens, it is often difficult to distinguish reentry from triggered activity by using the conventional criteria of electrophysiologic methods such as mode of induction and termination, effect of timed premature beats, overdriving, and the effect of automatic tone alteration on the tachycardia.[56] In this chapter, SA nodal reentrant tachycardia is classified and discussed separately.

Focal and reentrant mechanisms are both important as causative factors in this group of pure atrial arrhythmias

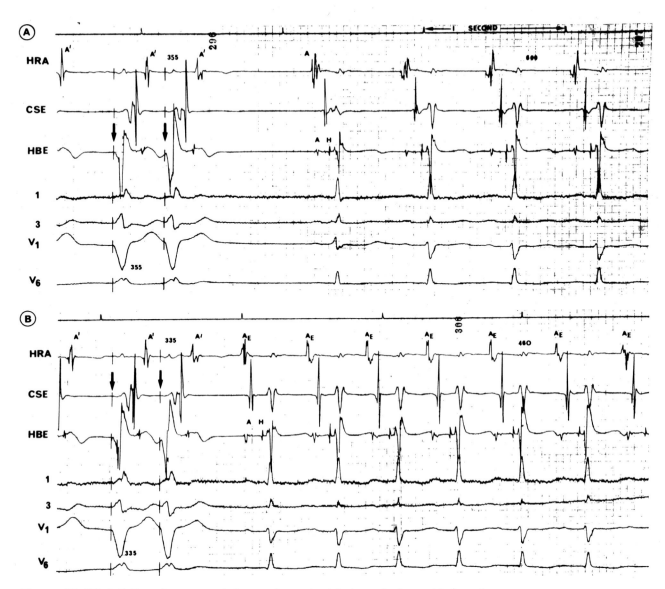

Figure 11-17. Initiation of paroxysmal sinus node reentrant tachycardia by ventricular extra-stimulation, with retrograde conduction to the atria occurring across a left-sided accessory atrioventricular pathway that is "latent" in sinus rhythm (*CSE*, left atrial electrogram from electrode in coronary sinus precedes atrial activity on other atrial leads during ventricular pacing). (**A**) Normal sinus rhythm after ventricular pacing. (**B**) Induced sinus node reentrant tachycardia.

that usually arise independently of abnormalities of either the sinus or AV nodes. The acronym PAT (*p*aroxysmal *a*trial *t*achycardia) has previously been widely applied but it is clear that true PAT is a comparatively rare or infrequently recognized arrhythmia and paroxysmal supraventricular tachycardia is a better and more accurate terminology.

Most often, the patient with paroxysmal or chronic atrial tachycardia is a child or young adult; alternatively, digoxin toxicity is causative.[57] We have observed few cases of chronic atrial tachycardia in children without any clinically detectable structural heart disease that were resistant

to virtually all available antiarrhythmic agents. Generally, however, most children with atrial tachycardia have structural cardiac disease. Perhaps in adult patients with atrial tachycardia structural heart disease is less common.

The symptoms are those of any regular paroxysmal supraventricular tachycardia in which the rate is about 150 to 200 beats per minute. Occasionally, atrial tachycardia appears to be incessant and if recurrent or chronic, it may result in tachycardia-induced cardiomyopathy. Generally, left ventricular function improves gradually after the elimination of the tachycardia.

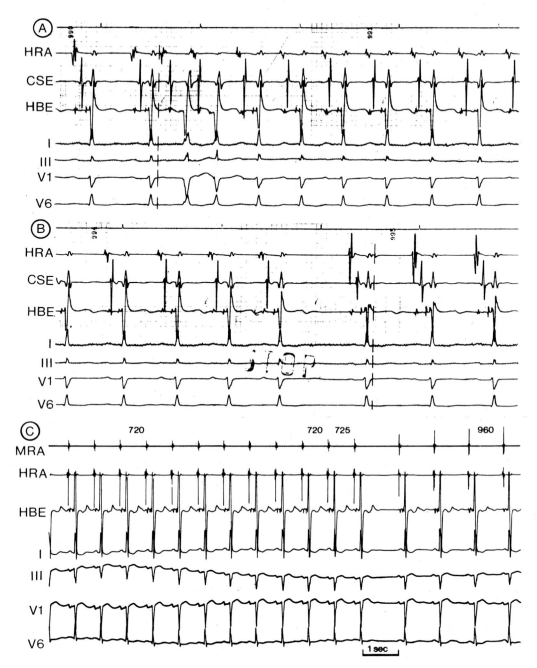

Figure 11-18. Examples of gradual slowing of paroxysmal sinus note reentrant tachycardia before spontaneously terminating. (**A**) Initiation. (**B**) Termination. (**C**) Abrupt termination in different patients.

The electrocardiographic features are often specific and include eccentric P-wave activity that in more than half the cases does *not* suggest an origin in the environs of either of the two nodal areas (Fig. 11-21). P-wave morphology during atrial tachycardia recorded on 12-lead ECG is useful in differentiating the site of origin of right from left atrial tachycardia. A positive P-wave vector in lead aV_L with a negative or isoelectric P-wave vector in lead V_1 is sensi-

tive and specific for atrial tachycardias arising from the right atrium, as is a positive P-wave vector in lead V_1 and a negative or isoelectric P-wave vector in lead aV_L for the left atrial tachycardias.[58] Additionally, the PR interval must be prolonged if the tachycardia arises remote from the AV node. A short PR interval suggests an origin within or with rapid access to the AV node.

Initiation usually occurs spontaneously and—in com-

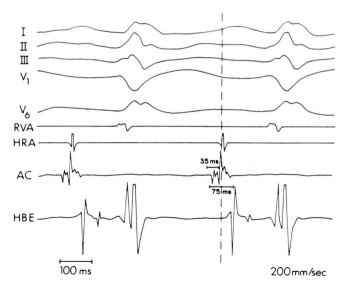

Figure 11-19. Surface and intracardiac recordings during sinoatrial node reentrant tachycardia. The ablation catheter (AC) is located at the site of successful radiofrequency current ablation of sinoatrial node reentrant tachycardia. Local atrial activation occurs 35 milliseconds before the surface P wave. The local atrial electrogram is markedly fractionated and has a duration of 75 milliseconds. (From Sanders WE, et al: Sinoatrial node reentrant tachycardia ablation. J Am Coll Cardiol 1994;23(4):926)

mon with paroxysmal sinus node reentrant tachycardia—without the need for antecedent premature extrasystoles. Sometimes, however, it appears to arise in association with a late-coupled atrial extrasystole but the P-wave configuration in tachycardia remains that of the extrasystole, suggesting either enhanced spontaneous focal activity or wide-zone reentrant tachycardia with atypical initiation.[49]

Spontaneous termination and duration of attacks are less predictable than for sinus node reentrant tachycardia. Perhaps automatic atrial tachycardia is relatively insensitive to the effects of alterations in vagal tone, a feature that is used in differential diagnosis (Table 11-3). Figure 11-22 illustrates a repetitive form of atrial tachycardia and Figure 11-23 shows an example of a incessant atrial tachycardia with occasional sinus beats in a young asymptomatic female. Holter monitoring is useful in investigating the characteristics of this tachycardia and its response to therapy.

Intracardiac Studies

Atrial tachycardia may be initiated in one of three ways: (1) after premature extrastimulation; (2) spontaneously, with late-coupled atrial extrasystoles whose P wave configura-

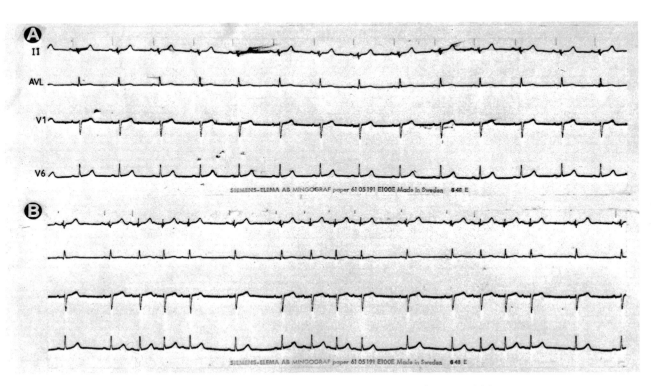

Figure 11-20. (**A**) Suppression of paroxysmal sinus node reentrant tachycardia after practolol (a beta blocking drug). (**B**) The effect wears off as time passes, although attacks are not so sustained.

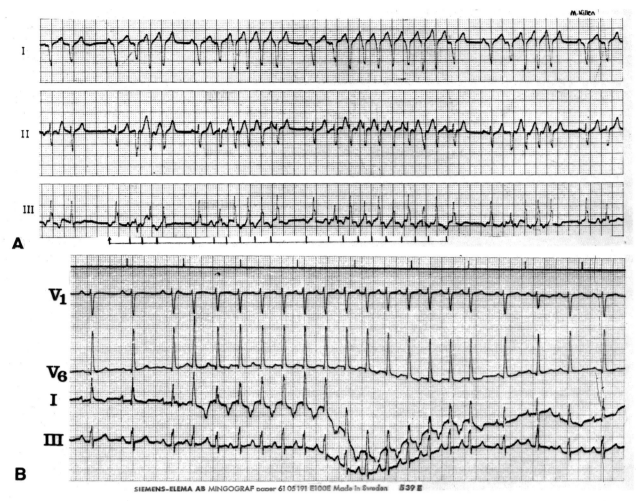

Figure 11-21. Two different examples of spontaneously occurring paroxysmal atrial tachycardia. Mild ventricular aberration in the upper electrocardiogram (ECG) strips compounds diagnosis, although careful scrutiny of the traces finds the P waves of the tachycardia. The negative P waves in tachycardia in ECG lead I of the lower example suggest that they are arising in the left atrium.

tion is identical to that seen during tachycardia; and (3) after sinus acceleration (Fig. 11-24). Initiation of atrial tachycardias with presumed abnormal automaticity (using either programmed extrastimulation or incremental pacing) is rarely reproducible, although we have experience of several cases with reentrant or triggered activity features (Fig. 11-25; see Fig. 11-21).[59, 60] A warm-up or acceleration phase often follows an initiation of the tachycardia.[61] Atrial mapping during the atrial tachycardia confirms the eccentric extranodal origin of such arrhythmias. Figure 11-26 illustrates differences in the sequence of activation during atrial tachycardia and sinus beats.

A reentrant atrial circuit is assumed to be the underlying mechanism of the paroxysmal atrial tachycardia if certain "capture phenomena" are obtained with *atrial* extrastimuli or if the tachycardia can be terminated with

this method from a pacing site that is remote from and later than sites of earliest activation during tachycardia. In effect, such impulses gain access to the reentrant circuit through the "back door" and closer to the "weak link" in the circuit, where the refractory period is longest (Fig. 11-27). On most occasions, however, persistent attempts with atrial overdrive pacing are required to suppress the tachycardia if it shows features of enhanced focal activity (Fig. 11-28).[45, 62]

In incessant forms of atrial tachycardia (probably due to automatic foci), overdrive pacing fails to terminate the tachycardia (Fig. 11-29). Even when atrial flutter was induced with rapid atrial pacing, on cessation of atrial flutter, atrial tachycardia resumed (Fig. 11-30).

Preliminary reports suggest that in adult patients, most atrial tachycardias are located in the right atrium,

TABLE 11-3. Characteristic Differences Between Paroxysmal Sinus Node Reentrant Tachycardia and Paroxysmal Pure Atrial Tachycardia

	Sinus Node Reentrant Tachycardia	Other Atrial Tachycardia
Rate (beats/min)	90–150	150–250
P wave	Similar to sinus rhythm	Different from sinus rhythm
Atrial mapping	Similar to sinus rhythm	Different from sinus rhythm
Initiation		
Sinus rhythm rate change	+ + +	0
Paced rate change	+ + +	+ +
Premature beat	+ + + (Effective zone in sinus rate is near sinoatrial node)	+ +
Duration	Short-lived	Often sustained
Termination		
Spontaneous with slowing	+ + +	+
Carotid sinus massage	+ + +	0 or +
Premature beat	+ + +	+
Drug Effects		
Atropine	+ + +	0
Verapamil	—	+ + or 0 or −
Beta blocker	—	—
Lanoxin	—	−
Quinidine-like drugs	—	—
Adenosine	—	— or 0
Independence of atrioventricular node	+	+
Cycle-length alternation	+ +	+

+, enhances; −, depresses; 0, not an important feature; more + or -, more specific effect.

whereas in children, most atrial tachycardias may originate from the left atrium.[18,19] The region of crista terminalis, located between the sinus node and AV node, has specific characteristics, such as high vagal innervation; inhomogeneity of muscle orientation, implying anisotropy; and inhomogeneity of repolarization and cell types. These specific properties of the crista terminalis may predispose this structure to various arrhythmias, and may explain the higher frequency of atrial tachycardias which have originated from the right atrium.

Management

Acute

Similar to acute clinical syndrome of supraventricular tachycardias, in acute presentation of atrial tachycardia, the main goal is to improve the patient's hemodynamics. Supine resting is essential for hemodynamic stability before considering vagal maneuvers such as Valsalva's or carotid sinus massage to facilitate tachycardia termination. Unless

REPETITIVE ATRIAL TACHYCARDIA (140 BPM)

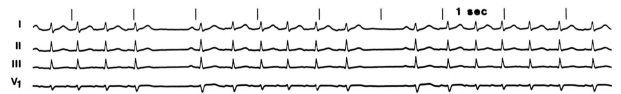

Figure 11-22. An example of repetitive atrial tachycardia in a patient without any clinically significant cardiac abnormality. Note that the PR interval during atrial tachycardia is longer than the occasional sinus beat. The QRS morphology is identical to those in sinus rhythm. The tachycardia initiates and terminates spontaneously.

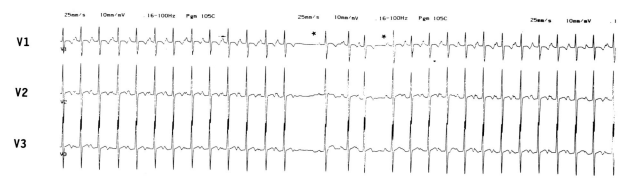

Figure 11-23. Three electrocardiograph leads from a patient having incessant atrial tachycardia with occasional sinus beats (asterisks). This patient has suffered from atrial tachycardia for several years and does not have any detectable cardiovascular abnormality.

the patient is in a hemodynamic collapse, a 12-lead surface ECG must be obtained to guide diagnosis and localize the tachycardia focus. Documentation of the tachycardia may prevent unnecessary invasive electrophysiologic testing. Almost all sinus node reentrant tachycardias slow significantly and terminate with a proper vagal maneuver.[22] Atrial tachycardias with other mechanisms may or may not be terminated with carotid sinus message. Rapid intravenous administration of 10 mg (after a test dose of 1 mg) edrophonium, a cholinestrase inhibitor, may terminate some cases of atrial tachycardia by enhancing the vagal tone (Fig. 11-31).

Rapid intravenous administration of exogenous adenosine terminates almost all episodes of SA nodal reentrant tachycardia, AV nodal reentrant tachycardia, AV reciprocating tachycardia (i.e., Wolff-Parkinson-White syndrome),

and some cases of atrial tachycardia (Figs. 11-32 through 11-34).[52] This may be the case for vagal maneuvers and edrophonium, although the relation of mechanism of atrial tachycardia to its response to vagal maneuvers and adenosine remains uncertain. The high efficacy of adenosine in terminating paroxysmal supraventricular tachycardias and its short half-life of less than 10 seconds make adenosine comparable or superior to intravenous verapamil in acute situations such as emergency room visits.

Verapamil has been most and safely used in acute presentations of narrow complex tachycardias. Care must be taken to prevent the potential vasodilatory effect of verapamil, which may further deteriorate hypotension. This is particularly important in wide-complex tachycardias, in which verapamil may cause hypotension in the

Text continues on p. 352

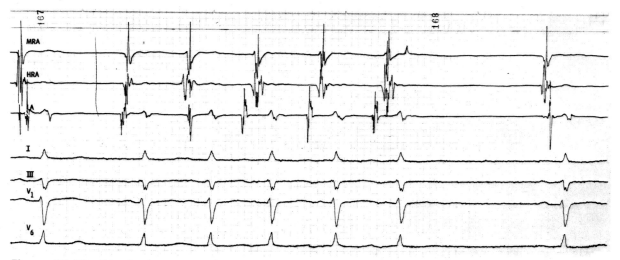

Figure 11-24. Short-lived spontaneously occurring atrial tachycardia, showing "shifting" activation sequence, with the left atrium finally winning the atrium on the last three beats. That the electrodes had not moved is shown by the comparable appearance of the atrial "map" in the two sinus beats that frame the tachycardia. *MRA*, mid-right atrium; *HRA*, high right atrium; *LA*, left atrium; *I*, *II*, *V₁*, and *V₆*, electrocardiogram leads.

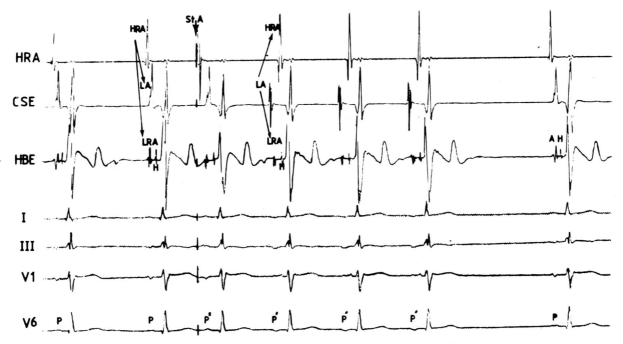

Figure 11-25. Short run of lower-left atrial tachycardia (*CSE* [coronary sinus electrode] activity precedes that of other leads), initiated by a right atrial extrastimulus (*StA*). The first two beats and the last beat are normal sinus beats.

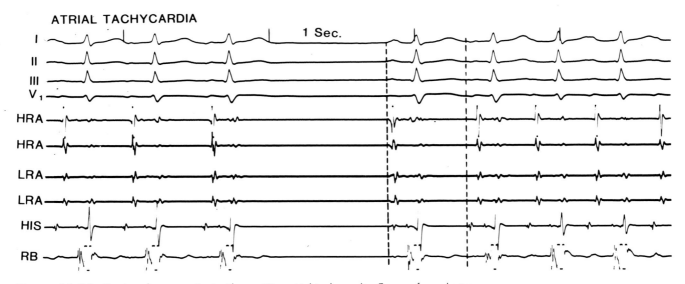

Figure 11-26. Tracings from a patient with repetitive atrial tachycardia. Four surface electrocardiographic leads are recorded, as are intracardiac electrograms from high right atrium (*HRA*), low right atrium (*LRA*), and *HIS*-bundle and right bundle (*RB*) electrogram. Note the difference in the sequence of activation from sinus beat, compared with the atrial tachycardia (*dotted lines*). During normal sinus rhythm, a sequence of activation is from high right atrium to low right atrium, whereas during atrial tachycardia, the earliest atrial activity is detected on the low right septal atrium recorded from the His-bundle electrograph.

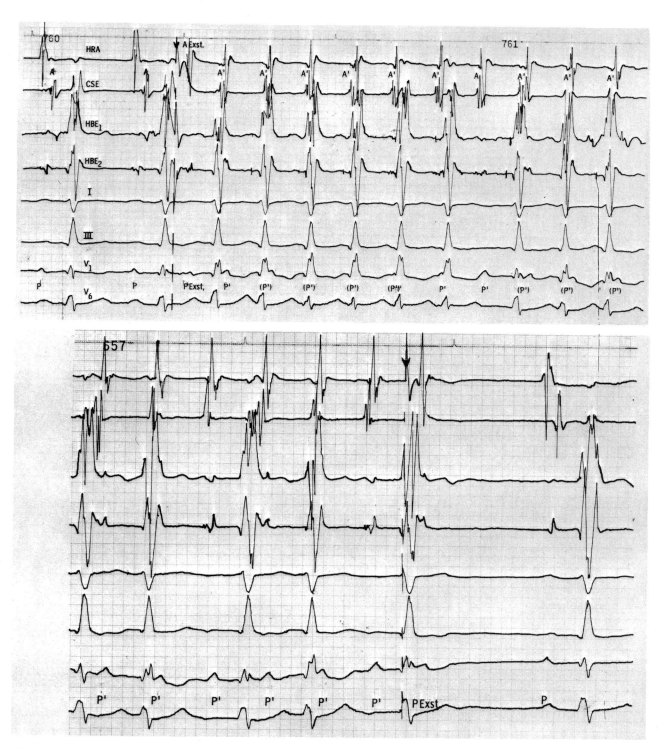

Figure 11-27. Initiation and termination of a mid-atrial paroxysmal tachycardia by programmed extra-atrial stimulation (*P Exst, arrowhead*). Variable atrioventricular (AV) conduction occurs during the attack, which excludes participation of the AV node in the arrhythmia mechanism.

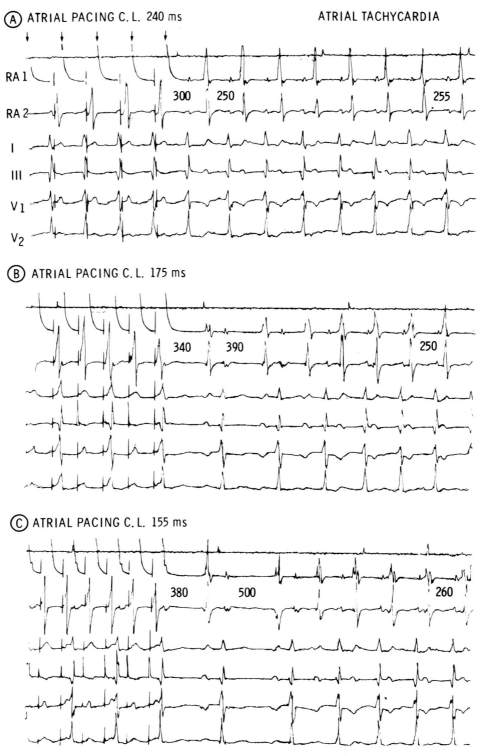

Figure 11-28. Overdrive atrial pacing at three different rates in an attempt to terminate paroxysmal atrial tachycardia. With higher-paced atrial frequencies, more suppression of the focus is obtained but it recovers before the sinus node on each occasion. Ajmaline was used successfully to stop the attack.

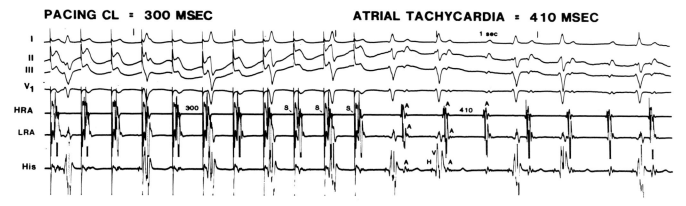

Figure 11-29. A patient with incessant atrial tachycardia, in whom atrial pacing is performed at the cycle length of 300 milliseconds, with a 1:1 atrial capture with variable degrees of atrioventricular (AV) conduction. On termination of pacing, the tachycardia resumes with cycle length of 410 milliseconds, with AV nodal Wenckebach-type.

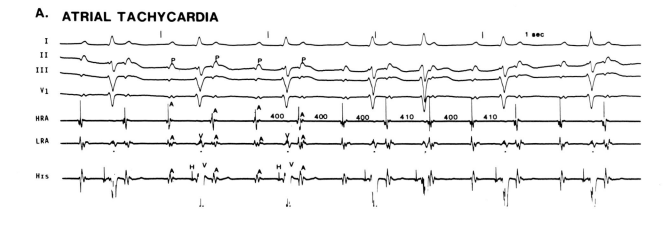

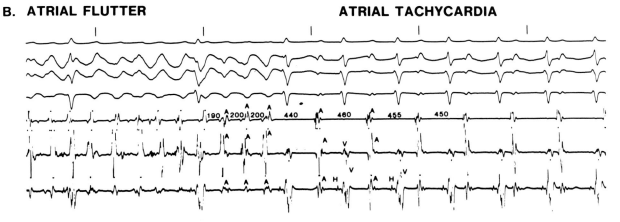

Figure 11-30. (**A**) From the same patient as in Figure 11-26, showing atrial tachycardia with variable degrees of atrioventricular conduction, which failed to terminate during atrial pacing, as was shown in Figure 11-26. (**B**) Finally, atrial flutter is induced with rapid atrial pacing; on termination of atrial flutter, atrial tachycardia resumes again.

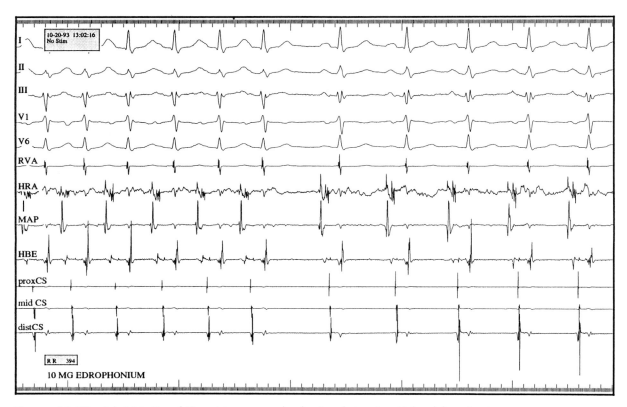

Figure 11-31. Administration of 10 mg intravenous edrophonium during sinoatrial nodal reentrant tachycardia in the same patient as in Figure 11-13. Note the prolongation of tachycardia cycle length before its termination. Atrial activation sequence during tachycardia is similar to that of sinus rhythm. Abbreviations are as in Figure 11-13.

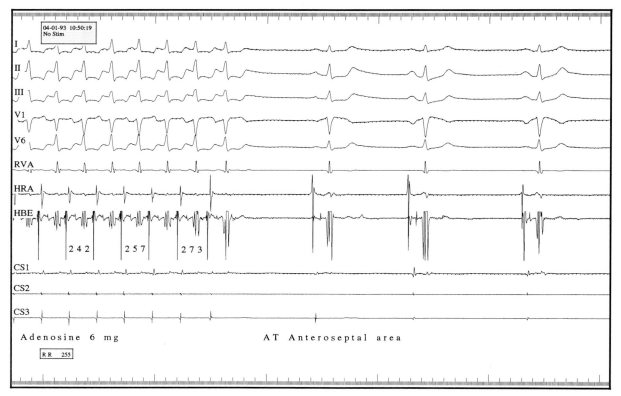

Figure 11-32. Effect of rapid intravenous administration of 6 mg of adenosine during sustained atrial tachycardia located in anteroseptal area of the right atrium. Note the prolongation of tachycardia cycle length before its termination. Abbreviations are as in Figure 11-13.

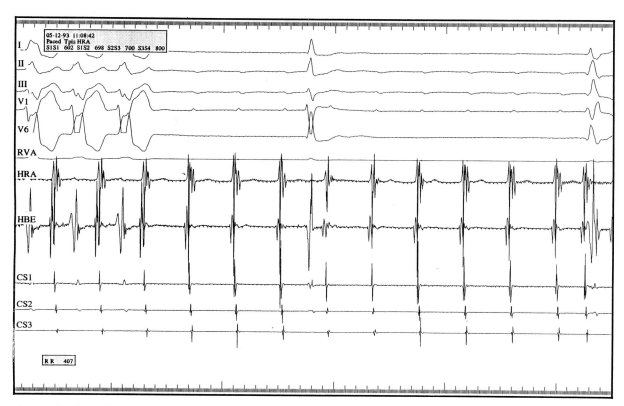

Figure 11-33. Effect of adenosine on an automatic atrial tachycardia arising in the His bundle. Note the presence of high-degree atrioventricular block without any alteration of tachycardia cycle length. Abbreviations are as in Figure 11-13. *CS1, CS2, CS3*, proximal, mid, and distal coronary sinus electrograms, respectively.

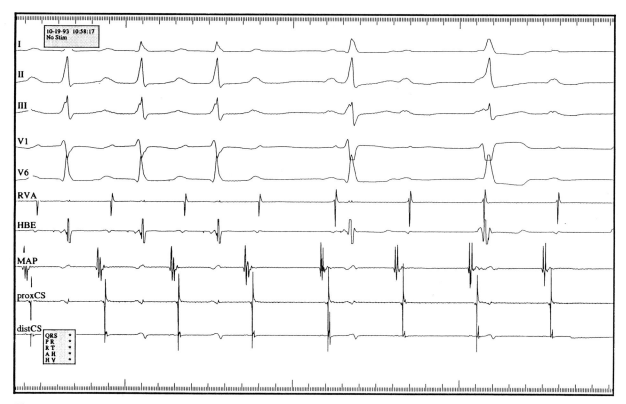

Figure 11-34. Effect of adenosine on sustained atrial tachycardia arising in the left atrium. Note the presence of high-degree atrioventricular block without affecting the tachycardia cycle length. Abbreviations are as in Figure 11-13.

presence of ventricular tachycardia, leading to hemo-dynamic collapse requiring electric cardioversion. In all likelihood, because verapamil has a longer half-life than adenosine, reinitiation of atrial tachycardia soon after its termination may be suppressed by verapamil. Intravenous procainamide (in the absence of hypotension) may be reserved for atrial tachycardias refractory to verapamil. Electric cardioversion of the tachycardia must be considered in unstable patient. Automatic atrial tachycardias are prone to immediate reinitiation after termination of these tachycardias. Therefore, pharmacologic management is more effective and is superior than electric cardioversion in these cases.

Chronic

PHARMACOLOGIC

To prevent attacks and chronic suppression of atrial tachycardia, the mostly practiced treatment is with a combination of digoxin (for ventricular protection) and a quinidine-like drug specifically targeting the arrhythmia as it arises within the working atrial myocardium. Disopyramide, propafenone, and flecainide are the most useful drugs in this latter category. This therapeutic regimen is based on the results of acute pharmacologic studies during intracardiac tests, in which it was found that verapamil effectively increased the protection afforded by the AV node against the transmission of rapid atrial impulses (Fig. 11-35) but sometimes had the paradoxical effect of accelerating the atrial rate. It is well known that verapamil may convert atrial flutter to atrial fibrillation, as does carotid sinus massage occasionally, presumably shortening the refractory period of the atrial myocardium. In contrast, ajmaline (a quinidine-like drug) slowed and finally stopped the tachycardia, restoring sinus rhythm (see Fig. 11-35). In one case, the tachycardia was terminated only after cessation of pacing-induced atrial flutter during administration of procainamide (Fig. 11-36). In this particular case, oral disopyramide failed to terminate tachycardia but it enhanced AV nodal conduction, causing 1:1 conduction during tachycardia (Fig. 11-37), whereas oral flecainide controlled the tachycardia and the patient re-

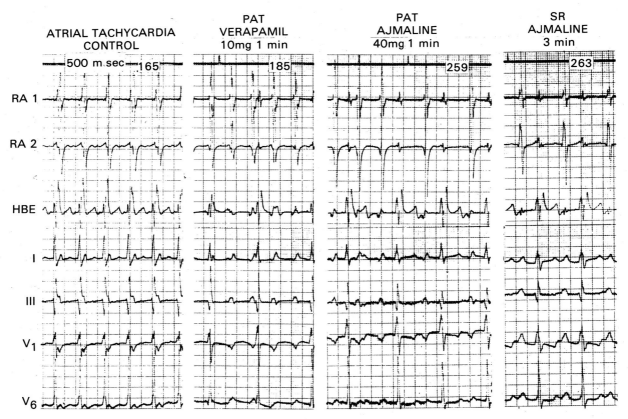

Figure 11-35. The relative sensitivity of paroxysmal "pure" atrial tachycardia (*control*) to (1) verapamil, which slows the ventricular rate through partial atrioventricular nodal block but increases the atrial rate, perhaps by vasodilation induced hypotension and beta adrenergic stimulation; and (2) ajmaline, which slows and finally terminates the tachycardia, restoring sinus rhythm (*last panel*). Carotid sinus massage had the same effect as verapamil in this case.

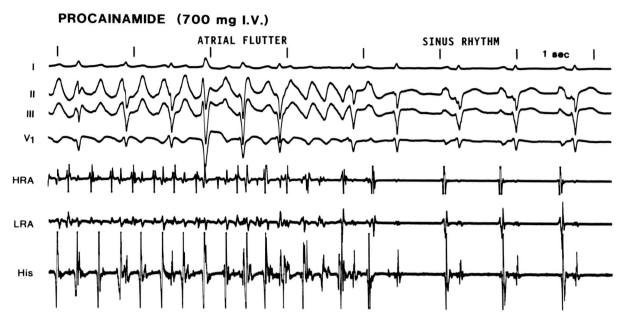

Figure 11-36. From the same patient as in Figure 11-29 and 11-30. Because the tachycardia did not terminate with atrial pacing and even after induction of atrial flutter, procainamide was administered intravenously and the tachycardia was terminated only after administration of procainamide when atrial flutter was terminated. Note the change in the P-wave morphology during sinus rhythm in this figure, compared with P-wave morphology during atrial tachycardia in Figure 11-29.

ORAL DISOPYRAMIDE

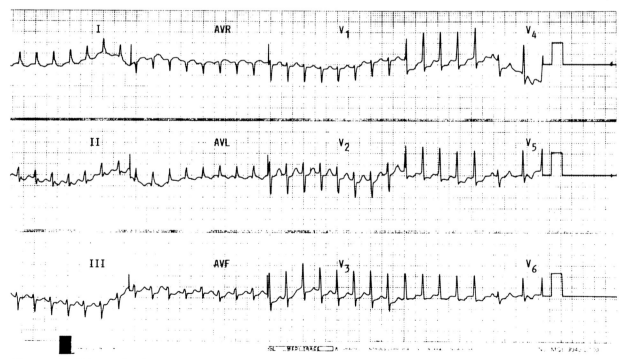

Figure 11-37. Atrial tachycardia with variable degrees of atrioventricular (AV) Wenckebach block. When oral disopyramide was administered, it did not terminate tachycardia; however, it enhanced AV nodal conduction time and the patient has a 1:1 atrioventricular response.

mained in sinus rhythm (Fig. 11-38). Amiodarone is most effective for such arrhythmias because it has properties of both of digoxin and a beta-blocking drug.[63,64] Drugs such as flecainide or propafenone may be worth trying, although further experience with these agents is needed to determine their efficacy and potential proarrhythmic effects. In our experience, propafenone and sotalol are effective and well tolerated. In cases where atrial tachycardia arises in a setting of possible digoxin toxicity, this drug should temporarily be withdrawn, pending results of a plasma digoxin assay. Verapamil can be used in the interim if an alternative is really needed.

NONPHARMACOLOGIC

Special pacing techniques are rarely needed on a long-term basis.[65] Even more rare is the need for surgery to ablate the refractory focus.[66,67] The safety and efficacy of radiofrequency catheter ablation of atrial tachycardia in medically refractory cases has been widely reported and has become a reasonable curative choice in some individuals.[68–71]

RADIOFREQUENCY CATHETER ABLATION

Radiofrequency catheter ablation has become increasingly more popular as the curative procedure for medi-

cally refractory paroxysmal supraventricular tachycardias, particularly AV nodal reentrant tachycardia and AV reentrant tachycardia involving an accessory pathway.

Transcatheter ablation of the site of origin of these tachycardias, using direct current, was favored over surgical ablation to avoid surgical morbidity of thoracotomy.[69–71] The finding that radiofrequency catheter ablation is safe and highly effective for the treatment of Wolff-Parkinson-White syndrome and AV nodal reentrant tachycardia led to the application of this technique for the curative treatment of other atrial arrhythmias, such as atrial tachycardia and atrial flutter. The limited experience with radiofrequency catheter ablation of medically refractory atrial tachycardia indicates this procedure is well tolerated and effective.[69–71] Nonetheless, reports on the electrophysiologic characteristics of the site of origin and the successful ablation site of these tachycardias are conflicting; therefore, further investigation is warranted. The reported success of radiofrequency ablation of atrial tachycardias is more than 90%, with a recurrence of up to 20% and permanent pacemaker requirement of 5%. The prolongation and fractionation of earliest atrial activation during atrial tachycardia are the most promising factors for successful ablation sites.[22] These approaches require further experience and long-term follow-up.

ORAL FLECAINIDE

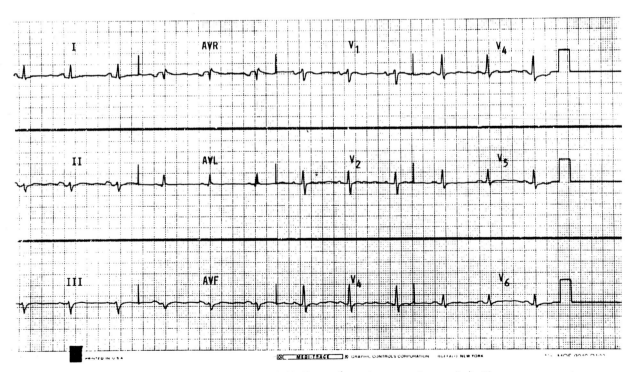

Figure 11-38. From the same patient as in Figure 11-30. This tachycardia was well controlled with oral flecainide and remained in sinus rhythm.

SURGICAL ABLATION

Surgical ablation of medically refractory atrial tachycardias has been reported, with a favorable outcome in the pre–catheter ablation era.[72, 73] It is worth mentioning that intraoperative mapping of atrial tachycardias during general anesthesia may be limited by the suppressant effects of anesthesia and hypothermia, which may further complicate the surgical procedure.[73]

Overall, the reported curative rate of surgical ablation of atrial tachycardias is about 70% to 90%, with a 20% risk of permanent pacemaker requirement.

CHAOTIC AND MULTIFOCAL ATRIAL TACHYCARDIA

Chaotic and multifocal atrial tachycardia is a moderately uncommon arrhythmia, usually seen with acute disturbances of atrial function or as a transitional atrial tachyarrhythmia in a natural history of atrial disease that culminates in atrial fibrillation.[1, 74–77] There appears to be a higher incidence of this arrhythmia in the elderly and in those with chronic pulmonary disease, although it is not known whether the chronic use of medications such as bronchodilators and β_2-adrenoreceptor stimulants is a causative factor in this latter group.[78] It is an unusual arrhythmia particularly when it occurs in patients with suspected digoxin toxicity.[79]

Electrocardiographic Features

The mean atrial rate during multifocal atrial tachycardia often exceeds 100 beats per minute but is rarely greater than 150 (Fig. 11-39). Random variation is seen in the PP interval, and P-wave morphology shows at least three different successive foci.[80] The different P waves occur in random arrangement, variously interspersed with periods of more normal atrial activity (sinus rhythm). Most atrial impulses are conducted so that the net hemodynamic and thereby the symptomatic effects are determined by the atrial arrhythmia more than by the AV node—a subtle distinction from the situation in atrial fibrillation. Most often, the resultant mean ventricular rate is tolerable; indeed, the patient may be unaware of the arrhythmia. Exercise is provocative, as is fever. Often, it is the underlying cardiovascular or respiratory disease that causes more symptoms than this arrhythmia.

Twenty-four hour ECG monitoring is appropriate for both the diagnosis and assessment of this arrhythmia. It is also appropriate for assessing any response to therapy, if needed. The need for intracardiac electrophysiologic studies is rare.

Management

Treatment is usually primarily directed toward the causative illness but a combination of digoxin with a quinidine-like drug tends to control the situation, pending spontaneous improvement or progression to chronic atrial

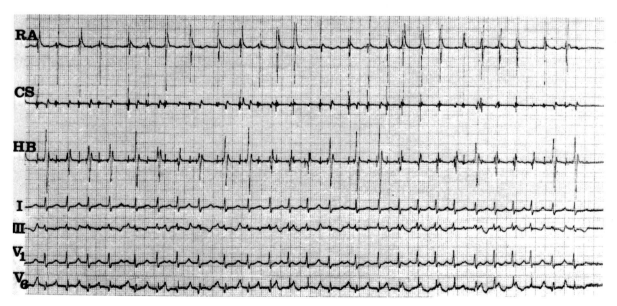

Figure 11-39. Multifocal atrial tachycardia.

fibrillation, when the quinidine-like agent can be discontinued. Fortunately, only a tenuous link exists between this arrhythmia and SA disease, so that further sinus node depression and the need for support pacing are not usually part of management of this disorder. Amiodarone is also effective in the management of this arrhythmia. When this arrhythmia becomes unresponsive to pharmacologic agents or when it is difficult to control the ventricular response during tachycardia, transvenous catheter ablation of the AV node and insertion of a permanent pacemaker may be required to control symptomatic attacks in these patients.[81]

ATRIAL FLUTTER

Atrial flutter is one of the most common causes of regular supraventricular tachycardia encountered clinically but unlike the situation that exists with paroxysmal reentrant AV tachycardia, atrial flutter usually occurs in association with atrial disease. Both atrial distention and intraatrial delay are predisposing factors.[82] Although still the subject of debate, the precise underlying abnormal electrophysiologic mechanism—whether reentrant or focal—is of little importance to those involved with the clinical management of such cases.[83–85] Most investigators

favor the reentry mechanism. What remains extremely important, however, is the atrial rate, its regularity, and the AV conduction ratio during this arrhythmia because practical management aims to affect these aspects, the priorities being in reverse order. Its differential diagnosis is when 2:1 conduction occurs in AV nodal reentrant tachycardia or orthodromic tachycardias. Carotid sinus massage may be useful to (1) induce transient high-degree AV block, (2) slow ventricular response, and (3) facilitate diagnosis of atrial flutter.

Most often occurring as an acute or transitory arrhythmia, atrial flutter may be chronic, paroxysmal, or repetitive, and sometimes without apparent cause (lone atrial flutter). It is a common complication of acute myocardial infarction and occurs in 14% of those with atrial arrhythmias and sick sinus syndrome but is uncommonly seen in children with cardiac disease.[15,30,86,87] It is a common feature after cardiac surgery and during digoxin toxicity.[88]

Characteristically, atrial rates in atrial flutter are in the range of 230 to 450 beats per minute, with the ventricular rate and ratio also varying in accordance with the refractory properties of the AV conducting system (Figs. 11-40 and 11-41). In new cases without antiarrhythmic agents, the 2:1 AV conduction is most common. In the presence of AV conduction abnormalities or antiarrhythmic drugs, a 3:1 or 4:1 ratio is seen. One-to-one conduction during atrial flutter produces perhaps one of the most serious

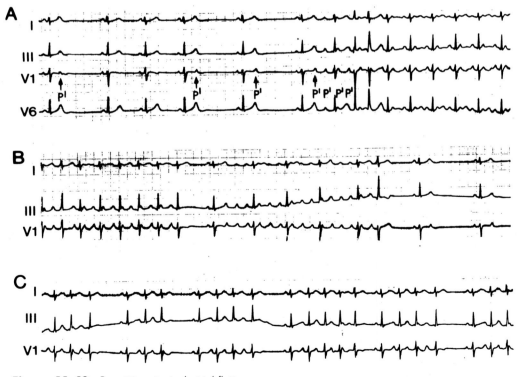

Figure 11-40. Repetitive atypical atrial flutter.

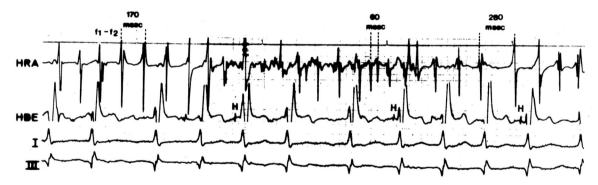

Figure 11-41. Atrial fibrillation among atrial flutter.

arrhythmias and may occur if AV refractoriness is short, as is the case with some patients who have either enhanced or anomalous AV conduction.[89] It may also occur if the atrial rate is slowed by a quinidine-like drug while AV conduction capacity remains enhanced. Cardiovascular reflex compensation is insufficient to avoid significant hypotension when ventricular rates exceed 250 beats per minute, even in those with otherwise normal cardiovascular systems.[61] Exercise and emotional stress increase the ventricular rate during atrial flutter but when the initial AV conduction ratio is only 4:1, the patient may be unaware of the arrhythmia. Increased vagal tone has varying effects. It may reduce the ventricular rate through its effects of increasing AV nodal refractoriness, a feature used in diagnosis to reveal underlying characteristic sawtoothed atrial flutter waves on the ECG. The atrial flutter frequency, however, may increase with maneuvers that increase vagal tone, sometimes precipitating atrial fibrillation.[11, 90, 91] Rarely, such maneuvers restore sinus rhythm but they may precipitate the arrhythmia when applied in sinus rhythm. This condition is called "vagally induced atrial flutter."

The discrete mechanical atrial activity that occurs during atrial flutter, even at rates of 340 beats per minute, may explain the relatively rare occurrence of both atrial thrombi and systemic emboli with this arrhythmia, as compared with atrial fibrillation. Tricuspid regurgitation is rarely seen. Symptoms depend mainly on the rate and regularity of the ventricular response. Restoring sinus rhythm in those with low cardiac output and atrial flutter improves cardiac output. In contrast, lone atrial flutter adversely affects only reserve cardiac output for exercise.[92]

During clinical electrophysiologic studies, atrial electrograms show that the flutter frequency varies both in rate and regularity (Figs. 11-42 and 11-43), especially with changing autonomic tone that occurs, for example, with carotid sinus massage (Fig. 11-44). Most often, rapid overdrive pacing is used to terminate the atrial flutter, either directly, when atrial entrainment must be achieved at an appropriate frequency and for an appropriate duration

(Fig. 11-45),[93] or to induce atrial fibrillation—more stable arrhythmia that has both a lower mean ventricular rate and a greater potential for spontaneous termination. Several comprehensive studies by Waldo describe the types and determinants of successful conversion of atrial flutter to sinus rhythm during atrial overdrive pacing.[94, 95] Acute pharmacologic studies may give results similar to those described for atrial tachycardia regarding relative responsiveness of the atrial arrhythmia and of the AV node. The main indications for intracardiac pacing studies are (1) therapeutic (overdrive termination), and (2) when this arrhythmia occurs as part of the sick sinus syndrome and the need both for pacing and antiarrhythmic drugs can be examined safely. Atrial pacing can also be used for the diagnosis of overt ventricular or junctional preexcitation in patients who present with syncope, one cause of which could be atrial tachyarrhythmia with rapid rates of 1:1 AV conduction across the accessory AV pathway. Transesophageal recording to document the type of atrial arrhythmias and the pacing has been used both in adults and children.[96, 97]

Advances in endocardial mapping of atrial flutter confirm reentry as being the mechanism of this arrhythmia. According to the direction of reentrant wavefront and mapping properties, atrial flutter is classified as typical (common type) and atypical.[98] In typical atrial flutter, the F wave on surface ECG is typically sawtoothed, with negative deflection in inferior leads, such as II, III, and aV$_F$ (Fig. 11-46). The sequence of atrial activation during typical atrial flutter is often from the posteroseptal space, toward the high right atrium, and downward to the lateral wall toward the orifice of inferior vena cava and tricuspid ring. During mapping of typical atrial flutter, a line of functional block along the region of crista terminalis has been observed. In its atypical (uncommon) form, broad flutter waves with inferior axis (positive F wave in inferior leads) are exhibited on surface ECG, and earliest atrial activation is mapped in the high postrolateral region of right atrium (Fig. 11-47; see Figs. 11-1 and 11-40).

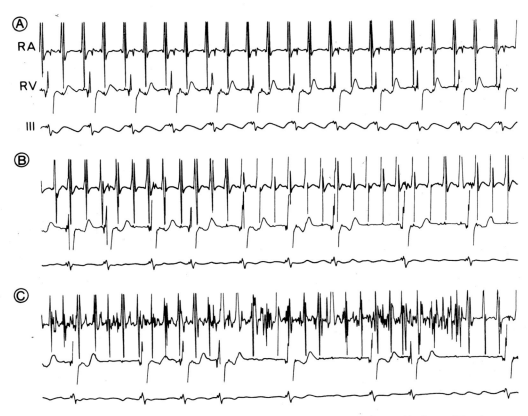

Figure 11-42. Differing atrial frequencies in atrial flutter (**A** and **B**) and in flutter/fibrillation (**C**) in the same patient.

Management

When possible, precipitation factors should be removed; otherwise, prophylaxis for attacks of atrial flutter is best achieved with the safe combination of quinidine or disopyramide with digoxin. Newer agents such as pro-

pafenone (class IC) or sotalol (class III) also can be initiated under electrocardiographic surveillance with favorable outcome. When class IC or III antiarrhythmic agents are used, digoxin should be discontinued or its dose reduced because these agents slow AV nodal conduction and may result in inappropriate slowing of ventricular

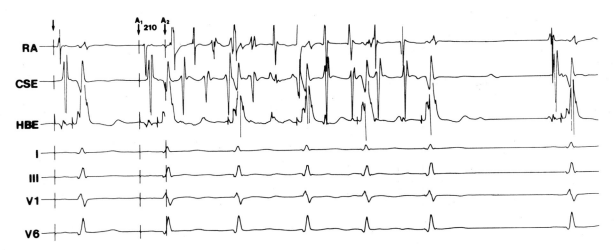

Figure 11-43. Initiation of irregular atrial flutter by programmed atrial extrastimulation during the atrial functional refractory (vulnerable) period.

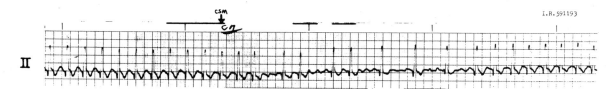

Figure 11-44. Transient conversion of atrial flutter to atrial fibrillation with carotid sinus massage (*CSM*).

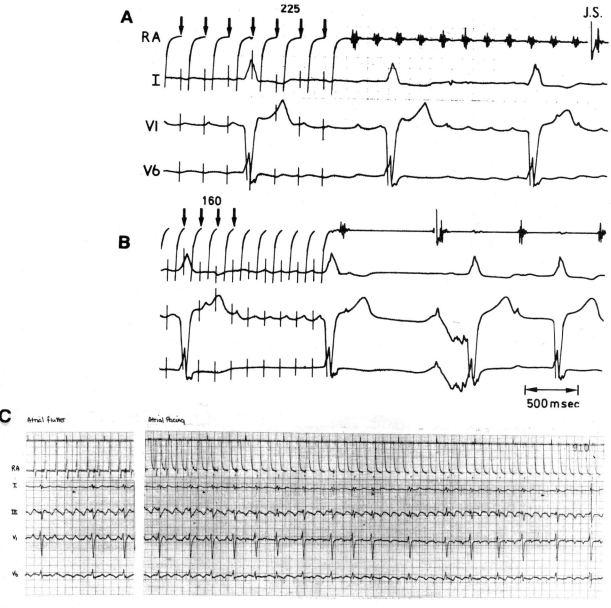

Figure 11-45. (**A**) Inadequate, then (**B**) successful atrial overdrive pacing to terminate atrial flutter. The lowest panel (**C**) shows that entrainment is best seen when more than one surface electrocardiogram lead is recorded during atrial overdrive pacing for atrial flutter.

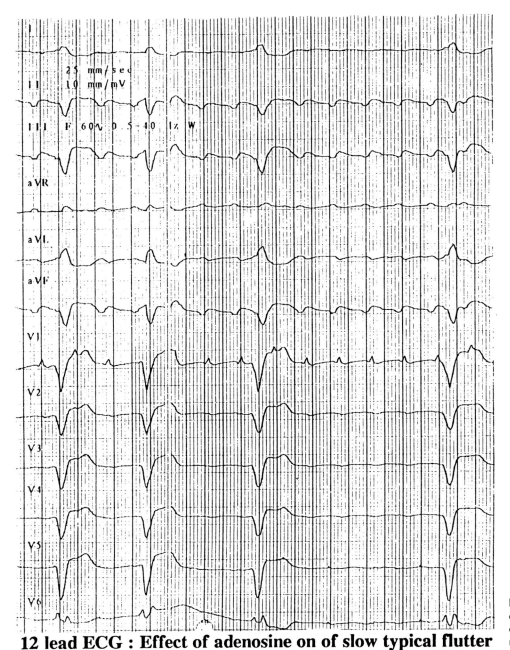

12 lead ECG : Effect of adenosine on of slow typical flutter

(on antiarrhythmic therapy)

Figure 11-46. Electrocardiogram of a patient with typical flutter during administration of adenosine. Slow rate of atrial flutter is related to the antiarrhythmic drug therapy. Note the typical sawtooth flutter waves, which are negative in inferior leads.

response. Amiodarone is used for refractory attacks.[99] Permanent pacing is also required if this arrhythmia occurs as part of the sick sinus syndrome. Quinidine-like drugs should never be given alone, either orally or intravenously, to patients with known 2:1 conduction during atrial flutter to avoid inducing a 1:1 AV response, but they may be safe for those with low ventricular rates.[100] Attacks of rapid atrial flutter can be treated with AV nodal agents such as intravenous esmolol, diltiazem, or verapamil, which readily controls the ventricular rate (at little cost to cardiovascular compensation unless heart failure is overt) and after which either atrial fibrillation or sinus rhythm can

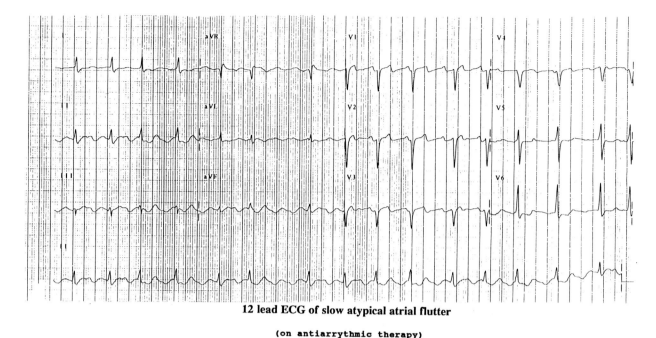

12 lead ECG of slow atypical atrial flutter

(on antiarrythmic therapy)

Figure 11-47. Electrocardiogram of a patient with atypical flutter. Slow rate of atrial flutter is related to the antiarrhythmic drug therapy. Note the absence of typical sawtooth flutter waves in inferior leads.

occur. When digoxin has caused the atrial flutter, digoxin should be withdrawn and consideration should be given to the method of overdrive pacing to stop the attack safely.[101] Newer antiarrhythmic agents such as propafenone, flecainide, and sotalol are also useful in acute management and long-term control of atrial flutter and fibrillation. In the presence of moderate to severe left ventricular dysfunction, however, flecainide should be avoided. Requirements for successful overdrive pacing have been well reported and consist of (1) ensuring good atrial contact; (2) effective atrial activation (entrainment), best followed electrocardiographically on three leads simultaneously; and (3) diligent atrial pacing, which should be gently increased once entrainment is obtained to steady rates that are initially 20, then 40, then 60 beats per minute (and so on) faster than the inherent flutter rate, which should have been recorded and measured before pacing commenced. Most successes are obtained when the initial atrial rhythm is regular. Conversely, flutter-–fibrillation is more difficult to capture. Atrial fibrillation is the more likely outcome of overdrive pacing in this latter group (but this is an acceptable outcome). Skill in this art comes only with experience, assisted by the use of the right equipment.[62,85,93,103,104] Temporary epicardial atrial electrodes are extremely useful in this context after heart surgery, both for diagnosis and management. Only "synchronized" cardioversion should be used if this alternative

is chosen to restore sinus rhythm. Long-term oral anticoagulants for those patients in whom rapid ventricular response produces hemodynamic embarrassment is advisable. Ablation of the AV node and implantation of a permanent pacemaker remains a suitable therapy.[81] Ablation of atrial tissue without AV nodal ablation has been reported.[105,106] These reports indicate that most atrial flutters could be safely and effectively ablated using radiofrequency catheter ablation technique, with a low incidence of pacemaker requirement.[105,106] Surgical ablation guided by intraoperative mapping of the atrium remains the last option in the drug refractory cases.

ATRIAL FIBRILLATION

Atrial fibrillation is a common condition associated with symptoms of varying severity, ranging from palpitation, fatigue, and dyspnea to more serious complications such as thromboembolic events leading to stroke, myocardial infarction, and congestive heart failure. Non-rheumatic atrial fibrillation affects 1.7% of persons aged 60 to 64 years and 11.6% of those older than 75 years.[107] The risk of stroke increases with age, from 1.5% in the fifth decade to 23.5% in the eighth decade.[108] As reported by the Framingham study group, most cases of chronic atrial fibrillation occur, in decreasing order, in patients with hypertensive heart disease, followed by no heart disease (lone atrial fibrillation), rheumatic heart disease, cardiac failure, and ischemic heart disease.[109] Complications of atrial fibrillation include (1) hemodynamic compromise related to lack of "atrial kick," resulting in reduction of cardiac output of about 25%; rapid ventricular rate may also reduce ventricular filling; (2) fast ventricular response, ventricular fibrillation, and sudden death in patients with accessory pathway with antegrade conduction, particularly those pathways with short refractory period (about 250 milliseconds or less); (3) increased risk for thromboembolic events (the relative risk in rheumatic atrial fibrillation is 18-fold in).[110] Resnekov and Abildskov and coworkers reported symptomatic and hemodynamic effects of atrial fibrillation.[116,117] Atrial fibrillation occurs in 7% to 10% of patients with acute myocardial infarction. Systemic emboli occur in up to 30% of those with chronic atrial fibrillation, whereas atrial fibrillation is present in 90% of those with both emboli and mitral stenosis.

Mechanism

The exact mechanism of atrial fibrillation is unknown; however, based on Moe's early studies and another contemporary investigation, most investigators believe it to be a multireentrant mechanism.[111,112] This was confirmed in human right atrium by high-density mapping of pacing-induced atrial fibrillation, which indicated that the right atrium is activated by one or multiple wavelets propagating in different directions.[113] Three types of propagation were described, depending on different numbers and dimensions of the intraatrial circuits.[113] Other investigators indicate that precipitating factors variously include (1) extent of atrial disease (which provides enhanced automaticity, slow intraatrial conduction, and heterogeneity in refractory properties); (2) autonomic imbalance; (3) sinus node dysfunction and atrial ischemia; and (4) provoked vulnerability.[3,11,12,14,16,87,91,114,115]

Management

Generally, the goal of management is (1) to maintain normal sinus rhythm as long as possible by chemical or electric cardioversion to optimize hemodynamic properties, without a significant increase in proarrhythmia; (2) to control ventricular rate response of atrial fibrillation by AV nodal medications, such as digoxin alone or in combination with antiarrhythmic agents; and (3) proper anticoagulation to minimize the risk of thromboembolic events. Pharmacologic and non-pharmacologic interventions may be applied to achieve these goals.

Pharmacologic Intervention

Maintainance of Sinus Rhythm

Concurrent use of a quinidine-like drug and digoxin helps to reduce the number of attacks in cases of paroxysmal atrial fibrillation. Although newer antiarrhythmic drugs, especially the class IC agents, are gaining widespread use, the results from the Cardiac Arrhythmia Suppression Trial raised serious concern, not only regarding the use of class IC antiarrhythmic agents in patients with left ventricular dysfunction and ventricular arrhythmias after myocardial infarction but also their use in other conditions, such as atrial fibrillation in patients with nonischemic structural heart disease.[119] In the same context, the report of a meta-analysis of six randomized studies on the efficacy and safety of quinidine therapy for maintenance of sinus rhythm after cardioversion of atrial fibrillation showed increased total mortality in patients receiving quinidine.[121] Nonetheless, few preliminary reports indicate efficacy and relative safety of class I agents, including flecainide, propafenone, and sotalol, for treatment of atrial fibrillation in patients with no evidence of structural heart disease. Further investigations and longer follow-up are required to establish the safety of antiarrhythmic agents for treatment of supraventricular tachycardias in patients without structural heart disease. At this time, most authors recommend in-hospital monitoring for initiation of antiarrhythmic agents, even in patients with otherwise normal heart. A report on meta-analysis of multiple studies indicates that low-dose amiodarone is supremely useful in this capacity, having a low risk of proarrhythmia, high efficacy to maintain sinus rhythm, and relatively low incidence of undesirable side effects when compared with patients treated with quinidine, warfarin, or no therapy.[120]

Control of Ventricular Response of Atrial Fibrillation

Digoxin is frequently prescribed to reduce the ventricular response of atrial fibrillation. Serum levels of digoxin do not always relate to therapeutic effect, especially when there is a concurrent febrile illness.[116] This is also true for some patients with enhanced AV nodal conduction when the sensitivity of the AV node may be reduced regarding depression of conduction by digoxin.[118] In both instances, improved control of the ventricular rate can be obtained either temporarily or in the long term with the concurrent use of verapamil.[117] Propafenone and flecainide are both effective against induced atrial fibrillation in the electrophysiology laboratory; however, their long-term effectiveness in chronic atrial fibrillation deserves further investigation.[122,123] Although oral flecainide therapy is effective in the management of atrial arrhythmias, in view of reports concerning its arrhythmogenic effect, it should be used cautiously.[124] Oral propafenone, however, is reported as having fewer arrhythmogenic events. Again, long-term studies are needed to confirm such conclusions.

Anticoagulation in Atrial Fibrillation

Several large randomized trials have shown the superior benefits of anticoagulation over placebo for reduction of thromboembolic stroke in patients with non-rheumatic atrial fibrillation.[129–133] Two studies tested placebo against aspirin: AFASAK found no positive results, whereas the Stroke Prevention in Atrial Fibrillation (SPAF) investigators found a statistically significant advantage for aspirin, compared with placebo.[129, 135] When the risk of major bleeding complications were weighed against the reduction of thromboembolic events in these patients, most studies revealed overall beneficial effects of anticoagulation. The SPAF group's results indicate that for patients younger than 75 years of age, either 325 mg of aspirin daily or warfarin therapy were superior to placebo in reduction of thromboembolic events. In published SPAF-II results, warfarin (prothrombin time ratio, 1.3 to 1.8; international normalized ratio, 2.0 to 4.5) was compared with aspirin (325 mg/day) in two group of patients: patients aged 75 year or younger and patients older than 75 years.[133] In low-risk patients (no history of hypertension, previous thromboembolism, and heart failure) younger than 75 years of age, aspirin was comparable in efficacy to warfarin. In high-risk and older patients, however, warfarin was superior to aspirin in reduction of thromboembolic events but had more bleeding complications. In summary, aspirin may be adequate for risk reduction in younger patients with lone atrial fibrillation; nonetheless, warfarin is recommended for all rheumatic atrial fibrillation, older individuals with lone atrial fibrillation, and high-risk younger patients.

Nonpharmacologic Management

Electric Cardioversion

Management of new cases is either with cardioversion or rapid digitalization. Reversion to sinus rhythm with digoxin is most likely to occur when the initial rate in atrial fibrillation is fast but usually occurs only after 4 to 8 hours. Digitalization and initiation of an antiarrhythmic agent is preferred if the precipitating stimulus is likely to last for more than a few hours because recurrence after successful electric cardioversion is a frequent event. It is recommended to avoid the risk of embolic event by proper anticoagulation if the duration of atrial fibrillation is more than a few days. Most authors suggest adequate anticoagulation with warfarin for a period of at least 4 to 6 weeks before and several days after cardioversion to allow endothelialization of thrombus, reducing the risk of its dislodgement. Electromechanical dissociation of atria after cardioversion has been well described as occurring and lasting up to several days.

With the emergence of implantable cardiodefibrillator devices for lethal medically refractory ventricular arrhythmias, the possibility of internal cardioversion for atrial flutter and fibrillation has been entertained.[125, 126]

It has been suggested that chronic atrial pacing may reduce or prevent attacks in patients with paroxysmal atrial fibrillation. There is no randomized study to support

Pre-ablation of slow pathway

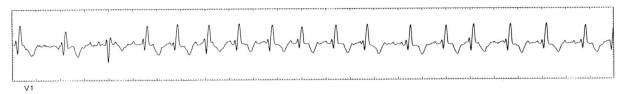

V1

Post-ablation of slow pathway

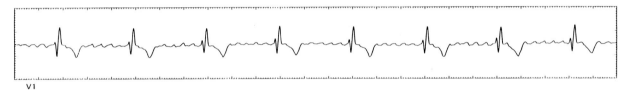

V1

Figure 11-48. Rhythm strip (VI) of atrial fibrillation pre- and postradiofrequency ablation of the atrioventricular nodal slow pathway. *Top panel* indicates faster and more irregular ventricular response during atrial fibrillation preablation than during postablation of the AV nodal slow pathway.

this hypothesis. Ongoing trials may answer questions regarding this matter, however.

His-Bundle Ablation

In refractory cases with poorly controlled ventricular response, ablation of the AV node is increasingly used.[81] Implantation of a permanent pacemaker is mandatory. This does not reduce the risk of thromboembolic events; therefore, chronic anticoagulation remains an important part of therapy.

Observations on the role of slow pathway in patients with dual AV nodal physiology and atrial fibrillation are promising. Because the refractory period of the slow pathway is usually shorter than that of the fast pathway of AV node, radiofrequency catheter ablation of the slow pathway may significantly reduce ventricular response during atrial fibrillation without significant bradycardia (Fig. 11-48).[128] About 15% to 25% of the general population have dual AV nodal physiology. It is therefore reasonable to assume that in selected patients who have refractory atrial fibrillation, slow pathway modification may prevent the need for His-bundle ablation and pacemaker implantation.

References

1. Katz LN, Pick A: Clinical electrocardiography. Part I: Arrhythmias with an atlas of electrocardiograms. Philadelphia: Lea & Febiger, 1956:595.
2. Legato MJ, Bull MB, Ferrer MI: Atrial ultrastructure in patients with fixed intra-atrial block. Chest 1974;65:252.
3. Kaplan BM, Langendorf R, Lev M, Pick A: Tachycardia-bradycardia syndrome (so called "sick sinus syndrome"). Pathology mechanisms and treatment. Am J Cardiol 1973;31:497.
4. Demoulin JC, Kulbertus HE: Pathological correlates of atrial arrhythmias. In: Kulbertus HE, ed. Re-entrant arrhythmias: mechanisms and treatment. Lancaster: MTP Press, 1977:99.
5. Hudson REB, ed: Cardiovascular pathology. London: Edward Arnold, 1965.
6. James TN: Arrhythmias and conduction disturbances in acute myocardial infarction. Am Heart J 1962;64:416.
7. Laas E: Das Arrhythmieherz. Zentrabl Allg Pathol 1962; 113:522.
8. Lippestad CT, Marton PF: Sinus arrest in proximal right coronary artery occlusion. Am Heart J 1967;74:551.
9. Davies MJ, Pomerance A: Pathology of atrial fibrillation in man. Br Heart J 1972;34:520.
10. Sims BA: Pathogenesis of atrial arrhythmias. Br Heart J 1972; 34:336.
11. El-Sherif N: Paroxysmal atrial flutter and fibrillation induced by carotid sinus compression and prevention by atropine. Br Heart J 1972;34:1024.
12. Loomis TA, Captain MC, Krop S: Auricular fibrillation induced and maintained in animals by acetylcholine or vagal stimulation. Circ Res 3:390 1955.
13. Friedberg CK, Donoso E: Arrhythmias and conduction disturbances due to digitalis. Prog Cardiovasc Dis 1960;2:408.
14. Burns JH: The cause of fibrillation. Br Med J 1960;1:1379.
15. Lindsay J, Hurst JW: The clinical features of atrial flutter and their clinical implications. Chest 1974;66:114.
16. Hecht HH: Mechanisms, causes and treatment of paroxysmal atrial fibrillation. In: Sandoe E, Flensted-Jensen E, Olesen KH eds. Symposium on cardiac arrhythmias. Sodertalje, Sweden, Elsinore Astra, 1970:747.
17. Narula OS: Sinus node re-entry: mechanism of supraventricular tachycardia (SVT) in man. Circulation 1972;46(Suppl 2):11.
18. Shenasa H, Merrill JJ, Hamer ME, Wharton JM: Distribution of ectopic atrial tachycardia along ctrista terminalis: an atrial ring of fire? Circulation 1993;88:II. Abstract.
19. Shenasa H, Kanter RJ, Sorrentino RA, Broughton A, Wharton JM: Different characteristics of left and right atrial tachycardias. Pacing Clin Electrophysiol April 1994. Abstract.
20. Chung EK: A reappraisal of atrial dissociation. Am J Cardiol 1971;28:111.
21. Wells JL, et al: Characterisation of atrial fibrillation in man: studies following open heart surgery. Pacing Clin Electrophysiol 1978;1:4.
22. Sanders WE, Sorrentino RA, Greenfield RA, Shenasa H, Hamer ME, Wharton JM: Catheter ablation of sinoatrial reentrant tachycardia. J Am Coll Cardiol 1994;23:926.
23. Allessie MA, Bonke FIM, Schopman FJG: Circus movement in rabbit atrial muscle as a mechanism of tachycardia. III. The "leading circle" concept: a new model of circus movement in cardiac tissue without the involvement of an anatomical obstacle. Circ Res 1977;41:9.
24. Warin JF, Fauchier JP: Les troubles de la conduction intra-auriculaire. In: Peuch P, Slama R, eds. Les troubles du rythme cardiaque. Paris: Roussel, 1978:95.
25. Hiss RG, Lamb LE: Electrocardiographic findings in 122,043 individuals. Circulation 1962;25:947.
26. Nagira S: Arrhythmias in children. Acta Med Jpn 1975;16:795.
27. Chung K-Y, Walsh TJ, Massie E: Atrial parasystole. Am J Cardiol 1964;14:255.
28. Chung EK: Diagnosis and clinical significance of parasystole. In: Sandoe E, Flensted-Jensen E, Olesen KH eds. Symposium on cardiac arrhythmias. Sodertalje, Sweden, Elsinore Astra, 1970:271.
29. Eliakim M: Atrial parasystole. Effect of carotid sinus stimulation, Valsalva maneuver, and exercise. Am J Cardiol 16:457 1965.
30. Shenasa M, Curry PVL, Sowton E: Comparison of atrial arrhythmias with atrial stimulation threshold and conduction times in patients with sick sinus syndrome. Br Heart J 1979; 42:237.
31. Scherf D, Yildiz M, DeArmas D: Atrial parasystole. Am Heart J 1959;57:507.
32. Goel BG, Han J: Atrial ectopic activity associated with sinus bradycardia. Circulation 1970;42:853.
33. Alicandri C, Fouad FM, Terazi RC, Castle L, Moraut V: Three cases of hypotension and syncope with ventricular pacing: possible role of atrial reflexes. Am J Cardiol 1978;42:137.
34. Maclean WAH, Karp RB, Kouchoukos NT, James TN, Waldo AL: P waves during ectopic atrial rhythms in man. A study utilizing atrial pacing with fixed electrodes. Circulation 1975;52:426.

35. Strauss HC, Geer MR: Sino-atrial node re-entry. In: Kulbertus HE, ed. Re-entrant arrhythmias: mechanism and treatment. Lancaster: MTP Press, 1977:27.

36. Marriott HJ: Tampa tracings. 1965:77.

37. Barker PS, Wilson FN, Johnson FD: The mechanism of auricular paroxysmal tachycardia. Am Heart J 1943;26:435.

38. Wallace AC, Daggett WM: Re-excitation of the atrium; the echo phenomenon. Am Heart J 1964;68:661.

39. Han J, Mallozzi AM, Moe GA: Sino-atrial reciprocation in the isolated rabbit heart. Circ Res 1968;22:355.

40. Allessie MA, Bonke FIM: Re-entry within the sinoatrial node as demonstrated by multiple micro-electrode recordings in the isolated rabbit heart. In: Bonke FIM, ed. The sinus node: structure, function and clinical relevance. The Hague, Netherlands: Martinus Nijhoff, 1978:409.

41. Josephson ME: Clinical cardiac electrophysiology: techniques and interpretations. Philadelphia: Lea & Febiger, 1993:181.

42. Wellens HJJ: Role of sinus node reentry in the genesis of cardiac arrhythmias. In: Bonke FIM, ed. The sinus node: structure function and clinical relevance. The Hague, Netherlands: Martinus Nijhoff, 1978:422.

43. Pahlajani DB, Millar RA, Serrato M: Sinus node re-entry and sinus node tachycardia. Am Heart J 1975;90:305.

44. Weisfogel GM, et al: Sinus node re-entrant tachycardia in man. Am Heart J 1975;90:295.

45. Gillette PG: The mechanisms of supraventricular tachycardia in children. Circulation 1976;54:133.

46. Curry PVL, Evans TR, Krikler DM: Paroxysmal reciprocating sinus tachycardia. Eur J Cardiol 1977;6:199.

47. Wu D, et al: Demonstration of sustained sinus node and atrial re-entry as a mechanism of paroxysmal supraventricular tachycardia. Circulation 1975;51:234.

48. Dhingra AC, et al: Sinus node response to atrial extrastimuli in patients without apparent sinus node disease. Am J Cardiol 1975;36:445.

49. Krikler DM, Curry PVL: Atypical initiation of reciprocating tachycardia in the Wolff-Parkinson-White syndrome. In: Kulbertus HE, ed. Re-entrant arrhythmias: mechanisms and treatment. Lancaster: MTP Press, 1977.

50. Curry PVL, Krikler DM: Significance of cycle length alternation during drug treatment of supraventricular tachycardia. Br Heart J 1976;38:882.

51. Shenasa H, Greenfield RA, Johnson EE, Sorrentino RA, Wharton JM: Does adenosine differentiate sinoatrial nodal reentrant tachycardia from ectopic atrial tachycardia? Circ 1993;88(II):4. Abstract.

52. Munsif AN, Liem LB, Young C, Lauer MR, Yu JCL, Sung RJ: Adenosine/verapamil sensitive atrial tachycardia: endocardial mapping and radiofrequency catheter ablation. J Am Coll Cardiol 1994;155A

53. Breithardt G, Seipel L: Sequence of atrial activation in patients with atrial echo beats. In: Bonke FIM, ed. The sinus node: structure, function and clinical reliance. The Hague, Netherlands: Martinus Nijhoff, 1978:389.

54. Reiffel JA, Bigger TJ Jr: Current status of direct recording of the sinus node electrogram in man. Pacing Clin Electrophysiol 1983;6:1143.

55. Lee JR, Grogin HR, Fitzpatrick AP, Epstein LM, Lesh MD, Scheinman MM: Sinus node modification for inappropriate sinus tachycardia. J Am Coll Cardiol 1994;882:155A.

56. Brugada P, Wellens HJJ: The role of triggered activity in clinical ventricular arrhythmias. Pacing Clin Electrophysiol 1984;7:260.

57. Keane JF, Plauth WH, Nadas AS: Chronic ectopic tachycardia of infancy and children. Am Heart J 1972;84:748.

58. Tang CY, Scheinman MM, Van Hare GF, et al: P wave morphology during automatic atrial tachycardia man. J Am Coll Cardiol 1994, 250 A. Abstract.

59. Scheinman MM, Basu D, Hollenberg M: Electrophysiologic studies in patients with persistent atrial tachycardia. Circulation 1974;50:266.

60. Goldreyer BN, Gallagher JJ, Damato AN: The electrophysiologic demonstration of atrial ectopic tachycardia in man. Am Heart J 1973;85:205.

61. Curry PVL: The haemodynamic and electrophysiological effects of paroxysmal tachycardia. In: Narula OS, ed. Cardiac arrhythmias: electrophysiology, diagnosis and management. Baltimore: Williams & Wilkins, 1979:579.

62. Pittman DE, Makar JS, Kooros KS, Joyner CR: Rapid atrial stimulation: successful method of conversion of atrial flutter and atrial tachycardia. Am J Cardiol 1973;32:700.

63. Gillette PG, Garson A Jr: Electrophysiologic and pharmacologic characteristics of automatic ectopic atrial tachycardia. Circulation 1977;56:571.

64. Haines DE, Lerman BB, Sellers TD, Dipparco JP: Intra-atrial reentrant tachycardia: clinical characteristics and response to chronic amiodarone therapy. Circulation 1985;72(Suppl III):III.

65. Arbel ER, Cohen HC Langendorf, R Glick, G: Successful treatment of drug resistant atrial tachycardia and intractable congestive heart failure with permanent coupled atrial pacing. Am J Cardiol 1978;41:336.

66. Coumel Ph, et al: Repérage et tentative d'exérèse chirurgicale d'un foyer ectopique avriculaire gauche avec tachycardie rebelle: évolution favorable. Ann Cardiol Angeiol (Paris) 1973;22:189.

67. Coumel Ph, Barold SS: Mechanisms of supraventricular tachycardias. In: Narula OS, ed. His bundle electrocardiography and clinical electrophysiology. Philadelphia: FA Davis, 1975:235.

68. Silka MJ, Gillette PC, Garson A Jr, Zinner A: Transvenous catheter ablation of a right atrial automatic ectopic tachycardia. J Am Coll Cardiol 1985;5:999.

69. Kay GN, Chong F, Epstein AE, Dailey SM, Plumb BJ: Radiofrequency ablation for primary atrial tachycardias. J Am Coll Cardiol 1993;21:910.

70. Tracy CM, Swartz JF, Fletcher RD, et al: Radiofrequency catheter ablation of ectopic atrial tachycardia using paced activation sequence mapping. J Am Coll Cardiol 1993;21:910.

71. Lesh MD, Van Hare GF, Epstein LM, et al: Radiofrequency catheter ablation of atrial arrhythmias. Results and mechanism. Circulation 1994;89:1974.

72. Ott DA, Gillette PC, Garson A, Cooly DA, Reul GJ, Mc Namara DG: Surgical management of refractory supraventricular tachycardia in infants and children. J Am Coll Cardiol 1985;5:124.

73. Olsson SB, Bloomstorm P, Sable KG, Williams Olsson G:

Incessant ectopic atrial tachycardia: successful surgical treatment with regression of dilated cardiomyopathy picture. Am J Cardiol 1984;53:1465.

74. Marriott HJ: Diagnosis of cardiac arrhythmias. GP 1964; 30:96.

75. Abrams DL, Eaddy JA: Repetitive multifocal paroxysmal atrial tachycardia with second degree AV block type I, and concealed and aberrant conduction. Am J Cardiol 1965;15:871.

76. Shine KI, Kastor JA, Yurchak PM: Multifocal atrial tachycardia. Clinical and electrocardiographic features in 32 patients. N Engl J Med 1968;279:344.

77. Lipson MJ, Naimi S: Multifocal atrial tachycardia (chaotic atrial tachycardia). Circulation 1970;42:397.

78. Corazza LJ, Pastor BH: Cardiac arrhythmias in chronic cor pulmonale. N Engl J Med 1958;258:862.

79. Berlinerblau R, Feder W: Chaotic atrial rhythm. J Electrocardiol 1972;5:135.

80. Phillips J, Spano J, Burch GE: Chaotic atrial mechanism. Am Heart J 1969;78:171.

81. Gallagher JJ, Svenson RH, Kasell JH, et al: Catheter technique for closed chest ablation of the atrioventricular conduction system: a therapeutic alternative for treatment of refractory supraventricular tachycardia. N Engl J Med 1982;306:194.

82. Leier CV, Meacham JA, Schaal SF: Prolonged atrial conduction; a major predisposing factor for the development of atrial flutter. Circulation 1978;57:213.

83. Hayden WG, Hurley EJ, Rytand DA: The mechanism of canine atrial flutter. Circ Res 1967;20:496.

84. Lewis T, Drury AN, Iliescu CC: A demonstration of circus movement in clinical flutter of the auricles. Heart 1921; 8:341.

85. Guiney TE, Lown B: Electrical conversion of atrial flutter to atrial fibrillation; flutter mechanism in man. Br Heart J 1972;34:1215.

86. Cristal N, Szwarcberg J, Gueron M: Supraventricular arrhythmias in acute myocardial infarction. Ann Intern Med 1975; 82:35.

87. Liberthson RR, Salisbury KW, Hutter AM, DeSanctis RW: Atrial tachycardias in acute myocardial infarction. Am J Med 1976;60:956.

88. Roberts NK, Yabek S: Arrhythmias following atrial and ventricular surgery. In: Roberts NK, Gelband H, eds. Cardiac arrhythmias in the neonate, infant and child. New York: Appleton-Century-Crofts, 1977:405.

89. Kennelly BM, Lane GK: Electrophysiological studies in four patients with 1:1 atrioventricular conduction. Am Heart J 1978;96:723.

90. Allessie R, Nusynowitz M, Abildskov JA, Moe GK: Non-uniform distribution of vagal effects on the atrial refractory period. Am J Physiol 1958;194:406.

91. Anbe DT, Rubenfire M, Drake EH: Conversion of atrial flutter to atrial fibrillation with carotid sinus pressure. J Electrocardiol 1969;2:377.

92. Ferret MI: Atrial flutter. Chest 1974;66:111.

93. Waldo AL, Maclean WAH, Karp RB, Kouchoukos NT, James TN: Entrainment and interruption of atrial flutter with atrial pacing. Studies in man following open heart surgery. Circulation 1977;56:737.

94. Waldo AL: Some observations concerning atrial flutter in man. Pacing Clin Electrophysiol 1983;6:1181.

95. Waldo AL, Henthorn RW, Plumb VJ: Atrial flutter, recent observations in man. In: Josephson ME, Wellens HJJ, eds. Tachycardias: mechanisms, diagnosis and treatment. Philadelphia: Lea & Febiger, 1984.

96. Benson DW Jr, Dunnigan A, Benditt DG: Follow-up evaluation of infant paroxysmal atrial tachycardia: transesophageal study. Circulation 1987;75(3):542.

97. Guarnerio M, Furlanello F, Del Greco M, Vergara G, Inama G, Disertori M: Transesophageal atrial pacing: a first choice technique in atrial flutter therapy. Am Heart J 1989;117:1241.

98. Waldo AL: Atrial flutter: new directions in management mechanism. Circulation 1990;81:1142.

99. Primeau R, Agha A, Giorgi C, Shenasa M, Nadeau R: Long-term efficacy and toxicity of amiodarone in the treatment of refractory cardiac arrhythmias. Can J Cardiol 1989;5(2):98.

100. Danahy DT, Aronow WS: Lidocaine-induced cardiac rate changes in atrial fibrillation and flutter. Am Heart J 1978; 95:474.

101. Schamroth L, Krikler DM, Garret G: Immediate effects of intravenous verapamil in cardiac arrhythmias. Br Med J 1972;1:660.

102. Das G, et al: Atrial pacing for conversion of atrial flutter digitalized patients. Am L Cardiol 1978;41:308.

103. Rosen KM, Sinno MZ, Gunnar RM, Rahimtools SH: Failure of rapid atrial pacing in the conversion of atrial flutter. Am J Cardiol 1972;29:524.

104. Preston TA: Atrial pacing to convert atrial flutter. Am J Cardiol 1973;32:737.

105. Calkins H, Leon AR, Deam G, Kalbfleisch SJ, Langberg JJ, Morady F: Catheter ablation of atrial flutter using radiofrequency energy. Am J Cardiol 1994;73:353.

106. Lesh MD, Van Hare GF, Epstein LM, Fitzpatrick AP, Scheinman MM: Radiofrequency catheter ablation of atrial arrhythmias, results and mechanisms. Circulation 1994;89:1074.

107. Lake FR, Cullen KJ, de Klerk NH: Atrial fibrillation and mortality in an elderly population. Aust NZ J Med 1989;19:321.

108. Wolf PA, Abbott R, Kannel W: Atrial fibrillation as an independent risk factor for stroke. Stroke 1991;22:983.

109. The Framingham study. Arch Intern Med 1987;147(9):1561.

110. Wolf PA, Dawber TR, Thomas HE, et al: Epidemiologic assessment of chronic atrial fibrillation and risk of stroke. The Framingham study. Neurology 1978;28:973.

111. Moe GK: On the multiple wavelet hypothesis of atrial fibrillation. Arch Int Pharmacodyn Ther 1962;140:732.

112. Allessie M, Lammers WJEP, Bonke RI, Hollen J: Experimental evaluation of Moe's multiple wavelet hypothesis of atrial fibrillation. In: Zipes DP, Jalife J, eds. Cardiac electrophysiology and arrhythmias. New York: Grune & Stratton, 1985.

113. Konings KTS, Kirchhof CJHJ, Smeets RLMJ, Wellens HJJ, Penn OC, Allessie MA: High-density mapping of electrically induced atrial fibrillation in humans. Circulation 1994;89:1665.

114. Scherf D: The mechanism of flutter and fibrillation. Am Heart J 1966;71:273.

115. Paulay KL, Varghese PJ, Damato AN: Atrial rhythms in response to an early atrial premature depolarization in man. Am Heart J 1973;85:323.

116. Resnekov L: Circulatory effects of cardiac dysrhythmias. Dreifus L, ed. Arrhythmias. Coardiovasc Clinics 1970; 2(2):27.

117. Abildskov JA, Millar K, Burgess MJ: Atrial fibrillation. Am J Cardiol 1971;28:263.

118. Kastor JA: Digitalis intoxication in patients with atrial fibrillation. Circulation 1973;47:888.

119. Cardiac Arrhythmia Suppression Trial (CAST) Investigators: Preliminary report: effect of encainide and flecainide on mortality in a randomized trial of arrhythmia suppression after myocardial infarction. The Cardiac Arrhythmia Suppression Trial. N Engl J Med 1989;321:406.

120. Disch DL, Greenberg ML, Holzberger PT, Malenka DJ, Birkmyer JD: Managing chronic atrial fibrillation: a Markov decision analysis comparing warfarin, quinidine, and low dose amiodarone. Ann Intern Med 1994;120:49.

121. Coplen SE, Antman EM, Berlin JA, Hewitt P, Chalmers TC: Efficacy and safety of quinidine therapy for maintenance of sinus rhythm after cardioversion. A meta-analysis of randomized control trials. Circulation 1990;82:1106.

122. Goldman S, Probst P, Selzer A, Cohn K: Inefficacy or "therapeutic" serum levels of digoxin in controlling the ventricular rate in atrial fibrillation. Am J Cardiol 1975;35:651.

123. Klein HO, Paugher H, DiSegni E, David D, Kaplinsky E: The beneficial effects of verapamil in chronic atrial fibrillation. Arch Intern Med 1979;139:747.

124. Shenasa M, Kus T, Fromer M, LeBlanc AR, Dubuc M, Nadeau R: Effect of intravenous and oral calcium antagonists (diltiazem and verapamil) on sustenance of atrial fibrillation. Am J Cardiol 1988;62:403.

125. Cooper RAS, Alferness CA, Smith WM, et al: Internal cardioversion of atrial fibrillation in sheep. Circulation 1993;87:1673.

126. Johnson EE, Yarger MD, Wharton JM: Monophasic and biphasic waveforms for low energy internal cardioversion of atrial fibrillation in human. Circulation 1993;88(II). Abstract.

127. Dubuc M, Kus T, Campa MA, Lambert C, Rosengarten M, Shenasa M: Electrophysiologic effects of intravenous propafenone in Wolff-Parkinson-White syndrome. Am Heart J 1989;117:370.

128. Blanck Z, Dhala A, Krum D, et al: Dramatic reduction in ventricular response during atrial fibrillation by ablating the atrioventricular nodal slow pathway: electrophysiologic and clinical implications. Circulation 1993;88:4,II,A.

129. Petersen P, Boysen G, Gotfredsen J, et al: Placebo controlled randomized trial of warfarin and aspirin for prevention of thromboembolic complications in chronic atrial fibrillation: the Copenhagen AFASAK study. Lancet 1989;1:175.

130. Boston Area Anticoagulation Trial for Atrial Fibrillation Investigators: The effect of low dose warfarin on the risk of stroke in patients with non-rheumatic atrial fibrillation. N Engl J Med 1990;323:1505.

131. Stroke Prevention in Atrial Fibrillation Investigators: Stroke prevention in atrial fibrillation study: final results. Circulation 1991;84:527.

132. Connolly SJ, Laupacis A, Gent M, et al: Canadian atrial fibrillation anticoagulation (CAFA) study. J Am Coll Cardiol 1991; 18:349.

133. Stroke Prevention in Atrial Fibrillation Investigators: Warfarin versus aspirin for prevention of thromboembolism in atrial fibrillation: stroke prevention in atrial fibrillation II study. Lancet 1994;343:687.

134. Kappenberger L, Fromer M, Shenasa M, Steinbrunn W, Gloor HO: Evaluation of flecainide in rapid atrial fibrillation complicating Wolff-Parkinson-White syndrome. Clin Cardiol 1985;8:321.

135. Falk RH: Flecainide-induced ventricular tachycardia and fibrillation in patients treated for atrial fibrillation. Ann Intern Med 1989;111:107.

136. Connolly SJ, Hoffert DL: Usefulness of propafenone for recurrent paroxysmal AF. Am J Cardiol 1989;63:817.

Cardiac Arrhythmias, 3rd edition, edited by William J. Mandel.
J. B. Lippincott Company, Philadelphia © 1995.

12

Robert A. Bauernfeind • Joseph J. Sarmiento Jr.

Paroxysmal Supraventricular Tachycardia

The purpose of this chapter is to discuss one class of cardiac arrhythmia: paroxysmal supraventricular tachycardia (PSVT). During the past 25 years, clinical cardiac electrophysiologic studies have elucidated the various mechanisms of PSVT. This delineation of mechanisms has led to more rational drug therapy and to development of ablative, surgical, and pacing therapies for PSVT. This chapter reviews the mechanisms of PSVT, discusses diagnosis of these mechanisms, and presents therapeutic approaches.

Paroxysmal supraventricular tachycardia (Fig. 12-1) has the following electrocardiographic characteristics:

1. There is sudden (paroxysmal) onset and termination, although the arrhythmia is occasionally persistent. Sudden onset and termination distinguish PSVT from non-PSVTs such as sinus tachycardia or nonparoxysmal junctional tachycardia.

2. The rhythm is usually regular, with only gradual changes of rate.

3. The atrial rate is 100 to 250 beats per minute and usually between 140 and 220 beats per minute. An atrial rate in excess of 250 beats per minute suggests a diagnosis of atrial flutter or fibrillation.

4. The ventricular rate equals the atrial rate or is less than the atrial rate (if there is atrioventricular [AV] block).

5. The QRS complexes are typically narrow but may be wide when aberrant conduction is present.[1]

MECHANISMS

There are several distinct varieties of PSVT. Most (90% to 95%) cases reflect reentrance. Reentrance using an anomalous AV pathway and AV nodal reentrance are most common.[2–5] Occasional cases reflect sinus node reentrance or atrial reentrance.[6,7] Rare cases of PSVT reflect increased automaticity and arise from an ectopic focus in the atria or in the AV node or His bundle.[4,8]

From HeartCare Midwest, S.C., and the Department of Medicine, University of Illinois College of Medicine, Peoria, Illinois.

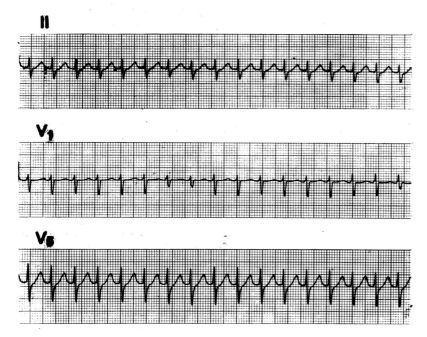

Figure 12-1. Paroxysmal supraventricular tachycardia.

Reentrance Using an Anomalous Atrioventricular Pathway

The conduction system of a patient with Wolff-Parkinson-White syndrome (manifest preexcitation) provides an ideal setting for reentrance: there is a proximal common pathway (the atria), a distal common pathway (the ventricles), and two connecting limbs (the normal AV conduction system and the anomalous AV pathway or Kent bundle). During sinus rhythm, there is antegrade conduction over both connecting limbs, resulting in fusion QRS complexes (Fig. 12-2). Reentrance, however, can be initiated in the following fashion.[2,9–11] An atrial premature beat finds the anomalous pathway refractory and conducts antegradely over only the normal pathway to the ventricles, resulting in a narrow QRS complex (see Fig. 12-2). During antegrade conduction over the normal pathway, the anomalous pathway recovers excitability, allowing the wavefront to conduct retrogradely over this pathway to the atria. The wavefront again conducts antegradely over the normal pathway to the ventricles and retrogradely over the anomalous pathway to the atria, creating a circus movement. This same circus movement can be initiated by a ventricular premature beat that blocks in the normal pathway and conducts retrogradely over the anomalous pathway to the atria.[2,9,12,13]

Reentrance using an anomalous pathway, as described above, sometimes occurs in patients who do not have manifest preexcitation. These patients have a concealed anomalous pathway that conducts in only the retrograde direction.[2,3,5,10,11] During sinus rhythm, there is antegrade conduction over only the normal pathway, so that QRS complexes are narrow.

In reentrance using an anomalous pathway, there is sequential depolarization of the atria and the ventricles. Because conduction to the ventricles is over the normal pathway, QRS complexes are narrow and PSVT is seen on the surface electrocardiogram.

Atrioventricular Nodal Reentrance

Goldreyer and coworkers suggested that reentrance in the region of the AV node is a common mechanism of PSVT.[14,15] Subsequent work suggests that the substrate for AV nodal reentrance is provided by functional longitudinal dissociation of the AV node into two pathways (dual AV nodal pathways).[16–19] It is not clear whether this dissociation has a structural basis or is a purely physiologic phenomenon.[20,21] Antegrade conduction over either pathway to the His bundle generally results in a narrow QRS complex. Thus, the two pathways are differentiated primarily by their relative conduction times and are referred to as "fast" and "slow" AV nodal pathways. Observations suggest that tissue that comprises the fast pathway lies just posterior to the His bundle, whereas tissue that comprises the slow pathway lies more inferiorly, extending toward the coronary sinus.[22,23] With respect to electrophysiologic properties and anatomic location, the fast pathway closely resembles the normal AV node.[22]

It has long been debated whether AV nodal reen-

A. Sinus rhythm

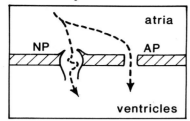

B. Premature atrial beat

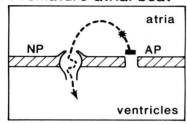

C. Reentrant tachycardia

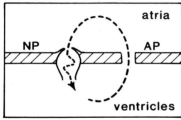

Figure 12-2. The conduction system in Wolff-Parkinson-White syndrome. (**A**) Sinus rhythm, with antegrade conduction over both pathways. (**B**) A premature atrial beat (*) blocks in the *AP* and conducts antegradely over only the *NP* to the ventricles. (**C**) The wavefront then conducts retrogradely over the *AP* to the atria and antegradely over the *NP* to the ventricles, creating a circus movement. *NP*, normal pathway; *AP*, anomalous pathway.

trance is confined to the AV node or involves atrial tissue at the proximal aspect or His-bundle tissue at the distal aspect. This debate continues, and its resolution may depend on where in a transition zone AV nodal tissue is arbitrarily deemed to have yielded to another variety of tissue.[22] Because it has been demonstrated that a wavefront can block between the proximal end of the reentrant pathway (proximal common pathway) and the bulk of atrial tissue or between the distal end of the reentrant pathway (distal common pathway) and the bulk of the His bundle, it seems practical to think of AV nodal reentrance as being confined to the AV node.[24–26]

During sinus rhythm, there is antegrade conduction over both AV nodal pathways. The wavefront conducting over the fast pathway reaches the His bundle first, resulting in a relatively short atrial-to-His (AH) interval, whereas conduction over the slow pathway is concealed. Reentrance can be initiated in the following fashion.[17–19,27] An atrial premature beat finds the fast pathway refractory and conducts antegradely over only the slow pathway, resulting in a relatively long AH interval. During antegrade conduction over the slow pathway, the fast pathway recovers excitability, allowing the wavefront to conduct retrogradely over this pathway to the proximal common pathway. The wavefront again conducts antegradely over the slow pathway and retrogradely over the fast pathway, creating a circus movement. This same circus movement can be initiated by a ventricular premature beat that blocks in the slow pathway and conducts retrogradely over the fast pathway.[28]

Atrioventricular nodal reentrance occasionally occurs in the opposite direction (i.e., the circus movement uses the fast pathway as the antegrade limb and the slow pathway as the retrograde limb).[29,30] This unusual variety of AV nodal reentrance can be initiated by an atrial premature beat that blocks in the slow pathway and conducts over the fast pathway or by a ventricular premature beat that blocks in the fast pathway and conducts over the slow pathway.

In most cases of AV nodal reentrance, each depolarization of the proximal common pathway is conducted retrogradely to the atria and each depolarization of the distal common pathway is conducted antegradely to the His bundle and the ventricles. Thus, PSVT is seen on the surface electrocardiogram.

Sinoatrial Reentrance

Sinus node reentrance is thought to be initiated in the following fashion.[6,7] An atrial premature beat finds one margin of the sinus node refractory (entrance block) but penetrates the node at a different site. While the wavefront slowly traverses the node, the right atrium recovers excitability, allowing the wavefront to exit from the node at the site of original entrance block. The wavefront again conducts into the node and out to the atrium, creating a circus movement. In atrial reentrance, the reentrant pathway is composed solely of atrial tissue.[6] Because sinus node reentrance and atrial reentrance both arise in structures above the AV node and frequently are difficult to differentiate, they are often considered together as being sinoatrial reentrant. Sinoatrial reentrance results in a rapid atrial rate and if the wavefronts are conducted to the ventricles, it results in a rapid ventricular rate. Unlike reentrance using an anomalous AV pathway, however, sinoatrial reentrance does not require antegrade conduction to the ventricles for its continuance.[6,7]

Automatic Tachycardias

The varieties of PSVT discussed to this point all reflect reentrance and differ only in the specific cardiac tissues comprising the reentrant pathways. Rare cases of PSVT do not reflect reentrance, however, but abnormal impulse formation.[4,8,31,32] Some automatic ectopic tachycardias—arising either in one of the atria or in the AV node or His bundle—are not initiated by premature beats but begin spontaneously, with the first beat being identical to subsequent beats of tachycardia. It is also possible that some cases of automatic ectopic atrial tachycardia, particularly those related to digitalis toxicity, reflect triggered activity due to late afterdepolarizations.[33] Automatic ectopic atrial tachycardia and sinoatrial reentrance are true examples of paroxysmal atrial tachycardia.

DIAGNOSIS OF MECHANISM

Treatment of PSVT often depends on the specific mechanism of the tachycardia. Although definitive diagnosis of mechanism usually requires performance of cardiac electrophysiologic studies, a tentative diagnosis can usually be made before these studies. In patients with manifest preexcitation, reentrance using an anomalous pathway is most common and should be suspected.[2] In patients without manifest preexcitation, AV nodal reentrance is most common.[4] Certain clinical features can suggest another diagnosis, however. For example, if a patient younger than age 35 years without apparent heart disease has PSVT with rate greater than 200 beats per minute, reentrance with a concealed anomalous pathway is likely.[4] Paroxysmal supraventricular tachycardia that is frequently repetitive (or incessant) is usually automatic ectopic atrial tachycardia or reentrance using a slowly conducting anomalous pathway.[34] Paroxysmal supraventricular tachycardia that occurs only in an acute clinical setting often is automatic ectopic atrial tachycardia.[31] Valuable information that may indicate a specific diagnosis can sometimes be derived by careful scrutiny of the surface electrocardiogram.[4,35,36] These electrocardiographic observations are also made during electrophysiologic studies and are discussed in this chapter in the context of these studies.

Electrophysiologic Studies

In most cases, the mechanism of PSVT can be accurately diagnosed during performance of invasive cardiac electrophysiologic studies.[2-5] The rare cases that reflect increased automaticity generally cannot be induced by cardiac pacing, so that evaluation of these tachycardias depends on persistence or fortuitous occurrence during the invasive procedure.[4,31,32] The tachycardias that reflect reentrance generally can be induced and terminated by pacing, however.[4] Because most cases of PSVT reflect reentrance, the usual problem addressed in the electrophysiology laboratory is differentiation between reentrance using an anomalous pathway, AV nodal reentrance, and sinoatrial reentrance.[4] In this regard, it is useful to consider the following sources of information: (1) programmed atrial stimulation, (2) programmed ventricular stimulation, (3) observations during paroxysmal tachycardia, and (4) administration of drugs. Each of these sources may yield important clues regarding the mechanism of reentrant tachycardia. In most cases, clues from two or more sources must be combined to arrive at a diagnosis.

Programmed Atrial Stimulation

Programmed atrial stimulation includes atrial extrastimulus testing and incremental atrial pacing. Extrastimulus testing is continued until atrial refractoriness is encountered, whereas incremental pacing is continued until second-degree AV block occurs. Stimulation is performed at the high right atrium and frequently at a second site, such as the coronary sinus. Programmed atrial stimulation combined with recording of a His-bundle electrogram may yield important information.

Programmed atrial stimulation may reveal ventricular preexcitation that is not apparent during sinus rhythm.[37] Closely coupled atrial beats usually encounter increased AV nodal refractoriness and conduct over the normal pathway with increased delay. There is little or no slowing of conduction over the anomalous pathway, however, so that the degree of ventricular preexcitation is increased. In rare cases, ventricular preexcitation may be revealed only when stimulation is performed at a particular atrial site, such as the coronary sinus.[37] Demonstration of ventricular preexcitation suggests a diagnosis of reentrance using an anomalous pathway.

Programmed atrial stimulation provides information regarding the quality of antegrade normal pathway conduction, which is usually excellent in patients with PSVT. In reentrance using an anomalous pathway, the normal pathway is the antegrade limb and must be capable of repetitive antegrade conduction at short cycle lengths.[38] In AV nodal reentrance, one of the AV nodal pathways (usually the slow pathway) is the antegrade limb and must be capable of repetitive antegrade conduction.[30,39] Although antegrade normal pathway conduction is not required in any of the varieties of paroxysmal atrial tachycardia, the most troublesome of these tachycardias are those associated with 1:1 AV conduction.

Antegrade dual AV nodal pathways are diagnosed

when atrial extrastimulus testing reveals discontinuous AV nodal (A_1–A_2, H_1–H_2 or A_1–A_2, A_2–H_2) conduction curves.[16-19] These discontinuous curves are generated when relatively late atrial extrastimuli conduct over the fast pathway (relatively short A_2–H_2 intervals) but slightly earlier atrial extrastimuli block in the fast pathway and conduct over the slow pathway, resulting in a sudden marked increase of A_2–H_2 intervals (Fig. 12-3). Discontinuous AV nodal conduction curves can be demonstrated in most patients with the usual variety of AV nodal reentrance.[40,41] In some patients with this variety of tachycardia, however, discontinuous curves cannot be demonstrated because of failure to achieve block in the fast pathway or because the fast and slow pathways have similar conduction times.[42] Thus, failure to demonstrate discontinuous AV nodal conduction curves does not exclude a diagnosis of AV nodal reentrance. Conversely, demonstration of discontinuous curves is not specific for a diagnosis of AV nodal reentrance; discontinuous curves are present in 5% to 10% of patients without AV nodal reen-

trance, including occasional patients with reentrance using an anomalous pathway or one of the varieties of paroxysmal atrial tachycardia.[41,43-45]

When paroxysmal tachycardia is induced during programmed atrial stimulation, it is important to determine whether induction is associated with a specific pattern of AV conduction. Induction of reentrance using an anomalous pathway by an atrial beat requires antegrade block in the anomalous pathway (normalization of the QRS complex in a patient with manifest preexcitation) and antegrade conduction to the ventricles over the normal pathway, with sufficient delay to allow the anomalous pathway to recover excitability.[2,9-11] The critical delay can occur in the AV node (prolongation of AH interval) or in the distal conduction system (prolongation of HV interval or functional block in the bundle branch ipsilateral to the anomalous pathway).[10,11,46] Induction of the usual variety of AV nodal reentrance requires antegrade block in the fast pathway and conduction over the slow pathway, with sufficient delay (critical AH interval) to allow the fast pathway

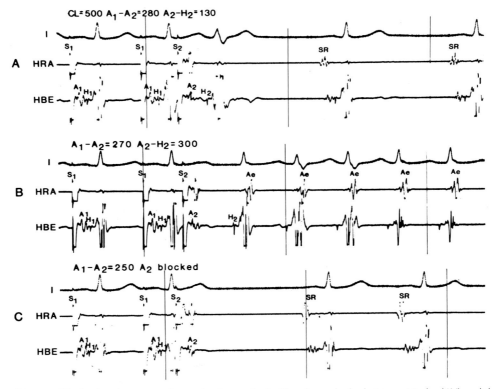

Figure 12-3. Atrial extrastimulus testing in a patient with antegrade dual atrioventricular (AV) nodal pathways and AV nodal reentrant tachycardia (usual variety). Shown in each panel are electrocardiographic lead I and high right atrial (*HRA*) and His-bundle (*HBE*) electrograms. Time lines are at 1-second intervals. (**A**) A_1–A_2 = 280 milliseconds. A_2 conducts over the fast pathway (A_2 − H_2 = 130 milliseconds), and sinus rhythm resumes. (**B**) A_1–A_2 = 270 milliseconds. A_2 blocks in the fast pathway, conducts over the slow pathway (A_2 − H_2 = 300 milliseconds) and induces reentrant tachycardia. (**C**) A_1–A_2 = 250 milliseconds. A_2 blocks in both the fast and slow pathways, and sinus rhythm resumes. A_e, atrial echo.

to recover excitability.[14, 15, 17–19, 27] Although there is usually antegrade conduction to the ventricles, AV nodal reentrance occasionally is induced by an atrial beat that blocks distal to the His bundle or even proximal to the His bundle (presumably in AV nodal tissue distal to the reentrant pathway).[24] Induction of the unusual variety of AV nodal reentrance requires antegrade block in the slow pathway and conduction over the fast pathway. In the presence of antegrade conduction over the fast pathway, antegrade block in the slow pathway is concealed and can only be inferred. Although sinoatrial reentrance usually can be induced by closely coupled atrial beats, the specific characteristics of intraatrial conduction required for induction generally cannot be identified using electrophysiologic techniques.[6, 7] The presence or absence of AV conduction is irrelevant to induction of sinoatrial reentrance.

The significance of specific patterns of tachycardia induction during programmed atrial stimulation can be summarized as follows. Induction of tachycardia by an atrial beat that blocks proximal to the His bundle strongly suggests a diagnosis of sinoatrial reentrance. This pattern is seen in only occasional patients with AV nodal reentrance and is incompatible with reentrance using an anomalous pathway. Induction of tachycardia by an atrial beat that blocks distal to the His bundle also excludes this latter diagnosis. Conversely, demonstration that conduction to the His bundle is required for induction of tachycardia excludes a diagnosis of sinoatrial reentrance and, if conduction to the ventricles is required, AV nodal reentrance can also be excluded, leaving a diagnosis of reentrance using an anomalous pathway. Similarly, demonstration that induction of tachycardia requires achievement of a critical AH interval suggests AV nodal reentrance or reentrance using an anomalous pathway; facilitation of induction by prolongation of the HV interval or occurrence of functional bundle branch block suggests reentrance using an anomalous pathway.

Although the above considerations are frequently useful and in some cases can indicate a specific diagnosis, their application can be difficult. The information provided by atrial extrastimulus testing is frequently of limited value.[15] Because patients with paroxysmal tachycardia usually have excellent antegrade normal pathway conduction, closely coupled atrial extrastimuli are usually conducted to the ventricles, with relatively long AH and AV intervals. Thus, it frequently is not clear whether induction of tachycardia by an atrial extrastimulus reflects achievement of a critical A_1–A_2 interval (suggesting sinoatrial reentrance), a critical A_2–H_2 interval (suggesting AV nodal reentrance), or a critical A_2–V_2 interval (suggesting reentrance using an anomalous pathway). Performance of rapid atrial pacing can be useful in this situation.[14] The rate of atrial pacing that results in type I second-degree AV block is determined and pacing at this rate is repeated,

frequently 30 to 40 times. When this is done, the A_1–A_1 interval remains constant, whereas conduction of the last atrial paced beat is variable; some of these beats block in the AV node, some are conducted with short AH and AV intervals, and some are conducted with long AH and AV intervals. This variability provides an opportunity to determine whether tachycardia can be induced by a blocked atrial beat or whether antegrade conduction (and a critical AH or AV interval) is required.

Programmed Ventricular Stimulation

Programmed ventricular stimulation includes ventricular extrastimulus testing and incremental ventricular pacing. Extrastimulus testing is continued until ventricular refractoriness is encountered, whereas incremental pacing is continued until second-degree VA block occurs. It is frequently useful to record electrograms from multiple atrial sites during programmed ventricular stimulation in patients having paroxysmal tachycardia.

Programmed ventricular stimulation provides information regarding the quality of VA conduction, which is usually excellent in patients with PSVT. In reentrance using an anomalous AV pathway, the anomalous pathway is the retrograde limb and must be capable of repetitive retrograde conduction at short cycle lengths.[38] In AV nodal reentrance, one of the AV nodal pathways (usually the fast pathway) is the retrograde limb and must be capable of repetitive retrograde conduction.[27, 39] VA conduction is not required for the occurrence of any of the varieties of paroxysmal atrial tachycardia.[6, 34] Thus, demonstration that VA conduction is absent or that VA block occurs at slow ventricular paced rates suggests a diagnosis of paroxysmal atrial tachycardia.

When VA conduction is intact, it is important to determine whether this conduction is over the normal conduction system or over an anomalous AV pathway. Determination of the sequence of retrograde atrial activation is often useful in this regard. When the normal pathway is used for retrograde conduction, the earliest atrial electrograms are recorded from the low septal right atrium (His-bundle electrogram) or at the os of the coronary sinus.[47] Thus, demonstration that retrograde activation begins at a different site suggests the presence of a retrogradely conducting anomalous pathway.[2, 11, 48] Conversely, a normal retrograde sequence is compatible with conduction over either the normal conduction system or a septal anomalous pathway.

It is also useful to examine the temporal relation between retrograde His-bundle depolarization and retrograde atrial depolarization. With closely coupled ventricular extrastimuli, the H_2 deflection frequently emerges after V_2.[49] If the V_2–A_2 interval prolongs parallel to the V_2–H_2 interval, it is likely that the His bundle is a part of the pathway used for VA conduction. Conversely, as the V_2–H_2 interval prolongs, if the V_2–A_2 interval remains relatively constant, so that that the H_2 deflection approaches or even appears later than the A_2 deflection, then the His bundle cannot be part of the pathway used for VA conduction, and a retrogradely conducting anomalous pathway must be present.[2, 50]

It might be expected that decremental VA conduction (manifest as a progressive increase of VA interval as the ventricular paced cycle length is decreased) would distinguish conduction over the normal AV pathway from conduction over an anomalous pathway. In practice, however, retrograde conduction over the normal conduction system frequently is not decremental; although retrograde conduction over an anomalous pathway usually is not decremental, exceptions have been noted.[51, 52] Moreover, occasional slowly conducting anomalous pathways manifest markedly decremental conduction.[53, 54]

Detection of a retrogradely conducting anomalous AV pathway in a patient with PSVT is important. When such a pathway is present, it is likely to be part of the reentrant pathway.

Discontinuous V_1–V_2 and V_2–A_2 conduction curves can be relevant to diagnosis of the mechanism of paroxysmal tachycardia. Sometimes, one portion (fast or slow) of the curve reflects conduction over an anomalous pathway and the other portion reflects conduction over the normal pathway.[11, 12, 50] In this situation, there frequently is a marked change in the sequence of retrograde atrial activation at the point of discontinuity. In other cases, discontinuous V_1–V_2 and V_2–A_2 curves reflect the presence of retrograde dual (fast and slow) AV nodal pathways.[29, 30] When retrograde conduction shifts from the fast to the slow AV nodal pathway, there generally is a subtle change in the sequence of atrial activation, with conduction over the slow pathway favoring relatively early activation near the os of the coronary sinus.[50, 55] In other cases, the discontinuous curves merely reflect a shift of ventriculo-His conduction from the right bundle branch to the left bundle branch, an occurrence that is not relevant to diagnosis of mechanism of tachycardia.[56]

It can be useful to analyze the specific events associated with induction of paroxysmal tachycardia during programmed ventricular stimulation. Occasional patients with sinoatrial reentrance have excellent VA conduction that allows critical A_1–A_2 intervals to be achieved during ventricular extrastimulus testing. In this situation, the characteristic pattern at the onset of tachycardia is that of A_2 being followed immediately by an atrial echo beat (A_3), which may or may not be conducted to the ventricles.[6] When reentrance using an anomalous pathway or AV nodal reentrance is induced during ventricular extrastimulus testing, the pattern is usually different: A_2 is followed immediately by a ventricular echo beat (V_3) and only then by

an atrial echo beat (A_3). Induction of the unusual variety of AV nodal reentrance requires retrograde block in the fast pathway and conduction over the slow pathway, with sufficient delay (critical VA interval) to allow the fast pathway to recover excitability.[29, 30] Therefore, demonstration of retrograde dual AV nodal pathways and a critical VA interval suggests this diagnosis. Repetitive performance of ventricular pacing at a rate that produces type I second-degree VA block is frequently useful in establishing that a critical VA interval is required for induction of tachycardia.

It is usually not possible to differentiate between reentrance using an anomalous pathway and the usual variety of AV nodal reentrance by scrutinizing the pattern of induction during programmed ventricular stimulation. In each of these situations, crucial events are concealed: induction of reentrance using an anomalous pathway requires retrograde conduction over the anomalous pathway and also retrograde block in the distal AV node or His-Purkinje system (a concealed event), whereas induction of the usual variety of AV nodal reentrance requires retrograde conduction over the fast pathway and also retrograde block in the slow pathway (a concealed event).[13, 28] Other clues, however, such as the sequence of retrograde atrial activation at the time of induction, are often useful in differentiating between these two varieties of tachycardia.[11, 53]

Observations During Paroxysmal Tachycardia

The ability to induce and examine paroxysmal tachycardia in the electrophysiology laboratory is crucial in establishing its mechanism. When tachycardia cannot be thus observed, clues such as the presence of a retrogradely conducting anomalous pathway or antegrade dual AV nodal pathways suggest only a probable (rather than definitive) diagnosis.

In examining paroxysmal tachycardia, it is useful to begin with the relation between P waves or (preferably, atrial electrograms) and QRS complexes (Fig. 12-4). In most cases, this relation is 1:1. In reentrance using an anomalous pathway, a 1:1 relation is obligatory. In AV nodal reentrance, the relation usually is 1:1 but this variety of tachycardia can continue despite block between the reentrant pathway and the bulk of atrial tissue (apparent VA block) or between the reentrant pathway and the ventricles (apparent AV block).[21, 24, 25, 57] In any of the varieties of paroxysmal atrial tachycardia, conduction to the ventricles is unnecessary and AV block is common (paroxysmal atrial tachycardia with block).[6, 7, 34] These considerations can be summarized as follows. Continuance of paroxysmal tachycardia despite occurrence of AV block suggests a diagnosis of paroxysmal atrial tachycardia but is compati-

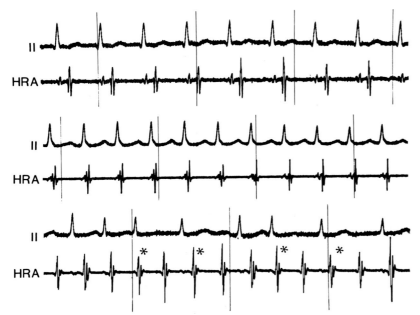

Figure 12-4. Three types of paroxysmal supraventricular tachycardia. Shown in each panel are electrocardiographic lead II and a high right atrial (*HRA*) electrogram. Time lines are at 1-second intervals. (**A**) Reentrance, using an anomalous pathway. Note the 1:1 relationship between atrial and ventricular depolarizations, with the former occurring in the first half of the RR interval (P after QRS). (**B**) Atrioventricular (AV) nodal reentrance (usual variety). Note that atrial depolarizations occur simultaneously with QRS complexes. (**C**) Paroxysmal atrial tachycardia that continues despite occurrence of AV block (* denotes blocked atrial beats).

ble with AV nodal reentry. This finding, however, excludes reentrance using an anomalous pathway. Continuance of paroxysmal tachycardia despite occurrence of VA block suggests a diagnosis of AV nodal reentrance or an automatic tachycardia arising in the AV node or His bundle.[8]

When paroxysmal tachycardia is characterized by a 1:1 relation between P waves and QRS complexes, it is useful to examine the relative timing of these events (see Fig. 12-4).[4,35] In reentrance using an anomalous pathway, antegrade conduction over the normal pathway characteristically takes longer than retrograde conduction over the anomalous pathway, so that P waves usually fall in the first half of the RR interval (P after QRS).[2-5] In occasional cases involving a slowly conducting anomalous pathway, retrograde conduction over the anomalous pathway takes longer than antegrade conduction over the normal pathway, and P waves are in the latter half of the RR interval (P before QRS).[50,53,54] In the usual variety of AV nodal reentrance, after antegrade conduction over the slow pathway to the distal common pathway, retrograde conduction over the fast pathway to the atria occurs simultaneously with antegrade conduction over the His-Purkinje system to the ventricles. Thus, P waves occur simultaneously with QRS complexes or slightly before or after.[4] In the unusual variety of AV nodal reentrance, after antegrade conduction over the fast pathway, antegrade conduction over the His-Purkinje system occurs more rapidly than retrograde conduction over the slow pathway, and P waves usually fall in the latter half of the RR interval (P before QRS).[29,30] In any of the varieties of paroxysmal atrial tachycardia, the relation between P waves and QRS complexes is a function of

atrial rate and PR interval: P waves are usually in front of QRS complexes but may fall after QRS complexes if atrial rate is fast or PR interval is long.[4,7] These considerations can be summarized as follows. If during paroxysmal tachycardia P waves occur simultaneously (or almost simultaneously) with QRS complexes, the likely diagnosis is the usual variety of AV nodal reentrance, although paroxysmal atrial tachycardia is also possible. If P waves follow QRS complexes, the likely diagnosis is reentrance using an anomalous pathway, although the usual variety of AV nodal reentrance or paroxysmal atrial tachycardia is possible. If P waves precede QRS complexes, the differential diagnosis includes paroxysmal atrial tachycardia, the unusual variety of AV nodal reentrance, and AV reentrance using a slowly conducting anomalous pathway.

It is also useful to examine the sequence of atrial activation during paroxysmal tachycardia. A normal retrograde sequence (low interatrial septum depolarized first) suggests a diagnosis of AV nodal reentrance but is compatible with reentrance using a septal anomalous pathway or paroxysmal atrial tachycardia arising in the interatrial septum.[11] In contrast, an abnormal sequence of retrograde atrial activation indicates reentrance using an anomalous pathway or paroxysmal atrial tachycardia. The sequence of atrial activation (and P-wave morphology) is also used to distinguish between sinus node reentrance and atrial reentrance.[6,7]

Appearance or disappearance of functional bundle branch block during paroxysmal tachycardia may provide clues that are diagnostic of reentrance using an anomalous AV pathway. In this variety of tachycardia, block in the bundle branch ipsilateral to the anomalous pathway is associated with an increment of VA interval.[10,58,59] This increment is less than 25 milliseconds when the anomalous pathway is septal and greater than 35 milliseconds when the anomalous pathway is located on the free wall.[60] The increment of VA interval may be partially compensated by the antegrade limb (AV node), so that there may be little or no corresponding increase in cycle length of tachycardia.[59,60] Block in the bundle branch contralateral to the anomalous pathway usually has little effect on VA interval or cycle length of tachycardia.[10,58,61] In AV nodal reentrance or paroxysmal atrial tachycardia, block in either bundle branch generally has no effect.

Performance of ventricular extrastimulus testing during paroxysmal tachycardia can also be useful in diagnosing reentrance using an anomalous AV pathway. In this variety of tachycardia, it is often possible to demonstrate that a ventricular extrastimulus, introduced at a time when the His bundle is being used for antegrade conduction, can reset the atria.[10,58,62] This finding suggests that an anomalous pathway has been used for retrograde conduction and is probably a part of the reentrant pathway. Inability to reset the atria with a ventricular extrastimulus is of limited diagnostic value; this is seen not only in AV nodal reentrance or paroxysmal atrial tachycardia but also in some cases of reentrance using an anomalous pathway, especially when the rate of tachycardia is fast or the site of ventricular stimulation is distant from the anomalous pathway.[63,64]

Administration of Drugs

Administration of drugs may be of value in diagnosing a specific variety of paroxysmal tachycardia. Adenosine may be helpful in determining whether VA conduction is over the normal conduction system or over an anomalous pathway.[65] This agent often markedly increases retrograde normal pathway refractoriness but usually has little effect on retrograde anomalous pathway refractoriness. This drug can be administered by rapid intravenous injection during ventricular pacing at a rate well below that at which second-degree VA block usually occurs. If this injection causes transient VA block, retrograde conduction over the normal pathway is suggested. This response, however, is also is consistent with retrograde conduction over a slowly conducting anomalous pathway.[54] Absence of VA block after injection of adenosine may reflect insufficient dosing, poor venous access, or prolonged circulation time and thus should be interpreted with extreme caution.[66] Other drugs generally have not been useful in delineating the route of VA conduction. Although digitalis, β-adrenergic blocking agents, or verapamil usually have little effect on

retrograde anomalous pathway refractoriness, they also usually have little effect on retrograde normal pathway refractoriness.[67–71] Although class I antiarrhythmic agents may markedly increase retrograde anomalous pathway refractoriness, they also may markedly increase retrograde normal pathway refractoriness.[71–74]

Administration of digitalis, a beta-blocking agent, or verapamil occasionally provides useful information by increasing antegrade AV nodal refractoriness. For example, this increased refractoriness may cause early atrial extrastimuli to block in the AV node, thus facilitating determination of whether antegrade conduction to the His bundle is required for induction of tachycardia. Intravenous adenosine may provoke transient AV block during paroxysmal atrial tachycardia.[75] The significance of these observations was discussed earlier.

Another situation in which administration of drugs can be useful is when despite the presence of an anomalous pathway or dual AV nodal pathways, paroxysmal tachycardia cannot be induced due to excessive AV nodal refractoriness. In this situation, intravenous isoproterenol or atropine may be used to decrease AV nodal refractoriness and thus facilitate induction of tachycardia.[76,77]

Strategies for Electrophysiologic Studies

The preceding section of this chapter has been a catalog of techniques that can be used to diagnose the common varieties of PSVT. Electrophysiologic studies in a patient with PSVT, however, should not be performed in a rigidly predetermined order. These studies should be flexible and aimed at providing the information most relevant to the differential diagnosis at a given point in time. For example, if the problem is to differentiate between sinoatrial reentrance and AV nodal reentrance, it is useful to perform repetitive atrial pacing at a rate that results in second-degree block in the AV node. In contrast, this technique is usually of limited value in distinguishing AV nodal reentrance from reentrance using an anomalous pathway.

Occasionally, the differential diagnosis cannot be narrowed before performance of electrophysiologic studies. In this situation, it is recommended to begin the studies with programmed ventricular stimulation. If VA conduction is absent, the likely diagnosis is paroxysmal atrial tachycardia. If VA conduction is intact, presence or absence of a retrogradely conducting anomalous pathway can be determined by noting the sequence of retrograde atrial activation and the temporal relation between depolarization of the His bundle and depolarization of the atria. If a retrogradely conducting anomalous pathway can be excluded, it is useful to perform rapid atrial pacing to differentiate between sinoatrial reentrance and AV nodal reentrance.

TREATMENT

Paroxysmal supraventricular tachycardia is generally not life-threatening unless severe underlying heart disease is present. It can have hemodynamic effects, however, and can produce symptoms.[78] Rapid ventricular rates limit diastolic filling, which can be further decreased by loss of AV coordination. This can result in decreased cardiac output, with hypotension and raised intraatrial pressures. Associated symptoms include palpitations, "pounding" in the neck, dyspnea, chest oppression, weakness, dizziness, and even syncope. The severity of symptoms varies markedly with rate of tachycardia, relative timing of atrial and ventricular contractions, presence or absence of heart disease, and duration of the attack. Chronic supraventricular tachycardia can cause tachycardia-induced cardiomyopathy.[79,80] Many patients with infrequent or well-tolerated attacks of PSVT do not need treatment. Some patients require therapy to achieve either of two goals: terminate an acute attack of PSVT or prevent recurrent or chronic attacks.

Treatment of PSVT should be tailored to the individual patient. Decision to treat; choice of medical, ablative, or surgical therapy; or selection of a specific antiarrhythmic drug often depends not only on the specific mechanism of tachycardia but also on severity of attacks, frequency of attacks, patient age, and presence of other cardiac abnormalities or medical conditions. Detailed discussion of individualization of therapy is generally beyond the scope of this chapter.

One situation that requires special mention is the patient with manifest preexcitation. Patients with preexcitation are predisposed not only to PSVT (reentrance using an anomalous AV pathway) but to paroxysmal atrial fibrillation also.[81] The basis for this latter predisposition appears to be that attacks of PSVT can initiate atrial fibrillation.[82] In patients with preexcitation, ventricular rates during atrial fibrillation often reflect antegrade refractoriness of the anomalous pathway rather than the AV node.[83] When anomalous pathway refractoriness is short, ventricular rates can be fast (sometimes more than 300 beats/minute) and this can lead to ventricular fibrillation and death.[84] Thus, in patients with manifest preexcitation, assessment of antegrade anomalous pathway refractoriness is crucial. When this refractoriness is short, addressing the mere possibility of a life-threatening arrhythmia (atrial fibrillation) often takes priority over treatment of actual attacks of symptom-producing PSVT. This consideration does not apply to patients with a concealed anomalous

pathway or an anomalous pathway that has long antegrade refractoriness.

Termination of an Acute Attack

The rationale for termination of an acute attack of PSVT can be exemplified by the situation in reentrance using an anomalous pathway. The circus movement (and therefore PSVT) continues as long as the circling wavefront finds the reentrant pathway excitable (Fig. 12-5). If the wavefront encounters refractory tissue and blocks, the circus movement is broken, and the tachycardia terminates (see Fig. 12-5). In a patient with an acute attack of reentrance using an anomalous pathway, the goal of therapy is to increase

A. Reentrant tachycardia

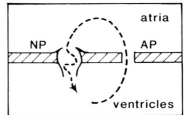

B. Block in normal pathway

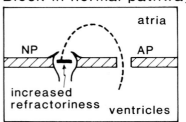

C. Block in anomalous pathway

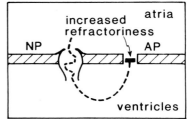

Figure 12-5. Conduction system in Wolff-Parkinson-White syndrome (see Fig. 11-2). (**A**) Reentrance, using an anomalous pathway. (**B**) The circus movement blocks in the antegrade limb because of increased atrioventricular nodal refractoriness. (**C**) The circus movement blocks in the retrograde limb because of increased anomalous pathway refractoriness.

refractoriness of either the antegrade limb (normal pathway) or the retrograde limb (anomalous pathway) sufficiently to cause the circling wavefront to block. These considerations are also applicable to the situation in AV nodal reentrance, in which the goal of therapy is to increase refractoriness of one of the AV nodal pathways.

Several modalities of treatment are available for termination of an acute attack of PSVT. Vagal maneuvers such as carotid sinus massage or Valsalva's maneuver often are tried first. These maneuvers may or may not increase AV nodal refractoriness sufficiently to terminate tachycardia.[85,86] Intravenous drugs can also be used to increase refractoriness of a limb of the reentrant pathway. Intravenous verapamil (5 to 10 mg) can convert about 90% of attacks of reentrance using an anomalous pathway or AV nodal reentrance within just a few minutes, with only rare adverse effects.[69,70] This agent should not be used in patients with hypotension or severe left ventricular dysfunction, however. Intravenous adenosine (6 to 12 mg injected rapidly into a peripheral vein or 3 to 6 mg injected through a central line) also can quickly convert about 90% of attacks of paroxysmal tachycardia that require conduction through the AV node, with only transient side effects.[75,87] This agent should be used with caution in patients with bronchial asthma. Either verapamil or adenosine is excellent therapy for conversion of an acute attack of PSVT. The efficacy of intravenous digitalis, β-adrenergic blocking agents, or procainamide in this situation is not well known. Even if effective, however, these agents usually do not act as quickly as verapamil or adenosine. It should be noted that in patients with manifest preexcitation, digitalis or verapamil can shorten antegrade anomalous pathway refractoriness.[88–90] It is reasonable to use these agents to terminate acute attacks of PSVT (in patients known to have preexcitation) in the setting of continuous ECG monitoring with resuscitative equipment nearby.

Single doses of oral antiarrhythmic drugs also can be used to convert acute attacks of PSVT.[91] For patients with sporadic attacks of well-tolerated tachycardia, this form of therapy can eliminate the inconvenience and expense of repeated Emergency Room visits. Before use of this therapy, however, the patient should be thoroughly evaluated and efficacy and safety of the oral drug assessed. Digitalis or verapamil should not be employed in the presence of an anomalous pathway with short antegrade refractoriness.[88–90]

Attacks of PSVT usually reflect reentrance and thus can be terminated by cardiac pacing.[9,15,92] If an appropriate pacing site and modality are selected, paced beats penetrate the reentrant pathway and render it refractory. Termination of a single attack of PSVT by pacing is cumbersome, requiring transvenous insertion of an electrode catheter or passage of an esophageal lead. The development of radiofrequency-triggered or automatic antitachycardia pacemakers has made it possible to use a permanent cardiac lead to terminate multiple attacks of PSVT.[93,94] Given the effectiveness and safety of radiofrequency catheter ablation techniques, however, there is little use for these antitachycardia devices. Finally, direct current countershock can be used to terminate attacks of PSVT that are poorly tolerated or refractory to other forms of therapy.

Relatively little is known about treatment of the less common varieties of PSVT. Sinoatrial reentrance usually can be terminated by carotid sinus massage.[6,7] Automatic ectopic atrial tachycardia is frequently resistant to antiarrhythmic drugs.[32] In this situation, however, administration of digitalis, verapamil, or a β-adrenergic blocking agent may increase AV nodal refractoriness sufficiently to produce second-degree AV block and thus slow ventricular rates. It should be kept in mind that paroxysmal atrial tachycardia with block can also be caused by digitalis excess, which requires elimination of this agent.

Chronic Oral Drug Therapy

Some patients with recurrent PSVT require therapy to prevent further attacks. In many cases, an oral antiarrhythmic drug is administered in an attempt to maintain increased refractoriness in a limb of the reentrant pathway so that a circus movement cannot be initiated. Drugs that might be used for this purpose are digitalis, verapamil, or a β-adrenergic blocking agent or a major antiarrhythmic agent such as procainamide, quinidine, disopyramide, flecainide, propafenone, sotalol, or amiodarone. Any of these drugs may or may not be effective, and none has emerged as the drug of choice.[71,95–101] Specifically, oral verapamil has not been as frequently effective in preventing recurrences of PSVT as intravenous verapamil has been in terminating acute attacks.[70]

When recurrent PSVT has not been productive of severe symptoms, it is reasonable to use the trial-and-error approach to therapy. Because any of the available antiarrhythmic agents may or may not be effective, it is recommended to start with digitalis, verapamil, or a β-adrenergic blocking agent.* These drugs generally are not proarrhythmic, are well-tolerated, and can be administered just once or twice daily. If these drugs are not effective, a major antiarrhythmic agent can be tried. Flecainide appears to have little proarrhythmic potential in patients with PSVT who do not have underlying heart disease, usually is well-tolerated, and can be administered just twice daily.[102,103] Thus, this agent often is used early. When the trial-and-error approach is used, a successful drug regimen usually can be delineated within a reasonable period.

Electrophysiologic testing of drugs can be performed

---

* Digitalis or verapamil should not be used in the presence of an anomalous pathway with short antegrade refractoriness.

in patients with PSVT (Fig. 12-6).[71,95,96] A control electrophysiologic study is performed first to delineate the mechanism of PSVT and confirm that the arrhythmia can be reliably induced by programmed cardiac stimulation. After this study, a hexapolar electrode catheter is positioned so that the distal two poles can be used for pacing the right ventricular apex and the proximal four poles can be used for recording and pacing from the right atrium. Available antiarrhythmic agents then are serially administered and tested for ability to prevent induction of sustained tachycardia. When a drug prevents induction of sustained tachycardia, it usually is possible to delineate the site of action. For example, procainamide may prevent induction of AV nodal reentrance by markedly increasing retrograde fast-pathway refractoriness. This increase of refractoriness can be confirmed by demonstration that the maximum ventricular paced rate that is associated with 1:1 VA conduction is markedly reduced.[72] Chronic oral therapy with an agent that prevents induction of sustained tachycardia usually is

effective in preventing spontaneous recurrences of sustained tachycardia.[71,95] Thus, electrophysiologic testing can be used to screen a new drug for effectiveness in the different varieties of PSVT or to systematically compare the effectiveness of several drugs in a series of patients with PSVT.[96] It also can be used to delineate one or more drugs that are likely to be effective therapy in an individual patient with severely symptomatic PSVT when the trial-and-error approach is unattractive.

It is important to note that chronic administration of a major antiarrhythmic agent is particularly unattractive in many patients with PSVT, who tend to be young and free of structural heart disease. Chronic drug therapy is inconvenient, frequently causes side effects, and can cause life-threatening proarrhythmia. Thus, radiofrequency catheter ablation procedures, which have been shown to be effective and safe in several of the varieties of PSVT, often provide an attractive alternative to the use of a major antiarrhythmic agent. The following would seem to be

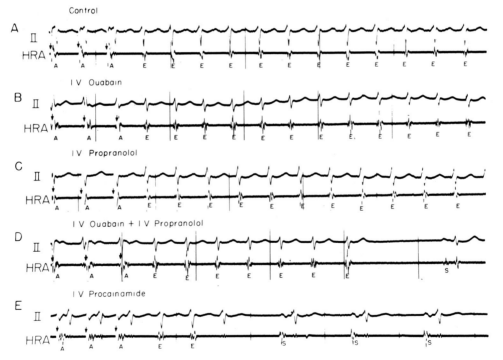

Figure 12-6. Serial electrophysiologic drug studies in a patient with paroxysmal supraventricular tachycardia due to atrioventricular nodal reentrance (usual variety). Shown in each panel are electrocardiograph lead II and a high right atrial (*HRA*) electrogram. Paroxysmal tachycardia was induced by atrial pacing (*arrows*). (**A**) Induced tachycardia was sustained in control studies, (**B**) after administration of ouabain, and (**C**) after administration of propranolol. (**D**) After administration of ouabain plus propranolol, induced tachycardia was nonsustained because of antegrade block in the slow pathway (the last atrial echo [*E*] is not followed by a QRS complex). (**E**) After administration of procainamide, induced tachycardia was also nonsustained but in this case because of retrograde block in the fast pathway (the last QRS complex is not associated with an atrial echo). (From Bauernfeind RA, Wyndham CR, Dhingra RC, et al: Serial electrophysiologic testing of multiple drugs in patients with atrioventricular nodal reentrant paroxysmal tachycardia. Circulation 1980;62:1341. By permission of the American Heart Association)

reasonable approaches for various subsets of patients with PSVT. When PSVT has been productive of severe symptoms or an anomalous pathway with short antegrade refractoriness renders the condition life-threatening, radiofrequency ablation should be considered as initial therapy because successful ablation provides the highest degree of protection. When PSVT produces more moderate symptoms (and an anomalous pathway with short antegrade refractoriness is not present), a therapeutic trial of digitalis, verapamil, or a β-adrenergic blocking agent would seem appropriate. If bothersome recurrences of PSVT continue, radiofrequency catheter ablation often is preferable to the use of a major antiarrhythmic agent. Finally, in drug-refractory cases of PSVT, radiofrequency catheter ablation usually is the procedure of choice.

Division or Ablation of Anomalous Atrioventricular Pathway

Delineation of the various mechanisms of PSVT and identification of specific tissues required for their occurrence have led to development of surgical and ablative therapies. The best example of such therapy is surgical excision or catheter ablation of an anomalous AV pathway.[104, 105] Successful elimination of the anomalous pathway prevents recurrences of reentrant tachycardia. It also eliminates rapid conduction over the pathway during bouts of atrial fibrillation and actually appears to prevent recurrences of atrial fibrillation, presumably by preventing the attacks of PSVT that initiate the arrhythmia.[106, 107]

The surgical or ablative approach begins with detailed cardiac electrophysiologic studies.[108] The presence of one or more anomalous AV pathways and their participation in reentrant tachycardia are confirmed. Catheters positioned in the right atrium and coronary sinus are then used to determine the location of the anomalous pathway or pathways. Commonly used techniques are:

1. Determination of the sequence of atrial activation during ventricular pacing or reentrant tachycardia, with retrograde conduction over the anomalous pathway[11, 37, 48]

2. Determination of the sequence of ventricular activation during sinus rhythm or atrial pacing, with antegrade conduction over the anomalous pathway[109]

3. Pacing the atria at multiple sites just above the AV ring and measuring intervals from atrial pacing spikes to onset of delta waves (the shortest stimulus–delta interval usually is obtained from the atrial site nearest the anomalous pathway)[110]

4. Noting the effect of functional bundle branch block on VA interval during reentrant tachycardia[60]

In addition, it usually is possible to record an electrogram reflecting conduction over the anomalous pathway by placing catheter electrodes in close proximity to the anomalous pathway.[111, 112]

Surgery is performed through a median sternotomy under general anesthesia. Epicardial wires are attached to the atrium and the ventricle near the suspected location of the anomalous pathway. These wires are used to record reference electrograms and for pacing. Either a hand-held probe or a nylon mesh band containing multiple bipolar button electrodes is used for mapping.[113, 114] The sequence of epicardial activation just below the AV groove is determined during antegrade conduction over the anomalous pathway. Similarly, the sequence of epicardial activation just above the AV groove is determined during retrograde conduction over the anomalous pathway. The anomalous pathway is localized to one of four anatomic spaces: left free wall, posteroseptal, anteroseptal, and right free wall.[115]

Two surgical approaches have been developed for division of anomalous pathways. The endocardial approach has been used more commonly.[115, 116] It is performed through an atriotomy on cardiopulmonary bypass. Left free wall pathways are approached by a left atriotomy in the cardioplegically arrested heart, whereas posteroseptal, anteroseptal, and right free wall pathways are approached by a right atriotomy in the normothermic beating heart. A supraannular incision is made, and a plane of dissection is developed between the AV groove fat pad and the ventricle. The epicardial approach is a closed-heart technique.[117, 118] Cardiopulmonary bypass is used for left free wall and anteroseptal pathways only. This approach establishes a plane of dissection between the AV groove fat pad and the atrium, thus severing the atrial end of the anomalous pathway. Some workers have added cryoablation of the underlying AV ring to the procedure.[117] Results with either the endocardial approach or the epicardial approach have been excellent. Regardless of anomalous pathway location, successful division has been achieved in almost 100% of cases, with an operative mortality of less than 1% for elective, uncomplicated cases.[107, 115–118] Despite its high degree of success and safety, surgical division has largely been replaced by catheter ablation procedures.

Catheter ablation procedures involve precise mapping of the anomalous pathway and careful positioning of the tip of a catheter at the identified site. The procedure originally employed a standard quadripolar electrode catheter and direct current energy.[119–122] The distal one or two poles of the catheter were connected to the cathodal output of a defibrillator, whereas a patch electrode on the chest wall was connected to the anode. Two or more shocks of 150 to 400 J typically were delivered. Tissue injury is thought to have resulted from thermal electrocoagulation. Most of the coronary sinus was unsuitable for delivery of direct current shocks because concussive waves could cause rupture and massive hemopericardium. Several groups of workers applied the shocks to anomalous pathways located near the os of the coronary sinus, with a reasonable rate of success (about two out of three patients).[119–121] Furthermore, at least one group of workers was able to apply the procedure to an anomalous pathway in any location by placing the catheter tip directly on the tricuspid or mitral annulus.[122, 123] The procedure was complicated by occasional instances of perforation, coronary artery spasm, or AV block.[120–123] Furthermore, direct current shocks produced heterogenous tissue damage that frequently caused transient ventricular arrhythmias and occasionally resulted in sudden death.[123]

Radiofrequency energy (frequency range, 150 to 1000 kHz) has been used for catheter ablation.[124] The high-frequency current does not stimulate neuromuscular fibers, so that general anesthesia is not required. A special steerable catheter with a bulbous-tip electrode has been developed to spread current over a larger surface.[125] The approach to the pathway varies from center to center and sometimes from patient to patient.[105, 126, 127] Pathways that traverse the tricuspid annulus are approached transvenously, whereas those that traverse the mitral annulus are approached either transarterially or transseptally. Some posteroseptal pathways have been ablated from inside the proximal coronary sinus or one of its branches.[105] The atrial insertion of the pathway can be addressed from above the AV ring, or the ventricular insertion can be approached from under the valve leaflets. The bulbous-tip electrode is connected to the cathodal output of a radiofrequency generator, and a patch electrode on the chest wall is connected to the anode. Energy is delivered at 45 to 60 V for a period of 20 to 60 seconds. The resulting lesion is small (less than 1 cm in diameter) and well demarcated.[124]

Several groups of workers have used radiofrequency energy to ablate anomalous pathways in large series of patients.[105, 126, 127] Initial success rates of 90% to 100% have been achieved with manifest or concealed pathways, regardless of location. Anomalous pathway conduction has recovered days, weeks, or months after the procedure in 5% to 10% of patients, but these pathways usually have been eliminated permanently in a second ablation session.[105, 126, 127] Complications have occurred in 3% to 4% of patients but have been minor and not productive of long-term disability. The well-demarcated lesions produced by radiofrequency energy generally have not been arrhythmogenic. Given its high rate of success and relative safety, radiofrequency ablation has become the treatment of choice for patients with AV reentrant tachycardia that is productive of severe symptoms or with an anomalous pathway that has short antegrade refractoriness. It also is an attractive alternative to chronic antiarrhythmic drug therapy for young patients with AV reentrant tachycardia.

Surgery or Ablation for Atrioventricular Nodal Reentry

Tissue that comprises the fast AV nodal pathway generally lies just posterior to the His bundle, whereas tissue that comprises the slow AV nodal pathway generally lies inferiorly, extending toward the coronary sinus.[22, 23] This anatomic relation has made it possible to selectively divide or ablate one or the other AV nodal pathways. Surgical dissection or cryosurgical ablation in the triangle of Koch, located inferior and posterior to the His bundle, prevented recurrence of AV nodal reentrant tachycardia without causing complete heart block in small series of patients.[128, 129] Later, some workers delivered direct current shocks just posterior to the His bundle in patients with AV nodal reentrant tachycardia, with reasonable success.[130]

The small discreet lesions produced by radiofrequency energy are particularly well-suited for selective ablation of the fast or slow AV nodal pathway; this form of energy has been used by several groups of workers in patients with AV nodal reentrant tachycardia.[23, 131, 132] Some workers have targeted the fast AV nodal pathway by delivering radiofrequency current just posterior to the His-bundle recording site.[23, 131] This procedure has prevented recurrence of paroxysmal tachycardia in most patients but has been associated with a 10% to 20% incidence of complete AV block. Most workers target the slow AV nodal pathway by delivering radiofrequency current in the region just anterior and superior to the coronary sinus.[23, 132] With this latter approach, success rates of 90% to 100% have been achieved, and the incidence of complete AV block has been low. Given a high rate of success and a low rate of serious complications, selective radiofrequency catheter ablation of the slow AV nodal pathway is the procedure of choice for patients with AV nodal reentrant tachycardia that is refractory to antiarrhythmic drugs. It is also an attractive alternative to chronic antiarrhythmic drug therapy for young patients with bothersome tachycardia.

Other Surgical or Ablative Procedures

New procedures have been applied to automatic ectopic atrial tachycardia. These require accurate mapping of the focus of tachycardia. Surgical approaches have been excision or cryoablation of implicated tissue.[133, 134] Catheter ablation employing direct current shocks has been attempted, with occasional success.[134] Radiofrequency energy has been employed in small series of patients, with good success.[135]

Other procedures have been used to unselectively ablate the AV node or His bundle. The usual surgical approach has involved direct recording of endocardial electrograms to localize the His bundle and cryoablation of the area that shows the largest deflection.[136] This surgery has been superseded by catheter ablation of the AV node, performed by delivering direct-current shocks or radiofrequency energy just posterior to the His-bundle recording site.[137–139] Catheter ablation has been completely or partially successful in about 90% of patients, with a low rate of unexpected complications. Successful ablation of the AV junction isolates the ventricles from tachycardias arising in the atria or the AV node. Unlike ablation of an anomalous pathway, however, or selective ablation of a slow AV nodal pathway, it does not restore normal physiology and leaves the patient with complete heart block and possible pacemaker dependency. Thus, ablation of the AV junction is a treatment of last resort for troublesome tachycardias that are refractory to drugs and not amenable to more specific procedures.

References

1. Katz LN, Pick A: Clinical electrocardiography. Part I: The arrhythmias. Philadelphia: Lea & Febiger, 1956:282.

2. Wellens HJJ, Durrer D: The role of an accessory atrioventricular pathway in reciprocal tachycardia: observations in patients with and without the Wolff-Parkinson-White syndrome. Circulation 1975;52:58.

3. Sung RJ, Gelband H, Castellanos A, Aranda JM, Myerburg RJ: Clinical and electrophysiologic observations in patients with concealed accessory atrioventricular bypass tracts. Am J Cardiol 1977;40:839.

4. Wu D, Denes P, Amat-y-Leon F, et al: Clinical, electrocardiographic and electrophysiologic observations in patients with paroxysmal supraventricular tachycardia. Am J Cardiol 1978;41:1045.

5. Farshidi A, Josephson ME, Horowitz LN: Electrophysiologic characteristics of concealed bypass tracts: clinical and electrocardiographic correlates. Am J Cardiol 1978;41:1052.

6. Wu D, Amat-y-Leon F, Denes P, Dhingra RC, Pietras RJ, Rosen KM: Demonstration of sustained sinus and atrial re-entry as a mechanism of paroxysmal supraventricular tachycardia. Circulation 1975;51:234.

7. Gomes JA, Hariman RJ, Kang PS, Chowdry IH: Sustained symptomatic sinus node reentrant tachycardia: incidence, clinical significance, electrophysiologic observations and the effects of antiarrhythmic agents. J Am Coll Cardiol 1985;5:45.

8. Ruder MA, Davis JC, Eldar M, et al: Clinical and electrophysiologic characterization of automatic junctional tachycardia in adults. Circulation 1986;73:930.

9. Durrer D, Schoo L, Schuilenburg RM, Wellens HJJ: The role of premature beats in the initiation and the termination of supraventricular tachycardia in the Wolff-Parkinson-White syndrome. Circulation 1967;36:644.

10. Neuss H, Schlepper M, Thormann J: Analysis of re-entry mechanisms in three patients with concealed Wolff-Parkinson-White syndrome. Circulation 1975;51:75.

11. Tonkin AM, Gallagher JJ, Svenson RH, Wallace AG, Sealy WC:

12. Wellens HJ, Durrer D: Patterns of ventriculo-atrial conduction in the Wolff-Parkinson-White syndrome. Circulation 1974;49:22.

13. Akhtar M, Lehmann MH, Denker ST, Mahmud R, Tchou P, Jazayeri M: Electrophysiologic mechanisms of orthodromic tachycardia initiation during ventricular pacing in the Wolff-Parkinson-White syndrome. J Am Coll Cardiol 1987;9:89.

14. Goldreyer BN, Damato AN: The essential role of atrioventricular conduction delay in the initiation of paroxysmal supraventricular tachycardia. Circulation 1971;43:679.

15. Goldreyer BN, Bigger JT: Site of reentry in paroxysmal supraventricular tachycardia in man. Circulation 1971;43:15.

16. Rosen KM, Mehta A, Miller RA: Demonstration of dual atrioventricular nodal pathways in man. Am J Cardiol 1974;33:291.

17. Denes P, Wu D, Dhingra RC, Chuquimia R, Rosen KM: Demonstration of dual A-V nodal pathways in patients with paroxysmal supraventricular tachycardia. Circulation 1973;48:549.

18. Touboul P, Huerta F, Porte J, Delahaye JP: Reciprocal rhythm in patients with normal electrocardiogram: evidence for dual conduction pathways. Am Heart J 1976;91:3.

19. Bissett JK, de Soyza N, Kane JJ, Murphy ML: Atrioventricular conduction patterns in patients with paroxysmal supraventricular tachycardia. Am Heart J 1976;91:287.

20. Bharati S, Bauernfeind R, Scheinman M, et al: Congenital abnormalities of the conduction system in two patients with tachyarrhythmias. Circulation 1979;59:593.

21. Scheinman MM, Gonzalez R, Thomas A, Ullyot D, Bharati S, Lev M: Reentry confined to the atrioventricular node: electrophysiologic and anatomic findings. Am J Cardiol 1982;49:1814.

22. Wu D, Yeh SJ, Wang CC, Wen MS, Chang HJ, Lin FC: Nature of dual atrioventricular node pathways and the tachycardia circuit as defined by radiofrequency ablation technique. J Am Coll Cardiol 1992;20:884.

23. Jazayeri MR, Hempe SL, Sra JS, et al: Selective transcatheter ablation of the fast and slow pathways using radiofrequency energy in patients with atrioventricular nodal reentrant tachycardia. Circulation 1992;85:1318.

24. Wellens HJJ, Wesdorp JC, Duren DR, Lie KI: Second degree block during reciprocal atrioventricular nodal tachycardia. Circulation 1976;53:595.

25. Josephson ME, Kastor JA: Paroxysmal supraventricular tachycardia: is the atrium a necessary link? Circulation 1976;54:430.

26. Miller JM, Rosenthal ME, Vassallo JA, Josephson ME: Atrioventricular nodal reentrant tachycardia: studies on upper and lower 'common pathways'. Circulation 1987;75:930.

27. Brugada P, Heddle B, Green M, Wellens HJJ: Initiation of atrioventricular nodal reentrant tachycardia in patients with discontinuous anterograde atrioventricular nodal conduction curves with and without documented supraventricular tachycardia: observations on the role of a discontinuous retrograde conduction curve. Am Heart J 1984;107:685.

28. Wu D, Kou HC, Yeh SJ, Lin FC, Hung JS: Determinants of tachycardia induction using ventricular stimulation in dual

Anterograde block in accessory pathways with retrograde conduction in reciprocating tachycardia. Eur J Cardiol 1975;3:143.

pathway atrioventricular nodal reentrant tachycardia. Am Heart J 1984;108:44.

29. Wu D, Denes P, Amat-y-Leon F, Wyndham CRC, Dhingra R, Rosen KM: An unusual variety of atrioventricular nodal reentry due to retrograde dual atrioventricular nodal pathways. Circulation 1977;56:50.

30. Strasberg B, Swiryn S, Bauernfeind R, et al: Retrograde dual atrioventricular nodal pathways. Am J Cardiol 1981;48:639.

31. Goldreyer BN, Gallagher JJ, Damato AN: The electrophysiologic demonstration of atrial ectopic tachycardia in man. Am Heart J 1973;85:205.

32. Scheinman MM, Basu D, Hollenberg M: Electrophysiologic studies in patients with persistent atrial tachycardia. Circulation 1974;50:266.

33. Waldo AL: Mechanisms of atrial fibrillation, atrial flutter, and ectopic atrial tachycardia—a brief review. Circulation 1987; 75(Suppl III):37.

34. Brugada P, Farre J, Green M, et al: Observations in patients with supraventricular tachycardia having a P-R interval shorter than the R-P interval: differentiation between atrial tachycardia and reciprocating atrioventricular tachycardia using an accessory pathway with long conduction times. Am Heart J 1984;107:556.

35. Bar FW, Brugada P, Dassen WRM, Wellens HJJ: Differential diagnosis of tachycardia with narrow QRS complex (shorter than 0.12 second). Am J Cardiol 1984;54:555.

36. Kay GN, Pressley JC, Packer DL, Pritchett ELC, German LD, Gilbert MR: Value of the 12-lead electrocardiogram in discriminating atrioventricular nodal reciprocating tachycardia from circus movement atrioventricular tachycardia utilizing a retrograde accessory pathway. Am J Cardiol 1987; 59:296.

37. Svenson RH, Miller HC, Gallagher JJ, Wallace AG: Electrophysiological evaluation of the Wolff-Parkinson-White syndrome: problems in assessing antegrade and retrograde conduction over the accessory pathway. Circulation 1975; 52:552.

38. Denes P, Wu D, Amat-y-Leon F, et al: Determinants of atrioventricular reentrant paroxysmal tachycardia in patients with Wolff-Parkinson-White syndrome. Circulation 1978; 58:415.

39. Denes P, Wu D, Amat-y-Leon F, Dhingra R, Wyndham CR, Rosen KM: The determinants of atrioventricular nodal reentrance with premature atrial stimulation in patients with dual A-V nodal pathways. Circulation 1977;56:253.

40. Neuss H, Schlepper M, Spies HF: Effects of heart rate and atropine on 'dual AV conduction.' Br Heart J 1975;37:1216.

41. Denes P, Wu D, Dhingra R, Amat-y-Leon F, Wyndham C, Rosen KM: Dual atrioventricular nodal pathways: a common electrophysiological response. Br Heart J 1975;37:1069.

42. Hess SG, Gallastegui J, Bauernfeind RA: Failure to demonstrate dual pathways in patients with atrioventricular nodal reentrant tachycardia. Circulation 1983;68(Suppl III):11. Abstract.

43. Sung RJ, Styperek JL: Electrophysiologic identification of dual atrioventricular nodal pathway conduction in patients with reciprocating tachycardia using anomalous bypass tracts. Circulation 1979;60:1464.

44. Pritchett ELC, Prystowsky EN, Benditt DG, Gallagher JJ: 'Dual atrioventricular nodal pathways' in patients with Wolff-Parkinson-White syndrome. Br Heart J 1980;43:7.

45. Bauernfeind RA, Swiryn S, Strasberg B, et al: Analysis of anterograde and retrograde fast pathway properties in patients with dual atrioventricular nodal pathways: observations regarding the pathophysiology of the Lown-Ganong-Levine syndrome. Am J Cardiol 1982;49:283.

46. Sung RJ, Castellanos A, Gelband H, Myerburg RJ: Mechanism of reciprocating tachycardia initiated during sinus rhythm in concealed Wolff-Parkinson-White syndrome. Circulation 1976;54:338.

47. Amat-y-Leon F, Dhingra RC, Wu D, Denes P, Wyndham C, Rosen KM: Catheter mapping of retrograde atrial activation: observations during ventricular pacing and AV nodal reentrant paroxysmal tachycardia. Br Heart J 1976;38:355.

48. Crossen KJ, Lindsay BD, Cain ME: Reliability of retrograde atrial activation patterns during ventricular pacing for localizing accessory pathways. J Am Coll Cardiol 1987;9:1279.

49. Akhtar M, Damato AN, Caracta AR, Batsford WP, Lau SH: The gap phenomena during retrograde conduction in man. Circulation 1974;49:811.

50. Brugada P, Bar FWHM, Vanagt EJ, Friedman PL, Wellens HJJ: Observations in patients showing A-V junctional echoes with a shorter P-R than R-P interval: distinction between intranodal reentry or reentry using an accessory pathway with a long conduction time. Am J Cardiol 1981;48:611.

51. Gomes JAC, Dhatt MS, Damato AN, Akhtar M, Holder CA: Incidence, determinants and significance of fixed retrograde conduction in the region of the atrioventricular node: evidence of retrograde atrioventricular nodal bypass tracts. Am J Cardiol 1979;44:1089.

52. Klein GJ, Prystowsky EN, Pritchett ELC, Davis D, Gallagher JJ: Atypical patterns of retrograde conduction over accessory atrioventricular pathways in the Wolff-Parkinson-White syndrome. Circulation 1979;60:1477.

53. Critelli G, Gallagher JJ, Monda V, Coltorti F, Scherillo M, Rossi L: Anatomic and electrophysiologic substrate of the permanent form of junctional reciprocating tachycardia. J Am Coll Cardiol 1984;4:601.

54. Lerman BB, Greenberg M, Overholt ED, et al: Differential electrophysiologic properties of decremental retrograde pathways in long RP′ tachycardia. Circulation 1987;76:21.

55. Sung RJ, Waxman HL, Saksena S, Juma Z: Sequence of retrograde atrial activation in patients with dual atrioventriuclar nodal pathways. Circulation 1981;64:1059.

56. Akhtar M, Gilbert C, Wolf FG, Schmidt DH: Reentry within the His-Purkinje system: elucidation of reentrant circuit using right bundle branch and His bundle recordings. Circulation 1978;58:295.

57. Bauernfeind RA, Wu D, Denes P, Rosen KM: Retrograde block during dual pathway atrioventricular nodal reentrant paroxysmal tachycardia. Am J Cardiol 1978;42:499.

58. Coumel P, Attuel P: Reciprocating tachycardia in overt and latent preexcitation: influence of functional bundle branch block on the rate of the tachycardia. Eur J Cardiol 1974;1:423.

59. Pritchett ELC, Tonkin AM, Dugan FA, Wallace AG, Gallagher JJ: Ventriculo-atrial conduction time during reciprocating tachycardia with intermittent bundle-branch block in Wolff-Parkinson-White syndrome. Br Heart J 1976;38:1058.

60. Kerr CR, Gallagher JJ, German LD: Changes in ventriculoatrial intervals with bundle branch block aberration during reciprocating tachycardia in patients with accessory atrioventricular pathways. Circulation 1982;66:196.

61. Baerman JM, Bauernfeind RA, Swiryn S: Shortening of ventriculoatrial intervals with left bundle branch block during orthodromic reciprocating tachycardia in three patients with a right-sided accessory atrioventricular pathway. J Am Coll Cardiol 1989;13:215.

62. Sellers TD, Gallagher JJ, Cope GD, Tonkin AM, Wallace AG: Retrograde atrial preexcitation following premature ventricular beats during reciprocating tachycardia in the Wolff-Parkinson-White syndrome. Eur J Cardiol 1976;4:283.

63. Benditt DG, Benson DW, Dunnigan A, et al: Role of extrastimulus site and tachycardia cycle length in inducibility of atrial preexcitation by premature ventricular stimulation during reciprocating tachycardia. Am J Cardiol 1987;60:811.

64. Miles WM, Yee R, Klein GJ, Zipes DP, Prystowsky EN: The preexcitation index: an aid in determining the mechanism of supraventricular tachycardia and localizing accessory pathways. Circulation 1986;74:493.

65. Belhassen B, Pelleg A, Shoshani D, Geva B, Laniado S: Electrophysiologic effects of adenosine-5'-triphosphate on atrioventricular reentrant tachycardia. Circulation 1983;68:827.

66. Lerman BB, Belardinelli L: Cardiac electrophysiology of adenosine: basic and clinical concepts. Circulation 1991;83:1499.

67. Denes P, Cummings JM, Simpson R, et al: Effects of propranolol on anomalous pathway refractoriness and circus movement tachycardias in patients with preexcitation. Am J Cardiol 1978;41:1061.

68. Dhingra RC, Palileo EV, Strasberg B, et al: Electrophysiologic effects of ouabain in patients with preexcitation and circus movement tachycardia. Am J Cardiol 1981;47:139.

69. Sung RJ, Elser B, McAllister RG: Intravenous verapamil for termination of re-entrant supraventricular tachycardias: intracardiac studies correlated with plasma verapamil concentrations. Ann Intern Med 1980;93:682.

70. Klein GJ, Gulamhusein S, Prystowsky EN, Carruthers SG, Donner AP, Ko PT: Comparison of the electrophysiologic effects of intravenous and oral verapamil in patients with paroxysmal supraventricular tachycardia. Am J Cardiol 1982;49:117.

71. Bauernfeind RA, Wyndham CR, Dhingra RC, et al: Serial electrophysiologic testing of multiple drugs in patients with atrioventricular nodal reentrant paroxysmal tachycardia. Circulation 1980;62:1341.

72. Wu D, Denes P, Bauernfeind R, Kehoe R, Amat-y-Leon F, Rosen KM: Effects of procainamide on atrioventricular nodal re-entrant paroxysmal tachycardia. Circulation 1978;57:1171.

73. Swiryn S, Bauernfeind RA, Wyndham CRC, et al: Effects of oral disopyramide phosphate on induction of paroxysmal supraventricular tachycardia. Circulation 1981;64:169.

74. Wu D, Hung JS, Kuo CT, Hsu KS, Shieh WB: Effects of quinidine on atrioventricular nodal reentrant paroxysmal tachycardia. Circulation 1981;64:823.

75. DiMarco JP, Sellers TD, Lerman BB, Greenberg ML, Berne RM, Belardinelli L: Diagnostic and therapeutic use of adenosine in patients with supraventricular tachyarrhythmias. J Am Coll Cardiol 1985;6:417.

76. Wu D, Denes P, Bauernfeind R, Dhingra RC, Wyndham C, Rosen KM: Effects of atropine on induction and maintenance of atrioventricular nodal reentrant tachycardia. Circulation 1979;59:779.

77. Brownstein SL, Hopson RC, Martins JB, et al: Usefulness of isoproterenol in facilitating atrioventriucular nodal reentry tachycardia during electrophysiologic testing. Am J Cardiol 1988;61:1037.

78. Goldreyer BN, Kastor JA, Kershbaum KL: The hemodynamic effects of induced supraventricular tachycardia in man. Circulation 1976;54:783.

79. Damiano RJ, Tripp HF, Asano T, Small KW, Jones RH, Lowe JE: Left ventricular dysfunction and dilation resulting from chronic supraventraicular tachycardia. J Thorac Cardiovasc Surg 1987;94:135.

80. Packer DL, Bardy GH, Worley SJ, et al: Tachycardia-induced cardiomyopathy: a reversible form of left ventricular dysfunction. Am J Cardiol 1986;57:563.

81. Newman BJ, Donoso E, Friedberg CK: Arrhythmias in the Wolff-Parkinson-White syndrome. Prog Cardiovasc Dis 1966;9:147.

82. Bauernfeind RA, Wyndham CR, Swiryn SP, et al: Paroxysmal atrial fibrillation in the Wolff-Parkinson-White syndrome. Am J Cardiol 1981;47:502.

83. Tonkin AM, Miller HC, Svenson RH, Wallace AG, Gallagher JJ: Refractory periods of the accessory pathway in the Wolff-Parkinson-White syndrome. Circulation 1975;52:563.

84. Klein GJ, Bashore TM, Sellers TD, Pritchett ELC, Smith WM, Gallagher JJ: Ventricular fibrillation in the Wolff-Parkinson-White syndrome. N Engl J Med 1979;301:1080.

85. Klein HO, Hoffman BF: Cessation of paroxysmal supraventricular tachycardias by parasympathomimetic interventions. Ann Intern Med 1974;81:48.

86. Josephson ME, Seides SE, Batsford WB, Caracta AR, Damato AN, Kastor JA: The effects of carotid sinus pressure in reentrant paroxysmal supraventricular tachycardia. Am Heart J 1974;88:694.

87. Belhassen B, Glick A, Laniado S: Comparative clinical and electrophysiologic effects of adenosine triphosphate and verapamil on paroxysmal reciprocating junctional tachycardia. Circulation 1988;77:795.

88. Sellers TD, Bashore TM, Gallaher JJ: Digitalis in the preexcitation syndrome: analysis during atrial fibrillation. Circulation 1977;56:260.

89. Gulamhusein S, Ko P, Carruthers SG, Klein GJ: Acceleration of the ventricular response during atrial fibrillation in the Wolff-Parkinson-White syndrome after verapamil. Circulation 1982;65:348.

90. Harper RW, Whitford E, Middlebrook K, Federman J, Anderson S, Pitt A: Effects of verapamil on the electrophysiologic properties of the accessory pathway in patients with the Wolff-Parkinson-White syndrome. Am J Cardiol 1982;50:1323.

91. Yeh SJ, Lin FC, Chou YY, Hung JS, Wu D: Termination of paroxysmal supraventricular tachycardia with a single oral dose of diltiazem and propranolol. Circulation 1985;71:104.

92. Massumi RA, Kistin AD, Tawakkol AA: Termination of recip-

rocating tachycardia by atrial stimulation. Circulation 1967; 36:637.

93. Peters RW, Shafton E, Frank S, Thomas AN, Scheinman MM: Radiofrequency-triggered pacemakers: uses and limitations. Ann Intern Med 1978;88:17.

94. Fisher JD, Johnston DR, Furman S, Mercando AD, Kim SG: Long-term efficacy of antitachycardia pacing for supraventricular and ventricular tachycardias. Am J Cardiol 1987; 60:1311.

95. Wu D, Amat-y-Leon F, Simpson RJ, et al: Electrophysiological studies with multiple drugs in patients with atrioventricular re-entrant tachycardias utilizing an extranodal pathway. Circulation 1977;56:727.

96. Bauernfeind RA, Swiryn S, Petropoulos AT, Coelho A, Gallastegui J, Rosen KM: Concordance and discordance of drug responses in atrioventricular reentrant tachycardia. J Am Coll Cardiol 1983;2:345.

97. Kim SS, Lal R, Ruffy R: Treatment of paroxysmal reentrant supraventricular tachycardia with flecainide acetate. Am J Cardiol 1986;58:80.

98. Hoff PI, Tronstad A, Oie B, Ohm OJ: Electrophysiologic and clinical effects of flecainide for recurrent paroxysmal supraventricular tachycardia. Am J Cardiol 1988;62:585.

99. Ludmer PL, McGowan NE, Antman EM, Friedman PL: Efficacy of propafenone in Wolff-Parkinson-White syndrome: electrophyisologic findings and long-term follow-up. J Am Coll Cardiol 1987;9:1357.

100. Hammill SC, McLaran CJ, Wood DL, Osborn MJ, Gersh BJ, Holmes DR: Double-blind study of intravenous propafenone for paroxysmal supraventricular reentrant tachycardia. J Am Coll Cardiol 1987;9:1364.

101. Kunze KP, Schluter M, Kuck KH: Sotalol in patients with Wolff-Parkinson-White syndrome. Circulation 1987;75:1050.

102. Pritchett ELC, Wilkinson WE: Mortality in patients treated with flecainide and encainide for supraventricular arrhythmias. Am J Cardiol 1991;67:976.

103. Hughes MM, Trohman RG, Simmons TW, et al: Flecainide therapy in patients treated for supraventricular tachycardia with near normal left ventricular function. Am Heart J 1992; 123:408.

104. Cobb FR, Blumenschein SD, Sealy WC, Boineau JP, Wagner GS, Wallace AG: Successful surgical interruption of the bundle of Kent in a patient with Wolff-Parkinson-White syndrome. Circulation 1968;38:1018.

105. Jackman WM, Wang X, Friday KJ, et al: Catheter ablation of accessory atrioventricular pathways (Wolff-Parkinson-White syndrome) by radiofrequency current. N Engl J Med 1991; 324:1605.

106. Sharma AD, Klein GJ, Guiraudon GM, Milstein S: Atrial fibrillation in patients with Wolff-Parkinson-White syndrome: incidence after surgical ablation of the accessory pathway. Circulation 1985;72:161.

107. Fischell TA, Stinson EB, Derby GC, Swerdlow CD: Long-term follow-up after surgical correction of Wolff-Parkinson-White syndrome. J Am Coll Cardiol 1987;9:283.

108. Gallagher JJ, Gilbert M, Svenson RH, Sealy WC, Kasell J, Wallace AG: Wolff-Parkinson-White syndrome: the problem, evaluation, and surgical correction. Circulation 1975;51:767.

109. Mitchell LB, Mason JW, Scheinman MM, Winkle RA, Burchell HB: Recordings of basal ventricular preexcitation from electrode catheters in patients with accessory atrioventricular connections. Circulation 1984;69:233.

110. Denes P, Wyndham CR, Amat-y-Leon F, et al: Atrial pacing at multiple sites in the Wolff-Parkinson-White syndrome. Br Heart J 1977;39:506.

111. Jackman WM, Friday KJ, Yeung-Lai-Wah JA, et al: New catheter technique for recording left free-wall accessory atrioventricular pathway activation: identification of pathway fiber orientation. Circulation 1988;78:598.

112. Calkins H, Kim YN, Schmaltz S, et al: Electrogram criteria for identification of approprite target sites for radiofrequency catheter ablation of accessory atrioventricular connections. Circulation 1992;85:565.

113. Gallagher JJ, Kasell J, Sealy WC, Pritchett ELC, Wallace AG: Epicardial mapping in the Wolff-Parkinson-White syndrome. Circulation 1978;57:854.

114. Kramer JB, Corr PB, Cox JL, Witkowski FX, Cain ME: Simultaneous computer mapping to facilitate intraoperative localization of accessory pathways in patients with Wolff-Parkinson-White syndrome. Am J Cardiol 1985;56:571.

115. Cox JL, Gallagher JJ, Cain ME: Experience with 118 consecutive patients undergoing operation for the Wolff-Parkinson-White syndrome. J Thorac Cardiovasc Surg 1985;90:490.

116. Lowe JE: Surgical treatment of the Wolff-Parkinson-White syndrome and other supraventricular tachyarrhythmias. J Cardiac Surg 1986;1:117.

117. Guiraudon GM, Klein GJ, Sharma AD, Jones DL, McLellan DG: Surgery for Wolff-Parkinson-White syndrome: further experience with an epicardial approach. Circulation 1986; 74:525.

118. Mahomed Y, King RD, Zipes DP, et al: Surgical division of Wolff-Parkinson-White pathways utilizing the closed-heart technique: a 2-year experience in 47 patients. Ann Thorac Surg 1988;45:495.

119. Ruder MA, Mead RH, Gaudiani V, Buch WS, Smith NA, Winkle RA: Transvenous catheter ablation of extranodal accessory pathways. J Am Coll Cardiol 1988;1245.

120. Bardy GH, Ivey TD, Coltorti F, Stewart RB, Johnson G, Greene HL: Developments, complications and limitations of catheter-mediated electrical ablation of posterior accessory atrioventricular pathways. Am J Cardiol 1988;61:309.

121. Morady F, Scheinman MM, Kou WH, et al: Long-term results of catheter ablation of a posteroseptal accessory atrioventricular connection in 48 patients. Circulation 1989;79:1160.

122. Warin JF, Haissaguerre M, Lemetayer P, Guillem JP, Blanchot P: Catheter albation of accessory pathways with a direct approach: results in 35 patients. Circulation 1988;78:800.

123. Warin JF, Haissaguerre M, D'Ivernois C, Le Metayer P, Montserrat P: Catheter ablation of accessory pathways: technique and results in 248 patients. Pacing Clin Electrophysiol 1990;13:1609.

124. Huang SKS: Radiofrequency catheter ablation of cardiac arrhythmias: appraisal of an evolving therapeutic modality. Am Heart J 1989;118:1317.

125. Jackman WM, Wang X, Friday KJ, et al: Catheter ablation of atrioventricular junction using radiofrequency current in 17 patients: comparison of standard and large-tip catheter electrodes. Circulation 1991;83:1562.

126. Calkins H, Langberg J, Sousa J, et al: Radiofrequency catheter ablation of accessory atrioventricular connections in 250 patients: abbreviated therapeutic approach to Wolff-Parkinson-White syndrome. Circulation 1992;85:1337.

127. Kuck KH, Schluter M: Single-catheter approach to radiofrequency current ablation of left-sided accessory pathways in patients with Wolff-Parkinson-White syndrome. Circulation 1991;84:2366.

128. Ross DL, Johnson DC, Denniss AR, Cooper MJ, Richards DA, Uther JB: Curative surgery for atrioventricular junctional ("AV nodal") reentrant tachycardia. J Am Coll Cardiol 1985; 6:1383.

129. Cox JL, Holman WL, Cain ME: Cryosurgical treatment of atrioventricular node reentrant tachycardia. Circulation 1987;76:1325.

130. Haissaguerre M, Warin JF, Lemetayer P, Saoudi N, Guillem JP, Blanchot P: Closed-chest ablation of retrograde conduction in patients with atrioventricular nodal reentrant tachycardia. N Engl J Med 1989;320:426.

131. Lee MA, Morady F, Kadish A, et al: Catheter modification of the atrioventricular junction with radiofrequency energy for control of atrioventricular nodal reentry tachycardia. Circulation 1991;83:827.

132. Wathen M, Natale A, Wolfe K, Yee R, Newman D, Klein G: An anatomically guided approach to atrioventricular node slow pathway ablation. Am J Cardiol 1992;70:886.

133. Seals AA, Lawrie GM, Magro S, et al: Surgical treatment of right atrial focal tachycardia in adults. J Am Coll Cardiol 1988;11:1111.

134. Gillette PC, Wampler DG, Garson A, Zinner A, Ott D, Cooley D: Treatment of atrial automatic tachycardia by ablation procedures. J Am Coll Cardiol 1985;6:405.

135. Walsh EP, Saul JP, Hulse JE, et al: Transcatheter ablation of ectopic atrial tachycardia in young patients using radiofrequency current. Circulation 1992;86:1138.

136. Klein GJ, Sealy WC, Pritchett ELC, et al: Cryosurgical ablation of the atrioventricular node-His bundle: long-term follow-up and properties of the junctional pacemaker. Circulation 1980;61:8.

137. Gallagher JJ, Svenson RH, Kasell JH, et al: Catheter technique for closed-chest ablation of the atrioventricular conduction system: a therapeutic alternative for the treatment of refractory supraventricular tachycardia. N Engl J Med 1982;306:194.

138. Scheinman MM, Evans-Bell T, the Executive Committee of the Percutaneous Cardiac Mapping and Ablation Registry: Catheter ablation of the atrioventricular junction: a report of the percutaneous mapping and ablation registry. Circulation 1984;70:1024.

139. Langberg JJ, Chin MC, Roesnqvist M, et al: Catheter ablation of the atrioventricular junction with radiofrequency energy. Circulation 1989;80:1527.

Cardiac Arrhythmias, 3rd edition, edited by William J. Mandel.
J. B. Lippincott Company, Philadelphia © 1995.

13

Hein J. J. Wellens • Joep L. R. M. Smeets
Anton P. M. Gorgels • Jerónimo Farré

Wolff-Parkinson-White Syndrome

More than 60 years ago, Wolff, Parkinson, and White described a clinical electrocardiographic entity in a series of 11 healthy young patients consisting of attacks of paroxysmal tachycardia in the presence of an electrocardiogram showing a bundle branch block-like pattern with a short PR interval.[1] Isolated cases showing the same features have been published previously and originally, this syndrome was considered to be an electrocardiographic curiosity.[2–5] Subsequently, however, it became clear that some patients with this condition suffer from incapacitating or even life-threatening arrhythmias.[6] After the introduction of intracavitary recordings and the technique of programmed stimulation of the heart, the mechanism of arrhythmias in these patients has become known, allowing a more rational approach to the management of Wolff-Parkinson-White (WPW) syndrome.[7]

In this chapter, we review present knowledge of WPW syndrome, as derived from clinical, electrocardiographic, and electrophysiologic data.

ANATOMIC BASIS OF WOLFF-PARKINSON-WHITE SYNDROME

Epicardial excitation mapping, electric stimulation studies, His-bundle recordings, intracavitary mapping techniques, and the outcome of ablative interventions show that in patients with WPW syndrome, two pathways are present between the atrium and ventricle.[8–15] Anatomic documentation of the existence of such an accessory atrioventricular (AV) connection in these patients is available.[16] Apart from the accessory pathways between the atrium and the ventricle, as found in patients with WPW syndrome, other abnormal connections between the atrium and the specific conduction system and between the specific conduction system and the ventricle are described.[17] Their electrophysiologic properties, diagnostic features, and clinical significance are discussed elsewhere.[18]

ELECTROCARDIOGRAM IN PATIENTS WITH WOLFF-PARKINSON-WHITE SYNDROME

The typical electrocardiogram of WPW syndrome (short PR interval with wide QRS complex, starting with a delta wave) is the result of fusion of ventricular activation through the normal atrioventricular connection (AV node–His-Purkinje axis) and the accessory pathway (AP). In these patients, the pattern of ventricular activation is determined by (1) location of the AP, (2) intraatrial conduction time, (3) conduction time over the AP, and (4) AV conduction time over the normal AV node–His-Purkinje pathway.

If, as shown in the left panel of Figure 13-1, the

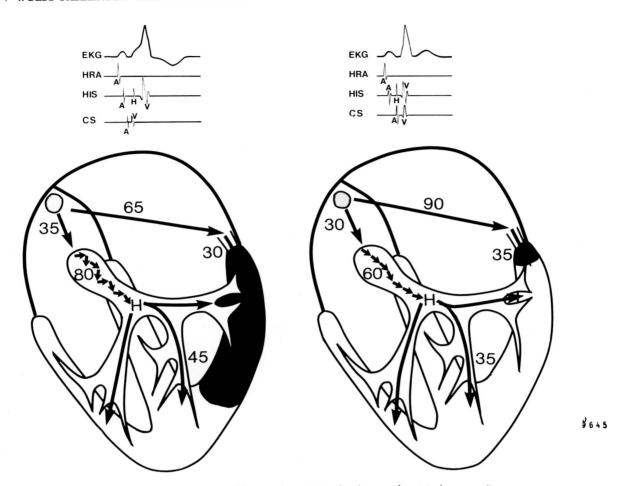

Figure 13-1. Schematic representation of factors determining the degree of ventricular preexcitation in the Wolff-Parkinson-White patient during sinus rhythm. The corresponding electrocardiogram and intracavitary recordings from the high right atrium (*HRA*), His-bundle region (*HIS*), and coronary sinus (*CS*) are shown in the upper part of the figure (*left*). The atrioventricular (AV) conduction time from the sinus node region over the normal AV pathway measures 160 milliseconds (the time required to travel from the sinus node to the AV node [PA interval] of 35 milliseconds; the transnodal conduction time [AH interval] of 80 milliseconds; and the time needed to travel through the bundle of His and the bundle branches to the ventricular myocardium [HV interval] of 45 msec). The time required to travel from the sinus node to the atrial insertion of the accessory pathway (AP) measures 65 milliseconds, and the conduction time over the AP measures 30 milliseconds. The total AV conduction time to travel from the sinus node to the ventricle using the AP is 95 milliseconds. Under these circumstances, the corresponding electrocardiogram shows a P-delta interval of 95 milliseconds and a wide QRS complex, with ventricular excitation starting 160 − 95 = 65 milliseconds earlier than expected (*right*). In this example, as compared with the left panel, there is (1) a longer conduction time from sinus node to the atrial insertion of the AP, (2) a longer conduction time over the AP, and (3) a shorter conduction time over the AV node (shorter PA, AH, and HV times). As a result of these differences, the AV conduction times over either the AP or the normal pathway are identical (both 125 milliseconds) and the electrocardiogram shows a PR interval of 125 milliseconds and a QRS complex that is not widened.

conduction time from the sinus node region to the ventricle over the AP is shorter than that over the normal AV node–His axis, ventricular excitation starts earlier than expected (preexcitation).[18] This results in the following electrocardiographic findings:

1. Shortening of the PR interval. If the total AV conduction time over the normal AV node–His pathway mea-

sures 160 milliseconds and the AV conduction time over the AP measures 95 milliseconds, the actual interval between the beginning of atrial and ventricular activation measures 95 milliseconds (Fig. 13-1, *left*).

2. Widening of the QRS complex with an initial delta wave. In most patients, the width of the QRS complex is determined by the degree of ventricular preexcitation. In the example shown (see Fig. 13-1, *left*) ven-

tricular excitation starts 65 milliseconds earlier than expected when only the normal AV pathway is present (160 − 95 = 65 milliseconds), resulting in a wider QRS complex. The initial forces of the QRS complex during preexcited beats represent ventricular activation of the slowly conducting ventricular working myocardium. In the electrocardiogram, this results in a low-frequency component called the delta wave.[19]

3. Secondary changes in the T wave. As a result of early asynchronous excitation of a part of the ventricle, the sequence of repolarization is different, leading to T-wave changes. These changes are related to the area and extent of preexcitation.

In some patients, the contribution of the AP to ventricular activation during sinus rhythm may be minimal, so that PR interval and QRS width are normal. An example of the latter situation is given in the right panel of Figure 13-1. If the atrioventricular conduction time (from the sinus node area) over the AP is not shorter than that over the normal AV node–His axis, the PR interval is not shortened and the QRS has a normal duration. This is the result of several factors acting alone or in combination in a given patient:

1. Location of the AP. The closer the AP is located to the sinus node, the less time it takes for the impulse to reach the atrial insertion of the AP, resulting in a greater amount of ventricular preexcitation during sinus rhythm. Conversely, in patients with laterally

located left-sided APs, contribution to ventricular excitation over the AP may be minimal during sinus rhythm. The importance of distance between the site of supraventricular impulse formation and the accessory pathway on preexcitation is shown in Figures 13-1 through 13-4.

2. Intraatrial conduction times. During sinus rhythm, two intraatrial conduction times are important: (1) the conduction time from the sinus node to the entrance of the AV node (which corresponds to the interval measured from the beginning of the P wave to the atrial deflection in the His-bundle lead or PA interval), and (2) the conduction time from the sinus node to the atrial insertion of the AP. The normal PA interval varies from 30 to 55 milliseconds but longer values can be observed under pathologic conditions.[20] Left atrial pathology prolongs the time required to reach a left-sided AP. Intraatrial conduction time can be affected by drugs, resulting in a lesser amount of preexcitation during sinus rhythm in patients with left lateral accessory pathways.

3. Conduction time over the AP. The conduction time over the AP depends on the conduction velocity and the length of the AP. Exact figures about conduction velocity in accessory atrioventricular pathways found in WPW syndrome are not available. Becker and co-workers report that the length of the accessory AV connection in patients with WPW syndrome varied

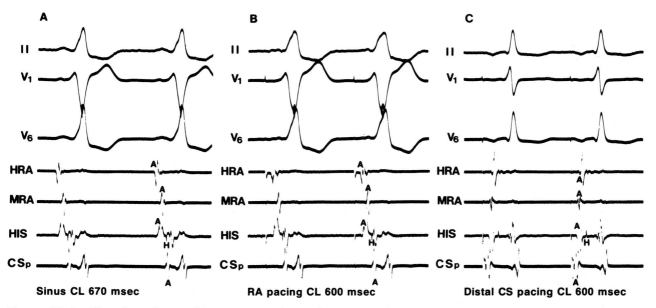

Figure 13-2. Effect of site of origin of the supraventricular impulse on ventricular excitation and the electrocardiogram in a patient with a right-sided accessory pathway. Leads II, V₁, and V₆ and intracardiac bipolar electrograms from the high right atrium (*HRA*), mid-right atrium (*MRA*), His-bundle region (*HIS*), and proximal coronary sinus (*CSp*) are simultaneously recorded. (**A**) Recordings obtained during sinus rhythm. (**B**) Right atrial pacing at a cycle length (*CL*) of 600 milliseconds, showing enhancement of ventricular preexcitation. (**C**) Pacing from the distal coronary sinus (*CS*) at a CL of 600 milliseconds results in disappearance of preexcitation.

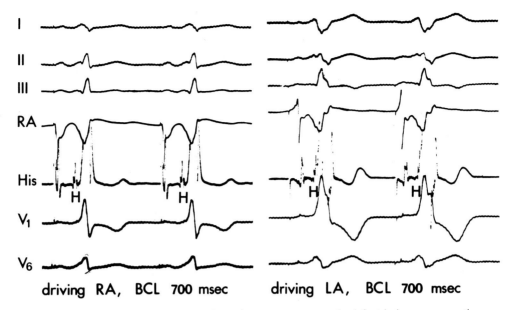

Figure 13-3. (*Left*) Right and left atrial stimulation in a patient with a left-sided accessory pathway. (*Right*) Atrial stimulation closer to the accessory pathway results in a greater amount of ventricular preexcitation, compared with atrial pacing at the same rate from the right atrium.

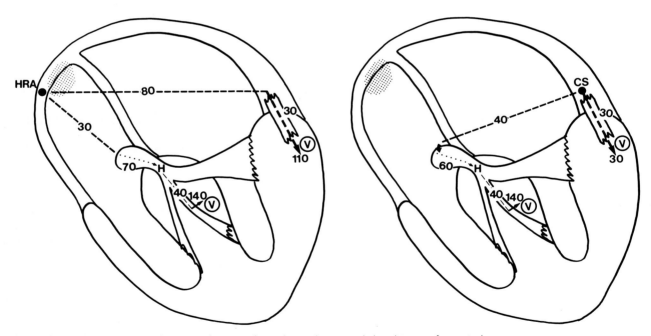

Figure 13-4. The relation between the site of atrial stimulation and the degree of ventricular preexcitation in patients with Wolff-Parkinson-White syndrome. A left-sided accessory pathway (AP) is shown. The upper diagram shows the effects of high right atrium (HRA) stimulation. The atrioventricular (AV) conduction time (from the site of stimulation over the normal AV node–His pathway measures 30 + 70 + 40 = 140 milliseconds, and over the AP, 80 + 30 = 110 milliseconds. In the lower diagram, atrial stimulation is performed from the coronary sinus, close to the location of the AP. The AV conduction time through the normal pathway measures 140 milliseconds (the postulated AH is 60, 10 msec shorter as compared to HRA pacing). The AV conduction time through the AP is 30 milliseconds resulting in a maximal amount of preexcitation.

from 1 to 10 mm.[16] This suggests that with the same conduction velocity of the impulse over the accessory pathway, conduction times over accessory pathways may vary by as much as a factor of 10 from one patient to another.

4. Conduction time over the AV node–His-Purkinje axis. Some patients with WPW syndrome have short intranodal conduction times (AH intervals of less than 60 milliseconds.[21] In these patients, especially when a left-sided AP is present, a lesser amount of ventricular preexcitation is observed during sinus rhythm.

In the right panel of Figure 13-1, atrioventricular conduction times through the AP and the AV nodal-His-Purkinje axis are equal (125 milliseconds). Therefore, the PR interval is normal (0.125 seconds) and no QRS widening is observed. The only abnormality encountered in such a patient is in the initial forces of the QRS because the ventricular muscle depolarizing early over the AV node–His-Purkinje axis is excited at the same time as the ventricular myocardium close to the insertion of the AP. This can result in QRS abnormalities; that is, abnormal Q waves, slurring in the ascending limb of the R wave, increased voltage in the R waves, and changes in the axis of the QRS complex. Therefore, QRS abnormalities mimicking myocardial infarction, ventricular hypertrophy, or intraventric-

ular conduction disturbances may be present in the electrocardiogram of these patients. Figure 13-5 shows an example of a patient with mitral valve prolapse and a left-sided AP, in which the electrocardiogram has been erroneously diagnosed as an old posteroinferior myocardial infarction.

Patients in whom the contribution of the AP to ventricular activation is minimal because of the coincidental arrival of the excitation wavefront to the ventricle over both the normal and the accessory pathway should not be diagnosed as having a so-called concealed accessory pathway.[22] Concealed APs are those accessory pathways that only conduct in the retrograde (ventriculoatrial) direction. Anterograde conduction through AP in these patients is absent because the refractory period of the AP in the anterograde direction is longer than the sinus cycle length. The clinical implications of the latter type of AP are discussed elsewhere in this volume.

INCIDENCE OF WOLFF-PARKINSON-WHITE SYNDROME

The true incidence of WPW syndrome is unknown, with the reported figures varying from 0.1 to 3 per 1000 electrocardiograms.[23,24] The WPW syndrome is undoubtedly

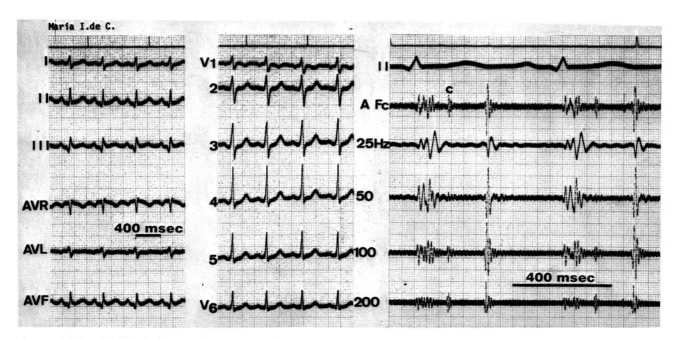

Figure 13-5. A 12-lead electrocardiogram and phonocardiogram, showing a mid-systolic click from a patient with mitral valve prolapse. The electrocardiogram was interpreted as being indicative of an old posteroinferior myocardial infarction. The PR interval measured 0.14 second and the QRS width was 0.08 second. Note that apart from the Q waves in the inferior wall leads and the tall broad R wave in lead V_1, slurring in the ascending limb of the R wave is present in leads V_4 and V_5.

underdiagnosed because many physicians require the presence of the typical electrocardiographic features (short PR interval and wide QRS complex with an initial delta wave) before making the diagnosis. Determination of the real incidence of the syndrome is hampered by (1) the existence of so-called intermittent preexcitation with inconstant AV conduction over the AP, and (2) the presence of left lateral APs, resulting (for reasons given above) in questionable or even normal electrocardiograms. Vidaillet and coworkers report that family members of patients with WPW syndrome have a fourfold greater chance of having the syndrome than do people without a family history.[25] The authors suggest that the WPW syndrome is inherited as an autosomal dominant trait.

Incidence of Tachyarrhythmias in Wolff-Parkinson-White Syndrome

The incidence of tachyarrhythmias in patients with WPW syndrome is also unknown. The reported figures vary from 12% to 80% and these figures are obviously affected by patients selection.[24,26] In our own series of patients with WPW syndrome who had undergone electrophysiologic study, electrocardiographic documentation of either supraventricular tachycardia or atrial fibrillation or both before the stimulation study was available in 97% of cases (Table 13-1).

Incidence of Wolff-Parkinson-White Syndrome in Patients With Paroxysmal Tachycardia

The WPW syndrome abnormality is probably the most important underlying cause of paroxysmal regular supraventricular tachycardia that is referred to hospital. In a

TABLE 13-1. Tachycardia Electrocardiographically Documented Before Stimulation Study in Patients With Wolff-Parkinson-White Syndrome

Type of Tachycardia	Patients (n)
CMT	410 (63%)
AF	119 (18%)
CMT plus AF	101 (15%)
No tachycardia documented	26 (4%)
Total	656

CMT, circus movement tachycardia; AF, Atrial Fibrillation.

series of 120 consecutive patients admitted to the hospital because of paroxysmal supraventricular tachycardia, an electrocardiogram diagnostic for WPW syndrome was found during sinus rhythm in 69 patients (57%). This high incidence of WPW syndrome is even more striking when considering the age of the patients. In 45 patients in whom the first attack of paroxysmal tachycardia occurred younger than age 21 years, 33 (73%) had WPW syndrome on the electrocardiogram recorded during sinus rhythm. In the 75 patients in whom the first attack of tachycardia occurred older than age 21 years, an electrocardiogram diagnostic for WPW was found in 36 (48%).[27]

ELECTROCARDIOGRAPHIC CLASSIFICATION OF WOLFF-PARKINSON-WHITE SYNDROME

In 1945, Rosenbaum and coworkers proposed a classification of WPW syndrome according to the QRS configuration in the precordial leads.[28] Type A WPW syndrome showed a predominant R wave in leads V_1, V_2, and V_E, whereas type B showed an S wave as the chief QRS deflection in the right precordial leads. Durrer and Roos demonstrated by epicardial mapping that type B WPW syndrome is caused by early activation of the lateral aspect of the right ventricle.[8] It was subsequently reported that in patients with type A WPW, early activation of the left ventricle is present.[29]

Extensive studies by the group from Duke University show that the accessory AV pathway responsible for this syndrome can insert not only in the ventricular free wall but also in the interventricular septum.[21] Therefore, Rosenbaum's classification of WPW syndrome into types A and B oversimplifies the electrocardiographic spectrum of this abnormality. Several authors presented tentative classifications of the location of the accessory pathway based on the initial forces of the QRS complex in both the precordial and extremity leads.[30–34] Determination of the location of the AP in WPW syndrome from the QRS configuration during sinus rhythm can be extremely difficult, however. It can only be done confidently during completely preexcited beats (i.e., when ventricular activation is exclusively or mostly over the accessory pathway.[21] As previously mentioned, some patients with WPW syndrome do not show much preexcitation during sinus rhythm, preventing analysis of the initial forces from ventricular excitation through the AP. Other factors hampering localization of the AP are (1) the existence of more than one AP in some patients, (2) the coexistence of congenital or acquired heart disease, (3) the occasional superposition of the terminal part of the P wave on the initial portion of the delta wave, and (4) differences in ventricular activation, depending on whether the AP is epicardially or endocardially located.[21]

ASSOCIATED CARDIOVASCULAR ABNORMALITIES

The most frequent forms of associated cardiovascular abnormalities found in patients with WPW syndrome are listed in Table 13-2. Right-sided accessory pathways are found in 5% to 25% of the reported cases of Ebstein's disease.[35] In patients with corrected transposition (L-transposition) of the great arteries, a few cases of WPW syndrome have been reported.[36,37] In those with tricuspid atresia, endocardial fibroelastosis, and double-inlet right ventricle, WPW syndrome has also been described.[35] Dextrocardia, even without cardiac abnormality, may also be associated with WPW syndrome.[38] Figure 13-6 illustrates a case of mirror-image dextrocardia without cardiac disease and type B WPW syndrome.

Association between WPW syndrome and various forms of cardiomyopathy has been noted.[21,35] Mitral valve prolapse and WPW syndrome (mainly left-sided) is another known association (see Fig. 13-5).[21]

Patients with rheumatic and nonrheumatic valve disease, coronary artery disease, and other pathologic conditions affecting the cardiovascular system may have WPW syndrome as a coincidental feature.

TABLE 13-2. Cardiovascular Abnormalities Associated With Wolff-Parkinson-White Syndrome

Ebstein's disease
Corrected transposition (L-transposition) of the great arteries
Tricuspid atresia
Endocardial fibroelastosis
Mitral valve prolapse
Cardiomyopathy
    Hypertrophic obstructive cardiomyopathy
    Hypertrophic nonobstructive cardiomyopathy
    Congestive cardiomyopathy

CLINICAL MANIFESTATIONS OF WOLFF-PARKINSON-WHITE SYNDROME

The clinical manifestations of WPW syndrome depend on the physiologic properties of the accessory pathway. The most important problems encountered in these patients are those caused by the development of paroxysmal regular supraventricular tachycardia or atrial fibrillation or

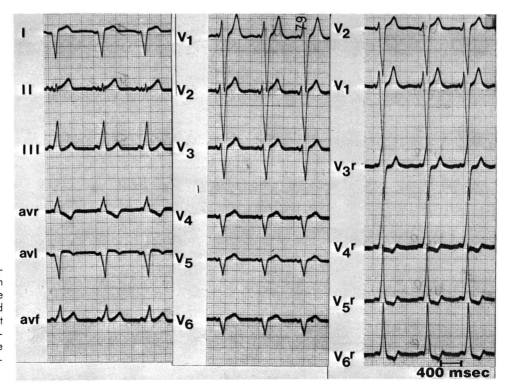

Figure 13-6. Wolff-Parkinson-White syndrome in a patient with mirror-image dextrocardia. Note the negative P wave in lead I and positive P wave in lead aV$_R$. The right precordial leads show the accessory pathway, located between the anatomic right atrium and right ventricle.

both. The occurrence of the latter arrhythmia may even result in sudden death.[6,39-44]

Paroxysmal Tachycardia in Wolff-Parkinson-White Syndrome

The combination of the technique of programmed electric stimulation of the heart with the recording of multiple intracardiac and surface electrocardiographic leads demonstrates that many circuits leading to paroxysmal tachycardia may be present in patients with WPW syndrome.[21,45] The most frequent form of paroxysmal tachycardia suffered by patients with WPW syndrome is a circus movement tachycardia (CMT), incorporating the AP in the tachycardia circuit.[21,46]

Circus Movement Tachycardia Incorporating the Accessory Pathway

Circus movement tachycardia incorporating the AP is based on a reentrant circuit that consists of the following structures: (1) AV node; (2) His-Purkinje system; (3) ventricular myocardium, from the terminal Purkinje network to the ventricular end of the AP; (4) the AP itself; and (5) atrial myocardium, from the atrial insertion of the AP to the AV node. This circuit can be used in both directions, resulting in two possible varieties of CMT using the accessory pathway (Table 13-3).[46]

1. Orthodromic CMT. This is the usual form of CMT in patients with WPW syndrome. Anterograde AV conduction occurs through the normal AV node–His pathway, ventriculo-atrial (VA) conduction through the AP. Thus, the QRS complex during tachycardia shows either normal intraventricular conduction or typical bundle branch block configuration (Fig. 13-7). Atrial activation during this type of tachycardia starts close to the AP after the ventricular myocardium and the AP have been activated (Fig. 13-8). In many of these patients, the retrograde P wave (P′) can be identified on the electrocardiogram after the QRS complex during tachycardia, the P′R interval usually being longer than the RP′ intervals (see Figs. 13-7 and 13-8).

2. Antidromic CMT. Much less frequently, the reversed (antidromic) form of CMT incorporating the AP has been observed in patients with WPW syndrome. During this type of CMT, anterograde AV conduction is through the AP, and retrograde VA conduction is through the normal His-AV node axis or a second AP. Therefore, the QRS during tachycardia shows maximal preexcitation (Fig. 13-9). The mechanisms of this form of CMT are discussed elsewhere.[45]

ELECTROPHYSIOLOGIC REQUIREMENTS.

In 1913, Mines suggested that tachycardia could be the result of an impulse circulating in a circuit consisting of atrium, AV node, ventricle, and an accessory AV connection.[47] Such a circuit is anatomically present in patients with the WPW syndrome. Essential for the development of a circus movement in this circuit is the creation of unidirectional block in one of the two AV connections, with conduction persisting over the other pathway. The conduction velocity of the impulse should be slow enough to

TABLE 13-3. Possible Types of Paroxysmal Regular Tachycardia in Wolff-Parkinson-White Syndrome and Differential Diagnoses

	Anterograde Pathway	Retrograde Pathway	Differential Diagnosis
CMT using AV-junctional structures			
Orthodromic CMT	AVN-His pathway	AP	AVN tachycardia with AV conduction over AP
Antidromic CMT	AP	AVN-His pathway	1. Atrial tachycardia
	AP	AP	2. AVN tachycardia with AV conduction over AP
			3. Ventricular tachycardia
AVN tachycardia	AVN slow pathway	AVN fast pathway	Orthodromic CMT
Atrial tachycardia with AV conduction over AP			1. Antidromic CMT
			2. Ventricular tachycardia
Ventricular tachycardia			1. Antidromic CMT
			2. Atrial tachycardia with AV conduction over AP

AP, accessory pathway; AVN, atrioventricular node; CMT, circus movement tachycardia.

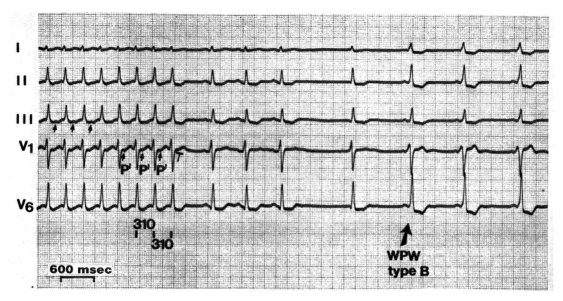

Figure 13-7. Spontaneous termination of circus movement tachycardia incorporating the AP in the retrograde direction in a patient with right-sided Wolff-Parkinson-White syndrome (WPW). Note that during tachycardia, the QRS complex indicates anterograde atrioventricular (AV) conduction over the normal AV node–His pathway. After termination of tachycardia and after a few beats that do not show preexcitation, right-sided WPW becomes evident during sinus rhythm. Retrograde P waves are identified during tachycardia (*small arrows*). This retrograde P wave is not present after the last QRS complex during tachycardia, suggesting that retrograde block in the accessory pathway was the mechanism of spontaneous termination of tachycardia.

find all parts of the circuit excitable. To use such an anatomic circuit in a reentrant tachycardia, the possibility of ventriculo-atrial (VA) conduction over at least one of the atrioventricular connections is essential. Therefore, patients without VA conduction over the AP can never develop orthodromic CMT.

The creation of unidirectional block in one of the limbs of the circuit requires differences in duration of the refractory periods of the normal and accessory pathway in AV (anterograde), VA (retrograde), or both directions.[48,49] Thus, a critically timed premature beat can be blocked in one of the pathways while still being conducted over the other. Figures 13-10 and 13-11 illustrate how the two forms of CMT incorporating the AP can be initiated by an atrial or ventricular premature beat, according to the electrophysiologic characteristics of the normal and accessory pathway in both anterograde and retrograde direction. Perpetuation of CMT requires that the time for the impulse to complete the whole circuit (the circulating time) is longer than the duration of the longest refractory period anywhere in the circuit.[48] This explains how circumstances (particularly drugs) that promote slow conduction in any of the components of the circuit can facilitate perpetuation of tachycardia if refractoriness is not prolonged in excess of conduction time.[46]

SYMPTOMS AND SIGNS

Some time ago, we studied the complaints of 69 consecutive patients with proven CMT incorporating the AP in the retrograde direction (orthodromic CMT) in the presence of WPW syndrome. As shown in Table 13-4, most of the patients were aware of attacks of rapid heart action starting and stopping abruptly. Anginal pain was common in the young patient but when present, it was associated with a high rate during tachycardia (more than 200 beats/minute. Polyuria during or after the attack was present in 26% of the patients. Frequently, patients with a long-standing history of paroxysmal tachycardia told us that polyuria tended to disappear gradually over the years.

Other Forms of Paroxysmal Tachycardia in Patients With Wolff-Parkinson-White Syndrome

Excepting a few patients in whom atrial tachycardia, AV node reentrant tachycardia, or ventricular tachycardia are induced during the programmed stimulation study, most patients have a CMT using the AP initiated during the study. Cases of CMT using two accessory pathways have been observed (Fig. 13-12).[45,50] It is of interest that most reported examples of intranodal reentrant tachycardias in

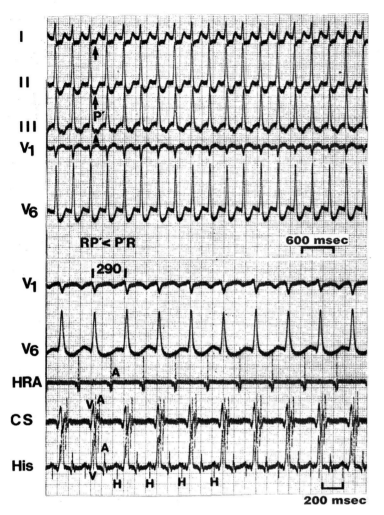

RP' < P'R   600 msec

290

Figure 13-8. The *upper panel* shows a 25 mm/second electrocardiographic recording of a tachycardia in a patient with a left-sided accessory pathway. QRS complexes during tachycardia show normal interventricular conduction. A retrograde P wave is identified (*arrows*), the RP' interval being shorter than the P'R interval. This finding suggests the incorportation of an accessory pathway in retrograde direction during tachycardia. In the *lower panel*, leads V₁ and V₆ plus intracardiac bipolar electrograms from the high right atrium (*HRA*), coronary sinus (*CS*), and His-bundle (*His*) region simultaneously recorded at a paper speed of 50 mm/second are shown. Note that retrograde atrial activation starts in the CS lead, indicating ventriculoatrial conduction through a left-sided accessory pathway.

200 msec

patients with WPW syndrome showed absence of ventricular preexcitation during tachycardia.[51] During AV nodal reentrant tachycardia, however, AV conduction may occur over an AP so-called "bystander" AV conduction. This results in a tachycardia with preexcited QRS complexes.[52]

Factors Influencing Clinical Manifestations of Tachycardia in Wolff-Parkinson-White Syndrome

The clinical consequences of paroxysmal tachycardia in patients with WPW syndrome depend on several factors: (1) heart rate during tachycardia (which in CMT depends on conduction velocity of the impulse, size, and functional refractory periods of the components of the circuit); (2) age of the patient (tolerance of the tachycardia tends to decrease with age); (3) presence of associated cardiovascular abnormalities; and (4) number and duration of the attacks of tachycardia.

Atrial Fibrillation in the Wolff-Parkinson-White Syndrome

Atrial fibrillation seems to be frequent in patients with WPW syndrome. As seen in Table 13-1, electrocardiographic documentation of at least one episode of atrial fibrillation was available in 220 of our 656 patients before the stimulation study. During atrial fibrillation, some patients with WPW syndrome may develop high life-threatening ventricular rates due to exclusive AV conduction over the AP (Fig. 13-13). Apart from markedly reducing cardiac output, these rapid ventricular rates may degenerate into ventricular fibrillation. It is important to realize that the presenting clinical problem is some patients who have WPW syndrome may be ventricular fibrillation.[43, 44]

Although the ventricular rate during atrial fibrillation in patients with WPW syndrome depends on several factors, a good correlation has been found between the shortest RR interval showing preexcitation during atrial

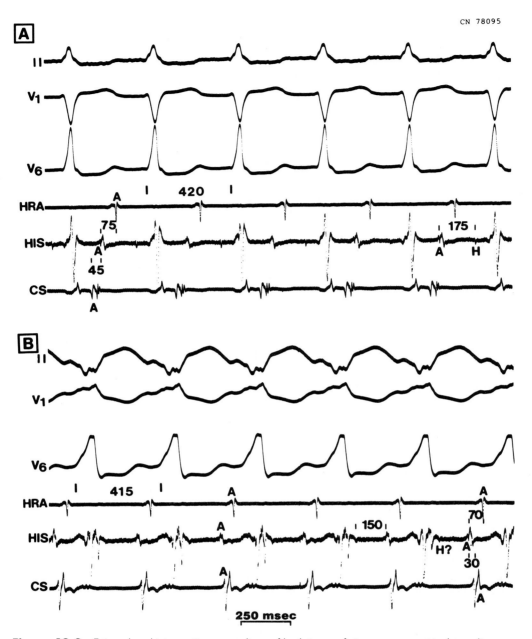

CN 78095

Figure 13-9. External and intracavitary recordings of both types of circus movement tachycardia (CMT) incorporating an accessory pathway. Leads II, V₁, and V₆ and bipolar electrograms from high right atrium (*HRA*), His-bundle (*HIS*), and coronary sinus (*CS*) regions are recorded simultaneously. Both types of tachycardia were induced in the same patient during programmed electric stimulation of the heart. (**A**) Type I A CMT. Note the arrow QRS, indicating normal intraventricular conduction. The RR interval during tachycardia measures 420 milliseconds. The sequence of retrograde atrial activation starts in the coronary sinus lead, indicating ventriculoatrial (VA) conduction over a left-sided accessory pathway (AP). As VA conduction occurs by the normal atrioventricular (AV) pathway, the QRS complex is preceded by a His-bundle electrogram. The AH interval during tachycardia is 175 milliseconds. (**B**) The reversed (antidromic) variety of CMT is illustrated. QRS complexes during tachycardia show maximal preexcitation because of AV conduction over the AP. No His-bundle potential precedes the QRS complex. Ventriculoatrial conduction is by the normal His–AV node pathway, resulting in a different sequence of retrograde atrial activation. The cycle length during tachycardia is 415 milliseconds.

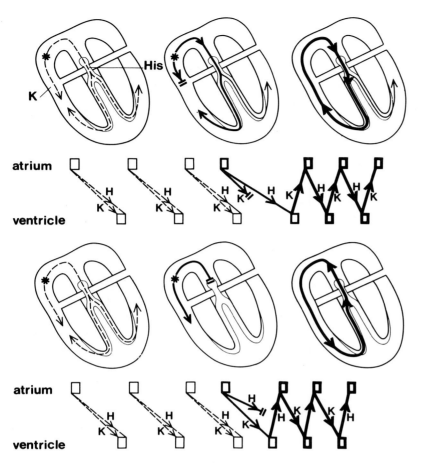

Figure 13-10. Representation of the modes of initiation of circus movement tachycardia (CMT) incorporating the accessory pathway (AP) by an atrial premature beat during atrial pacing. As seen in the *upper panel*, if the refractory period of the AP is longer than that of the atrioventricular (AV) node–His axis, a precisely timed atrial premature beat is blocked in the AP (*K*) while still being conducted through the normal pathway (*H*). After activation of the ventricle, the impulse is conducted to the ventricle through the AV node and CMT is initiated. The *lower panel* illustrates the AV node; CMT is initiated. The *lower panel* illustrates the much rarer situation in which the refractory period of the AP is shorter than that of the AV node–His pathway, and an appropriately timed atrial premature beat is blocked in the normal pathway while still being conducted over the AP to the ventricles. After activation of the ventricle, this impulse can be conducted in the ventriculoatrial direction over the His–AV node pathway, resulting in initiation of the antidromic form of CMT.

fibrillation and the effective refractory period of the AP, as determined by the single test stimulus technique.[53]

Figure 13-13 shows an example of atrial fibrillation and high ventricular rate because of exclusive conduction over the AP in a patient with WPW syndromemple of atrial fibrillation and high ventricular rate because of exclusive conduction over the AP in a patient with WPW syndrome. Frequently, one can observe runs of short RR intervals alternating with groups of RR intervals showing a slower rate. A decrease in refractoriness of both the AP and ventricular muscle with increasing rates may play an important role in this phenomenon.[53]

The group from Duke University reports a series of 16 of 135 patients with WPW syndrome who presented with ventricular fibrillation.[43] The only important marker for the development of ventricular fibrillation in this series was the occurrence of RR intervals equal to or less than 205 milliseconds during atrial fibrillation. This observation might be of relevance in selecting the best mode of therapy in these patients. Note that the degree of ventricular preexcitation observed in the electrocardiogram during sinus rhythm bears no relation to the risk of developing life-threatening ventricular rates during atrial fibrillation. This is illustrated in the electrocardiogram in Figure 13-14

from a patient in whom the AP did not markedly contribute to ventricular excitation during sinus rhythm. As seen in the lower panel, the patient presented with high ventricular rates due to AV conduction through the AP during atrial fibrillation (shortest RR interval, 200 milliseconds). In Figure 13-15, which was recorded in the same patient, an atrial premature beat during sinus rhythm brings out clear-cut ventricular preexcitation for reasons discussed earlier in this chapter. This again stresses the importance of distinguishing patients with little contribution to ventricular excitation through the AP from those having so-called concealed accessory pathways. The latter group of patients are projected against life-threatening ventricular rates if atrial fibrillation develops.

ELECTROPHYSIOLOGIC INVESTIGATIONS IN WOLFF-PARKINSON-WHITE SYNDROME

Since 1967, many patients with WPW syndrome have undergone electrophysiologic investigations.[21, 46, 49, 51] The apparatus used and the protocol followed during these

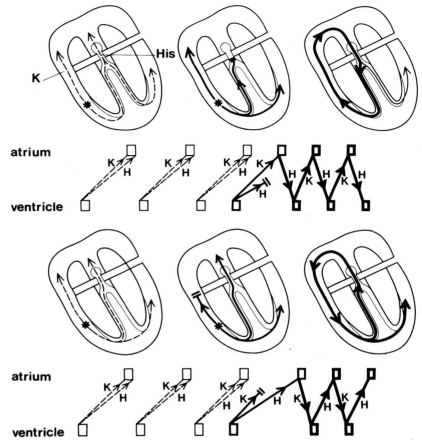

Figure 13-11. Modes of initiation of circus movement tachycardia CMT incorporating the AP by a ventricular premature beat during ventricular pacing. In the *upper panel*, the accessory pathway (AP) (*K*) is postulated to have a shorter refractory period than that of the normal atrioventricular (AV) node–His pathway (*H*). As shown, an appropriately timed ventricular premature beat is blocked in the AV node–His pathway while still being conducted over the accessory pathway to the atrium. If this impulse returns to the ventricles over the normal AV node–His pathway, CMT is initiated. The *lower panel* illustrates the exceptional situation in which an antidromic CMT incorporating the AP is initiated. To initiate this type of tachycardia, the refractory period of the AP must be longer than that of the AV node. An appropriately timed ventricular premature beat can then be blocked in the AP while being conducted to the atrium over the His–AV node pathway (*H*). If on reaching the atrium this impulse is conducted back to the ventricles over the AP, antidromic CMT is initiated.

studies are reviewed elsewhere.[49] The purpose of the studies (49) was to:

1. determine the location and number of the accessory pathways

2. determine the mechanism and pathway of tachycardia

3. establish the diagnosis of WPW syndrome in patients with a questionable electrocardiogram

4. identify a low-risk group

5. evaluate the effect of drugs on the electrophysiologic properties of the heart, especially on mechanisms of tachycardia and ventricular rates during atrial fibrillation

6. choose the correct therapy for a patient or for a group of patients with similar electrocardiophysiologic finding

7. select candidates for ablation of accessory pathways

8. evaluate postablation or postoperatively the effect of the intervention on conduction over the accessory pathways and mechanism of the tachycardia

Electrophysiologic investigations have become an important tool in diagnosis and management of the patient with WPW syndrome. Their value is examined during the discussion of our approach to the patient with WPW syndrome in relation to the problem he or she presents.

DIAGNOSTIC AND THERAPEUTIC APPROACH TO THE PATIENT WITH WOLFF-PARKINSON-WHITE SYNDROME

A patient with WPW syndrome can be examined by a physician for at least one of the following reasons: (1) a history of palpitations without an electrocardiographically

TABLE 13-4. Symptoms During Paroxysmal Circus Movement Tachycardia Incorporating the Accessory Pathway in 69 Patients With Wolff-Parkinson-White Syndrome

Symptom	Patients (n)
Palpitations	67 (97%)
Dyspnea	40 (58%)
Anginal pain	39 (56%)
Perspiration	38 (55%)
Fatigue	28 (41%)
Anxiety	20 (29%)
Dizziness	20 (29%)
Polyuria	18 (26%)

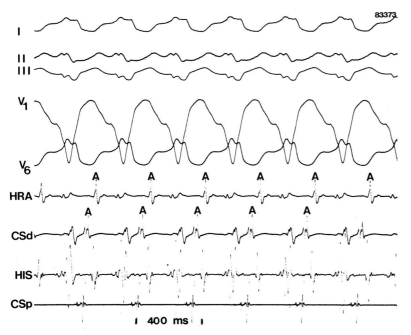

Figure 13-12. Antidromic circus movement tachycardia with atrioventricular (AV) conduction over a right free-wall accessory pathway. The intracardiac recordings reveal that ventriculoatrial conduction occurs over a left free-wall accessory pathway. Atrial activation starts in the coronary sinus (*CS*), followed by activation in the His-bundle recording and the high right atrial (*HRA*) recording. These findings indicate the presence of two accessory atrioventricular (AV) pathways, one (right free-wall) is used for AV and the other (left free-wall) is used for ventriculoatrial conduction during the tachycardia.

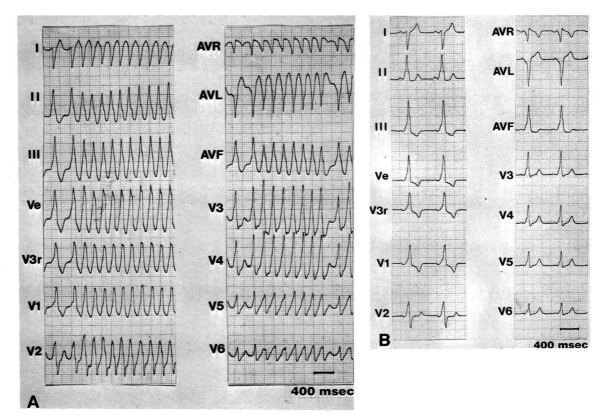

Figure 13-13. Atrial fibrillation in the presence of an accessory pathway with a short refractory period. **(A)** The typical features of this arrhythmia: (1) irregular RR interval, (2) marked widening of the QRS complex, and (3) a ventricular rate reaching 300 beats/minute **(B)** The electrocardiogram of the same patient during sinus rhythm.

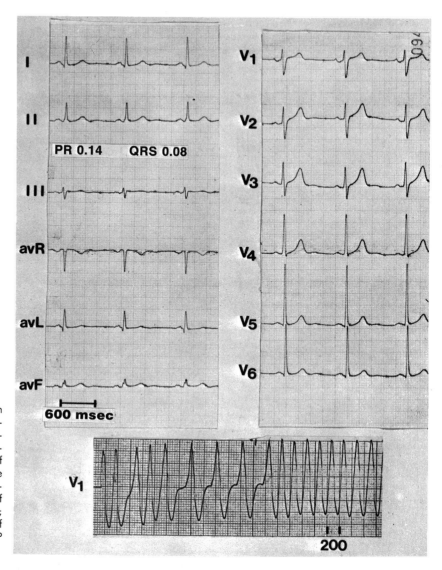

Figure 13-14. Example of a patient with Wolff-Parkinson-White syndrome with (during sinus rhythm) little contribution to ventricular activation by atrioventricular conduction over the accessory pathway (AP). As seen in the *upper part* of the figure, the PR interval and QRS width were both normal (0.14 and 0.08 seconds, respectively). The patient was admitted with an attack of atrial fibrillation (with a high ventricular rate; shortest RR interval, 200 milliseconds) because of conduction from atrium to ventricle over the AP (lower panel).

documented tachyarrhythmia, (2) an ongoing attack of palpitations, (3) an electrocardiographic diagnosis of WPW syndrome, and (4) an electrocardiogram with questionable signs of ventricular preexcitation. In the latter two instances, patients are usually referred to the cardiologist after recording of a routine electrocardiogram or because of an electrocardiogram for evaluation of complaints related to the cardiovascular system. Patients with palpitations are frequently seen for the first time by their general practitioner.

Patients With Palpitations

Patients Seen After an Attack of Palpitations

The general practitioner tends to misdiagnose complaints of patients suffering from paroxysmal tachycardias when the patient is seen after an attack of tachycardia. In a series of 69 consecutive patients with WPW syndrome admitted to the hospital for evaluation of attacks of paroxysmal supraventricular tachycardia, 39 were first seen by their general practitioner after an attack of tachycardia. We found that in only a few patients, the correct diagnosis was suspected by the general practitioner. In 25 patients, a diagnosis was made of "functional" complaints such as nervousness and fatigue. Various diagnoses such as "heart murmur" were made in six patients, whereas six other patients were told that their physician could find no abnormalities.[27]

Improvement in diagnosis by the general practitioner can be accomplished by (1) a careful history taking; (2) the recording of an electrocardiogram (if the WPW electrocardiographic pattern is observed, the patient must be considered as probably suffering from tachyarrhythmias

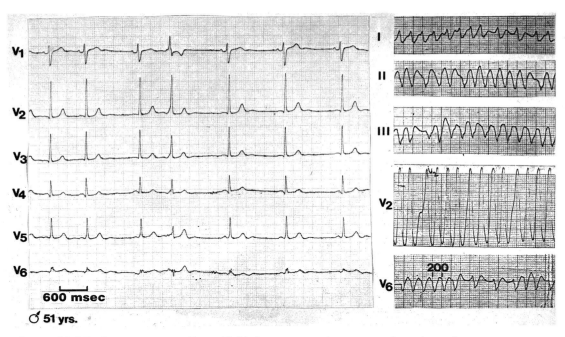

Figure 13-15. Same patient as in Figure 13-14. A supraventricular premature beat shows clear-cut left-sided preexcitation. On the *right*, several electrocardiographic leads during atrial fibrillation are seen.

until proved otherwise); (3) instructing the patient to have an electrocardiogram recorded as soon as a tachycardia occurs; and (4) the use of 24-hour electrocardiogram recordings.

As mentioned previously, rapid heart action in patients with WPW syndrome is most frequently the result of either paroxysmal CMT or atrial fibrillation. The presence of accompanying symptoms (see Table 13-4) supports the existence of arrhythmias, either CMT or atrial fibrillation. Abrupt onset and termination of the attack favor the existence of a paroxysmal tachyarrhythmia. Palpitations are regular during CMT and irregular during atrial fibrillation. Patients with WPW paroxysmal CMT frequently observe that at least some of their attacks could be stopped by vagal maneuvers. Patients with WPW syndrome and atrial fibrillation with a very rapid ventricular rate frequently suffer from dizziness or syncope during the arrhythmia. In patients with palpitations and an electrocardiogram showing WPW syndrome, the following steps should be taken:

1. Take careful history evaluating the frequency and length of the attacks, accompanying symptoms during tachycardia, physical and psychological tolerance of the attacks, and a physical examination with chest radiograph studies and echocardiogram to assess the presence or absence of concomitant heart disease. The latter may affect tolerance of the attacks of tachycardia and influence therapeutic decisions.

2. Record a 24-hour electrocardiogram, which gives information on the nature of the rhythm disturbance when the patient experiences palpitations and it enables confirmation of the existence of tachyarrhythmias and determination of their type (CMT or atrial fibrillation) and mode of initiation

3. Perform a stimulation study if the patient's quality of life is affected and the 24-hour electrocardiogram is negative. Inability to induce CMT during the stimulation study makes it very unlikely that the patient suffers from this type of arrhythmia outside the hospital. In a study by Denes and coworkers, none of their 22 patients with WPW syndrome in whom CMT could not be induced during the stimulation study had electrocardiographic documentation of paroxysmal supraventricular tachycardia.[54] In this group of patients, 50% were asymptomatic and the other 50% complained of paroxysmal palpitations. Because inability to induce CMT does not exclude atrial fibrillation as a cause of palpitations, we specifically induce this arrhythmia during the stimulation study, asking the patient whether he recognizes the symptoms. Denes and coworkers also report 28 patients with WPW syndrome in whom CMT was induced during the stimulation study.[54] Only one of these patients had no symptoms of tachycardia, 19 patients (68%) had electrocardiographic documentation of a similar type of tachycardia

outside the cardiac laboratory, and eight patients (28%) had a history of paroxysmal palpitations without electrocardiographic verifications.

Patients Seen During an Attack of Palpitations

As discussed previously, patients with WPW syndrome usually suffer from either a CMT incorporating the AP or atrial fibrillation or both.

PAROXYSMAL SUPRAVENTRICULAR TACHYCARDIA

Any patient presenting with a supraventricular tachycardia is first approached by vagal maneuvers (carotid sinus massage, elevation of the lower extremities, immersion of the face into cold water). If successful, the vagal maneuver terminates the CMT incorporating the AP by creating block in the AV node (Fig. 13-16). If vagal maneuvers do not easily terminate tachycardia, the following information should be obtained: (1) what the electrocardiogram shows during sinus rhythm, and (2) whether the patient was receiving medication; if so, what has been the success of intravenously and orally given antiarrhythmics in the past. If the patient is known to have WPW syndrome, the supraventricular tachycardia most likely is a CMT incorporating the AP in the retrograde direction. If no information on the electrocardiogram during sinus rhythm is available, this type of tachycardia is still the most likely on a statistical basis. In 120 consecutive hospital admissions because of supraventricular tachycardia, we found that during subse-

quent electrophysiologic evaluation, a CMT incorporating an AP in the retrograde direction could be induced in 79 patients (66%)—69 patients having the WPW syndrome and 10 patients having a concealed accessory pathway. In 32 patients (27%), a reentrant tachycardia confined to the AV node was demonstrated. In patients with a tachycardia incorporating an AP, one is often able to identify retrograde P waves (P') after the QRS, with a $P'R$ interval longer than the RP' interval (see Fig. 13-8).

As shown in Table 13-5, intravenous adenosine or verapamil is the first antiarrhythmic drug used in patients with a regular supraventricular tachycardia. Both drugs can terminate CMT incorporating the AP by creating block in the AV node. Digitalis has also been used in the treatment of patients with this arrhythmia. Because some patients may develop atrial fibrillation during CMT, which is an unpredictable event, digitalis may worsen the situation by abbreviating the refractory period of the AP, resulting in higher ventricular rates during atrial fibrillation.[55, 56] Therefore, we do not recommend the use of digitalis in these patients. Occasionally, atrial fibrillation may develop during the administration of adenosine for treatment of a CMT.[57] This may be dangerous in the case of a short anterograde refractory period of the AP. It stresses the necessity of having a defibrillator available when termination of CMT by adenosine is attempted in a patient with the WPW syndrome.

If drugs acting on the AV node do not terminate the tachycardia, antiarrhythmic agents known to affect the properties of the accessory pathway should be given intra-

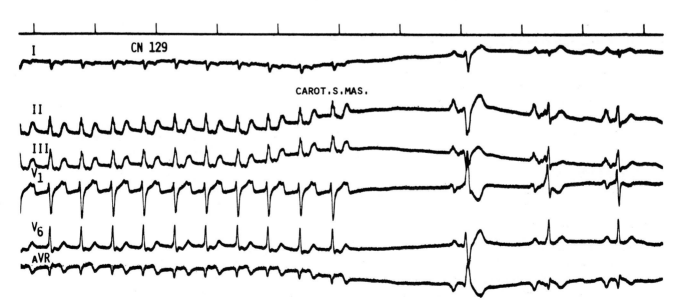

Figure 13-16. Termination of a circus movement tachycardia incorporating the accessory pathway in ventriculoatrial direction by carotid sinus massage. Retrograde P waves are identified after the QRS complex during tachycardia. Note that termination of tachycardia is the result of block in the atrioventricular node.

TABLE 13-5. Treatment of Circus Movement Tachycardia in Patients With Wolff-Parkinson-White Syndrome

TREATMENT DURING AN ATTACK OF CMT

Vagal maneuvers
Verapamil, 10 mg IV over 3 minutes
Adenosine, 6–12 mg IV; may be repeated at 1-minute intervals
Ajmaline, 1 mg/kg IV
Procainamide, up to 10 mg/kg IV
Pacing
DC shock

PROPHYLAXIS OF CMT

Sotalol
Long-acting quinidine
Long-acting quinidine plus propranolol
Class IC drugs
    Propafenone
    Flecainide
    Encainide
Amiodarone

CMT, circus movement tachycardia.

venously. Ajmaline, procainamide, disopyramide, and class IC agents are used for this purpose.[58–62] If these methods fail to terminate the tachycardia, or if the patient is tolerating the arrhythmia poorly, electrical methods (direct current cardioversion or pacing) should be employed.[63] Pacing techniques are safer in patients who are receiving drugs that might endanger direct current cardioversion (i.e., digitalis, verapamil, beta-blocking agents, and amiodarone). Electric stimulation techniques creating block in the tachycardia circuit are preferred in those patients in whom termination of tachycardia is rapidly followed by reinitiation of tachycardia.

ATRIAL FIBRILLATION

Patients with high ventricular rates during atrial fibrillation because of AV conduction over an AP with a short refractory period deserve special attention. In these patients, mean ventricular rates range from 160 to 300 beats per minute. During these high ventricular rates, there usually is not only severe hemodynamic impairment but also the risk of ventricular fibrillation. As a rule, digitalis should be avoided in these patients. During episodes of atrial fibrillation with fast ventricular rates, cardioversion is the treatment of choice. If the patient is receiving drugs that may promote asystole after electric cardioversion (e.g., verapamil, beta-blocking agents, and probably amiodarone), a temporary pacing lead is positioned in the right ventricle before direct current shock. If the ventricular rate during atrial fibrillation is not excessively high (below 200 beats/minute), drugs such as procainamide, ajmaline, disopyramide, and quinidine (which prolong the duration

of the refractory period of the AP) can be given (Table 13-6).

Drug Prophylaxis in Patients With Proved Tachyarrhythmias

Patients with WPW syndrome should receive prophylactic drug treatment when the arrhythmia is physically and psychologically poorly tolerated. In our experience, amiodarone is the most effective drug in the prevention of attacks of paroxysmal tachycardia in patients with WPW syndrome.[64–66]

Amiodarone acts on most of the components of the reentrant circuit in these patients.[65] Sotalol, long-acting quinidine, and class IC drugs may also be used. For reasons already mentioned, digitalis should be avoided whenever possible in patients with WPW syndrome. In view of the current results of radiofrequency ablation of APs and its low risk, indications for this type of therapy are changing. Originally, they consisted of refractoriness to a disabling arrhythmia, intolerance to drug therapy, unacceptable side effects of antiarrhythmic drugs, and lack of patient compliance. An increasing number of less-symptomatic patients are benefiting from radiofrequency ablative interventions that result in permanent cure.[67,68]

Patients with documented atrial fibrillation and high ventricular rates because of a short refractory period of the AP should be electrophysiologically evaluated to establish the correct treatment. If the patient refuses radiofrequency ablation of the AP, the necessity of such an evaluation is indicated by the observation that the effect of a drug on the duration of the refractory period of the AP is related to the length of the refractory period of the AP before drug administration.[69] We have shown that the duration of the refractory period of the AP may shorten during sympa-

TABLE 13-6. Drug Treatment of Atrial Fibrillation in Patients With Wolff-Parkinson-White Syndrome

Treatment during the attack:
  Hemodynamically not tolerated DC shock
  Hemodynamically tolerated intravenous administration of:
    Procainamide
    Ajmaline
    Disopyramide
    Flecainide
    Propafenone
Prophylaxis of atrial fibrillation
  Amiodarone
  Sotalol
  Long-acting quinidine plus propranolol
  Class IC drugs

thetic stimulation.[70] This occurred even in patients receiving amiodarone. Patients with symptomatic atrial fibrillation are now preferably treated with radiofrequency ablation of their accessory pathway.

APPROACH TO THE PATIENT WITH AN ELECTROCARDIOGRAPHIC DIAGNOSIS OF WOLFF-PARKINSON-WHITE SYNDROME

Patients with an electrocardiographic diagnosis of WPW syndrome should be divided into two groups according to the presence or absence of complaints suggestive of arrhythmias. If a history of palpitations is present, we approach the patients as discussed previously.

As mentioned, the presenting symptom in patients with WPW syndrome may be ventricular fibrillation.[42] Therefore, in the patients with an electrocardiogram showing the WPW abnormality, one should like to identify the group of patients who seem to be protected against sudden death if atrial fibrillation supervenes.

In patients with WPW syndrome, the development of life-threatening ventricular rates during atrial fibrillation (possibly leading to ventricular fibrillation) is related to the value of the anterograde effective refractory period of the accessory pathway.[53] We have observed that failure to achieve complete anterograde block in the AP after the intravenous administration of 50 mg of ajmaline is highly suggestive of an anterograde effective refractory period of the AP with a duration of less than 270 milliseconds.[58] This also holds for procainamide given intravenously in a dose of 10 mg/kg over a 5-minute period.[71]

Therefore, in patients with WPW syndrome and no previous complaints of palpitations, a positive ajmaline or procainamide test (induction of anterograde block over the AP, as demonstrated in Figures 13-17 and 13-18, indicates that the patient has a relatively long duration of the refractory period of the AP and that no further investigations are required. Using a modified ajmaline test, Chimienti and coworkers showed that the amount of ajmaline required to block conduction over the accessory pathway correlates with the duration of the anterograde refractory period of the accessory pathway.[72] Because both ajmaline and procainamide also prolong the refractory period of His-Purkinje system, these tests should be conducted in an area where the possible complication of complete AV block can be appropriately managed.

There are two other noninvasive tests that indicate a long duration of the refractory period of the accessory pathway in anterograde direction. First, the finding of intermittent preexcitation indicates a long anterograde refractory period of the accessory pathway.[73] Secondly, as shown by Levy and coworkers, disappearances of preexcitation during exercise indicate a long anterograde refractory period of the AP.[74] One should be careful, however, because sympathetic stimulation during exercise speeds up trans-AV node conduction and might thereby diminish the area of the ventricles preexcited over the accessory pathway. Several electrocardiogram leads should therefore be recorded simultaneously, and special attention should be given to the electrocardiogram after exercise, when exercise-induced block in the AP may show a sudden marked change in the QRS complex on resumption of AV conduction over the accessory pathway.

Although patients at low risk can be identified relatively easily, the asymptomatic patient in whom results of noninvasive testing suggest a short anterograde refractory period of the accessory pathway presents more difficulty. The European multicenter study reported by Torner shows that in six of 23 patients with WPW syndrome

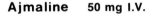

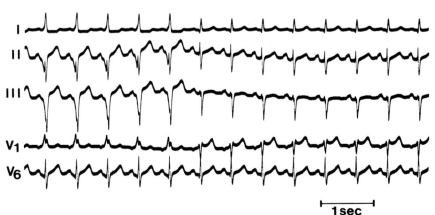

Figure 13-17. Creation of complete atrioventricular block in the accessory pathway by the intravenous administration of 50 mg of ajmaline.

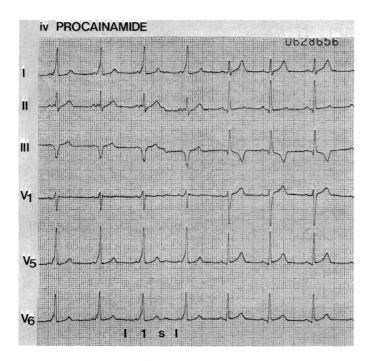

Figure 13-18. Disappearance of preexcitation (*middle* of the figure) after the intravenous injection of 300 mg of procainamide.

resuscitated from ventricular fibrillation, the (lethal) arrhythmia was the first symptomatic arrhythmia they ever experienced.[44]

Other studies, however, such as those by Sharma and coworkers and Beckman and associates suggest that asymptomatic patients with a short anterograde refractory period of their AP and not treated with antiarrhythmic drugs have a good prognosis.[75,76] Our current policy is to withhold antiarrhythmic drug therapy in the asymptomatic patient with a short anterograde refractory period of the accessory pathway. In selected asymptomatic patients with a short anterograde refractory period of the AP, we have interrupted conduction over that structure only for professional reasons (e.g., license to fly a commercial airliner or to be insured as a professional football player).

APPROACH TO THE PATIENT WITH A QUESTIONABLE ELECTROCARDIOGRAM

In patients with questionable evidence of WPW syndrome because of little contribution of the AP to ventricular activation during sinus rhythm, resulting in a normal PR interval and normal QRS width, the clinician faces the problem of making the correct diagnosis of preexcitation. In some patients, the diagnosis can be made by the following noninvasive procedures: (1) increasing AV node delay or creating AV node block, thereby enhancing ventricular excitation over the AP by carotid sinus massage or the administration of adenosine; and (2) giving drugs such as ajmaline or

procainamide, which by causing block in the AP may cause QRS abnormalities to disappear secondary to preexcitation (see Figs. 13-17 and 13-18). Both tests are only of diagnostic value when positive. The effect of carotid sinus massage on AV node conduction depends on many variables, and some patients with WPW syndrome may have a short intra-AV node conduction time. The ability to induce block over the AP after the administration of drugs such as ajmaline and procainamide depends on the initial value of the effective refractory period of the accessory pathway.[69]

If both of the aforementioned noninvasive tests are negative, the only way of making the correct diagnosis of WPW syndrome is by (1) atrial pacing at increasing rates, or (2) applying atrial test stimuli with increasing prematurity.[51] Both modes of atrial stimulation result in progressive prolongation of the AV node conduction time, without changing the AV conduction time over the AP, and brings out preexcitation.

MAHAIM FIBERS

In 1938 Mahaim described islands of tissue acting as a connection between the AV node and the ventricular myocardium.[77] Subsequent studies have suggested the presence of nodo-ventricular and fasciculo-ventricular fibers.[78–82] The presence of these anomalous connections would allow for the development of a form of AV reentrant tachycardia which was in fact observed in these patients. Electrophysiologic studies as early as 1971 focused attention on this condition supporting the concept of a nodo-ventricular fiber as the key component in this syndrome.[83] Subsequent studies added further data supporting the concepts initiated by Mahaim's observations.[84-94] It was not until 1982 that data from Gillette and colleagues identified that some of these patients had atrio-fascicular pathways which could be ablated surgically.[95] These observations were subsequently verified by other investigators' intraoperative mapping studies.[96,97] In patients with this entity, tachycardia may occur with either: 1) anterograde conduction over the Mahaim connection and retrograde conduction over the His-Purkinje system; or 2) the Mahaim tract acting as an "innocent bystander" producing a wide QRS tachycardia whose etiology may be AV nodal reentry, atrial fibrillation, etc.[84,97-103]

Clinically, Epstein's anomaly is relatively common and multiple accessory pathways are also observed with an increased frequency.[84]

Electrocardiographically, normal or short PR intervals may be seen but Delta waves are rarely observed. If Delta waves are present, multiple accessory pathways must be considered.

The electrocardiogram during supraventricular tachycardia with this entity has characteristic features such as: 1) left bundle branch block morphology; 2) superior axis deviation; 3) a QRS duration generally equal to or less than 150 milliseconds; and 4) a QRS transition at or after V_4.

Electrophysiologic studies have demonstrated: 1) more prominent conduction abnormalities with right versus left (coronary sinus) atrial pacing; 2) progressive AH prolongation and HV abbreviation with increasing atrial pacing rates associated with progressive QRS conduction delay; 3) that once maximal preexcitation is present, further atrial rate increases do not result in any further increases in the V-H interval; 4) incremental ventricular pacing results in a mid-line (septal) activation sequence with decremental conduction characteristics;

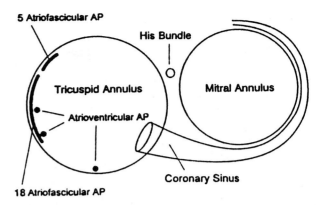

Figure 13-19. Schematic of the mitral and tricuspid annulus as seen in the left anterior oblique view. Site of successful ablation of Mahaim tracts are shown. (From McClelland JH, Wang X, Beckman KJ, et al: Radiofrequency catheter ablation of right atriofascicular [Mahaim] accessory pathways guided by accessory pathway activation potentials. Circulation 1994;89:2655.)

5) anterograde conduction occurs through the anomalous connection but may have decremental (AV nodal–like) properties; and 6) during antidromic tachycardia, single late atrial prematures advance the next QRS and reset the tachycardia.

These electrophysiologic studies have obtained evidence which suggests that these patients do in fact have a pathway which connects the lateral right atrium to either the right ventricular apex or the right bundle branch (Figs. 13-19 and 13-20).[95-102]

Electrograms recorded at the tricuspid annulus near the accessory pathway have demonstrated characteristic findings of: 1) an isoelectric interval between the atrial and accessory pathway potential; 2) an atrial–accessory pathway interval of 63 ± 12 milliseconds (40–85 milliseconds); 3) an accessory pathway −V interval of 83 ± 23 milliseconds (50–150 milliseconds); and 4) a ventricular

Figure 13-20. Schematic of a right atrio-fasacular accessory pathway. The distal end of the accessory pathway might insert in the apex of the right ventricle (**A**) or might insert into the distal right bundle branch (**B**). *AVN,* AV node; *HB,* His bundle; *LBB,* left bundle branch; *RBB,* right bundle branch. (From McClelland JH, Wang X, Beckman KJ, et al: Radiofrequency catheter ablation of right atrio-fascicular [Mahaim] accessory pathways guided by accessory pathway activation potentials. Circulation 1994;89:2655.)

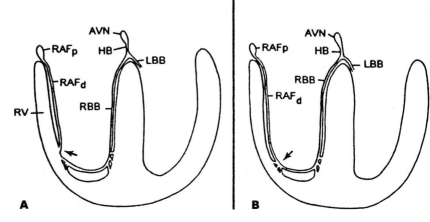

electrogram, (with fully preexcited QRS complexes), recorded at the tricuspid annulus and inscribed *after* the onset of the QRS by 21 ± 7 milliseconds (10–38 milliseconds).[100]

Radiofrequency catheter ablation techniques have been successfully used to cure patients with this form of anomalous AV conduction.[99–102]

ASYMPTOMATIC PATIENTS WITH A WOLFF-PARKINSON-WHITE ANOMALY

Some interest has been directed at electrophysiologic investigation of the asymptomatic Wolff-Parkinson-White patient. The interest in such studies relates to the possibility of a first episode of tachycardia being atrial fibrillation associated with very rapid ventricular rates and, therefore, the possibility of sudden cardiac death. This may be of special importance in patients with high risk occupations or vocations (e.g., airplane pilots, high voltage line workers, athletes, etc.)

Prospective electrophysiologic studies have demonstrated that there is a very low risk for the development of tachycardia (i.e. less than 10%) thereby negating the importance of such studies for prognostication. There were no clinical or electrophysiologic characteristics that clearly identify patients who might subsequently develop supraventricular tachycardia, atrial fibrillation and, potentially, sudden cardiac death.[104, 105]

References

1. Wolff J, Parkinson J, White PD: Bundle branch block with short P-R interval in healthy young people prone to paroxysmal tachycardia. Am Heart J 1930;5:685.
2. Wilson FN: A case in which vagus influenced the form of ventricular complex of the electrocardiogram. Arch Intern Med 1915;16:1008.
3. Wedd AM: Paroxysmal tachycardia. With reference to nomotopic tachycardia and the role of the extrinsic cardiac nerves. Arch Intern Med 1921;27:571.
4. Bach F: Paroxysmal tachycardia of forty-eight years duration and right bundle branch block. Proc R Soc Med 1929;22:412.
5. Hamburger WW: Bundle branch block. Four cases of intraventricular blocks showing some interesting and unusual clinical features. Med Clin North Am 1929;13:343.
6. Dreifus LS, Hairat R, Watanabe Y, et al: Ventricular fibrillation, a possible mechanism of sudden death in patients with the Wolff-Parkinson-White syndrome. Circulation 1971;43:520.
7. Wellens HJJ: Contribution of cardiac pacing to our understanding of the Wolff-Parkinson-White syndrome. Br Heart J 1975;37:231.
8. Durrer D, Roos JP: Epicardial excitation of the ventricles in a patient with Wolff-Parkinson-White syndrome (type B). Circulation 1967;35:15.
9. Durrer D, Schoo J, Schuilenburg RM, Wellens HJJ: The role of premature beats in the initiation and termination of supraventricular tachycardia in the Wolff-Parkinson-White syndrome. Circulation 1967;36:644.
10. Castellanos A Jr, Chapunoff E, Castillo CA, et al: His-bundle electrograms in two cases of WPW (pre-excitation) syndrome. Circulation 1970;41:399.
11. Gallagher JJ, Sealy WC, Wallace AG, Kasell J: Correlation between catheter electrophysiological studies and findings on mapping of ventricular excitation in the WPW syndrome. In: Wellens HJJ, Lie KI, Janse MJ, eds. The conduction system of the heart. Philadelphia: Lea & Febiger, 1976:588.
12. Cox JL: The status of surgery for cardiac arrhythmias. Circulation 1985;71:412.
13. Klein GJ, Guiraudon GM, Perkins DG: Surgical correction of the Wolff-Parkinson-White syndrome in the closed heart using cryosurgery: a simplified approach. J Am Coll Cardiol 1984;3:405.
14. Weber H, Schmitz L: Catheter technique for closed chest ablation of an accessory pathway. N Engl J Med 1983;308:654.
15. Morady F, Scheinman MM: Transvenous catheter ablation of a posteroseptal accessory pathway in a patient with the Wolff-Parkinson-White syndrome. N Eng J Med 1984;310:705.
16. Becker AE, Anderson RH, Durrer D, Wellens HJJ: The anatomical substrates of Wolff-Parkinson-White syndrome. Circulation 1978;57:870.
17. Anderson RH, Becker AE, Brechemacher C, et al: Ventricular pre-excitation. A proposed nomenclature for its substrates. Eur J Cardiol 1975;3:27.
18. Durrer D, Schuilenburg RM, Wellens HJJ: Preexcitation revised. Am J Cardiol 1970;25:690.
19. Segers M, Lequime J, Denolin H: L'activation ventriculaire précoce de certain coeurs hyperexcitables. Etude de l'onde delta de l'electrocardiogramme. Cardiologia 1944;8:113.
20. Puech P, Grolleau R. L'activité du faisceau de His normale et pathologique. Paris, edition Sandoz, 1972.
21. Gallagher JJ, Pritchett ELC, Sealy WC, Kasell J, Wallace AG: The preexcitation syndromes. Prog Cardiovasc Dis 1978; 20:285.
22. Coumel Ph, Attuel P: Reciprocating tachycardia in overt and latent preexcitation. Eur J Cardiol 1974;1:423.
23. Chung KY, Walsh T, Massie E: Wolff-Parkinson-White syndrome. Am Heart J 1965;69:1.
24. Bellet S: Clinical disorders of the heart beat. 3rd ed. Philadelphia: Lea & Febiger, 1971:506.
25. Vidaillet HJ, Pressley JC, Henke E, et al: Familial occurrence of accessory atrioventricular pathways (pre-excitation syndrome). N Engl J Med 1987;34:65.
26. Averill KM, Fosmoe RJ, Lamb LE: Electrocardiographic findings in 67,375 asymptomatic subjects. IV. Wolff-Parkinson-White syndrome. Am J Cardiol 1960;6:108.
27. Wellens HJJ: Paroxysmal supraventricular tachycardia. Recognition by the general practitioner. Rev Lat Cardiol 1980;1:51.
28. Rosenbaum FF, Hecht HH, Wilson FN, Johnston FD: Potential variations of the thorax and the esophagus in anomalous atrioventricular excitation (Wolff-Parkinson-White syndrome). Am Heart J 1945;29:281.
29. Wallace AG, Sealy WC, Gallagher JJ, et al: Surgical correction

of anomalous left ventricular preexcitation: Wolff-Parkinson-White (type A). Circulation 1974;49:206.

30. Tonkin AM, Wagner GS, Gallagher JJ, Wallace AG: Initial forces of ventricular depolarization in the Wolff-Parkinson-White syndrome. Circulation 1975;42:1020.

31. Lemery R, Hammill SC, Wood DL, et al: Value of the resting 12 lead electrocardiogram and vectorcardiogram for locating the accessory pathway in patients with the Wolff-Parkinson-White syndrome. Br Heart J 1987;58:324.

32. Milstein S, Sharma AD, Guiraudon GM, et al: An algorithm for the electrocardiographic localization of accessory pathways in the Wolff-Parkinson-White syndrome. Pacing Clin Electrophysiol 1987;10:555.

33. Reddy GV, Schamroth L: The localization of bypass tracts in the Wolff-Parkinson-White syndrome from the surface electrocardiogram. Am Heart J 1987;113:984.

34. Lindsay BD, Crossen KJ, Cain ME: Concordance of distinguishing electrocardiographic features during sinus rhythm with the location of accessory pathways in the Wolff-Parkinson-White syndrome. Am J Cardiol 1987;57:1096.

35. Wellens HJJ, Lubbers JC, Losekoot TG: Preexcitation. In: Roberts J, Gelband H, eds. Cardiac arrhythmias in children. New York: Appleton-Century-Croft, 1977:231.

36. Schiebler GL, Edwards JE, Burchell HB: Congenital corrected transposition of the great vessels. A study of 33 cases. Pediatrics 1960;27:11.

37. Ellis K, Morgan BS, Blumenthal S, Anderson DH: Congenital corrected transposition of the great vessels. Radiology 1962; 79:35.

38. Schliebler GL, Adams P, Anderson RC: The Wolff-Parkinson-White syndrome in infants and children. A review and a report of 28 cases. Pediatrics 1959;24:585.

39. Ahlinger S, Granath A, Holmer S: Wolff-Parkinson-White syndrome med paroxysmalt atrieflimmer overgaende i ventrikelflimmer. Nord Med 1963;70:1336.

40. Castillo-Fenoy A, Goupil A, Offenstadt G: Syndrome de Wolff-Parkinson-White et mort subite. Ann Med Interne (Paris) 1973;124:871.

41. Martin-Noel P, Denis B, Grunwald D, Buisson M: Deux cas mortels de syndrome de Wolff-Parkinson-White. Arch Mal Coeur 1970;63:1647.

42. Touche M, Jouvet M, Touche S: Fibrillation ventriculaire au coeurs d'un syndrome de Wolff-Parkinson-White. Réduction par choc électrique externe. Arch Mal Coeur 1966;59:1122.

43. Klein GJ, Bashore T, Sellers TD, Gallagher JJ, Wallace AG: Ventricular fibrillation in the Wolff-Parkinson-White syndrome. N Engl J Med 1979;301:1080.

44. Torner PM, the European Registry on Sudden Death in the Wolff-Parkinson-White syndrome: Ventricular fibrillation in the Wolff-Parkinson-White syndrome. Eur Heart J. 1991; 12:144.

45. Wellens HJJ, Atie J, Penn OC, Gorgels APM, Brugada P, Smeets JLRM: Diagnosis and treatment of patients with accessory pathways. In: Scheinman MM, ed. Cardiology clinics. Philadelphia: WB Saunders, 1990:503.

46. Wellens HJJ: The electrophysiological properties of the accessory pathway in the Wolff-Parkinson-White syndrome. In: Wellens HJJ, Janse MJ, Lie KI, eds. The conduction system of the heart. Philadelphia: Lea & Febiger, 1976:567.

47. Mines GR: On dynamic equilibrium in the heart. J Physiol 1913;46:23.

48. Wellens HJJ: Value and limitations of programmed electrical stimulation of the heart in the study and treatment of tachycardias. Circulation 1978;57:845.

49. Wellens HJJ, Brugada P: Value of programmed stimulation of the heart in patients with the Wolff-Parkinson-White syndrome. In: Josephson ME, Wellens HJJ, eds. Tachycardias. Philadelphia: Lea & Febiger, 1984:199.

50. Gallagher JJ, Sealy WC, Kasell J, Wallace AG: Multiple accessory pathways in patients with the preexcitation syndrome. Circulation 1976;54:571.

51. Wellens HJJ, Farré J, Bär FW: Stimulation studies in the Wolff-Parkinson-White syndrome. In: Narula O, ed. Clinical electrophysiology. Philadelphia: FA Davis, 1979.

52. Smith WM, Broughton A, Reiter MJ, et al: Bystander accessory pathway during AV node reentrant tachycardia. Pacing Clin Electrophysiol 1983;6:537.

53. Wellens HJJ, Durrer D: Relation between refractroy period of the accessory pathway and ventricular frequency during atrial fibrillation in patients with the Wolff-Parkinson-White syndrome. Am J Cardiol 1974;33:178.

54. Denes P, Wu D, Amat-y-Leon F, et al: Determination of atrioventricular reentrant paroxysmal tachycardia in patients with Wolff-Parkinson-White syndrome. Circulation 1978;58: 415.

55. Wellens HJJ, Durrer D: Effect of digitalis on atrioventricular conduction and circus movement tachycardia in patients with the Wolff-Parkinson-White syndrome. Circulation 1973;47:1229.

56. Sellers TD, Bashore TM, Gallagher JJ: Digitalis in the preexcitation syndrome: analysis during atrial fibrillation. Circulation 1977;56:260.

57. Cowell RPW, Paul VE, Ilsley CD: Hemodynamic deterioration after treatment with adenosine. Br Heart J 1994;71:569.

58. Wellens HJJ, Bär FW, Gorgels AP, Vanagt EJ: Use of ajmaline in identifying patients with short refractory period of their accessory pathway in Wolff-Parkinson-White syndrome. Am J Cardiol 1980;45:130.

59. Wellens HJJ, Durrer D: Effect of procainamide, quinidine and ajmaline on the Wolff-Parkinson-White syndrome. Circulation 1974;50:114.

60. Mandel WJ, Laks MM, Obayashi K: The Wolff-Parkinson-White syndrome: pharmacological effects of procainamide. Am Heart J 1975;90:744.

61. Sellers TD, Campbell RW, Bashore TM, Gallagher JJ: Effects of procainamide and quinidine sulfate in the Wolff-Parkinson-White syndrome. Circulation 1977;55:15.

62. Spurrell RAJ, Thorburn CW, Camm J, et al: Effects of disopyramide on electrophysiological properties of specialized conduction system in man on accessory atrioventricular pathway in the Wolff-Parkinson-White syndrome. Br Heart J 1975;37:861.

63. Den Dulk K, Bertholet M, Brugada P, et al: A versatile pacemaker system for termination of tachycardias. Am J Cardiol 1983;52:731.

64. Rosenbaum MB, Chiale PA, Ryba D, Elizari MV: Control of tachyarrhythmias associated with Wolff-Parkinson-White syndrome by amiodarone hydrochloride. Am J Cardiol 1974;34:215.

65. Wellens HJJ, Lie KI, Bär FW, et al: Effect of amiodarone in the Wolff-Parkinson-White syndrome. Am J Cardiol 1976;38:189.

66. Wellens HJJ, Brugada P, Abdollah H: Effect of amiodarone in paroxysmal supraventricular tachycardia with or without Wolff-Parkinson-White syndrome. Am Heart J 1983;106:876.

67. Jackman WM, Wang W, Friday KJ, et al: Catheter ablation of accessory atrioventricular pathways (Wolff-Parkinson-White syndrome) by radiofrequency current. N Engl J Med 1991; 324:1605.

68. Calkins H, Souza J, El-Atassi R, et al: Diagnosis and cure of the Wolff-Parkinson-White syndrome of paroxysmal supraventricular tachycardia during a single electrophysiologic test. N Engl J Med 1991;324:1612.

69. Wellens HJJ, Bär FW, Gorgels AP: Effect of drugs in WPW syndrome. Importance of initial length of effective refractory period of accessory pathway. Am J Cardiol 1980;46:665.

70. Wellens HJJ, Brugada P, Roy D, et al: Effects of isoproterenol on the anterograde refractory period of the accessory pathway in patients with the Wolff-Parkinson-White syndrome. Am J Cardiol 1982;50:180.

71. Wellens HJJ, Braat SHJG, Brugada P, et al: Use of procainamide in patients with the Wolff-Parkinson-White syndrome to disclose a short refractory period of the accessory pathway. Am J Cardiol 1982;50:921.

72. Chimienti M, Moizi M, Klersy C, et al: A modified ajmaline test for prediction of the effective refractory period of the accessory pathway in the Wolff-Parkinson-White syndrome. Am J Cardiol 1987;59:164.

73. Wellens HJJ: The Wolff-Parkinson-White syndrome. Part I. Modern concepts of cardiovascular disease 1983;52:53.

74. Levy S, Broustet JP, Clemency J: Syndrome de Wolff-Parkinson-White. Correlations entre l'exploition electrophysiologique et 'effet de l'épreuve d'effort sur l'aspect electrocardiographique de pre-excitation. Arch Mal Coeur 1979;72: 634.

75. Sharma AD, Yee R, Guiraudon G, et al: Sensitivity and specificity of invasive and noninvasive testing for risk of sudden death in Wolff-Parkinson-White syndrome. J Am Coll Cardiol 1987;10:373.

76. Beckman KJ, Gallastegui JL, Bauman JL, Hariman RJ: The predictive value of electrophysiologic studies in untreated patients with Wolff-Parkinson-White syndrome. J Am Coll Cardiol 1990;15:640.

77. Mahaim I, Benatt A: Nouvelles recherches sur les connexions superieures de la branche gauche du faisceau de His-Tawara avec cloison interventriculaire. Cardiologia 1938;1:61.

78. Lev M, Fox SM, Bharati S, Greenfield JC Jr, Rosen KM, Pick A: Mahaim and James fibers as a basis for a unique variety of ventricular preexcitation. Am J Cardiol 1975;36:880.

79. Brechenmacher C, Courtadon M, Jourde M, Yermia JC, Cheynee J, Voegtlin R. Syndrome de Wolff-Parkinson-White par association de fibres atrio-hisiennes et de fibres de Mahaim. Arch Mal Coeur Vaiss 1976;69:1275.

80. Becker AE, Anderson RH: Morphology of the human atrioventricular junctional area. In: Wellens HJJ, Lie KI, Janse MJ, eds. The Conduction System of the Heart. Leiden, the Netherlands: HE Stenfert Kroese BV 1976:263.

81. Becker AE, Bouman LN, Janse MJ, Anderson RH: Functional anatomy of the cardiac conduction system. In: Harrison DC, ed. Cardiac Arrhythmias. A Decade of Progress. Boston, Mass: GK Hall Medical Publishers 1981:3.

82. Anderson RH, Becker AE, Brechenmacher C, Davies MJ, Rossi L: Ventricular preexcitation: a proposed nomenclature for its substrates. Eur J Cardiol 1975;3:27.

83. Wellens HJJ: The preexcitation syndrome. In: Wellens HJJ, ed. Electrical stimulation of the heart in the study and treatment of tachycardias. Baltimore, MD: University Park Press 1971:97.

84. Ellenbogen KA, Ramirez NM, Packer DL, et al: Accessory nodoventricular (Mahaim) fibres: a clinical review. Pacing Clin Electrophysiol 1986;9:868.

85. Motte G, Brechenmacher C, Davy JM, Belhassen B: Association de fibres nodoventriculaires et atrio-ventriculaires a l'origine de tachycardies reciproques. Arch Mal Coeur Vaiss 1980;73:737.

86. Gmeiner R, Ng CK, Hammer I, Becker AE: Tachycardia caused by an accessory nodoventricular tract: a clinicopathologic correlation. Eur Heart J 1984;5:233.

87. Ward DE, Camm AJ, Spurrell RAJ: Ventricular preexcitation due to anomalous nodoventricular pathways: report of 3 patients. Eur J Cardiol 1979;9:111.

88. Bardy GH, German LD, Packer DL, Coltorti F, Gallagher JJ: Mechanism of tachycardia using a nodoventricular Mahaim fiber. Am J Cardiol 1984;54:1140.

89. Touboul P, Vexler RM, Chatelain MT: Re-entry via Mahaim fibres as a possible basis for tachycardia. Br Heart J 1978;40:806.

90. Tchou P, Lehmann MH, Jazayeri M, Akhtar M: Atriofascicular connection or a nodoventricular Mahaim fiber? Electrophysiologic elucidation of the pathway and associated reentrant circuit. Circulation 1988;77:837.

91. Castellanos A, Sung RJ, Castillo CA, Agha AS, Befeler B, Myerburg RJ: His bundle recordings in diagnosis of impulse formation in Kent and Mahaim tracts. Br Heart J 1976;38:1173.

92. Coumel P, Waynberger M, Fabiato A, Slama R, Aigueperse A, Bouvrain Y. Wolff-Parkinson-White syndrome: problems in evaluation of multiple accessory pathways and surgical therapy. Circulation 1972;45:1216.

93. Gallagher JJ, Smith WM, Kasell JH, Benson DW Jr, Sterba R, Grant AO. Role of Mahaim fibers in cardiac arrhythmias in man. Circulation 1981;64:176.

94. Tonkin AM, Dugan FA, Svenson RH, Sealy WC, Wallace AG, Gallagher JJ: Coexistence of functinal Kent and Mahaim-type tracts in the pre-excitation syndrome: demonstration by catheter techniques and epicardial mapping. Circulation 1975;52:193.

95. Gillette PC, Garsoh A Jr, Cooley DA, McNamara DG: Prolonged and decremental antegrade conduction properties in right anterior accessory connections: wide RS antidromic tachycardia of left bundle branch block pattern without Wolff-Parkinson-White configuration in sinus rhythm. Am Heart J 1982;103:66.

96. Ross DL, Johnson DC, Koo CC, et al: Surgical treatment of supraventricular tachycardia without the WPW syndrome:

current indications, techniques and results. In: Brugada P, Wellens HJJ, eds. Cardiac Arrhythmias: Where to Go From Here? Mount Kisco, NY: Futura Publishing Co 1987; 591.

97. Klein GJ, Guiraudon GM, Kerr CR, et al: Nodoventricular accessory pathway: evidence for a distinct accessory atrioventricular pathway with atrioventricular node-like properties. J Am Coll Cardiol 1988;11:1035.

98. Leitch JW, Klein GJ, Yee R, Murdock CJ: New concepts on nodoventricular accessory pathways. J Cardiovasc Electrophysiol 1990;1:220.

99. Haissaguerre J-FW, Le Metayer P, Maraud L, et al: Catheter ablation of Mahaim fibers with preservation of atrioventricular nodal conduction. Circulation 1990;82:418.

100. McClelland JH, Wang X, Beckman KJ, et al: Radiofrequency catheter ablation of right atriofascicular (Mahaim) accessory pathways guided by accessory pathway activation potentials. Circulation 1994;89:2655.

101. Cappato R, Schluter M, Weib C, et al: Catheter-induced mechanical conduction block of right-sided accessory fibers with Mahaim-type preexcitation to guide radiofrequency ablation. Circulation 1994;90:282.

102. Grogin HR, Lee RJ, Kwasman M, et al: Radiofrequency catheter ablation of atriofascicular and nodoventricular Mahaim tracts. Circulation 1994;90:272.

103. Deng Z, Gang ES, Rosenthal ME, Oseran D, Mandel WJ, Peter T: Wide QRS tachycardia due to AV nodal reentry and a bystander bypass tract with slow conduction properties. PACE 1986;9:1.

104. Beckman KJ, Gallastegui JL, Bauman JL, Hariman RJ: The predictive value of electrophysiologic studies in untreated patients with Wolff-Parkinson-White syndrome. J Am Coll Cardiol 1990;15:640.

105. Leitch JW, Klein GJ, Yee R, Murdock C: Prognostic value of electrophysiology testing in asymptomtic patients with Wolff-Parkinson-White pattern. Circulation 1990:82:1718.

Appendix 13-1

The surface electrocardiogram has been used as a guide by many investigators to localize accessory pathway positions initially for surgical, and subsequently for RF, ablation procedures.[1-7] Figures 13-21 and 13-22 show two diagrams identifying locations of accessory pathways utilizing standard annotations for pathway locations. Multiple algorithms have been developed to relate electrocardiographic findings to accessory pathway locations which have been verified by surgical or ablation data.[8-11]

Figures 13-23 through 13-25 show representative samples from such studies. These and other studies are clearly useful for preliminary localization of accessory pathway sites especially in patients who are expected to undergo radiofrequency ablation.

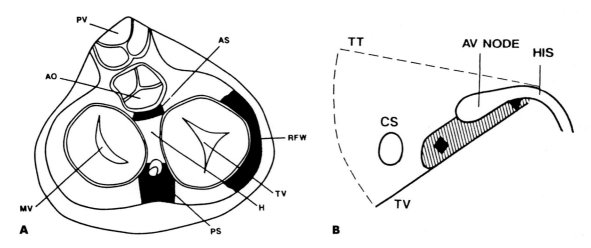

Figure 13-21. (**A**) A cross section schematic of the heart at the level of the AV rings identifying location of various accessory pathway types. (**B**) A schematic of the triangle Koch (cross-hatched area). AS, anteroseptal; Ao, Aorta; CS, coronary sinus; H, His bundle; MV, mitral valve; PS, true posteroseptal; PV, pulmonary valve; RFW, right free wall; TT, tendon of Todaro; TV, tricuspid valve. (From Rodriguez LM, Smeets JLMR, de Chillou C, et al: The 12-lead electrocardiogram in midseptal, anteroseptal, posteroseptal and right free wall accessory pathways. Am J Cardiol 1993;72:1274.)

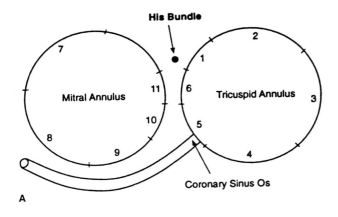

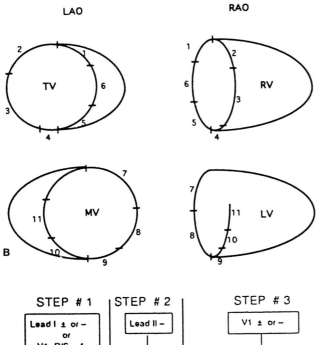

Figure 13-22. Diagram of the locations of accessory pathways. Schematic cross-section of the ventricles at the level of the atrioventricular valve rings (**A**) and schematic left and right anterior oblique projection (**B**). *LV*, left ventricle; *MV*, mitral valve annulus; *RAO*, 30 right anterior oblique projection; *RV*, right ventricle; *TV*, tricuspid valve annulus; 1, right anteroseptal; 2, right anterior; 3, right lateral; 4, right posterior; 5, right posteroseptal; 6, right midseptal; 7, left anterolateral; 8, left posterolateral; 9, left posterior; 10, left posteroseptal; 11, left midseptal. (From Xie B, Heald SC, Bashir Y, et al: Localization of accessory pathways from the 12-lead electrocardiogram using a new algorithm. Am J Cardiol 1994;74:161.)

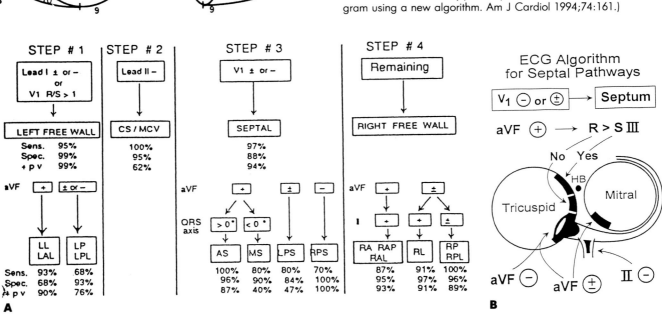

Figure 13-23. (**A**) Algorithm to locate accessory pathway. (**B**) Algorithm for septal pathway location. (From Arruda M, Wang X, McClelland J, et al: ECG algorithm for predicting sites of successful radiofrequency ablation of accessory pathways. PACE 1993;16:II-865.

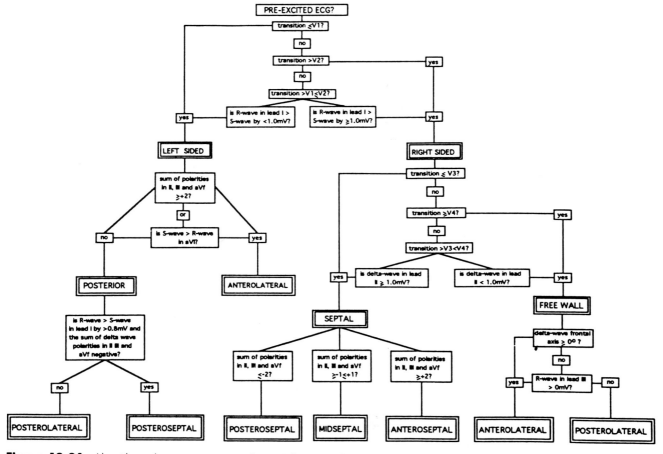

Figure 13-24. Algorithm to locate accessory pathway. Follow steps from the top downward. (From Fitzpatrick AP, Gonzales RP, Lesh MD, Modin GW, Lee RJ, Scheinman MM: New algorithm for the localization of accessory atrioventricular connections using a baseline electrocardiogram. J Am Coll Cardiol 1994;23:107.)

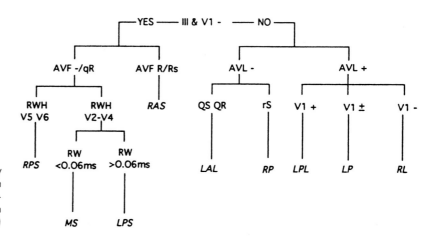

Figure 13-25. Algorithm to locate accessory pathway. Follow steps from the top downward. (From Xie B, Heald SC, Bashir Y, et al: Localization of accessory pathways from the 12-lead electrocardiogram using a new algorithm. Am J Cardiol 1994;74:161.)

Of additional importance is the use of the electrocardiogram in identifying patients with multiple accessory pathways. Several clues have been identified: 1) more than one P wave morphology during orthodromic supraventricular tachycardia; 2) a mismatch between the location of the atrial and ventricular ends of the accessory pathway; 3) atrial fibrillation with QRS complexes with more than one preexcitation pattern; 4) spontaneous changes from orthodromic to antidromic tachycardia; 5) changes from one type of antidromic tachycardia to another; and 6) change in the preexcitation pattern after drug administration.[12]

References

1. Gallagher JJ, Pritchett ELC, Sealy WC, et al: The preexcitation syndromes. Proc Cardiovasc Dis 1978;20:285.

2. Iwa T, Kawasuji M, Misaki T, et al: Localization and interruption of accessory conduction pathway in the Wolff-Parkinson-White syndrome. J Thorac Cardiovasc Surg 1980;80:271.

3. Lindsay BD, Crossen KJ, Cain ME: Concordance of distinguishing electrocardiographic features during sinus rhythm with the location of accessory pathways in the Wolff-Parkinson-White syndrome. Am J Cardiol 1987;59:1093.

4. Epstein AE, Kirklin JK, Holman WL, Plumb VJ, Kay GN: Intermediate septal accessory pathways: electrocardiographic characteristics, electrophysiologic observations and their surgical implications. J Am Coll Cardiol 1991;17:1570.

5. Boineau JP: Intermediate septal accessory pathways: electrocardiographic localization of pre-excitation. JACC 1991;17:579.

6. Yuan S, Iwa T, Tsubota M, Bando H: Comparative study of eight sets of ECG criteria for the localization of the accessory pathway in Wolff-Parkinson-White syndrome. J Electrocardiology 1992;25:203.

7. Rodriguez L-M, Smeets JLMR, de Chillou C, et al: The 12-Lead electrocardiogram in midseptal, anteroseptal, posteroseptal and right free wall accessory pathways. Am J Cardiol 1993;72:1274.

8. Milstein S, Sharma AD, Guiraudon GM, Klein GJ: An algorithm for the electrocardiographic localization of accessory pathways in the Wolff-Parkinson-White syndrome. PACE 1987;10:555.

9. Arruda M, Wang X, McClelland J, et al: ECG algorithm for predicting sites of successful radiofrequency ablation of accessory pathways. PACE 1993;16:II-865.

10. Fitzpatrick AP, Gonzales RP, Lesh MD, Modin GW, Lee RJ, Scheinman MM: New algorithm for the localization of accessory atrioventricular connections using a baseline electrocardiogram. J Am Coll Cardiol 1994;23:107.

11. Xie B, Heald SC, Bashir Y, et al: Localization of accessory pathways from the 12-Lead electrocardiogram using a new algorithm. Am J Cardiol 1994;74:161.

12. Wellens HJJ, Atie J, Smeets JLRM, Cruz FES, Gorgels AP, Brugada P: The electrocardiogram in patients with multiple accessory atrioventricular pathways. J Am Coll Cardiol 1990;16:745.

Cardiac Arrhythmias, 3rd edition, edited by William J. Mandel.
J. B. Lippincott Company, Philadelphia © 1995.

14

Yoshio Watanabe • Leonard S. Dreifus • Todor Mazgalev

Atrioventricular Block: Basic Concepts

An abundance of information is available concerning the anatomy, pathology, electrophysiology, and clinical significance of disturbances of atrioventricular (AV) conduction. Interest in this subject apparently began in 1827 with a description by Adams of syncope associated with a slow heart rate, which was followed two decades later by observations by Stokes (1846).[1,2] Wenckebach (1899) and Hay (1906) described AV conduction block, ushering in the era of eponyms and synonyms in the classification of AV conduction disturbances.[3,4] In 1924, Mobitz classified AV block according to rather precise criteria.[5] Since then, numerous clinical and experimental studies have appeared in the medical literature.

More recent studies indicate that the clinical course, prognosis of, and mode of therapy for AV block depend predominantly on localization of the conduction disturbance within the AV conducting system (for example, within the AV node or the His–Purkinje system).[6] It has become increasingly apparent that AV block should be classified by the level of propagation failure rather than by constancy or fluctuations of the PR interval.[7,8]

Precise determination of the site of conduction block may sometimes be difficult, even in experimental studies using microelectrodes.[9,10] The total AV conduction time contains the following three components: intra-atrial conduction time, intra-AV nodal conduction time, and His–Purkinje (subnodal) conduction time. Experimental studies using microelectrode techniques have shown that the total AV conduction time in isolated perfused rabbit hearts under normal experimental conditions measures between 90 and 100 milliseconds, of which, intra-atrial, intranodal, and His–Purkinje conduction times measure 30, 30 to 35, and 30 milliseconds, respectively.[11,12] Therefore, each of the three components roughly corresponds to one third of the total AV interval.

In routine clinical electrocardiograms, these intervals cannot be determined separately, and the AV conduction time is measured from the beginning of the P wave (atrial excitation) to the onset of the QRS complex (ventricular excitation). However, with the use of His bundle electrocardiography, the three conduction times can be approximately measured (Fig. 14-1). Based on several clinical electrophysiologic studies, individual components of the total AV conduction time in the presence of a PR interval between 0.14 and 0.18 second (140 to 180 milliseconds) are as follows: intra-atrial conduction time, 0.04 to 0.05 second (40 to 50 milliseconds); intranodal conduction time, 0.05 to 0.07 second (50 to 70 milliseconds); and

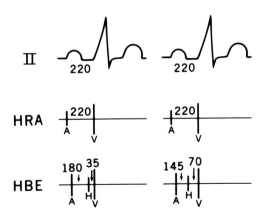

Figure 14-1. Schematic diagrams showing first degree atrioventricular block with the three components of atrioventricular interval. The left side of this figure shows conduction delay between the atria and the His bundle. The right side shows subjunctional conduction delay. The duration of the His electrogram is 5 milliseconds.

His–Purkinje conduction time, 0.05 to 0.06 second (50 to 60 milliseconds).[13–15] Thus, the ratios among these three components in human hearts may not be grossly different from those in rabbit hearts. Even when both the intranodal conduction time and the His–Purkinje conduction time measure 60 milliseconds, the distance that an impulse travels during this time is much shorter for the intranodal conduction. This indicates that the conduction velocity is slowest in the AV node and much higher in the His–Purkinje system. The AV node is said to constitute the weakest point in the entire AV conducting system, although AV conduction block does not occur exclusively within the AV nodal tissue.

CLASSIFICATION OF ATRIOVENTRICULAR BLOCK

Atrioventricular block is divided into first, second, and third (or high grade) degrees according to the severity of conduction disturbance.[16–18] First degree AV block represents a prolongation of the AV conduction time (the PR interval in the electrocardiogram) beyond the normal range. Experimental studies and His bundle electrocardiography have shown that such prolongation of the AV conduction time may result from a conduction delay within the atria, AV node, or His–Purkinje system, or from any combination thereof (see Fig. 14-1).[19–22] Second degree AV block is diagnosed when some of the impulses originating either in the sinus node or within the atria die out in certain portions of the AV conducting system and fail to reach the ventricles. Third degree AV block represents conditions in which impulse transmission from the atria to the ventricles is almost entirely blocked and the ventricles are controlled by a subsidiary pacemaker. Although third

degree or high grade AV block has classically been called complete AV block, an occasional occurrence of successful AV conduction is often observed with continuous electrocardiographic monitoring. Again, failure of propagation of impulses in cases with second degree or third degree AV block could occur within the atria, AV node, or in the His–Purkinje system, in both the experimental and clinical settings.[9, 10, 23–27]

Second degree AV block has been further subdivided into two types depending on the sequence of PR intervals in conducted supraventricular beats. This classification is based on the original observations of Wenckebach and of Mobitz and is simply stated as follows: when the AV conduction times in several successive beats are progressively prolonged, culminating in the dropping out of one ventricular depolarization, type I is diagnosed; a sudden failure of AV conduction after the maintenance of a constant PR interval is designated type II.[3, 5, 28] This classification can be used only when more than two sinus or supraventricular impulses are consecutively conducted to the ventricles in the presence of second degree AV block, and the classification is not applicable in third degree AV block.

For clinical purposes, identification of the site of block either within the AV node or in the His–Purkinje system or either above or below the bifurcation of the His bundle is desirable and probably sufficient. This information can be obtained with the use of His bundle electrocardiography.[13–15, 24, 27] However, it is our opinion that His bundle electrocardiography should not be used routinely in every patient with AV block because it is an invasive technique and because the level of conduction disturbance can roughly be estimated by studying the QRS duration or the mode of ventricular excitation in the electrocardiogram in most clinical cases.[18, 29]

The electrophysiologic events responsible for AV transmission disorders have received less attention than their classification. However, it is the site and electrophysiologic behavior of the conduction disorder that provide the most clinical information for prognosis of the patient.[6–8, 24, 25, 30, 31]

The following outline summarizes the factors controlling AV conduction. The physiology of AV transmission should be reviewed for an in-depth understanding of the nature and mechanisms of AV conduction block. Some of the more common electrophysiologic mechanisms of AV block that have clinical significance are cited.

FACTORS CONTROLLING IMPULSE TRANSMISSION

    I. Primary determinants of conductivity
        A. Physiologic factors
            1. Effectiveness of stimuli produced by depolarization of upstream fibers

2. Excitability of responding downstream fibers
3. Temporal fluctuation of the above physiologic factors
B. Anatomic factors
   1. Fiber diameter
   2. Geometric arrangement of fibers
II. Abnormal conduction phenomena resulting from alterations in the primary determinants of conductivity
A. Decremental conduction
B. Inhomogeneous conduction
C. Electrotonic transmission
D. Summation or inhibition
E. Conduction delay and block
F. Unidirectional block
G. Reentry and reflection
III. Abnormal conduction phenomena secondarily affecting conductivity
A. Conduction delay and block
   1. Effects of conduction delay on the action potential duration (prolongation)
   2. Effects of conduction block on the action potential duration of fibers proximal to the site of propagation failure (shortening)
   3. Effects of conduction block on the action potential duration of fibers distal to the site of propagation failure (prolongation)
   4. Effects of conduction delay or block on excitability of the downstream fibers
   5. Conduction delay or block causing impulse formation in the downstream fibers
B. Reentry and reflection
   1. Collision of reentrant impulse with the more slowly advancing anterograde wave of excitation resulting in cancellation of both wavefronts
   2. Further disorganization of the excitation front (increased inhomogeneity) in subsequent impulse transmission
   3. Reorganization of the excitation front (decreased inhomogeneity) in subsequent impulse transmission

FIRST DEGREE ATRIOVENTRICULAR BLOCK

Because the normal range of AV conduction time (PR interval) in an adult is between 0.12 and 0.21 second, PR intervals longer than 0.22 second (220 milliseconds) indicate a first degree AV block. These criteria can be applied only in the presence of regular sinus mechanism (or atrial rhythm). If an atrial premature systole is conducted to the ventricles with a PR interval longer than 0.22 second, it is not called a first degree AV block as long as all the sinus

beats show a normal PR interval. Thus, the diagnosis of first degree AV block should not be difficult, except in those cases with sinus tachycardia and a markedly prolonged PR interval in which the P waves are superimposed on the T waves of the preceding beats.

In clinical cases of simple first degree AV block, the area of conduction delay responsible for the prolonged PR interval is usually disregarded. However, when first degree AV block is associated with subjunctional block (e.g., right bundle branch block or a combination of fascicular blocks), His bundle studies may be required to identify those patients at high risk of developing complete heart block because primary conduction disorders of the remaining fascicle may be present. Figure 14-1 shows that His bundle electrograms can localize the conduction delay either above or below the His bundle in the presence of an identical PR interval of 0.22 second.

COMPARISON OF THE TWO TYPES OF SECOND DEGREE ATRIOVENTRICULAR BLOCK

The original classification of second degree AV block into type I (Wenckebach periodicity) and type II (so-called Mobitz type II) depended on the behavior of the PR interval in successive beats.[3, 5, 28] Such classification cannot be made unless several regularly occurring atrial impulses are consecutively conducted to the ventricles. For example, 2:1 or 3:1 AV conduction, AV conduction block in the presence of atrial fibrillation, and complete AV block cannot be categorized by using this classification. Conversely, by studying the QRS duration, the site of conduction failure can be roughly estimated, even in cases of higher degrees of AV block.[18, 29, 31] More specifically, QRS duration of 0.11 second or shorter most probably indicates block above the bifurcation of the His bundle, whereas that of 0.12 second or longer suggests a conduction block below the AV junction.[18, 29, 31] Therefore, in the following discussion, second degree AV block with narrow QRS complexes is discussed first, followed by second degree AV block with wide QRS complexes.

SECOND DEGREE ATRIOVENTRICULAR BLOCK WITH NARROW QRS COMPLEXES

In Figure 14-2, a group of three P-QRS complexes is seen in the middle portion of lead II with progressive prolongation of the PR interval, and a fourth P wave (P4) fails to be conducted to the ventricles, producing a long pause. This pause is terminated by a P wave (P5) that is conducted to the ventricles with a shorter PR interval. Because three of

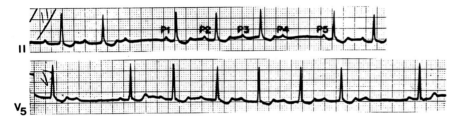

Figure 14-2. A typical Wenckebach cycle (type 1) with a 4:3 conduction ratio.

the four sinus impulses are transmitted to the ventricles, this is called a 4:3 conduction ratio, and the sequence is called the Wenckebach phenomenon.[3,16-18] Similarly, in lead V_5, six consecutive P waves are conducted to the ventricles, followed by blockage of the seventh P wave (7:6 conduction). The QRS complexes show normal duration; therefore, no intraventricular conduction disturbance is present. Characteristics of typical Wenckebach phenomenon (type I block) include the following: (1) the PR interval is progressively prolonged in consecutively conducted beats, (2) the R-R intervals gradually shorten before a pause (long R-R interval), and (3) the duration of this pause is shorter than twice the sinus interval (or any R-R interval between two successively conducted beats; see Fig. 14-2).

The mechanism of gradual shortening of the R-R cycle in the presence of progressive prolongation of the AV conduction time is shown in Figure 14-3. If the PR interval of two consecutively conducted sinus beats remains constant in the presence of a sinus cycle of 800 milliseconds (0.80 second), the R-R interval also measures 800 milliseconds. In type I block, however, the AV conduction time in the second beat is prolonged compared with that of the first beat. If the PR interval is prolonged from 180 milliseconds to 300 milliseconds, the R-R interval becomes longer than the sinus interval by a difference of 120 milliseconds and attains a value of 920 (800 + 120) milliseconds. If the PR interval of the third beat remains at 300 milliseconds, an R-R interval of 800 milliseconds is again obtained. Because the PR interval is further prolonged, the increment of the PR interval must again be added to the sinus cycle of 800 milliseconds (not to the preceding R-R interval of 920 milliseconds). The increment of the PR interval

between the second and third conducted beats usually is smaller than that between the first and second conducted beats and may amount to 60 (360 − 300) milliseconds. Therefore, an R-R interval of 860 (800 + 60) milliseconds is obtained, which is shorter than the preceding R-R interval of 920 milliseconds. Such decreasing increments of AV conduction time produce a gradual shortening of the ventricular cycle despite the progressive increase in the PR intervals. Figures 14-3 and 14-4 show that the duration of a pause is shorter than two sinus cycles. Such a typical Wenckebach phenomenon is most often noted in the presence of relatively low conduction ratios such as 4:3 or 5:4 conduction, whereas higher conduction ratios are often associated with atypical patterns of conduction as shown in Figure 14-5. Therefore, demonstration of a prolonged AV interval in at least any two consecutive beats has recently been advocated by some investigators as a criterion for the Wenckebach periodicity.

Figure 14-4 shows a record of typical Wenckebach phenomenon obtained in an isolated perfused rabbit heart in which membrane action potentials from the N (nodal) region of the AV node (N1) and from the proximal portion of the His bundle (N2) were recorded, together with an atrial electrogram (A) from the sinus nodal region and a ventricular electrogram (V) obtained between the left ventricular apex and right ventricular base.[9] The figure shows that a period of 4:3 conduction is followed by a 3:2 conduction ratio and that, in both sequences, the AV conduction time is progressively prolonged, from 206 to 252 to 275 milliseconds and from 230 to 273 milliseconds. Therefore, a typical type I block is present. Furthermore, progressive prolongation of the conduction time from the sinus nodal region to nodal fiber N1 and between nodal

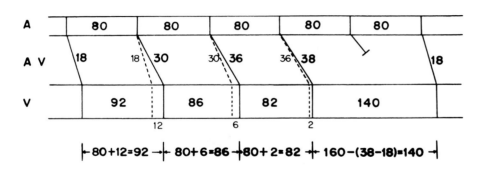

Figure 14-3. Diagrammatic representation of the typical Wenckebach cycle. Numbers are in hundredths of a second.

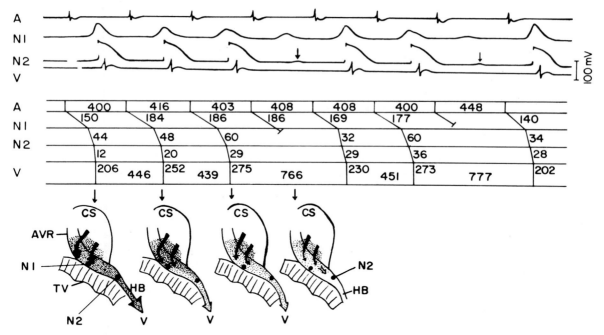

Figure 14-4. Type I second degree atrioventricular block in an isolated perfused rabbit heart. *A,* atrial electrogram; *N1* and *N2,* transmembrane potentials from two fibers located in the N region; *V,* ventricular electrogram; *CS,* ostium of coronary sinus; *AVR,* fibrous atrioventricular ring; *HB,* His bundle; *TV,* tricupid valve.

fibers N1 and N2 suggests the presence of intranodal conduction delay. The transmembrane potentials from the N region of the AV node (N1) reveal a gradual decrease in the amplitude and upstroke velocity in successive beats, culminating in an incomplete depolarization (so-called local response) that is associated with failure of propagation to the His bundle (N2, *arrows*) and the ventricles. The reduction in the action potential amplitude as well as the rate of depolarization in fiber N1 may suggest decremental conduction and a decreased efficacy of the excitation front.

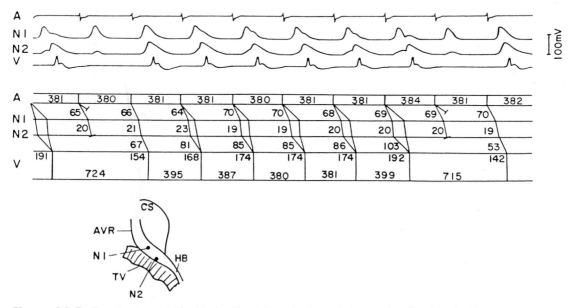

Figure 14-5. Type I atrioventricular block with a 7:6 conduction ratio in an isolated perfused rabbit heart. (See Fig. 14-4 for key to abbreviations.)

Although a slight prolongation of the conduction time is also noted below fiber N2 (subnodal), major conduction delay is localized within the AV node. Other records showed a constant conduction time from the sinus node to the atrial muscle fibers adjacent to the AV node (not shown).

An example of atypical Wenckebach periodicity with a higher conduction ratio of 7:6 is shown in Figure 14-5. In this figure, fibers N1 and N2 are considered to be located in the proximal and distal portions of the node–His (NH) region, respectively. The first conducted beat in this group shows the shortest AV conduction time of 154 milliseconds. The increment of AV conduction time is large in the second conducted beat (168 − 154 = 14 milliseconds) and becomes smaller in the third beat (174 − 168 = 6 milliseconds). The AV conduction time in two subsequent beats remains constant until another significant increase (192 − 174 = 18 milliseconds) is noted in the last conducted beat. As a result, the ventricular cycle is slightly shortened initially (from 395 to 387 milliseconds), then remains constant at approximately 380 milliseconds, and is finally prolonged to 399 milliseconds before the pause. A similar sequence is often seen in clinical cases of Wenckebach periodicity with relatively high conduction ratios. One of the most significant findings in this record (see Fig. 14-5) is probably the development of steplike potentials preceding the upstroke of the action potential from fiber N2 and associated with a gradual prolongation of the AV interval. The duration of such steplike potentials is progressively prolonged from 28 to 63 milliseconds, whereas the interval from the atrial electrogram to the onset of these steplike potentials is relatively constant (87 to 89 milliseconds). At the same time, the action potential from the upstream fiber (N1) gradually develops a second peak during its repolarization phase, finally producing an almost separate waveform in the last conducted beat. During the transmission of the next impulse, the action potential of fiber N1 loses the second peak and shows a much shorter action potential duration, which is associated with the appearance of only the initial steplike potential in fiber N2 without causing phase 0 depolarization. Thus, propagation of this impulse to the ventricles fails.

These peculiar changes in the action potential contour may result from disorganization of the wavefront of excitation invading the NH region, with an increased degree of inhomogeneous conduction occurring in the N region of the AV node.[9,32] Then, the first excitation front may cause depolarization of fiber N1 as well as the steplike potential in fiber N2, whereas the second wavefront may generate a second peak in the N1 action potential and cause a rapid depolarization of fiber N2. When such disorganization of the wavefront becomes more marked with progressive decrement, the efficacy of the excitation front as a stimulus to downstream fibers is decreased, engendering failure of propagation.[30,33] The analytical diagram in Figure 14-5 illustrates this concept. However, these experimental records must be analyzed carefully because reexcitation of these fibers caused by intra-AV nodal reentry cannot be definitely eliminated.[10,19,32] Based on observations made with His bundle electrocardiography, it has been suggested that reentry movement may play a role in the production of Wenckebach phenomenon.[34]

A different mechanism has more recently been proposed to explain those peculiar action potential configurations. For instance, experimental studies using sucrose gap techniques in canine Purkinje fiber preparations have indicated that the steplike potentials most likely represent an electrotonic spread across a region of depressed conduction.[35] When such an electrotonus barely succeeds in bringing the membrane potential of downstream fibers to the threshold level, a more rapid action potential upstroke (or phase 0) results. This, in turn, may produce the hump on the repolarization phase of the action potential of upstream fibers, as seen in fiber N1 in Figure 14-5.[35]

Nevertheless, the studies showed that experimentally produced type I AV block in the presence of normal QRS duration was usually associated with a conduction disturbance within the AV node.

In certain cases showing atypical Wenckebach phenomenon, especially in the presence of higher conduction ratios such as 8:7 conduction, the R-R interval immediately preceding a pause often becomes longer than that after the pause because of an increasing increment of the PR interval. Identification of a pause, and hence the diagnosis of type I second degree AV block, may be difficult in these cases.

It has been shown that, except for those patients with 2:1 conduction, most patients with second degree AV block with narrow QRS complexes show type I or Wenckebach periodicity. Occasionally, exceptions are noted (Fig. 14-6). In the two strips of lead I, sinus rhythm with slight sinus arrhythmia ranging from 65 to 70 beats per minute is present. The bottom record shows a regular 2:1 conduction and cannot be classified as either type I or type II. However, in the top record, an initial pause caused by 2:1 block is followed by the consecutive appearance of four P waves with associated QRS complexes and failure of conduction of the fifth P wave. Therefore, a 5:4 conduction ratio is seen. The PR interval in these four beats is constant at 0.16 second, satisfying the criteria for Mobitz type II AV block. An episode of 3:2 conduction toward the end of this strip is also accompanied by a constant AV conduction time. The sudden dropping out of a QRS complex, as seen in this case with a narrow QRS complex, suggests intra-Hisian block.

A question then arises as to the location of the site of propagation failure in these instances. Recordings of His

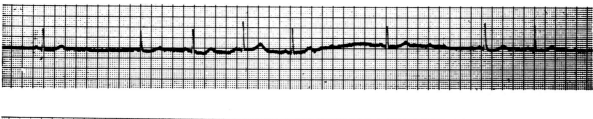

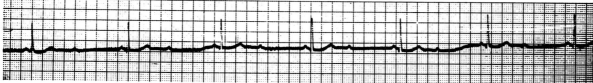

Figure 14-6. Type II atrioventricular block with normal QRS duration.

bundle potentials are the most likely means to provide such information. His bundle studies carried out in several similar cases suggested a concealed-premature depolarization of the His bundle or AV junctional tissue as the cause of this type of block.[33,36] Whether such premature depolarization is caused by automatic impulse formation, concealed reciprocal movement, or local reentry cannot be determined even with His bundle electrocardiography.[9,32,37] Nevertheless, impulses above the bifurcation of the His bundle are usually blocked.

As discussed, the original classification of types I and II cannot be applied to cases showing regular 2:1 conduction. When transmembrane potentials are recorded from numerous fibers of the AV node in similar instances, regular alternation of the action potential amplitude and upstroke velocity in individual fibers is usually demonstrated. Figure 14-7 summarizes the results of such a study in the presence of regular 2:1 AV conduction in an isolated rabbit heart by plotting both the action potential configuration and the conduction time (in milliseconds) from the sinus node for individual recording sites. The spread of AV nodal excitation during conducted beats is shown in Figure 14-7A and that during the blocked beats is shown in Figure 14-7B. In the blocked beats, the action potential becomes gradually smaller along the pathway of excitation (*tapering arrows*), culminating in small fluctuations in the membrane potential within the NH region. When the action potentials from two fibers (those with activation times of 17 and 27 milliseconds) are compared between Figure 14-7A and B, the N fiber activated at 27 milliseconds maintains a more normal action potential contour than the upstream fiber showing an activation time of 17 milliseconds. This illustrates unequal degrees of decrement of conduction in different portions of the AV node or increased inhomogeneity of conduction.[32] Nevertheless, the occurrence of a major conduction disturbance within the N region of the AV node is evident.[9]

SECOND DEGREE ATRIOVENTRICULAR BLOCK WITH WIDE QRS COMPLEXES

Second degree AV block in the presence of intraventricular conduction delay (QRS ≥ 0.12 second) usually shows the Mobitz type II variety and appears to be associated with a more serious prognosis than AV block with narrow QRS complexes. Therefore, the diagnosis and behavior of this variety of AV block must be fully understood.[7,8,10,30,31] A typical example of second degree AV block, type II, is shown in Figure 14-8. Lead I shows successful transmission of six consecutive sinus impulses, with the seventh P wave not being followed by a QRS complex (7:6 conduction). In this case, the PR interval remains constant in this group of six beats and in those beats occurring after a pause. In other words, a dropped ventricular complex is not preceded by a progressive prolongation of the AV conduction time. This characterizes the classic second degree AV block of Mobitz type II variety, which often is simply called type II block.[5,16–18,28] In this electrocardiogram, the QRS duration is prolonged and has a pattern of left bundle branch block.

Occasionally, similar type II AV block, which does not appear in clinical electrocardiograms, may be produced by a premature depolarization of the AV junctional tissue. An experimental record demonstrating this mechanism is shown in Figure 14-9.[9,32] Fibers N1 and N2 in this record were considered to be located within the NH region close to the His bundle, and fiber N1 was slightly upstream to fiber N2. The presence of marked conduction delay below fiber N2 is readily noted. The first two atrial impulses are successfully conducted to the ventricles, and the action potential configuration in fibers N1 and N2 as well as the conduction time in each subdivision of the AV interval remains constant in these two beats. However, this is followed by a premature depolarization of fibers N1 and N2, occurring almost at the same time as the second

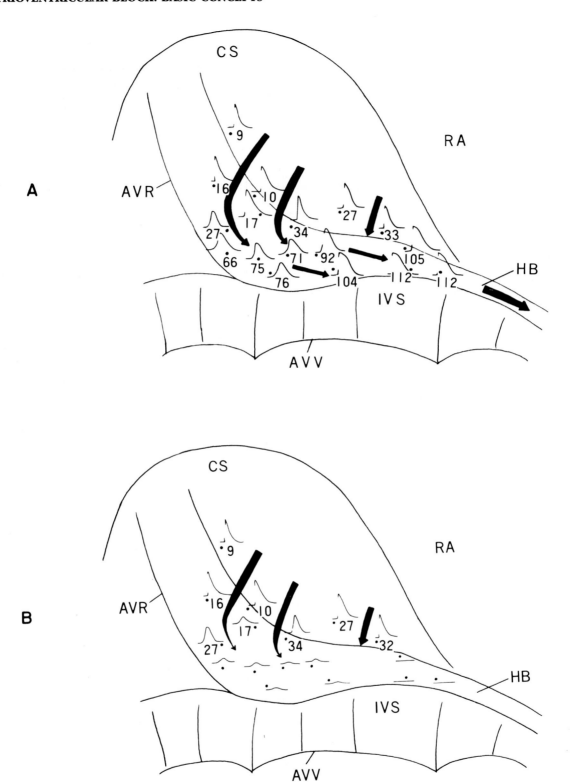

Figure 14-7. Spread of excitation in the atrioventricular nodal region of the rabbit heart in the presence of 2:1 conduction. Time of activation in milliseconds and action potential contour at individual recording sites are shown in conducted (**A**) and blocked (**B**) beats. *AVV*, atrioventricular Valve; *IVS*, interventricular septum; *RA*, right atrium. (See Fig. 14-4 for an additional key to abbreviations.)

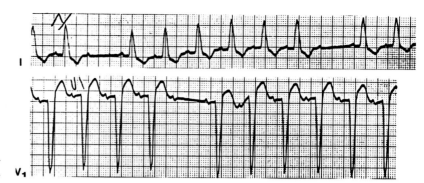

Figure 14-8. Type II second degree atrioventricular block in the presence of wide QRS complexes.

ventricular excitation in which the downstream fiber N2 is depolarized slightly earlier than the upstream fiber N1. This indicates retrograde activation of the AV nodal tissue, which does not reach the atria. The third atrial impulse, occurring on time, produces only a small potential change or a local response in fiber N1 (*arrows*) and is not transmitted to fiber N2 and the ventricles. Thus, a sudden dropping out of the ventricular complex without a preceding progressive prolongation of the AV conduction time, or typical type II block, was produced by a concealed depolarization of the AV node. The presence of a significant conduction delay below the AV node in this experiment may suggest the development of a reciprocal movement in the His–Purkinje system. Similar examples of apparent type II AV block could be produced by a new impulse formation within the AV junction due to automaticity or any other cause, as long as such impulses depolarize only a portion of the AV conducting system and are not con-

ducted to the ventricles. A clinical example of such concealed AV junctional premature systole causing first degree and second degree AV block patterns was reported in 1947, and more recent studies using His bundle electrocardiography have confirmed these observations.[35–37] It is our opinion that many cases of type II AV block without associated intraventricular conduction disturbances, such as that shown in Figure 14-6, may result from such concealed ectopic impulse formation in the AV junction. Nevertheless, the experiment shown in Figure 14-9 was clearly associated with abnormal intraventricular conduction.

Second degree AV block with a wide QRS may not always show the type II conduction pattern. The electrocardiogram in Figure 14-10 reveals type I block (Wenckebach phenomenon) associated with wide QRS complexes. Lead II shows persistent 3:2 conduction, with the PR interval of the second conducted beat being significantly prolonged over that of the first beat. Periods of 2:1 block are

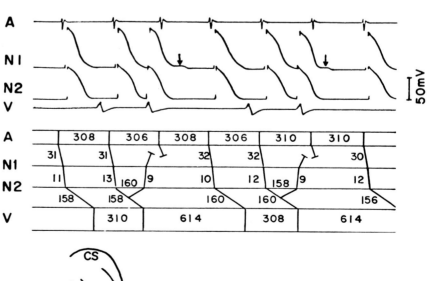

Figure 14-9. Type II atrioventricular block produced by concealed reciprocation with premature discharge of the atrioventricular junction. Time in milliseconds. (See Fig. 14-4 for key to abbreviations.)

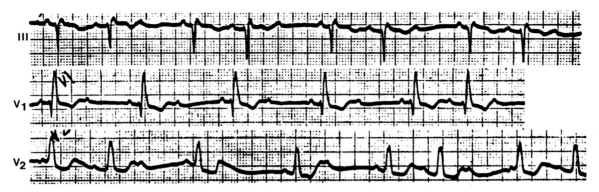

Figure 14-10. Wenckebach conduction associated with wide QRS complexes.

noted in leads V_1 and V_2 as is a similar 3:2 AV response. The QRS duration measures 0.14 second with a right bundle branch block configuration. Two levels of block (i.e., AV nodal and subjunctional) must be considered in this case.

Occasional interruption of typical Wenckebach sequence by an atrial reciprocal beat has often been observed in the presence of second degree AV block with narrow QRS complexes.[29] A similar phenomenon occurring in a case with wide QRS complexes is shown in Figure 14-11. Not all cases of premature P waves appearing in the course of a Wenckebach sequence can be attributed to atrial reciprocation, and premature impulse formation within the atria may interrupt the progression of type I AV block.

The Wenckebach phenomenon, or a progressive prolongation of the conduction time followed by blockage of an impulse, can be observed in any portion of myocardial tissue where conductivity is depressed and a state of decremental conduction exists. In other words, this phenomenon does not occur only in the AV node; it could be demonstrated even in Purkinje fibers or between contig-

uous ventricular muscle fibers.[7,38–40] His bundle recordings in clinical cases have also shown the occurrence of such conduction phenomena below the AV node or in the His–Purkinje system.[27] Furthermore, occasional cases have been observed in which gradual changes in the QRS morphology suggest progressive conduction delay in one of the bundle branches or fascicles, culminating in complete blockage of transmission, although a Wenckebach type of PR prolongation is not usually seen in these cases.[18,31] In most cases, then, second degree AV block of the type I variety first suggests a conduction delay within the AV node, as has been shown experimentally.[9] In Figure 14-10, the Wenckebach periodicity suggests a conduction disturbance within the AV node, whereas the right bundle branch block pattern indicates abnormal intraventricular conduction.[29] When His bundle electrocardiography is not available in these cases, two levels of conduction disorder can be assumed, which is probably both sufficient and safe in the clinical management of these arrhythmias.[18,29,31]

A His bundle electrogram obtained in a case of 2:1 AV conduction with wide QRS complexes is shown in Figure

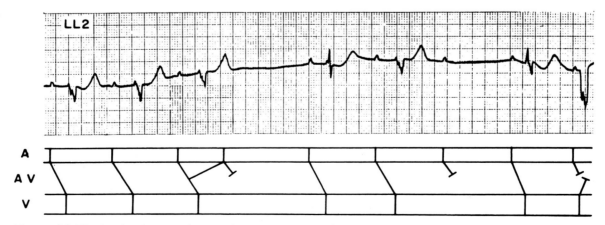

Figure 14-11. Lead II electrocardiogram showing interruption of a Wenckebach cycle by an atrial reciprocal complex (*left side*) and a second degree block type I with 3:2 conduction ratio (*right side*).

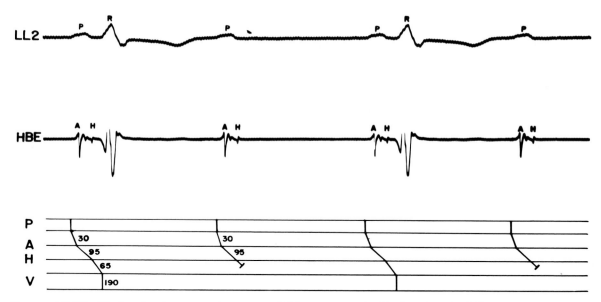

Figure 14-12. His bundle electrogram in a case of 2:1 atrioventricular block with wide QRS complexes. *P*, P wave; *A*, atria; *H*, His bundle; *V*, ventricles.

14-12. Every other sinus impulse is conducted to the ventricles with a PR interval of 190 milliseconds, of which the PA interval (from the onset of the P wave to excitation of the lower right atrium recorded on the His bundle electrogram), representing intra-atrial conduction time, measures 30 milliseconds; the AH interval, representing AV nodal conduction time, measures 95 milliseconds; and the HV interval (from the H deflection to the onset of ventricular depolarization), representing His–Purkinje conduction time, measures 65 milliseconds. Although this HV interval shows only a slight prolongation over the normal range, the blocked impulses are always accompanied by a His deflection, indicating successful propagation at least to the portion of the His bundle located beneath the recording electrode. Therefore, the site of conduction block must be below this portion of the His bundle. (The portion of the His bundle that lies closest to the recording electrode cannot be precisely determined.) Whether these impulses are blocked below the bifurcation of the His bundle or between the recording site and the bifurcation is difficult to determine, although the presence of wide QRS complexes indicating intraventricular conduction disturbances would probably favor the bundle branch or fascicular level.

Experimental studies indicate that two levels of block with so-called concealed conduction are most likely responsible for alternation of the PR interval in the presence of persistent 2:1 AV conduction (Fig. 14-13).[10,30] In this experiment on an isolated perfused rabbit heart, an atrial electrogram from the sinoatrial nodal region (SA), a ventricular electrogram (V), and transmembrane potentials of the NH region of the AV node (NH) were simultaneously recorded. The sinus cycle measures 530 milliseconds, corresponding to a rate of 113 beats per minute. In the top record (see Fig. 14-13A), every atrial impulse is associated with depolarization of the NH fiber with normal amplitude as well as upstroke velocity of the action potential, suggesting a 1:1 conduction across the N region of the node. However, every other NH action potential is not followed by a ventricular excitation, and a 2:1 conduction block below the AV node or in the His–Purkinje system is indicated. Intraventricular conduction disturbance is evident from the wide and abnormal ventricular electrogram as well as from the marked increase in the subnodal conduction time to 160 milliseconds compared with the normal value of 30 to 35 milliseconds. The conduction time from the sinus node to this distal NH fiber is between 102 and 104 milliseconds. Because a normal intra-atrial conduction time of 35 milliseconds was demonstrated from other records, the intranodal conduction time also was prolonged to 67 to 69 milliseconds. These observations indicate the presence of conduction disturbance both within the AV node and in the His–Purkinje system, although failure of propagation occurs only in the His–Purkinje system.

In the bottom record (see Fig. 14-13B), which was obtained 3 minutes after the top record, persistence of 2:1 block is noted on the ventricular electrogram. However, the AV conduction time shows an alternation of long (262 to 264 milliseconds) and short (234 milliseconds) intervals, causing alternation of short and long ventricular cycles. The mechanism for such alternation becomes appar-

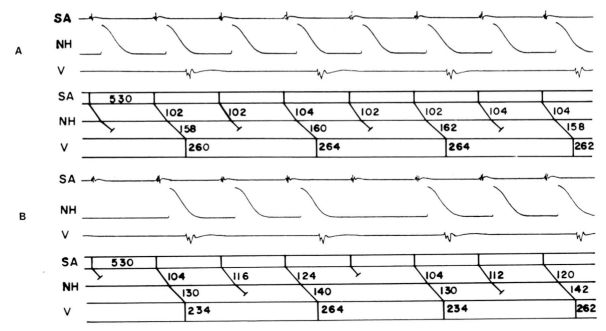

Figure 14-13. Action potentials recorded from rabbit heart showing 2:1 atrioventricular block with alternation of long and short atrioventricular conduction times. *SA,* sinoatrial node; *NH,* node–His region. Time in milliseconds.

ent from studying the action potential record from the NH region where every fourth sinus impulse fails to depolarize the NH fiber, indicating a 4:3 conduction across the N region of the AV node. This intranodal block shows typical Wenckebach periodicity with progressive prolongation of the SA to NH interval from 104 to 116 to 124 milliseconds. Of the three sinus impulses that successfully traverse the AV node, the second one is blocked below the NH region as in Figure 14-13A, whereas the first and third sinus impulses reach the ventricles. The AV conduction time in beat 3 is much longer than that in beat 1. This prolongation resulted not only from a greater delay in the intranodal conduction but also from a prolongation of the His–Purkinje conduction time from 130 to 140 milliseconds. Such an increase in the His–Purkinje conduction time is caused by the partial penetration of the second atrial impulse into the His–Purkinje system, which leaves a refractory tissue in its wake. After blockage of the sinus impulse above the NH region of the AV node, both the intranodal and His–Purkinje conduction times are shortened, causing a return of a shorter conduction time of 234 milliseconds. Thus, 2:1 AV block with alternation of the AV conduction time was caused by the presence of two levels of conduction disturbance and an alternation of subnodal and intranodal block.

Although the longer AV interval seen in Figure 14-13B is almost identical to the persistently long AV interval in Figure 14-13A, in which failure of propagation always oc-

curs below the AV node, the ratio of intranodal and His–Purkinje conduction times is significantly different between the two records. This illustrates the fact that the PR interval in the clinical electrocardiogram is the total of intra-atrial, intranodal, and subnodal conduction times, and the role played by each component cannot be simply evaluated. Nevertheless, these experimental findings are similar to some of the clinical electrocardiograms, supporting the concept of concealed conduction in explaining the mechanism underlying such clinical cases.[7] Also, a 2:1 AV block with alternation of short and long AV conduction times may be seen mostly in the presence of a 4:3 conduction ratio in the intranodal transmission. When 3:2 conduction is present across the AV node, the ventricular response shows either a 3:2 or a 3:1 AV conduction ratio (Fig. 14-14).

Type I or type II classification cannot be applied to this record. The classification and clinical course depend on the lowermost level of block in these cases. On the other hand, alternation of short and long PR intervals in the presence of 2:1 conduction may also be explained by assuming the existence of two functionally (or anatomically) independent conducting fiber groups, a concept termed *dual pathways.*[41–43] Several clinical and experimental reports have shown possible roles of dual pathways in AV conduction and intra-atrial or interatrial conduction.[44] However, microelectrode studies indicate that the conduction patterns seen with dual pathways can be

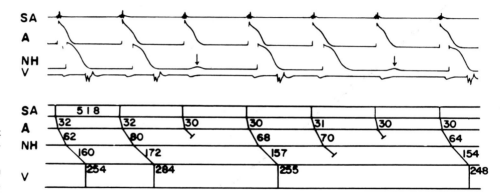

Figure 14-14. Two levels of block (atrioventricular node and His–Purkinje system) causing 3:2 and 3:1 atrioventricular conduction ratios in the rabbit heart. Time in milliseconds.

explained by different degrees of inhomogeneous conduction, several levels of conduction delay (Fig. 14-15; see Fig. 14-13), and the relative contributions of the two principal inputs to the AV node, which can produce either summation or cancellation of the wavefront invading the AV node.

ADVANCED SECOND DEGREE AND THIRD DEGREE ATRIOVENTRICULAR BLOCK

Advanced second degree AV block refers to conditions in which more than two consecutive supraventricular impulses are blocked.[10] Differentiation between advanced second degree and third degree AV block is sometimes difficult. In the presence of third degree AV block, most of the ventricular complexes are produced by impulses originating from a subsidiary automatic focus, whereas ventricular excitation in the presence of advanced second degree AV block is predominantly controlled by conducted supraventricular impulses.

When one sinus impulse is conducted to the ventricles and is followed by the blockage of two consecutive impulses, it is called a 3:1 conduction, whereas successful transmission of one out of four P waves is termed a 4:1 conduction. The term 3:1 (or 4:1) block is not used because it may give an impression that one out of three (or four) impulses is blocked, corresponding to a 3:2 (or 4:3) conduction. Advanced second degree and third degree AV block can be seen in the presence of either narrow or wide

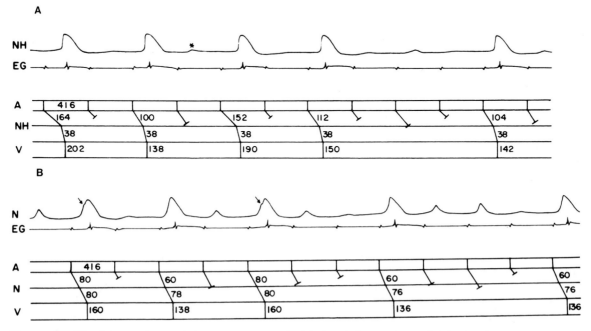

Figure 14-15. Advanced second degree atrioventricular block with fluctuations in the depth of penetration into the atrioventricular node. *EG*, electrogram. Time in milliseconds.

QRS complexes; examples of these varieties of AV block are discussed.

Figure 14-15 shows transmembrane action potentials from the NH region, an electrocardiogram, and analytical diagrams. Figure 14-15A shows several periods of 2:1 AV block in which the AV interval shows alternation of short and long conduction times measuring 202, 138, 190, and 150 milliseconds. Failure of propagation always occurs above this NH fiber, and the His–Purkinje or subnodal conduction time remains constant and almost within the normal range. The ventricular complexes in the electrocardiogram show no intraventricular conduction disturbances. Thus, there appears to be only one level of block. However, fluctuations in the size of local responses in this NH fiber suggest that the alternation of the AV conduction time results from different depths of penetration into the AV node by these blocked impulses. For instance, the second and sixth atrial excitation waves (the small diphasic deflections in the electrocardiogram) produce little change in the membrane resting potential of this NH fiber, whereas the fourth atrial impulse is accompanied by a slightly greater potential change or a local response (*asterisk*), indicating a slightly deeper penetration. This causes a prolongation of the AV conduction time of the fifth atrial impulse (or the third conducted beat) compared with the second and fourth conducted beats, an effect of concealed conduction. A period of 4:1 AV response follows the period of 2:1 conduction. During this 4:1 conduction, the second of the three consecutively blocked atrial impulses produces a slightly greater potential change in the NH fiber, suggesting a deeper penetration of this particular impulse. A similar phenomenon is commonly seen in the presence of 4:1 conduction.

In Figure 14-15B,, which was recorded 3 minutes after Figure 14-15A, three periods of 2:1 AV conduction are followed by 3:1 and 4:1 responses. The transmembrane potentials recorded from the N region of the AV node during the periods of 2:1 conduction again demonstrate fluctuations in the levels of propagation failure, with resultant alternation of the AV conduction time. When a blocked impulse penetrates deeper into the AV node, the subsequent action potential from this N fiber shows a decreased upstroke velocity, with slurring or notching of phase 0 (*arrows*). This finding suggests the occurrence of either decremental or inhomogeneous conduction. From the sequence of alternating levels of concealment during the periods of 2:1 conduction, the sixth atrial impulse is expected to be blocked at a relatively proximal portion of the AV node, but the amplitude of the local response shows that it apparently penetrates again deeper. Intranodal blockage of the subsequent seventh atrial impulse and the production of a 3:1 conduction ratio most likely result from deeper concealment of the sixth impulse. A period of 4:1 AV conduction is then observed, with failure of conduc-

tion of three successive atrial impulses in which the second impulse penetrates deepest into the node, the first penetrates less deep, and the third is blocked most proximally. Thus, in advanced second degree AV block, the depth of penetration appears to vary, even when failure of propagation always occurs within the AV nodal tissue.

Other mechanisms, such as concealed reentry movement, could also contribute to the development of higher degrees of AV conduction block.[10] The experimental record shown in Figure 14-14 was obtained several minutes after those shown in Figure 14-13. In Figure 14-14, transmembrane potentials from an atrial fiber adjacent to the AV node (A) and from the NH region of the AV node (NH) are shown together with an electrogram from the sinus node area (SA) and a ventricular electrogram (V). In the left part of this figure, two consecutive atrial impulses fully depolarize the NH fiber and are conducted to the ventricles, but both the intranodal and His–Purkinje conduction times become prolonged in the second beat. The third atrial impulse causes only incomplete depolarization of the NH fiber (*first arrow*) and fails to propagate to the ventricles. Therefore, a 3:2 conduction with Wenckebach periodicity is diagnosed. Subsequently, two atrial impulses again produce normal action potentials in this NH fiber, indicating a successful intra-AV nodal conduction. However, only the first impulse is transmitted to the ventricles while the second impulse is blocked below the NH region, most likely within the His–Purkinje system. Failure of propagation of the third atrial impulse occurs above this NH fiber as in the initial sequence (*second arrow*), thus resulting in a 3:1 AV response. The development of two levels of block, one within and one below the AV node, was associated with an intraventricular conduction disturbance as suggested by the wide ventricular complexes and markedly prolonged His–Purkinje conduction time. In contrast to the 4:3 intranodal conduction observed in Figure 14-13, the 3:2 ratio in the record in Figure 14-14 may suggest further depression of the intranodal conduction; a 2:1 intranodal block developed some time after Figure 14-14 was recorded.

Nevertheless, in this record, the second of the two atrial impulses was conducted to the ventricles successfully at one time but was blocked within the His–Purkinje system at another time, even though the intra-AV nodal conduction maintained a constant conduction ratio of 3:2.

It is possible that the His–Purkinje conductivity shows temporal fluctuations; thus, a slight improvement causes a 3:2 response, whereas a lowering of conductivity results in a 3:1 conduction (as seen in the right half of Figure 14-14).[10,30] On the other hand, blockage of the third atrial impulse within the AV node in the presence of a 3:2 ratio results in a reduced frequency of excitation in the His–Purkinje system. Therefore, the first conducted beat after such a pause (third QRS complex) would be associated with a marked prolongation of the action potential duration and the refractory period of those Purkinje fibers. Because of such prolonged refractoriness, the second atrial impulse after the pause may be blocked at the His–Purkinje level, a mechanism often referred to as phase 3 block. In this record, an effective refractory period lasting longer than 500 milliseconds must be postulated in the Purkinje system to invoke this latter mechanism. Although this duration may seem long, such values of action potential duration in the Purkinje fibers can be observed under certain experimental conditions. Furthermore, it has been shown in experiments using canine Purkinje fibers that a sudden prolongation of the cycle length after a shorter one shifted the restitution curves, resulting in effective refractory periods that were markedly longer than those predicted from the diastolic interval alone.[45] Of these two mechanisms, depression of conduction below the AV node probably plays a greater role in determining the clinical significance. It is possible that when intraventricular conduction disturbances cause AV block, the same pathophysiologic mechanism involves the AV nodal region as well.

OTHER MECHANISMS CONTRIBUTING TO ATRIOVENTRICULAR CONDUCTION DISORDERS

There are several abnormal conduction phenomena resulting from alterations in the primary determinants of conductivity. First, *decremental conduction* refers to a gradual decrease in both the effectiveness of stimuli and the magnitude of response along the pathway of conduction in anatomically uniform but functionally depressed tissue.[30,46,47] Decremental conduction is more easily produced in the N region of the AV node where the action potentials show inherently slow upstroke and reduced amplitude even under physiologic conditions. The sequential changes in the action potential characteristics from the atrial fiber to the so-called AN region and then to the N region of the AV node may superficially mimic decremental conduction in the absence of any pathophysiologic factors depressing conductivity. However, the changes probably result from nonuniform anatomic structures and associated differences in their membrane characteristics, and the action potential characteristics in a given fiber would show little beat-to-beat fluctuations as contrasted to the records shown in Figures 14-4 and 14-5. Therefore, it is our opinion that such changes should not be regarded as decremental conduction.

The second abnormal conduction phenomenon, or *inhomogeneous conduction*, is explained as follows: when decremental conduction develops nonuniformly at one portion of the conducting pathway, the wavefront of

excitation becomes irregular.[9,32] The overall effectiveness of stimuli is then decreased compared with that in the presence of a smoother excitation front and a synchronous depolarization of neighboring fibers. As a result, conductivity is further depressed, leading to either delay in or failure of propagation.[48] In a strand of conducting tissue in which fibers run parallel to and in close contact with one another, there is less chance for inhomogeneous conduction. Conversely, when small fibers are sparsely distributed or show frequent ramifications and anastomoses to form a complex network as in the AV node, fragmentation of the wavefront is more readily produced.

Several experimental observations supporting this concept include collision of two impulses within the AV node, producing a greater amplitude and upstroke velocity of action potential.[49] It has also been demonstrated that, when excitation waves originating from two different portions of the right atrium invade the AV nodal tissue almost simultaneously, transnodal conduction either proceeds more rapidly or becomes successful, whereas arrival of only one wavefront results in much slower conduction or blockage in the node.[10,30,31] Thus, the significance of inhomogeneous conduction in this tissue must be emphasized. Furthermore, the mode of invasion of impulses into the AV node appears important in determining the difficulty or ease of intra-AV nodal conduction.[10,30,32]

When inhomogeneity of conduction is markedly increased, failure of propagation may occur in one side of the AV node, while a slow but successful conduction occurs in the other side.[32] This phenomenon is called *functional longitudinal dissociation* and has been cited as the cause for reciprocal beating and reciprocal tachycardia (paroxysmal AV junctional tachycardia). However, whether this condition could produce electrophysiologic characteristics of so-called dual AV nodal pathways and allow the development of sustained reentrant tachycardia is unknown.[42,43] Such longitudinal dissociation is reported to develop in other cardiac tissues, including the His bundle and bundle branches. Nevertheless, inhomogeneous conduction is considered a parallel (transverse) expression and decremental conduction is considered a series (longitudinal) expression of depressed conductivity.[10,30,31]

Other manifestations of AV conduction disturbance, such as unidirectional conduction, are shown in Figures 14-16 and 14-17. In Figure 14-16, high grade AV block is diagnosed from the regular appearance of ventricular complexes at the rate of 37 per minute without any fixed relationship with P waves. In lead aVF, for example, the first four P waves appear at constant P-P intervals, showing a rate of 70 per minute. The fifth P wave appears prematurely and is considered an atrial extrasystole, which also fails to be conducted to the ventricles. Thus, the forward (or AV) conduction is always blocked. Conversely, more than half of the ventricular complexes are imme-

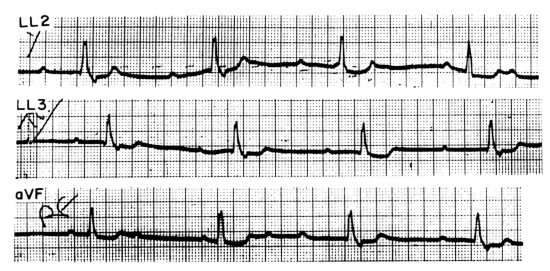

Figure 14-16. High-grade atrioventricular block with unidirectional retrograde conduction to the atria in the presence of wide QRS. *LL2,* lead II; *LL3,* lead III; *aVF,* lead aVF.

diately followed by inverted P waves (beats 1 and 2 in lead II, or LL 2; beats 1, 2, and 4 in lead III, or LL 3; and beats 3 and 4 in lead aVF), which clearly reset the sinus rhythm and produce the phenomenon of return cycle. Therefore, atrial excitation by retrograde (VA) conduction or the presence of unidirectional AV conduction can be diagnosed.[18] A closer examination of the time relationships between the QRS complexes and the P waves reveals that those ventricular complexes terminating relatively short PR intervals (these do not represent AV conduction time because the P waves are not conducted to the ventricles) are not followed by retrograde conduction. More precisely, retrograde conduction to the atria appears to be permitted when a QRS complex occurs at least 0.38 second after the

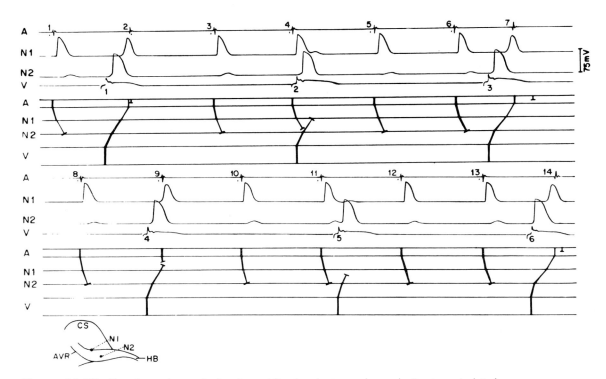

Figure 14-17. Experimental records showing unidirectional retrograde conduction in an isolated perfused rabbit heart (See Fig. 14-4 for key to abbreviations.)

attempted invasion of the AV conducting system by the blocked sinus impulses. This indicates that after the expiration of the refractory period of the AV conducting system caused by concealed forward conduction, retrograde impulses may successfully traverse the site of block and reach the atria.

In Figure 14-16, the third beat in lead III is not followed by a retrograde P wave even though its interval from the preceding sinus P wave appears to be sufficiently long. This finding can be explained by collision of a retrograde impulse in the AV junctional tissue with attempted forward conduction of an atrial premature systole, which occurred simultaneously with this particular QRS complex. The findings that support this interpretation are as follows: (1) the interval between the third QRS complex and the preceding P wave (0.44 second) is almost identical to the coupling intervals of atrial premature beats seen in other portions of the record (0.44 to 0.46 second) and (2) if an ectopic P wave were hidden in this QRS complex, the interval from this P wave to the following sinus P wave would measure approximately 1.04 seconds, the same value as other return cycles following retrograde P waves.[18]

Some investigators deny the possibility of a retrograde conduction through the site of orthograde block and believe that a mechanical effect of ventricular contraction somehow facilitates impulse formation in the automatic AV junctional fibers above the site of block.[50,51] Another theory states that the electrotonic spread of a retrograde impulse jumps over the site of block and excites the atria.[52] It is our opinion that the most likely explanation is different degrees of decrement in forward versus retrograde conduction.[30,31] Figure 14-17 shows an experimental record of unidirectional conduction within the AV junctional tissue that is similar to the clinical observation in Figure 14-16.[18,48]

In Figure 14-17, the action potentials from the AN region (N1) and the NH region (N2) of the AV node are recorded together with the atrial (A) and ventricular (V) electrograms. The stimulus artifacts seen in these electrograms indicate that the atria and the ventricles are electrically stimulated at different rates. The action potentials of fiber N1, except for those numbered 2, 7, 9, and 14, always follow the atrial excitation, but they cause only partial depolarization of fiber N2 and fail to be conducted to the ventricles. Thus, high grade block in a forward direction is present. In contrast, the ventricular impulses always fully depolarize fiber N2 in the NH region. When an N2 action potential occurs immediately after depolarization of fiber N1 caused by atrial impulses (ventricular complexes numbered 2 and 5), a local response in fiber N1 is produced and the retrograde conduction does not proceed further. This suggests that the success or failure of retrograde activation of fiber N1 depends on the excitability or

refractoriness in this area. Later appearance of the N2 action potentials with reference to the previous depolarization of fiber N1 (numbers 1, 3, 4, and 6) is followed by an action potential in N1, which, although showing a slow upstroke velocity, is successfully transmitted to the atria to cause atrial excitation (atrial numbers 2, 7, and 14). When such a retrograde impulse encounters the atrial refractory period (numbered 9), it is probably blocked between this fiber N1 and the site of the atrial recording electrode. This is considered an example of unidirectional conduction within the N region of the AV node. It is likely that those clinical cases of high grade AV block in which ventricular pacing produces a 1:1 retrograde conduction are associated with similar mechanisms.[53,54]

On the other hand, a group of clinical phenomena called *supernormal AV conduction* (Figs. 14-18 and 14-19) is still controversial.[16,53-55] Some investigators even deny its presence. Although several different varieties of supernormal AV conduction have been identified, only part of this complex problem is discussed here. Supernormal AV conduction refers to an unexpected improvement in conduction in the presence of depressed conductivity (either in AV conduction or in conduction in any other portion of the myocardium). For example, successful conduction when failure of propagation is expected or the occurrence of a shorter conduction time when its prolongation is more likely is called supernormal, although it does not represent a condition better than or superior to normal.

Figure 14-18 shows an experimental record from an isolated, perfused rabbit heart. During the period of 4:3 AV conduction seen in the middle portion of this record, the AV conduction time is initially increased from 190 to 210 milliseconds and then again shortened to 197 milliseconds. Such findings contradict the classic type I block (Wenckebach phenomenon), and the paradoxical shortening of the AV interval, instead of a further prolongation, may be interpreted as supernormal conduction. When the action potentials from the N region of the AV node (N) are examined, the first beat of the 4:3 conduction shows a normal action potential contour, whereas the second atrial impulse produces a doubly peaked action potential with a markedly decreased rate of phase 0 depolarization resulting in a prolongation of the conduction time from this N fiber to the ventricles (from 78 to 100 milliseconds). The action potential in the N fiber caused by the third atrial impulse shows a smoother upstroke of phase 0, although the rate of depolarization is not significantly greater, and the conduction time to the ventricles is again shortened to 85 milliseconds. The last (fourth) atrial impulse depolarizes the N fiber only incompletely and is not conducted to the ventricles. These findings may be explained by our concept of inhomogeneous conduction as follows: a marked inhomogeneity of intranodal conduction in the

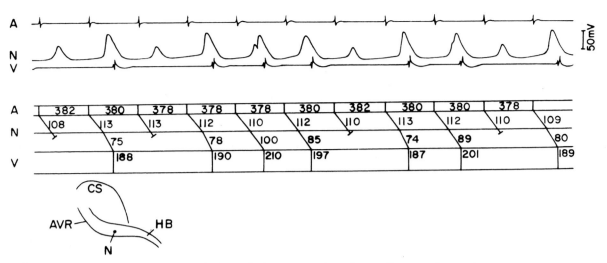

Figure 14-18. An experimental record of so-called supernormal conduction. Time in milliseconds.

second beat resulted in decreased efficacy of its excitation wave, thus delaying conduction below this N region. In contrast, the third beat was somehow associated with a more homogeneous excitation front within the AV node, and its greater efficacy as a stimulus caused a better subnodal conduction. Thus, slight fluctuations of conductivity within the AV junction may produce this type of supernormal conduction, although the reason for such fluctuations cannot be readily determined.[10, 29, 31]

A different type of supernormal conduction is illustrated in a clinical electrocardiogram shown in Figure 14-19. Because both limb lead II (LL2, top) and lead aVF (bottom) show identical conduction phenomena, only lead aVF is discussed here. The P waves appear regularly at the rate of 140 per minute, suggesting sinus tachycardia as the basic mechanism. The ventricular complexes appear irregularly, showing two different QRS contours. The com-

plexes having a wide rS pattern terminate a long pause measuring 1.50 seconds without any fixed time relationships with the preceding P waves. Therefore, these beats most likely represent either AV junctional or ventricular rhythm caused by a high grade AV block. On the other hand, beats 2 and 5 with narrow QRS of the R type are preceded by a P wave at an interval of 0.18 second. Exactly the same findings are noted in lead II, which suggests that these narrow QRS complexes are produced by propagation of atrial impulses. Furthermore, these conducted sinus P waves show a constant time relationship with the preceding QRS of the escape rhythm. The P waves are never conducted to the ventricles unless they appear immediately after the T wave. It has been postulated that invasion of the AV junction by concealed retrograde conduction of the impulses from the subsidiary pacemaker somehow improves the conduction in the forward direc-

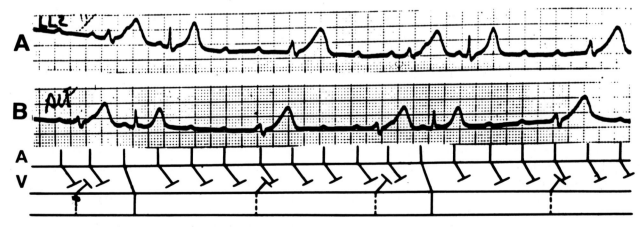

Figure 14-19. Successful atrioventricular conduction of atrial impulses only after the discharge of a subsidiary pacemaker at an appropriate time. This is one type of so-called supernormal conduction.

tion. Because the conducting tissues are ordinarily rendered refractory after their invasion by an impulse and the recovery of excitability is supposed to proceed with time, such improved conductivity immediately after a preceding excitation is considered a type of supernormal conduction.

With the use of microelectrode techniques, several investigators have explained this phenomenon as follows. A concealed orthograde conduction of atrial impulses into the AV node leaves a long refractory period in this tissue, which prevents transmission of the next impulse. When a retrograde impulse arrives at this area with an appropriate timing (retrograde conduction of the first ventricular impulse in the diagram in Figure 14-19), it depolarizes the AV nodal tissue prematurely, preventing invasion of the second atrial impulse into the region. Because of such early depolarization, repolarization is terminated earlier at the site of conduction block (so-called pealing back of the refractory barrier), thus allowing the third sinus impulse to be conducted to the ventricles.[56, 57] However, this theory can be challenged, and it is not the only explanation.

An alternative explanation is based on the concept of so-called phase 4 block.[58] When significant diastolic depolarization is present in the His–Purkinje system, causing a decreased membrane potential (but not reaching the threshold potential) and resultant depression of conductivity, propagation of impulses through these fibers becomes more difficult toward later diastole, whereas arrival of an impulse immediately after an action potential, when the membrane potential is the most negative, may be associated with improved conduction.[59] Because the QRS complexes of the escape rhythm in Figure 14-19 are wide, suggesting the site of impulse formation (and consequently the site of block) to be below the bifurcation of the His bundle, the second theory invoking phase 4 block at the His–Purkinje level may be the preferred explanation in this case.[60] Another explanation invoking the mechanism of supernormal periods of excitability is also possible.[61]

Finally, there is a phenomenon that has classically been considered a type of supernormal conduction, but we disagree.[31, 62] This phenomenon is a regular alternation of the PR interval in the presence of 1:1 conduction. In the experimental records shown in Figure 14-20, alternation of long and short AV conduction times is noted in the presence of almost regular sinus rhythm, causing an alternation of the ventricular cycle. In contrast to the several examples of alternating PR intervals in 2:1 AV block (Figs. 14-13, 14-15), every sinus impulse is transmitted to the ventricles in Figure 14-20. The argument for calling this type of rhythm supernormal conduction is as follows. The second atrial impulse in the top record of Figure 14-20 (marked P) follows the first ventricular excitation (R) with a relatively long interval (178 milliseconds), yet its conduction to the ventricles takes a longer time (124 + 87 = 211 milliseconds). On the other hand, the third atrial

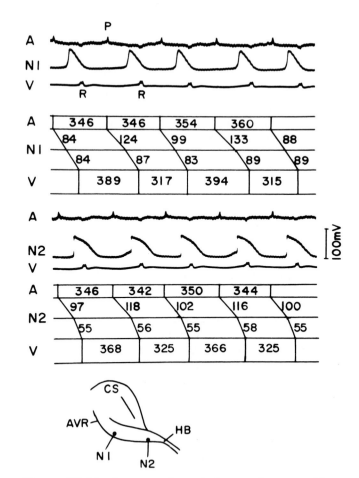

Figure 14-20. Experimental records showing alternation of short and long atrioventricular conduction times in the presence of 1:1 response. Time in milliseconds.

impulse appears only 135 milliseconds after the second ventricular depolarization (R) but is conducted with a shorter AV conduction time (99 + 83 = 182 milliseconds), which is an apparently paradoxical conduction pattern. In other words, if the AV transmission takes 211 milliseconds when the recovery of excitation of the AV conducting system is considered to be better after a longer RP interval, then conduction of the next impulse in the presence of poorer recovery of the conducting system after a shorter RP interval should be associated with a further prolongation of the PR interval. Thus, the paradoxical shortening of PR interval to 182 milliseconds may satisfy the criteria for supernormal conduction. However, Figure 14-20 clearly indicates that the RP interval would have no effect on the recovery of excitability in the conducting system. The second atrial impulse (P) as well as the third atrial impulse try to invade the AV node with the same cycle length of 346 milliseconds, not after 178 or 135 milliseconds. The effects of such RP intervals must be considered only when impulses originating in a subsidiary pacemaker control the ventricles and invade the AV junction in a retrograde fashion as in the example of Figure 14-19. Such values have no meaning when ventricular excitation is caused by supraventricular impulses alone. For this reason, it is our opinion that this phenomenon should not be called a supernormal conduction.[30]

The question then is how to explain these findings. In this regard, the action potentials from fiber N1 in the top record in Figure 14-20 appear to show slight diastolic depolarization, whereas the N2 potential in the bottom record develops a prominent prepotential or step formation when the conduction time is prolonged. These changes suggest that the intra-AV nodal conduction of every other atrial impulse becomes inhomogeneous, and the decreased effectiveness of an irregular excitation front causes depression of conductivity. It may further be postulated that there is functional longitudinal dissociation of the AV junctional tissue in which one fiber group maintains a 1:1 response while the other fiber group is in a condition of 2:1 block.[30] Although this latter mechanism may appear similar to the so-called dual AV conducting system in which two anatomically separate conducting pathways are often postulated, a functional duality or inhomogeneity is probably sufficient to cause these phenomena.[42, 43] In either case, when the intranodal conduction is delayed, the membrane potential of certain downstream fibers may become less negative due to phase 4 depolarization, which could further delay conduction below the AV node.[58, 59] Conversely, if the next sinus impulse traverses the AV node faster, it reaches those downstream fibers showing diastolic depolarization after a shorter interval, sustains a lesser degree of phase 4 block, and is associated with a significantly shorter subnodal conduction time. Alternation of the PR interval (as well as the RR interval) would thus be exaggerated.

The explanation of even apparently simple conduction disorders may often involve diverse electrophysiologic mechanisms. Recent studies have further demonstrated the important role of the two limbs of the autonomic nervous system (vagal and sympathetic) in the regulation of impulse transmission through the AV node.[63, 64] Vagal control is characterized by its dynamics because, normally, vagal discharges appear in short volleys (bursts) of nerve impulses synchronized with the arterial pulse wave and the baroreceptor response.[65] Consequently, a beat-by-beat regulation of AV nodal conduction can be expected to result from the periodic repetitive vagal discharges. Furthermore, the vagal effect is phase-dependent: each vagal burst produces transient hyperpolarization predominantly of the cells in the N region of the AV node, and the absolute value of this hyperpolarization (at given vagal intensity) depends on the timing of the vagal burst in the cardiac cycle.[64] The larger the vagal-induced hyperpolariz-

ation, the greater the depression of conduction through the N region of the AV node, a consequence of the slow-channel properties of these cells. The phasic nature of such vagal effects on AV nodal conduction can be responsible for the development of AV nodal gap, a phenomenon bordering with a supernormal behavior, because, in this case, conduction of atrial impulses with shorter cycle lengths would be permitted, whereas the conduction of atrial impulses with longer cycles would be blocked.[66] The tracings in Figure 14-21 show this behavior in an experimental model using rabbit atrial-AV nodal preparation instrumented for the application of short bursts of postganglionic vagal stimulation. The bipolar surface electrograms were recorded from crista terminalis (CrT) and the bundle of His (H), and action potentials (AP) were recorded with a microelectrode from a cell in the N region of the AV node. In all panels (A through H), the vagal burst (short horizontal bar) was applied at a fixed interval of

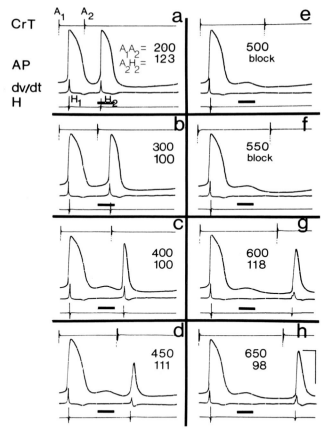

Figure 14-21. Atrioventricular nodal gap when the coupling interval of $A_1 A_2$ is decreased from 650 to 500 milliseconds (h-f) after a vagal burst (*bar*). Further shortening of the $A_1 A_2$ interval to 450, 400, 300, and 200 milliseconds (d-a) permits atrioventricular conduction to continue. Conduction is related to the degree of prematurity and the time of the vagal burst determining the degree of hyperpolarization of the atrioventricular nodal cells.

300 milliseconds after the preceding beat (A_1). Extra-stimuli (A_2) were given at progressively longer coupling intervals of 200 to 650 milliseconds. The extrastimuli with shorter coupling intervals of 200, 300, 400, and 450 milliseconds were successfully conducted, whereas extra-stimuli with intermediate coupling intervals of 500 and 550 milliseconds were blocked before the conduction resumed at still longer coupling intervals of 600 and 650 milliseconds. It can be seen that this behavior is based on the combination of two factors: the prematurity of the extrastimulus and the degree of accompanying vagal-induced hyperpolarization. Thus, the intermediate extra-stimuli in panels *E* and *F* arrived in the N region at the time of maximal vagal-induced hyperpolarization and failed to be conducted. In contrast, the earlier extrastimuli (panels *A* through *D*) were associated with lesser vagal-induced hyperpolarization at the moment of their arrival in the N region, and the net depressive effect (i.e., the combination of short recovery period and relatively small hyperpolariz-ation) was accordingly smaller. Similarly, the latest extra-stimuli (panels *G* and *H*) arrived not only after a significant recovery time had elapsed but also at the "tail" of vagal-induced hyperpolarization. This resulted predictably in successful AV nodal conduction.

If the situation discussed in relation to Figure 14-21 was observed in vivo, phasic vagal discharges might be considered responsible for the alternating PR intervals. The mechanism would be similar to the one just described for the AV nodal gap. If each R wave (see Fig. 14-20) was followed by a short burst of vagal discharge and the maxi-mal vagal-induced hyperpolarization in the N region of the AV node was observed about 250 milliseconds after the R wave (*upward arrows*), then the second sinus impulse in Figure 14-20 (marked P) would arrive in the N region at the moment of maximal vagal depression and would be conducted slower. In contrast, the next sinus impulse, which occurs after a shorter RP interval, would arrive in the N region of the AV node before the maximal vagal-induced hyperpolarization develops. Consequently, the

conduction of this beat would be less depressed and the AV interval would be shortened.

The difficulty in reaching a conclusion about super-normal AV conduction in many cases might rest on the lack of adequate information about the physiologic mecha-nisms involved in the observed phenomena. One charac-teristic example, which illustrates the role of the sympa-thetic nerve in modulating AV nodal conduction, is shown in Figure 14-22. In this case, a brief postganglionic sympa-thetic stimulation (PGSS) applied in the sinus node area was used to produce transient sinus tachycardia (shorten-ing of the interval CrT–CrT between the successive crista terminalis electrograms, *lower left panel*). This tachycar-dia was initially accompanied by an expected prolonga-tion of the CrT–H interval (*middle left panel*, between the broken lines a and b). Slightly later, however, an unex-pected or paradoxical shortening of the CrT–H interval persisted despite the continuing tachycardia (between the broken lines b and c). A period of alternating short and long CrT–H intervals was also evident (around the broken line d). The simultaneous recording of the interval be-tween the CrT and interatrial septum (IAS) electrograms (i.e., CrT–IAS) in this case revealed that, after PGSS, there was a significant shortening of this interval (line b), and, ultimately, the IAS was depolarized earlier than CrT (note the negative CrT–IAS values around line c). The alterna-tion in the CrT–H interval coincided with alternation in the sequence of activation of CrT and IAS (line d). Thus, shift of the major input to the AV node from CrT to IAS induced by sympathetic stimulation was responsible for the unusual pattern of AV nodal conduction. When feed-back pacing was used and identical tachycardia was pro-duced without a CrT–IAS alternation, the pattern of the response of AV nodal conduction was exactly as predicted (see Fig. 14-22B, *right panels*).

The gap phenomena have been explained by differ-ences in the duration of refractory period or in conducting properties between consecutive units of the AV conduct-ing system, that is, between the atrium and the AV node,

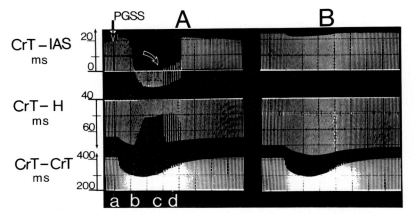

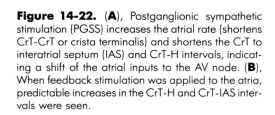

Figure 14-22. (**A**), Postganglionic sympathetic stimulation (PGSS) increases the atrial rate (shortens CrT-CrT or crista terminalis) and shortens the CrT to interatrial septum (IAS) and CrT-H intervals, indicat-ing a shift of the atrial inputs to the AV node. (**B**), When feedback stimulation was applied to the atria, predictable increases in the CrT-H and CrT-IAS inter-vals were seen.

the AV node and the bundle of His, and the bundle of His and the Purkinje system.[61,65] More specifically, the prerequisite for the development of gap phenomena, in most cases, was considered to be the existence of a distal unit with an effective refractory period longer than the functional refractory period of the proximal unit. The aforementioned studies[66] indicate that another mechanism or nonuniform recovery of excitability caused by phasic vagal discharge may lead to the development of AV nodal gaps.

In summary, (1) often, no single electrophysiologic mechanism can explain even apparently simple conduction disorders, and (2) identification of the site of block and pathophysiologic mechanisms involved appears essential to better clinical management of conduction disorders. More detailed experimental studies are needed to elucidate the mechanisms causing these complex AV conduction phenomena.[31]

References

1. Adams R: Dublin Hospital Report. 1827;4:353.
2. Stokes W: Dublin Q J Med Sci 1846;2:73.
3. Wenckebach KF: Zur Analyse des unregelmässigen Pulses. Z Klin Med 1899;37:475.
4. Hay J: Bradycardia and cardiac arrhythmia produced by depression of certain functions of the heart. Lancet 1906;1:139.
5. Mobitz W: Über die unvollständige Störung der Erregungsüberleitung zwischen Vorhof und Kammer des Menschlichen Herzens. Z Gesamte Exp Med 1924;41:180.
6. Haiat R, Dreifus LS, Watanabe Y: Fate of AV block. An electrocardiographic study. In: Han J, ed. Cardiac arrhythmias. A symposium. Springfield, IL: Charles C Thomas, 1972:73.
7. Dreifus LS, Watanabe Y, Haiat R, Kimbiris D: Atrioventricular block. Am J Cardiol 1971;28:371.
8. Dreifus LS, Watanabe Y: Localization and significance of atrioventricular block. Am Heart J 1971;82:435.
9. Watanabe Y, Dreifus LS: Second degree atrioventricular block. Cardiovasc Res 1967;1:150.
10. Watanabe Y, Dreifus LS: Levels of concealment in second degree and advanced second degree AV block. Am Heart J 1972;84:330.
11. Watanabe Y, Dreifus LS: Sites of impulse formation within the atrioventricular junction of the rabbit. Circ Res 1968;22:717.
12. Watanabe Y: Atrioventricular conduction disturbance and electrophysiology. Igaku no Ayumi (In Japanese) 1969;69:339.
13. Damato AN, Lau SH: Clinical value of the electrogram of the conduction system. Prog Cardiovasc Dis 1970;13:119.
14. Narula OS, Scherlag BJ, Samet P, Javier RP: Atrioventricular block. Localization and classification by His bundle recordings. Am J Med 1971;50:146.
15. Puech P, Grolleau R: L'Activite de Faisceau de His Normale et Pathologique. Paris: Editions Sandoz, 1972.
16. Katz LN, Pick A: Clinical electrocardiography, Part I. The arrhythmias. Philadelphia: Lea & Febiger, 1956.
17. Bellet S: Clinical disorders of the heart beat. 3rd ed. Philadelphia: Lea & Febiger, 1971.
18. Watanabe Y: Cardiac arrhythmias. Electrophysiologic and clinical aspects. (In Japanese) Tokyo: Bunkodo, 1973.
19. Watanabe Y, Dreifus LS: Electrophysiologic effects of digitalis on A-V transmission. Am J Physiol 1966;211:1461.
20. Watanabe Y, Dreifus LS: Interactions of quinidine and potassium on atrioventricular transmission. Circ Res 1967;20:434.
21. Watanabe Y, Dreifus LS: Interactions of lanatoside C and potassium on atrioventricular conduction in rabbits. Circ Res 1970;27:931.
22. Rosen KM, Rahimtoola SH, Chuquimia R, Loeb HS, Gunnar RM: Electrophysiological significance of first degree atrioventricular block with intraventricular conduction disturbance. Circulation 1971;43:491.
23. Damato AN, Lau, Helfant R, et al: A study of heart block in man using His bundle recordings. Circulation 1969;39:297.
24. Narula OS, Cohen LS, Samet P, Lister JW, Scherlag B, Hildner FJ: Localization of A-V conduction defects in man by recording of the His bundle electrogram. Am J Cardiol 1970;25:228.
25. Narula OS, Scherlag BJ, Javier RP, Hildner FJ, Samet P: Analysis of the A-V conduction defect in complete heart block utilizing His bundle electrogram. Circulation 1970;41:437.
26. Massumsi RA, Ali N: Determination of the site of impaired conduction in atrioventricular block. J Electrocardiol 1970;30:193.
27. Narula OS, Samet P: Wenckebach and Mobitz type II AV block due to block within the His bundle and bundle branches. Circulation 1970;41:947.
28. Mobitz W: Über den partiellen Herzblock. Z Klin Med 1928;107:449.
29. Watanabe Y: Atrioventricular block. Saishin Igaku (In Japanese) 1970;25:799.
30. Watanabe Y, Dreifus LS: Factors controlling impulse transmission with special reference to AV conduction. Am Heart J 1975;89:790.
31. Watanabe Y, Dreifus LS: Cardiac arrhythmias: Electrophysiologic basis for clinical interpretation. New York: Grune & Stratton, 1977:153.
32. Watanabe Y, Dreifus LS: Inhomogeneous conduction in the AV node. A model for re-entry. Am Heart J 1965;70:505.
33. Rosen KM, Rahimtoola SH, Gunnar RM: Pseudo A-V block secondary to premature nonpropagated His bundle depolarizations. Documentation by His bundle electrocardiography. Circulation 1970;42:367.
34. Damato AN, Varghese PJ, Lau SH, Gallagher JJ, Bobb GA: Manifest and concealed reentry: A mechanism of AV nodal Wenckebach phenomenon. Circ Res 1972;30:283.
35. Jalife J: The sucrose gap preparation as a model of AV nodal transmission: Are dual pathways necessary for reciprocation and AV nodal "echoes"? PACE 1983;6:1106.
36. Fisch C, Zipes DP, McHenry P: Electrocardiographic manifestations of concealed junctional ectopic impulses. Circulation 1976;53:217.
37. Langendorf R, Mehlman JS: Blocked (nonconducted) A-V

nodal premature systoles imitating first and second degree A-V block. Am Heart J 1947;34:500.

38. Rosenbaum MB, Nau GJ, Levi RJ, Halpern MS, Elizari MV, Lazzari JO: Wenckebach periods in the bundle branches. Circulation 1969;40:79.

39. Kretz A, DaRuos HO: Experimental Luciani-Wenckebach phenomenon in the anterior and posterior divisions of the left bundle of the canine heart. Am Heart J 1972;84:513.

40. Wennemark JR, Bandura JP: Microelectrode study of Wenckebach periodicity in canine Purkinje fibers. Am J Cardiol 1974;33:390.

41. Moe GK, Preston JB, Burlington H: Physiologic evidence for a dual A-V transmission system. Circ Res 1956;4:357.

42. Wu D, Denes P, Dhingra R, Wyndham C, Rosen KM: Determinants of fast and slow pathway conduction in patients with dual atrioventricular nodal pathways. Circ Res 1975;36:782.

43. Noy Y, Fleischmann P: Electrocardiographic manifestations of dual pathways of retrograde impulse conduction in the human heart. Am J Cardiol 1975;35:293.

44. Ogawa S, Dreifus LS: Longitudinal dissociation of Bachmann's bundle as a mechanism of paroxysmal supraventricular tachycardia. Am J Cardiol 1977;40:915.

45. Watanabe M, Zipes DP, Gilmour RF Jr: Oscillations of diastolic interval and refractory period following premature and postmature stimuli in canine cardiac Purkinje fibers. PACE 1989;12:1089.

46. Hoffman BF, Paes de Carvalho A, de Mello WC, Cranefield PF: Electrical activity of single fibers of the atrioventricular node. Circ Res 1959;7:11.

47. Hoffman BF, Cranefield PF: The electrophysiology of the heart. New York: McGraw-Hill, 1960.

48. Watanabe Y, Dreifus LS: Newer concepts in the genesis of cardiac arrhythmias. Am Heart J 1968;76:114.

49. Iinuma H, Dreifus LS, Mazgalev T, et al: Role of the perinodal region in atrioventricular nodal reentry: Evidence in an isolated rabbit heart preparation. J Am Coll Cardiol 1983;2:465.

50. Cullis WC, Dixon WE: Excitation and section of the auriculoventricular bundle. J Physiol 1911;42:156.

51. Cohn AE, Fraser PR: The occurrence of auricular contractions in a case of incomplete heart block due to stimuli received from the contracting ventricles. Heart 1913;5:141.

52. Scherf D: Retrograde conduction in complete heart block. Dis Chest 1959;35:320.

53. Mack I, Langendorf R, Katz LN: The supernormal phase of recovery of conduction in the human heart. Am Heart J 1947;34:374.

54. Fisch C, Steinmetz EF: Supernormal phase of atrioventricular (A-V) conduction due to potassium. A-V alternans with first degree AV block. Am Heart J 1961;62:211.

55. Pick A, Langendorf R, Katz LN: The supernormal phase of atrioventricular conduction. I. Fundamental mechanisms. Circulation 1962;26:388.

56. Moe GK, Childers RW, Merideth J: An appraisal of "supernormal" A-V conduction. Circulation 1968;38:5.

57. Moore EN, Spear JF: Experimental studies on the facilitation of A-V conduction by ectopic beats in dogs and rabbits. Circ Res 1971;29:29.

58. Elizari MV, Lazzari JO, Rosenbaum MB: Phase 3 and phase 4 intermittent left anterior hemiblock. Report of first case in the literature. Chest 1972;63:673.

59. Singer DH, Lazzara R, Hoffman BF: Interrelationships between automaticity and conduction in Purkinje fibers. Circ Res 1967;20:537.

60. Watanabe Y: How to read arrhythmia electrocardiograms. VII. High grade AV block, unidirectional AV conduction and supernormal AV conduction. Clinic All-round (In Japanese) 1975;24:492.

61. Spear JF, Moore EN: Supernormal excitability and conduction in the His Purkinje system of the dog. Circ Res 1974;35:782.

62. Ashman R, Herrmann G: A supernormal phase in conduction and a recovery curve for the human junctional tissue. Am Heart J 1926;1:594.

63. Mazgalev T, Dreifus LS, Michelson EL, Pelleg A, Price R: Phasic effects of postganglionic vagal stimulation on atrioventricular nodal conduction. Am J Physiol 1986;251:H619.

64. Mazgalev T, Dreifus LS, Michelson EL, Pelleg A: Vagally induced hyperpolarization in atrioventricular node. Am J Physiol 1986;251:H631.

65. Kaneta PG, Poitras TW, Barnett GO, Terry BS: Cardiac vagal efferent activity and heart period in the carotid sinus reflex. Am J Physiol 1970;218:1030.

66. Mazgalev T, Dreifus LS, Michelson EL: A new mechanism for atrioventricular nodal gap-vagal modulation of conduction. Circulation 1989;79:417.

Cardiac Arrhythmias, 3rd edition, edited by William J. Mandel.
J. B. Lippincott Company, Philadelphia © 1995.

15

Onkar S. Narula

Clinical Concepts of Spontaneous and Induced Atrioventricular Block

The term *heart block* was first introduced by Gaskell almost a century ago in 1882.[1,2] In the following two decades, various portions of the specialized atrioventricular conducting system (i.e., atrioventricular [AV] node, His bundle, and bundle branches) were identified.[3–6] The first electrocardiogram showing experimental and clinical heart block was published by Einthoven in 1906.[7] Numerous histopathologic, experimental, and clinical studies have demonstrated that AV block may be due to lesions in any portion of the conducting system.[8–15] Although the standard electrocardiogram may indicate AV block or damage to the conduction system, it is limited in identifying the precise site or sites of a lesion(s) and the degree of damage to each region. The therapy and prognosis of AV block not only depends on diagnosing AV block but are also related to the site of lesion in the specialized conducting system. During the early 1970s, the development of His-bundle electrocardiography was valuable in enhancing the understanding of normal and abnormal AV-impulse transmission.[16] Complete AV block has been induced for therapeutic purposes in the management of selected patients with supraventricular tachyarrhythmias. Ongoing investigations are directed toward therapeutic induction of desired degrees of AV delays or AV block

through various catheter techniques. Some of these methods appear promising.

DEFINITION OF TERMS

The PR interval is broken into its three components by the recording of a His-bundle electrogram: (1) *PA* is an approximation of intraatrial conduction time and is measured from the high right atrial electrogram or the onset of the P wave on the standard electrocardiogram to the first rapid deflection of the A wave on the bipolar His bundle lead (Fig. 15-1); (2) *AH* represents the AV nodal conduction time and is measured from the first rapid deflection of the A wave (in the His-bundle lead) to the earliest onset (rapid or slow) of the His-bundle (*BH*) potential; and (3) *HV* represents the conduction time through the His-Purkinje system (HPS) and is measured from the onset of the BH potential to the earliest onset of ventricular activation recorded on either the intracardiac bipolar His-bundle lead or any of the multiple surface electrocardiogram leads.[17] RBV represents the condition from the right bundle depolarization to the onset of ventricular depolarization.

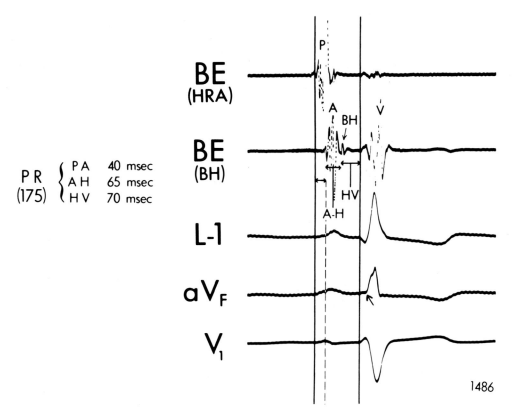

$$PR \atop (175) \left\{ \begin{array}{lll} P\,A & 40 & msec \\ A\,H & 65 & msec \\ H\,V & 70 & msec \end{array} \right.$$

Figure 15-1. Simultaneous bipolar recordings (*BE*) from the high right atrium (*HRA*) and the His-bundle (*BH*) region along with three electrocardiographic leads show the components of the PR interval. The *solid vertical lines* demarcate the earliest onset of the P wave and the QRS complex. (PA, intraatrial conduction time; AH, the time interval from the A wave to the BH, representing AV nodal conduction time; HV, the time interval from the BH to the ventricle, V.) (From Narula OS: Current concepts of A-V block. In: Narula OS, ed. His-bundle electrocardiography and clinical electrophysiology. Philadelphia. FA Davis, 1975:134.)

NORMAL ATRIOVENTRICULAR CONDUCTION

The normal range and mean, plus or minus standard deviation, for various conduction intervals in our laboratory are as follows: PA, 25 to 45 milliseconds (37 ± 7); AH, 50 to 120 milliseconds (77 ± 16); and HV, 35 to 45 milliseconds (40 ± 3).[18] The His-bundle duration is 15 to 20 milliseconds. The RBV times normally range from 20 to 25 milliseconds.[19] The range of conduction values reported by others is essentially similar to ours, except for the difference in the upper limit of normal HV interval, which others consider to be 55 milliseconds.[20-23] The reasons for these differences in the normal values reported by various groups have been previously discussed in detail.[24] The PA and HV intervals are not affected by sympathetic or parasympathetic influences and therefore remain constant from day to day. The AH interval, however, is influenced by changes in parasympathetic and sympathetic activity and may vary during the same study.

Normally, the AH interval lengthens with an increase in the atrial pacing rate, whereas the PA and HV intervals remain constant. During atrial pacing, 1:1 AV conduction may be noted up to a rate of 150 to 220 beats per minute; however, physiologic second-degree type I AH block may be manifest at rates of 130 beats per minute or more. Because these observations are based on studies without autonomic blockade, they cannot be applied with certainty to diagnose an abnormal AV node in cases manifesting second-degree AH block at rates less than 130 beats per minute. In addition, the phenomenon of "AV nodal accommodation" also influences the Wenckebach point, which is related to the size of increment in atrial pacing rate and the duration of pacing between incremental steps.[25] Development of second-degree AV block distal to the His-bundle potential with atrial pacing rates less than 150 beats per minute is considered abnormal.[24, 26]

SPONTANEOUS ATRIOVENTRICULAR BLOCK

First-Degree Atrioventricular Block

First-degree AV block (PR, ≧ 0.21 second) may result from conduction delays in the atrium, AV node, His bundle, or bundle branches (Fig. 15-2).[27] In 79% of our patients with a prolonged PR interval, the conduction delays were localized at more than one site, although the AV node was the dominant site of delay in most (83%). Conduction delays at a single site were noted in only 21% of patients (AV node in 11%, atrium in 3%, and HPS in 7%).[28] Patients with a wide QRS complex, especially those with a left bundle branch block, have a high incidence (50% to 90%) of abnormal HV intervals superimposed on a prolonged AH time.[29-32] Usually, with severe intraatrial delays, the P-wave amplitude is markedly diminished and in some, the P waves may be completely absent on the surface electrocardiogram and may fallaciously simulate a junctional rhythm with silent atria.[32] A notched and wide P wave, however, does not necessarily indicate an intraatrial conduction defect because it may also result from interatrial delays.[32]

In patients with first-degree AV block, the response to atrial pacing depends primarily on the site of delay. Patients with PA delays usually show 1:1 AV conduction at rapid pacing rates. The PA time may lengthen and occasionally, type I block may be manifest within the atrium.[33] In patients with AV nodal (AH) delays, second-degree type I block is usually manifest at slower atrial pacing rates (less than 130 beats/minute). Patients with a prolonged HV time usually exhibit 1:1 conduction at rapid pacing rates and only occasionally is second-degree block manifest distal to the His bundle.

Prognosis and therapy are determined not only by the degree of block but also by the site of the block. Patients with intraatrial conduction defects are usually prone to multiple atrial arrhythmias (i.e., atrial fibrillation, atrial flutter, or atrial tachycardia).[34] Conduction delays in the atrium or the AV node are usually stable and slowly progress to higher degrees of AV block. The symptoms of

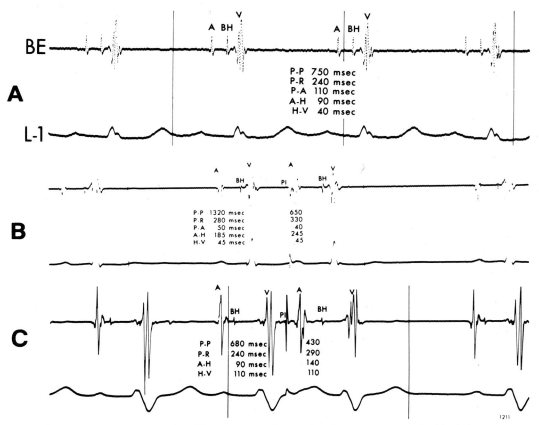

Figure 15-2. Recordings from three different patients showing first degree atrioventricular block due to delays at various sites. The PR interval is prolonged because of (**A**) intraatrial conduction delay (PA, 110 milliseconds), in which the AH and HV times are normal; (**B**) AV nodal delay (AH, 185 milliseconds); and (**C**) His-Purkinje system delay (HV, 110 milliseconds).

syncope are less likely to be due to intermittent complete heart block if the first-degree AV block is localized in the atrium or the AV node. First-degree AV block in the HPS usually progresses to Mobitz type II block or complete heart block (CHB) over a relatively shorter period. Therapy with digitalis is not contraindicated in patients with a prolonged PA or HV interval but the drug should be administered with caution in patients with a prolonged AH time. Conversely, quinidine or procainamide should be administered with caution in patients with a severely diseased HPS and a prolonged HV interval because these drugs may further lengthen the HV interval. Atrioventricular block due to antiarrhythmic therapy with quinidine or procainamide is rare.

Second-Degree Atrioventricular Block

Second-degree AV block is generally divided into two types: Wenckebach I (Mobitz I) and Wenckebach II (Mobitz II).[35,36] High-grade AV block with higher conduction ratios (2:1, 3:1) may be type I or type II.

Wenckebach Type I Block

The classic type I block (also known as Mobitz type I) is characterized by a progressive lengthening of the PR interval until a P wave is blocked (Fig. 15-3). The maximum PR increment occurs between the first and second conducted beats of the Wenckebach cycle. The PR interval is usually longest in the beat preceding the blocked P wave and shortest after the dropped beat. The RR intervals progressively decrease. The pause produced by the nonconducted P wave is equal to the difference between the last PR (before the pause) and the first PR (after the pause) intervals subtracted from twice the PP interval.[37] This classic pattern of Wenckebach cycles is seen infrequently (14%).[38,39] During spontaneous type I block, atypical cycles are seen commonly and their frequency increases with conduction ratios greater than 4:3. The atypical cycles

are as frequent with lesions in the AV node as in the HPS block.[40] In atypical cycles, various differing patterns of PR intervals may be noted because the PR interval may decrease before the dropped beat or may increase in equal steps; however, the PR interval after the dropped beat is always the shortest (Fig. 15-4). Chronic spontaneous type I block was localized in the AV node in 72% of our patients and in the His bundle or the bundle branches in 28%.[28] Others have reported a similar frequency of block at these sites.[29] In most cases with type I HPS block, the progressive and total increment in the PR interval (or HV) is usually smaller than that seen during AV nodal block (Fig. 15-5). During sinus rhythm, spontaneous type I block has not been documented within the atrium. Intraatrial block has been demonstrated during atrial pacing, however.[33]

Wenckebach periods of alternate beats have also been reported. These atypical cycles result from simultaneous occurrence of block at two different sites (i.e., His bundle and bundle branches, AV node and the HPS, or atrium and the AV node).[41–43] Wenckebach cycles may also be modified by the occurrence of other phenomena (i.e., supernormal conduction and bradycardia-dependent conduction delays or block). In addition, complete AV dissociation may be simulated by the simultaneous occurrence of second-degree block at multiple sites.[44] In rare cases, two consecutive P waves may be blocked in a Wenckebach cycle. Some of these cases may be explained by the occurrence of block at two different sites, whereas in others, only a single site of block has been documented.

Electrocardiographic findings of type I second-degree AV block and the resultant bradycardia may have different implications, depending on the clinical settings. Twenty-four-hour Holter-monitor recordings in healthy male medical students without apparent heart disease reveal a 6% incidence of spontaneous occurrences of second-degree type I AV block during sleep.[45] In athletes, a 9% incidence of second-degree type I AV block has been reported during periods of complete rest and in the recumbent position. This is considered to be a physiologic phenomenon related to heavy physical training because

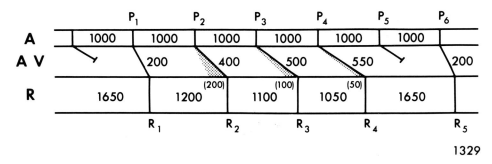

Figure 15-3. Diagrammatic representation of classic Wenckebach type I atrioventricular block. All the intervals are in milliseconds. The shaded area and the numbers in parentheses indicate the amount of the PR interval increment over that of the preceding PR interval (Narula OS: 1974;6(3):137.)

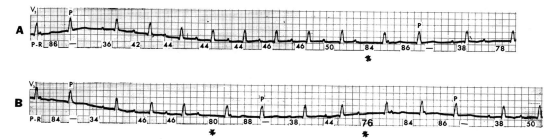

Figure 15-4. Second-degree type I atrioventricular block, with atypical Wenckebach cycles. The PR interval increases between the first and second conducted beats; however, maximum increment occurs abruptly in the later cycles (*asterisks*). In some of the consecutive beats, the PR interval remains unchanged. All the numbers are given in tenths of a second.

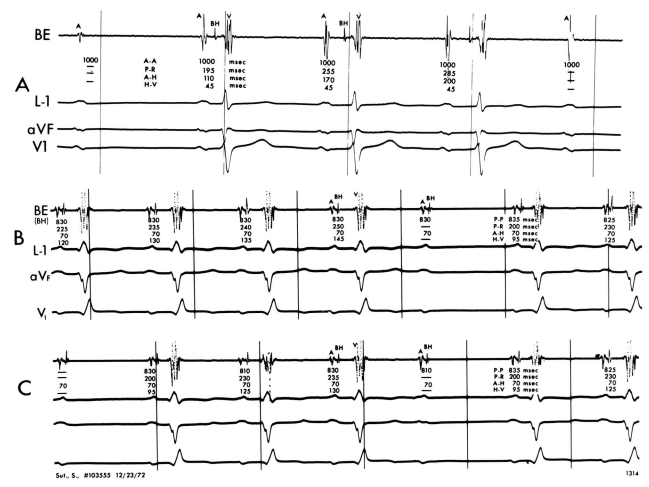

Figure 15-5. Second degree type I atrioventricular (AV) block is shown in the AV node and in the His–Purkinje system. (**A**) The AH time progressively lengthens from 110 to 200 milliseconds before an A wave (fifth) is blocked proximal to the BH (i.e., in the AV node). (**B** and **C**) The HV time progressively lengthens until an A wave is blocked distal to the BH deflection. This typical example of type I AV block in the His–Purkinje system also demonstrates that the increments in conduction delay (PR or HV) are minimal. This is in contrast to the larger delays seen in the AV nodal block in **A**.

follow-up observations over 6 years showed no symptoms or progression of block.[46] In another study, however, it was suggested that type I block in children should not be considered benign because during prospective observations, seven of the 16 children progressed to CHB, and one experienced dizzy spells.[47]

Wenckebach Type II Block

In Mobitz type II second-degree AV block (Wenckebach type II), the PR intervals preceding the dropped beats are always constant. This author has previously emphasized that in type II block the PR interval remains constant *throughout* (i.e., even after the dropped beat).[44, 48] Although in his original description Mobitz did not comment on this, the Lewis diagram in his paper clearly shows a constant PR interval, even after the dropped beat.[36] In cases consistent with the latter criteria, the type II block is limited to the HPS (35% in His bundle and 65% in the distal HPS).[18, 29, 32, 44] Each nonconducted P wave is transmitted through the AV node and is blocked distal to the recorded His-bundle deflection (Fig. 15-6). In the conducted beats, a single or "split" His-bundle potential may be recorded, depending on block in the distal or the middle portion of the His bundle, respectively. In rare cases with block in the uppermost portion of the His bundle, the A wave may not be followed by a recordable His-bundle deflection and thus may fallaciously simulate AV nodal block.[18, 49, 50] The PR interval in the conducted beats is usually normal and is less often prolonged.[44] The QRS complex is narrow in more than a third of patients (35%) and wide in the others (65%).[28]

Some workers indicate that in type II block, the PR interval after the pause may be slightly shorter ($\leqq 20$ milliseconds) than that of the remaining conducted beats.[49] Such a modified interpretation or definition of type II block appears unwarranted. Second-degree AV block with a shortening of the PR interval, even by 20 milliseconds, should be classified as type I block. A few reports claim the demonstration of second-degree type II block in the AV node.[51, 52] A detailed analysis of these reports, however, suggests atypical type I sequences because the PR interval was variable and shortened after the dropped beat. Some cases with type I block and atypical Wenckebach cycles may simulate type II block in the AV node. In these cases, however, the PR interval is always shortened after the dropped beat and long rhythm strips reveal changing PR intervals (Fig. 15-7).

The ability to diagnose the site of block on a standard electrocardiogram is of great clinical value because prog-

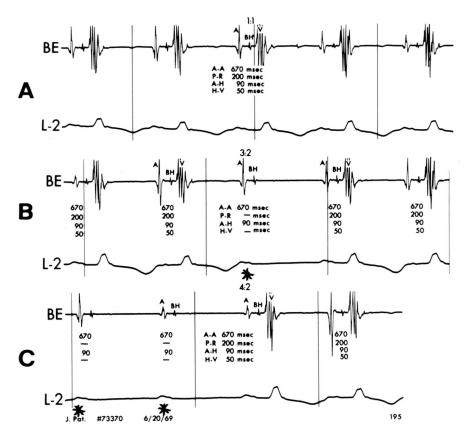

Figure 15-6. Mobitz type II atrioventricular block. His bundle recordings show that the nonconducted P waves (*asterisks*) are blocked distal to the BH deflection. The PR interval remains constant throughout.

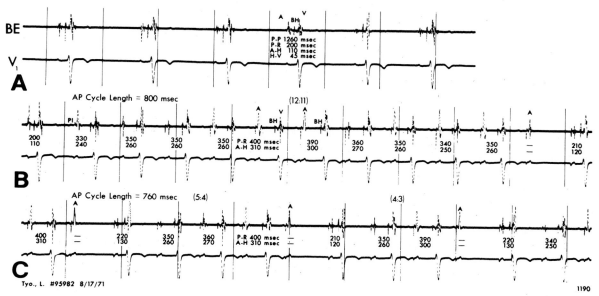

Figure 15-7. Type I atrioventricular (AV) block, with atypical Wenckebach cycles simulating type II block. (**A**) Recordings during sinus rhythm show 1:1 AV conduction. (**B**) Atrial pacing (*AP*) at a cycle length of 800 milliseconds shows second-degree AV block (12:11). The PR and AH intervals in the four consecutive beats immediately preceding the dropped beat do not lengthen and thus fallaciously simulate type II AV block. A comparison of the PR intervals in the beats preceding and following the dropped beat shows a marked shortening of the PR interval, diagnostic of type I block. (**C**) AP at a slightly faster rate (cycle length, 760 milliseconds) shows classic Wenckebach cycles, with a progressive prolongation of the PR interval.

nosis and therapy depend on the site of block. It is generally considered that second-degree blocks in the HPS often progress to CHB and Adams-Stokes attacks (Fig. 15-8) and require pacemaker implantation. In contrast, second-degree blocks in the AV node have a relatively benign course and do not lead to sudden asystole.[53] The electrocardiographic diagnosis of type II block is always indicative of an HPS lesion, whereas type I block is not predictive of the site of lesion. Cases with type I block require His-bundle recordings for the localization of site of lesion. Although minimal increments in the PR interval may suggest block in the HPS, they are not diagnostic. For these reasons, the classification of second-degree AV block into types I and II is clinically valuable because it eliminates the need for His-bundle recordings in those classified as type II. The clinical importance of this electrocardiographic classification was not accepted by all investigators but newer data have produced more widespread acceptance.[40,54] In our series, almost a third of patients with chronic second-degree AV block fulfilled the strict electrocardiogram definition of type II block, and these cases failed to reveal a shortening of either the PR interval or the HV interval by as much as 5 milliseconds after the dropped beat. Considering these facts, the clinical need for strict adherence to the definition of type II block is self-evident.[48]

2:1 or 3:1 Atrioventricular Block

Cases of 2:1 and 3:1 AV block cannot be classified into type I or type II unless the PR intervals are observed in two consecutively conducted beats during periods of changing conduction ratios (3:2 or 1:1).[53] With a change in conduction ratio, the constancy of the PR interval indicates type II block, whereas varying PR intervals are compatible with type I block. A minimal change in conduction delay secondary to a slight alteration in the number of impulses or vagal influences may readily change conduction ratios from 3:2 to 2:1 or vice versa.[32] Irrespective of type I or type II block, an increase in atrial rate, usually by 10 beats per minute, changes the conduction ratio from 3:2 to 2:1; however, an increase of 40 to 50 beats per minute is required to change the conduction ratios from 2:1 to 3:1. Although a change in AV block from 3:2 to 2:1 may not reflect a progression of the conduction defect, an increase from 2:1 to 3:1 *does* indicate a significant progression. Spontaneous fixed 2:1 block is localized in the AV node in a third of patients and in the HPS in the other two thirds (17% in His bundle, 50% in the distal HPS).[28,29] The QRS complex may be narrow or wide.

Carotid massage, if applied with caution, may be clinically useful in suggesting the site of block because the effect of vagal influences is usually limited to the AV node.

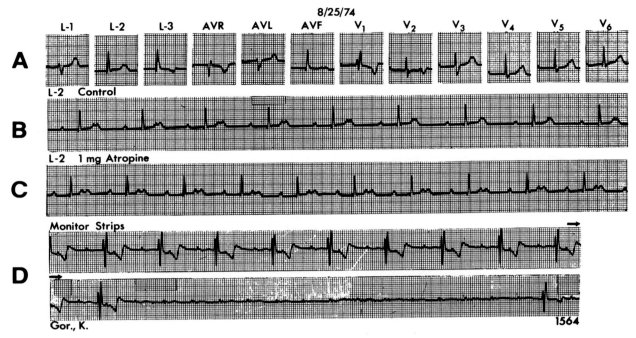

Figure 15-8. Electrocardiographic recordings from a patient with second-degree AV block (2:1) localized in the His–Purkinje system show a sudden development of asystole (**D**). This type of an occurrence is usual in patients with Mobitz type II or HPS block.

After carotid massage, the degree of block is likely to increase or decrease, depending on whether the lesion is in the AV node or the HPS, respectively. In case of a lesion in the HPS, slowing of the sinus rate with vagal stimulation results in improved AV conduction (1:1 or a decrease in block) due to fewer impulses arriving at the abnormal HPS. In rare patients with bradycardia-dependent HPS block, carotid massage may aggravate or aid in the manifestation of second-degree AV block, and atropine may abolish it.[55, 56] Generally, however, atropine increases HPS block due to an increase in atrial rate and may improve conduction in AV nodal block. Exercise may also be helpful in differentiating the two types of block. A change in conduction ratios by the above maneuvers may permit classification of 2:1 or 3:1 block into type I or type II.[32, 48]

Complete Heart Block

Complete heart block may be localized at three sites.[27, 29, 57, 58] In different series, the incidence of CHB ranges from 16% to 25% in the AV node, 14% to 20% in the His bundle, and 56% to 68% in the bundle branches. Complete heart block may occur due to congenital or acquired lesions. All congenital CHBs are not necessarily localized in the AV node because some have been documented within the His bundle, especially the middle portion of the His bundle.[58–63] Histologic studies indicate that

congenital CHB in otherwise anatomically normal hearts may result from a failure of the atrial myocardium to contact the AV node or may be due to congenital separation of the AV node from the ventricular conducting tissue.[64–66]

The most common cause of CHB is probably bilateral bundle branch block. The block is localized distal to the His-bundle deflection, and the escape rhythm shows a wide QRS complex. Each P wave is followed by a His-bundle deflection. The heart rate may range from 25 to 58 beats per minute and does not accelerate with atropine.[32, 59] These subsidiary pacemakers are readily suppressed by ventricular stimulation (mechanical or electric) and are prone to long periods of asystole.

Complete heart block may be localized in any portion of the His bundle (i.e., proximal, middle, or distal). In cases with middle and distal His-bundle blocks, split His-bundle potentials may be documented and the escape rhythm may either show a narrow or wide QRS complex identical to that seen during intact AV conduction (Fig. 15-9). His-bundle recordings may not differentiate a proximal His-bundle block from an AV nodal block because in both instances, the P waves are not followed by a His-bundle deflection and the QRS complexes are preceded by a His-bundle potential. After atropine administration, an acceleration in heart rate suggests AV nodal block, and a lack of increase suggests a His-bundle block.[32, 67] The latter, however, does not necessarily indicate block in the uppermost portion of the His bundle because His-bundle pace-

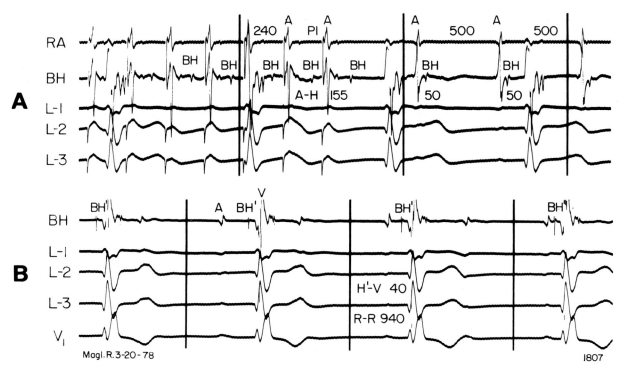

Figure 15-9. A patient with complete heart block localized within the His bundle. His-bundle recordings show "split" BH potentials. (**A**) Each A wave is blocked distal to a BH deflection (proximal His bundle). (**B**) Each QRS complex is preceded by a BH' deflection at an H'V interval of 40 milliseconds. The QRS complex is wide and shows a pattern of right bundle branch block, with right axis deviation.

makers may escape despite a localization of block in the AV node. The heart rate usually ranges from 30 to 50 beats per minute and may rarely exceed 70 beats per minute, especially in a surgically induced block.[28, 29, 58] A minimal variation in heart rate over a 24-hour period or from day to day may be noted (Fig. 15-10).[68] After atropine administration or with exercise, the heart rate may remain unchanged or may increase slightly and reach a maximum heart rate of 56 beats per minute.[56, 59–63, 67–69] With carotid stimulation or beta blockade, the heart rate may decrease by one or two beats per minute.[28, 56] Most of these patients have symptoms of syncope or dizziness, and an occasional patient may be asymptomatic.[69] Elderly women are more prone to His-bundle lesions because of degenerative calcific infringement of this region, which occurs three times more often in women than in men.[70, 71]

In patients with AV nodal CHB, the P waves are not followed by a His-bundle deflection and the escape QRS complexes may be preceded by a His-bundle deflection (with an HV interval $\geq$ 35 milliseconds) if the subsidiary pacemaker originates from the His bundle. The QRS complexes are usually narrow but may be wide in 20% to 50% of patients.[29, 32, 59] The heart rate usually ranges from 37 to 57 beats per minute and in most patients, a significant

acceleration in rate is noted after atropine administration or exercise.[27, 67, 68, 72]

Clinically, it is apparent that symptoms of syncope or dizziness cannot be reliably predicted based on electrocardiographic findings. Adams-Stokes attacks have been considered to occur most commonly in those patients with an escape rhythm showing a wide QRS complex, presumably due to complete interruption of both the bundle branches, and less commonly in those patients with escape rhythms showing a narrow QRS complex and an AV nodal block. After the introduction of His-bundle electrocardiography, it was suggested that the presence or absence of symptoms may be correlated to the site of block in the HPS (His bundle or bundle branches) or the AV node, respectively.[32, 59, 73]

Subsequent observations, however, suggest that patients with acquired or congenital CHB localized in the AV node (or proximal to the His-bundle deflection) are not a homogenous group because in some cases, the subsidiary pacemaker is unstable and requires management with an artificial pacemaker (Figs. 15-11 and 15-12).[69] Our data suggest that the criteria based on (1) localization of the site of origin, (2) the resting heart rates, and (3) the chronotropic responses to atropine are not sufficient for clinical

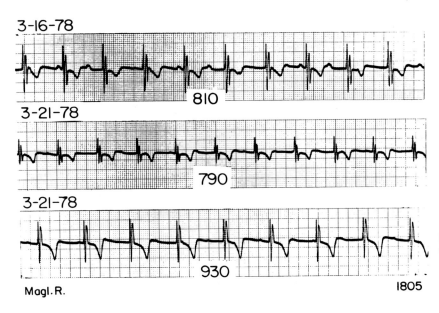

3-16-78

810

3-21-78

790

3-21-78

930

Magl. R.

1805

Figure 15-10. Minor day-to-day fluctuations in the heart rate or cycle length of a subsidiary pacemaker located within the His bundle in a patient with intra–His-bundle block (same patient as in Figure 15-9).

and therapeutic purposes.[69] Despite a significant increase in heart rate after atropine administration (≧ 72 beats/minute), some of the patients with subsidiary pacemakers located proximal to the His-bundle deflection were symptomatic. In addition to the above considerations, the response to overdrive suppression is an important determinant in a patient's clinical course. It was suggested that patients with subsidiary junctional pacemakers may be separated into those patients at risk and those less likely to have syncopal attacks based on electrophysiologic studies consisting of response to overdrive suppression and a measurement of junctional recovery time (JRT), with and without parasympathetic and beta blockade.

The JRT is measured with ventricular pacing at different rates (70 to 150 beats/minute). It is the interval between the last paced QRS complex and the first escape QRS complex. The corrected JRT (CJRT) is derived by deducting the basic control cycle length of the subsidiary rhythm from the JRT. In symptomatic patients with a subsidiary junctional pacemaker but without documentation of the cause of syncope or dizziness, the diagnosis may be confirmed or rendered less likely by the findings of a CJRT greater or less than 200 milliseconds, with or without atropine, respectively.[69] The measurements of the recovery interval of an escape pacemaker during CHB are of greater value than the mere localization of the site of block in determining the necessity of pacemaker therapy. Contrary to previous clinical views, our report documents that an asymptomatic patient with an intra–His-bundle block and an escape pacemaker located within the His bundle is not automatically a candidate for a prophylactic pacemaker insertion (Fig. 15-13).[59, 69, 73] Note, however, that most of the patients with an intra–His-bundle block have

unstable escape His-bundle rhythms, are symptomatic, and do require an artificial pacemaker (Fig. 15-14).

Congenital Heart Block

The incidence of congenital heart block is about 1 in every 25,000 live births but there is an increased incidence in children with congenital heart disease (0.4% to 0.9%).[74, 75] There have been studies that suggest that isolated CHB occurs more frequently in children whose mothers have connective tissue disorders. This has especially been the case in mothers with autoantibodies to the SS-A/RO and SS-B/La antigens.[76, 77] The neonatal outcome of the affected children is not influenced by the presence of these antibodies.[78]

In one study, the incidence of structural heart disease in fetuses with heart block was as high as 53%. In other studies evaluating infants (only after delivery) with heart block, only a 30% to 39% incidence of structural heart disease was noted. In the children who survived delivery and were followed-up long-term, between 58% and 70% of these patients survived long-term.[74, 79–82]

In the patients without structural heart disease, the long-term prognosis is good, with most patients remaining asymptomatic. Some patients, however, develop syncope and need permanent pacing.[83, 84]

Pathologic studies suggest that CHB may result from the failure of a hypoplastic AV node to develop connections with the internodal pathway or pathways, absence of a portion of the His bundle or bundle branches, or failure of the His bundle to link to the AV node.[85, 86]

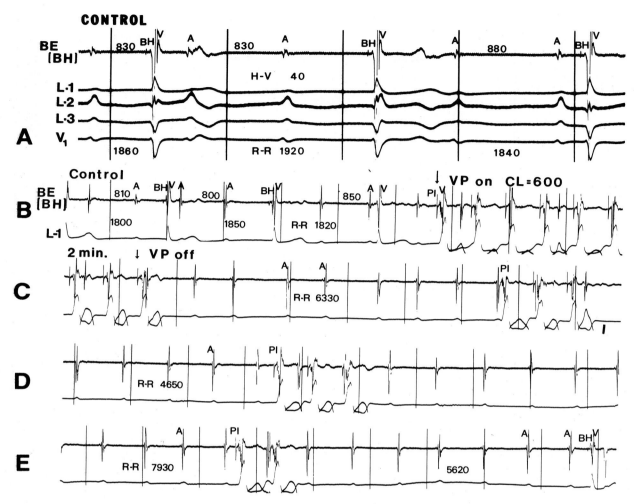

Figure 15-11. Severely prolonged junctional recovery time in a patient with complete heart block localized in the atrioventricular node. (**A**) Control recordings show that the A waves are not followed by a BH deflection. Each QRS is preceded by a BH potential at an HV interval of 40 milliseconds. (**B**) Onset of ventricular pacing (*VP*) at a cycle length (*CL*) of 600 milliseconds. (**C** to **E**) Termination of VP after 2 minutes followed by a long asystole (6330 milliseconds), indicating a severely prolonged junctional recovery time. The VP was intermittently resumed to prevent Adams-Stokes attacks, and the spontaneous subsidiary pacemaker escapes after 27 seconds (last beat, **E**). Recordings in panels **C** to **E** are continuous. Time lines are at 1-second intervals. (PI, pacing impulse). (Narula OS, Narula JT: Junctional pacemakers in man: response to overdrive suppression with and without parasympathetic blockade. Circulation 1978;57:880. By permission of the American Heart Association.)

Heart Block Associated With Acute Myocardial Infarction

Second-Degree Atrioventricular Block

INFERIOR MYOCARDIAL INFARCTION. In inferior myocardial infarction, the reported incidence of Mobitz type I second-degree AV Block (Wenckebach type I) is about 6%. This finding was not associated with increased immediate or long-term mortality when compared with a similar infarct group without second-degree AV block.[87-89]

The presence of Mobitz type II second-degree AV block is extremely rare.[90] The site of block in inferior myocardial infarction has been reported to be in the supra-Hisian area.

Complete Heart Block

INFERIOR MYOCARDIAL INFARCTION. In inferior myocardial infarction, the reported incidence of heart block is about 11%. The incidence is higher in women and in patients older than 70 years of age. The hospital course generally is more complicated than that of their coun-

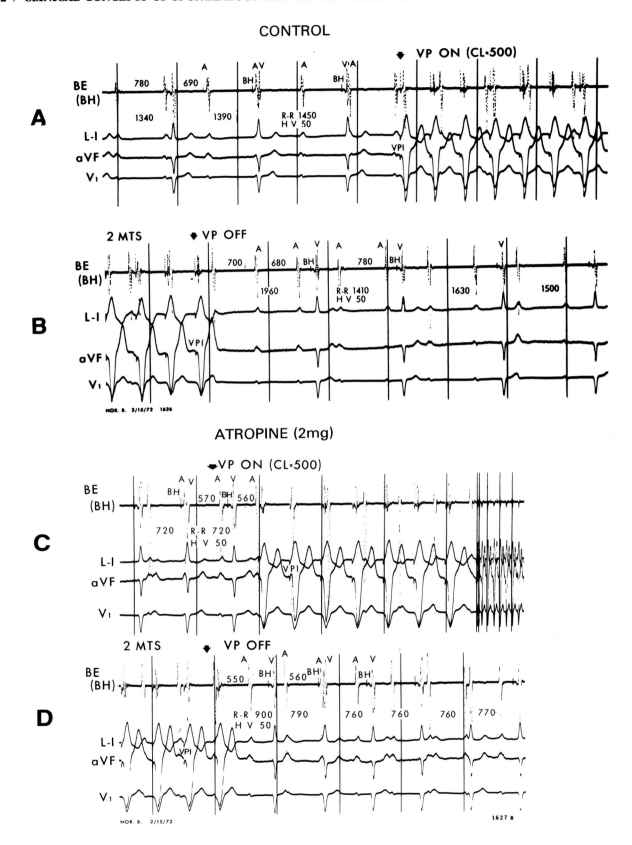

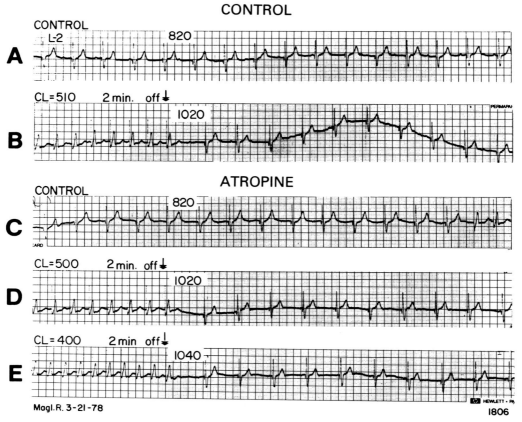

CONTROL

ATROPINE

Figure 15-13. Normal junctional recovery time in a patient with intra–His-bundle block and subsidiary pacemaker (same patient as in Fig. 15-9). This patient was not given a permanent pacemaker. (**A**) During control, the ventricular cycle length (*CL*) is 820 milliseconds. (**B**) Control junctional recovery time after VP at a CL of 510 milliseconds is only 1020 milliseconds. (**C**) After atropine administration, the ventricular CL remains unchanged (820 milliseconds). (**D**) and **E**) After atropine administration, the junctional recovery time is again normal at both the pacing CLs (500 and 400 milliseconds).

terparts without advanced AV block and inferior myocardial infarction, leading to a mortality rate that of more than three times that of the control group (37% versus 11%).[91–93] The long-term prognosis in patients discharged from the hospital, however, was only minimally different than that for the control group.[91–94]

Pre- and postthrombolytic therapy groups with inferior myocardial infarction have been compared, and the incidence for CHB has been found to be similar.[95]

Using electrophysiologic studies, the site of block

has been found to be supra-Hisian.[96] Early onset of AV block appears to be related to increased parasympathetic tone. Late onset of AV block usually does not respond to atropine, however, and alternative mechanisms have been suggested.[96–101] Anatomic studies have demonstrated the absence of major necrosis in the AV conducting system in numerous patients with inferior infarction.[96–100]

In inferior myocardial infarction, temporary pacing may be needed if the escape rate is low (i.e., equal to or

Figure 15-12. Normalization of junctional recovery time after atropine administration in a patient with complete heart block localized in the atrioventricular node. (**A** and **B**) Recordings during control, with onset (**A**) and termination (**B**) of ventricular pacing (*VP*). The junctional recovery time is 1960 milliseconds. (**C** and **D**) After atropine administration, the heart rate accelerates as the RR interval is shortened from 1450 to 720 milliseconds (**A** and **C**). In addition, the junctional recovery time is markedly shortened from 1960 to 900 milliseconds (**B** and **D**). (VPI, ventricular pacing impulse). (Narula OS, Narula JT: Junctional pacemakers in man: response to overdrive suppression with and without parasympathetic blockade. Circulation 1978;57:880. By permission of the American Heart Association.)

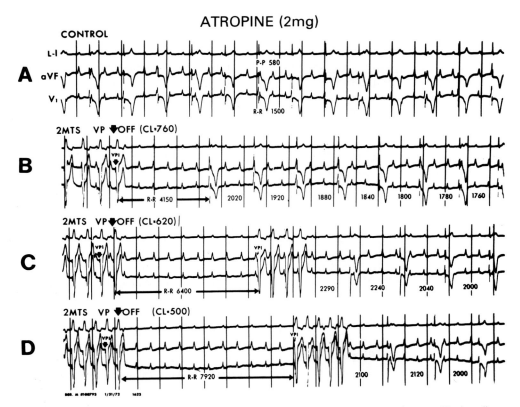

Figure 15-14. Severely prolonged junctional recovery time in a patient with intra–His-bundle complete heart block. The heart rate and the junctional recovery time remained unchanged after atropine administration. The junctional recovery time was directly related to the ventricular pacing (*VP*) rate and exceeded 7.9 seconds after VP at 120 beats/min (**D**).

less than 40 beats/minute) or hemodynamic compromise is observed. Permanent pacing may be needed in the few (i.e., equal to or less than 10%) patients whose block is localized to the His-bundle region.

ANTERIOR MYOCARDIAL INFARCTION. Complete heart block after anterior myocardial infarction is generally associated with ischemic damage to the bundle branches.[96–100] The resultant rhythm is usually less than 40 beats per minute and is generally unstable, requiring temporary (and permanent?) pacing in many patients.

Miscellaneous Entities Associated With Heart Block

Transient CHB may be inadvertently produced in patients undergoing cardiac catheterization. This appears most commonly in patients with left bundle branch block undergoing right heart catheterization but may rarely be observed in patients with right bundle branch block during left ventricular angiography.[102, 103] Most such events are temporary but temporary pacing may be needed.

Heart block is also occasionally observed after aortic and mitral valve replacement and after correction of a ventricular septal defect.[104, 105] Permanent pacing may be required in these patients but should be withheld as long as clinically feasible. Patients with aortic or mitral valve disease who have heavy calcification of the annulus may also develop heart block spontaneously.[106, 107]

There are a number of entities that are infrequently associated in varying degrees with the development of advanced heart block, such as Chagas' disease, Lyme disease, sarcoidosis, rheumatoid arthritis, hemochromatosis, neuromuscular disorders, and cardiac tumors.[108–115]

ATRIOVENTRICULAR BLOCK TRIGGERED BY ARRHYTHMIAS

All three degrees of AV block may be triggered by an atrial or ventricular arrhythmia. This is generally seen in patients with an abnormal or pathologic conduction system and is rare in those with normal AV conduction. Resetting of the AV node by an atrial or ventricular extrasystole may terminate or induce a sustained PR prolongation.[28] An atrial extrasystole, when conducted with a marked prolongation of the AH (or the PR) interval, may in turn prolong the AH time in the subsequent sinus impulses.[116] The partial compensatory atrial pause may not be long enough to permit complete recovery of the AV node. A sustained prolongation of the PR (AH) interval or induction of second-degree AV nodal block after a single extrasystole (atrial or ventricular) is seen only in patients with prolonged AV nodal refractoriness.

Concealed AV junctional extrasystoles may also simulate first- or second-degree AV block (type I or II) in the absence of true AV block.[18, 45, 117–120] Concealed His-bundle extrasystoles, when conducted in the retrograde direction to the atrium, may simulate ectopic atrial extrasystoles.[18, 32] In patients with concealed His-bundle extrasystoles, the HV time is usually prolonged and these patients generally exhibit second-degree block in the HPS, independent of the extrasystoles, either during sinus rhythm or with atrial pacing (Fig. 15-15).[48, 119] The presence of His-bundle extrasystoles is probably another manifestation of a disease process in the His bundle. Cases with pseudo–second-degree AV block should not be discounted because their prognosis may not be benign and may be similar to that of true Mobitz type II block.[32]

Paroxysmal AV block may be triggered after a properly timed premature atrial beat or rapid driving of the heart.[48, 121] The block is localized in the HPS—that is, proximal to the His bundle (upper His bundle), within the His bundle, or distal to the His bundle.[48] Paroxysmal AV block is a manifestation of pathologic HPS, indicated by a prolonged HV time or refractory period of the HPS and by the occurrence of spontaneous Mobitz type II AV block. The underlying mechanism may be related to (1) bradycardia-dependent AV block, which may result from a longer PP or HH interval noted after atrial stimulation; (2) supernormal conduction, which is responsible for maintenance of 1:1 AV conduction (atrial stimulation may lead to AV block due to an alteration in the self-perpetuating zone of supernormal conduction); and (3) the "fatigue" phenomenon encountered in the abnormal HPS.[18, 25, 50, 55, 121, 122] Thus far, fatigue phenomenon has not been seen in the normal conduction system.

ATRIOVENTRICULAR DELAYS WITH A NORMAL ELECTROCARDIOGRAM

The demonstration of a normal PR interval ($\leqq$ 200 milliseconds) and a narrow QRS complex does not exclude significant AV conduction defects.[18, 32] Lesions in the main His bundle, proximal to its bifurcation into bundle branches, do not prolong the QRS duration; also, the PR interval may not exceed 0.20 second. First-degree AV block may be noted, however, when marked intra–His-bundle delays (more than 40 milliseconds) are associated with PA (45 milliseconds) and AH (120 milliseconds) intervals at upper limits of normal. Intra–His-bundle conduction defects are frequently encountered in cases with a normal electrocardiogram and are diagnosed based on (1) a wide His-bundle deflection (more than 25 milliseconds); (2) split His-bundle potentials; and (3) a prolonged HV time with a narrow QRS complex. A mild degree of intraatrial conduction delays (PA more than 45 milliseconds) may exist despite a normal PR interval if both the AH (50 milliseconds) and HV (35 milliseconds) times are at lower limits of normal. Therefore, in a symptomatic patient, AV conduction defects cannot be ruled out based on a normal electrocardiogram.

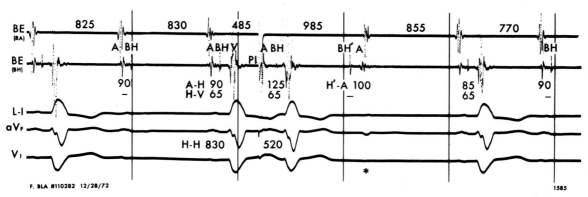

Figure 15-15. Association of concealed His-bundle extrasystoles with spontaneous second-degree atrioventricular block distal to the His bundle. In addition, in the conducted beats, the HV time is prolonged (65 milliseconds). The concealed His-bundle extrasystole (BN′) is blocked in anterograde direction but results in retrograde atrial depolarization, as indicated by the inverted P wave (*asterisk*) and the sequence of atrial depolarization (*fifth A wave*).

THERAPY

Each patient should be evaluated individually, and other possible causes of syncope besides conduction abnormalities must be excluded before implantation of a permanent pacemaker. Treatment and prognosis of a patient depend on many factors, including the patient's history, symptoms, electrocardiogram, and electrophysiologic factors. The following guidelines are suggested:

1. A significantly prolonged HV time in patients with syncope and without documented AV block is an indication for pacemaker therapy when other possible causes for syncope have been excluded.

2. Asymptomatic patients with first-degree delays in the HPS should be clinically followed-up at frequent intervals because of the possibility of a sudden development of type II block or CHB.

3. Irrespective of the site of block, symptomatic patients with second-degree AV block are candidates for therapy. Artificial pacing is indicated in patients with HPS lesions and when drugs are ineffective in AV nodal block. Asymptomatic patients with second-degree AV nodal block usually do not require therapy. Asymptomatic patients with second-degree HPS block (type I or II) should be considered for artificial pacing because these blocks are associated with sudden asystole and eventually progress to CHB.

4. Symptomatic patients with CHB, irrespective of the site of lesion, are candidates for pacemaker therapy. Asymptomatic patients with CHB localized in the AV node or in the His bundle may not require a permanent pacemaker if the subsidiary pacemaker has an adequate rate, is stable, and does not exhibit an abnormal suppression after overdrive pacing, both with and without autonomic blockade.[69] In addition, in asymptomatic patients with congenital CHB, Holter electrocardiographic recordings should be obtained to exclude other serious arrhythmias.[68]

5. Patients with CHB during acute myocardial infarction, irrespective of anterior or inferior wall infarction and a narrow or wide escape QRS complex, should be treated with a temporary pacemaker.[123]

References

1. Gaskell WH: On the rhythm of the heart of the frog and the nature of the action of the vagus nerve. Philos Trans R Soc Lond 1882;17:993.
2. Gaskell WH: On the innervation of the heart, with special reference to the heart of the tortoise. J Physiol (Lond) 1883; 4:43.
3. His W Jr: Die Thatigkeit des embroyonalen Herzens und deren Bedeutung für die Lehre von der Herzbewegung beim Erwachsenen. Arb Med Klin (Leipzig) 1893:14.
4. Kent AFS: Researches on the structure and function of the mammalian heart. J Physiol (Lond) 1893;15:233.
5. Tawara S: Das Reizleitungssystem des Saugetierherzens. Jena: Fischer, 1906.
6. Aschoff L, Tawara S: Die heutige Lahre von den pathologisch-anatomischen Grundlagen der Herzschwache. Jena: Fisher, 1906.
7. Einthoven W: L'electrocardiogramme. Arch Int Physiol 1906;4:132.
8. Erlanger J, Blackman JR: Further studies in the physiology of heart block in mammals: chronic auriculoventricular heart block in the dog. Heart 1909;1:177.
9. Eppinger H, Rotherberger J: Ueber die Folgen der Durchschneidung der Tawaraschen Schenkel des Reizleitungssystems. Z Klin Med 1910;70:1.
10. Mathewson GD: Lesions of the branches of the auriculoventricular bundle. Heart 1912;4:385.
11. Scherf D, Schookhoff C: Reizleitungsstorungen im Bundel: II. Mitteilung. Wien Arch Inn Med 1926;11:425.
12. Mahaim I: Les Maladies Organiques du Faisceau de His-Tawara. Paris: Masson et Cie, 1931.
13. Yater WM, Cornell VH, Clayton T: Auriculoventricular heart block due to bilateral bundle branch lesions. Arch Intern Med 1936;57:132.
14. Lenegre J: Bilateral bundle branch block. Cardiologia 1966; 48:134.
15. Lepeschkin E: The electrocardiographic diagnosis of bilateral bundle branch block in relation to heart block. Prog Cardiovasc Dis 1964;6:445.
16. Narula OS: His bundle electrocardiography and clinical electrophysiology. Philadelphia: FA Davis, 1975.
17. Narula OS, Cohen LS, Scherlag BJ, et al: Localization of A-V conduction defects in man by recording of the His bundle electrogram. Am J Cardiol 1970;25:228.
18. Narula OS: Conduction disorders in the A-V transmission system. In: Dreifus LS, Likoff W, eds. Cardiac arrhythmias, 25th Hahnemann Symposium. New York: Grune & Stratton, 1973:259.
19. Narula OS, Javier RP, Samet P, Maramba LC: Significance of His and left bundle recordings from the left heart in man. Circulation 1970;42:385.
20. Bekheit S, Morton P, Murtagh JG, Fletcher E: Comparison of sino-ventricular conduction in children and adults using bundle of His electrograms. Br Heart J 1973;35:507.
21. Damato AN, Gallagher JJ, Schnitzler RN, et al: Use of His bundle recordings in understanding A-V conduction disturbances. Bull NY Acad Med 1971;47:905.
22. Dhingra RC, Rosen KM, Rahimtoola SH: Normal conduction intervals and responses in sixty-one patients using His bundle recording and atrial pacing. Chest 1973;64:55.
23. Castellanos A, Castillo CA, Agha AS: Contribution of His bundle recording to the understanding of clinical arrhythmias. Am J Cardiol 1971;28:499.
24. Narula OS: Validation of His bundle electrograms: limitations of the catheter technique. In: Narula OS, ed. His bundle electrocardiography. Philadelphia: FA Davis, 1975:65.
25. Narula OS, Runge M: A-V nodal accommodation and fatigue

phenomenon in the His-Purkinje system. In: Wellens HJJ, Lie KI, Janse M, eds. The conduction system of the heart. Leiden: HE Stenfert Kroese, 1976:529.

26. Rosen KM: Evaluation of cardiac conduction in the cardiac catheterization laboratory. Am J Cardiol 1972;30:701.

27. Narula OS, Scherlag BJ, Samet P, Javier RP: Atrioventricular block: localization and classification by His bundle recordings. Am J Med 1971;50:146.

28. Narula OS: Atrioventricular block. In: Narula OS, ed. Cardiac arrhythmias: electrophysiology, diagnosis and management. Baltimore: Williams & Wilkins, 1979.

29. Peuch P, Grolleau R, Guimond C: Incidence of different types of A-V block and their localization by His bundle recordings. In: Wellens HJJ, Lie KI, Janse M, eds. The conduction system of the heart. Leiden: HE Stenfert Kroese, 1976: 467.

30. Haft JI, Levites R: Significance of first degree heart block (prolonged P-R interval) in bifascicular block. Am J Cardiol 1974;34:257.

31. Narula OS, Samet P: Significance of first degree AV block. Circulation 1971;43:772.

32. Narula OS: Current concepts of A-V block. In: Narula OS, ed. His bundle electrocardiography and clinical electrophysiology. Philadelphia: FA Davis, 1975:139.

33. Narula OS, Runge M, Samet P: Second degree Wenckebach type A-V block due to block within the atrium. Br Heart J 1972;34:1127.

34. Leier CV, Meacham JA, Schall SF: Prolonged atrial conduction: a major predisposing factor for the development of atrial flutter. Circulation 1978;57:213.

35. Wenckebach KF: Beitrage zur Kenntis der menschlichen Herztatigkeit. Arch Anat Physiol 1906:297.

36. Mobitz W: Über die unvollstandinge Storung der Erregungsüberleitung zwischen Vorhof und Kammer des menschlichen Herzens. Z Gesamte Exp Med 1924;41:180.

37. Wenckebach KF, Winterberg H: Die Unregelmassige Herztatigkeit. Leipzig: Wilhem Engelman, 1927:305.

38. Denes P, Levy L, Pick A, Rosen KM: The incidence of typical and atypical A-V Wenckebach periodicity. Am Heart J 1975; 88:26.

39. Friedman HS, Gomes JAC, Haft JI: An analysis of Wenckebach periodicity. J Electrocardiol 1975;8:307.

40. El-Sherif N, Aranda J, Befler B, Lazzara R: Atypical Wenckebach periodicity simulating Mobitz II A-V block. Br Heart J 1978;40:1376.

41. Halpern MS, Nau GJ, Levi RJ, et al: Wenckebach periods of alternate beats: clinical and experimental observation. Circulation 1973;48:41.

42. Amat-y-Leon F, Chuquimia R, Wu D, et al: Alternating Wenckebach periodicity: a common electrophysiologic response. Am J Cardiol 1975;36:757.

43. Castellanos A, Sung RJ, Mallon SM, et al: Effects of proximal intra-atrial Wenckebach on distal atrioventricular nodal and His-Purkinje block. With special reference to the theory of alternating Wenckebach periods. Am Heart J 1978;95:228.

44. Narula OS, Samet P: Wenckebach and Mobitz type II A-V blocks due to lesions within the His bundle and bundle branches. Circulation 1975;41:947.

45. Brodsky M, Wu D, Denes P, et al: Arrhythmias documented by 24 hour continuous electrocardiographic monitoring in 50 male medical students without apparent heart disease. Am J Cardiol 1977;39:390.

46. Meyles I, Kaplinsky E, Yahini J, et al: Wenckebach A-V block: a frequent feature following heavy physical training. Am Heart J 1974;90:426.

47. Young D, Eisenberg R, Fisch B, Fischer JD: Wenckebach AV block (Mobitz I) in children and young adults. Am J Cardiol 1977;40:393.

48. Narula OS: Wenckebach type I and type II atrioventricular block (revisited). Cardiovasc Clin 1974;6(3):137.

49. Langendorf R, Cohen H, Gozo EG: Observations on second degree atrioventricular block, including new criteria for the differential diagnosis between type I and type II block. Am J Cardiol 1972;29:111.

50. Goodfriend MA, Barold SS: Tachycardia dependent and bradycardia dependent Mobitz type II atrioventricular block within the bundle of His. Am J Cardiol 1974;33:908.

51. Rosen KM, Loeb HS, Gunnar RM, Rahimtoola SH: Mobitz type II block without bundle branch block. Circulation 1971;44:1111.

52. Yeh BK, Tao P, DeGuzman N: Mobitz type II A-V blocks as a manifestation of digitalis toxicity. J Electrocardiol 1972;5:74.

53. Langendorf R, Pick A: Atrioventricular block type II (Mobitz): its nature and clinical significance. Circulation 1968;38:819.

54. Scherlag BJ, El-Sherif N, Lazzara R: Experimental study of model for Mobitz type II and paroxysmal atrioventricular block. Am J Cardiol 1974;34:309.

55. Jonas EA, Kosowsky BD, Ramaswamy K: Complete His-Purkinje block produced by carotid sinus massage: report of a case. Circulation 1974;50:192.

56. Schuilenberg RM, Durrer D: Problems in recognition of conduction disturbances in the His bundle. Circulation 1975;51:68.

57. Narula OS, Scherlag BJ, Javier RP, et al: Analysis of the A-V conduction defect in complete heart block utilizing His bundle electrograms. Circulation 1970;41:437.

58. Guimond C, Puech P: Intra-His bundle blocks (102 cases). Eur J Cardiol 1976;4:481.

59. Rosen KM, Dhingra RC, Loeb HS, Rahimtoola SH: Chronic heart block in adults. Arch Intern Med 1973;131:663.

60. Gupta PK, Lichstein E, Chadda K: Electrophysiological features of complete A-V block within the His bundle. Br Heart J 1973;35:610.

61. Tricot R, Guerot C, Valere P, Coste A: Etude de la conduction auriculoventriculaire par enregisterment du faisceau de His dans 60 cas de block auriculoventriculaire. Arch Mal Coeur 1972;65:441.

62. Nasarallah AT, Gillette PC, Mullins CE: Congenital and surgical atrioventricular block within the His bundle. Am J Cardiol 1965;36:916.

63. Rosen KM, Mehta A, Rahimtoola SH, Miller RA: Sites of congenital and surgical heart block as defined by His bundle electrocardiography. Circulation 1971;44:833.

64. Anderson RH, Wenick ACG, Losekoot TG, Becker AE: Congenital complete heart block: developmental aspects. Circulation 1977;56:90.

65. Lev M, Silverman J, Fitzmaurice FM, et al: Lack of connection between the atria and the more peripheral conduction

system in congenital atrioventricular block. Am J Cardiol 1971;27:481.

66. Lev M, Candros H, Paul MH: Interruption of the atrioventricular bundle with congenital atrioventricular block. Circulation 1971;43:703.

67. Narula OS, Samet P: Effect of atropine and glucagon on A-V nodal and His bundle pacemakers in man. Circulation 1971;44(suppl):II.

68. Levy AM, Camm AJ, Keane JF: Multiple arrhythmias detected during nocturnal monitoring in patients with congenital complete heart block. Circulation 1977;55:247.

69. Narula OS, Narula JT: Junctional pacemakers in man: response to overdrive suppression with and without parasympathetic blockade. Circulation 1978;57:880.

70. Narula OS, Samet O: Predilection of elderly females for intra His bundle (BH) blocks. Circulation 1974;50(suppl):III.

71. Pomerance A: Pathological and clinical study of calcification of the mitral valve ring. J Clin Pathol 1970;23:354.

72. Kelly DT, Brodsky SJ, Mirowski M, et al: Bundle of His recordings in congenital heart block. Circulation 1972; 45:277.

73. Rosen KM: Catheter recordings of His bundle electrograms. Mod Concepts Cardiovasc Dis 1973;42:23.

74. McHenry MM, Cayler GG: Congenital complete heart block in newborns, infants, children and adults. Med Times 1969; 97:113.

75. Michaëlsson M, Engle MA: Congenital complete heart block: an international study of the natural history. Cardiovasc Clin 1972;4:85.

76. Scott JS, Maddison PJ, Taylor PV, Esscher E, Scott O, Skinner RP. Connective-tissue disease, antibodies to ribonucleoprotein, congenital heart block. N Engl J Med 1983;309:209.

77. Buyon JP, Ben-Chetrit E, Karp S, et al: Acquired congenital heart block: pattern of maternal antibody response to biochemically defined antigens of the SSA/Ro-SSB/La system in neonatal lupus. J Clin Invest 1989;84:627.

78. Ramsey-Goldman R, Hom D, Deng JS, et al: Anti-SS-A antibodies and fetal outcome in maternal systemic lupus erythematosus. Arthritis Rheum 1986;29:1269.

79. Schmidt KG, Ulmer HE, Silverman NH, Kleinman CS, Copel JA: Perinatal outcome of fetal complete atrioventricular block: a multicenter experience. J Am Coll Cardiol 1991; 17:1360.

80. Crawford D, Chapman M, Allan L: The assessment of persistent bradycardia in prenatal life. Br J Obstet Gynaecol 1985; 92:941.

81. Machado MVL, Tynan MJ, Curry PVL, Allan LD: Fetal complete heart block. Br Heart J 1988;60:512.

82. Pinsky WW, Gillette PC, Garson A, McNamara DG: Diagnosis, management, and long-term results of patients with congenital complete atrioventricular block. Pediatrics 1982; 69:728.

83. Karpawich PP, Gillette PC, Garson A, Hesslein PS, Porter C, McNamara DG: Congenital complete atrioventricular block: clinical and electrophysiologic predictors of need for pacemaker insertion. Am J Cardiol 1981;48:1098.

84. Esscher EF: Congenital complete heart block in adolescence and adult life. A follow-up study. Eur Heart J 1981; 2:281.

85. Lev M: Pathogenesis of congenital AV block. Prog Cardiovasc Dis 1972;15:145.

86. Carter JB, Blieden LC, Edwards JE: Congenital heart block. Anatomic correlations and review of literature. Arch Pathol 1974;97:51.

87. Bigger JT, Dresdale RN, Heissenbuttel RH, Weld FM, Wit AL: Ventricular arrhythmias in ischemic heart disease, mechanisms, prevalence, significance and management. Prog Cardiovasc Dis 1977;19:255.

88. Lamas GA, Muller JE, Turi ZG, et al: A simplified method to predict occurrence of complete heart block during acute myocardial infarction. Am J Cardiol 1986;57:1213.

89. Behar S, Zissman E, Zion M, et al: Prognostic significance of second-degree atrioventricular block in inferior wall acute myocardial infarction. Am J Cardiol 1993;72:831.

90. Barold SS: Narrow QRS Mobitz type II second-degree atrioventricular block in acute myocardial infarction: true or false? Am J Cardiol 1991;67:1291.

91. Friedberg CK, Cohen H, Donoso E: Advanced heart block as a complication of acute myocardial infarction: role of pacemaker therapy. Prog Cardiovasc Dis 1968;10:466.

92. Nicod P, Gilpin E, Dittrich H, Polikar R, Henning H, Ross J Jr: Long-term outcome in patients with inferior myocardial infarction and complete atrioventricular block. J Am Coll Cardiol 1988;12:589.

93. Behar S, Zissman E, Zion M, et al: Complete atrioventricular block complicating inferior acute wall myocardial infarction: short- and long-term prognosis. Am Heart J 1993; 125:1622.

94. Sugiura T, Iwasaka T, Takahashi N, et al: Factors associated with late onset of advanced atrioventricular block in acute Q wave inferior infarction. Am Heart J 1990;119:1008.

95. Clemmensen P, Bates ER, Califf RM, et al: Complete atrioventricular block complicating inferior wall acute myocardial infarction treated with reperfusion therapy. Am J Cardiol 1991;67:225.

96. Rosen KM, Loeb HS, Chuquimia R, Sinno MZ, Rahimtoola SH, Gunnar RM: Site of heart block in acute myocardial infarction. Circulation 1970;42:925.

97. Hunt D, Lie JT, Vohra J, Sloman G: Histopathology of heart block complicating acute myocardial infarction. Circulation 1973;48:1252.

98. Sutton R. Davies M: The conduction system in acute myocardial infarction complicated by heart block. Circulation 1968;38:987.

99. Hackel DB, Wagner G, Ratliff NB, Cies A, Estes EH Jr: Anatomic studies of the cardiac conducting system in acute myocardial infarction. Am Heart J 1972;83:77.

100. Bilbao FJ, Zabalza IE, Vilanova JR, Froufe J: Atrioventricular block in posterior acute myocardial infarction: a clinicopathologic correlation. Circulation 1987;75:733.

101. Wesley RC, Lerman BB, DiMarco JP, Berne RM, Belardinelli L: Mechanism of atropine-resistant atrioventricular block during inferior myocardial infarction: possible role of adenosine. J Am Coll Cardiol 1986;8:1232.

102. Gupta PK, Haft JI: Complete heart block complicating cardiac catheterization. Chest 1972;61:185.

103. Abernathy WS: Complete heart block caused by the Swan-Ganz catheterization. Chest 1974;65:349.

104. Sayed HM: Complete heart block following open heart surgery. J Cardiovasc Surg 1965;6:426.

105. Sondheimer HM, Izukawa T, Olley DM, et al: Conduction disturbances after total correction of tetralogy of Fallot. Am Heart J 92:278 1976.

106. Rytand DA, Lipsitch LS: Clinical aspects of calcification of mitral annulus. Arch Intern Med 1946;78:544.

107. Narula OS, Samet P: Predilection of elderly females for intra-His bundle (BH) blocks. Circulation 1974;50(Suppl):III.

108. Rosenbaum MB: Chagasic myocardiopathy. Prog Cardiovasc Dis 1964;7:199.

109. Fawcett FJ, Goldberg MJ: Heart block resulting from myocardial sarcoidosis. Br Heart J 1974;36:220.

110. Hoffman FG, Leight L: Complete AV block associated with rheumatoid disease. Am J Cardiol 1965;16:585.

111. Aronow WS, Meister L, Kent JR: AV block in familial hemochromatosis treated by permanent synchronous pacemaker. Arch Intern Med 1969;133:433.

112. Schellhammer PF, Engle M, Hagstrom JW: Histochemical studies of the myocardium and conduction system in acquired iron storage disease. Circulation 1967;35:631.

113. Perloff JK: Cardiac involvement in heredofamilial neuromyopathic diseases. Cardiovasc Clin 1972;4:33.

114. Prystowsky EN, Pritchett EL, Roses AD, Gallagher JJ: The natural history of conduction system disease in mytonic muscular dystrophy as determined by serial electrophysiologic studies. Circulation 1979;60:1360.

115. Burucúa JE, Bellido CA, Vazquez ST, Casas JG, et al: Mesothelioma of AV node. N Engl J Med 1973;289:753.

116. Billette J: Preceding His-atrial interval as a determinant of atrioventricular nodal conduction time in the human and rabbit heart. Am J Cardiol 1976;38:889.

117. Langendorf R, Mehlman JS: Blocked (nonconducted) A-V nodal premature systoles imitating first and second degree A-V block. Am Heart J 1947;34:500.

118. Rosen KM, Rahimtoola SH, Gunnar RM: Pseudo A-V block secondary to premature non-propagated His bundle depolarizations: documentation by His bundle electrocardiography. Circulation 1970;42:367.

119. Grolleau R, et al: Les depolarizations hisiennes ectopiques non propagees. Arch Mal Coeur 1972;65:1069.

120. Fisch C, Zipes DP, McHenry PL: Electrocardiographic manifestations of concealed junctional ectopic impulses. Circulation 1976;53:217.

121. Coumel P, Fabiato A, Waynberger M, et al: Bradycardia dependent atrioventricular block. J Electrocardiol 1977; 4:168.

122. Rosenbaum MB, Elizari MV, Levi RJ, et al: Paroxysmal atrioventricular block related to hypopolarization and spontaneous diastolic depolarization. Chest 1973;63:678.

123. Lie KI, Durrer D: Conduction disturbances in acute myocardial infarction. In: Narula OS, ed. Cardiac arrhythmias: electrophysiology, diagnosis and management. Baltimore: Williams & Wilkins, 1979.

Cardiac Arrhythmias, 3rd edition, edited by William J. Mandel.
J. B. Lippincott Company, Philadelphia © 1995.

16

Donald H. Singer • Howard C. Cohen

Aberrancy: Electrophysiologic Mechanisms and Electrocardiographic Correlates

The character of the QRS complex is a function of the sequence of ventricular activation, with alterations in QRS contour reflecting deviations from normal in the path of spread. This may occur in one of two general ways: (1) shift in the site of cardiac impulse formation to an ectopic focus in the ventricles or to certain types of atrioventricular (AV) nodal bypass tracts, or (2) altered ventricular spread of supraventricular impulses. The latter may result from congenital or acquired impairment of the conduction system. Alternatively, it may be functional in character, due to impulse conduction during periods of refractoriness.

Since their initial introduction by Lewis early in this century, the terms *aberrancy, aberration,* and *aberrant ventricular conduction* have come to be principally applied to functional intraventricular conduction disturbances, particularly those occurring in conjunction with changes in cycle length.[1–7] They apply with equal logic to the other types of intraventricular conduction disturbances, however. In this chapter and in the next chapter, aberrancy is considered within this broader context. Elec-

trophysiologic mechanisms and clinical aspects and implications of the different types of aberrancy are reviewed.

SPECIALIZED CONDUCTING SYSTEM OF THE HEART

It is convenient to consider the heart as consisting of two general types of tissue (Fig. 16-1A): (1) ordinary atrial and ventricular myocardium, which is responsible for contractile work and for inscription of the P and QRS deflections of the standard electrocardiogram; and (2) a chain of "specialized" tissues (see Chap. 2), including the sino-atrial node (SA) and atrio-ventricular (AV) nodes and the ramifications of the His-Purkinje system.[8–13] Atrioventricular nodal bypass tracts and specialized atrial internodal tracts also have been described.[9,14,15]

The specialized tissues are responsible for normal impulse formation and for the rapid and orderly distribution of the cardiac impulse from its site of origin to the remainder of the heart. Changes in impulse formation or conduction in the specialized tissues underlie changes in heart rate in response to changing physiologic conditions and also give rise to many dysrhythmias and conduction disturbances. The electrophysiologic characteristics of the

The work for this chapter was supported in part by grants-in-aid to Dr. Singer by the Reingold Estate, the Brinton Trust, the Deborah M. Cooley Charitable Trust.

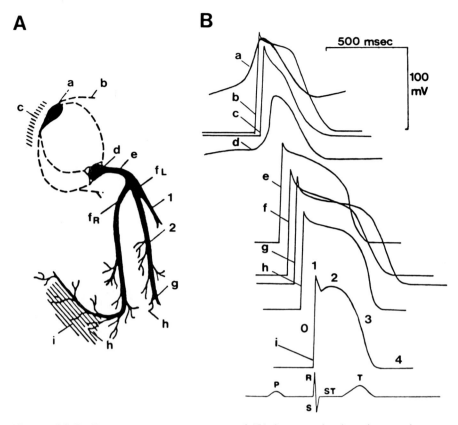

Figure 16-1. Diagrammatic representation of (**A**) the specialized cardiac conduction system, and (**B**) transmembrane potentials from ordinary and specialized tissues of the dog heart, illustrating differences in action-potential characteristics at the several sites. The relation between records indicates sequence of activation. A standard body-surface electrocardiogram (ECG) lead also is shown. Lowercase letters refer to a, sinoatrial node; b, Bachmann's bundle and other specialized atrial internodal tracts (see dashed lines connecting sinoatrial and atrioventricular nodes); c, ordinary atrial myocardium; d, atrioventricular node; e, bundle of His; f, bundle branches; f_R, right bundle branch; f_L, left bundle branch; anterior (1) and posterior (2) divisions of the left bundle branch; g, Purkinje fiber; h, terminal Purkinje fiber at Purkinje-ventricular muscle junction; and i, ventricular muscle. The phases of the ventricular muscle action potential (i) are designated by arabic numerals (0) through (4); the deflections of the surface ECG lead are identified by the letters P, R, S, and T.

specialized tissues are a principal determinant of aberrancy. Activity of the specialized tissues is not readily defined from the standard surface leads because of the small mass of these tissues relative to ordinary myocardium—a factor that has hampered electrocardiographic assessment of the mechanisms underlying the development of conduction disturbances, including aberrancy and dysrhythmias. The introduction of intracavitary catheter–recording techniques, which allow specialized tissue activity recording, has been helpful in this regard.[16,17]

Electrophysiologic Aspects

As noted, abnormalities of QRS configuration can result from several causes. This chapter focuses on the subgroup that was originally described by Lewis, for which the term aberrancy was coined—namely, altered QRS contour of supraventricular beats occurring in conjunction with cycle length–dependent changes in excitability and conduction.[1,2] Aberrancy represents one aspect of a larger group of cycle length–dependent conduction disturbances, which includes such varied entities as concealed conduction, supernormal conduction, and rate-related AV block.[3–5,16–22] Unidirectional block and reentrant excitation are in a sense also manifestations of this phenomenon.[3–7]

Aberrancy is considered in terms of cycle length dependency of the QRS changes, as proposed by Singer and Ten Eick.[23] The discussion is based on correlations between electrocardiographic material and transmembrane potential data from microelectrode studies on cardiac tissues from animals and from patients undergoing open-heart surgery.

Electrical Activity of Cardiac Cells

Understanding of the mechanisms of aberrancy depends on an understanding of the electrophysiologic basis of impulse formation and conduction in the heart and of the changes in these variables underlying development of conduction disturbances. A brief review of concepts follows. The reader is referred to other textbooks of physiology, reviews, and monographs on cardiac electrophysiology for a more comprehensive exposition.[24-38]

NORMAL TRANSMEMBRANE POTENTIAL

Insertion of a glass microelectrode into an excitable cell permits the recording of the potential difference between the cell interior and an indifferent electrode located outside the cell.[39] Figure 16-1B shows idealized transmembrane potential records from different parts of the heart with a simultaneously recorded surface electrocardiogram. The phases of the action potential are designated by Arabic numerals 0 to 4. During electric diastole (phase 4), the cell interior is negative, with respect to the extracellular fluid. In most normal cardiac fibers, including the ordinary atrial and ventricular myocardial cells, the potential difference during phase 4 remains constant until excitation occurs (resting potential), normally averaging between -85 and -95 mV. On excitation, the cell undergoes rapid depolarization (phase 0), with a transient reversal of polarity, followed by a gradual repolarization process (phases 1, 2, and 3), during which membrane potential is restored to resting levels. Comparison with the surface electrocardiogram shows that phases 0 and 1 of the ventricular action potential correspond to the R and S waves, and phases 2 and 3, to the ST segment and T wave, respectively (see Fig. 16-1B).

Transmembrane potentials recorded from ordinary and specialized fibers in different parts of the heart may differ from each other in several respects, including level of diastolic potential, action potential amplitude, maximum rate of depolarization during phase 0 ($\dot{V}_{max}$), time course of repolarization, and action potential duration (see Fig. 16-1B).[30] Differences in excitability, conductivity, and pacemaker capabilities (automaticity) also occur. Local differences in electrophysiologic properties within the His-Purkinje system may represent an important consideration with respect to aberrancy, as may local differences in response to a variety of physiologic and pharmacologic factors (e.g., temperature, pH, rate, pCO$_2$, hypoxia, isch-

emia, inorganic cations, and many important cardioactive ions and drugs, the latter including a variety of antiarrhythmic agents).[28,30,40-49]

Membrane Mechanisms

Cardiac electric activity originates in the movements of ions across the cell membrane.[24-27,30-38,50] Physiologic interventions and pharmacologic agents that influence impulse formation and conduction in the heart do so largely by their ability to influence these ionic currents.[28,30,32-34,36,40-48,49] Figure 16-2 depicts the important ionic currents thought to underlie inscription of the action potential in Purkinje fibers. A simplified explanation for specific phenomena pertinent to considerations of aberrancy follows.

Resting Membrane Potential

The potential difference across the cardiac cell membrane results from differences in ionic composition that exist between the cell interior and the extracellular fluid.[30-36,38,50,51] In the intracellular fluid, K$^+$ is the principal cation, and phosphate and the organic acid radicals are the dominant anions. The latter are largely polyvalent ions, often associated with proteins, to which the cell membrane is impermeable. In the extracellular fluid, Na$^+$ and Cl$^-$ predominate. To-and-fro transmembrane movements of these ions through specialized pores or channels in response to changes in electrochemical gradients constitute the membrane currents, which underlie inscription of the action potential.[30,31-36,38,50,52,53] The resting cell membrane is principally permeable to K$^+$ and relatively impermeable to the other intra- and extracellular ions.[30-33,35,36,38,50,51] The potential difference across the resting membrane is accordingly largely determined by the K$^+$ concentration gradient. Maintenance of the resting ionic and voltage differences is made possible by several factors: (1) the permeability characteristics *or* conductance (g) of the membrane to these ions, which in turn reflects availability of membrane channels for use by a given ion species; and (2) the operation of various ion pumps and exchange mechanisms,[54-59] including the well-documented energy-dependent Na$^+$–K$^+$ ion exchange pump,[57,58] which transports Na$^+$ out of and K$^+$ into the cell against their concentration gradients, and Na$^+$–Ca^{2+} exchange mechanism.[59]

Action Potential

DEPOLARIZATION. When the cell is stimulated and membrane potential is lowered to a critical level, the threshold potential (i.e., the potential at which a net inward current is just generated), a sequential series of changes in membrane ionic conductances and currents occurs, giving rise to in-

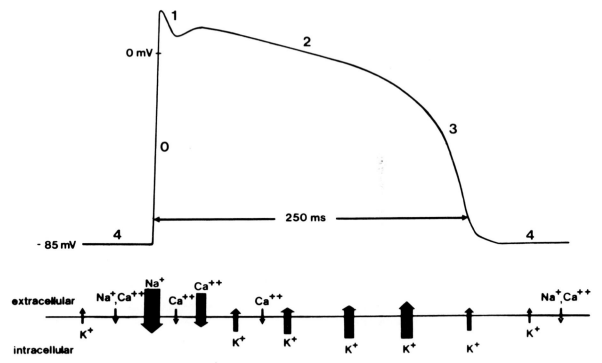

Figure 16-2. Schematic representation of the action potential in normal ventricle, depicting the direction, strength, and period of flow of the principal ionic currents underlying the action potential. Direction and size of the *arrows* indicate whether current is directed inward or outward and relative current strength, respectively, of the involved ion. The horizontal position of the arrow corresponds to the same moment in the time course of the action potential. (Modified from Ten Eick RE, Baumgarten CM, Singer DH: Ventricular dysrhythmia: membrane basis of currents, channels, gates, and cables. Prog Cardiovasc Dis 1981;24:157–188.)

scription of the action potential (see Fig. 16-2).[30–33,36,38,51] In normal well-polarized cardiac fibers, exclusive of SA and AV nodal cells, depolarization (phase 0) results primarily from an explosive increase in membrane conductance to Na^+ (g_{Na}) and in a rapid inward-directed ionic current carried by Na^+ (I_{Na}; the fast inward Na^+ current or fast inward current) in conjunction with opening of the fast Na^+ channels.[24,30–33,36–38,50,60] The ability of the membrane to undergo an increase in g_{Na} (i.e., to activate [open] closed Na^+ channels) is related to the level of membrane potential at excitation.[60,61] Generally, the availability of Na^+ channels is maximal, and a maximum fast inward Na^+ current is generated when membrane potential is at the level of the normal resting potential, (i.e., average: -85 to -95 mV). When membrane potential is less negative than normal, the maximum possible increase in Na^+ permeability and the magnitude of the fast Na^+ current are diminished because of decreased channel availability. If membrane potential is reduced to a low enough level, the increase in fast inward Na^+ current may be inadequate to produce a regenerative response or any response, so that the fiber becomes inexcitable.

The amplitude and $\dot{V}_{max}$ during phase 0 (the upstroke) are functions of the fast inward Na^+ current. It follows that they are dependent on the level of membrane potential. The amplitude of well-polarized Purkinje fiber action potentials averages up to 130 mV, and $\dot{V}_{max}$ is rapid; values of 500 to 1000 V/second are reported. Both decrease with decreases in the level of potential. Figure 16-3A shows the progressive decrease in amplitude and rising velocity of Purkinje fiber action potentials initiated at successively lower levels of membrane potential. The curves in Figure 16-3B depict the relation between membrane potential at excitation and $\dot{V}_{max}$ of the response for two ventricular myocardial cells. This relation, which was first defined for cardiac fibers by Weidman and subsequently confirmed by Hoffman and coworkers, is often termed the responsiveness relation, and the curve is termed the responsiveness curve.[61–63] Such curves are sometimes used as a rough measure of the availability of the Na^+ channels.

There is a second inward current in heart tissue that is activated only at low levels of membrane potential, about -35 to -45 mV.[34,64–68] This current is carried primarily by

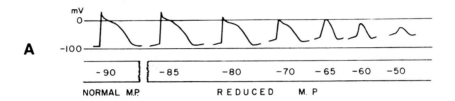

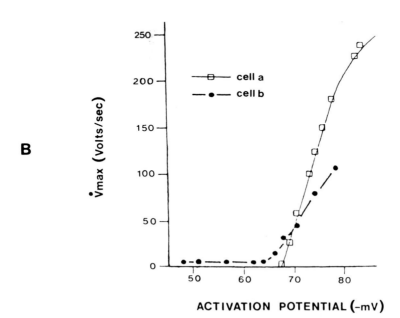

Figure 16-3. (**A**) Schematic representation of the changes in the characteristics of an action potential as it propagates from a normally polarized region into one in which membrane potential is progressively reduced. The level of membrane potential, in millivolts, is indicated for selected sites along the fiber. Action potentials initiated at these sites are shown. Note particularly the progressive diminution in amplitude and maximum rate of depolarization ($\dot{V}_{max}$) which would be expected to be accompanied by progressive slowing of conduction. Also note changes in time course of repolarization and in action-potential duration. (**B**) Curves depicting the relation between the level of membrane potential, in millivolts, at excitation (*abscissa*) and $\dot{V}_{max}$ in $\dot{V}$/sec (ordinate) of action potentials initiated in well-polarized human ventricular muscle cells (*a*, $E_m = -90$ mV; and *b*, $E_m = -79$ mV), from patient with coronary heart disease and ventricular aneurysm. Determinations were made on action potentials that were initiated at selected levels of membrane potential by stimulating the preparation at intervals during repolarization and during phase 4. The curve relating these variables is designated the "responsiveness curve." Note that the curve for cell *b* is shifted down and to the right in the mid-range of potential and up and to the left at the low end of the potential range.

Ca^{2+} ions and is of lower density (about 10%) than the fast Na^+ current. The calcium channel activates (turns on) and inactivates (turns off) more slowly than does the fast Na^+ channel, so that the current is slower and of longer duration than the fast Na^+ current.[68] Recovery from inactivation also takes longer. This current has accordingly been designated the slow inward current (I_{si}). Channels carrying the fast and slow inward currents are separable pharmacologically.[67,68] Tetrodotoxin (TTx) principally blocks

the fast inward Na^+ channel. Conversely, the slow channel is blocked by multivalent inorganic ions, including the divalent cations cadmium, cobalt, manganese, and nickel, as well as by many organic compounds such as the phenylalkylamines (D-600 and verapamil), the 1–4 dihydropyridines (nifedipine, nitrendipine) and the benzothiazepines (diltiazen). In normal well-polarized cells, the slow current influences the latter portion of the upstroke—more so in working myocardial cells than in Purkinje fibers—but contributes principally to phase 2 (the plateau) of repolarization. Depolarization of low-potential SA and AV nodal cells and muscle fibers in the AV-valve leaflets and coronary sinus appears largely to depend on the slow inward current.[34,69-75] It also becomes more important to the depolarization of non-nodal fibers, in which membrane potential is sufficiently reduced (i.e., to the vicinity of -45 mV or less).[33,34,36,76,77] This latter assumes particular importance when considering findings that specimens of experimentally infarcted dog heart[78-87] and human heart from patients with heart disease[33,88-107] contain large numbers of partially depolarized fibers.

The electrophysiologic properties of slow inward current–dependent fibers (slow response fibers) differ in many respects from those of fast inward current–dependent (fast response) fibers.[34,36,64,65,67] Generally, slow inward current–dependent fibers are characterized by (1) low diastolic potential, (2) low amplitude and slowly rising action potentials, (3) diminished excitability, (4) altered responsiveness, (5) prolongation of refractoriness, and (6) slow conduction. Such fibers also are often automatic. Indeed, even normally nonautomatic fibers may become capable of spontaneous impulse formation if membrane potential is reduced to levels at which the slow current becomes operative (Fig. 16-4*I*). Most of the peculiarities of SA and AV nodal activity appear explicable in terms of the behavior of the slow inward current.[30,34,36,67] This also appears to be true of at least some of the altered electrophysiologic properties of the partially depolarized cells in tissues from ischemic and diseased hearts.

REPOLARIZATION. Overall, the increase in the conductance (openings) of the fast inward Na^+ channels (activation process) that underlies depolarization is rapid, self-limited, of brief duration, and followed by inactivation. Most normal Na^+ channels inactivate quite rapidly. Findings of a slow component of the inactivation process suggest that a second smaller population of slowly inactivating channels also may be present.[108] Inactivation of the Na^+ channels and the consequent reduction in the fast inward Na^+ current usher in repolarization, a more prolonged (up to several hundred milliseconds) and complex process involving principally the Na^+, K^+, Ca^{2+} and Cl^- ions (see Fig. 16-2).[30,32,33,39,108-110] The specific ionic mechanisms underlying the several components of the repolarization process have not yet been completely clarified. Regardless, for repolarization to occur, there must be a decrease in intracellular positive charge. In Purkinje fibers, three clear-cut phases have been defined. The initial stage (phase 1) is rapid and results from the inactivation of the Na^+ current and the development of a transient outward current carried by K^+ and possibly also by Cl^- ions.[111,112] After phase 1, repolarization markedly slows (the plateau, or phase 2). There is an overall reduction in

membrane conductance during this phase, with the small currents that do occur more or less balancing each other, (i.e., the repolarizing effects of the inactivation of the inward Na^+ current and of activation of an outward K^+ current are counterbalanced by the depolarizing effects of the slow inward current).[36,109,110] The slowly inactivating component of the Na^+ current also is thought to contribute to the plateau phase.[112] The K^+ current, principally the delayed rectifier K^+ current (I_k), gradually increases in conjunction with time- and voltage-dependent increases in g_k.[33,109,110] This together with the waning of the inward currents results in an increasing net loss of positive charge, culminating in the stage of rapid repolarization (phase 3). As repolarization progresses, g_k becomes even larger, favoring additional K^+ efflux and further acceleration of repolarization. This is additionally favored by accumulation of the K^+ efflux in the restricted extracellular space, which further increases g_k, as well as by the activity of the electrogenic Na^+-K^+ pump.[113-115] Once membrane potential is restored to about -40 to -45 mV, it falls rapidly to resting values.

Impulse Formation

Excitation and inscription of the action potential result from a flow of sufficient depolarizing current across the cell membrane to rapidly lower (i.e., make less negative) the transmembrane potential to the threshold potential. The threshold potential differs for different cell types and is related to the level of maximum diastolic potential.[34,63,116] Excitatory (depolarizing) currents may be supplied by an external source or may arise spontaneously. Normally, they derive from local potential differences created by the propagating action potential. Certain cells, termed automatic, are capable of generating such currents spontaneously and thus may undergo self-excitation and initiate impulses spontaneously (automaticity).[30]

Automaticity normally results from the cyclic occurrence of spontaneous depolarization during phase 4 in the specialized tissues of the heart (see Fig. 16-1*B*; SA nodal cell potential).[30,33,35,36] Cells with the fastest rates of spontaneous diastolic (phase 4) depolarization (normally those in the SA node) serve as the primary pacemaker; the remainder act as latent pacemakers. Ordinarily, probably only SA nodal cells actually exhibit phase 4 depolarization (see Fig. 16-1*B*), with latent (escape) pacemakers developing the requisite changes in response to factors such as sinus slowing or AV block.

Spontaneous impulse formation can result from causes other than slow diastolic depolarization of specialized automatic cells. Because such alternate causes are not thought to be present under normal physiologic conditions, they are considered abnormal causes of automaticity, and the resultant spontaneous activity is called ab-

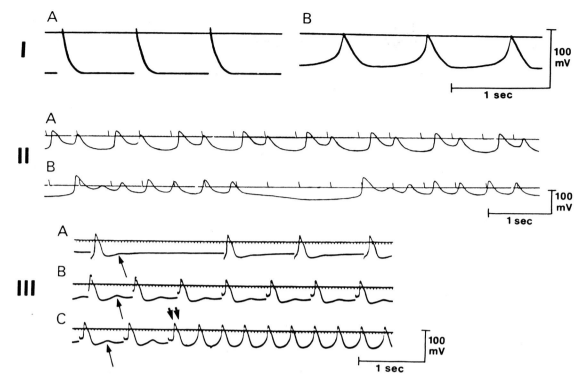

Figure 16-4. Transmembrane potentials recorded from specimens of human atrium (*Panels I, III*) and ventricle (*Panel II*) to show different types of abnormal automaticity in cardiac tissues from a patient with heart disease. *Panel I*: (**A**) Transmembrane potentials from well-polarized "fast response," and (**B**) low-potential "slow response" fibers in human right atrial appendage. Maximum diastolic potential (and amplitude) exhibited by cells A and B are −72 mV (80 mV) and 55 mV (−55 mV), respectively. Contrast the large-amplitude rapidly rising potentials elicited from the well-polarized fiber with the low-amplitude slowly rising potentials from the depolarized cell. Also, note that the slow-response cell begins to spontaneously depolarize as soon as repolarization is complete; that is, it has become automatic (depolarization induced automaticity). *Panel II*: Transmembrane potentials from partially depolarized, spontaneously active human papillary muscle cell from a patient with rheumatic heart disease complicated by atrial fibrillation, high-grade ventricular ectopy, and variable-rate–dependent conduction disturbance. In *Panel II, row A*, repolarization of each basic automatic beat is interrupted by a single early afterdepolarization-type oscillation, giving rise to a bigeminal pattern. In *Panel II, row B*, each basic beat is interrupted by a small oscillation, followed by five larger repetitive oscillations, with resultant marked prolongation of repolarization. The runs are terminated by low-amplitude oscillation, which further delays completion of repolarization of the basic beats. *Panel III*: Induction of late afterdepolarization-type oscillations and triggered activity in an initially quiescent specimen of human atrium. The first oscillation in each panel is indicated by *arrows. Rows A and B* and the initial part of *Row C* show development of oscillations in conjunction with stimulation at increasing rates. Note the gradual increase in oscillation amplitude with rate increases. Eventually, oscillations reached threshold, and repetitive triggered activity ensued (mid-portion, [**C**]), which persisted even after discontinuation of stimulation. Although each of the examples shown occurred in partially depolarized cells, similar phenomena have been observed in well-polarized cells. (Modified from Singer DH, Baumgarten CM, Ten Eick RE: Cellular electrophysiology of ventricular and other dysrhythmias: studies on diseased and ischemic heart. Prog Cardiovasc Dis 1981;24:97–156.)

normal automaticity.[117, 118] The term encompasses several diverse phenomena. Spontaneously occurring, cyclic, pacemaker-like oscillations of the diastolic potential unrelated to a prior initiating event represent one major grouping. This type of activity is largely a phenomenon of depressed, partially depolarized fibers, in which membrane potential has been reduced to levels at which the slow inward current becomes operative: hence the designation depolarization-induced automaticity. It appears to be evocable in most cells, including ordinary atrial and ventricular myocardial cells, by lowering the diastolic potential.[119–121] The phenomenon appears to be common in specimens of ischemic and diseased heart.[31, 78–101, 104–107] The records in Figure 16-4*I*, showing a partially depolarized, automatic, human atrial myocardial cell, are representative.

There are other types of oscillations that depend on the occurrence of a prior initiating action potential for their existence (i.e., triggered automaticity).[122, 123] They may originate during or after completion of repolarization of the initiating event (see Fig. 16-4*II* and *III*). These oscillations have been accorded many designations, of which the most widely used is that proposed by Cranefield, who referred to them as "early" and "delayed" afterdepolarizations, respectively.[34] Early afterdepolarizations most commonly interrupt phase 2 of repolarization at plateau-level potentials of −20 to −25 mV but also may occur during phase 3. They prolong repolarization and refractoriness, sometimes for many seconds (see Fig. 16-4*II*). Conversely, delayed afterdepolarizations (see Fig. 16-4*III*) occur during phase 4 at more or less normal (−70 to −85 Mv) as well as at reduced levels of diastolic potential. Afterdepolarizations that reach thresholds result in initiation of triggered rhythms (see Fig. 16-4*III*), of which the best known are those due to the digitalis glycosides.[122, 123]

Slow diastolic (phase 4) depolarization results from a progressive net increase in intracellular positive charge.[32–36] Specific membrane mechanisms underlying the inscription of the pacemaker potential in S-A nodal and subsidiary pacemaker cells are not entirely clarified, however.[33, 35, 36, 124] Phase 4 depolarization theoretically could result from (1) a time-dependent decrease in outward (K^+) current in the presence of steady background inward current; (2) a time-dependent increase in an inward current (e.g., the pacemaker current [I_f] carried by Na^+ in the present of a steady background outward current); or (3) combinations thereof.[125–128] A slowly decreasing I_k appears to be involved, as does an interaction between I_k and the inward Ca^{2+} current.[129, 130] The pacemaker current (I_f), which operates in the voltage range of −90 to −50 mV, appears to best fit the activity of normal Purkinje fibers. Because the maximum diastolic potential of SA nodal cells is generally −65 mV or lower, the contribution of this current to sinus automaticity is equivocal. An inward Ca^{2+} appears to be more important in this regard.[131] The ionic mechanisms underlying the pacemaker potential are even less well-defined for the specialized atrial tissues than for the sinus node. There is evidence suggesting that the pacemaker potential in these cells may result principally from a hyperpolarization-activated time- and voltage-dependent I_f current, with contributions by a gradually increasing I_{si} and a declining I_k.[132] Automaticity of partially depolarized myocardial cells and of afterdepolarization-type oscillations is only poorly understood. With respect to the former, a pacemaker current carried by Na^+ and similar to the I_f current in Purkinje fibers has been reported in both atrial

and ventricular myocardial cells but is unlikely to be operative normally.[133–135] Insofar as afterdepolarizations are concerned, different types appear to depend on different mechanisms. Some have identified a transient inward current (I_{ii}) as the cause of delayed afterdepolarizations.[136, 137] The Na^+–Ca^{2+} exchange mechanism also has been implicated as the source of the oscillatory current.[138] Irrespective of type, however, delayed afterdepolarizations are associated with an overload of free intracellular Ca^{2+}.[123] In contrast, the occurrence of early afterdepolarizations is generally associated with prolongation of the early stages of repolarization due to a decrease in outward K^+ current or to an increase in the inward current carried by Ca^{2+} and possibly also by Na^{2+}.[123]

Conduction

Conduction of the cardiac impulse (action potential) is a highly complex and only imperfectly understood phenomenon. A number of recent textbooks,[24, 25, 27] as well as monographs and reviews by Jack and coworkers, Fozzard, Spach and Kootsey, and Cranefield[34, 37, 139–141] highlight the complexities. Conduction is considered to result from sequential depolarization of contiguous areas of cell membrane by local currents, which arise as a result of potential differences between adjacent segments of resting (polarized) and active (depolarized) membrane and flow from cell to cell by low-resistance electric connections. The rate at which this process proceeds (i.e., conduction velocity) depends on many interrelated variables including the fast and slow inward currents and their determinants, excitability, passive cable properties of cardiac fibers, and fiber diameter and geometry.

INWARD CURRENTS AND CONDUCTION. For normal well-polarized cardiac cells outside the SA and AV nodes, the ability of the propagating action potential to excite adjacent regions of resting membrane and therefore to conduct, as well as the rate of impulse spread (conduction velocity), critically depend on the fast inward Na^+ current and $\dot{V}_{max}$, which serves as an indirect measure of this current. This relation is particularly clear-cut for cells in the His-Purkinje system, which have relatively few slow inward current channels and therefore a small slow inward current. As previously noted, the magnitude of the inward current and $\dot{V}_{max}$ are in turn related to membrane potential at excitation. It follows that conduction velocity also depends on the membrane potential of cells in the path of impulse spread.[37, 61–63, 140, 142]

Other factors being equal, the fast inward Na^+ current, $\dot{V}_{max}$, and conduction velocity are optimal in fibers in which membrane potential is at or near the level of the normal resting potential, about −85 to −95 mV. Reduction in membrane potential is associated with a decrease in the fast inward Na^+ current and $\dot{V}_{max}$ and with slowing of conduction. Conduction impairment is voltage-dependent, with significant slowing usually first appearing at potential levels of less than -70 to -65 mV and failure of conduction at -50 mV or below. At such low levels of potential, the fast Na^+ current is largely inactivated and depolarization becomes increasingly slow current–dependent. Dependence of depolarization on the slow inward current is the norm in the low-potential cells of the SA and AV nodes, regions known for slow conduction. Figure 16-3A shows a schematic representation of the deterioration of the action potential during propagation from a normally polarized region into one that is progressively more depolarized. Spread into the partially depolarized region is depicted as resulting in progressive reduction of amplitude and rising velocity, changes that would be expected to be associated with increasingly marked slowing of conduction.

Conduction also is influenced by the character of the relation between membrane potential at excitation and the magnitude of the inward current, defined in terms of the $\dot{V}_{max}$ of responses elicited at that potential level (responsiveness). Changes in the relation, such that the normal curve (see Fig. 16-3B, cell *a* curve) is shifted down and to the right (see Fig.16-3B, cell *b* curve), depress responsiveness and slow conduction because the availability of the fast inward Na^+ current, defined in terms of $\dot{V}_{max}$ of evoked responses, would be decreased at any given potential relative to normal. Because such a shift would predispose to slowing of conduction at all levels of potential, it may be expected to (1) accentuate conduction disturbances resulting from reduction in membrane potential, and (2) facilitate development of conduction disturbances at more normal (i.e., more negative levels of potential than usual). Changes in the relation such that the curve shifts up and to the left in the high and middle ranges of potential exert the opposite effect. Paradoxically, leftward shifts in the low range of potential (see Fig. 16-3B, cell *b* curve) may predispose to the development of conduction disturbances because they would facilitate generation of slowly rising slow-conducting responses at potential levels that would otherwise be too low to support any activity.

Numerous cardioactive drugs, including many of the standard antiarrhythmic agents, influence conduction by virtue of their effects on responsiveness.[30,34,40–49] Depressant effects of quinidine and procainamide result primarily from their action in displacing the curve down and to the right.[143,144] Ischemia and disease also may affect this relation.[38,78,79,83,86,87,106,145–147] Studies on infarcted dog ventricle and on multicellular specimens of diseased human heart indicate that the curve for at least some cells appears to be shifted down and to the right in the upper and middle regions of the voltage range *and* up and to the left at the low end of the range (see Fig. 16-3B, cell *b* curve).[38,78,79,83,86,106]

The latter most probably reflects activation of the slow inward current at low potentials. Regardless, both types of shift would be expected to predispose to an increase in conduction disturbances and aberrancy. Paradoxically, studies on isolated human atrial and ventricular myocytes have not demonstrated alterations in the voltage dependence of the fast inward Na^+ current similar to those noted in multicellular preparations.[148–150] This may simply be due to diseased cells being less robust than normal cells and being destroyed by the enzymatic cell separation process. Cell recovery in the well-oxygenated superfusate represents a second possible cause for the discrepancy.[148]

EXCITABILITY AND CONDUCTION. Conduction also depends on membrane excitability.[37,139,151–153] The term "excitability" refers to the current required to lower membrane potential from levels extant at the moment of stimulation to the threshold potential and to initiate an action potential. It also is a complex function and depends on numerous factors, including the level of membrane potential and the threshold potential. A decrease in excitability is synonymous with an increase in current requirements for excitation and other factors being equal, would be expected to be associated with slowing of conduction. Conversely, increases in excitability (i.e., decreased current requirements for excitation) have the opposite effect. Speeding of conduction in response to moderate depolarization has been explained on this basis.[151,152] In a similar vein, cycle length–dependent changes in excitability of depressed cells in the His-Purkinje system have been suggested as a possible cause of intermittent bundle branch block.[154] Several physiologic and pharmacologic factors that influence conduction are thought to do so (at least partly) by their effects on excitability. Potassium is an example, with increases in extracellular K^+ between 2.7 to 4 mmol being associated with increases in excitability and in conduction velocity. Further increases in extracellular K^+ to more than 7 mmol depress excitability and conduction.[152] Depressant effects on conduction of lidocaine and procainamide may be related to their action in decreasing excitability.[155,156] Ischemia and disease also may depress excitability and influence conduction on this basis.

CABLE PROPERTIES AND CONDUCTION. Cardiac fibers are considered to exhibit many of the electric properties characteristic of a linear coaxial cable.[24,25,27,30,37,38,139,157] Individual cells are electrically coupled by low-resistance specializations of the membrane, the nexus or gap junction,[158,159] which facilitate cell-to-cell current flow and the creation of functionally long cables. The electric properties associated with such a structure, termed "passive" or "cable" properties, include membrane resistance (the reciprocal of conduction) and capacitance *and* internal longitudinal resistance (the sum of the resistance of the cytoplasm and of the gap junction). They govern cell-to-cell current spread and are therefore also principal determinants of conduction.[24,37,38,139,157,160] Modifications of these parameters can profoundly influence conduction. Much attention has focused on the gap junction, a unit consisting of a parallel array of closely packed ion channels.[159] Factors—principally H^+, Ca^{2+}, and the transjunctional and transmembrane voltages—that regulate the opening and closing of the gap junctional channels (gating processes), are probably of major import with respect to considerations of conduction and the development of conduction disturbances.

There is evidence suggesting drug- and disease-related changes in the cable properties may contribute to conduction disturbances in a clinical setting. Findings that toxic doses of ouabain, acidosis, decreases in intracellular pH, and hypoxia and simulated ischemia (all of which are associated with conduction abnormalities in vivo) appear to increase gap-junction resistance are consistent with this possibility.[161–166] Simulation studies suggest that sufficient increases in internal resistance could result in complete conduction block due to electric uncoupling.[167] There is also evidence of electric uncoupling in diseased human ventricular myocardium.[106] The exact mechanism underlying electric uncoupling is uncertain but appears to involve increases in ionized Ca^{2+} in the cytosol, as evidenced by findings that internal resistance increases when calcium is injected intracellularly.[168] Many interventions that magnify hypoxia- or ischemia-induced increases in internal resistance (e.g., increases in frequency of stimulation) also increase intracellular Ca^{2+}.[169]

CONDUCTION DISTURBANCES IN THE HEART

Cardiac conduction disturbances are attributable to a multiplicity of causes. Congenital or acquired abnormalities of the specialized tissues and their actual disruption by disease are well known.[8,170–175] In normal heart, probably the most common cause is impulse propagation in fibers in which membrane potential is low. The electrophysiologic properties of partially depolarized slow-response fibers and the changes in ischemic and diseased ventricle appear to be pertinent, with respect to the increased incidence of aberrancy in patients with heart disease.[34,38,67,68,83,85–87,89,91,94–100,105–107] Alterations in excitability and in the cable properties of cardiac fibers due to such factors as (1) drugs and disease, (2) peculiarities of fiber geometry, and (3) temporal and spatial convergence of impulses also are important.[37,38,106,139,143,151,157,160,176,177] This discussion focuses on the membrane potential–dependence of conduction disturbances. Conduction distur-

bances due to low potential can occur anywhere in the heart. Numerous electrocardiographic patterns are possible, the particular pattern in a given instance reflecting the location of the depolarized fibers and the extent of membrane depolarization. For example, if the site of involvement is the His bundle, AV block may be expected to ensue. Conversely, if the depolarized cells are located below the bifurcation, conduction disturbances would be more likely to be manifest as various types of intraventricular conduction defects.

The timing of the reduction in membrane potential also is critical, with respect to the nature of a conduction disturbance and its electrocardiographic representation. Two general categories can be defined. First and most common, low potential is associated with incomplete repolarization. Figure 16-5A shows a Purkinje fiber action potential with five premature responses initiated at different times during repolarization. The changes in action potential characteristics and conduction during repolarization combined with accompanying changes in threshold current requirements (excitability; see Fig. 16-5B) and in threshold potential comprise what is usually defined as refractoriness. It can be seen in Figure 16-5A that stimulation does not result in an active response until membrane potential has been restored to the vicinity of − 50 mV. The earliest response (a) thus defines the end of the absolute refractory period and the beginning of the relative refractory period. The earliest responses (a and b) are, however, so small and slowly rising that they may not propagate (local or graded responses). The first propagated impulse (c) defines the end of the effective refractory period (i.e., the period during which a propagated response does not occur). Amplitude, $\dot{V}_{max}$, and duration of responses initiated at successively more negative levels of membrane potential increase progressively, with associated improvement in conduction. An optimal response (e) occurs only after restoration of membrane potential to − 85 to − 95mV. Conduction disturbances resulting from impulse spread in incompletely repolarized fibers are common in both the normal and diseased heart (e.g., the altered conduction of premature responses during phase 3 of repolarization).[62,142,178] Nonconducted and aberrantly conducted atrial premature complexes in Figure 16-5C represent the electrocardiographic equivalents.

The foregoing presumes that the recovery of excitability and conduction (i.e., functional recovery) is strictly voltage-dependent and parallels repolarization. This had been thought to be more or less true for most normal cardiac fibers, except nodal cells, in which functional recovery lags behind completion of repolarization (i.e., the recovery process exhibits time- and voltage-dependence).[30,34,67,70,72,73] Newer findings indicate that this is true even for non-nodal fibers.[179,180] The disparity is normally small, however, becoming appreciable only in cells with

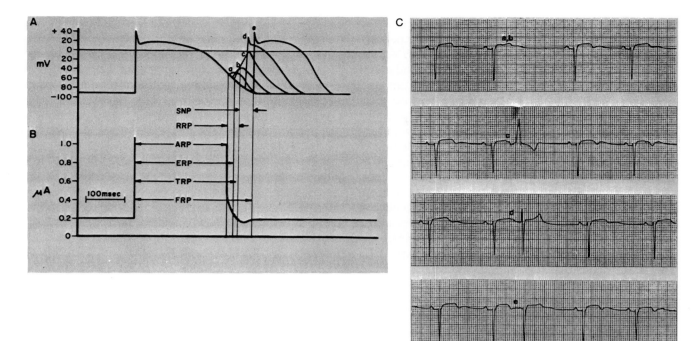

Figure 16-5. (**A**) Schematic representation of normal Purkinje fiber transmembrane action potential and of the responses elicited by premature stimulation at selected times during repolarization. The level of the threshold potential also is shown. Note that the amplitude and maximum rate of depolarization (V_{max}) of the responses are related to the level of membrane potential at the time of stimulation. The earliest responses (*a* and *b*) arise at such low levels of membrane potential and are so small and slowly rising that they cannot propagate (graded or local responses). Subsequent responses (*b–e*) show progressive increase in amplitude, velocity, and duration until completion of repolarization. The earliest propagated response (*c*) defines the end of the effective refractory period (ERP). The first normal response (*e*) defines the end of the full recovery time (FRT). Although response (*d*) arises during the end of supernormal period (SNP) of excitability, it is still smaller and more slowly rising than response (*e*). (**B**) Schematic representation of the usual relationship between membrane potential and cathodal excitability. Threshold-current requirements are indicated in microamperes (μA). The fiber becomes inexcitable coincident with the inscription of phase 0 of the action potential. Recovery of excitability, indicated by changes in threshold, progresses slowly during phase 3. The diagram also illustrates the approximate duration of the absolute refractory period (ARP), the ERP, relative refractory period (RRP), total refractory period (TRP), FRT, and the period of SNP. Vertical lines, which connect parts *A* and *B*, indicate the relation between the time course of repolarization and refractoriness and excitability. Threshold potential, which becomes infinite in conjunction with rapid depolarization, is also restored to normal values during repolarization (not shown). (**C**) Four V_1 rhythm strips with isolated atrial premature beats initiated at different times during repolarization. The record represents an electrocardiographic "analog" of the trace in *A*, atrial premature beats *a, b, c, d,* and *e*, corresponding to similarly labeled responses in *A*. The earliest atrial premature beats (*a* and *b*) reach the atrioventricular conducting system so early during repolarization that they either do not conduct at all or else give rise to locally propagated responses, which would be appreciated as a nonconducted atrial premature beat. The next two atrial premature beats (*c* and *d*) reach the conducting system somewhat later during recovery and conduct to the ventricles. Conduction is still depressed, however, as evidenced by the prolonged PR and altered (aberrant) QRS contour. Beat *e* is inscribed after completion of repolarization and conducts normally.

diminished levels of diastolic potential. The disparity between voltage and functional recovery has been termed postrepolarization refractoriness.[181]

Differences between recovery of excitability in normal and low-potential fibers may be explicable in terms of differences in ionic mechanisms underlying depolariza-

tion. Depolarization of most normal well-polarized fibers depends on the activation of the fast inward Na^+ channels. Depolarization in turn inactivates the channels, with resultant inexcitability. Removal of inactivation must occur before the channel can again respond. By the time repolarization has progressed to about -40 to $-50mV$, a sufficient number of channels have recovered to allow the cell to respond (end of the absolute refractory period). Normally, by the time the cell has repolarized to -85 to -95 mV, recovery of the fast Na$^+$ channels—and therefore of excitability and conduction—is virtually complete. Conversely, depolarization of normally low-potential fibers in the SA and AV nodes and in the AV-valve leaflet and coronary sinus largely depends on the slow inward current.[34,36,69–75] This also holds true to a variable degree for partially depolarized fibers in experimentally infarcted and chronically diseased heart muscle.[34,38,42,83,85–87,93–95,97–100,104–107] Recovery of slow channels occurs more slowly than that of the fast channels, so that refractoriness may outlast completion of repolarization by up to hundreds of milliseconds. Figure 16-6*I* and *II*

compares recovery in well-polarized and partially depolarized right bundle branch fibers. In the well-polarized fiber, voltage and functional recovery approximate each other. In contrast, in the partially depolarized fiber, recovery is depicted as exhibiting marked time-dependency. Full functional recovery does not occur until almost middiastole. Findings of Na$^+$ channels with slow recovery from inactivation suggest that under some circumstances, significant postrepolarization refractoriness can occur, even in well-polarized cells.[108] Exposure to certain drugs that slow recovery of the fast N$^+$ channels also may induce this phenomenon.[40,48,49,182–184] Figure 16-6*III*, showing examples of the phenomenon in reasonably well-polarized human ventricular muscle cell from a patient with ventricular dysrhythmia, suggests that disease may exert simi-

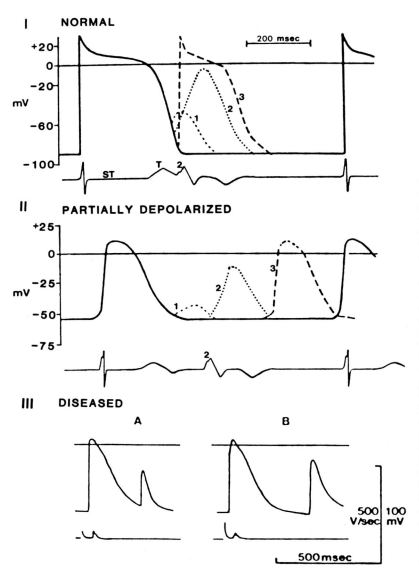

Figure 16-6. Schematic representation of transmembrane potentials and simultaneously recorded bipolar electrograms from normal (**Panel I**) and partially depolarized (**Panel II**) canine Purkinje fibers to show time-dependent prolongation of refractoriness in the latter. Responses *1, 2,* and *3* result from premature stimulation at selected times during the cycle. Response *1* is the earliest that could be elicited and defines the end of the "absolute" refractory period; *2* is the latest response, exhibiting sufficient reduction in amplitude and $\dot{V}_{max}$ and resulting in an altered (aberrant) QRS contour in the electrogram; and *3* is the earliest normally configured response, defining the time at which full recovery was achieved. In the normal fiber, recovery of excitability and conduction and disappearance of refractoriness virtually coincide with completion of repolarization. Conversely, in the partially depolarized fiber, refractoriness appears to outlast repolarization—in this instance, to a quite marked degree. Time-dependent prolongation of refractoriness would increase the predisposition to aberration of even late extrasystoles. (**Panel III**) An example of post repolarization refractoriness in a specimen of human papillary muscle obtained from a patient with chronic rheumatic heart disease complicated by congestive failure and high-grade atrial and ventricular ectopy, the former exhibiting both right and left bundle-branch block aberrancy. (Modified from Singer DH, Baumgarten CM, Ten Eick RE: Cellular electrophysiology of ventricular and other dysrhythmias: studies on diseased and ischemic heart. Prog Cardiovasc Dis 1981;24:97–156.)

lar effects. The changes in question would predispose to aberrant conduction of premature responses initiated during the latter stages of repolarization during diastole.

Second, membrane potential also may be reduced during electric diastole (phase 4) because of lowering of resting potential or spontaneous diastolic depolarization of automatic cells. As may be predicted from the responsiveness curves in Figure 16-3B, reduction in diastolic potential results in changes in action potential characteristics and conduction similar to those noted during repolarization.[61,63,142] Impulse propagation in fibers with low diastolic potential could therefore be associated with slow conduction and aberrancy.

Low levels of diastolic potential (less than −75 to −80 mV) do not occur normally except in SA and AV nodal cells, where they presumably contribute to slow conduction.[30,34] In contrast, low resting potential is commonly observed in experimentally infarcted hearts and in diseased human heart.[83,85–102,104–107] Figure 16-7 shows examples of reduced diastolic potential and slow conduction in human ventricle. Many physiologic and pharmacologic interventions to which the heart may be exposed (including stretch, ischemia, hypoxia, changes in pH, altered ionic milieu, and high concentrations of antiarrhythmic agents) also act to lower resting potential and may cause conduction disturbances on this basis.[30–38,40–47] Hyperkalemia-induced intra-atrial and intraventricular conduction disturbances represent a well-documented example.

Conversely, phase 4 depolarization of automatic cells occurs even in normal heart. Automaticity of SA nodal cells is best known and may contribute to slow conduction in this tissue. Experiments on Purkinje fibers show that enhancement of automaticity of latent pacemaker fibers can cause a broad spectrum of conduction disturbances, ranging from simple slowing to complete block.[63] In addition, development of phase 4 depolarization proximal to regions of preexisting local block may act to further depress conduction in the latter.[154] The widespread distribution of latent pacemaker cells and the numerous environmental factors and drugs that enhance phase 4 depolarization make it tempting to think that this mechanism may be a factor in human conduction disturbances.[28,30,34–36,40–49] Previously alluded–to findings that ordinary myocardial cells also may become automatic (see

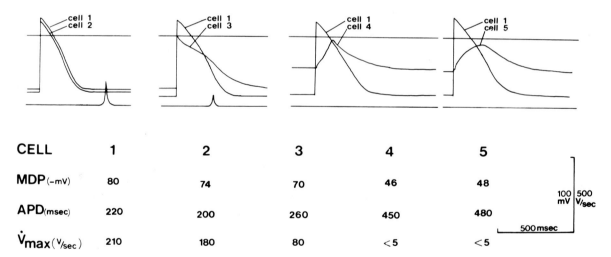

Figure 16-7. Transmembrane potentials from five cells in a papillary muscle specimen from a patient with rheumatic heart disease show variability in diastolic potential and in action-potential characteristics, together with occurrence of slow conduction and local block. Preparation was stimulated at cycle length, 800 milliseconds. Records were obtained around the margin of a small region of scar (old microinfarct of fibrosed Aschoff bodies). Each panel shows simultaneous records from a well-polarized fiber (cell 1) and from one of four partially depolarized fibers (cells 2–5) to permit comparisons of action potential characteristics and interelectrode conduction time. Maximum velocity ($\dot{V}_{max}$) of second cell of each pair is indicated by differentiated spike on trace of each panel. $\dot{V}_{max}$ of cells 4 and 5 is too low to result in appreciable deflection. Values for maximum diastolic potential (MDP) and action potential duration (APD), taken as time to repolarize to −40 mV, and $\dot{V}_{max}$ of phase 0 are indicated. Note prolongation of interelectrode conduction time between cell 1 and cells 4 and 5, compared with that between cell 1 and cells 2 and 3, as evidenced by increased separation of upstrokes of responses recorded from these cells. Time and voltage calibrations are in the lower right-hand corner. (Modified from Singer DH, Baumgarten CM, Ten Eick RE: Cellular electrophysiology of ventricular and other dysrhythmias: studies on diseased and ischemic heart. Prog Cardiovas Dis 1981;24:97–156.)

Fig. 16-4) due to factors such as drug effects, ischemia, and disease are pertinent because it would further predispose to conduction disturbances.

The low diastolic potential of diseased human atrium and ventricle is of interest mechanistically. Partially depolarized human atrial cells generally exhibit a marked insensitivity to changes in extracellular K^+ over a broad concentration range.[92,95,96] Ten Eick and Singer showed that the low diastolic potential exhibited by many such cells primarily reflected a low membrane conductance to K^+ (g_k).[95] This was subsequently supported by K^+ ion–specific electrode studies showing that intracellular K^+ activity of partially depolarized automatic human atrial cells was normal and did not change in conjunction with acetylcholine and cooling-induced suppression of phase 4 depolarization and consequent increases in maximum diastolic potential.[96] Thus, the low potential could not have been due to changes in intracellular K^+. Findings by Sato and coworkers that human atrial myocytes have fewer acetylcholine-sensitive K^+ channels than do normal cells from other mammalian species and that channels are less sensitive to the effects of acetycholine are also pertinent because such changes could contribute to the reduction in g_k and to the depolarized state.[185]

The Ten Eick and Singer data also make it unlikely that low potential was due to a depolarizing steady state inward current leak carried by Na^+ or Ca^{2+}.[95] Findings from the same study that the fast Na^+ channel–blocking agent tetrodotoxin and the slow channel blocker D600 did not affect the diastolic potential of the partially depolarized cells are also supportive.[95] Imanishi and Arita further confirmed the importance of the reduced membrane g_k.[186] They thought, however, that an increased Na^+ influx by background or TTX-sensitive channels also contributed significantly to the depolarization and in addition, that an outward electrogenic pump current prevented even more marked degrees of depolarization. Findings in ultrastructural studies of depressed sarcomal Na^+-K^+-ATPase activity in diseased human atrial tissues detract from the latter possibility.[187]

McCullough and associates found that the low-potential levels of partially depolarized human ventricular myocardial cells also were primarily due to reduced g_k.[100] The characteristics of the diastolic potential differed somewhat from atrium, with respect to K^+ sensitivity. Although the diastolic potential of most of the cells was quite stable, there were sizable numbers of cells that spontaneously hyperpolarized and then either remained at the new level of potential or depolarized again. This sequence sometimes repeated itself three or four times during an experiment (DH Singer, unpublished observations by the author). The pattern could be mimicked experimentally by varying bath K^+ concentration.[100] There were three response patterns. Most of the cells exhibited the same insensitivity to K^+ described for atrium, with the diastolic potential remaining substantially unchanged over a K^+ range of 4 to 40 mmol. A second group of cells depolarized still further in response to increases in bath K^+. In a third group, increases in bath K^+ from 4 to 7 mmol hyperpolarized the cells (average: 26 mV). If the tissue was returned to bath K^+ equal to 4 mmol, the original depolarized potential levels were usually restored. Increases beyond 10 mmol resulted in progressive depolarization.

Figure 16-8 shows a representative experiment.[100] The diastolic potential hyperpolarized 22 mV when K^+ was increased from 4 to 7 mmol. Intracellular K^+ activity was normal (106.7 ± 4.4 mmol at bath K^+ equal to 4 mmol) and did not change with changes in extracellular K^+ concentration and diastolic potential. The hyperpolarization could be prevented by Ba^{2+} (which blocks the inward rectifying K^+ current) but not by acetylstrophanthidin (which blocks the Na^+-K^+ exchange pump), suggesting that the increase in diastolic potential was due to an increase in K^+ conductance and that electrogenic Na^+ pumping did not contribute significantly.[188,189] The depolarization that ensued when bath K^+ was subsequently decreased to 4 mmol could be blocked by Mn^{2+} but not by tetrodotoxin, suggesting that the depolarizing current was carried by Ca^{2+}. Considering evidence that the inward rectifier is blocked by depolarization and requires a critical extracellular K^+ concentration for normal function, these findings suggest that a weak inward rectifier may contribute to low levels of potential and that the K^+-induced hyperpolarization may be because of the resultant improvement in rectifier function. The findings also are consistent with the existence of two stable levels of diastolic potential ($\sim -78 \pm 4$ mV and -45 ± 5 mV) similar to those reported in sheep and canine Purkinje fibers.[190–192] Whereas the changes in diastolic potential in Purkinje fibers were only observed under extreme experimental conditions, the phenomenon in diseased human ventricle occurred under conditions emulating the physiologic state.

It is tempting to think that the variable response of the diastolic potential of partially depolarized human ventricular cells to changes in extracellular K^+ may have important implications to the development of conduction disturbances and dysrhythmia in patients with heart disease.[100] For example, the small increases in interstitial K^+ concentration associated with increases in heart rate could lead to hyperpolarization of some partially depolarized cells and to the depolarization of others.[113] Variable depolarization of normally polarized cells also would ensue. Insofar as diastolic potential is an important determinant of conduction, changes in interstitial K^+ that may be too small to effect conduction significantly in the normal ventricle (i.e., one composed only of well-polarized cells) could cause dramatic changes in a diseased heart contain-

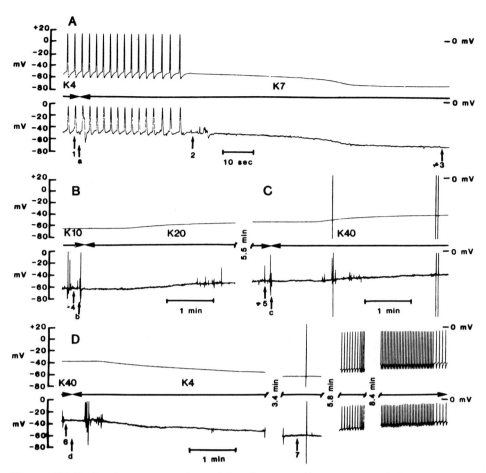

Figure 16-8. Simultaneous recordings of diastolic potential (*top tracing*) and of K$^+$-ion activity (*bottom tracing*) in a specimen of human papillary muscle during sequential changes in bath K$^+$ concentration (*lettered arrows*): a, 4–7 mM; b 10–20 mM; c$_1$ 20–40 mM; and d, 40–4 mM. The increase in bath K$^+$ concentration from 4 to 7 mm resulted in a 22-mV hyperpolarization of the diastolic potential (measured from the arrest of spontaneous activity to attainment of steady-state hyperpolarization). Further increases in bath K$^+$ (from 7 to 40 m) were associated with a progressive depolarization of the diastolic potential. Diastolic potential at the several bath K$^+$ concentrations is 4 mM, −61 mV (spontaneous activity); 7 mM, −52 mV (arrest of spontaneous activity and before hyperpolarization); 10 mM, −66 mV; 20 mM, −51 mV; and 40 mM, −38 mV. In contrast, note that intracellular K$^+$ activity remained constant at all bath K$^+$ concentrations tested. Internal K$^+$ activities (in mM) at the numbered arrows were (*1*) 117.3; (*2*) 113.1; (*3*) 114.5; (*4*) 116.2; (*5*) 113.1; (*6*) 118.8; and (*7*) 114.5. (Reproduced with permission from McCullough JR, Chua WT, Rasmussen HH, Ten Eick RE, Singer DH: Two stable levels of diastolic potential at physiological K$^+$ in human ventricular myocardial cells Circ Res 1990;66:199–201.)

ing admixtures of well-polarized and partially depolarized cells. The rate-dependence of the K$^+$-induced potential changes could in turn result in variable cycle length–dependent changes in conduction (aberrancy). Local differences in potential, resulting from cell-to-cell variability in the response to rate-related changes in interstitial K$^+$, also could predispose to fragmentation of excitation and reentry. Conversely, depending on the propor-tion of cells exhibiting a hyperpolarizing response to the K$^+$-induced potential changes, rate increases could result in abolition of already established conduction disturbances and dysrhythmias. In a similar vein, the initiation and termination of conduction disturbance and dysrhythmia associated with coronary insufficiency also could be influenced by the variable response to ischemia-related changes in extracellular K$^+$.

MECHANISMS OF ABERRANCY

Aberrancy is considered primarily in terms of impulse propagation in fibers in which membrane potential is reduced relative to normal, with the character of the disturbance being related to (1) the location of the involved cells, (2) the level of membrane potential in the path of impulse spread, and (3) the mechanism of membrane potential reduction (i.e., incomplete repolarization, low resting potential, phase 4 depolarization, or combinations thereof). The effects of altered electrophysiologic properties due to factors such as disease and cardiac drugs are considered in relation to these mechanisms. Other possible causes of altered QRS configuration of supraventricular complexes, including (1) impulse spread along anomalous AV communications,[3-7, 170-173] (2) disruption of the AV conducting system due to disease,[174, 175] (3) longitudinal dissociation of conduction within the AV conducting system,[194-197] (4) asynchronous activation of the AV junction,[198] (5) abnormalities of the gating mechanism of the His-Purkinje system,[199, 200] (6) impedance mismatch between fibers in different portions of the His-Purkinje system at the Purkinje-papillary muscle junction,[201] and (7) drug- and disease-induced alterations in excitability and in cable properties are outside the scope of this discussion.[24-27, 37, 38, 106, 139, 141, 151, 157, 160]

Aberrancy is classified by the cycle length–dependency of the QRS changes.[23] Four major groups can be defined: (1) short-cycle aberrancy, which occurs in conjunction with shortening of the cardiac cycle and increases in heart rate; (2) long-cycle aberrancy, which is associated with prolongation of the cardiac cycle and slowing of the heart rate; (3) aberrancy without significant cycle length changes; and (4) mixed aberrancy.

Short-Cycle Aberrancy

Short-cycle aberrancy, exemplified by the altered QRS contour of early supraventricular extrasystoles and of the complexes of rapid supraventricular tachyarrhythmias, is the entity for which the term was originally introduced.[1, 2] Aberrancy of premature supraventricular complexes is the best known and most common form, occurring in people with clinically normal hearts as well as in those with heart disease.[3-7] The incidence of spontaneous short-cycle aberrancy is not known. Atrial pacing studies, however, suggest that it can be induced in virtually everyone.[201-203] Aberrant complexes exhibit a right bundle branch block (RBBB) contour in 70% to 85% of reported clinical cases[11, 203, 211] and in the normal dog heart.[178, 212] Left bundle branch and nonspecific intraventricular conduction defect–type aberration comprise the remainder and appear to be more common in the diseased heart, as do admixtures of the several types.[213]

The clinical importance of short-cycle aberration stems from the fact that aberrant premature supraventricular complexes, including both isolated premature complexes and bursts of tachycardia, can closely mimic isolated ventricular premature complexes and repetitive ventricular firing, including runs of ventricular tachycardia.[11, 203-211, 214] Aberrancy always must be considered in any differential diagnosis of wide QRS beats of undetermined type.

Figure 16-9 shows Holter-monitoring records (modified V_2 surface and intra-atrial leads) obtained from a 27-year-old male who had cardiomyopathy complicated by wide QRS tachycardias (see Fig. 16-9I, beats 4–12), which were initially suspected of being ventricular in origin, considering the LBBB contour; the presence of intermediate (fusional type) complexes (see Fig. 16-9I, beat 12); and findings of clear-cut ventricular premature beats (VPBs) with a similar contour (see Fig. 16-9I, beat 4). That the run was preceded by a supraventricular extrasystole that was normally configured despite the long preceding cycle (see Fig. 16-9I, beat 3), and that the coupling interval of this beat to the preceding sinus beat differed markedly from the interval between it and the first wide QRS beat also supported a ventricular origin for the tachycardia. Findings that clear-cut supraventricular extrasystoles exhibit RBBB aberrancy was supportive (see Fig. 16-9I, beat 14). Analysis of the intra-atrial lead clearly documents the supraventricular origin of the wide QRS tachycardia, each QRS complex being preceded by an atrial spike. This contrasts with the similarly configured VPB in Figure 16-9II, in which initiation of QRS precedes the atrial electrogram.

Numerous efforts have been made to define criteria for distinguishing aberrant supraventricular beats from ventricular ectopic beats.[11, 204-210, 214] No clear-cut distinctions have been found, particularly in the case of supraventricular dysrhythmias without clear-cut P waves (e.g., early atrial premature beats in which the P is superimposed on the T wave of the preceding sinus beat; certain types of junctional rhythms; and atrial fibrillation).[204, 208, 209] The latter is a particular problem. Although differential diagnostic guidelines have been suggested, clear-cut distinctions may be difficult to make from the standard electrocardiogram.[205, 207-209, 214] Use of esophageal or intracardiac leads may be of diagnostic import in questionable cases (Fig. 16-10).

Although some regard this type of aberrancy as a strictly normal phenomenon,[215, 216] others suggest that under certain circumstances, it may be indicative of latent conduction-system disease.[11, 201-203, 217, 218] The question is complicated by the observation that the absence of clinical signs of heart disease does not necessarily preclude localized disease in a portion of the conduction system. Our experience coincides with that of Chung—that occasional aberration of early supraventricular premature complexes

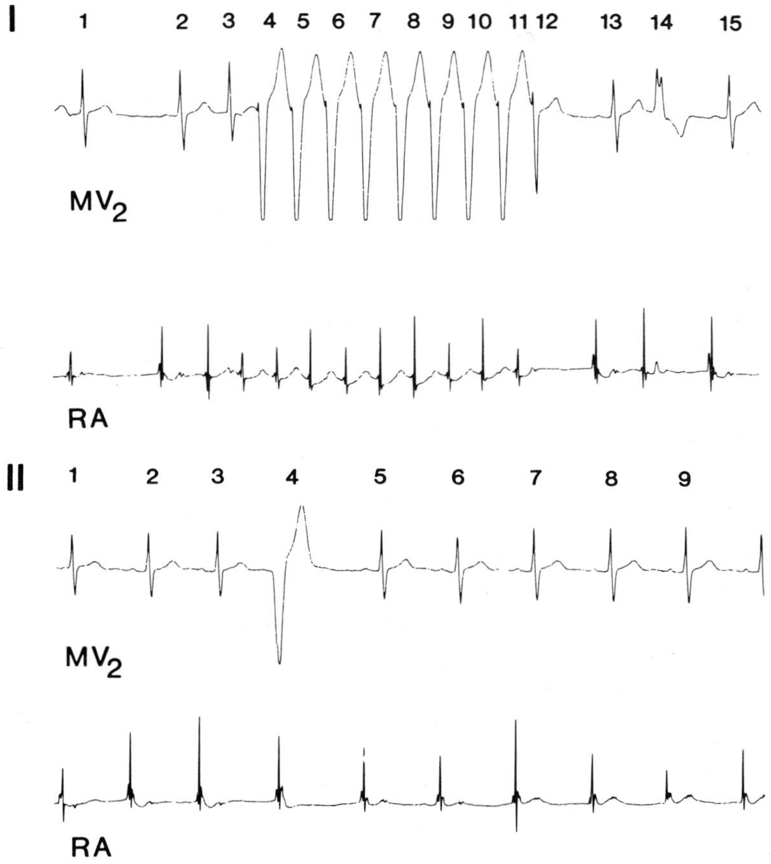

Figure 16-9. Holter-monitoring records from a 27-year-old male with suspect ventricular tachycardia in a setting of cardiomyopathy. Each panel consists of simultaneously recorded modified V$_2$ surface (MV$_2$) and intra-atrial (RA) leads. (**Panel I**) Lead MV$_2$ shows a nine-beat run of left bundle-branch block–(LBBB) type wide QRS tachycardia of unknown origin (4–11), which was preceded by a normally configured supraventricular premature beat (3) and terminated by an intermediate form (?fusion) beat (12). Note that beat 3 did not exhibit aberrancy, despite the fact that it closed a short cycle following a long cycle and that the coupling interval of the first wide QRS beat (4) was shorter (0.25 seconds) than the interval between the last wide QRS beat and the fusional form that terminates the run (0.35 seconds). In addition to the beats of the tachycardia, there also are isolated premature beats, exhibiting right bundle-branch block (RBBB) (panel I, 14) and LBBB (panel II, 4) configurations. The intracardiac lead shows that the wide QRS beats during the tachycardia and beat 14 (panel I) were preceded by atrial deflections, thus identifying them as being supraventricular, with LBBB and RBBB aberration, respectively. In contrast, the onset of the QRS of LBBB-type beat 4 (panel II) precedes the atrial spike, indicating a ventricular origin.

or of rapid supraventricular tachycardias is physiologic.[7] In contrast, an unusually high incidence of aberrant beats or the occurrence of aberration at long coupling intervals is highly suggestive of underlying conduction-system disease. Findings of left bundle branch block (LBBB) or mixed LBBB and RBBB aberrancy further increase the likelihood of underlying disease. In addition, there is suggestive evidence of an association between short-cycle aberrancy and an increased predisposition to ventricular ectopy.[220] Such an association would not be surprising from a mechanistic point of view because impulse spread in regions of slow conduction could theoretically instigate reentry as well as aberrancy. High degrees of short-cycle aberrancy thus may serve as a harbinger of ventricular dysrhythmia.

Electrophysiologic Mechanisms

In normal heart, short-cycle aberrancy is best explained in terms of altered conduction in incompletely repolarized fibers of the His-Purkinje system, with the character of the aberration being related to the location of the involved fibers and the extent to which they had repolarized by the time the impulse arrived. Generally, affected fiber groups

would be expected to be infra-His bundle in location, although suggestive evidence that the AV conducting system may function as a longitudinally partitioned system could be interpreted to imply that aberrancy also may result from His bundle and possibly even AV nodal lesions.[193–196]

Assume, for example, that the affected group of cells is located in the main right bundle branch. If the propagating action potential arrives before restoration of membrane potential to about -50 mV, it may not be able to excite the cells of the right bundle branch at all or only a local response may ensue, with resultant high-degree block in the region. The right ventricle would have to be depolarized circuitously by the left bundle branch, the left ventricular Purkinje system and myocardium, and finally, the right ventricular Purkinje system and myocardium. The resultant delay in right ventricular activation would be manifest as complete RBBB-type aberrancy. If repolarization progressed somewhat further before arrival of the impulse, conduction through the region would be slowed rather than completely blocked and incomplete RBBB aberrancy would ensue. In a similar vein, lesions in the left bundle branch system could result in LBBB-type conduction disturbances and so forth. Because the rapid repolar-

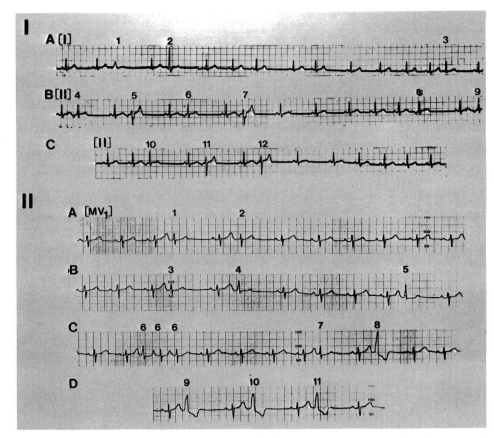

Figure 16-10. Electrocardiogram (ECG) records show varying aberrancy of atrial extrasystoles and cycle length–dependence of the phenomenon. (**Panel I**) Lead I (*A*) and lead II (*B and C*) ECGs from a 43-year-old woman with sarcoidosis. There are 12 numbered supraventricular premature beats. Beat *1* exhibits left bundle-branch block aberrancy; beats *2, 5, 7, 11,* and *12* exhibit variable right bundle-branch block aberrancy. The remainder of the beats are configured normally. Note the dependency of aberration in coupling interval and preceding cycle length. (**Panel II**) Modified (Holter) V₁ rhythm strip from a 54-year-old man with ischemic heart disease and high-grade atrial ecy, showing the spectrum of QRS changes due to cycle length–dependent variations in short-cycle aberrancy. Records contain 11 isolated atrial extrasystoles, designated by numerals *1* to *11*, and a single triplet (*6, 6a,* and *6b*). Extrasystoles *2, 6a,* and *6b* exhibit a normal QRS contour; the remainder exhibit varying RBBB aberration. Generally, as was true for the records in *panel I*, aberration is a function of prematurity and preceding cycle length. Examination of beats 8 to 11 underscores difficulties in distinguishing between aberrant supraventricular and ventricular extrasystoles in instances in which no clear-cut ecic P wave is discernible—due (as in this case) to superimposition on the preceding T wave or to other causes. The run of bigeminy in *row D* is particularly striking.

ization phase of the action potential is designated phase 3, short-cycle aberrancy also has been called phase 3 aberrancy or phase 3 block.[11]

Aberrancy of Supraventricular Premature Beats

Altered QRS configuration of early supraventricular premature beats is the most common form of short-cycle aberrancy. Figure 16-10 shows examples of normal and aberrantly conducted complexes in records from a 43-

year-old woman with systemic sarcoidosis (see Fig. 16-10*I*) and a 54-year-old man with ischemic heart disease (see Fig. 16-10*II*). With one exception (see Fig. 16-10*I,A,1*), aberrant complexes exhibit the characteristic RBBB contour. Comparisons between the normally conducted and aberrant complexes demonstrate the dependence of aberration on the prematurity of the complex and the duration of the preceding cycle.[201, 204–206, 221, 222] Generally, the earlier the premature complex and the longer the preceding cycle, the more likely aberrancy is to occur and the more marked the deviation is from normal. This relation, which was described many years ago by Lewis and Master and by Scherf, is best exemplified by differences in QRS contour of complexes of comparable prematurity in Figure 16-10I.[221, 222] That complexes 1 and 2 in Figure 16-10I,A are aberrant, whereas complex 3 exhibits a normal QRS despite its somewhat greater prematurity also is explicable in terms of differences in preceding cycle length. Beats 8 to 11 in Figure 16-10II,C and D, the most aberrant in the record, deserve comment because at first glance they appear to be inscribed later than many of the nonaberrant complexes. More careful analysis shows that the complexes are actually the earliest in the record but that the premature P waves are buried in the T wave of the preceding sinus complex, with prolongation of PR. In a sense, PR prolongation of such early complexes represents aberration of AV nodal–His-bundle conduction.

In Figure 16-10I, even the most bizarre complexes are readily identifiable as being supraventricular rather than ventricular by virtue of the clear-cut preceding abnormal P waves. In contrast, in Figure 16-10II, the most aberrant complexes are difficult to distinguish from ventricular ectopic complexes, particularly during the period of bigeminy (see Fig. 16-10D, beats 9–11), with the diagnosis resting on findings in the same record of other more clear-cut atrial premature complexes exhibiting intermediate degrees of aberrancy (see Fig. 16-10II,A–C, beats 1–7). The less than compensatory pauses after the aberrant complexes also suggest supraventricular origin.[3–7] This distinction, however, is not absolute because atrial premature complexes may produce fully compensatory or even longer pauses.[223–225]

Electrophysiologic Determinants

Given the relation between membrane potential and conduction, it follows that factors that influence the level of potential encountered by the propagating premature impulse, in addition to the relation between membrane potential and $\dot{V}_{max}$, should affect the occurrence of aberrancy.

COUPLING INTERVAL. The relation among prematurity, coupling interval, and conduction has been alluded to previously (see Fig. 16-5A and C). Other factors being equal, the earlier the complex and the shorter the coupling interval, the greater the likelihood that a given premature complex will encounter incompletely repolarized tissues in its course of spread through the His-Purkinje system.[62, 142, 178, 212] Thus, short coupling intervals predispose to aberrancy. Early premature complexes may be blocked, however, if membrane potential has not yet repolarized to sufficiently negative levels to permit development of a regenerative response (see Fig. 16-5C,a and b). Varying aberrancy of atrial premature complexes in Figure

16-5C and Figure 16-10I and II) is largely explicable in terms of degree of prematurity.

PRECEDING CYCLE LENGTH. The relation between preceding cycle length and aberrancy is usually equally clear-cut, at least in normal heart. With the exception of the SA and AV nodes, time course, duration of repolarization, and refractoriness are a function of the frequency of stimulation.[30, 178, 212, 226] To a point, decreases in cycle length shorten repolarization. Cycle length prolongation exerts the opposite effect. It follows that the longer the preceding cycle, the longer the action potential duration of the basic beat and the greater the likelihood that a complex of given prematurity will encounter incompletely repolarized fibers and conduct abnormally.

Figure 16-11 shows the effects of cycle length on action potential duration in a normal transitional Purkinje fiber (see Fig. 16-11A) as well as the relations among preceding cycle length, action potential duration and membrane potential encountered by a hypothetical complex of constant prematurity (see Fig. 16-11B). On the one hand, action potential duration at the longest cycle (2000 milliseconds) is so long that the premature stimulus would occur at levels of membrane potential too low to result in a propagated response, and conduction would fail. Conversely, action potential duration after the shortest preceding cycle (200 milliseconds) is so short that the premature response would not be inscribed until just before or immediately after completion of repolarization and would therefore conduct normally. Action potential durations at intermediate cycles (400 milliseconds and 630 milliseconds) are such that the premature response would exhibit reduced amplitude and $\dot{V}_{max}$ and altered conduction. Thus, long preceding cycles predispose to aberration of premature complexes. Conversely, short preceding cycles diminish the likelihood of aberrancy.

Figure 16-12I,A shows a transmembrane potential analogue of the interrelations between cycle length and QRS configuration of premature complexes (B). Depressed action potential characteristics and conduction of the premature response initiated at cycle length 260 milliseconds, as compared with those at 190 milliseconds (A), are due to the longer preceding cycle—as is the more aberrant QRS contour of complexes initiated at cycle length 500 milliseconds, as compared with those initiated at cycle length 420 to 460 milliseconds (B). Figure 16-12I, A also depicts how identically coupled premature responses may differ with respect to amplitude, $\dot{V}_{max}$, and conduction because of differences in preceding cycle length. Compare the first and third premature responses in Figure 16-12I,A, both initiated at a coupling interval equal to 260 milliseconds. Diminished amplitude and $\dot{V}_{max}$ and depressed conduction of the first response are attributable to the longer preceding cycle. Differences in QRS contour between the

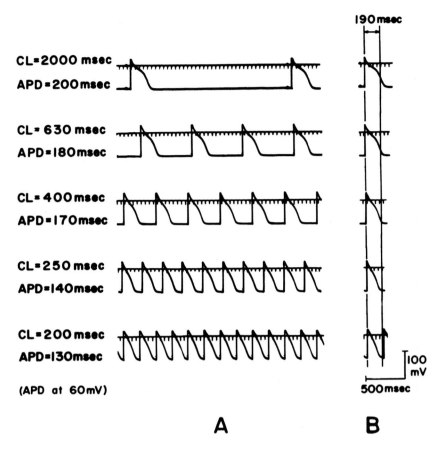

CL = 2000 msec
APD = 200 msec

CL = 630 msec
APD = 180 msec

CL = 400 msec
APD = 170 msec

CL = 250 msec
APD = 140 msec

CL = 200 msec
APD = 130 msec

(APD at 60 mV)

A

190 msec

100 mV

500 msec

B

Figure 16-11. Transmembrane potentials recorded from a normal canine Purkinje fiber, showing interrelationships among cycle length (*CL*), action potential duration (*APD*), and level of membrane potential encountered by a hypothetical extrasystole of constant prematurity. (**Panel A**) Effects of successive abrupt rate increases from CL 2000 milliseconds to 200 milliseconds on action-potential characteristics, including APD. The CL at which the preparation was stimulated and APD, measured as the time required to repolarize to −60 mV, are indicated in milliseconds. Note progressive shortening of APD, with increases in rate. (**Panel B**) The normal relation between preceding CL and membrane potential encountered by premature response. A representative action potential at each rate is shown. The upstrokes are aligned to allow better comparisons of APD. A vertical line is drawn to show level of membrane potential that would be encountered by an extrasystole having constant coupling interval of 190 milliseconds. Time lines are 50 milliseconds apart. Time and voltage calibrations are in the lower right-hand corner. (Modified from Singer DH, Ten Eick RE: Aberrancy: electrophysiologic aspects. Am J Cardiol 1971; 28:381–401.)

two complexes initiated at coupling interval equals 500 milliseconds (*B*) are similarly explicable. The records also show how differences in preceding cycle length can explain why even early premature complexes sometimes conduct more normally than those with longer coupling intervals.

Exceptions to the preceding cycle length rule do occur, however, particularly in diseased heart and in hearts exposed to selected pharmacologic agents, including the standard antiarrhythmic agents.[211,213] This may partly reflect diminished cycle length dependence of action potential duration and of refractoriness, which has been observed in vitro in tissues from animal models of ischemia and from human heart and clinically.[38,83,86,106,203,213] Spontaneous variation in action potential duration at constant cycle lengths, which also has been observed in human heart muscle, represents an additional possible factor. Figure 16-12*II*, showing a schematic representation of two atrial premature complexes, is an example in this regard. Despite identical coupling and preceding RR intervals, the two complexes differ; *A* exhibits an aberrant QRS complex and *B* exhibits a normal QRS complex. Transmembrane potentials from human ventricular muscle fiber (located above each electrocardiographic sequence) seek to ex-

plain the changes in terms of differences in preceding cycle length due to spontaneous alternation of action potential duration. This provides one possible cause of cycle length–independent alternation of normal and aberrant beats. Alternation of the QT interval of the surface electrocardiogram is the only clue to the underlying mechanism.

MEMBRANE POTENTIAL, ACTION POTENTIAL DURATION, AND REFRACTORINESS. Numerous physiologic interventions and pharmacologic agents to which the heart is exposed influence (i.e., frequently lower) diastolic potential, either directly or in the case of automatic cells, by effects on spontaneous phase 4 depolarization.[30,33–36,40–49,63] Ischemia and disease also may lower diastolic potential.[38,83,85–88,92,95,104–107]

The significance of these findings with respect to short-cycle aberrancy is that duration of repolarization and refractoriness are influenced by the level of membrane potential. Action potentials initiated at reduced levels of membrane potential are usually characterized by shortening of the early stages of repolarization (phase 2 and early phase 3). In contrast, the terminal stage of phase 3 is relatively prolonged. This could affect conduction of premature responses in at least two ways. Shortening of

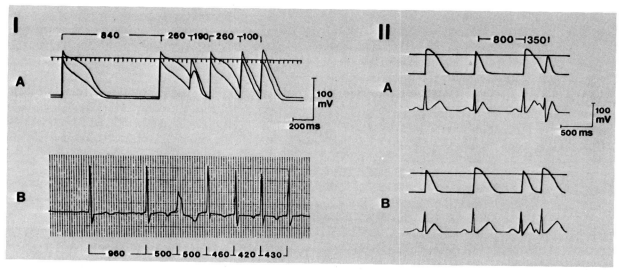

Figure 16-12. (Panel I) Transmembrane potentials simultaneously recorded from two sites in a Purkinje fiber (*row A*) and rhythm strip from a 42-year-old man with high-grade atrial ectopy and short-cycle right bundle-branch block aberrancy (*row B*), further illustrating the normal interrelation among coupling interval, preceding cycle length, and conduction of premature beats. The interval between beats is indicated in milliseconds. Time and voltage calibrations for transmembrane potentials are on the lower right of each panel. *Row A* shows the effects of premature stimulation on Purkinje fiber action-potential characteristics and represents a transmembrane potential analog of the cycle length–dependent changes in QRS configuration of supraventricular premature beats in *row B*. **(Panel II)** Schematic surface electrocardiogram rhythm strip, showing atrial extrasystoles (*A and B*; trace, fourth beat), which appear to exhibit alterations in the usual relation between QRS contour, coupling interval, and preceding cycle length. Despite identical coupling and preceding R-R intervals, the extrasystole in row A is inscribed before completion of repolarization and is aberrant, whereas the extrasystole in *row B* occurs after repolarization is over and conducts normally. The top trace shows transmembrane potentials from a specimen of diseased human papillary muscle which seek to explain the phenomenon in terms of spontaneous alternation of action-potential duration. Associated alternation in the QT interval of the surface electrocardiogram would provide the only real clue to the nature of the underlying electrophysiologic mechanisms.

phase 2 and early phase 3 may be expected to decrease the number of premature impulses that block completely. Prolongation of the terminal portion of phase 3 increases the likelihood of any propagated premature response encountering incompletely repolarized fibers in its path of spread. Both predispose to an overall increase in short-cycle aberrancy. Prolongation of phase 3 particularly favors development of aberrancy at longer than normal coupling intervals.

As previously noted, the level of membrane potential influences refractoriness and conduction in still other ways that may be expected to predispose to conduction disturbances and aberrancy in conjunction with premature stimulation. Development of automaticity and slow conduction in low-potential cells represents one such mechanism. Prolongation of refractoriness beyond voltage recovery and alterations in the normal cycle length dependence of action potential duration also occur. These are considered in relation to disease because, excepting SA and AV nodal cells and possibly also cells in the AV-valve

leaflets and the vicinity of the coronary sinus, low diastolic potential is not seen in normal heart.

Changes in Diseased Heart

Ischemia[34, 83–87, 227–229] and other experimental[228] and clinical disease states[38, 92, 97–99, 104–107] appear to profoundly influence the time course of repolarization and refractoriness, both directly and by causing variable reduction in diastolic potential. Aside from the early stages of ischemia, during which repolarization shortens, these conditions are generally associated with prolongation of both repolarization and refractoriness.

The observed changes partly reflect previously alluded–to findings that specimens of experimentally infarcted animal heart and spontaneously diseased human heart contain large numbers of partially depolarized cells, many of which exhibit slow-response characteristics. In addition, there are reports of relatively well-polarized fibers in such specimens exhibiting similar type changes in repolarization and refractoriness.[83,106,230,231] The extent to which such changes occur in well-polarized cells is not known. However, given the vast preponderance of well-polarized cells in even a diseased heart, the potential implication of such changes with respect to the increased frequency and altered patterns of aberration in patients with heart disease, could be considerable.

Duration of Repolarization

Figure 16-7 shows records from five deep intramural cells in a papillary muscle from a patient with short-cycle RBBB and LBBB aberrancy in a setting of rheumatic heart disease complicated by atrial and ventricular ectopy. In contrast to normal (cell 1), there is considerable local variability in both diastolic potential and action potential characteristics (including amplitude, $\dot{V}_{max}$ and time course of repolarization), as well as high-grade local block. In particular, note the marked prolongation of terminal phase 3 in the partially depolarized fibers. Figure 16-15 shows similar findings. Prolongation of repolarization may be even further accentuated by early afterdepolarization type oscillatory activity; increases of up to many seconds having been observed.[78–80,83,106,122,123,230,231] Figure 16-4II shows examples in human ventricular muscle cell.

Postrepolarization Refractoriness and Altered Responsiveness

Partially depolarized and well-polarized fibers in infarcted dog ventricle and diseased human ventricle also may exhibit postrepolarization refractoriness and alterations in responsiveness of the type depicted by the curve for cell b in Figure 16-3B.[23,38,83,84,86,89–91,106,181,227,230,231]

Figure 16-6III shows postrepolarization refractoriness in a slightly depolarized human ventricular muscle fiber (resting potential, − 70 mV). In Figure 16-6III,A, note that stimulation just before the end of repolarization results in a deteriorated response, even though the level of potential had been restored to nearly resting levels. In Figure 16-6III,B, a second and later response initiated after completion of repolarization, still exhibits marked reduction in amplitude in $\dot{V}_{max}$ at a time when full recovery should have been achieved. Similar changes in the postextrasystolic beats in Figure 16-13 are even more striking given the long time lapse (about 570 to 580 milliseconds) between premature and postextrasystolic beats. That the cell in question also was only slightly depolarized (− 78 mV) shows that the phenomenon is not confined to low-potential slow-response cells. The membrane mechanisms underlying this phenomenon are not yet defined for well-polarized cells. It is tempting to think that the phenomenon could reflect (at least partly) disease-related alterations in the recovery of the normally or slowly inac-

tivating Na⁺ channels. Voltage-clamp studies from our laboratory on human atrial and ventricular myocytes have not shown evidence of this or other types of abnormalities of the kinetics of either activation or inactivation of the Na⁺ current.[148–150] As previously noted, it is possible that this could be due partly to (1) the diseased cells not surviving the rigors of the enzymatic dissociation process, leaving mostly normal cells for study; and (2) only normal appearing cells being chosen for study purposes.[148] Further study is required.

The effects of alterations in responsiveness are more complex, involving displacement of the curve downward and to the right in the mid-range of potential and upward and to the left at low levels of potential (see Fig. 16-3B). The rightward displacement would be expected to result in increased generation of slowly conducting (aberrant) responses at more negative levels of potential and, therefore, later during the cycle than normal. In contrast, the leftward displacement at the low end of the range may increase aberration during early recovery by facilitating generation of slowly conducting responses at potentials ordinarily too low to support any activity. Here the underlying mechanism or mechanisms also require clarification because available studies of human cardiac myocytes have not revealed alterations in the Na⁺ current consistent with this phenomenon.[148–150]

Altered Cycle Length Dependence of Action Potential Duration

Also pertinent are findings that the usual relation between cycle length and action potential duration do not necessarily hold for partially depolarized and well-polarized fibers in experimentally infarcted dog ventricle and in human heart muscle.[23,38,78,79,83–86,89–92,106,230–232] Some fibers may exhibit a qualitatively normal relation but the degree of shortening may be less than normal and may take longer to accomplish (Fig. 16-14). In other fibers, action potential duration may not change significantly with changes in cycle length, whereas in still others it may change in the opposite direction to that which normally occurs (Fig. 16-15). Sometimes, spontaneous beat-to-beat changes in duration occur even in the absence of cycle length changes (see Fig. 16-12II).

Implications of Incidence and Patterns of Aberrancy of Supraventricular Extrasystoles in Diseased Heart

The foregoing changes, alone or in combination, in critical regions of the His-Purkinje system would be expected to predispose to an overall increase in aberrant conduction

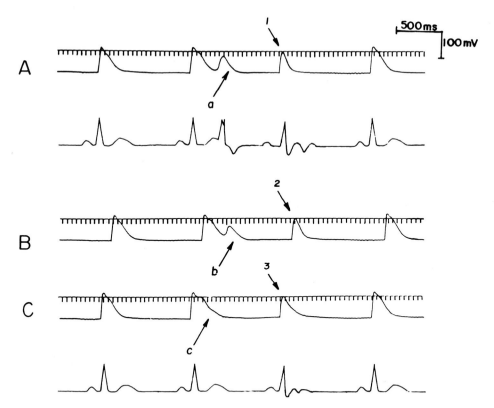

Figure 16-13. Transmembrane potentials from human papillary muscle or transitional Purkinje fiber, in a specimen from a patient with chronic rheumatic heart disease, together with schematic surface electrocardiogram, showing how nonpropagated premature responses could result in aberration of the post-ectopic beat, even in the absence of cycle-length changes of the basic beats. The preparation was regularly stimulated at cycle-length 1000 milliseconds (60/minute). **(Panels A–C)** The basic beats were interrupted by three spontaneous early premature responses (a, b, and c). Premature response (a) was initiated sufficiently late to result in a propagated extrasystole, which is depicted as exhibiting typical short-cycle aberrancy. Conversely, premature impulse (c) occurred so early that only a small, nonpropagated, local (concealed) response ensued. The same was probably true of b. Note that postextrasystole beats 1, 2, and 3 exhibit marked diminution in amplitude and $\dot{V}_{max}$, as compared with the other basic beats, changes that could result in aberration. In the case of postextrasystolic beat 3, aberration would be perceived as occurring in the absence of perceptible changes in cycle length because preceding nonpropagated local response (c) would not be noted eletrocardiographically. Beats 1, 2, and 3 also exhibit variable alterations in time course of repolarization, which would be appreciated as post-ectopic T-wave changes. Gross changes in amplitude and $\dot{V}_{max}$ do not persist beyond the first postextrasystolic beat. In contrast, changes in repolarization persist for several beats. Time markers are 50 milliseconds apart. Time and voltage calibrations are shown on the right. (Modified from Singer DH, Ten Eick RE: Aberrancy: Electrophysiologic Aspects. Am J Cardiol 1971;28:381–401.)

of premature beats, particularly those initiated during the terminal phase of repolarization and electric diastole. They also would favor altered patterns of aberrancy. For example, to the extent that disease affects the left ventricle more than the right, the changes would favor an increase in LBBB and mixed aberrancy in diseased hearts, compared with normal hearts. In addition, the changes in question may be expected to alter the usual relation between preceding cycle length and development of aberrancy in such a fashion as to make occurrence of the latter less predictable than normal and therefore more difficult to distinguish from ventricular ectopy.

The foregoing appears to correlate well with findings in patients with organic heart disease studied by atrial pacing and His-bundle recording techniques, to the effect that refractory periods were found not to change and even to increase with increases in rate. In addition, aberrancy was largely of the LBBB or mixed variety and its development appeared unrelated to preceding cycle length.[203, 211, 213] Finally, insofar as disease-related changes are non-

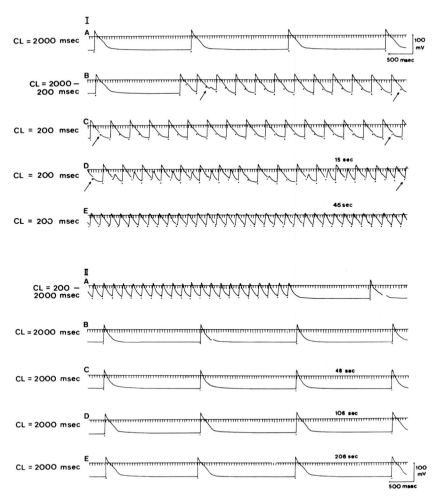

Figure 16-14. Transmembrane potentials from well-polarized human ventricular muscle fiber in a specimen of left ventricular free wall from a patient with ventricular aneurysm, showing altered cycle length (*CL*)–dependence of action-potential duration (APD) and increased time requirements to achieve new steady-state duration after rate changes. (**Panel I**) Effects of an abrupt rate increase. (Row *A*) records during stimulation at CL 2000 milliseconds (30/minute). (Rows *B–D*) Continuous record just before and after an abrupt increase in stimulation frequency to Cl 200 milliseconds (300/minute). Dots (•) designate stimulus artifacts. Initially, except for one local response (first *arrow, row B*), capture occurred with every other stimulus. *Arrows* at end of row *B*, the beginning and end of row *C*, and the beginning of row *D* indicate representative ineffective stimuli. Sufficient shortening of the APD needed to achieve a 1:1 response did not occur until 15 seconds after the rate increase (row *D*, end). Note initial alternation of large and small responses due to differences in membrane potential at excitation. Variability persisted until APD shortened sufficiently to permit excitation of successive beats to occur at the same level of potential (row *E*). Achieving a new steady-state required an additional 30 seconds, for a total of 45 seconds (190 complexes). Also, note more pronounced decrease in maximum rising velocity of the action-potential upstroke at CL 200 milliseconds than in fiber from normal dog ventricle (see Fig. 16-11). (**Panel II**) Effect of subsequent decrease in the frequency of stimulation to CL 2000 milliseconds (30/minute). Records in row *A* were obtained very shortly after those in panel *I*, row *E* and show steady-state action potentials at CL 200 milliseconds, as well as the first beat after the rate decrease. Records in rows *A* and *B* are continuous; those in rows *C–E* were obtained 48, 106, and 206 seconds, respectively, after the rate decrease. Comparisons with panel *I*, row *A* show that action potentials did not return to their control configuration until 206 seconds (103 beats) after decrease. Time and voltage calibrations are shown at right. Time lines are 50 milliseconds apart.

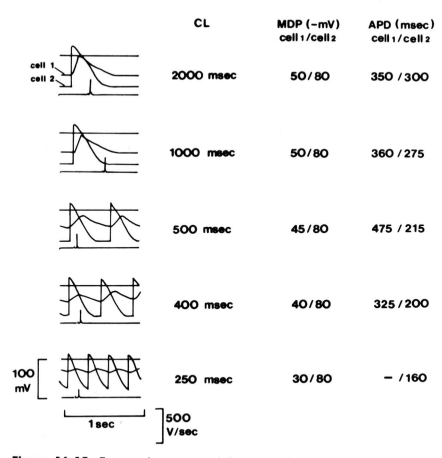

Figure 16-15. Transmembrane potentials from well-polarized (cell *2*) and partially depolarized (cell *1*) fibers, in specimen of human papillary muscle from patient with severe rheumatic heart disease, showing cycle length (*CL*)–dependent changes in action-potential characteristics, including amplitude, $\dot{V}_{max}$ time course of repolarization, and duration (*APD*). Cycle length of stimulation, maximum diastolic potential (*MDP*), and ADP (75% repolarization) are indicated. Amplitude of differentiated spike on trace of each panel is measurement of $\dot{V}_{max}$ of cell *2*. Note that whereas the APD of the well-polarized fiber decreases rapidly as rate is increased, that of the depolarized cell not only does not decrease significantly but actually increases, with the result that action potentials begin to impinge on each other at much lower rates than normal (CL = 1000 milliseconds (60/minute), as opposed to a CL = 250 milliseconds (240/minute). Progressive decrease in MDP and in action-potential amplitude and $\dot{V}_{max}$ as well as progressive slowing of conduction ensues. The fact that cell *2* is actually not entirely normal, despite reasonable levels of diastolic potential, is suggested by the progressive reduction in $\dot{V}_{max}$ with increase in rate in the absence of changes in MDP.

uniform, they increase electric inhomogeneity and the predisposition to fragmentation of excitation and reentry, thus providing an additional basis for the association between aberrancy and dysrhythmia.[86,88,91,97–100,106,230]

Characteristics of the His-Purkinje System

The electrophysiologic characteristics of the His-Purkinje system represent an additional important determinant of short-cycle aberrancy. The likelihood that a supraventricu-

lar premature impulse will traverse incompletely repolarized fibers and conduct aberrantly is facilitated by the progressive increase in action potential duration between the proximal portion of the bundle of His and the peripheral Purkinje fibers (see Fig. 16-1*B*).[19,30,178,198,233] As a result, early premature impulses entering the His-Purkinje system from the AV node are likely to encounter progressively less-polarized fibers during the course of distal spread, with resultant deterioration of the propagating action potential and development of conduction abnormalities. It is actually surprising that aberration does not occur more frequently than it does, even in the normal heart. Presumably, many impulses that may conduct aberrantly undergo complete decrement and block as they propagate into successively less-polarized regions.[19,30,178,233,234]

The predominance of RBBB aberration has been pointed out. Many explanations have been offered.[11,212,233-238] Rosenbaum and coworkers attribute it to the greater length of the right bundle branch.[11] They postulate that although an early supraventricular premature complex may conduct at equal speeds in both left and right bundle branches, the greater length of the latter may result in delayed activation of the right ventricle. Peculiarities in anatomy of the right bundle branch, which may render it unusually susceptible to the effects of stretch in conjunction with right ventricular dilation, also have been implicated. Most investigators, however, interpret the findings as reflecting differences in repolarization or refractoriness between the two sides. Experimental findings are controversial, with some workers failing to find consistent differences between the right and left sides at comparable levels (DH Singer, unpublished observations by author).[187-192] The weight of evidence from in vitro studies on the dog His-Purkinje system, studies on the in situ dog heart, and clinical electrophysiologic studies indicate that the duration of repolarization or refractoriness is actually somewhat longer on the right.[198,199,203,212,237,238] Findings in some of the same studies that action potential duration was sometimes longer on the left than on the right and that sometimes no consistent differences could be found between the two sides may explain the occasional occurrence of LBBB and mixed aberrancy in the normal heart.[198]

Reasons for the increase in LBBB and mixed aberrancy in patients with organic heart disease are not yet entirely defined. One possible explanation may be the relatively greater involvement of the left ventricle by disease, with resultant lowering of the diastolic potential and development of electrophysiologic changes that characterize depressed fibers. To the extent that these processes prolong action potential duration or refractoriness of one or more portions of the left-sided conduction system more than those on the right, they would increase LBBB and mixed type aberrancy.

The question of the possible site or sites at which functional conduction disturbances responsible for aberrancy occur has been extensively studied. Theoretically, block could occur anywhere in the conducting system proximal to or at the site of maximum action potential duration in the peripheral Purkinje fibers (see Fig. 16-1B). Most workers implicate the bundle branches and their principal proximal subdivisions.[11,19,178,212,235-240] Others, including Lewis, and Myerburg and coworkers, suggest that the block is peripheral.[1,2,198,199] Findings that an incision into the right ventricular muscle mass results in a RBBB pattern also support a peripheral site of block; such lesions presumably damage the subendocardial Purkinje net.[241] Based on findings by Moore and coworkers that lesions in the proximal and distal portions of the right bundle branch system cause complete and incomplete RBBB patterns, respectively; still others have postulated two or more sites of block.[202,242]

Kaufmann and Rothberger in 1919 and subsequently Scherf and James proposed that the AV conducting system exhibits functional longitudinal dissociation, so that individual fiber bundles in the His bundle and possibly even the AV node communicate with specific portions of the right bundle branch system and others communicate with the left bundle branch system.[193,194] This theory complicates the matter further because it implies that AV nodal or His-bundle lesions may result in intraventricular conduction disturbances. Electrophysiologic findings suggesting the existence of dual AV nodal conduction paths in both the dog and in man are pertinent, as are findings that His-bundle lesions and electric stimulation of the His bundle may sometimes result in electrocardiographic patterns typical of bundle branch block, fascicular block, or both.[195,243-248] Observations in man by Narula and by El-Sherif and coworkers that distal His-bundle stimulation resulted in abolition of various types of preexisting intraventricular conduction defects also are supportive.[196,249] Histologic studies of the His-bundle, showing separation of the longitudinally arranged cells by poorly conducting fibrous septa with only sparse transverse connections, provide a possible anatomic basis for this phenomenon.[250] Counterarguments have been presented, however, based on in vitro electrophysiologic studies to the effect that the transverse connections, sparse though they may be, are nevertheless adequate to ensure uniform activation of the AV conducting system under normal conditions.[251] It may be inferred that the occurrence of dissociation should be principally confined to instances in which the connections are damaged or destroyed by disease or environmental changes to which the diseased heart may be exposed. The preponderance of reported cases of longitudinal dissociation in patients with overt heart disease accords with this view.[196,245]

Distinctions with respect to specific sites of block and specific mechanisms of block may be illusory, however. Considering the numerous variables that influence conduction and the extent to which they in turn may be affected by local environmental factors, it would not be surprising if the site and possibly even the mechanism or mechanisms of block varied with changing conditions.

Aberrancy of Supraventricular Tachycardias

Alterations in QRS contour during supraventricular tachyarrhythmias constitute the second major type of short-cycle aberrancy. Normally, this type of aberrancy is less common than aberrancy of isolated supraventricular premature beats. It also is predominantly RBBB in character. Conversely, LBBB, nonspecific, and multiform aberrancy appear more frequently in patients who have underlying heart or conduction-system disease. Aberrancy may be confined to only a few beats of a tachycardia (usually the initial beats) or it may persist until the rate decreases again. Variations in the degree of aberrancy during a bout of tachycardia also occur, as do differences in the rates at which QRS changes appear and disappear.[203,211,213,252] Variable, usually minor, degrees of aberration may sometimes persist for brief periods after the rate has slowed. This too appears more common in patients with overt heart or conduction-system disease than in those with clinically normal hearts. Aberration also occurs at lower rates and with lesser degrees of cycle length shortening in the former and may eventually appear even at normal rates and with only minimal shortening.[3-6,23,211]

Figure 16-16A and B shows examples of atrial tachycardia at rates of 150 to 180 per minute from two patients,

aged 19 and 51 years, respectively, with a history of paroxysmal rapid heart action but without other evidence of heart disease. Despite the rapid rates (150 to 180/minute), the first patient did not develop aberrancy. In the second patient, the initial six beats exhibited right bundle branch aberration. Subsequent beats were normally configured. Records in Figure 16-16C and D were obtained from patients who had coronary artery disease and show appearance of aberrancy at successively lower rates (90/minute and 60/minute), with minimal cycle length shortening. In Figure 16-16D, aberrancy is of the LBBB type. Figure 16-17 shows records from a 35-year-old woman with a history of paroxysmal atrial tachyarrhythmias in a setting of rheumatic heart disease. The electrocardiograms in Figure 16-17A were obtained during a bout of atrial tachycardia at a rate of 140 per minute. Despite the rate of tachycardia being slower than those shown in Figure 16-16A and B, note that all of the complexes exhibit RBBB aberrancy. Records in Figure 16-17B, which were obtained about a half hour after restoration of sinus rhythm, show persistence of minor degrees of aberration. Aberrancy was no

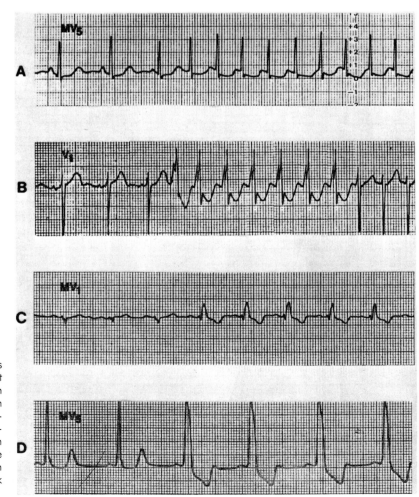

Figure 16-16. Rhythm strips from four patients showing a predisposition of aberration to occur at lower rates and with lesser degrees of cycle-length shortening in patients with overt heart–conduction system disease rather than in individuals with clinically normal hearts. Eventually, aberration may appear even at more or less normal rates and with minimal or imperceptible cycle length shortening. The latter is generally associated with left bundle-branch block, as opposed to right bundle-branch block aberrancy.

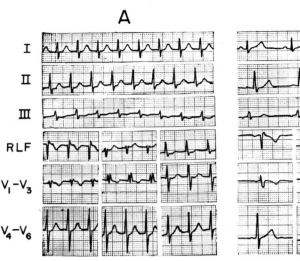

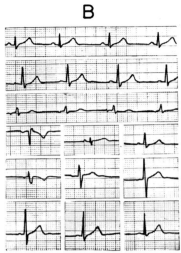

Figure 16-17. Twelve-lead electrocardiograms from a 35-year-old patient with recurrent paroxysmal supraventricular tachycardias. (**Panel A**) During tachycardia at rate of 140/minute. Note right bundle-branch block configuration. (**Panel B**) Shortly after reversion to sinus rhythm. Persistent broad S waves in limb and left chest leads represent a residual right-sided conduction delay, which disappeared shortly after the record was obtained.

longer noted on a tracing obtained the following morning at comparable rates. The Holter-monitor records in Figure 16-18, which were obtained from the same patient as those in Figure 16-9*II*, show the wide variation in the rates at which aberrancy can occur in the same individual during a 24-hour period. Aberrancy is LBBB in type. Figure 16-18*A* shows an 18-beat burst of rapid (185/minute) paroxysmal supraventricular tachycardia (beats *3–18*), of which the first seven beats (beats *3–7*) exhibit varying LBBB aberrancy and the last nine beats exhibit normal intraventricular conduction, even though the rate is substantially unchanged. In Figure 16-18*B, 2*, development of aberrancy by two atrial premature beats (beats *3* and *4*) occurs at coupling intervals (0.64 to 0.68 seconds) equivalent to rates of 90 to 95/minute. In Panel B, Row 1, aberration occurs at still longer intervals (0.76 to 0.80 seconds) (rates, 75/minute) and in conjunction with only minimal shortening of the sinus cycle. In Figure 16-18*A*, also note differences in coupling intervals at which aberrancy appears (0.44 seconds) and disappears (0.32 seconds). At other times, the patient exhibited RBBB aberrancy.

Electrophysiologic Determinants

Aberration during supraventricular tachyarrhythmias is generally explicable on the same basis as isolated premature beats; namely, conduction in incompletely repolarized fibers. The likelihood that a given rate increase will result in aberrancy as well as the magnitude and duration of the conduction disturbance depends on several interrelated factors, including (1) the nature of the relation between cycle length and action potential duration and refractoriness, (2) the magnitude and abruptness of the rate change, and (3) the characteristics of the His-Purkinje system.

Cycle Length Dependence of Action Potential Duration

Relationships between cycle length dependence of action potential duration and aberrancy of supraventricular premature complexes have been previously described. Aberration of the initial one or two beats of a supraventricular tachycardia is readily explicable on the same basis as that for isolated premature complexes. In contrast, perpetuation of aberration for sustained periods is more difficult to explain because increases in rate are normally associated with progressive shortening of the action potential. The extent to which action potential duration can shorten is limited, however. As rate increases beyond a certain limit, shortening becomes progressively less effective in compensating for the decrease in diastole. Initiation of new action potentials before completion of the previous repolarization eventually ensues, with resultant reduction in amplitude and V_{max} and development of both intermittent and sustained conduction abnormalities, including aberrancy.

The cycle length at which action potentials begin to impinge on each other and exhibit changes associated with development of conduction disturbances is variable. With the notable exceptions of SA and AV nodes, increases to quite high rates are usually required before significant deterioration of the action potential and depression of conduction occurs normally.[30, 34, 63, 64] Figure 16-11 demonstrates the effects of stepwise rate increases on action potential duration in a normal Purkinje fiber. An increase in the frequency of stimulation from 30 to 300 beats per minute was required for demonstrable diminution in action potential amplitude and rising velocity. Even at this rate, the changes were still quite minimal and would not be expected to give rise to significant aberration.

The normally pronounced cycle length–dependent

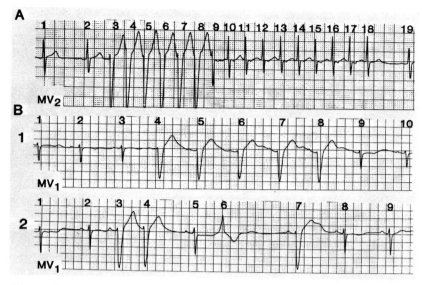

Figure 16-18. Holter-monitor records, obtained to show multiple types of aberrancy during a single 24-hour monitoring period from the same patient as those in Figure 15-8. (**Panel A**) A 16-beat run of rapid supraventricular tachycardia (*3–18*). The first seven beats exhibit varying left bundle-branch block (LBBB) aberrancy (*3–9*). The remainder are similar to the dominant beats. Note that both the coupling interval (0.52 seconds) and duration of the preceding cycle (0.92 seconds) preceding the first aberrant beat are longer than the corresponding intervals for the last aberrant beat (0.36 seconds and 0.34 seconds, respectively). (**Panel B, row 1**) Record obtained early in the morning during a period of rest–sleep, showing appearance and disappearance of LBBB-type aberrancy in conjunction with small cycle-length changes associated with a sinus arrhythmia. Note that the interval at which aberrancy appears (0.88 seconds) and disappears (1.0 second) differ. (**Panel B, row 2**) Records obtained 2 hours after those in *row 1* showing examples of both short-cycle LBBB aberrancy of two atrial premature beats (*3, 4*) and long-cycle LBBB-type aberrancy of a post-ectopic sinus beat (*7*). Note that the ventricular premature beat (*6*) exhibits a right bundle-branch block contour suggestive of a left-sided origin.

shortening of action potential duration makes it necessary to invoke mechanisms other than simple initiation of aberrant beats before completion of repolarization of the preceding beat in the involved region to explain perpetuation of aberrancy during supraventricular tachycardias. One view is that it reflects the effects of concealed trans-septal conduction of the tachycardia impulses, followed by retrograde activation of the involved bundle branch, which would maintain the latter in a refractory state.[212] Thus, repetitive RBBB aberrancy would be explained in terms of concealed left-to-right trans-septal conduction and retrograde activation of the right bundle branch, with the result that impulses propagating into the latter in the orthograde direction would consistently find the tissue refractory. Conversely, termination of aberrancy would be explicable in terms of block of trans-septal conduction and of retrograde activation, arrival of the orthogradely conducting impulses at the bundle branch before retrograde activation, or cycle length–dependent shortening of repolarization or refractoriness. This mechanism has been implicated in numerous published cases of repetitive aberration

and documented by intracardiac electrogram and in vitro microelectrode studies.[253–258] Irrespective, high rates are still probably required for the mechanism to operate normally.

Achieving New Steady-State Action Potential Duration After Rate Changes

Achievement of new steady-state action potential duration after abrupt rate changes is usually not immediate, even in normal fibers, but takes place gradually over several cycles.[30, 259] Similar observations have been made with respect to rate-dependent changes in refractoriness in the in situ heart.[260] It may be inferred that the likelihood of premature responses being initiated before completion of repolarization and disappearance of refractoriness due to the previous beat (and therefore the likelihood of aberration) is maximal immediately after the rate change and diminishes with each complex at the new rate. This provides a reasonable explanation for instances in which the initial complex or complexes of a tachycardia are aberrant and in which aberrancy subsequently diminishes or disappears (see Fig. 16-16*B*). The number of beats needed to achieve the new steady-state action potential duration after rate increases varies, with some investigators indicating that it may normally require up to 40 to 50 beats.[259] Differences may exist in the number of beats required for equilibration after increases and decreases in rate for the same fiber (see Fig. 16-14) and for the whole heart (see Fig. 16-18). The bulk of the change normally takes place over relatively few beats, however.

Changes In Diseased Heart

Considerations similar to those noted in relation to aberrancy of isolated supraventricular beats in the normal heart probably also apply to patients with heart disease. Two factors deserve additional comment, however.

Altered Cycle Length Dependence of Action Potential Duration

Findings that both partially depolarized and well-polarized fibers in specimens of ischemic and diseased heart may exhibit diminished action potential shortening for a given increase in rate (see Fig. 16-15) represent one such factor.[23, 83, 86, 89, 91, 106, 232] Other considerations being equal, this would result in (1) a greater than expected diminution in action potential amplitude and $\dot{V}_{max}$ for any given rate increase, and (2) development of aberrancy at lower than expected rates and to its perpetuation during bouts of tachycardia. Increased action potential duration (see Figs. 16-4 and 16-7), altered responsiveness (see Fig. 16-3*B*), and time-dependent prolongation of refractoriness beyond completion of repolarization (see Fig. 16-6*III*), which also characterize many fibers in diseased heart, would further accentuate this tendency. Comparisons between action potentials at comparable rates in a normal dog Purkinje fiber (see Fig. 16-11) and normal and partially depolarized fibers in diseased human ventricle (Figs. 16-14 and 16-15) are illustrative. Note that in contrast to normal, the human ventricular muscle fibers exhibit a longer action potential duration than the Purkinje fiber at comparable cycles. Also note that although the partially depolarized fiber in Figure 16-15 exhibited greater diminution of action potential amplitude and $\dot{V}_{max}$ in conjunction with cycle length shortening than did the well-polarized fiber in the same figure, the latter also experienced a progressive decrease in $\dot{V}_{max}$, suggesting postrepolarization refractoriness. It is tempting to think that this may be due to disease-related delay in recovery from inactivation or use-dependent block of the Na^+ channel. Single-channel recordings on isolated human cardiac myocytes do not support these possibilities, however. Dif-

ferential sensitivity of normal and diseased cells to the rigors of the enzymatic isolation process may have killed most of the latter, so that studies were conducted on relatively normal cells.[149]

Increased Time to Achieve Steady-State Action Potential Duration After Rate Changes

Findings that it may take considerably longer than normal to achieve steady-state action potential after rate changes in ischemic and diseased heart muscle represent the second factor.[23, 38, 106] Figure 16-14 shows sequential changes in action potential duration in response to an abrupt tenfold increase (see Fig. 16-14*I*) and decrease (see Fig. 16-14*II*) in stimulation frequency in a well-polarized human ventricular muscle fiber from the margin of a ventricular aneurysm. Figure 16-14*I,A* shows records during stimulation at cycle length 2000 milliseconds (30/minute). Stimulation frequency was then increased to cycle length 200 milliseconds (300/minute; Figure 16-14*I,B*). An initial 2:1 response ensued. It was not until 14 seconds after the rate change that sufficient shortening of duration occurred to permit even an abortive 1:1 response (Figure 16-14*I,D*). After establishment of a stable 1:1 response (Figure 16-14*I,E*), action potential characteristics continued to change for an additional 30 seconds before achievement of the new steady-state duration (Figure 16-14*II,A*). In total, equilibration required 45 seconds and 190 complexes. Also note the more pronounced decrease in $\dot{V}_{max}$ at cycle length 200 milliseconds than in a fiber from a normal dog heart (see Fig. 16-11).

Figure 16-14*II* shows the effects of a subsequent abrupt reduction in frequency of stimulation back to 30 per minute. The first few complexes after the rate decrease exhibited variable prolongation of action potential duration, with subsequent complexes exhibiting shortening—followed by gradual prolongation—of duration until the new steady state was reached. Equilibration time was again long: 206 seconds (103 complexes).

Implications of Incidence and Patterns of Aberrancy of Supraventricular Tachycardias in Diseased Heart

It may be inferred from the foregoing that persistent aberration during supraventricular tachycardias is unlikely to occur normally except at high rates, although not necessarily as high as those suggested by the records in Figure 16-11. Conversely, the electrophysiologic changes exhibited by fibers in ischemic and diseased heart muscle appear to provide the necessary basis both for an overall increase in aberrancy and for its appearance at lower rates than normal. Probably, aberration of supraventricular tachycardia at physiologic rates implies that the electrophysiologic properties of the conduction system, the geometry of impulse spread, or both have been altered by ischemia, disease, drugs, or other factors. In addition, as noted for extrasystoles, the observed changes also favor changing patterns of aberrancy. In particular, because disease generally affects the left ventricle more than the right, the changes favor an increase in LBBB and mixed aberrancy, compared with the RBBB ordinarily observed in normal heart. The changes also may be expected to alter the cycle length dependency of repolarization and refractoriness, making occurrence of aberrancy less predictable than normal and therefore more difficult to distinguish from ventricular ectopy.

Observations that achievement of a new steady-state action potential duration after abrupt rate changes may be a more gradual process than normal in ischemic or diseased heart has other implications with respect to patterns of aberrancy. For example, local differences in equilibration time after rate decreases may be a factor in persistence of aberration for brief periods after cessation of tachycardia. In a similar vein, persistence of rate-related changes in action potential duration after rate slowing provide a possible explanation for posttachycardia ST-T changes. Variability in action potential duration after abrupt rate increases and before achieving the new steady state also may explain other peculiarities. For example, alternation of normally configured and aberrant complexes may occur in instances in which the rate change results in an action potential alternans of the type seen in Figure 16-14B and C. In addition, delay in achieving a 1:1 response in conjunction with abrupt cycle length shortening provides a possible basis for increases in the rate of initially slow supraventricular tachycardias and for onset of aberrancy at times other than at the beginning of a run.

Findings that the number of complexes required to reach a new steady-state action potential duration may differ after increases and decreases in rate in the same fiber (see Fig. 16-14) may underlie instances in which appearance and disappearance of short-cycle aberrancy occur at different rates (see Fig. 16-18). Differences in preceding cycle length duration between the first aberrant (see Fig. 16-18A, beat 3) and non-aberrant (see Fig. 16-18A, beat 10) beats of a tachycardia also may be contributory. Hoffman[261] suggests a third possible explanation based on studies on impulse spread in partially depolarized regions of local block: (1) slowing of conduction in a depressed region is associated with prolongation of action potential duration at its proximal margin, and (2) conversely, failure of conduction is associated with marked shortening of duration proximally.[176, 200] Under such circumstances, abrupt rate increases would result in the generation of action potentials that are prolonged out of proportion to

cycle length at the proximal margin. Rate-related block would occur at a particular cycle length. Once block develops, action potential duration shortens. On subsequent rate slowing, normal conduction resumes at shorter cycles than those at which block appeared during the prior period of acceleration. This could permit onset of aberration at lower rates than offset in conjunction with abrupt rate increases and decreases, respectively.

Abruptness of Cycle Length Change

The abruptness of a rate change also may influence aberrancy. Generally, aberrancy appears more likely to occur in response to abrupt increases in rate between any two levels than if the same rate increase were made in stepwise fashion. Gradual stepwise rate increases allow more time for shortening of action potential duration and thus decrease the likelihood that the initial complexes at the new rate will be inscribed before completion of repolarization of the previous complex. This represents one possible explanation for observations that the beats of a sinus tachycardia appear less likely to become aberrant than the complexes of a paroxysmal supraventricular tachycardia, even at comparable rates, because rate changes usually occur more gradually in the former. The phenomenon is likely to be more pronounced in normal than in diseased hearts because changes observed in the latter, including diminished cycle length dependence of action potential duration and increased time requirements for achievement of the new steady-state after rate changes would minimize differences due to abruptness of the rate change.

Electrophysiologic Characteristics of the His-Purkinje System

Certain of the conduction-system characteristics that predispose to aberration of supraventricular premature complexes also would be expected to favor its development during supraventricular tachycardias.

That aberration of supraventricular tachycardias is not common normally is best explained in terms of the action potential shortening and concomitant reduction in the disparity of action potential duration, both between comparable levels of the right and left ventricular components of the His-Purkinje system and different levels of the system that accompany cycle length shortening.[199, 200, 212, 233] In addition, Han and associates have shown that the extent of temporal dispersion of the recovery of ventricular muscle excitability is inversely related to the rate.[262] Figure 16-12I,A shows an example of decreased disparity in duration between action potentials simultaneously recorded from two normal Purkinje fibers on cycle length shortening. Conversely, the increased aberration of supraventricular tachyarrhythmias in the diseased heart also could reflect diminution in the usual rate-related decreases in disparity of action potential duration in different parts of the conduction system due to factors such as the previously alluded to decrease in cycle length dependence of action potential duration and development of postrepolarization refractoriness and alterations in the responsiveness relations of the type depicted in Figures 16-6 and 16-3B). That the effects of ischemia and disease are not uniform tends to support this interpretation. Figure 16-15 shows an example of increased dispersion of repolarization in a specimen of human ventricle in conjunction with cycle length shortening.

Antiarrhythmic Agents and Short-Cycle Aberrancy

Many pharmacologic agents used in the treatment of heart disease, including several major antiarrhythmic agents (digitalis, the slow channel and β-adrenergic blocking agents) and the antianginal agents, influence time course of repolarization and refractoriness, independent of their effects on diastolic potential.[25–30,40–49] The class I antiarrhythmic agents including procainamide and quinidine[144] and class III agents e.g., amiodarone[263,264] are well known for their ability to slow repolarization due to blocking effects on both the outward K^+[266,267] and inward Ca^{2+}[267–269] currents. Observations that these agents may increase aberrancy date back many years.[215] Conversely, agents such as diphenylhydantoin and propranolol, which act to shorten repolarization, may diminish aberrancy.[270–272]

Although prolongation of repolarization by the class I agents contributes to antiarrhythmic efficacy, it is thought that their principal action is to block the fast inward Na^+ channel in both a voltage- and time-dependent manner.[40–46,182,273] Other antiarrhythmic agents, including the important class III agent amiodarone, also block this current.[267,274] Observations by Hoffman that quinidine and procainamide alter the responsiveness relation in such a way that the normal curve depicted in Figure 16-3B (cell a) is shifted downward and to the right in the middle and low ranges of potential date back many years.[144] Depressant effects on the Na^+ channel are voltage-dependent, being more pronounced in low-potential as compared with well-polarized cells.[41,49,143,144,273] The selectivity of these agents for partially depolarized cells is probably principally because they have a higher affinity for the inactivated Na^+ channel than for the resting channel. Depolarization increases the number of channels in the inactivated state, so that higher degrees of block are achieved. In addition, because the availability of drug-associated channels for activation is shifted to more negative potential levels, activation-induced removal of block diminishes

in conjunction with depolarization.[49] As previously noted, sodium channel block induced by these agents also exhibits time dependence, with the result that functional recovery may be prolonged beyond completion of repolarization (postrepolarization refractoriness). Other factors being equal, this would be expected to further increase the likelihood that premature responses initiated during repolarization, including those initiated during late phases and possibly even during diastole, will conduct aberrantly. Findings that the class I agents and other types of antiarrhythmic agents, including amiodarone, also cause use-dependent (rate-dependent) block of the fast Na^+ channel are pertinent because this action would further increase aberration in conjunction with increases in heart rate.[46,49,182,273,274] In addition, the voltage dependence of the drug-induced blockade of the Na^+ channels suggests that the increase in aberrancy should be particularly prone to occur in ischemic and diseased hearts, with their large numbers of partially depolarized cells. This would be expected to facilitate development of aberrancy at lower rates than normal and possibly also in association with gradual (as opposed to abrupt) rate increases in patients with heart disease. Findings that ischemia and disease also may shift the responsiveness curve downward and to the right in the high and middle ranges of potential (see Fig. 16-3B; compare curves for cell a and b) in the absence of drug effect further accentuate this tendency.[38,78,79,83,86,87,106,145–147]

LONG-CYCLE ABERRANCY

Alterations in QRS contour that appear in conjunction with cycle length prolongation and diminish or disappear on cycle length shortening represent a second major type of aberrancy. Although not as common as the short-cycle variety, long-cycle aberrancy is nevertheless a well-documented entity,[11,193,211,275–302] which was initially described by Kaufmann and Rothberger in 1919,[193] by Wilson in 1915,[275] and was produced experimentally by Drury and McKenzie in 1934[297] and by Elizari and coworkers in 1974.[293] It is best exemplified by development of bundle branch block patterns on slowing of the sinus rate and by the altered QRS contour of supraventricular escapes. Although aberrant complexes may frequently exhibit a RBBB contour, this does not appear to be as characteristic as with short-cycle aberration.[11,211,282,285,295,296] In addition, whereas short-cycle aberrancy is common in patients with both normal and impaired hearts, long-cycle aberrancy appears to be more strictly confined to those with underlying conduction-system pathology.[11,222,285,290,291]

The overall significance of long-cycle aberrancy is in many ways similar to that described for the short-cycle variety. Aberrant supraventricular complexes closing long-cycles can closely mimic isolated ectopic ventricular escapes, including fusional complexes and runs of slow ventricular tachycardia. The distinction is a particular problem in rhythms without P waves, including slow atrial fibrillation and junctional escape rhythms. Even more importantly, occurrence of this type of aberrancy should imbue a high degree of suspicion regarding the possibility of intrinsic conduction-system disease or functional abnormalities due to such causes as ischemia, toxic drug effects, and severe electrolyte imbalance. Suggestions that at least some types of long-cycle aberrancy may be due to phase 4 depolarization of latent pacemaker cells underscores an association with increased ventricular ectopy.

Figure 16-18*B,2* shows a typical example of long-cycle LBBB aberrancy of a sinus beat (beat 7) closing a 1.8-second pause after a ventricular premature beat (beat *6*). Sinus beats closing pauses less than 1.4 seconds did not exhibit the phenomenon, emphasizing long-cycle dependency. Figure 16-18*A* and *B*, row *1*, also shows examples of short-cycle LBBB aberration from the same patient for comparison purposes.

The record in Figure 16-19 shows an example of long-cycle RBBB aberrancy in a 78-year-old woman hospitalized for acute anteroseptal infarction. The case differs from that depicted in Figure 16-18 and is atypical in that aberration occurs with only slight prolongation in cycle length. There is prominent alternation in cycle length due to intermittent atrial bigeminy. QRS complexes closing cycles shorter than 0.76 second in duration are normal; those closing longer cycles exhibit varying degrees of RBBB aberrancy. The degree of aberration is cycle length–dependent: the longer the cycle, the wider the QRS complex. The phenomenon appeared on the third hospital day and persisted for an additional four days, during which time scattered early supraventricular extrasystoles exhibiting RBBB type aberration also were noted. Both were superseded by fixed RBBB. The latter disappeared three days later, by which time all traces of long-cycle aberrancy also were noted to be gone. Variably coupled LBBB VPBs, which also had initially been present, also disappeared.

Mechanistic Considerations

In contrast to short-cycle aberrancy, the long-cycle variety cannot be explained in terms of impulse spread in incompletely repolarized fibers because there is more than

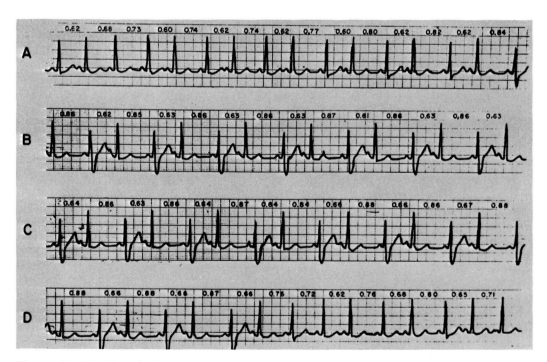

Figure 16-19. (Panels A–D) A continuous electrocardiographic record (modified monitor lead II), obtained from a 78-year-old patient during the initial stage of acute anteroseptal myocardial infarction. QRS complexes have been retouched. R-R intervals are indicated in seconds. Atrial bigeminy is present throughout most of the record. Note varying right bundle-branch block (RBBB) aberrancy of beats (closing cycles ≥ 0.76 seconds in duration), the degree of aberration generally being related to the degree of cycle-length prolongation. **(Panel D)** Also note that of the beats closing two identical cycles of 0.76 seconds, one exhibits an incomplete RBBB contour, whereas the other is normal.

adequate time for completion of recovery before inscription of the aberrant complex. Many alternatives have been suggested.

Preferential Atrioventricular Junctional Transmission of Aberrant Beats

Initial interest focused on aberration of junctional escapes. The earliest hypotheses sought to explain differences in QRS contour between normally configured sinus and aberrant junctional complexes in terms of differences in path of AV junctional spread.[193, 279, 286, 298] Kaufmann and Rothberger attribute the phenomenon to selective activation by the sinus and aberrant junctional complexes of different portions of the bundle of His, a concept that implies anatomic or functional longitudinal dissociation within this structure or within the larger AV conducting system, as visualized by Scherf and James.[193, 194, 298] Wellens also invokes functional dissociation within the bundle branch system.[300] It is unclear, however, why aberration due to this should be bradycardia-dependent. In addition, to the extent that dissociation occurs, it would be expected to be a reasonably common phenomenon, particularly in patients with AV conduction–system pathology. Because sinus bradycardia and junctional escape complexes are frequent occurrences, long-cycle aberration also should be common. Its relative rarity, therefore, further detracts from this explanation.

Pick and others implicate spread along the paraspecific fibers of Mahaim (which run from the AV node, His bundle, and left bundle branch to septal myocardium) as the cause of junctional aberration.[171, 172, 279, 283, 286] Findings that Mahaim fibers appear to decrease with age, whereas aberration of junctional escapes is most commonly observed in older subjects, detract from this possibility, as does the lack of clear-cut electrophysiologic evidence for their functional significance.[303] Still, the possibility that at least some instances of long-cycle aberrancy may reflect impulse spread along one or the other of the AV bypass tracts cannot be excluded.

Altered Site of Origin of Aberrant Complexes

Aberration of junctional escape complexes also could be explicable in terms of an abnormal site of origin. Pick implicates the Mahaim fibers.[279] Massumi and coworkers and Lie and coworkers conclude that many such complexes are fascicular rather than junctional, originating in the anterior or posterior fascicles of the left bundle branch.[289, 295] Such complexes would be expected to exhibit a relatively narrow QRS with an incomplete RBBB pattern, so this represents one possible cause of RBBB junctional aberration. It would not explain LBBB and non-

specific types of aberration, however. More importantly, it leaves unanswered questions concerning mechanisms of long-cycle aberrancy of sinus complexes.

Vagal Mediation

Because many of the early reported cases of aberration occurred in conjunction with vagally mediated sinus slowing, the possibility that QRS prolongation resulted from direct depressant acetylcholine effects on conduction in the His-Purkinje system also was suggested.[275, 276, 282] Findings that acetylcholine does not depress the normal His-Purkinje system and that it may actually improve conduction in depressed tissues appear to obviate this explanation.[30, 304] In a different vein, Dressler proposed that increased vagal activity resulted in an altered QRS contour by means of a vagally mediated coronary vasoconstrictor reflex.[280] This could not, however, explain instances of aberration in which vagal mediation could not be readily invoked; for example, aberration of supraventricular complexes closing postextrasystolic pauses of short duration, such as those depicted in Figure 16-16.

Phase 4 Depolarization

Latent Pacemaker Cells

That the His-Purkinje system is comprised of numerous latent pacemaker cells capable of undergoing spontaneous diastolic depolarization suggests a fourth possible mechanism for long-cycle aberrancy of both slow sinus beats and junctional escapes, based on the previously cited interrelations between automaticity and conduction (Fig. 16-20).[63, 291–294]

The cyclic lowering of diastolic potential that phase 4 depolarization entails results in a voltage- and time-dependent reduction in $\dot{V}_{max}$ and amplitude of action potentials and in development of conduction disturbances more or less comparable with those occurring in incompletely repolarized fibers (see Fig. 16-20).[63] Considering the widespread distribution of latent pacemaker cells, enhancement of phase 4 depolarization in the His-Purkinje system could theoretically result in virtually any type of AV and intraventricular conduction disturbance, the specific nature of the abnormality being related to the location of the involved fibers and the rate and extent of depolarization. In instances in which the involved cells are located in the bundle branches, QRS contour changes defined as aberrancy may be expected to ensue. Insofar as longitudinal dissociation of the AV conducting system occurs, it is possible that enhancement of automaticity in the distal segment (N-H region) of the AV node or the His bundle, which ordinarily would be expected to result in AV block, also may give rise to intraventricular conduction

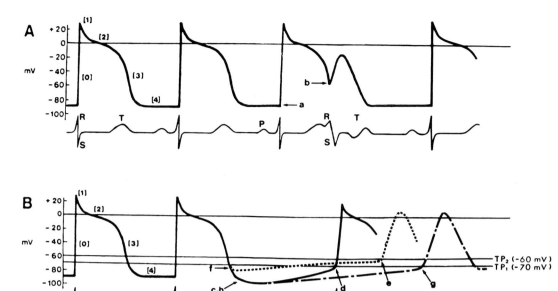

Figure 16-20. Schematic transmembrane potentials from a latent pacemaker cell in the His–Purkinje system and simultaneous surface electrocardiogram (ECG), illustrating interrelationship between automaticity and conduction. Action-potential phases are designated by arabic numerals 0–4; ECG deflections by the letters P, R, S, and T. (**Panel A**) During the first three beats, stimulation is sufficiently fast to suppress phase 4 depolarization, a situation analogous to that occurring during sinus rhythm. Membrane potential is normal and remains constant during diastole (phase 4). The action potentials, which are initiated at −90 mV (*a*), also are normal, as is the ECG. Repolarization of the third beat is interrupted by a premature response initiated at −60 mV (*b*), which exhibits marked diminution in amplitude and maximum velocity ($\dot{V}_{max}$) and depressed conduction, as evidenced by aberrant QRS contour of ECG. (**Panel B**) The initial two beats were recorded during stimulation at the same rate as in *panel A*. Action potentials and ECG are normal. The third through fifth beats were evoked after development of phase 4 depolarization, in response to a decrease in frequency of stimulation to a low rate. The *third action potential* is depicted as arising at a time when maximum diastolic potential (−90 mV; *c*) and threshold potential (−70 mV; *d*; TP$_1$) are still both normal. Because the depolarization process cannot lower diastolic potential to below the threshold potential, the resultant decrease in amplitude and $\dot{V}_{max}$ is not sufficient to depress conduction significantly and the ECG remains normal. The *fourth action potential* depicts the effect of a shift in TP to a less negative level (TP$_2$). The shift allows the fourth action potential to be initiated at a much lower diastolic potential (−60 mV; *e*) than normal. Diminution in amplitude and $\dot{V}_{max}$ and depression of conduction are correspondingly more marked. The QRS complex of the ECG is aberrant. Note similarities to premature response in *panel A*, which also was initiated at −60 mV. Also note that the shift in TP is associated with a decrease in MDP (*f*). The *fifth action potential* shows how responsiveness changes of the type depicted in *Figure 16-3, panel B* could predispose to aberrancy due to phase 4 depolarization at more negative potentials than usual and in cells with a normal TP. Note that although this beat is initiated at −70 mV (*g*), amplitude and $\dot{V}_{max}$ are sufficiently reduced to depress conduction and cause aberration of the QRS complex. It thus resembles the fourth response, which arises at −60 mV (*e*), more than it does the third, even though the latter also is initiated at −70 mV (*d*). The greater than expected decrease in amplitude and $\dot{V}_{max}$ and depression of conduction for level of potential reflect the responsiveness change. (Modified from Singer DH, Lazarra R, Hoffman DS: Interrelationships between automaticity and conduction of Purkinje fibers Circ Res 1967;21:537–558.)

disturbances and aberrancy. Because aberrancy due to this results from lowering of membrane potential during phase 4 of the action potential, it has been designated phase 4 block or phase 4 aberrancy.[11,291] This designation is not sufficiently specific, however, because it also would apply to aberrancy due to low resting potential.

Massumi lists electrocardiographic characteristics of long-cycle aberrancy.[287] Given the nature of phase 4 depolarization, increases in cycle length prolongation should be associated with increasing degrees of aberration. The records in Figure 16-19 are illustrative. Conversely, factors that decrease the rate and extent of phase 4 depolarization would be expected to prevent development of and diminish or abolish preexisting long-cycle aberrancy. Shortening of the sinus cycle in conjunction with activity or by use of such agents as atropine *and* increasing base heart rate by pacemaker implantation in instances of bradyarrhythmia represent examples, as does pharmacologic suppression of phase 4 depolarization. Interventions that manipulate sinus rate should prove useful in elucidating suspect occult cases.

In addition, it may be expected that patients with aberrancy due to phase 4 depolarization also should exhibit ventricular ectopic complexes originating in the region of enhanced automaticity; patients with RBBB aberration should develop premature complexes exhibiting a LBBB contour and vice versa. Findings of the appropriate type of extrasystoles would support conclusions that a given case of long-cycle aberration was due to enhanced automaticity. In the case of the patients whose records are shown in Figures 16-18B,2 and 16-19, development of left and RBBB aberrancy was associated with the presence of right and LBBB ventricular ectopic beats, respectively. In addition, in the case depicted in Figure 16-19, both aberrancy and ventricular ectopy disappeared coincidentally.

Electrophysiologic Determinants

Aberrancy due to phase 4 depolarization would be likely to occur under circumstances that enhance automaticity of latent pacemaker cells in the His-Purkinje system. Two sets of conditions are of principal importance. (1) Reduction in heart rate due to sinus slowing or to other causes, such as high-grade AV block or nonconducted atrial premature complexes. Long diastoles provide more time for phase 4 depolarization to develop, with consequent reduction in the level of diastolic membrane potential and in the availability of Na^+ channels encountered by the propagating impulse (see Fig. 16-20B). This represents one possible explanation for aberration occurring in conjunction with decreases in heart rate to the vicinity of the intrinsic firing rate of latent AV junctional or His-Purkinje pacemakers or below (40 to 55 per minute) (see Fig. 16-18B,2). (2) Direct enhancement of latent pacemaker

automaticity, numerous physiologic interventions act to increase the rate of phase 4 depolarization of latent His-Purkinje pacemaker cells, including changes in pH, pCO_2, and temperature; ischemia; stretch in dilated hearts; alterations in extracellular ionic concentrations; and many pharmacologic agents, including digitalis.[30,40-48] Direct enhancement of latent pacemaker automaticity provides one possible explanation for instances such as those illustrated in Figure 16-19 in which aberrancy occurs with only modest prolongation in cycle length and at sinus rates that do not normally permit significant phase 4 depolarization of latent pacemaker cells.

It may reasonably be inferred from the widespread distribution of automatic cells and the numerous physiologic and pharmacologic factors that act to depress sinus activity or enhance latent pacemaker automaticity that this type of aberrancy should be quite common. Published reports do not support this inference. This is particularly true of patients with clinically normal hearts, with most reported cases occurring in a setting of organic heart disease.

Analysis of the relation between membrane potential and conduction provides a possible explanation for this apparent paradox.[63,142] As noted, conduction is usually well maintained and may even improve slightly with depolarization until membrane potential is reduced to less than -70 mV, a finding that has been attributed to (1) decreased current requirements for excitation (i.e., increase in excitability) as membrane potential is brought closer to the threshold potential; and (2) increased space constant, which results from the increase in membrane resistance associated with phase 4 depolarization. Both enhance the effectiveness of electrotonic current spread and compensate for the voltage-dependent decrease in $\dot{V}_{max}$.[63] Because the threshold potential of normal His-Purkinje fibers approximates -70 mV, phase 4 depolarization cannot reduce diastolic membrane potential to less negative levels because spontaneous firing and an ectopic ventricular beat would ensue.[143] Phase 4 depolarization is therefore unlikely to result in slow conduction and aberrancy normally (see Fig. 16-20B, beat 3).

Phase 4 depolarization could, however, theoretically cause sufficient reduction in diastolic potential to result in significant aberration under special circumstances, one of which may operate normally. Figure 16-21 presumes that the rate of phase 4 depolarization in a latent pacemaker cell has increased to the point that its spontaneous firing rate is only fractionally lower than that of the sinus. Given a close similarity in rates, it is theoretically possible for the sinus impulse to reach the latent pacemaker cell at the time when its diastolic potential had been lowered to the vicinity of the threshold potential. Because the threshold potential is the transition between diastole (phase 4) and the upstroke (phase 0) of the next action potential, a rapid

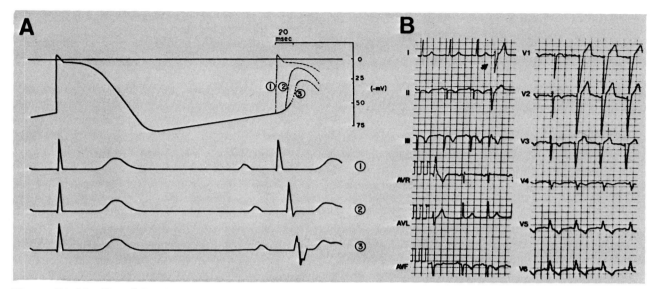

Figure 16-21. (Panel A) Schematic transmembrane potentials from latent pacemaker cell in the right bundle branch (RBB), showing how phase 4 depolarization may result in both long-cycle aberration and aberration in the absence of perceptible changes in sinus rate, even in the normal heart. The rate of phase 4 depolarization in the RBB cells is presumed to have increased to a level just lower than that of the sinus. The close similarity in rates makes it possible for the propagating sinus impulse to reach the bundle branch cells at a time when diastolic potential had been lowered to the vicinity of the threshold potential. This period, the transition between phase 4 and the upstroke of the next action potential, is characterized by a rapid increase in the rate of depolarization and a large decrease in potential over a brief time (20 milliseconds). Even slight changes in the time of arrival of the propagated impulse, due either to changes in sinus rate or in rate of diastolic depolarization of the latent pacemaker cell, would, therefore associate with marked differences in the level of potential encountered by the impulse, with resultant variability in the character and conduction of the response. Note progressive reduction in amplitude and $\dot{V}_{max}$ of the three responses (*1, 2,* and *3*) initiated successively later during the 20-millisecond period, together with depressive effects on conduction (indicated by QRS changes in electrocardiogram (ECG). Response *1* is initiated just before inscription of the threshold potential and conducts normally. Response *2* and *3* exhibit increasing right bundle-branch block aberration due to activation of the RBB at successively lower potentials. The small differences in time would not be noticeable on a standard ECG, so variations in QRS contour would be appreciated as occurring in the absence of rate changes. This mechanism also provides a reasonable explanation for beat-to-beat changes in QRS contour of the type seen in Figure 16-18. **(Panel B)** Standard 12 lead ECG from a 68-year-old male with coronary heart disease, status postinferior and anterior myocardial infarction, showing appearance and disappearance of left bundle-branch block aberrancy in the absence of clear-cut changes in sinus rate (leads V_1–V_6). Findings of variably coupled, automatic-type ventricular extrasystoles exhibiting characteristics indicative of a left-sided site of origin (beats designated by *arrow* in leads I–III) suggest that aberration may have been due to accelerated phase 4 depolarization of latent pacemakers in the left bundle branch.

increase in the rate of depolarization and a large decrease in membrane potential take place over a brief time (10 to 20 milliseconds). Under such circumstances, even small variations in the time of arrival of the propagated impulse, due either to changes in sinus rate or in the rate of diastolic depolarization of latent pacemaker cells, could result in marked changes in the level of membrane potential encountered by (and therefore in conduction of) the impulse. Accordingly, slight prolongation of the sinus cycle could result in development of considerable aberrancy. Conversely, minimal shortening may normalize conduction. In a similar vein, small changes in the rate of phase 4

depolarization of the latent pacemaker cells could affect conduction in the absence of any change in sinus rate. This mechanism would allow virtual complex-to-complex changes in conduction and provide a possible explanation for intermittent aberration of supraventricular escapes and differences in contour of beats occurring at closely similar escape intervals (see Fig. 16-19*D*).

Of the other circumstances that may be expected to facilitate development of conduction disturbances and aberrancy, two deserve special mention in light of findings in ischemic and diseased heart muscle: (1) a shift in threshold potential to less than −70 mV, so that the depolarization process can lower membrane potential to levels at which conduction is significantly impaired; and (2) alterations in the responsiveness relation similar to that depicted in Figure 16-3B, which would lessen the extent to which automatic cells must depolarize before slow conduction and block ensue.[63] In Figure 16-19B, for example, significant conduction disturbances may make an appearance on depolarization to −70 rather than at −60 mV. Lesser degrees of cycle length prolongation also may suffice. It is pertinent that the experimental production of conduction disturbances due to progressive phase 4 depolarization in isolated Purkinje fibers was generally associated with changes in the voltage time course of repolarization, such that maximum diastolic potential decreased (i.e., generalized hypopolarization ensued)[63] by shifts in take-off potential toward zero potential. Figure 16-20B (beats 4 and 5) illustrates these possibilities. Figure 16-22 (top and middle panels) seeks to explain the changes in QRS configuration seen in the records of Figure 16-19 in terms of cycle length–dependent changes in diastolic potential in latent pacemaker cells in the right bundle branch. Given the small changes in cycle length associated with the appearance and disappearance of aberrancy, the diagram presumes that phase 4 depolarization was accelerated by ischemia or other causes and that depolarization-induced shifts in threshold potential toward zero potential or the aforementioned changes in responsiveness also have occurred. El-Sherif and co-workers, based on their studies of conduction disturbance in the dog His-Purkinje system after coronary ligation, further underscore the importance of these factors in the development of long-cycle aberrancy.[305] Still others emphasize the role of cycle length–dependent changes in excitability in this regard.[154]

Oscillatory Activity

It is also suggested that depolarization-induced and other types of oscillatory activity may give rise to conduction disturbances.[34,306] The only requirement is that the cyclic changes in membrane potential be at a sufficiently slow rate to allow membrane properties to follow. Thus, the relatively slow oscillations associated with digitalis may be expected to allow cyclic changes in $\dot{V}_{max}$ and conduction velocity during diastole similar to those during phase 4 depolarization.[306] In contrast, rapid oscillations may result in a more uniform depression of membrane properties to levels commensurate with the average potential during the oscillatory activity. This would result in changes in excitability and conduction more typical of those associated with low resting potential than with enhanced automaticity. Findings of relatively slow oscillatory activity in many specimens of ischemic and diseased myocardium (see Fig. 16-4) and that many of the spontaneously active cells appear to exhibit changes in take-off potential and in responsiveness, which would be expected to facilitate development of slow conduction, underscore the potential importance of such activity as a cause of conduction disturbances.[83,86,92,106] The reported association between oscillatory activity and variable local block in such specimens also is pertinent.[83,85,86,92,104–106]

Antiarrhythmic Agents and Long-Cycle Aberrancy

Therapeutic concentrations of all antiarrhythmic agents in current use act to suppress phase 4 depolarization of latent pacemaker cells and thus may be expected to influence long-cycle aberrancy. Certain caveats are in order, however. The actions of quinidine and procainamide are illustrative and present an interesting paradox with respect to their effects on phase 4 conduction disturbances.[41,42,307,308] In one instance, therapeutic concentrations decrease or abolish automaticity of latent pacemakers, preventing development of or reversing established long-cycle aberrancy. Conversely, the direct Na^+ channel blocking actions of these agents may be expected to facilitate development of or accentuate already existing aberrancy.[40–46,144,182] The net effect on conduction and aberration would depend on the extent to which the beneficial effects of decreasing phase 4 depolarization would outweigh direct depressant effects. With low concentrations, direct depressant effects on conduction may be so minimal that the decrease in phase 4 depolarization results in improved conduction and decreased aberrancy. In contrast, with high drug concentration, depressant effects may prevail. In addition, in the case of quinidine and procainamide, high drug concentrations also may act to lower resting potential, thus facilitating development of depolarization-induced automaticity.[40–42]

To the extent that the increase in phase 4 aberrancy in ischemic and diseased hearts is due to the altered electrophysiologic properties of the large numbers of partially depolarized spontaneously active fibers contained therein, restoration of maximum diastolic potential toward more normal levels may suppress automaticity and decrease aberrancy. The catecholamines are an example of agents that act in this manner.[41,42,63,309,310] That they concomitantly enhance automaticity of normal latent pacemaker cells detracts from their usefulness, however.

Supernormal Conduction

The concept of supernormal intraventricular conduction also has been invoked to explain at least some instances of long-cycle aberrancy.[288,299–301] The term refers to the ap-

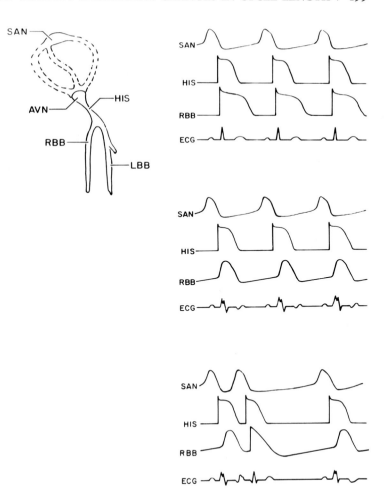

Figure 16-22. Diagram showing an alternate mechanism whereby enhanced phase 4 depolarization of latent pacemaker cells could cause aberration in the absence of significant changes in sinus rate. A possible mechanism for supernormal intraventricular conduction also is shown. A simplified representation of the conduction system is shown at left: the abbreviations are the same as those used in Figure 1 (A). Traces show transmembrane potentials from sinoatrial node, His bundle, and latent pacemaker in right bundle branch, together with lead II electrocardiogram (ECG; **top panel**) control conditions. The sinus rate is normal. Latent pacemakers in the His bundle and right bundle branch are not undergoing phase 4 depolarization. The ECG is normal. (**Middle panel**) Sinus rate unchanged. Automaticity of latent pacemakers in right bundle branch is enhanced to just less than in the sinoatrial node. Shift in threshold potential to less negative than normal levels and depressed responsiveness are assumed. As a result, amplitude and $\dot{V}_{max}$ of response initiated in right bundle-branch cells are markedly diminished and conduction depressed. The ECG shows right bundle-branch block (**Bottom panel**) A premature atrial extrasystole reaches the involved right bundle-branch cells at the point of maximum diastolic potential. Therefore, amplitude and $\dot{V}_{max}$ of the premature response are greater than those of the dominant beats, with corresponding improvement of conduction in the right bundle branch relative to that of dominant beats. QRS is correspondingly less aberrant than in dominant beats (i.e., supernormal intraventricular conduction).

parently paradoxical improvement in conduction that may occur early during recovery in patients with underlying conduction disturbances.[3–7, 21, 22, 291, 294, 301] Explanations have been offered for the phenomenon, which in a sense is the reverse of aberrancy.[3–5, 21, 22, 291, 294, 301] Paradoxically, phase 4 depolarization in latent pacemaker cells in the His-Purkinje system represents one possible cause of supernormality.[63, 291–294, 301, 311]

Because automatic cells begin to depolarize immediately on completion of repolarization, membrane potential is maximal early in the cycle and declines progressively thereafter. Action potentials initiated during the terminal phase of repolarization and immediately after its completion may therefore exhibit a greater amplitude and $\dot{V}_{max}$ and also conduct more rapidly than those initiated later in the cycle. Thus, in instances in which enhanced phase 4 depolarization causes impaired intraventricular conduction, QRS configuration of early premature beats may be more normal than those of the dominant beats. Occurrence of similar changes in the His bundle would give rise to supernormal AV conduction. Figure 16-22

(*bottom*) depicts schematically how phase 4 depolarization could produce supernormality of intraventricular conduction and the appearance of long-cycle aberrancy. With respect to the latter, notice that whereas the supernormally conducted early atrial premature complex appears normally configured, sinus complexes closing the long cycles exhibit RBBB.

ABERRANCY WITHOUT SIGNIFICANT CHANGES IN CYCLE LENGTH

Aberrancy also may occur with only minimal or even without perceptible changes in cycle length and at normal or low heart rates. The first case was probably reported in 1913 by Lewis, who designated the entity "unstable bundle branch block."[312] Intermittent bundle branch block, transient bundle branch block, inconstant bundle branch block, reversible bundle branch block, rate-dependent bundle branch block, and rate-dependent aberrancy are other designations.[203, 211, 218, 276, 277, 313–316] Although precise figures are not available, it is undoubtedly common, at least in diseased heart. Both RBBB and LBBB aberration have been reported.[203, 211, 218, 276, 277, 313–316] In contrast to the short- and long-cycle varieties, however, LBBB aberration predominates overwhelmingly. The significance of this type of aberration is substantially similar to that described for the others, except that it is even more indicative of significant conduction-system pathology than long-cycle aberrancy and is a forerunner of fixed bundle branch block. Virtually all reported cases have occurred in patients with clinical heart disease.[203, 211, 213, 218, 276, 277, 313–316]

Figures 16-16D, 16-18B,1, 16-19C and D, 16-21A; and Figure 16-23B show representative examples of intermittent LBBB and RBBB, occurring with only minimal changes in basic cycle length and at physiologic heart rates. As noted in previous cases, the cycle length of appearance and disappearance differed.[211, 213] In addition, the full-blown bundle branch block pattern usually appeared immediately, the degree of aberration varying only minimally (see Figs. 16-16D, 16-16-21A, and 16-23B). In some cases, however, variations in aberration may be considerable. For example, of the two 0.76-second cycles in Figure 16-19D, one is closed by a normally configured complex, the other by a complex exhibiting a slightly delayed terminal S wave, indicative of incomplete RBBB. Cycle length prolongation beyond 0.76 seconds resulted in further increases in aberration, culminating in a complete RBBB pattern (see Fig. 16-19A to C).

Electrophysiologic Determinants

The occurrence of aberrancy with only minimal or even without perceptible changes in cycle length implies that the propagating impulse encounters tissues that exhibit variable refractoriness throughout much or all of the cardiac cycle. This is difficult to explain simply in terms of cycle length–dependent changes in repolarization or in diastolic potential.

The major physiologic and pharmacologic factors that affect membrane potential and refractoriness independent of cycle length have been enumerated. Given the preponderant occurrence of this type of aberrancy in patients with clinical heart or conduction-system disease, alterations in electrophysiologic properties associated with ischemic and other types of disease would appear particularly relevant. Overall, the changes observed in ischemic and diseased cardiac tissues would be expected to increase refractoriness throughout the cardiac cycle. Findings of large populations of cells exhibiting reduced diastolic potential, enhanced automaticity, and variable prolongation of repolarization are representative because such changes would facilitate traversal by the propagating

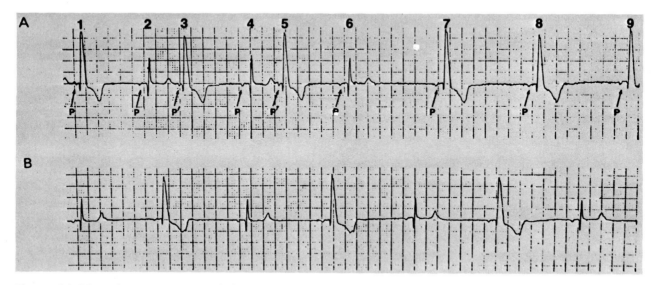

Figure 16-23. Holter-monitoring records from a 70-year old patient with hypertensive cardiovascular disease complicated by atrial ectopy and multi-type right bundle-branch block (RBBB) aberrancy. (**Panel A**) There is a basic sinus bradyarrhythmia and arrhythmia interrupted by three atrial premature beats (1, 3, 5) in the bigeminal pattern. The beats closing the shortest cycles (1, 3, 5) and those closing the longest cycles (7, 8, 9) exhibit complete RBBB. Beats closing the post-ecic cycles (2, 4, 6), which are intermediate in length, exhibit incomplete RBBB. (**Panel B**) The sinus beats, exhibit alternating incomplete and complete RBBB patterns, which are not clearly cycle length–dependent with differences between cycles averaging 0.04 seconds or less.

impulse of regions of low potential during all phases of the cardiac cycle, irrespective of cycle length. Prolongation of refractoriness beyond completion of repolarization (see Fig. 16-6) represents an additional factor. This, together with diminished cycle length dependency of action potential duration (see Figs. 16-14 and 16-15) and an increase in the time required for establishment of new steady-state duration (see Fig. 16-14), could accentuate and prolong depressant effects on conduction and refractoriness associated with repolarization and magnify the effects of even small rate changes. Altered responsiveness characteristics of the type depicted in Figure 16-3B also could be a factor because they may predispose to development of slow conduction in conjunction with even slight lowering of membrane potential, without regard to timing in the cycle.

Drug effects also are important. Several major cardio-active drugs—including particularly high concentrations of the antiarrhythmic agents, including amiodarone and the quinidine-procainamide group—act to induce changes in action potential duration, responsiveness, and conduction and diastolic potential, which may be expected to predispose to aberration, both during repolarization and phase 4. Waxing and waning of such changes in conjunction with varying drug concentrations could result in variations in QRS configuration independent of cycle length. That these agents are principally used in patients with heart disease underscores their potential importance because drug- and disease-related electrophysiologic changes may act synergistically.

Figures 16-20B, beat 5; 16-21A; 16-22 show schematic diagrams of two possible mechanisms whereby phase 4 depolarization can initiate aberration, independent of cycle length. Both have been discussed in relation to long-cycle aberrancy. The first involves accelerated rates of phase 4 depolarization of latent pacemaker cells in the involved tissues in combination with depressed responsiveness (see Figs. 16-20B, beat 5; and 16-22). The second presumes excitation of latent pacemaker cells at a time when they undergo large, rapid voltage changes over a brief time (i.e., in the vicinity of the threshold potential; see Fig. 16-21) and may be operative even normally. Because these mechanisms allow development of conduction abnormalities in the absence of significant changes in the dominant cycle, they could explain differences in QRS contour of the two complexes closing cycles of 0.76 second in Figure 16-19D. That the increases in cycle length beyond 0.76 second resulted in progressively more marked aberration (see Fig. 16-19A–C) and that the patient also exhibited premature ventricular complexes with an LBBB contour support contentions that differences in QRS contour between the two complexes in Figure 16-19D reflect changing levels of diastolic potential in the right bundle branch due to variable phase 4 depolarization. Findings

that the case of intermittent LBBB shown in Figure 16-20B was associated with premature ventricular complexes exhibiting an RBBB contour suggest that it too could have been due to variable enhancement of automaticity, this time in the left bundle branch system.

The records in Figure 16-13, which were obtained from a specimen of human papillary muscle regularly stimulated at a cycle length of 1000 milliseconds, show an unusual example of how altered electrophysiologic properties of diseased heart may cause aberration without changes in cycle length. Phase 3 of repolarization of the second beat in each of the three panels is interrupted by a spontaneously occurring premature depolarization (see Fig. 16-13, beats a–c). Premature response a is depicted as producing an aberrantly conducted propagated response (short-cycle aberrancy); conversely, b and c occur at such low levels of potential that they result in nonpropagated local responses. The postextrasystolic complexes (1, 2, and 3) show diminished amplitude and $\dot{V}_{max}$ and may be expected to exhibit depressed conduction. If comparable changes were to occur in appropriate portions of the conducting system, aberrancy would ensue. Because premature responses b and c would not propagate to the rest of the heart and produce extrasystoles that would disturb the basic rhythm, alterations in QRS contour of postextrasystolic complexes 2 and 3 would be perceived as occurring in the absence of cycle length changes.

Altered QRS contour due to this is probably a variant of short-cycle aberrancy because the first postectopic cycle is actually shorter than the interval between the basic complexes because of the occurrence of the premature response. Although reasons for the altered characteristics of the postectopic complexes are not entirely clarified, that refractoriness may considerably outlast completion of repolarization in diseased heart muscle appears to provide the best explanation because the premature responses would prolong the recovery process still further.

MIXED-TYPE ABERRANCY

The foregoing presumes that the principal types of aberrancy are explicable in terms of a unique mechanism or at least a unique primary mechanism. This generalization may hold true for most cases of short-cycle aberrancy, particularly in normal heart. It probably does not apply to the general run of cases occurring in the absence of significant cycle length changes and to instances in which more than one type of aberration occurs in the same patient (see Figs. 16-18 and 16-23). Simultaneous operation of more than one mechanism is required.

The complex interrelations between the several electrophysiologic variables appear to facilitate the simultaneous operation of multiple mechanisms of aberration. The interrelations among phase 4 depolarization of automatic cells, diastolic potential, action potential duration, and conduction are representative.[63] Phase 4 depolarization reduces end-diastolic potential of automatic cells, with resultant decrease in amplitude and $\dot{V}_{max}$ of action potentials initiated in the involved fibers and variable depression of excitability and conduction, changes that predispose to long-cycle aberrancy.[63, 291–294] Because the time course of repolarization and action potential duration are also voltage-dependent (see Figs. 16-3A, 16-8, and 16-15), it follows that reduction of diastolic potential by phase 4 depolarization may also affect these variables (see Fig. 16-20B) and thus influence development of short-cycle aberration. More specifically, because impulses initiated in partially depolarized fibers exhibit foreshortening of the early phases and prolongation of the terminal phases of repolarization, enhancement of phase 4 depolarization also may create conditions favorable to short-cycle aberrancy. If phase 4 depolarization is allowed to proceed unchecked and end-diastolic potential is reduced to sufficiently low levels, a change in voltage time course of repolarization may develop, so that maximum diastolic potential becomes reduced and generalized cell hypopolarization may ensue.[63] Impulses initiated in such fibers would be expected to develop slow-response characteristics, with respect to regarding depression of responsiveness and conduction, time-dependent prolongation of refractoriness, and diminished cycle length dependence of action potential duration. Different types of oscillatory activity also may develop. This combination of changes would expand the portion of the cycle during which aberration can occur. Conversely, the zone of normal conduction would increasingly be encroached. As the zone of normal conduction is reduced, aberration becomes increasingly independent of timing in the cycle and cycle length. Occurrence of aberrancy, with only minimal or even without significant cycle length changes and eventually, fixed bundle branch block, represents the culmination of this process.

Numerous other examples can be cited of how the interrelations between the several electrophysiologic parameters result in changes that may be expected to predispose to simultaneous operation of multiple cellular mechanisms of aberrancy. Occurrence of independent changes in two or more electrophysiologic parameters in the same or different portions of the AV conducting system (e.g., due to cardioactive drugs, ischemia, other types of disease, stretch) represents an additional predisposing factor, as would changes in the cable properties of cardiac fibers. The role of the cable properties of cardiac fibers in conduction has already been mentioned. Changes in gap junctional properties, membrane resistance and capaci-

tance, and core resistance could cause major changes in conduction velocity during all phases of the cardiac cycle. The extent to which conduction disturbances actually result from changes in the cable properties is uncertain. For the reasons cited previously, however, it is not unreasonable to suppose that changes in one or more of these properties could represent significant factors underlying altered conduction caused by stretch, changes in autonomic tone, alterations in transmembrane ionic gradients, exposure to selected cardioactive drugs, and most importantly, ischemia and disease.

The concept that multiple mechanisms of aberrancy may be simultaneously operative is useful in explaining peculiarities of conduction that are otherwise difficult to understand, including (1) occurrence of aberration at unusual times during the cardiac cycle, (2) aberration at normal heart rates and with minimal or no clear-cut evidence of cycle length dependency, and (3) multiple types (see Figs. 16-18 and 16-23) and multiform (see Figs. 16-9 and 16-10) aberrancy in a single patient at a given point in time. Rosenbaum and coworkers invoke the interrelations between automaticity and conduction to explain cases of intermittent bundle branch block and paroxysmal AV block exhibiting both long- and short-cycle–length dependency characteristics and transient development of fixed block.[291–294] Observations by this group that many of the patients with long-cycle aberrancy also exhibit the short-cycle variety are readily explicable on this basis. Our own experience accords with Rosenbaum's in this regard because we also find the combination of short- and long-cycle aberrancy in a single patient to be common. Records in Figures 16-18 and 16-23, which show both short- and long-cycle aberrancy, are representative. The patient whose records are shown in Figure 16-19 represents a third case. She originally presented with typical long-cycle RBBB aberrancy in conjunction with acute anterior infarction and went on to develop short-cycle RBBB aberration and ultimately demonstrated a period of fixed RBBB.

Finally, it is pertinent to recall findings from in vitro studies showing that specimens of ischemic and diseased human cardiac tissues are characterized by a wide spectrum of electrophysiologic changes, which may be expected to predispose to aberration in several ways because they underscore the applicability of the multiple-mechanism hypothesis to considerations of clinical aberrancy.

Acknowledgements

The authors wish to express their appreciation to Ruth H. Singer for her critical contributions and outstanding editorial services as well as for her patience with the whole endeavor.

References

1. Lewis T: The mechanism and graphic registration of the heart beat 3rd ed. London: Shaw & Sons, 1925:91.

2. Lewis T: Observations upon disorders of the heart's action. Heart 1911;3:279.

3. Pick A, Langendorf R: Interpretation of complex arrhythmias. Philadelphia: Lea & Febiger, 1979.

4. Scherf D, Schott A: Extrasystoles and allied arrhythmias. London: William Heinemann, 1973.

5. Schamroth L: Disorders of cardiac rhythm. Oxford: Blackwell Scientific Publications, 1971.

6. Bellet S: Clinical disorders of the heart beat. 3rd ed. Philadelphia: Lea & Febiger, 1971.

7. Chung EK: Principles of cardiac arrhythmias. Baltimore: Williams & Wilkins, 1971.

8. Lev M: The conduction system. In: Gould SF, ed. Pathology of the heart and blood vessels. 3rd ed. Springfield, IL: Charles C Thomas, 1968:180.

9. Truex RC: Comparative anatomy and functional considerations of the cardiac conduction system. In Paes de Carvalho A, De Mello WC, Hoffman BF, eds. The specialized tissues of the heart. Amsterdam: Elsevier, 1961:22.

10. Davies MJ: Pathology of conducting tissue of the heart. New York: Appleton-Century-Crofts, 1971.

11. Rosenbaum MB, Elizari MO, Lazzari JO: The hemiblocks. Oldsmar, FL: Tampa Tracings, 1970.

12. Demoulin JC, Kulbertus HE: Left hemiblocks revisited from the histopathological viewpoint. Am Heart J 1973;86:712.

13. Massing GK, James TN: Anatomical configuration of the His bundle and bundle branches in the human heart. Circulation 1976;53:609.

14. James TN: The connecting pathways between the sinus node and A-V node and between the right and the left atrium in the human heart. Am Heart J 1963;66:498.

15. Wagner ML, Lazzara R, Weiss RM, Hoffman BF: Specialized conducting fibers in the interatrial band. Circ Res 1966; 18:502.

16. Scherlag BJ, Lau S, Helfant R, Berkowitz W, Stein E, Damato AN: Catheter technique for recording His bundle activity in man. Circulation 1969;39:13.

17. Damato AN, Lau SH: Clinical value of the electrogram of the conduction system. Prog Cardiovasc Dis 1970;13:119.

18. Langendorf R: Concealed A-V conduction: the effect of blocked impulses on the formation and conduction of subsequent impulses. Am Heart J 1948;35:542.

19. Hoffman BF, Cranefield PF, Stuckey JH: Concealed conduction. Circ Res 1961;9:194.

20. Moe GK, Abildskov JA, Mendez C: An experimental study of concealed conduction. Am Heart J 1964;67:338.

21. Pick A, Langendorf R, Katz L: The supernormal phase of atrioventricular conduction. I. Fundamental mechanisms. Circulation 1962;26:388.

22. Moe GK, Childers RW, Merideth J: An appraisal of "supernormal" A-V conduction. Circulation 1968;38:5–28.

23. Singer DH, Ten Eick RE: Aberrancy: electrophysiologic aspects. Am J Cardiol 1971;28:381.

24. Aidley DJ: The physiology of excitable cells, 3rd ed. Cambridge: Cambridge University Press, 1989.

25. Sperelakis N, ed: Physiology and pathophysiology of the heart, 3rd ed. Boston: Kluwer, 1994.

26. Zipes DP, Jalife J, eds: Cardiac electrophysiology, from cell to bedside. Philadelphia: WB Saunders, 1990.

27. Fozzard HA, Haber E, Jennings RB, Katz AM, Morgan HE, eds: The heart and cardiovascular system. Scientific foundations, 2nd ed. New York: Raven Press, 1991.

28. Rosen MR, Janse MJ, Wit AL, eds: Cardiac electrophysiology: a textbook. Mount Kisco, NY: Futura Publishing, 1990.

29. Gilman AG, Rall TW, Nies, AS, Taylor P, eds: The pharmacologic basis of therapeutics. 8th ed. New York: McGraw-Hill, 1990.

30. Hoffman BF, Cranefield PF: Electrophysiology of the heart. New York: McGraw-Hill, 1960.

31. Singer DH, Ten Eick RE: Electrophysiology of the heart and genesis of cardiac arrhythmias. In: Conn HL Jr, Horwitz O, eds. Cardiac and vascular diseases, vol 1. Philadelphia: Lea & Febiger, 1971:182.

32. Weidmann S: Heart: electrophysiology. Annu Rev Physiol 1974;36:155.

33. Noble D: The initiation of the heart beat, 2nd ed. Oxford: Clarendon Press, 1979.

34. Cranefield PF: The conduction of the cardiac impulse. The slow response and cardiac arrhythmias. Mt. Kisco, NY: Futura Publishing, 1975.

35. Baumgarten CM, Fozzard HA: Cardiac resting and pacemaker potentials. In Fozzard HA, Haber E, Jennings RB, Katz AM, Morgan HE, eds. The heart and cardiovascular system. Scientific foundations. New York: Raven Press, 1991:963.

36. Carmeliet E, Vereecke J: Electrogenesis of the action potential and automaticity. In: Berne RM, Sperelakis N, Geiger SR, eds. Handbook of physiology, section 2. The cardiovascular system, vol 1. Baltimore, Williams & Wilkins, 1979:269.

37. Fozzard HA: Conduction of the action potential. In: Berne RM, Sperelakis N, Geiger SR, eds. Handbook of physiology, section 2. The cardiovascular system, vol 1. Baltimore: Williams & Wilkins, 1979:335.

38. Ten Eick RE, Baumgarten CM, Singer DH: Ventricular dysrhythmias: membrane basis or of currents, channels, gates, and cables. Prog Cardiovasc Dis 1981;24:157.

39. Ling G, Gerard RW: The normal membrane potential of frog sartorius fibers. J Cell Comp Physiol 1949;34:383.

40. Trautwein W: Generation and conduction of impulses in the heart as affected by drugs. Pharmacol Rev 1963;15:277.

41. Singer DH: Possible modes of pharmacologic regulation of disturbances of cardiac rate and rhythm. In:Manning GW, ed. Electrical activity of the heart. Springfield, IL: Charles C Thomas, 1968:163.

42. Singer DH, Ten Eick RE: Pharmacology of cardiac arrhythmias. Prog Cardiovasc Dis 1969;11:488.

43. Bassett AL, Hoffman BF: Antiarrhythmic drugs: electrophysiological actions. Annu Rev Pharmacol 1971;11:143.

44. Rosen MR, Hoffman BF: Mechanisms of action of antiarrhythmic drugs. Circ Res 1973;32:1.

45. Hauswirth O, Singh BN: Ionic mechanisms in heart muscle

in relation to the genesis and the pharmacologic control of cardiac arrhythmias. Pharmacol Rev 1978;30:5.

46. Singh BN, Courtney KR: The classification of antiarrhythmic mechanisms of drug action: experimental and clinical considerations. In: Zipes DP, Jalife J, eds. Cardiac electrophysiology, from cell to bedside. Philadelphia: WB Saunders, 1990:882.

47. Coraboeuf E, Deroubaix E, Coulombe A: Acidosis-induced abnormal repolarization and repetitive activity in isolated dog Purkinje fibers. J Physiol (Paris) 1980:76:97.

48. Carmeliet E: Selectivity of anti-arrhythmic drugs and ionic channels. A historical overview. Ann NY Acad Sci 1984;427:1.

49. Snyder Dirk J, Bennett PD, Hondeghem LM: Mechanisms of drug channel interaction. In: Fozzard HA, Haber E, Jennings RB, Katz AM, Morgan HE, eds. The heart and cardiovascular system scientific foundations, vol 2. New York: Raven Press, 1991:2115.

50. Hodgkin AL: The ionic basis of electrical activity in nerve and muscle. Biol Rev 1951;26:339.

51. Sperelakis N: Electrical properties of cells at rest and maintenance of the ion distribution. In: Sperelakis N, ed. Physiology and pathophysiology of the heart. Boston: Martinus Nijhoff, 1984:59.

52. Hille B: Ionic channels in nerve membranes. Prog Biophys Mol Biol 1970;21:1.

53. Catrell WA: Mollecular properties of voltage-gated ion channels in the heart. In: Fozzard HA, Haber E, Jennings RB, Katz AM, Morgan HE, eds. The heart and cardiovascular system. Scientific foundations., New York: Raven Press, 1991:945.

54. Mullins LJ: Ion transport in heart. New York: Raven Press, 1981.

55. Page E, Storm SR: Cat heart muscle in vitro. VIII. Active transports of sodium in papillary muscles. J Gen Physiol 1965;48:957.

56. Glitsch HG: Electrongenic Na pumping in the heart. Am Rev Physiol 1982;44:389.

57. Gadsby DC: The Na/K pump of cardiac cells. Am Rev Biophys Bioeng 1984;13:373.

58. Eisner DA, Smith TW: The Na-K pump and its effectors in cardiac muscle. In: Fozzard HA, Haber E, Jennings RB, Katz AM, Morgan HE, eds. The heart and cardiovascular system. Scientific foundations. New York: Raven Press, 1991:863.

59. Shey-shing S, Blaustein MP: Sodium/calcium exchange and control of cell calcium and contractility in cardiac and vascular smooth muscles. In: Fozzard HA, Haber E, Jennings RB, Katz AM, Morgan HE, eds. The heart and cardiovascular system. Scientific foundations. New York: Raven Press, 1991:903.

60. Fozzard HA, Hanck DA: Sodium channels. In: Fozzard HA, Haber E, Jennings RB, Katz AM, Morgan HE, eds. The heart and cardiovascular system. Scientific foundations. New York: Raven Press, 1991:1091.

61. Weidmann S: The effect of the cardiac membrane potential on the rapid availability of the sodium carrying system. J Physiol 1955;127:213.

62. Hoffman BF, Kao CY, Suckling EE: Refractoriness in cardiac muscle. Am J Physiol 1957;190:473.

63. Singer DH, Lazzara R, Hoffman BF: Interrelationships between automaticity and conduction in Purkinje fibers. Circ Res 1967;21:537.

64. Reuter H: The dependence of slow inward current in Purkinje fibers on the extracellular calcium-concentration J Physiol 1967;192:479.

65. Reuter H: Divalent cations as charge carriers in excitable membranes. Prog Biophys Mol Biol 1973;26:1.

66. Kohlhardt M, Bauer B, Krause H, et al: Differentiation of the transmembrane Na and Ca channels in mammalian cardiac fibers by the use of specific inhibitors. Pflugers Arch 1972; 335:309.

67. Zipes DP, Bailey JC, Elharrar V, eds. The slow inward current and cardiac arrhyythmias. Boston: Martinus Nijhoff, 1980.

68. Pelzer D, Pelzer S, McDonald TF: Calcium channels in heart. In: Fozzard HA, Haber E, Jennings RB, Katz AM, Morgan HE, eds. The heart and cardiovascular system. Scientific foundations. New York: Raven Press, 1991:1049.

69. Paes de Carvalho A, Hoffman BF, de Paula Carvalho M: Two components of the cardiac action potential. I: Voltage-time course and the effect of acetylcholine on atrial and nodal cells of the rabbit heart. J Gen Physiol 1969;54:607.

70. Wit AL, Cranefield PF: Effect of verapamil on the sinoatrial and atrioventricular nodes of the rabbit and the mechanism by which it arrests reentrant atrioventricular nodal tachycardia. Circ Res 1974;35:413.

71. Zipes DP, Fischer JC: Effects of agents which inhibit the slow channel on sinus node automaticity and atrioventricular conduction in the dog. Circ Res 1974;34:184.

72. Merideth J, Mendez C, Mueller WJ, Moe GK: Electrical excitability of atrioventricular nodal cells. Circ Res 1968;23:69.

73. Mendez C, Moe GK: Atrioventricular transmission. In: De Mello WC, ed. Electrical phenomena in the heart. New York: Academic press, 1972:263.

74. Wit AL, Fenoglio JJ Jr, Wagner BM, Bassett AL: Electrophysiological properties of cardiac muscle in the anterior mitral valve leaflet and the adjacent atrium in the dog: possible implications for the genesis of atrial dysrhythmias. Circ Res 1973;32:31.

75. Wit AL, Cranefield PF: Triggered and automatic activity in the canine coronary sinus. Circ Res 1977;41:435.

76. Cranefield PF, Wit AL, Hoffman BF: Conduction of the cardiac impulse. IV. Characteristics of very slow conduction. J Gen Physiol 1972;59:227.

77. Cranefield PF, Aronson RS, Wit AL: Effect of verapamil on the normal action potential and on a calcium dependent slow response of canine cardiac Purkinje fibers. Circ Res 1974; 34:204.

78. Solberg LE, Singer DH, Ten Eick RE: Electrophysiological study of myocardial infarction in dog. Fed Proc 31:387, 1972. Abstract.

79. Solberg L, Ten Eick RE, Singer DH: Electrophysiological basis of arrhythmia in infarcted ventricle (abstr.). Circulation 1972;46(Suppl II):116.

80. Lazzara R, El-Sherif N, Scherlag BJ: Electrophysiological properties of canine purkinje cells in one-day old myocardial infarction. Circ Res 1973;33:722.

81. Lazzara R, El-Sherif N, Scherlag BJ: Early and late effects of coronary artery occlusion on canine purkinje fibers. Circ Res 1974;35:391.

82. Friedman PL, Stewart JR, Fenoglio JJ Jr, Wit AL: Survival of subendocardial Purkinje fibers after extensive myocardial infarction in dogs; in vitro and in vivo correlations. Circ Res 1973;33:597.

83. Ten Eick RE, Singer DH, Solberg LE: Coronary occlusion. Effects on cellular electrical activity of the heart. Med Clin North Am 1976;60:49.

84. Downar E, Janse MJ, Durrer D: The effect of acute coronary artery occlusion on subepicardial transmembrane potentials in the intact porcine heart. Circulation 1977;56:217.

85. Lazzara R, Scherlag B: Role of the inward current in the genesis of arrhythmias in ischemic myocardium. In: Zipes DP, Bailey JL, Elharrar V, eds. The slow inward current and cardiac arrhythmias. Boston: Martinus Nijhoff, 1980:399.

86. Lazzara R, Scherlag R: Cellular electrophysiology and ischemia. In: Sperelakis N, ed. Physiology and pathophysiology of the heart. Boston: Martinus Nijhoff, 1984:443.

87. Gettes LS, Cascio WE: Effect of acute ischemia on cardiac electrophyysiology. In: Fozzard HA, Haber E, Jennings RB, Katz AM, Morgan HE, eds. The heart and cardiovascular system. Scientific foundations. New York: Raven Press, 1991:2021.

88. Trautwein W, Kassebaum DG, Nelson RM, Hecht HH: Electrophysiological study of human heart muscle. Circ Res 1962;10:306.

89. Ten Eick RE, Singer DH, Solberg LE, DeBoer AA: Alterations in the electrophysiological characteristics of diseased human ventricle. Circulation 1972;46(Supp III):9. Abstract.

90. Singer DH, Ten Eick RE, DeBoer AA: Possible electrophysiologic basis of chronic dysrhythmia. Circulation 1972;46 (Suppl II):90.

91. Singer DH, Ten Eick RE: Electrophysiologic correlates of aberrancy in diseased hearts. Am J Cardiol 1972;29:293. Abstract.

92. Singer DH, Ten Eick RE, DeBoer AA: Electrophysiologic correlates of human atrial tachyarrhythmias. In: Dreifus L, Likoff W, eds. Cardiac arrhythmias. New York: Grune & Stratton, 1973:97.

93. Hordof AJ, Edie R, Malm JR, Hoffman BF, Rosen MR: Electrophysiologic properties and response to pharmacologic agents of fibers from diseased human atria. Circulation 1976;54:774.

94. Talano JV, Singer DH, Ten Eick RE, et al: Intractable ventricular tachyarrhythmia in post-infarction aneurysm: clinical, electrophysiologic and electropharmacologic studies. Clin Res 1976;24:242A.

95. Ten Eick RE, Singer DH: Electrophysiologic properties of diseased human atrium. I. Low diastolic potential and altered cellular response to potassium. Circ Res 1979;44:545.

96. McCullough JR, Baumgarten CM, Singer DH: Intra- and extracellular potassium activities and the potassium equilibrium potential in partially depolarized human atrial cells. J Mol Cell Cardiol 1987;54:65.

97. Spear JF, Horowitz LN, Hodess AB, MacVaugh H III, Moore EN: Cellular electrophysiology of human myocardial infarction. I. Abnormalities of cellular activation. Circulation 1979;59:247.

98. Dangmann KH, Danilo P, Hordof A, Mary-Rabine L, Reder RF, Rosen MR: Electrophysiologic characteristics of human ventricular and Purkinje fibers. Circulation 1982;65:362.

99. Gilmour RF, Heger JJ, Prystowsky N, Zipes DP: Cellular electrophysiologic abnormalities of diseased human ventricular myocardium. Am J Cardiol 1983;51:137.

100. McCullough JR, Chua WT, Rasmussen HH, Ten Eick RE, Singer DH: Two stable levels of diastolic potential at physiological K^+ in human ventricular myocardial cells. Circ Res 1990;66:199.

101. Mary-Rabine L, Albert A, Pham TD, et al: The relationship of human atrial cellular electrophysiology to clinical function and ultrastructure. Circ Res 1983;52:188.

102. Wit A, Rosen MR, Hoffman BF: Electrophysiology and pharmacology of cardiac arrhythmias. II. Relationship of normal and abnormal electrical activity of cardiac fibers to the genesis of arrhythmias. A: Automaticity. Am Heart J 1974;88:515.

103. Wit A, Rosen MR, Hoffman BF: Electrophysiology and pharmacology of cardiac arrhythmias. II. Relationship of normal and abnormal electrical activity of cardiac fibers to the genesis of arrhythmias. B: Re-entry. Am Heart J 1974;88:664.

104. Rosen MR, Hordof AJ: The slow response in human atrium In: Zipes DP, Bailey JC, El Harrar V, eds. The slow inward current and cardiac arrhythmias. Boston: Martinus Nijhoff, 1980:295.

105. Spear JF, Horowitz LN, Moore EN: The slow response in human ventricle. In: Zipes DP, Bailey JC, Elharrar V, eds. The slow inward current and cardiac arrhythmias. Boston: Martinus Nijhoff, 1980:309.

106. Singer DH, Baumgarten CM, Ten Eick RE: Cellular electrophysiology of ventricular and other dysrhythmias: studies on diseased and ischemic heart. Prog Cardiovasc Dis 1981;24:97.

107. Singer DH: Automaticity in human cardiac tissue. In: Rosen MR, Janse MJ, Wit AL, eds. Cardiac dlectrophysiology: a textbook. Mount Kisco, NY: Futura Publishing, 1990:247.

108. Gintant GA, Datyner NB, Cohen IS: Slow inactivation of a tetrodotoxin sensitive current in cardiac Purkinje fibers. Biophys J 1984;45:509.

109. Noble D, Tsien RW: The repolarization process of heart cells. In: DeMello WC, ed. Electrical phenomena in the heart. New York: Academic Press, 1972:133.

110. Gintant GA, Cohen IS, Datyner NB, Kline RP: Time dependent outward currents in the heart. In: Fozzard HA, Haber E, Jennings RB, Katz AM, Morgan HE, eds. The heart and cardiovascular system. Scientific foundations. New York: Raven Press, 1991:1121.

111. Kenyon JL, Gibbons WR: Influence of chloride potassium, and tetraethylammonium on the early outward current of sheep cardiac Purkinje fibers. J Gen Physiol 1979;73:117.

112. Ebihara L, Shigeto NL, Lieberman M, et al: A note on the reactivation of a fast sodium current in spherical clusters of embryonic chick heart cells. Biophys J 1983;42:191.

113. Baumgarten CM, Isenberg G: Depletion and accumulation of potassium in the extracellular clefts of cardiac Purkinje fibers during voltage clamp hyperpolarization and depolarization. Pflugers Arch 1977;368:19.

114. Dant J, Rudel R: The electrogenic sodium pump in guinea-

pig ventricular muscle: inhibition of pump current by cardiac glycosides. J Physiol 1982;330:243.

115. Gadsby DC, Cranfield PF: Effects of electrogenic sodium extrusion on the membrane potential of cardiac Purkinje fibers. In: Paes de Carvalho AP, Hoffman BF, Lieberman M, eds. Normal and abnormal conduction in the heart. Mt. Kisco, New York: Futura Publishing, 1982:225.

116. Ten Eick RE, Singer DH: Effect of membrane potential and potassium on threshold potential. Fed Proc 1969;28:270. Abstract.

117. Hoffman BF, Cranefield PF: Physiologic basis of cardiac arrhythmias. Am J Med 1964;37:670.

118. Surawicz B: Normal and abnormal automaticity. In: Rosen MR, Janse MJ, Wit AL, eds. Cardiac electrophysiology: a textbook. Mount Kisco, NY: Futura Publishing, 1990:159.

119. Katzung BG, Hondeghem LM, Grant AO: Cardiac ventricular automaticity induced by current of injury. Pflugers Arch 1975;360:193.

120. Katzung BG, Morgenstern JA: Effects of extracellular potassium on ventricular automaticity and evidence for a pacemaker current in mammalian ventricular myocardium. Circ Res 1977;40:105.

121. Imanishi S, Surawicz B: Automatic activity in depolarized guinea pig ventricular myocardium. Characteristics and mechanisms. Circ Res 1976;39:751.

122. Wit AL, Cranefield PF, Gadsby DC: Triggered activity. In: Zipes DP, Bailey JC, Elharrar V, eds. The slow inward current and cardiac arrhyythmias. Boston: Martinus Nijhoff, 1980:437.

123. Wit AL, Rosen MR: Afterdepolarization and triggered activity: distinction from automaticity as an arrhyythmogenic mechanism. In: Fozzard HA, Haber E, Jennings RB, Katz AM, Morgan HE, eds. The heart and cardiovascular system. Scientific foundations. New York: Raven Press, 1991:2113.

124. Brown HF: Electrophysiology of the sinoatrial node. Physiol Rev 1982;62:505.

125. Vassale M: Analysis of the cardiac pacemaker potential using "voltage clamp" technique. Am J Physiol 1966;210:1335.

126. Noble D, Tsien RW: The kinetic and rectifier properties of the slow potassium current in cardiac Purkinje fibers. J Physiol 1968;195:185.

127. DiFrancesco D: A new interpretation of the pace-maker current in calf Purkinje fibers. J Physiol 1981;314:359.

128. DiFrancesco D: A study of the ionic nature of the pace-maker current in calf Purkinje fibres. J Physiol 1981;314:377.

129. Noma A, Irisawa H: A time and voltage dependent potassium current in the rabbit sinoatrial node. Pflugers Arch 1976; 366:251.

130. Brown HF, DiFrancesco D: Voltage clamp investigations of membrane currents underlying pacemaker activity in rabbit S-A node. J Physiol 1980;308:331.

131. Noma A, Kotake H, Irisawa H: Slow inward current and its role mediating the chronotropic effect of epinephrine in the rabbit sino-atrial node. Pflugers Arch 1980;388:1.

132. Rubenstein ES, Lipsius SL: Mechanisms of automaticity in subsidiary pacemakers from cat right atrium. Circ Res 1989; 64:648.

133. Katzung BG, Morgenstern JA: Effect of extracellular potassium on ventricular automaticity and evidence for a pacemaker current in mammalian ventricular myocardium. Circ Res 1977;40:105.

134. Carmeliet E: Evidence of pacemaker current, I_f, in human atrial appendage fibers. J Physiol 1984;357:125.

135. Malecot C, Coraboeuf E, Coucombe A: Automaticity of ventricular fibers induced by low concentrations of barium. Am J Physiol 1984;247:H429.

136. Lederer WJ, Tsien RW: Transient inward current underlying arrhythmic effect of cardiotonic steroids in Purkinje fibers. J Physiol (Lond) 1976;263:73.

137. Hiraoka M: Membrane current changes induced by acetylstrophanthidin in cardiac Purkinje fibers. Jpn Heart J 1977;18:851.

138. El-Sherif N, Gough WB, Zeiler RH, Mehra R: Triggered ventricular rhythms in 1-day-old myocardial infarction in the dog. Circ Res 1983;52:566.

139. Jack JJB, Noble D, Tsien RW: Electric current flow in excitable cells. Oxford: Clarendon, 1975.

140. Fozzard HA: The roles of membrane potential and inward Na^+ and Ca^{++} currents in determining conduction. In: Rosen MR, Janse MJ, Wit AL, eds. Cardiac electrophysiology: a textbook. Mount Kisco, NY: Futura Publishing, 1990:415.

141. Spach MS, Kootsey JM: The nature of electrical propagation in cardiac muscle. Am J Physiol 1983;244:H3.

142. Van Dam RT, Moore EN, Hoffman BF: Initiation and conduction of impulses in partially depolarized cardiac fibers. Am J Physiol 1963;204:1133.

143. Weidmann S: Effects of calcium ions and local anesthetics on electrical properties of Purkinje fibers. J Physiol 1955;129:568.

144. Hoffman BF: The action of quinidine and procainamide on single fibers of dog ventricle and specialized conduction systems. Ann Acad Bras Cienc 1958;29:365.

145. Morena H, Janse MJ, Fiolet JWT, Krieger WJG, Crijns H, Durrer D: Comparison of the effects of regional ischemia, hypoxia, hperkalemia, and acidosis on intracellular and extracellular potentials and metabolism in the isolated porcine heart. Circ Res 1980;46:634.

146. Vleugels A, Carmeliet E: Refractory period in hypoxia and in high extracellular potassium in the embryonic heart. Arch Int Physiol Biochim 1975;83:152.

147. McDonald TF, MacLeod DP: Metabolism and the electrical activity of anoxic ventricular muscle. J Physiol 1973;229:559.

148. Sakakibara Y, Wasserstrom JA, Furukawa T, et al: Characterization of the sodium current in single human atrial myocytes. Circ Res 1992;71:535.

149. Sakakibara Y, Furukawa T, Singer D, et al: Sodium current in isolated human ventricular myocytes. Am J Physiol 1993; 265:H1301.

150. Furukawa T, Sakakibara Y, Backer C, Eager S, Wasserstrom A, Singer DH: Age related changes in lidocaine effects on sodium current in isolated human atrial and ventricular myocytes. Circulation 1992;86(4):I.

151. Peon J, Ferrier GR, Moe GK: The relationship of excitability to conduction velocity in canine Purkinje tissue. Circ Res 1978;43:125.

152. Dominguez G, Fozzard HA: Influence of extracellular K^+ concentration on cable properties and excitability of sheep cardiac Purkinje fibers. Circ Res 1970;26:565.

153. Spear JF, Moore EN: Supernormal excitability and conduction in the His-Purkinje system of the dog. Circ Res 1974; 35:782.

154. Jalife J, Antzelevitch C, Lamanna V, Moe GK: Rate-dependent changes in excitability of depressed cardiac Purkinje fibers as a mechanism of intermittent bundle branch block. Circulation 1983;67:912.

155. Arnsdorf MF, Bigger JT Jr: The effect of procainamide on components of excitability in long mammalian cardiac Purkinje fibers. Circ Res 1976;38:115.

156. Arnsdorf MF, Bigger JT Jr: The effect of lidocaine on components of excitability in long mammalian cardiac Purkinje fibers. J Pharmacol Exp Ther 1975;195:206.

157. Weidman S: Passive properties of cardiac fibers. In: Rosen MR, Janse MJ, Wit AL, eds. Cardiac electrophysiology: a textbook. Mount Kisco, NY: Futura Publishing, 1990:29.

158. Weingart R, Imanaga I, Weidmann S: Low resistance pathways between myocardial cells. In: Fleckenstein A, Dhalla NS, eds. Basic functions of cations in myocardial activity. Baltimore: University Park Press, 1975:227.

159. Page E: Cardiac gap junctions. In: Fozzard HA, Haber E, Jennings RB, Katz AM, Morgan HE, eds. The heart and cardiovascular system. Scientific foundations. New York: Raven Press, 1991:1003.

160. Cranefield PF: Channels, cables, networks, and the conduction of the cardiac impulse. Am J Physiol 1983;245:H901.

161. Weingart R: The actions of ouabain on intercellular coupling and conduction velocity in mammalian ventricular muscle. J Physiol (Lond) 1977;264:341.

162. Turin L, Warner A: Carbon dioxide reversibly abolishes ionic communications between cells of early amphibian embryo. Nature 1977;270:56.

163. Weingart R, Reber W: Influence of internal pH on r_i of Purkinje fibers from mammalian heart. Experientia 1979; 35:928.

164. Janse MJ, VanCapelle FJL, Morsink H, et al: Flow of "injury" current and patterns of excitation during early ventricular arrhythmias in acute regional myocardial ischemia in isolated porcine and canine hearts. Evidence for two different arrhythmogenic mechanisms. Circ Res 1980;47:151.

165. Hoffman H: Interaction between a normoxic and a hypoxic region of guinea pig and ferret papillary muscles. Circ Res 1985;56:876.

166. Kleber AG, Riegger CB, Janse MJ: Electrical uncoupling and increase of extracellular resistance after induction of ischemia in isolated, artificially perfused rabbit papillary muscle. Circ Res 1987;61:271.

167. Lieberman M, Kootsey JM, Johnson EA, Sawanobori T: Slow conduction in cardiac muscle. Biophys J 1973;13:37.

168. DeMello WC: Effect of intracellular injection of calcium and strontium on cell communication in heart. J Physiol (Lond) 1975;250:231.

169. Wojtczak J: Contractures and increase in internal longitudinal resistance of cow ventricular muscle induced by hypoxia. Circ Res 1978;44:88.

170. Wood FC, Wolferth CC, Geckeler GD: Histologic demonstration of accessory muscular connections between auricle and ventricle in a case of short P-R interval and prolonged QRS complex. Am Heart J 1943;25:454.

171. Mahaim I: Kent's fibers and the A-V paraspecific conduction through the upper connections of the bundle of His-Tawara. Am Heart J 1947;33:651.

172. Lev M, Lerner R: The theory of Kent. A histologic study of the normal atrioventricular communications of the human heart. Circulation 1955;12:176.

173. James TN: Morphology of the human atrioventricular node, with remarks pertinent to its electrophysiology. Am Heart J 1961;62:756.

174. Lenegre J: Etiology and pathology of bilateral bundle branch block in relation to complete heart block. Prog Cardiovasc Dis 1964;6:409.

175. Lev M: The pathology of complete atrioventricular block. Prog Cardiovasc Dis 1964;6:317.

176. Cranefield PF, Klein HO, Hoffman BF: Conduction of the cardiac impulse. I. Delay, block, and one-way block in depressed Purkinje fibers. Circ Res 1971;28:199.

177. Cranefield PF, Hoffman BF: Conduction of the cardiac impulse. II. Summation and inhibition. Circ Res 1971;28:220.

178. Hoffman BF, Moore EN, Stuckey JH, Cranefield PF: Functional properties of the atrioventricular conduction system. Circ Res 1963;13:308.

179. Gettes LS, Reuter H: Slow recovery from inactivation of inward currents in mammalian myocardial fibers. J Physiol 1974;240:703.

180. Saikawa T, Carmeliet E: Slow recovery of the maximal rate of rise (Vmax) of the action potential in sheep cardiac Purkinje fibers. Pflugers Arch 1982;394(Suppl):90.

181. Lazzara R, El-Sherif N, Scherlag BT: Disorders of cellular electrophysiology produced by ischemia of the canine His bundle. Circ Res 1975;36:444.

182. Chen C-M, Gettes LS, Katzung BG: Effect of lidocaine and quinidine on steady-state characteristics and recovery kinetics of (dv/dt)max in guinea pig ventricular myocardium. Circ Res 1974;37:20.

183. Weld FM, Bigger JT: Effect of lidocaine on the early inward transient current in sheep cardiac Purkinje fibers. Circ Res 1975;37:630.

184. Bean BP, Cohen CJ, Tsien RW: Lidocaine block of cardiac sodium channels. J Gen Physiol 1983;81:613.

185. Sato R, Hisatome I, Wasserstorm JA, Arentzen CE, Singer DH: Acetylcholine-sensitive K^+ channel in human atrial myocytes. Am J Physiol 1990;259:H1730.

186. Imanishi S, Arita N: Factors relating to the membrane potentials of diseased human atrial muscle. Jpn J Physiol 1987; 37:393.

187. Lee YS: Pathophysiologic mechanisms of altered transmembrane potentials in diseased human atria. J Electrocardiol 1986;19:41.

188. Cranefield PF, Aronson RS: Initiation of sustained rhyythmic activity by single propagated action potentials in canine cardiac Purkinje fibers exposed to sodium-free solution or to ouabain. Circ Res 1974;34:477.

189. Sakmann B, Trube E: Voltage dependent inactivation of inward-rectifying single channel currents in the guinea pig heart cell membrane. J Physiol (Lond) 1984;347:659.

190. Carmeliet E: Chloride ions and the membrane potential of Purkinje fibers. J Physiol (Lond) 1961;156:375.

191. Carmeliet E: Induction and removal of inward-going rectification in sheep cardiac Purkinje fibers. J Physiol (Lond) 1982;327:285.

192. Gadsby DC, Cranefield PF: Two levels of resting potential in cardiac Purkinje fibers. J Gen Physiol 1977;70:725.

193. Kaufmann R, Rothberger CJ: Beitrage zur Entstehungsweise extrasystolischer Allorhythmien (Zweite Mitteilung). Z Gesamte Exp Med 1919;7:199.

194. Sherf L, James TN: A new electrocardiographic concept: synchronized sinoventricular conduction. Dis Chest 1969; 55:127.

195. Moe GK, Preston JB, Burlington H: Physiologic evidence for a dual A-V transmission system. Circ Res 1956;4:357:375.

196. Narula O: Longitudinal dissociation in the His bundle. Bundle branch block due to asynchronous conduction within the His bundle in man. Circulation 1977;56:996.

197. Janse MJ: Influence of the direction of the atrial wave front on A-V nodal transmission in isolated hearts of rabbits. Circ Res 1969;25:439.

198. Myerburg RJ, Stewart JW, Hoffman BF: Electrophysiological properties of the canine peripheral A-V conducting system. Circ Res 1970;26:361.

199. Myerburg RJ, Gelband H, Hoffman BF: Functional characteristics of the gating mechanism in the canine A-V conducting system. Circ Res 1971;28:136.

200. Mendez C, Mueller WJ, Merideth JT, Moe GK: Interaction of transmembrane potentials in canine Purkinje fibers and at Purkinje fiber-muscle junctions. Circ Res 1969;24:361.

201. Cohen SI, Lau SH, Haft JI, Damato AN: Experimental production of aberrant ventricular conduction in man. Circulation 1967;36:673.

202. Cohen SI, Lau SH, Stein E, Young MW, Damato AN: Variations of aberrant ventricular conduction in man: evidence of isolated and combined block within the specialized conduction system. Circulation 1968;38:899.

203. Denes P, Wu D, Dhingra RC, Amat-y-Leon F, Wyndham C, Rosen KM: Electrophysiological observations in patients with rate dependent bundle branch block. Circulation 1975;51:244.

204. Ashman RC, Byer E: Aberration in the conduction of premature ventricular impulses. J La State Univ School Med 1946; 8:62.

205. Gouaux JL, Ashman R: Auricular fibrillation with aberration simulating ventricular paroxysmal tachycardia. Am Heart J 1947;34:366.

206. Langendorf R: Aberrant ventricular conduction. Am Heart J 1951;41:700.

207. Langendorf R: Differential diagnosis of ventricular paroxysmal tachycardia. Exp Med Surg 1950;8:228.

208. Sandler IA, Marriott HJL: The differential morphology of anomalous ventricular complexes of RBBB type in lead V1. Ventricular ectopy versus aberration. Circulation 1965; 31:551.

209. Marriott HJL, Sandler IA: Criteria, old and new, for differentiating between ectopic ventricular beats and aberrant ventricular conduction in the presence of atrial fibrillation. Prog Cardiovasc Dis 1966;9:18.

210. Kistin AD: Problems in the differentiation of ventricular

211. Fisch C, Zipes DP, McHenry PL: Rate dependency aberrancy. Circulation 1973;48:714.

212. Moe GK, Mendez C, Han J: Aberrant A-V impulse propagation in the dog heart: a study of functional bundle branch block. Circ Res 1965;16:261.

213. Neuss H, Thormann J, Schlepper M: Electrophysiological findings in frequency dependent left bundle branch block. Br Heart J 1974;36:888.

214. Wellens HJJ, Bar FWHM, Lie KI: The value of the electrocardiogram in the differential diagnosis of a tachycardia with a wide QRS complex. Am J Med 1978;65:27.

215. Berliner K, Lewithin L: Auricular premature systole. I. Aberration of the ventricular complex in the electrocardiogram. Am Heart J 1945;29:449.

216. White PD: Heart disease. New York: Macmillan, 1951:867.

217. Carter JB: The fundamentals of electrocardiographic interpretation. JAMA 1932;99:1345.

218. Shearn MA, Rytand DA: Intermittent bundle branch block. Observations with special reference to the critical heart rate. Arch Intern Med 1953;91:448.

219. Cooksey JD, Dunn M, Massie E: Clinical vectorcardiography and electrocardiography. Chicago: Year Book Publishers, 1977:528.

220. Guerot CL, Valere PE, Castillo-Fenoy A, Tricot R: Tachycardie par re-entree de branche a branch. Arch Mal Coeur 1974;67:1.

221. Lewis T, Master AM: Observations upon conduction in the mammalian heart: A-V conduction. Heart 1925;12:209.

222. Scherf D: Uber intraventrikulare Storungen der Erregungsausbreitung bei den Wenckebachschen Perioden. Wein Arch Inn Med 1929;18:403.

223. Klein H, Singer D, Hoffman B: Alterations of sinus rhythm by atrial premature systoles. Circulation 1966;34(Suppl III):145.

224. Klein HO, Singer DH, Hoffman BF: Effects of atrial premature systoles on sinus rhythm in the rabbit. Circ Res 1973; 32:480.

225. Bonke F, Bouman L, Schopman F: Effects of an early atrial premature beat on activity of the sinoatrial node and atrial rhythm in the rabbit. Circ Res 1971;29:704.

226. Moe GK, Mendez C: Functional block in the intraventricular conduction system. Circulation 1971;43:949.

227. Brooks C, McGilbert JL, Greenspan ME, Lange G, Mazzella HM: Excitability and electrical response of ischemic heart muscle. Am J Physiol 1960;198:1143.

228. Ten Eick RE, Basset AL: Cardiac hypertrophy and altered cellular electrical activity of the myocardium. In: Sperelakis N, ed. Physiology and pathophysiology of the heart. Boston: Martinus Nijhoff, 1984: 521.

229. Mayuga RD Singer DH: Effects of intravenous amiodarone on electrical disperson in normal and ischemic tissues and on arrhythmia inducibility: monophasic action potential studies. Cardiovasc Res 1992;26:571.

230. Chua WT, Singer DH, Ten Eick RE: Ventricular dysrhythmia in man: cellular electrophysiologic aspects. Clin Res 1981; 29:181. Abstract.

231. Chua W, Singer D, Ten Eick R, Moran J, Hagelstein E: Well

polarized but abnormal cells: a cause of increased heterogeneity in diseased human ventricle. Fed Proc 1982;41:1385. Abstract.

232. Singer DH, Ten Eick RE, Elson J, Bonnar J: Electrophysiologic properties of diseased human atrium. Fed Proc 1977; 36:3.

233. Moore EN, Preston JB, Moe GK: Durations of transmembrane action potentials and fuctional refractory periods of canine false tendon and ventricular myocardium: comparisons in single fibers. Circ Res 1965;17:259.

234. Moore EN: Microelectrode studies on concealment of multiple premature atrial responses. Circ Res 1966;18:660.

235. Elizari MV, Greenspan K, Fisch C: Electrophysiologic studies on intraventricular aberrant conduction. Adv Cardiol 1975; 14:115

236. Toyami J: Responses of the His-Purkinje conducting system to supraventricular premature beats—in vitro and in vivo canine experiments on ventricular aberrant conduction. Jpn Circ J 1976;40:1401.

237. Bailey JC, Lathrop DA, Pippenger DL: Differences between proximal left and right bundle branch block action potential durations and refractoriness in the dog heart. Circ Res 1977;40:464.

238. Zipes DP, Knope RF, Mendez C, Moe GK: The site of functional right bundle branch block in the intact canine heart. Adv Cardiol 1975;14:105.

239. Damato AM, Lau SH, Berkowitz WD, Rosen KM, Lisi KP: Recording of specialized conducting fibers (A-V nodal, His bundle, and right bundle branch) in man using an electrode catheter technique. Circulation 1965;16:261.

240. Rosen KM, Ahahbudin H, Rahimtoola MB, Sinno MZ, Gunnar RM: Bundle branch and ventricular activation in man. Circulation 1971;43:193.

241. Krongrad E, Hefler SE, Bowman FO Jr, Malm JR, Hoffman BF: Further observations on the etiology of the right bundle branch block pattern following right ventriculotomy. Circulation 1974;50:1105.

242. Moore EN, Hoffman BF, Patterson DF, Stuckey JH: Electrocardiographic changes due to delayed activation of the wall of the right ventricle. Am Heart J 1964;68:347.

243. Rosen KM, Mehta M, Miller RA: Demonstration of dual atrioventricular nodal pathways in man. Am J Cardiol 1974; 33:291.

244. Sciacca A, Sangiorgi M: Trouble de la conduction intraventriculaire droite du a la lesion du tronc common du faisceau de His. Acta Cardiol 1957;12:486.

245. Fabregas RA, Tse WW, Han J: Conduction disturbances of the bundle branches produced by lesions in the nonbranching portion of the His bundle. Am Heart J 1976;92:356.

246. El-Sherif N, Scherlag BJ, Lazzara R: Conduction disorders in the canine proximal His-Purkinje system following acute myocardial ischemia. II. The pathology of bilateral bundle branch block. Circulation 1974;49:848.

247. Scherlag BJ, El-Sherif N, Lazzara R: Bundle branch block due to His bundle lesions. Am J Cardiol 1974;33:169.

248. Han J, Fabregas RA: Can His bundle lesions produce the electrocardiographic pattern of bundle branch block? J Electrocardiol 1977;10:205.

249. El-Sherif N, Amat-Y-Leon F, Schonfield C, et al: Normalization of bundle branch block patterns by distal His bundle pacing. Clinical and experimental evidence of longitudinal dissociation in the pathologic His bundle. Circulation 1978; 57:473.

250. James TN, Sherf L: Fine structure of the His bundle. Circulation 1971;44:9.

251. Bailey JC, Spear JF, Moore EN: Functional significance of transverse conducting pathways within the canine bundle of His. Am J Cardiol 1979;34:790.

252. Kinoshita S: Variations in the critical cycle length inducing rate dependent bundle branch block. Am Heart J 1978;96:54.

253. Wellens HJJ, Durrer D: Supraventricular tachycardia with left aberrant conduction due to retrograde invasion into the left bundle branch. Circulation 1968;38:474.

254. Spurrell RAJ, Krikler DM, Sowton E: Retrograde invasion of the bundle branches producing aberration of the QRS complex during supraventricular tachycardia. Studies by programmed electrical stimulation. Circulation 1974;50:487.

255. Slama R, Motte A, Coumel PH, Guerin F: Bloc de branche fonctionnel et conduction retrograde cachee sur la branche bloquee. Arch Mal Coeur 1970;63:1317.

256. Cohen SI, Lau SH, Sherlag BJ, Damato AN: Alternate patterns of premature ventricular excitation during induced atrial bigeminy. Circulation 1969;39:819.

257. Castellanos A, Embi A, Aranda J, Befeler B: Retrograde His bundle deflection in bundle branch re-entry. Br Heart J 1967;38:301.

258. Bandura JP, Brody DA: Microelectrode study of alternating responses to repetitive premature excitation. Circ Res 1974; 34:406.

259. Carmeliet E: Influence du rhythme sur la duree du potentiel d'action ventriculaire cardiaque. Arch Int Physiol 1955; 63:222.

260. Janse MJ, van der Steen ABM, van Dam R Th, Durrer D: Refractory periods of the dog's ventricular myocardium following changes in the frequency. Circ Res 1969;24:251.

261. Hoffman BF: Electrophysiologic mechanisms for conduction abnormalities. Chest 1973;63:651.

262. Han J, Millet D, Chizzonotti B, Moe GK: Temporal dispersion of recovery of excitability in atrium and ventricle as a function of heart rate. Am Heart J 1966;71:481.

263. Rosenbaum MB, Chiale PA, Halpern MS, et al: Clinical efficacy of amiodarone as an antiarrhythmic agent. Am J Cardiol 1976;38:934.

264. Singh BN, Vaughan Williams EM: The effect of amiodarone, a new antianginal drug, on cardiac muscle. Br J Pharmacol 1970;39:657.

265. Aomine M, McCullough J, Mayuga R, Morrone W, Singer D: Cellular electrophysiologic effects of acute exposure to amiodarone on guinea pig heart. Fed Proc 1984;43(4):961.

266. Sato R, Singer DH, Hisatome I, Jia H, Eager S, Wasserstrom JA: Amiodarone blocks the inward rectifier potassium channel in isolated guinea pig ventricular cells. J Pharmacol and Exp Therap 1994;269(3):1213.

267. Aomine M, McCullough J, Morrone W, Cigan A, Singer DH: Inhibition by amiodarone of steady-state Na current and slow inward current in guinea pig heart. Fed Proc 1985; 44(4):900.

268. Nishimura M, Follmer CH, Singer DH: Amiodarone blocks calcium current in the single ventricular myocyte of the guinea pig. J Pharmacol Exp Ther 1989;251(2):650.

269. Nishimura M, Follmer CH, Singer DH: Calcium current in single adult human atrial myocytes. J Mol Cell Cardiol. Submitted.

270. Bigger JT, Bassett AL, Hoffman BF: Electrophysiological effects of diphenylhydantoin on canine Purkinje fibers. Circ Res 1968;22:221.

271. Davis LD, Temte JV: Effects of propranolol on the transmembrane potentials of ventricular muscle and Purkinje fibers of the dog. Circ Res 1968;22:661.

272. Bissett JK, De Soyza NDB, Kane JJ, Doherty JE: Effect of diphenylhydantoin on induced aberrant conduction. J Electrocardiol 1974;7:65.

273. Johnson EA, McKinnon MC: The differential effect of quinidine and pyrilamine on the myocardial action potential at various rates of stimulation. J Pharmacol Exp Ther 1957; 120:460.

274. Follmer CH, Aomine M, Yeh JZ, Singer DH: Amiodarone-induced block of sodium current in isolated cardiac cells. J Pharmacol Exp Ther 1987;243(1):187.

275. Wilson FN: A case in which the vagus influenced the form of the ventricular complex of the electrocardiogram. Arch Intern Med 1915;16:1008.

276. Comeau WJ, Hamilton JGM, White PD: Paroxysmal bundle branch block associated with heart disease. A review and analysis of literature, with thirteen new cases and notes upon the influence of the vagus. Am Heart J 1938;15:276.

277. Vesell H: Critical rates in ventricular conduction. Unstable bundle branch block. Am J Med Sci 1941;202:198.

278. Hwang W, Langendorf R: Auriculoventricular nodal escape in the presence of atrial fibrillation. Circulation 1950;1:930.

279. Pick A: Aberrant ventricular conduction of escaped beats. Preferential and accessory pathways in the A-V junction. Circulation 1956;13:702.

280. Dressler W: Transient bundle branch block occurring during slowing of heart beat and following gagging. Am Heart J 1959;58:760.

281. Goodman RM, Pick A: An unusual type of intermittent A-V dissociation in acute rheumatic myocarditis. Am Heart J 1961;61:259.

282. Wallace AG, Lazlo J: Mechanisms influencing conduction in a case of intermittent bundle branch block. Am Heart J 1961; 61:548.

283. Walsh TJ: Ventricular aberration of A-V nodal escape beats. Comments concerning the mechanism of aberration. Am J Cardiol 1962;10:217.

284. Vessel H, Lowen G: Bundle branch block on cardiac slowing at a critical slow heart rate. Am Heart J 1963;66:329.

285. Bauer GE, Julian DG, Valentine PA: Bundle branch block in acute myocardial infarction. Br Heart J 1965;27:724.

286. Kistin AD: Atrioventricular junctional premature and escape beats with altered QRS and fusion. Circulation 1966;34:740.

287. Massumi RA: Bradycardia-dependent bundle branch block. A critique and proposed criteria. Circulation 1968;38:1066.

288. Sarachek NS: Bradycardia-dependent bundle branch block. Relation to supernormal conduction and phase 4 depolarization. Am J Cardiol 1970;25:727.

289. Massumi RA, Erten GE, Vera Z: Aberrancy of junctional escape beats. Evidence for origin in the fascicles of the left bundle branch. Am J Cardiol 1972;29:351.

290. Gay R, Brown DF: Bradycardia dependent bundle branch block in acute myocardial infarction. Chest 1973;64:114.

291. Rosenbaum MB, Elizari MV, Lazzari JO, Halpern MS, Nau GJ, Levi RJ: The mechanism of intermittent bundle branch block: relationship to prolonged recovery, hypopolarization, and spontaneous diastolic depolarization. Chest 1973; 63:666.

292. Rosenbaum MB, Elizari MV, Levi RJ, Nau GJ: Paroxysmal atrioventricular block related to hypopolarization and spontaneous diastolic depolarization. Chest 1973;63:678.

293. Elizari MV, Nau GJ, Levi RJ, Lazzari J, Halpern S, Rosenbaum M: Experimental production of rate dependent bundle branch block in the canine heart. Circ Res 1974;34:730.

294. Rosenbaum MB, Elizari MV, Chaiale P: Relationship between increased automaticity and depressed conduction in the main intraventricular conducting fascicles of the human and canine heart. Circulation 1974;49:818.

295. Lie KI, Wellens HJ, Schuilenburg RM, Durrer D: Mechanism and significance of widened QRS complexes during complete atrioventricular block in acute inferior myocardial infarction. Am J Cardiol 1974;33:833.

296. Cohen HC, D'Cruz I, Arbel ER, Langendorf R, Pick A: Tachycardia and bradycardia-dependent bundle branch block alternans. Clinical observations. Circulation 1976;55:242.

297. Drury AM, Mackenzie DW: Aberrant ventricular beats in the dog during vagal stimulation. QJ Exp Physiol 1934;24:237–247.

298. Scherf L, James TN: The mechanism of aberration in late atrioventricular junctional beats. Am J Cardiol 1972;29:529.

299. Pick A: Mechanisms of cardiac arrhythmias: from hypothesis to physiologic fact. Am Heart J 1973;86:249.

300. Wellens H: Unusual occurrence of nonaberrant conduction in patients with atrial fibrillation and aberrant conduction. Am Heart J 1969;77:158.

301. Pick A, Fishman AP: Observations in heart block. Supernormality of A-V and intraventricular conduction and ventricular parasystole under the influence of epinephrine. Acta Cardiol 1950;5:270.

302. Scherf D, Scharf MM: Supernormal phase of intraventricular conduction. Am Heart J 1948;36:621.

303. James TN: Cardiac conduction system: fetal and post natal development. Am J Cardiol 1970;25:213.

304. Bailey JC, Greenspan K, Elizari MV, Anderson GJ, Fisch C: Effects of acetylcholine on automaticity and conduction in the proximal portion of the His-Purkinje specialized conduction system of the dog. Circ Res 1972;30:210.

305. El-Sherif N, Scherlag BJ, Lazzara R, Samet P: Pathophysiology of tachycardia and bradcardia dependent block in the canine proximal His-Purkinje system after acute myocardial ischemia. Am J Cardiol 1974;33:529.

306. Saunders JH, Ferrier GR, Moe GK: Conduction block associated with transient depolarizations induced by acetylstrophanthidin in isolated canine Purkinje fibers. Circ Res 1967;32:610.

307. Strauss HC, Singer DH, Hoffman BF: Biphasic effects of

procainamide on cardiac conduction (Abstract). Bull NY Acad Med 1967;43:1194. Abstract.

308. Singer DH, Strauss HC, Hoffman BF: "New" mode of action of antiarrhythmic agents. Am J Cardiol 1967;19:151. Abstract.

309. Hoffman BF, Singer DH: Appraisal of the effects of catecholamines on cardiac electrical activity. Ann NY Acad Sci 1967;139:914.

310. Ten Eick RE, Singer DH, Parameswaran R, Drake F: Effect of catecholamines on electrical diastole in normal, acutely and chronically depolarized cardiac tissues. Fed Proc 1971; 30:393. Abstract.

311. Hoffman BF: Physiology of atrioventricular transmission. Circulation 1961;24:506.

312. Lewis T: Certain physical signs of myocardial involvement. Br Med J 1913;1:484.

313. Baker BM Jr: The effect of cardiac rate and the inhalation of oxygen on transient bundle branch block. Arch Intern Med 1930;45:814.

314. Sandberg AA, Wener J, Master AM, Scherlis L: Intermittent and transient bundle branch block. A clinical and electrocardiographic study. Ann Intern Med 1951;35:1085.

315. Bauer GE: Transient bundle branch block. Circulation 1964;29:730.

316. Schuilenburg RM, Durrer D: Rate dependency of functional block in the human His bundle and bundle branch Purkinje system. Circulation 1973;48:526–540.

Cardiac Arrhythmias, 3rd edition, edited by William J. Mandel.
J. B. Lippincott Company, Philadelphia © 1995.

17

Howard C. Cohen • Donald H. Singer

Bundle Branch Block and Other Forms of Aberrant Intraventricular Conduction: Clinical Aspects

The contour of the QRS complex reflects the direction and magnitude of the electric potentials produced by the depolarizing cells of the ventricles. The possible number of different patterns of QRST complexes in patients is infinite, with no two patients having precisely the same 12-lead electrocardiogram. Certain similarities, however, allow electrocardiographic patterns of aberrant intraventricular conduction to be divided into groups by recognizable characteristics. This chapter discusses the groups that include bundle branch blocks (BBB), fascicular blocks, mural blocks, conduction defects associated with spontaneous or pacemaker-induced ectopic ventricular beats, and several types of ventricular preexcitation.

A discussion of these intraventricular conduction defects must incorporate the specialized conduction system of the heart, including (1) the sinus node and a specialized endocardial atrial conduction system; (2) the atrioventricular (AV) node; (3) the His bundle (HB), which may be nonhomogenous; (4) the main left bundle branch (LBB); (5) the anterior, posterior, and possibly septal fascicles or divisions of the LBB, which are probably not entirely discrete; (6) the right bundle branch (RBB); and (7) the Purkinje system, which spreads throughout the endocardium and is in contact with the working myocardium.[1–7] The nonhomogeneity of the HB has been proved by normalization of BBB with distal HB pacing.[8]

BUNDLE BRANCH BLOCK AND FASCICULAR BLOCK

Incidence, Etiology, and Prognosis

Bundle branch block occurs in about 0.6% of the population, in 1% to 2% of the population older than 60 years of age, and less in men from 35 to 65 years of age with a negative history and physical examination.[9] Organic heart disease is present in up to 80% of these patients, with

The work for this chapter was supported in part by grants-in-aid to Drave Cohen by United States Public Health Service (HL-176648) and by Cardiac Consultants of Chicago and to Dr. Singer by the American Heart Association (74-1065), the Chicago Heart Association (B74-73), and the Reingold Estate.

513

coronary artery disease being present in up to 50%.[10] Conduction defects in bundle branches and fascicles, diagnosed by electrocardiogram, are frequently associated with pathologic changes in the suspected locations.[11] Patients with such chronic conduction defects have a higher mortality if significant cardiac disease is present and develop AV block and sudden death with greater frequency than patients without such defects.[12,13] Mortality is also higher if premature ventricular contractions are present; the predominant cause of sudden death in these patients is ventricular arrhythmia, including fibrillation.[14,15] The good prognosis in asymptomatic patients with BBB is related to the absence of progressive disease and perhaps to the finding that BBB per se, at least in animals, does not decrease the fibrillation threshold.[16] In middle-aged men, the 5-year mortality in those shown to have a conduction defect on a 6-hour electrocardiogram is about 33%.[17] Almost 33% of asymptomatic patients with intraventricular conduction defects develop clinical evidence of coronary artery disease in an average of 8 years.[18] Most patients with chronic BBB who die suddenly have coronary artery disease, and the presence of left bundle branch block (LBBB) with coronary artery disease predicts higher long-term mortality than other forms of BBB.[19,20] Patients with BBB and coronary artery disease have more extensive disease and worse left ventricular function than patients without BBB. Patients with BBB also are more prone to hypertension, cardiomegaly, and heart failure.[21] Some studies to predict prognosis, including electrode catheter recordings from the HB to diagnose the location of AV block in the presence of BBB, show that if conduction from the HB to the ventricles (HQ interval) is markedly prolonged, the rate of progression to second-degree type II AV block is high.[21,22] The prognosis is poor in terms of progression of the conduction defect and of cardiac failure if clinically significant symptoms of cardiac disease are present when BBB is diagnosed.[15,23-29] The PR intervals may or may not be good predictors of longer HQ intervals or of survival.[23,30,31] Patients with LBBB are more likely to have long HQ intervals than patients with right bundle branch block (RBBB), at least partly because RBB conduction is normally longer than LBB conduction.[32,33]

Drugs In Patients With Bundle Branch Block

Although one study suggests that intravenous quinidine does not cause increased infranodal conduction time in patients with BBB, intravenous procainamide, disopyramide, and ajmaline have caused such increases, and drugs such as quinidine, procainamide, amiodarone, ajmaline, and possibly lidocaine must be used with caution

in these patients, especially when HQ intervals are long, to avoid producing AV block.[34-41]

Atria-to-His Bundle and HQ Intervals

High degrees of HQ block may occur in patients with BBB, even when conducted beats have normal or almost normal HQ intervals.[42] Patients with syncope and BBB frequently have either inducible ventricular tachycardia or inducible HQ block.[37]

Additional studies indicate that patients with chronic BBB and prolonged conduction from the atria to the His-bundle (AH) interval are more likely to have significant congestive failure but have no greater mortality than patients with normal AH intervals.[43]

Chronic Bundle Branch Block

In the aging heart, BBB appears to be a remarkably stable pattern.[44] Between 3% and 4% of patients with chronic bifascicular block develop high-degree AV block during a 5-year average follow-up.[45] Most deaths are due to progression of congestive heart failure.[46]

The type and degree of AV block may indicate the most likely location of block and the general prognosis. Patients with second-degree type I (Wenckebach) AV block usually have block in the AV node and have a better prognosis than patients with second-degree type II AV block, which is usually in the HB or the bundle branches, although type I block may also occur in the HB or bundle branches (Figs. 17-1 through 17-3).[47-50] The electrocardiogram and the HB recording together give an even better indication of the location of conduction defects.[51] In the absence of BBB associated with acute myocardial infarction (MI) or second-degree AV block, however, there is no general agreement that any other information allows conclusions on the need for prophylactic artificial pacing. If patients with chronic bifascicular block develop block below the HB during atrial pacing at rates of 130 beats per minute or less, they are likely to develop spontaneous AV block. The absence of such block during pacing, however, may be found in patients with long HV intervals.[52] The rate at which second-degree AV block occurs may be altered by sympathetic or parasympathetic tone, as shown by studies with propranolol and atropine.[53] Asymptomatic patients who have or develop BBB with no obvious heart disease are likely to have an excellent prognosis, even when HV intervals are significantly prolonged.[29,54-56] Even in patients who demonstrate RBBB and LBBB at different times,

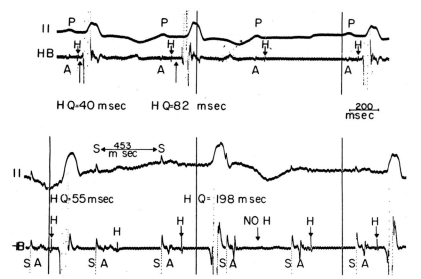

Figure 17-1. The *top panel* shows lead II and a His bundle (HB) electrogram. The QRS is of left bundle-branch block. the first two complexes are conducted but with a gradually prolonging His-to-QRS (HQ) interval going from 40 to 82 milliseconds. The third atrial (*A*) wave is followed by an HB potential (*H*) but no QRS complex. Thus, left bundle-branch block with type I second-degree HQ blocks exists, possibly occurring in the right bundle branch. In the *lower panel*, lead II and an HB electrogram are also seen. Here, with atrial pacing (*S*, pacing spike) at a rate more rapid than seen in the top panel, 2:1 atrioventricular (AV) block is seen; the first complex is conducted, the second is not, and the third is conducted again. On the conducted beats, the HQ interval prolongs from 55 to 198 milliseconds. The next complex that should have conducted, after the fifth pacing spike, does not reach the ventricles, although the HB potential is seen. Thus, alternate-beat type I second-degree HQ block exists. Also, the fourth paced atrial beat is the only one not followed by an His potential. This beat follows the long HQ interval (198 milliseconds) and could be missing because there has been intra-Hisian reentry, with concealed conduction moving retrogradely into the AV node, causing the subsequent atrial-to-His bundle (AH) block. (Abbreviations remain the same in all the figures in this chapter unless otherwise indicated.)

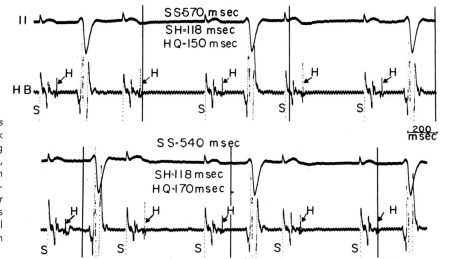

Figure 17-2. Both the *top* and *bottom panels* show artificial pacing of the atria with 2:1 block below the His bundle. At the shorter pacing interval of 540 milliseconds in the lower panel, however, the HQ interval has lengthened from 150 milliseconds in the upper panel to 170 milliseconds in the lower panel. This tendency for increasing conduction time as the rate increases is a feature of tissue capable of displaying type I second-degree atrioventricular block, as shown in Figure 17-3.

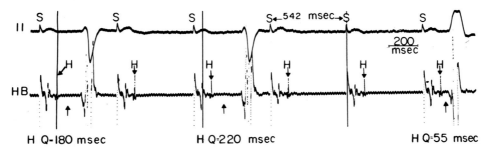

Figure 17-3. Lead II shows left anterior fascicular block. (Lead V₁, not shown, indicated right bundle-branch block simultaneously.) In the first four beats, there is a 2:1 block below the His bundle, so that the first and third *H* are followed by QRS complexes but the second and fourth are not. The HQ interval of the first conducted beat is 180 milliseconds, however, and the HQ interval of the second conducted beat is 220 milliseconds. The fifth *H* is not followed by the expected QRS complex, so that the pattern of alternate-beat type I second-degree HQ block is seen. The sixth beat is again conducted but now, after the long pause, the right bundle branch is recovered. Although the right bundle branch has a longer refractory period, having been blocked in previous beats, it has shorter conduction time, so that the HQ in the last beat is 55 milliseconds and the pattern of left bundle-branch block appears.

prognosis is more strongly related to associated heart disease than to the degree of AV block.[57]

Neurologic Symptoms and Bundle Branch Block

Patients with BBB who have neurologic symptoms must be followed-up closely. Syncope in patients with bifascicular block is usually not due to complete heart block, however.[27,58] Atrioventricular block in these patients is likely to be associated with long HQ intervals, whereas neurologic symptoms without AV block are likely to be associated with nearly normal HQ intervals.[59,60] Prophylactic permanent pacing may or may not protect these patients from sudden death.[19,60]

Chronic Bundle Branch Block and Pacemakers

Patients who have definite second-degree type II AV block need permanent pacemakers.[61] The prognosis in patients with Mobitz type II AV block is probably similar to that of those with third-degree AV block. In younger patients, complete heart block is frequently congenital and although the risk of syncope is about 5% over 15 years, the risk of sudden death is probably not increased.[62] Patients with second or third-degree AV block who get pacemakers are unlikely to die from pacemaker failure but they do have an increased mortality compared with the general population, mainly because of progression of underlying heart disease.[63]

Acute Myocardial Infarction and Bundle Branch Block

Perhaps 20% of patients admitted to a coronary care unit with definite MI have or develop conduction defects. Of patients with definite acute MI, complete AV block may occur in 6% of those without conduction defects, in 50% of those with RBBB, in 40% of those with RBBB and left anterior fascicular block (LAFB) or left posterior fascicular block (LPFB), and in 20% of those with LBBB.[64] Development of LBBB, RBBB, or RBBB with fascicular block acutely at the time of a MI indicates a poorer prognosis than does the infarction without these conduction defects.[65-67] Patients with RBBB are more likely to develop cardiogenic shock, AV block, or ventricular asystole, whereas those with LBBB tend to develop ventricular arrhythmias.[68] Thirty-six percent of patients with acute MI and BBB develop late in-hospital ventricular fibrillation.[69] Both in-hospital and out-of-hospital risk of sudden death is higher in postinfarction patients with BBB.[70,71] Ventricular tachycardia may be initiated by bundle branch reentry, and such reentrant tachycardias may sometimes be treated with catheter ablation.[72-75] Even if second-degree or high-degree AV block is transient, permanent pacing should be strongly considered.[27,72] Patients with acute conduction defects after anterior MI have a high risk of developing complete AV block and a temporary artificial pacemaker should be inserted despite some evidence that such treatment may have little effect on survival.[65,67,76-81]

Prognosis is better for patients with a normal HQ interval and transient BBB.[82,83] The combination of BBB and congestive heart failure suggests a poor prognosis. The prevalence of late sudden death may be high, even if the BBB is transient.[27] If AV block develops and then regresses, patients are more likely to have coronary artery disease and they have a poorer prognosis than patients with stable chronic AV block.[84] When etiologies are compared, patients with LBBB who develop AV block are likely to have coronary artery disease, whereas patients with RBBB and LAFB who develop AV block are more likely to have primary conduction system disease.[85]

Coronary Artery Bypass and Bundle Branch Block

Intraventricular conduction defects develop in from 17% to 30% of patients undergoing coronary artery bypass surgery.[86,87] In Chu and coworkers' study slightly less than half of the conduction defects were persistent.[87] Right bundle branch block, LAFB, and incomplete right bundle branch block (IRBBB) were the most frequent patterns. Right bundle branch block occurred more than twice as frequently as any other pattern in the transient blocks but each of these three patterns occurred in about 30% of the persistent examples. Bundle branch block was more likely to have been diagnosed recently and in older patients. Perioperative development of intraventricular conduction defects had little effect on prognosis. The presence of LBBB before surgery was associated with a significantly higher 1-year mortality during and after surgery. Caspi and associates found that patients who developed BBB at surgery had a higher incidence of left main coronary artery disease and previous MI.[86] Patients with postoperative BBB had a higher perioperative MI rate (7.3% versus 1.9%), higher incidence of low cardiac output (16.4% versus 2.7%), and a higher mortality (5.5% versus 0.8%). New LBBB had the worst outlook.

In a third study, slightly more than 20% of patients undergoing coronary artery bypass surgery developed an intraventricular conduction defect.[88] This development correlated with long-standing hypertension, older age, left main coronary artery disease, posterior descending coronary artery disease, preoperative use of digitalis, and longer pump and cross-clamp times. There was no effect on prognosis.

Production of Bundle Branch Block by Drugs

Class IA drugs such as quinidine may cause intraventricular conduction defects, sometimes but not usually suggestive of BBB. During supraventricular tachycardia, class IC drugs such as flecainide may be associated with QRS patterns compatible with RBBB with right or right superior axis or LBBB with left axis deviation.[89]

Rate- and Exercise-Related Bundle Branch Block

Bundle branch block and fascicular block may be persistent or intermittent.[57,90] These conduction defects may be tachycardia-, bradycardia-, or non–rate-dependent and they may occur on alternate beats or as a BBB Wenckebach phenomenon.[91–94] In one study, exercise-induced BBB has a high correlation with coronary artery disease, with a high prevalence of proximal left anterior descending narrowing, whereas in another study, no coronary artery disease was found.[95,96]

LEFT BUNDLE BRANCH BLOCK

Incidence and Etiology

Left bundle branch block almost always develops after birth, occasionally with no clinical evidence of heart disease and is most common in males.[62,97] The incidence is 1 in 100 to 1 in 10,000 in various studies, with the 10-year Icelandic study showing an incidence of 0.43% in men and 0.28% in women.[98,99] Usually, LBBB is associated with hypertensive heart disease, coronary artery disease, myocarditis, or aortic valvular disease, including bacterial endocarditis and aortic root abscess formation.[97,100,101,102,103] Routine exercise tests may not differentiate between patients with and patients without obstructive coronary disease in the presence of LBBB but potassium and rubidium scans of the heart during exercise show defects compatible with unsuspected old anteroseptal MI; thallium scans, especially with dipyridamole or adenosine, may show transient ischemia, thereby delineating the possible etiology of LBBB.[104–107] Also, the space–time analysis of the interventricular septum by Fourier transform, using radionuclide imaging, may differentiate anteroseptal MI from cardiomyopathy as a cause of LBBB.[108]

Left bundle branch block is not uncommon in patients with cardiomyopathies—both the dilated and the hypertrophic obstructive type.[109,110] The site of LBBB in dilated cardiomyopathies may be peripheral rather than in the left bundle.[111] Myocarditis may also be associated with LBBB.[112] Less frequently, LBBB may be associated with other cardiac or generalized conditions such as hyperkalemia, rarely myotonic dystrophy, bacterial endocarditis, or even digitalis toxicity.[113–117] Pathologic correlations suggest that LBBB is usually associated with fibrosis in the main LBB, although electrophysiologic studies suggest that the pattern of LBBB may occur as a result of an HB lesion.[8,118] Left bundle branch block occurs rarely as a congenital lesion with unknown pathology.[119]

Clinical Findings

The discovery of LBBB on the electrocardiogram is often associated with symptoms, signs, or a history compatible with clinical heart disease such as angina, old MI, hypertension, cardiac failure, or cardiomegaly. Left bundle branch block may occur only with increased heart rate associated with exercise and chest pain and may respond to physical training, even in the absence of coronary artery disease.[120] Quantitative analysis of radionuclide ventriculograms may show abnormalities even in patients at rest, who have only exercise-induced LBBB and no other obvious disease.[121] There may be a 3-year cumulative mortality of 17% in patients with chronic LBBB and organic heart disease.[122] On physical examination, there may be evidence of aortic valvular disease, diastolic gallops associated with heart failure, or a paradoxically split second heart sound, produced by prolongation of left ventricular isometric contraction because of left ventricular dysfunction or because of delay of onset of mechanical systole secondary to the LBBB.[123] Also, the first heart sound may be diminished and the preejection period may be prolonged.[124] His-bundle recordings in patients with LBBB may show prolonged HQ intervals (more commonly with hypertension than with ischemic heart disease) or second-degree AV block (Fig. 17-4).[30, 32, 125, 126] The catheter used to record HB potentials in patients with LBBB may damage the RBB and produce complete AV block and balloon-tipped pulmonary artery catheters may do the same.[127–129] Generally, patients with LBBB do not have as good a prognosis as patients with normal electrocardiograms because of the cardiac diseases frequently associated with this conduction abnormality. Left axis deviation may or may not worsen this prognosis but additional nonspecific intraventricular conduction defects, sometimes after MI, are independently associated with excess mortality to a significant degree.[31, 41, 55, 130, 131] Left ventricular dysfunction

is more likely to be present with coronary artery disease if LBBB is present.[1] New-onset LBBB in adults probably carries a poor prognosis.[62] The general experience is mixed, however. Patients with chronic LBBB and first-degree AV block have a 33% yearly mortality.[16]

Acute Myocardial Infarction and Left Bundle Branch Block

Left bundle branch block associated with acute MI may or may not affect prognosis acutely but the 1-year mortality with LBBB after an acute MI is worse than without LBBB, and programmed ventricular stimulation to produce ventricular tachycardia probably identifies a higher risk group.[132–136] If new first-degree AV block is associated with LBBB and acute MI, the incidence of development of sudden AV block is higher.[137] Temporary pacemakers are usually used when new LBBB occurs with acute anteroseptal MI, although the indication is in dispute; however, complete AV block may develop. Left bundle branch block existing before an MI indicates an even worse prognosis, increasing the mortality to 57% acutely, compared with 29% in patients who sustain an acute MI after having had a previously normal electrocardiogram, but the cause of death is usually not AV block.[138]

Left Bundle Branch Block Without Associated Heart Disease

In the absence of associated heart disease, LBBB may be benign and without obvious hemodynamic effect, even though septal motion may be abnormal on echocardiography.[139, 140] This abnormal septal motion may produce falsely positive thallium scans in patients with LBBB.[141] Chronic LBBB not associated with acute MI carries a low

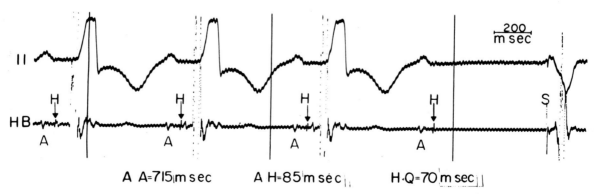

Figure 17-4. Lead II and an His bundle recording during sinus rhythm with left bundle-branch block. Atrial-to-His (AH) intervals are normal at 85 milliseconds. (His-to-QRS (HQ) intervals are prolonged at 70 milliseconds. Both AH and HQ intervals are fixed in the first three beats. In the fourth beat, there is no QRS complex. Thus, there is second-degree type II block within or below the bundle of His.

incidence of development of AV block and does not warrant a prophylactic permanent pacemaker.[30] Exercise-induced LBBB in the absence of coronary artery disease or LV (left ventricular) dysfunction carries a good prognosis, with little or no incidence of development of complete AV block.[142]

Arrhythmias and Left Bundle Branch Block

Left bundle branch block has some implications with respect to ventricular arrhythmias. For example, LBBB may obscure QT prolongation caused by quinidine, so that the risk of torsades de pointes is not recognized.[143]

Electrocardiogram

The electrocardiogram of LBBB (Tables 17-1 and 17-2) is generally characteristic (Fig. 17-5), with QRS complexes widening to at least 0.12 second but averaging 0.07 seconds more than normal, showing slurring throughout, prolongation of the intrinsicoid deflection, and ST-segment and T-wave deviation away from the direction of the major QRS depolarization. QT intervals are prolonged by 0.062 seconds beyond normal.[144] The axis is usually normal but is sometimes leftward or even rightward, perhaps in association with LAFB or LPFB.[145, 146] (The diagnosis of LAFB and LPFB, however, is generally not used simultaneously with the diagnosis of LBBB.) There is loss of the normal Q waves in some or all of the left-sided leads (I, aV_L, V_5, and V_6) because the direction of the interventricular septal depolarization is reversed from its normal left-to-right to right-to-left orientation.[147] More details are apparent on the signal-averaged electrocardiogram.[148] Left bundle branch block may be constant (see Fig. 17-5), intermittent (Fig. 17-6), or alternating and may occur in a Wenckebach pattern.[92–94] Left bundle branch block on the electrocardiogram may in part mimic or conceal other electrocardiographic diagnoses such as MI, although iso-integral mapping or dipole analysis may allow diagnosis of MI even in the presence of this conduction abnormality.[149–152] Certain ECG criteria are said to correlate with MI in the presence of LBBB. Some of these, such as Q waves in leads I, aV_L, V_5, or V_6 are problematic because many electrocardiographers do not diagnose LBBB in the presence of these Q waves.[153] Other criteria, such as notching of the upstroke of the S waves in two of V_3, V_4 or V_5 and R-wave

(*text continues on page 522*)

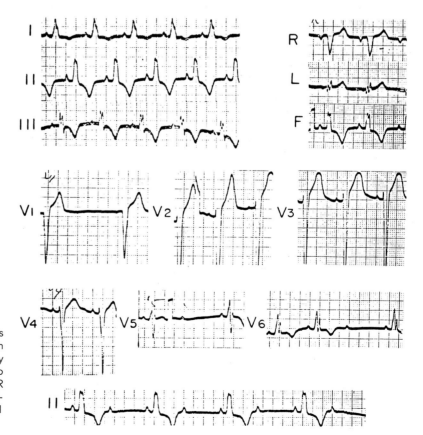

Figure 17-5. Left bundle-branch block at a sinus rate of 76 beats/min. QRS complexes are upright in lead I, with no Q wave in leads I, V_5, and V_6, and they are wide and slurred throughout. Long pauses due to blocked P waves are seen in leads V_1, V_5, and V_6. PR intervals are constant in V_6. The block is second-degree, type II. In the bottom strip showing lead II, 2:1 block develops at a sinus rate of 81 beats/minute.

TABLE 17-1. Effects of Bundle Branch and Fascicular Block on QRS Contour

	LBBB	RBBB	IRBBB	ILBBB	LAFB	LPFB	LSFB	RBBB + LAFB	RBBB + LPFB
QRS in leads I, aVL	Loss of Q wave	Terminal slurred S wave	Small terminal S wave	Loss of Q wave	Small Q, tall R waves	Small R, deep S waves		Small Q, tall R, terminal slurred S wave	Small R, deep slurred S wave
QRS in leads II, III, aVF		Terminal slurred S or R wave			Small R, deep S waves	Small Q, tall R waves		Small R, deep slurred S waves	Small Q, tall R wave, slurred S wave
QRS in lead aVR		Terminal slurred R wave	Terminal R wave		Terminal R wave	Terminal S or R wave		Terminal slurred R wave	Terminal slurred R wave
QRS in lead V1	Mainly negative	Terminal slurred R wave	Terminal R wave	Mainly negative	May have initial Q wave		Tall R wave	Terminal slurred R wave	Terminal slurred R wave
QRS in leads V5, V6	Loss of Q wave	Terminal slurred S wave	Terminal S wave	Loss of Q wave	Biphasic RS wave			Biphasic R wave and slurred S	Terminal slurred S wave
May mimic RVH	No	No	No	No	No	No	No	No	Yes
May mimic LVH	Occasionally	No	No	No	Yes	No	no	Yes	No
May hide LVH	Yes	No	No	No	No	Yes	No	No	Yes
QRS duration	At least 0.12 sec or 0.07 sec greater than normal	At least 0.12 sec or 0.06 sec greater than normal	Classically 0.1–0.11 sec	0.1–0.11 sec	25 ms greater than normal (also see text)	See text		≥0.12 sec	≥0.12 sec
QRS axis	No effect	No major effect	No effect	No effect	More negative than −30°	+100° or greater	No effect	More negative than −30°	+100° or more

*RVH, right ventricular hypertrophy; LVH, left ventricular hypertrophy; LBBB left bundle branch block, RBBB, right bundle branch block; IRBBB, incomplete right bundle branch block; ILBBB, incomplete left bundle branch block; LAFB, left anterior fascicular block; LPFB, left posterior fascicular block; LSFB, left septal fascicular block.

TABLE 17-2. Effects of Bundle Branch and Fascicular Block on Patterns of Myocardial Ischemia

	LBBB	RBBB	ILBBB	IRBBB	LAFB	LPFB	LSFB	RBBB + LAFB	RBBB + LPFB
May mimic anteroseptal MI	Yes	No	Yes	No	Yes	No	No	Yes	No
May mimic inferior MI	Yes	No	No	No	No	Yes	No	No	Yes
May mimic lateral MI	No	No	No	No	Yes	No	No	Yes	No
May mimic true posterior MI	No	Sometimes	No	No	No	No	Yes	Sometimes	Sometimes
May hide inferior MI	Sometimes	No	Sometimes	No	Yes	No	No	Yes	No
May hide lateral MI	Yes	No	Yes	No	No	Yes	No	No	Yes
May hide true posterior MI	Yes	No	Yes	No	No	No	No	No	No
May mimic anteroseptal ischemia	No	Yes	No	Yes	No	No	Yes	Yes	Yes
May mimic inferior ischemia	Yes	No	Yes	No	No	Yes	No	No	Yes
May mimic lateral ischemia	Yes	No	Yes	No	Yes (leads I, aV$_L$)	No	No	No	No
May hide anteroseptal ischemia	Yes	No	Yes	No	No	No	No	No	No
May hide inferior ischemia	Sometimes	Sometimes	No	No	Yes	No	No	Yes	No
May hide lateral ischemia	No	Yes	No	Yes	Yes (leads V$_5$, V$_6$)	Yes	No	Yes (leads V$_5$, v$_6$)	Yes
May hide high lateral ischemia	No	Yes	No	Yes	No	Yes	No	Yes	Yes

LBBB, left bundle branch block; RBBB, right bundle branch block; ILBBB, incomplete left bundle branch block; IRBBB, incomplete right bundle branch block; LAFB, left anterior fascicular block; LSFB, left septal fascicular block; MI, myocardial infarction.

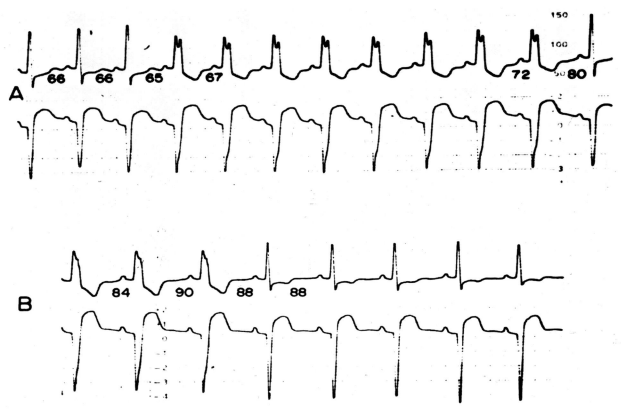

Figure 17-6. (**A**) A lateral and an anterior lead during sinus arrhythmia. RP intervals are indicated in hundredths of a second. PR intervals are constant. As the RR interval decreases from 66 to 65 hundredths of a second, left bundle-branch block develops and persists because of concealed transseptal retrograde conduction, even as the rate slows and RR intervals gradually change from 67 to 72 hundredths of a second. When the RR interval prolongs further, to 80 hundredths of a second, left bundle-branch block disappears. (**B**) Left bundle-branch block disappears when the RR interval goes from 90 to 88 hundredths of a second. Thus, in the *upper panel*, left bundle-branch block is tachycardia-dependent, although the rate at which it appears and the rate at which it disappears are not the same. In the *lower panel* the changes suggest bradycardia-dependent left bundle-branch block.

regression from V_1 to V_4 with LBBB are easier to accept.[154] Other investigators have found that in the presence of LBBB produced by right ventricular pacing, Q waves in V_5 and V_6 do not have sufficient specificity or predictive accuracy.[155] They found that notching of the upstroke of the S wave in V_3, V_4, and V_5 was more often with MI than without and more often with anterior than with posterior MI. Notching of the R wave in leads I, aV$_L$, and V$_6$ were more common without MI than with MI. Notching in leads II, III and aV$_F$ was not useful to diagnose MI. Certain electrocardiograms clearly show qR complexes in II, III and aV$_F$, in anterolateral leads, or both, and intraventricular conduction defects.[156] These QRS complexes may be 0.12 seconds in duration but do not fulfill the usual criteria for a conduction defect in the LBB. Cardiac surface isoarea maps, however, may be of greater benefit in the diagnosis and localization of myocardial ischemia and infarction in the presence of LBBB.[157] The reciprocal changes associated with the absence of Q waves in the left precordial leads are

Q waves in the right precordial leads, usually in V_1 and sometimes in V_1 through V_3. Occasional cases of intermittent LBBB are associated with electrocardiograms that have QS complexes in leads V_1 through V_3 during LBBB but R waves in leads V_1 through V_3 during normal conduction. Thus, in the presence of LBBB, abnormal Q waves in leads V_1 through V_3 may be suggestive but not diagnostic of anteroseptal MI. Inferior and anterolateral MIs may be disguised by the pattern of LBBB; that is, Q or QS waves in leads II, III, and aV$_f$ associated with inferior myocardial infarction[150] and Q waves in anterolateral precordial leads associated with anterolateral infarction may disappear with the development of LBBB. Left bundle branch block may be associated with QS complexes in leads II, III, and aV$_f$ that truly[151] or falsely[152] suggest inferior myocardial infarction. Left bundle branch block itself produces ST segment depression and T wave inversion in leads in which QRS complexes mainly are upright and ST segment elevation in leads in which QRS complexes mainly are inverted. The superimposition of myocardial injury, ischemia, or infarction may be recognized by a changing pattern over two or several electrocardiograms and by clinical correlation[153] even in the absence of diagnostic Q waves. When LBBB is present, ST segment elvations of 8 mm or more in right precordial leads or ST segment depression in right precordial leads or ST segment elevation in left precordial leads suggest myocardial injury.[154] Thallium exercise tests falsely may suggest anteroseptal ischemia in patients with LBBB, but no coronary artery disease.[69, 70, 155, 155a] The changes of left ventricular hypertrophy (LVH) are also affected by the development of LBBB. Frequently, a decrease in voltage occurs, causing the search for voltage criteria of LVH to be falsely negative.[165] Much less frequently voltage increases, producing false-positive criteria for LVH.[166] A horizontal plane QRS-T angle $\geq 150°$,[167] or monomorphic R waves in leads I and V6[168] for the diagnosis of LVH in the presence of LBBB were excellent criteria.

The review of LBBB by Flowers should be studied for its profusion of additional details.[169]

RIGHT BUNDLE BRANCH BLOCK

Incidence and Etiology

The incidence of RBBB (see Tables 17-1 and 17-2) ranges from about 1 in 1300 to 1 in 4000.[62, 170] This conduction abnormality may appear as a congenital defect unassociated with other cardiac abnormalities or after surgery for pulmonary stenosis, tetralogy of Fallot, or a large ventricular septal defect (VSD).[171, 172] Surgery for VSD in the presence of increased pulmonary vascular resistance produces less of a decrease in heart size if RBBB has developed.[173] Surgically induced RBBB may regress up to 12 years after the procedure.[174] In one study, right ventriculotomies in steps of three to seven small incisions were performed during repair of various congenital defects. Right bundle branch block developed at the time of one incision, regardless of the order of the incision, suggesting that the conduction defect was caused by disruption of a distal branch or branches of the right bundle within the right ventricle.[175] Thus, RBBB may occur with right ventricular damage. Right bundle branch block may be associated with right ventricular cardiomyopathy.[176] The pattern of RBBB may appear with premature supraventricular beats (Fig. 17-7), or it may be caused by hyperkalemia, chest trauma, or anteroseptal MI.[113, 177–179] Inferior MI may produce RBBB because a portion of the RBB is supplied by the right coronary artery.[26, 64] Anteroseptal ischemia; anteroseptal infarction; fibrosis of the ventricular conduction system (Lenegre's disease); calcification of the root of the aorta (Lev's disease); generalized cardio-

myopathy, including the hypertrophic obstructive type; positive-pressure ventilation; tumor invasion of the heart; myotonic dystrophy; radiation therapy; Chagas' disease; lesions within the HB; and even digitalis toxicity may produce RBBB.[8, 110, 114, 180–186] Right bundle branch block may occur with coronary artery bypass graft surgery.[87, 88] In patients with asymptomatic RBBB, there is a 17% incidence of coronary artery disease.[62] Patients with acquired RBBB without evidence of other disease may have a benign course, although in one study, most had elevated left ventricular end-diastolic pressure, suggesting the presence of diffuse myocardial disease.[187, 188]

Clinical Findings

Right bundle branch block, which sometimes develops at the time of acute anteroseptal MI or pulmonary embolus, frequently causes widely but physiologically split second heart sounds. Hemodynamic studies show right ventricular contraction to be delayed and less efficient.[189] Right bundle branch block may produce changes in the multiple-gated blood-pool angiogram.[190]

Right bundle branch block in children and young adults usually has no effect on prognosis when not associated with other cardiac disease but rarely, it may progress to complete AV block.[191] Intermittent AV block associated with RBBB may be tachycardia- or bradycardia-dependent.[192] In older adults, RBBB accompanying pulmonary disease suggests high pulmonary pressures. The vectorcardiogram may help in the presence of RBBB by demonstrating patterns either likely or unlikely to be associated with pulmonary disease or cardiac failure.[193] Right bundle branch block associated with deterioration of the specialized ventricular conduction system or with ischemic heart disease, especially at the time of acute MI, may be the first step toward complete AV block. If RBBB is present at the time of an acute anteroseptal MI, a temporary artificial pacemaker is indicated, even if the RBBB is old.[132, 194] Patients with preexisting RBBB who sustain acute MI are at increased risk of late sudden death.[132]

When chronic RBBB is associated with significant coronary artery disease, hypertension, or rheumatic heart disease, survival is significantly decreased.[195] Chronic RBBB found randomly is associated with a 9% progression rate to complete heart block.[196]

Electrocardiogram

Electrocardiographic changes produced by RBBB (see Tables 17-1 and 17-2) are manifest by delayed rightward and anterior forces (Fig. 17-8), producing a slurred terminal S wave in left-sided leads (I, aV$_L$, V$_5$, and V$_6$).[197–199] Lead

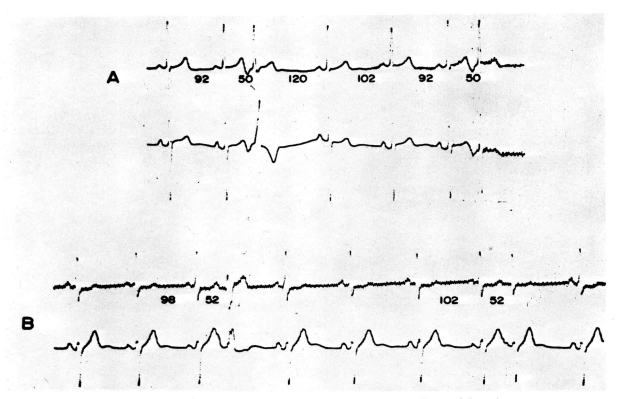

Figure 17-7. Each panel has a lateral and an anterior lead. (**A**) A premature atrial beat is followed by right bundle-branch block–type of aberrant conduction to the ventricles. Later in **A**, the same intervals are associated with normal conduction to the ventricles. (**B**) In a different patient, a premature atrial beat first does and then does not produce aberrant conduction, although the immediate cycle lengths are the same. The premature atrial beat associated with the shorter preceding cycle length of 98 hundredths of a second is the one that produces aberrant ventricular conduction. This reversal of the usual circumstances is found only in patients with significant myocardial disease.

V_1 shows terminal slurred R waves. Occasionally, such changes occur as an indication of MI scar without real RBBB.[200] The QRS duration is at least 0.12 seconds but averages 0.06 seconds longer than normal.[144] Right axis deviation in the presence of RBBB suggests chronic pulmonary disease, right ventricular hypertrophy (RVH), associated LAFB, loss of lateral forces secondary to MI, or that the patient is young. Thus, ordinarily, the R wave in lead I is taller than the slurred terminal S wave is deep. Occasionally, RBBB causes the QRS to be entirely upright in lead V_1, even in the absence of RVH.

Right Ventricular Hypertrophy and Bundle Branch Block

The criterion that R or R′ wave in lead V_1 must be greater than 15 mm in the presence of RBBB produces a high false-negative rate for RVH because with RVH, RBBB decreases R-wave voltage in lead V_1.[201] On the vectorcardiogram, RVH should be suspected if (1) the 0.04-second vector and the maximum QRS vector are to the right in the horizontal plane, (2) the initial vector is to the left and posterior, (3) the maximum QRS vector in the frontal plane is greater than $+110°$, and (4) the right QRS area is greater than the left.[202] A review of vector criteria versus electrocardiogram criteria for RVH in the presence of RBBB enumerates other advantages of the vector.[203]

Left Ventricular Hypertrophy and Right Bundle Branch Block

The usual criteria for left ventricular hypertrophy (LVH) used in the presence of RBBB have low sensitivity. The multiple-dipole electrocardiogram may increase this sensitivity.[98] Eight criteria for the diagnosis of LVH in the presence of RBBB were reviewed; a net positivity in lead I plus a net negativity in lead III of or greater than 17 mm (Lewis index) and R in lead aV_L of or greater than 11 mm were neither sensitive nor specific.[204, 205] A mean QRS axis of or greater than 30° had a sensitivity of 52% and P-wave

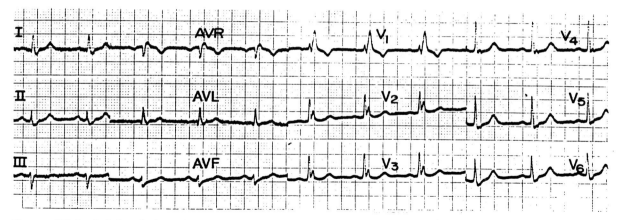

Figure 17-8. Right bundle-branch block shows terminal slurred S waves in leads I, II, aV_L, V_5, and V_6 and tall, wide, slurred R' waves in right precordial leads V_1, V_2, and V_3 QRS duration is 0.12 second.

terminal force of or greater than 0.04 seconds and 1 mm in depth was 28% sensitive.[206, 207] The Sokolow index of (1) S in V_1 and R in V_5 or V_6 of or greater than 35 mm, (2) R wave in V_5 or V_6 of or greater than 25 mm, (3) R wave in I plus S wave in lead III of or greater than 25 mm, and (4) intrinsicoid deflection in V_5 or V_6 of or greater than 0.05 seconds had specificities of 100%, 96.3%, 92.6%, and 88.5% respectively.[208]

Ischemic Disease and Right Bundle Branch Block

In most cases, RBBB alone does not disturb the pattern of diagnostic Q waves due to MI. Cor pulmonale, however, may be associated with RBBB and Q waves in right precordial or inferior leads that mimic MI. Right bundle branch block alone does not lower the specificity of the exercise thallium scan for the diagnosis of coronary artery disease.[209]

ST-T Changes With Right Bundle Branch Block

With RBBB, T waves and ST segments tend to deviate in a direction opposite that of the slurred delayed terminal forces. Thus, in leads I, aV_L, V_5, and V_6, development of RBBB may cause inverted T waves to become upright, depressed ST segments to return to baseline, and normal ST segments to become elevated. In the right precordial leads, upright T waves may become inverted, inverted T waves more inverted, elevated ST segments normal, normal ST segments depressed, and depressed ST segments more depressed. QT intervals average 0.05 seconds longer than normal with RBBB.[144]

INCOMPLETE RIGHT BUNDLE BRANCH BLOCK

Incidence and Etiology

The pattern of IRBBB may occur as a variant of normal, especially in young adults.[198,199,210] In 7685 male flying personnel, the prevalence was 3.4%. The highest prevalence was between the ages of 20 and 29 years. Among 261 cases, 66 were permanent, 94 had or developed left axis deviation, and 12 evolved to become complete RBBB.[211] If the QRS complex is prolonged to 0.10 seconds or more, IRBBB is more likely to represent a real conduction abnormality. Such abnormalities may occur with ostium secundum–type atrial septal defects (ASD) or anomalous pulmonary venous drainage. This pattern may represent late depolarization of the crista supraventricularis in these conditions or any conditions that produce right-sided hypertension or RVH, such as pulmonary hypertension or pulmonary stenosis. When IRBBB occurs with ostium primum–type ASD, and especially with endocardial cushion defects that include VSD, there is associated LAFB.[212] Incomplete right bundle branch block may also occur as a congenital abnormality unassociated with other lesions.[213] Examination of intervals from HB potentials to right ventricular apex potentials in ASD suggests that the associated pattern of IRBBB does not represent delay in the RBBB; in animals, the pattern of IRBBB may be due to variations in the thickness of the right ventricular free wall or may be produced by incising the internal subdivision of the RBB (the false tendon).[214–216]

Clinical Findings

When IRBBB is associated with ASD, splitting of the heart sound tends to be wide and fixed. These findings may be related to the large shunt flow rather than to electric events. The prognosis of patients with IRBBB is associated with the natural history or surgical intervention for the pathologic condition (if one exists).

Electrocardiogram

In patients with IRBBB, there is usually a terminal S wave in some or all of the left-sided leads (leads I, aV_L, V_5, and V_6) and an R′ in right precordial leads V_1 and sometimes V_2 (see Tables 17-1 and 17-2). Right ventricular hypertrophy differs because QRS is narrow, right axis deviation is seen, and lead V_1 usually shows a qR, a qRs, or an Rs rather than an RSR′. QRS complex duration in patients with IRBBB is sometimes in the normal range but classically is 0.1 seconds or more but less than 0.12 seconds. T waves tend to be upright and therefore opposite the abnormal S waves in the left-sided leads and are sometimes secondarily inverted and opposite the R′ waves in the right precordial leads. T-wave changes in the left precordial leads and leads I and aV_L tend to disguise T waves that are small or slightly inverted from other causes and in the right precordial leads may falsely suggest an active or ischemic myocardial process.

INCOMPLETE LEFT BUNDLE BRANCH BLOCK

Etiology

Incomplete left bundle branch block (ILBBB) may represent an intermediate step toward "complete" LBBB. As such, it may be seen in the elderly without clinical evidence of other heart disease or it may be associated with coronary artery disease, hypertensive heart disease, aortic valvular disease, or cardiomyopathy. Frequently, ILBBB is seen in association with LVH and is used by some clinicians as one electrocardiographic criterion for this diagnosis.[217]

Clinical Findings

The clinical findings and the prognosis of ILBBB are those related to the associated cardiac disease, such as hypertension with LVH.

Electrocardiogram

QRS complexes are prolonged, being 0.1 seconds or more but less than 0.12 seconds, and left-sided Q waves are absent or significantly decreased in leads I, aV_L, V_5, and V_6

(Fig. 17-9; see Tables 17-1 and 17-2). The QRS complex is minimally slurred throughout but especially during the intrinsicoid deflection. T waves become abnormally small or inverted in left-sided leads (I, aV_L, V_5, and V_6) and sometimes abnormally upright in right precordial leads. The inverted T waves in the left-sided leads may mimic the changes of anterolateral ischemia, and the changes in the right precordial leads may obliterate the electrocardiographic findings of anteroseptal ischemia (see Table 17-2).

LEFT ANTERIOR FASCICULAR BLOCK

Etiology

Left anterior fascicular block unassociated with block in other fascicles may occur with aging, without evidence of other specific cardiac disease. This conduction defect may occur secondary to a conduction defect in the HB. Associated diseases include anterior ischemia, anterior MI, Chagas' disease, sclerodegenerative disease, cardiomyopathy, calcific aortic valve disease, hyperkalemia, myocarditis, infiltrative and degenerative diseases, trauma, myotonic dystrophy, hypertension, Ehlers-Danlos syndrome, and aortic regurgitation.[113–115,218–220] The disorder is usually considered a relatively benign abnormality in adults but one study has shown that patients with LAFB who were undergoing coronary angiography, and therefore already suspected of having coronary artery disease, had a 50% chance of having 95% or greater occlusion of the left anterior descending coronary artery.[221] Occasionally, LAFB is congenital and in an infant, it often indicates either ostium primum atrial septal defect (usually with IRBBB or RBBB) or tricuspid atresia.[222] Right bundle branch block and LAFB may be acquired conduction defects with ostium primum.[223] Left anterior fascicular block may occur in 5% of hospitalized patients. Pathologically, fibrosis has been found at autopsy in the branching portion of the LBB in patients who had LAFB. In one study, fibrosis was always present in the anterior fibers but frequently was widely distributed over the anterior, middle, and posterior fibers of the LBB.[224]

Clinical Findings

The physical findings associated with LAFB are those of associated abnormalities. The prognosis of LAFB depends on the associated cardiac diseases. There is no apparent effect on prognosis in young asymptomatic men or when LAFB occurs with aging, especially in the eighth decade of life, in the absence of other obvious cardiac diseases.[225]

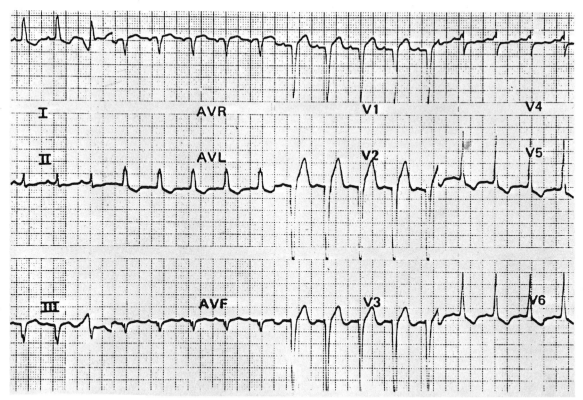

Figure 17-9. This 12-lead electrocardiogram taken during sinus tachycardia at a rate of 114 beats/minute shows incomplete left bundle-branch block associated with left ventricular hypertrophy. There are no Q waves in leads I and aV$_L$ or in the left precordial leads. R waves are absent or minimal in leads V$_1$ and V$_2$. QRS complexes are slurred in all leads. T waves are inverted in leads I and aV$_L$ and in the left precordial leads. ST segments are depressed in the same leads and elevated in right precordial leads. QRS duration in 0.1 second.

The incidence of progression to bifascicular block is 7% and to complete AV block, 3%.[196] Also, the presence or development of LAFB does not increase mortality or complicate the course of an acute MI.[132, 226, 227]

Electrocardiogram

The changes of LAFB frequently find expression in most of the 12 electrocardiogram leads (Fig. 17-10; see Tables 17-1 and 17-2). In leads II, III, and aV$_F$, complexes tend to be rS; in leads I and aV$_L$, complexes tend to be qR.[228] These deep terminal S waves in leads II, III and aV$_F$ and terminal R waves in aV$_R$ almost always mean anterior fascicular block, even in the presence of the QS complexes of inferior MI. If leads II, III, and aV$_F$ show QS complexes, inferior MI should be diagnosed. Terminal R waves in aV$_R$ indicate the simultaneous presence of LAFB. In the presence of LAFB, even a small Q wave in leads II, III or aV$_F$ indicates probable inferior infarction.[229] QRS complexes frequently become biphasic in the left precordial leads V$_4$ through V$_6$, of

the RS type; occasionally, small new Q waves may appear in the right precordial leads.[90, 230] Thus, LAFB may mimic lateral or anteroseptal infarction, and new initial r waves in inferior leads may hide inferior MI.[26, 231] LAFB may even obscure RBBB.[232] The axis is usually between −30° and −90° but may cross over into the right upper quadrant of the frontal plane, perhaps as far as −110°.[122, 228, 233–235] Between −30° and −59°, the LAFB may be incomplete.[228, 236] R waves tend to become taller in leads I and aV$_L$, so that the usual criteria for LVH in these leads may not be valid in the presence of LAFB.[26] A new index, however—S in lead III plus the largest R and S in a single precordial lead, equaling 30 mm—appears to have high specificity, high sensitivity, and high positive and negative predictive value.[237] T waves may become inverted in leads I and aV$_L$ and tend to be upright in leads II, III, and aV$_F$, sometimes hiding otherwise inverted T waves in the inferior leads. Likewise, T waves tend to become more upright in the left precordial leads in which the QRS complexes have become biphasic. Associated ST- and T-wave changes may help to differentiate between the right precordial Q waves

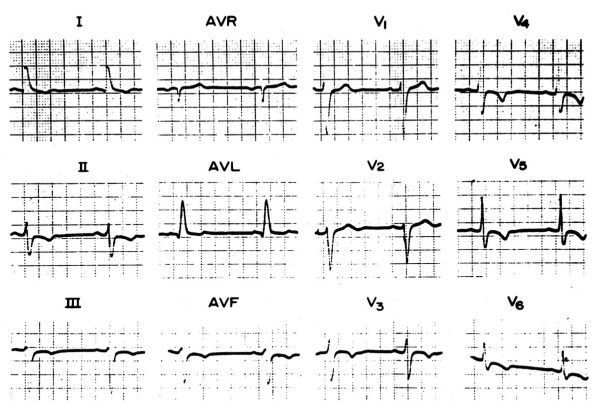

Figure 17-10. Sinus bradycardia with left anterior fascicular block. Terminal forces are inverted in leads II, III, and aV$_F$ with S-wave voltage greater than R-wave voltage. R waves are tall in lead aV$_L$. There are terminal S waves in left precordial leads. QRS duration is prolonged to 0.12 second. In addition, this electrocardiogram shows inferior and anterolateral ischemia.

of anteroseptal infarction and Q waves that sometimes appear in the right precordial leads secondary to LAFB. Also, the Q waves of infarction tend to be wider (0.04 seconds or more) and more slurred.

The development of LAFB is associated with slight prolongation of the QRS complex (average increase, 25 milliseconds). The more marked the left axis deviation, the greater the QRS prolongation.[238] A prolonged time of inscription of the intrinsicoid deflection in lead aV$_L$ (greater than 50 milliseconds); a 10-millisecond longer time of inscription of the intrinsicoid deflection in lead aV$_L$, compared with lead V$_6$; the peak of the r wave in lead III coming later than the peak in lead II; and a shift of the initial 0.02-second forces inferiorly and to the right have been used as criteria for LAFB.[239-241] If the intraventricular conduction delay exceeds 20 to 25 milliseconds or if the total QRS is 120 or more milliseconds, there must be an associated left ventricular focal block if BBB is not present.[240] Such a delay in the posteroinferior wall may obscure the LAFB, and LAFB with an anterior focal block may obscure IRBBB.

Right axis deviation associated with the superior axis

of LAFB may occur because of concomitant RVH, lateral MI, or some types of RBBB.[240]

LEFT POSTERIOR FASCICULAR BLOCK

Etiology

Left posterior fascicular block may occur unassociated with block of other fascicles as a result of a chronic degenerative or fibrotic process of the specialized conduction system of the ventricles, hyperkalemia, or an ischemic process affecting the posterior fascicle itself or perhaps the Purkinje system or myocardium, for which the posterior fascicle ordinarily serves as the specialized conduction pathway. The ischemia may occur because of obstruction in the posterior descending or circumflex coronary arteries; it may occur acutely when the left anterior descending obstructs, if it has collaterals to an obstructed posterior descending.[242] Myocarditis, infiltrative disease, Chagas' disease, myotonic dystrophy, and possibly acute cor pulmonale may cause LPFB.[115, 243] A pattern suggesting LPFB may occur as a congenital electrocardiogram abnormality, without heart disease.[244]

Electrocardiogram

Left posterior fascicular block usually produces a right axis deviation of greater than +90° such that in lead I and usually in lead aV_L, there is a small R wave and a deep S wave, whereas in leads II, III and aV_F, there are small Q waves and tall R waves (see Tables 17-1 and 17-2).[52, 245, 246] An axis less than +120° may represent incomplete LPFB.[219] The pattern of LPFB may mimic an inferior MI or hide a lateral MI.[26] Some observers, however, suggest that right axis deviation is unusual and that the diagnosis should be made based on the other described changes, including initial and terminal slurring of the QRS and delayed onset of R-wave intrinsicoid deflection greater than 45 milliseconds in lead aV_F.[247] Left precordial leads such as V_5 and V_6 sometimes display biphasic QRS complexes. The QRS complex in lead V_1 is mainly negative and thus does not suggest RVH. If LPFB is associated with a positive QRS in lead V_1 due to RBBB, RVH must be ruled out clinically. When right axis deviation is the result of the positional changes that occur with chronic pulmonary disease, R waves in leads II, III, and aV_F are not tall (as they are with LPFB) and generally, the voltage of complexes in most of the 12 leads is decreased. In children and young adults, right axis deviation is frequently normal, and differentiation between a juvenile pattern and LPFB is difficult.

T waves tend to be more upright in leads I and aV_L, and this tendency may mask pathologically small or slightly inverted T waves that would appear in these leads in the absence of the conduction defect. T waves may become inverted in leads II, III, and aV_F in patients with LPFB and may mimic an active or ischemic inferior myocardial process.

Acute cor pulmonale or anterolateral MI may produce changes similar to those of LPFB. Thus, clinical correlation and close attention to other electrocardiographic details are necessary before LPFB can be diagnosed.

LEFT SEPTAL FASCICULAR BLOCK

Etiology

Left septal fascicular block (LSFB) has been anatomically demonstrated[248, 249] and is most commonly found in patients with ischemic heart disease, especially when angina pectoris and papillary muscle dysfunction are present. Other etiologies include diabetes mellitus and hyper-

trophic cardiomyopathy. The disorder is associated with fibrosis of the septal fascicle of the LBB.[250]

Clinical Findings

Symptoms and signs in patients with left septal fascicular block are those found with the primary diseases. The cardiac findings often include a systolic murmur when papillary muscle dysfunction is associated.

Electrocardiogram

Descriptions of the electrocardiogram changes in LSFB are varied. The electrocardiogram may show prominent R waves in the right precordial leads similar to those found in "true" posterior MI or may show Q waves in these leads. The RS ratio in V_1 should be more than two and R in V_1 5 mm or more; or the RS ratio in V_2 should be more than two and R in V_2 15 mm or more; or the S in V_2 should be less than 5 mm.[250–252]

RIGHT BUNDLE BRANCH BLOCK AND LEFT ANTERIOR FASCICULAR BLOCK

Etiology

Among the major causes of RBBB with LAFB are (1) sclerodegenerative disease of the specialized conduction system of the ventricles, mainly in the elderly; (2) ischemic heart disease, especially MI involving the interventricular septum; (3) hypertension; and (4) Chagas' disease.[219, 253, 254] Right bundle branch block with LAFB may occur as a congenital abnormality alone or associated with progressive ophthalmoplegia.[213, 255, 256] There is also a familial form associated with syncope and a high incidence of sudden death.[257–259] This conduction defect may also be associated with chest trauma; hyperkalemia; myocarditis; aortic valve disease; cardiomyopathy, including hypertrophic cardiomyopathy associated with myotonic dystrophy; or granulomatous disease of the ventricles such as sarcoidosis.[113, 219, 260–263] Pathologically, many patients show fibrosis, calcification, and fatty changes in the central fibrous body, the HB, both proximal bundle branches, the intermediary portions of the RBB, and the anterior fibers of the LBB.[3, 11, 23, 264, 265] The disorder may also occur as a result of surgical repair of tetralogy of Fallot or of VSD. Right-sided intracardiac conduction-time studies show that RBBB with LAFB in these circumstances indicates damage to the specialized conduction system, whereas RBBB alone indicates only a surgically induced lesion in the peripheral Purkinje system.[266] Surgically induced RBBB with LAFB may be an ominous sign, requiring permanent pacing: however, without evidence of fixed or transient residual trifascicular block, the prognosis may be good even without pacing, at least for several years.[267–269] Some investigators have found no increase in mortality, with or without chronic coronary artery disease, in the absence of fixed or transient AV block.[62]

Clinical Findings

On physical examination, RBBB with LAFB may produce the same change in heart sounds as RBBB alone, that is, widening of the second heart sound. Phonocardiogram, carotid pulse tracings, and cardiograms show late onset and slow rise of ventricular ejection.[270] Otherwise, physical findings are related to the etiologic disease. Chronic RBBB with LAFB may carry a rate of progression to advanced AV block of 10% or higher in patients followed-up for various times and 19% in patients followed-up for 5 years.[62, 271, 272] If organic heart disease is present, the rate of progression to higher degrees of AV block ranges from 14% to 100%.[78, 271, 273]

Acute Myocardial Infarction and Right Bundle Branch Block With Left Anterior Fascicular Block

Right bundle branch block with LAFB that develops at the time of acute anteroseptal MI significantly changes the patient's prognosis for surviving the acute episode, especially if the HV interval on an HB recording is prolonged.[25, 274, 275] Complete AV block may develop and because bifascicular block suggests that a large portion of myocardial tissue has been destroyed, the incidence of cardiogenic shock is higher than in similar patients without bifascicular block. An artificial transvenous pacemaker may not change the survival rate of patients with acute anteroseptal MI with RBBB and LAFB. Many cardiologists recommend insertion of a temporary ventricular pacemaker in such circumstances, even if RBBB was previously present, although the need for a prophylactic pacemaker if the BBB is old is more controversial.[73, 132, 276] If bifascicular block precedes the acute MI, the 1-year mortality is 65%, although sudden death is unlikely.[45] If the intraventricular conduction defect persists and especially if transient second- or third-degree AV block occurs, permanent pacing may prolong life.[64, 82, 83, 203, 204, 205, 277–279] These recommendations apply also to the development of LBBB (less strongly) and to the development of RBBB alone; they do not apply to the development of LAFB or LPFB alone at the time of MI.

HQ Intervals and Prognosis in Right Bundle Branch Block With Left Anterior Fascicular Block

Asymptomatic ambulatory patients with chronic RBBB and LAFB have a good prognosis, whereas similar hospitalized patients have a significant risk of sudden death or development of complete AV block, especially if HQ intervals are markedly prolonged.[254, 275, 280, 281] Although there is some correlation between prolonged PR intervals and long HQ intervals, most long HQ intervals are associated with normal PR intervals in the presence of RBBB and LAFB.[28, 282, 283] Patients with RBBB and LAFB who have long HQ intervals are more likely to have more severe cardiac disease with cardiomegaly and congestive heart failure, compared with patients with normal HQ intervals.[288] Pacemakers for patients with chronic RBBB and LAFB have not been shown to change statistically the risk of sudden death unless second-degree AV block is present. For example, ventricular fibrillation rather than AV block is the cause of death in many patients who have Chagas' disease with BBB.[284] If it is not already present, second-degree HQ block is not likely to occur with rapid atrial pacing or during anesthesia in patients with RBBB and LAFB without cardiac symptoms, although in one study, one patient of 44 with RBBB and LAFB developed transient AV block during intubation.[58, 125, 285, 286] One group reports a 12% 3-year cardiovascular mortality in patients with bifascicular block.[122] The exceptions to the lack of benefit from prophylactic pacemakers may be in patients with RBBB and LAFB and long HQ intervals, in whom permanent pacemakers decreased the incidence of sudden death.[287] Another investigative group, however, found a high incidence of sudden death (10% the first year, 13% the second year, and 16% the third year) in patients with chronic bifascicular block and reported that monitored deaths were due to ventricular fibrillation rather than to AV block.

Electrocardiogram

Right bundle branch block and LAFB each produce their own changes of QRS and T contour, some of which are superimposed (Fig. 17-11; see Tables 17-1 and 17-2). Usually, there is a tall R wave and a terminal slurred S wave in leads I and aV$_L$. A small Q wave may be present or absent in these two leads. In leads II and aV$_F$, small R waves and deep, widened S waves are usually seen. Lead III and sometimes leads II and aV$_F$ show a small R wave and either

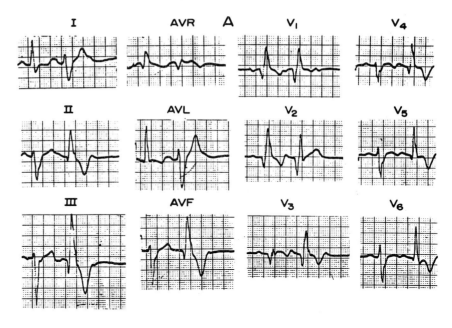

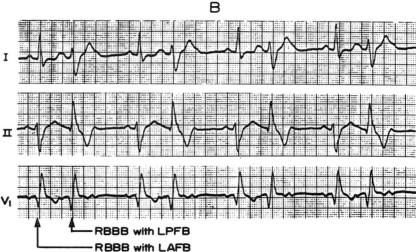

Figure 17-11. (A) The 12-lead electrocardiogram shows two conducted P waves and one blocked P wave in each lead. (The bigeminal rhythm is best seen in the tracings in *B*.) In *A*, the first QRS complex of each pair shows right bundle-branch block (RBBB) with left anterior fascicular block (LAFB). The second of each pair of QRS complexes shows RBBB with left posterior fascicular block (LPFB). The Q waves in right precordial leads in both beats indicate anteroseptal myocardial infarction. Q waves are present only in the second of each pair of beats in leads II, III, and aV$_F$, however, implying that LPFB may mimic inferior myocardial infarction or that LAFB may hide this abnormality. Overall, there is constant RBBB and 3:1 block in both the left anterior fascicle and the left posterior fascicle but occurring out of phase by one beat, producing the alternate QRS pattern and the 3:2 atrioventricular block.

a deep, widened S wave or a small r wave, a deep S wave and a terminal slurred R' wave. T waves tend to be more upright in leads I, aV$_L$ and sometimes leads II, III, and aV$_F$, sometimes obscuring small or inverted T waves that might otherwise be present. In lead V$_1$ and sometimes in leads V$_2$ and V$_3$, there is a terminal slurred R wave. T waves tend to be inverted, sometimes mimicking anteroseptal ischemia. Right precordial leads may also show a small Q wave and a tall, wide, slurred R or RR' wave, with an inverted T wave; recent anteroseptal MI must be ruled out based on other clinical or electrocardiographic findings, such as the presence of only narrow Q waves or the disappearance of RBBB and LAFB simultaneously with the disappearance of anteroseptal Q waves and T wave inversions. Left pre-

cordial leads are biphasic, with terminal slurred S waves. The frontal plane axis based on voltage of R and S is leftward.

RIGHT BUNDLE BRANCH BLOCK WITH LEFT POSTERIOR FASCICULAR BLOCK

Etiology

Right bundle branch block with LPFB may occur as a result of sclerosis of the specialized conduction system of the ventricles or, as with all the other bundle branch and fascicular blocks, as a result of calcium impingement on the conduction system in the aortic valve or the mitral valve ring, extensive acute anteroseptal MI, or significant chronic obstructive coronary artery disease.[288] It may occur as a result of trauma to the chest, myocarditis, cardiomyopathy, infiltrative diseases of the myocardium, scleroderma, or hyperkalemia.[113, 289, 290]

Clinical Findings

On physical examination, a widely split second heart sound is heard secondary to the RBBB. Other physical findings are related to the causative pathologic process. When RBBB with LPFB is due to ischemic heart disease, extensive damage to the interventricular septum is likely. Ischemic damage from inferior MI involving the right ventricle and posterior left ventricular damage may also cause this pattern. The incidence of development of complete AV block is high when RBBB with LPFB is associated with acute anteroseptal MI, a situation requiring placement of an artificial pacemaker.[291] Patients with chronic RBBB and LPFB are at high risk of developing complete AV block.[292] Such block is usually preceded by second-degree AV block and associated with symptoms and progression of the causative pathologic process.[29]

Electrocardiogram

Leads I and aV_L show terminal slurred S waves with voltage greater than the initial small R waves, producing a right axis deviation in the frontal plane (see Fig. 17-11; see Tables 17-1 and 17-2). Usually, leads II, III, and aV_F display a small Q wave, as is seen with LPFB alone. The R waves are usually not as tall, however, as those seen with LPFB alone, and there may be terminal slurred S waves in one or more of these leads. The previously described changes of RBBB are present. Right bundle branch block with LPFB should be diagnosed only if RVH or lateral infarction are unlikely to have produced the right axis deviation.

Right bundle branch block with LAFB may change to RBBB with LPFB (see Fig. 17-11) suddenly or gradually, the latter suggesting a Wenckebach phenomenon in the left posterior fascicle.[293, 294]

MURAL DELAYS

Etiology

Left- and right-sided intraventricular conduction defects may occur because of damage to the muscle or the Purkinje system produced by coronary artery obstruction, cardiomyopathy, infiltrative diseases such as sarcoidosis or amyloidosis, hyperkalemia, or right ventriculotomy during cardiac surgery.[295]

Clinical Findings

Left-sided mural conduction defects may cause paradoxical splitting of the second heart sounds; the right-sided mural conduction defects may produce wide but physiologic splitting of the second heart sound.

Electrocardiogram

Left-sided mural conduction defects may produce loss of the Q wave in leads I, aV_L, V_5, and V_6 similar to LBBB but with extreme widening of the QRS, frequently to 160 milliseconds and greater. Such a pattern is compatible with LBBB *and* a mural conduction defect. There may also be widening of the QRS without loss of left-sided Q waves but with forces that are mainly left and posterior. T waves tend to be opposite in direction to the main QRS forces, sometimes obscuring normal or abnormal T waves. With right-sided mural conduction defects, the electrocardiogram is frequently indistinguishable from RBBB but has been shown to differ in QRS duration being greater than with RBBB alone.[29] Myocardial infarction may produce intramural conduction defects that are not similar to any BBB (Fig. 17-12).[296] Hyperkalemia and classes IA, IC, and III antiarrhythmic drugs may do the same. Intraventricular conduction defects may produce late forces, appearing as late as the T wave and, in a reported case of right ventricular myopathy, may represent epsilon potentials.[297]

VENTRICULAR PREEXCITATION

Etiology

Several bypass tracts in the human heart have been described, any one of which may cause the ventricle to be depolarized earlier than normal; all but one group produces a change in the QRS contour. These tracts must be operative and must demonstrate anterograde, retrograde, or bidirectional conduction to be recognized. The bundles of Kent directly connect atrial muscle to either the left ventricular free wall or posterior septum (type A), the right ventricular free wall or the anterior septum (type B), or to a fascicle, producing ventricular preexcitation.[298] It is appropriate to refer to variations of accessory pathways according to location, such as right atrium to left or right ventricular free wall; or to left or right or anterior or

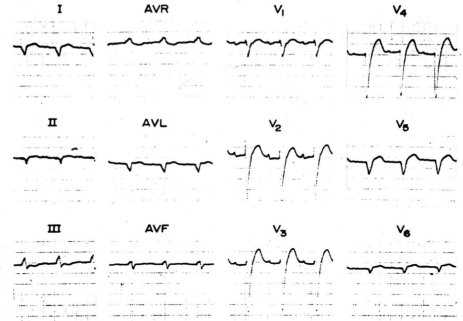

Figure 17-12. QS complexes in leads I, II, aV$_L$, V$_5$, and V$_6$ are compatible with lateral myocardial infarction. QRS complexes are slightly widened and slurred but the intraventricular conduction defect does not suggest any of the usual patterns of bundle-branch block or fascicular block and is therefore a nonspecific intraventricular conduction defect secondary to the myocardial infarction.

posterior septum; and even to designate high or low or anterior, posterior, or lateral ventricular wall. James fibers connect the atrium to the HB or the AV node, bypassing, or partially bypassing, the AV node, allowing short PR intervals but normal QRS complexes. When this type of bypass is associated with LBBB, however, a Kent bypass may be mistakenly suspected.[299] Also, AV nodal-like (decremental conduction) qualities may allow preexcitation by James fibers to show PR intervals in the normal range.[300,301] Mahaim fibers connect the HB or AV node to the ventricular muscle or a fascicle directly and when operative, produce abnormal QRS contour without marked PR interval shortening. Kent and Mahaim fibers may both be present simultaneously.[302]

Classic Wolff-Parkinson-White (WPW) syndrome is associated with an operating bundle of Kent on the right or left side that at least intermittently produces early depolarization of the ventricles associated with an initial slurred wave on the QRS (delta wave). The incidence may be as high as 0.2% in the total population.[62] Patients with WPW syndrome have episodes of tachycardia, produced either by a circus movement (using the normal and accessory pathways) or by one or several rapidly conducted or reentry beats through the accessory or the normal pathway, producing an early atrial or ventricular depolarization that provokes atrial, reciprocating junctional, or rarely, ventricular tachycardia.

The diagnosis of the WPW syndrome type of ventricular preexcitation may be made with greater certainty after HB recordings show short HQ intervals (Fig. 17-13) asso-

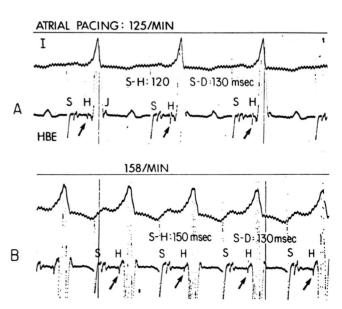

Figure 17-13. A case of ventricular preexcitation. Lead I and a His-bundle electrogram (HBE) are shown. SH intervals are 120 milliseconds at an atrial pacing rate of 125 beats/minute in *A* and 150 milliseconds at a pacing rate of 158 beats/minute in *B*. The pacing spike to the beginning of the delta wave (SD) interval remains the same at 130 milliseconds. Thus, the conduction time through the accessory pathway remains constant at both pacing rates. Because SH is longer at the faster pacing rate, the relationship of the H and the beginning of the delta wave changes. In *A*, H is almost simultaneous with the delta wave; in *B*, H occurs clearly after the beginning of the delta wave.

ciated with delta waves, especially in patients who have demonstrated paroxysmal syupraventricular tachycardias.

Clinical Findings

Wolff-Parkinson-White syndrome represents the most typical set of clinical circumstances found in patients with recognized ventricular preexcitation. There is early depolarization of the ventricles through the bundle of Kent, causing a delta wave. On the physical examination, the second heart sound may be paradoxically split if the patient has ventricular preexcitation to the right ventricle. The second heart sound in left-sided ventricular preexcitation is physiologically but widely split because of early depolarization of the left ventricle. Ventricular preexcitation is congenital and tends to be hereditary. One congenital lesion with a significant simultaneous occurrence is Ebstein's anomaly, in which the displacement of the tricuspid valve frequently causes a systolic murmur of tricuspid regurgitation.

Supraventricular tachycardias occur in 79% of patients with WPW syndrome, with atrial fibrillation being found in 17% and atrial flutter in 40%. Long-term morbidity is slightly increased, and death may occur from rapid rates associated with paroxysmal atrial fibrillation or development of ventricular fibrillation.[62] This is more likely to occur in patients on digitalis or calcium channel blockers.[303] If arrhythmias are symptomatic, especially if they are life-threatening and resistant to medication, catheter fulguration should be considered.[304] If this is unsuccessful, surgery should be considered.[305] Patients with ventricular rates of 200 beats per minute or greater during atrial fibrillation should be considered for fulguration or surgery.[306] Such high rates are more likely to be found in patients with persistent rather than intermittent preexcitation.[307] At surgery, epicardial mapping must be performed to delineate the bypass location. Certain information should be obtained even before surgery, however. The 12-lead electrocardiogram may suggest the general location of the bypass tract. Ventriculoatrial conduction times may be helpful.[308] During reciprocating tachycardias using the normal conduction pathway as the anterograde tract (orthodromic) and a free-wall bypass as the retrograde tract, if BBB occurs on the side of the bypass, the ventriculoatrial interval increases because the ventricular depolarization starts in the ventricle opposite the bypass and must cross the septum before reaching the bypass.[309,310] If LBBB occurs with a right-sided accessory pathway, the HV becomes longer, the ventriculoatrial time becomes shorter but the His-to-atrium conduction time stays the same.[311] Also, with orthodromic tachycardias, functional LAFB prolongs ventriculoatrial conduction time but only when the accessory pathway is in the left lateral wall of the LV.[312] Rarely, if the bypass cannot be selectively interrupted and arrhythmias have been unacceptably symptomatic or life-threatening, complete AV block is surgically produced and a ventricular pacemaker is inserted.

Electrocardiogram

In patients with an accessory pathway, preexcitation is sometimes intermittent, sometimes absent, sometimes constant, and sometimes found on alternate beats (Figs. 17-14 and 17-15).[313]

The electrocardiogram in patients with type A (atrium to posterior left ventricular septum or free-wall bypass) WPW syndrome (Fig. 17-16) shows a slurred initial upward deflection (delta wave) in lead V_1 and usually an upright delta wave in left-sided leads such as I, aV_L, V_5, and V_6 (Table 17-3). Occasionally, the delta wave is upright in lead V_1 but inverted in leads I and aV_L (Fig. 17-17), suggesting a more superior and lateral left ventricular insertion of the accessory pathway. In type B (atrium to anterior septum or right ventricular free wall) WPW syndrome, the delta wave is downward in lead V_1 and upward in leads I, aV_L, V_5 and V_6 (Fig. 17-18). Table 17-3 indicates additional patterns produced by pathways, the location of which are better determined by vectorcardiograms and body surface potential mapping.[314] In patients with WPW syndrome, the QRS complex usually represents a fusion beat in which a portion of the ventricle is depolarized through the accessory pathway and the rest through the normal pathway. If conduction through the normal pathway is prolonged or absent, however, the ventricle is completely depolarized through the accessory pathway, producing complete ventricular preexcitation (Fig. 17-19A), either type A or type B, and complete AV block in the normal pathway may be obscured.[315] If anterograde conduction in the accessory pathway fails (see Fig. 17-19B) and if no conduction occurs through the normal pathway, complete AV block becomes manifest (Fig. 17-20).[316] Complete preexcitation type A, with the accessory pathway going to the left ventricle, usually mimics RBBB, whereas complete ventricular preexcitation type B, with the accessory pathway going to the right ventricle, usually mimics left bundle branch block (Table 17-4). Catheter ablation of accessory pathways requires better localization.[317] An analysis of about the first 40 milliseconds of the QRS (the delta wave) allows a modest estimate of the location of the accessory pathway insertion (see Table 17-3).[318] New criteria for such localization have been proposed.[319] A newer algorithm is transferred to table form (Table 17-5) and may represent a method for more precise localization of accessory pathways, if verified by prospective studies.[320]

(*text continues on page 539*)

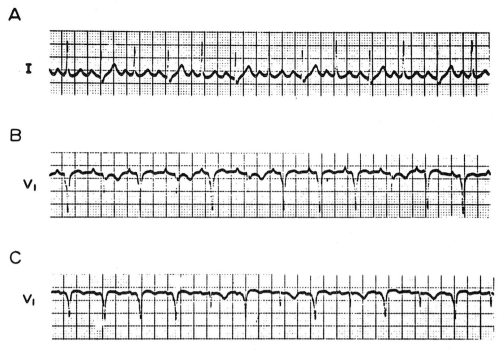

Figure 17-14. (**A**) Lead I during electrical alternans. Half the QRS complexes have a terminal slurred S wave and suggest incomplete right bundle-branch block. Alternate complexes show disappearance of the small initial Q waves, a slightly shorter PR interval, and no terminal S wave. This occurred in a known case of ventricular preexcitation, type B. The accessory pathway goes to the right ventricle and depolarizes the area responsible for the terminal S waves in incomplete right bundle-branch block. Thus, type B Wolff-Parkinson-White syndrome eliminates the findings of incomplete right bundle-branch block. (**B** and **C**) Lead V₁ shows clearly the shorter PR intervals associated with beats that display type B Wolff-Parkinson-White syndrome. Especially in *C,* the very small R' wave suggesting incomplete right bundle-branch block disappears on beats with ventricular preexcitation. The tracings in *B* and *C* are from two different patients.

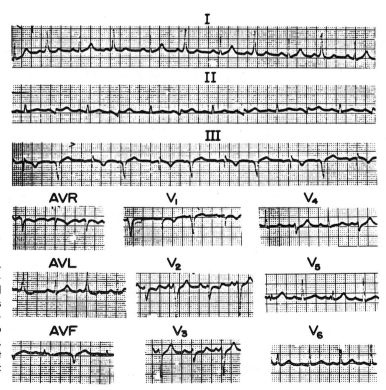

Figure 17-15. Alternate beats are widened and slurred, especially in their initial portions, and have a short PR interval. Initial slurring is upward in leads I and aV_L and in all precordial leads but in leads II, III, and aV_F, slurring is downward, producing wide Q waves. These features suggest ventricular preexcitation with a bypass from the atria to the left ventricle, with an insertion that is to the left, posterior, and relatively inferior, so that initial forces proceed from left to right, anteriorly, and superiorly. Leads II, II, and aV_F mimic the pattern of inferior myocardial infarction.

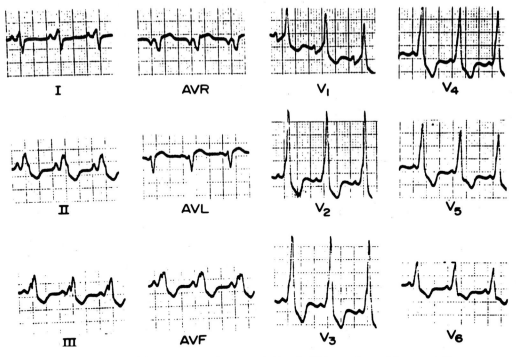

Figure 17-16. Upright delta waves in right precordial leads. PR intervals are 0.1 second. The very wide QRS complexes, most clearly seen in leads II, III, and aV$_F$, the terminal S waves in lead I, and the entirely upright QRS complex in lead V$_1$ suggest the possibility of complete ventricular preexcitation, type A.

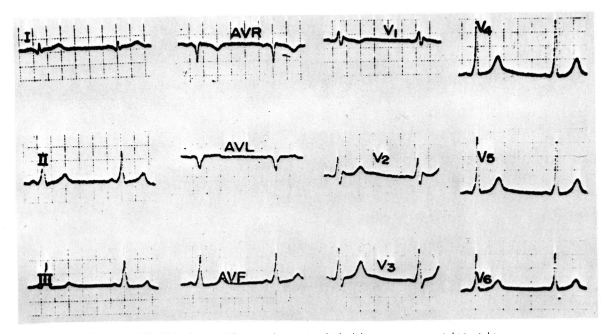

Figure 17-17. Type A Wolff-Parkinson-White syndrome, in which delta waves are upright in right precordial leads and in leads, II, III, and aV$_F$ but inverted in leads I and a V$_L$ mimicking high lateral myocardial infarction. There may also be incomplete right bundle-branch block.

TABLE 17-3. Delta Waves in Ventricular Preexcitation

	Delta Waves in Type A: Accessory Pathway to					Delta Waves in Type B: Accessory Pathway to			
	Anterior LV	Posterior Septum	Posterior Superior LV	Posterior Inferior LV	Postero-lateral LV	Anterior RV	Anterior Septum	Lateral RV	Posterior RV
Leads I, aVL	Up in 1 Down in aV$_L$	Up	Up	Up	Down	Usually up	Up	Up	Up
Leads II,III,aV$_F$	Up	Down	Up	Down	Usually up	Usually up	Up	Up	Down
Lead V$_1$	Up	Up	Up	Up	Up	Down	Down	Down	Down
Lead V$_5$, V$_6$	Up	Up or down	Up	Up	Down	Up	Up	Up	Up

*The variation in ventricular preexcitation is greater than indicated here; these are common patterns.

LV, left ventricle; RV, right ventricle.

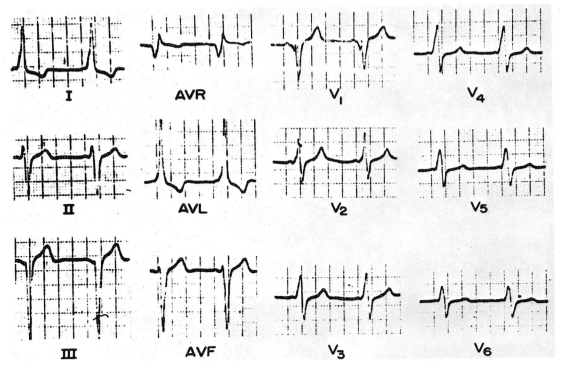

Figure 17-18. Type B Wolff-Parkinson-White syndrome, with downward-pointing delta waves in lead V₁. QRS complexes are mainly inverted in leads II, III, and aV_F, a pattern suggestive of left anterior fascicular block.

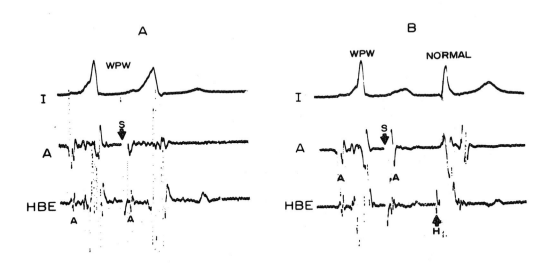

Figure 17-19. Lead I, an intraatrial electrogram (*A*), and a His bundle electrogram (HBE). The first of each pair of complexes is a spontaneous sinus beat and shows the delta wave of ventricular preexcitation; the second is an artificially induced premature atrial beat. (**A**) The premature atrial beat produces prolongation of conduction through the normal pathway so much that ventricular preexcitation increases on the second beat, probably becoming complete. The terminal S wave in the second beat suggests that this is type A Wolff-Parkinson-White syndrome, with a bypass to the left ventricle. (**B**) The atrial beat is more premature and the wave of polarization finds the accessory pathway completely refractory, whereas the atrioventricular node is still relatively refractory, so that although the AH interval becomes markedly prolonged, the QRS complex is normal in contour.

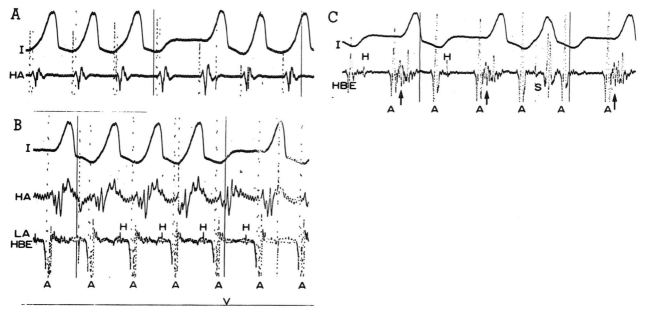

Figure 17-20. (**A**) Lead I and an atrial recording from the high right atrium (HA) show a regular spontaneous atrial tachycardia, with slightly irregular ventricular responses, each of which shows an initial delta wave. One QRS but no atrial complex is missing, suggesting that although ventricular preexcitation may be present, the tachycardia is not the reciprocating type that uses the normal pathway for one leg and the accessory pathway for the other. That type of reciprocation requires involvement of the ventricles to complete the circuit and if one ventricular beat is missing, the circuit would have been broken. (**B**) Lead I and recordings from the HA and the low right atrium (LA) recorded at the usual location for the His bundle electrogram (HBE). Note that the His bundle appears to depolarize first, the LA second, the HA third, and the ventricles last. This is compatible with a focal or reciprocating His-bundle tachycardia, using the normal atrioventricular (AV) conduction pathway retrogradely to the atria and only then using an accessory pathway anterograde to the ventricles (through a Kent bundle). The QRS complexes in lead I all show delta waves, and the RR intervals in B progressively shorten until there is a long pause. This configuration suggests type I second-degree block in the accessory pathway. Again, the pause is not associated with interruption of the atrial tachycardia. Therefore, the tachycardia cannot require the ventricle to complete the circuit. (**C**) Lead I and an HBE. An *H* follows each *A*, except the one that is next to last. Alternate *A* waves are followed by QRS complexes, except for interruption by a premature ventricular beat (*V*). Additional deflections (*upward-point arrows*) represent depolarization of the accessory pathway in this patient with ventricular preexcitation. The atrial rhythm is not interrupted by absence of ventricular response on alternate beats or after an artificial pacemaker spike (*S*). In this patient, with AV conduction did not occur by the accessory pathway, it did not occur at all, suggesting complete block below the His bundle.

Preexcitation may eliminate the classic features of BBB. In type B preexcitation, with a rapidly conducting bypass to the right ventricle, the portion of the heart that is last to depolarize in the presence of RBBB or IRBBB alone is depolarized first, so that RBBB of IRBBB may not be recognized.[321,322] Right bundle branch block or IRBBB may be diagnosed in the presence of type A WPW syndrome by showing prolongation of conduction time from the HB to the right ventricular apex or by showing that the terminal portion of the QRS suggests RBBB or IRBBB and is the same both with and without the preexcitation (Fig. 17-21).[323] Likewise, in type A preexcitation, with a bypass to the left side of the heart, that portion of the heart depolarized last in the presence of LBBB alone is depolarized first. Thus, type A ventricular preexcitation may obscure LBBB (Fig. 17-22), suggesting that the LBBB is a discrete rather than a diffuse process.[324,325]

If secondary T-wave changes occur with ventricular preexcitation, they tend to be in the opposite direction of the delta waves (Table 17-6). Occasionally, downward-pointing delta waves are diagnosed as MI (e.g., in atrial fibrillation, where short PR intervals cannot be recognized). Preexcitation may produce ST-segment depression, especially with exercise testing. Thallium scans may be falsely abnormal and therefore not differentiate true from false abnormal stress tests.[326]

TABLE 17-4. Delta-QRS Patterns in Ventricular Preexcitation*

	Type A Accessory Pathway					Type B Accessory Pathway			
	Anterior LV	Posterior Septum	Posterior Superior LV	Posterior Inferior LV	Postero-lateral LV	Anterior RV	Anterior Septum	Lateral RV	Posterior RV
May mimic anteroseptal MI	No	No	No	No	No	Yes	Yes	Yes	Yes
May mimic inferior MI	No	Yes	No	Yes	No	No	No	No	Yes
May mimic lateral MI	Sometimes	No	No	No	Yes	No	No	Yes	No
May mimic true posterior MI	Yes	Yes	Yes	Yes	Yes	No	No	Yes	No
May mimic LBBB	No	Yes	No	No	No	Yes	Yes	Yes	Yes
May mimic RBBB	No	No	Yes	Yes	Yes	No	No	No	No
May hide anteroseptal MI	Yes	Yes	Yes	Yes	Yes	No	No	No	No
May hide inferior MI	Yes	No	Yes	No	Usually no	No	Yes	Yes	No
May hide lateral MI	Sometimes	Yes	Yes	Yes	No	Yes	Yes	Yes	Yes
May hide true posterior MI	No	Yes	No	No	No	Yes	Yes	Yes	Yes
May hide LBBB	Yes	No	Yes	Yes	Yes	No	No	No	No
May hide RBBB	No	No	No	No	No	Yes	Yes	Yes	Yes
May mimic LAFB	No	Yes	Yes	No	No	No	No	No	Yes

*The variation in ventricular preexcitation is greater than indicated here. These are common patterns. LV, left ventricle; RV, right ventricle; MI, myocardial infarction; LBBB, left bundle branch block; RBBB, right bundle branch block; LAFB, left anterior fascicular block.

TABLE 17-5. Electrocardiogram Criteria for Diagnosis of Insertion of Accessory Pathway

Left Ventricle	Right Ventricle
Anterolateral—1 or 2 and 2, 4, or 5	Anterolateral—7 or 2 and 8, 10 or 11 and 13, 14, or 15
Posterolateral—1 or 2 and 3	Posterolateral—7 or 2 and 8, 10 or 11 and 13
Posteroseptal—1 or 2 and 3, 6	Posteroseptal—7 or 2 and 8, 9 or 11 and 12, 16
	Midseptal—7 or 2 and 8, 9 or 11 and 12, 17
	Anteroseptal—7 or 2 and 8, 9 or 11 and 12, 18
Left sided—1 through 6	Right sided—2 and 8 through 18

1, Transition at or before V1; 2, transitions after V1 and at or before V_2; 3, R wave in lead I > S wave by < 1.0 mV; 4, two or three of II, III, and AVF positive; 5, S wave > R wave in V_1; 6, R wave > S wave in lead I by > 0.8 mV and two or three deltas in II, III, and AVF negative; 7, transition after V_2; 8, R wave in lead I > S wave by 1.0 mV or more; 9, transition before or at V_3; 10, transition at or after V_4; 11, transition between V_3 and V_4; 12, deltawave in lead II 1.0 mV or more; 13, deltawave in lead II less than 1.0 mV; 14, delta-wave in frontal axis 0° or more; 15, R wave in lead III more than 0 mV; 16, two or three of II, III, AVF negative; 17, two or fewer of II, III, AVF negative and two or fewer positive; 18, two or more of II, III, AVF positive.

SPONTANEOUS ECTOPIC VENTRICULAR COMPLEXES

Etiology

When the spontaneous pacemaker of the ventricles lies within the Purkinje system or the ventricular muscle or even in a bundle branch or a fascicle, depolarization of the ventricle takes place without full use of the specialized conduction system, and aberrant conduction occurs.[327]

Ectopic ventricular complexes occur because of increased automaticity of ventricular cells, triggered responses, or reentry requiring microreentry or macroreentry circuits, the two legs of which must have different conduction times, different refractory periods, or both and must be functionally or anatomically separate. Ven-

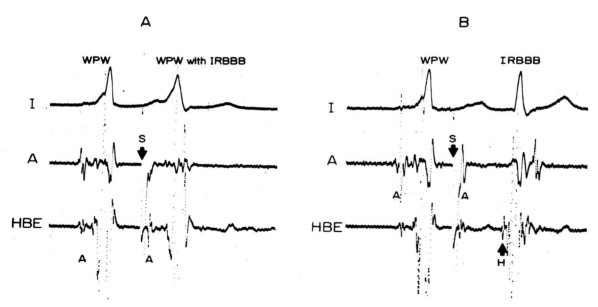

Figure 17-21. Lead I, an intraatrial electrogram (A), and a His bundle electrogram (HBE). **(A)** the artificially induced premature atrial beat prolongs conduction through the normal pathway, leading to an increased degree of ventricular preexcitation. The terminal S wave is probably not related to complete ventricular preexcitation because the QRS is less wide than the one seen in Figure 17-19A (same patient). This terminal S wave is probably related to incomplete right bundle branch block (IRBBB). **(B)** The artificially induced atrial beat is more premature, occurring when the accessory pathway is refractory. A long AH interval is seen. However, the QRS complex shows a terminal S wave, indicating IRBBB but no ventricular preexcitation.

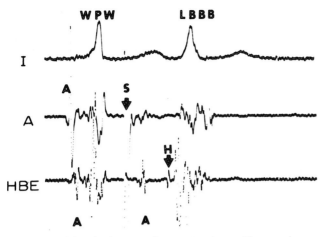

Figure 17-22. The first complex is a sinus beat with some degree of ventricular preexcitation, type A. The artificially induced premature atrial beat again finds the accessory pathway refractory. The AH interval is less long; therefore, the RR interval is shorter and instead of incomplete right bundle branch, there is left bundle-branch block.

tricular tachycardia with LBBB pattern is frequently entrained from the LV, whereas ventricular tachycardia with RBBB is frequently entrained from the RV.[328] Entrainment is considered evidence of reentry and occurs when a portion of the reentrant circuit is captured by a pacing stimulus, perpetuating the tachycardia contour at the stimulus rate. Ventricular ectopy may occur in patients with almost every significant cardiac disease, especially when there is marked cardiomegaly. Ectopic ventricular beats are found on Holter-monitor recordings in more than 50% of clinically normal persons, however, and in such a setting these beats have minimal prognostic significance. Complex ventricular ectopy with exercise in these clinically normal patients may require limitation of the highest levels of stress.[62] Excessive numbers of ectopic ventricular complexes are especially ominous in patients with ischemic heart disease, particularly after acute MI. Ectopic beats are frequent and may indicate successful throm-

bolysis after acute MI.[329] Ectopic ventricular complexes may be extremely difficult to control when there is marked cardiomegaly. They are common with cardiomyopathy; with infiltrative cardiac disease such as sarcoidosis; with inflammatory diseases, including viral myocarditis; and with mitral valve prolapse syndrome, even without cardiomegaly.[263,330] Ventricular rhythms that occur with right ventricular dysplasia may be rapid and life-threatening or slow and bradycardia-dependent.[331]

Clinical Findings

Patients with ectopic ventricular complexes may complain of palpitations. During auscultation of the heart or palpation of the pulse, irregularities may be recognized. Frequently, neither the patient nor the observer feels or hears the premature complexes themselves. It is the sinus beat after the pause that usually causes palpitation in the patient and a strong pulse felt by the observer. Also, a loud first heart sound is produced by the postectopic beat. During ventricular tachycardia, however, the pulse may be regular in timing. With AV dissociation, because of the changing relation between atrial and ventricular contraction, intermittent loud first heart sounds and cannon waves in the veins of the neck may be appreciated. With slow to moderate rates of ventricular tachycardia, patients may complain of palpitations. Rapid ventricular tachycardia may produce palpitation, dyspnea due to congestive heart failure, lightheadedness, syncope, or even death.

Electrocardiogram: Location of Ectopic Focus by Contour

If the ectopic ventricular pacemaker or reentry circuit lies in or near the posterior or anterior fascicle of the LBBB, the QRS complex shows the pattern of RBBB and LAFB or LPFB

TABLE 17-6. T-Wave Changes in Ventricular Preexcitation*

	Type A Accessory Pathway					Type B Accessory Pathway			
	Anterior LV	Posterior Septum	Posterior Superior LV	Posterior Inferior LV	Postero-lateral LV	Anterior RV	Anterior septum	Lateral RV	Posterior RV
May mimic anterior ischemia	Yes	No	Yes	Yes	Yes	No	No	Yes	No
May mimic inferior ischemia	Sometimes	No	Yes	No	Yes	Yes	Yes	No	No
May mimic lateral ischemia	Yes	Yes	Yes	Yes	No	Yes	Yes	No	Yes
May hide anterior ischemia	No	Sometimes	No	No	No	Yes	Yes	No	Yes
May hide inferior ischemia	No	Yes	No	Yes	No	No	No	Yes	Yes
May hide lateral ischemia	No	No	No	No	Yes	No	No	Yes	No

*The variation in ventricular preexcitation is greater than indicated here. These are common patterns. LV, left ventricle; RV, right ventricle.

(Fig. 17-23). If the pacemaker or reentry circuit lies in or near the main LBB, the QRS complex demonstrates RBBB and if the pacemaker or reentry circuit lies in or near the RBB, the contour of the QRS complex is that of LBBB.[332,333] Premature ventricular beats and ventricular tachycardia, however, can and often do arise from the left side of the interventricular septum and do not necessarily show RBBB.[334-336] The location of the origin of ectopic ventricular beats can frequently be designated to an area of the heart by attention to details of the QRS contour on the 12-lead electrocardiogram during the ventricular tachycardia. Six patterns have been shown to allow such a designation.[336] With an LBBB pattern and a left superior axis, QS complexes in V_1 through V_6 or R waves only in V_6 suggest an inferoapical septum location, whereas gradual increase of R waves across the precordial leads suggest an inferobasal septum location. The patterns of LBBB with a left or right inferior axis suggest an anteroapical septum location. With the pattern of RBBB and a right inferior axis, dominant R waves from V_1 through V_6 suggest an anteroapical septum location for the origin of the ventricular tachycardia, whereas dominant S waves in only V_5 or in V_5 and V_6 suggest an inferolateral free-wall location. A pattern of RBBB with a left or right superior axis and a change from dominant R to dominant S waves going from right precordial to left precordial leads suggest an inferobasal free-wall location for the origin of the ventricular tachycardia.[336] The location of ischemia and therefore the vessel involved can frequently be designated by ectopic ventricular beat contour.[337]

QRS complexes tend to be less widened if the ectopic ventricular pacemakers lie more proximal in the fascicles. Ectopic ventricular pacemakers arising in the distal Pur-

kinje system, away from insertions of the fascicles, produce QRS complexes with contours that may not fit well into the aforementioned categories. Pacemakers in the left ventricle away from the septum, however, usually produce slurred complexes with late rightward forces, whereas ectopic pacemakers arising in the right ventricle produce slurred leftward forces.

Differentiation of Ventricular Beats From Supraventricular Beats With Aberrant Conduction

Premature ventricular complexes that do not penetrate retrogradely to the atrium but that reach the AV node cause block of the next sinus complex, so that the time between the two conducted sinus P waves that encompass the ectopic ventricular beat is equal to two sinus cycles. The pause after the ectopic ventricular beat in these circumstances is said to be compensatory. If an ectopic ventricular complex conducts back to the atrium, however, the sinoatrial (SA) node may be reset and no compensatory pause occurs. Thus, ectopic ventricular complexes do not necessarily have compensatory pauses. Premature junctional and even atrial complexes *may* not reset the SA node and thus may be followed by compensatory pauses and also may be early enough to cause aberrant conduction. They may therefore appear to be ventricular because of the contour and the presence of a compensatory pause. If wide complexes do not fit the pattern of bundle branch or fascicular block, they are more likely to be ventricular. If difficulty arises in differentiating ventricular from supra-

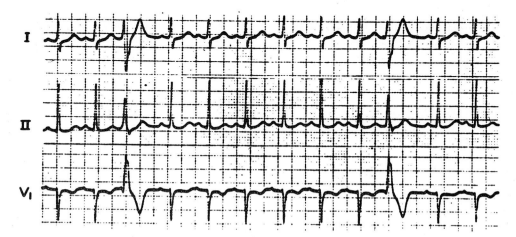

Figure 17-23. Simultaneously recorded leads I, II, and V_1 show two premature beats. Neither is preceded by P waves, and the first has a definite compensatory pause. The pause after the second premature beat is slightly longer than compensatory. These beats are mainly inverted in lead I, upright in lead II, and upright in lead V_1, having the contour of right bundle-branch block and left posterior fascicular block. If these are ventricular beats, they arise in or near the anterior fascicle of the left bundle branch.

ventricular tachycardia with aberrant conduction, HB recordings may be necessary to differentiate one from the other.[338] At rapid rates, supraventricular tachycardia tends to be either absolutely regular or markedly irregular, whereas ventricular tachycardia, even when all complexes have the same contour, tends to be slightly irregular but usually not precisely regular or markedly irregular. Occasionally, various degrees of exit block may cause ventricular tachycardia to be irregular. During wide complex tachycardias, certain details suggest a ventricular origin, such as AV dissociation; positive QRS concordance (positive QRS complexes in all precordial leads); a northwest axis; LBBB with right axis deviation; QRS duration of greater than 140 milliseconds with RBBB; QRS greater than 160 milliseconds with LBBB; and a different QRS configuration during the tachycardia compared with preexisting BBB.[339] To diagnose ventricular tachycardia in the absence of preexisting BBB, Wellens and colleagues used a monophasic wide R wave in V_1; a biphasic or triphasic R wave in V_1, with the initial R tallest (biphasic or triphasic left); RS less than 1 in V_6; and LBBB pattern with Q waves in V_6.[340] In the presence of preexisting BBB, Kremers and coworkers found that precordial concordance, monophasic R wave in V_1, a right superior axis, and a greater than 30 milliseconds R wave in V_1 or V_2 with LBBB pattern suggest ventricular tachycardia.[341] The differentiation of ectopic ventricular beats and aberrancy during atrial fibrillation is also difficult but certain criteria may be highly specific for ectopic ventricular beats.[342] These include LBBB morphology; RBBB morphology, with monophasic R in V_1 or RS or QS in V_6; a pause after the ectopic beat significantly longer than the average cycle length of the ten preceding RR intervals (taught to be called a compensatory-like pause by Pick more than 30 years ago); a frontal plane axis directed superiorly and to the right; and a short–long cycle sequence. Findings specific for aberrancy include RBBB with a triphasic qRs in V_1 or qRs pattern in V_6 and concordance of the initial vector with the normally conducted beats in V_1 or in two or more electrocardiogram leads.

Kindwall and associates found that an R wave in V_1 or V_2 of greater than 30 milliseconds duration, a Q wave in V_6 greater than 60 milliseconds from the beginning of the QRS to the nadir of the S wave in V_1 or V_2, and notching on the downstroke of the S wave in V_1 and V_2 to have high predictive accuracy (96% to 100%) and specificity (94% to 100%) for ventricular beats.[343] The sensitivity was low for any one of these criteria alone but the sensitivity was 100% using any of the four as an indication of ventricular beats (specifically during ventricular tachycardia with LBBB morphology). One of these criteria, a Q wave in V_6, was also associated with MI (mainly anterior), even when it occurred on ventricular beats.

ARTIFICIALLY INDUCED VENTRICULAR RHYTHMS

Etiology

Artificially induced ventricular rhythms are produced by artificial pacemakers implanted on the epicardium, into the myocardium through the epicardium, or by reaching the endocardium of the ventricles transvenously. Pacemakers are used in patients who have or have the potential for life-threatening or symptomatic bradycardia or AV block and in patients in whom tachycardias need to be broken or suppressed. Discussion of the causes of these abnormalities and the indications for placement and type of pacemaker are beyond the scope of this chapter.

Clinical Findings

The clinical findings in patients with artificial pacemakers are the same as those in patients with idioventricular rhythms at similar rates. Occasionally, patients develop unacceptable palpitation when ventricular pacemakers cause AV dissociation. This problem can be solved by the use of AV sequential pacemakers.

Electrocardiogram

Ventricular aberrancy caused by an artificial pacemaker can almost always be recognized if the artificial-pacemaker spikes at the beginning of each paced QRS complex are visible (Fig. 17-24). Implanted pacemakers on the left ventricle produce complexes with RBBB similar to some of the spontaneous left ventricular pacemakers, whereas transvenous pacemakers pace the right ventricle and produce a pattern of LBBB similar to that seen with spontaneous right ventricular pacemakers (see Fig. 17-24). Usually, this pattern of LBBB is associated with left axis deviation (Fig. 17-25), although a normal axis or a right axis deviation may occur. Rarely, there is alternation of the axis (Fig. 17-26), supporting the postulation that a single ectopic ventricular focus may produce QRS complexes of varying contour.

Pacemakers in the coronary sinus may pace the atria, the right ventricle, or the left ventricle and thus may produce normal QRS complexes or LBBB or RBBB pattern.[344]

CONDITIONS UNDER WHICH INTRAVENTRICULAR CONDUCTION DEFECTS OCCUR

The electrophysiologic mechanisms involved in aberrant conduction are discussed in detail in Chapter 15, which brings up to date a prior edition.[345] These mechanisms and

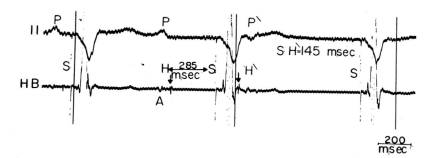

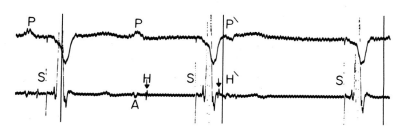

Figure 17-24. Both panels illustrate antegrade block below the bundle of His. Each *A* is followed by an anterograde *H* but no ventricular complex. Ventricular deflections are each initiated by an artificial pacemaker spike (*S*), and when the His bundle, atrioventricular node, and atria are not refractory, they are followed by a retrograde His deflection (*H′*) and a retrograde P wave (*P′*). Thus, there is unidirectional block below the bundle of His.

certain additional variations are reviewed here to complete this clinical section.

Tachycardia- or Short-Cycle–Dependent Intraventricular Conduction Defects

A premature supraventricular complex may fail to depolarize a group of cells because of the refractory period produced by the preceding depolarization. If this refractory period is shortened by isoproterenol, the conduction defect may regress.[346] If such a group of cells is strategically located, for instance in the LBB, the QRS complex produced displays the features of LBBB (Fig. 17-27). In normal hearts, this is more likely to occur in the RBB because of the longer action potential durations in the proximal RBB than the proximal LBB or because the RBB is longer than the LBB.[347] In addition, fibers more distal are more likely to be refractory because of their longer functional refractory periods.[348] The refractory period of the strategically located group of cells may be such that RBBB occurs as the rate increases, even without premature complexes, or the refractory period may be so long that persistent abnormal conduction occurs at all rates. Persistent BBB because of a

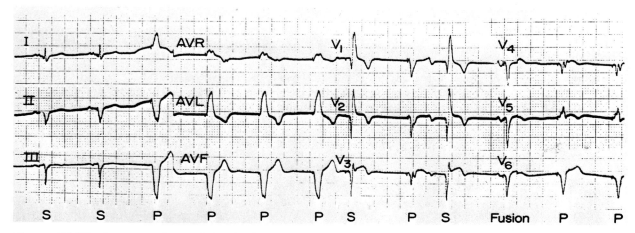

Figure 17-25. A continuously recorded 12-lead electrocardiogram. Sinus beats are marked *S* and ventricular paced beats are marked *P*. Sinus beats show the contour of right bundle-branch block, left anterior fascicular block, anteroseptal myocardial infarction, and possibly inferior infarction. Paced beats are wide, slurred, and entirely upright in leads I and aV_L and therefore pacing is in the right ventricle. Paced complexes are mainly inverted in leads II, III, and aV_F as is usually the case with transvenous ventricular pacing.

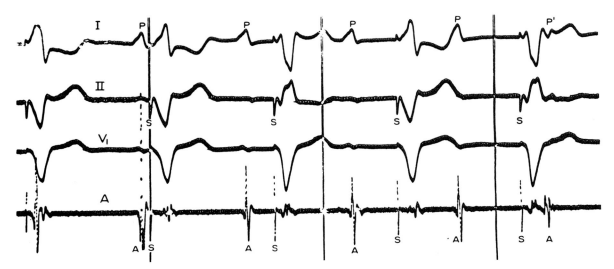

Figure 17-26. Leads I, II, and V₁ and an intra-atrial electrogram (A) are recorded simultaneously. There is no antegrade conduction, all the atrial beats (P) being blocked. Retrograde conduction occurs on the last beat, with the retrograde P wave (P') seen at the end of the QRS complex. All ventricular beats begin with a pacing spike (S). QRS complexes are inverted in lead V₁. In leads I and II, they are alternately mainly upright and mainly inverted. Thus, artificial right ventricular pacing with a pacing catheter tip in the apex of the right ventricle produces a pattern similar to the left bundle-branch block but with alternating left and right axis deviation, beginning with the second QRS complex in this tracing. This suggests that a single ventricular pacemaker may produce QRS complexes varying contours.

long refractory period implies concealed conduction (see section Concealed Conduction Within a Portion of the Ventricles Producing Persistent or Intermittent Intraventricular Conduction in this chapter).

The aberrancy produced by short cycle (phase III block) is generally considered to partly depend on the previous cycle length because refractory periods in the bundle branches appear to prolong at slower rates and shorten at faster rates.[26,349,350] In a group of patients with intermittent LBBB studied with pacing and HB recordings, however, LBB refractory periods were found not to change or to lengthen at faster pacing rates. Also, the rates at which LBBB disappeared as the atrial pacing rate slowed and the rate at which LBBB appeared as the atrial pacing frequency was increased were markedly different.[351–353] Others have found that LBBB appearing with spontaneous increases in rate appears at a slower and narrower range of rates and with less hysteresis than with exercise, indicating the probable effect of catecholamines on the conduction system.[354]

The rate of change of pacing frequency also was a factor, determining the rates at which the LBBB appeared and disappeared. Also, paradoxical improvement in conduction occurred in several instances as the rate increased, possibly related to type I, II, or III gap phenomenon.[252,355–357] Aberrancy sometimes does not depend on the previous cycle length.[358] Thus, tachycardia-dependent

ventricular aberrancy depends on complex phenomenon (see Chap. 15).

Bradycardia- or Long-Cycle–Dependent Aberrant Ventricular Conduction

A strategically located group of cells in a ventricle may fail to conduct a wave of depolarization in a normal manner late after its last depolarization. Such bradycardia-dependent conduction defects occur at slow rates or after long pauses and may be associated with anterior or inferior MI, sclerodegenerative disease, and other diseases affecting the conduction system.[91,359,360] Bradycardia-dependent intraventricular conduction defects may be more common than tachycardia-dependent defects after acute MI.[361] The phenomenon of bradycardia-dependent conduction defect may depend on the presence of diastolic depolarization.[362] If isoproterenol accelerates the diastolic depolarization, bradycardia-dependent BBB may appear.[346,363] Also, BBB may be present in late complexes but may disappear in early complexes as a manifestation of supernormal conduction.[364,365] It has also been suggested that RBBB seen after long cycles may disappear after short cycles because of Wedensky facilitation.[357] Occasionally, patients are reported in whom there is both tachycardia- and bradycardia-dependent BBB.[91,94,365–369] Bradycardia-

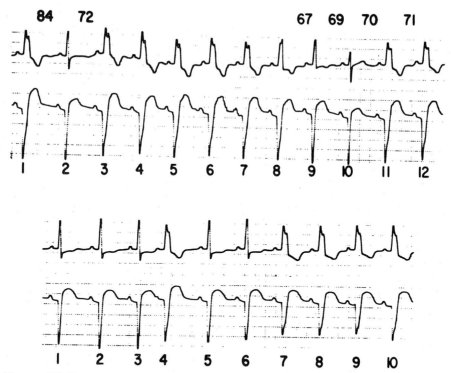

Figure 17-27. Two panels of a consecutive electrocardiogram showing a modified lead V$_5$ and a modified lead V$_1$. The relatively long pause of 84 hundredths of a second between complexes 1 and 2 ends with a normal complex, and the next interval of 72 hundredths of a second between complexes 2 and 3 ends with tachycardia-dependent left bundle-branch block. Complex 9, however, ending an interval of 67 hundredths of a second, shows only incomplete left bundle-branch block. The narrowing of complex 9 may be a result of the gradual shortening of the refractory period of the left bundle branch during the more rapid rhythm from complex 3 through 9, and the further decrease of left bundle-branch block in complex 10 may be a result of the sudden slight sinus slowing. These findings are still compatible with tachycardia-dependent left bundle-branch block. Complex 11, however, follows an even longer interval of 70 hundredths of a second yet displays left bundle-branch block. This could represent non–rate-dependent left bundle-branch block, tachycardia-dependent left bundle-branch block occurring because of a lengthened refractory period of the left bundle branch after the slight slowing seen between complexes 9 and 10 or bradycardia-dependent left bundle-branch block. Complex 12, ending an interval of 71 hundredths of a second, could manifest left bundle-branch block because late depolarization of the left bundle branch has occurred after concealed transseptal retrograde conduction during complex 11. In the bottom panel, a premature atrial beat is followed by left bundle-branch block that is apparently tachycardia-dependent and a slight shortening of the RR interval between complexes 6 and 7 produces left bundle-branch block in complex 7. Therefore, analysis of this rhythm strip requires at least a consideration of tachycardia-dependent bundle-branch block, bradycardia-dependent bundle-branch block, non–rate-dependent bundle-branch block, concealed transseptal retrograde depolarization of a bundle branch, and the effect of changes of rate on the refractory period of a bundle branch.

dependent block may occur in both bundle branches simultaneously and thus cause AV block.[370] Once bradycardia-dependent AV block has occurred, it continues until the area of block is repolarized. If the AV block is unidirectional, an ectopic ventricular escape complex may fully depolarize the cells in the areas of block, allowing them to repolarize fully and once again conduct in the antero-grade direction or the cells may depolarize spontaneously to threshold potential, fire in a concealed manner, repolarize, and conduct again.[371]

Non–Rate-Dependent or Non–Cycle-Length–Dependent Aberrant Ventricular Conduction

If strategically located cells have been destroyed, aberrant conduction is unrelated to rate. This may occur congenitally because of disease or trauma or secondary to a surgical procedure.

Aberrant ventricular conduction may also occur intermittently, regardless of the direction of change in cardiac rate (see Fig. 17-7 and Chap. 15).[372]

ELECTRIC ALTERNANS

Tachycardia- or Short-Cycle Length–Dependent Electric Alternans

If an area of the ventricles has a refractory period longer than one but shorter than two cycle lengths of a given rhythm, there is no depolarization of the cells in this area on alternate beats.[92] If this area lies in a strategic location, such as a bundle branch, alternate beats have BBB. This BBB alternans is tachycardia-dependent because it depends on beats falling into phase III refractory period of a

portion of the ventricles. The refractory period may even be longer than two cycle lengths but shorter than three, so that block occurs in two out of every three complexes (Fig. 17-28D). Bundle branch block alternans may occur even with irregular rhythms (Fig. 17-29).

Bradycardia-Initiated Electric Alternans

An intraventricular conduction defect that occurs only after a long pause, possibly related to spontaneous diastolic depolarization, is bradycardia- or long-cycle–dependent and may initiate electric alternans, sometimes of the BBB type. Sudden bradycardia may initiate BBB alternans by prolonging the refractory period of a bundle branch.[92] The BBB that occurs is actually tachycardia-dependent.

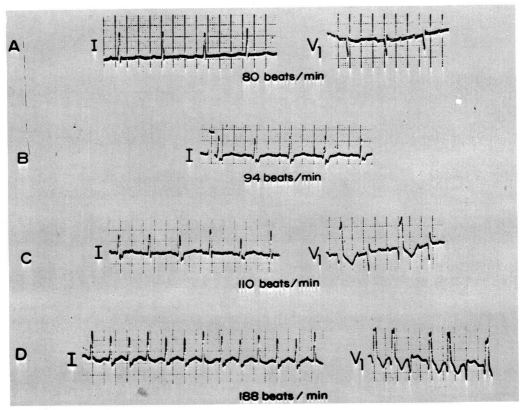

Figure 17-28. (**A**) Leads I and V₁ show QRS complexes of normal duration. Small terminal R waves in lead V₁ suggest the possibility of incomplete right bundle-branch block. Sinus rate is 89 beats/minute. (**B**) The sinus rate is 94 beats/minute and constant right bundle-branch block is seen in lead I. It must be assumed that there is transseptal retrograde conduction into the right bundle with each complex. (**C**) Leads I and V₁ show right bundle-branch block alternans. At 110 beats/minutes both anterograde and retrograde refractory periods are longer than one interval but shorter than the two RR intervals, so that anterograde conduction and retrograde conduction are blocked on alternate beats. (**D**) Leads I and V₁ show right bundle-branch block in two out of every three complexes at a sinus rate of 188 beats/minute. We assume that the right bundle-branch refractory period is longer than two intervals but shorter than three. This figure shows pseudo–bradycardia-dependent bundle-branch block alternans because in *B* there is right bundle-branch block on only every other beat.

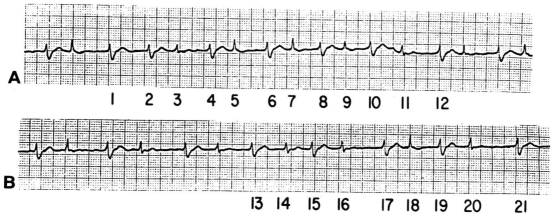

Figure 17-29. Lead I during atrial fibrillation. Frequent complexes show right bundle-branch block, producing irregular bundle-branch block alternans. All longer pause—such as those between complexes 1 and 2, 11 and 12, 16 and 17, and 20 and 21—show right bundle-branch block, suggesting that the block is bradycardia-dependent. All shorter intervals end with complexes differing from the immediately preceding complex; for example, complexes 7, 9, and 18 have no right bundle-branch block, whereas complexes 8, 10, and 15 show right bundle-branch block. Thus, there appears to be right bundle-branch block alternans that is recognizable even though the rhythm is irregular. The alternans appears to be tachycardia-dependent, whereas the right bundle-branch block is bradycardia-dependent. The only two consecutive long intervals end with complexes 1 and 2, both of which have right bundle-branch block.

Pseudo-Bradycardia–Dependent Electric Alternans

Occasionally, electric alternans, especially of the BBB type, changes to persistent BBB on every beat when the rate slows (see Figs. 17-28B and C).[92] This initially suggests that the BBB is bradycardia-dependent. With further slowing of the rate, however, the BBB disappears entirely (see Fig. 17-28). Under these circumstances, the electric alternans is actually tachycardia-dependent. At the faster rate, there is both anterograde and retrograde block in the abnormal bundle branch on alternate beats. At the slightly reduced rate, the "blocked" bundle branch is kept in a refractory state because of retrograde penetration on every beat. Thus, although the pattern of BBB becomes persistent, there is retrograde conduction into the abnormal bundle branch on every beat, and conduction into this bundle branch has changed from 2:1 to 1:1 (improved). With further slowing of the rate, each consecutive beat falls beyond both the anterograde and retrograde refractory periods, so that all complexes are normal.

Etiology

All the diseases that produce intermittent BBB may be associated with BBB alternans, except that complete anatomic interruption of a bundle branch does not allow BBB alternans. Diseases that have been specifically associated with BBB alternans include sclerodegenerative disease of

the conduction system, hypertension, ischemic heart disease, and bacterial endocarditis.[95]

CONCEALED CONDUCTION WITHIN A PORTION OF THE VENTRICLES PRODUCING PERSISTENT OR INTERMITTENT INTRAVENTRICULAR CONDUCTION

Concealed Retrograde Conduction With Subsequent Intraventricular Conduction Defect

The pattern of persistent BBB may occur when the apparently blocked bundle is depolarized on every complex (see Figs. 17-4 and 17-30). For instance, if an early supraventricular complex finds the RBB still refractory, it produces anterograde RBBB. The refractory period of the RBB may be over by the time there is conduction down the LBB and across the septum, allowing retrograde conduction into the RBB to occur. This concealed transseptal retrograde conduction causes the RBB to remain refractory for the next regular supraventricular complex. Thus, once anterograde RBBB has occurred, retrograde conduction into that same bundle may cause the conduction defect to persist.[373,374] This phenomenon may also occur with LBBB, LAFB, LPFB, or complete ventricular preexcitation. Transseptal retrograde concealed conduction caus-

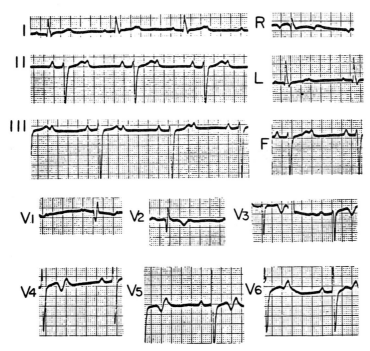

Figure 17-30. Same patient as in Figure 17-2, at a more rapid sinus rate. In leads II, III, and aV$_F$, QRS complexes are mainly inverted and there is an R' wave in lead V$_1$. QRS duration is 0.12 second. These changes are compatible with right bundle-branch block and left anterior fascicular block. Also, alternate beats are blocked and PR intervals are prolonged. In the absence of digitalis, these changes suggest that the only remaining conducting fascicle (the left posterior fascicle) conducts with a prolonged interval on alternate beats and is blocked on alternate beats. Thus, conduction, although prolonged, goes through the main left bundle and the left posterior fascicle on alternate beats. Although there is the pattern of right bundle-branch block, the right bundle branch must be able to conduct, as it did in the tracing in Figure 17-2 (taken several minutes earlier). Likewise, although left bundle-branch block is evident in Figure 17-2, the left bundle is able to conduct, as it does in this figure. Thus, given time for recovery, either bundle can and does conduct, either in an obvious or in a concealed slow anterograde or retrograde manner. After several ventricular cycles, either bundle would have surely recovered had it not been kept refractory by concealed conduction. At this slow ventricular rate (43 beats/minute), the absence of conduction down the right bundle branch (with left bundle-branch block pattern and a normal PR, as seen in the first portion of Figure 17-2) must be explained on the basis of a right bundle-branch refractory period that has prolonged during the slow ventricular rate seen at the bottom of Figure 17-2 and in this figure.

ing BBB at longer intervals than expected has been called the linking phenomenon and may even cause unexpected loss of BBB because of supernormal conduction.[375] Moreover, such a circuit, when complete, may produce macroreentrant ventricular tachycardia and may be treated by electric catheter ablation of a bundle branch.[376,377]

Concealed retrograde conduction in these circumstances may also be a step in the reentry process whereby two anatomically or functionally dissociated pathways are present, so that conduction may occur in one direction in one pathway and at a later time, in the opposite direction in the other pathway. Reentry may be manifest or concealed and may occur through large pathways or small ones (microreentry). Microreentry could be responsible for most coupled premature ventricular beats. Reentry has

been clinically shown to occur in a ventricular fascicle (see Fig. 17-10), and the conditions for reentry have been experimentally shown to be present in the RBB.[49,374]

Concealed Anterograde Conduction

An intraventricular conduction defect may occur not only when anterograde conduction is interrupted down a pathway into or within the ventricles but also when there is marked delay of anterograde conduction down one of these pathways. For instance, if anterograde conduction down the RBB is slow, both ventricles may be depolarized through the LBB. This slow, delayed, anterograde conduction could also cause the RBBB to be in a refractory state

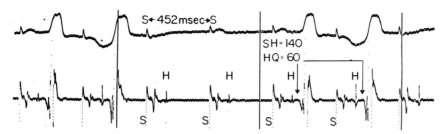

Figure 17-31. Type II block below the bundle of His. All HQ intervals are the same in the conducted beats. Suddenly, there is no conduction below the His potential after the third and fourth pacing spikes but conduction resumes after the fifth and sixth pacing spikes, with no change in HQ intervals. This 4:2 ratio can be explained by two levels of type II sub-Hisian block, the upper being 4:3 and the lower being 3:2.

for the next supraventricular complex, so that persistent intraventricular conduction defect may occur, at least for several complexes, because of concealed slow antergrade conduction. Concealed anterograde conduction discharging a bundle branch but not any other part of the ventricles may cause a subsequent conducted complex to display BBB or may shorten the bundle branch cycle length and refractory period, so that a subsequent short interval does not produce BBB, or it may discharge a fascicular pacemaker without reaching the rest of the ventricle.[49,378] Also, concealed anterograde conduction may be responsible for intermittent penetration of a proximal portion of the AV conduction system, causing curious ratios of AV conduction (Fig. 17-31).

CONCLUSION

In this chapter and in Chapter 15, we have examined the electrophysiologic, electrocardiographic, and clinical aspects of abnormal intraventricular conduction.[379] The cellular membrane mechanisms that mainly control single-cell action potentials and impulse formation are discussed. The effects of changes at the cellular level are, in a series of steps, related to clinical examples and to implications of aberrant intraventricular conduction.

Discussion of abnormal intraventricular conduction is divided into short and long cardiac-cycle-length–dependent, and non–cycle-length–dependent aberrancy. The role of drugs as a factor in all types of aberrant conduction is included.

Finally, we have set forth a clinical compendium of the various electrocardiographic expressions of aberrant intraventricular conduction, including bundle branch and fascicular blocks, ventricular preexcitation, and spontaneous and artificial ventricular rhythms.[345]

Descriptions and clinical implications of aberrant intraventricular conduction, such as the effect of left axis deviation on the prognosis of LBBB, accompany examples of the primary and secondary electrocardiographic changes.[380]

Most of the principles included in this chapter and in Chapter 15 have been proved. Many of the explanations that accompany clinical examples of aberrant intraventricular conduction are speculative. The mechanistic background in these chapters and in the references, however, should provide the tools with which to approach and most often understand each electrocardiogram in which intraventricular aberrancy comes into question.

References

1. Fabregas RA, Tse WW, Han J: Conduction disturbances of the bundle branches produced by lesions in the non-branching portion of the His bundle. Am Heart J 1976;92:356.
2. James TN, Sherf L: Fine structure of the His bundle. Circulation 1971;44:9.
3. Sciacca A, Sangiorgi M: Trouble de la conduction intraventriculaire droite de la lesion du tronc commun du faisceau de His. Acta Cardiol 1957;12:486.
4. El-Sherif N, Scherlag BJ, Lazzara R: Conduction disorders in the canine proximal His-Purkinje system following acute myocardial ischemia. II. The pathophysiology of bilateral bundle branch block. Circulation 1974;49:848.
5. Massing GK, James TN: Anatomical configuration of the His bundle and bundle branches in the human heart. Circulation 1976;53:609.
6. Demoulin JC, Kulbertus HE: Left hemiblocks revisited from the histopathological viewpoint. Am Heart J 1973;86:712.
7. Lazzara R, Yeh BK, Samet P: Functional transverse interconnections within the His bundle and the bundle branches. Circ Res 1973;32:509.
8. El-Sherif N, Amat-Y-Leon F, Schonfield C, et al: Normalization of bundle block patterns by distal His bundle pacing. Clinical and experimental evidence of longitudinal dissociation in the pathologic His bundle. Circulation 1978;57:473.
9. Selvester RH, Velasquez DW, Elko PP, Cady LD: Intraventricular conduction defect (IVCD), real or fancied, QRS dura-

tion in 1,254 normal adult white males by a multilead automated algorithm. J Electrocardiol 1990;23(Suppl):118.

10. McAnulty J, Rahimtoola S: Prognosis in bundle branch block. Ann Rev Med 1981;32:499.

11. Bharati S, Lev M, Dhingra R, et al: Pathologic correlations in three cases of bilateral bundle branch (block) disease with unusual electrophysiologic manifestations in two cases. Am J Cardiol 1976;38:508.

12. Singer RB: Mortality in 966 life insurance applications with bundle branch block or wide QRS. Trans Assoc Life Insur Med Dir Am 1968;52:94.

13. Lister JW, Kline RS, Lesser ME: Chronic bilateral bundle branch block. Long-term observations in ambulatory patients. Br Heart J 1977;39:203.

14. Denes P, Dhingra RC, Wu D, et al: Sudden death in patients with bifascicular block. Arch Intern Med 1977;137:1005.

15. Scheinman MM, Peters RW, Morady F, et al: Electrophysiologic studies in patients with bundle branch block. Pace 1983;6:1157.

17. Yoon MS, Han J, Fabregas RA: Effect of ventricular aberrancy on fibrillation threshold. Am Heart J 1975;89:599.

17. Hinkle LE Jr, Carver ST, Stevens M: The frequency of asymptomatic disturbances of cardiac rhythm and conduction in middle-aged men. Am J Cardiol 1969;24:629.

18. Kannel WB, Kagan A, Dawber RT, et al: Epidemiology of coronary heart disease. Geriatrics 1962;17:675.

19. Peters RW, Scheinman MM, Modin GM, et al: Prophylactic permanent pacemakers for patients with chronic bundle branch block. Am J Med 1979;66:978.

20. Freedman RA, Alderman EL, Sheffield LT, Saporito M, Fisher LD, et al: Bundle branch block in patients with chronic coronary artery disease: angiographic correlates and prognostic significance. J Am Coll Cardiol 1987;10:73.

21. Puech P: Contribution of the His bundle recording to the diagnosis of bilateral bundle branch conduction defects. Adv Cardiol 1975;14:178.

22. Aronson AL: Evaluation of surface ECG findings as prodromata of type II complete heart block. Circulation 1973;48(Suppl IV):122.

23. Scheinman MM, Peters RW, Modin G, et al: Prognostic value of infranodal conduction time in patients with chronic bundle branch block. Circulation 1977;56:240.

24. Scheinman M, Brenman BA: Clinical and anatomic implications of intraventricular conduction blocks in acute myocardial infarction. Circulation 1972;46:753.

25. Gould L, Venkataraman K, Mohammad N, Gomprecht RF: Prognosis of right bundle branch block in acute myocardial infarction. JAMA 1972;219:502.

26. Fisch GR, Zipes DP, Fisch C: Bundle branch block and sudden death. Prog Cardiovasc Dis 1980;23:187.

27. Scheinman MM, Golschlager NF, Peters RW: Bundle branch block. Cardiovasc Clin 1980;11:57.

28. Denes P, Dhingra RC, Wu D, et al: HV interval in patients with bifascicular block (right bundle branch block and left anterior hemiblock). Clinical, electrocardiographic, and electrophysiologic correlations. Am J Cardiol 1975;35:23.

29. Dhingra RC, Denes P, Wu D, et al: Prospective observations in patients with chronic bundle branch block and marked HV prolongation. Circulation 1976;53:600.

30. Rosen KM, Ehsani A, Rahimtoola SH: H-V intervals in left bundle branch block. Clinical and electrocardiographic correlations. Circulation 1972;46:717.

31. McAnulty JH, Kauffman S, Murphy E, et al: Survival in patients with intraventricular conduction defects. Arch Intern Med 1978;128:30.

32. Berkowitz WD, Lau SH, Patton RD, Rosen KM, Damato AN: The use of His bundle recordings in the analysis of unilateral and bilateral bundle branch block. Am Heart J 1971;81:340.

33. Castellanos A Jr: HV intervals in LBBB. Circulation 1973;47:1133.

34. Hirschfeld DS, Ueda CT, Rowland M, et al: Clinical and electrphysiologic effects of intravenous quinidine in man. Br Heart J 1977;39:309.

35. Scheinman MM, Weiss AN, Shaftom E, et al: Electrophysiologic effects of procainamide in patterns with intraventricular conduction delay. Circulation 1974;49:522.

36. Desai JM, Scheinman MM, Peters TE, et al: Electrophysiologic effects of disopyramide in patients with bundle branch block. Circulation 1979;59:215.

37. Kaul U, Dev V, Narula J, Malhotra A, Talwar KK, Bhatia ML: Evaluation of patients with bundle branch block and "unexplained" syncope: a study based on comprehensive electrophysiologic testing and ajmaline stress. Pace 1988;11:289.

38. Santinelli V, Chiariello M, Ambrosio G, et al: Further observations on the electrophysiologic effects of oral amiodarone therapy. Chest 1982;82:117.

39. Chaile PA, Przybylski J, Laino RA, et al: Usefulness of the ajmaline test in patients with latent bundle branch block. Am J Cardiol 1982;49:21.

40. Kunkel F, Rowland M, Scheinman MM: The electrophysiologic effects of lidocaine in patients with intraventricular conduction defects. Circulation 1974;49:894.

41. Gupta PK, Lichstein E, Chadda KD: Lidocaine-induced heart block in patients with bundle branch block. Am J Cardiol 1974;33:487.

42. DeJoseph RL, Zipes DP: Normal H-V time in a patient with right bundle branch block, left anterior hemiblock and intermittent complete distal His block. Chest 1973;63:564.

43. Dhingra RC, Wyndham C, Amat-Y-Leon F, et al;: Significance of A-H interval in patients with chronic bundle branch block. Clinical electrophysiologic and follow-up observations. Am J Cardiol 1976;37:231.

44. Bhat PK, Watanabe K, Rao DB, et al: Conduction defects in the aging heart. J Am Geriatr Soc 1974;22:517.

45. Wiberg TA, Richman HG, Gobel FL: The significance and prognosis of chronic bifascicular block. Chest 1977;71:329.

46. Graybiel A, Sprague HB: Bundle branch block: an analysis of 395 cases. Am J Med Sci 1933;185:395.

47. Langendorf R, Cohen H, Gozo EG Jr: Observations on second degree atrioventricular block including new criteria for the differential diagnosis between type I and type II block. Am J Cardiol 1972;29:111.

48. Dhingra RC, Denes P, Wu D, et al: The significance of second degree atrioventricular block and bundle branch block. Observations regarding site and type of block. Circulation 1974;49:638.

49. Cohen HC, D'Cruz I, Pick A: Concealed intraventricular

conduction in the His bundle electrogram. Circulation 1976;53:766.

50. Gray R, Kaushik VS, Mandel WJ: Wenckebach phenomenon occurring in the distal conduction system in a young adult. Br Heart J 1976;38:204.

51. Akhtar M, Damato AN: Clinical uses of His bundle electrocardiography. Am Heart J 1976;91:520.

52. Dhingra RC, Denes P, Wu D, et al: Chronic right bundle branch block and left posterior hemiblock. Clinical electrophysiologic and prognostic observations. Am J Cardiol 1975;36:867.

53. Markel ML, Miles WM, Zipes DP, Prystowsky EN: Parasympathetic and sympathetic alterations of Mobitz type II heart block. J Am Coll Cardiol 1988;11:271.

54. Smith RF, Jackson DH, Harthorne JW, Sanders CA: Acquired bundle branch block in a healthy population. Am Heart J 1970;80:746.

55. Rotman M, Triebwasser JHG: A clinical and follow-up study of right and left bundle branch block. Circulation 1975; 51:477.

56. Canaveris G, Nau GJ: Intraventricular conduction disturbances in flying personnel: development and prognosis of bifascicular blocks. Aviat Space Environ Med 1987;58:683.

57. Wu D, Denes P, Dhingra RC, et al: Electrophysiological and clinical observations in patients with alternating bundle branch block. Circulation 1976;53:456.

58. Rooney SM, Gondiner PL, Muss E: Relationship of right bundle branch block and marked left axis deviation in complete heart block during general anesthesia. Anesthesiology 1976;44:64.

59. Scheinman M, Weiss A, Kunkel F: His bundle recordings in patients with bundle branch block and transient neurologic symptoms. Circulation 1973;48:322.

60. Altschuler H, Fisher JD, Furman S: Significance of isolated H-V interval prolongation in symptomatic patients without documented heart block. Am Heart J 1979;97:19.

61. Rotman M, Wagner GS, Wallace AJ: Bradyarrhythmias in acute myocardial infarction. Circulation 1972;45:703.

62. Barrett PA, Peter CT, Swan HJC, Singh BN, Mandel WJ: The frequency and prognostic significance of electrocardiographic abnormalities in clinically normal individuals (review article). Prog Cardiovasc Dis 1981;23:299.

63. Simon AB, Zloto AE: Atrio-ventricular block. Natural history after permanent ventricular pacing. Am J Cardiol 1978; 41:500.

64. Kones RJ, Phillips JH: Review: Bundle branch block in acute myocardial infarction: Current concepts and indications. Acta Cardiol 1980;35:469.

65. Nimetz AA, Shubrooks SJ, Hutter AM, DeSanctis RW: The significance of bundle branch block during acute myocardial infarction. Am Heart J 1975;90:439.

66. Riley CP, Jackson DH, Russell RO, Rackley CE: Partial bilateral bundle branch block in acute myocardial infarction. Chest 1973;63:342.

67. Godman MJ, Lassers BW, Julian DG: Complete bundle branch block complicating acute myocardial infarction. N Engl J Med 1970;282:237.

68. Scheidt S, Killip T: Bundle-branch block complicating acute myocardial infarction. JAMA 1972;222:919.

69. Lie KI, Liem KL, Schuilenburg RM, et al: Early identification of patients developing late in-hospital ventricular fibrillation after discharge from the coronary care unit. A 5 1/2 year retrospective and prospective of 1897 patients. Am J Cardiol 1978;41:674.

70. Hindman MC, Wagner GS, JaRo M, et al: The clinical significance of bundle branch block complicating acute myocardial infarction. I. Clinical characteristics hospital mortality and one-year follow-up. Circulation 1978;58:679.

71. Hindman MC, Wagner GS, JaRo M, et al: The clinical significance of bundle branch block complicating acute myocardial infarction. II. Indications for temporary and permanent pacemaker insertion. Circulation 1978;58:689.

72. Touboul P, Kirkorian G, Atallah G, Moleur P: Bundle branch reentry: a possible mechanism of ventricular tachycardia. Circulation 1983;67:674.

73. Rosenfeld LE: Bradyarrhythmias, abnormalities of conduction, and indications for pacing in acute myocardial infarction. Cardiol Clin 1988;6:49.

74. Caceres J, Jazayeri M, McKinnie J, et al: Sustained bundle branch reentry as a mechanism of clinical tachycardia. Circulation 1989;79:256.

75. Volkmann H, Kuhnert H, Dannberg G, Heinke M: Bundle branch reentrant tachycardia treated by transvenous catheter ablation of the right bundle branch. Pace 1989;12:258.

76. Fenig S, Lichstein E: Incomplete bilateral bundle branch block and A-V block complicating acute anterior wall myocardial infarction. Am Heart J 1972;84:38.

77. Rao MS, Antani J: Prognostic profile of fascicular blocks in myocardial infarction. Jpn Heart J 1977;18:406.

78. DePasquale NP, Bruno MS: Natural history of combined right bundle branch block and left anterior hemiblock (bilateral bundle branch block). Am J Med 1973;54:297.

79. Hunt D, Sloman G: Bundle branch block in acute myocardial infarction. Br Med J 1969;1:85.

80. Waters DD, Mizgala HF: Long-term prognosis of patients with incomplete bilateral bundle branch block complicating acute myocardial infarction. Role of cardiac pacing. Am J Cardiol 1974;34:1.

81. Lichstein E, Gupta PK, Chadda KD: Long-term survival of patients with incomplete bundle branch block complicating acute myocardial infarction. Br Heart J 1975;27:924.

82. Resnekov L: Pacemaking and acute myocardial infarction Impulse 1978;11:1.

83. Lichstein E, Gupta PK, Chadda KD, et al: Findings of prognostic value in patients with incomplete bilateral bundle branch block complicating acute myocardial infarction. Am J Cardiol 1973;32:913.

84. Lichstein E, Ribas-Meneclier C, Naik D, et al: The natural history of trifascicular disease following permanent pacemaker implantation. Significance of continuing changes in atrioventricular conduction. Circulation 1978;54:780.

85. Siegman-Igra Y, Yahini JH, Goldbourt U, et al: Intraventricular conduction disturbances. A review of prevalence, etiology, progression for 10 years within a stable population of Israeli adult males. Am Heart J 1978;96:699.

86. Caspi Y, Safadi T, Ammar R, Elamy A, Fishman NH, Merin G: The significance of bundle branch block in the immediate postoperative electrocardiograms of patients undergoing

coronary artery bypass. J Thorac Cardiovasc Surg 1987; 93:442.

87. Chu A, Califf RM, Pryor DB, et al: Prognostic effect of bundle branch block related to coronary artery bypass grafting. Am J Cardiol 1987;59:798.

88. Wexelman W, Lichstein E, Cunningham JN, Hollander G, Greengart A, Shani J: Etiology and clinical significance of new fascicular conduction defects following coronary bypass surgery. Am Heart J 1986;111:923.

89. Crijns HJ, vanGelder IC, Lie KI: Supraventricular tachycardia mimicking ventricular tachycardia during flecainide treatment. Am J Cardiol 1988;62:1303.

90. Rosenbaum MB, Elizari MV, Levi RJ, et al: Five cases of intermittent left anterior hemiblock. Am J Cardiol 1969;24:1.

91. Rosenbaum MB, Elizari MV, Lazzari JO, et al: The mechanisms of intermittent bundle branch block. Relationship to prolonged recovery, hypopolarization and spontaneous diastolic depolarization. Chest 1973;63:666.

92. Cohen HC, D'Cruz I, Arbel ER, et al: Tachycardia and bradycardia-dependent bundle branch block alterans. Clinical observations. Circulation 1977;55:242.

93. Friedberg HD, Schamroth L: The Wenckebach phenomenon in left bundle branch block. Am J Cardiol 1969;24:591.

94. Friedberg HD: Mechanisms of the Wedensky phenomena in the left bundle branch. Am J Cardiol 1971;27:698.

95. Williams MA, Esterbrooks DJ, Nair CK, Sailors MM, Sketch MH: Clinical significance of exercise-induced bundle branch block. Am J Cardiol 1988;61:346.

96. LaCanna G, Giubbini R, Metra M, et al: Assessment of myocardial perfusion with thallium-201 scintigraphy in exercise-induced left bundle branch block: diagnostic value and clinical significance. Eur Heart J 1992;13(7):942.

97. Lev M, Unger PN, Rosen KM, Bharati S: The anatomic base of the electrocardiographic abnormality of left bundle branch block. Adv Cardiol 1975;14:16.

98. Holt JH Jr, Barnard ACL, Kramer JO Jr: A study of the human heart as a multiple dipole source. IV. Left ventricular hypertrophy in the presence of right bundle branch block. Circulation 1977;56:391.

99. Hardarson T, Arnason A, Eliasson GJ, Palsson K, Eyjolfsson K, Sigfusson, N: Left bundle branch block: prevalence, incidence, follow-up and outcome. Eur Heart J 1987;8:1075.

100. Herbert WH: Left bundle branch block and coronary artery disease. J Electrocardiol 1975;8:317.

101. Sugiura M, Okada R, Ohkawa S, Shimada H: Pathohistological studies on the conduction system in 8 cases of complete left bundle branch block. Jpn Heart J 1970;11:5.

102. Brake CM: Complete left bundle branch block and asymptomatic airmen. Aero Med 1969;40:781.

103. Cripps T, Joy M: Aortic root abscess in *Actinobacillus actinomycetemcomitans* endocarditis: Non invasive diagnosis and successful outcome following early surgery. Eur Heart J 1986;7:632.

104. Whinnery JE, Froelicher VF, Stewart AJ, et al: The electrocardiographic response to maximal treadmill exercise of asymptomatic men with left bundle branch block. Am Heart J 1977;94:316.

105. McGowan RL, Welch TG, Zaret BL, et al: Noninvasive myocardial imaging with potassium^{-43} and rubidium^{-81} in patients with left bundle branch block. Am J Cardiol 1976;38:422.

106. O'Keefe JH Jr, Bateman TM, Barnhart CS: Adenosine thallium-201 is superior to exercise thallium-201 for detecting coronary artery disease in patients with left bundle branch block. J Am Coll Cardiol 1993;21(6):1332.

107. Burns RJ, Galligan L, Wright LM, Lawand S, Burke RJ, Gladstone PJ: Improved specificity of myocardial thallium-201 single-photon emission computed tomography in patients with left bundle branch block by dipyridamole. Am J Cardiol 1991;68(5):504.

108. Henze E, Hildebrand P, Hellwig D, et al: Differentiation between infarction and cardiomyopathy in left bundle branch block by parametric radionuclide imaging. Am J Physiol Imaging 1988;3:121.

109. Aoki T, Motoyasu M, Simizu Y, et al: A case of dilated cardiomyopathy manifested by exercise-induced left bundle branch block. Jpn Circ J 1993;57(6):573.

110. Chen CH, Sakurai T, Fujita M, et al: Transient intraventricular conduction disturbances in hypertrophic obstructive cardiomyopathy. Am Heart J 1981;101:672.

111. Rahko PS, Shaver JA, Salerni R: Evaluation of mechanical events and systolic function in dilated cardiomyopathy: comparison between patients with and without left bundle branch block. Acta Cardiol 1988;43:179.

112. Morgera T, Di-Lenarda A, Dreas L, et al: Electrocardiography of myocarditis revisited: clinical prognostic significance of electrocardiographic changes. Am Heart J 1992;124(2):455.

113. Cohen H, Rosen KM, Pick A: Disorders of impulse conduction and impulse formation caused by hyperkalemia in man. Am Heart J 1975;89:501.

114. Olofsson B, Forsberg H, Andersson S, Bjerle P, Henriksson A, Wedin I: Electrocardiographic findings in myotonic dystrophy. Br Heart J 1988;59:47.

115. Hiromasa S, Ikeda T, Kubota K, et al: Myotonic dystrophy: ambulatory electrocardiogram, electrophysiologic study, echocardiographic evaluation. Am Heart J 1987;113:1482.

116. Fenichel NM, Jimenez FA, Polachek AA: 2:1 left bundle branch block in acute bacterial endocarditis with septal abscess. J Electrocardiol 1977;10:287.

117. Singh RB, Agrawal BV, Somani PN: Left bundle branch block: A rare manifestation of digitalis intoxication. Acta Cardiol 1976;31:175.

118. Bharati S, Lev M, Dhingra RC, Chuquimia R, Towne WD, Rosen KM: Electrophysiologic and pathologic correlations in two cases of chronic second degree atrioventricular block with left bundle branch block. Circulation 1975;52:221.

119. Steenkamp WFJ: Familial trifascicular block. Am Heart J 1972;84:758.

120. Heinsimer JA, Skelton TN, Califf RM: Rate-related left bundle branch block with chest pain and normal coronary arteriograms treated by exercise training. Am J Med Sci 1986;292:317.

121. Schultz DA, Wahl RL, Juni JE, et al: Diagnosis of exercise-induced left bundle branch block at rest by scintigraphic phase analysis. Eur J Nucl Med 1986;11:434.

122. Dhingra RC, Wyndham C, Bauernfeind R, et al: Significance of chronic bifascicular block without apparent organic heart disease. Circulation 1979;60:33.

123. Shaver JA, Rahko PS, Grines CL, Boudoulas H, Wooley CF: Effects of left bundle branch block on the events of the cardiac cycle. Acta Cardiol 1988;43:459.

124. D'Cunha GF, Friedberg HD, Jaume F: The first heart sound

in intermittent left bundle branch block. Am J Cardiol 1971; 27:447.

125. Haft JI, Weinstock M, DeGuia R, et al: Assessment of atrioventricular conduction in left and right bundle branch block using His bundle electrogram and atrial pacing. Am J Cardiol 1971;27:474.

126. Shah KD, Daxini BV: Non-invasive and invasive evaluation of left bundle branch block (LBBB). Acta Cardiol 1990;45(2):125.

127. Jacobson LB, Scheinman M: Catheter-induced intra-Hisian and intrafascicular block during recording of His bundle electrograms. A report of two cases. Circulation 1974;49:579.

128. Patton RD, Bordia A, Ballantyne F, et al: Bundle-of-His recording of complete heart block during cardiac catheterization: Electrophysiologic documentation of bilateral bundle branch block. Am Heart J 1971;81:108.

129. Morris D, Mulvihill D, Lew WYW: Risk of developing complete heart block during bedside pulmonary artery catheterization in patients with left bundle-branch block. Arch Intern Med 1987;147:2005.

130. Haft JI, Herman MV, Gorlin R: Left bundle branch block. Etiologic, hemodynamic, ventriculographic considerations. Circulation 1971;43:279.

131. Coronary Drug Project Research Group: The prognostic importance of the electrocardiogram after myocardial infarction Experience in the coronary drug project. Ann Intern Med 1972;77:677.

132. Gann D, Balachandran PK, Sherif NE, Samet P: Prognostic significance of chronic versus acute bundle branch block in acute myocardial infarction. Chest 1975;67:298.

133. Friedman RA, Alderman EL, Sheffield LT, et al: Bundle branch block in patients with chronic coronary disease. Angiographic correlates and prognostic significance. J Am Coll Cardiol 1987;10:73.

134. Kulbertus HE: The magnitude of risk of developing complete heart block in patients with LAD-RBBB. Am Heart J 1973;86:278.

135. Tibbits PA, Evaul JE, Goldstein RE, et al: Serial acquisition of data to predict one-year mortality rate after acute myocardial infarction. Am J Cardiol 1987;60:451.

136. Twidale N, Tonkin AL, Tonkin AM: Programmed stimulation after anterior myocardial infarction complicated by bundle branch block—late ventricular tachyarrhythmias and outcome. Pace 1988;11:1024.

137. Waugh RA, Wagner GS, Harvey TL, et al: Immediate and remote prognostic significance of fascicular block during acute myocardial infarction. Circulation 1973;47:765.

138. Pell S, D'Alonso CA: Immediate mortality and five-year survival of employed men with a first myocardial infarction. N Engl J Med 1964;270:915.

139. Wong B, Rinkenberger R, Dunn M, Goodyer A: Effect of intermittent left bundle branch block on left ventricular performance in the normal heart. Am J Cardiol 1977;39:459.

140. Dillon JC, Chang S, Feigenbaum H: Echocardiographic manifestations of left bundle branch block. Circulation 1974; 49:876.

141. Huerta EM, Rodriguez Padial L, Castro Beiras JM, Illera JP, Asin Cardiel E: Thallium-201 exercise scintography in patients having complete left bundle branch block with normal coronary arteries. Int J Cardiol 1987;16:43.

142. Heinsimer JA, Irwin JM, Basnight LL: Influence of underlying coronary artery disease on the natural history and prognosis of exercise-induced left bundle branch block. Am J Cardiol 1987;60:1065.

143. Fields CD, Ezri MD, Denes P: "Quinidine syncope" without lengthening of Q-Tc interval in the presence of left bundle branch block: role of programmed ventricular stimulation studies. Chest 1988;94:111.

144. Talbot S: QT interval in right and left bundle branch block. Br Heart J 1973;35:288.

145. Hancock EW: Left bundle branch block with right axis deviation. Hosp Pract Dec 1988;23:17.

146. Vera Z, Ertem G, Cheng TO: Left bundle branch block with intermittent right axis deviation. Evidence for left posterior hemiblock accompanying predivisional left bundle branch block. Am J Cardiol 1972;30:896.

147. Cannom DS, Wyman MG, Goldreyer BN: Initial ventricular activation in left-sided intraventricular conduction defects. Circulation 1980;62:621.

148. Fontaine JM, Rao R, Henkin R, Sunega R, Ursell SN, El-Sherif N: Study of the influence of left bundle branch block on the signal-averaged electrocardiogram: a qualitative and quantitative analysis. Am Heart J 1991;121(Pt 1):494.

149. Goldman MJ, Pipberger HV: Analysis of the orthogonal electrocardiogram and vectorcardiogram in ventricular conduction defects with and without myocardial infarction. Circulation 1969;39:243.

150. Pryor R: Recognition of myocardial infarction in the presence of bundle branch block. Cardiovasc Clin 1974;6:255.

151. Igarashi A, Kubota I, Ikeda K, Tsuiki K, Yasui S: Determination of the site of myocardial infarction by QRST isointegral mapping in patients with abnormal ventricular activation sequence. Jpn Heart J 1987;2:165.

152. Tsunakawa H, Nishiyama G, Kanesaka S, Harumi K: Application of dipole analysis for the diagnosis of myocardial infarction in the presence of left bundle branch block. J Am Coll Cardiol 1987;10:1015.

153. Havelda CJ, Sohi GS, Flowers NC, et al: The pathologic correlates of the electrocardiogram: complete left bundle branch block. Circulation 1982;65:445.

154. Hands ME, Cook EF, Stone PH, et al: Electrocardiographic diagnosis of myocardial infarction in the presence of complete left bundle branch block. Am Heart J 1988;116:23.

155. Kindwall KE, Brown JP, Josephson ME: Predictive accuracy of criteria for chronic myocardial infarction in pacing-induced left bundle branch block. Am J Cardiol 1986;57:1255.

156. Hancock EW: Myocardial infarct, left bundle branch block, or both? Hosp Pract 1988;23:61.

157. Hirai M, Burgess MJ, Haws CW: Effects of coronary occlusion on cardiac and body surface PQRST isoarea maps of dogs with abnormal activation simulating left bundle branch block. Circulation 1988;77:1414.

158. DeKock J, Schamroth L: Left bundle branch block associated with acute inferior wall myocardial infarction. S Afr Med J 1975;49:397.

159. Horan LG, Flowers NC, Tolleson WJ, Thomas JR: The significance of diagnostic Q waves in the presence of bundle branch block. Chest 1970;58:214.

160. Timmis GC, Gangadharan V, Ramos RG, Gordon S: Reassessment of Q waves in left bundle branch block. J Electrocardiol 1976;9:109.

161. Chung EK: Electrocardiogram of the month. Acute myocardial infarction in the presence of left bundle branch block. W V Med J, 1970;66:20.

162. Kuhn M: ECG diagnosis of acute myocardial infarction in patients with bundle branch block. Ann Emerg Med 1988; 17:633.

163. DePuey EG, Guertler-Krawczynska E, Robbins WL: Thallium-201 SPECT in coronary artery disease patients with left bundle branch block. J Nucl Med 1988;29:1479.

164. Delonca J, Camenzind E, Meier B, Righetti A: Limits of thallium-201 exercise scintigraphy to detect coronary disease in patients with complete and permanent bundle branch block: a review of 134 cases. Am Heart J 1992;123(5): 1201.

165. Petersen GV, Tikoff G: Left bundle branch block and left ventricular hypertrophy: Electrocardiographic pathologic correlations Chest 1971;59:174.

166. Chung DK, Panitch NM, Chung EK: A comparison of the conventional criteria for left ventricular hypertrophy before and after the development of complete left bundle branch block. Jpn Circ J 1969;33:19.

167. Rohatgi R, Mittal S, Bhardwaj B, Gupta M: Electrocardiographic diagnosis of left ventricular hypertrophy in the presence of left bundle branch block: an electrocardiographic correlation. Int J Cardiol 1993;39(2):147.

168. Komsuoglu B, Ulusoy S, Duman EL: Electrocardiographic criteria of left ventricular hypertrophy in the presence of left bundle branch block. Jpn Heart J 1989;30(1):47.

169. Flowers NC: Left bundle branch block: a continuously evolving concept. J Am Coll Cardiol 1987;9:684.

170. Manning GW: An historical review of the electrocardiogram of right bundle branch block in the Royal Canadian Air Force. Can J Cardiol 1987;3:375.

171. Simonsen EE, Madsen EG: Four cases of right-sided bundle branch block and one case of atrioventricular block in three generations of a family. Br Heart J 1970;32:501.

172. Gelband H, Waldo AL, Kaiser GA, Bowman FO Jr, Hoffman BF: Etiology of right bundle branch block in patients undergoing total correction of Tetralogy of Fallot. Circulation 1971;44:1022.

173. Yasui H, Takeda Y, Yamauchi S, et al: The deleterious effects of surgically induced complete right bundle branch block on long-term follow-up results of closure of ventricular septal defect. J Thorac Cardiovasc Surg 1977;74:210.

174. Mehran-Pour M, Borkat G, Liebman J, Ankeney J: Resolution of surgically induced right bundle branch block. Ann Thorac Surg 1977;23:139.

175. Krongrad E, Hefler SE, Bowman FO Jr, Malm JR, Hoffman BF: Further observations on the etiology of the right bundle branch block pattern following right ventriculotomy. Circulation 1974;50:1105.

176. Martini B, Nava A, Buja GF: Complex arrhythmias in a patient with predominantly right ventricular cardiomyopathy. Int J Cardiol 1988;19:268.

177. Harris LK: Transient right bundle branch block following blunt chest trauma Am J Cardiol 1969;23:884.

178. Kumpuris AG, Casale TB, Mokotoff D, et al: Right bundle branch block. JAMA 1979;242:172.

179. Schamp DJ, Plotnick GD, Croteau D, Rosenbaum RC, Johnston GS, Rodriguez A: Clinical significance of radionuclide angiographically-determined abnormalities following acute blunt chest trauma. Am Heart J 1988;116:500.

180. Okabe M, Fukuda K, Nakashima Y, Hiroki T, Arakawa K, Kikuchi M: Pathological extent of interventricular septal infarction in patients with acute anteroseptal myocardial infarction with and without right bundle branch block. Jpn Heart J 1993;34(2):121.

181. MacLennan BA, Tsoi EY, Maguire C, Adgey AA: Familial idiopathic congestive cardiomyopathy in three generations: a family study with eight affected members. Q J Med 1987; 63:335.

182. Parker JS, deBoisblanc BP: Case report: intermittent positive pressure ventilation-dependent right bundle branch block. Am J Med Sci 1991;302(6):380.

183. Wadler S, Chahinian P, Slater W, Goldman M, Mendelson D, Holland JF: Cardiac abnormalities in patients with diffuse malignant pleural mesothelioma. 1986;Cancer 58:2744.

184. Pohjola-Sintonen S, Totterman KJ, Salmo M, Siltanen P: Late cardiac effects of mediastinal radiotherapy in patients with Hodgkin's disease. Cancer 1987;60:31.

185. Maguire JH, Hoff R, Sherlock I, et al: Cardiac morbidity and mortality due to Chagas' disease: prospective electrocardiographic study of a Brazilian community. Circulation 1987;75:1140.

186. Gould L, Patel C, Betzu R, Judge D, Lee J: Right bundle branch block: a rare manifestation of digitalis toxicity—case report. Angiology 1986;37:543546.

187. Massing GK, Lancaster MC: Clinical significance of acquired complete right bundle branch block in 59 patients without overt cardiac disease. Aero Med 1969;40:967.

188. Lancaster MC, Schechter E, Massing GK: Acquired complete right bundle branch block without overt cardiac disease. Am J Cardiol 1972;30:32.

189. Fernandez F, Baragan J, Benaim R, Seebat L, Lénègre J: Right ventricular hemodynamics in intermittent complete right bundle branch block in man. Catheterization study of one case. Acta Cardiol 1968;23:569.

190. Bahar RH, Abdel-Dayem HM, Ziada G, Al-Suhali AR, Constantinides C, Nair KM: Phase abnormalities in right heart studies. Demonstration of six different patterns. Clin Nucl Med 1987;12:185.

191. Van Mieghem W, Ector H, Classens J, DeDeest H: Acquired complete heart block in young adults. Acta Clin Belg 1972; 27:506.

192. Denes P, Murabit I, Ezri M: Tachycardia- and bradycardia-dependent atrioventricular block: observations regarding the mechanism of block. J Am Coll Cardio 1987;9:446.

193. Fedor JM, Walston A II, Wagner GS, Starr J: The vectorcardiogram in right bundle branch block. Correlation with cardiac failure and pulmonary disease. Circulation 1976;53:926.

194. Norris RM, Croxson MS: Bundle branch block in acute myocardial infarction. Am Heart J 1970;79:728.

195. Shreenivas S, Messer AL, Johnson RP, et al: Prognosis in bundle branch block. II. Factors influencing the survival period in right bundle branch block. Am Heart J 1950;40:891.

196. Schneider JF, Thomas HE Jr, Kreger BE, et al: Newly acquired left bundle branch block. The Framingham study. Ann Intern Med 1979;90:303.

197. Alboni P: Intraventricular conduction disturbances. The Hague, The Netherlands: Martinus Nijhoff, 1981.

198. Blondeau M, Hiltgen M: Electrocardiographie clinique. Paris: Masson, 1980.

199. Lénégre J, Carouso G, Chevalier H: Electrocardiographie clinique. Paris: Masson et Cie, 1954.

200. Varriale P, Chryssos BE: The RSR' complex not related to right bundle branch block: diagnostic value is a sign of myocardial infarction scar. Am Heart J 1992;123(2):369.

201. Belleti DA, Gould L: Evaluation of the magnitude of the R' in V1 and detecting right ventricular hypertrophy in the presence of complete right bundle branch block. Aero Med 1969;40:896.

202. Gandhi MJ, Rao YC, Desai JM: Diagnosis of right ventricular hypertrophy in complete RBBB and electrophysiologic implications. Indian Heart J 1974;26:110.

203. Sodi-Pallares D: Electrocardiografia Y vectocardiografia dedictivas. Mexico: La Prensa Medica Mexicana, 1964.

204. DeLeonardis V, Goldstein SA, Lindsay J Jr: Electrocardiographic diagnosis of left ventricular hypertrophy in the presence of complete right bundle branch block. Am J Cardiol 1988;62:590.

205. Scott RC, Seivert VJ, Simion DL, McGuire J: Left ventricular hypertrophy: a study of the accuracy of current echocardiographic criteria when compared with autopsy findings in 100 cases. Circulation 1955;11:89.

206. Romhilt DW, Estes EH: A point score system for the ECG diagnosis of left ventricular hypertrophy. Am Heart J 1968;75:752.

207. Morris JJ, Estes EH Jr, Whalen RE, Thompson HK Jr, McIntosh HD: P wave analysis in valvular heart disease. Circulation 1964;29:242.

208. Sokolow M, Lyon PP: The ventricular complex in left ventricular hypertrophy as obtained by unipolar precordial and limb leads. Am Heart J 1949;37:161.

209. Tawarahara K, Kurata C, Taguchi T, Kobayashi A, Yamazaki N: Exercise testing and thallium-201 emission computed tomography in patients with intraventricular conduction disturbances. Am J Cardiol 1992;69(1):97.

210. Chou T: When is the vectorcardiogram superior to the Scalar electrocardiogram? J Am Coll Cardiol 1986;8:791.

211. Canaveris G, Halpern MS: Intraventricular conduction disturbances in flying personnel: incomplete right bundle branch block. Aviat Space Environ Med 1988;59:960.

212. MacDonald D, Behrendt DM, Jochim KE, et al: Electrophysiologic delineation of the intraventricular His bundle in two patients with endocardial cushion type of ventricular septal defect. Circulation 1981;63:225.

213. Husson GS, Blackman MS, Rogers MS, Bharati S, Lev M: Familial congenital bundle branch system disease. Am J Cardiol 1973;32:365.

214. Sung RJ, Tamer DM, Agha AS, et al: Etiology of the electrocardiographic pattern of "incomplete right bundle branch block" in atrial septal defect: an electrophysiologic study. J Pediatr 1975;87:1182.

215. Moore EN, Boineau JP, Patterson DF, et al: Incomplete right bundle branch block. An electrocardiographic enigma and possible misnomer. Circulation 1971;44:678.

216. Hishida H: IRBBB pattern after incising a subdivision of the right bundle branch. Jpn Heart J 1969;10:350.

217. Terasawa F Kuramochi M, Yazaki Y, et al: Clinical and patho-logical studies on incomplete left bundle branch block in the aged. Isr J Med Sci 1969;5:732.

218. Chandrashekhar Y, Kalita HC, Anand IS: Left anterior fascicular block: an ischaemic response during treadmill testing. Br Heart J 1991;65(1):51.

219. Rosenbaum MB: The hemiblocks: diagnostic criteria and clinical significance. Mod Concepts Cardiovasc Dis 1970;39:141.

220. DiMario C, Zanchetta M, Maiolino P: Coronary aneurysms in a case of Ehlers-Danlos syndrome. Jpn Heart J 1988;29:491.

221. Kenedi P, O'Reilly MV, Goldberg E: Association between intraventricular conduction defects, coronary artery disease and left ventricular function. Adv Cardiol 1976;16:504.

222. Schatz J, Krongrad E, Malm JR: Left anterior and left posterior hemiblock in tricuspid atresia and transposition of the great vessels. Observations and electrocardiographic nomenclature and electrophysiologic mechanisms. Circulation 1976;54:1010.

223. Eckberg DL, Ross J Jr, Morgan JR: Acquired right bundle branch block and left anterior hemiblock in ostium primum atrial septal defect. Circulation 1972;45:658.

224. Demoulin JC, Simar LJ, Kulbertus HE: Quantitative study of left bundle branch fibrosis in left anterior hemiblock: a sterologic approach. Am J Cardiol 1975;36:751.

225. Krivisky M, Aberbouch L, Shochat I, Ribak J, Tamir A, Froom P: Left anterior hemiblock in otherwise healthy pilots. Aviat Space Environ Med 1988;59:651.

226. Kincaid DT, Botti RE: Significance of isolated left anterior hemiblock and left axis deviation during acute myocardial infarction. Am J Cardiol 1972;30:797.

227. Sugiura T, Iwasaka T, Takayama Y, Takahashi N, Matsutani M, Inada M: The factors associated with fascicular block in acute anteroseptal infarction. Arch Intern Med 1988;148:529.

228. Jacobson LB, Lafollette L, Cohn K: An appraisal of initial QRS forces in left anterior fascicular block. Am Heart J 1977;94:407.

229. Cooper MJ, Reid GC, Barrett PA, Lyons NR: Diagnosis of inferior myocardial infarction in the presence of left anterior hemiblock. Aust NZ J Med 1987;17:47.

230. McHenry PL, Phillips JF, Fisch C, et al: Right precordial QRS pattern due to left anterior hemiblock. Am Heart J 1971;81:498.

231. Brown J, King A: Left anterior fascicular block and masking of inferior wall infarction. Am J Med 1987;82:563.

232. Ortega-Carnicer J, Malillos M, Mûoz L, Rodriguez-Garcia J: Left anterior hemiblock masking the diagnosis of right bundle branch block. J Electrocardiol 1986;19:97.

233. Castellanos A, Lemberg L: Diagnosis of isolated and combined block in the bundle branches and the divisions of the left branch. Circulation 1971;43:971.

234. Kulbertus HE, DeLeval-Rutten F, Dubois M, Petit JM: Sudden death in subjects with intraventricular conduction defects. In: Kulbertus HE, Wellens HJJ, eds. Sudden death. The Hague, The Netherlands: Martinus Nijhoff, 1980:379.

235. Ross DL: Approach to the patient with bundle branch block. In: Wellens HJJ, Kulbertus HE, eds. What's new in electrocardiography The Hague, The Netherlands: Martinus Nijhoff, 1981:110.

236. Grayzel J, Neyshaboori M: Left-axis deviation: etiologic factors in one-hundred patients. Am Heart J 1975;89:419.

237. Gertsch M, Theler A, Foglia E: Electrocardiographic detec-

tion of left ventricular hypertrophy in the presence of left anterior fascicular block. Am J Cardiol 1988;61:1098.

238. Gopal D: Left axis deviation. A spectrum of intraventricular conduction block. Circulation 1976;53:917.

239. Horwitz S, Lupi E, Hayes J, Frishman W, Cárdenas M, Killip T: Electrocardiographic criteria for the diagnosis of left anterior fascicular block. Left axis deviation and delayed intraventricular conduction. Chest 1975;68:317.

240. Castellanos A, Pina IL, Zaman L, Myerburg RJ: Recent advances in the diagnosis of fascicular blocks. Cardiol Clin 1987;5:469.

241. Rosenbaum MB, Shabetai R, Peterson KL, O'Rourke RA: Nature of the conduction disturbance in selective coronary arteriography in left heart catheterization. Am J Cardiol 1972;30:334.

242. Sclarovsky S, Sagie A, Strasberg B, Lewin RF, Rehavia E, Agmon J: Transient right axis deviation during acute anterior wall infarction or ischemia: electrocardiographic and angiographic correlation. J Am Coll Cardiol 1986;8:27.

243. Scott RC: The S_1Q_3 (McGinn-White) pattern in acute cor pulmonale: a form of transient left posterior hemiblock? Am Heart J 1971;82:135.

244. Lorber A, Maisuls E, Naschitz J: Hereditary right axis deviation: electrocardiographic pattern of pseudo left posterior hemiblock and incomplete right bundle branch block Int. J Cardiol 1988;20:399.

245. Criteria Committee of the New York Heart Association: Nomenclature and Criteria for diagnosis of diseases of the heart and great vessels. 8th ed. Boston: Little, Brown, 1979.

246. Schneider JF, Emerson TH Jr, Sorlie P, Kreger BE, McNamara PM, Kannel WB: Comparative features of newly acquired left and right bundle branch block in the general population: The Framingham study. Am J Cardiol 1981;47:931.

247. Medrano GA, Brenes C, Micheli A, Sodi-Pallares D: Clinical electrocardiographic and vectorcardiographic diagnosis of left posterior subdivision block isolated or associated with RBBB. Am Heart J 1972;84:727.

248. Demoulin JC, Kulbertus HE: Histopathological examination of concept of left hemiblock. Br Heart J 1972;34:807.

249. Uhley HN: Some controversy regarding the peripheral distribution of the conduction system. Am J Cardiol 1972;30:919.

250. Nakaya Y, Hiasa Y, Murayama Y, et al: Prominent anterior QRS force as a manifestation of left septal fascicular block. J Electrocardiol 1978;11:39.

251. Mori H, Kobayashi S, Mohri S: Electrocardiographic criteria for the diagnosis of the left septal fascicular block and its frequency among primarily elderly hospitalized patient. Nippon Ronen Igakkai Zasshi 1992;29(4):293.

252. Gambetta M, Childers RA: Rate-dependent right precordial Q waves: "septal focal block." Am J Cardiol 1973;32:196.

253. Wei-Min H, Cheng-Lang T: Bilateral bundle branch block. Right bundle branch block associated with left anterior fascicular block. Cardiology 1977;62:35.

254. Watt TB Jr, Pruitt RD: Character, cause and consequence of combined left axis deviation and right bundle branch block in human electrocardiograms. Am Heart J 1969;77:460.

255. Schaal SF, Seidensticker J, Goodman R, Wooley CF: Familial right bundle branch block, left axis deviation, complete heart block, early death. A heritable disorder or cardiac conduction. Ann Intern Med 1973;79:63.

256. Morriss JH, Eugster GS, Nora JJ, Pryor R: His bundle recording in progressive external opthalmoplegia. J Pediatr 1972; 81:1167.

257. Brink AJ, Torrington M: Progressive familial heart block—two types. S Afr Med J 1977;52:6.

258. Stephen E: Hereditary bundle branch system defect A new genetic entity? Am Heart J 1979;97:708.

259. Evans W: Familial cardiomegaly. Br Heart J 1949;11:68.

260. Gozo EG Jr, Cohen HC, Pick A: Traumatic bifascicular intraventricular block. Chest 1972;61:294.

261. Chuquimia R, Ramadurai TS, Towne W, Rosen K: Bifascicular block due to penetrating wound of the heart: electrophysiology studies. Chest 1974;66:195.

262. Pandullo C, Nicolosi GL, Scardi S: Hypertrophic cardiomyopathy associated with myotonic muscular dystrophy (Steinert's disease). Int J Cardiol 1987;16:205.

263. Gozo EG Jr, Cosnow I, Cohen HC, Okun L: The heart in sarcoidosis. Chest 1971;60:379.

264. Sugiura M, Okada R, Hiraoka K, Ohkawa S: Histological studies on the conduction system in 14 cases of right bundle branch block associated with left axis deviation. Jpn Heart J 1969;10:121.

265. Ohmae M: Correlative studies on electrocardiogram and histopathology of the conduction system. I. Right bundle branch block with left axis deviation and prolonged PR interval. Jpn Circ J 1977;41:677.

266. Sung RJ, Tamer DM, Garcia OL, Castellanos A, Myerburg RJ, Gelband H: Analysis of surgically-induced right bundle branch block pattern using intracardiac recording techniques. Circulation 1976;54:442.

267. Wolff GS, Rowland TW, Ellison RC: Surgically induced right bundle branch block with left anterior hemiblock. An ominous sign in postoperative tetralogy of Fallot. Circulation 1972;46:587.

268. Yabek SM, Jarmakani JM, Roberts N: Postoperative trifascicular block complicating tetralogy of Fallot repair. Pediatrics 1976;58:236.

269. Cairns JA, Dobell ARC, Gibbons JE, Tessler I: Prognosis of right bundle branch block and left anterior hemiblock after intracardiac repair of tetralogy of Fallot. Am Heart J 1975; 90:549.

270. Baragan J, Fernandez F, Coblence B, Saad Y, Lénégre J: Left ventricular dynamics in complete right bundle branch block with left axis deviation of QRS. Circulation 1970;42:797.

271. Lasser RP, Haft JI, Friedberg CK: Relationship of right bundle branch block and marked left axis deviation (with left parietal or peri-infarction block) to complete heart block and syncope. Circulation 1968;37:429.

272. Ranganathan N, Dhurandhur R, Phillips JH, et al: His bundle electrogram in bundle branch block. Circulation 1972; 45:282.

273. Scanlon PJ, Pryor R, Blount SG Jr: Right bundle branch block associated with left superior and inferior intraventricular block. Circulation 1970;42:1123.

274. Lamas GA, Muller JE, Turi ZG, et al: A simplified method to predict occurrence of complete heart block during acute myocardial infarction. Am J Cardiol 1986;57:1213.

275. Lie KI, Wellens HJ, Schuilenburg RM, et al: Factors influencing prognosis of bundle branch block complicating acute antero-septal infarction. Circulation 1974;50:935.

276. Aranda J, Befeler B, Castellanos A: His bundle recordings, bundle branch block, myocardial infarction. Ann Intern Med 1977;86:106.

277. Atkins JM, Leshin SJ, Blomqvist G, Mullins CB: Prognosis of right bundle branch block and left anterior hemiblock: a new indication for permanent pacing. Am J Cardiol 1970; 26:624. Abstract.

278. Atkins JM, Leshin SJ, Blomqvist G, Mullins CB: Ventricular conduction blocks and sudden death in acute myocardial infarction. N Engl J Med 1973;288:281.

279. Ritter WS, Atkins JM, Blomqvist CG: Permanent pacing in patients with transient trifascicular block during acute myocardial infarction: long-term prognosis. Am J Cardiol 1976; 38:205.

280. Kulbertus HE: Reevaluation of the prognosis of patients with LAD-RBBB. Am Heart J 1976;92:665.

281. Gupta P, Lichstein E, Chadda KD: Follow-up studies in patients with right bundle branch block and left anterior hemiblock: significance of HV interval. J Electrocardiol 1977; 10:221.

282. Levites R, Haft JI: Significance of first degree block (prolonged P-R interval) in bifascicular block. Am J Cardiol 1974;34:259.

283. Narula OS, Samet P: Right bundle branch block with normal, left, or right axis deviation. Am J Med 1971;51:432.

284. Rosenbaum MB: Chagasic myocardiopathy. Prog Cardiovasc Dis 1964;7:199.

285. Venkataraman K, Madias JE, Hood WB Jr: Indications for prophylactic preoperative insertion of pacemakers in patients with right bundle branch block and left anterior hemiblock. Chest 1975;68:501.

286. Pastore JO, Yurchak PM, Jamis KM, et al: The risk of advanced heart block in surgical patients with right bundle branch block and left axis deviation. Circulation 1978;57:677.

287. Narula O, Qazi N, Samet P, et al: Ten-year prospective observations based on H-V internal in patients with right bundle branch block (RBBB) and left axis deviation (LAD). Circulation 1978;58(Suppl II):197.

288. Sugiura M, Hiraoka K, Ohkawa S: A histological study on the conduction system in 16 cases of right bundle branch block associated with right axis deviation. Jpn Heart J 1974;15:113.

289. Harris R, Siew S, Lev M: Smoldering myocarditis with intermittent complete AV block and Stokes-Adams syndrome. A histopathologic and electrocardiographic study of "trifascicular" bundle branch block. Am J Cardiol 1969;24:880.

290. Loperfido F, Fiorilli R, Santarelli P, et al: Severe involvement of the conduction system in a patient with sclerodermal heart disease. An electrophysiological study. Acta Cardiol 1982;37:31.

291. Varriale P, Kennedy RJ: Right bundle branch block and right axis deviation in patients with coronary artery disease. Am Heart J 1971;81:291.

292. Castellanos A Jr, Maytin O, Arcebal AG, et al: Significance of complete right bundle branch block with right axis deviation in absence of right ventricular hypertrophy. Br Heart J 1970;32:85.

293. Thomsen PEB, Sterndorff B, Gøtzsche H: Intraventricular trifascicular block verified by His bundle electrocardiography. Am Heart J 1976;92:497.

294. Cerquira-Gomez M, Teixeira A: Wenckebach phenomenon in the posterior division of the left branch. Am Heart J 1971;82:377.

295. Hassan ZU, Mendoza RA, Steinke WE, Propert DB: Multiple conduction defects with markedly prolonged vertricular depolarization in cardiomyopathy. J Electrocardiol 1977; 10:275.

296. Barnhill JE, Tendera M, Cade H, Campbell WB, Smith RF: Depolarization changes early in the course of myocardial infarction: significance of changes in the terminal portion of the QRS complex. J Am Coll Cardiol 1989;14:143.

297. Angelini P, Springer A, Sulbaran T, Livesay WR: Right ventricular myopathy with an unusual intraventricular conduction defect (epsilon potential). Am Heart J 1981;101:680.

298. Kou WH, Morady F, DeBuitleir M, Nelson SD: Electrophysiologic demonstration of an atriofascicular accessory pathway. Pace 1988;11:166.

299. Befeler B, Castellanos A, Aranda J, et al: Intermittent bundle branch block in patients with acessory atrio-His or atrio-AV nodal pathways. Variants of the Lown-Ganong-Levine syndrome. Br Heart J 1976;38:173.

300. Klein GJ, Guiraudon GM, Kerr CR, et al: "Nodoventricular" accessory pathway: evidence for a distinct accessory atrioventricular pathway with atrioventricular node-like properties. J Am Coll Cardiol 1988;11:1035.

301. Tchou P, Lehmann MH, Jazayeri M, Akhtar M: Atriofascicular connection or a nodoventricular Mahaim fiber? Electrophysiologic elucidation of the pathway and associated reentrant circuit. Circulation 1988;77:837.

302. Abbott JA, Scheinman MM, Morady F, et al: Coexistant Mahaim and Kent accessory connections: diagnostic and therapeutic implications. J Am Coll Cardiol 1987;10:364.

303. Gulamhusein S, Ko P, Klein GJ: Ventricular fibrillation following verapamil in the Wolff-Parkinson-White syndrome. Am Heart J 1983;106:145.

304. Warin JF, Haissaguerre M: Fulguration of accessory pathways in any location: report of seventy cases. Pace 1989;12:215.

305. Mahomed Y, King RD, Zipes DP, Miles WM, Prystowsky EN, Heger JJ, Brown JW: Surgical division of Wolff-Parkinson-White pathways utilizing the closed-heart technique: a 2-year experience in 47 patients. Ann Thorac Surg 1988; 45:495.

306. Morady F, Sledge C, Shen E, et al: Electrophysiologic testing in the management of patients with the Wolff-Parkinson-White syndrome and atrial fibrillation. Am J Cardiol 1983; 51:1623.

307. Klein GJ, Gulamhusein SS: Intermittent preexcitation in the Wolff-Parkinson-White syndrome. Am J Cardiol 1983;52:292

308. Weiss J, Brugada P, Roy D, et al: Localization of the accessory pathway in the Wolff-Parkinson-White syndrome from the ventriculo-atrial conduction time of right ventricular apical extrasystoles. Pace 1983;6:260.

309. Pritchett ELC, Tonkin AM, Dugan FA, et al: Ventriculo-atrial conduction time during reciprocating tachycardia with intermittent bundle branch block in Wolff-Parkinson-White syndrome. Br Heart J 1976;38:1058.

310. Kremers MS, Wheelan KR: The effect of fascicular block on ventriculoatrial conduction during AV reentrant tachycardia. Pace 1987;10:916.

311. Baerman JM, Bauernfeind RA, Swiryn S: Shortening of ventriculoatrial intervals with left bundle branch block during orthodromic reciprocating tachycardia in three patients with a right-sided accessory atrioventricular pathway. J Am Coll Cardiol 1989;13:215.

312. Jazayeri MR, Caceres J, Tchou P, Mahmud R, Denker S, Akhtar M: Electrophysiologic characteristics of sudden QRS axis deviation during orthodromic tachycardia. Role of functional fascicular block in localization of accessory pathway. J Clin Invest 1989;83:952.

313. Lichstein E, Goyal S, Chadda K, Gupta PK: Alternating Wolff-Parkinson-White-(preexcitation) pattern. J Electrocardiol 1978;11:81.

314. Giorgi C, Ackaoui A, Nadeau R, Savard P, Primeau R, Pagé P: Wolff-Parkinson-White VCG patterns that mimic other cardiac pathologies: a correlative study with the preexcitation pathway localization. Am Heart J 1986;111:891.

315. Seipel L, Both A, Breithardt G, Loogen F: His bundle recordings in a case of complete atrioventricular block combined with preexcitation syndrome. Am Heart J 1976;92:623.

316. Massumi RA: His bundle recordings in bilateral bundle branch block combined with Wolff-Parkinson-White syndrome. Antegrade type II (Mobitz) block and 1:1 retrograde conduction through the anomalous bundle. Circulation 1970;42:287.

317. Jackman WM, Xunzhang W, Friday KJ, et al: Catheter ablation of accessory atrioventricular pathways (Wolff-Parkinson-White syndrome) by radiofrequency energy. N Engl J Med 1991;324:1605.

318. Gallagher JJ, Pritchett ELC, Sealy WC, Kasell J, Wallace AG: The preexcitation syndromes. Prog Cardiovasc Dis 1978; 20:285.

319. Yuan S, Iwa T, Tsubota M, Bando H: Comparative study of eight sets of ECG criteria for the localization of the accessory pathway in Wolff-Parkinson-White syndrome. J Electrocardiol 1992;25:203.

320. Fitzpatrick A, Gonzales R, Lesh M, Modin G, Lee R, Scheinman M: New algorithm for the localization of accessory atrioventricular connections using a baseline electrocardiogram. J Am Coll Cardiol 1994;23:107.

321. Gersony WM, Ekery DD: Concealed-right bundle branch block in the presence of type B ventricular preexcitation. Am Heart J 1969;77:668.

322. Sobrino JA, Mate I, Mũnoz JE, Sobrino N: Disappearance of right bundle branch block with left anterior hemiblock when associated with a type B preexcitation syndrome. Am Heart J 1974;87:497.

323. Castillo CA, Castellanos A Jr, Befeler B, et al: Arrival of excitation of right ventricular apical endocardium on Wolff-Parkinson-White syndrome type A, with and without right bundle branch block. Br Heart J 1973;35:594.

324. Denes P, Goldfinger P, Rosen KM: Left bundle branch block and intermittent type A preexcitation. Chest 1975;68:356.

325. Robinson K, Davies MJ, Krikler DM: Type A Wolff-Parkinson-White syndrome obscured by left bundle branch block associated with a vascular malformation of the coronary sinus. Br Heart J 1988;60:352.

326. Archer S, Gornick C, Grund F, Shafer R, Weir EK: Exercise thallium testing in ventricular preexcitation. Am J Cardiol 1987;59:1103.

327. Nalos PC, Mandel WJ, Cang ES, Cain RP, Massumi RA, Peter T: Intermittent fascicular extrasystoles producing pseudo AV block: electrophysiologic effects of beta agonists and antagonists. Pace 1987;10:1160.

328. Rosenthal ME, Stamato NJ, Almendral JM, Gottlieb CD, Josephson ME: Resetting of ventricular tachycardia with electrocardiographic fusion: incidence and significance. Circulation 1988;77:581

329. Gorgels AP, Vos MA, Letsch IS, et al: Usefulness of the accelerated idioventricular rhythm as a marker for myocardial necrosis and reperfusion during thrombolytic therapy in acute myocardial infarction. Am J Cardiol 1988;61:231.

330. Olshausen KV, Stienen U, Schwarz F, Kubler W, Meyer J: Long-term prognostic significance of ventricular arrhythmias in idiopathic dilated cardiomyopahty. Am J Cardiol 1988;61:146.

331. Martini B, Nava A, Theine G, et al: Accelerated idioventricular rhythm of infundibular origin in patients with a concealed form of arrhythmogenic right ventricular dysplasia. Br Heart J 1988;59:564.

332. Blanck Z, Akhtar M: Ventricular tachycardia due to sustained bundle branch reentry: diagnostic and therapeutic considerations. Clin Cardiol 1993;16:619.

333. Blanck Z, Jazayeri M, Dhala A, Deshapande S, Sra J, Akhtar M: Bundle branch reentry: mechanism of ventricular tachycardia in absence of myocardial or valvular dysfunction. J Am Coll Cardiol 1993:122(6):1718.

334. Josephson ME, Horowitz Ln, Farshidi A, et al: Recurrent sustained ventricular tachycardia. 4. Pleomorphism. Circulation 1979;59:459.

335. Josephson ME, Horowitz LN, Farshidi A, et al: Recurrent sustained ventricular tachycardia. 2. Endocardial mapping. Circulation 1978;57:440.

336. Miller JM, Marchlinski FE, Buxton AE, Josephson ME: Relationship between the 12-lead electrocardiogram during ventricular tachycardia and endocardial site of origin in patients with coronary artery disease. Circulation 1988;77:759.

337. Holt P, Brennand-Roper D, Curry PV, Maisey MN: Can the site of origin of ventricular extrasystoles enhance the localization of exercise-induced ischaemia? Int J Cardiol 1986; 13:185.

338. Brugada P, Wylick AV, Abdollah H: Identical QRS complexes during atrial fibrillation with aberrant conduction and ventricular tachycardia. The value of a His bundle recording. Pace 1983;6:1057.

339. Akhtar M, Shenasa M, Jazayeri M, Caceres J, Tchou PJ: Wide QRS complex tachycardia: reappraisal of a common clinical problem. Ann Intern Med 1988;109:905.

340. Wellens HJJ, Bar FW, Lie KI: The value of the electrocardiogram in the differential diagnosis of a tachycardia with a widened QRS complex. Am J Med 1978;64:27.

341. Kremers MS, Black WH, Wells PJ, Solodyna M: Effect of preexisting bundle branch block on the electrocardiographic diagnosis of ventricular tachycardia. Am J Cardiol 1988;62:1208.

342. Gulamhusein S, Yee R, Ko PT, Klein GJ: Electrocardiographic criteria for differentiating aberrancy and ventricular extra-

systole in chronic atrial fibrillation: validation by intracardiac recordings. J Electrocardiol 1985;18:41.

343. Kindwall KE, Brown J, Josephson ME: Electrocardiographic criteria for ventricular tachycardia in wide complex left bundle branch block morphology tachycardias. Am J Cardiol 1988;61:1279.

344. Colvard MC Jr, Whalen RE, Johnsrude I, Oldham N: Transvenous pacing, alternate bilateral bundle branch block, syncope. Arch Intern Med 1973;132:411.

345. Singer DH, Ten Eick RE: Aberrancy: electrophysiological aspects. Am J Cardiol 1971;28:381.

346. Halpern MS, Chiale PA, Nau GJ, et al: Effects of isoproterenol on abnormal intraventricular conduction. Circulation 1980; 62:1357.

347. Bailey JC, Lathrop DA, Pippenger DL: Differences between proximal left and right bundle branch block action potential durations and refractoriness in the dog heart. Circ Res 1977;40:464.

348. Moore EN, Preston JB, Moe GK: Durations of transmembrane action potentials and functional refractory periods of the canine false tendons and ventricular myocardium: comparisons in single fibers. Circ Res 1965;17:259.

349. Elizara MV, Novakosky A, Quinteiro RA, et al: The experimental evidence of phase 3 and phase 4 block in the genesis of AV conduction disturbances. In: Wellens HJJ, Lie KI, Janse MJ, eds. The conduction system of the heart: structure function and clinical implications. Philadelphia: Lea & Febiger, 1976:360.

350. Moe GK, Mendez C, Han J: Aberrant A-V impulse propagation in the dog heart: a study of functional bundle branch block. Circ Res 1965;16:261.

351. Hoffman BF: Electrophysiologic mechanisms for conduction abnormalities. Chest 1973;63:651.

352. Cranefield PF, Klein HO, Hoffman BF: Conduction of the cardiac impulse. I. Delay, block, one way block in depressed Purkinje fibers. Circ Res 1971;28:199.

353. Mendez C, Muller WJ, Merideth J, Moe GK: Interaction of transmembrane potentials in canine Purkinje fibers and at Purkinje fiber-muscle junctions. Circ Res 1969;24:361.

354. Koito H, Spodick DH: Physiologic differences in rate-related versus exercise-induced left bundle branch block. Am J Cardiol 1988;62:316.

355. Neuss H, Thormann J, Schlepper M: Electrophysiological findings in frequency-dependent left bundle branch block. Br Heart J 1974;36:888.

356. Agha AS, Castellanos A, Wells D, et al: Type I, type II and type III gaps in the bundle branch block. Circulation 1973;47:325.

357. Gallagher JJ, Damato AN, Varghese PJ, et al: Gap in AV conduction in man: type I and type II. Clin Res 1972;20:373.

358. Fisch C, Zipes DP, McHenry PL: Rate dependent aberrancy. Circulation 1973;48:714.

359. Gay R, Brown DF: Bradycardia-dependent bundle branch block in acute myocardial infarction. Chest 1973;64:114.

360. Massumi RA: Bradycardia-dependent bundle branch block. A critique and proposed criteria. Circulation 1968;38:1066.

361. Travazzi L, Salerno JA, Chimienti M, et al: Tachycardia-dependent and bradycardia-dependent intraventricular conduction defects in acute myocardial infarction: electrocardiographic electrophysiologic and clinical correlates. Am Heart J 1981;102:675.

362. Singer DH, Lazzara R, Hoffman BF: Interrelationships between automaticity and conduction in Purkinje fibers. Circ Res 1967;21:537.

363. Suarez L, Kreta A, Alarez JA, et al: Effects of isoproterenol on bradycardia-dependent intra-His and left bundle branch blocks. Circulation 1981;64:427.

364. Massumi RA, Amsterdam EA, Mason DT: Phenomenon of supernormality in the human heart. Circulation 1972;46:264.

365. Sarachek NS: Bradycardia-dependent bundle branch block. Relation to supernormal conduction and phase 4 depolarization. Am J Cardiol 1970;25:727.

366. Barold SS, Schamroth L: Tachycardia-dependent left bundle branch block associated with bradycardia-dependent variable left bundle branch block. A case report. Circulation 1973;48:216.

367. El-Sherif N: Tachycardia-dependent versus bradycardia-dependent intermittent bundle branch block. Br Heart J 1972;34:167.

368. Tanaka H, Nuruki K, Toyama Y, et al: Tachycardia- and bradycardia-dependent left bundle branch block associated with first degree AV block. A study using His bundle electrogram during carotid sinus compression. Jpn Heart J 1976;17:717.

369. El-Sherif N.: Tachycardia- and bradycardia-dependent bundle branch block after acute myocardial ischemia. Br Heart J 1974;36:291.

370. Corrado G, Levi RF, Nau GJ, Rosenbaum MB: Paroxysmal atrioventricular block related to phase 4 bilateral bundle branch block. Am J Cardiol 1974;33:553.

371. Rosenbaum MB, Elizari MV, Chiale P, et al: Relationships between increased automaticity and depressed conduction in the main intraventricular conducting fascicles of the human and canine heart. Circulation 1974;49:818.

372. Patton RD, Roberts JS: Simultaneous intermittent right and partial left bundle branch block. Am Heart J 1971;81:255.

373. Langendorf R, Pick A: Concealed intraventricular conduction in the human heart. Adv Cardiol 1975;14:40.

374. Walston A II, Boineau JP, Alexander JA, Sealy WC: Dissociation and delayed conduction in the canine right bundle branch. Circulation 1976;53:605.

375. Luzza F, Oreto G, Donato A, Satullo G, Scimone IM: Supernormal conduction in the left bundle branch unmasked by the linking phenomenon. Pacing Clin Electrophysiol 1992; 15(9):1248.

376. Tchou P, Jazayeri M, Denker S, Dongas J, Caceres J, Akhtar M: Transcatheter electrical ablation of right bundle branch: A method of treating macroreentrant ventricular tachycardia attributed to bundle branch reentry. Circulation 1988;78: 246.

377. Blanck Z, Akhtar M: Ventricular tachycardia due to sustained bundle branch reentry: diagnostic and therapeutic considerations. Clin Cardiol 1993;16:619.

378. Mazzoleni A, Johnson D, Fletcher E, Class RN: Concealed conduction in left bundle of His. Br Heart J 1972;34:365.

379. Dhingra RC, Amat-Y-Leon F, Wyndham C, et al: Significance of left axis deviation in patients with chronic left bundle branch block. Am J Cardiol 1978.42:551.

380. Fisher ML, Mugmon MA, Carliner HH, et al: Left anterior fascicular block: electrocardiographic criteria for its recognition in the presence of inferior myocardial infarction. Am J Cardiol 1979;44:645.

Cardiac Arrhythmias, 3rd edition, edited by William J. Mandel.
J. B. Lippincott Company, Philadelphia © 1995.

18

Hrayr S. Karagueuzian • William J. Mandel

Electrophysiologic Mechanisms of Ischemic Ventricular Arrhythmias: Experimental and Clinical Correlations

HISTORY

Sudden cardiac death due to coronary artery obstruction appears to be an ancient disease. According to von Bissing, a German Egyptologist, sudden death was depicted in scenes on an ancient Egyptian tomb relief during the Sixth Dynasty (2625 to 2475 B.C.) (Fig. 18-1).[1] Later documentation of the presence of atherosclerotic plaque in Egyptian mummies suggests to many that ischemic heart disease may have caused sudden cardiac death in ancient civilizations.[1,2]

An early experimental attempt to document the relation between interruption of blood supply to the myocardium and sudden cardiac arrest was made by Chirac in 1698 in a dog.[3] Unfortunately, however, this important pioneering experimental work did not capture the interest or the imagination of the physicians and intelligentsia of his day. As a result, the work remained an isolated finding until almost 150 years later, when interest in this field was renewed. In 1842, Dr. Marshall Hall, in his Gulstonian lecture series *On the Mutual Relations Between Anatomy, Physiology, Pathology and Therapeutics* (read at the British Association for the Advancement of Science), attributed the cause of sudden death in many instances to an interruption of the coronary circulation. In that same year, Ericksen experimentally verified Hall's contention.[4] He

occluded coronary arteries in dogs and rabbits and reached the following conclusion:

> Any circumstance that may interfere with the passage of the blood through the coronary arteries, either directly, as in ossification of the coats of those vessels, or indirectly, by there not being sufficient blood sent out of the left ventricle, as in cases of extreme obstruction or regurgitant disease of the aortic or mitral valves, may occasion the fatal event.

In 1894, the effects of experimental coronary artery occlusion on cardiac rhythm were described in greater detail by Porter.[5] He observed irregularities of cardiac rhythm after coronary artery occlusion that commonly preceded terminal ventricular fibrillation. In 1909, Lewis, in a series of elaborate experimental studies, demonstrated the relation of paroxysmal ventricular tachycardia and coronary artery occlusion (Fig. 18-2).[6] He later made a "curious" electrophysiologic observation that he correctly interpreted and ascribed as a "natural" symptom, characteristic of an overly stressed heart.[7] He wrote the following:

> Heart alternation (R and T wave) occurs under two circumstances. It is seen when the cardiac muscle is not of necessity altered structurally, as an accompaniment of great acceleration of the rate of rhythm. It is also

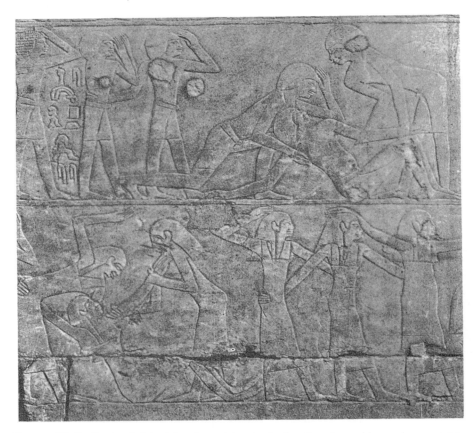

Figure 18-1. Tomb relief depicting the sudden death of an Egyptian nobleman (*upper right*), who collapses in the midst of his family. Two servants busy themselves with the dead noble, while others show their grief with the characteristic gesture—hands to the forehead—expressing sorrow in ancient Egypt. *Below*, the wife, overcome by emotion, has fainted and sunk to the floor. She is being attended by two women who are trying to revive her. To the *right*, the wife, holding on to two servants, is being led from the scene. Tomb of Sesi at Sakkara. (Sixth Dynasty 2625–2475 B.C.). (Reproduced from Plate 18B, "Plötzlicher Tod" (Sudden Death), in FW von Bissing: Denkmäler Ägyptischer Sculptur. Plates I, 1-57, München: F Bruckmann, 1914.)

found when the pulse is of normal rate, and under such circumstances the muscle is either markedly degenerate or the heart shows evidence of embarrassment as a result of poisoning or some other factor.

Lewis further wrote in his paper (which appears to be the first description of electric alternans in medical literature):

The electrocardiographic curves obtained in clinical heart alternation are similar to those obtained experimentally; there is a divergence between the heights of R and T and the amplitude of the radial upstrokes. These facts demonstrate the identity of the clinical and experimental conditions.[7]

In the parlance of present day nonlinear dynamics, such an alternance is the first state of dynamic transition to more complex dynamic states that emerge as a result of greater degrees of applied stress.[8]

In 1921, Robinson and Herrman extended the relation between ischemia and arrhythmias to the clinical level and established such a relation in man.[9] The increased vulnerability of the ischemic myocardium to electric stimuli was discovered by Wiggers and associates in 1941.[10] These investigators found that ischemia caused by coronary occlusion lowered the amount of current required to induce ventricular fibrillation (reduced fibrillation threshold?) and broadened the period of the cardiac cycle during which fibrillation occurred (vulnerable period). Yet another novel observation of cardiac arrhythmias related to coronary occlusion was made by Harris in 1950.[11] This investigator discovered the presence of two distinct time periods (phases) after coronary occlusion in which ventricular arrhythmias occurred within minutes of coronary artery occlusion and often degenerated to ventricular fibrillation. The delayed or second phase of arrhythmias began 6 to 8 hours after occlusion and lasted for 2 to 4 days. Harris and associates speculated that the electro-

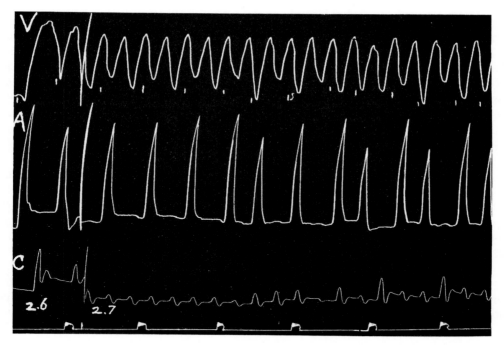

Figure 18-2. Initiation of paroxysmal ventricular tachycardia 2 hours 6 minutes after right coronary artery occlusion in the dog. Upper recording (*V*) is ventricular muscle shortening; middle recording (*A*) is atrial muscle shortening. Both were made by special myocardiographic levers. The lower recording (*C*) is carotid artery pressure. The bottom tracing is time marker with 1-second intervals. The first two beats appear normal; thereafter, a paroxysm of approximately 220 beats/min is initiated. Alteration is well seen in both the atrial and ventricular curves but is less marked in the carotid. At first, the atrium responds to every second beat and later to two in three. With the 2:3 rhythm, a periodic variation in the carotid tracing and a variation in the Vs–As intervals are seen. (Lewis T: The experimental production of paroxysmal tachycardia and the effects of ligation of the coronary arteries. Heart 1909;1:98.)

physiologic mechanisms of these arrhythmias that were operating during these two phases may differ—a speculation supported by later evidence.[12]

The early demonstration of cardiac-rhythm irregularities after experimental coronary artery occlusion, establishment of similar relations in humans, and demonstration of increased vulnerability of the ischemic myocardium to ventricular fibrillation during electric stimulation of the heart laid the groundwork for studies of the last two decades in the area of ischemic arrhythmias. Perhaps as a result of better understanding and appreciation of the various settings in which sudden cardiac death occurs during ischemia, it is encouraging to see that a significant decline in the rate of sudden coronary death occurred during the period 1980–1985, both out-of-hospital and in the emergency room.[13]

In this chapter, we review various electrophysiologic mechanisms of ventricular arrhythmias after experimental coronary artery occlusion and briefly evaluate the role of pharmacologic interventions designed to control these arrhythmias. Most of these studies were made in dogs. Clinicians' general understanding of pathophysiologic mechanisms of ventricular arrhythmias during various

phases of evolving myocardial ischemia and infarction are primarily derived from the canine model of infarction introduced by Harris, in which the left anterior descending (LAD) coronary artery is permanently occluded.[11] Later experiments with the swine model, in which the LAD coronary artery was occluded, also provide important insights. We make every attempt, whenever evidence permits, to extrapolate experimental findings to clinical results, recognizing that experimental models may often differ from clinical conditions in an important way.

PHASE ONE OR EARLY VENTRICULAR ARRHYTHMIAS

Occlusion Arrhythmias

Ventricular arrhythmias that occur within minutes after complete occlusion of the LAD coronary artery (the early arrhythmic phase) appear to depend primarily on the immediate effects of ischemia on working myocardial muscle cells.[14] Ventricular muscle cells depend completely on their coronary artery blood for proper supply of nutrients and oxygen; coronary occlusion therefore has a pronounced and immediate effect on the electrophysiologic, metabolic, and ultrastructural fate of the affected myocardial cells. The etiologic factors involved in alteration of the electrophysiologic properties of acutely ischemic myocardial cells include hypoxia, acidosis, elevated levels of extracellular potassium ions and intracellular calcium ions, depletion of cellular energy stores, and release of catecholamines and various mediators. The electrophysiologic consequences of the various ischemia-induced stigma on ventricular muscle cells are loss of resting membrane potential; alteration in refractoriness and excitability; and slowing of conduction, with possible emergence of various mechanisms of automatic impulse initiation and various complex patterns of conduction slowing and conduction block.

The various cellular electrophysiologic abnormalities may eventually lead to ventricular ectopic activity or ventricular tachycardia, which may degenerate into ventricular fibrillation.

Immediately after coronary occlusion, ischemia of the ventricular muscle causes the extracellular potassium ion concentration to rise.[14] Such a rise in potassium ion in the extracellular space can decrease resting membrane potential, inactivating the fast inward excitatory sodium current.[14] Depending on the level of loss of resting potential, some myocardial cells manifest depressed fast inward currents, whereas others only show slow-response action potentials, the results of which are variable delay and block of myocardial activation in the ischemic zone.[14-16] Hill and Gettes, using a potassium-sensitive electrode, studied the relation between extracellular potassium rise in ischemic zones immediately after LAD occlusion in

intact in situ porcine hearts and the pattern of myocardial activation (Fig. 18-3).[15] Changes in myocardial activation during the early minutes of acute ischemia were heterogenous and these changes in ventricular activation paralleled the rise of extracellular potassium ion. Nonhomogenous distribution of extracellular potassium ion concentration during regional acute ischemia was emphasized by Coronel and associates.[17,18] It is suggested that during regional ischemia (as opposed to global ischemia), a border zone about 1 cm wide exists, having a large degree of inhomogeneity, and that it is with total and not partial occlusion that an appreciable elevation of extracellular potassium concentration is reached.[17,18] Temporal changes in extracellular potassium during partial and total coronary occlusion were further related to regional conduction and electrogram morphologies.[18] After complete occlusion of the LAD coronary artery during two-stage ligation, conduction (activation) block in the ischemic zone occurred about 6 minutes earlier than during one-stage ligation, even though the average potassium concentrations at which block occurred were identical. Such a level of $[K]_o$ during total ischemia was achieved earlier during two-stage ligation than during one-stage ligation.[18] These authors suggest that early activation block that occurs during two-stage ligation may explain the reduced incidence of ventricular fibrillation during two-stage occlusion of the LAD coronary artery.[18] The importance of heterogenous extracellular potassium ion distribution, with emphasis on the rate of change of $[K]_o$ (dK/dt) at a given site (temporal heterogeneity), was further advanced as a possible mechanism of ventricular arrhythmia genesis during acute ischemia.[19,20] The evaluation of the mechanism of extracellular accumulation of potassium ion during acute ischemic episodes has been the subject of

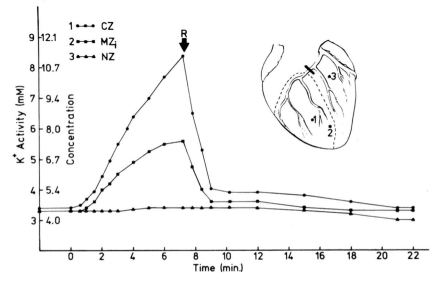

Figure 18-3. Time course of change in mid-myocardial extracellular K+ activity (ak+), recorded after acute occlusion of the left anterior descending (LAD) coronary artery at time zero. The diagram of the anterior surface of the heart illustrates electrode positions (*symbol* and *number*), point of LAD occlusion (*bar*), and resulting margin of cyanosis (*dashed line*). Electrode 1 was in the center of the ischemic zone (*CZ*), electrode 2 was within 5 mm of the inside margin of the ischemic zone (*MZi*), and electrode 3 was in the nonischemic zone (*NZ*). Release of the occlusion is indicated by the arrow (*R*). The ordinate shows both the measured ak+ and the calculated K+. (Hill JL, Gettes LS: Effect of acute coronary artery occlusion on local myocardial extracellular K+ activity in swine. Circulation 1980;61:768. By permission of the American Heart Association.)

intense interest. An important role for the opening of adenosine triphosphate (ATP)-sensitive potassium channel has been ascribed to the observed accumulation of potassium ions in the extracellular space.[21-23] Blocking of the ATP-sensitive potassium current with the specific ATP-sensitive channel blocker glibenclamide was shown to prevent hypoxia-induced shortening of the action potential duration and reduce the rate of extracellular accumulation of potassium ion during the first minute of ischemia.[22,23] Potassium loss did not appear to influence the rate and extent of extracellular acidification.[22] It is suggested that the activation of the ATP-sensitive potassium channel by intracoronary pinacidil infusion in the dog mimics the ST-segment elevation that is typically seen during acute ischemic episode in the intact ventricle after occlusion of the LAD coronary artery.[24] In a subsequent section, we describe dynamic concepts and methods that allow quantification and characterization of the degree of "heterogeneity" of ventricular excitability and impulse propagation.[25,26,28]

A complex pattern of intramyocardial conduction slowing in an acutely ischemic segment of the canine myocardium was observed by Hamamoto and associates.[29,30] These investigators found that the acute effects of ischemia caused by coronary occlusion were highly variable and that conduction times varied, depending on whether the impulse was directed toward the epicardium or the endocardium.[29] Furthermore, these authors demonstrated a disparity between anterograde and retrograde conduction times at both epicardial and endocardial ischemic sites.[30] Based on these observations, these investigators suggest that nonhomogenous abnormalities in conduction time in various regions of the ischemic myocardium can set the stage for reentrant premature excitation of the ventricles.[27]

In an attempt to shed some light on the cellular mechanism or mechanisms of ventricular tachyarrhythmias during the first 10 minutes after complete coronary artery occlusion, Downar and coworkers recorded subepicardial transmembrane potentials from an ischemic zone after complete LAD coronary artery occlusion in intact porcine hearts.[16] During the initial 5 minutes, acute ischemia shortened action potential duration and decreased resting membrane potential, action potential amplitude, and upstroke velocity of phase 0.[16] As the duration of occlusion progressed from 5 to 10 minutes, greater loss of resting membrane potential occurred, with long delays (100 milliseconds) occurring between electric stimulation and ischemic myocardial cell response (Fig. 18-4). Furthermore, before complete inexcitability of these cells was attained (10 to 12 minutes after occlusion), alternation in the amplitude of action potential progressed to 2:1 responses. These local changes in electric response reflected the phenomenon of postrepolarization refractoriness, indicat-

ing a lengthening of the effective refractory period that exceeds the duration of the basic cycle length of stimulation.[16,26,243] These local cellular electrophysiologic changes coincided with the emergence of ventricular arrhythmias. These cellular changes (conduction delays, presence of heterogenous local cellular responsiveness with variable lengthening of ischemic zone refractoriness) suggest that the early arrhythmias were caused by a reentry mechanism.[16,31]

Fujimoto and associates suggest that the faster the rate of conduction slowing in an acutely ischemic segment of the myocardium, the higher the incidence of spontaneous initiation of ventricular fibrillation during the initial 30 minutes of complete coronary artery occlusion.[32] These authors further suggest that conduction delay and the rate of change of conduction delay in an acutely ischemic myocardium may be used as reliable electrophysiologic markers of whether early ischemic ventricular fibrillation will develop.[32] Such an association may be caused by the rate of dK/dt in the ischemic and border zones.[19]

The relation of more complete and rapid reduction of myocardial blood flow to the incidence of ventricular fibrillation during the early postocclusion period was explored by Meesmann.[33] This investigator found that the greater the intensity of ischemia in a given region of the myocardium (i.e., absence of collateral flow), the higher the incidence of ventricular fibrillation.[33] It is tempting to postulate that with more intense ischemia, electrophysiologic properties would deteriorate more rapidly—an event shown to be associated with a higher incidence of early postocclusion ventricular fibrillation.[32] In line with this suggestion are the early findings of Harris, showing that gradual occlusion of the LAD coronary artery (two-stage occlusion) was associated with a lesser incidence of ventricular fibrillation when compared with sudden occlusion of the same artery.[11] It is of note that studies designed to elucidate this issue suggest that early activation block with two-stage ligation was associated with faster elevation of $[K]_o$.[18]

The relation of slow conduction and unidirectional conduction block to the emergence of reentrant ventricular arrhythmias during the first few minutes after coronary artery occlusion was demonstrated by Janse and associates.[34,35] These investigators, by simultaneously recording from 60 ischemic and nonischemic sites, delineated the direction and sequence of the spread of excitation during ventricular premature depolarizations. They demonstrated that the cardiac impulse was blocked when it reached the center of the ischemic zone and that two wavefronts bypassed the zone of block and invaded it retrogradely to reexcite the site of original conduction block (Fig. 18-5). This event coincided with the emergence of ventricular premature depolarizations and subsequent ventricular tachycardia.[35] Furthermore, it was also

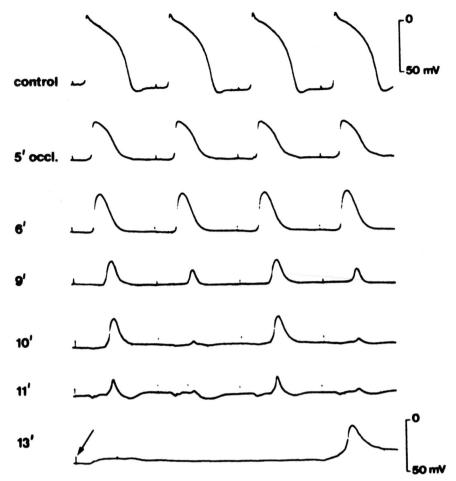

Figure 18-4. Transmembrane action potentials recorded from the subepicardium of the left ventricle of an *in situ* pig heart before and after occlusion of the proximal left anterior descending coronary artery. (Downar E, Janse MJ, Durrer D: The effects of acute coronary artery occlusion on subepicardial transmembrane potentials in the intact porcine heart. Circulation 1977;56:217. By permission of the American Heart Association.)

reported that when ventricular tachycardia degenerated to ventricular fibrillation, multiple wavelets were present, which collided with each other and inscribed microcircus movements.[34,35] These studies established that within minutes after coronary artery occlusion, many of the ventricular tachycardias are caused by a macroreentrant mechanism (about 2 cm in diameter) and that ventricular fibrillation that may later develop is caused by multiple smaller microreentrant circuits (about 0.5 cm or less in diameter).[34,35] The mechanism or mechanisms of acute ischemia-induced alterations of ventricular impulse propagation in the intact ventricle were investigated by many.[36–40] Acute ischemia causes an increase in internal longitudinal resistance—probably by cellular uncoupling, an effect that slows impulse conduction irrespective of transmembrane potential properties.[41] Cellular uncoupling depends on heart rate and on myocardial fiber orien-

tation, with respect to the direction of impulse propagation (anisotropy).[42,43] An increase in the rate of stimulation from 0.5 to 2 Hz was found to be associated with an increase in conduction slowing from 12% to 24%.[42] Using heptanol as a specific agent to induce cellular uncoupling, Balke and coworkers observed that conduction slowing was greater in the transverse direction than in the longitudinal because more junctional resistances were encountered per unit distance in the transverse than in the longitudinal direction.[43] The increase in longitudinal resistance associated with cellular uncoupling during acute ischemia appears to be caused by an elevation of intracellular calcium ion concentration because verapamil was found to modulate ischemia-induced conduction slowing in an important manner.[42,44,45] A positive correlation was found to exist between the heart rate and the occurrence of ventricular tachyarrhythmias during acute myocardial

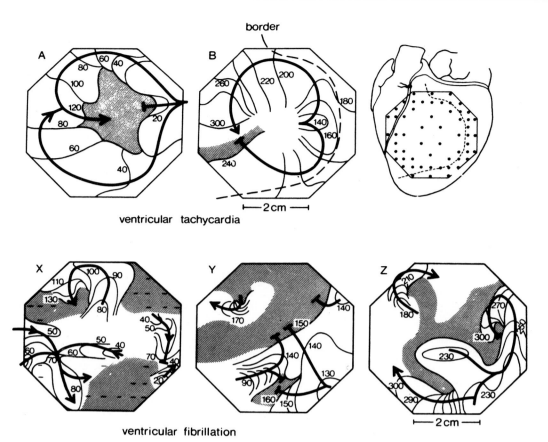

Figure 18-5. Patterns of activation during a spontaneously occurring ventricular tachycardia that degenerated into ventricular fibrillation 4 minutes after occlusion of the left anterior descending coronary artery in an isolated pig heart. The electrode configuration is shown on the *upper right panel*, each dot indicating an electrode terminal. Direct current extracellular electrograms from these 60 terminals were recorded simultaneously. A recording period lasted for 2 seconds, during which complexes were digitalized and stored in a computer. The *dotted line* delineates the electrophysiologic border zone; that is, the zone where TQ-segment potentials of normally propagated beats became negative. In the first two ectopic beats (not shown), earliest activity was recorded in the normal myocardium close to the border. (**A** and **B**; *upper row*) The third and fourth ectopic beats; t = 0 was arbitrarily chosen, and isochronic lines separate areas activated within the same 20 millisecond interval. *Shaded areas* represent areas of conduction block. *Arrows* indicate general direction of spread of excitation; the symbol T stands for block. In **A**, the earliest activity is found in the normal side of the border; this wavefront is blocked in the center of the ischemic zone but two wavefronts bypass the zone of block and invade it retrogradely to reexcite the site of origin at **B** after 140 milliseconds. In **B**, again two semicircular wavefronts are set up but because the 2-second recording periods ended here, it is not known how the arrhythmia continued. One second later, when the heart was fibrillating, **X**, **Y**, and **Z** were recorded. Multiple wavelets then were present, fusing and colliding with each other and describing microcircus movements; in the upper part of the area covered by the electrode, the reentrant wavefront describes a figure-8–shaped circus movement between 80 and 210 milliseconds in beats **X**, **Y**, and **Z**. (Janse MJ, Kleber AG: Electrophysiological changes and ventricular arrhythmias in the early phase of regional myocardial ischemia. Circ Res 1981;49:1069. By permission of the American Heart Association.)

ischemia in the anesthetized open-chest canine LAD coronary artery occlusion model.[46, 47] As the heart rate was increased by pacing, a significantly higher incidence of ventricular tachyarrhythmias was observed than during pacing at slower rates.[46, 47] Furthermore, it was found in these studies that after complete LAD coronary artery

occlusion, the incidence of acute ischemic arrhythmias were positively correlated with the amount of myocardium at risk.[46, 47] The importance of relatively faster heart rate in the genesis of ventricular arrhythmias during the initial 20 to 30 minutes of coronary artery occlusion has been stressed by Scherlag and associates.[48] It is also worth mentioning that the incidence of ventricular fibrillation during acute ischemia also depends on the presence or absence of previous healed myocardial infarction. Acute ischemia superimposed on an old infarct is associated with significantly greater occurrence of ventricular arrhythmias in the canine model.[49, 50]

The possibility exists that some sort of automatic mechanism or mechanisms may also exist during the early postocclusion period, thus causing some of the acute ischemic ventricular arrhythmias. Conditions simulating ischemia and using the microelectrode technique to record transmembrane potentials in isolated tissues, it is suggested that delayed afterdepolarization (DAD) and triggered activity can be induced by both α- and β-adrenergic–receptor stimulation.[51] In another study on canine Purkinje fibers, a specific α_1-adrenergic–receptor subtype was advanced as a responsible link for the induction of DAD and triggered activity in conditions stimulating ischemia and reperfusion.[52] The significance of these in vitro studies to the mechanism of early ventricular tachyarrhythmias in the in situ ischemic ventricles remains undefined. Furthermore, because the occurrences of both the DADs and triggered activity were not always uniform (percentage of the times or the tissues) and the agonist and the antagonists of the adrenergic receptors used are not "strictly clean" in their action, assigning strict receptor type or subtype for the induction of either DAD or triggered activity seems unwarranted at the present time. An automatic mechanism may also be caused by the flow of an injury (depolarization) current between ischemic and normal zones.[34] When differences in action potential duration in adjacent areas exist, current flows from the site of the longest action potential duration to that of the shorter duration.[34, 35] When the intensity of such a depolarizing current is large enough, it may induce threshold depolarization in adjacent cells with shorter action potential duration, causing ectopic activity.[54] The induction of pacemaker-like activity by depolarizing current pulses, both in ventricular myocardial cells and in Purkinje fibers, are well documented.[20, 55] Katzung termed this phenomenon depolarization-induced automaticity (DIA) and Cranefield called it automaticity caused by early afterdepolarizations (EAD).[55, 56] These descriptions simply state that if the free-running course of repolarization is interrupted by an applied depolarizing current, pacemaker-like activity is induced during the entire period of applied depolarizing current. Furthermore, Katzung and colleagues showed that in in vitro preparations of guinea pig papillary muscle, the current that flows between cells depolarized by 145-mmol potassium ion and normal cells superfused with 4-mmol potassium ion may induce transient spontaneous activity in the normal cells, especially in the presence of epinephrine.[57] The probable mechanism of the induction of pacemaker-like activity by current

of injury is as follows. The membrane potentials of cells exposed to 145-mmol potassium ion is zero or nearly zero and the membrane potential of cells exposed to normal potassium ion is about −80 mV. This potential gradient sets up an "injury" depolarizing current, which flows between the intracellular compartments of depolarized cells toward normal cells.[57] That such depolarizing current may be responsible for at least the initial beats of ventricular tachycardia and ventricular fibrillation in the intact canine and porcine hearts immediately after coronary artery occlusion is suggested by Janse and colleagues.[34] These authors estimated the intensity of the injury current and found it to be about 2 μA per cubic millimeter at the site of current generation (current source) and 5 μA per cubic millimeter at the site of current disappearance (current sink).[34] Interestingly, ventricular premature beats were observed when injury currents were maximal, with the earliest activity always arising in the normal zone adjacent to an ischemic zone.

In addition to injury currents, DIA or EAD may also be induced by acidosis due to elevated CO_2 tension (Fig. 18-6).[61, 62] Myocardial ischemia induced by coronary artery occlusion decreases both extracellular and intracellular pH of affected myocardial cells.[63, 64] This most probably occurs because of elevated CO_2 tension and accumulated acidic metabolites or both. Coraboeuf and associates showed, in isolated Purkinje fibers, that elevation of the partial pressure of CO_2 in Tyrode's gas mixture from 3% to 20% was associated with a decrease of pH from 7.4 to 6.6.[61] This acidosis slowed the repolarization process (induction of humps), which was often associated with triggering of pacemaker-like activity by a mechanism similar to that seen with applied depolarizing (injury) currents, described both in isolated ventricular muscle cells and in Purkinje fibers.[54–57] Whether ventricular muscle cells are also susceptible to acidosis-induced pacemaker-like activity and whether such a mechanism—involving either ventricular muscle cells of Purkinje fibers or both cells types—plays a role in the genesis of early postocclusion ventricular arrhythmias in the intact heart remains to be seen. Furthermore, it is also unknown whether the mechanism of triggered automaticity has any role in the early postocclusion ventricular arrhythmias.[65, 66] Such a mechanism may be operative because it appears to be related to an elevation of intracellular calcium ion concentration in both Purkinje fibers and ventricular muscle fibers.[67–69] One of the major consequences of myocardial ischemia and hypoxia is depressed oxidative metabolism and depletion of myocardial cellular energy stores, which leads to an accumulation of intracellular calcium ions, among other things.[70] This in turn may cause oscillatory afterpotentials (also known as DAD) and triggered automaticity to emerge.[67–69] Proof, however, of such an arrhythmogenic mechanism during the immediate

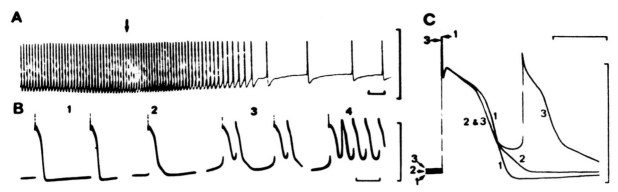

Figure 18-6. Effect of CO_2-rich gas mixture (CO_2, 20%; O_2, 80%) on canine cardiac Purkinje fiber. The pH of Tyrode's superfusion solution decreases from 7.4 to 6.6. (**A**) Acid solution is admitted at the time indicated by the *vertical arrow*. In this example, the fiber depolarizes and its rhythm slows but no humps and reexcitation occur. (**B**) Acidosis-induced humps and reexcitation occur. The fiber is bathed in acid solution for 2 minutes in *1*, for 6 minutes in *2*, for 7 minutes in *3*, and for 8 minutes 30 seconds in *4*. (**C**) Superimposed normal action potential (*1*) and action potential with hump (*2*) and reexcitation (*3*). Vertical scales, 100 mV for **A**, **B**, and **C**; horizontal scales, **A**, 10 second; **B**, 1 second; **C**, 400 milliseconds. (Coraboeuf E, Deroubaix E, Coulombe A: Acidosis-induced abnormal repolarization and repetitive activity in isolated dog Purkinje fibers. J Physiol (Paris) 1980;76:97.)

postocclusion period is lacking. The possibility that DADs may cause acute ischemic ventricular arrhythmias was investigated in isolated guinea pig ventricles.[71] Although during simulated acidosis DADs were readily induced in the ventricular myocardial cells, when acidosis, high potassium levels, and hypoxia were simultaneously applied, no DADs were induced.[71] Based on these ischemia-simulated studies on isolated ventricular cells, these authors suggest that DADs are unlikely to occur during severe ischemia.[71] It is likely, however, that other agents may also accumulate in the acutely ischemic myocardium, with the potential of inducing DADs. One such class of agents, lysophosphoglycerides, has been proposed as a putative mediator of ventricular ischemia.[72] At relevant concentrations, these agents (including lysophosphatidyl ethanolamine and lysophosphatidyl choline) induced DADs and subsequent triggering in isolated canine Purkinje fibers, an effect that persisted even during hyperkalemia and acidosis.[72] Proof of such an arrhythmogenic mechanism during the immediate postocclusion period in the intact in situ heart is still lacking. Elevated free fatty acids, which often accompany acute myocardial ischemia, can induce cellular electrophysiologic changes that can lead to the emergence of both automatic and reentrant arrhythmias.[53,93] Karagueuzian and associates report that high concentrations of palmitate can delay the repolarization process of Purkinje fibers in a manner that may be heterogenous, thus setting the stage for reentrant arrhythmias (Fig. 18-7).[93] Furthermore, elevated free fatty acid levels promote abnormal automaticity in partially depolarized Purkinje fibers (see Fig. 18-7).[93] The prolongation of action potential duration of subendocardial Purkinje

fibers 1 day after either LAD or right coronary artery occlusion in the dog has been ascribed to excessive intracellular lipid accumulation.[126,135] Stimulation of α-receptors and β-receptors has also been proposed as a possible determinant of both occlusion (acute ischemia) and reperfusion ventricular arrhythmias.[74]

Clusin and associates suggest that calcium overload may cause fibrillatory electric and mechanical activity similar to that recorded from fibrillating hearts (Fig. 18-8).[73] These investigators hypothesize that a calcium-dependent ionic current may mediate ischemic ventricular fibrillation. It is also important to note that an elevated level of intracellular calcium ions can cause an increase in myoplasmic resistance to impulse propagation, thus slowing conduction velocity and causing various degrees of conduction block due to eventual cellular uncoupling.[41,42,60,63,70,74] Kleber and associates suggest that in the early reversible phase of ischemia, the increase in the extracellular longitudinal resistance contributes to a small but significant extent to the slowing of conduction and that after 15 to 20 minutes of ischemia, the rapid cellular uncoupling is reflected by an increase in intracellular longitudinal resistance.[60] In a newer study, these investigators stress that cellular uncoupling occurs only under severe conditions of ischemia and with a delay of more than 10 minutes.[63] Furthermore, marked action potential shortening precedes uncoupling.[63] In addition to these electrophysiologic changes induced by elevated levels of intracellular calcium concentrations, calcium current restitution (recovery) is altered in a complex manner, which may eventually alter action potential duration and recovery of excitability, leading to reentrant ventricular tachyarrhythmias.[75]

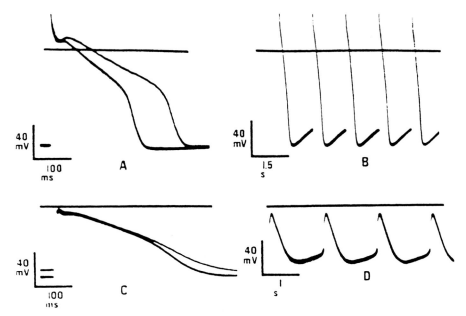

Figure 18-7. Sheep Purkinje fiber transmembrane potential characteristics after superfusion with palmitate/albumin = 10. (**A**) Action potential properties during control (*inner trace*) and after 4 h of superfusion with palmitate-albumin = 10 (*outer trace*). Impalement was maintained in the same cell. Note the considerable prolongation of action potential duration. At this point, the preparation became spontaneously active (**B**), with evidence of enhanced spontaneous diastolic depolarization. (**C** and **D**) Obtained from a depressed preparation: In **C**, effects of 2 hours of superfusion with normal oxygenated Tyrode's solution is shown (note a slight further diminution of the resting potential). (**D**) (same cell as in **C**), the effect of palmitate/albumin = 10 (45 min) is shown. Spontaneous activity, with enhanced spontaneous diastolic depolarization, is evident. (Karagueuzian HS, Pennec JP, Deroubaix E, de Leiris J, Corabeuf E: Effects of excess free acids on the electrophysiological properties of ventricular specialized conducting tissue. A comparative study between the sheep and the dog. J Cardiovasc Pharmacol 1982;4:462.)

Clinical Implications

One important observation from occluding the coronary artery of dogs is the relation between continuous electric activity in the ischemic myocardium, as recorded by either bipolar extracellular electrograms (Fig. 18-9) or composite electrograms, and the occurrence of ventricular arrhythmias.[36,37] Although it has not been possible to record this sort of electric activity in human ventricular myocardium within the first few minutes after the onset of acute ischemia that causes ventricular arrhythmias, such activity has been recorded from chronic ischemic regions in aged ventricular infarcts and aneurysms. This raises the possibility that abnormal electric activity leading to arrhythmia genesis may also occur in human ischemic ventricular myocardium immediately after the onset of acute ischemia. A favored hypothesis for continuous electric activity is reentry, and this is based on the following interpretations. Continuous, low-amplitude, fragmented activity is caused by slowly conducting impulses in one or multiple reentrant circuits in the ischemic myocardium, probably because muscle cells lose resting membrane

potential and generate slowly conducting action potentials. If this is the mechanism, continuous electric activity spanning the entire diastolic interval could be recorded. The induction of this sort of continuous electric activity is usually associated with the appearance of ventricular premature complexes and tachycardia.[36,37] Although attractive, this hypothesis does not prove that reentry is occurring. Early afterdepolarization caused by injury currents or triggered automatic activity induced by intracellular elevation of calcium ions in the ischemic myocardium may show a series of low-amplitude depolarizations with rapid rates that may show continuous electric activity on an extracellular electrograms.[76] This may especially be the case when catecholamine levels are high, which occurs after acute coronary artery occlusion.[39] Therefore, the cellular electrophysiologic basis for cardiac electrograms showing continuous electric activity may involve more than one mechanism.[76]

Alterations in neural activity and neurohumoral factors have long been implicated in the genesis of sudden cardiac death in man.[77] In a swine model of acute ischemia, the

A

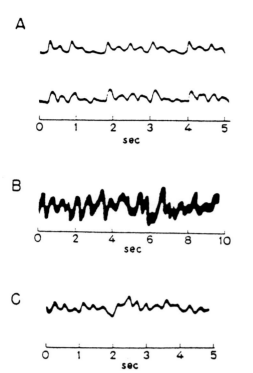

Figure 18-8. Intracellular calcium overload causes fibrillation in small embryonic myocardial cell clusters. (**A**) Two simultaneous intracellular recordings from a small specimen of embryonic rat myocardium intoxicated with strophanthidin (3 × 10⁻⁵ M). The specimen was between 500 and 800 μm in diameter, and the interelectrode distance was 540 μm. Although this recording resembles those obtained during in vivo fibrillation, the synchrony of deflections at opposite sides of the preparation suggests that this activity does not arise from reentrant conduction. (**B** and **C**) Fibrillatory electric and mechanical activity in chick embryonic myocardial cell aggregates intoxicated with veratrine (5 × 10⁻⁵ g/mL). (**B**) An intracellular recording, from a 120 μm diameter aggregate; (**C**) An optical recording of fibrillatory mechanical activity in a similar aggregate. The mean intracellular potential in **B** is −42 mV. The vertical calibration represents 50 mV in **A** and 2 mV in **B**. (Clusin WT, Bristow MR, Karagueuzian HS, et al: Do calcium-dependent ionic currents mediate ischemic ventricular fibrillation. Am J Cardiol 1982;491-606.)

incidence of ventricular fibrillation was significantly decreased in chronically denervated heart when compared with intact innervated hearts.[78] Similarly, both right and left stellate ganglionectomy significantly reduced acute ischemic ventricular fibrillation in a canine model induced by left circumflex coronary occlusion.[79] This finding strengthens the link between adrenergic activation and ventricular arrhythmogenesis during acute ischemia. Adrenergic activation by left stellate ganglion stimulation induced DADs in intact cat preparations.[80] Left-side sympathetic nerve activation can precipitate life-threatening ventricular arrhythmias during acute ischemia.[81] There is some preliminary evidence that suggests a significant reduction in sudden death

in high-risk patients with postmyocardial infarction who are treated with surgical high-thoracic left sympathectomy.[82]

REPERFUSION ARRHYTHMIAS

Tennant and Wiggers reported in 1935 that ventricular fibrillation could occur when coronary blood flow was suddenly restored to an occluded coronary artery in the dog (reperfusion or release ventricular fibrillation).[40] This early laboratory observation gained intense clinical and experimental interest when it was found that victims of sudden cardiac death (ventricular fibrillation), after resuscitation and careful follow-up, did not uniformly show evidence of myocardial damage and infarction.[83] It is suggested that sudden death in victims with no evidence of myocardial cell necrosis is precipitated by the phenomenon of reperfusion-induced ventricular fibrillation, most likely triggered by dissolution of platelet plugs or sudden resolution of coronary artery spasm. Although the relevance of these findings to humans is uncertain, the sudden nature of reperfusion-induced ventricular fibrillation in the canine heart suggests that this model may help clinicians understand sudden cardiac death in humans. Consequently, release arrhythmias have become the subject of experimental studies to assess the mechanisms of reperfusion-induced ventricular fibrillation and to design effective antiarrhythmic drug regimens to prevent recurrence of sudden cardiac death. It has become clear that the duration of coronary artery occlusion before release (reperfusion) is one major factor in the induction of ventricular fibrillation. Balke and associates have studied this parameter and found that reperfusion-induced ventricular fibrillation is most likely to occur in the LAD coronary artery occlusion model when the duration of occlusion is 20 to 30 minutes.[84] That the incidence of reperfusion-induced ventricular fibrillation peaks at this time may relate to the reversibly induced ischemic myocardial damage.[85]

Another important parameter that influences the occurrence of ventricular fibrillation is the amount of myocardium at risk (i.e., ischemic) that becomes reperfused. Using the logistic risk regression model, Austin and associates described the relation between the occurrence of ventricular fibrillation and the amount of myocardium at risk after coronary artery occlusion (Fig. 18-10).[86] Their model predicted uniformly low and uniformly high probability of ventricular fibrillation with small and large amounts (mass) of myocardium at risk, respectively, with direct correlation for mid-range values of myocardium at risk. This study largely explains the great variability in the incidence of reperfusion-induced ventricular fibrillation that occurs as a result of variation in the amount of myocardium at risk due to variation in the degree of collateral blood flow to the ischemic zone. In a later study, the possible role of heart rate accelera-

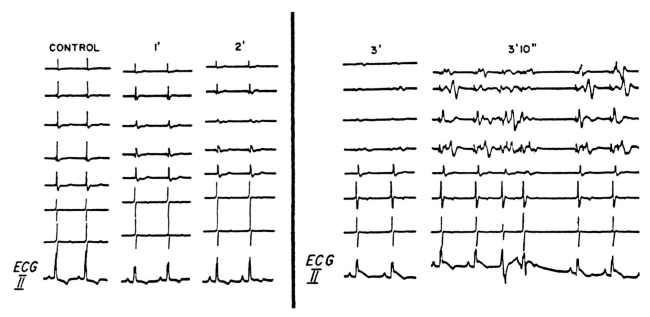

Figure 18-9. The immediate effects of coronary artery occlusion on bipolar electrograms recorded from the epicardium of the canine heart. In each panel, bipolar electrogram recordings from seven different regions are shown in the first seven traces. The bottom trace is a lead II electrocardiogram. The top five electrograms were recorded from the region that became ischemic after the left anterior descending (LAD) coronary artery was occluded; the sixth and seventh electrograms were recorded from nonischemic myocardium. At the left, recordings taken before coronary artery occlusion are shown (control). At all sites, electrograms appear as large-amplitude spikes of short duration. To the right of the control records are records obtained 1 minute, 2 minutes, 3 minutes, and 3 minutes 10 seconds after complete occlusion of the LAD near its origin. There is a progressive decrease in amplitude and increase in duration of the electrograms recorded from the ischemic region and no change in the electrograms recorded from the nonischemic regions. ST segment changes on the electrocardiogram can be seen after 3 minutes. At 3 minutes 10 seconds, the signals recorded from the ischemic region have increased amplification. Discrete spikes of electric activity are no longer evident. In the top four traces, the electrograms have become fragmented, and continuous electric activity is evident. This is associated with the occurrence of ventricular premature depolarizations. (Waldo AL, Kaiser GA: A study of ventricular arrhythmias associated with acute myocardial infarction in the canine heart. Circulation 1973;47:1222.)

tion on outcome during reperfusion was systemically evaluated.[46] Pacing-induced heart rate acceleration in dogs having LAD coronary artery occlusion and reperfusion had a higher incidence of ventricular arrhythmias than in dogs that had slower heart rate, even though both groups had similar amounts of myocardium at risk.[46] In an attempt to delineate the mechanism or mechanisms of reperfusion ventricular tachycardia and fibrillation, Pogwizd and Corr simultaneously recorded from 232 intramural sites in a feline model of a 10-minute LAD occlusion followed by reperfusion using a three-dimensional computerized mapping system.[88] These authors suggest that the initiation of nonsustained ventricular tachycardia during reperfusion was caused by nonreentrant mechanisms (75% of cases; Fig. 18-11) and that in 61% of the cases, nonreentrant mechanisms maintained the tachycardia, the remainder being maintained by intramural reentry and at times involving both nonreentrant and

reentrant mechanisms.[88] The nature of the nonreentrant mechanism causing transition to ventricular fibrillation remains undefined. Such a transition to ventricular fibrillation was associated with multiple small reentrant circuits and multiple simultaneous wavefronts characteristic of ventricular fibrillation.[88]

The cellular electrophysiologic mechanisms and the immediate inciting causes of reperfusion ventricular tachyarrhythmias remain a question of of extreme interest and intense research. A possible explanation of reperfusion arrhythmias is that both chemical and electric gradients (caused by washout of various ions and metabolites that have accumulated in the ischemic zone) may be responsible for inducing reperfusion arrhythmias. Massive washout of lactate and potassium ions may occur soon after reperfusion.[12, 17, 18] The output of potassium ions into neighboring normal myocardial cells can cause partial depolarization and

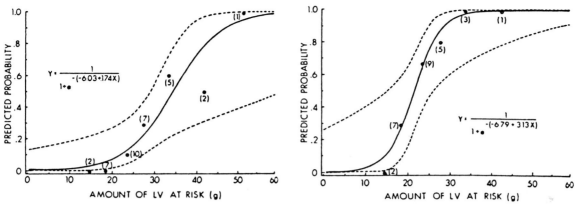

Figure 18-10. Relation between myocardium "at risk" and likelihood of ventricular fibrillation during occlusion (*left panel*) and after release of a 20-minute occlusion (*right panel*). *Solid line* is defined by equation; *hatched lines* describe 95% confidence limits. Observed incidence of ventricular fibrillation for each 5-g increment of myocardium at risk is shown with *dots*. Number of animals in each group is given in parentheses. (Austin M, Wenger TL, Harrell FE Jr, et al: Effect of myocardium at risk on outcome after coronary artery occlusion and release. Am J Physiol 1982;243:H340.)

pacemaker-like repetitive activity of the sort described by Cranefield and by Katzung and associates.[55,57] Such activity, if present in the intact canine myocardium, may cause runs of ventricular tachycardia and ventricular fibrillation. Furthermore, the output of acidic metabolites may cause abnormal repolarization with humps during phase 3 (an event described by Coraboeuf and associates) that can cause repetitive depolarizations, leading to ventricular arrhythmias in the intact heart.[61] These possibilities, however, remain just that and await experimental verification. In addition, potassium-induced partial depolarization of affected myocardial cells may inactivate the fast-response action potentials and leave the slow-response action potentials for impulse conduction. Such impulses conduct slowly and can lead to unidirectional conduction block. Once these events occur, it is possible that reentrant premature ventricular depolarizations could emerge.[38,65] Experimental studies have introduced the concept that reactive oxygen intermediates such as the superoxide O_2- and hydroxyl radicals (OH), which are formed during reperfusion or reoxygenation of ischemic or hypoxic myocardial tissue, may be responsible for the induction of electrophysiologic alterations that lead to the development of ventricular fibrillation.[89] The association between free radical production and arrhythmia genesis has been questioned, however.[90,91] These studies failed to demonstrate electrophysiologic changes arising from free radical production, and inhibition of their generation failed to alter the course of arrhythmia generation.[90,91] In newer studies, the production of transient bursts of reactive oxygen intermediates caused relatively fast electrophysiologic changes with subsequent arrhythmia development in isolated perfused rat hearts.[92] The addition of a quenching agent in this model significantly delayed the occurrence of the electro-

physiologic changes and arrhythmias.[92] The possible cellular electrophyisologic mechanisms of reperfusion arrhythmias with various reactive free radicals remain to be elucidated. As with ischemic ventricular tachyarrhythmias, both mechanisms of reentry and a type of automatic activity may also be operative during reperfusion.[34] It is suggested that all etiologic factors that precipitate the occurrence of ischemic ventricular arrhythmias also exacerbate the initiation of these arrhythmias during reperfusion.[96] These include myocardium at risk, heart rate, severity of ischemia, and duration of the antecedent period of ischemia.[46,87,94]

Akiyama recorded transmembrane potentials from subepicardial ventricular muscle cells in the reperfused region during reperfusion-induced ventricular fibrillation (Fig. 18-12).[97] He found that cells in the reperfused region had depressed resting membrane potentials and were sensitive to verapamil (a slow-channel blocker) but not to tetradotoxin (a fast-channel blocker). The results of this study suggest that myocardial cells in the reperfused zone have action potentials of the slow-response type.[97] Downar and colleagues found that cells in the reperfused region had highly heterogenous transmembrane potential configurations (Fig. 18-13); some cells were inexcitable and others were fully excitable.[16] These properties indicate that such a heterogenous electrophysiologic substrate may lead to reentrant-type arrhythmias. Although automaticity was not documented in these microelectrode studies, its absence does not imply that some sort of automatic mechanism cannot be operative during the period of reperfusion ventricular arrhythmias.[16,97] In a preliminary report, Ten Eick and colleagues contend that deep myocardial cells within the ischemic zone can initiate automatic impulses, suggesting that reperfused isch-

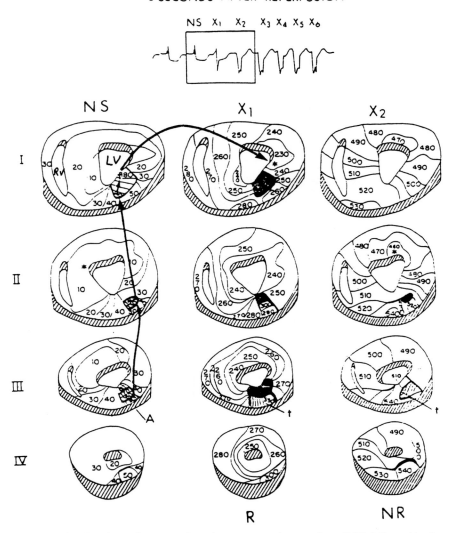

Figure 18-11. Three-dimensional isochronic maps of a sinus beat (*NS*), followed by the first 2 beats (*X₁, X₂*) of a 6-beat run of nonsustained ventricular tachycardia 3 seconds after reperfusion in which the tachycardia initiates by intramural reentry, shown by the dark arrow from *NS* to *X₁*, but is maintained by a nonreentrant mechanism. The seconds are oriented with the base on top and the apex on the bottom. The right ventricular and left ventricular cavities are labeled on the most basal slice for the control nonischemic beat. Areas of conduction block are indicated by the thickened lines and the blackened areas. Asterisks (*) denote the sites of initial activation for each beat, and daggers (†) denote the sites of latest activation for each beat. The numbers within the isochrones indicate the time in milliseconds from the initiation of each beat. (Pogwizd SM, Corr PB: Electrophysiological mechanisms underlying arrhythmias due to reperfusion of ischemic myocardium. Circulation 1987;76:404.)

emic myocardial cells can generate an automatic mechanism.[98] Oscillatory afterpotentials and automaticity at low membrane potential were reported by Ferrier and colleagues and by others to occur in isolated canine ventricular tissues during conditions simulating ischemia and reperfusion.[99,52,62]

Levine and associates constructed strength-interval curves for both anodal and cathodal modes of stimulation within a few minutes after acute coronary artery occlusion in the dog and immediately after reperfusion during the peak incidence of ventricular arrhythmias.[100] These authors found increased myocardial excitability that correlated well with both early occlusion and reperfusion-induced ventricular arrhythmias. Furthermore, anodal ex-

Time after
VF (min)

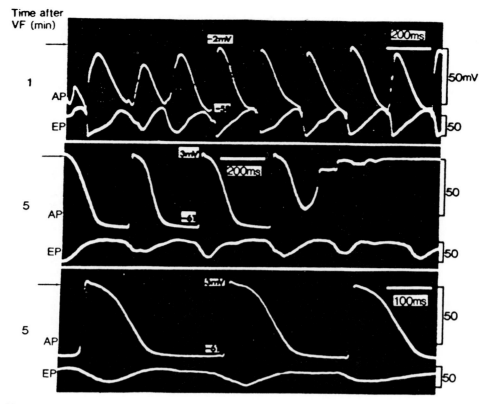

Figure 18-12. Recording of transmembrane action potentials of subepicardial ventricular cells during ventricular fibrillation induced by reperfusion of ischemic areas. Action potentials (*AP*) and unipolar epicardial electrocardiograms (*EP*) were simultaneously recorded from reperfused areas 1 minute (*upper panel*) and 5 minutes (*middle panel* at a slower speed and *lower panel* at a faster speed) after onset of ventricular fibrillation. Zero reference level for membrane potential (*arrows*, left) is determined by withdrawing a micropipette into a thin film of Tyrode's solution covering epicardial surface inside the well (*middle plate*). At onset of ventricular fibrillation, ventricular cells discharged panel action potentials of various amplitudes at a fast rate of over 300 beats/min. As noted, one action potential had a maximum diastolic potential of–58 mV and overshoot potential of–2 mV (*upper panel*). Later, during ventricular fibrillation, local excitation rate slowed and remained relatively stable at about 150 beats/min, allowing membrane potential to reach a stable level during diastole. In this instance, resting potential was–61 mV and overshoot potential was 3 mV. Note increase in overshoot potential (3 mV) when local excitation rate was slower and diastolic potential before onset of upstroke reached a more negative value of–61 mV (*tracings, middle*, and *lower panel*). (Akiyama T: Intracellular recording of in situ ventricular cells during ventricular fibrillation. Am J Physiol 1981;240:H465.)

citability correlated better with the incidence of arrhythmias than did cathodal excitability.[100] Alterations in the excitability threshold and refractoriness were also demonstrated by Elharrar and associates.[101] The prolongation of postrepolarization refractoriness (i.e., inability of the cell to initiate an action potential for up to 200 milliseconds after full repolarization) in ischemic myocardial fibers was described by Lazzara and associates, as was the phenomenon of time-dependent recovery of myocardial excitability, which may have an anomalous relation with heart rate (i.e., the duration of postrepolarization refractoriness may increase as heart rate increases).[102, 103] Such an event may slow conduction velocity, favoring the emergence of reentrant premature excitation.

Although complex multiple mechanisms may operate during the early postocclusion and reperfusion periods, differences exist in the mechanism of ventricular arrhythmias in these two different conditions.[104] Coker and Parratt found that intracoronary administration of prostacyclin markedly reduced the incidence of ventricular fibrillation induced by reperfusion after a 40-minute occlusion of the LAD coronary artery in dogs.[106] These authors suggest that the release of endogenous prostacyclin may have a protective effect during reperfusion of an ischemic myocardium but may exhibit different action during occlusion arrhythmias. Pretreatment with nisoldipine, a calcium channel blocker, diminished reperfusion-induced ventricular arrhythmias in chronically instrumented conscious ba-

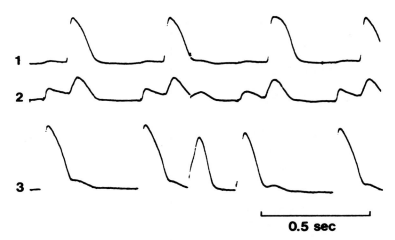

Figure 18-13. Transmembrane action potentials recorded from the subepicardium of the left ventricle (within 1 mm of each other) of an in situ pig heart after left anterior descending coronary artery occlusion. Cells *1* and *2* were at the same location but cell *1* was deeper. Action potentials from cells *3* and *1* and from cells *3* and *2* were recorded simultaneously only 1 minute apart, while stimulation pattern remained the same. Stimulating electrode was close to cell *3*. All three cells were located within 1 mm of each other. Note the delay and block of the premature impulse between cells *3* and *1*. (Downar E, Janse MJ, Durrer D: The effects of acute coronary artery occlusion on subepicardium transmembrane potentials in the intact porcine heart. Circulation 1977;56:217.)

boons.[107] The ability of free radical scavengers to afford arrhythmia protection during reperfusion is suggested in some studies; however, other studies failed to demonstrate such an efficacy.[90–92,108] Both species and methodological approaches may influence the outcome with free radical scavengers. More work is needed to elucidate this issue and to determine the clinical usefulness of the role of free radical scavengers in the prevention of reperfusion arrhythmias.

In isolated perfused feline left ventricular preparations, verapamil and not procainamide was capable of preventing reperfusion-induced rapid repetitive activity.[109] Furthermore, superfusion with calcium-free media before reperfusion prevented reperfusion-induced arrhythmias without affecting action potential changes during ischemia.[109] We have shown that a metoprolol-quinidine combination significantly reduced the incidence of reperfusion-induced ventricular fibrillation in a closed-chest anesthetized canine model of LAD coronary artery occlusion reperfusion model.[110] Neither drug was effective when given alone. During occlusion arrhythmias, however, these drugs, when given singly, afforded significant protection to the ventricle.[110] These studies suggest that different mechanisms may be operative during ischemia and reperfusion arrhythmias.[87,105] More studies are needed to unravel cellular electrophysiologic differences and precipitating factors in the induction of these potentially lethal arrhythmias in these two different settings. The role of ATP-sensitive potassium channel activity in the

mechanism of reperfusion ventricular fibrillation and ventricular tachycardia was evaluated in a guinea pig model of global ischemia.[111] When the ATP-sensitive potassium channel was blocked with glibenclamide, the incidence of reperfusion-induced ventricular fibrillation and ventricular tachycardia was reduced in a concentration-dependent manner.[111] In contrast, however, when the APD-sensitive channel opener cromakalim was used, no arrhythmia or an actual aggravation of arrhythmias was observed despite an anti-ischemic potential effect of cromakalim.[111,112]

Pharmacologic Considerations

Pharmacologic therapy and management of early acute ischemic ventricular arrhythmias present a unique and formidable problem because drugs have limited or no access to the site of origin of the arrhythmia. Wit and Bigger suggest that if the drug can reach the site of arrhythmia origin, two mutually exclusive mechanisms must be operative for successful antiarrhythmic action: (1) the drug must completely block conduction in the ischemic region, and (2) the drug must restore normal conduction.[113] Furthermore, in light of newer findings, a potentially useful antiarrhythmic agent must also suppress abnormal automaticity—possibly caused by EAD (Table 18-1).[57,61] Wenger and associates injected procainamide intravenously in dogs 40 minutes after complete left circumflex coronary artery occlusion and found pro-

TABLE 18-1. The Nature, Time Course, Mechanisms, Site of Origin, and Response to Drugs of Ventricular Arrhythmias After Coronary Artery Occlusion

	Phase I	Phase II	Phase III
Nature	VT/VF	VT	VT/VF
Time course	15–30 min	6–72 h	3–12 d
Site of origin	Ischemic myocardial cells Purkinje fibers? Normal zone bordering the ischemic zone	Subendocardial Purkinje fibers in infarct zone Subepicardial muscle overlying the infarct	Subepicardial muscle cells overlying the infarct Surviving intramural muscle cells Purkinje fibers?
Mechanism(s)	Reentry Automaticity (early after depolarization)?	Abnormal automaticity Triggered automaticity Reentry?	Reentry Triggered automaticity?
Response to drugs	Usually resistant	Usually suppressed	Usually resistant

VT, ventricular tachycardia; VF, ventricular fibrillation, ?, evidence uncertain. Time course refers to postocclusion period.

gressively decreasing myocardial drug concentrations, depending on the severity of myocardial ischemia.[114] Most severely ischemic myocardial areas had the lowest myocardial drug concentrations. Zito and colleagues found lower myocardial lidocaine concentrations in ischemic zones in dogs given lidocaine 2 hours after LAD occlusion.[115] Nevertheless, it appears that even such lowered levels of drug delivery to severely ischemic sites may still cause electrophysiologic effects during the early postocclusion period. The studies of Kupersmith and colleagues show that lidocaine administered 2 hours after complete LAD occlusion caused a preferential increase in myocardial refractoriness in the infarcted zone, thus decreasing the disparity of refractoriness between normal and infarcted zones that was present before lidocaine administration.[116] Furthermore, lidocaine increased the activation time in the infarcted zone but had no effect on the normal zone. In this study, however, the antiarrhythmic consequences of such local electrophysiologic effects of lidocaine on an acutely ischemic region of the myocardium were not evaluated. Moreover, the role of diminished antiarrhythmic drug delivery to an acutely ischemic zone in arrhythmia suppression is still undefined. Nattel and associates show that introducing an antiarrhythmic agent (aprinidine) to a potentially arrhythmic region before coronary artery occlusion may lead to different regional myocardial distribution and different electrophysiologic actions and antiarrhythmic efficacy.[117] Based on the frequency of arrhythmias, these authors suggest that further drug-induced slowing in conduction in ischemic zones is likely to increase the incidence of early ventricular tachycardia and ventricular fibrillation.[117] This study demonstrates that drugs can actually exacerbate early postocclusion arrhythmias if their concentration is sufficiently

raised in the ischemic zone. Further studies of this type are needed to elaborate this important point. Reduction of extracellular potassium ion concentration in the ischemic zone with insulin–glucose infusion was reported to improve intramyocardial conduction, thus providing a potential for antiarrhythmic efficacy during the acute ischemic phase.[118] It is postulated that glucose in the presence of insulin increases the glycolytic flux, thereby providing adequate ATP for suppressing ATP-sensitive potassium channels, which may be at least partially responsible for the extracellular potassium ion rise in the early phase of ischemia.[22,23,24,118]

For reperfusion-induced ventricular fibrillation, most antiarrhythmic agents were found to be ineffective.[119,120] In one study, however, bretylium was found to reduce the incidence of reperfusion-induced ventricular fibrillation when the amount of myocardium at risk (ischemic) was considered during statistic computation.[121] We found that the combination of metoprolol-quinidine was effective in preventing reperfusion-induced ventricular fibrillation in the closed-chest anesthetized dog model and that when given singly, these drugs were ineffective.[110] It is important to note that it is possible to introduce pharmacologic agents to an acutely ischemic region of the myocardium by the coronary venous retrograde perfusion (retroperfusion) system.[122,123] Meerbaum and associates lysed a thrombus in the LAD coronary artery with streptokinase, administered through the great cardiac vein, which drains the perfusion bed of the LAD coronary artery.[122,124] Whether delivery of antiarrhythmic drugs to an acutely ischemic zone by retroinfusion through cardiac veins prevents or reduces the incidence of early arrhythmias remains to be seen. This approach, however, seems promising.[123]

Data on the mechanism or mechanisms of early postocclusion arrhythmias in humans are difficult to study because of the extraordinary conditions under which they occur. In a preliminary report, Cinca and associates compared precordial electrocardiogram (ECG) recordings during the first minutes of acute myocardial infarction in humans with experimental coronary occlusion (Fig. 18-14).[125] These authors suggest that the cellular electrophysiologic changes in humans may be similar to those in experimental animals. If so, pharmacologic management of the early-phase arrhythmias will be extremely difficult. The possibility, however, that similar cellular electrophysiologic abnormalities may exist in humans and in experimental ischemic models emphasizes that experimental studies designed to elucidate the mechanisms and pharmacologic effects of drugs may help in the management and prophylaxis of early-phase arrhythmias in humans.

PHASE TWO VENTRICULAR ARRHYTHMIAS

If the dog survives the early arrhythmic phase after permanent occlusion of the LAD coronary artery, a relatively quiescent period ensues that may last up to 10 hours. After this nonarrhythmic period is another prolonged interval of spontaneously occurring rapid ventricular tachycardia that may last up to 72 hours.[12, 14, 83, 102] In the following sections, we present experimental findings that the site or sites of origin, the cellular electrophysiologic mechanism or mechanism, and the response of these arrhythmias to pacing and antiarrhythmic drug therapy differ from those tachycardias that occur immediately after occlusion or after transient occlusion followed by reperfusion. Furthermore, we attempt to present pertinent data showing that these arrhythmias are similar in many respects to the in-hospital phase of ventricular arrhythmias that occur in humans during the first few days after the onset of acute symptoms indicative of myocardial infarction.

The persistence of myocardial ischemia after the LAD coronary artery occlusion in the dog causes myocardial cell necrosis that may involve the entire left anteroseptal structures.[126, 127] Usually, the lateral, superior, and inferior margins of the infarct are well defined. On the epicardial surface, a rim of cells (reaching in some cases a third of the left ventricular wall thickness) remain viable (epicardial border zone).[126–128] The margins at these epicardial sites are irregular and are not sharply defined and occasionally, small areas of infarcted myocardium are separated from the main infarcted core by noninfarcted viable tissue.[127]

On the endocardial surface underlying the infarcted

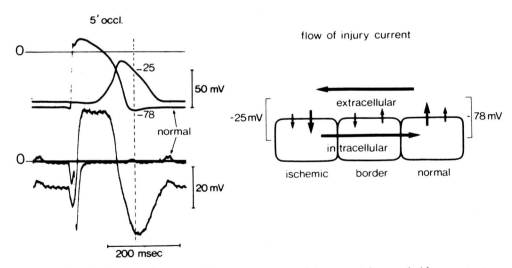

Figure 18-14. Transmembrane and direct current extracellular potentials recorded from an in situ dog heart. Potentials before and 5 minutes after left anterior descending coronary artery occlusion are superimposed, using as time reference the stimulus artifact on the atrium. Note extreme delay in activation of the epicardial ischemic cell, which is depolarized when normal cells are already repolarized. The negative T wave in the local electrogram recorded from the ischemic zone represents the intrinsic deflection caused by the delayed activity. In the diagram, the flow of injury current at the moment, indicated by the *dotted line* is schematically depicted. At the moment of the cardiac cycle, the injury current produces current sources at the nonischemic side of the border and current sinks on the ischemic side. (Cinca J, Janse MJ, Morena H, et al: Mechanism and time course of the early electrical changes during acute coronary occlusion. An attempt to correlate the early ECG charges in man to cellular electrophysiology in pigs. Chest 1980;77:499.)

zone, two to four layers of myocardial cells, identified as Purkinje fibers, remain viable.[126, 127] The core of the infarcted myocardium (i.e., within the wall of the left ventricle) manifests relatively homogenous necrosis throughout the entire zone of infarction. In contrast, myocardial infarct structure produced by transient LAD coronary artery occlusion followed by reperfusion differs from that produced by permanent LAD coronary artery occlusion. In infarcts caused by temporary occlusions, regions of noninfarcted myocardium are found throughout. These regions of noninfarcted myocardium are either completely surrounded by infarcted myocardium or continuous, with noninfarcted myocardium bordering the infarct.[127] The lateral margins of the infarct are extremely irregular, however; on both the epicardial and endocardial edges of the infarct, variable layers of myocardial cells remain viable. Between four and 15 cell layers remain viable on the endocardial surface of the infarct, as does up to a third of the epicardium.[127] The anatomy and pattern of myocardial cell necrosis of right ventricular infarcts caused by permanent occlusion of the right coronary artery in the dog are similar to infarcts caused by transient LAD coronary artery occlusion; necrosis is heterogenous, with irregular margins, often including viable muscle bundles within the general zone of infarction.[129] The structure of myocardial infarcts, especially infarct caused by transient LAD occlusion, demonstrates in many respects close resemblance to the structure of infarcts that occur in patients with ischemic heart disease and myocardial infarction.[130–132] The similar characteristics include (1) the presence on the endocardial surface of the infarct of a zone of myocardial fibers (15 to 20 cell layers), retaining normal staining qualities; and (2) the presence of normal-staining bundles of myocardial cells scattered in the infarcted left ventricular wall. Such features are reported to occur in many human autopsy specimens, more so in cases with nonocclusive coronary insufficiency involving infarction of the inner endocardial half of the wall.[130–133] Similarly, the structure and pattern of myocardial cell necrosis in human right ventricular infarction? has many similarities to canine right ventricular infarction because the necrosis is heterogenous and subendocardial fibers survive beneath the infarcts.[129, 134, 135]

To determine the site of origin of spontaneous ventricular arrhythmias during the late phase, El-Sherif and associates made multiple simultaneous bipolar recordings from the entire epicardial surface and from selected endocardial and intramural sites using a computerized multiplexing technique.[136] The arrhythmia had a focal origin in the surviving subendocardial Purkinje network underlying the infarct and that frequent shift of the ectopic pacemaker occurred. Earlier experimental studies using a limited number of biopolar recordings electrodes also indicate the subendocardial Purkinje network is a site of

origin of these tachyarrhythmias for both left and right ventricular myocardial infarcts.[53, 135, 137, 138] Furthermore, Scherlag and coworkers found that many of ectopic beats originated from the epicardium in the infarcted zone because electric activity at this site preceded the Q wave of the tachycardia.[48] Newer studies also reiterate these earlier findings of both subendocardial and epicardial sites being involved in arrhythmogenesis.[128, 139–141]

Sugi and associates also suggest both endocardial and epicardial sites of origin for late-phase spontaneous ventricular tachyarrhythmia in the canine model during myocardial infarction limited exclusively to the right ventricle (Fig. 18-15).[135] As reported by these authors, ventricular arrhythmia also occurs 24 hours after permanent right coronary artery occlusion in the dog, which produces ventricular myocardial infarction that is exclusively limited to the right ventricle.[135] In addition to the spontaneous form of ventricular arrhythmia, pacing at rates above 300 beats per minute may induce still another form of ventricular tachyarrhythmias in the same dogs at rates of 230 to 450 beats per minute (average, 345 beats/minute), which was faster than the spontaneous tachycardia (average, 154 beats/minute).[142, 143] The computerized isochronal mapping studies of El-Sherif and colleagues suggest that these induced rapid ventricular tachyarrhythmias arise by a reentrant mechanism in the surviving epicardial layers of the infarcted left ventricle.[143] Furthermore, these induced rapid ventricular tachyarrhythmias easily degenerated into ventricular fibrillation, especially when the rapid induced rhythm had pleomorphic characteristics of the torsades de pointes type.[143]

In an attempt to determine the mechanism or mechanisms of spontaneous ventricular arrhythmia, Scherlag and associates exposed ventricular automaticity after inducing atrial slowing by vagal stimulation.[48] Vagal stimulation revealed a ventricular automatic rhythm of an average of 166 beats per minute, as opposed to 39 beats per minute in control dogs.[48] Furthermore, such ventricular rhythms may be suppressed by rapid atrial pacing. These authors suggest the existence of an enhanced ventricular automatic mechanism as a cause for these spontaneous arrhythmias.[48] Dangman and coworkers recorded transmembrane action potentials from these surviving subepicardial muscle cells (epicardial border zone) isolated from dogs 2 to 4 days after LAD occlusion.[128] The authors showed that these surviving cells were capable of generating DADs and triggered activity during rapid pacing in the presence of catecholamines.[128] It is suggested that the subepicardial border zone may the site of origin of both abnormal and triggered automatic arrhythmias during phase 2 arrhythmias.[128] Transmembrane potential recordings from partially depolarized subendocardial Purkinje fibers isolated from the infarcted left ventricle during late-phase arrhythmias show the presence of spontaneous

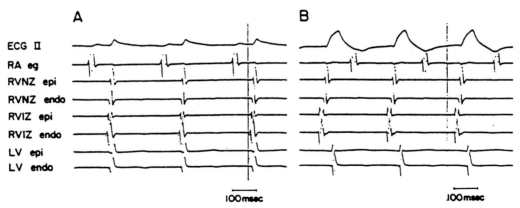

Figure 18-15. Intramural bipolar electrograms recorded from normal and infarcted zones in an open-chest dog 24 hours after right coronary artery occlusion. (**A**) Recordings are during normal sinus rhythm. (**B**) Recordings during spontaneous uniform ventricular tachycardia. Recordings are, from top to bottom: electrocardiogram (*ECG II*), right atrial electrogram (*RA eg*), right ventricular normal zone epicardial (*RVNZ epi*), and endocardial (*RVNZ endo*), respectively; left ventricular (apex) epicardial (*LV epi*) and endocardial (*LV endo*) sites (which are not involved in infarction). Note that earliest activity during spontaneous uniform ventricular tachycardia (but not during normal sinus rhythm) occurs in the infarcted zone of the right ventricle. (Sugi K, Karagueuzian HS, Fishbein MC, et al: Spontaneous ventricular tachycardia associated with isolated right ventricular infarction, one day after right coronary artery occlusion in the dog: studies on the site of original and mechanism. Am Heart J 1985;109:232.)

diastolic depolarizations, initiating automatic impulses (abnormal automaticity) that may propagate and excite adjoining normal myocardial tissue (Fig. 18-16).[137,144,145] El-Sherif and colleagues show that surviving subendocardial Purkinje fibers in the infarct zone (average resting potential, −60 mV) can develop DAD and subsequent triggered automaticity, which is normally present during this arrhythmic period (Fig. 18-17).[137,145] Similar conclusions were also drawn with respect to site of origin and arrhythmia mechanism in a newer study.[140] Dresdner and associates evaluated the ionic basis of partial depolarization of these surviving subendocardial Purkinje fibers using ion-sensitive microelectrodes.[146,147] Using pH and potassium ion–sensitive microelectrodes, intracellular ac-

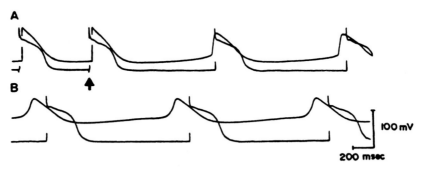

Figure 18-16. Transmembrane potentials recorded from subendocardial Purkinje fibers in an isolated preparation of infarcted canine myocardium. The *top trace* in each panel shows action potentials recorded from a fiber on the endocardial surface of the infarct and the *bottom trace* in each panel shows action potentials recorded from a fiber in an adjacent noninfarcted region. (**A**) The first two impulses are elicited by electric stimulation of the preparation. The stimulus is turned off at the *arrow*. Spontaneous diastolic depolarization develops in the Purkinje fiber in the infarct and results in automatic firing. (**B**) Recordings from the same two cells several minutes later; impulses are arising in the automatic Purkinje fibers in the infarct (*top trace*) and conducting into the noninfarcted region. (Friedman PL, Stewart JR, Fenoglio JJ Jr, Wit AL: Survival of subendocardial Purkinje fibers after extensive myocardial infarction: in vitro and in vivo correlations. Circ Res 1973;33:612.)

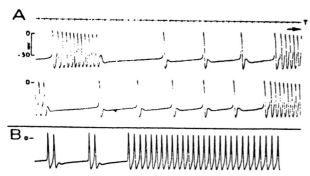

Figure 18-17. Initiation of triggered automaticity by background slow Purkinje fiber automaticity isolated from a canine preparation 24 hours after permanent left anterior descending coronary artery occlusion. (**A** and **B**) Transmembrane recordings from Purkinje fibers in two different infarcted endocardial preparations. The time scale (*T*) designates 1-second intervals. (El-Sherif N, et al: Triggered ventricular rhythm in one day old myocardial infarction in the dog. Circ Res 1983;52:566.)

idification did not appear to be the cause of partial depolarization and only a portion of the maximum diastolic potential changes can be explained by a reduction of the potassium equilibrium potential.[146, 147] Alteration of membrane Na–K pump activity and membrane conductance of ions are suggested as additional likely mechanisms.[146] The passive electric properties of surviving subendocardial Purkinje fibers 1 day after LAD coronary artery occlusion in the dog were evaluated.[148] This study suggests electric uncoupling between adjacent cells, which increases internal resistivity. The significance of this study remains to be defined because the conduction velocity, membrane length constant, membrane time constant, and the time constant and capacitance of the foot of the action potential all remained unchanged.[148] Significant increases in input resistance, membrane resistance, and axial resistance (with a significant decrease in membrane capacitance) were observed in the surviving reported.[148]

The mechanistic conclusions drawn from these isolated canine infarcted tissue studies with single-cell recordings were largely corroborated with results obtained in intact in vivo canines ventricles with LAD coronary artery occlusion by employing pacing protocol and analyzing the various rhythmic pattern of the infarcted ventricle.[149] Some of the ventricular tachycardia could not be overdrive-suppressed nor could it be terminated by premature pacing with applied single premature stimuli (Fig. 18-18), a mechanism that is not consistent with reentry but is consistent with abnormal automaticity.[127, 129, 135] In other cases, ventricular ectopy was induced by pacing, a mechanism consistent with triggered activity.[149] Although the subendocardium may be the seat of various automatic arrhythmogenic mechanisms, this site has also been implicated in the genesis of reentrant activity.[150, 139] Abnormal

automatic foci may be surrounded by variable impairment of impulse conduction, which may set the stage for reflected reentrant activity.[139, 150]

Isolated tissue studies from dogs having right ventricular infarction during the 24-hour arrhythmic period also show enhanced automatic activity in the surviving subendocardial Purkinje fiber network, suggesting that enhanced automaticity at this site may be responsible for the arrhythmias seen during this arrhythmic period.[135] Therefore, microelectrode studies support the idea that some sort of automatic mechanism—abnormal, triggered, or both—may be responsible for at least many of the ectopic ventricular beats that occur during late-phase arrhythmias.

Fujimoto and associate found no apparent relation between intramyocardial conduction slowing in the ischemic zone and the emergence of late-phase ventricular arrhythmias in dogs having permanent LAD coronary artery occlusion.[151] These authors suggest abnormal automaticity as a mechanism for late-phase ventricular arrhythmias.[151] The mechanism of induced rapid ventricular rhythm, which arises in the surviving subepicardial muscle cells, appears to be caused by a reentrant mechanism, although a triggered automatic mechanism is possible.[136, 142, 143] The considerable prolongation of subendocardial Purkinje fiber action potential duration and the ability of premature stimuli to undergo conduction delay and to subsequently induce rapid nondriven repetitive activity in in vitro preparation suggest that reentry at subendocardial sites remains a distinct potential mechanism, independent of subepicardial sites.[144, 152] It is therefore apparent that the mechanism or mechanisms of 24-hour arrhythmias are more complex than originally thought.[11, 12]

When spontaneously depolarizing Purkinje cells initiate an automatic impulse and propagate to adjacent normal ventricular muscle cells, ventricular ectopic beats and rhythms are expected to result. At times, various degrees of exit block may exist around the infarct.[152, 150] Therefore, the rhythm that may be expected to result from at least an abnormal automatic or even a triggered mechanism could include accelerated idioventricular rhythm, nonparoxysmal ventricular tachycardia, and noncoupled ventricular premature depolarizations; all are common in the first few days after acute myocardial infarction in humans.[83] For instance, accelerated idioventricular rhythm occurs in as many as 30% to 40% of patients with acute myocardial infarction and may correspond to the abnormal automaticity seen in experimental infarction.[83]

Furthermore, histologic and ultrastructural studies show intact Purkinje fibers surviving on the endocardial surface of some anteroseptal human infarcts.[153] Moreover, these surviving fibers contain lipid droplets similar to those seen in the Purkinje fibers in canine infarcts.[126, 137, 144]

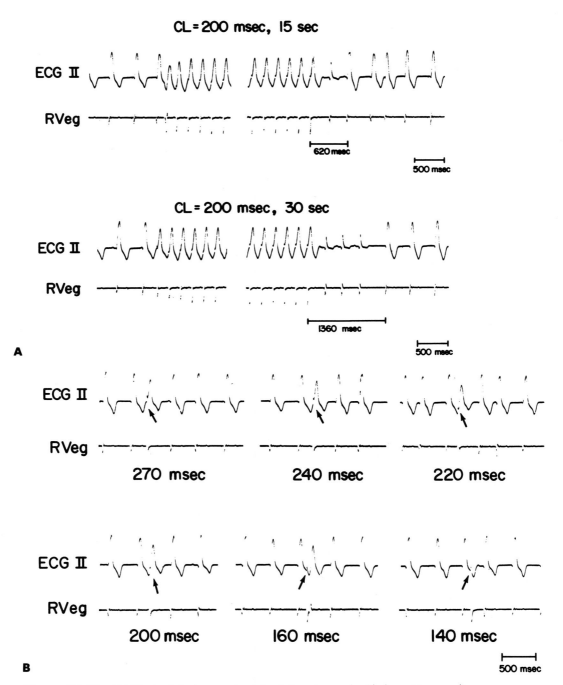

Figure 18-18. (**A**) Effects of single premature stimulations (*arrows*), with decreasing coupling intervals on spontaneously occurring ventricular tachycardia in a closed-chest dog, one day after permanent occlusion of the right coronary artery. Note the inability of the premature stimulus to terminate the tachycardia. (**B**) Effects of overdrive pacing at 200-milliseconds cycle length for 15 seconds (*top panel*) and for 30 seconds (*lower panel*) on spontaneously occurring ventricular tachycardia in a closed-chest dog one day after permanent occlusion of the right coronary artery (same dog as in the top panel). Note that after the termination of the overdrive, one beat (*top panel*) and two beats (*lower panel*) of sinus origin are followed by the resumption of the tachycardia.

In addition to these experimental-clinical similarities, it is interesting that electrophysiologic studies in the catheterization laboratory suggest that many of the ventricular tachycardias that occur on the first day after the onset of symptoms of infarction are caused by automaticity.[154] These findings indicate that despite the differences between experimentally and clinically occurring myocardial infarction, studies on animal models can provide meaningful information on the mechanisms of clinical arrhythmias.

Pharmacologic Considerations

Changes in myocardial site of origin and mechanisms of ventricular arrhythmias during late-phase as opposed to early-phase arrhythmia can have important pharmacologic consequences. For example, Nattel and associates found that when aprinidine was administered 24 hours after LAD coronary artery occlusion, it had markedly different effects on the arrhythmias than when given just after occlusion, despite similar aprinidine concentrations in different myocardial zones.[117] These authors suggest that aprinidine is more effective against 24-hour arrhythmias than against early-phase arrhythmias because it suppresses enhanced ventricular automaticity, a mechanism at least partly responsible for late-phase arrhythmias.[117] Similarly, other studies found that lidocaine and procainamide were effective against 24-hour arrhythmias.[155] This is also the case with the newer investigational agents ethmozine and propafenone.[156,157] Similarly, ventricular tachycardias that occur 24 hours after right coronary artery occlusion are also effectively suppressed with lidocaine and verapamil in combination because these arrhythmias are thought to be caused by both abnormal automatic and enhanced normal automatic mechanisms.[156,158] Similar pharmacologic response patterns were also seen in the left ventricular infarction model 1 day after the occlusion of the LAD coronary artery model.[159] It would appear that the surviving subendocardial fibers (partially ischemic?) during the fist few days after LAD coronary artery occlusion appear to show differential sensitivity to various antiarrhythmic drugs.[160,161] and Cardinal and Sasyniuk showed that bretylium prolonged action potential duration of normal subendocardial Purkinje fibers more than that of partially ischemic fibers in the infarct zone where the action potential duration was already considerably prolonged (due to prolonged ischemia) before bretylium superfusion.[141] Such a differential effect on action potential duration (and presumably on refractoriness) decreases the dispersion, thereby decreasing the likelihood of reentrant premature excitation.[141]

It is worth mentioning that the response of 24-hour experimental ventricular tachycardia to antiarrhythmic drugs is similar in many respects to the effects of these drugs on humans.[83] Antiarrhythmic drugs usually control and suppress ventricular tachycardia in coronary care unit patients who have had a recent myocardial infarction.[83] Meesmann and associates failed to show beneficial effects of enhanced vagal activity against 24-hour ventricular tachycardias that occur in the canine model of permanent LAD coronary artery occlusion.[162] Such a lack of beneficial effect was independent of background sympathetic activity or delivery of cholinergic agents to ischemic sites because both beta blockade and great cardiac vein injections of the cholinergic agents to ischemic sites failed to impart significant antiarrhythmic activity.[162]

PHASE THREE VENTRICULAR ARRHYTHMIAS

Recurrent sustained ventricular tachycardia may occur in humans who have a history of chronic ischemic heart disease and myocardial infarcts or ventricular aneurysms.[163,164] Ventricular tachycardia similar to that occurring spontaneously can be induced in these patients by programmed electric stimulation applied to the ventricle through an electrode catheter. Similarly, once tachycardia is initiated, it can also be terminated by electric stimulation. It has been concluded from these clinical studies that these tachycardias that can be initiated and terminated by stimulating the ventricles are caused by reentry because it was shown in isolated preparations of cardiac tissue that reentry can be initiated and terminated in this manner.[165,166] Definite proof for such a hypothesis, however, requires detailed mapping of the excitation pattern of the ventricles during the arrhythmia. Therefore, more detailed electrophysiologic and pharmacologic studies on ventricular tachycardias initiated and terminated by premature depolarizations are important because such tachycardias lead to ventricular fibrillation and sudden death and may respond to antiarrhythmic drugs differently than other types of ventricular arrhythmias. Studies designed to determine the mechanism and inciting factors of this arrhythmia can be best accomplished in animal models because electric recordings can be readily obtained from all regions of the ventricles and a variety of experimental interventions can be undertaken that cannot be performed in humans.[167]

The use of experimental canine models of myocardial ischemia and infarction greatly enhances our understanding of the pathophysiologic and pharmacologic mechanisms involved in the induction of ventricular tachyarrhythmias by programmed electric stimulation in humans. In the following section, we discuss some of the advances made in this field, being fully aware that the present state of knowledge is by no means complete.

The importance of the structure and geometry of myocardial infarction in the induction of sustained ventricular tachycardia by a critically timed premature stimulus was stressed by Karagueuzian and associates.[127,168] These authors found that a critical mass of infarcted and ischemic myocardium, averaging 35% of the left ventricle, was needed for arrhythmia induction, a finding corroborated later by other investigators.[169] Furthermore, for sustained ventricular tachycardia to occur, the structure of the infarct had to be heterogenous; that is, myocardial cell death within the zone of the infarction must not be uniform or homogenous but numerous viable myocardial cells must be in close proximity with necrotic cells. Such structural ischemic damage conducive to arrhythmia induction may be produced by temporary coronary artery occlusion followed by reperfusion.[127,144,168] Such structural requirements for arrhythmia induction with greater ease (i.e., single premature stimulus; Fig. 18-19) and reproducibility were contrasted to myocardial infarction caused by permanent coronary artery occlusion, in which myocardial cell death is relatively homogenous and induction of sustained ventricular tachycardia is less frequent.[127,167,168] In dogs having infarcts involving homogenous myocardial cell necrosis, only the nonsustained (fewer than 10 seconds duration) form of ventricular tachycardia were induced with ease. Furthermore, because these studies were conducted serially in awake dogs and each dog was studied over several consecutive days, the temporal relation between the age of the infarct and arrhythmia induction was emphasized.[127,167,168] It was found that as the infarct aged, the arrhythmia could no longer be induced by premature stimuli beyond the first week of infarction, probably reflecting changing electrophysiologic properties of myocardial cells in an ischemic zone (stabilization of the irritable ventricle). Note, however, that in studies conducted on open-chest preparations, arrhythmia induction is possible from 3 weeks to up 4 years.[170,171] This is probably caused by elevated circulating catecholamine levels in the open-chest model, which are known to facilitate arrhythmia induction in both experimental and clinical settings.[156,172] A relation between infarct size and the nature of the induced rhythm was also evaluated with single strong premature stimuli.[173] Using a strong premature stimulus of 5 milliseconds duration and strengths of 10 to 100 mA, it was found that when the transmural infarct extent was 80%, only sustained ventricular tachycardia could be induced; when the size was 63% of the left ventricle, both tachycardia and fibrillation could be induced; and finally, when the extent of the infarct was 15%, only ventricular fibrillation could be

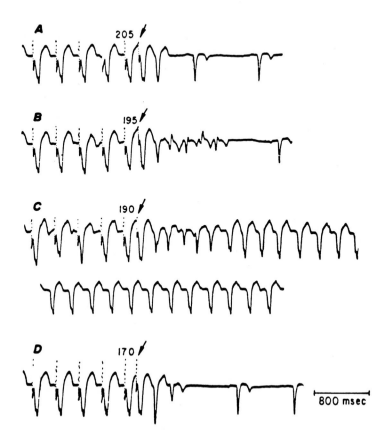

Figure 18-19. Initiation of protracted ventricular tachycardia in a dog on the third day of reperfusion after a transient (2 hours) occlusion of the left anterior descending coronary artery. The electrocardiogram is shown in each panel. (**A** to **D**) The ventricles are being driven at a cycle length of 350 milliseconds and a single premature stimulus (*arrow*) is applied to the ventricle. (**A**) The coupling interval of the stimulated premature impulse is 205 milliseconds; this is followed by five nondriven impulses. The QRS morphology and the cycle length of the nondriven impulses are variable. After a pause of 720 milliseconds, sinus rhythm reoccurs. (**C**) The coupling interval of the stimulated premature impulse is 190 milliseconds; this is followed by 10 minutes of tachycardia. The lower trace in **C** shows the electrocardiogram 8 minutes after initiation of tachycardia. (**D**) A single stimulated premature impulse induced at a coupling interval of 170 milliseconds is followed by two nondriven impulses. Sinus rhythm occurs after a pause of 760 milliseconds. (Karagueuzian HS, Fenoglio JJ Jr, Weiss MB, Wit AL: Protracted ventricular tachycardia induced by premature stimulation of the canine heart after coronary artery occlusion and reperfusion. Circ Res 1979;44:833. By permission of the American Heart Association.)

induced.[173] A critically timed single strong premature stimulus induced a figure-eight reentry pattern by the mechanism of graded-response propagation.[174,175] It is suggested that with thicker transmural infarcts, the thinner (i.e., two-dimensional) the spared rime of the myocardium (border zone) becomes, the more likely is the induction of a stable single figure-eight reentry wavefront of activation, thus resulting in ventricular tachycardia rather than ventricular fibrillation.[173] Ventricular infarction limited exclusively to the right ventricle is also susceptible to inducible sustained ventricular tachycardia and ventricular fibrillation during the chronic phase of infarction.[129] The inducibility of these tachyarrhythmias with an applied single premature stimulus was found to be reproducible (Fig. 18-20). We found that these types of infarcts may be produced by permanent occlusion of the right coronary artery in the dog and that both the structure of the infarct and the time course of tachyarrhythmia inducibility paralleled that of the left-sided ventricular infarction caused by occlusion and reperfusion.[129]

It is worth mentioning that the myocardial infarction model in cats (caused by coronary artery occlusion) is associated with spontaneous ventricular arrhythmias lasting for up to 6 months after healing from acute injury.[176] Such arrhythmias may be related at least partly to subendocardial surviving fibers remaining abnormal for several months after coronary occlusion.[177,178] Whether ventricular tachycardia could also be induced for such a long period in the feline model remains to be seen.

The importance of the size of myocardial infarction in arrhythmia induction in the coronary artery occlusion and reperfusion model was further pursued by Gang and associates.[179] In large-sized myocardial infarcts, a lowered fibrillation threshold and greater ease of induction of sustained ventricular tachycardia was found.[179] The proarrhythmic potentials of heterogenous myocardial infarcts in the canine model caused by coronary artery occlusion and reperfusion were emphasized by Michelson and colleagues.[180] These authors measured myocardial excitability and refractoriness within the heterogenous infarcted zone and found a great disparity in both excitability and refractoriness, suggesting that such disparity may be conducive to arrhythmia induction by programmed electric stimulation.[180] Furthermore, these authors demonstrated that the site of electric stimulation in relation to the infarct location was important in arrhythmia induction.[181] For example, intramyocardial sites within 2 cm of the infarct had the highest success rate in arrhythmia induction with electric stimulation.[181] Microelectrode studies were also conducted on infarcted myocardial tissues isolated from canine hearts having myocardial infarction caused by occlusion and reperfusion of the LAD coronary artery. Karagueuzian and colleagues studied the transmembrane potential properties of subendocardial cardiac fibers in the infarct zone.[144] During the period of susceptibility for tachycardia induction by electric stimulation in the intact dog, surviving suendocardial Purkinje fibers and ventricular muscle fibers were normal or nearly so, and premature impulses did not undergo conduction delay at this site.[144] Delayed afterdepolarization and subsequent triggered automatic activity also were not seen.[144] These authors concluded that the surviving subendocardial cardiac fibers underlying the infarct could not be implicated as primary sites for arrhythmia induction.[144] Therefore, other sites (namely, the intramural and subepicardial muscle cells overlying the infarct) may possibly

Figure 18-20. Induction of rapid ventricular tachycardia (**A** and **B**) and ventricular fibrillation (**C** and **D**) in a conscious dog 6 days after permanent right coronary artery occlusion. Single premature stimulus (*arrow*) applied during regular right ventricular pacing induces the tachyarrhythmia in a reproducible manner. All the tachyarrhythmias were induced within 15 minutes. After successful defibrillation the rhythms were reinduced after 8 minutes of "stabilization." The recordings are from lead II. (Karagueuzian HS, previously unpublished.)

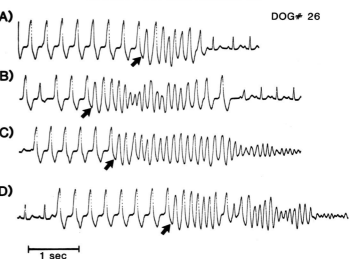

RIGHT VENTRICULAR INFARCTION
(6 DAYS POST RCA OCCLUSION)

DOG# 26

A)

B)

C)

D)

1 sec

be involved in arrhythmia genesis.[167] Spear and colleagues studied the transmembrane potential properties of subepicardial muscle overlying infarcts isolated from dogs having transient coronary artery occlusion and reperfusion.[182] The resting potential, action potential amplitude, maximal rate of depolarization, and action potential duration at 30% repolarization were significantly reduced in the infarcted region. Furthermore, conduction velocity in the infarcted region was slowed from 0.54 millisec in normal to 0.15 millisec in the infarct zone.[182] Also, a reduced space constant in the epicardial infarct zone was another important factor (in addition to reduced membrane responsiveness) in causing slowing of conduction velocity.[183,184] Slow conduction and depressed transmembrane potential properties of epicardial muscle cells in the infarcted zone in dogs having permanent LAD occlusion was also reported by Gessman and associates.[185]

In addition to transmembrane cellular changes at the epicardial border zone, important structural changes take place that may change the anisotropic properties in these regions in a nonuniform manner, which may have implication in arrhythmogenesis.[186–189] The mechanism of induced ventricular tachycardia by electric stimulation in the late myocardial infarction phase has been studied by several investigators, using computer-assisted cardiac mapping algorithms.[190–194] In these studies, isochronal maps of ventricular activation were constructed by computerized technique during the tachycardia with bipolar electrograms recorded from multiple ventricular sites. These studies attempted to identify the pattern and sequence of activation of the ventricle during the tachycardia to determine the mechanism and site of origin of the arrhythmia.

El-Sherif and colleagues presented evidence that reentry occurring at the epicardial surface of the infarct was the cause of some 21% of the induced beats.[190] Furthermore, these authors presented evidence for the presence of a zone of functional conduction block in the in situ heart, around which the activation front advanced by radial spread to cause reexcitation of the ventricle.[190]

The authors also suggest that epicardial recordings were of limited value in analyzing induced ventricular beats, indicating that sites other than the epicardial infarct zone may be involved in the process of arrhythmia induction (i.e., intramural surviving muscle cells in the zone of infarction).[127,167,168] During the chronic phase of the myocardial ischemia, a nonuniform spatial distribution of epicardial refractory periods with steep gradients of refractoriness between them occur, suggesting that such an electrophysiologic milieu constitutes a substrate for the induction of reentrant tachycardias.[193] Furthermore, these authors terminated reentrant arrhythmias by modifying the spatial distribution of recovery times by appropriate dual-site stimulation.[194] Nonuniform epicardial activation can cause nonuniform repolarization that in turn may initiate reentrant ventricular tachyarrhythmias.[195–198] The

studies of Wit and associates, using 192 simultaneous recordings from various epicardial sites, also indicate that reentry is the most likely mechanism of these induced ventricular beats.[191] Regarding the site of origin of these induced tachycardias, these authors suggest that the nonsustained form of tachycardia occurred on the anterior left ventricle at the border of the infarcted region and in epicardial muscle surviving over the infarcted region because circuitous conduction patterns in the epicardial muscle was demonstrated. In contrast, however, during the sustained form of induced tachycardia, circuitous conduction pattern leading to reentry was not seen in the surviving epicardial muscle, implying the involvement of other sites.[167,191] The studies by Kramer and associates indicate that intramural cells in the infarcted left ventricle may constitute the site of origin of these reentrant ventricular tachycardias in dogs.[199] Cooling of the reentrant circuits involved in the maintenance of induced tachycardia on the epicardial surface abruptly terminated the arrhythmia.[185,200] In a newer study, Dillon and coworkers (using 192 epicardial recording sites) suggest that during the chronic phase of infarction, ventricular tachycardia induced by electric stimulation may be caused by the anisotropic tissue structure on the epicardial site, irrespective of dispersion of refractory periods.[192] These authors propose that the parallel orientation of muscle bundles at the epicardial border zone may be the site of functional conduction block because activation transverse to myocardial fiber is sufficiently slow to permit recovery and the occurrence of reentry.[192] The role of surviving subendocardial fibers overlying isolated right ventricular infarction was investigated by Sugi and associates.[201] The cellular electrophysiologic properties of the surviving network remained unchanged and were independent of temporal changes of tachycardia inducibility.[201] Perhaps, as in the left-sided ventricular infarction, both epicardial border zone and intramural sites may be involved in the inducibility of ventricular tachyarrhythmias during the chronic phase of myocardial infarction and ischemia.

The transmembrane potential properties of surviving epicardial muscle cells, manifesting depressed action potential properties and slowed conduction velocity, can offer adequate explanation for some of the reentrant beats induced at this particular site. The cellular electrophysiologic basis and the precise anatomic location of induced ventricular beats not occurring at the epicardial surface remain to be determined, as in the case of induced sustained ventricular tachycardia. Earlier studies of El-Sherif and associates, using composite electrodes to record from large areas of epicardium, interpreted the presence of continuous electric activity bridging the entire cardiac cycle during tachycardia as evidence that reentry was occurring, even though the sequence of electric activation of the ventricle was not determined.[202,203] Wit and associates, however, suggest that such electric activity recorded at a given site should not be taken as evidence for reentry.[38,191] These authors presented evidence from simultaneous multiple recordings and isochronal map construction that electric activity could be recorded during the entire cardiac cycle in the absence of obvious reentry at that site.[191] Similar findings were also made by Janse and associates during the early postocclusion period.[34] Therefore, it seems reasonable—as suggested by Wit and associates and shown in isolated endocardial preparations—*not* to accept the occurrence of continuous electric activity as proof of reentry, although such activity should be present in an area where reentry is occurring.[38,76,191]

The issue sympathetic denervation supersensitivity of ventricular refractoriness and the ease of inducibility of ventricular arrhythmias during sympathetic stimulation in denervated ventricle was raised.[204,205] Supersensitivity in the area apical to transmural myocardial infarction was manifest by an exaggerated shortening of effective refractory period during infusion with catecholamines.[204] Such a differential change in the refractoriness may enhance non-uniform ventricular recovery and may cause reentrant arrhythmias.[193,195,205]

Clinical Implication

A cardiac mapping study in patients (in the operating room) having chronic ischemic heart disease and sustained ventricular tachycardia suggests that reentry may be a mechanism for the VT (see Table 18-1).[206] By simultaneously recording from 64 endocardial sites during tachycardias, De Bakker and associates,[206] suggest that the apparent focal origin of reentrant tachycardia may be caused by exit from a circuitous pathway that consists of two separated zones of surviving myocardium (Fig. 18-21). One of these zones being the tract of surviving myocardial fibers at the border of the infarction, and the second being the subendocardial muscle mass. This study confirms that at least some of the ventricular tachycardias, occurring during the chronic phase of myocardial infarction are

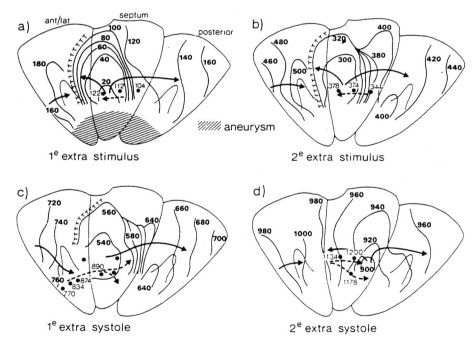

Figure 18-21. Activation patterns of four beats in the induction phase of a ventricular tachycardia induced in a patient with medically intractable arrhythmias. (**A** and **B**) Activation maps of the last two stimulated complexes. (**C** and **D**) Activation sequences of the first two spontaneously occurring beats. Isochrones are in milliseconds and are timed with respect to the first extrastimulus. *Arrows with solid lines* indicate spread of endocardial activation. *Arrows with dashed lines* indicate spread of secondary activation fronts, the signals of which are recorded at the *black dots; numbers next to the dots* indicate activation times in milliseconds. The first spontaneously occurring extrasystole (**C**) arises from macroreentry through the subendocardial muscle. The second and following ectopic beats are also due to macroreentry but this time, return of activation toward the site of earliest endocardial activation occurs by isolated pathways of surviving muscle fibers. (De Bakker JMT, Van Capelle FJL, Janse MJ, et al: Reentry as a cause of ventricular tachycardia in patients with chronic ischemic heart disease: electrophysiological and anatomic correlation. Circulation 1988; 77:589.)

caused by reentry, as in the canine model of chronic infarction. Endocardial site of origin for reentrant ventricular tachycardia (macroreentry) in the infarcted human heart was emphasized by De Bakker and colleagues.[207] These investigators found that human tachycardia is based on reentry in a macrocircuit comprising a tract of surviving tissue traversing the infarct and the remaining healthy tissue. The absence of late potentials during sinus rhythm does not guarantee the absence of arrhythmogenic pathways.[207] In addition to an endocardial site for reentry in human infarcted ventricles, intramural and epicardial sites of origin for reentrant ventricular tachycardias in the human infarcted ventricles are also suggested.[208, 209] The characteristics of premature stimulus for the induction of ventricular tachycardia and ventricular fibrillation in humans appear to be related to the presence of late potentials.[210] The coupling intervals of the premature stimulus needed to induce ventricular tachycardia or fibrillation are longer in patients with than in those without an abnormal signal-averaged ECG.[210] More studies of this nature are needed in humans to further refine the microstructural basis of reentrant tachycardias. Furthermore, the role of nonuniformity in activation and excitability of a chronically infarcted left ventricle in the susceptibility to inducible ventricular tachycardia in humans is also emphasized.[211] As in the canine model, the greater the dispersion of total recovery times, the greater the occurrence of tachycardia inducibility.[193, 195, 211, 212] In another clinical study involving patients with myocardial infarction, as the infarct aged from 2 to 20 weeks, the inducibility of ventricular tachycardia was reduced.[213] This suggests, as in the canine model, that the changing pattern of the cellular electrophysiologic properties of affected myocardial cells changes the inducibility of ventricular tachycardia as infarct ages. Functional evidence of slow conduction at infarcted endocardial sites showing fractionated electric activity in patients who have chronic myocardial infarction and are susceptible to inducible ventricular tachycardia is presented by Stevenson and co-

workers.[231] Pacing from areas with fractionated activity was associated with longer stimulus-QRS durations. The potential important contribution of stimulus-latency was not evaluated in this study.[231]

Almost all the cellular electrophysiologic abnormalities seen in the canine model of myocardial infarction were also observed in chronic infarcted and ischemic tissues isolated from human ventricular myocardium. This indicates that the cellular electrophysiologic mechanisms of ventricular tachyarrhythmias in humans may be analogous to canine ischemic ventricular arrhythmias.

Spear and associates recorded transmembrane potentials from cardiac fibers on the endocardial surface of preparations isolated from human infarcts and aneurysms (Fig. 18-22).[214] Although some of these potentials appear to be characteristic of Purkinje fibers, others may have been recorded from ventricular muscle cells. Some of the surviving fibers manifest phase 4 depolarization and automatic impulse initiation. These action potentials conducted slowly and were sensitive to verapamil. Furthermore, variable-amplitude action potentials—ranging from normal, fast-depressed, and slow-response—were present in these aneurysmal tissues. These authors suggest that the heterogenous electrophysiologic profile of these surviving cells may lead to ventricular tachyarrhythmias in these patients.[214] Dangman and colleagues demonstrated that human Purkinje fibers, isolated from the hearts of five patients undergoing cardiac transplantation, manifested DAD and triggered automaticity when exposed to ouabain and catecholamine, suggesting that triggered automatic mechanism can also occur in human ventricle.[215]

Pharmacologic Considerations

The response of inducible ventricular tachyarrhythmias to antiarrhythmic drugs during the chronic phase of myocardial infarction (phase 3) differs from that seen during 24-

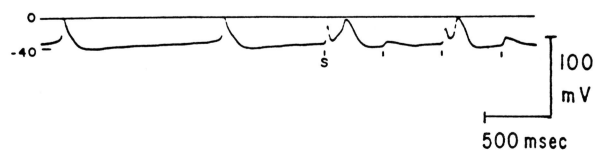

Figure 18-22. Transmembrane potentials recorded from the endocardial surface of a human infarct. At the left, the fiber is spontaneously active and phase 4 depolarization is evident. At S, stimulation at a basic cycle length of 450 milliseconds is begun. The first and third stimuli excite the fiber. From these records, it is not possible to determine whether this is a Purkinje fiber or a ventricular muscle fiber. (Spear JF, Horowitz LN, Hodess AB, et al: Cellular electrophysiology of human myocardial infarction. I. Abnormalities of cellular activation. Circulation 1979;59:247.)

hour spontaneous ventricular arrhythmias. The chronic-phase tachyarrhythmia often manifests resistance to most pharmacologic agents.[155,180,216,217] This is in sharp contrast to the 24-hour arrhythmias, which were ultimately controlled by a given antiarrhythmic agent (see Table 18-1).[155-157,159] The cause or causes of refractoriness to drugs remain largely undefined. In broadest terms, it is not known whether the drug fails to reach the arrhythmic site and adjoining myocardial region in sufficiently high concentration (four to 10 times that of serum levels) or whether refractoriness is a property of the site itself, relatively independent of drug concentration.[218] The results obtained by Karagueuzian and associates indicate that raising the myocardial concentration of procainamide by close coronary injection terminates an established induced sustained ventricular tachycardia (Fig. 18-23) and prevents its reinducibility (Fig. 18-24).[219] These tachycardias were otherwise resistant to procainamide when given intravenously (see Figs. 18-23 and 18-24). In these studies, procainamide was injected through a specially designed autoinflatable balloon catheter in the great cardiac vein in dogs 3 to 8 days after permanent occlusion of the LAD coronary artery.[219] Procainamide administered by the great cardiac vein (5 to 20 mg/kg) was more effective that intravenous procainamide (35 mg/kg) in preventing and terminating inducible tachycardias (see Figs. 18-23 and 18-24). Procainamide given by the great cardiac vein had 15 to 20 times higher myocardial procainamide concentration than that obtained after intravenous injection. The need for excess levels of plasma steady-state disopyramide to terminate inducible ventricular tachyarrhythmia during the chronic phase of infarction in the canine heart was demonstrated by Patterson and associates.[220] It was also interesting to note that bretylium was fairly effective in suppressing inducible ventricular tachycardia in the canine model, an effect that may be at least partly caused by the ability of bretylium to concentrate in the myocardium and achieve myocardial levels 14 times higher than in plasma levels.[221,222] It is tempting to suggest that the greater efficacy of amiodarone in suppressing ventricular tachyarrhythmias (sevenfold higher in the right ventricle than in plasma) may be related to the ability of this drug to be concentrated in the myocardium.[223] Elevation of myocardial drug concentration alone may not be sufficient to terminate the arrhythmia, however. It appears that a preferential increase of drug concentration at critical myocardial sites (based on the site of origin of the arrhythmia) or at low-pressure hypoperfused sites (which usually occur with great cardiac vein injection in a setting of myocardial ischemia) may be important determinant factors of whether the arrhythmia will be suppressed.[219,224] These consideration, however, need further clarification and experimental verification. In a newer study, Meesmann and associates failed to demonstrate beneficial effects of both systemic and great cardiac vein retroinfusion of various cholinergic agents against inducible ventricular tachycardia in a conscious canine model of chronic myocardial ischemia and infarction.[253]

It is important to note that many similarities exist in the response to antiarrhythmic drugs in experimental and clinical settings. In patients with ischemic heart disease, Myerburg and associates observed that higher levels of plasma procainamide concentrations were needed to control ventricular arrhythmias during the chronic phase of myocardial infarction than during the acute phase, indicating (as in canine models) a different mechanism or different site operative for arrhythmia induction during various phases of myocardial infarction.[225] Furthermore, in other studies it was found that inducible ventricular tachyarrhythmias often manifest resistance to both standard and new antiarrhythmic agents. In five reports totaling 250 patients (most of whom had coronary artery disease and ventricular aneurysm), refractoriness to drugs ranged from 9.5% to 47.5% (mean, 26.3%).[226-230] This response appears to differ from the response of ventricular tachyarrhythmias seen during the acute in-hospital phase, in which most ventricular arrhythmias can ultimately be controlled.

NONLINEAR DYNAMICS AND VENTRICULAR ARRHYTHMIAS

The experimental demonstration that cardiac excitability, cardiac impulse propagation, and cardiac automaticity manifest beat-to-beat variability in the response pattern that is nonlinear with respect to time has prompted a whole new perspective in the understanding of ventricular stability and its vulnerability to various rhythm disorders, including ventricular fibrillation.[28,232-236] It is proposed that such temporal changes, which usually occur under abnormal conditions, be called dynamic diseases (i.e., abnormal temporal organization).[8] The importance and diagnostic, prognostic, and therapeutic usefulness of time-dependent behavior, in both experimental and clinical settings, are based on the general premise that variations—or more correctly, transitions from one dynamic state to another—follow a well-defined rule that is characteristic of the nonlinear system in question. Glass and Mackey propose three types of qualitative changes in dynamics that all have actually been observed: (1) the appearance of regular oscillation in a physiologic control system that is otherwise absent under normal conditions, (2) new periodicities that may arise in an already periodic process, and (3) the disappearance of periodicities and their replacement by constant dynamics or, perhaps more importantly, by aperiodic (chaotic) dynamics.[8] The relevance of such dynamic behavior to the genesis of reentrant premature ventricular excitation follows. First, the electro-

EFFECT OF GCV PROCAINAMIDE
ON ESTABLISHED INDUCED SUSTAINED VENTRICULAR TACHYCARDIA

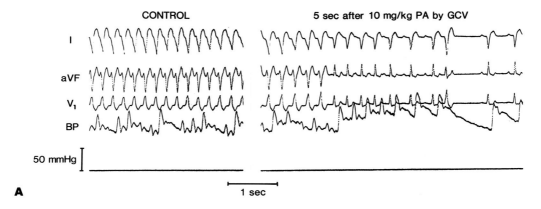

EFFECT OF I.V. PROCAINAMIDE ON ESTABLISHED
INDUCED SUSTAINED VENTRICULAR TACHYCARDIA

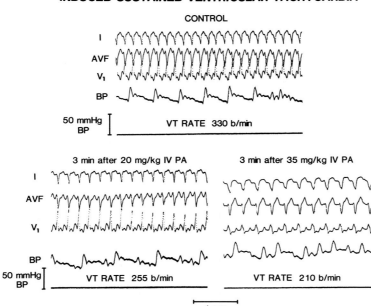

Figure 18-23. Termination of established monomorphic sustained ventricular tachycardia by the administration of 10 mg/kg of procainamide (*PA*) into the great cardiac vein (*GCV*) in a dog 6 days after permanent left anterior descending coronary artery occlusion (*left panel*). In the *right panel*, the last 4 seconds of the tachycardia is shown, just before tachycardia termination and resumption of normal sinus rhythm. In each panel *I, aV$_F$* and V$_1$ are electrocardiographic leads. AoP is aortic blood pressure with 50 mmHg calibration. (**B**) Inability of intravenous procainamide (35 mg/kg) to terminate established induced sustained ventricular tachycardia in a dog 6 days after permanent left anterior descending coronary artery occlusion. *Top panel* (control) shows monomorphic sustained ventricular tachycardia (*VT*) 3 minutes after administration of 20 mg/kg intravenous (IV) procainamide (*PA*) (*bottom left panel*); the rate of the tachycardia was decreased from 330 to 255 beats/min. An additional 20 mg/kg (total, 35 mg/kg) of procainamide further decreased the tachycardia rate (210 beats/min) without termination. (Karagueuzian HS, Ohta M, Drury KJ, et al: Coronary venous retroinfusion of procainamide: a new approach for the management of spontaneous and inducible sustained ventricular tachycardia during myocardial infarction. J Am Coll Cardiol 1986;7:551.)

EFFECT OF CORONARY RETROVENOUS INFUSION OF PROCAINAMIDE ON INDUCIBLE SUSTAINED VENTRICULAR TACHYCARDIA

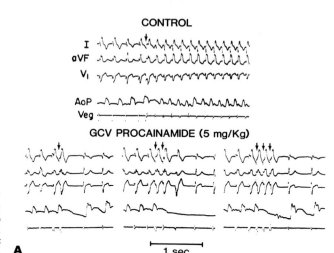

EFFECT OF INTRAVENOUS PROCAINAMIDE ON INDUCIBLE SUSTAINED VENTRICULAR TACHYCARDIA

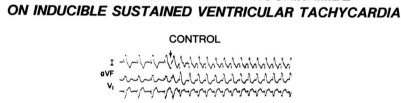

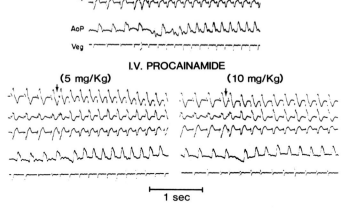

Figure 18-24. (**A**) Induction of sustained ventricular tachycardia with a single premature stimulation (*arrow*) during regular ventricular drive in a dog 5 days after left anterior descending coronary occlusion (control, *top panel*). After the interruption of tachycardia by ventricular overdrive (not shown), 5 mg/kg of procainamide injected into the great cardiac vein (*GCV*) (*bottom panels*) prevented reinduction of ventricular tachycardia by single, double, and triple extrastimuli (*arrows*). VEg, right ventricular electrogram; other abbreviations as in Figure 18-23. (**B**) Induction of sustained ventricular tachycardia with a single premature stimulus (*arrow*) during regular ventricular drive in a dog 5 days after permanent left anterior descending artery occlusion (*top panel*, control) and 3 hours after great cardiac vein injection of procainamide. After interruption of the tachycardia by ventricular overdrive (not shown), 5 mg/kg of procainamide was administered intravenously (*I.V.*); tachycardia, however, was still inducible, although at a slower rate (*bottom left panel*). Despite an additional 10 mg/kg of procainamide (total, 15 mg/kg), tachycardia was again induced with a single premature stimulus (*arrow; bottom right panel*). Abbreviations as in Figure 18-23. (Karagueuzian HS, Ohta M, Drury KJ, et al: Coronary venous retroinfusion of procainamide: a new approach for the management of spontaneous and inducible sustained ventricular tachycardia during myocardial infarction. J Am Coll Cardial 1986;7:551.)

physiologic properties of the ventricular myocardium manifest typical nonlinear response patterns when subjected to stress (i.e., fast rates of drive; catecholamine ischemia; drug intoxication), as in other nonlinear physical systems.[7,8,25,26,28,236–239,240,241,246] These include period-two alternans (also known in the jargon of nonlinear dynamics as *period-doubling bifurcation*) and higher-order periodicities, finally terminating in an aperiodic dynamic state as the level of applied stress is continuously increased.[7,8,25,28,241] Second, an important mechanism of reentrant arrhythmias is thought to result from dispersion of

refractoriness, excitability, and conduction.[16,38,83,139,166,193,195] The concept of electrophysiologic heterogeneity has been an accepted tenet for the initiation of reentrant arrhythmias for a long time, and most of the newer experimental studies provide evidence to support this old idea. For example, the presence of electric alternans in both the QRS complexes and the ST-T wave was associated with greater incidence of inducible ventricular tachycardia in patients with ischemic heart disease.[237] This finding corroborated earlier clinical findings by Salerno and associates in patients with myocardial ischemia.[238] These authors

POST LAD OCCLUSION PERIODS

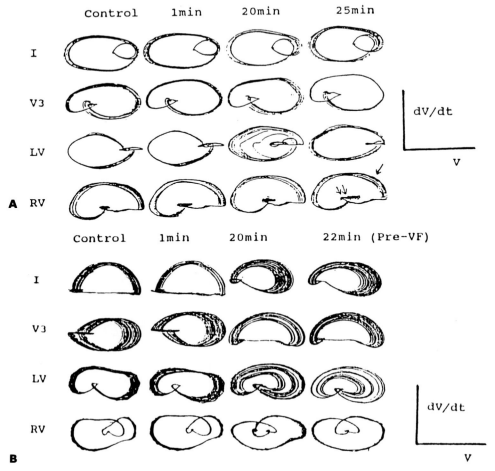

Figure 18-25. Phase plane plot (rate of change [dV/dt] versus volt [V]) of various electrocardiographic leads; *I, V₃,* bipolar left ventricular (*LV*), and right ventricular, (*RV*) electrograms respectively, in two dogs (**A** and **B**) at increasing time after complete occlusion of the left anterior descending (*LAD*) coronary artery. All recordings in both dogs are made in the closed-chest anesthetized state during sinus rhythm. (**A**) Left anterior descending occlusion with intracoronary balloon inflation for up to 1 hour failed to manifest ventricular fibrillation (*VF*). The trajectories at all recording sites show reasonable degree of homogeneity for depolarization (larger loops, *single arrow*) and repolarization (smaller loops, *double loops*). This indicates beat-to-beat homogenous electric response pattern.[8,25,254] In contrast, in the dog that degenerated to spontaneous VF at the 23rd minute postocclusion period (**B**), the surface electrocardiograms (*I* and *V₃*) and in particular, the LV bipolar electrograms from the left ventricular ischemic sites, manifest distinct dynamic characteristics (banding of the trajectories), indicative of temporal heterogeneity that is typically seen in stressed nonlinear dynamic systems.[8,25,254] In addition, the differential thickening of the trajectories is a sign of sensitive dependence on initial conditions, a hallmark of chaotic dynamics.[8,25,254] Note the absence of such dynamic behavior in the RV bipolar electrogram (a recording made near the outflow tract, remote from the ischemic LV site) as the trajectories remain tightly bound together throughout the entire duration of occlusion. See text for further discussion and significance for prediction and monitoring for ventricular electrical stability. (Karagueuzian HS, previously unpublished observations.)

suggest that ST-segment alternans should be considered a reliable marker of the possible occurrence of ventricular arrhythmias during myocardial ischemia.[238] That stress alone, (i.e., in our case, fast heart rate, with or without ischemia) can cause transient electric alternans was alluded to at the turn of the century by Lewis.[7] This was later documented to occur both in the dog model and in man, a phenomenon that clearly reflects the nonlinear dynamic property of the ventricle.[239, 240, 242] The simultaneous occurrence of fast heart rate and ischemia (greater stress) is bound to even further increase the degree of nonlinearity, causing the emergence of higher-order periodicities culminating in aperiodic dynamics (i.e., heterogeneity). Such a phenomenon in the ventricle may culminate in reentrant ventricular tachyarrhythmias. Experimental evidence demonstrates that the major determinants of ischemic ventricular tachycardia and ventricular fibrillation are directly linked to the intensity and size of the ischemic insult and to the heart rate.[42-44] The incidence of arrhythmias was greater with faster rates and more intense ischemia.[42-44] This was presumably caused by increased degrees of heterogeneity. Although direct experimental proof of such ventricular electric heterogeneity before the initiation of ventricular fibrillation is still lacking, our preliminary experimental data indicate that such heterogeneity may indeed be present during what appears to be a "normal sinus rhythm" destined to degenerate to ventricular fibrillation. Figure 18-25 depicts phase plane plots of various electrocardiographic leads recorded at increasing times after LAD coronary artery occlusion in two closed-chest anesthetized dogs. Phase plane plot is constructed by plotting dV/dt versus V (rate of change of voltage versus voltage) of the digitized signal of interest the same way left ventricular pressure dP/dt is plotted against pressure. Such a method of plot is often used in the study and analysis of dynamic systems.[234, 235, 244, 245, 253] The superimposition of 20 to 25 consecutive beats of normal sinus origin is shown in the two dogs. Note that the dog that does not develop ventricular fibrillation has homogenous profiles of ventricular depolarization and repolarization on all leads, as indicated by neatly packed trajectories in the phase plane plot. In contrast, the dog that developed ventricular fibrillation manifests highly irregular trajectories on the phase plane, especially in the left ventricular electrogram that is within the ischemic zone. This reflects a beat-to-beat electric heterogeneity that can be clearly appreciated and quantified by such a dynamic method of analysis. Furthermore, the effect of a given intervention on the degree of heterogeneity can be evaluated by comparing phase plane plots at specified pre- and postintervention intervals. The new method provides a new approach for evaluating cardiac electric stability during sinus rhythm, independent of ectopy or arrhythmias suppression. By comparing the geometry of the rhythms under various

conditions, one can determine the efficacy or lack thereof of a given intervention (pharmacologic or otherwise) with a reasonable degree of certainty.[8]

The usefulness of dynamic analysis in the analysis and characterization of atrial fibrillation has been demonstrated.[252] In a comprehensive review, Denton and associates describe the potential application of theory based on nonlinear dynamics (chaos) in cardiology and cardiac arrhythmias.[253] The future seems to hold much promise in this newly evolving field of nonlinear dynamics.

CONCLUSION

Although the experimental animal model of ischemic heart disease differs in many respects from its parallel in humans, it nevertheless has provided important information and improved clinicians' understanding of potentially lethal ventricular arrhythmias. Although the experimental work provides new insights into events in the clinical settings, many important questions raised in the clinical cardiac catheterization laboratory provide a stimulus for experimental work. We have outlined a few of these pathophysiologic and pharmacologic interrelations. Surely many more important discoveries are forthcoming. The nonlinear dynamic approach to the study of ventricular arrhythmias appears particularly promising.

References

1. Bruetsch WL: The earliest record of sudden death possibly due to atherosclerotic coronary occlusion. Circulation 1959;20:438.
2. Shattock SG: A report upon the pathologic condition of the aorta of King Menephtah, traditionally regarded as the pharaoh of the exodus. Proc R Soc Med 1908;2:122.
3. Chirac P: De motu cordis. Adversaria Analytica 1698:121. Cited by See, Bochefontaine, Roussy.
4. Ericksen JE: On the influence of the coronary circulation on the action of the heart. Lond Med Gaz 1842;2:561.
5. Porter WT: On the results of ligation of the coronary arteries. J Physiol 1894;15:121.
6. Lewis T: The experimental production of paroxysmal tachycardia and the effects of ligation of the coronary arteries. Heart 1909;1:98.
7. Lewis T: Notes upon alternation of the heart. Q J Med 1911;4:141.
8. Glass L, Mackey MC: From clocks to chaos. The rhythms of life. Princeton, NJ: Princeton University Press, 1988.
9. Robinson GC, Herrman GR: Paroxysmal tachycardia of ventricular origin, and its relation to coronary occlusion. Heart 1921;8:59.
10. Wiggers CJ, Wegria R, Pinera B: The effects of myocardial ischemia on fibrillation threshold-mechanism of sponta-

neous ventricular fibrillation following coronary artery occlusion. Am J Physiol 1941;133:651.

11. Harris AS: Delayed development of ventricular ectopic rhythms following experimental coronary occlusion. Circulation 1950;1:1318.

12. Harris AS, Bisteni A, Russel RA, et al: Excitatory factors in ventricular tachycardia resulting from myocardial ischemia. Potassium, a major excitant. Science 1954;119:200.

13. Gillum RF: Sudden coronary death in the United States. 1980–1985. Circulation 79:756.

14. Wit AL, Friedman PL: The basis for ventricular arrhythmias accompanying myocardial infarction: alterations in electrical activity of ventricular and Purkinje fibers after coronary artery occlusion. Arch Intern Med 1975;135:459.

15. Hill JL, Gettes LS: Effect of acute coronary artery occlusion on local myocardial extracellular K^+ activity in swine. Circulation 1980;61:768.

16. Downar E, Janse MJ, Durrer D: The effects of acute coronary artery occlusion on subepicardial transmembrane potentials in the intact porcine heart. Circulation 1977;56:217.

17. Coronel R, Fiolet JWT, Wims-Scopman FJG, et al: Distribution of extracellular potassium in relation to electrophysiologic changes during acute myocardial ischemia in the isolated perfused porcine heart. Circulation 1988;77:1125.

18. Coronel R, Fiolet JWT, Wilms-Schopman FJG, Opthof T, Schaapherder AFM, Janse JM: Distribution of extracellular potassium and electrophysiologic changes during two-stage coronary ligation in the isolated perfused canine heart. Circulation 1989;80:165.

19. Pelleg A, Mitamura H, Price R, Kaplinsky E, Menduke H, Dreifus LS, Michelson EL: Extracellular potassium ion dynamics and ventricular arrhythmias in the canine heart. J Am Coll Cardiol 1989;13:941.

20. David D, Michelson EL, Naito M, Dreifus LS, Schaffenburg M, Nielands J: Extracellular potassium dynamics in the border zone during acute myocardial ischemia in a canine model. J Am Coll Cardiol 1988;11:422.

21. Nichols CG, Lederer WJ: Adenosine triphosphate-sensitive potassium channels in the cardiovascular system. Am J Physiol 1991;261:H1675.

22. Wilde AAM, Escande D, Schumacher CA, Mestre TM, Fiolet JWT, Janse MJ: Potassium accumulation in globally ischemic mammalina heart. A role for the ATP-sensitive potassium channel. Circ Res 1990;67:835.

23. Venkatesh N, Stuart JS, Lamp ST, Alexander LD, Weiss JN: Activation of ATP-sensitive K^+ channels by cromakalim. Effects on cellular K^+ loss and cardiac function in ischemic and reperfused mammalian ventricle. Circ Res 1992;71:1324.

24. Kubota I, Yamaki M, Shibata T, Ikeno E, Hosoya Y, Tomoike H: Role of ATP-sensitive K^+ channel on ECG ST segment elevation during a bout of myocardial ischemia. A study on epicardial mapping in dogs. Circulation 1993;88:1845.

25. Chialvo DR, Jalife J: On the nonlinear equilibrium of the heart: Locking behavior and chaos in Purkinje fibers. In: Zipes DP, Jalife J, eds. Cardiac electrophysiology an cardiac arrhythmias. From the cell to bedside. Philadelphia: WB Saunders, 1990:201.

26. Delmar M, Michaels D, Jalife J: Slow recovery of excitability and Wenckebach phenomenon in the single guinea pig ventricular myocyte. Circ Res 1989;65:761.

27. Fujimoto T, Peter T, Hamamoto H, Mandel WJ: Electrophysiologic observations during the spontaneous initiation of ischemia induced ventricular fibrillation. Am Heart J 1983;105:189.

28. Dante RC, Jalife J: Non-linear dynamics of cardiac excitation and impulse propagation. Nature 1987;330:749.

29. Hamamoto H, Peter T, Mandel WJ: Characteristics of conduction of premature impulses during acute myocardial ischemia and reperfusion: a comparison of epicardial and endocardial activation. Circulation 1981;64:190.

30. Hamamoto H, Peter T, Fujimoto T, Mandel WJ: Characteristics of conduction of premature impulses during acute myocardial ischemia and reperfusion: a comparison between antegrade and retrograde activation. Am J Cardiol 1982;49:307.

31. Han J, Goel BG, Hanson CS: Re-entrant beats induced in the ventricle during coronary occlusion. Am Heart J 1970;80:778.

32. Fujimoto T, Hamamoto H, Peter T, Mandel WJ: Relation between conduction delay and ventricular fibrillation: characteristics of conduction of premature impulses during acute myocardial ischemia. Am J Cardiol 1981;48:287.

33. Meesmann W: Early arrhythmias and primary ventricular fibrillation after acute myocardial ischemia in relation to pre-existing coronary collaterals. In: Parratt JR, ed. Early arrhythmias resulting from myocardial ischemia. London: McMillan, 1982:93.

34. Janse MJ, van Capelle FJ, Morsink H, et al: Flow of injury current and patterns of excitation during early ischemia in isolated porcine and canine hearts. Evidence for two different arrhythmogenic mechanisms. Circ Res 1980;47:151.

35. Janse MJ, Kleber AG: Electrophysiological changes and ventricular arrhythmias in the early phase of regional myocardial ischemia. Circ Res 1981;49:1069.

36. Waldo AL, Kaiser GA: A study of ventricular arrhythmias associated with acute myocardial infarction in the canine heart. Circulation 1973;47:1222.

37. Williams DO, Scherlag BJ, Hope RR, et al: The pathophysiology of malignant ventricular arrhythmias during acute myocardial ischemia. Circulation 1974;50:1163.

38. Wit AL, Cranefield PL: Reentrant excitation as a cause of cardiac arrhythmias. Am J Physiol 1978;235:H1.

39. Ceremuzynaki L, Staszewska-Barczak J, Herbaezynska-Cedro K: Cardiac rhythm disturbances and the release of catecholamines after acute coronary occlusion in dogs. Cardiovasc Res 1969;3:190.

40. Tennant R, Wiggers CJ: The effect of coronary occlusion on myocardial contraction. Am J Physiol 1935;112:351.

41. Kleber AG, Riegger CB, Janse MJ: Electrical uncoupling and increase of extracellular resistance after induction of ischemia in isolated, arterially perfused rabbit papillary muscle. Circ Res 1987;61:271.

42. Hiramatsu Y, Buchanan JW Jr, Knisley SB, Koch GG, Kropp S, Gettes LS: Influence of rate-dependent cellular uncoupling on conduction change during simulated ischemia in guinea pig papillary muscles: effect of verapamil. Circ Res 1989;65:95.

43. Balke CW, Lesh MD, Spear JF, Kadish A, Levine JH, Moore EN: Effects of cellular uncoupling on conduction in anisotropic canine ventricular myocardium. Circ Res 1988;63:879.

44. Kabell G: Modulation of conduction slowing in ischemic

rabbit myocardium by calcium-channel activation and blockade. Circulation 1988;7:1385.

45. Fleet WF, Johnson TA, Graebner CA Engle CL, Gettes LS: Effects of verapamil on ischemia-induced changes in extracellular K^+, pH, and local activation in the pig. Circulation 1986;73:837.

46. Lederman SN, Wenger TL, Harrell FE, Strauss HC: Effects of different paced heart rates on canine coronary occlusion and reperfusion arrhythmias. Am Heart J 1987;113:1365.

47. Bolli R, Fisher DJ, Entman ML: Factors that determine the occurrence of arrhythmias during acute myocardial ischemia. Am Heart J 1986;111:261.

48. Scherlag BJ, El-Sherif N, Hope R, Lazzara R: Characterization and localization of ventricular arrhythmias resulting from myocardial ischemia and infarction. Circ Res 1974;35:372.

49. Garan H, McComb JM, Ruskin JN: Spontaneous and electrically induced ventricular arrhythmias during acute ischemia superimposed on 2 week old canine myocardial infarction. J Am Coll Cardiol 1988;11:603.

50. Sakai T, Ogawa S, Miyazaki T, et al: Electrophysiological effects of acute ischemia on electrically stable myocardial infarction. Cardiovasc Res 1989;23:169.

51. Priori SG, Yamada KA, Corr PB: Influence of hypoxia on adrenergic modulation of triggered activity in isolated adult canine myocytes. Circulation 1991;83:248.

52. Molina-Viamonte V, Anyukhovsky EP, Rosen MR: An alpa-1 adrenergic receptor subtype is responsible for delayed afterdepoalrizations and triggered activity during simulated ischemia and reperfusion of isolated canine Purkinje fibers. Circulation 1991;84:1732.

53. Kurien VA, Yates PA, Oliver MF: The role of free fatty acids in the production of ventricular arrhythmias after acute coronary artery occlusion. Eur J Clin Invest 1971;1:225.

54. Katzung B: Electrically induced automaticity in ventricular myocardium. Life Sci 1974;14:1133.

55. Cranefield PE: The conduction of the cardiac impulse. Mt. Kisco, NY: Futura Publishing, 1975.

56. Katzung BG: Effects of extracellular calcium and sodium on depolarization induced automaticity in guinea pig papillary muscle. Circ Res 1975;37:118.

57. Katzung BG, Hondeghem LM, Grant AO: Cardiac ventricular automaticity induced by current of injury. Pflugers Arch 1975;360:193.

58. Kleber AG, Janse MJ, van Capelle FJL, Durrer D: Mechanism and time course of S-T and T-Q segment changes during acute regional myocardial ischemia in the pig heart determined by extracellular and intracellular recordings. Circ Res 1978;42:603.

59. Katzung BG, Morgenstern JA: Effects of extracellular potassium on ventricular automaticity and evidence for a pacemaker current in mammalian ventricular myocardium. Circ Res 1977;40:105.

60. Kleber AG, Riegger CB, Janse MJ: Electrical uncoupling and increase of extracellular resistance after induction of ischemia in isolated, arterially perfused rabbit papillary muscle. Circ Res 1987;61:271.

61. Coraboeuf E, Deroubaix E, Coulombe A: Acidosis-induced abnormal repolarization and repetitive activity in isolated dog Purkinje fibers. J Physiol (Paris) 1980;76:97.

62. Rozanki GJ, Witt RC: Early afterdeplarization and triggered activity in rabbit cardiac Purkinje fibers recovering from ischemic-like conditions. Role of acidosis. Circulation 1991; 83:1352.

63. Riegger CB, Alperovich G, Kleber AG: Effect of oxygen withdrawal on active and passive electrical properties of arterially perfused rabbit ventricular muscle. Circ Res 1989; 64:532.

64. Khuri SF, Flaherty JT, O'Riordan J, et al: Changes in intramyocardial ST segment voltage and gas tensions with regional myocardial ischemia in the dog. Circ Res 1975;37:455.

65. Hoffman BF, Rosen ME: Cellular mechanisms for cardiac arrhythmias. Circ Res 1981;49:1.

66. Wit AL, Cranefield PL: Triggered activity in cardiac muscle fibers of the simian mitral valve. Circ Res 1976;38:85.

67. Tsien RW, Kass RS, Weingart R: Cellular and subcellular mechanisms of cardiac pacemaker oscillation. J Exp Biol 1979;81:205.

68. Karagueuzian HS, Katzung BA: Voltage-clamp studies of transient inward current and mechanical oscillations induced by ouabain in ferret papillary muscle. J Physiol 1982; 327:255.

69. Matsuda H, Noma A, Kurachi Y, Irisawa H: Transient depolarization and spontaneous voltage fluctuations in isolated single cells from guinea pig ventricles. Calcium-mediated membrane potential fluctuations. Circ Res 1982;51:142.

70. De Mello WC: Intercellular communication in cardiac muscle. Circ Res 1982;51:1.

71. Coetzee WA, Opie LH: Effects of components of ischemia and metabolic inhibition on delayed afterdepolarizations in guinea pig papillary muscle. Circ Res 1987;61:157.

72. Pogwizd SM, Onufer JR, Kramer JB, Sobel BE, Corr PB: Induction of delayed afterdepolarizations and triggered activity in canine Purkinje fibers by lysophosphogycerides. Circ Res 1986;59:416.

73. Clusin WT, Bristow MR, Karagueuzian HS, et al: Do calcium-dependent ionic currents mediate ischemic ventricular fibrillation. Am J Cardiol 1982;49:606.

74. Hiramatsu Y, Buchanan JW, Knisley SB, Koch GG, Kropp S, Gettes LS: Influence of rate-dependent cellular uncoupling on conduction change during simulated ischemia in guinea pig papillary muscles: effects of verapamil. Circ Res 1989; 65:95.

75. Tseng GN: Calcium current restitution in mammalian ventricular myocytes is modulated by intracellular calcium. Circ Res 1988;63:468.

76. Ino T, Karagueuzian HS, Meesmann M, McCullen A, Mandel WJ, Peter T: Mutiple cellular electrophysiologic correlates of low amplitude fracionated activity in bipolar electrograms. (Abstract) Circulation 1986;74:(Suppl)II:II.

77. Lown B, Verrier RL: Neural activity and ventricular fibrillation. N Engl J Med 1976;104:1165.

78. Cinca J, Bardaji A, Caudevillaa AS: Ventricular arrhythmias and local electrograms after chronic regional denervation of the ischemic area in the pig heart. J Am Coll Cardiol 1989;11:414.

79. Puddu PE, Jouve R, Langlet F, Guillen JC, Lanti M, Reale A: Prevention of postischemic ventricular fibrillation late after right or left stellate ganglionectomy in dogs. Circulation 1988;77:935.

80. Priori SG, Mantica M, Schwartz PJ: Delayed afterdepolariza-

tions eleicited in vivo by left stellate ganglion stimulation. Circulation 78:178.

81. Corr PB, Yamada KA, Witkowsky FX: Mechanisms controlling cardiac autonomic function and their relation to arrhythmogenesis. In: Fozzard HA, Haber E, Jennings RB, Katz AM, Morgan HE, eds. The heart and the cardiovascular system. New York: Raven Press, 1986:1343.

82. Schwartz PJ, Motolese M, Pollovini G, Malliani A, Bartorelli C, Zanchetti A: Surgical and pharmacological antiadrenergic interventions in the prevention of sudden death after a first myocardial infarction. Circulation 1985;72:(Suppl III):III.

83. Bigger JT Jr, Dresdale RJ, Heissenbuttel RH, et al: Ventricular arrhythmias in ischemic heart disease: Mechanism, prevalence, significance, and management. Cardiovasc Dis 1977; 19:255.

84. Balke CW, Kaplinsky EL, et al: Reperfusion ventricular tachyarrhythmias: Correlation with antecedent coronary artery occlusion tachyarrhythmias and duration of myocardial ischemia. Am Heart J 1981;101:449.

85. Jennings RB, Sommers HM, Smyth GA, et al: Myocardial nectrosis induced by temporary occlusion of a coronary artery in the dog. Arch Pathol 1960;70:68.

86. Austin M, Wanger TL, Harrell FE Jr, et al: Effect of myocardium at risk on outcome after coronary artery occlusion and release. Am J Physiol 1982;243:H340.

87. Corbalan R, Verrier RL, Lown B: Differing mechanisms for ventricular vulnerability during coronary artery occlusion and release. Am Heart J 1976;92:223.

88. Pogwizd SM, Corr PB: Electrophysiologic mechanisms underlying arrhythmias due to reperfusion of ischemic myocardium. Circulation 1987;76:404.

89. Bernier M, Hearse DJ, Manning AS: Reperfusion-induced arrhythmias and oxygen-derived free radicals: studies with "anti-free radical" interventions and a free radical generating system in the isolated perfused rat heart. Circ Res 1986; 58:331.

90. Parratt JR, Wainwright CL: Failure of allopurinol and a spin trapping agent N-t-butyl-alpha-phenylnitrone to modify significantly ischaemia- and reperfusion-induced arrhythmias. Br J Pharmacol 1987;91:49.

91. Podzuweit T, Braun W, Muller A, Schaper W: Arrhythmias and infarction in the ischemic pig heart are not mediated by xanthine oxidase-derived free oxygen radicals. Basic Res Cardiol 1987;82:493.

92. Hearse DJ, Kusama Y, Bernier M: Rapid electrophysiological changes leading to arrhythmias in the aerobic rat heart. Circ Res 1989;65:146.

93. Karagueuzian HS, Pennec JP, Deroubaix E, de Leiris J, Corabeuf E: Effects of excess free acids on the electrophysiological properties of ventricular specialized conducting tissue. A comparative study between the sheep and the dog. J Cardiovasc Pharmacol 1982;4:462.

94. Bolli R, Patel B: Factors that determine the occurrence of reperfusion arrhythmias. Am Heart J 1988;115:20.

95. Penny WJ, Sheridan DJ: Arrhythmias and cellular electrophysiological changes during myocardial "ischemia" and reperfusion. Cardiovasc Res 1983;17:363.

96. Bolli R, Fisher DJ, Entman ML: Factors that determine the occurrence of arrhythmias during acute myocardial ischemia. Am Heart J 1986;111:261.

97. Akiyama T: Intracellular recording of in situ ventricular cells during ventricular fibrillation. Am J Physiol 1981;240:H465.

98. Ten Eick R, Singer DH, Solberg LE: Coronary occlusion. Effect on cellular electrical activity of the heart. Med Clin North Am 1976;60:49.

99. Ferrier GR, Moffat MP, Lukas A: Possible mechanisms of arrhythmias elicited by ischemia followed by reperfusion. Studies on isolated canine ventricular tissues. Circ Res 1985; 56:184.

100. Levine HJ, Avitall B, Pauker SG, Naimi S: Sequential unipolar strength-interval curves and conduction times during myocardial ischemia and reperfusion in the dog. Circ Res 1978; 43:63.

101. Elharrar V, Foster PR, Tirak TL, et al: Alterations in canine myocardial excitability during ischemia. Circ Res 1977; 40:98.

102. Lazzara R, El Sherif N, Hope RR, Scherlag HJ: Ventricular arrhythmias and electrophysiological consequences of myocardial ischemia and infarction. Circ Res 1978;42:740.

103. Lazzara R, El Sherif N, Schlerlag HJ: Disorders of cellular electrophysiology produced by ischemia of the canine His bundle. Circ Res 1975;36:444.

104. Penkoske PA, Sobel BE, Corr PB: Disparate electrophysiological alterations accompanying dysrhythmia due to coronary occlusion and reperfusion in the cat. Circulation 1978; 58:1023.

105. Podzuweit T, Binz KH, Nennstiel P, Flaig W: The antiarrhythmic effects of myocardial ischaemia. Relation to reperfusion arrhythmias. Cardiovasc Res 1989;23:81.

106. Coker SJ, Parratt JE: Prostacyclin-antiarrhythmic or arrhythmogenic? Comparison of the effects of intravenous and intracoronary prostacyclin and ZK36374 during coronary artery occlusion and reperfusion in anesthetized greyhounds. J Cardiovasc Pharmacol 1983;5:557.

107. Vatner SF, Patrick TA, Knight DR, Manders WT, Fallon JT: Effects of calcium channel blocker on responses of blood flow, function, arrhythmias, extent of infarction following reperfusion in conscious baboons. Circ Res 1988;62:105.

108. Hearse DJ, Tosake A: Free radicals and reperfusion-induced arrhythmias: Protection by spin trap agent PBN in the rat heart. Circ Res 1987;60:375.

109. Kimura S, Bassett AL, Saoudi NC, Cameron JS, Kozlovskis PL, Myerburg RJ: Cellular electrophysiologic changes and "arrhythmias" during experimental ischemia and reperfusion in isolated cat ventricular myocardium. J Am Coll Cardiol 1986;7:833.

110. Karagueuzian HS, Liu ZW, Yao F, Fishbein MC, Mandel WJ: Suppression of reperfusion ventricular fibrillation by metoprolol-quinidine combination. Rev Biomed Int 1990;12:69. Abstract.

111. Tosaki A, Hellegouarch A: Adenosine triphosphate-sensitive potassium channel blocking agent ameliorates, but the opening agent aggravates ischemia/reperfusion-induced injury. Heart function studies in nonfibrillating isolated hearts. J Am Coll Cardiol 1994;23:487.

112. Grover GJ, McCullough JR, Henry DE, Conder ML, Sleph PG: Anti-ischemic effects of the potassium channel activators Pinacidil and Cromakalim and the reversal of these effects with the potassium channel blocker gyburide. J Pharmacol Exp Ther 1989;251:98.

113. Wit AL, Bigger JT Jr: Electrophysiology of ventricular arrhythmias accompanying myocardial ischemia and infarction. Postgrad Med J 1977;53(Suppl):98.

114. Wenger TL, Browning DJ, Masterton CE, et al: Procainamide delivery to ischemic canine myocardium following rapid intravenous administration. Circ Res 1980;46:789.

115. Zito RA, Caride VJ, Holford T, et al: Regional myocardial lidocaine concentration following continuous intravenous infusion early and late after myocardial infarction. Am J Cardiol 1982;50:497.

116. Kupersmith J, Antman EM, Hoffman BF: In vivo electrophysiological effects of lidocaine in canine acute myocardial infarction. Circ Res 1975;36:84.

117. Nattel S, Pederson DH, Zipes DP: Alterations in regional myocardial distribution and arrhythmogenic effects of aprinidine produced by coronary artery occlusion in the dog. Cardiovasc Res 1981;15:80.

118. Bekheit S, Isber N, Jani H, Butros G, Boutjdir M, El-Sherif N: Reduction of ishemia-induced electrophysiologic abnormalities by glucose-insulin infusion. J Am Coll Cardiol 1993; 22:1214.

119. Naito M, Michelson EL, Kmetzo JJ, et al: Failure of antiarrhythmic drugs to prevent experimental reperfusion ventricular fibrillation. Circulation 1981;63:70.

120. Rosenfeld J, Rosen MR, Hoffman BF: Pharmacologic and behavioral effects on arrhythmias that immediately follow abrupt coronary occlusion: a canine model of sudden coronary death. Am J Cardiol 1978;41:1075.

121. Wenger TL, Lederman S, Starmer FC, et al: A method for quantitating anti-fibrillatory effects of drugs after coronary reperfusion in dogs: improved outcome with bretylium. Circulation 1984;69:142.

122. Meerbaum S, Lang TW, Povzhitkov M, et al: Retrograde lysis of coronary artery thrombus by coronary venous streptokinase administration. J Am Coll Cardiol 1983;1:1262.

123. Corday E, Meerbaum S: Introduction: symposium on the present status of reperfusion of the acutely ischemic myocardium. I J Am Coll Cardiol 1983;1:1031.

124. Friesinger GC, Schaefer J, Gaestner RA, Ross RS: Coronary sinus drainage and measurement of left coronary artery flow in the dog. Am J Physiol 1964;206:57.

125. Cinca J, Janse MJ, Morena H, et al: Mechanism and time course of the early electrical changes during acute coronary occlusion. An attempt to correlate the early ECG changes in man to cellular electrophysiology in the pig. Chest 1980; 77:499.

126. Fenoglio JJ Jr, Karagueuzian HS, Friedman PL, et al: Time course of infarct growth toward the endocardium after coronary occlusion. Am J Physiol 1979;236:H356.

127. Karagueuzian HS, Fenoglio JJ Jr, Weiss MB, Wit AL: Protracted ventricular tachycardia induced by premature stimulation of the canine heart after coronary artery occlusion and reperfusion. Circ Res 1979;44:833.

128. Dangman KH, Dresdner KP, Zaim S: Automatic and triggered impulse initiation in canine subepicardial ventricular muscle cells from border zones of 24-hour transmural infarcts. New mechanisms for malignant cardiac arrhythmias. Circulation 1988;78:1020.

129. Karagueuzian HS, Sugi K, Ohta M, et al: Inducible sustained ventricular tachycardia and ventricular fibrillation in con-

130. Braunwald E, Moroko PR, Libby P: Reduction of infarct size following coronary occlusion. Circ Res 1974;34(Suppl)III: 192.

131. Edwards JE: What is myocardial infarction? Circulation 1969;39(Suppl IV):5.

132. Mallory GK, White PD, Salcedo-Salazar J: The speed of healing of myocardial infarction. A study of the pathologic anatomy in seventy-two cases. Am Heart J 1939;18:647.

133. Miller RD, Burchell HB, Edwards JE: Myocardial infarction with and without coronary occlusion. Arch Intern Med 1951;88:597.

134. Wade WG: The pathogenesis of infarction of the right ventricle. Br Heart J 1959;21:545.

135. Sugi K, Karagueuzian HS, Fishbein MC, et al: Spontaneous ventricular tachycardia associated with isolated right ventricular infarction, one day after right coronary artery occlusion in the dog: studies on the site of origin and mechanism. Am Heart J 1985;109:232.

136. El-Sherif N, Gough WB, Zieler RH, et al: Triggered ventricular rhythms in one day old myocardial infarction in the dog. Circ Res 1983;52:566.

137. Friedman PL, Stewart JR, Fenoglio JJ Jr, Wit AL: Survival of subendocardial Purkinje fibers after extensive myocardial infarction: In vitro and in vivo correlations. Circ Res 1973; 33:612.

138. Horowitz LN, Spear JF, Moore EN: Subendocardial origin of ventricular arrhythmias in 24-hour old experimental myocardial infarction. Circulation 1976;53:56.

139. Rosenthal JE: Reflected reentry in depolarized foci with variable conduction impairment in 1 day old infarcted canine cardiac tissue. J Am Coll Cardiol 1988;12:404.

140. Le Marec H, Dangman KH, Danilo P, Rosen MR: An evaluation of automaticity and triggered activity in the canine heart one to four after myocardial infarction. Circulation 1985; 71:1224.

141. Cardinal R, Sasyniuk B: Electrophysiological effects of bretylium tosylate on subendocardial Purkinje fibers from infarcted canine heart. J Pharmacol Exp Ther 1978;204:159.

142. Scherlag BJ, Kabell G, Brachmann J, et al: Mechanisms of spontaneous and induced ventricular arrhythmias in the 24-hour infarcted heart. Am J Cardiol 1983;51:207.

143. El Sherif N, Mehra R, Gough WB, et al: Ventricular activation patterns of spontaneous and induced ventricular rhythms in canine one-day old myocardial infarction. Circ Res 1982; 51:152.

144. Karagueuzian HS, Fenoglio JJ Jr, Weiss MB, Wit AL: Coronary occlusion and reperfusion: effects on subendocardial fibers. Am J Physiol 1980;238:H581.

145. Lazzara R, El Sherif N, Sherlag BJ: Electrophysiological properties of canine Purkinje cells in one-day old myocardial infarction. Circ Res 1973;33:722.

146. Dresdner KP, Kline RP, Wit AL: Intracellular K^+ activity, intracellular Na^+ activity and maximum diastolic potential of canine subendocardial Purkinje cells from one-day old infarcts. Circ Res 1987;60:122.

147. Dresdner KP, Kline RP, Wit AL: Intracellular pH of canine subendocardial Purkinje cells surviving in 1-day-old myocardial infarcts. Circ Res 1989;65:554.

148. Argentieri TM, Frame LH, Colatsky TJ: Electrical properties of canine subenedocardial Purkinje fibers surviving in 1-day-old experimental myocardial infarction. Circ Res 1990;66:123.

149. Malfatto G, Rosen TS, Rosen MR: The response to overdrive pacing of triggered atrial and ventricular arrhythmias in the canine heart. Circulation 1988;77:1139.

150. Rosenthal JE: Contribution of depolarized foci with variable conduction impairement to arrhthmogenesis in 1 day old infarcted canine cardiac tissue. J Am Coll Cardiol 1986;8:648.

151. Fujimoto T, Peter T, Katoh T, et al: The relationship between ventricular arrhythmias and ischemia induced conduction delay in closed-chest animals within 24 hours of myocardial infarction. Am Heart J 1984;107:201.

152. Friedman PL, Stewart JR, Wit AL: Spontaneous and induced cardiac arrhythmias in subendocardial Purkinje fibers surviving extensive myocardial infarction in dogs. Circ Res 1973;33:612.

153. Fenoglio JJ Jr, Albala A, Silva FG, et al: Structural basis of ventricular arrhythmias in human myocardial infarction: a hypothesis. Hum Pathol 1976;7:547.

154. Wellens HJJ, Lie KI, Durrer D: Further observations on ventricular tachycardia as studied by electrical stimulation of the heart. Chronic recurrent ventricular tachycardia and ventricular tachycardia during acute myocardial infarction. Circulation 1974;49:647.

155. Davis J, Glassman R, Wit AL: Method for evaluating the effects of antiarrhythmic drugs on ventricular tachycardia with different electrophysiological characteristics and different mechanisms in the infarcted canine heart. Am J Cardiol 1982;49:1176.

156. Danilo P Jr, Langan WB, Rosen MR, Hoffman BF: Effects of phenothiazine analog, EN-313, on ventricular arrhythmias in the dog. Eur J Pharmacol 1977;45:127.

157. Karagueuzian HS, Fujimoto T, Katoh T, et al: Suppression of ventricular arrhythmias by propafenone, a new antiarrhythmic agent, during acute myocardial infarction in the conscious dog. A comparative study with lidocaine. Circulation 1982;66:1190.

158. Karagueuzian HS, Sugi K, Ohta M, Mandel WJ, Peter T: The efficacy of lidocaine and verapamil in combination on spontaneously occurring automatic ventricular tachycardia in conscious dogs one day after right coronary artery occlusion. Am Heart J 1986;111:438.

159. Vos MA, Gorgels APM, Leunissen JDM, et al: Programmed electrical stimulation and drugs identify two subgroups of ventricular tachycardia occurring 16–24 hours after occlusion of the left anterior descending coronary artery. Circulation 1992;85:747.

160. Gough WB, Hu D, El Sherif N: Effects of clofilium on ischemic subendocardial Purkinje fibers 1 day postinfarction. J Am Coll Cardiol 1988;11:431.

161. Dersham GH, Han J, Cameron JS, O'Connell DP: Effects of tocainide on Purkinje fibers from normal and infarcted ventricular tissues. J Electrocardiol 1986;19:355.

162. Meesmann M, Karagueuzian HS, Ino T, Mcgrath MF, Mandel WJ: The role of enhanced vagal activity on ischemic ventricular tachycardia. Pharmacologic basis of inefficiency. Am Heart J 1991;121:1703.

163. Wellens HJJ, Durrer DR, Lie KI: Observations on mechanisms of ventricular tachycardia in man. Circulation 1976; 54:237.

164. Josephson ME, Horowitz LN, Farshidi A, Kastor JA: Recurrent sustained ventricular tachycardia in man. Circulation 1978; 57:431.

165. Wit AL, Cranefield PF, Hoffman BF: Slow conduction and reentry in the ventricular conducting system. I. Return extrasystole in canine Purkinje fibers. Circ Res 1972;30:1.

166. Sasyniuk BI, Mendez C: A mechanism for reentry in canine ventricular tissue. Circ Res 1971;28:3.

167. Karagueuzian HS, Wit AL: Studies on ventricular arrhythmias in animal models of ischemic heart disease. What can we learn? In: Kulbertus HE, Wellens HJJ eds. Sudden death. The Hague: Martinus Nijhoff, 1980:69.

168. Karagueuzian HS, Fenoglio JJ Jr, Hoffman BF, Wit AL: Sustained ventricular tachycardia induced by electrical stimulation after myocardial infarction, relation to infarct structure. Circulation 1977;55:111. Abstract.

169. Garan H, Ruskin JN, McGovern B, Grant G: Serial analysis of electrically induced ventricular arrhythmias in a canine model of myocardial infarction. J Am Coll Cardiol 1985;5: 1095.

170. Garan H, Fallon JT, Ruskin JN: Sustained ventricular tachycardia in recent canine myocardial infarction. Circulation 1980;62:980.

171. Hanish RF, De Langen CDJ, Kadish AH, Michelson AL, Levine JH, Spear JF, Moore EN: Inducible sustained ventricular tachycardia 4 years after experimental canine myocardial infarction: electrophysiologic and anatomic comparisons with early healed infarcts. Circulation 1988;77:445.

172. Reddy CR, Gettes LS: Use of isoproteronol as an aid to electric induction of chronic recurrent ventricular tachycardia. Am J Cardiol 1979;44:705.

173. Kavanagh KM, Kabas JS, Rollins DL, Melnick SB, Smith WM, Ideker RE: High-current stimuli to the spared epicardium of a large infarct induce ventricular tachycardia. Circulation 1992;85:680.

174. Chen P-S, Wolf PD, Dixon EG, Danieley ND, Frazier DW, Smith WM, Ideker RE: Mechanism of ventricular vulnerability to single premature stimuli in open-chest dogs. Circ Res 1988;62:1191.

175. Gotoh M, Chen P-S, Mandel WJ, Karagueuzian HS: Graded responses and induction of ventricular rotors by a premature stimulus. Circulation 1993;88:4(Pt 2):I. Abstract.

176. Myerburg RJ, Gelband H, Nilsson K, et al: Long-term electrophysiological abnormalities resulting from experimental myocardial infarction in cats. Circ Res 1977;41:73.

177. Kimura S, Bassett AL, Kohya T, Kozlovskis PL, Myerburg RJ: Automaticity, triggered activity, and responses to adrenergic stimulation in cat subendocardial Purkinje fibers after healing of myocardial infarction. Circulation 1987;75:651.

178. Kimura S, Bassett AL, Cameron JS, Huikuri H, Kozlovskis PL, Myerburg RJ: Cellular electrophysiological changes during ischemia in isolated, coronary perfused cat ventricle with healed myocardial infarction. Circulation 1988;78:401.

179. Gang ES, Bigger JT Jr, Livelli ED Jr: A model of chronic ischemic arrhythmias: the relation between electrically inducible tachycardia, ventricular fibrillation threshold and myocardial infarct size. Am J Cardiol 1982;50:469.

180. Michelson EL, Spear JF, Moore EN: Strength-interval rela-

tions in a chronic canine model of myocardial infarction. Implications for the interpretation of electrophysiologic studies. CIrculation 1981;63:1158.

181. Michelson EL, Spear JF, Moore EN: Initiation of sustained ventricular tachyarrhythmias in canine model of chronic myocardial infarction. Importance of the site of stimulation. Circulation 1981;63:776.

182. Spear JF, Michelson EL, Moore EN: Cellular electrophysiological characteristics of chronically infarcted myocardium in dogs susceptible to sustained ventricular tachyarrhythmia. J Am Coll Cardiol 1983;1:1099.

183. Spear JF, Michelson EL, Moore EN: Reduced space constant in slowly conducting regions of chronically infarcted canine myocardium. Circ Res 1983;53:176.

184. Gardner PI, Ursell PC, Fenoglio JJ, Wit AL: Electrophysiologic and anatomic electrograms recorded from healed myocardial infarcts. Circulation 1985;72:596.

185. Gessman LJ, Agarwal JB, Endo T, Helfant RM: Localization and mechanism of ventricular tachycardia by ice mapping one-week after the onset of myocardial infarction in dogs. Circulation 1983;68:657.

186. Ursell PC, Gardner PI, Albala A, Fenoglio JJ Jr, Wit AL: Structural and electrophysiological changes in the epicardial border zone of canine myocardial infarcts during infarct healing. Circ Res 1985;56:436.

187. Spach MS, Dolber PC, Heidlage JF: Influence of the passive anisotropic properties on directional differences in propagation following modification of the sodium conductance in human atrial muscle. Circ Res 1988;62:811.

188. Osaka T, Kodama I, Tsuboi N, Toyama J, Yamada K: Effects of activation sequence and anisotropic cellular geometry on the repolarization phase of action potential of dog ventricular muscle. Circulation 1987;76:226.

189. Cardinal R, Vermeulen M, Shenasa M, et al: Anisotropic conduction and functional dissociation of ischemic tissue during reentrant ventricular tachycardia in canine myocardial infarction. Circulation 1988;77:1162.

190. El Sherif N, Smith RA, Evans K: Canine ventricular arrhythmias in the late myocardial infarction period. VIII. Epicardial mapping of reentrant circuits. Circ Res 1981;49:255.

191. Wit AL, Allessie MA, Bonke FIM, et al: Electrophysiologic mapping to determine the mechanism of experimental ventricular tachycardia initiated by premature impulses. Experimental approach and initial results demonstrating reentrant excitation. Am J Cardiol 1982;49:166.

192. Dillon SM, Allessie MA, Ursell PC, Wit AL: Influences of anisotropic tissue structure on reentrant circuits in the epicardial border zone of subacute canine infarcts. Circ Res 1988;63:182.

193. Gough WB, Mehra R, Restivo M, Zeiler RH, El Sherif N: Reentrant ventricular arrhythmias in the late myocardial infarction period in the dog. 13. Correlation of activation and refractory maps. Circ Res 1985;57 3:432.

194. Restivo M, Gough WB, El Sherif N: Reentrant ventricular rhythms in the late myocardial infarction period: prevention of reentry by dual stimulation during basic rhythm. Circulation 1988;77:429.

195. Burgess MJ, Steinhaus BM, Spitzer KW, Ershler PR: Nonuniform epicardial activation and repolarization properties of in vivo canine pulmonary conus. Circ Res 1988;62:233.

196. Ogawa S, Furuno I, Satoh Y, et al: Quantitative indices of dispersion of refractoriness for identification of propensity to re-entrant ventricular tachycardia in a canine model of myocardial infarction. Cardiovsc Res 1991;25:378.

197. Zuanetti G, Hoyt RH, Corr PB: Beta-adrenergic-meidated influences on micoscopic conduction in epicardial regions overlying infarcted myocardium. Circ Res 1990;67:284.

198. Butrous GS, Gough WB, Restivo M, Yang H, El-Sherif N: Adrenergic effects on reentrant ventricular rhythms in subacute myocardial infarction. Circulation 1992;86:247.

199. Kramer JB, Saffitz JE, Witkowski FX, et al: Intramural reentry as a mechanism of ventricular tachycardia during evolving canine myocardial infarction. Circ Res 1985;56:736.

200. El Sherif N, Mehra R, Gough WB, Zeiler RH: Reentrant ventricular arrhythmias in the late myocardial infarction period. Interruption of reentrant circuits by cryothermal techniques. Circulation 1983;644.

201. Sugi K, Karagueuzian HS, Fishbein MC, Mandel WJ, Peter T: Cellular electrophysiologic characteristic of surviving subendocardial fibers in chronically infarcted right ventricular myocardium susceptible to inducible sustained ventricular tachycardia. Am Heart J 1987;114:559.

202. El Sherif N, Hope RR, Scherlag BJ, Lazzara R: Reentrant ventricular arrhythmias in the late myocardial infarction period. I. Conduction characteristics in the infarction zone. Circulation 1977;55:686.

203. El Sherif N, Hope RR, Scherlag BJ, Lazzara R: Reentrant arrhythmias in the late myocardial infarction period. II. Patterns of initiation and termination. Circulation 1977; 55:702.

204. Kammerling JJ, Green FJ, Watanabe AM, et al: Denervation supersensitivity of refractoriness in noninfarcted areas apical to transmural myocardial infarction. Circulation 1987; 76:383.

205. Herre JM, Wetstein L, Lin YL, Mills AS, Dae M, Thames MD: Effects of transmural versus nontransmural myocardial infarction on inducibility of ventricular arrhythmias during sympathetic stimulation in dogs. J Am Coll Cardiol 1988; 11:414.

206. De Bakker JMT, van Capelle FJL, Janse MJ, et al: Reentry as a cause of ventricular tachycardia in patients with chronic ischemic heart disease: electrophysiologic and anatomic correlation. Circulation 1988;77:589.

207. De Bakker J, van Capelle FJL, Janse MJ, et al: Macroreentry in the infarcted human heart: the mechanism of ventricular tachycardias with a "focal" activation patterns. J Am Coll Cardiol 1991;18:1005.

208. Pogwizd SM, Hoyt RH, Saffitz JE, Corr PB, Cox JL, Cain ME: Reentrant and focal mechanisms underlying ventricular tachycardia in the human heart. Circulation 1992;86:1872.

209. Kaltenbrunner W, Cardinal R, Dubuc M, et al: Epicardial and endocardial mapping of ventricualr tachycardia in patients with myocardial infarction. Is the origin of the tachycardia always subendocardially localized? Circulation 1991;84:1058.

210. Martinez-Rubio A, Shenasa M, Borggrefe M, Chen X, Benning F, Breithardt G: Electrophysiologic variables characterizing the induction of ventricular tachycardia versus ventricular fibrillation after myocardial infarction: relation between ventricualr alte potentials and coupling intervals

for the induction of sustained ventricular tachyarrhythmais. J Am Coll Cardiol 1993;21:1624.

211. Vassallo JA, Cassidy DM, Kindwall E, Marchlinsky FE, Josephson ME: Nonuniform recovery of excitability in the left ventricle. Circulation 1988;78:1365.

212. Agarwal JB, Naccarella FF, Weintraub WS, Helfant RH: Sinus rhythm mapping in healed experimental myocardial infarction: contrasting activation pattern for inducing ventricular tachycardia versus fibrillation. Am J Cardiol 1985;55:1601.

213. Bhandari AK, Au PK, Rose JS, Kotlewski A, Blue S, Rahimtoola SH: Decline in inducibility of sustained ventricular tachycardia from two to twenty weeks after acute myocardial infarction. Am J Cardiol 1987;59:284.

214. Spear JF, Horowitz LN, Hodess AB, et al: Cellular electrophysiology of human myocardial infarction. I. Abnormalities of cellular activation. Circulation 1979;59:247.

215. Dangman DH, Danilo P Jr, Hordoff AJ, et al: Electrophysiologic characteristics of human ventricular and Purkinje fibers. Circulation 1982;65:362.

216. Glassman RD, Davis JC, Wit AL: Effects of antiarrhythmic drugs on sustained ventricular tachycardia induced by premature stimulus in dogs after coronary artery occlusion and reperfusion. Fed Proc 1978;37:730. Abstract.

217. Kragueuzian HS, Sugi K, Ohta M, Meesmann M, Ino T, Peter T, Mandel WJ: The efficacy of cibenzoline and propafenone against inducible sustained and nonsustained ventricular tachycardia in conscious dogs with isolated chronic right ventricular infarction: a comparative study with lidocaine. Am Heart J 1986;112:1173.

218. Saxon LA, Sherman T, Stevenson WG, Yeatman LA, Wiener I: Ventricular tachycardia after infarction: sources of coronary blood flow to the infarct zone. Am Heart J 1992;124:84.

219. Karagueuzian HS, Ohta M, Drury KJ, et al: Coronary venous retroinfusion of procainamide: a new approach for the managemnet of spontaneous and inducible sustained ventricular tachycardia during myocardial infarction. J Am Coll Cardial 1986;7:551.

220. Patterson E, Gibson JK, Lucchesi BR: Electrophysiologic effects of disopyramide phosphate on reentrant ventricular arrhythmia in concsious dogs after myocardial infarction. Am J Cardiol 1980;46:792.

221. Patterson E, Gibson JK, Lucchesi BR: Prevention of chronic canine ventricular tachyarrhythmias with bretylium tosylate. Circulation 1981;64:1045.

222. Anderson JL, Patterson E, Conlon M, et al: Kinetics of antifibrillatory effects of bretylium: Correlation with myocardial drug concentrations. Am J Cardiol 1980;46:583.

223. Patterson E, Ella BT, Abrams GD, et al: Ventricular fibrillation in a conscious canine preparation of sudden coronary death—prevention by short and long-term amiodarone administration. Circulation 1983;68:857.

224. Meesmann M, Karagueuzian HS, Takeshi I, et al: Selective perfusion of ischemic myocardium during coronary venous retroinjection: a study of the causative role of venoarterial and venoventricular pressure gradients. J Am Coll Cardiol 1987;10:887.

225. Myerburg RJ, Kesseler KM, Kiem I, et al: Relationship between plasma levels of procainamide, suppression of premature ventricular complexes and prevention of recurrent ventricular tachycardia. Circulation 1981;64:280.

226. Winkle RA, Alderman EL, Fitzgerald JW, Harrison DC: Treatment of symptomatic ventricular tachycardia. Ann Intern Med 1976;85:107.

227. Denes P, Wu D, Wyndham C, et al: Chronic long-term electrophysiologic study of paroxysmal ventricular tachycardia. Chest 1980;77:478.

228. Rinkenberger RL, Prystowsky EN, Jackman WM, et al: Drug conversion of non-sustained ventricular tachycardia to sustained ventricular tachycardia during serial electrophysiologic studies: Identification of drugs that exacerbate tachycardia and potential mechanisms. Am Heart J 1982;103:177.

229. Mason JW, Winkle RA: Electrode-catheter arrhythmia induction in the selection and assessment of antiarrhythmic drug therapy for recurrent ventricular tachycardia. Circulation 1978;58:971.

230. Waxman HL, Buxton AE, Sadowski IM, Josephson ME: The response to procainamide during electrophysiologic study for sustained ventricular tachyarrhythmias predicts the response to other medications. Circulation 1983;67:30.

231. Stevenson WG, Weiss JN, Wiener I, et al: Fractionated endocardial electrograms are associated with slow conduction in humans: evidence from pace-mapping. J Am Coll Cardiol 1989;13:369.

232. Shrier A, Dubasky H, Rosengarten M, et al: Prediction of complex atrioventricular conduction rhythms in humans with the use of the atrioventricular nodal recovery curve. Ciculation 1987;76:1196.

233. Guevara MR, Shtier A, Glass L: Phase-locked rhythms in periodically stimualted heart cell aggregate. Am J Physiol 1988;254:H1.

234. Goldberger AL, Bhargava V, Wesr BJ, Mandell AJ: Some obsevation on the question: is ventricular fibrillation "CHAOS"? Physica D 1986;19:282.

235. Kaplan DT: Nonlinear dynamics and cardiac electrical instability. Cambridge, MA: Massachussetts Institue of Technology, 1988. PhD dissertation.

236. Garfinkel AG, Karagueuzian HS, Khan SS, Diamond GA: Is the proarrhythmic effect of quinidine a chaotic phenomenon? (Abstr) J Am Coll Cardiol 1989;13(2):186A.

237. Smith JM, Clancy EA, Valeri RC, Ruskin JN, Cohen RJ: Electrical alternans and cardiac electrical inatability. Circulation 1988;77:110.

238. Salerno JA, Previtali M, Pancirolic, et al: Ventricular arrhythmias during acute myocardial ischemia in man. The role and significance of R-ST-T alternans and the prevention of ischaemic sudden death by medical treatment. Eur Heart J 1986; 7(Suppl A):63.

239. Janse MJ, van der Steen ABM, van Dam RTH, Durrer D: Refractory period of the dog's ventricular myocardium following sudden changes in frequency. Circ Res 1969;26:251.

240. Marchlinsky FE: Characterization of oscillations in ventricular refractoriness in man after an abrupt increment in heart rate. Circulation 1987;75:550.

241. Ritzenberg AL, Adam DR, Cohen RJ: Period multupling: evidence for nonlinear behaviour of the canine heart. Nature 1984;307:159.

242. Saitoh H, Bailey JC, Surawicz B: Alternans of action potential duration after abrupt shortening of cycle length: differences between dog Purkinje and ventricular muscle fibers. Circ Res 1988;6F2:1027.

243. Davidenko JM, Antzelevitch C: Electrophysiological mechanisms underlying rate-dependent changes of refractoriness in normal and segmentally depressed canine Purkinje fibers: the characteristics of post-repolarization refractoriness. Circ Res 1986;58:257.

244. May RM: Simple mathematical models with very complicated dynamics. Nature 1976;261:459.

245. Abraham AM, Shaw C: Dynamics: the geometry of behavior, part 2: chaotic behavior. Santa Cruz, CA: Aerial Press, 1983.

246. Karagueuzian HS, Khan SS, Mandel WJ, Hong K, Diamond GA: Nonlinear dynamic analysis of temporally heterogeneous action potential characteristics. Pacing Clin Electrophysiol 1990;13:2113 1990.

247. Willems AR, Tijssen JGP, van Capelle, et al: Determinants of prognosis in symptomatic ventricular tachycardia or ventricular fibrilaltion late after myocardial infarction. J Am Coll Cardiol 1990;16:521.

248. Richards DAB, Byth K, Ross DL, Uther JB: What is the best predictor of spontaneous ventricular tachycardia and sudden death after myocardial infarction? Circulation 1991;83:756.

249. Bhandari AK, Widerhorn J, Sagar PT, et al: Prognostic significance of programmed ventricular stimulation in patients surviving complicated acute myocardial infarction: a prospective study. Am Heart J 1992;124:87.

250. Bourke JP, Young AA, Richards DAB, Uther JB: Reduction in incidence of inducible ventricular tachycardia after myocardial infarction by treatment with strptokinase during infarct evolution. J Am Coll Cardiol 1990;16:1703.

251. Mitrani RD, Biblo LA, Carlson MD, Gatzoylis KA, Henthorn RW, Waldo AL: Multiple monomophic tachycardia configurations predict failure of antiarrhythmic drug therapy guided by electrophysiologic study. J Am Coll Cardiol 1993;22:1117.

252. Karagueuzian HS, Khan SS, Peters W, Mandel WJ, Diamond GA: Nonhomogeneous local atrial activity during acute atrial fibrillation. Spectral and dynamic analysis. Pacing Clin Electrophysiol 1990;13:1937.

253. Denton TA, Diamond GA, Khan SS, Kraragueuzian HS: Fascinating rhythm: a primer on chaos theory and its application to cardiology. Am Heart J 1990;120:1419.

Cardiac Arrhythmias, 3rd edition, edited by William J. Mandel.
J. B. Lippincott Company, Philadelphia © 1995.

19

Nabil El-Sherif • Gioia Turitto

Ventricular Premature Complex: Risk Stratification and Management

Sudden cardiac death is the major contributor to overall cardiovascular mortality in the modern world. It comprises about 60% of all coronary heart disease fatalities that occur annually.[1] The need for a systematic approach to identify the high-risk patient, aid in initiating appropriate therapy, and prevent the occurrence of sudden cardiac death is paramount. It has been amply documented that patients with sustained ventricular tachyarrhythmias, including those resuscitated from cardiac arrest, have a high incidence of sudden cardiac death.[2–6] Those patients, however, represent only a small proportion of the total population with complex ventricular arrhythmias. The relation of complex ventricular arrhythmias (excluding sustained ventricular tachycardia [VT]–ventricular fibrillation [VF]) to sudden cardiac "arrhythmic" death remains controversial. Several studies suggest that complex ventricular arrhythmias in the postinfarction patient are independent markers for risk of sudden cardiac arrest but there is general agreement that sensitivity and specificity are relatively low.[7–10]

In the last several years, many studies investigated the role of programmed electrical stimulation (PES) as a means of classifying patients with complex ventricular arrhythmias into groups at low or high risk for sudden cardiac death.[11–40] This chapter reviews the role of PES and the noninvasive technique of signal-averaged electrocardiogram (ECG) in risk stratification and management of patients with complex ventricular arrhythmias. Although complex ventricular arrhythmias are usually defined as frequent, multiform, and repetitive ventricular premature complexes (VPCs), the role of nonsustained VT (defined as three or more consecutive VPCs that are less than 30 seconds in duration at a rate of more than 100/minute) is particularly emphasized.

COMPLEX VENTRICULAR ARRHYTHMIAS AND SUDDEN DEATH IN THE PRESENCE OF NORMAL HEART OR ORGANIC HEART DISEASE, WITH OR WITHOUT IMPAIRED VENTRICULAR FUNCTION

Complex ventricular arrhythmias are uncommon in the absence of organic heart disease, and their presence does not increase the risk of either cardiac death or sudden

Supported by the National Institutes of Health Grant HL36680 and Veterans Administration Medical Research Funds death.[41] A long-term follow-up (average, 6.5 years) of 73 asymptomatic subjects who had frequent and complex ventricular arrhythmias, including nonsustained VT, showed no increased risk of death, compared with that of the healthy United States population.[42]

The incidence of complex ventricular arrhythmias increases in the presence of heart disease. In the absence of impaired ventricular function, however, the arrhythmia does not seem to be associated with an increased incidence of sudden death. Of 92 patients with normal left ventricular ejection fraction who were studied after coronary artery bypass surgery, 57% had complex ventricular arrhythmias, including 21.5% who had nonsustained VT. The incidence of complications in patients with complex ventricular arrhythmias was not higher than that found in those with no arrhythmias, and there were no cardiac or sudden deaths during an average follow-up period of 16 months.[43] In another series of 130 patients with chronic stable angina pectoris, complex ventricular arrhythmias were not associated with an increased risk of sudden cardiac death.[44]

In the presence of impaired left ventricular function, complex ventricular arrhythmias may be an independent risk for sudden cardiac death. This view is not without controversy.[41] In the first quantitative study of the relation between impaired left ventricular function and complex ventricular arrhythmias after myocardial infarction, cardiac death was strongly associated with a low left ventricular ejection fraction, and the independent role of the arrhythmia could not be established.[45] The interrelation between impaired ventricular function, complex ventricular arrhythmias, and sudden cardiac death was systematically analyzed later in two groups of patients: (1) patients with congestive heart failure, commonly the result of ischemic or idiopathic dilated cardiomyopathy; and (2) patients who survived the early phase of myocardial infarction. Packer summarized the results of seven studies comprising 891 patients with congestive heart failure.[46] The incidence of nonsustained VT ranged from 39% to 60%. The total mortality averaged 37.4% and the rate of sudden cardiac death 14.3% per year. Surawicz reviewed eight additional studies comprising 398 patients with congestive heart failure.[41] The incidence of nonsustained VT ranged from 49% to 100% and averaged 65%, whereas total mortality and sudden cardiac death averaged 42.4% and 21.4%, respectively, during a follow-up period of 18.5 months (range, 11 to 34 months). In most of the above studies, sudden cardiac death was unrelated to nonsustained VT. The role of complex ventricular arrhythmias in predicting sudden cardiac death in patients with dilated cardiomyopathy has been reviewed by Larsen and coworkers and Tamburro and Wilber.[37,47] Larsen and associates summarized seven studies on the prevalence of ventricular arrhythmias during 24-hour ambulatory ECGs

obtained in 343 patients with dilated cardiomyopathy and concluded that the identification of patients at risk for sudden cardiac death based on the finding of frequent VPCs or nonsustained VT is difficult and unreliable. This may be partly because bradyarrhythmias may play an important role in the pathogenesis of sudden death in some patients with dilated cardiomyopathy and congestive heart failure. Conversely, Tamburro and Wilber concluded that most evidence available in the literature confirms the prognostic significance of frequent VPCs and nonsustained VT in patients with idiopathic dilated cardiomyopathy. According to these authors, however, data are insufficient to establish which criterion of spontaneous arrhythmia frequency or severity may provide the optimum indicator of high risk. That these two reviews reached almost opposite conclusions illustrates the ongoing controversy regarding the prognostic value of spontaneous complex ventricular arrhythmias in the setting of dilated cardiomyopathy.

In survivors of myocardial infarction, three studies addressed the interrelation between impaired ventricular function, complex ventricular arrhythmias, and sudden cardiac death in large series of patients.[7-9] All three studies suggested that complex ventricular arrhythmias are an independent risk factor for sudden cardiac death. The multicenter postinfarction research group was a nine-hospital natural history study of patients younger than age 70 years who had a proved myocardial infarction.[7] In 766 patients, 86 deaths occurred during a 3-year follow-up period. When multivariate survivorship techniques were used to evaluate the independent contribution of ventricular arrhythmias and impaired left ventricular function to postinfarction mortality, VPC frequency, VPC runs, and left ventricular ejection fraction were each independently associated with both total mortality and arrhythmia-specific mortality. The Multicenter Investigation of the Limitation of Infarct Size Study was a five-hospital intervention study of the effect of hyaluronidase, propranolol, or both in patients younger than age 76 years who had acute myocardial infarction.[8] Five hundred thirty-three patients who survived 10 days after infarction were followed-up for a mean of 18 months. Frequent VPCs (more than 10/hour) and left ventricular ejection fraction of less than 40% were independently significant markers of risk for subsequent sudden death believed to be the result of primary ventricular arrhythmia. The incidence of sudden death was 18% in patients with both left ventricular dysfunction and frequent VPCs, an 11-fold increase when compared with patients in whom neither risk factor was present; 79% of all sudden deaths occurred within 7 months after the index infarction. Maisel and colleagues studied 191 survivors of non–Q-wave myocardial infarction and 586 survivors of Q-wave infarction.[9] Complex ventricular arrhythmia at the time of hospital discharge was an important predictor of mortality only in patients with non–Q-wave infarction. The 10% incidence of sudden cardiac death in this group was higher than in patients with Q-wave infarction and higher than the incidence of sudden death reported in most other studies. This was explained by the presence of an unstable ischemic state in these patients.

The prognostic significance of VT (three or more complexes) detected with ambulatory electrocardiographic recording during the postinfarction period has been investigated by Bigger and coworkers in 430 patients who survived the cardiac care–unit phase of acute myocardial infarction.[48] The prevalence of spontaneous VT was 11.6%. Patients with tachycardia had a significantly greater prevalence of previous myocardial infarction, left ventricular failure in the cardiac care unit, atrial fibrillation, VT or VF in the cardiac care unit, and significantly more frequent use of digitalis, diuretics, and antiarrhythmic drugs at the time of hospital discharge. Ventricular tachycardia was strongly associated with 1-year mortality (odds ratio, 4.7). This association was still significant when other important risk variables were controlled statistically, using a multiple logistic regression model. One- and 3-year mortality rates were 38% and 54%, respectively, in the group with VT, whereas they were 12% and 19%, respectively, in the group without VT.

Although several multicenter studies show that complex ventricular arrhythmias are an independent risk factor for sudden cardiac death, in survivors of myocardial infarction, the corollary observation that suppression of these arrhythmias reduces the incidence of sudden death has not been demonstrated. Yusuf and associates reviewed data from various randomized trials that evaluated the effects of several antiarrhythmic drugs in postinfarction patients.[49] Eighteen trials evaluated class IA drugs (quinidine, procainamide, disopyramide, imipramine, and moricizine) in a total of 6582 patients. There were 253 deaths among 3292 treated patients, compared with 217 deaths among 3290 control patients. Thirty-two trials evaluated class IB drugs (lidocaine, tocainide, phenytoin, and mexiletine) in a total of 14,013 patients. There were 306 deaths among 7068 treated patients, compared with 275 deaths among 6945 control subjects. There have been eight trials of class IC agents (aprindine, encainide, and flecainide) in a total of 2538 patients. There were 97 deaths among 1303 treated patients, compared with 74 deaths among 1235 control patients. Therefore, individually and collectively, there was no evidence that class I drugs reduce the risk of death in postinfarction patients. The results of a large multicenter study sponsored by the National Institutes of Health, the Cardiac Arrhythmia Suppression Trial (CAST), deserve additional comments.[50–53] The goal of CAST was to determine whether suppression of asymptomatic ventricular arrhythmias reduces the incidence of sudden cardiac death in patients at moderate risk.

This trial was carried out at 27 sites in the United States, Canada, and Sweden; candidates for enrollment were patients with previous myocardial infarction, asymptomatic ventricular arrhythmias, and reduced left ventricular function. Patients whose arrhythmias were suppressed by antiarrhythmic drugs were randomly assigned to receive either placebo or effective suppressant therapy during follow-up; the incidence of sudden death in the two groups was compared. The CAST trial was prematurely terminated in April 1989 after 2309 patients had been recruited for the initial drug-titration phase of the study: 1727 (75%) had initial suppression of their arrhythmia (as assessed by Holter recording) through the use of one of the three study drugs (encainide, flecainide, and moricizine) and had been randomly assigned to receive active drug or placebo. Among the randomized patients, 857 were assigned to receive encainide or its placebo (432 to active drug and 425 to placebo) and 641 were assigned to receive flecainide or its placebo (323 to active drug and 318 to placebo). After an average of 10 months of follow-up, 89 patients had died: 59 of arrhythmia (43 receiving drug versus 16 receiving placebo; $p = .0004$), 22 of nonarrhythmic cardiac causes (17 receiving drug versus five receiving placebo; $p = .01$), and eight of noncardiac causes (three receiving drug versus five receiving placebo). The cardiac arrhythmia suppression trial demonstrated that the use of encainide or flecainide to treat asymptomatic or mildly symptomatic ventricular ectopy in patients with mild to moderate left ventricular dysfunction after myocardial infarction carries an excessive mortality risk. Thus, the suppression of VPCs alone in this population is not an adequate indication that a drug will be helpful to prolong survival. At the time of discontinuation of the encainide–flecainide portion of the CAST, only 320 patients were being treated with moricizine or its placebo, and an insignificant but favorable trend in mortality was observed among patients treated with moricizine (11 deaths in the placebo group versus four deaths in the moricizine group). Therefore, it was decided to continue the study as CAST-II, with moricizine alone. There were several changes in the study protocol. The upper limit of eligible values for left ventricular ejection fraction was lowered from 0.55 or less (the original cut-off point in CAST-I) to 0.40 or less. Second, the length of time from the qualifying myocardial infarction to the qualifying ambulatory electrocardiographic recording was shortened from 2 years or less—the interval used in CAST-I—to 90 days or less. Third, disqualifying VT was redefined to exclude from the trial patients with any runs lasting 30 or more seconds at a rate 120 or more per minute but to allow the enrollment of patients with VT of 15 or more beats and lasting up to 30 seconds without symptoms (these patients were excluded from CAST-I). These changes were implemented to enroll a group at higher risk of events relative to the original CAST population. Cardiac arrhythmia suppression trial II was divided into two blinded, randomized phases: an early 14-day exposure phase that evaluated the risk of starting treatment with moricizine after myocardial infarction (1325 patients), and a long-term phase that evaluated the effect of moricizine on survival after myocardial infarction in patients whose VPCs were either adequately suppressed by moricizine (1155 patients) or only partially suppressed (219 patients). Cardiac arrhythmia suppression trial II was stopped in July 1991 because the first 14-day period of treatment with moricizine was associated with excess mortality (17 of 665 patients died or had cardiac arrest) compared with no treatment or placebo (three of 660 patients died or had cardiac arrest); and estimates of conditional power indicated that it was highly unlikely (less than 8% chance) that a survival benefit from moricizine would be observed if the trial were completed. At the completion of the long-term phase, there were 49 deaths or cardiac arrests due to arrhythmias in patients assigned to moricizine and 42 in patients assigned to placebo (adjusted $p = .40$). Thus, as with the antiarrhythmic agents used in CAST-I (flecainide and encainide), the use of moricizine in CAST-II to suppress asymptomatic or mildly symptomatic VPCs to try to reduce mortality after myocardial infarction proved to be not only ineffective but also harmful. Suppression of ventricular arrhythmias by type I antiarrhythmic drugs has not been linked to improved survival in the CAST studies. Initial data on the effect of amiodarone on survival in postinfarction patients appear to be more encouraging.[49, 54, 55] In the Basel Antiarrhythmic Study of Infarct Survival (BASIS), patients with asymptomatic complex ventricular arrhythmias after myocardial infarction were prospectively randomized to treatment with class I antiarrhythmic drugs (amiodarone, 200 mg/day) or no antiarrhythmic therapy.[54] During the 1-year follow-up, there were only five deaths in the amiodarone group, with 12 deaths in the class I group and 15 deaths in the control group. Thus, this study showed a significantly improved 1-year survival in postinfarction patients with ventricular ectopy treated with amiodarone. Later analysis of the BASIS data found that the benefits of amiodarone were limited to patients with preserved left ventricular function (left ventricular ejection fraction more than 40%).[56] Ceremuzynski and colleagues reported the results of the Polish amiodarone study.[55] The rationale of this study differed from that of other trials because the presence of complex ventricular arrhythmias was not a prerequisite for enrollment. Eligible patients (confirmed acute myocardial infarction, contraindications to beta-blockade) were randomized between the 5th and 7th postinfarction day to amiodarone (800 mg daily for the first week, and 200 to 400 mg daily thereafter for 1 year) or placebo. When the data were analyzed on an intention-to-treat basis, there were 19 cardiac deaths among amiodarone patients, compared with 33 in the placebo group

(44% reduction in cardiac mortality; odds ratio, 0.55; $p = .048$). The Spanish study on sudden death was designed to assess the efficacy of amiodarone versus metoprolol or no antiarrhythmic treatment in suppressing asymptomatic ventricular ectopy and improving survival in patients with myocardial infarction, left ventricular ejection fraction of 20% to 45%, and three or more VPCs per hour (pairs or runs).[57] A total of 368 patients were enrolled and randomly assigned to receive amiodarone (200 mg/day), metoprolol (100 to 200 mg daily), or no antiarrhythmic treatment 10 to 60 days after acute myocardial infarction. After a median follow-up of 2.8 years, mortality in the amiodarone-treated patients did not differ significantly from that of control subjects (3.5% versus 7.7%; $p = .19$) but was lower than that of the metoprolol treated group (15%; $p = .006$). The question of whether prophylactic amiodarone improves survival after myocardial infarction in patients with ventricular ectopy or depressed left ventricular function is also being addressed by several other studies: the Canadian amiodarone myocardial infarction arrhythmia trial and the European myocardial infarct amiodarone trial.[58, 59]

Even if the CAST study had shown that suppression of complex ventricular arrhythmias significantly decreased the incidence of sudden cardiac death in survivors of myocardial infarction, a risk stratification strategy other than the mere presence of complex ventricular arrhythmias on ambulatory monitoring would still be required. This is because of the low sensitivity and specificity of Holter monitoring alone as a marker of sudden cardiac death in these patients. Because of the low sensitivity, many patients with no complex ventricular arrhythmias but who still may be at risk for sudden cardiac death may be deprived of appropriate therapy. Furthermore, the low specificity of this marker may lead to unnecessary chronic therapy in a large percentage of patients. This would be of relatively less concern if antiarrhythmic drugs (and other forms of antiarrhythmic therapy) were consistently effective, affordable, and without serious side effects. None of these premises are in sight. Because of this and similar arguments, the role of PES and of the signal-averaged ECG in risk stratification and management of patients with complex ventricular arrhythmias has received considerable interest.

PROGRAMMED ELECTRICAL STIMULATION IN PATIENTS WITH COMPLEX VENTRICULAR ARRHYTHMIAS

Several studies investigated the role of PES in identifying subsets of patients with complex ventricular arrhythmias at low and high risk for sudden cardiac death.[11–40] Patients in whom PES fails to induce sustained VT may have a low risk of sudden cardiac death. In those patients, antiarrhythmic therapy may not be warranted. In contrast, patients with inducible sustained VT may be at increased risk of sudden cardiac death. It is possible that antiarrhythmic therapy guided by the results of PES may decrease the risk of sudden death in this group.

Stimulation Protocols

The incidence and type of ventricular arrhythmias induced by PES depend on the stimulation protocol. The stimulation protocol may vary with regard to the following factors:

1. The nature of the basic drive (sinus or ventricular paced rhythm)
2. The cycle length of the basic paced drive
3. The current strength of the stimulus
4. The nature of the stimulating train (basic drive followed by one or more extrastimuli, burst pacing, and alternation of short and long cycle)
5. The site of stimulation
6. The use of drugs such as isoproterenol to facilitate induction of VT
7. What constitutes a specific end point for the stimulation protocol

The introduction of a single ventricular extrastimulus during sinus rhythm rarely resulted in the induction of VT, which most often required two or more extrastimuli in patients with spontaneous nonsustained VT. In the studies of Estes and coworkers and Prystowsky and associates, about 20% of all episodes of VT (sustained or nonsustained) were induced by one to three extrastimuli delivered during sinus rhythm.[60,61] Spielman and colleagues report that only 13% of all induced sustained VT was induced by triple extrastimuli during sinus rhythm.[15] Extrastimuli applied during ventricular pacing were consistently more effective in inducing ventricular tachyarrhythmias. The optimal duration and cycle length of the pacing drive are not clearly established, however.[62] Based on results obtained in patients with spontaneous sustained ventricular tachyarrhythmias and in those with nonsustained VT, it seems advisable to use more than one pacing drive, with cycle lengths between 600 and 400 milliseconds.[15,63,64] In these studies, the yield of induced sustained VT with up to three extrastimuli increased by about 20% with the use of a second pacing drive and by an additional 20% when a third drive was included in the protocol. In a study by Breithardt and colleagues, shortening the cycle length of the basic drive allowed induction of sustained VT by extrastimuli with longer coupling intervals.[65] This finding was not reproduced by other groups, however.[66]

The incidence of inducible ventricular tachyarrhythmias varied directly with the number of extrastimuli applied during basic ventricular pacing, both in patients with spontaneous sustained and with nonsustained VT. In patients with spontaneous sustained VT, the probability of inducing sustained monomorphic VT ranged from 22% to 33% (mean, 27%) with one extrastimulus; from 47% to 73% (mean, 66%) with two extrastimuli; and from 72% to 94% (mean, 88%) with three extrastimuli.[63,64,67–70] Thus, the introduction of a second and a third extrastimulus increased the sensitivity of the stimulation protocol for sustained monomorphic VT by an average of 45% and 23%, respectively. The same phenomenon was reported in patients with spontaneous nonsustained VT. Four studies that used a similar stimulation protocol (three extrastimuli, one or two right ventricular pacing sites, and multiple basic drives) and similar end points (induction of sustained ventricular tachyarrhythmias) reported their data according to the number of extrastimuli required for induction.[15,21,23,70] The fraction of patients who had sustained monomorphic VT induced by one extrastimulus was low (0% to 3%) but rose substantially with two extrastimuli (9% to 24%) and showed further increase with three extrastimuli (21% to 39%). A similar trend was described for the induction of VF, which increased from 0% with one extrastimulus to 2% to 7% with two extrastimuli and to 10% to 14% with three extrastimuli.[15,21,70]

Burst pacing was used by several authors to induce ventricular tachyarrhythmias in patients with spontaneous nonsustained VT. The additional yield of this mode of stimulation above the use of two extrastimuli ranged from 3% to 11%.[60,61,67] Similar results were reported in patients with spontaneous sustained VT.[60,67,71,72] Burst pacing may have no advantage over the use of three extrastimuli, however.[61] Furthermore, animal studies show that the technique of burst pacing depends on the number of beats in the paced train and the cycle length of stimulation in a manner that makes it difficult to standardize or to reproduce in the clinical setting.[73] A protocol employing an abrupt short–long sequence of the basic drive before the introduction of one or more extrastimuli was reported to initiate sustained VT in patients not otherwise inducible with conventional protocols.[74] When the efficacy of such technique was compared with the use of triple extrastimuli, however, no significant difference was found.[75]

Programmed stimulation is usually limited to right ventricular sites. In patients with spontaneous nonsustained VT, there was little advantage of stimulating a second right ventricular site (usually the outflow tract or the septum) after three extrastimuli applied at the right ventricular apex had failed to induce VT. In the studies by Turitto and coworkers and Kharsa and colleagues, VT initiated at the outflow tract represented 0% to 4% of all induced sustained VT.[23,24] Similarly, Zheutlin and coworkers (using up to two extrastimuli and VT lasting six or more complexes as the end point) found that only 3% of inductions occurred during stimulation at the outflow tract.[17] Spielman and associates report that stimulation at the outflow tract was effective in 14% of patients and comprised 53% of induced sustained VT.[15]

Specificity of Induced Tachyarrhythmias

In patients with recurrent sustained monomorphic VT, the sensitivity of the technique of programmed stimulation is defined as the ability to reproduce the clinical arrhythmia. Such a definition is not applicable in patients with spontaneous nonsustained VT. In these patients, programmed stimulation may induce nonsustained VT, sustained monomorphic or polymorphic VT, or VF. There is some evidence that the induction of sustained monomorphic VT, rather than that of nonsustained VT or VF, should be considered as the specific end point of PES in patients with spontaneous nonsustained VT. Nonsustained VT was as commonly induced in patients with heart disease as in those without (34% and 21%, respectively).[76-79] Induced nonsustained VT was polymorphic in 80% of the cases.[63,75,76,78] Polymorphic nonsustained VT induced in patients without organic heart disease did not differ in cycle length and mode of initiation from those elicited in postinfarction patients with spontaneous sustained ventricular tachyarrhythmias.[79] These data strongly suggest that the specificity of induced nonsustained VT is low. Although some authors try to improve the specificity of induced nonsustained VT by comparing its QRS configuration or cycle length to the spontaneous arrhythmia, this approach is fraught with difficulties.[11,14,61] Careful comparison between the QRS configuration of spontaneous and induced rhythms may be difficult to accomplish because of limitations on the number of simultaneously recorded ECG leads. It is almost impossible to adequately compare the QRS configuration of polymorphic nonsustained VT. Furthermore, there is usually little correlation between the cycle length of spontaneous and induced VT.[15,80-82]

The induction of VF may be a nonspecific response to programmed stimulation in patients with nonsustained VT. Ventricular fibrillation was induced with comparable frequency in patients with spontaneous sustained ventricular tachyarrhythmias (3% to 13%), survivors of myocardial infarction without documented sustained VT–VF (1% to 14%), and in patients with spontaneous nonsustained VT (0% to 15%).[11,13-15,17,18,20,21-24,32-34,38,60,61,67,70,72,76,77,80,83-88] The frequency of induced VF was related to the aggressiveness of the stimulation protocol.[15,23,77,78]

Conversely, sustained monomorphic VT was not induced by PES in patients without organic heart disease; thus its specificity is close to 100%.[76-79] The arrhythmia

was considered to be a marker for an electrophysiologic substrate of reentry and may not be induced in the absence of such substrate.[87] Sustained monomorphic VT, however, was inducible in patients with heart disease, regardless of the presence of spontaneous sustained VT. Its prevalence was less than 3% in studies on miscellaneous populations but was higher in patients with spontaneous nonsustained VT and in survivors of myocardial infarction.[11,13-15,17,18,20,21-24,26,30,32-34,38,39,60,61,63,67,70,72,76,77,80,88] In the latter, sustained monomorphic VT was inducible in 28% to 51% of patients with spontaneous nonsustained VT and in 11% to 45% of those without documented arrhythmias.[23,33,39,70,85,86,88-90]

The induction of sustained monomorphic VT in patients with spontaneous nonsustained runs may be interpreted as demonstration of the ability of programmed stimulation to expose a fixed electrophysiologic substrate. Such abnormality may be implicated in the high risk of sudden cardiac death in these patients.

Results of Programmed Stimulation

This section summarizes the results of PES in patients with complex ventricular arrhythmias and nonsustained VT in 25 studies published between 1983 and 1994.[11,13-15,17,18,20,21-24,26,30,32-34,38,39,60,61,70,72,76,88,91] This includes an early study by Gomes and colleagues and a more recent series by Turitto and coworkers.[13,23,91]

Programmed stimulation initiated sustained monomorphic VT in 23% of patients (range, eight to 49); VF in 4% (range, two to 14); and nonsustained VT in 23% (range, 10 to 64). Fifty percent of patients (range, 18 to 73) did not have any inducible ventricular arrhythmias. Induced nonsustained VT was monomorphic in 49% of cases and polymorphic in the remaining 51%. The difference in the results of the reported studies may be partly related to the characteristics of the enrolled population as well as to the use of differing stimulation protocols and end points. The proportion of patients with induced sustained monomorphic VT was lower (11%) when a maximum of two extrastimuli and burst pacing were delivered and higher (29%) when three extrastimuli were used. The use of three extrastimuli was associated with a proportional but not greater increase in the induction of VF. In studies from Turitto and associates and Wilber and colleagues, VF represented 31% and 11%, respectively, of sustained tachyarrhythmias induced by two extrastimuli, compared with 45% and 15% of those induced by three extrastimuli, with no statistically significant differences.[23,32]

The cycle length of induced sustained monomorphic VT was relatively short, ranging between 190 to 280 milliseconds in most studies.[14,15,18,22,23,70,89] These cycle lengths were shorter than those induced in patients with spontaneous sustained VT (285 to 370 milliseconds).[63,65,66,68,70,80,82,83] This may at least partly be because the induction of sustained monomorphic VT usually required more extrastimuli in patients without spontaneous sustained VT than in those with spontaneous sustained VT.[70] The cycle length of induced VT tended to shorten as the number of extrastimuli necessary for induction increased. This was demonstrated in patients with spontaneous nonsustained VT as well as in those with sustained VT.[16,17,63]

Noninvasive Predictors of the Results of Programmed Stimulation

Because only a fraction of patients with spontaneous nonsustained VT had inducible sustained monomorphic VT on PES, several noninvasive determinants of VT inducibility have been investigated as a means to screen patients for the invasive electrophysiologic procedure (Table 19-1). The presence and type of heart disease (in addition to other clinical variables), ECG characteristics of the spontaneous arrhythmia, and left ventricular function indices have been investigated separately or in combination. The value of the signal-averaged ECG has also been assessed.

CLINICAL VARIABLES. Induction of VT was more common in patients with heart disease than in those without.[11,13,14,22-24,38,61,92] In most studies, patients with induced sustained VT or induced nonsustained or sustained VT had structural heart disease.[13,14,22,24] In some reports, the incidence of induced nonsustained or sustained VT in patients with apparently normal heart ranged from 12% to 17% to 40%.[11,61,92] Observed differences reach statistical significance when data from several reports are pooled, even though this approach may not be entirely satisfactory because of the different design of individual studies. Eight investigative groups subjected to PES a total of 483 patients with heart disease and 112 subjects with apparently normal hearts.[11,13,14,22-24,61,92] When inducible nonsustained and sustained VT were considered together, they were significantly more frequent in patients with heart disease than in those without (48% versus 30%, respectively; $p < .05$). When inducible sustained monomorphic VT was considered alone, the difference between its incidence in patients with or without organic heart disease (20% versus 2%, respectively) became more statistically significant ($p < .01$). Organic heart disease was present in 86% of patients with induced nonsustained or sustained VT and in 98% of those with induced sustained VT.[11,13,14,22-24,61,92]

The relation between the type of heart disease and inducibility can be demonstrated by combining data from six groups that studied both patients with coronary artery disease (n = 326) and patients with idiopathic dilated cardiomyopathy (n = 178), using similar protocols and endpoint for PES.[13,14,17,23,38,91] Induction of nonsustained

or sustained ventricular tachyarrhythmias was more frequent in the group with coronary artery disease, compared with the group with idiopathic dilated cardiomyopathy (42% versus 25%; $p < .0001$). When only induction of sustained monomorphic VT was considered, the percentage difference between the two groups was also significant. Sustained monomorphic VT was induced in 30% of patients with coronary artery disease and in 14% of those with dilated cardiomyopathy ($p < .001$). Induction of sustained monomorphic VT in other types of organic heart disease was rare. In the study from Kadish and coworkers, sustained VT was induced in 13% only of 24 patients with miscellaneous heart disease.[38]

A previous myocardial infarction was documented more often in patients with induced VT than in those without induced VT in studies by Gomes and associates (85% versus 43%; $p < .01$) and Kharsa and colleagues (88% versus 44%; $p < .05$), whereas the difference was not significant in the report from Zheutlin and coworkers (73% versus 53%).[13,17,24] In a study by Sulpizi and associates, all patients with recent myocardial infarction (within 3 months of programmed stimulation) had inducible sustained or nonsustained VT, yielding a higher inducibility rate than in the remaining population (100% versus 54%; $p < .007$).[22] This variable, however, was not considered to be independently related to VT inducibility by multivariate analysis. In contrast, old myocardial infarction was a significant variable in multivariate models published by Schoenfeld and colleagues ($p < .001$) and Nalos and coworkers ($p < .0002$).[72,90] The influence of the site of prior myocardial infarction on induction of sustained monomorphic VT was studied by Zehender and associates in 106 postinfarction patients.[70] In the group with spontaneous nonsustained VT or no documented VT, inducibility was 34% for inferior infarction, compared with 65% for anterior infarction ($p < .05$).

Symptoms were significantly related to VT induction only in the series by Turitto and colleagues.[23] A history of syncope–presyncope was present in 50% of patients with induced sustained monomorphic VT and in 22% of those without induced sustained monomorphic VT ($p < .05$). Other investigators did not find any significant difference in the frequency of syncope between patients with or without inducible VT.[11,15,22,34,39]

ELECTROCARDIOGRAPHIC VARIABLES. In a study by Gradman and associates, three quantitative variables that were derived from 24-hour ambulatory ECG were found to be significantly related to the induction of VT by PES: a mean VPC frequency of 100 or more per 1000 normal beats, a mean couplet frequency of 1 or more per 1000 normal beats, and a repetition-index value of 15 or more per 1000 VPCs.[93] The repetition index was defined as the ratio of the number of couplets to the total number of VPCs. These

TABLE 19-1. Determinants of Ventricular Tachyarrhythmia Inducibility by Programmed Stimulation in Patients With Non-sustained Ventricular Tachycardia and/or Complex Ventricular Ectopy

Author and Predicted Arrhythmia → Variables ↓	Buxton,[11,12] VT	Spielman,[15] S-VT/VF	Veltri,[14] VT	Sulpizi,[22] S-VT,m	Turitto,[23] S-VT,m	Gomes,[13] VT/VF	Zheutlin,[17] VT	Gradman,[93] VT	Schoenfeld,[72] VT/VF	Nalos,[90] S-VT,m	Vatterott,[94] S-VT,m	Winters,[39] VT	Turitto,[91] S-VT,m
Age	—	no	—	—	no	—	no	—	no	yes	no	no	no
Sex	—	no	—	—	no	—	no	—	yes	no	no	—	no
Presence of HD†	yes	—	yes	no	no	—	—	—	—	—	—	—	—
Ischemic HD	yes	no	—	no	no	yes	no	—	no	yes	no	—	—
Prior MI†	—	—	—	no	no	yes	no	—	yes	yes	yes	—	—
Syncope	no	no	—	—	yes	—	—	—	yes	yes	—	no	no
VPCs†/h	—	—	—	—	no	—	—	yes	—	—	no	—	no
Couplets/24 h	—	—	—	—	no	—	—	yes	—	—	yes	—	no
Repetition index	—	—	—	—	no	—	—	yes	—	—	—	—	no
VT† runs/24 h	no	no	no	—	no	—	—	—	—	—	yes	—	no
VT duration	no	no	no	—	no	—	—	—	—	—	—	—	no
VT rate	—	no	—	—	no	—	—	—	—	—	—	—	no
VT morphology	—	no	—	—	no	—	no	—	—	—	—	—	no
Ejection fraction	yes	no	no	yes	yes	yes	—	—	no	yes	yes	no	no
LV† dyskinesia	yes	yes	—	no	no	—	—	—	no	yes	—	no	—
Signal-averaged ECG†	—	—	—	yes	yes	—	—	—	—	yes	yes	yes	yes

Study population included only patients with (1) spontaneous nonsustained VT in the reports from Buxton, Spielman, Veltri, Sulpizi, Turitto, Winters, et al; (2) nonsustained VT, complex ventricular ectopy, or both in the reports from Gomes and Zheutlin et al; and (3) various clinical presentations (sustained VT, cardiac arrest, nonsustained VT, syncope) in the reports from Gradman, Schoenfeld, Nalos, Vatterott, et al.

*Indicates studies in which multivariate methods to predict inducibility of the index arrhythmia were used; univariate methods were used in the remaining studies.

†Yes, significant variable; no, variable not significantly related to inducibility; —, variable not studied; ECG, electrocardiogram; h, hours; HD, heart disease; LV, left ventricle; MI, myocardial infarction; VF, ventricular fibrillation; VPCs, ventricular premature complexes; VT, ventricular tachycardia; S, sustained, m, monomorphic.

data are at variance with other studies, in which ECG characteristics of the spontaneous arrhythmia did not predict VT inducibility.[11,14,15,23,91]

LEFT VENTRICULAR FUNCTION INDICES. Several studies found that patients with ejection fraction of less than 40% had a greater frequency of induced sustained monomorphic VT, compared with those with ejection fraction of more than 40%. This difference was significant in studies by Turitto and coworkers (86% versus 36%; $p < .0001$); Hammill and colleagues (28% versus 11%; $p < .03$); and Kadish and associates (40% versus 18%; $p < .05$).[23,30,38] Ejection fraction was a significant predictor of inducibility in multivariate analysis models reported by Turitto and associates, Nalos and colleagues, and Vatterott and coworkers.[23,90,94] In a study by Sulpizi and associates, impairment of left ventricular function (defined as an ejection fraction lower than 0.35 or functional class III–IV, with cardiomegaly on chest x-ray) was identified as the only variable independently related to sustained VT induction.[22] Conversely, the degree of left ventricular dysfunction was similar in patients with or without induced VT in other reports, including a study by Turitto and colleagues, enrolling only subjects with dilated cardiomyopathy.[14,15,17,34,91]

Besides left ventricular ejection fraction, the relation of wall motion abnormalities to inducibility was considered by several studies. Spielman and coworkers found that induced sustained VT–VF was more frequent in patients with at least one akinetic or dyskinetic left ventricular segment, as shown by radionuclide angiography, compared with those without such abnormalities (69% versus 29%; $p < .01$).[15] Buxton and associates report that among patients with coronary artery disease, sustained VT was induced more often in the presence of left ventricular aneurysm than in its absence (69% versus 20%; $p < .01$).[11] This finding, however, was not corroborated by subsequent studies from the same authors or other groups.[21,23,26]

SIGNAL-AVERAGED ELECTROCARDIOGRAM. The signal-averaged ECG is recorded by amplifying, averaging, and filtering the signal recorded on the body surface by orthogonal leads.[95] The recording detects low-amplitude cardiac electrical signals in the late QRS–ST segment that may represent delayed activation of abnormal myocardial tissue.[96] These signals are usually called late potentials. The signal-averaged ECG was initially found to accurately predict the results of PES in patients with spontaneous sustained VT.[97-99] The predictive value of the signal-averaged ECG for the induction of sustained VT was initially confirmed in a study by Nalos and colleagues in patients with miscellaneous presenting arrhythmias and by Buxton and coworkers in patients with spontaneous nonsustained VT after healing of myocardial infarction.[88,90]

The first prospective study of the value of the signal-averaged ECG as a predictor of the results of programmed stimulation in patients with nonsustained VT, using stepwise discriminant function analysis, was published by Turitto and associates.[23] The study found that the signal-averaged ECG is the single most accurate screening test to predict the inducibility of sustained VT in patients with spontaneous nonsustained VT. A consecutive series of 105 patients with spontaneous nonsustained VT on 24-hour ambulatory ECG was studied. The study population consisted of 60 patients with coronary artery disease, 26 with idiopathic dilated cardiomyopathy, and 19 with no identifiable heart disease. Patients were divided into three groups according to the results of programmed stimulation (three extrastimuli, two right ventricular sites): group 1 included 22 patients with induced sustained monomorphic VT (Fig. 19-1); group 2 included 14 patients with induced VF; and group 3 included 69 patients without induced sustained ventricular tachyarrhythmias (Fig. 19-2).

Table 19-2 shows the characteristics of patients in the groups. Group 1 patients showed a significantly higher frequency of syncope–presyncope, left ventricular ejection fraction of less than 40%, and late potentials on the signal-averaged ECG, compared with group 3. Late potentials were defined as low-amplitude signals in the terminal part of the QRS, with duration of more than 38 milliseconds and root mean square voltage of less than 25 microvolts. The etiology of underlying heart disease, the ECG characteristics of the spontaneous arrhythmia (number, duration, and cycle length of nonsustained VT runs), and the prevalence of left ventricular wall motion abnormalities were not significantly different in groups 1 and 3. In contrast, when patients with induced VF (group 2) were compared with patients without induced sustained VT–VF (group 3), none of the variables showed significant differences. Further analysis of group 3 patients revealed no significant differences in clinical and ECG variables, left ventricular function indices, and the signal-averaged ECG between patients in whom monomorphic nonsustained VT, polymorphic nonsustained VT, or no VT were induced. Late potentials were recorded in 23 patients (22%): 14 in group 1, three in group 2, and six in group 3. The sensitivity, specificity, and positive, negative, and total predictive accuracy of late potentials for the induction of sustained monomorphic VT were, respectively: 64%, 89%, 61%, 90%, and 84%. In other words, the probability of inducing sustained monomorphic VT was 61% in patients with late potentials and declined to 10% in those without late potentials. The frequency of late potentials was similar in patients with coronary artery disease (25%) and in those with idiopathic dilated cardiomyopathy (23%). Their predictive accuracy was also comparable in the two groups: 85% in coronary artery disease and 81% in cardiomyopathy patients. Among the 43 patients with prior myo-

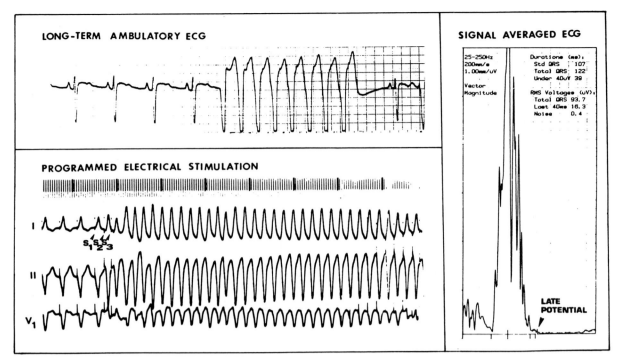

Figure 19-1. Recordings of ambulatory electrocardiogram (ECG), programmed electrical stimulation, and signal-averaged ECG from a 56-year-old man with coronary artery disease. A 24-hour ambulatory ECG showed frequent ventricular premature complexes and runs of nonsustained ventricular tachycardia. The signal-averaged ECG showed late potentials (the root mean square (RMS) voltage of the last 40 milliseconds of the filtered QRS = 16.3 μV and the duration of the low-amplitude signal under 40 μV = 39 milliseconds). Programmed electrical stimulation using an $S_1S_2S_3$ protocol from the right ventricular apex induced a sustained monomorphic tachycardia.

cardial infarction, late potentials showed high predictive accuracy both in anterior infarction (73%) and in inferior infarction (88%). Using stepwise discriminant function analysis, late potentials proved to be the variable most strongly correlated ($p < .00001$) with the induction of sustained monomorphic VT, with an overall predictive accuracy of 84%. No combination between late potentials and other significant variables (ejection fraction and symptoms) provided an improvement in predicting sustained VT inducibility in comparison with late potentials alone. When late potentials were removed from the analysis, the combination of other variables provided a predictive accuracy of 71%. Late potentials were still able to enter the model, with a probability of improving it less than 0.05. Thus, the signal-averaged ECG offered predictive information above that found in clinical variables and other noninvasive tests. Conversely, no single variable or combination of variables predicted the induction of VF.

In our series of 105 patients, concurrence between the results of PES and those of the signal-averaged ECG was observed in 84% of cases. The largest subgroup consisted of patients who had no late potentials and no induced sustained monomorphic VT (70%). In these patients, it is reasonable to speculate that the spontaneous

arrhythmia may be due to mechanisms other than reentry (e.g., abnormal automaticity or triggered activity).[100, 101] Patients with both late potentials and induced sustained monomorphic VT comprised 14% of cases. The results of the two tests were discordant in the remaining 16% of cases. Nine patients had late potentials but failed to develop sustained monomorphic VT at PES. This may be explained by electrophysiologic limitations of both PES and signal-averaging techniques.[62, 96] The relation between myocardial zones with delayed conduction during sinus rhythm and the occurrence of reentrant arrhythmias is complex. Zones showing conduction delay (i.e., late potentials) during basic rhythm may completely block during premature stimulation and not participate in a reentrant pathway.[96] In eight patients, a sustained VT was induced in the absence of late potentials. Again, limitations of the signal-averaged ECG (e.g., inability to detect delayed activation potentials with a dynamic Wenckebach's sequence) and the possibility that some induced VT may have represented a nonspecific response to PES can be invoked. In this regard, four of the eight patients in this group had a cycle length of induced sustained monomorphic VT of 190 to 195 milliseconds.

Our observation that patients with induced VF were

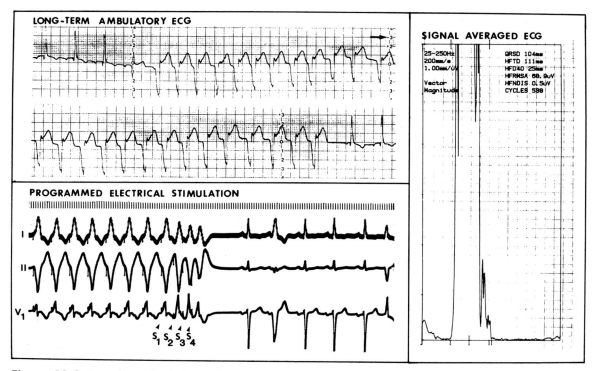

Figure 19-2 Recordings of ambulatory electrocardiograms (ECGs), programmed electrical stimulation, and signal-averaged ECG from a 41-year-old man with idiopathic dilated cardiomyopathy. The patient had no history of syncope–presyncope. The ejection fraction by radionuclide ventriculography was 16%. A 24-hour ambulatory ECG showed frequent ventricular premature complexes (average 240/hour) and six runs of nonsustained monomorphic ventricular tachycardia; the longest is shown in the figure. It comprised 26 beats and had an averaged cycle length of 452 milliseconds. The signal-averaged ECG was normal. There was no inducible arrhythmia on programmed electrical stimulation. (Turitto G, Fontaine JM, Ursell SN, Caref EB, Henkin R, El-Sherif N: Value of the signal-averaged electrocardiogram as a predictor of the results of programmed stimulation in non-sustained ventricular tachycardia. Am J Cardiol 1988;61:1272.)

TABLE 19-2. Characteristics of 105 Patients With Spontaneous Nonsustained Ventricular Tachycardia With or Without Induced Ventricular Tachyarrhythmias

	Group 1 (n, 22)	Group 2 (n, 14)	Group 3 (n, 69)	Probability	
	(n) (%)	(n) (%)	(n) (%)	Group 1 vs Group 3	Group 2 vs Group 3
Heart disease					
Ischemic;	16 (73)	7 (50)	37 (54)	NS	NS
with prior MI*	12	5	26		
Dilated CMP*	5 (23)	3 (21)	18 (26)	NS	NS
None	1 (5)	4 (29)	14 (20)	NS	NS
Syncope/presyncope	11 (50)	7 (50)	15 (22)	<0.05	NS
LV* ejection fraction <0.40	19 (86)	5 (36)	25 (36)	<0.0001	NS
LV segmental a/dyskinesia	11 (50)	3 (21)	16 (23)	NS	NS
Late potentials on the signal averaged ECG*	14 (64)	3 (21)	6 (9)	<0.00001	NS

Group 1, induced sustained monomorphic VT; group 2, induced VF; group 3, no induced sustained ventricular tachyarrhythmias.

*CMP, cardiomyopathy; ECG, electrocardiogram; LV, left ventricle; MI, myocardial infarction; NS, not significant.

indistinguishable from patients with no induced VT–VF, by the signal-averaged ECG or any other variables, suggests that the induction of VF may represent a nonclinical response to PES in this group of patients.[102, 103] Furthermore, that the induction of sustained monomorphic VT rather than that of VF or nonsustained VT was correlated to the presence or absence of late potentials on the signal-averaged ECG provides evidence for the hypothesis that late potentials represent abnormal myocardial zones with delayed activation potentials capable of providing the electrophysiologic substrate for reentrant rhythms.[96] It also emphasizes the specificity of induced sustained monomorphic VT, rather than induced nonsustained VT or VF, as the end point of PES in patients with spontaneous nonsustained VT.

The best criteria to define an abnormal signal-averaged ECG for predicting VT induction are still debated. This is related at least partly to the lack of standardization of recording equipment and to the use of different filter settings and criteria for normality in different studies. A study from Caref and colleagues defined normal values for signal-averaged ECG parameters in 100 normal subjects, examined the effect of different high-pass filters on these values, and used multivariate analysis to identify the best parameter or parameters to predict induction of sustained monomorphic VT in 80 patients with spontaneous nonsustained VT and normal QRS duration on the conventional ECG.[104] A computer program was written, in which the three signal-averaged ECG parameters (QRS duration, duration of low-amplitude signals less than 40 microvolts [LAS40], and root mean square voltage of last 40 milliseconds of QRS [RMS40]) were analyzed at 11 high-pass filter settings (10, 20, 25, 30, 40, 50, 60, 70, 80, 90, and 100 Hz) and combined in 6017 combinations of singles, pairs, and triplets of parameters to improve prediction of the results of PES. Among the study subjects, 28 had induced sustained monomorphic VT, whereas 52 did not. This approach allowed for comparison of the three parameters across all high-pass filter settings. There were 32 combinations that provided the highest total predictive accuracy of 89%. Only two combinations were pairs: RMS40 at 20 or 25 Hz, combined with RMS40 at 40 Hz; the remaining 30 were composed of triplets, which included values for LAS40 and RMS40 at different filter settings. None of the top combinations included QRS duration. Thus, it was concluded that optimization of prediction of the outcome of PES in patients with spontaneous nonsustained VT may be achieved by combining values of RMS40 obtained at 25- and 40-Hz filter settings. These are the most commonly used high-pass filters in clinical practice and in studies reported in the literature. An example of the prospective application of these criteria to predict PES results is a study by Turitto and coworkers, which included 70 patients presenting with spontaneous nonsustained VT and idiopathic

dilated cardiomyopathy.[91] In this study, sustained monomorphic VT was induced in nine patients (13%). An abnormal signal-averaged ECG had a high predictive accuracy of 86% for the results of PES.

New techniques for the analysis of the signal-averaged ECG in the frequency domain have been used to predict the outcome of PES in patients with spontaneous nonsustained VT.[91, 105] Frequency domain analysis or spectral turbulence analysis of the signal-averaged ECG was found to be superior to time domain analysis in its prediction of induced sustained monomorphic VT in patients with coronary artery disease and spontaneous nonsustained VT.[105] In contrast, in patients with dilated cardiomyopathy, the opposite was true.[91]

Use of Programmed Electrical Stimulation for Risk Stratification

In patients with no documented sustained ventricular tachyarrhythmias, the induction of sustained monomorphic VT by PES may either represent a mere laboratory finding or indicate patients at high risk for future serious arrhythmic events. The latter hypothesis was tested by many investigators (Table 19-3), discussed in a series of editorials, and is the basis for several ongoing multicenter studies on the prognostic role of PES in patients with coronary artery disease and spontaneous nonsustained VT.[12–14, 16, 17, 19–22, 24–28, 30–34, 36–40, 106–108] Available published reports on the prognostic significance of ventricular tachyarrhythmias induced by PES in patients with complex ventricular arrhythmias and nonsustained VT may be criticized for:

1. Small sample size[12–14, 17, 21, 22, 24, 26, 34, 39, 106]

2. Retrospective data collection[14, 21–23]

3. Study population not representative of the overall population with nonsustained VT (selection was based on the absence of symptoms in most studies)[13, 14, 17, 33, 106]

4. Lack of standardization of the stimulation protocol and its endpoint

5. Lack of uniform therapeutic approach

The indication for antiarrhythmic therapy varied in different studies. Authors subjected to treatment patients with induced sustained VT and those with induced nonsustained VT and induced VF.[13, 14, 17, 21, 24, 26, 30, 33, 34, 38, 39] In some studies, therapy was defined by means of repeat PES, whereas in other studies, this was not always the case.[14, 17, 21, 24, 30–34, 38, 106] Conversely, guidelines for the management of patients without induced VT were disparate; in some instances, these subjects did not receive any antiarrhythmic treatment, whereas in other studies, there were subgroups followed-up or off antiarrhythmic

TABLE 19-3. Outcome of Patients With Spontaneous Nonsustained Ventricular Tachycardia or Complex Ventricular Ectopy Studied with Programmed Electrical Stimulation

Author	Heart disease	PES End Point	PES+/ PES− (n)	Follow-up (months)	Sudden death or Major Arrhythmia (PES+/PES−) [%]	Relation of PES+ to Sudden Death	Patients Treated With Drugs (n)	Role of Therapy	Risk Factors for Sudden Death
Gomes[13]	CAD, 77%; other, 23%	VT/VF	20/53	30 ± 15	32/2	P < .001	PES+, 17; PES−, 26		Baseline PES+ LVEF < .40
Buxton[12]	CAD, 40%; CM, 18%; other, 42%	VT/VF	15/68	33	27/9	P < .00001 for sustained VT			Baseline PES+ LVEF < .40
Veltri[14]	CAD, 58%; other, 42%	VT	14/19	23 ± 16	21/21	NS	PES+, 12; PES−, 11		Low LVEF
Zheutlin[17]	CAD, 65%; CM, 26%; other, 9%	VT	33/55	22 ± 17	12/0	P < .02	Only PES+		Baseline PES+
Buxton[21]	CAD, 100%	Sustained VT	28/34	28	25/12	Among all pts, higher SD rate with empiric therapy than with therapy guided by PES (P < .001)	PES+, 24; PES−, 15	Lower SD rate with therapy guided by PES, compared with empiric therapy	Therapy not guided by PES results
Sulpizi[22]	CAD, 62%; CM, 15%; none, 23%	VT	9/52	26	11/6	NS	Not specified		Low LVEF
Kharsa[24]	CAD, 53%; other, 47%	Sustained VT, mono	8/32	16	0/0	Low risk of SD, both in PES− pts and PES+ pts on therapy guided by PES	Only PES+		
Winters[26]	CAD, 50%; other, 50%	VT	13/40	15 ± 10	15/5	NS	Not specified		
Klein[106]	CAD, 100%	VT	22/18	14	41/0	P < .01	Only PES+	Lower SD rate with therapy guided by PES, compared with empiric therapy (P < .01)	Therapy not guided by PES results
Turitto[25]	CAD, 70%; CM, 30%	Sustained VT, mono	22/68	30 ± 10	19/8	Low risk of SD, both in PES− pts and PES+ pts on therapy guided by PES	Only PES+		

(continued)

TABLE 19-3. Outcome of Patients With Spontaneous Nonsustained Ventricular Tachycardia or Complex Ventricular Ectopy Studied with Programmed Electrical Stimulation *(Continued)*

Author	Heart disease	PES End Point	PES+/PES- (n)	Follow-up (months)	Sudden death or Major Arrhythmia (PES+/PES-) [%]	Relation of PES+ to Sudden Death	Patients Treated With Drugs (n)	Role of Therapy	Risk Factors for Sudden Death
Hammill[30]	CAD, 78%; CM, 22%	Sustained VT, mono	21/89	15	10/13		Only PES+		Low LVEF, NYHA class III–IV; high event rate in pts with CM and PES– (33%); low inducibility (11%), low event rate (4%) in pts with CAD and LVEF >0.40; high inducibility (50%), high event rate (21%) in pts with CAD and LVEF <.40
Wilber[32]	CAD, 100% (LVEF < 0.40)	Sustained VT/VF	43/57	17	PES–; 6% PES+; 11% if PES– on drugs; 50% if PES+ on drugs	$P < .001$ for PES+ on drugs	Only PES+		PES+ on drugs
Kowey[33]	CAD, 100%	VT/VF	130/75	18	19/27	NS	PES+, 66; PES– 57		LVEF
Manolis[34]	CAD, 100%	VT/VF	21/31	21 ± 17	0/3	NS	Only PES+		
Kadish[38]	CAD, 48%; CM, 15%; other, 9%; none, 28%	Sustained VT, mono	52/228	20 ± 14	PES+: 0 if PES– on drugs; 11% if PES+ on drugs; PES–: 5% on no therapy; 4% on empirical therapy	$P < .01$ for PES+ on drugs	PES+, 50; PES– 89		LVEF, PES+ on drugs
Winters[39]	CAD, 100%	VT	16/41	22 ± 27	34/16	NS	Only PES+		VT induced at baseline, LVEF < .30, nonadherence to PES-guided therapy

CAD, coronary artery disease; *CM*, cardiomyopathy; *LVEF*, left ventricular ejection fraction; *mono*, monomorphic; *NS*, not significant; *SD*, sudden death; *VF*, ventricular fibrillation; *VT*, ventricular tachycardia.

drugs.[13, 14, 17, 21, 24, 26, 30, 32–34, 38, 106] In none of the published reports was treatment randomized.

Most studies reported a low risk of sudden cardiac death in patients with nonsustained VT who had no induced VT (see Table 19-3).[12–14, 17, 21, 22, 24, 25, 32, 34, 38, 106] The risk of sudden death was equally low in patients with induced nonsustained VT in studies by Turitto and associates, Wilber and colleagues, and Kharsa and coworkers.[24, 25, 32] In our series (Table 19-4) the 3-year sudden death rate was 9% in 56 patients with no induced sustained VT–VF followed-up off antiarrhythmic therapy.[25] The 3-year sudden death rate was the same (7%) in patients with left ventricular ejection fraction of less than 40% or 40% or more. In contrast, the 3-year total cardiac mortality was significantly higher in those patients with ejection fraction of less than 40%, compared with those with an ejection fraction of 40% or more (27% versus 7%, respectively; $p < .05$) (Figs. 19-3 and 19-4). A review of the studies summarized in Table 19-3 reveals that the risk of serious arrhythmic events in the noninducible group was similar both in the presence and absence of antiarrhythmic therapy.[12, 13, 17, 24, 32, 38] It seems reasonable to conclude that subjects with spontaneous nonsustained VT and no induced sustained VT may be managed safely without the use of antiarrhythmic drugs.[13, 17, 24, 30, 32, 34, 38, 106]

There are few follow-up studies of patients with induced VF. In our series, all patients with spontaneous nonsustained VT who had induced VF remained alive off antiarrhythmic therapy during a follow-up of 30 ± 10 months.[25] These findings are consistent with the findings of DiCarlo and associates and Mahmud and colleagues.[102, 103] These authors report no major arrhythmic events in a total of 27 patients without documented spontaneous sustained VT–VF and with induced VF who were followed-up for more than 2 years. The arrhythmia was considered a nonclinical response to PES in patients without clinical sustained ventricular tachyarrhythmias.

Conversely, VT inducibility seems to carry an increased risk of sudden death in patients with spontaneous nonsustained VT. The induced arrhythmia that portends a poor prognosis was identified as sustained VT by Buxton and coworkers, Wilber and associates, Kadish and colleagues, and as VT (sustained or nonsustained) by Gomes and coworkers, Zheutlin and associates, and Winters and colleagues (see Table 19-3).[12, 13, 17, 21, 32, 38, 39] In one study by Buxton and coworkers, sudden death occurred in four of 15 patients (27%) with induced sustained VT, in two of 37 (5%) with induced nonsustained VT, and in four of 31 (13%) without induced VT during a follow-up of 33 months.[12] Sudden death occurred only in patients with left ventricular ejection fraction of less than 40%. Using multivariate analysis, patients with one poor prognostic marker (induced sustained VT or low ejection fraction) were characterized by a threefold increased risk of sudden death, whereas patients with both markers had a sevenfold increased risk. In the study by Gomes and associates, actuarial survival curves revealed that at one year, 75% of patients with induced VT–VF and 100% of those

TABLE 19-4. Cardiac Mortality Rate in Patients With Organic Heart Disease and Spontaneous Nonsustained Ventricular Tachycardia, Subgrouped by Ejection Fraction, Signal-averaged Electrocardiogram and Arrhythmias Induced at Electrophysiologic Study[25]

Ejection Fraction (%)	Signal-Averaged ECG	Arrhythmia Induced at EPS*	Patients (n)	Cardiac Mortality	
				Number	Rate (%)
<40	Positive	No sustained VT/VF*	4	1	25
		VF	2	0	0
		Sustained VT	13	2	15
	Negative	No sustained VT/VF	20	5	25
		VF	7	0	0
		Sustained VT	7	3	43
≥40	Positive	No sustained VT/VF	1	0	0
		VF	1	0	0
		Sustained VT	2	0	0
	Negative	No sustained VT/VF	33	2	6
		VF	0	0	0
		Sustained VT	0	0	0
		Total	90	13	14

*EPS, electrophysiologic study; VT, ventricular tachycardia; VF, ventricular fibrillation.

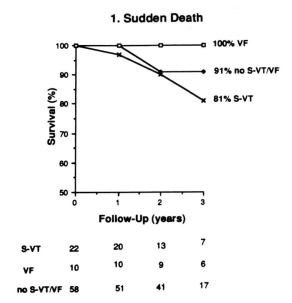

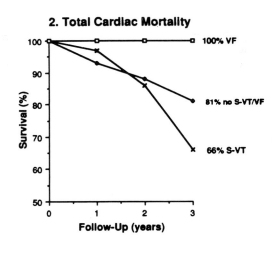

Figure 19-3. Three-year actuarial survival curves for sudden death and total cardiac mortality in patients with organic heart disease and spontaneous nonsustained ventricular tachycardia, classified by the outcome of programmed stimulation. The number of patients followed-up at each interval is indicated on the bottom of the figure. (*VF, ventricular fibrillation; S-VT, sustained ventricular tachycardia.*)

without it were alive, whereas at 2 years, the probability of survival declined to 65% and 97%, respectively (*p* < .001).[13]

Few studies failed to find a correlation between the inducibility of VT and high risk for sudden cardiac death in patients with spontaneous nonsustained VT. Most of these studies were retrospective.[14,22,33] In the study by Sulpizi and colleagues, the overall probability of sudden death was low (7% during a follow-up of 26 months) and was not influenced by VT inducibility.[22] In contrast, poor left ven-

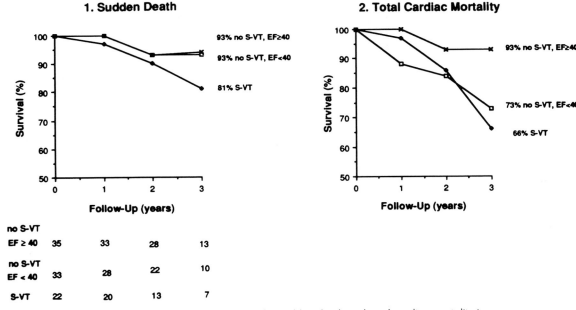

Figure 19-4. Three-year actuarial survival curves for sudden death and total cardiac mortality in patients with organic heart disease and spontaneous nonsustained ventricular tachycardia (VT) who had no induced sustained VT (S-VT), classified by left ventricular ejection fraction (EF). The survival curves for all patients with induced VT are also shown for comparison. The number of patients followed-up at each interval is indicated on the bottom of the figure.

tricular function was an important predictor of mortality. Similar findings were reported by Veltri and coworkers.[14] In their study, a 21% incidence of serious arrhythmic events was documented over a follow-up period of about 2 years. Ejection fraction was significantly lower in the group with arrhythmic events than in the group without (0.49 ± 0.18 versus 0.31 ± 0.17; $p < .04$), whereas the ability to induce VT was not correlated to outcome.

The available literature on the effects of empiric antiarrhythmic therapy or therapy guided by PES on survival of patients with spontaneous nonsustained VT and induced VT is controversial. Some of the reported studies fail to demonstrate that PES-guided therapy improves survival of patients with induced VT or is superior to empiric therapy.[12,13,18] Patients with induced VT treated with drug regimens selected by PES maintained an excess mortality relative to those without induced VT in studies by Gomes and associates and Zheutlin and colleagues.[13,17] A study by Buxton and coworkers that only used historical controls suggested that therapy guided by PES in this group was associated with a lower rate of sudden cardiac death, compared with empiric therapy.[21] A similar conclusion was reached by studies from Klein and associates, Wilber and colleagues, and Kadish and coworkers.[32,38,106] Conversely, the significance of the finding that PES-guided therapy in patients with induced sustained VT was associated with a low risk of sudden death in our study and others is limited by the lack of a controlled group not on antiarrhythmic therapy.[24,25,34]

The hypothesis that the induction of ventricular tachyarrhythmias in patients with spontaneous nonsustained VT identifies a subset of patients with increased risk of sudden cardiac death is being tested by several multicenter randomized studies.[40,108] These studies are comparing the incidence of sudden death in different groups of patients: patients without the index arrhythmia during PES and inducible patients, randomized to no therapy or to therapy guided by PES.[108]

RECOMMENDED PROTOCOL FOR RISK STRATIFICATION AND MANAGEMENT OF PATIENTS WITH NONSUSTAINED VENTRICULAR TACHYCARDIA

A study from our laboratory strongly suggests that an optimal protocol for risk stratification and management of patients with organic heart disease and spontaneous nonsustained VT should be based on the results of the signal-averaged ECG, left ventricular ejection fraction, and PES as follows (Fig. 19-5):[25]

1. Patients with no late potentials in the signal-averaged ECG and with an ejection fraction of more than 40% do not require testing by PES nor long-term antiar-

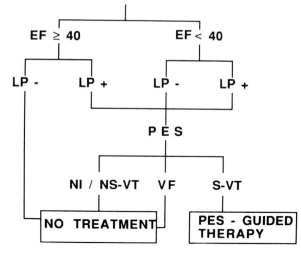

Figure 19-5. A suggested management protocol for patients with organic heart disease and spontaneous nonsustained ventricular tachycardia. (*EF*, left ventricular ejection fraction); *LP*, no late potentials in the signal-averaged electrocardiogram; *LP+*, late potentials in the signal-averaged electrocardiogram; *PES*, programmed electrical stimulation; *NI*, not inducible; *NS-VT* inducible nonsustained ventricular tachycardia; *VF* inducible ventricular fibrillation; *S-VT*, inducible sustained monomorphic ventricular tachycardia.)

rhythmic therapy because the incidence of inducible sustained monomorphic VT and the risk of sudden death are low in this group of patients. There was no instance of induced sustained VT in 33 consecutive patients in this group.

2. Patients with no late potentials but with ejection fraction of less than 40% and patients with late potentials should be recommended for electrophysiologic evaluation. The incidence of inducible sustained monomorphic VT was 21% in the former group and 65% in the latter group.

In patients with late potentials, the high incidence of inducible VT was independent of the etiology of heart disease and the degree of ejection fraction (50% with ejection fraction of more than 40% versus 68% with ejection fraction of less than 40%). Based on the results of PES, patients with no inducible tachyarrhythmia and those with inducible nonsustained VT or VF may be followed-up off antiarrhythmic therapy with a low risk of sudden death. If sustained monomorphic VT is induced, however, these patients should be enrolled in one of the ongoing randomized studies to assess the value of antiarrhythmic drug therapy in preventing sudden death. If this is not possible, patients with induced sustained monomorphic VT probably should receive antiarrhythmic therapy guided by PES criteria, with the understanding that the value of antiarrhythmic therapy has yet to be definitely established.

References

1. Lown B: Sudden cardiac death—1978. Circulation 1979; 60:1593.
2. Mason J, Winkle R: Electrode-catheter arrhythmia induction in the selection and assessment of antiarrhythmic drug therapy for recurrent ventricular tachycardia. Circulation 1978;58:971.
3. Horowitz L, Josephson M. Farshidi A, Spielman SR, Michelson EL, Greenspan AM: Recurrent sustained ventricular tachycardia. 3. Role of the electrophysiologic study in selection of antiarrhythmic regimens. Circulation 1978;58:986.
4. Swerdlow CD, Winkle RA, Mason JW: Determinants of survival in patients with ventricular tachyarrhythmias. N Engl J Med 1983;308:1436.
5. Myerburg RJ, Kessler KM, Estes D, et al: Long-term survival after prehospital cardiac arrest: analysis of outcome during an 8 year study. Circulation 1984;70:538.
6. Goldstein S, Landis JR, Leighton R, et al: Predictive survival models for resuscitated victims of out-of-hospital cardiac arrest with coronary heart disease. Circulation 1985;5:873.
7. Bigger JT Jr, Fleiss JL, Kleiger R, Miller JP, Rolnitzky LM, The Multicenter Post-Infarction Research Goup: The relationships among ventricular arrhythmias, left ventricular dysfunction, and mortality in the 2 years after myocardial infarction. Circulation 1984;69:250.
8. Mukharji J, Rude RE, Poole WK, et al: Risk factors for sudden death after acute myocardial infarction: two-year follow-up. Am J Cardiol 1984;54:31.
9. Maisel AS, Scott N, Gilpin E, et al: Complex ventricular arrhythmias in patients with Q wave versus non-Q wave myocardial infarction. Circulation 1985;72:963.
10. Josephson ME: Treatment of ventricular arrhythmias after myocardial infarction. Circulation 1986;74:653.
11. Buxton AE, Waxman HL, Marchlinski FE, Josephson ME: Electrophysiologic studies in nonsustained ventricular tachycardia: relation to underlying heart disease. Am J Cardiol 1983;52:985.
12. Buxton AE, Marchlinski FE, Waxman HL, Flores BT, Cassidy DM, Josephson ME: Prognostic factors in nonsustained ventricular tachycardia. Am J Cardiol 1984;53:1275.
13. Gomes JAC, Hariman RI, Kang PS, El-Sherif N, Chowdhry I, Lyons J: Programmed electrical stimulation in patients with high-grade ventricular ectopy: electrophysiologic findings and prognosis for survival. Circulation 1984;70:43.
14. Veltri EP, Platia EV, Griffith LSC, Reid PR: Programmed electrical stimulation and long-term follow-up in asymptomatic, nonsustained ventricular tachycardia. Am J Cardiol 1985; 56:309.
15. Spielman SR, Greenspan AM, Kay HR, et al: Electrophysiologic testing in patients at high risk for sudden cardiac death. 1. Nonsustained ventricular tachycardia and abnormal ventricular function. J Am Coll Cardiol 1985;6:31.
16. Meinertz T, Treese N, Kasper W, et al: Determinants of prognosis in idiopathic dilated cardiomyopathy as determined by programmed electrical stimulation. Am J Cardiol 1985;56:337.
17. Zheutlin TA, Roth H, Chua W, et al: Programmed electrical stimulation to determine the need for antiarrhythmic therapy in patients with complex ventricular ectopic activity. Am Heart J 1986;111:860.
18. Breithardt G, Borggrefe M, Podczeck A: Electrophysiology and pharmacology of asymptomatic nonsustained ventricular tachycardia. Clin Progr Electrophysiol Pacing 1986;4:81.
19. Das SK, Morady F, DiCarlo L Jr, et al: Prognostic usefulness of programmed ventricular stimulation in idiopathic dilated cardiomyopathy without symptomatic ventricular arrhythmias. Am J Cardiol 1986;58:998.
20. Poll DS, Marchlinski FE, Buxton AE, Josephson ME: Usefulness of programmed stimulation in idiopathic cardiomyopathy. Am J Cardiol 1986;58:992.
21. Buxton AE, Marchlinski FE, Waxman HL, et al: Nonsustained ventricular tachycardia in patients with coronary artery disease: role of electrophysiologic study. Circulation 1987; 75:1178.
22. Sulpizi AM, Friehling TD, Kowey PR: Value of electrophysiologic testing in patients with nonsustained ventricular tachycardia. Am J Cardiol 1987;59:841.
23. Turitto G, Fontaine JM, Ursell SN, Caref EB, Henkin R, El-Sherif N: Value of the signal-averaged electrocardiogram as a predictor of the results of programmed stimulation in non-sustained ventricular tachycardia. Am J Cardiol 1988; 61:1272.
24. Kharsa MH, Gold RL, Moore H, Yazaki Y, Haffajee C, Alpert JS: Long-term outcome following programmed electrical stimulation in patients with high-grade ventricular ectopy. Pace 1988;11:603.
25. Turitto G, Fontaine JM, Ursell S, Caref EB, Bekheit S, El-Sherif N: Risk stratification and management of patients with organic heart disease and non-sustained ventricular tachycardia. Role of programmed stimulation, left ventricular ejection fraction and the signal averaged electrocardiogram. Am J Med 1990;88(1):35N.
26. Winters SL, Stewart D, Targonski A, Gomes JA: Role of signal averaging of the surface QRS complex in selecting patients with nonsustained ventricular tachycardia and high grade ventricular arrhythmias for programmed ventricular stimulation. J Am Coll Cardiol 1988;12:1481.
27. Kron J, Hart M, Schual-Berke S, Niles NR, Hosenpud JD, McAnulty JH: Idiopathic dilated cardiomyopathy: role of programmed electrical stimulation and Holter monitoring in predicting those at risk of sudden death. Chest 1988; 93:85.
28. Stevenson WG, Stevenson LW, Weiss J, Tillisch JH: Inducible ventricular arrhythmias and sudden death during vasodilator therapy of severe heart failure. Am Heart J 1988;116:1447.
29. Fauchier JP, Cosnay P, Moquet B, Balleh H, Rouesnel P: Late ventricular potentials and spontaneous and induced ventricular arrhythmias in dilated or hypertrophic cardiomyopathies. A prospective study about 83 patients. Pace 1988;11:1974.
30. Hammill SC, Trusty JM, Wood DL, et al: Influence of ventricular function and presence or absence of coronary artery disease on results of electrophysiologic testing for asymptomatic nonsustained ventricular tachycardia. Am J Cardiol 1990;65:722.
31. Gossinger HD, Jung M, Wagner L, et al: Prognostic role of

inducible ventricular tachycardia in patients with dilated cardiomyopathy and asymptomatic nonsustained ventricular tachycardia. Int J Cardiol 1990;29:215.

32. Wilber DJ, Olshansky B, Moran JF, Scanlon PJ: Electrophysiological testing and nonsustained ventricular tachycardia: use and limitations in patients with coronary artery disease and impaired ventricular function. Circulation 1990;82:350.

33. Kowey PR, Waxman HL, Greenspon A, et al: Value of electrophysiologic testing in patients with previous myocardial infarction and nonsustained ventricular tachycardia. Am J Cardiol 1990;65:594.

34. Manolis AS, Estes NAM: Value of programmed ventricular stimulation in the evaluation and management of patients with nonsustained ventricular tachycardia associated with coronary artery disease. Am J Cardiol 1990;65:201.

35. Brembilla-Perot B, Donetti J, Terrier de la Chaise A, Sadoul N, Aliot E, Juilliere Y: Diagnostic value of ventricular stimulation in patients with idiopathic dilated cardiomyopathy. Am Heart J 1991;121:1124.

36. Kowey PR, Taylor JE, Marinchak RA, Rials SJ: Does programmed stimulation really help in the evaluation of patients with nonsustained ventricular tachycardia? Results of a meta-analysis. Am Heart J 1992;123:481.

37. Tamburro P, Wilber D: Sudden death in idiopathic dilated cardiomyopathy. Am Heart J 1992;124:1035.

38. Kadish A, Schmaltz S, Calkins H, Morady F: Management of nonsustained ventricular tachycardia guided by electrophysiological testing. PACE 1993;16:1037.

39. Winters SL, Ip J, Deshmukh P, et al: Determinants of induction of ventricular tachycardia in nonsustained ventricular tachycardia after myocardial infarction and the usefulness of the signal-averaged electrocardiogram. Am J Cardiol 1993;72:1281.

40. Pires LA, Huang SKS: Nonsustained ventricular tachycardia: identification and management of high-risk patients. Am Heart J 1993;126:189.

41. Surawicz B: Prognosis of ventricular arrhythmias in relation to sudden cardiac death: therapeutic implications. J Am Coll Cardiol 1987;10:435.

42. Kennedy HL, Whitlock JA, Sprague MK, Kennedy LJ, Buckingham TA, Goldberg RJ: Long-term follow-up of asymptomatic healthy subjects with frequent and complex ventricular ectopy. N Engl J Med 1985;312:193.

43. Rubin DA, Nieminski KE, Monteferrante JC, Mages T, Reed GE, Herman MV: Ventricular arrhythmias after coronary artery bypass graft surgery: incidence, risk factors and long-term prognosis. J Am Coll Cardiol 1985;6:307.

44. DeSoyza N, Murphy ML, Bissett JK, Kane JJ, Doherty JE: Ventricular arrhythmia in chronic stable angina pectoris with surgical or medical treatment. Ann Intern Med 1978;89:10.

45. Schultze RA Jr, Strauss HW, Pitt B: Sudden death in the year following myocardial infarction. Relationship to ventricular premature contractions in the late hospital phase and left ventricular ejection fraction. Am J Med 1977;62:192.

46. Packer M: Sudden unexpected death in patients with congestive heart failure: a second frontier. Circulation 1985;72:681–685.

47. Larsen L, Markham J, Haffajee CL: Sudden death in idiopathic dilated cardiomyopathy: role of ventricular arrhythmias. Pace 1993;16:1051.

48. Bigger JT Jr, Weld FM, Rolnitzky LM: Prevalence, characteristics and significance of ventricular tachycardia (three or more complexes) detected with ambulatory electrocardiographic recording in the late phase of acute myocardial infarction. Am J Cardiol 1981;48:815.

49. Yusuf S, Venkatesh G, Teo KK: Critical review of the approaches to the prevention of sudden death. Am J Cardiol 1993;72:51F.

50. Cardiac Arrhythmia Suppression Trial (CAST) Preliminary report: effect of encainide and flecainide on mortality in a randomized trial of arrhythmia suppression after myocardial infarction. N Engl J Med 1989;321:406.

51. Ruskin JN: The cardiac arrhythmia suppression trial (CAST). N Engl J Med 1989;321:386.

52. Echt DS, Liebson PR, Mitchell LB, et al: Mortality and morbidity in patients receiving encainide, flecainide, or placebo. The cardiac arrhythmia suppression trial. N Engl J Med 1991;324:781.

53. Cardiac Arrhythmia Suppression Trial II: Effect of the antiarrhythmic agent moricizine on survival after myocardial infarction. N Engl J Med 1992;327:227.

54. Burkart F, Pfisterer M, Kiowski W, Follath F, Burckhardt D: Effect of antiarrhythmic therapy on mortality in survivors of myocardial infarction with asymptomatic complex ventricular arrhythmias: Basel antiarrhythmic study of infarct survival (BASIS). J Am Coll Cardiol 1990;16:1711.

55. Ceremuzynski L, Kleczar E, Krzeminska-Pakula M, et al: The effect of amiodarone on mortality after myocardial infarction: a double blind, placebo controlled, pilot study. J Am Coll Cardiol 1992;20:1056.

56. Pfisterer M, Kiowski W, Burckhardt D, Follath F, Burkart F: Beneficial effect of amiodarone on cardiac mortality in patients with asymptomatic complex ventricular arrhythmias after acute myocardial infarction and preserved but not impaired left ventricular function. Am J Cardiol 1992;69:1399.

57. Navarro-Lopez F, Cosin J, Marrugat J, Guindo J, Bayes de Luna A: Comparison of the effects of amiodarone versus metoprolol on the frequency of ventricular arrhythmias and on mortality after acute myocardial infarction. Am J Cardiol 1993;72:1243.

58. Cairns JA, Connolly SJ, Roberts R, Gent Michael: Canadian amiodarone myocardial infarction arrhythmia trial (CAMIAT): Rationale and protocol. Am J Cardiol 1993;72:87F.

59. Camm AJ, Julian D, Janse G, Munoz A, Schwartz P, Simon P, Frangin G: The European myocardial infarct amiodarone trial (EMIAT). Am J Cardiol 1993;72:95F.

60. Estes NAM III, Garan H, McGovern B, Ruskin JN: Influence of drive cycle length during programmed stimulation on induction of ventricular arrhythmias: analysis of 403 patients. Am J Cardiol 1986;57:108.

61. Prystowsky EN, Miles WM, Evans JJ, et al: Induction of ventricular tachycardia during programmed electrical stimulation: analysis of pacing methods. Circulation 1986;73(Suppl II):II-32.

62. Mason JW, Anderson KP, Freedman RA: Techniques and

criteria in electrophysiologic study of ventricular tachycardia. Circulation 1987;75(Suppl III):III-125.

63. Buxton AE, Waxman HL, Marchlinski FE, Unterker WJ, Waspe LE, Josephson ME: Role of triple extrastimuli during electrophysiologic study of patients with documented sustained ventricular tachyarrhythmias. Circulation 1984;69:532.

64. Brugada P, Wellens HJJ: Comparison in the same patient of two programmed stimulation protocols to induce ventricular tachycardia. Am J Cardiol 1985;55:380.

65. Breithardt G, Borggrefe M, Podczeck A, Budde T: Influence of the cycle length of basic drive on induction of sustained ventricular tachycardia associated with coronary artery disease. Am J Cardiol 1987;60:1306.

66. Morady F, DiCarlo LA Jr, Baerman JM, de Buitleir M: Comparison of coupling intervals that induce clinical and nonclinical forms of ventricular tachycardia during programmed stimulation. Am J Cardiol 1986;57:1269.

67. Vandepol CJ, Farshidi A, Spielman SR, Greenspan AM, Horowitz LN, Josephson ME: Incidence and clinical significance of induced ventricular tachycardia. Am J Cardiol 1980;45:725.

68. Morady F, DiCarlo L, Winston S, Davis JC, Scheinman MM: A prospective comparison of the role of triple extrastimuli and left ventricular stimulation in studies of ventricular tachycardia induction. Circulation 1984;70:52.

69. Gottlieb C, Josephson ME: The preference of programmed stimulation guided therapy for sustained ventricular arrhythmias. In: Brugada P, Wellens HJJ, eds. Cardiac arrhythmias: where to go from here? Mount Kisco, NY: Futura Publishing, 1987:421.

70. Zehender M, Brugada P, Geibel A, Waldecker B, Stevenson W, Wellens HJJ: Programmed electrical stimulation in healed myocardial infarction using a standardized ventricular stimulation protocol. Am J Cardiol 1987;59:578.

71. Platia EV, Greene HL, Vlay SC, Werner JA, Gross B, Reid PR: Sensitivity of various extrastimulus techniques in patients with serious ventricular arrhythmias. Am Heart J 1983; 106:698.

72. Schoenfeld MH, McGovern B, Garan H, Kelly E, Grant G, Ruskin JN: Determinants of the outcome of electrophysiologic study in patients with ventricular tachyarrhythmias. J Am Coll Cardiol 1985;6:298.

73. El-Sherif N, Mehra R, Gough WB, Zeiler RH: Reentrant ventricular arrhythmias in the late myocardial infarction period. 11. Burst pacing versus multiple premature stimulation in the induction of reentry. J Am Coll Cardiol 1984;4:295.

74. Denker S, Lehmann M, Mahmud R, Gilbert C, Akhtar M: Facilitation of ventricular tachycardia induction with abrupt changes in ventricular cycle length. Am J Cardiol 1984; 53:508.

75. Rosenfeld LE, McPherson CA, Kennedy EE, Stark SI, Batsford WP: Ventricular tachycardia induction: comparison of triple extrastimuli with an abrupt change in ventricular drive cycle length. Am Heart J 1986;111:868.

76. Livelli FD Jr, Bigger JT Jr, Reiffel JA, et al: Response to programmed ventricular stimulation: sensitivity, specificity and relationship to heart disease. Am J Cardiol 1982;50:452.

77. Brugada P, Green M, Abdollah H, Wellens HJJ: Significance of ventricular arrhythmias initiated by programmed ventricular stimulation: the importance of the type of ventricular arrhythmia induced and the number of premature extrastimuli required. Circulation 1984;69:87.

78. Morady F, Shapiro W, Shen E, Sung RJ, Scheinman MM: Programmed ventricular stimulation in patients without spontaneous ventricular tachycardia. Am Heart J 1984; 107:875.

79. Stevenson WG, Brugada P, Waldecker B, Zehender M, Wellens HJJ: Can potentially significant polymorphic ventricular arrhythmias initiated by programmed stimulation be distinguished from those that are nonspecific? Am Heart J 1986;111:1073.

80. Mann DE, Luck JC, Griffin JC, et al: Induction of clinical ventricular tachycardia using programmed stimulation: value of third and fourth extrastimuli. Am J Cardiol 1983; 52:501.

81. Kim SG, Mercando AD, Fisher JD: Comparison of characteristics of nonsustained ventricular tachycardia on Holter monitoring and sustained ventricular tachycardia observed spontaneously or induced by programmed stimulation. Am J Cardiol 1987;60:288.

82. Kammerling JM, Miles WM, Zipes DP, et al: Characteristics of spontaneous nonsustained ventricular tachycardia poorly predict rate of sustained ventricular tachycardia (abstract). Clin Res 1986;34:312A.

83. Doherty JU, Kienzle MG, Waxman HL, Buxton AE, Marchlinski FE, Josephson ME: Programmed ventricular stimulation at a second right ventricular site: an analysis of 100 patients, with special reference to sensitivity, specificity and characteristics of patients with induced ventricular tachycardia. Am J Cardiol 1983;52:1184.

84. Lin H-T, Mann DE, Luck JC, et al: Prospective comparison of right and left ventricular stimulation for induction of sustained ventricular tachycardia. Am J Cardiol 1987;59:559.

85. Denniss RA, Richards DA, Cody DV, et al: Prognostic significance of ventricular tachycardia and fibrillation induced at programmed stimulation and delayed potentials detected on the signal-averaged electrocardiograms of survivors of acute myocardial infarction. Circulation 1986;74:731.

86. Roy D, Arenal A, Godin D, et al: The Canadian experience on the identification of candidates for sudden cardiac death after myocardial infarction. In: Brugada P, Wellens HJJ, eds. Cardiac arrhythmias: where to go from here? Mount Kisco, NY: Futura Publishing, 1987:343.

87. Wellens HJJ, Brugada P, Stevenson WG. Programmed stimulation of the heart in life-threatening ventricular arrhythmias: what is the significance of induced arrhythmias and what is the correct stimulation protocol? Circulation 1985; 72:1.

88. Buxton, AE, Simson MS, Falcone RA, Marchlinski FE, Doherty JU, Josephson ME: Results of signal-averaged electrocardiography and electrophysiologic study in patients with nonsustained ventricular tachycardia after healing of acute myocardial infarction. Am J Cardiol 1987;60:80.

89. Marchlinski FE, Buxton AE, Waxman HL, Josephson ME: Identifying patients at risk of sudden death after myocardial infarction: value of the response to programmed stimulation, degree of ventricular ectopic activity and severity of left ventricular dysfunction. Am J Cardiol 1983;52:1190.

90. Nalos PC, Gang ES, Mandel WJ, Ladenheim ML, Lass Y, Peter T: The signal-averaged electrocardiogram as a screening test for inducibility of sustained ventricular tachycardia in high risk patients: a prospective study. J Am Coll Cardiol 1987; 9:539.

91. Turitto G, Ahuja RK, Bekheit S, Caref EB, Ibrahim B, El-Sherif N: Incidence and prediction of induced ventricular tachyarrhythmias in idiopathic dilated cardiomyopathy. Am J Cardiol 1994;73:770.

92. Naccarelli GV, Prystowsky EN, Jackman WM, Heger JJ, Rahilly GT, Zipes DP: Role of electrophysiologic testing in managing patients who have ventricular tachycardia unrelated to coronary artery disease. Am J Cardiol 1982;50:165.

93. Gradman AH, Batsford WP, Rieur EC, Leon L, Van Zetta AM: Ambulatory electrocardiographic correlates of ventricular inducibility during programmed electrical stimulation. J Am Coll Cardiol 1985;5:1087.

94. Vatterott PJ, Bailey KR, Hammill SC: Improving the predictive ability of the signal-averaged electrocardiogram with a linear logistic model incorporating clinical variables. Circulation 1990;81:797.

95. Simson MB: Use of signals in the terminal QRS complex to identify patients with ventricular tachycardia after myocardial infarction. Circulation 1981;64:235.

96. El-Sherif N, Gomes JAC, Restivo M, Mehra R: Late potentials and arrhythmogenesis. Pacing Clin Electrophysiol 1985; 8:440.

97. Denes P, Uretz E, Santarelli P: Determinants of arrhythmogenic ventricular activity detected on the body surface QRS in patients with coronary artery disease. Am J Cardiol 1984;53:1519.

98. Freedman RA, Gillis AM, Keren A, Soderholm-Difatte V, Mason JW: Signal-averaged electrocardiographic late potentials in patients with ventricular fibrillation or ventricular tachycardia: correlation with clinical arrhythmia and electrophysiologic study. Am J Cardiol 1985;55:1350.

99. Lindsay BD, Ambos HD, Schechtman KB, Cain ME: Improved selection of patients for programmed ventricular stimulation by frequency analysis of signal-averaged electrocardiograms. Circulation 1986;73:675.

100. Hoffman BF, Rosen MR: Cellular mechanisms for cardiac arrhythmias. Circ Res 1981;49:1.

101. El-Sherif N, Gough WB, Zeiler RH, Mehra R: Triggered ventricular rhythms in 1-day-old myocardial infarction in the dog. Circ Res 1983;52:566.

102. DiCarlo LA Jr, Morady F, Schwartz AB, et al: Clinical significance of ventricular fibrillation-flutter induced by ventricular programmed stimulation. Am Heart J 1985;109:959.

103. Mahmud R, Denker S, Lehmann MH, Tchou P, Dongas J, Akhtar M: Incidence and clinical significance of ventricular fibrillation induced with single and double ventricular extrastimuli. Am J Cardiol 1986;58:75.

104. Caref EB, Turitto G, Ibrahim BB, Henkin R, El-Sherif N: Role of band-pass filters in optimizing the value of the signal-averaged electrocardiogram as a predictor of the results of programmed stimulation. Am J Cardiol 1989;64:16.

105. Kelen GJ, Henkin R, Starr A-M, Caref EB, Bloomfield D, El-Sherif N: Spectral turbulence analysis of the signal-averaged electrocardiogram and its predictive accuracy for inducible sustained monomorphic ventricular tachycardia. Am J Cardiol 1991;67:965.

106. Klein RC, Machell C: Use of electrophysiologic testing in patients with nonsustained ventricular tachycardia: prognostic and therapeutic implications. J Am Coll Cardiol 1989;14:155.

107. Wiener I, Stevenson W, Weiss J, Nademanee K: Are electrophysiologic studies indicated in nonsustained ventricular tachycardia? Am J Cardiol 1990;66:642.

108. Buxton AE, Fisher JD, Josephson ME, et al: Prevention of sudden death in patients with coronary artery disease: The multicenter unsustained tachycardia trial (MUSTT). Prog Cardiovasc Dis 1993;36:215.

Cardiac Arrhythmias, 3rd edition, edited by William J. Mandel.
J. B. Lippincott Company, Philadelphia © 1995.

20

Mary L. Dohrmann • Nora Goldschlager

Exercise-Induced Ventricular Arrhythmias: An Overview

Ventricular ectopic activity after acute myocardial infarction is considered to be an important prognostic indicator of subsequent mortality, especially in patients with depressed left ventricular function.[1–4] The Coronary Drug Project Research Group noted a twofold increase in mortality in a 3-year follow-up study of 235 patients with ventricular extrasystoles who survived 3 months after myocardial infarction.[1] Frequent ventricular ectopic activity (e.g., pairs or runs of extrasystoles) quadruples the expected mortality in the first 3 years after infarction.[2] A similar relation of ventricular ectopic activity to risk of sudden death and the development of symptomatic coronary disease is also suggested by the results of the Tecumseh epidemiologic study of more than 5000 subjects.[4] In contrast, a long-term epidemiologic study of risk factors for arrhythmic death failed to demonstrate a relation between prior ventricular dysrhythmias and risk of sudden death in 301 men followed-up for 20 years.[5] Another large study of 3351 patients, of whom 1.5% developed ventricular tachycardia during exercise testing, failed to show an impact of this rhythm disturbance on 2-year mortality.[6] Similarly, a study of 1160 healthy volunteers ranging in age from 21 to 96 years found no difference in incidence of any cardiac event in the 6.9% of subjects who developed ventricular arrhythmias, compared with age- and gender-matched controls.[7] The Coronary Artery Surgery Study found no relation of ventricular arrhythmias induced by exercise to survival in patients who have either minimal or significant (more than 70% luminal obstruction) coronary artery disease and stable angina; similar results have been reported by others.[8,9] These somewhat disparate observations, mostly explained by differing methodologies and population groups, have led to the question of whether and under which circumstances ventricular arrhythmias induced by exercise have diagnostic or prognostic importance.

GENERAL CONSIDERATIONS

Prevalence

The reported prevalence of exercise-induced ventricular arrhythmias varies from 7% to 60%.[7,10–19] Exercise-related ventricular arrhythmias increase in frequency with advancing age and their prevalence approaches 50% in subjects older than 50 years of age.[6,20] The age-related increase in ventricular ectopy is especially common in men.[6]

Prevalence of exercise-induced ventricular arrhythmias is also greater in patients with symptomatic coronary disease, compared with normal subjects (Table 20-1); 7% to 38% of healthy subjects develop ventricular arrhythmias during exercise, compared with 36% to 50% of patients with coronary disease.[7, 10, 14, 18, 21] Exercise-induced ventricular arrhythmias in patients who have coronary artery disease are commonly but not necessarily associated with ischemic ST-segment shifts during exercise and have been correlated (albeit to varying degrees) with the extent and severity of disease documented angiographically.[11-13, 21-25] Although there is usually a higher prevalence of exercise-induced ventricular arrhythmias in patients who have multi-vessel compared with single-vessel coronary artery disease, these arrhythmias may be a better marker of greater extent of left ventricular wall motion abnormality and depressed ejection fraction than they are of extent of arteriographic pathology.[21, 25, 26]

High grades of ventricular ectopy—in particular, multiform extrasystoles and ventricular tachycardia—are uncommon in a healthy person undergoing exercise testing (see Table 20-1), although they occasionally do occur (Fig. 20-1).[10-15, 17] The clinical entity of nonischemic exercise-induced ventricular tachycardia has been defined and characterized in the exercise and electrophysiology laboratories.[11] This tachycardia, often involving the right ventricular outflow tract, is considered to be idiopathic because it occurs in subjects without structural heart disease, as assessed by the usual means of physical examination, echocardiography, ventriculography, and coronary arteriography. It is often catecholamine-sensitive, thus explaining its occurrence during exercise. Ventricular tachycardia occurring during exercise is more frequent in patients who have known coronary artery disease, with a reported prevalence of about 6%.[14] Patients with documented ventricular tachycardia after myocardial infarction have an 11% incidence of ventricular tachycardia on exercise testing.[11]

The definition of ventricular tachycardia (including exercise-induced ventricular tachycardia) has not been uniform; thus, criteria for this arrhythmia vary among published studies. Ventricular tachycardia is generally defined as three or more consecutive ventricular extrasystoles occurring at a rate greater than 100 per minute. Nonsustained (less than 30 seconds duration) and sustained (greater than 30 seconds duration) ventricular arrhythmias have not been thus identified until recently.[11] It does seem, however, that sustained ventricular tachycardia is decidedly uncommon in clinical practice. Ventricular tachycardia resembling accelerated tachycardia (Fig. 20-2) is similarly uncommon.

The exercise test performed in the standard manner may underestimate the true prevalence of exercise-induced ventricular arrhythmias. Studies in trained athletes have shown that exercise-induced ventricular arrhythmias are more frequently provoked during active sport participation (for example, distance running and squash) than during an exercise test performed in standard fashion.[15, 19] In one study, exercise-induced ventricular arrhythmias occurred in 27% of well-trained runners during maximal exercise testing but in a full 60% during an actual distance run.[15] Moreover, complex ventricular ectopy (couplets, multiform complexes) were observed more commonly (10% and 5%, respectively) in distance running, compared with exercise testing (3%).[15] These observations have obvious relevance to the predictive value for sudden death of laboratory-related exercise-induced arrhythmias.

Arrhythmias provoked during an exercise test do not predict an increased risk of complications during stress testing.[6, 7] A review of the safety of exercise tests conducted by various laboratories demonstrates that the risk of exercise-induced ventricular arrhythmias that are sufficiently serious to require intervention was 4.78 per 10,000 tests, with only 0.5 deaths per 10,000 tests.[27] A study of 71,914 subjects evaluated between 1971 and 1987 reports only 0.8 complications per 10,000 maximal treadmill tests, which included only two persons having ventricular tachycardia or fibrillation, both of whom were successfully resuscitated.[28] Even patients with a known history of ventricular tachycardia or fibrillation can be exercised with little risk of sequelae.[29, 30] In one study of 263 patients having prior documented ventricular tachycardia or fibrillation during exercise, only 24 (9%) had dysrhythmia during the exercise test, and all were successfully resuscitated.[29]

Reproducibility

The incidence of ventricular arrhythmias during serially performed stress tests in the same patient varies.[31, 32] In patients with known or suspected cardiovascular disease and those with exercise-induced or nonischemic ventricular tachycardia, reproducibility of arrhythmias is consistent enough to be considered more than random.[20, 31] In consecutively performed exercise tests, high grades of ventricular ectopy, especially ventricular tachycardia, appear to be more reproducible than lower grades, having a reported reproducibility of 50% to 79%.[14, 33, 34] The change in frequency of ventricular arrhythmias during exercise, compared with their resting baseline frequency, is a more reproducible finding in serially performed exercise tests than is the absolute number of ventricular extrasystoles developing during exercise.[34] In patients with frequent ventricular extrasystoles only, reproducibility is reported to be only 30%.[14] This inherent variation in exercise-induced ventricular arrhyth-

TABLE 20-1. Exercise Induced Ventricular Ectopic Activity

	Any VEA (%)	Frequent VEA (%)	Serious VEA (Pairs, triplets, VT, VF) (%)
Normal subjects	7–38	3–11	1–6
Patients with coronary artery disease	38–50	23–37	6–35

VEA, ventricular ectopic activity; VT, ventricular tachycardia; VF, ventricular fibrillation.

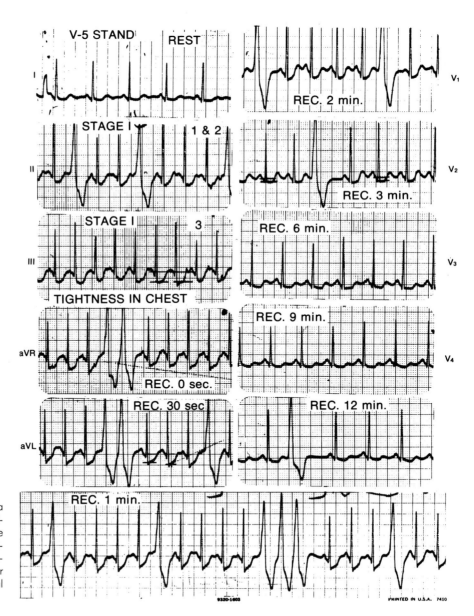

Figure 20-1. Stress test obtained in a woman 61 years of age complaining of palpitations, with pairs and trios of premature ventricular beats. Selective coronary arteriography and left ventriculography were entirely normal, and there was no clinical or echographic evidence of prolapsing mitral valve.

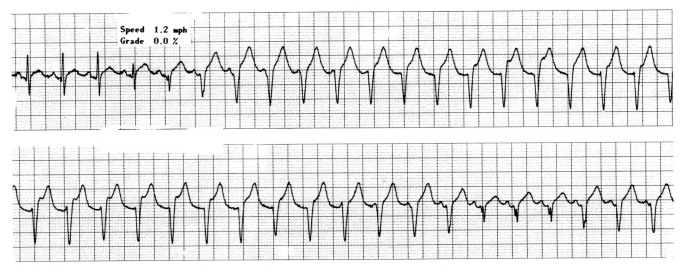

Figure 20-2. Continuously recorded lead V₅ in a 72-year-old patient with ischemic cardiomyopathy. The slow ventricular tachycardia, which has its onset and offset by fusion complexes, is suggestive of accelerated ventricular rhythm, although slowing of sinus rate before the tachycardia is not present. It is unusual to see this rhythm during exercise.

mias in a given person makes interpretation of efficacy of anti-ischemic or antiarrhythmic therapy difficult.[35]

COMPARISON OF EXERCISE STRESS TESTING AND AMBULATORY ELECTROCARDIOGRAPHIC MONITORING FOR DETECTION OF VENTRICULAR ARRHYTHMIAS

Except in patients with "idiopathic" exercise-induced ventricular tachycardia, ventricular tachycardia and other forms of high-grade ventricular ectopy are more frequently documented by ambulatory electrocardiographic monitoring than by exercise stress testing.[36] This is especially true in patients who have cardiomyopathy.[37] Patients with prior myocardial infarction are reported to be more likely to have ventricular ectopy noted on both exercise stress testing and ambulatory electrocardiographic monitoring, whereas patients with angina pectoris but without past infarction often demonstrate ventricular ectopy only with the latter technique.[36] In one series of 64 patients with known prior ventricular tachycardia or fibrillation, only 8% had ventricular tachycardia provoked during an exercise stress test, whereas 72% of patients demonstrated nonsustained ventricular tachycardia on 24-hour ambulatory electrocardiographic monitoring.[30]

Some studies suggest that the exercise test does not simulate effort to the same degree that occurs randomly during a 24-hour monitoring period or ambulatory monitoring during specific exertional activities.[15,19] In one study of athletes (squash players), 67% had ventricular arrhythmias during a game but only 25% had ventricular arrhythmias provoked during an exercise stress test.[19] In another study of well-conditioned athletes, 57% of runners who had ventricular ectopy on ambulatory electrocardiographic monitoring had no ectopy on an exercise stress test.[15] The issue of correlation between the two techniques remains controversial, however, with some studies showing greater equivalence among their findings.[38] Ventricular tachycardia can occasionally be induced by exercise testing when it has not been documented by ambulatory electrocardiographic monitoring.[36,38]

In patients with ischemic heart disease, ventricular arrhythmias noted during ambulatory electrocardiographic monitoring and those occurring during exercise stress testing appear to be independently predictive of sudden death; however, the ST-segment response during exercise is probably of greater value in predicting overall cardiac morbidity and mortality.[9,11,25,39,40,41] In this regard, it is worth emphasizing that the definition of sudden death was not uniform among the published studies and cannot be assumed to have been arrhythmic. In a report of 163 patients studied before hospital discharge after acute myocardial infarction, although 12% and 15% (respectively) of patients had ventricular arrhythmias provoked on exercise testing and ambulatory electrocardiographic monitoring, the subsequent risk of sudden death was best predicted by exercise-induced ventricular arrhythmias during the predischarge symptom-limited stress test; this risk was greatest in the first 12 weeks after infarction.[43] During a 2-year follow-up period, sudden death occurred in 5 of 20 postmyocardial infarction patients (25%) with ventricular arrhythmias on exercise testing, compared with 1 of 25 patients (4%) with ventricular ectopy detected by ambulatory electrocardiographic monitoring.[42]

In addition to detecting ventricular arrhythmias in patients recovering from myocardial infarction, ambulatory electrocardiographic monitoring is also used to detect silent myocardial ischemia.[44-46] Although both silent myocardial ischemia and ventricular arrhythmias seem to predict a poor outcome after myocardial infarction, the prevalence of ventricular arrhythmias on 24-hour ambulatory electrocardiographic monitoring is no greater in patients with silent myocardial ischemia than in patients with symptomatic angina pectoris, averaging about 20% in each of these groups.[44,45,46] Similarly, when complex ventricular ectopic activity and depressed left ventricular ejection fraction (less than 40%) are considered together, the combination is not observed more frequently in patients with silent than with overt ischemia.

From the available literature and knowledge of the techniques, it seems clear that exercise testing and ambulatory electrocardiography are looking at different aspects of the issue of ventricular arrhythmias and thus cannot be compared directly. Whereas ambulatory electrocardiographic monitoring provides information regarding ambient ventricular ectopy during the activities of daily life, exercise testing provides data on the cardiovascular response to vagolysis, increases in sympathetic tone and circulating catecholamine levels, electrolyte and pH shifts, and myocardial ischemia—the latter not always or even often achieved during average daily activity.[43]

Characteristics of Exercise-Induced Ventricular Arrhythmias

Ventricular arrhythmias induced by exercise testing frequently occur only during the postexercise recovery period, usually within the first 3 minutes.[14,22,47,48] It is suggested that ventricular ectopy occurring in the recovery phase is more often observed in patients with coronary artery disease, whereas healthy persons are more likely to have ectopy during exercise, especially with maximal exercise and peak heart rates above 173 beats per minute.[14,17,48,49] In one study of 5842 patients without and with heart disease, of whom 1% (mostly with coronary artery disease) developed ventricular tachycardia, nonsustained ventricular tachycardia occurring in the recovery period was characterized as following short-long-short RR intervals (Fig. 20-3), whereas those occurring during exercise occurred both with and without this RR sequence.[48] The initiating mechanism was reproducible in these patients, suggesting specific mechanisms, possibly bradycardia-dependent afterdepolarization triggering.

The disappearance of resting ventricular extrasystoles

with exercise (Fig. 20-4) does not imply that they are innocuous; in one report, eight of 10 such patients had triple vessel coronary artery disease.[22] Exertional hypotension frequently precedes ventricular tachycardia and fibrillation (Fig. 20-5) and occurred in almost half of the 34 patients in one study.[50] Although marked elevations of blood pressure (systolic pressure greater than 200 mmHg) that were produced by intravenously administered metaraminol provoked ventricular arrhythmias, this phenomenon has not been consistently observed during clinical exercise testing at similarly high systemic pressures.[51]

Ventricular tachycardia tends to occur at sinus rates of less than 150 per minute in patients who have coronary artery disease. In contrast, sinus rates are considerably higher—at or near voluntary maximum—in patients who have nonischemic ventricular tachycardia. Among patients with known coronary artery disease, exercise-induced ventricular arrhythmias, particularly ventricular tachycardia, tend to be associated with more severe degrees of coronary artery stenosis; double- and triple-vessel disease; significant left ventricular dysfunction; ischemic ST-segment depression (Fig. 20-6); or less commonly, elevation (Fig. 20-7) and transient reversible perfusion defects on isotopic imaging, even if electrocardiographic evidence of ischemia is not present.[13,22-26,52-55] In patients with known coronary artery disease, ischemic episodes identified by ambulatory electrocardiographic monitoring are greater in frequency, magnitude (assessed by severity of ST-segment displacement), and duration when accompanied by ventricular arrhythmias, compared with ischemic episodes unassociated with ventricular arrhythmias.[56] Similar correlations have not been consistently observed during exercise testing.

In patients with coronary artery disease, ST-segment elevation reflecting transmural ischemic injury that develops during an exercise stress test is frequently associated with ventricular arrhythmias, suggesting that increases in coronary artery vasomotor tone or frank spasm may cause or contribute to the precipitation of ischemia and resultant arrhythmias.[18] Ambulatory electrocardiographic monitoring in patients who have vasospastic angina pectoris demonstrates that early cycle (R on T) ventricular extrasystoles are more likely to initiate ventricular tachycardia when they follow an episode of ST-segment elevation than are ventricular extrasystoles that occur late in the cardiac cycle.[57]

EXERCISE-INDUCED VENTRICULAR TACHYCARDIA

Sustained ventricular tachycardia that develops during exercise (Figs. 20-8 and 20-9) occurs less frequently than lower grades of ventricular ectopic activity. In one large

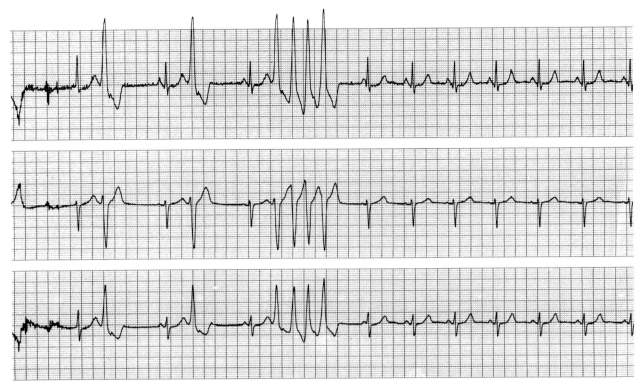

Figure 20-3. Simultaneously recorded leads II, V$_1$, and V$_5$, illustrating a burst of monomorphic ventricular tachycardia, occurring for the first time at seven minutes into the recovery period in a 48-year-old man with frequent ventricular ectopy but no symptoms of cerebral hypoperfusion. The treadmill test showed no evidence of ischemia. The premature ventricular depolarizations and this burst of tachycardia suggest a right ventricular outflow tract origin (left bundle-branch block pattern with inferior frontal plane QRS axis). Note that the burst occurs after a postextrasystolic pause.

series of 5730 consecutive patients undergoing treadmill testing, 47 patients (0.8%) developed episodes of ventricular tachycardia.[50] In another series of 713 consecutive patients undergoing submaximal exercise testing, 12 (1.7%) developed ventricular tachycardia; a fourth of these were thought to have no evidence of underlying heart disease.[47] In a newer study of 3351 subjects undergoing routine treadmill testing, only 0.1% developed sustained ventricular tachycardia.[6] Right ventricular tachycardia (ventricular tachycardia often originating from the right ventricular outflow tract and demonstrating left bundle branch block morphology with a normal or inferior and rightward frontal plane axis) is a common form of exercise-induced ventricular tachycardia and may be the most common form of ventricular tachycardia not related to ischemia, although exercise-induced left ventricular tachycardia (right bundle branch block pattern with leftward frontal plane QRS axis) does occur.[58, 59] In one series of 23 patients having ventricular tachycardia with the morphologic characteristics of right ventricular site of origin, tachycardia was provoked by exercise in 14.[58] In a newer

and larger study, 70% of 53 patients with idiopathic nonischemic ventricular tachycardia developed the arrhythmia during exercise.[23] The reproducibility of nonischemic ventricular tachycardia induced by exercise is reported to be as high as 62%, in marked contrast to reproducibility in patients who have coronary artery disease.[23, 24]

Mechanisms

Three mechanisms are generally accepted as underlying most cardiac arrhythmias: reentry, abnormal automaticity, and triggered activity.[60–64] These same mechanisms are thought to explain exercise-induced ventricular tachycardia and it is entirely possible that the tachycardia mechanisms of onset and maintenance are not the same.[65–68]

The requirements for *reentry* are unidirectional block in one area and delay in impulse conduction in another. Regional myocardial ischemia provoked by exercise could result in slow conduction through the ischemic

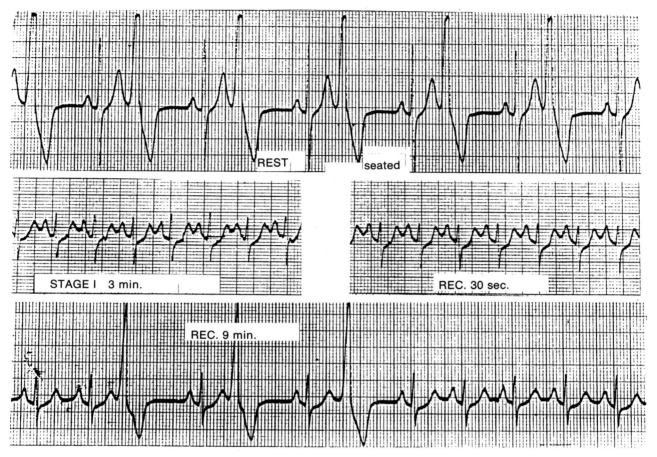

Figure 20-4. Portions of a treadmill test performed on a man aged 57 years, in whom premature ventricular complexes, occurring in a bigeminal fashion at rest, are completely suppressed during the sinus tachycardia induced by exercise and recur well into the recovery period after deceleration of sinus rate has been achieved. The patient, despite borderline ST-segment alterations during exercise at a submaximal attained heart rate, had 75% stenoses in all three coronary arteries. Many patients who have ischemic cardiac pain and in whom ventricular extrasystoles are suppressed by exercise have severe coronary disease.

region; in this connection, variation in refractory periods of isolated Purkinje fibers occurs after experimental coronary artery occlusion.[69]

Enhanced automaticity may develop during exercise for several reasons. Experimentally induced myocardial ischemia may result in a reduction of maximum diastolic potential to between -60 and -50 mV in both Purkinje fibers and myocardium, thereby enhancing phase 4 depolarization in these tissues.[60] High circulating catecholamine levels occurring during exercise and increased sympathetic tone can cause myocardial ischemia through increases in heart rate and blood pressure. In addition, sympathetic stimulation can also be arrhythmogenic by enhancing phase 4 depolarization and possibly by provoking afterdepolarizations.[63] In experimental animals, both stellate ganglion stimulation and adrenal medullary secre-

tion through splanchnic nerve stimulation cause enhanced ventricular automaticity.[70, 71] Plasma concentrations of norepinephrine are significantly higher in patients with coronary artery disease during and after exercise testing, compared with normal subjects—especially in those with an increase in blood pressure in the recovery period.[72] Plasma epinephrine levels are higher in patients with exercise-induced ventricular arrhythmias, compared with those without arrhythmias.[72]

Triggered activity refers to arrhythmias that arise from oscillations in membrane potential (early and delayed afterdepolarizations) during cell repolarization. These membrane oscillations have two special properties: (1) they do not occur spontaneously but depend on previous depolarizations, and (2) they are rate-dependent, usually developing within a critical range of cycle

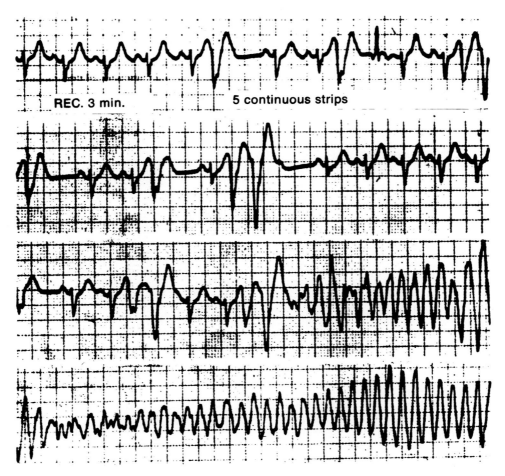

Figure 20-5. Onset of ventricular fibrillation 3 minutes into the postexercise recovery period in a man aged 55 years, with exertional hypotension 1 month after he suffered an acute inferior wall myocardial infarction. After successful defibrillation, selective coronary and left ventricular angiography were performed, revealing severe triple-vessel coronary disease. Aortocoronary bypass graft surgery was accomplished, after which ventricular arrhythmias did not occur on repeat treadmill exercise testing.

lengths.[61] The amplitude of afterdepolarizations increases in the presence of catecholamines.[60] In addition, afterdepolarizations are calcium-dependent and their appearance in vitro can be prevented by calcium channel blocking agents such as verapamil. Clinical responsiveness to verapamil has been used by some investigators as proof that triggered activity is the underlying mechanism for exercise-induced ventricular tachycardia.[67,68] Afterdepolarizations and triggered activity may be provoked during exercise as a result of heightened catecholamine state and increased heart rate. Considering the effects of catecholamines in provoking myocardial ischemia, enhanced automaticity, and afterdepolarizations, beta blockade would theoretically be the most effective medical therapy for prevention of exercise-induced ventricular tachycardia.

In addition to myocardial ischemia and catecholamine effects underlying the three recognized mechanisms for cardiac arrhythmia production, postexercise fluctuations in arterial potassium levels may contribute to arrhythmogenesis.[73,74] During exercise, as plasma catecholamine levels rise, potassium is released from skeletal muscle. The degree of rise in arterial potassium during exercise parallels venous lactate levels, suggesting that anaerobic rather than aerobic metabolism is responsible for potassium release.[42,73] Arterial potassium levels decrease rapidly postexercise; this decrease is most profound in patients who have an elevated lactate threshold and in patients with ischemic heart disease, with limited aerobic capacity.[73,75] Hypokalemia decreases the ventricular fibrillation threshold in ischemic myocardium.[76] The observation that ventricular arrhythmias can occur for the first time in the postexercise recovery phase in patients with coronary

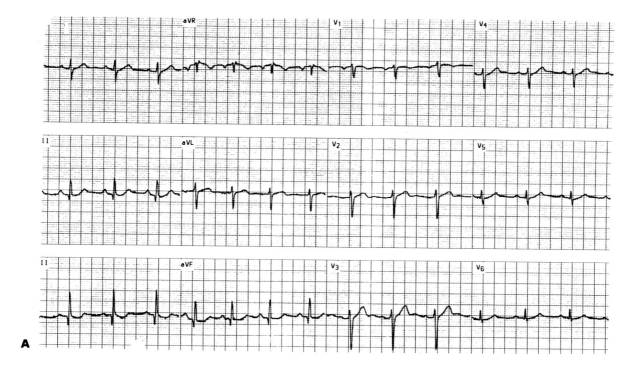

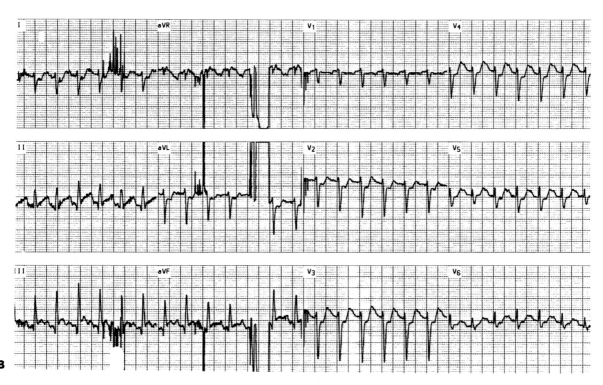

Figure 20-6. Spontaneously terminating polymorphic ventricular tachycardia associated with exercise-induced ischemia in a 63-year-old man. The resting tracing (**A**) suggests the presence of old inferior wall myocardial infarction. The tracing recorded during exercise (**B**) shows marked ischemic changes in the anterior and lateral leads and ST elevation in the inferior leads (consistent with past Q-wave infarction). Polymorphic ventricular tachycardia develops at peak effort   (*continued*)

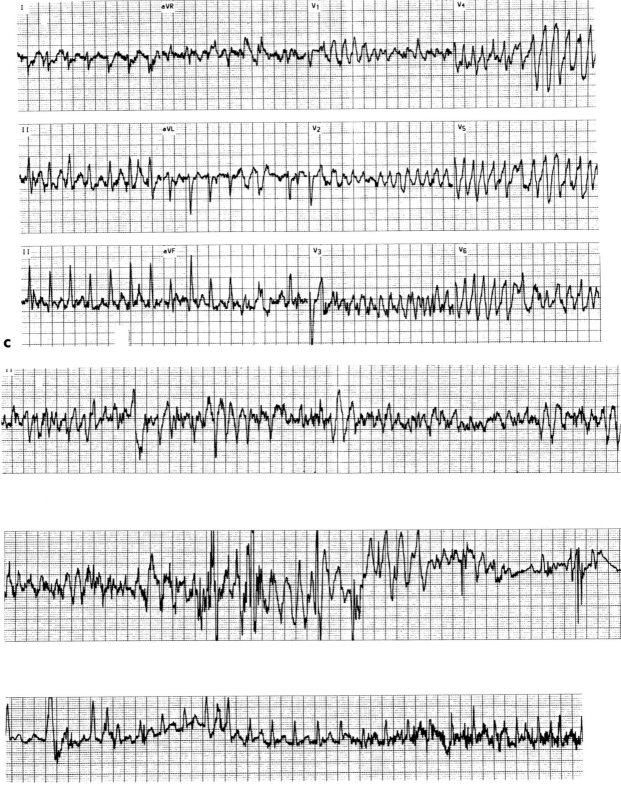

Figure 20-6. (*continued*) (**C**); the patient continues to exercise (**D**; continuously recorded lead II) because the arrhythmia was not recognized. The patient eventually fell on the treadmill, after which the rhythm is noted to be sinus. The fall presumably caused a form of thumpversion of the arrhythmia.

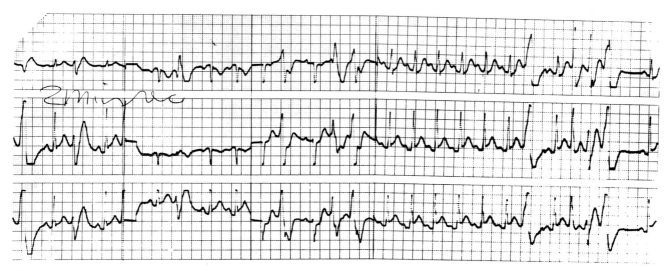

Figure 20-7. Multiform ventricular doublets, developing during transmural ischemic injury (indicated by ST-segment elevation) in a 58-year-old patient with three-vessel coronary artery disease, including a high-grade obstruction of the left anterior descending coronary artery.

artery disease can be partly explained by these marked potassium fluctuations.[73] Hypertensive patients chronically treated with diuretics constitute another subset of patients in whom potassium fluctuations after exercise may be arrhythmogenic. In one study, exercise-induced ventricular arrhythmias occurred in 57% of patients who had mild hypertension treated with diuretics, compared with 38% of age-matched normotensive control subjects.[77] These results have not been confirmed in all studies, however.[78]

Electrophysiologic Studies

Electrophysiologic studies performed in patients who had exercise-induced ventricular tachycardia have yielded provocative, if not entirely definitive, information. During electrophysiologic testing, a reentry mechanism as the basis for ventricular tachycardia is suggested by initiation or termination of ventricular tachycardia using extrastimulus techniques. Catecholamine-sensitive automaticity is suggested by the ability to provoke ventricular

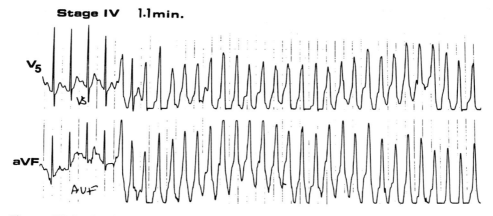

Figure 20-8. Simultaneously recorded leads V₅ and aVF, showing the onset of ventricular tachycardia during stage IV (Bruce protocol) in a healthy man aged 18 years. The tachycardia rate is 190 beats/minute and the sinus rate at its onset is 150 beats/minute. The patient was treated with low doses of nadolol, which prevented the exercise-induced ventricular tachycardia.

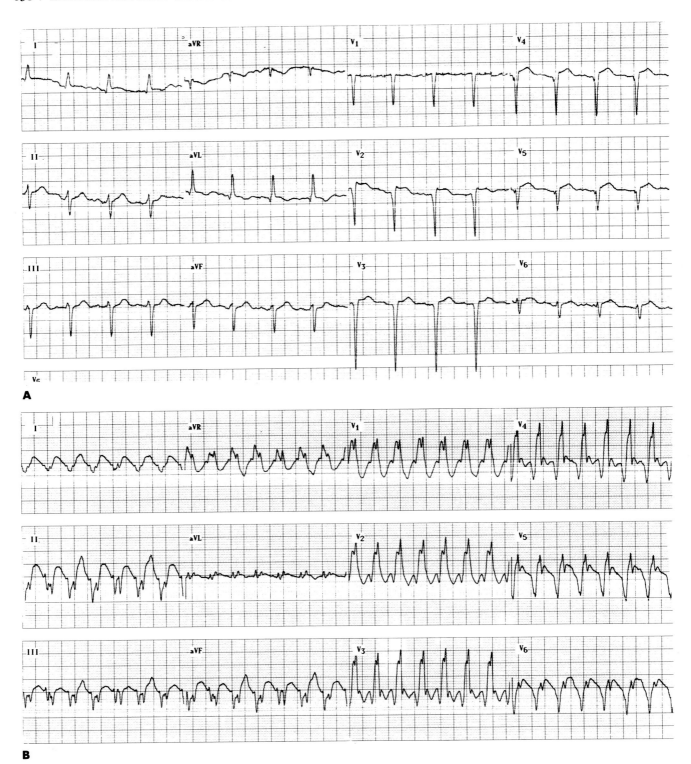

Figure 20-9. Twelve-lead electrocardiograms recorded at rest and during exercise in a 68-year-old woman with recent anterior wall myocardial infarction. The resting tracing (**A**) shows the Q-wave infarction, with ST-segment elevation. At the sixth minute of exercise (modified Bruce protocol), monomorphic ventricular tachycardia developed (**B**), which terminated spontaneously during the first minute of recovery without specific intervention. Perfusion scintigraphy revealed ischemia remote from the infarcted area, and the patient underwent revascularization. Electrophysiologic study was not performed. A subsequent maximal exercise test was performed without incident.

tachycardia during or after intravenous isoproterenol infusion; abnormal automaticity is unaffected by ventricular extrastimuli. Triggered activity usually occurs only within a critical range of heart rates, and the rate of the ventricular tachycardia tends to increase as the underlying heart rate increases. Catecholamines may play a role in triggered rhythms by increasing heart rate and causing afterdepolarizations. Triggered activity is assumed to be operative if the calcium entry blocker verapamil can prevent the initiation of ventricular tachycardia.

Sung and associates performed electrophysiologic studies in 12 patients who had exercise-induced sustained ventricular tachycardia, provoking ventricular tachycardia morphologically similar to the clinical tachycardia in 10.[66] Seven of the 10 had findings consistent with a reentry mechanism, and three had ventricular tachycardia that was inducible only with isoproterenol infusion. In another study of three patients, the ventricular tachycardia that was induced with isoproterenol infusion was prevented by propranolol administration and terminated with verapamil.[65]

In one series of 33 patients who had documented sustained ventricular tachycardia and underwent electrophysiologic studies, 14 had had previously documented exercise-induced ventricular tachycardia.[67] Of the 14 patients who had exercise-induced ventricular tachycardia, two (14%) demonstrated reentry during electrophysiologic testing; five (36%) had catecholamine-sensitive ventricular tachycardia, which was suppressed with beta blockade; and seven (50%) had triggered activity as the cause. In this last group, inducibility of ventricular tachycardia was prevented in all patients with verapamil.[67]

Some investigators suggest delineating the mechanism of exercise-induced ventricular tachycardia by electrophysiologic studies because the documentation would help guide therapy, especially in the verapamil-responsive and catecholamine-sensitive categories.[67,79] Patients displaying reentry during electrophysiologic studies are more likely to have underlying heart disease (particularly coronary artery disease and cardiomyopathy), whereas patients with verapamil-responsive and catecholamine-sensitive ventricular tachycardia frequently have no evidence of underlying heart disease.[67] Tachycardia mapping during electrophysiologic study allows detection of the optimal site for radiofrequency ablative procedures, which are used with increasing frequency as a therapy for nonischemic exercise-induced symptomatic ventricular tachycardia.

ASSOCIATED CLINICAL CONDITIONS

The most common etiology underlying exercise-related ventricular tachycardia is coronary artery disease. Other disease processes that may be associated with increased occurrence of exercise-related ventricular arrhythmias include mitral valve prolapse, hypertrophic and congestive cardiomyopathy, infiltrative diseases such as sarcoidosis, valvular aortic stenosis, presence of digitalis or hypokalemia, syndromes associated with prolonged QT interval (Fig. 20-10), arrhythmogenic right ventricular dysplasia and other congenital abnormalities, and pulmonary disease (Table 20-2).[52,66,80-100] It is also possible that patients with nonischemic exercise-induced ventricular tachycardia who have apparent structurally "normal" hearts actually have abnormalities of function or structure, the latter evidenced on magnetic resonance imaging. A study suggests that selective denervation of the myocardium, assessed by tomographic γ-scanning using ^{123}I meta-iodo-benzyl-guanidine, was present in 47% of such patients, compared with a 0% incidence in normal controls.[101]

The fairly common syndrome of mid-systolic click—late-systolic murmur (due to myxomatous degeneration of mitral valve leaflet tissue, leading to prolapse of one or both leaflets) is frequently associated with ventricular ectopic activity at rest, after exercise, or both. The prevalence of exercise-related ventricular arrhythmias ranges from 11% to 75%, with advanced forms of ventricular irritability often being present.[80-85,102,103] Ventricular tachycardia reportedly occurs in 6.3% of patients with mitral valve prolapse.[80] Pairs and runs of ventricular extrasystoles occurred in 20% of individuals in a Framingham study cohort evaluated with 24-hour ambulatory electrocardiographic monitoring and M-mode echocardiography; however, the frequency of ventricular arrhythmias in asymptomatic persons with mitral valve prolapse is probably no different from that in normal control subjects.[104] Ventricular extrasystoles present at rest may disappear, persist, or worsen during exercise and ventricular arrhythmias may develop de novo during exercise. Sudden death in patients having this syndrome, occurring only rarely, is presumably due to ventricular fibrillation. In a series of 300 patients with mitral valve prolapse, three patients died suddenly during long-term follow-up—two with documented ventricular fibrillation.[103] In one report, sudden death occurred without prior evidence of either rest- or effort-related ventricular arrhythmias.[102] A prolonged QT interval was present in 47% of patients, potentially contributing to arrhythmogenesis; QT-interval prolongation may develop or be enhanced by exercise in this patient subset.[80-82]

Sudden death is a frequent complication of sarcoid involvement of the heart. In one large clinicopathologic study, sudden death occurred in 67% of 89 patients and was the first manifestation of the disease in 17% of patients who died.[87] Most patients with cardiac sarcoidosis who die suddenly have antecedent ventricular arrhythmias—in particular, ventricular tachycardia or complete atrioventricular block; sudden death is frequently precipitated by exertion.[87]

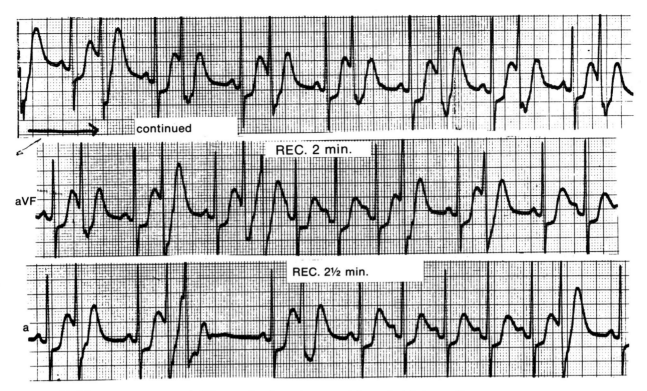

Figure 20-10. Woman patient with QT-interval prolongation, especially marked during and immediately after exercise. The QT interval measures 0.4 second, with a sinus rate of 100 beats/minute.
J-point depression (2 mm) with slowly upsloping ST segments is present failing to meet criteria for a
positive stress test. Ventricular ectopic activity occurs frequently, and there are occasional pairs with a
short-coupling interval. Exercise-induced ventricular arrhythmias in patients with long QT intervals not
due to quinidine or hypokalemia may respond favorably to propranolol.

TABLE 20-2. Conditions Associated With Exercise-Induced Arrhythmias

Normal cardiovascular status
Coronary artery disease
Mitral valve prolapse
Digitalis administration and toxicity
Hypokalemia
Cardiomyopathy (hypertrophic, dilated)
Left ventricular outflow obstruction
  Aortic valvular stenosis
  Hypertrophic obstructive cardiomyopathy
Prolonged-QT–interval syndromes
  Idiopathic
  Type 1 antiarrhythmic medication (e.g., quinidine, flecainiole)
  Phenothiazine administration
Congenital cardiac abnormalities
  Anomalous origin left coronary artery
  Congenital complete heart block
  Postrepair tetralogy of Fallot
  Arrhythmogenic right ventricular dysplasia
  Myocardial bridge
Pulmonary disease

In individuals under age 40 years—in particular, young athletes—sudden death most commonly reflects structural or congenital heart disease (e.g., hypertrophic cardiomyopathy or anomalous origin of the left coronary artery) and most likely occurs during or immediately after strenuous exertion.[90] Although 14 of 19 athletes in one series who died suddenly had hypertrophic cardiomyopathy demonstrated at autopsy, it is uncertain whether routine screening for this condition, using echocardiography before participation in competitive sports, is warranted.[90] Conversely, if the diagnosis of hypertrophic cardiomyopathy is known and because ventricular arrhythmias occur so frequently during 24-hour ambulatory electrocardiographic monitoring in patients with this condition (more than 50% of patients have high-grade ventricular arrhythmias and 19% have nonsustained ventricular tachycardia), it has been recommended that ambulatory electrocardiographic monitoring be routinely performed to assess risk of a given patient for sudden death.[105,106] Sudden death in this condition, especially in its familial form, is usually precipitated during or after effort and is attributed to ventricular tachycardia or ventricular fibrillation.[107,108] Abnormally thickened, small intramural coronary arteries that have been described in hypertrophic cardiomyopathy may provide the anatomic condition that provokes ischemia and in turn, ventricular arrhythmias.[109]

Patients with diabetes mellitus, although prone to atherosclerotic coronary artery disease, may have changes in myocardial composition that make them more susceptible to arrhythmias, especially if subjected to strenuous exertion when they have not been physically conditioned.[110,111] Deconditioned diabetic dogs have increased sensitivity to catecholamine stimulation; physical reconditioning of the diabetic animal decreases ventricular irritability in response to catecholamines.[111]

Digitalis preparations may contribute both to the manifestation of latent arrhythmias and to de novo arrhythmogenesis. The expected clinical signs and symptoms of digitalis toxicity may not be apparent, and ventricular arrhythmias occurring during and after exercise may be the only clue.[92] Hypokalemia not only aggravates ventricular arrhythmias in patients with digitalis toxicity but also may be implicated in the increased rate of sudden death that occurs in some hypertensive patients treated long-term with diuretics.[112] One study demonstrated an increased prevalence of exercise-induced isolated ventricular extrasystoles in hypertensive patients receiving diuretic therapy, compared with normotensive control subjects (57% versus 38%); the prevalence of high-grade exercise-related ventricular arrhythmias was no different between the two groups.[77] Postexercise decreases in arterial potassium, especially in deconditioned patients with ischemic heart disease, may also contribute to exercise-induced ventricular arrhythmias.[73,75] Patients receiving antiarrhythmic agents, particularly class I drugs, may manifest proarrhythmic effects of these drugs only during exercise; however, routine exercise testing to evaluate proarrhythmia is not common in clinical practice.[98] Exercise-related proarrhythmia is likely due to the interaction of the drug with pH and electrolyte shifts, heightened sympathetic state, and the cellular effects of myocardial ischemia in some patients. Exercise-induced proarrhythmia is not predictable but does appear to be relatively rare, although the small number of patients who routinely undergo such testing likely leads to underestimation of the actual prevalence. One study suggests a possible use of exercise testing in patients receiving class IA antiarrhythmic agents to evaluate the behavior of the QT interval as a marker for development of polymorphic ventricular tachycardia unrelated to exercise.[113] In that investigation, 10 of 11 patients who developed polymorphic ventricular tachycardia while receiving the offending drug had an unexpected increase in corrected QT interval during exercise despite an increase in heart rate, compared with only one of 11 control patients. Lack of QT-

interval shortening with exercise has also been described in patients with structural heart disease and exercise-induced ventricular tachycardia but not in patients with idiopathic exercise-induced ventricular tachycardia.[114]

PROGNOSIS

The prognosis of patients who have ventricular arrhythmias that occur during exercise relates to their underlying disease and to the use of specific treatment aimed at preventing the dysrhythmia. Coronary artery disease (and in particular, evidence of myocardial ischemia on exercise stress testing) and left ventricular dysfunction appear to be the most important prognostic indicators for risk of sudden death.[25,26,39,40] Some studies indicate that exercise-induced ventricular arrhythmias in patients with coronary artery disease do not significantly contribute to the risk of sudden death once the extent of coronary artery disease and of left ventricular dysfunction is considered.[25,26,115,116] In one study of patients undergoing exercise testing before hospital discharge after myocardial infarction, patients with high-grade exercise-induced ventricular arrhythmias were more likely to have had extensive infarctions and lower left ventricular ejection fractions than patients without these arrhythmias.[116] In this study, 1-year mortality was 15% in patients with exercise-induced ventricular arrhythmias, compared with 7% in patients without exercise arrhythmias, but the increase in mortality was best predicted by markers of left ventricular dysfunction (evidence of congestive heart failure or inadequate blood pressure rise with exercise) than by the arrhythmia per se.[116] These observations have been generally confirmed by most, but not all, investigators.

In survivors of cardiac arrest who undergo subsequent exercise stress testing, failure of the blood pressure to rise and development of angina appear to have a stronger relation to subsequent risk of recurrent cardiac arrest than does the appearance of exercise ventricular arrhythmias, although the point is controversial.[11,117] The development of exercise ventricular tachycardia occurs in a minority (10% to 15%) of patients who survive cardiac arrest and is unaccompanied by evidence of myocardial ischemia in many patients.[11] In patients who undergo coronary artery bypass surgery, the incidence of exercise-induced ventricular arrhythmias is reported to be unchanged at 1 and 5 years after surgery or increased.[118,119] The first-time appearance of exercise-induced ventricular tachycardia in surgically treated patients, however, might be predictive of recurrent sudden death.[118] In a large study of 200 patients undergoing coronary artery bypass graft surgery, exercise-induced ventricular ectopy was more frequent at 3 months after surgery (25%) than before

(16%).[119] This finding was not related to subsequent sudden cardiac deaths, all of which occurred in patients having no exercise ventricular arrhythmias.

The prognosis of apparently healthy persons who experience ventricular tachycardia during exercise is better than that of patients with symptomatic coronary artery disease. In one study of 10 asymptomatic persons who had exercise-related nonsustained ventricular tachycardia, none had perfusion defects on thallium scintigraphy, and no heart disease, syncope, or sudden death occurred during an average 2-year follow-up period.[17] Similar observations were made in a larger, newer study of 37 patients with exercise-induced ventricular tachycardia (none of whom died suddenly) and in a study of 52 patients followed-up for 96 months.[23, 120] It appears, therefore, that prognosis of patients with exercise-induced ventricular tachycardia may depend at least partly on the development of exercise-induced ischemia.

The prognosis for subjects with effort-related ventricular tachycardia in conditions other than normal or coronary artery disease remains virtually unknown but may depend on the clinician's ability to provide definitive antiarrhythmic therapy.

THERAPY

When exercise-induced ventricular tachycardia occurs in the setting of myocardial ischemia, the primary treatment should be directed toward preventing the ischemia. Medical therapy, with long-acting nitrates or beta- or calcium channel blocking agents, or revascularization therapy can be offered. Intravenous nitroglycerin is reported to significantly reduce the prevalence of reproducible exercise-induced ventricular arrhythmias in a small study of 20 patients and was equally effective in reducing total ventricular ectopy, ventricular doublets, and runs of ventricular tachycardia.[121] The investigators suggest that a favorable response to intravenous nitrates may be used to guide therapy of exercise-induced ventricular arrhythmias toward anti-ischemic medications and away from antiarrhythmic agents in such patients. In patients with mild to moderate heart failure who have exercise-induced ventricular arrhythmias, angiotensin-converting–enzyme inhibitor therapy has resulted in reduction of these rhythms. In one study in 14 patients having reproducible ventricular arrhythmias during exercise testing, benazepril reduced the number of tachycardia episodes by 66% and total ventricular extrasystolic episodes by 61%.[122] It is not clear whether this favorable effect on ventricular ectopic activity is direct or results from improved ventricular functional dynamics.

Although coronary artery bypass grafting does not appear to decrease the overall frequency of exercise-induced ventricular arrhythmias and may even be associated with an increase, there are reports of successful arrhythmia management by this means, with no recurrence of arrhythmias for up to 2 years postoperatively.[118, 119, 123, 124] Importantly, exercise-induced ventricular arrhythmias can worsen or even develop de novo after coronary artery bypass grafting.[125–127] Most patients who develop exercise-induced ventricular arrhythmias for the first time after coronary artery bypass grafting have had prior myocardial infarctions.[125, 126] In one study, persistence of exercise-induced ventricular arrhythmias after surgery was related either to preoperative left ventricular wall motion abnormalities or to the persistence of myocardial ischemia, as demonstrated by ST-segment depression during a postoperative exercise stress test.[128] Graft patency has not been found to be different in patients who develop new exercise-induced ventricular arrhythmias, compared with those who do not.[119, 125]

If exercise-induced ventricular tachycardia cannot be specifically related to myocardial ischemia, treatment should be directed at the mechanism underlying the arrhythmia if this can be documented. Electrophysiologic testing is of value because lack of reproducibility of exercise-induced arrhythmias generally precludes serial stress testing to guide efficacy of pharmacologic antiarrhythmic therapy. In the series of Sung and colleagues, in which electrophysiologic testing was used to guide therapy, all patients with catecholamine-sensitive automaticity responded to propranolol administered intravenously and subsequently administered orally.[66] Patients with reentry as the mechanism of their exercise-induced arrhythmia can be treated successfully with procainamide or amiodarone.[66] The combination of a beta blocker with a type I antiarrhythmic agent such as procainamide may be especially useful in abolishing exercise-induced ventricular tachycardia, even when either agent alone has been ineffective.[129] Amiodarone is also effective in patients with heart failure who have exercise-induced ventricular tachycardia and in patients with hypertrophic cardiomyopathy.[130, 131]

Failure to abolish exercise-induced ventricular arrhythmias in patients without underlying cardiac disease by using pharmacologic means alone is frequent and often frustrating (Fig. 20-11). Ablative procedures using radiofrequency energy may be curative in appropriately selected patients.

Beta-blocking agents are of specific benefit in patients who demonstrate a relation between the onset of exercise-induced tachycardia and a critical sinus rate. In one study of 11 patients having reproducible exercise-induced ventricular tachycardia, eight had a consistent sinus rate at the onset of ventricular tachycardia; in all eight, ventricular tachycardia was prevented by administration of acute and

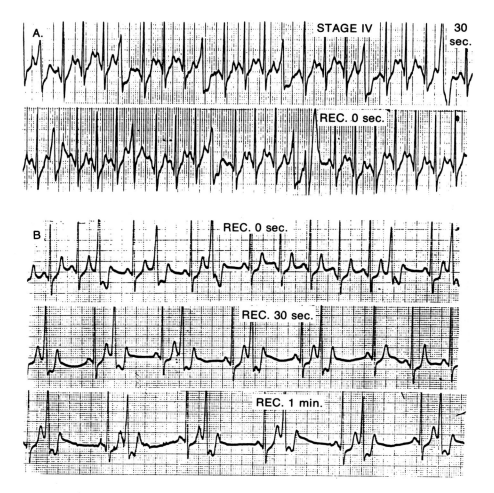

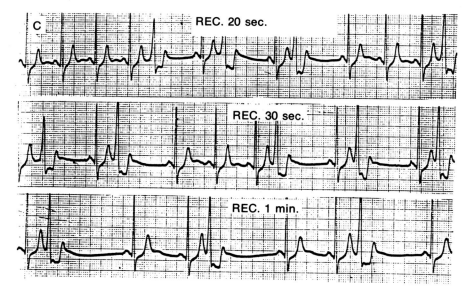

Figure 20-11. Exercise-induced ventricular premature beats in an asymptomatic man aged 55 years, whose effort tolerance was excellent. (**A**) Baseline treadmill stress test, illustrating closely coupled ventricular extrasystoles appearing at the height of exercise and persisting into the early recovery period, in which a single pair of ventricular beats is recorded. The treadmill test is negative for myocardial ischemic changes. Although the patient had no symptoms, this rhythm disturbance was thought to merit suppressant treatment. (**B**) Repeat treadmill test performed 2 weeks later, with the patient having received propranolol, 20 mg 4 times daily. Maximum heart rate achieved is now only about 110 beats/minute. Ventricular premature beats are still present and occur more frequently. (**C**) A third treadmill test performed 2 weeks after that shown in *B*, with the patient now receiving procainamide, 375 mg every 8 hours, in addition to propranolol, 40 mg 4 times daily. Maximum attained heart rate at this time is only about 95 beats/minute. This combination of antiarrhythmic medications failed to suppress the patient's ventricular ectopy.

subsequently chronic beta-blockade medications.[33] In another study of 10 patients who had reproducible exercise-induced ventricular tachycardia, nine patients had no recurrence of ventricular tachycardia during exercise after acutely receiving 0.2 mg/kg propranolol, intravenously.[132] The abolition of exercise-induced ventricular tachycardia by propranolol is associated with a measurable decrease in plasma norepinephrine level.[132] Chronic therapy with oral nadolol is similarly effective. In a report of 64 patients with reproducible exercise-induced ventricular arrhythmias, 48 (75%) had significant reductions in exercise ventricular arrhythmias and 18 (38%) of these 48 had total arrhythmia suppression after 3 to 6 months of therapy.[133]

Suppression or elimination of exercise-induced ventricular arrhythmias may have little direct import on morbidity and total cardiac and sudden death mortality because these rhythm disturbances are not reliable predictors of death. In this regard, the Coronary Artery Surgery Study showed no beneficial effect of beta blockade on survival in patients with exercise-induced ventricular arrhythmias.[8]

Propranolol is also reported to be efficacious in patients with exercise-induced ventricular tachycardia occurring in the long QT-interval syndrome, although its efficacy appears to be unrelated to the measured QT interval.[134] Propranolol has also been successfully used in patients with mitral valve prolapse and exercise-induced ventricular tachycardia.[83]

Intravenous verapamil may be highly effective in the management of patients with exercise-induced ventricular tachycardia because it both terminates and prevents the arrhythmia.[65, 135] Not all patients who respond to intravenous verapamil respond to oral verapamil, however. In a study by Woelfel and colleagues, intravenous loading with verapamil (0.2 mg/kg) prevented exercise-induced ventricular tachycardia in 12 of 16 patients, and oral verapamil (160 to 320 mg every 8 hours for 48 hours) prevented exercise-induced ventricular tachycardia in 8 of 12 patients who were previously responsive to intravenous verapamil.[135] Continued oral therapy with verapamil, however, appears to be only moderately effective in preventing exercise-induced ventricular tachycardia when compared with chronic beta blockade; all patients found to be unresponsive to verapamil subsequently responded to beta blockade.[135] This difference in responsiveness of exercise-induced ventricular tachycardia to calcium channel blocking agents compared with beta-blockade underscores the observation that the mechanisms of exercise-induced ventricular tachycardia vary among patients and may even vary in the same patient at different times in the clinical course.[67] The effect of verapamil in patients with ventricular tachycardia associated with mitral valve prolapse has not been investigated; because afterdepolarizations have

been noted in fibers from isolated simian mitral valves, this would be of interest.[63]

Finally, it should be mentioned that proarrhythmic effects of antiarrhythmic agents have not been described in the exercise setting, although systematic investigation has not been undertaken.

Implications for Exercise Rehabilitation Programs

The popularity of cardiac rehabilitation programs has raised two relevant issues regarding patients with exercise-induced ventricular arrhythmias: (1) what is the risk of exercise conditioning in these patients, and (2) what is the response of the arrhythmia to physical conditioning?

The risk of cardiac arrest is low in physician-directed cardiac rehabilitation programs, although it appears to be higher in patients with coronary disease during exercise training sessions than during routine daily activities.[136–139] A survey of 167 cardiac rehabilitation programs between 1980 and 1984 demonstrated only 8.9 cardiac arrests and 1.3 fatalities per million exercise-hours in 51,303 patients.[138] The low occurrence rate of cardiac arrest in physician-directed cardiac rehabilitation programs was independent of the size of the program or the extent of on-site continuous electrocardiographic monitoring capability but may relate partly to avoidance of excessive exercise heart rates.[49, 137, 138] Because the risk of sudden death in patients with cardiac disease (usually due to atherosclerotic processes) relates primarily to the extent and severity of coronary artery disease and to the degree of underlying left ventricular dysfunction, patients with poor left ventricular function or ongoing myocardial ischemia (during formal exercise testing or ambulatory electrocardiographic monitoring) who have documented exercise-induced ventricular tachycardia should not undertake a vigorous exercise program.[140]

Physical conditioning appears to diminish the frequency of exercise-induced ventricular ectopy in an asymptomatic population according to one report.[49] Nonetheless, there have been reports of sudden death in apparently healthy persons during jogging, although in asymptomatic individuals older than age 40 years, sudden death during this sort of activity most commonly reflects previously undetected coronary artery disease.[141–144] The risk of death during unsupervised jogging is reported in one study to be one death per 7620 joggers per year.[141]

Screening for ventricular arrhythmias of the asymptomatic person who undertakes sporadic vigorous exercise, with either exercise stress testing or ambulatory electrocardiographic monitoring, is probably of little overall benefit and not cost-effective, although screening for risk factors for coronary artery disease, such as hypertension or hypercholesterolemia, may be useful in predicting the individual at risk for exercise-related sudden death.[5, 144]

References

1. Coronary Drug Project Research Group: Prognostic importance of premature beats following myocardial infarction. JAMA 1973;223:1116.
2. Weld FM, Chu KL, Bigger JT, et al: Risk stratification with low level exercise testing two weeks after myocardial infarction. Circulation 1981;64:306.
3. Kron RJ, Gillespie JA, Weld FM, et al: Multicenter postinfarction research group. Low-level exercise testing after myocardial infarction: usefulness in enhancing clinical risk stratification. Circulation 1985;71:80.
4. Chiang BN, Perlman LV, Ostrander LD Jr, Epstein FH: Relationship of premature systoles to coronary heart disease and sudden death in the Tecumseh epidemiologic study. Ann Intern Med 1969;70:1159.
5. Hinkle LE Jr, Thaler HT, Merke DP, Renier-Berg D, Morton NE: The risk factors for arrhythmic death in a sample of men followed for 20 years. Am J Epidemiol 1988;127:500.
6. Yang JC, Wesley RC Jr, Froelicher VF: Ventricular tachycardia during routine treadmill testing. Risk and prognosis. Arch Intern Med 1991;151:349.
7. Busby MJ, Shefrin EA, Fleg JL: Prevalence and long-term significance of exercise-induced frequent or repetitive ventricular ectopic beats in apparently healthy volunteers. J Am Coll Cardiol 1989;14:1659.
8. Sami M, Chaitman B, Fisher L, Holmes D, Fray D, Alderman E: Significance of exercise-induced ventricular arrhythmia in stable coronary artery disease: a coronary artery surgery study project. Am J Cardiol 1984;54:1182.
9. Weiner DA, Levine PR, Klein MD, et al: Ventricular arrhythmias during exercise testing: mechanism, response to coronary bypass surgery, prognostic significance. Am J Cardiol 1984;53:1553.
10. McHenry PL, Fisch C, Jordan JW, Corya BR: Cardiac arrhythmias observed during maximal treadmill exercise testing in clinically normal men. Am J Cardiol 1972;29:331.
11. O'Hara GE, Brugada P, Rodriguez L-M, et al: Incidence, pathophysiology and prognosis of exercise-induced sustained ventricular tachycardia associated with healed myocardial infarction. Am J Cardiol 1992;70:875.
12. Anderson MT, Lee GB, Campion BC, et al: Cardiac dysrhythmias associated with exercise testing. Am J Cardiol 1972;30:763.
13. Marieb MA, Beller GA, Gibson RS, Lerman BB, Kaul S: Clinical relevance of exercise-induced ventricular arrhythmias in suspected coronary artery disease. Am J Cardiol 1990;66:172.
14. Jelinek MV, Lown B: Exercise stress testing for exposure of cardiac arrhythmia. Prog Cardiovasc Dis 1974;16:497.
15. Pantano JA, Oriel RJ: Prevalence and nature of cardiac arrhythmias in apparently normal well-trained runners. Am Heart J 1982;104:762.
16. Pilcher GF, Cook AJ, Johnston BL, Fletcher GF: Twenty-four-hour continuous electrocardiography during exercise and free activity in 80 apparently healthy runners. Am J Cardiol 1983;52:859.
17. Fleg JL, Lakatta EG: Prevalence and prognosis of exercise-induced nonsustained ventricular tachycardia in apparently healthy volunteers. Am J Cardiol 1984;54:762.
18. Specchia G, La Rovere MT, Falcone C, et al: Cardiac arrhythmias during exercise-induced myocardial ischemia in patients with coronary artery disease. Eur Heart J 1986;7 (Suppl A):45.
19. Visser FC, Mihciokur M, Van Dijk CN, et al: Arrhythmias in athletes: comparison of stress test, 24 h Holter and Holter monitoring during the game in squash players. Eur Heart J 1987;8(Suppl D):29.
20. Ekblom B, Hartley LH, Day WC: Occurrence and reproducibility of exercise-induced ventricular ectopy in normal subjects. Am J Cardiol 1979;43:35.
21. De Caprio L, Duomo S, Vigorito C, et al: Exercise induced ventricular arrhythmias: angiographic correlation with the severity of coronary artery disease. Jpn Heart J 1983;24:489.
22. Goldschlager N, Cake D, Cohn K: Exercise-induced ventricular arrhythmias in patients with coronary artery disease. Am J Cardiol 1973;31:434.
23. Mont L, Seixas T, Brugada P, et al: Clinical and electrophysiologic characteristics of exercise-related idiopathic ventricular tachycardia. Am J Cardiol 1991;68:897.
24. Klein GJ, Millman PJ, Yee R: Recurrent ventricular tachycardia responsive to verapamil. Pacing Clin Electrophysiol 1984;7:938.
25. Califf RM, McKinnis RA, McNeer JF, et al: Prognostic value of ventricular arrhythmias associated with treadmill exercise testing in patients studied with cardiac catheterization for suspected ischemic heart disease. J Am Coll Cardiol 1983; 2:1060.
26. Nair CK, Thomson W, Aronow WS, et al: Prognostic significance of exercise-induced complex ventricular arrhythmias in coronary artery disease with normal and abnormal left ventricular ejection fraction. Am J Cardiol 1984;54:1136.
27. Stuart RJ Jr, Ellestad MH: National survey of exercise stress testing facilities. Chest 1980;77:94.
28. Gibbons L, Blair SN, Kohl HW, Cooper K: The safety of maximal exercise testing. Circulation 1989;80:846.
29. Young DZ, Lampert S, Graboys TB, Lown B: Safety of maximal exercise testing in patients at high risk for ventricular arrhythmia. Circulation 1984;70:184.
30. Allen BJ, Casey TP, Brodsky MA, et al: Exercise testing in patients with life-threatening ventricular tachyarrhythmias: results and correlation with clinical and arrhythmia factors. Am Heart J 1988;116:997.
31. Faris JV, McHenry PL, Jordan JW, Morris SN: Prevalence and reproducibility of exercise-induced ventricular arrhythmias during maximal exercise testing in normal men. Am J Cardiol 1976;37:617.
32. Sheps DS, Ernst JC, Briese FR, et al: Decreased frequency of exercise-induced ventricular ectopic activity in the second of two consecutive treadmill tests. Circulation 1977;55:892.
33. Woelfel A, Foster JR, Simpson RJ Jr, Gettes LS: Reproducibil-

ity and treatment of exercise-induced ventricular tachycardia. Am J Cardiol 1984;53:751.

34. Saini V, Graboys TB, Towne V, Lown B: Reproducibility of exercise-induced ventricular arrhythmia in patients undergoing evaluation for malignant ventricular arrhythmia. Am J Cardiol 1989;63:697.

35. Podrid PJ: Treatment of ventricular arrhythmia: application and limitations of noninvasive vs invasive approach. Chest 1985;88:121.

36. Ryan M, Lown B, Horn H: Comparison of ventricular ectopic activity during 24-hour monitoring and exercise testing in patients with coronary heart disease. N Engl J Med 1975; 292:224.

37. Fauchier JP, Cosnay P, Moquet B, et al: Late ventricular potentials and spontaneous and induced ventricular arrhythmias in dilated or hypertrophic cardiomyopathies: a prospective study about 83 patients. Pacing Clin Electrophysiol 1988;11:1974.

38. Kosowsky BD, Lown B, Whiting R, Guiney T: Occurrence of ventricular arrhythmias with exercise as compared to monitoring. Circulation 1971;44:826.

39. Ivanova LA, Mazur NA, Smirnova TM, et al: Electrocardiographic exercise testing and ambulatory monitoring to identify patients with ischemic heart disease at high risk of sudden death. Am J Cardiol 1980;45:1132.

40. Kennedy HL: Comparison of ambulatory electrocardiography and exercise testing. Am J Cardiol 1981;47:1359.

41. Froelicher VF Jr, Thomas MM, Pillow C, Lancaster MC: Epidemiologic study of asymptomatic men screened by maximal treadmill testing for latent coronary artery disease. Am J Cardiol 1974;34:770.

42. Henry RL, Kennedy GT, Crawford MH: Prognostic value of exercise-induced ventricular ectopic activity for mortality after acute myocardial infarction. Am J Cardiol 1987;59:1251.

43. Coplan NL, Gleim GW, Nicholas JA: Exercise-related changes in serum catecholamines and potassium: effect of sustained exercise above and below lactate threshold. Am Heart J 1989;117:1070.

44. Mathes P: Arrhythmogenic potential of silent myocardial ischemia following transmural myocardial infarction. Adv Cardiol 1986;34:186.

45. Reinke A, Michel D, Mathes P: Arrhythmogenic potential of exercise-induced myocardial ischaemia. Eur Heart J 1987;8 (Suppl G):119.

46. Gottlieb SO, Gottlieb SH, Achuff SC, et al: Silent ischemia on Holter monitoring predicts mortality in high-risk postinfarction patients. JAMA 1988;259:1030.

47. Gooch AS, McConnell D: Analysis of transient arrhythmias and conduction disturbances occurring during submaximal treadmill exercise testing. Prog Cardiovasc Dis 1970;13:293.

48. Tuininga YS, Crijns HJGM, Wiesfeld ACP, Van Veldhuisen DJ, Hillege HL, Lie KI: Electrocardiographic patterns relative to initiating mechanisms of exercise-induced ventricular tachycardia. Am Heart J 1993;126:359.

49. Blackburn H, Taylor HL, Hamrell B, et al: Premature ventricular complexes induced by stress testing. Am J Cardiol 1973;31:441.

50. Codini MA, Sommerfeldt L, Eybel CE, Messer JV: Clinical significance and characteristics of exercise-induced ventricular tachycardia. Cathet Cardiovasc Diagn 1981;7:227.

51. Sideris DA: The importance of blood pressure in the emergence of arrhythmias. Eur Heart J 1987;8(Suppl D):129.

52. Helfant RH, Pine R, Kabde V, Banka VS: Exercise-related ventricular premature complexes in coronary heart disease. Ann Intern Med 1974;80:589.

53. McHenry PL, Morris SN, Kavalier M, Jordan JW: Comparative study of exercise-induced ventricular arrhythmias in normal subjects and patients with documented coronary artery disease. Am J Cardiol 1976;37:609.

54. Levine SR, Weiner DA, Klein MD, Ryan TJ: Significance of ventricular arrhythmias during exercise testing. Circulation 1983;68:III.

55. Hilton TC, Ira GH Jr, Bolena W, Stowers SA: Myocardial perfusion imaging during stress-induced sustained ventricular tachyarrhythmia. Am Heart J 1993;125:539.

56. Carboni GP, Lahiri A, Cashman PMM, Raftery EB.: Mechanisms of arrhythmias accompanying ST-segment depression on ambulatory monitoring in stable angina pectoris. Am J Cardiol 1987;60:1246.

57. Turitto G, Dini P, Prati PL: The R on T phenomenon during transient myocardial ischemia. Am J Cardiol 1989;63:1520.

58. Buxton AE, Waxman HL, Marchlinski FE, et al: Right ventricular tachycardia: clinical and electrophysiologic characteristics. Circulation 1983;68:917.

59. Lemery R, Brugada P, Della Bella P, et al: Nonischemic ventricular tachycardia. Clinical course and long-term followup in patients without clinically overt heart disease. Circulation 1989;79:990.

60. Hoffman BF, Rosen MR: Cellular mechanisms for cardiac arrhythmias. Circ Res 1981;49:1.

61. Rosen MR, Reder RF: Does triggered activity have a role in the genesis of cardiac arrhythmias? Ann Intern Med 1981; 94:794.

62. Spear JF, Moore EN: Mechanisms of cardiac arrhythmias. Ann Rev Physiol 1982;44:485.

63. Cranefield PF, Wit AL: Cardiac arrhythmias. Ann Rev Physiol 1979;41:459.

64. Josephson ME, Horowitz LN, Farshidi A, Kastor JA: Recurrent sustained ventricular tachycardia. Circulation 1978;57:431.

65. Wu D, Kou H, Hung J: Exercise-triggered paroxysmal ventricular tachycardia. Ann Intern Med 1981;95:410.

66. Sung RJ, Shen EN, Morady F, et al: Electrophysiologic mechanism of exercise-induced sustained ventricular tachycardia. Am J Cardiol 1983;51:525.

67. Sung RJ, Keung EC, Nguyen NX, Huycke EC: Effects of beta-adrenergic blockade on verapamil-responsive and verapamil-irresponsive sustained ventricular tachycardias. J Clin Invest 1988;81:688.

68. Sung RJ, Huycke EC, Lai W, et al: Clinical and electrophysiologic mechanisms of exercise-induced ventricular tachyarrhythmias. Pacing Clin Electrophysiol 1988;11:1347.

69. Sasyniuk BI, Mendez C: A mechanism for reentry in canine ventricular tissue. Circ Res 1971;28:3.

70. Vassalle M, Levine MJ, Stuckey JH: On the sympathetic control of ventricular automaticity. Circ Res 1968;23:249.

71. Vassalle M, Stuckey JH, Levine MJ: Sympathetic control of

ventricular automaticity: role of the adrenal medulla. Am J Physiol 1969;217:930.

72. Miyakoda H, Noguchi N, Matsumoto T, et al: Plasma catecholamine responses to dynamic exercise in patients with coronary artery disease—the relationship between sympathetic activity and systolic blood pressure and exercise-induced ventricular arrhythmias Jpn Circ J 1992;56:1115.

73. Thomson A, Kelly DT: Exercise stress-induced changes in systemic arterial potassium in angina pectoris. Am J Cardiol 1989;63:1435.

74. Coester N, Ellio JC, Luft UC. Plasma electrolytes, pH, and ECG during and after exhaustive exercise. J Appl Physiol 1973;34:677.

75. Coplan NL, Gleim GW, Nicholas JA: Relation of potassium flux during incremental exercise to exercise intensity. Am J Cardiol 1988;62:334.

76. Hohnloser SH, Verrier RL, Lown B, Raeder EA: Effect of hypokalemia on susceptibility to ventricular fibrillation in the normal and ischemic canine heart. Am Heart J 1986; 112:32.

77. Bause GS, Fleg JL, Lakatta EG: Exercise-induced arrhythmias in diuretic-treated patients with uncomplicated systemic hypertension. Am J Cardiol 1987;59:874.

78. Papademetriou V, Notargiacomo A, Heine D, Fletcher RD, Freis ED: Effects of diuretic therapy and exercise-related arrhythmias in systemic hypertension. Am J Cardiol 1989; 64:1152.

79. Vlay SC: Catecholamine-sensitive ventricular tachycardia. Am Heart J 1987;114:455.

80. Swartz MH,a Teichholz LE, Donoso E: Mitral valve prolapse. Am J Cardiol 1977;62:377.

81. Garza LA, Vick RL, Nora JJ, McNamara DG: Heritable QT prolongation without deafness. Circulation 1970;41:39.

82. Moss AJ, Schwartz PJ, Crampton RS, Locati E, Carleen E: The long QT syndrome: a prospective international study. Circulation 1985;71:17.

83. Pocock WA, Barlow JB: Postexercise arrhythmias in the billowing posterior mitral leaflet syndrome. Am Heart J 1970; 80:740.

84. Sloman G, Wong M, Walker J: Arrhythmias on exercise in patients with abnormalities of the posterior leaflet of the mitral valve. Am Heart J 1972;83:312.

85. Gooch AS, Vicencio F, Maranhao V, Goldberg H: Arrhythmias and left ventricular asynergy in the prolapsing mitral leaflet syndrome. Am J Cardiol 1972;29:611.

86. Broustet JP, Douard H, Mora B: Exercise testing in arrhythmias of idiopathic mitral valve prolapse. Eur Heart J 1987;8 (Suppl D):37.

87. Roberts WC, McAllister HA Jr, Ferrans VJ: Sarcoidosis of the heart. Am J Med 1977;63:86.

88. Voigt J, Agdal N: Lipomatous infiltration of the heart. Arch Pathol Lab Med 1982;106:497.

89. Thiene G, Nava A, Corrado D, et al: Right ventricular cardiomyopathy and sudden death in young people. N Engl J Med 1988;318:129.

90. Maron BJ, Roberts WC, McAllister HA, et al: Sudden death in young athletes. Circulation 1980;62:218.

91. Morales AR, Romanelli R, Boucek RJ: The mural left anterior descending coronary artery, strenuous exercise and sudden death. Circulation 1980;62:230.

92. Gooch AS, Natarajan G, Goldberg H: Influence of exercise on arrhythmias induced by digitalis-diuretic therapy in patients with atrial fibrillation. Am J Cardiol 1974;33:230.

93. Virmani R, Robinowitz M, Clark MA, McAllister HA Jr: Sudden death and partial absence of the right ventricular myocardium. Arch Pathol Lab Med 1982;106:163.

94. Winkler RB, Freed MD, Nadas AS: Exercise-induced ventricular ectopy in children and young adults with complete heart block. Am Heart J 1980;99:87.

95. Garson A Jr, Gillette PC, Gutgesell HP, McNamara DG: Stress-induced ventricular arrhythmia after repair of tetralogy of Fallot. Am J Cardiol 1980;46:1006.

96. Feld H, Guadanino V, Hollander G, Greengart A, Lichstein E, Shani J: Exercise-induced ventricular tachycardia in association with a myocardial bridge. Chest 1991;99:1295.

97. Gosselink ATM, Cruns HJGM, Wiesfeld ACP, Lie KI: Exercise-induced ventricular tachycardia: a rare manifestation of digitalis toxicity. Clin Cardiol 1993;16:270.

98. Nazari J, Bauman J, Pham T, Ivanovich L, Kehoe RF: Exercise induced fatal sinusoidal ventricular tachycardia secondary to moricizine. Pacing Clin Electrophysiol 1992;15:1421.

99. Sellers DT, Di Marco JP: Sinusoidal ventricular tachycardia associated with flecainide Acetate. Chest 1984;5:647.

100. Falk RH: Flecainide induced ventricular tachycardia and fibrillation in patients treated for atrial fibrillation. Ann Intern Med 1989;111:107.

101. Gill JS, Hunter GJ, Gane J, Ward DE, Camm AJ: Asymmetry of cardiac [^{123}I] meta-iodobenzyl-guanidine scans in patients with ventricular tachycardia and a "clinically normal" heart. Br Heart J 1993;69:6.

102. Shappell SD, Marshall CE, Brown RE, Bruce TA: Sudden death and the familial occurrence of mid-systolic click, and late systolic murmur syndrome. Circulation 1973;48:1128.

103. Duren DR, Becker AE, Dunning AJ: Long-term follow-up of idiopathic mitral valve prolapse in 300 patients: a prospective study. J Am Coll Cardiol 1988;11:42.

104. Savage DD, Levy D, Garrison RJ, et al: Mitral valve prolapse in the general population. Am Heart J 1983;106:582.

105. Savage DD, Seides SF, Maron BJ, et al: Prevalence of arrhythmias during 24-hour electrocardiographic monitoring and exercise testing in patients with obstructive and nonobstructive hypertrophic cardiomyopathy. Circulation 1979; 59:866.

106. Maron BJ, Savage DD, Wolfson JK, Epstein SE: Prognostic significance of 24 hour ambulatory electrocardiographic monitoring in patients with hypertrophic cardiomyopathy: a prospective study. Am J Cardiol 1981;48:252.

107. Maron BJ, Lipson LC, Roberts WC, et al: "Malignant" hypertrophic cardiomyopathy: identification of a subgroup of families with unusually frequent premature death. Am J Cardiol 1978;41:1133.

108. Nicod P, Polikar R, Peterson KL: Hypertrophic cardiomyopathy and sudden death. N Engl J Med 1988;318:1255.

109. Maron BJ, Wolfson JK, Epstein SE, Roberts WC: Intramural ("small vessel") coronary artery disease in hypertrophic cardiomyopathy. J Am Coll Cardiol 1986;8:545.

110. Regan TJ, Lyons MM, Ahmed SS, et al: Evidence for cardio-myopathy in familial diabetes mellitus. J Clin Invest 1977; 60:885.

111. Bakth S, Arena J, Lee W, et al: Arrhythmia susceptibility and myocardial composition in diabetes. J Clin Invest 1986; 77:382.

112. Multiple Risk Factor Intervention Trial Research Group: Multiple risk factor intervention trial. JAMA 1982;248:1465.

113. Kadish AH, Weisman HF, Veltri EP, Epstein AE, Slepian MJ, Levine JH: Paradoxical effects of exercise on the QT interval in patients with polymorphic ventricular tachycardia receiving type 1a antiarrhythmic agents. Circulation 1990; 81:14.

114. Gill JS, Baszko A, Xia R, Ward DE, Camm AJ: Dynamics of the QT interval in patients with exercise-induced ventricular tachycardia in normal and abnormal hearts. Am Heart J 1993;126:1357.

115. Nair CK, Aronow WS, Sketch MH, et al: Diagnostic and prognostic significance of exercise-induced premature ventricular complexes in men and women: a four year follow-up. J Am Coll Cardiol 1983;1:1201.

116. Fioretti P, Deckers J, Baardman T, et al: Incidence and prognostic implications of repetitive ventricular complexes during pre-discharge bicycle ergometry after myocardial infarction. Eur Heart J 1987;8(Suppl D):51.

117. Weaver WD, Cobb LA, Hallstrom AP: Characteristics of survivors of exertion- and nonexertion-related cardiac arrest: value of subsequent exercise testing. Am J Cardiol 1982; 50:671.

118. Lehrman KL, Tilkian AG, Hultgren HN, Fowles RE: Effect of coronary arterial bypass surgery on exercise-induced ventricular arrhythmias. Am J Cardiol 1979;44:1056.

119. Yli-Mäyry S, Huikuri HV, Korhonen UR, et al: Prevalence and prognostic significance of exercise-induced ventricular arrhythmias after coronary artery bypass grafting. Am J Cardiol 1990;66:1451.

120. Lemery R, Brugada P, Della Bella P, Dugernier T, van den Dool A, Wellens HJJ: Nonischemic ventricular tachycardia. Clinical course and long-term follow-up in patients without clinically overt heart disease. Circulation 1989;79:990.

121. Margonato A, Bonetti F, Mailhac A, Vicedomini G, Cianflone D, Chierchia SL: Intravenous nitroglycerin suppresses exercise-induced arrhythmias in patients with ischaemic heart disease: implications for long-term treatment. Eur Heart J 1991;12:1278.

122. Nordrehaug JE, Vollset SE: Reduction of exercise-induced ventricular arrhythmias in mild symptomatic heart failure by benazepril. Am Heart J 1993;125:771.

123. Bryson AL, Parisi AF, Schechter E, Wolfson S: Life-threatening ventricular arrhythmias induced by exercise. Am J Cardiol 1973;32:995.

124. Codini MA, Sommerfeldt L, Eybel CE, et al: Efficacy of coronary bypass grafting in exercise-induced ventricular tachycardia. J Thorac Cardiovasc Surg 1981;81:502.

125. Huikuri HV, Korhonen UR, Takkunen JT: Ventricular arrhythmias induced by dynamic and static exercise in relation to coronary artery bypass grafting. Am J Cardiol 1985;55:948.

126. Anastassiades LC, Antonopoulos AG, Petsas AA: The effect of coronary revascularization on exercise-induced ventricular ectopic activity. Eur Heart J 1987;8(Suppl D):75.

127. Mathes P: The effect of coronary revascularization on exercise-induced ventricular arrhythmias. Eur Heart J 1987;8 (Suppl D):79.

128. Weiner DA, Levine SR, Klein MD, Ryan TJ: Ventricular arrhythmias during exercise testing: mechanism, response to coronary bypass surgery and prognostic significance. Am J Cardiol 1984;53:1553.

129. Hirsowitz G, Podrid PJ, Lampert S, et al: The role of beta blocking agents as adjunct therapy to membrane stabilizing drugs in malignant ventricular arrhythmia. Am Heart J 1986;111:852.

130. Cleland JGF, Dargie HJ: Ventricular arrhythmias during exercise in patients with heart failure: the effect of amiodarone. Eur Heart J 1987;8(Suppl D):65.

131. McKenna WJ, Oakley CM, Krikler DM, Goodwin JF: Improved survival with amiodarone in patients with hypertrophic cardiomyopathy and ventricular tachycardia. Br Heart J 1985;53:412.

132. Sokoloff NM, Spielman SR, Greenspan AM, et al: Plasma norepinephrine in exercise-induced ventricular tachycardia. J Am Coll Cardiol 1986;8:11.

133. Sung RJ, Olukotun AY, Baird CL, et al: Efficacy and safety of oral nadolol for exercise-induced ventricular arrhythmias. Am J Cardiol 1987;60:15D.

134. Alpert BS, Boineau J, Strong WB: Exercise-induced ventricular tachycardia. Ped Cardiol 1982;2:51.

135. Woelfel A, Foster JR, McAllister RG Jr, et al: Efficacy of verapamil in exercise-induced ventricular tachycardia. Am J Cardiol 1985;56:292.

136. Rothfield D, Werres R, Rommer TC, Pongpoonsuksri V: Cardiac arrest in a physician-directed cardiac rehabilitation program: a clinical and angiographic profile of two cases. Angiology 1980;31:576.

137. Boone T: Exercise prescription for cardiac patients. Sports Med 198;3:157.

138. Van Camp SP, Peterson RA: Cardiovascular complications of outpatient cardiac rehabilitation programs. JAMA 1986; 256:1160.

139. Cobb LA, Weaver WD: Exercise: a risk for sudden death in patients with coronary heart disease. J Am Coll Cardiol 1986;7:215.

140. Jelinek VM: Exercise induced arrhythmias: their implications for cardiac rehabilitation programs. Med Sci Sports Exerc 1980;12:223.

141. Thompson PD, Funk EJ, Carleton RA, Sturner WQ: Incidence of death during jogging in Rhode Island from 1975 through 1980. JAMA 1982;247:2535.

142. Virmani R, Robinowitz M, McAllister HA Jr: Nontraumatic death in joggers. Am J Med 1982;72:874.

143. Thompson PD, Stern MP, Williams P, et al: Death during jogging or running. JAMA 1979;242:1265.

144. Waller BF, Roberts WC: Sudden death while running in conditioned runners aged 40 years or over. Am J Cardiol 1980;45:1292.

Cardiac Arrhythmias, 3rd edition, edited by William J. Mandel.
J. B. Lippincott Company, Philadelphia © 1995.

21

Dennis M. Krikler • Michael Perelman
Edward Rowland • William J. Mandel

Ventricular Tachycardia and Ventricular Fibrillation

It clearly was difficult for our predecessors to distinguish one arrhythmia from another until graphic methods were introduced; even then—a century or so ago—sphygmography was insufficiently precise to allow differentiation of various tachycardias.[1] Undoubtedly, Brunton recognized (albeit without defining the cause) that under chloroform anesthesia, some patients developed a rapid heart rate with shock and died.[2] This observation was particularly important in relation to the subsequent demonstration by Levy and Lewis that ventricular tachycardia and fibrillation could be induced by chloroform.[3] The term *paroxysmal tachycardia* can be found in a monograph by Hoffmann, and in his first book, Wenckebach refers to the disorder generally, only distinguishing ventricular tachycardia from the atrial and junctional forms a decade later.[4,5,6] Although Mackenzie used the term paroxysmal tachycardia and described cases, it is impossible to identify any of these cases as being due to paroxysmal ventricular tachycardia, and Mackenzie did not attempt to distinguish the site of impulse formation.[7] In the meantime, Lewis provided the essential background information to permit recognition of ventricular tachycardia, which he induced in dogs by coronary artery ligation.[8] In his experiments, such aspects as atrioventricular (AV) dissociation, the presence or absence of ventriculoatrial conduction, lack of response to vagal maneuvers, and the development of ventricular fibrillation were carefully discussed and illustrated with electrocardiographic tracings.

Ventricular fibrillation and ventricular tachycardia are presumably the same arrhythmia as the "tremulous motion" and "tumultuous" action of the heart described under these circumstances by Erichsen.[9] Allessie recounts the experimental production and recordings of ventricular fibrillation by Hoffa and Ludwig, using electric currents, and also the more definitive description of ventricular fibrillation by McWilliam.[10,11] A clinical example by Lewis in 1911 showed AV dissociation and numerous clinical and electrocardiographic reports appeared thereafter.[12] Better understanding of the mechanisms and causes of ventricular tachycardia and fibrillation has come sporadically as the importance of ischemic heart disease has become appreciated (both generally and in relation to ventricular arrhythmias) and as electrophysiologic techniques applied to animal preparations and those used in patients have enhanced clinicians' understanding of the mechanisms of these arrhythmias.

DEFINITIONS

Although the terms *paroxysmal ventricular tachycardia* and *ventricular fibrillation* refer to disorders of rhythm affecting and located in the ventricles, a more specific definition is required. Arrhythmias associated with disturbances in the bundle of His proximal to its bifurcation are conventionally classed as supraventricular, even though this is anatomically imprecise. This is not only because they usually have narrow QRS complexes because some focal arrhythmias arising in the bundle of His may do so eccentrically or may be conducted less well into one bundle branch than into the other, producing the appearances of aberration (Fig. 21-1). The same consideration applies to those few cases of tachycardia in which reciprocation occurs between an infranodal accessory pathway, a so-called Mahaim tract, and one of the bundle branches.[13] The term *ventricular tachycardia* is generally meant to indicate an arrhythmia that arises within the ventricles distal to the subdivision of the bundle of His, involving either rapid discharge from an ectopic focus or reentry at a Purkinje-myocardial junction or between bundle branches or fascicles or solely within the myocardium.

Accelerated idioventricular rhythm describes the development of an independent ventricular rhythm more rapid than sinus that becomes manifest only intermittently. Semantically, the arrhythmia in Figure 21-1 could be placed in this category in which the rate is only marginally faster than sinus. Schamroth suggests a rate range of 55 to 108 beats per minute.[14] Such arrhythmias often occur during acute myocardial infarction but are probably benign. Accelerated indioventricular rhythm is closely linked with the lower rate limit, defined by Scherf and Schott as low as 110.[15]

ELECTROPHYSIOLOGY

Arrhythmias may arise by any of several mechanisms: enhanced automaticity at a focal ectopic site, reentry, or triggered activity (see Chap. 3). Most early electrocardiographers believed that paroxysmal ventricular tachycardia was usually due to enhanced automaticity, but newer evidence suggests that reentry is the major cause.[14] Intraventricular reentry is well established in animal models, and modern electrophysiologic techniques have suggested that even in humans, reentry is the most com-

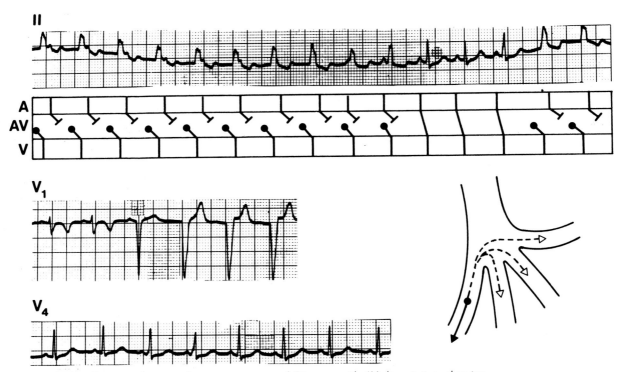

Figure 21-1. Electrocardiograms from a woman aged 24 years with AV dissociation, showing intermittent rapid discharge from an area apparently located within the proximal right bundle branch, producing in those complexes appearances consistent with incomplete left bundle branch block. The arrhythmia is terminated when the sinus rate increases and captures the ventricles and manifests as the sinus rate slows.

mon mechanism.[16–18] Under appropriate circumstances, one can initiate and terminate a tachycardia by suitably timed electric impulses, suggesting a reentry loop, but contemporary techniques may not be able to differentiate between a focal origin and reentry. The former may be due to a localized microreentry circuit occurring within an area of 30 mm² if studies on isolated atria can be extrapolated to the ventricles, and the role of triggered activity adds a further element that is not yet well-defined clinically.[19, 20]

Propagated action potentials from myocardial cells can be induced by changes in electrolyte and acid–base balance (especially a decrease in potassium concentration) or in extracellular and intracellular pH, and the preliminary studies of Bouvrain and Coraboeuf may have therapeutic implications in cardiac infarction.[21] Furthermore, the development of a stable animal model permits mapping of reentrant ventricular arrhythmias.[22] Such studies have been conducted on dogs 3 to 7 days after ligation of the anterior descending coronary artery. A specially designed composite electrode permits reentrant impulses to be mapped during their course through the infarction zone. This model has been used to study the patterns of initiation and termination of reentry ventricular arrhythmias and to show that ventricular fibrillation may be related to a marked delay in the reentrant pathway conduction of the beat before that which is apparently coupled to the premature beat (see Chaps. 13 and 18).[23] Using intracellular and extracellular recordings in the dog heart in situ, Russell and colleagues showed the conditions that can give rise to arrhythmias, notably slow conduction.[24] When this is accompanied by alternans of the action potential (affecting amplitude, duration, and morphology), ventricular fibrillation could be produced by occlusion of the left anterior descending coronary artery. Similar results were reported with observations on subepicardial membrane potentials recorded from intact pig hearts by Downar and associates.[25] Both groups noted that varying degrees of localized conduction blocks (e.g., 2:1 responses) and alternation were important precursors of fibrillation; highly relevant to this is the way in which reentrant extrasystoles can be noted in the model by El-Sherif and coworkers.[26]

The precise importance of focal tachycardia, as opposed to macroreentry, requires reevaluation not only in persons with acute myocardial infarction but also in persons in whom other causes exist. Intracardiac studies by Brechenmacher and colleagues revealed that even though surface electrocardiograms (ECGs) failed to disclose any evidence of reentry during sinus rhythm, a late potential could be identified with endocavitary recordings, which activated the bundle of His retrogradely and the right bundle branch anterogradely; from this localized area, obvious macroreentry developed, with typical reciprocat-

ing ventricular tachycardia.[27] Operative endocardial and epicardial recordings show both continuous activity and late potentials in patients with ventricular tachycardia.[28, 29] This may also have applications to ventricular fibrillation, although focal automaticity may play a role, and different electrophysiologic mechanisms may exist. Recognition of the importance of reentry in this field is growing.[30] Our own studies show that in those patients with underlying disorders of repolarization, electric stimulation may lead to the form of reentry ventricular tachycardia called torsades de pointes, a potential forerunner of ventricular fibrillation.[31] This appears to be the mechanism for sudden death noted during ambulatory monitoring.[32]

It is not yet appropriate in the clinical context to do more than allude to the possible role of triggered activity, a mechanism of arrhythmia well demonstrated in vitro.[33] Such behavior, in which a focus becomes rhythmically active only if driven at a given rate or by a critically timed premature stimulus, is thus distinguished from spontaneous automaticity; its occurrence after phase 4 depolarization due to an afterpotential is different from that seen in the usual models for reentry. Although triggered automaticity may be responsible for experimental canine atrial arrhythmias, it has not been linked with clinical ventricular arrhythmias, although this is an attractive explanation.[34, 20] Indeed, Rozanski and coworkers showed in vitro that delayed reflection (type II) can result in an extrasystole at the point of origin without the presence of pacemaker elements.[35] This work may provide an explanation for microreentry in ischemic myocardium.

It remains to be seen whether triggered automaticity is responsible for initiating one particular variety of ventricular tachycardia that can be terminated by verapamil.[36] Further support for the role of triggered automaticity comes from Coumel, who examined the effect of calcium channel blockers such as verapamil on ventricular extrasystoles.[37] Finally, the role of the autonomic nervous system in relation to the induction and termination of ventricular tachycardia and fibrillation needs reappraisal. Apparently benign chronic recurrent ventricular tachycardia can be terminated by phenylephrine, and vagal stimulation may prevent ventricular arrhythmias, particularly in situations with high sympathetic tone (e.g, after acute anterior myocardial infarction). That endogenous catecholamines may also be important (perhaps in increasing transmembrane calcium influx) may likewise be relevant to the initiation of ventricular arrhythmias.[38–41]

In ventricular fibrillation, the disorganized morphologic appearances on the ECG probably reflect incoordinate localized reentry processes rather than diffuse ectopic hyperactivity and may (1) follow sustained ventricular tachycardia of the uniform variety, (2) occur with the R-on-T phenomenon in previous sinus rhythm, or (3) develop after a few beats of tachycardia (Fig. 21-2). Un-

II

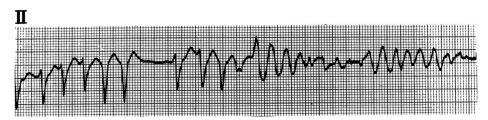

Figure 21-2. Lead II electrocardiogram recorded from a patient with acute myocardial infarction soon after admission to the coronary care unit. Two ventricular extrasystoles, a single sinus beat, and two further ventricular extrasystoles culminate in ventricular fibrillation.

treated torsades de pointes and multifocal ventricular tachycardia (Fig. 21-3) may degenerate into ventricular fibrillation, with which they tend to be confused.

ELECTROCARDIOGRAPHIC FEATURES

Descriptions of the characteristics of ventricular tachycardia are given differently by various authorities. These should clearly be based on the existence of a rapid ar-

rhythmia arising or existing within the ventricles distal to the bifurcation of the bundle of His, whether based on enhanced automaticity or microscopic or macroscopic reentry. Ventricular activity is independent of that of the atria because the atria may continue to respond to the influence of the sinus node or they may respond to retrograde stimulation from the ventricles or be the seat of a supraventricular arrhythmia (e.g., atrial fibrillation). Generally, the QRS complex is both wider than normal and altered in appearance, more so if the mechanism of the arrhythmia is seated further away from the bundle of His.

V₄   C. Walf.

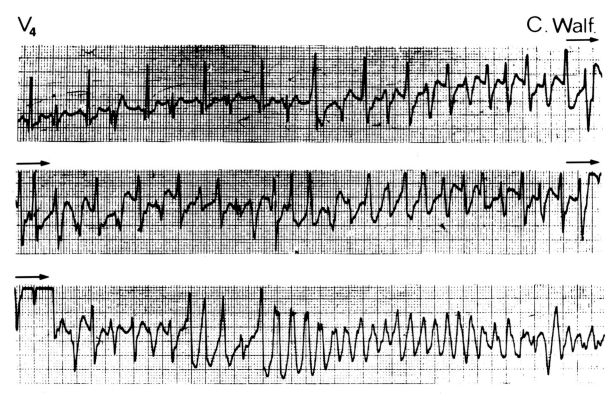

Figure 21-3. Continuous electrocardiographic recordings (V₄) showing, at first, sinus rhythm with bigeminy due to ventricular extrasystoles. During the second part of the *upper panel*, ventricular tachycardia develops, with variability in the QRS complexes that becomes grossly evident in the *second panel*. In the middle of the *third panel*, this multiform tachycardia degenerates into ventricular fibrillation, for which direct current electric defibrillation was required.

Precisely what constitutes tachycardia in terms of number of successive complexes (Bellet requires four to six, Schamroth and Anderson and coworkers are satisfied with three) is less important than identification of the site of the sustained rhythm disturbance; the relevance of nonsustained tachycardia must always be assessed.[14, 42, 43]

Although some ventricular tachycardias have features that may enable them to be recognized as benign, conversely, ventricular fibrillation can never be pronounced benign. Ventricular fibrillation is a disorder that leads to death unless the arrhythmia is arrested by external means, and its presence implies disease even though the precise nature may not be defined. So-called self-limited attacks of "ventricular fibrillation" usually represent torsades de pointes.

Characteristically, ventricular tachycardia has a uniform aspect consisting of a series of widened QRS complexes, usually regular (Fig. 21-4) but sometimes moderately irregular (Fig. 21-5), with appearances different from those of the basic sinus rhythm. As can be seen in Figures 21-4 and 21-5, the initial vector of the QRS complex is usually different from those in sinus impulses. The QRS vector may indicate that part of the ventricle first depolarized (as with total anomalous conduction in patients

with the Wolff-Parkinson-White syndrome) by the forces that appear to emanate from it.[44] Thus, in Figure 21-6, one may infer from the marked superior axis deviation in the frontal plane and the positive R in lead V_1 a posteroseptal origin for the ventricular tachycardia, compatible with the clinical diagnosis of mitral valve prolapse that was confirmed at operation and epicardial mapping.[45] Even though basically uniform, the QRS complexes show some variability in morphology.

Where evident, the hallmark of ventricular tachycardia is AV dissociation. Atrial activity cannot be discerned during tachycardia in Figure 21-4 but is easier to identify in lead III in Figure 21-6 as sharper peaking of alternate T waves, possibly representing 2:1 ventriculoatrial conduction. Discrete sinus P waves, unrelated to ventricular activation, more clearly indicate AV dissociation in Figures 21-5 and 21-7, but it is sometimes necessary to record a simultaneous right atrial electrogram to display this phenomenon (Fig. 21-8B). When the P wave falls in the appropriate part of the cycle, capture and fusion complexes may be seen (see Fig. 21-7). In the absence of sinus rhythm (e.g., when atrial fibrillation is the basic rhythm), AV dissociation cannot be defined in this way.

A subgroup within uniform ventricular tachycardia in

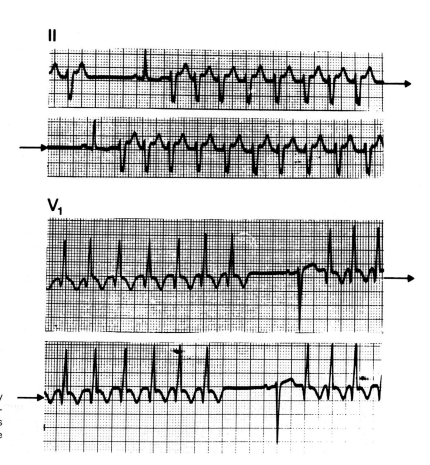

Figure 21-4. Electrocardiograms from a healthy man 22 years of age with repetitive regular ventricular tachycardia interrupted for single sinus impulses only. The paroxysms start late at the end of or after the T waves of sinus complexes.

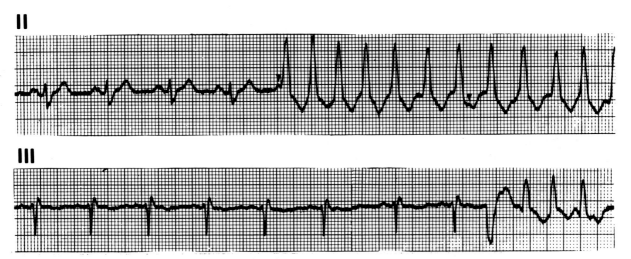

Figure 21-5. Leads II and III are electrocardiographic tracings from a patient with diffuse chronic ischemic fibrosis of the left ventricle after repeated myocardial infarcts. Uniform wide QRS complexes represent ventricular tachycardia. The arrhythmia is slightly irregular and in lead III, initial vectors of the QRS complex in tachycardia and sinus rhythm point in opposite directions. Selected P waves (*arrows*) help reveal the atrioventricular dissociation. In lead III, the tachycardia appears to be initiated by a QRS complex opposite in direction to its successors; its causative role is uncertain.

which the QRS complexes and T waves become fused in a regular and more rapid oscillation is sometimes called ventricular flutter and is exemplified in Figure 21-9.[15] This type of ventricular tachycardia is generally held to indicate a poor prognosis, although in the patient shown in Figure 21-9, resuscitation and subsequent oral drug prophylaxis were successful, albeit only in the short term.

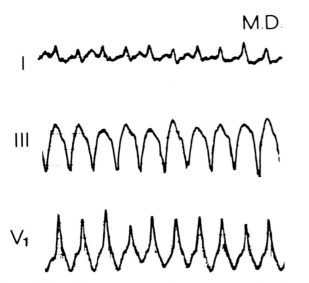

Figure 21-6. Electrocardiograms from a patient with a floppy mitral valve, showing ventricular tachycardia with marked left axis deviation, tall R waves in lead V_1, and probable intermittent 2:1 ventriculoatrial conduction (best seen in lead III).

As with ventricular extrasystoles in uniform tachycardias the QRS configuration may suggest a right or left ventricular origin, inferred when there is a pattern suggestive of contralateral bundle branch block (see Fig. 21-8), although this is by no means specific.[28,46] Epicardial mapping confirms this in some cases but right ventricular tachycardia diagnosed by these criteria may be associated with a left ventricle aneurysm, raising the possibility that the reentry circuit actually arose in the diseased left ventricle and initially depolarized the healthy right ventricle.[46–48] In the experience of Pietras and coworkers and from their review of the literature, left ventricular tachycardia is more consistently associated with serious organic heart disease than is right ventricular tachycardia.[48] Our own observations, however, are mixed. More of our patients with apparently benign ventricular tachycardia have the characteristics of right ventricular arrhythmia (Fig. 21-10), but this is by no means invariable (see Fig. 21-4). Ventricular tachycardia arising in the right ventricular outflow tract (Fig. 21-11*B*) is often benign but ventricular tachycardia associated with a dilated right ventricular usually has malignant features. T-wave inversion in the right precordial leads (see Fig. 21-11*A*) tends to indicate the presence of underlying structural right ventricle disease.[51]

In another subgroup of uniform ventricular tachycardia, the QRS complex during tachycardia shows right bundle branch block pattern and left axis deviation.[36]

Classic ventricular tachycardia, defined as above, often begins in response to a ventricular extrasystole falling during repolarization of the preceding impulse (whether

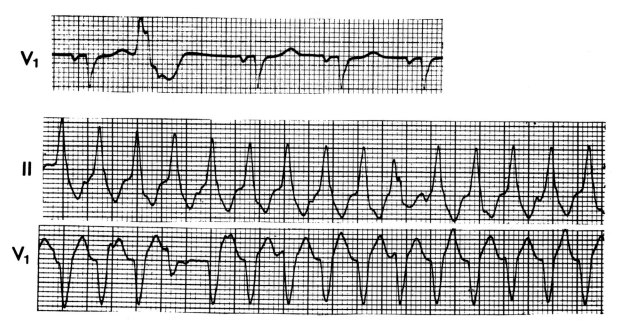

Figure 21-7. Electrocardiograms showing (*upper panel*, lead V₁) sinus rhythm with ventricular extrasystole that does not disturb it (normal P wave in its T). *Lower panels* (leads II and V₁) show tachycardia with broad QRS complexes; independent P waves can be discerned in some areas. The tenth QRS in lead II appears to reflect fusion; the fourth in lead V₁, capture (note similarity of latter to QRS complexes of sinus origin in *upper panel* of lead V₁).

of sinus or other origin), the so-called R-on-T phenomenon.[50] When this occurs, the ventricular extrasystole usually interrupts the apex of that T wave and a uniform tachycardia ensues in which the QRS morphology is maintained. The extrasystole or first complex of the tachycardia may be late (see Fig. 21-5) or have its effect at varying times of repolarization but it also may not depend on this effect at all, especially in repetitive tachycardias (see Fig. 21-4). Clinically, the precise initiation sometimes cannot be defined or may vary from time to time or it may have no relation to a preceding T wave. Initiation (and termination) by spontaneous ventricular extrasystoles favors a reentry mechanism, especially if the QRS complexes in tachycardia are of a somewhat different morphology from the extrasystoles (Fig. 21-12).[51]

Not only may spontaneous ventricular extrasystoles (early or late) initiate ventricular tachycardias (reproducible in electrophysiologic studies), but, albeit more rarely, suitably timed atrial extrasystoles can also be transmitted through the AV node with critical relation and reach the ventricles when these are vulnerable and able to respond by reentry.[31,52,53] Although this is uncommon, we have observed it and have also noted its special importance in the presence of accessory AV tracts.[45] Here, its significance is in the induction of ventricular fibrillation by conducted impulses from the fibrillating atria in patients with the Wolff-Parkinson-White syndrome.[54] In keeping with what

we observed when rapid atrial stimulation induced ventricular tachycardia, the short RR intervals in atrial fibrillation complicating this disorder may reflect branch-to-branch reentry, the initiation of ventricular arrhythmia.[45]

Not all ventricular tachycardias are uniform and there is confusion regarding the significance and terminology of such disorders. The definition of torsades de pointes has clarified much of this confusion and enabled clinicians to recognize what was previously called by a variety of names: transient ventricular fibrillation, paroxysmal ventricular fibrillation, transient recurrent ventricular fibrillation, and cardiac ballet.[55–62]

Torsades de pointes has important morphologic and etiologic facets that we have reviewed.[57,58] On the ECG, short runs of tachycardia are seen in which the form and axis of the QRS complex undulate in a sinusoidal fashion around the isoelectric line (often best displayed on simultaneous tracings of several leads). Characteristically, the initiating extrasystole occurs late, at the end of a prolonged QT interval (Fig. 21-13). Important etiologic factors include high-degree AV block, sinoatrial depression, electrolyte deficits, congenital QT-prolongation syndromes, drugs, and extreme dietary restriction. The association with a prolonged QT interval is an important diagnostic pointer; if the QT interval is normal, then the episode, although multiform, should be considered to be in the same category as the more usual uniform variety of ven-

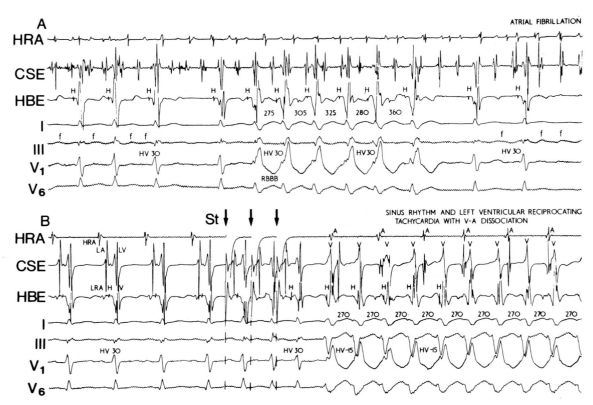

Figure 21-8. Simultaneous intracardiac and surface electrograms from a patient with idiopathic congestive cardiomyopathy, recorded at a paper speed of 25 mm/second. (**A**) During spontaneous atrial fibrillation, the HV time is normal (30 milliseconds) whether intraventricular conduction shows a normal pattern or right bundle branch block. (**B**) Sinus rhythm, with normal sequence of atrial activation in a craniocaudal right-to-left direction and normal HV interval. Reciprocating ventricular tachycardia at a cycle length of 270 milliseconds was established after three successive right atrial stimuli. In tachycardia, the bundle of His was activated after the ventricle (HV is − 15 millisecond), and AV dissociation was evident. *CSE,* coronary sinus (left atrial) electrogram; *HBE,* His bundle electrogram; *HRA,* high right atrial electrogram: A, atrial activation: LA, left atrial activation: LRA, low right atrial activation: H, His bundle activation; *V,* ventricular action; *LV,* left ventricular activation; HV, intraventricular conduction time: *St* and *arrows,* high right atrial stimuli.

tricular tachycardia.[56] One cannot always assign cases into one group or the other, desirable though this may be, because of the different treatment that may be required.[56–58]

Torsades de pointes can easily be misdiagnosed if only a single lead is recorded when the arrhythmia is multifocal ventricular tachycardia (see Fig. 21-3), which

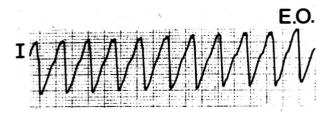

Figure 21-9. Electrocardiogram (lead I) showing sawtooth QRS complexes merging with T waves, reflecting ventricular flutter.

is sometimes seen in patients with hypersensitivity to catecholamines.[84]

In the rate definition of ventricular tachycardia, accelerated idioventricular rhythm (also known as idioventricular tachycardia and less correctly as slow ventricular tachycardia—a somewhat contradictory statement) can be defined as the occurrence of an independent ventricular rhythm that is more rapid than the sinus rate and manifests as the dominant cardiac rhythm for varying lengths of time. Semantically, it may be justifiable to describe the distal junctional right bundle branch tachycardia illustrated in Figure 21-1 in this way; a more definite example is illustrated in Figure 21-14, with a rate a little greater than that observed in sinus rhythm. It may be sustained for long periods or, as in Figures 21-1 and 21-14, may be intermittent. Often seen during acute myocardial infarction—at which time it is of uncertain significance

II

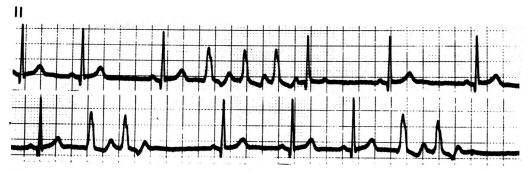

Figure 21-10. Continuous electrocardiographic tracings (lead II) showing sinus rhythm interrupted by ventricular couplets (*lower panel*) and a three-complex episode of ventricular tachycardia (*upper panel*). The QRS complexes of the tachycardia show features consistent with what would be seen in left bundle branch block with normal conduction. There is second-degree retrograde ventriculoatrial block (type I), during tachycardia, with sinus capture terminating the episode in the *upper panel*.

A   Sinus Rhythm

I   III   V1   V2   V3   V4

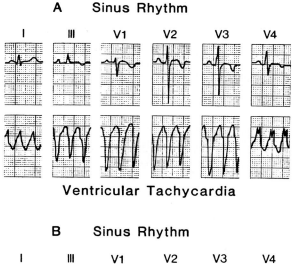

Ventricular Tachycardia

B   Sinus Rhythm

I   III   V1   V2   V3   V4

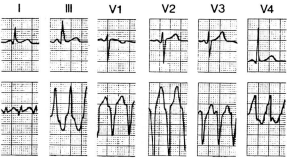

Ventricular Tachycardia

Figure 21-11. Selected leads taken from the 12-lead electrocardiograms recorded during sinus rhythm and ventricular tachycardia in two patients who show a left bundle branch block configuration during ventricular tachycardia, suggesting a right ventricular origin. (**A**) From a patient with a dilated right ventricle. During sinus rhythm, there is T-wave inversion in V_1 to V_4. The rate of ventricular tachycardia is 250 beats/minute and the QRS complex shows left axis deviation. (**B**) From a patient with a normal right ventricle. The electrocardiogram in sinus rhythm is normal, and during ventricular tachycardia there is right axis deviation, suggesting that the tachycardia originates in the outflow tract of the right ventricle.

(i.e., by no means indicative of progression to more sinister arrhythmias)—it may also occur for no good reason, as in the patients whose ECGs are shown in Figures 21-1 and 21-14. In this case, it falls into the category of idiopathic repetitive ventricular tachycardias. This particular arrhythmia is difficult to classify and in any context appears to have a benign prognosis. Its existence is closely linked with the lower limit of the rate defined as ventricular tachycardia of the more usual variety.

Morphologically intermediate between these uniform and "nonuniform" arrhythmias is bidirectional ventricular tachycardia. Earlier, doubt had been cast on the existence of this entity and it was considered to be a concept of historical significance only.[14] Its reality can be confirmed not only by deductive analysis of surface electrocardiographic tracings (Fig. 21-15) but also by intracardiac recordings (Fig. 21-16). When this pattern is seen, hypokalemia (perhaps with digitalis intoxication) should be suspected. Bidirectional ventricular tachycardia may be the forerunner of other forms of ventricular tachycardia (e.g., torsades de pointes).[64]

Wide QRS Tachycardia

In the ECG, a frequent diagnostic difficulty is the distinction between supraventricular arrhythmias complicated by both intraventricular aberration and ventricular tachycardia. The criteria of Sandler and Marriott and of Wellens and associates are usually helpful; for example, characteristic right bundle branch block appearance (RSR′ in lead V_1) favors the former and a broad complex (more than 140 milliseconds) favors the latter.[65, 66] Figure 21-7A shows atrial fibrillation with a run of conducted QRS complexes showing right bundle branch block; identical changes were seen in lead V_1 in this patient when left ventricular reciprocating tachycardia was induced by electric stimulation during sinus rhythm—the diagnosis being confirmed

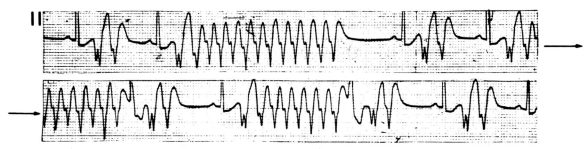

Figure 21-12. Continuous electrocardiographic tracings from a patient during the second week after myocardial infarction. Ventricular extrasystoles interrupt T waves of sinus beats and either occur in pairs or result in runs of ventricular tachycardia with relatively narrow QRS complexes. These stopped spontaneously or were interrupted by fusion beats followed by two further extrasystoles. The appearances suggest intraventricular reentry.

by the presence of AV dissociation (see Fig. 21-7B). When other criteria prove inadequate, intracardiac electrography (as in Fig. 21-7B) may be essential to establish the diagnosis of ventricular tachycardia by showing absence of activation of the ventricles from the atria.

Significant concern exists in the emergency room setting when a patient presents with rapid regular tachycardia with a prolonged QRS duration. In one study by Akhtar and colleagues, 122 of 150 such patients were documented to have ventricular tachycardia.[67]

The patient who presents with wide QRS tachycardia may be a significant diagnostic dilemma because the differentiation of supraventricular tachycardia with aberration from ventricular tachycardia may not be easily made.

A wide variety of criteria have been established to define a ventricular origin, including:

1. Superior axis deviation

2. AV dissociation

3. QRS duration of more than 140 milliseconds or morphologic changes of the QRS

Studies by Wellens and coworkers emphasize a variety of key points that aid the clinician in differentiating these two entities.[66]

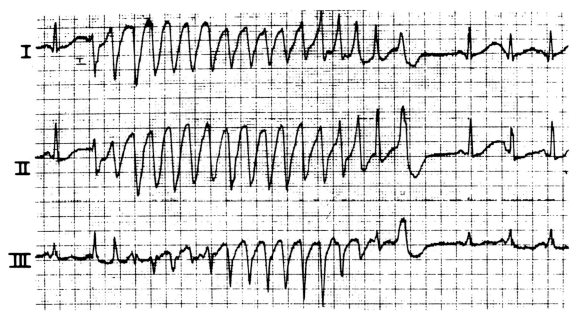

Figure 21-13. Simultaneous recordings of leads I, II, and III from a patient with chronic hypokalemia. Sinus complexes show marked QT prolongation: note the onset of the arrhythmia toward the end of the first T waves and the alterations in the QRS axes during tachycardia.

aVF

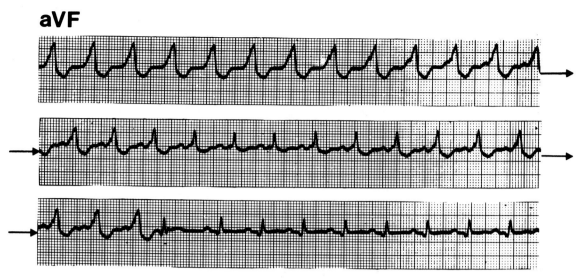

Figure 21-14. Continuous electrocardiogram (lead aV$_f$), showing accelerated idioventricular rhythm only slightly faster than the inherent sinus rate in the *upper panel*, first and last thirds of the *middle panel*, and first third of the *lower panel*. In the *second panel*, transition between "idioventricular tachycardia" and sinus rhythm shows fusion but in the *third panel*, the tachycardia appears to be terminated by a narrow extrasystole.

These criteria were subsequently modified by Brugada and colleagues to improve their sensitivity and specificity, with a sensitivity and specificity for ventricular tachycardia of 0.965 and 0.965 as applied to the diagnosis of supraventricular tachycardia with aberration.[68]

These authors held as a major premise that the intrinsic deflection should be longer in ventricular tachycardia than in supraventricular tachycardia, regardless of the morphology (e.g., right or left bundle branch block). They used an algorithm having a sensitivity of 0.987 and a specificity of 0.965 (Fig. 21-17).

Of additional importance is the observation that spontaneous premature ventricular complexes may only occa-

sionally have a similar morphology to the QRS morphology during ventricular tachycardia.[69]

Ventricular Tachycardia With Preexisting Bundle Branch Block

In patients with preexisting bundle branch block, the electrocardiographic manifestations of ventricular tachycardia may be different from those in patients with ventricular tachycardia but without an underlying conduction defect.[70] The presence of the following, however, may be relatively specific of ventricular tachycardia, even in patients with underlying bundle branch block:

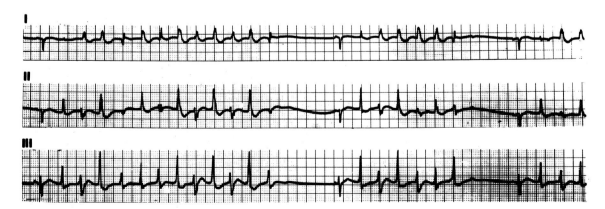

Figure 21-15. Simultaneous electrocardiograms (leads I, II, and III) from a patient with hypokalemia due to familial periodic paralysis, showing runs of bidirectional ventricular tachycardia (most obvious in lead II).

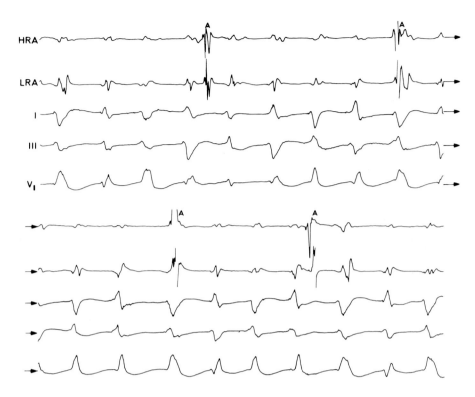

Figure 21-16. Intracardiac and surface electrocardiograms from the same patient as in Figure 21-16. The paper speed is 100 mm/seconds. Independent atrial activity (A) can be seen in the atrial electrograms.

1. Monomorphic R wave in V_1
2. QRS concordance
3. Right superior axis deviation in the frontal plane
4. More than 30 milliseconds R in V_1, V_2 (left bundle branch block)

More significant problems occur with left bundle branch morphology and ventricular tachycardia. Kindwall and colleagues, using four criteria, attempted to establish the diagnosis of ventricular tachycardia in patients with left bundle branch block morphology and ventricular tachycardia.[71] These criteria included the presence of *all* four of the following:

1. R wave in V_1 and V_2 of more than 30 milliseconds
2. Q wave in V_6
3. More than 60 milliseconds from the onset of the QRS to the nadir of the S wave V_1 or V_2
4. Notching of the S wave in V_1 and V_2

These criteria have a high predictive accuracy (equal to or greater than 0.96) and specificity (equal to or greater than 0.94).

Narrow QRS and Ventricular Tachycardia

Rarely, patients may have ventricular tachycardia but have an ECG that demonstrates a narrow QRS configuration.

Hayes and coworkers identified five of 106 patients with documented ventricular tachycardia who had narrow QRS configuration.[72] They suggest that if a baseline ECG shows a QRS change in the first 40 milliseconds in addition to the criteria listed above, one should consider the diagnosis of ventricular tachycardia, especially in patients with an underlying history of heart disease and a poor response to routine therapy for supraventricular tachycardia.

Surface ECG and Endocardial Location of Ventricular Tachycardia

The 12-lead surface ECG during ventricular tachycardia has been used by some investigators as a tool to estimate the approximate endocardial site of origin.[73, 74] The surface ECG data is apparently less useful for localization in patients with prior myocardial infarcts *with* wall motion abnormalities. Several authors feel that one can use the ECG to determine an "area" where the tachycardia may arise in most cases.[61, 62] (Figs. 21-18 and 21-19).

ENDOCARDIAL MAPPING TECHNIQUES

Ventricular endocardial mapping was developed initially for identification of potential "foci" of ventricular tachycardia origins in anticipation of surgical ablation. Subse-

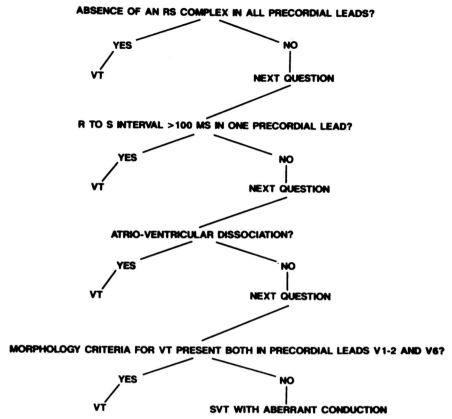

Figure 21-17. Algorithm for the diagnosis of a wide complex tachycardia. When an RS complex can not be identified in any precordial lead, the diagnosis of ventricular tachycardia is certain. If an RS complex is present in more than one precordial lead, the longest RS interval is measured. If the RS interval is greater than 100 milliseconds, ventricular tachycardia is established. If the RS complex is less than 100 milliseconds, move to the next step of the algorithm. The stepwise decision-making follows. (From Brugada P, Brugada J, Mont L, Smeets J, Andries EM: A new approach to the differential diagnosis of a regular tachycardia with a wide QRS complex. Circulation 1991;83:1649.)

quently, the technique has been expanded as catheter ablative techniques developed.

It is generally necessary to be able to induce reproducibly the index arrhythmia or have it occur spontaneously to allow adequate endocardial mapping. A major problem with mapping ventricular arrhythmias is the frequent hemodynamic instability. Therefore, antiarrhythmic drug administration such as intravenous procainamide has been used to slow the ventricular tachycardia, allowing the patient to tolerate hemodynamically longer episodes of ventricular tachycardia. In addition, endocardial mapping during sinus rhythm has been used to identify abnormal electrograms.

Mapping techniques require recording of multiple sites using close bipolar (2 to 5 mm) or unipolar recordings. It may be necessary to obtain data from sites in both ventricles (Fig. 21-20).[63]

During stable ventricular tachycardia, the earliest site of ventricular activation is the point of major interest. Other significant findings include (1) early electrograms with systolic and diastolic components, (2) continuous diastolic activity, and (3) double potentials, the significance of which is debated (Figs. 21-21 and 21-22)[78–81]

Sinus Rhythm Mapping

If ventricular tachycardia cannot be initiated or if the tachycardia is hemodynamically unstable, endocardial catheter mapping during sinus rhythm may be of value (see Figs. 21-21 and 21-22).[81] The major abnormalities are marked fractionation of the electrograms or late electrograms. The correlation between these abnormal electrograms and successful tachycardia termination (either with

Text continues on p. 664

PRECORDIAL R—WAVE PROGRESSION PATTERNS

PATTERN (NO.)	V_1	V_2	V_3	V_4	V_5	V_6
INCREASING (30)						
NONE OR LATE (27)						
REGRESSION/GROWTH (NOT QS) (18)						
REGRESSION/GROWTH (QS) (15)						
DOMINANT (15)						
ABRUPT LOSS (20)						
LATE REVERSE (41)						
EARLY REVERSE (16)						

A

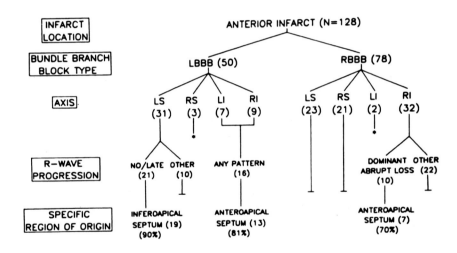

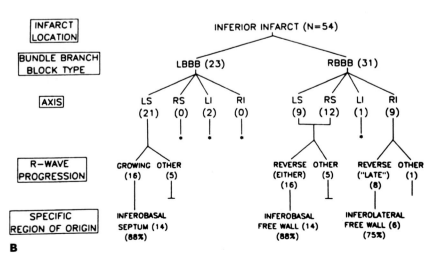

B

Figure 21-18. (**A**) Precordial R-wave progression patterns, associated with various types of ventricular tachycardia. Relation between the 12-lead electrocardiogram during ventricular tachycardia and endocardial site of origin in patients with coronary artery disease. (**B**) Algorithm relating regions of origin of ventricular tachycardia to the QRS morphology of ventricular tachycardia on a 12-lead electrocardiogram. The basic features relate to the major QRS morphology. (From Miller JM, Marchlinski FE, Buxton AE, Josephson ME: Relatioship between 12-lead electrocardiogram during ventricular tachycardia and endocardial site of origin in patients with coronary artery disease. Circulation 1988;71:759.)

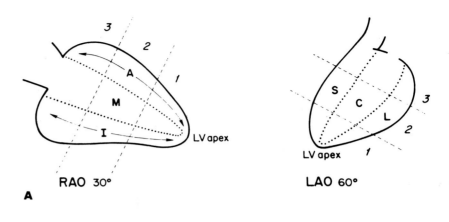

A

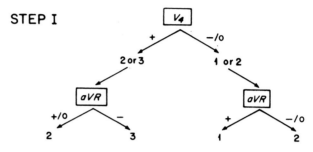

STEP I

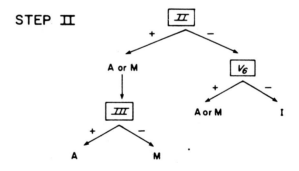

STEP II

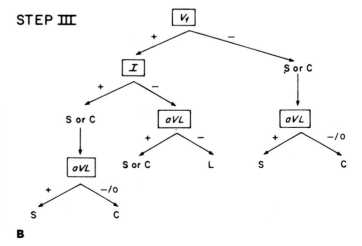

STEP III

Figure 21-19. (**A**) Left ventricular endocardial map grid. A, anterior; C, central; I, inferior; L, lateral; LAO, left anterior oblique projection; M, middle; RAO, right anterior oblique projection; S, septal; 1, 2, 3, three regions along the long axis of the left ventricle (apical, mid-ventricular, and basal.) (**B**) Flow chart for predicting the endocardial site of origin of ventricular tachycardia using QRS morphology and electrocardiographic leads. The electrocardiogram leads are in boxes and the endocardial sites are in bold type. (From Kuchar DL, Ruskin JN, Garan H: Electrocardiographic localization of the site of orgin of ventricular tachycardia in patients with myocardial infarction. J Am Coll Cardiol 1989;13:893.)

B

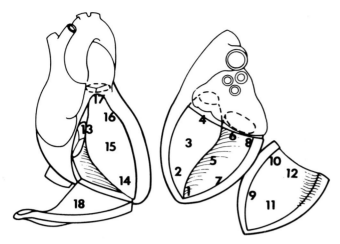

Figure 21-20. Mapping sites for for endocardial recordings from right and left ventricle. Sites 13–17 are right ventricular sites. (From Josephson ME: Clinical cardiac electrophysiology. 2nd ed. Philadelphia: Lea & Febiger, 1992.)

catheter ablation or endocardial resection techniques) has been poor, essentially negating this recording modality as a useful tool.

Pace Mapping

Pace mapping is another method of localizing the site of ventricular tachycardia. Pacing is performed at multiple locations in an effort to produce a QRS morphology, which is identical to this spontaneous ventricular tachycardia.[82, 83] This technique has been used effectively in tachycardias originating in the outflow tract of the right ventricle in anticipation of catheter ablation (Fig. 21-23).[70]

NONSUSTAINED VENTRICULAR TACHYCARDIA

The most accepted definition for nonsustained ventricular tachycardia is three or more consecutive ventricular premature complexes at a rate greater than 120 per minute and lasting less than 30 seconds (Fig. 21-24; see Figs. 21-3 and 21-11).

In Patients With Ischemic Heart Disease

In patients who have ischemic heart disease, nonsustained ventricular tachycardia has been shown by many investigators to be a marker for sudden cardiac death.[85–94] Nevertheless, medical management has been tempered by the Cardiac Arrhythmia Suppression Trial data and subsequent fears by the clinicians relative to potential proarrhythmic effects of antiarrhythmic drugs.[95]

Possible markers used in an attempt to identify the

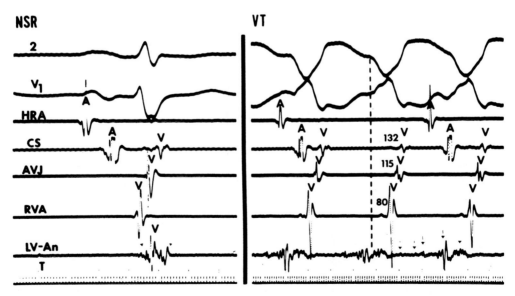

Figure 21-21. Electrogram (ECG) recordings during sinus rhythm and during ventricular tachycardia. In the *right panel*, an electrogram recorded just inside a left ventricular aneurysm demonstrates continues electric activity during ventricular tachycardia. During sinus rhythm, this electrogram is markedly abnormal, with electric activity extending beyond the end of the QRS, as seen on the surface ECG. (From Josephson ME: Clinical cardiac electrophysiology. 2nd ed. Philadelphia: Lea & Febiger, 1992.)

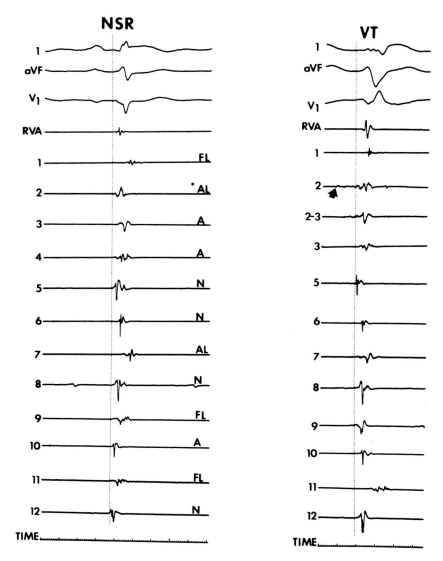

Figure 21-22. Electrograms recorded from a patient during sinus rhythm (*left panel*) and during ventricular tachycardia (*right panel*). Surface leads *1*, *aVf* and V₁ and recordings from 12 standard left ventricular (LV) sites and from the right ventricular apex (see Fig. 21-20). Fractionated abnormal or late electric activity is noted at multiple left ventricular sites. The earliest site during the ventricular tachycardia is LV site 2. It is important to note that during sinus rhythm, left ventricular site 2 is neither late nor abnormal. (From Josephson ME: Clinical cardiac electrophysiology. 2nd ed. Philadelphia: Lea & Febiger, 1992.)

high-risk patient with nonsustained ventricular tachycardia include:

1. Left ventricular ejection fraction
2. Signal-averaged ECGs
3. Programmed ventricular stimulation

Meta-analysis of 12 studies composed of 926 patients who underwent electrophysiologic studies and who had nonsustained ventricular tachycardia has been reported.[96] In this retrospective analysis of the literature, 302 patients (33% of the total) had inducible ventricular tachycardia. Of this inducible group, 264 had monomorphic ventricular tachycardia that was initiated at the time of electrophysiologic studies. The noninducible group (624 patients) had a 93% chance of remaining event-free in follow-up of at least 18 months. Nevertheless, electro-physiologic testing in this group having nonsustained ventricular tachycardia remains controversial. As a result of this continued controversy, the National Institutes of Health has initiated a multicenter unsustained tachycardia trial to evaluate patients having nonsustained ventricular tachycardia with an ejection fraction of less than 40% in an effort to determine the role of electrophysiologic guided therapy. A further study has been designed to enroll patients with nonsustained ventricular tachycardia; those having a left ventricular ejection fraction of less than 35% will get an implantable cardioverter defibrillator if they remain inducible on procainamide therapy.

One group of investigators suggests a risk-stratification approach to patients who have nonsustained ventricular tachycardia. Use of this algorithm (Fig. 21-25) appears to be a reasonable approach until further data are forthcoming.[98]

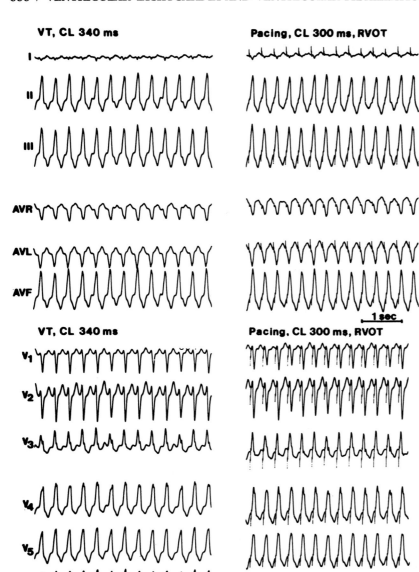

Figure 21-23. Pace mapping in a patient who has ventricular tachycardia originating from the right ventricular outflow tract. The *left panel* demonstrates the 12-lead electrocardiogram during sustained ventricular tachycardia. In the *right panel*, pacing from the right ventricular outflow tract at a cycle length of 300 milliseconds demonstrates a QRS morphology virtually identical to that seen during the sustained clinical tachycardia. (From Morady F, Kadish AH, DiCarlo L, et al: Long-term results of catheter ablation of idiopathic right ventricular tachycardia. Circulation 1990;82:2093.)

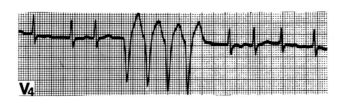

Figure 21-24. Electrocardiogram showing atrial fibrillation as the basic rhythm. This was interrupted by four consecutive broad QRS complexes, constituting ventricular tachycardia. The patient had digitalis intoxication.

In Patients Without Ischemic Disease

The importance of nonsustained ventricular tachycardia in this group has been less clearly defined than in those having ischemic heart disease. Therefore, risk stratification is clearly more difficult in this patient population.

Hypertrophic Cardiomyopathy

In patients with hypertrophic cardiomyopathy, nonsustained ventricular tachycardia appears to be an important marker for sudden cardiac death. The incidence of nonsustained ventricular tachycardia in these patients approaches

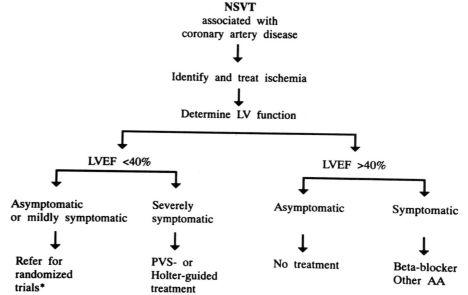

Figure 21-25. An algorithm for risk stratification and management of patients with nonsustained ventricular tachycardia who have underlying ischemic heart disease. *AA,* antiarrhythmic agent; *LVEF,* left ventricular ejection fraction; *NSVT,* nonsustained ventricular tachycardia; *PVS,* programmed ventricular stimulation. (From Pires LA, Huang SKS: Nonsustained ventricular tachycardia: identification and management of high-risk patients. Am Heart J 126:189, 1993.)

25%, with a higher incidence related to increasing degrees of hypertrophy.[98–100] Electrophysiologic studies do not appear to define clearly who is at high risk for sudden cardiac death (ie. the inducibility of monomorphic ventricular tachycardia, even in patients with hypertrophic cardiomyopathy with a documented episode of sudden cardiac death).[101,102] Conventional therapy has not clearly reduced the incidence of sudden cardiac death.[103,104] Initially, only amiodarone was thought to offer significant benefits but this observation has been challenged.[103–109]

Dilated Cardiomyopathy

Nonsustained ventricular tachycardia has been found in up to 80% of patients who have idiopathic dilated cardiomyopathy.[109–114] There is, however, some debate regarding the significance of this finding. One study identifies only 38% of cardiac arrests in such patients as being due to ventricular tachyarrhythmias.[115] There is also controversy whether electrophysiologic studies clearly identify patients with nonsustained ventricular tachycardia who are at high risk.[117–121] In addition, there appears also to be significant disagreement regarding the benefits of amiodarone in this group.[122–126]

Mitral Valve Prolapse

This entity is associated with an incidence of nonsustained ventricular tachycardia as high as 21%, with a purported higher incidence in patients with greater degrees of mitral regurgitation.[127] Electrophysiologic studies do not appear helpful in determining those patients who are at high risk because the incidence of sudden cardiac death appears

low.[128–130] Therefore, therapy appears to be indicated only in the symptomatic patient, using beta blockade or moricizine as drugs of first choice.[131]

Hypertension

Patients with untreated hypertension have a higher incidence of ventricular arrhythmias than do normal subjects.[132] Furthermore, there appears to be a correlation between the degree of left ventricular hypertrophy and the incidence of arrhythmias such as nonsustained ventricular tachycardia.[133,134] There is, however, no clear evidence that reduction in ventricular premature complexes or decreased left ventricular hypertrophy improves survival.[13]

ETIOLOGIC FACTORS OF VENTRICULAR TACHYCARDIA AND FIBRILLATION

For convenience, ventricular tachycardia (uniform or variable) and fibrillation are considered as a single entity for the purpose of classifying underlying disease processes that may cause either or both.

Ischemic Heart Disease

Acute Myocardial Infarction

The importance of ventricular fibrillation as a cause of sudden death or death within the first few hours after the onset of pain is well recognized and constitutes a major therapeutic challenge that still awaits resolution. From animal studies, it is possible to assess the time course of changes in ventricular fibrillation threshold and to observe its abrupt reduction immediately after acute coronary occlusion, with a return to previous levels 30 minutes later.[135] Extrapolation to the clinical situation appears reasonable but variations among patients in disease process preclude more categorical statements.

In this context, ventricular tachycardia in humans during the first 24 hours after myocardial infarction has been judged by electrophysiologic techniques to be compatible with enhanced automaticity by Wellens and Lie, but these authors emphasize the relatively crude nature of the studies that can be carried out in humans and do not exclude local reentry phenomena.[52,136] The clinical demonstration by Wellens and Lie of reentry ventricular tachycardia late after myocardial infarction is consistent with the elegant animal mode in which this has been shown by El-Sherif and colleagues.[23,52] Other supporting evidence was cited earlier in the discussion of electrophysiologic mechanisms. Whether triggered activity plays a role is not established.

Variant Angina

It is increasingly recognized that variant angina can produce ventricular tachycardia, sometimes associated with paroxysmal AV block, although this is not the major factor.[137] Ventricular tachycardia may be related to coronary spasm and suggest torsades de pointes, although some investigators believe that such resemblance may not be of pathogenetic significance but may reflect multifocal (multiform) tachycardia, perhaps similar to idiopathic catecholamine-induced arrhythmias.[63,138,139]

Chronic Ischemic Heart Disease

Cardiac aneurysm forms a well-recognized anatomic basis for reentry ventricular tachycardia (Figs. 21-26 and 21-27); in sinus rhythm, the characteristic signs (usually present but not pathognomonic of aneurysm) are deep QS complexes with persistent ST-segment elevation or T-wave inversion after recovery from the acute infarct. The mechanism of the arrhythmia is reentry, with slowed conduction across the interface between healthy and scarred myocardium. During intracardiac studies, induced extrasystoles can activate the latent circuit.[140]

Exactly similar arrhythmias may be seen with localized dyskinesia short of aneurysm formation or indeed without any clinically manifest scarring.[52] Strong evidence in favor of reentry has been adduced by Josephson and coworkers in three cases of recurrent ventricular tachycardia after infarction; one patient had an aneurysm and the other two suffered from diffuse hypokinesia.[28] Local electric activity was recorded from the affected area and when it became continuous, tachycardia developed—the termination of which necessitated suppression of this activity. These findings are consistent with the phenomenon noted experimentally by Durrer and colleagues many years ago.[141] Others have found discrete late potentials with surface electrocardiographic signal-averaging techniques and during operative endocardial mapping in patients with ventricular tachycardia.[29,142] Residual fibrosis after myocardial infarction may be an important factor in subsequent ventricular arrhythmias; it is essential that anatomic factors be included in any assessment of the possible significance of apparent "warning arrhythmias," which may indicate an increased risk of sudden death because of ventricular fibrillation.[143,144] This does not contradict the observations of Wellens and Lie because the areas of

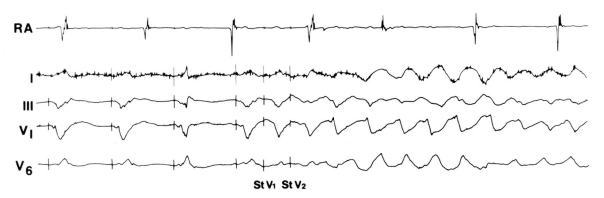

Figure 21-26. Simultaneous right atrial (*RA*) electrogram and surface electrocardiographic leads from a patient with left ventricular aneurysm after myocardial infarction. Basic right ventricular pacing is being carried out (*unlabeled spikes*). The introduction of two ventricular extrastimuli (StV₁, StV₂) leads to ventricular tachycardia but the atrial activation (*RA* lead) remains undisturbed (i.e., ventricular tachycardia has been induced with atrioventricular dissociation).

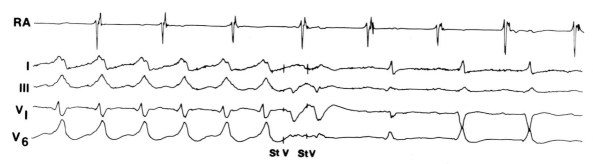

Figure 21-27. Same patient as illustrated in Figure 21-12. At the commencement of the tracing, the patient is in ventricular tachycardia, with atrioventricular dissociation. Two ventricular extrastimuli (StV) terminate the tachycardia, and the ventricles now respond to the sinus rhythm.

fibrosis in their patients may have been insufficiently extensive to have been clinically detectable.[52] In this context, repolarization abnormalities in those who survive ventricular fibrillation appear to indicate a risk of recurrence.[145] Ventricular extrasystoles and their importance (see Chap. 19) in relation to tachycardias and fibrillation are not discussed in this chapter. Myocardial ischemia and infarction offer an electrophysiologic milieu that is especially favorable for the initiation and maintenance of ventricular tachycardia.

The pioneering work of Harris and Rojas has been followed-up by studies that established a time course of electrophysiologic events associated with the onset of ischemia.[146–149] Ventricular arrhythmia in the earliest stages of acute myocardial infarction is generally attributed to reentry, whereas after 6 to 8 hours the mechanism of ventricular arrhythmia is attributed to abnormal automaticity. Late arrhythmias appear again to be related to a reentrant mechanism.

Nevertheless, most sustained ventricular tachycardias occur distant to the acute infarction and appear to be mechanistically related to reentry, although triggered automaticity must be considered.[150,151] The characteristic features of reentry—a reentrant pathway, dispersion of refractoriness, and an area of slow conduction—can be demonstrated in patients having old infarction and sustained ventricular tachycardia. Furthermore, intraoperative mapping has demonstrated apparent reentrant circuits.[152–154] Pressure or myocardial lesions at the site of mid-diastolic activity has resulted in termination of tachycardia, supporting the concept of a reentrant mechanism of ventricular tachycardia in the human heart with old infarction. Slow conduction has been demonstrated frequently in the setting of old infarction. Endocardial catheter mapping in sinus rhythm has demonstrated the presence of markedly fractionated low amplitude potentials in some areas.[155–158] Signal-averaged ECGs have also demonstrated the presence of "late potentials," again consistent with areas of slow conduction in the infarcted ventricle.[159,160] Dispersion of refractoriness has been demonstrated in the intact ventricle, but only a few limited studies have been undertaken on dispersion in local areas thought to be near the reentrant circuit.

Ventricular tachycardia in patients with old infarctions is characterized by a low ejection fraction (less than 40%), with aneurysm formation and a history of acute complications 48 or more hours after myocardial infarction (i.e., congestive heart failure, bundle branch block, ventricular fibrillation, and hypotension).[161–163]

Although most patients develop ventricular tachycardia less than 1 year after myocardial infarction, many patients experience the first episode 5 or more years after the index event.

Clinical documentation of ventricular tachycardia has been enhanced by Holter monitoring, which may demonstrate late coupled ventricular premature complexes with morphology similar to sustained ventricular tachycardia, but these data have been questioned.

Studies in patients having old infarction demonstrate other electrophysiologic features consistent with reentry, including initiation and termination of ventricular tachycardia with programmed stimulation and resetting responses.[52,53,150,155]

An important subgroup of patients are those subjects with sudden cardiac death. Extensive studies have identified that a significant number (i.e., approximately 1/3) of these patients have no inducible ventricular tachycardia.[164–169] These patients have been the subject of intense investigation including serial electrophysiologic studies, implantation of cardiac defibrillators, and other cardiac surgical procedures.

Nonischemic Anatomic Lesions

Although posttraumatic cardiac infarction is rare, we have seen several examples of ventricular asynergy resulting from this and one case of a discrete aneurysm. This last patient was a fit young man (aged 18 years) who presented with ventricular tachycardia experienced while playing sports. His resting ECG showed appearances typical for cardiac aneurysm; retrospectively, a history was obtained of an extremely severe closed-chest injury 15 years earlier. During one episode of palpitation, an ECG confirmed ventricular tachycardia (Fig. 21-28), and the aneurysm was confirmed angiographically. This study also revealed the coronary arteries to be normal. During the operation in which the aneurysm was successfully resected, epicardial mapping during tachycardia confirmed the presence of a reentry mechanism. Similar tachycardias have also been seen in patients with a history of chest trauma but without definable cardiac aneurysm. In addition, dyskinetic areas or aneurysms may develop because of inflammatory disease or no underlying cause may be found by full investigation of those rare patients who present with ventricular tachycardia (Figs. 21-29 and 21-30).

Mitral Valve Prolapse

Although ventricular extrasystoles and other arrhythmias are common in mitral valve prolapse, they are usually benign.[169] We are aware of several cases of catastrophic ventricular arrhythmias that were not controlled by available antiarrhythmic agents but were controlled by mitral valve replacement (Yu PN, personal communication).[170] Indeed, we have such a patient, whose tachycardia was previously illustrated (see Fig. 21-6). Although this patient tolerated well his mild mitral incompetence during sinus rhythm, he developed syncope during attacks of ventricular tachycardia, undoubtedly because under these circumstances, the mitral incompetence was grossly exaggerated and transaortic blood flow was minimal. At operation, reentry ventricular tachycardia identical to that seen clinically could be elicited from the posterior papillary muscle. Eight years after mitral valve replacement, the patient has remained symptom-free, although he subsequently required a pacemaker. The reported incidence of this entity

has burgeoned since the development of echocardiography. The relation between mitral valve prolapse and ventricular arrhythmias is well recognized, but the spectrum of arrhythmias described is large.[171] Electrophysiologic investigation in these patients has resulted in disparate results, with no uniform opinion regarding who is at risk. For life-threatening ventricular arrhythmias, inducible sustained monomorphic ventricular tachycardia has been documented, but this arrhythmia appears to be uncommon.[172–174]

The mechanism of ventricular arrhythmias in these patients has been hypothesized to be partly related to mechanical trauma. Other possible mechanisms include mitral embolization and autonomic dysfunction.

The use of electrophysiologic testing appears justified only in a few patients but includes those with documented monomorphic sustained or nonsustained ventricular tachycardia or syncope.

Cardiomyopathy and Myocarditis

Cardiomyopathy and myocarditis are relatively uncommon causes of ventricular tachycardia. When the inflammatory disorder is active, arrhythmias may occur.

Hypertrophic Cardiomyopathy

Ventricular tachycardia is a strong positive marker for sudden death in adults with hypertrophic cardiomyopathy.[175] Typically, such episodes are slow (mean rate, 142 beats/minute) and nonsustained (mean duration, eight beats) and tend to occur at night.[176] Sudden death has been attributed to sustained ventricular arrhythmia, but we have full documentation of an episode of "sudden death" and successful resuscitation in one patient who remained in sinus rhythm throughout.[177] Children with hypertrophic cardiomyopathy who die suddenly have particularly marked fiber disarray, a likely milieu for arrhythmias.[178]

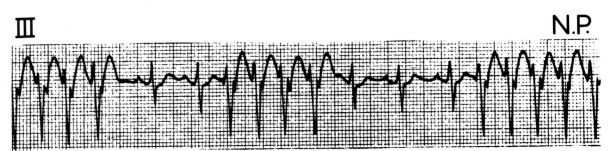

Figure 21-28. Electrocardiogram (lead III) from a patient aged 18 years with a posttraumatic left ventricular aneurysm. Runs of ventricular tachycardia are seen at the commencement, in the middle, and at the end of the strip. There are two intervening sinus complexes between the first two episodes and three between the second.

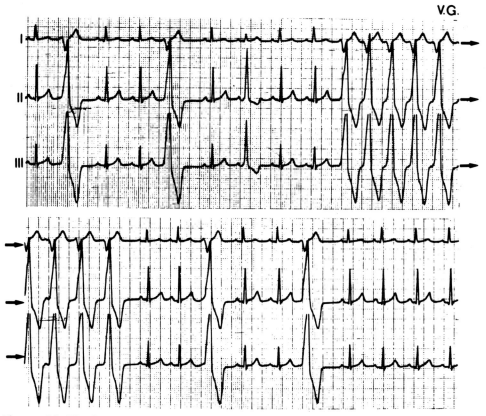

Figure 21-29. Continuous electrocardiographic (leads I, II, and III), showing sinus rhythm with late ventricular ectopic complexes, probably parasystolic, the third of which shows fusion with the sinus activation. The fourth ectopic complex is the first of nine consecutive impulses constituting ventricular tachycardia.

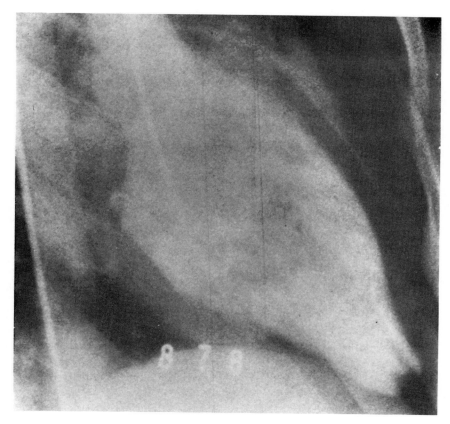

Figure 21-30. Left ventricular angiogram (recorded in systole) from the same patient whose electrocardiogram was shown in Figure 21-29. Note dyskinetic area at the apex.

We have also seen one patient with hypertrophic cardiomyopathy who had a concealed accessory pathway linking the right atrium and ventricle. This patient died as a result of ventricular tachycardia initiated by atrial stimuli during a diagnostic electrophysiologic study.[45] Although this experience has led us to avoid electrophysiologic studies in patients with hypertrophic cardiomyopathy, we would consider such studies if therapeutic value could be demonstrated; thus far, this has not been the case and ambulatory monitoring provides the only satisfactory guide in identifying those at risk.[176]

Symmetric or asymmetric hypertrophy of the left ventricle without dilation is the hallmark of this disease. Although the hemodynamic consequences of disease appear to be slowly progressive, unexpected sudden death occurs, with reported frequency of up to 3% per year.[179] This relation is especially important for the young patient with hypertrophic cardiomyopathy.[180] The incidence of monomorphic ventricular tachycardia appears to be low but only a few patients have undergone electrophysiologic studies.[181–183] Many of these latter patients, however, had initiation of polymorphic ventricular tachycardia.

The mechanism of the arrhythmia is speculative, but marked muscular fiber disarray lends itself to the development of reentry.[184] Some experimental data suggest that triggered activity may also play a role.[185]

Drug therapy appears to have two potential benefits: arrhythmia reduction or prevention and reduction in hypertrophic and obstructive phenomenon. Drugs having some benefits include beta blockers, disopyramide, sotalol, and amiodarone.[179,183] The latter appears to be the most effective therapy for ventricular arrhythmias.

Dilated Cardiomyopathy

Ventricular arrhythmias are common in patients with dilated cardiomyopathy but their prognostic significance is uncertain because in many cases death is not sudden but occurs from a gradual decline related to cardiac pump performance.[186] After the first year from diagnosis, sudden death becomes more common and may be arrhythmogenic; whether drug treatment to suppress ventricular arrhythmias improves prognosis remains undetermined. In isolated cases, we have seen severe ventricular arrhythmias that are not controlled by conventional medication (Fig. 21-31) respond to amiodarone, with concomitant improvement in cardiac performance and decrease in heart size. Right ventricular dysplasia may represent that part of the spectrum of dilated cardiomyopathy in which the right ventricle bears the brunt of the disease.

These patients are thought to be at high-risk by many investigators.[187–189] The sudden death incidence may be as high as 50%, but most deaths are associated with ventricular fibrillation.

Generally, patients with dilated cardiomyopathy and sustained ventricular tachycardia have abnormal signal-averaged ECGs.[190] Most patients who have inducible sustained monomorphic ventricular tachycardia on electrophysiologic studies have had similar arrhythmias spontaneously.[191] Bundle branch reentry is a common finding in these patients. Endocardial mapping studies in these patients document abnormal electrograms but not to the level (i.e., number and degree) seen in patients with coronary artery disease and ventricular tachycardia.[192]

Based on the following, the most common mecha-

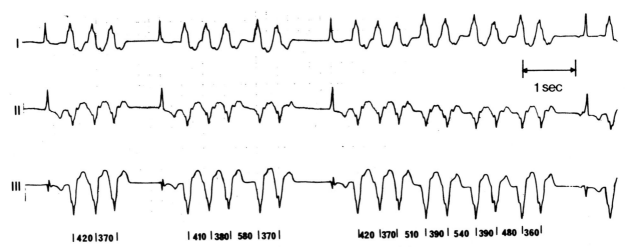

Figure 21-31. Electrocardiogram (simultaneous recordings of leads I, II, and III) showing repetitive ventricular tachycardia interrupted by a single junctional and one atrial impulse. The numbers at the bottom indicate the RR intervals in milliseconds. These tracings were recorded from a patient with congestive cardiomyopathy.

nism for ventricular tachycardia in these patients appears to be reentry:

1. Abnormal signal-averaged electrograms
2. Abnormal endocardial electrograms
3. Inducibility by standard electrophysiologic protocols[193]

Many patients with recurrent ventricular tachycardia and cardiomyopathy are ultimately candidates for cardiac transplantation, which may be performed for recurrent ventricular tachycardia not responsive to drug therapy or for progressive cardiac failure.

In these patients, implantation of a cardiac defibrillator as a "bridge" to transplantation has been considered. The defibrillator is especially useful because it potentially would allow significant reduction or elimination of antiarrhythmic agents that have potential negative hemodynamic effects.[195]

BUNDLE BRANCH REENTRY. In this arrhythmia, seen almost exclusively in patients with an underlying cardiomyopathy, the surface QRS morphology is left bundle branch block, generally with superior axis deviation. The tachycardia uses the right bundle branch as the anterograde limb and the left bundle branch as the retrograde limb of this reentrant arrhythmia.[195–198] The following characteristic features of this tachycardia are also shown in Figures 21-32 and 21-33:

1. Presence of a His-bundle deflection before each QRS
2. Tachycardia cycle-length changes (i.e., RR interval changes) are *preceded* by changes in the His-His interval

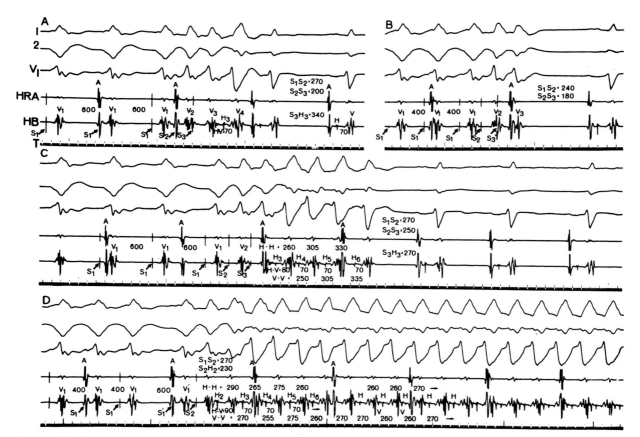

Figure 21-32. Tracings at the onset of sustained bundle branch reentrant tachycardia. Each panel shows surface electrocardiogram leads 1, 2, V₁, a high right atrial electrogram recording and His-bundle recording. Premature complexes initiated in **A**, **B** and **C** with two extrastimuli (S₂, S₃) failed to initiate a sustained tachycardia. (**D**) There is a long-short cycle sequence followed by a single ventricular extrastimulus (S₂), which initiates a sustained monomorphic ventricular tachycardia with left bundle branch block and superior axis deviation morphology. Note the presence of atrioventricular dissociation. Of importance, when there is a change in the cycle length of the tachycardia, the HH-interval change precedes the VV-interval change. (From Caceres J, Jazayeri M, McKinnie J, Avitall B, et al: Sustained bundle branch reentry as a mechanism of clinical tachycardia. Circulation 1989;79:256.)

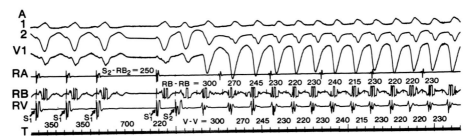

Figure 21-33. Tracing of His-Purkinje activation during bundle branch reentrant tachycardia. The panels demonstrate electrocardiogram leads 1, 2, and V_1, high right atrial, and His-bundle recordings respectively. A sustained bundle branch reentrant tachycardia was initiated by a long-short sequence change terminated by a single extrastimulus (S_2). Note the prolonged right bundle branch to ventricular interval of 45 milliseconds (sinus beat interval was 20 milliseconds). This RB–V interval remains unchanged despite variations in cycle length of the tachycardia. RB–RB interval changes precede VV-interval changes when the cycle length is altered. (From Caceres J, Jazayeri M, McKinnie J, Avitall B, et al: Sustained bundle branch reentry as a mechanism of clinical tachycardia. Circulation 1989;79:256.)

3. HV (intraventricular conduction time) intervals are equal to or greater than the HV intervals in sinus rhythm

4. Critical V-H delay is needed to initiate the tachycardia

5. His-bundle deflection precedes the right bundle deflection, with an H-RB interval greater in sinus rhythm than during ventricular tachycardia

6. Right ventricular activation must precede left ventricular activation

The incidence of this tachycardia is uncertain but depends largely on the population studied. It is interesting to note that a relatively high incidence of bundle branch reentry of brief duration (1 to 2 complexes) has been observed by many investigators during routine electrophysiologic studies, but the incidence of *sustained* bundle branch reentry appears to be low.

Recognition of this form of ventricular tachycardia has become clinically significant since the advent of radiofrequency ablation. This tachycardia appears to be highly amenable to "cure" with ablation of the proximal right bundle branch.[198–201] Some patients may require permanent pacing in the presence of preexisting disease of the remainder of the intraventricular conduction system.

QT Prolongation Syndrome

Hereditary Long-QT Syndrome

There are two important and usually distinct syndromes in which a prolonged QT interval is associated with a tendency to ventricular arrhythmias. In the syndrome described first by Jervell and Lange-Nielsen, there is associated deafness and inheritance is recessive. In the other form (Romano-Ward syndrome, first described by Romano and coworkers), there is no associated loss of hearing and the syndrome has a dominant pattern of inheritance.[202, 203] Patients having either variety may show uniform ventricular tachycardia (Fig. 21-34) or torsades de

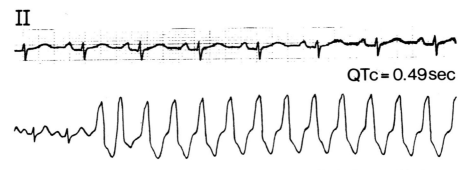

Figure 21-34. Electrocardiogram recorded from a patient with the Romano-Ward syndrome (lead II). The *upper panel* shows sinus rhythm with a prolonged QTc interval (0.49 milliseconds). The *lower panel* shows the development of ventricular tachycardia of uniform character.

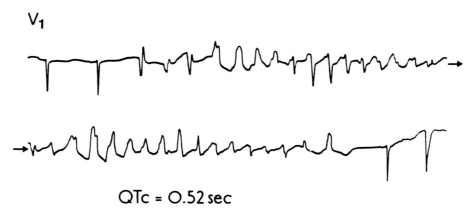

V_1

QTc = 0.52 sec

Figure 21-35. Continuous electrocardiogram (lead V_1) from another patient with the Romano-Ward syndrome, showing QTc prolongation and the development of a short run of tachycardia in which the axes of the QRS complexes appeared to rotate in keeping with torsades de pointes.

pointes (Fig. 21-35). Physiologically, the QT interval usually shortens with exercise; a third subset has been described in which this fails to occur and in which the QT interval lengthens with exercise.[204] Unless this possibility is considered in otherwise inexplicable cases of ventricular tachycardia, the mechanism may not be appreciated. Figure 21-36 shows ECGs recorded from a 40-year-old man in whom attacks of ventricular tachycardia were usually noted on exercise. As can be seen in the upper panel, the QT interval was slightly prolonged at rest but more obviously so during exercise (when it should have decreased); this was accompanied by the development of ventricular tachycardia (see Fig. 21-36B).

The prognosis for patients with these syndromes is unpredictable and sudden death is a recognized risk. There is only one report of a clear-cut extrinsic autonomic defect in one member of such an affected family, with undue QT-interval lengthening in response to small doses of isoproterenol.[205] Schwartz, through a registry of persons having long-QT syndrome, documented that prognosis is improved dramatically by left stellate sympathectomy, whereas beta blockade also offers some benefit.[207]

Acquired Long-QT Syndrome

As with the congenital forms of QT-interval prolongation, the acquired QT-interval prolongation syndromes are associated with ventricular arrhythmias and torsades de

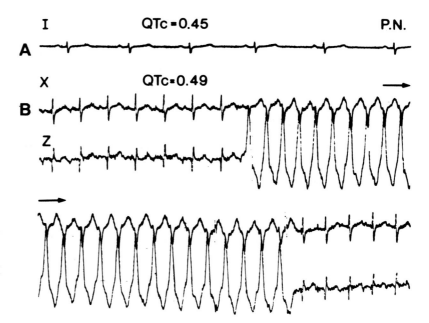

Figure 21-36. Electrocardiograms recorded from a patient with a history of palpitations. (**A**) Lead I shows sinus rhythm with modest QTc prolongation. (**B**) Continuous recordings of orthogonal, X, and Z leads, showing lengthening of the QT interval during exercise, with the development of a self-limited episode of ventricular tachycardia.

pointes.[56] Acquired QT-interval prolongation occurs with electrolyte disturbances (hypokalemia and apparently also hypomagnesemia and hypocalcemia), liquid protein diets, and most commonly with drugs—particularly class I antiarrhythmic agents, phenothiazines, and tricyclic antidepressants.

Catecholamine-Induced Ventricular Tachycardias

The hypothesis that ventricular arrhythmias could be induced by sensitization to epinephrine by chloroform was the subject of work culminating in the confirmation published by Levy and Lewis; numerous instances of the direct effect of catecholamines in producing ventricular arrhythmias have subsequently appeared.[3] Several years ago, we studied a family (Krikler D, Perelman M, Rowland E; unpublished data) and other sporadic cases in which sensitivity to endogenous catecholamines appeared to be the mechanism for ventricular arrhythmias, in some instances fatal (see Fig. 21-23); their arrhythmias were reproducible by the infusion of small amounts of isoproterenol.[63] Therapeutic assessment is facilitated by noting the response to prophylactic beta blockers, with the dose being increased until measured exercise no longer reinduces the arrhythmia; Coumel and colleagues believe that nadolol in particular has definite benefits in these patients.[207]

Exercise-Related Ventricular Tachycardia

Exercise-related ventricular tachycardia is of special interest because this entity frequently arises from the right ventricular outflow tract and may be easily evaluated using catheter mapping techniques. Invariably, the patients have no recognizable heart disease. This arrhythmia is usually precipitated by exercise, with a young female preponderance. An ECG during the episodes generally manifests left bundle branch block configuration with a right inferior axis deviation (see Fig. 21-23). The pathologic explanation for this arrhythmia is not known; one must be certain that a variant of right ventricular dysplasia is not present. Detailed cardiologic studies, including signal-averaged ECGs and anatomic studies of the right ventricle (angiography, magnetic resonance imaging [MRI], two-dimensional echocardiograms), generally do not reveal any significant abnormality.[208–212]

The mechanism of this tachycardia is speculative but most opinions favor triggered activity due to delayed afterdepolarizations. Several features favor such a mechanism, including:

1. Initiation depends on catecholamines
2. Events mainly occur in waking hours

3. Prevention is with beta-blocking and calcium channel blocking agents[213]
4. Difficulty in initiation with stimulation protocols
5. Adenosine administration can terminate the tachycardia[214–217]

Previously, the primary therapy for this arrhythmia was beta-blocking drugs. This treatment had a high success rate and generally was well tolerated. The use of calcium channel blocking drugs has not been as well studied. Nevertheless, in the last several years, many investigators have reported excellent success rates for "curing" this tachycardia using radiofrequency ablation techniques.[217–219] The long-term follow-up, however, remains to be evaluated.

Arrhythmogenic Right Ventricular Dysplasia

This entity was first described by Fontaine and colleagues in 1977.[220] The pathologic abnormality is severe muscular displacement with fat and fibrous tissue, involving only the right ventricle. The findings are similar but pathologically different from Uhl's anomaly, in which the right ventricular wall is described as having a parchment-like quality without fatty deposition.[221] The right ventricle functions reasonably well in arrhythmogenic right ventricular dysplasia, but congestive heart failure is frequently seen in Uhl's anomaly.

Clinically, the entity has a male preponderance, with an average age of 40 years. Electrocardiograms frequently show T-wave inversion in the right-side precordial leads, with many patients having incomplete right bundle branch block during sinus rhythm (Fig. 21-37).[220, 222–225]

Cardiac MRI studies are helpful in establishing the diagnosis of arrhythmogenic right ventricular dysplasia but generally require special imaging techniques to obtain high quality data (Fig. 21-38).[226]

Other studies are useful to evaluate or diagnose patients with suspected right ventricular dysplasia, including:

1. Transthoracic echocardiography, which may demonstrate an increase in right ventricular diastolic diameter and aneurysmal abnormalities[227]
2. Right ventricular angiography, which may demonstrate a large right ventricle with segmental wall abnormalities or aneurysmal abnormalities[228]
3. Right ventricular wall motion studies (nuclear imaging techniques), which may demonstrate a depressed right ventricular ejection fraction of about 25% (Fig. 21-39)[225]
4. Left ventricular wall motion, which is generally normal by routine testing procedures[228]

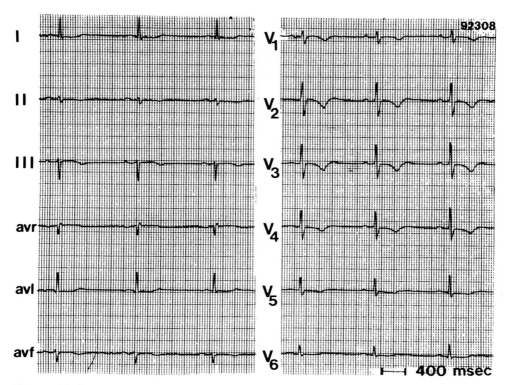

Figure 21-37. Twelve-lead electrocardiogram during sinus rhythm in a patient with arrhythmogenic right ventricular dysplasia and recurrent ventricular tachycardia. Note the prominent T-wave abnormalities in the precordial leads. (From Metzger JT, de Chillou C, Cheriex E, Rodriguez L-M, Smeets JLRM, Wellens HJJ: Value of the 12-lead electrocardiogram in arrhythmogenic right ventricular dysplasia, and absence of correlation with echocardiographic findings. Am J Cardiol 1993;72:964.)

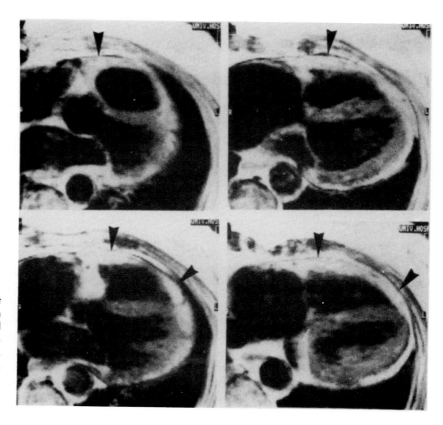

Figure 21-38. Spin-echo images in a patient with right ventricular dysplasia. Four axial slices in which significant apparent fatty infiltration is noted from the pericardium (*arrowheads*) to the endocardium, which is apparent in the tricuspid area, apex, and right ventricular outflow tract. (From Ricci C, Lango R, Pagnan L, et al: Magnetic resonance imaging in right ventricular dysplasia. Am J Cardiol 1992;70:1589.)

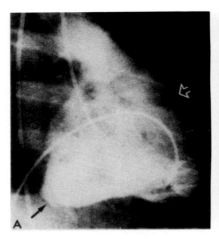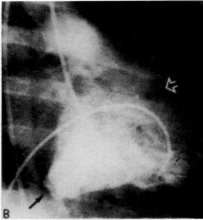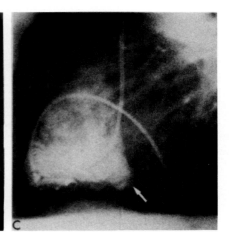

Figure 21-39. Right ventricular angiogram (anteroposterior projection in diastole and systole (**A** and **B**) and a lateral projection (**C**). The right ventricle is dilated and less trabeculated than usual. Aneurysms are shown in the outflow tract (*open arrow*) and below the tricuspid valve (*closed arrow*). (From Peters S, Hartwig CA, Reil GH: Risk assessment in nonischemic ventricular arrhthymia by left and right ventriculography. Am Heart J 1992;124:116.)

The ECG during tachycardia is usually of a left bundle branch block morphology, with superior or inferior axis deviation. Depending on the degree of right ventricular abnormality, multiple ECG morphologies may be observed. The signal-averaged ECG is usually abnormal and frequently correlates with a fragmented prolonged right ventricular electrogram during endocardial mapping (Fig. 21-40).[229]

This tachycardia is usually easily initiated with ventricular pacing and extrastimulation, supporting reentry as the predominant mechanism.

These patients frequently present as a management problem. Their tachyarrhythmias may not respond to any antiarrhythmic drug therapy, including amiodarone.[223, 225, 226, 231] A surgical approach has been suggested, which may require "autotransplantation" of the right ventricular free wall.[231–233] Radiofrequency ablation has been attempted; however, the diffuse nature of the disease may not allow a high success rate.[234] The use of an implantable defibrillator may be necessary in resistant cases. Some patients may be considered for cardiac transplantation.

Drug-Induced Tachycardias

Digitalis is the agent likely to produce ventricular arrhythmias because it is administered so frequently. These tachycardias are often heralded by systemic symptoms of toxicity but the cardiac effects may come first. Occasionally, bigeminy due to regular ventricular extrasystoles may be the first indication, but bidirectional tachycardia may be another warning sign. Conversely, ventricular tachycardia may be seen without any other clinical indication of intoxication, and it may be sustained (Fig. 21-41) rather than episodic (see Fig. 21-17). A host of other agents may be responsible, however, including those prone to cause torsades de pointes.[57, 58] In some cases, the effect is indirect (e.g., diuretics that produce hypokalemia); in other cases, the effect is direct (e.g., cardioactive agents and major tranquilizers that prolong repolarization). In our experience, the most likely offenders are quinidine, procainamide, flecainide, disopyramide, phenothiazines, and tricyclic antidepressants. Whenever torsades de pointes is seen, careful inquiry should be made concerning the possible consumption of such medications. The calcium antagonist bepridil may cause this tachycardia, especially when given to elderly hypokalemic women or if the recommended dose is exceeded.[235] Other agents have been implicated as possible causes of ventricular tachycardia but in many cases reported in the literature, only single instances have been cited and the direct relevance is not always clear.[15]

Disturbances of Impulse Formation in Conduction

The most important ventricular arrhythmia associated with either sinoatrial disease or AV block is torsades de pointes. This appears to occur in relation to the consequent disturbance of repolarization and may be one of the mechanisms whereby Adams-Stokes attacks occur in either form of heart block.[57]

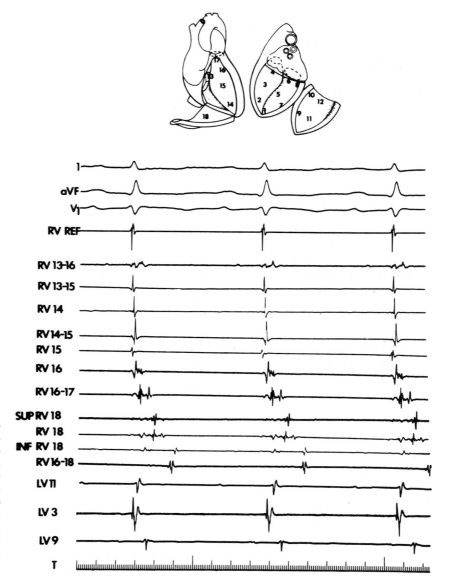

Figure 21-40. Sinus rhythm mapping in a patient with right ventricular dysplasia. Surface electrograms leads 1, aV$_f$ and V$_1$ are shown with multiple electrograms from the right and left ventricle. Note the marked abnormality of electrograms recorded from the right ventricular free wall. Electrical activity is recorded nearly 200 milliseconds beyond the end of QRS (i.e., sites 18 and 16–18). The left ventricular electrograms are normal. (From Josephson ME: Clinical cardiac electrophysiology. 2nd ed. Philadelphia: Lea & Febiger, 1992.)

Miscellaneous Causes

Numerous disorders may be listed as miscellany, including collagen diseases, electrolyte disturbances, and carbon monoxide poisoning, which we have not investigated personally. The ventricular arrhythmias that occur have no specific features, and the subjects have been well reviewed elsewhere.[15] Cardiac tumors are rare but potentially treatable causes.[236]

Cardiovascular involvement in sarcoidosis has been well recognized for at least 60 years, with an autopsy incidence of at least 20%.[237,238] Sustained ventricular tachycardia has only rarely been described, however.[239] Treatment with antiarrhythmic drugs has not been successful

and the use of implantable cardioverter defibrillators has been advocated.[239] Conventional therapy has had poor success.[240]

Idiopathic Causes

Several investigators have identified a subset of patients with no apparent structural heart disease and recurrent ventricular tachycardia.[225,241–244] In some patients, detailed cardiovascular testing has identified evidence of minor abnormalities of right ventricular function.[244] Therefore, the suspicion exists that many of these patients having no evident heart disease actually have some form of arrhyth-

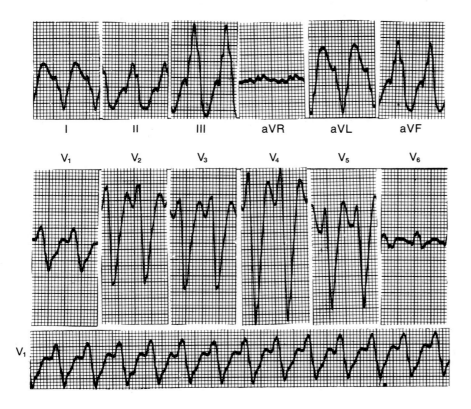

I II III aVR aVL aVF

V₁ V₂ V₃ V₄ V₅ V₆

V₁

Figure 21-41. Electrocardiogram showing ventricular tachycardia in a patient suffering from digitalis intoxication.

mogenic right ventricular dysplasia. Follow-up studies indicate that less than 60% respond to antiarrhythmic drug therapy.[244–246]

A small but important group of cases can be classified as being idiopathic. Short of careful pathologic examination of the heart, however, it may not be possible to uphold such a diagnosis except in the short term. Moreover, pathologic examination may not be helpful because ventricular tachycardia usually is seen in patients with QT-interval prolongation syndromes (Davies MJ; personal communication), although Rossi and Matturri note non-specific abnormalities of the conduction system in patients with this disorder.[247]

Gallavardin and Parkinson and Papp describe patients with repetitive ventricular tachycardias in whom the prognosis has been benign in the long term.[248,249] One such case is illustrated in Figure 21-8, showing ECGs from a woman aged 38 years in whom the arrhythmia was noted at birth. She is totally unaware of palpitation and leads a normal life. Electrophysiologic study and cardiac catheterization were normal in her case, as they usually are in others investigated in this manner. Figure 21-3 shows a more impressive tachycardia, in which the episodes of ventricular arrhythmia were interrupted only by single sinus complexes; the patient was asymptomatic and the arrhythmia was discovered when he was 22 years old and examined for life-insurance purposes. As is often the case with those affected by this disorder, the arrhythmia was not suppressed by medications and in this patient also, electrophysiologic studies showed no underlying abnormality. Conversely, the patient aged 19 years whose ECG is depicted in Figure 21-42 and who was otherwise indistinguishable from the two previous cases, died in his sleep; electrophysiologic studies had revealed no abnormality and pathologic investigation was entirely negative.

A more serious view was taken in the case of the man aged 18 years whose ECG is shown in Figure 21-43. The patient had a negative family history and presented with recurrent ventricular tachycardia. He was taking no medication, and no clinical evidence of cardiac disorder was apparent. At electrophysiologic study (Fig. 21-44), the sole abnormal feature was the finding of prolonged intraventricular conduction. He was untreated and suddenly died a year later. Again, necropsy revealed no cardiac abnormalities. In both this patient and the patient discussed in Figure 21-42, the cardiac conduction system was carefully examined, but because both patients died out of hospital, autopsy was not performed sufficiently soon after death to permit useful electron-microscope or other detailed investigations to be performed.

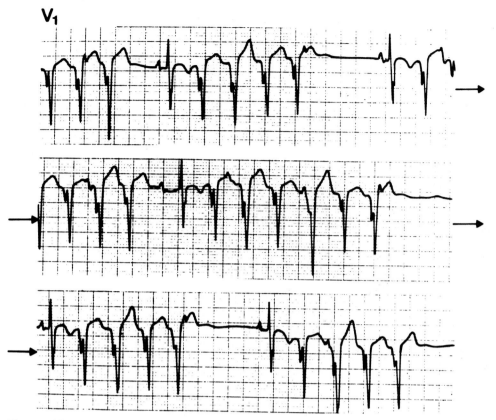

Figure 21-42. Electrocardiogram recorded from a young man with apparently benign ventricular tachycardia (lead V₁). In tachycardia, the QRS complexes have appearances consistent with what would be seen in sinus rhythm complicated by left bundle branch block, suggesting a right ventricular origin for the tachycardia. The episodes of tachycardia are interrupted by no more than one or two sinus complexes; if two, the first one shows atrioventricular (AV) block due to concealed conduction into the AV node, which is also seen in the sinus complex interrupting the tachycardia shown in the *second panel* (PR prolongation). Atrioventricular dissociation is evident from the independent P waves.

Figure 21-43. Electrocardiogram recorded from an otherwise healthy young man suffering from ventricular tachycardia with episodes of syncope. He was not taking any medications. His electrocardiogram showed PR prolongation and broad bizarre QRS complexes with gross disturbance of the ST segment and T waves. Leads V₁, V₂, and V₃ were recorded at half voltage. (From Brugada P, Brugada J: Right bundle branch block, persistent ST segment elevation and sudden cardiac death: a district clinical and electrocardiographic syndrome. A multicenter report. J Am Coll Cardiol 1992;20:1391.)

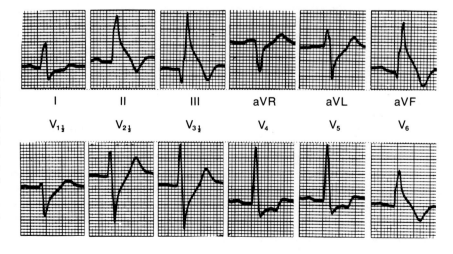

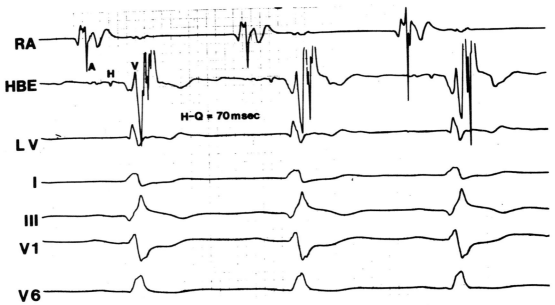

Figure 21-44. Intracardiac and surface electrocardiograms, including left ventricular electrogram (LV) recorded at a paper speed of 100 mm/second from the same patient as in Figure 21-43. The sole abnormality noted on the intracardiac leads was HQ (HV) prolongation (70 milliseconds; upper limit of normal, 55).

Left Ventricular Tachycardia Without Evident Heart Disease

This clinical arrhythmia occurs with a young male preponderance. The characteristic ECG features are a right bundle branch branch block morphology, with superior axis deviation. In contrast to the tachycardia arising from the right ventricular outflow tract, this arrhythmia generally is readily initiated with ventricular (and occasional atrial) pacing or extrastimulation. Detailed diagnostic studies demonstrate no significant cardiac abnormalities.[250-254]

The mechanism of this tachycardia appears to be reentry, possibly involving the posterior division of the left bundle branch.[255]

Activation mapping during the tachycardia suggests the earliest activation may be in the inferior mid-septal region in the left ventricle. There are, however, no fragmented electrograms recorded, in contrast to studies of a similar nature in patients with coronary artery disease. Signal-averaged ECGs are generally negative.[254-257]

Most interesting is the observation that this tachycardia is often sensitive to verapamil or other calcium channel blocking agents. Therefore, this is the therapy of choice. Generally, beta-blocking therapy is not useful. There may be a need for type I antiarrhythmic drug therapy, however.[250, 253, 254, 257, 258]

Limited data are available but radiofrequency ablation may have a role when energy is delivered to the area of earliest activation in the left ventricle (ie, the interior mid-septal region; Fig. 21-45).[256]

MEDICAL MANAGEMENT OF PATIENTS WITH VENTRICULAR TACHYCARDIA

Initially, the management strategy for patients with recurrent ventricular tachycardia was empiric antiarrhythmic drug therapy because only a limited number of drugs were available. Subsequently, with the development of additional antiarrhythmic agents, an empiric noninvasive approach was suggested, including the use of inpatient monitoring, serial stress testing, and Holter-monitor recordings. With the advent of electrophysiologic studies designed to test the ability to induce ventricular tachycardia, patients were subjected to serial electrophysiologic testing, with pharmacologic challenges. Extensive publications from multiple laboratories confirmed the short- and long-term benefit of such invasive evaluation technique.[259-263] Multiple therapeutic agents were used in the myriad reported studies. Attempts were made to use the effects of one agent to predict the outcome of others of the same category; those studies generally proved unsuccessful.[264-266] Also, adjunctive therapies were studied, with beta blockade and mexiletine being popular agents for evaluation.[268] Furthermore, serial studies found that elec-

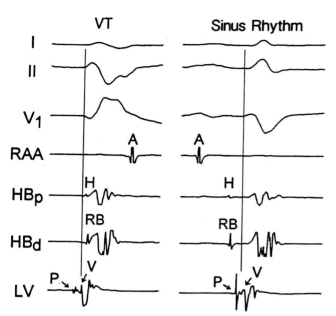

Figure 21-45. Purkinje potentials recorded during ventricular tachycardia and sinus rhythm at a successful radiofrequency ablation site in a patient having ventricular tachycardia with left axis deviation and right bundle branch block configuration. (From Nakagawa H, Beckman K, McClelland J, et al: Radiofrequency catheter ablation of idiopathic left ventricular tachycardia guided by a Purkinje potential circulation 1993;88:2607.)

implications are potentially far-reaching and the final word has not been heard.

Conclusion

Many reviews of ventricular tachycardia have appeared since the disorder was identified, and two aspects need consideration in determining those points arising from the large amount of data that offer scope for the future. At the clinical level, the greatest difficulty in patients with chronic recurrent ventricular tachycardia is the significance and reliability of reinitiation during electrophysiologic studies.[277] (This contentious point is discussed in further detail elsewhere in this volume.) This probably reflects the crude nature of contemporary tools in conjunction with the need to focus on what may be a restricted area of potential reentry. The other aspect is the question of triggered activity and whether this may have implications regarding the genesis of arrhythmias.[17] One can only speculate that triggered activity may be important in some focal tachycardias, perhaps associated with the effects of catecholamines and drugs such as digoxin. We do not, however, have the evidence that would enable us to correlate the interesting experimental electrophysiologic findings with ventricular arrhythmias that are little or not understood.

trophysiologic studies may not predict the efficacy of agents such as amiodarone.[268–271] These studies also revealed the importance of achieving a pharmacologic steady state before using invasive testing.

Debate existed concerning the criteria for declaring a test as being successful or unsuccessful (i.e., inducible or noninducible). Arguments raised questions about the importance of intermediate results for predicting long-term success or failure. Studies determined that agents showing only partial electrophysiologic success may occasionally have long-term benefit, with limited or no recurrences of the index ventricular arrhythmia.[272]

Nevertheless, controversy continued regarding the benefits and risks of serial electrophysiologic testing. It was decided that a multicenter trial be organized to address the question of the benefits of invasive versus noninvasive therapeutic evaluation of patients with recurrent ventricular tachycardia. The ESVEM trial (*E*lectrophysiologic *S*tudy *v*ersus *E*lectrocardiographic *M*onitoring) was organized and initially described in 1989.[273] The results of this trial have been reported; in the study, there were no significant differences in the success of drug therapy selected by these two methods.[274–275] Results of the ESVEM trial are the subject of debate concerning the merits and demerits of this large multicenter trial.[276] The

References

1. Lorain T: Etude de Médecine Clinique Faites avec l'Aide de la Methode Graphique et des Appareils Enregistreurs. Le Pouls, ses Variations et ses Formes Diverses dan les Maladies. Paris: JB Baillière, 1870.
2. Brunton L: One of the causes of death during the extraction of teeth under chloroform. Br Med J 1875;2:695.
3. Levy AG, Lewis T: Heart irregularities, resulting from the inhalation of low percentages of chloroform vapour, and their relationship to ventricular fibrillation. Heart 1911;3:99.
4. Hoffmann A: Die paroxysmale Tachycardie. Anfälle von Herzjagen. Wiesbaden: Bergmann, 1900.
5. Wenckebach KF: Die Arrhythmie als Ausdruck bestimmter Funktionsstorungen des Herzens. Eine physiologisch-klinische Studie. Leipzig: Wilhelm Engelmann, 1903.
6. Wenckebach KF: Die unreglmassige Herztätigkeit und ihre klinische Bedeutung. Leipzig: Wilhelm Engelmann, 1914.
7. Mackenzie J: Diseases of the heart. London: Henry Frowde & Hodder & Stoughton, 1908.
8. Lewis T: The experimental production of paroxysmal tachycardia and the effects of ligation of the coronary arteries. Heart 1909;1:98.
9. Erichsen JE: On the influence of the coronary circulation on the action of the heart. Lond Med Gaz 1842;2:561.
10. Allessie MA: Circulating excitation in the heart. Maastricht, The Netherlands: Drukkerij RU Limburg, 1977:21.

11. McWilliam JA: Cardiac failure and sudden death. Br Med J 1889;1:6.
12. Lewis T: The mechanism of the heart neat. London: Shaw & Sons, 1911.
13. Coumel P, Attuel P, Flammang D: The role of the conduction system in supraventricular tachycardias. In: Wellens HJJ, Lie KI, Janse MJ, eds. Structure, function and clinical implications. Leiden: HE Stenfert Kroese, 1976:424.
14. Schamroth L: The disorders of cardiac rhythm. London: Blackwell Scientific Publications, 1971:13.
15. Scherf D, Schott A: Extrasystoles and allied rrhythmias. 2nd ed. London: William Heinemann, 1973.
16. Schmitt FA, Erlanger J: Directional differences in the conduction of the impulse through heart muscle and their possible relation to extrasystolic and fibrillatory contractions. Am J Physiol 1928;65:125.
17. Wit AL, Hoffman BF, Cranefield PF: Slow conduction and reentry in the ventricular conducting system. I. Return extrasystole in canine Purkinje fibers. Circ Res 1972;30:1.
18. Wellens HJJ: Value and limitations of programmed electrical stimulation of the heart in the study and treatment of tachycardia. Circulation 1978;57:845.
19. Allessie MA, Bonke FIM, Schopman FJG: Circus movement in rabbit atrial muscle as a mechanism of tachycardia. III. The "leading circle" concept: a new model of circus movement in cardiac tissue without the involvement of an anatomical obstacle. Circ Res 1977;41:9.
20. Brugada P, Wellens HJJ: The role of triggered activity in clinical ventricular arrhythmias. Pacing Clin Electrophysiol 1984;7:260.
21. Bouvrain Y, Coraboeuf E: Pathogénie des troubles du rythme de l'infarctus aigu due myocarde. Arch Mal Coeur 1976;69:873.
22. El-Sherif N, Scherlag BJ, Lazzara R, Hope RR: Reentrant ventricular arrhythmias in the late myocardial infarction period. I. Conduction characteristics in the infarction zone. Circulation 1977;55:686.
23. El-Sherif N, Hope RR, Scherlag BJ, Lazzara R: Reentrant ventricular arrhythmias in the late myocardial infarction period. II. Patterns of initiation and termination of re-entry. Circulation 1977;55:702.
24. Russell DC, Oliver MF, Wojtczak J: Combined electrophysiological technique for assessment of the cellular basis of early ventricular arrhythmias. Experiments in dogs. Lancet 1977;2:686.
25. Downar E, Janse MJ, Durrer D: The effect of acute coronary occlusion on subepicardial transmembrane potentials in the intact porcine heart. Circulation 1977;56:217.
26. El-Sherif N, Lazzara R, Hope RR, Scherlag BJ: Re-entrant ventricular arrhythmias in the late myocardial infarction period. III. Manifest and concealed extrasystolic grouping. Circulation 1977;56:225.
27. Brechenmacher C, Moussard JM, Voegtlin R: Réentree ventriculaire permanente cachée et tachycardie ventriculaire paroxystique par mouvement circulaire. Arch Mal Coeur 1977;70:61.
28. Josephson ME, Horowitz LN, Farshidi A: Continuous local electrical activity. A mechanism of recurrent ventricular tachycardia. Circulation 1978;57:659.
29. Klein H, Karp RB, Kouchoukos NT, et al: Intraoperative electrophysiologic mapping of the ventricles during sinus rhythm in patients with a previous myocardial infarction. Identification of the electrophysiologic substrate of ventricular arrhythmias. Circulation 1982;66:847.
30. Antoni H: Electrophysiological mechanisms underlying pharmacological models of cardiac fibrillation. Arch Pharmacol 1971;269:177.
31. Evans TR, Curry PVL, Fitchett DH, Krikler DM: "Torsade de pointes" initiated by electrical ventricular stimulation. J Electrocardiol 1976;9:255.
32. Gradman AH, Bell PA, DeBusk RF: Sudden death during ambulatory monitoring. Clinical and electrocardiographic correlations. Report of a case. Circulation 1977;55:210.
33. Cranefield PF: Action potentials, afterpotentials and arrhythmias. Circ Res 1977;41:415.
34. Wit AL, Cranefield PF: Triggered and automatic activity in the canine coronary sinus. Circ Res 1977;41:435.
35. Rozanski GJ, Jalife J, Moe GK: Reflected reentry in non homogeneous ventricular muscle as a mechanism of cardiac arrhythmias. Circulation 1984;69:163.
36. Lin FC, Finley CD, Rahimtoola SH, Wu D: Idiopathic paroxysmal ventricular tachycardia with a QRS pattern of right bundle branch block and left axis deviation: a unique clinical entity with specific properties. Am J Cardiol 1983;52:95.
37. Coumel Ph, Leclercq JF, Attuel P, et al: Tachycardies ventriculaires en salves. Etude electro-physiologique et theraputique. Arch Mal Coeur 1980;73:153.
38. Waxman MB, Wald WR: Termination of ventricular tachycardia by an increase in cardiac vagal drive. Circulation 1977;56:385.
39. Rosen MR, Hoffman BF: The vagus and ventricles. Circ Res 1978;42:1.
40. Rardon DP, Bailey JC: Parasympathetic effects on electrophysiologic properties of cardiac ventricular tissue. J Am Coll Cardiol 1983;6:1200.
41. Pollack GH: Cardic pacemaking: an obligatory role of catecholamines? Science 1977;196:731.
42. Bellet S: Clinical disorders of the heart beat. 3rd ed. Philadelphia: Lea & Febiger, 1971:532.
43. Anderson KP, DeCamilla J, Moss AJ: Clinical significance of ventricular tachycardia (3 beats or longer) detected during ambulatory monitoring after myocardial infarction. Circulation 1978;57:890.
44. Frank R, Fontaine G, Guiraudon G, et al: Corrélation entre l'orientation de l'onde delta et la topographie de la préexcitation dans le syndrome de Wolff-Parkinson-White. Arch Mal Coeur 1977;70:441.
45. Krikler D, Davies MJ, Goodwin JF, et al: Sudden death in hypertrophic cardiomyopathy: associated accessory pathways. Br Heart J 1980;43:245.
46. Pietras RJ, Mautner R, Denes P, et al: Chronic recurrent right and left ventricular tachycardia: comparison of clinical, hemodynamic and angiographic findings. Am J Cardiol 1977;40:32.
47. Gallagher JJ, Oldham HN, Wallace AG, et al: Ventricular aneurysm with ventricular tachycardia. Report of a case with epicardial mapping and successful resection. Am J Cardiol 1975;35:696.

48. Fontaine G, Guiraudon G, Frank R, et al: Stimulation studies and epicardial mapping in ventricular tachycardia. Study of mechanisms and selections for surgery. In: Kulbertus HE, ed. Reentrant arrhythmias. Lancaster: MTP Press, 1976:334.

49. Rowland E, McKenna WJ, Sugrue D, et al: Ventricular tachycardia of left bundle branch block configuration in patients with isolated right ventricular dilatation. Br Heart J 1984; 51:15.

50. Smirk FH: R waves interrupting T waves. Br Heart J 1949; 11:23.

51. Krikler DM, Curry PVL: The paroxysmal supraventricular arrhythmias. In: Yu PN, Goodwin JF, eds. Progress in cardiology 5. Philadelphia: Lea & Febiger, 1976:291.

52. Wellens HJJ, Lie KI: Ventricular tachycardia: the value of programmed electrical stimulation. In: Krikler DM, Goodwin JF, eds. Cardiac arrhythmias, the modern electro-physiological approach Philadelphia: WB Saunders, 1975:182.

53. Wellens HJJ, Schuilenburg RM, Durrer D: Electrical stimulation of the heart in patients with ventricular tachycardia. Circulation 1972;46:216.

54. Dreifus LS, Haiat R, Watanabe Y, et al: Ventricular fibrillation, a possible mechanism of sudden death in patients with the Wolff-Parkinson-White syndrome. Circulation 1971;43:250.

55. Dessertenne F: La tachycardie ventriculaire à deux foyers opposes variables. Arch Mal Coeur 1966;59:263.

56. Slama R, Coumel Ph, Motté G, et al: Tachycardies ventriculaires et torsades de pointes: frontières morphologiques entre les dysrhythmies ventriculaires. Arch Mal Coeur 1973;66:1401.

57. Krikler DM, Curry PVL: Torsade de pointes, an atypical ventricular tachycardia. Br Heart J 1976;38:117.

58. Perelman M, Rowland E, Krikler DM: Torsade de pointes: a review. Intern Med 1983;11:126.

59. Schwartz SP, Orloff J, Fox C: Transient ventricular fibrillation. I. The prefibrillary period during established auriculoventricular dissociation with a note on the phonocardiograms obtained at such times. Am Heart J 1949;37:21.

60. Loeb HS, Pietras RJ, Gunnar RM, Tobin JR Jr: Paroxysmal ventricular fibrillation in two patients with hypomagnesemia. Treatment by transvenous pacing. Circulation 1968;37:210.

61. Tamura K, Tamura T, Yoshida S, et al: Transient recurrent ventricular fibrillation due to hypopotassemia with special note on the U wave. Jpn Heart J 1967;8:652.

62. Smirk FH, Ng J: Cardiac ballet: repetitions of complex electrocardiographic patterns. Br Heart J 1969;31:426.

63. Coumel P, Fidelle J, Lucet V, et al: Catecholamine-induced severe ventricular arrhythmias with Adams-Stokes syndrome in children. Report of four cases. Br Heart J 1978;40 (Suppl):28.

64. Curry P, Fitchett D, Stubbs W, Krikler D: Ventricular arrhythmias and hypokalaemia. Lancet 1976;1:231.

65. Sandler IA, Marriott HJL: The differential morphology of anomalous ventricular complexes of right bundle branch block type in lead VI. Ventricular ectopy versus aberration. Circulation 1965;31:551.

66. Wellens HJJ, Bär FWHM, Lie KI: The value of the electrocardiogram in the differential diagnosis of a tachycardia with a widened QRS complex. Am J Med 1978;64:27.

67. Akhtar M, Shenassa M, Jazayeri M, Caceres J, Tchou P: Wide QRS complex tachycardia: reappraisal of a common clinical problem. Ann Intern Med 1988;109:905.

68. Brugada P, Brugada J, Mont L, Smeets J, Andries EM: A new approach to the differential diagnosis of a regular tachycardia with a wide QRS complex. Circulation 1991;83:1649.

69. Anderson KP, Lux RA, Dustman T: Comparison of QRS morphologies of spontaneous premature ventricular complexes and ventricular tachycardia induced by programmed stimulation. Am Heart J 1990;119:1302.

70. Kremers MS, Black WH, Wells PJ, Solodyna M: Effect of preexisting bundle branch block on the electrocardiographic diagnosis of ventricular tachycardia. Am J Cardiol 1988;62:1208.

71. Kindwall KE, Brown J, Josephson ME: Electrocardiographic criteria for ventricular tachycardia in wide complex left bundle branch block morphology tachycardias. am j cardiol 1988;61:1279.

72. Hayes JJj, Stewart RB, Greene HS, Bardy GH: Narrow QRS ventricular tachycardia. Ann Intern Med 1991;114:460.

73. Miller JM, Marchlinski FE, Buxton AE, Josephson ME: Relationship between 12-lead electrocardiogram during ventricular tachycardia and endocardial site of origin in patients with coronary artery disease. Circulation 1988;71:759.

74. Kuchar DL, Ruskin JN, Garan H: Electrocardiographic localization of the site of origin of ventricular tachycardia in patients with prior myocardial infarction. J Am Coll Cardiol 1989;13:893.

75. Josephson ME: Clinical cardiac electrophysiology. 2nd ed. Philadelphia: Lea & Febiger, 1992.

76. Kuchar DL, Ruskin JN, Garan H: Electrocardiographic localization of the site of origin of ventricular tachycardia in patients with myocardial infarction. J Am Coll Cardiol 1989; 13:893.

77. Josephson ME, Horowitz LN, Farshidi A, Spear JF, Kastor JA, Moore EN: Recurrent sustained ventricular tachycardia. 2. Endocardial mapping. Circulation 1978;57:440.

78. Gardner PI, Ursell PC, Fenoglio JJ Jr, Wit AL: Electrophysiologic and anatomic basis for fractionated electrograms recorded from healed myocardial infarcts. Circulation 1985; 72:596.

79. Stevenson WG, Weiss JN, Wiener I, et al: Fractionated endocardial electrograms are associated with slow conduction in humans: evidence from pace-mapping. J Am Coll Cardiol 1989;13:369.

80. Olshansky B, Moreira D, Waldo AL: Characterization of double potentials during ventricular tachycardia studies during transient entrainment. Circulation 1993;87:373.

81. Cassidy DM, Vassallo JA, Buxton AE, Doherty JU, Marchlinski FE, Josephson ME: The value of catheter mapping during sinus rhythm to localize site of origin of ventricular tachycardia. Circulation 1984;69:1103.

82. Josephson ME, Waxman HL, Cain ME, Gardner MJ, Buxton AE: Ventricular activation during ventricular endocardial pacing II. Role of pace-mapping to localize origin of ventricular tachycardia. Am J Cardiol 1982;50:11.

83. Holt PM, Smallpiece C, Dedverall PB, Yates AK, Curry PVL: Ventricular arrhythmias: a guide to their localizations. Br Heart J 1985;53:417.

84. Morady F, Kadish AH, DiCarlo L, et al: Long-term results of catheter ablation of idiopathic right ventricular tachycardia. Circulation 1990;82:2093.

85. Moss AJ, Davis HT, Decamilla J, Bayer LW: Ventricular ectopic beats and their relation to sudden and nonsudden cardiac death after myocardial infarction. Circulation 1979;60:998.

86. Bigger JT, Fleiss JL, Kleiger R, Miller JP, Rolnitzky LM: The relationships among ventricular arrhythmias, left ventricular dysfunction and mortality in the 2 years after myocardial infarction. Circulation 1984;69:250.

87. Mukharji J, Rude FE, Poole K, the Myocardial Infarction LIS Study Group. Risk factors for sudden death after acute myocardial infarction: two-year follow-up. Am J Cardiol 1984; 54:31.

88. Anderson KP, DeCamilla J, Moss AJ: Clinical significance of ventricular tachycardia (3 beats or longer) detected during ambulatory monitoring after myocardial infarction. Circulation 1978;57:890.

89. Bigger JT, Weld FM, Rolnitzky LM: Prevalence, characteristics and significance of ventricular tachycardia (3 or more complexes) detected with ambulatory electrocardiographic recording in the late hospital phase of acute myocardial infarction. Am J Cardiol 1981;48:815.

90. Kleiger RE, Miller JP, Thanavaro S, Province MA, Martin TF, Oliver GC: Relationship between clinical features of acute myocardial infarction and ventricular runs 2 weeks to 1 year after infarction. Circulation 1981;63:64.

91. Follansbee WP, Michelson EL, Morganroth J: Nonsustained ventricular tachycardia in ambulatory patients: characteristics and association with sudden cardiac death. Ann Intern Med 1980;92:741.

92. Chakko CS, Gheorghiade M: Ventricular arrhythmias in severe heart failure: incidence, significance, and effectiveness of antiarrhythmic therapy. Am Heart J 1985;109:497.

93. Holmes J, Kubo SH, Cody RJ, Kligfield P: Arrhythmias in ischemic and nonischemic dilated cardiomyopathy: prediction of mortality by ambulatory electrocardiography. Am J Cardiol 1985;55:146.

94. Wilson JR, Schwartz JS, St. John Sutton M, et al: Prognosis in severe heart failure: relation to hemodynamic measurements and ventricular ectopic activity. J Am Coll Cardiol 1983;2:403.

95. Echt DS, Liebson PR, Mitchell B, et al: Mortality and morbidity in patients receiving encainide, flecainide or placebo. The cardiac arrhythmia suppression trial. New Engl J Med 1991;324:781.

96. Kowey PR, Taylor JE, Marinchak RA, Rials SJ: Does programmed stimulation really help in the evaluation of patients with nonsustained ventricular tachycardia? Results of a meta-analysis. Am Heart J 1991;123:481.

97. Pires LA, Huang SKS: Nonsustained ventricular tachycardia: identification and management of high-risk patients. Am Heart J 1993;126:189.

98. Savage DD, Seides SF, Maron BJ, Meyers DM, Epstein SE: Prevalence of arrhythmia during 24-hour electrocardiographic monitoring and exercise testing in patients with obstructive and nonobstructive hypertrophic cardiomyopathy. Circulation 1979;59:866.

99. McKenna WJ, England D, Doi YL, Deanfield JE, Oakley C, Goodwin JF: Arrhythmias in hypertrophic cardiomyopathy: influence on prognosis. Br Heart J 1981;46:168.

100. Spirito P, Watson RM, Maron BJ: Relation between extent of left ventricular hypertrophy and occurrence of ventricular tachycardia in hypertrophic cardiomyopathy. Am J Cardiol 1987;1137.

101. Fananapazir L, Tracy CM, Leon MB, et al: Electrophysiologic abnormalities in patients with hypertrophic cardiomyopathy: a consecutive analysis in 155 patients. Circulation 1989; 80:1259.

102. Kuck KH, Kunze KP, Schluter M, Nienaber CA, Costard A: Programmed electrical stimulation in hypertrophic cardiomyopathy: results in patients with and without cardiac arrest or syncope. Eur Heart J 1988;9:177.

103. McKenna WJ, Krikler DM, Goodwin JF: Arrhythmias in dilated and hypertrophic cardiomyopathy. Med Clin North Am 1984;54:802.

104. McKenna WJ, Harris L, Perez G, Krikler DM, Oakley C, Goodwin JF: Arrhythmia in hypertrophic cardiomyopathy. II. Comparison of amiodarone and verapamil in treatment. Br Heart J 1981;46:173.

105. McKenna WJ, Harris L, Rowland E, et al: Amiodarone for long term management of patients with hypertrophic cardiomyopathy. Am J Cardiol 1984;54:802.

106. McKenna WJ, Oakley CM, Krikler DM, Goodwin JF: Improved survival with amiodarone in patients with hypertrophic cardiomyopathy and ventricular tachycardia. Br Heart J 1985;53:412.

107. Fananapazir L, Leon MB, Bonow RO, Tracy CM, Cannon RO, Epstein SE: Sudden death during empiric amiodarone therapy in symptomatic hypertrophic cardiomyopathy. Am J Cardiol 1991;67:169.

108. Fananapazir L, Epstein SE: Value of electrophysiologic studies in hypertrophic cardiomyopathy. Am J Cardiol 1991;67:175.

109. Holmes J, Kubo SH, Cody RJ, Kligfield P: Arrhythmias in ischemic and nonischemic dilated cardiomyopathy: prediction of mortality by ambulatory electrocardiography. Am J Cardiol 1985;55:146.

110. Huang SK, Messer JV, Denes P: Significance of ventricular tachycardia in idiopathic dilated cardiomyopathy: observations in 35 patients. Am J Cardiol 1983;51:507.

111. Meinertz T, Hoffmann T, Kasper W, Treese N, Bachtold H, Stoenen V: Significance of ventricular arrhythmias in idiopathic dilated cardiomyopathy. Am J Cardiol 1984;53:902.

112. Unverferth DV, Magorien RD, Moeschberger ML, Baker PB, Fetters JK, Leier CV: Factors influencing the one-year mortality of dilated cardiomyopathy. Am J Cardiol 1984;54:147.

114. Von Olhausen K, Stienen U, Schwarz F, Kobler W, Meyer J: Long term prognostic significance of ventricular arrhythmias in idiopathic dilated cardiomyopathy. Am J Cardiol 1988;61:146.

115. Luu M, Stevenson WG, Stevenson LW, Baron K, Walden J: Diverse mechanisms of unexpected cardiac arrest in advanced heart failure. Circulation 1989;80:1675.

116. Das SK, Morady F, DiCarlo L, et al: Prognostic usefulness of programmed ventricular stimulation in idiopathic dilated cardiomyopathy without symptomatic ventricular arrhythmias. Am J Cardiol 1986;58:998.

117. Poll DS, Marchlinski FE, Buxton AE, Josephson ME: Usefulness of programmed stimulation in idiopathic dilated cardiomyopathy. Am J Cardiol 1986;58:992.

118. Meinertz T, Treese N, Kasper W, et al: Determinants of prognosis in idiopathic dilated cardiomyopathy as determined by programmed electrical stimulation. Am J Cardiol 1985;56:337.

119. Stamato N, O'Connell JB, Murdock DK, Moran JF, Loeb HS, Scanlon PJ: The response of patients with complex ventricular arrhythmias secondary to dilated cardiomyopathy to programmed electrical stimulation. Am Heart J 1986;112:505.

120. Gossinger HD, Jung M, Wagner L, et al: Prognostic role of inducible ventricular tachycardia in patients with dilated cardiomyopathy and asymptomatic nonsustained ventricular tachycardia. Int J Cardiol 1990;29:215.

121. Kron J, Hart M, Schual-Berke S, Niles NR, Hosenpud JD, McAnulty JH: Idiopathic dilated cardiomyopathy: role of programmed electrical stimulation and Holter monitoring in predicting those at risk of sudden death. Chest 1988; 93:85.

122. Cleland JGF, Dargie HJ, Findlay IN, Wilson JT: Clinical, hemodynamic and antiarrhythmic effects of long term treatment with amiodarone of patients in heart failure. Br Heart J 1987;57:436.

123. Neri R, Mestroni L, Salvi A, Pandullo C, Camerini F: Ventricular arrhythmias in dilated cardiomyopathy: efficacy of amiodarone. Am Heart J 1987;113:707.

124. Dargie HJ, Cleland JGF, Leckie BJ, Inglis CG, East BW, Ford I: Relation of arrhythmias and electrolyte abnormalities to survival in patients with severe chronic heart failure. Circulation 1987;75(Suppl IV):98.

125. Simonton CA, Daly PA, Kereiakes D, Modin G, Chatterjee K: Survival in severe left ventricular failure treated with the new nonglycosidic, nonsympathomimetic oral inotropic agents. Chest 1987;92:118.

126. Nicklas JM, McKenna WJ, Stewart RA, et al: Prospective, double-blind, placebo-controlled trial of low-dose amiodarone in patients with severe heart failure and asymptomatic frequent ventricular ectopy. Am Heart J 1991;122:1016.

127. Winkle RA, Lopes MG, Fitzgerald JW, Goodman DJ, Schroeder JS, Harrison DC: Arrhythmias in patients with mitral valve prolapse. Circulation 1975;52:73.

128. Boudoulas H, Kligfield P, Wooley CF: Mitral valve prolapse: sudden death. In: Boudoulas H, Wooley CF, eds. Mitral valve prolapse and the mitral valve prolapse syndrome. Mt. Kisco, NY: Futura Publishing, 1988:591.

129. Morady F, Shen E, Bhandari A, Schwartz A, Scheinman MM: Programmed ventricular stimulation in mitral valve prolapse: analysis of 36 patients. Am J Cardiol 1984;53:135.

130. Rosenthal ME, Hamer A, Gang ES, Oseran DS, Mandel WJ, Peter T: The yield of programmed ventricular stimulation in mitral valve prolapse patients with ventricular arrhythmias. Am Heart J 1985;110:970.

131. Pratt CM, Young JB, Wierman AM, et al: Complex ventricular arrhythmias associated with the mitral prolapse syndrome. Am J Med 1986;80:626.

132. James MA, Jones JV: Ventricular arrhythmia in untreated newly presenting hypertensive patients compared with matched normal population. J Hypertens 1989;7:409.

133. Mclenachan JM, Dargie HJ: A review of rhythm disorders in cardiac hypertrophy. Am J Cardiol 1990;65(Suppl G):42.

134. Ghali JK, Kadakia S, Cooper RS, Liao Y: Impact of left ventricular hypertrophy on ventricular arrhythmias in the absence of coronary artery disease. J Am Coll Cardiol 1991; 17:1277.

135. Meesmann W, Gülker H, Krämer B, Stephan K: Time course of changes in ventricular fibrillation threshold in myocardial infarction: characteristics of acute and slow occlusion with respect to the collateral vessels of the heart. Cardiovasc Res 1976;10:446.

136. Scherlag BJ, Helfant RH, Haft JI, Damato AN: Electrophysiology underlying ventricular arrhythmias due to coronary ligation. Am J Physiol 1970;219:1665.

137. Chiche P, Haiat R, Steff P: Angina pectoris with syncope due to paroxysmal atrioventricular block: role of ischaemia. Report of two cases. Br Heart J 1974;36:577.

138. Benaim R, Calvo J, Seban C, et al: Les aspects anatomiques de l'Angine de Prinzmétal: à propos d'une observation anatomoclinique. Arch Mal Coeur 1975;68:189.

139. Maseri A, Mimmo R, Chierchia S, et al: Coronary artery spasm as a cause of acute myocardial ischaemia in man. Chest 1975;68:625.

140. Hartzler GO, Maloney JD: Programmed ventricular stimulation in management of recurrent ventricular tachycardia. Mayo Clin Proc 1977;52:731.

141. Durrer D, et al: Human cardiac electrophysiology. In: Dickinson CJ, Marks J, eds. Developments in cardiovascular medicine, Lancaster: MTP Publishers, 1978:53.

142. Breithardt G, Borggrefe M, Quantus B, et al: Ventricular vulnerability assessed by programmed ventricular stimulation in patients with and without late potentials. Circulation 1983;68:275.

143. Califf RM, Burkes JM, Behar VS, et al: Relationships among ventricular arrhythmias, coronary artery disease, and angiographic and electrocardiographic indicators of myocardial fibrosis. Circulation 1978;57:725.

144. Vismara LA, Amsterdam EA, Mason DT: Relation of ventricular arrhythmias in the late hospital phase of acute myocardial infarction to sudden death after hospital discharge. Am J Med 1975;59:6.

145. Haynes RE, Hallstrom AP, Cobb LA: Repolarisation abnormalities in survivors of out-of-hospital ventricular fibrillation. Circulation 1978;57:654.

146. Harris AS, Rojas AG: The initation of ventricular fibrillation due to coronary occlusion. Exp Med Surg 1943;1:105.

147. Janse MJ, Wit AI: Electrophysiological mechanisms of ventricular arryythmias resulting from mycardial ischemia and infarction. Physiol Rev 1989;69:1049.

148. El-Sherif N, Scherlag BJ, Lazzara R: Electrode catheter recordings during malignant ventricular arrhythmia following experimental acute myocardial ischemia. Circulation 1975; 51:1003.

149. Pogwizd SM, Corr PB: Reentrant and nonreentrant mechanisms contrribute to arrhythmogenesis during early myocardial ischemia: results using three-dimensional mapping. Circ Res 1987;61:352.

150. de Bakker JM, van Capelle FJL, Janse MJ, et al: Reentry as a cause of ventricular tachycardia in patients with chronic

ischemic heart disease: electrophysiologic and anatomic correlation. Circulation 1988;77:589.

151. Gorgels APM, Vas MA, Brugada P, Wellens HJJ: The clinical relevance of abnormal automaticity and triggered activity. In: Brugada PP, Wellens HJJ, eds. Cardiac arrhythmias: where to go from here? Mt. Kisco, NY: Futura Publishing, 1987:147.

152. Josephson ME, Harken AH, Horowitz LN: Endocardial excision: A new surgical technique for the treatment of recurrent ventricular tachycardia. Circulation 1979;60:1430.

153. Downar E, Harris L, Mickelborough LL, Shaikh NA, Parson ID: Endocardial mapping of ventricular tachycardia in the intact human ventricle: evidence for reentrant mechanisms. J Am Coll Cardiol 1988;11:783.

154. Littman L, Svenson RH, Gallagher JJ, et al: Functional role of the epicardium in postinfaction ventricular tachycardia, Observations derived from computerized epicadial activation mapping, entrainment, and epicardial laser photoablation. Circulation 1991;83:1577.

155. Stevenson WG, Weiss J, Wiener I, Nademanee K: Slow conduction in the infarct scar: relevance to the occurrence detection, and ablation of ventricular reentry circuits resulting from myocardial infarction. Am Heart J 1989;117:452.

156. Wiener I, Mindich B, Pitchon R: Fragmented endocardial electrical activity in patients with ventricular tachycardia: a new guide to surgical therapy. Am Heart J 1984;107:86.

157. Josephson ME, Wit AI: Fractionated electrical activity and continuous electrical activity: fact or artifact? Circulation 1984;70:529.

158. Ideker RE, Lofland GK, Bardy GH, et al: Late fractionated potentials and continuous electrical activity caused by electrode motion. Pacing Clin Electrophysiol 1983;6:908.

159. Simson MB: Use of signals in the terminal QRS complex to identify patients with ventricular tachycardia after myocardial infarction. Circulation 1981;64:235.

160. Hall PA, Atwood JE, Myers J, Froelicher VF: The signal averaged surface electrocardiogram and the identification of late potentials. Prog Cardiovasc Dis 1989;31:295.

161. Marchlinski FE, Buxton AE, Waxman HL, Josephson ME: Identifying patients at risk of sudden death after myocardial infarction: value of the response to programmed stimulation, degree of ventricular ectopic activity and severity of left ventricular dysfunction. Am J Cardiol 1983;52:1190.

162. Gomes JA, Winters SL, Martinson M, Machac J, Stewart D, Targonski A: The prognostic significance of quantitative signal-averaged variables relative to clinical variables, site of myocardial infarction, ejection fraction and ventricular premature beats: a prospective study. J Am Coll Cardiol 1989;13:377.

163. Kuchar DL, Thornburn CW, Sammel NL: Prediction of serious arrhythmic events after myocardial infarction: signal-averaged electrocardiogram, Holter monitoring, and radionuclide ventriculography. J Am Coll Cardiol 1987;9:531.

164. Roy D, Waxman HL, Kienzle MG, Buxton AE, Marchlinski FE, Josephson ME: Clinical characteristics and long-term follow-up in 119 survivors of cardiac arrest: relation to inducibility at electrophysiologic testing. Am J Cardiol 1983;51:85.

165. Skale BT, Miles WM, Heger JJ, Zipes DP, Prystowsky EN: Survivors of cardiac arrest; prevention of recurrence by drug therapy as predicted by electrophysiologic testing or electrocardiographic monitoring. Am J Coll Cardiol 1986; 57:113.

166. Eldar M, Sauve MJ, Scheinman MM: Electrophysiologic testing and follow-up of patients with aborted sudden death. J Am Cardiol 1987;10:291.

167. Wilber DJ, Garan H, Finkelstein D, et al: Out-of-hospital cardiac arrest: use of electrophysiologic testing in the prediction of long-term outcome. N Engl J Med 1988;318:19.

168. Fogoros RN, Bonnet CA, Chendarides JG: Long-term outcome of survivors of cardiac arrest whose therapy is guided by electrophysiologic testing. J Am Coll Cardiol 1992;19:780.

169. Winkle RA, Lopes MG, Fitzgerald JW, et al: Arrhythmias in patients with mitral valve prolapse. Circulation 1975;52:73.

170. Cobbs BW Jr, King SB: Ventricular buckling: a factor in the abnormal ventriculogram and peculiar hemodynamics associated with mitral valve prolapse. Am Heart J 1977;93:741.

171. Duren DR, Becker AE, Dunning AJ: Long-term follow-up of idiopathic mitral valve prolapse in 300 patients: a prospective study. J Am Coll Cardiol 1988;11:42.

172. Rosenthal ME, Hamer A, Gang ES, Oseran DS, Mandel WJ, Peter T: The yield of programmed ventricular stimulation in mitral valve prolapse patients with ventricular arrhythmias. Am Heart J 1985;110:970.

173. Winkle RA, Lopes MG, Fitzgerald JW, Goodman DJ, Schroeder JS, Harrison DC: Arrhythmias in patients with mitral valve prolapse. Circulation 1975;52:73.

174. Morady F, Shen E, Bhandari A, Schwartz A, Scheinman MM: Programmed ventricular stimulation in mitral valve prolapse: analysis of 36 patients. Am J Cardiol 1984;5:135.

175. McKenna WJ, England D, Doi Y, et al: Arrhythmia in hypertrophic cardiomyopathy. I. Influence on prognosis. Br Heart J 1981;46:168.

176. McKenna WJ: Arrhythmia and prognosis in hypertrophic cardiomyopathy. Eur Heart J 1983;4(Suppl F):225.

177. McKenna WJ, Harris L, Deanfield J: Syncope in hypertrophic cardiomyopathy. Br Heart J 1982;47:177.

178. Maron BJ, Roberts WC: Quantitative analysis of cardiac muscle cell disorganisation in the ventricular septum of patients with hypertrophic cardiomyopathy. Circulation 1979;59:689.

179. Watson RM, Schwartz JL, Maron BJ, Tucker E, Rosing DR, Josephson ME: Inducible polymorphic ventricular tachycardia and ventricular fibrillation in a subgroup of patients with hyperthrophic cardiomyopathy at high risk for sudden death. J Am Coll Cadiol 1987;10:761.

180. Teare D: Asymmetrical hypertrophy of the heart in young patients. Br Heart J 1958;20:1.

181. Fananapazir L, Tracey CM, Leon MB, et al: Electrophysiologic abnormalities in patients with hypertrophic cardiomyopathy. Circulation 1989;80:1259.

182. Jansson K, Dahlstrom U, Karlsson E, Nylander E, Walfrissdon H, Sonnhag C: The value of exercise test, Holter monitoring and programmed electrical stimulation in detection of ventricular arrhythmias in patients with hypertrophic cardiomyopathy. Pacing Clin Electrophysiol 1990;13:1261.

183. Fananapazir L, Epstein SE: Value of electrophysiologic studies in hypertropic cardiomyopathy treated with amiodarone. Am J Cardiol 1991;67:175.

184. Schiavone WA, Maloney JD, Lever HM, Castle LW, Sterba R, Morant V: Electrophysiologic studies of patients with hyper-

trophic cardiomyopathy presenting with syncope of undertermined etiology. Pacing Clin Electrophysiol 1986;9:476.

185. Aronson RS: Afterpotentials and triggered activity in hypertrophied myocardium from rates with renal-hypertension. Circ Res 1981;48:720.

186. Oakley CM: Prognosis in dilated cardiomyopathy related to left ventricular function, conduction defects and arrhythmia. In: Goodwin JF, Hjalmarson A, Olsen EGJ, eds. Congestive cardiomyopathy. Kiruna: AB Hassle, 1980:249.

187. Huang SK, Messer JV, Denes P: Significance of ventricular tachycardia in idiopathic dilated cardiomyopathy. Observation in 35 patients. Am J Cardiol 1983;51:507.

188. Meinertz T, Hofman T, Kasper W, et al: Significance of ventricular arrhythmias in idiopathic dilated cardiomyopathy. Am J Cardiol 1984;53:902.

189. DeMaria R, Gavazzi A, Caroli A, Ometto R, Biagini A, Camerini F: Ventricular arrhythmias in dilated cardiomyopathy as an independent prognostic hallmark. Am J Cardiol 1992; 69:1451.

190. Poll DS, Marchlinski FE, Falcone RA, Josephson ME, Simson MB: Abnormal signal-averaged electrocardiograms in patients with nonischemic congestive cardomyopathy: relationship to sustained ventricular tachyarrhythmias. Circulation 1985;72:1308.

191. Martins JB, Constantin L, Brownstein SL, Kienzle MG, Ashoff A: Entrainment of sustained ventricular tachycardia in patients with dilated cardiomyopathy suggests a reentry mechanism. Pacing Clin Electrophysiol 1989;12:682.

192. Poll DS, Marchlinski FE, Buxton AE, Josephson ME: Usefulness of programmed stimulation in idopathic dilated cardiomyopathy. Am J Cardiol 1986;58:992.

193. Brembilla-Perrot B, Donetti J, Terrier de la Chaise A, Sadoul N, Aliot E, Juilliere Y: Diagnostic value of ventricular stimulation in patients with idiopathic dilted cardiomyopathy. Am Heart J 1991;121:1124.

194. Lehmann MH, Steinman RT, Schuger CD, Jackson K: The automatic implantable cardioverter defibrillator as antiarrhythmic treatment modality of choice of survivors of cardiac arrest unrelated to acute myocardial infarction. Am J Cardiol 1988;62:803.

195. Reddy CP, Stack JD: Recurrent sustained ventricular tachycardia: Report of a case with His-bundle branches reentry as the mechanism. Eur J Cardiol 1980;11:23.

196. Lloyd EA, Zipes DP, Heger JJ, Prystowsky EN: Sustained macroreentrant ventricular tachycardia. Am Heart J 1982; 104:166.

197. Touboul P, Kirkorian G, Atallah G, Moleur P: Bundle branch reentry: a possible mechanism of ventricular tachycardia. Circulation 1983;67:674.

198. Touboul P, Kirkorian G, Atallah G, Lavaud P, Moleur P, Lanraud M, Mathiev M: Bundle branch reentrant tachycardia treated by electrical ablation of the right bundle branch. J Am Coll Cardiol 1986;7:1404.

199. Tchou P, Jzayeri M, Kenker S, Dongas J, Caceres J, Akhtar M: Transcatheter electrical ablation of the right bundle branch: a method of treating macro-reentrant ventricular tachycardia due to bundle branch reentry. Circulation 1988;78: 246.

200. Caceres J, Jazayeri M, McKinnie J, Avitall B, Denker ST, Tchou P, Akhtar M: Sustained bundle branch reentry as a mechanism of clinical tachycardia. Circulation 1989;79:256.

201. Cohen TD, Chien WW, Lurie KG, et al: Radiofrequency catheter ablation for treatment of bundle branch reentrant ventricular tachycardia: results and long-term follow-up. J Am Coll Cardiol 1991;18:1767.

202. Jervell A, Lange-Nielson F: Congenital deaf-mutism, functional heart disease with prolongation of the QT interval and sudden death. Am Heart J 1957;54:59.

203. Romano C, Gemme G, Pongiglione R: Aritmie cardiocha rare dell' eta' pediatrica. Clin Pediat (Bologna) 1963;45:656.

204. Von Bernuth G, Belz GG, Evertz W, Stauch M: QTU-abnormalities, sinus bradycardia and Adams-Stokes attacks due to ventricular tachyarrhythmia. Acta Paediatr Scand 1973; 62:675.

205. Curtiss EI, Heibel RH, Shaver JA: Autonomic maneuvers in hereditary QT interval prolongation (Romano-Ward) syndrome. Am Heart J 1978;95:420.

206. Schwartz PJ: The idiopathic long QT syndrome: the need for a prospective registry. Eur Heart J 1983;4:529.

207. Coumel PH, Rosengarten MD, Leclercq JF, Attuel P: Role of sympathetic nervous system in non-ischaemic ventricular arrhythmias. Br Heart J 1982;47:137.

208. Wu D, Kou HC, Hung JS: Exercise-triggered paroxysmal ventricular tachycardia: a repetitive rhythmic activity possibly related to afterdepolarization. Ann Intern Med 1981; 95:410.

209. Palileo EV, Ashley WW, Swiryn S, et al: Exercise provacable right ventricular outflow tract tachycardia. Am Heart J 1982; 104:185.

210. Sung RJ, Shen EN, Morady F, Scheinman MM, Hess D, Botvinick EH: Electrophysiologic mechanism of exercise-induced sustained ventricular tachycardia. Am J Cardiol 1983; 51:525.

211. Mont L, Seixas T, Brugada P, et al: Clinical and electrophysiologic characteristics of exercise-related idiopathic ventricular tachycardia. Am J Cardiol 1991;68:897.

212. Prociemer A, Ciani R, Fergulio GA: Right ventricular tachycardia with left bundle branch block and inferior axis morphology: Clinical and arrhythmological characteristics in 15 patients. Pacing Clin Electrophysiol 1989;12:977.

213. Gill JS, Blasyzk K, Ward DE, Camm AJ: Verapamil for the suppression of idiopathic ventricular tachycardia of left bundle branch block-like morphology. Am Heart J 1993;126:1126.

214. Lerman BB, Belardinelli L, West GA, Berne RM, DiMarco JP: Adenosine-sensitivie ventricular tachycardia: Evidence suggesting cyclic AMP-mediated triggered activity. Circulation 1986;74:271.

215. Wilber DJ, Baerman J, Olshansky B, Kall J, Kopp D: Adenosine-sensitive ventricular tachycardia: Clinical characteristics and response to catheter ablation. Circulation 1993; 87:126.

216. Lerman BB: Response of nonreentrant catecholamine-mediated ventricular tachycardia to endogenous adenosine and acetylcholine: Evidence for myocardial receptor-mediated effects. Circulation 1993;87:382.

217. Stevenson WG, Nademanee K, Weiss JN, Weiner I: Treatment of catecholamine-sensitive right ventricular tachycardia by catheter ablation. J Am Coll Cardiol 1990;16:752.

218. Morady F, Kadish AH, DiCarlo L, et al: Long-term results of catheter ablation of idiopathic right ventricular tachycardia. Circulation 1990;82:2093.

219. Breithardt G, Borggrefe M, Wichter T: Catheter ablation of idiopathic right ventricular tachycardia. Circulation 1990; 82:2273.

220. Fontaine G, Guiraudon G, Frank R: Stimulation studies and epicardial mapping in ventricular tachycardia: study of mechanisms and selection for surgery. In: Kulbertus H, ed. Reentrant arrhythmias Lancaster: MTP Publishing, 1977;334.

221. Child JS, Perloff JK, Franconz R, et al: Uhl's anomaly (parchment right ventricle): clinical, echocardiographic, radionuclear, hemodynamic and angiocardiographic features. Am J Cardiol 1984;53:635.

222. Marcus FI, Fontaine GH, Guiraudon G, et al: Right ventricular dysplasia: a report of 24 adult cases. Circulation 1982; 65:384.

223. Manyari DE, Klein GJ, Gulamhusein S, et al: Arrhythmogenic right ventricular dysplasia: a generalized cardiomyopathy? Circulation 1983;68:251.

224. Rossi P, Massumi A, Gillette P, Hall RJ: Arrhythmogenic right ventricular dysplasia: clinical features, diagnostic techniques and current management. Am Heart J 1982;103:415.

225. Lemery R, Brugada P, Janssen J, Cheriex E, Dugernier T, Wellens HJJ: Nonischemic sustained ventricular tachycardia: clinical outcome in 12 patients with arrhythmogenic right ventricular dysplasia. J Am Coll Cardiol 1989;14:96.

226. Ricci C, Longo R, Pagnan L, Palma LD, Pinamonti B, Camerini F, Bussani R, Silvestri F: Magnetic resonance imaging in right ventricular dysplasia. Am J Cardiol 1992;70:1589.

227. Baran A, Nanda NC, Falkoff M, Barold SS, Gallagher JJ: Two-dimensional echocardiographic detection of arrhythmogenic right ventricular dysplasia. Am Heart J 1982;103:1066.

228. Peters S, Hartwig CA, Reil GH: Risk assessment in nonischemic ventricular arrhythmia by left and right ventriculography. Am Heart J 1992;124:116.

229. Metzger JT, de Chillou C, Cheriex E, Rodriguez L-M, Smeets JLRM, Wellens HJJ: Value of the 12-lead electrocardiogram in arrhythmogenic right ventricular dysplasia, and absence of correlation with echocardiographic findings. Am J Cardiol 1993;72:964.

230. Wichter T, Borggrefe M, Haverkamp W, Chen X, Breithardt G: Efficacy of antiarrhythmic drugs in patients with arrhythmogenic right ventricular disease: Results in patients with inducible and noninducible ventricular tachycardia. Circulation 1992;86:29.

231. Guiraudon GM, Klein GJ, Gulamhusein SS, et al: Total disconnection of the right ventricular free wall: surgical reatment of right ventricular tachycardia associated with right ventricular dysplasia. Circulation 1983;67:463.

232. Cox JL, Bardy GH, Damiano RJ, et al: Right ventricular islation procedures or nonischemic ventricular tachycardia. J Thorac Cardiovasc Surg 1985;90:212.

233. Nimkhedkar K, Hilton CJ, Furniss SS, et al: Surgery for ventricular tachycardia associated with right ventricular dysplasia: disarticulation of right ventricle in 9 of 10 cases. J Am Coll Cardiol 1992;19:1079.

234. Leclercq JF, Chouty F, Couchemez B, Leenhardt A, Coumel P, Slama R: Results of electrical fulguration in arrhythmogenic right ventricular dysplasia. Am J Cardiol 1988;62:220.

235. Leclercq JF, Kural S, Valere PE: Bepridil et torsades de pointes. Arch Mal Coeur 1983;76:341.

236. Simcha A, Wells BG, Tynan MJ, Waterston DJ: Primary cardiac tumours in childhood. Arch Dis. Child 1971;46:508.

237. Bernstein M, Konzelmann FW, Sidlick DM: Boeck's saccoid: report of a case with visceral involvement. Arch Intern Med 1929;44:721.

238. Silverman KJ, Hutchins GM, Bulkley BH: Cardiac sarcoid: a clinicopathologic study of 84 selected patients with syustemic sarcoidosis. Circulation 1978;58:1204.

239. Winters SL, Cohen M, Greenberg S, et al: Sustained ventricular tachycardia associated with sarcoidosis: assessment of the underlying cardiac anatomy and the prospective utility of programmed ventricular simulation, drug therapy and an implantable antitachycardia device. J Am Coll Cardiol 1991; 18:937.

240. Belhassen B, Pines A, Laniado S: Failure of corticosteroid therapy to prevent induction of ventricular tachycardia in sarcoidosis. Chest 1989;95:918.

241. Naccarelli GV, Prystowsky EN, Jackman WM, et al: Role of electrophysiologic testing in managing patients who have ventricular tachycardia unrelated to coronary artery disease. Am J Cardiol 1982;50:165.

242. Buxton AE, Waxman HL, Marchlinski FE, Simson MB, Cassidy D, Josephson ME: Right ventricular tachycardia: clinical and electrophysiologic characteristics. Circulation 1983; 68:917.

243. Foale RA, Nihoyannopoulos P, Ribeiro P, et al: Right ventricular abnormalities in ventricular tachycardia of right ventricular origin: relation to electrophysiological abnormalities. Br Heart J 1986;65:45.

244. Brodsky MA, Orlov MV, Winters RJ, Allen BJ: Determinants of inducible ventricular tachycardia in patients with clinical ventricular tachyarrhythmia and no apparent structural heart disease. Am Heart J 1993;126:113.

245. Herre JM, Mann DE, Luck JC, et al: Effect of increased current multiple pacing sites and number of extrastimuli on induction of ventricular tachycardia. Am J Cardiol 1981;47:244.

246. Oseran DS, Gang ES, Hamer AW, et al: Mode of stimulation versus response: Validation of a protocol for induction of ventricular tachycardia. Am Heart J 1985;110:646.

247. Rossi L, Matturri L: Histopathological findings in two cases of torsade de pointes with conduction disturbances. Br Heart J 1976;38:1312.

248. Gallavardin L: Extrasystolic ventriculaire a paroxysmes tachycardiques prolonges. Arch Mal Coeur 1922;15:298.

249. Parkinson J, Papp C: Repetitive paroxysmal tachycardia. Br Heart J 1947;9:241.

250. Belhassen B, Rotmensch HH, Laniado S: Response of recurrent sustained ventricular tachycardia to verapamil. Br Heart J 1981;46:679.

251. Lin FC, Finley CD, Rahimtoola SH, Wu D: Idiopathic paroxysmal ventricular tachycardia with a QRS pattern of right bundle branch block and left axis deviation. A unique clinical entity with specific properties. A unique clinical entity with specific properties. Am J Cardiol 1983;52:95.

252. German LD, Packer DL, Bardy GH, Gallagher JJ: Ventricular tachycardia induced by atrial stimulation in patients without symptomatic cardiac disease. Am J Cardiol 1983;52:1202.

253. Belhassen B, Shapira I, Pelleg A, Copperman I, Kauli N,

Laniado SH: Idiopathic recurrent sustained ventricular tachycardia responsive to verapamil: an ECG-electrophysiologic entity. Am Heart J 1984;108:1034.

254. Mont L, Seixas T, Brugada P, et al: The electrocardiographic, clinical, and electrophysiologic spectrum of idiopathic monomorphic ventricular tachycardia. Am Heart J 1992; 124:746.

255. Okumura K, Matsuyama K, Miyagi H, Tsuchiya T, Yasue H: Entrainment of idiopathic ventricular tachycardia of left ventricular origin with evidence for reentry with an area of slow conduction and effect of verapamil. Am J Cardiol 1988; 62:727.

256. Nakagawa H, Beckman K, McClelland J, et al: Radiofrequency Catheter ablation of idiopathic left ventricular tachycardia guided by a Purkinje potential. Circulation 1993; 88:2607.

257. Ohe T, Simomura K, Aihara N, et al: Idiopathic sustained left ventricular tachycardia: clinical and electrophysiologic characteristics. Circulation 1988;77:560.

258. Sung RJ, Shapiro WA, Shen EN, Morady F: Effects of verapamil on ventricular tachycardia possibly caused by reentry, automaticity and triggered activity. J Clin Invest 1983; 72:350.

259. Mason JW, Winkle RA: Electrode-catheter arrhythmia induction in the selection and assessment of antiarrhythmic drug therapy for recurrent ventricular tachycardias. Circulation 1978;89:971.

260. Horowitz LN, Josephson ME, Kastor JA: Intracardiac electrophysiologic studies as a method for the optimizaton of drug therapy in chronic ventricular arrhythmia. Prog Cardiovasc Dis 1980;23:81.

261. Doherty JU, Josephson ME: Role of electrophysiologic testing in the therapy of ventricular arrhyuthmias. Pacing Clin Electrophysiol 1983;6:1070.

262. Breithardt G, Borggrefe M, Seipel L: Selection of optimal drug treatment of ventricular tachycardia by programmed electrical stimulation of the heart. Ann NY Acad Sci 1984; 427:49.

263. Reddy CP, Chen TJ, Guillory WR: Electrophysiologic studies in selection antiarrhythmic agents: use with ventricular tachycardia. Pacing Clin Electrophysiol 1986;9:759.

264. Waxman HL, Buston AE, Sadowski LM, et al: The response to procainamide during electrophysiologic study for sustained ventricular tachyarrhythmias predicts the response to other medication. Circulation 1982;67:30.

265. Oseran DS, Gang E, Rosenthal ME, et al: Electropharmacologic testing patients with sustained ventricular tachycardia: value of the response to intravenous procainamide in predicting the response to oral procainamide and oral quinidine. Am J Cardiol 1985;56:883.

266. Pires LA, Wagshal AB, Greene TO, Mittleman RS, Huang SKS: Usefulness of the response to intravenous procainamide during electrophysiologic study in predicting the response to oral quinidine in patients with inducible sustained monomorphic ventricular tachycardia associated with coronary artery disease. Am J Cardiol 1993;72:908.

267. Brodsky MA, Chough SP, Allen BJ, Caparell EV, Orlov MV, Caudillo G: Adjuvant metoprolol improves efficacy of class 1 arrhythmic drugs in patients with inducible sustained mnomorphic ventricular tachycardia. Am Heart J 1992; 124:629.

268. Hamer AN, Finerman WB, Peter T, Mandel WJ: Disparity between the clinical and electrophysiologic effects of amiodarone in the treatment of recurrent ventricular tachyarrhythmias. Am Heart J 1981;102:992.

269. McGovern B, Garan H, Malacoff R, et al: Long-term clinical outcome of ventricular tachycardia or fibrillation treated with amiodarone. Am J Cardiol 1984;53:1558.

270. Horowitz LN, Greenspan A, Spielman SR, et al: Usefulness of electrophysiologic testing in evaluation of 1miodarone therapy for sustained ventricular tachycardias associated with coronary heart disease. Am J Cardiol 1985;55:367.

271. Borggrefe M, Breithardt G: Predictive value of electrophysiologic testing in the treatment of drug-refactory ventricular arrhythmias with amiodarone. Eur Heart J 1986; 7:735.

272. Borggrefe M, Trampisch HJ, Breithardt G: Reappraisal of criteria for assessing drug efficacy in patients with ventricular tachyarrhythmias: complete versus partial suppression of inducible arrhuythmias. J Am Coll Cardiol 1988;12:140.

273. The ESVEM Investigators: The ESVEM trial: electrophysiologic study versus electrocardiographic monitoring for selection of antiarrhythmic therapy of ventricular tachyarrhythmias. Circulation 1989;79:1354.

274. Mason JW: A comparison of electrophysiologic testing with holter monitoring to predict antiarrhythmic-drug efficacy for ventricular tachyarrhythmias. N Engl J Med 1993;329:445.

275. The ESVEM Investigators: Determinnts of predicted efficacy of antiarrhythmic drugs in the electrophysiologic study versus electrocardiographic monitoring trial. Circulation 1993;87:323.

276. Greenspan AM: Determinants of antiarrhythmic drug efficacy of ventricular tachyarrhythmias using ambulatory monitoring and electrophysiological techniques. Circulation 1993;87:643.

277. Brugada P, Green M, Abdullah H, Wellens HJJ: Significance of ventricular arrhythmias initiated by programmed ventricular stimulation: the importance of the type of ventricular arrhythmia induced and the number of premature stimuli required. Circulation 1984;69:87.

278. Naccarelli GV, Prytowsky EN, Jackman WM, et al: Repetitive ventricular response. Prevalence and prognostic significance. Br Heart J 1981;46:152.

279. Gomes JAC, Kang PS, Khan R, et al: Repetitive ventricular response. Its incidence, inducibility, reproducibility, mechanism, and significance. Br Heart J 1981;46:159.

Cardiac Arrhythmias, 3rd edition, edited by William J. Mandel.
J. B. Lippincott Company, Philadelphia © 1995.

22

G. Michael Vincent

Inherited Long-QT Syndrome

The inherited long-QT syndrome is characterized by prolongation of the QT interval on the electrocardiogram (ECG; Fig. 22-1) and by syncope and sudden death due to ventricular tachyarrhythmias, particularly torsades de pointes (Fig. 22-2).[1-6] Although once thought to be rare, the syndrome is not and is a frequent cause of sudden unexpected death in children and young adults. Two forms of the syndrome have been recognized: the Jervell and Lange-Nielsen and the Romano-Ward varieties.[1-6] In addition to the inherited syndrome, sporadic cases have been identified with similar clinical findings but in whom no familial occurrence is evident. Furthermore, other forms of heart disease and many drugs cause prolongation of the QT interval and an acquired long-QT syndrome.[7-8]

JERVELL AND LANGE-NIELSEN SYNDROME

The first clear recognition of an inherited long-QT syndrome was provided in 1957 by Jervell and Lange-Nielsen, who described a Norwegian family characterized by congenital deaf mutism, recurrent "fainting attacks," QT-interval prolongation on the ECG, and sudden death in children. Although Jervell and Lange-Nielsen are credited with recognition of the syndrome, earlier descriptions were likely given by Meissner in 1856, who described a deaf female student who died suddenly while being reprimanded by the school director and who had two sibs who had died suddenly after emotional outbursts; Morquio, who in 1901 reported a Uruguayan family in which five of eight children had recurrent syncope, with sudden death occurring in four; and Moller in 1953.[9-11] QT-interval prolongation was not identified in the reports of Meissner and Morquio because the ECG was not developed by Einthoven until 1903 but it was present in the case described by Moller. In Jervell and Lange-Nielsen's report, the familial nature of the syndrome was evident and autosomal recessive transmission was suspected. The parents and two of six children had normal hearing and no fainting episodes. The other four children were deaf and had recurrent episodes of sudden loss of consciousness, which began around the age of 3 to 5 years, occurring during exercise and anxiety. Their history was otherwise unremarkable, as were their physical examinations, chest x-rays, and laboratory studies, including serum potassium and calcium. Prominent QT-interval prolongation was

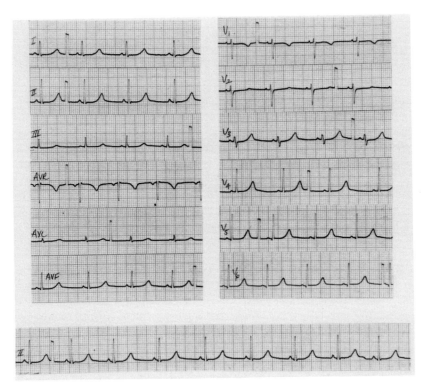

Figure 22-1. Twelve-lead electrocardiogram from an H-*ras*-1 gene carrier. QTc is 0.49, T waveform is normal.

noted on the resting ECGs, with QTc (QT interval corrected for heart rate, typically by Bazett's formula) intervals ranging from 0.49 to 0.53 sec$^{1/2}$. Three of the four affected children died during an attack at the ages of 4, 5, and 9 years, respectively. An autopsy on one child disclosed no evidence of structural heart disease. The au-

thors found that the QT interval was further lengthened by exercise, quinidine administration, and injection of adrenaline.

In 1958, Levine and Woodworth provided the second report of this syndrome and confirmed the new entity.[2] They reported an 8-year-old boy with congenital deafness,

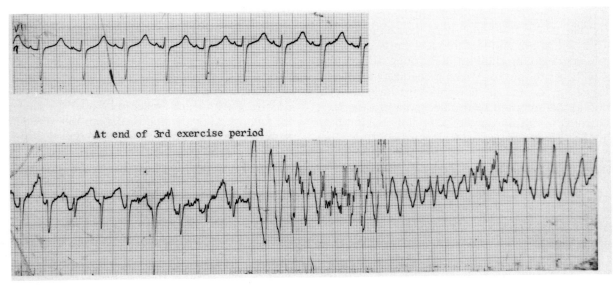

Figure 22-2. Torsade de pointes, which occurred during an exercise test in a 15-year-old symptomatic male. The V$_1$ strip at the top was taken during early exercise, and the arrhythmia occurred at near maximal exercise.

QT-interval prolongation, variable but sometimes bizarre T waves, and a history of syncope during fright, anger, or swimming. The clinical examination, including electrolytes, was normal. QT interval duration and T-wave morphology were variable, and notching of the T wave, particularly in the lateral precordial leads, was noted. Unlike the cases of Jervell and Lange-Nielsen, in which epinephrine further lengthened the QT interval, the QT interval was not changed by administration of epinephrine, insulin, or neostigmine nor by carotid artery massage, hyperventilation, or exposure to anxiety-provoking stimuli.

This autosomal recessive form of the syndrome, with congenital deafness, was initially called the cardioauditory syndrome or the surdocardiac syndrome but is referred to as the Jervell and Lange-Nielsen syndrome or the autosomal recessive form of long-QT syndrome. Relatively few cases have been described over the years, and this form of the inherited long-QT syndrome appears to be rare.

ROMANO-WARD SYNDROME

An autosomal dominant form, with normal hearing, was described in 1963 independently by Romano and co-workers in Italy and by Ward in Ireland.[4–6] In the few years thereafter, several cases and family studies were reported.[12–28] Except for the absence of deafness, the clinical features are similar to those of the autosomal recessive form, with syncope and sudden death occurring most often during exercise and emotional stimuli, although deaths during sleep are not uncommon. As in the Jervell and Lange-Nielsen form, the physical and laboratory examinations are normal. This autosomal dominant form of the syndrome is often referred to as the Romano-Ward syndrome. It has been identified in essentially all races and ethnic groups. As discussed in the next section, this form of the syndrome appears to be common.

FREQUENCY OF LONG-QT SYNDROME

The frequency is unknown but almost certainly it is more prevalent than commonly believed. It is likely that just the tip of the iceberg of this syndrome has been identified. Initially, the syndrome was thought to be rare. This appears to be the case for the autosomal recessive form of Jervell and Lange-Nielsen. Even the authors of early reports of the autosomal dominant form of Romano-Ward syndrome suggested it was more unrecognized than rare, and observations support this concept. For example, when a new case is identified, usually a few or no other family members have been studied, even though it is a familial condition. This mistake obviously limits the number of recognized cases. In addition, this approach only identifies the symptomatic, more severe, and blatant cases, skewing the observations and characterization of the syndrome, affecting both diagnosis and treatment decisions. Many readers recall such an experience with hypertrophic cardiomyopathy, which was initially referred to as idiopathic hypertrophic subaortic stenosis (IHSS) because of the early finding of subaortic obstruction. Subsequently, it has become apparent that this is only one and not necessarily the most frequent manifestation of the disease. Therefore, the terminology has shifted from IHSS to familial hypertrophic cardiomyopathy. Ongoing genetic studies demonstrate substantial genotypic and phenotypic heterogeneity, showing a wide variety of clinical and echocardiographic manifestations of the disease. Patients are identified as gene carriers who never would have been diagnosed as having IHSS based on initial limited understanding of the disease. This same phenomenon is occurring with the inherited long-QT syndrome. With respect to frequency of diagnosis, the following experience is illustrative. In 1973, we began to study an autosomal dominant long-QT syndrome family of Danish ancestry. Desiring to identify as many affected family members as possible, we used a proactive approach to case finding; we used family and other genealogy records to find the members and over many years constructed a nine-generation pedigree, consisting of more than 1500 members. Most of the family groups do not know they are related. We estimate that our pedigree to date represents about half of the members of this large family. As the members were identified, they were contacted and a history and ECG were obtained from as many as possible. We have screened more than 1000 individuals and more than 150 members affected with long-QT syndrome have been identified. Had we stopped our investigation with the proband of this family, only a single case would have been identified and reported, as opposed to the 150 (and growing) cases, all from just one family. Many of the affected members were identified in the presymptomatic stage and might never have been correctly identified or would have shown up as a sudden death of unknown cause. We have subsequently used this approach on several other (albeit smaller) families, with similar success in identification of affected members.

Other observations also suggest that long-QT syndrome is not uncommon. In 1985, Moss, Schwartz, and Crampton established the International Long QT Syndrome Registry in an attempt to study several long-QT syndrome patients over a protracted period.[29,30] No attempt has been made to collect all long-QT syndrome patients in the registry, yet about 2000 known or suspected long-QT syndrome patients have been entered. A nonprofit charitable foundation, the Sudden Arrhythmia Death Syndromes Foundation (SADS Foundation, Salt

Lake City, UT), was formed to assist in research and education regarding long-QT syndrome and to help prevent the tragic sudden deaths of children and young adults affected by the syndrome. The foundation has invested considerable effort in a public-awareness campaign and in increased physician education regarding long-QT syndrome. As physicians and the lay public have become more aware of the condition, the number of newly identified cases has markedly increased. For example, over the 9-month period from April to December 1993, more than 9000 individuals called the foundation expressing concern over unexplained syncope or sudden death in family members. During that time, many ECGs were sent by these callers to the foundation for review. About 1000 ECGs, exercise tests, and ambulatory recordings from 311 individuals have been reviewed; 61 people have been newly identified as long-QT syndrome patients, representing an astounding 20% of those screened. Thus, whereas the frequency of the inherited long-QT syndrome is unknown, it is clear that it is more frequent than commonly believed and it appears to be a common cause of unexplained syncope and sudden death in children and young adults.

GENETICS OF LONG-QT SYNDROME

The inherited nature of the syndrome was recognized in the initial reports of the syndrome.[1-6] Over many years, little additional information regarding the genetics of the syndrome was added. Now, however, using the numerous tools for studying molecular biology, the genetic basis of the syndrome is being unraveled. It is clear that at least four genes can cause long-QT syndrome. No specific disease genes have been identified but one responsible gene is located on chromosome 11. This was identified in our large autosomal dominant long-QT syndrome family of Danish origin, described earlier in this chapter. Using the technique of linkage analysis, Keating and associates identified tight linkage with the Harvey-ras-1 (H-ras-1) gene on the short arm of chromosome 11 at 11p15.5.[31] Subsequently, additional families were found to link to the H-ras-1 locus.[32] The H-ras-1 gene is apparently not the disease gene because sequencing of the H-ras-1 gene has proved it to be normal; yet the tight linkage with H-ras-1 confirms that the disease gene is in close proximity to this locus, although it has not yet been identified. Linkage studies in additional families reveal that about 50% do not link to the H-ras-1 locus.[33-36] The genetic abnormality in these families is therefore on another portion of chromosome 11 or on a different chromosome. Recently, some of these families have been linked to markers at two other loci, and some families do not link to any of these three

loci, demonstrating that at least four genes can cause the long QT syndrome. It is not known whether families with the recessive form of Jervell and Lange-Nielsen syndrome link to H-ras-1. One study of two children showed no linkage but the small number of study subjects precludes accurate linkage-analysis interpretation.[37]

The syndrome demonstrates reduced penetrance and variable expressivity.[38] Reduced penetrance means that not all the affected individuals show the clinical manifestations (phenotype) of the disease. This was demonstrated in a study of 199 members of three autosomal dominant long-QT syndrome families, which included 83 H-ras-1 gene carriers.[38] The prolonged QT interval and syncope are the principle phenotypic manifestations of this syndrome. A third of H-ras-1 gene carriers had no history of syncope or presyncope, and 5% of gene carriers had a normal QT interval, demonstrating the reduced penetrance. Variable expressivity refers to a variable expression of a phenotype. The same study showed a wide range of resting QTc intervals in the 83 gene carriers, ranging from 0.41 to 0.59.[38] The reduced penetrance and variable expressivity have important ramifications for diagnosis and treatment.

CLINICAL CHARACTERISTICS OF LONG-QT SYNDROME

Symptoms

Syncope and sudden death are the characteristic events in this syndrome. They usually occur during or less commonly just after physical exertion or at times of emotional stress such as anger or fright. Sudden vigorous exercise or sudden emotional stimulation seems most likely to precipitate these events, although they may occur during more protracted exercise and emotional upset. The combination of emotional factors (i.e., excitement) and exercise, as may occur with sports competition, is a common set of precipitating circumstances. Running, frightening experiences, arguing, entry into a swimming pool, and swimming are common precipitating factors. Symptoms rarely occur while awake and at rest. Occasionally, sudden death occurs during sleep. Some patients experience syncope when exposed to a loud or unexpected noise (e.g., an alarm clock, siren). Some patients recognize premonitory feelings, usually consisting of palpitations or presyncope, and can abort the syncopal attack if they stop exercising or remove themselves from a stressful circumstance. Frequent premature ventricular beats or brief and episodic bursts of ventricular tachycardia have been recorded during these presyncopal symptoms in some patients. More commonly, the syncope occurs without warning and the patient has no ability to prevent the event. Sudden death may occur with the first or second episode in a significant number of patients, and this influences the treatment of asymptomatic patients. Those patients who have sudden death during sleep usually have only one or two or no prior episodes. Some patients experience many—even hundreds—of syncopal events without sudden death. About a third of affected individuals never have syncope.

The symptoms most often begin about age 8 to 14 years—earlier, on average, in males than in females. The symptoms may first occur as early as the first weeks of life or as late as 20 to 30 years of age but uncommonly begin at ages older than 30 to 40 years. When symptoms first occur after this age, there are often concurrent aggravating factors such as hypokalemia or the use of drugs that prolong the QT interval; some of the more common drugs are listed in Table 22-1. Combinations of drugs such as terfenedine and ketoconazole or terfenedine and erythromycin seem to be particularly problematic. Also, the use of these drugs may be a factor in some of the patients who experience sudden death during sleep.

In many patients, the frequency of symptoms decreases over time, particularly as the patient enters the second and third decade. Some patients have just a few syncopal episodes as a child and none throughout the remainder of a normal life span.

Physical Examination

The physical examination is normal. Numerous reports describe autopsy findings, and both gross and microscopic examination of the heart are usually normal.[39-45] Bharati and colleagues reviewed the findings in the conduction system of the heart.[39] In a few cases, a variety of abnormalities were found, without consistency of the findings from one case to another. The abnormalities include inflammation of the myocardium, the perisinoatrial nerves, and the specialized conduction pathways of the atria in addition to patchy fibrosis, fibroelastosis, and pathologic changes in the sinoatrial node, bundle of His, the left bundle, and the Purkinje cells. Electron microscopy in one case showed shortened sarcomeres in the myocardium. Although some of the findings may influence the predisposition to ventricular arrhythmias, none easily explain the QT-interval prolongation, and the relation of these findings to the pathophysiology of the syndrome is unclear.

ELECTROCARDIOGRAM

The ECG has been the principle diagnostic tool in this syndrome but the limitations of this test have become apparent, making the diagnosis of the syndrome more difficult and challenging.

The ECG is similar in the recessive and dominant forms of the syndrome. A typical ECG is shown in Figure 22-1. No consistent abnormalities of the PR interval, P-wave morphology, QRS duration, or QRS morphology have been identified. Syncope and sudden death are due to torsades de pointes, as shown in Figure 22-2.

Heart Rate

On average, the resting heart rate is lower than normal in long-QT syndrome patients up to the age of about 5 years.[51] The overlap with normal patients is large, and this finding has limited diagnostic use. At ages older than 5 years, the resting heart rate is usually normal but a chronotropic abnormality is still evident during exercise, manifest by a maximal heart rate that is lower than normal.[52] Again, the overlap with normal patients is significant and the exercise heart rate abnormality has limited diagnostic use. The heart rate findings are important to the considerations of pathophysiology, however, and are discussed further in that section.

QT Interval

Prolongation of the QT interval is the hallmark of the syndrome but it is not always present. The ability to identify patients by gene carrier status rather than by QT-interval prolongation has allowed study of the distribution of QT-interval durations in genetically proved long-QT patients.[38] From these studies, it is known that the QTc interval at rest is normal in a percentage of long-QT patients—about 5% in the H-ras-1 gene carrier studies. In many other patients, the QT-interval is only modestly prolonged and the overlap with normal patients is substantial. These observations have important ramifications

TABLE 22-1. Drugs That Prolong the QT Interval

Quinidine and similar class IA antiarrhythmic drugs
Erythromycin
Terfenedine
Astemizole
Ketoconazole
Fluconazole
Phenothiazines
Tricyclic antidepressants
Diuretics with potential to reduce potassium

for diagnosis. The average QTc interval is about 0.49, with a range from 0.41 to 0.65 or higher.[38, 53] The duration of the QTc interval is related to risk of syncope and sudden death, with longer QTc intervals indicating a greater risk.[53] At particularly long QTc intervals (e.g., more than 0.60), the risk appears to be high but over a wide range of lower QTc intervals, the relation cannot be used to predict individual risk with certainty. Syncope and sudden death occur in patients with normal to borderline QTc prolongation. The most recent death in the families we follow up occurred in a 15-year-old male with a QTc of 0.45 on his resting ECG. In contrast, other patients with QTc intervals greater than 0.50 have no symptoms over a long life (Fig. 22-3). In most patients, the QT interval is persistently prolonged, although it varies in duration from one time to another. In other patients, the QT interval may be normal at times and prolonged at other times. In perhaps 5% of patients, the QT interval is consistently normal to borderline. An example is shown in Figure 22-4 from an H-*ras*-1 gene carrier. This patient had received the gene from his father and had transmitted the syndrome to his children. He had several typical exercise-induced syncopal episodes as a child, before treatment with beta blockers. He has been asymptomatic on medication.

An abnormal relation between QT-interval duration

and exercise-induced changes in cycle length is a characteristic feature of the syndrome. Although in normal patients the QT interval shortens with decreases in cycle length, patients with long-QT syndrome may have a paradoxical lengthening of the QT interval or inadequate QT-interval shortening relative to the cycle length. Figure 22-5A shows the normal exercise relation between QT interval and the QS_2 interval, which is used as a gold standard for QT response. The two variables track essentially the same. Contrast this response to that of long-QT patients (see Fig. 22-5B). The QT interval does not shorten as much as does QS_2, demonstrating the abnormal response of the QT interval to exercise. The dramatic paradoxical QT lengthening during exercise was described in the initial report of the syndrome by Jervell and Lange-Nielsen and the observation has been confirmed subsequently by several authors.[1] An example of this type of ECG response is shown in Figure 22-6. More commonly, the QT interval shortens with increasing heart rate but the decrease is less than normal; this can be identified by an increase in QTc during and shortly after exercise (Fig. 22-7). These observations have diagnostic and possibly prognostic significance.

The repolarization properties of long-QT syndrome patients have also been evaluated by QT-dispersion mea-

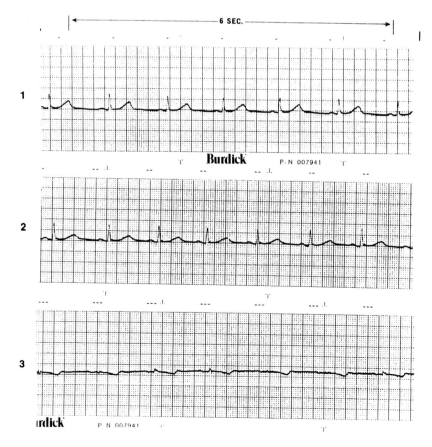

Figure 22-3. A three-lead electrocardiogram (ECG) from a 37-year-old asymptomatic female with QTc of 0.56. Serial ECGs over a number of years all showed QTc prolongation of this degree, yet she has remained asymptomatic through her current age of 43 years.

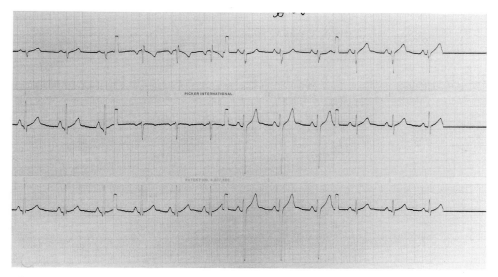

Figure 22-4. An electrocardiogram (ECG) during early exercise from an H-*ras*-1 gene carrier, showing a QTc of 0.45. Some resting ECGs showed QTc intervals as low as 0.41. The patient was symptomatic with syncope at the time this ECG was taken.

surements[54–56] and by body surface mapping techniques.[54–59] Dispersion is evaluated by measuring the QT or QTc interval in each of the 12 leads of the ECG. The difference between the longest and shortest intervals has been termed the QT or QTc dispersion measurement. An increase in QT–QTc dispersion measurement is thought to reflect increased regional disparity of recovery and increased vulnerability to ventricular arrhythmias and

sudden death.[60–62] QTc dispersion is larger at rest in long-QT syndrome patients than in normal patients and becomes more abnormal during exercise, perhaps reflecting the increased vulnerability to arrhythmias that accompanies exercise in these patients.[54] Beta-blocking medications and left cervicothoracic ganglionectomy decrease the dispersion at rest, and beta blockers prevent or limit the increase with exercise.[54,55] The reduced dispersion

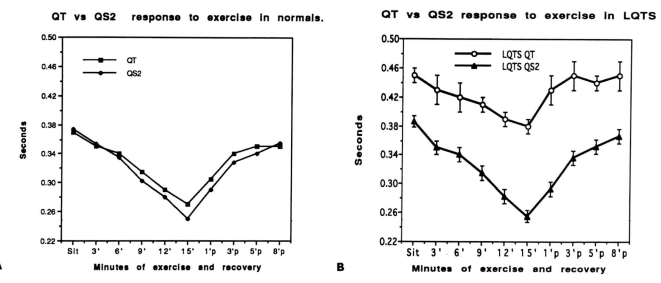

Figure 22-5. In this figure, the QT-interval response to exercise in long-QT syndrome (LQTS) patients and normal subjects is compared. The QS_2 interval is used as a "gold standard" for QT-interval response. In normal subjects, (**A**) 5a the QT and QS_2 respond nearly identically. (**B**) In the long-QT patient group, however, the QT does not shorten to the same degree as the QS_2, demonstrating the defect in QT response to exercise.

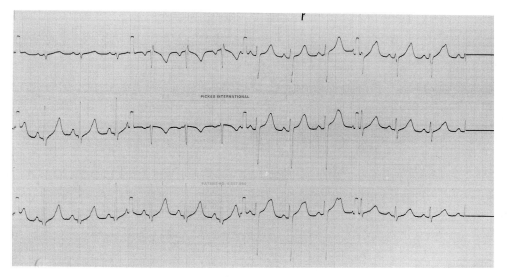

Figure 22-6. An electrocardiogram from the same patient as in Figure 22-4, taken at one minute after exercise. The QTc is now 0.54, compared with 0.45 in early exercise. Note also the development of the two-component bifid T wave, particularly in V$_3$ and V$_4$.

produced by these interventions may indicate a reduction of vulnerability, observations that may be useful for predicting the efficacy of treatment. Mapping of body surface potentials from multiple sites shows complex and multipolar distributions that are consistent with increased regional disparity of recovery, and prominent negative potentials on the anterior thorax, consistent with delayed recovery in the anterior regions of the heart.[57–59]

T-Wave Morphology

The T-wave morphology is dynamic in this syndrome; in a given patient, changes in morphology from one recording to another are common. Often, the T-wave morphology is normal (see Fig. 22-1). In other patients, the T waves may be large, biphasic, or inverted. In many patients, there are bifid or two-component T waves (see Fig. 22-6). In some

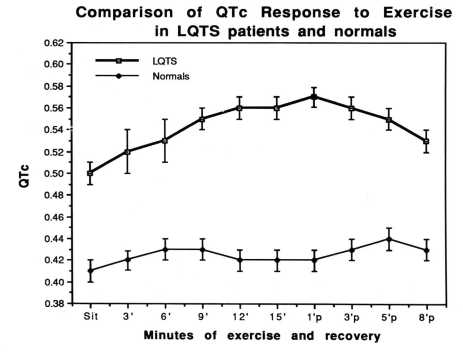

Comparison of QTc Response to Exercise in LQTS patients and normals

Figure 22-7. The QTc response to exercise in patients with long-QT syndrome (LQTS). Because the QT interval does not shorten appropriately with increases in heart rate (see Fig. 22-5), the QTc-interval increases, with a further increase in the early recovery period.

patients, bifid T waves are present in resting ECGs. In others, these T-wave changes are seen during exercise. Bifid T waves are normal in leads V_2 and V_3 in children because T-wave transition from inverted to upright occurs. In long-QT syndrome patients, however, the bifid T waves are present in limb or lateral precordial leads also. A less common but characteristic T-wave abnormality is T-wave alternans, in which the T wave is alternately upright and inverted in the most blatant cases and of variable amplitude on alternate beats in the less dramatic cases. This pattern, as is the case in other cardiac disease states, reflects increased electric instability and usually indicates a high risk of arrhythmias. It is often seen in the periarrhythmia period.

LABORATORY EXAMINATION

Blood Studies

No abnormalities are evident on usual laboratory examination. Specifically, the usual hematologic and chemistry examinations are normal. Because of the QT-interval prolongation, abnormalities of potassium, calcium, or magnesium have been specifically considered as the possible cause of this syndrome; however, the blood levels of these ions are normal. Muscle enzymes and isoenzymes are normal.

X-Ray Studies

The chest x-ray shows a normal heart size and configuration, normal pulmonary examination, and normal bony and soft-tissue structures.

Echocardiography

Cardiac structure and function are normal by usual analytic techniques. The incidence of mitral valve prolapse is similar to that of the general population. One study demonstrated peculiar left ventricular wall motion abnormalities using novel analytic methods.[46] Two mechanical abnormalities were identified; more rapid early contraction of the ventricular wall and a longer time at a low thickening rate just before fast relaxation. These observations are important because they represent the first evidence of structural or functional impairment of the heart and therefore may have particular bearing on understanding the pathophysiology of the syndrome. The findings have not yet been confirmed by other investigators and cannot be

recommended for routine use but may become important for diagnosis and prognosis in the future.

^{123}I-Metaiodobenzylguanidine and Positron Emission Tomography Imaging

It has become possible to noninvasively examine cardiac sympathetic innervation using two catecholamine analogues, ^{123}I-metaiodobenzylguanidine (MIBG) and ^{11}C-hydroxyephedrine (HED). These agents are taken up by sympathetic nerve terminals and their distribution in the heart can be evaluated by single-photon emission computed tomography for MIBG and by positron emission tomography (PET) for HED. An abnormality of the sympathetic nervous system has been proposed for the pathophysiology of long-QT syndrome, specifically implicating diminished right cardiac sympathetic effect with reflex overactivity of the left system. It may be expected that the right sympathetic deficiency proposed for the syndrome would result in reduced numbers of the sympathetic nerve terminals and catecholamine concentrations, as demonstrated in animal models with sympathetic denervation. These abnormalities may be demonstrated by these imaging techniques. The few human studies reported have produced variable and conflicting results. Three studies using MIBG imaging have been reported.[47–49] One showed normal and homogenous distribution, similar to normal subjects.[47] Two showed regional disparities of tracer uptake but found the abnormality to be in different areas within the heart. In one, the decreased uptake was generally in the anterior and lateral walls near the apex but a variety different patterns was seen among the patients in the study.[49] The other study examined 12 members of a family having five symptomatic patients, four with long-QT intervals. All five showed decreased activity in the inferior and septal areas of the left ventricle. Scans on seven asymptomatic members with normal QT intervals showed a similar inferior defect in three, raising concern about the specificity of the scan result.[48] Positron emission tomography scintigraphy with ^{11}C HED is considered to be more accurate than single-photon emission computed tomography imaging and may clarify the discrepancy seen in these MIBG studies. A study of nine patients with the syndrome showed normal uptake and distribution of HED, thus, cardiac sympathetic innervation was normal as assessed by HED. Given the variability of the MIBG results and the normal HED results, the weight of evidence suggests that no abnormalities of sympathetic innervation are demonstrable in long-QT syndrome patients by these imaging techniques. They have no diagnostic or prognostic use at the present time but may have importance for further investigational studies.

PATHOPHYSIOLOGY OF LONG-QT SYNDROME

The pathophysiology of the syndrome is still unknown. Interestingly, several early reports on patients with the autosomal recessive form of Jervell and Lange-Nielsen described episodes of pallor, sweating, abdominal and chest pain associated with marked QT- and T-wave changes but a normal pulse, and a normal rhythm on ECG.[3,63,64] Similarly, the pulse was normal during a syncopal spell in the Romano-Ward patient described by Levine and Woodworth.[2] These observations suggest a systemic response, such as intense sympathetic stimulation, rather than an arrhythmia as a cause for the symptoms. Subsequently, it was evident that the symptoms were regularly associated with arrhythmias, particularly torsades de pointes.[4,6,64-66] Uncommonly, the syncope is precipitated by asystole.[64-66] Perhaps the observations of a normal pulse during episodes were due to a delay in examining the patient, with a brief episode of torsades de pointes or asystole occurring before the examination.

A variety of pathophysiologic mechanisms have been considered over the years. A cardiac metabolic abnormality involving potassium or calcium was suggested in the initial reports of the Jervell and Lange-Nielsen form. Also, the earliest reports of this syndrome made it evident that the symptoms and sudden death occur most commonly during times of sympathetic stimulation such as exercise or fright. This observation led Jervell and Lange-Nielsen to suspect that an abnormality of the adrenergic nervous system was responsible for the syndrome.[1] These two hypotheses—an intracardiac abnormality or sympathetic imbalance—remain the principal considerations. They have been discussed extensively elsewhere and are only presented in overview here.[67-70] There are several characteristic findings of long-QT syndrome that must be explained by any hypothesis. These include:

1. Prolonged QT interval
2. Abnormal response of the QT interval to exercise
3. Bifid T waves
4. T-wave alternans
5. Abnormally slow resting heart rate or impaired exercise heart rate response
6. Vulnerability to torsades de pointes arrhythmias
7. Failure to induce the arrhythmias by programmed electric stimulation at catheterization
8. Apparent presence of afterdepolarizations on intracardiac recordings
9. Common precipitation of syncope by events that stimulate the sympathetic nervous system.

Sympathetic Imbalance Hypothesis

It is well known that abnormalities of the sympathetic nervous system can affect cardiac electrophysiology, resulting in QT-interval prolongation on the ECG and arrhythmias.[71-75] Armed with these observations and an extensive body of animal experiment data linking the sympathetic system with QT-interval prolongation and arrhythmias, Schwartz and coworkers advanced the sympathetic imbalance hypothesis.[76] This proposes a deficiency of the right cardiac sympathetic nervous system as the fundamental defect, accompanied by reflex overactivity of the left sympathetic system. The resultant right–left imbalance causes regional disparity of sympathetic effects on recovery properties, manifest as QT-interval prolongation, T-wave morphology changes, and vulnerability to ventricular arrhythmias. This is an attractive hypothesis because it seems to explain most of the findings of the syndrome and is supported by many experimental animal studies. The MIBG and positron emission tomography studies discussed above, which in aggregate show no evidence of sympathetic denervation or regional disparity of sympathetic mediator concentration, may cast some doubt on this hypothesis. The inability to precipitate torsades de pointes by programmed electric stimulation in patients with the syndrome suggests that disparity of recovery and reentry are not the mechanism of the arrhythmias in these patients. Also, the sympathetic imbalance hypothesis does not explain the occasional sporadic cases of long-QT syndrome nor the marked similarity of drug-induced QT-interval prolongation syndromes to the inherited form. Recent studies, however, suggest that congenital sympathetic deficiency may adversely influence the development of cardiac ion channels; thus, the sympathetic imbalance and intracardiac hypotheses may be unified by these observations.[77,78]

Intracardiac Abnormality Hypothesis

An abnormality of cardiac cellular function, particularly potassium, calcium, or magnesium metabolism, was suspected in the initial reports of Jervell and Lange-Nielson and Romano and Ward because of the long known relation of these ions to QT-interval prolongation and ventricular arrhythmias. Serum levels of these ions have been evaluated in many cases and found to be normal. The contemporary hypothesis proposes that an abnormality of an ion channel is present and leads to early afterdepolarization (EAD) and triggered activity, which are the cause of the repolarization abnormalities and torsades de pointes. An abnormality of the delayed rectifier potassium current may be the most likely culprit.

Both clinical observations and animal experimental data provide support for this hypothesis. Many drugs lengthen the QT interval and predispose patients to torsades de pointes arrhythmias.[7,8] Quinidine and other class IA antiarrhythmic drugs, the macrolide antibiotic erythromycin, the nonsedating antihistaminics terfenedine and astemizole, and the antifungal drugs ketoconazole and fluconazole are examples. One effect of these drugs is to block the delayed rectifier potassium current, producing QT-interal prolongation and torsades de pointes arrhythmias in some patients. Only a few patients exposed to these drugs develop torsades de pointes, suggesting variable susceptibility. This may be due to variable P-450 system metabolism of the drugs but also may suggest that subclinical abnormalities of delayed rectifier potassium channel function exist (i.e., subclinical or atypical cases of long-QT syndrome). In either case, patients who are electrophysiologically compensated in the absence of these drugs may develop QT-interval prolongation and torsades de pointes when exposed to the agents. A similar inhibition of the delayed rectifier current in animal models by such drugs and also cesium chloride produces a clinical picture similar to the inherited long-QT syndrome, including prolongation of the QT interval, bifid T waves, EADs, and torsades de pointes. Recordings of monophasic action potentials in long-QT syndrome patients show apparent EADs similar to those seen in some of the drug-induced models.[79-83] Sympathetic stimulation increases the amplitude of the afterdepolarizations, producing triggered automaticity and torsades de pointes arrhythmias. Beta blockers and verapamil diminish the EAD amplitude and occurrence of torsades de pointes. The QT-interval prolongation and bifid T waves appear to correspond to the presence and size of the EADs. Thus, the hypothesis of impaired delayed rectifier potassium current seems to explain the clinical characteristics of the inherited long-QT syndrome, including long-QT interval, bifid T waves, afterdepolarizations, the propensity to torsades de pointes, and the relation to the sympathetic nervous system. The proposal for afterdepolarizations as the mechanism of the arrhythmia is also consistent with inability to induce torsades de pointes by programmed electrical stimulation at electrophysiologic study. The one clinical characteristic that is not so obviously explained by the potassium channel hypothesis is the low heart rate at rest or during exercise in these patients. A refinement of the hypothesis explains this finding. The "G protein hypothesis" proposes that the long-QT gene encodes for a G protein, which is responsible for signaling in ion channels and also in β-adrenergic pathways—specifically, the pacemaker channel of the sinus node. If the gene mutation leads to an abnormal G protein, with reduced signal transduction ability, impaired function of ion channels affected by this protein and reduced sinus node responsiveness to sympathetic tone would result, manifest as the repolarization abnormalities and heart rate abnormalities, respectively. The G protein hypothesis was stimulated by the genetic linkage studies mentioned earlier, in which the H-ras-1 gene, a G protein, was identified as the marker gene. Ras proteins are intermediaries in some potassium channels and participate in heart rate regulation by receptor–effector coupling in the pacemaker channel.[84,85] Thus, it appears that an abnormal G protein affecting ion channel and pacemaker channel function could explain all the features of the syndrome.

Evidence has also been presented to suggest that M cells are involved in the pathogenesis of the QT-interval prolongation and torsades de pointes and may represent an alternate or cofactor explanation to a disorder of potassium conductance.[86]

In summary, much remains to be done to elucidate the molecular physiology of long-QT syndrome and the mechanism of QT-interval prolongation and torsades de pointes arrhythmias. Evidence suggests that both EADs and dispersion of recovery participate in the pathophysiology of the syndrome; a potential explanation that combines these mechanisms may be that EADs produce the QT-interval prolongation, T-wave morphology changes, and the initiating mechanism for torsades de pointes, whereas increased dispersion of recovery and reentry are the substrate for sustaining the torsades de pointes.

DIAGNOSIS

The diagnosis of the syndrome is straightforward in a patient with exercise-induced syncope, documented torsades de pointes, a family history of long-QT syndrome, and a markedly prolonged QTc interval (e.g., 0.60 seconds). Most of the time, however, not all of these features are present and not infrequently, the diagnosis is difficult and complex.

History

The history is important. As mentioned, the symptoms usually occur in children and young adults, most often during physical exertion or emotional stress, sometimes during sleep, but not often during rest or usual daily activities. A syncopal episode occurring during physical activity or precipitated by a sudden fright or loud noise should immediately raise the possibility of long-QT syndrome. Recurrent syncope under these conditions is particularly an indicator for this syndrome. The most common misdiagnoses are vasovagal episodes and seizures. The factors that are commonly associated with vasovagal syncope (e.g., pain, nausea, squeamish situations) are generally absent. Vagal events generally do not occur during physical activity because this is a time of sympathetic stimulation and vagal withdrawal. Furthermore, the usual progression over a few or more seconds of the vagal symptoms of lightheadedness and sweating before syncope is absent. In contrast, the syncope of long-QT syndrome is abrupt, usually without warning. In addition, the patient having vasovagal syncope generally regains consciousness within seconds after becoming supine, whereas the patient experiencing syncope due to torsades de pointes (actually a cardiac arrest) is often unconscious for 30 to 60 seconds; this time differential is usually apparent from the history if an observer can be questioned. Therefore, a careful history is of great importance in differentiating between vagal and long-QT causes of syncope. With respect to the misdiagnosis as seizures, a careful history is clarifying in most instances. In long-QT syndrome, there is usually no aura; no motor movements, focal or generalized; no incontinence or tongue biting; and no postictal mental changes. Absence of these findings usually excludes a primary seizure event. Occasionally, a protracted episode of torsades leads to a hypoxic seizure. This can complicate the history if a careful description of the sequence of events is not obtained from an observer. If available, the history reveals that the patient's syncope was initially not accompanied by seizure stigmata but that the seizure occurred after the onset of syncope and usually after the patient became noticeably cyanotic.

The family history may also be important. Syncope occurring in a member of a family with diagnosed long-QT syndrome should lead to immediate concern. A family history of unexplained childhood sudden death also raises suspicion. The absence of a family history of sudden death or long-QT syndrome does not exclude the diagnosis.

QT Prolongation

Although QT-interval prolongation on the resting ECG is the hallmark of the syndrome, it is not always present and is not absolutely necessary for the diagnosis. It has been suspected for some years that there may be long-QT syndrome patients with normal or borderline QT intervals. Discovery of the H-ras-1 genetic marker allows diagnosis of the syndrome to be made independently of the QT interval in H-ras-1 linked families and provides an opportunity to evaluate the range of QT intervals in gene carriers.[38] In 199 members of three long-QT syndrome families, including 83 gene carriers, we confirmed that some gene carriers have normal QT intervals on their resting ECG. In this study, 5% of gene carriers had QTc intervals of

0.44 or less (range, 0.41 to 0.44). Also, a significant percentage of gene carriers had QTc values that were borderline prolonged and overlapped with those of normal patients. The overlap range was 0.41 to 0.47, and 62% of all study subjects had QTc intervals in this overlap range. The QT interval, therefore, must be interpreted with some caution; a normal QTc interval does not exclude the diagnosis and for many patients, the QTc-interval value is not a sufficient diagnostic tool to allow a definite diagnosis or exclusion. Based on available evidence, a QTc-interval value of less than 0.41 would exclude the diagnosis with a high likelihood, whereas a QTc-interval value of 0.47 or more in males and 0.48 or more in females in the absence of drugs or other heart disease that may prolong the QT interval indicates a high probability of the syndrome. The QTc-interval cutpoint of 0.46 or more appears to provide the best overall predictive value.[38] For the large group of patients whose QTc-interval values fall in the overlap range, a multivariable point-scoring system that includes history and several physiologic variables (including QTc) has been proposed as a strategy to enhance diagnostic accuracy (Table 22-2).[87] Also, several other approaches to diagnosis may be employed if the history and ECG are confusing. These include (1) evaluation of several resting EGGs (many patients having a borderline QT interval on one EGG show a distinctly prolonged QT interval on others); (2) evaluation of other family members for evidence of a long QT interval; and (3) evaluation of the QT interval during an exercise or ambulatory ECG. As mentioned earlier, it has been recognized that the QT interval may prolong during exercise. This is attributed to the increase in sympathetic tone that occurs with exercise because similar prolongation of the QT interval has been seen in patients experiencing frightening or anxiety-provoking situations. Actual prolongation during exercise, although not uncommon, appears to be the exception rather than the rule and more commonly, the QT-interval shortens but does not shorten appropriately for the cycle length change.[52] This is detected by an increase in the QTc interval to 0.48 or greater, with the most prominent increase in QTc often occurring in the early stages of recovery. Figure 22-7 contrasts the increase of QTc of long-QT patients with that of normal patients in whom the QTc interval remains constant throughout exercise and recovery. The ambulatory ECG recording can also be used to identify intermittent prolongation of the QT interval but may be more difficult to interpret than the exercise ECG. Many physiologic variables occur during the course of a 24-hour Holter-monitor recording, some of which may influence QT interval (e.g, sleep during which the QT interval is longer than in the awake state). It is not clear that these variables have been carefully identified; thus, the intermittent prolongation of QT interval on the ambulatory recording should be interpreted cautiously. Clearly

TABLE 22-2. Multivariable Point-Scoring System for Diagnosis of Long-QT Syndrome

	Points
ECG FINDINGS*	
QT$_c$†	
$\geq$ 480 msec$^{1/2}$	3
460–470 msec$^{1/2}$	2
450 msec$^{1/2}$ (in males)	1
Torsades de pointes‡	2
T-wave alternans	1
Notched T wave in three leads	1
Low heart rate for age§	
CLINICAL HISTORY	
Syncope‡	2
With stress	1
Without stress	1
Congenital deafness	0.5
FAMILY HISTORY‖	
Family members with definite LQTS¶	1
Unexplained sudden cardiac death below age 30 years among immediate family members	0.5

LQTS, long-QT syndrome.
* In the absence of medications or disorders known to affect these electrocardiographic features.
† QT$_c$ calculated by Bazett's formula.
‡ Mutually exclusive.
§ Resting heart rate below the second percentile for age.[25]
‖ The same family member cannot be counted in both A and B.
¶ Definite LQTS is defined by an LQTS score $\geq$ 4.
Scoring: $\leq$ 1 point, low probability of LQTS; 2 to 3 points, intermediate probability of LQTS; $\geq$ 4 points, high probability of LQTS.

prolonged QT intervals (e.g., QTc-interval values of more than 0.50) would be more suspicious than lesser degrees of prolongation. Another concern with ambulatory monitor recordings is the potential influence on QT interval of a limited low-frequency response. Although current recorders reportedly have the same low-frequency response as that required of diagnostic ECG machines, it is not certain that all devices are periodically checked and maintained to assure continued appropriate low-frequency response. Also of potential diagnostic value on ambulatory ECG or exercise studies are T-wave morphology changes such as bifid T waves, T alternans, or episodes of torsades de pointes. Another proposed diagnostic method that has received some attention is the QT-interval response to isoproterenol and epinephrine infusion. It has been presumed that the QT prolongs in LQTS patients, but not in others. The sensitivity and specificity of such pharmacologic provocation interventions have not been carefully identified and infusion of catacholamines in LQTS patients may involve some element of risk, so the use of these

studies may be best left until further data are available in a research environment. Also, the novel echocardiographic abnormalities mentioned above may become useful for diagnosis if subsequent studies confirm these findings.

A reasonable index of suspicion is important to the proper diagnosis. Children and young adults who have sudden loss of consciousness during physical activity or during fear or fright are particular candidates for investigation and should have, at minimum, a resting ECG. Computed tomography scans, magnetic resonance imaging scans, electroencephalograms, and laboratory examinations are commonly performed in young persons having syncope (at considerable expense), whereas the ECG (the least costly) is omitted or the QT interval is not carefully evaluated if the ECG is obtained. The presymptomatic diagnosis of this syndrome is particularly important if sudden deaths are to be prevented. Therefore, once an affected individual is identified, screening of as many family members as possible is necessary to identify the asymptomatic patients.

PROGNOSIS

It is difficult to predict risk and prognosis with accuracy. Frequent syncope or cardiac arrest; onset of symptoms early in life; a particularly long-QT interval (e.g., more than 0.60); T-wave alternans; prominent bifid T waves; and a family history of sudden death all indicate an important risk.[53] Unfortunately, sudden death occurs frequently in the absence of these factors, reminding us that risk stratification is difficult in this syndrome; for many patients, risk prediction is imprecise.

TREATMENT

There are four treatment options for consideration, including medications, left cervicothoracic sympathectomy, pacemakers, and the implantable internal defibrillator.

Medications

Beta-blocking medications are the mainstay of therapy and should be the initial treatment choice in most patients. In Ward's initial description in 1964,[6] he treated one child who was having daily attacks with a then experimental drug, Inderal. It prevented the attacks for 1 week but the medication was then discontinued by the parents; the child died of an attack 18 hours after the last dose. Over the ensuing 30 years, the effectiveness of beta-blocking agents has been demonstrated by considerable anecdotal but compelling experience and by several observational studies.[53,69,88,89] All beta blockers appear to be effective, although no comparative trials have been reported. In children old enough to swallow pills and in adults, our preferences are nadolol and long acting propranolol because they allow once a day dosing and have been effective in our hands. Generally, a dose of 1 to 3 mg/kg suffices to completely relieve the symptoms. In smaller children, a pleasantly flavored syrup (raspberry works well) can be delivered by dropper or teaspoon. The goal of therapy is complete resolution of symptoms. Failure to achieve that goal indicates that additional therapy should be initiated.[69,88,89] In addition, the reduction of the exercise-induced QT-interval and T-wave abnormalities and QTc dispersion by beta blockers may be useful markers of therapeutic efficacy and an end point of therapy.[52,54]

Left Cervicothoracic Sympathectomy

Left cervicothoracic sympathectomy was first employed by Moss and McDonald in 1971.[24] The procedure has met with mixed success.[90,91] Schwartz prefers the term "high-thoracic left sympathectomy" to emphasize that the excision must include the upper four or five thoracic ganglia, with only the caudal portion of the stellate ganglion.[69] Sparing of the cephalic portion of the stellate ganglia avoids the complication of Horner's syndrome and does not lessen the effectiveness of the intervention. Using this approach, the effectiveness of sympathectomy has been good.[91] Left sympathectomy is warranted when beta-blocking medication alone fails to control symptoms or in the patient who cannot tolerate the medication (e.g., because of severe asthma or intolerable fatigue). If possible, it seems desirable to continue beta blockers after left sympathectomy to increase therapeutic effectiveness.[91]

Pacemakers

Pacemakers also exert a beneficial effect.[92–94] They are indicated in patients with symptomatic bradycardia or those in whom the treatment with beta-blocking agents produces adverse effects such as asthma or symptomatic bradycardia. Another indication is the presence of 2:1 atrioventricular block in the young child.[87,95–97] There are no controlled data to suggest that pacemakers should be the initial therapy for other patients but pacemakers plus beta-blocking medications have been suggested as primary therapy.[94] Furthermore, in those patients who fail or cannot tolerate beta-blocking agents, it is unclear whether pacemaker therapy or left sympathectomy is the next appropriate intervention. Based on sympathectomy results

at different centers, it appears that the technique and experience of the surgeon play an important role in success and these factors should be considered when deciding between pacemaker and sympathectomy therapy.

Implantable Defibrillator

There are no studies indicating which patients may do best with an automatic implantable cardiac defibrillator (AICD) device. Patients with recurrent cardiac arrest despite the above therapy are clear choices. Which other patients deserve this treatment is unclear. One group having high mortality is children who develop symptoms early in life (in the first weeks or months), particularly if they also have a very long QT-interval and T-wave alternans.

References

1. Jervell A, Lange-Nielsen F: Congenital deaf mutism, functional heart disease with prolongation of the Q-T interval and sudden death. Am Heart J 1957;54:59.
2. Levine S, Woodworth C: Congenital deaf mutism, prolonged Q-T interval, syncopal attacks and sudden death. N Engl J Med 1958;259:412.
3. Fraser GR, Froggatt P, James TN: Congenital deafness associated with electrocradiographic abnormalities, fainting attacks and sudden death. J Med 1964;33:361.
4. Romano C, Genrme G, Pongiglione R: Aritmie Cardiache rare dell'eta pediatrica. II. Assessi sincopali per fibrillozione ventricolare parossistics. (Presentazione del primo case della letteratura pediatrica Italiana.) Clin Paediate 1963;45:656.
5. Ward O: Report Council Royal Acadamy of Medicine in Ireland, 1963.
6. Ward O: A new familial cardiac syndrome in children. J Ir Med Assoc 1964;54:103.
7. Jackman WM, Friday KJ, Anderson JL, et al: The long QT syndromes: a critical review, new clinical observations and a unifying hypothesis. Prog Cardiovasc Dis 1988;2:115.
8. Surawicz B: Electrophysiologic substrate of torsade de pointes: dispersion of repolarization or early afterdepolarizations? J Am Coll Cardiol 1989;14:172.
9. Meissner FL: Taubstummheit und Taubstummenbildung. Leipzig and Heidelberg. 1856;119.
10. Morquio L: Sur une maladie infantile et familiale characterisee par des modifications permanentes du pouls, des attaques epilepitformes et la morte subite. Arch Med Enf 1901;4:467.
11. Barlow J, Bosman C, Cochrane J: Congenital cardiac arrhythmia. Lancet 1964;2:531.
12. Gamstorp I, Nilsen R, Westling H: Congenital cardiac arrhythmia. Lancet 1964;2:965.
13. Combrink JM, Kloppers PJ: Hartsiekte by n'besondere familie. S Afr Med J 1965;39:308.
14. Ward O: The electrocardiographic abnormality in familial cardiac arrhythmia. Ir J Med Sci 1966;6:553.

15. James T: Congenital deafness and cardiac arrhythmias. Am J Cardiol 1967;19:627.

16. Kallfelz HC: Ueber ein neues EKG syndrom bei Kindern mit syncopalen Anfallen und plotzlichem Tod. Dtsch Med Wochenschr 1968;93:1046.

17. Garza L, McNamara D, Nora J, et al: Familial repolarization myocardiopathy. Am J Cardiol 1969;23:112.

18. Garza LA, Vick RL, Nora JJ, et al: Heritable Q-T prolongation without deafness. Circulation 1970;41:39.

19. Gale GE, Bosman CK, Tucker RBK, et al: Hereditary prolongation of the Q-T interval (study of 2 families). Br Heart J 1970;32:505.

20. Motte G, Coumel P, Abitol G, et al: The long Q-T interval and syncope caused by spike torsades. Arch Mal Coeur 1970; 63:831.

21. Phillips J, Ichinose H: Clinical and pathologic studies in the heriditary syndrome of a long Q-T interval, syncopal spells and sudden death. Chest 1970;58:236.

22. Lipp H, Pitt A, Anderson ST, et al: Recurrent ventricular tachyarrhythmias in a patient with a prolonged Q-T interval. Med J Aust 1970;I:1296.

23. Karhunen P, Luomanmaki K, Heikkila J, et al: Syncope and Q-T prolongation without deafness. The Romano-Ward syndrome. Am Heart J 1970;80:820.

24. Moss AJ, McDonald J: Unilateral cervicothoracic sympathetic gangionectomy for the treatment of long Q-T interval syndrome. N Engl J Med 1971;285:903.

25. Ratshin RA, Hunt D, Russell RO, et al: Q-T interval prolongation, paroxysmal ventricular arrhythmias, and convulsive syncope. Ann Intern Med 1971;75:919.

26. Lubbers P: Hereditary syndrome of Q-T elongation with syncopes. Z Kreislauforsch 1972;61:907.

27. Csanady M, Kiss Z: Hereditary protraction of the Q-T distance in the ECG without congenital deafness (Romano-Ward syndrome). Orv Hetil 1972;113:2840.

28. Mathews EC Jr, Blount AW Jr, Townsend I: Q-T prolongation and ventricular arrhythmias, with and without deafness, in the same family. Am J Cardiol 1972;29:702.

29. Moss AJ, Schwartz PJ: The idiopathic long QT syndrome: the need for prospective registry. Eur Heart J 1983;4:529.

30. Moss AJ, Schwartz PJ, Crampton RS, Locati E, Carleen E: The long QT syndrome: a prospective international study. Circulation 1985:71:17.

31. Keating M, Atkinson D, Dunn C, Timothy K, Vincent GM, Leppert M: Linkage of a cardiac arrhythmia, the long QT syndrome, and the Harvey ras-1 gene. Science 1991;252:704.

32. Keating M, Atkinson D, Dunn C, Timothy K, Vincent GM, Leppart M: Consistent linkage of the long QT syndrome to the Harvey ras-1 locus on chromosome 11. Am J Hum Genet 1991;49:1335.

33. Towbin JA, Pagotto L, Siu B, et al: Romano-Ward long QT syndrome (RWLQTS): evidence of genetic heterogeneity. Pediatr Res 1992;31:23A. Abstract.

34. Curran M, Atkinson D, Timothy K, et al: Locus heterogeneity of autosomal dominant long QT syndrome. J Clin Invest 1993;92:799.

35. Benhorin J, Kalman YM, Medina A, et al: Evidence of genetic heterogeneity in the long QT syndrome. Science 1993; 260:1960.

36. Akimoto K, Matsuoka R, Kasanuki H, Takao A, Hayakawa K, Hosoda S: Linkage analysis in a Japanese long QT syndrome family. Kokyu To Junkan 1993;41:463.

37. Jeffrey S, Jamieson R, Patton MA, Till J: Long QT and Harvey-ras. Letter to the Editor. Lancet 1993;339:255.

38. Vincent GM, Timothy K, Leppert M, Keating M: The spectrum of symptoms and QT interval in carriers of the gene for the long-QT syndrome. N Engl J Med 1992;327:846.

39. Bharati S, Dreifus L, Bucheleres G, et al: The conduction system in patients with a prolonged QT interval. J Am Coll Cardiol 1985;6:1110.

40. Mathews EC Jr, Blount AW Jr, Townsend JI: Q-T prolongation and ventricular arrhythmias, with and without deafness in the same family. Am J Cardiol 1972;29:702.

41. Andersson P, Lundkvist L: The Q-T syndrome—a family description. Acta Med Scand 1979;206:73.

42. Frazer GR, Froggatt P, James TN: Congenital deafness associated with electrocardiographic abnormalities, fainting spells and sudden death. A recessive syndrome. Q J Med 1964;33:361.

43. Hashiba K: Hereditary Q-T prolongation syndrome in Japan: genetic analysis and pathological findings of the conduction system. Jpn Circ J 1978;42:1133.

44. Phillips J, Ichinose H: Clinical and pathologic studies in the hereditary syndrome of a long Q-T interval, syncopal attacks and sudden death. Chest 1970:58:236.

45. James TN, Froggatt P, Atkinson WJ Jr, et al: De subitaneis mortibus. Observations on the pathophysiology of the long Q-T syndromes with special reference to the neuropathology of the heart. Circulation 1978;57:1221.

46. Nador F, Beria G, De Ferrari GM, et al: Unsuspected echocardiographic abnormality in the long Q-T syndrome: diagnostic, prognostic, and pathogenetic implications. Circulation 1991;84:1530.

47. Zipes DP: Influence of myocardial ischemia and infarction on autonomic innervation of the heart. Circulation 1990; 82:1095.

48. Gohl K, Feistel H, Weikel A, et al: Congenital myocardial sympathetic dysinnervation (CMSD)—a structural defect of idiopathic long QT syndrome. Pacing Clin Electrophysiol 1991;14:1544.

49. Muller KD, Jakob J, Neunzer SF, Frebe M, Schlepper, Pitchner HF: I-metaiodobenzygluanidine scintigraphy in the detection of irregular regional sympathetic innervation in long QT syndrome. Eur Heart J 1993;14:316.

50. Calkins H, Lehmann M, Allman K, Wieland D, Schwaiger M: Scintigraphic pattern of regional cardiac sympathetic innervation in patients with familial long QT syndrome using positron emission tomography. Circulation 1993;87: 1616.

51. Vincent GM: The heart rate of Romano-Ward syndrome patients. Am Heart J 1986;112:61.

52. Vincent GM, Jaiswal D, Timothy KW: Effects of exercise on heart rate, QT, QTc and QT/QS2 in the Romano-Ward inherited long QT syndrome. Am J Cardiol 1991;68:498.

53. Moss AJ, Schwartz PJ, Crampton RS, et al: The long QT syndrome; prospective longitudinal study of 328 families. Circulation 1991;84:1136.

54. Fu Z, Timothy K, Fox J, Vincent GM: Beta-blockers markedly

affect QT dispersion during exercise in long QT syndrome patients. J Am Coll Cardiol 1993;21:93A.

55. Linker NJ, Colonna P, Kekwick A, Till J, Camm AJ, Ward DE: Assessment of QT dispersion in symptomatic patients with congenital long QT syndromes. Am J Cardiol 1992;69:634.

56. Day CP, McComb JM, Campbell RWF: QT dispersion: an indication of arrhythmic risk in patients with long QT intervals. Br Heart J 1990;63:342.

57. Abildskov JA, Vincent GM, Evan K, Burgess MJ: Distribution of body surface ECG potentials in familial QT interval prolongation. Am J Cardiol 1981;47:480.

58. De Ambroggi L, Bertoni T, Locati E, Stramba-Badiale M, Schwartz PJ: Mapping of body surface potentials in patients with the idiopathic long QT syndrome. Circulation 1986; 74:1334.

59. Kinoshita O, Takabayashi Y, Tanaka M, Hongo M, Sekiguchi M: QRST isointegral maps in patients with Romano-Ward syndrome. Am Heart J 1992;124:1631.

60. Linker NJ, Nunain SO, Colonna P, Camm AJ, Ward DE: Relationship between QT interval dispersion and arrhythmic events in patients with congenital long QT syndrome. Pacing Clin Electrophysiol 1991;14:657.

61. Day CP, McComb JM, Matthews J, Campbell RWF: Reduction in QT dispersion by sotalol following myocardial infarction. Eur Heart J 1991;12:423.

62. Hii JTY, Wyse DG, Billis AM, Duff HJ, Solyo MA, Mitchell LB: Precordial QT interval dispersion as a marker of torsade de pointes. Disparate effects of class Ia antiarrhythmic drugs and amiodarone. Circulation 1992;86:1376.

63. Jervell A, Thingstad R, Endsjo TO: The surdo-cardiac syndrome. Am Heart J 1966;72:582.

64. Jervell A, Sivertssen E: Surdo-cardiac syndrome. Nord Med 1967;78:1433.

65. VanBruggen H, Sebus J, VanHeyst A: Convulsive syncope resulting from arrhythmia in a case of deafness with ECG abnormalities. Am Heart J 1969;78:81.

66. Olley PM, Fowler RS: The surdo-cardiac syndrome and therapeutic observations. Br Heart J 1970;32:467.

67. Schwartz PJ, Locati E, Priori SG, Zaza A: The long QT syndrome. In Zipes DP, Jalife J, eds. Cardiac electrophysiology: from cell to bedside. Philadelphia: WB Saunders, 1990:589.

68. Zipes DP: The long QT interval syndrome. A rosetta stone for sympathetic related ventricular tachy arrhythmias. Circulation 1991;84:1414.

69. Schwartz PJ, Bonazzi O, Locati E, Napolitano C, Sala S: Pathogenesisis and therapy of the idiopathic long QT syndrome. Ann NY Acad Sci 1992;644:112.

70. Vincent GM: Hypothesis for the molecular physiology of the Romano-Ward long QT syndrome. J Am Coll Cardiol 1992; 20:500.

71. Burch GE, Meyers R, Abildskov JA: A new electrocardiographic pattern observed in cerebrovascular accidents. Circulation 1954;9:719.

72. Hugenholtz P: Electrocardiographic abnormalities in cerebral disorders, report of six cases, and a review of the literature. Am Heart J 1963;63:451.

73. Yanowitz F, Preston JB, Abildskov JA: Functional distribution of right and left stellate innervation to the ventricles. Produc-

tion of neurogenic electrocardiographic changes by unilateral alterations of sympathetic tone. Circ Res 1966;18:416.

74. Attar H, Gutierrez M, Bellet S, et al: Effect of stimulation of hypothalamus and reticular activating system on production of cardiac arrhythmias. Circ Res 1963;12:14.

75. Mauck HD, Hockman CH: Central nervous system mechanisms mediating cardiac rate and rhythm. Am Heart J 1967; 74:96.

76. Schwartz PJ, Periti M, Malliani: The long QT syndrome. Am Heart J 1975;89:378.

77. Malfatto G, Sun LS, Rosen TS: Bradycardia and long QT interval in neonate rats with delayed cardiac sympathetic inervation. J Auton Nerv Syst 1990;30:101.

78. Ogawa S, Barnett JV, Sen L, Galper JB, Smith TW, Marsh JD: Direct contact between sympathetic neurons and rat cardiac myocytes in vitro increases expression of functional calcium channels. J Clin Invest 1992;89:1085.

79. Schechter E, Greeman CC, Lazzara R: After depolarizations as a mechanism for the long QT syndrome: Electrophysiologic studies of a case. J Am Coll Cardiol 1984;3:1556.

80. Gavrilescu S, Luca C: Right ventricular monophasic action potential in patients with long QT syndrome. Br Heart J 1978;40:1014.

81. Bonatti V, Rolli A, Botti G: Monophasic action potential studies in human subjects with prolonged ventricular repolarization and long QT syndromes. Eur Heart J 1985; 6:131.

82. Ohe T, Kurita T, Aihara N, Kamakura S, Matsuhisa M, Shimomura K: Electrocardiographic and electrophysiologic studies in patients with torsades de pointe: role of monophasic action potentials. Jpn Circ J 1990;54:1323.

83. Zhou JT, Zheng LR, Liu WY: Role of early after depolarization in familial long QTU syndrome and torsade de pointes. Pacing Clin electrophysiol 1992;15:2164.

84. Yatani A, Okabe K, Codina J, Birnbaumer L, Brown AM: Heart rate regulation by G proteins acting on the cardiac pacemaker channel. Science 1990;249:1163.

85. Yatani A, Okabe K, Polakis P, Halenbeck R, McCormick F, Brown AM: Ras p21 and GAP inhibit coupling of muscarinic receptors to atrial K⁺ channels. Cell 1990;61:769.

86. Antzelevitch C, Sicouri S: Clinical relevance of cardiac arrhythmias generated by after depolarizations. Role of M cells in the generation of U waves, triggered activity and torsades de pointes. J Am Coll Cardiol 1994;23:259.

87. Schwartz PJ, Moss AJ, Vincent GM, Crampton RS: Diagnostic criteria for the long QT syndrome. An update. Circulation 1993;88:782.

88. Weintraub RG, Gow RM, Wilkinson JL: The congenital long QT syndromes in childhood. J Am Coll Cardiol 1990;16:674.

89. Garson A, Dick M, Fournier A, et al: The long QT syndrome in children. An international study of 287 patients. Circulation 1993;87:1866.

90. Bhandari AK, Scheinman MM, Morady F, Svinarich J, Mason J, Winkle R: Efficacy of left cardiac sympatectomy in the treatment of patients with the long QT syndrome. Circulation 1984;70:1018.

91. Schwartz PJ, Locati EH, Moss AJ, Crampton RS, Trazzi R, Ruberti R: Left cardiac sympathetic denervation in the ther-

apy of congenital long QT syndrome. Circulation 1991; 84:503.

92. Eldar M, Griffin JY, Abbott JA, et al: Permanent cardiac pacing in patients with the long QT syndrome. J Am Coll Cardiol 1987;10:600.

93. Moss AJ, Liu JE, Gottlieb S, Locati EH, Schwartz PJ, Robinson JL: Efficacy of permanent cardiac pacing in the management of high risk patients with long QT syndrome. Circulation 1991;84:1526.

94. Eldar M, Griffin JC, Van Hare GF, et al: Combine use of beta-adrenergic blocking agents and long term cardiac pacing for patients with the long QT syndrome. J Am Coll Cardiol 1992;20:830.

95. Scott WA, Dick MA: Two:one atrioventricular block in infants with congenital long QT syndrome. Am J Cardiol 1987; 60:1409.

96. Sharma S, Nair KG, Gadekar HA: Romano-Ward prolonged QT syndrome with intermittent T wave alternans and atrioventricular block. Am Heart J 1981;101:500.

97. Gascho JA, Schieken R: congenital complete heart block and long Q-T syndrome requiring ventricular pacing for control of refractory ventricular tachycardia and fibrillation. J Electrocardiol 1979;12:331.

Cardiac Arrhythmias, 3rd edition, edited by William J. Mandel.
J. B. Lippincott Company, Philadelphia © 1995.

23

William G. Stevenson • Holly R. Middlekauff

Electrophysiologic Evaluation of Ventricular Tachycardia

In 1972, Wellens and coworkers demonstrated that ventricular tachycardia could be initiated by critically timed electric stimuli applied to the ventricle.[1] Programmed electric stimulation is widely used to initiate and terminate ventricular tachycardia in susceptible patients. Information derived from electrophysiologic studies (Table 23-1) is useful in guiding therapeutic decisions, including patient eligibility for implantable antitachycardia devices, arrhythmia surgery, and catheter ablation.

Patients undergoing programmed electric stimulation usually fall into one of two groups. The first are those who have had a spontaneous sustained arrhythmia, requiring diagnosis or therapy. This includes patients resuscitated from a cardiac arrest in the absence of acute myocardial infarction and those who present with sustained wide-QRS tachycardia. The second group are patients at risk for life-threatening arrhythmias but in whom sustained ventricular tachycardia or ventricular fibrillation have not yet occurred. This includes patients with syncope of unknown etiology, nonsustained ventricular tachycardia, depressed ventricular function, and palpitations. In the first group, the goal of programmed stimulation is initiation of the previously documented arrhythmia, a clear end point. In the second group, the significance of the arrhythmias initiated is often less clearly defined or controversial.

TECHNICAL CONSIDERATIONS

Procedures for performing electrophysiologic studies are discussed in Chapter 5 and are only briefly reviewed here. Studies are performed in a cardiac catheterization laboratory or procedure room equipped with fluoroscopy, an emergency cart, and defibrillator. The patient is in the postabsorptive state. Sedation may decrease sympathetic tone, rendering arrhythmias more difficult to induce.[2] Most laboratories, however, sedate patients to some degree and in children, general anesthesia is often employed. Local anesthesia should be sufficient to alleviate pain but not excessive because injection of more than 2.5 mg/kg of lidocaine (17.5 mL of a 1% solution in a 70-kg patient) can produce systemic blood levels greater than 1 mg/L and affect arrhythmia inducibility.[3] Alternatives to lidocaine may also be used. Multipolar electrode catheters are positioned in the His-bundle position, right ventricle, and in some cases at other atrial sites, the coronary sinus, or in the left ventricle. Typically, the distal electrode pair of the ventricular catheter is used for stimulation and a ventricular electrogram is recorded from a proximal electrode pair. Intracardiac electrograms are usually filtered and recorded simultaneously with three or more surface electrocardiogram leads. Obtain-

TABLE 23-1. Potential Information Derived From Electrophysiologic Studies

Presence or absence of inducible VT

Hemodynamic consequences of induced VT

Effects of pacing on VT
  Ease of termination
  Risk of pacing induced acceleration

Effect of antiarrhythmic drugs on VT
  Inducibility
  VT rate
  Hemodynamic tolerance
  Pacing termination/acceleration

VT origin (mapping)

VT, ventricular tachycardia.

TABLE 23-2. Controllable Variables in Programmed Stimulation Protocols

Stimulation site

Stimulus current strength

Stimulus mode—unipolar or bipolar

Number and timing of extrastimuli

Basic drivetrain or sinus rhythm: pacing site, number of stimuli, duration of intertrain pause

Patient sedation

ment of a 12-lead electrocardiogram of induced arrhythmias is strongly desirable.

The safety of electrophysiologic studies is well established. In a survey of 8545 electrophysiology studies in 4015 patients, death occurred in 0.06% of those studied.[4] Major complications included cardiac perforation (0.2%), hemorrhage (0.05%), and venous thrombosis (0.2%).

STIMULATION PROTOCOLS AND INDUCED ARRHYTHMIAS

During programmed electric stimulation, many factors that affect induction of arrhythmias are under the control of the physician (Table 23-2). Stimulation protocols vary greatly among electrophysiology laboratories. Typically, stimulation is performed at the right ventricular apex, initially with stimuli of two to five times the late diastolic threshold in strength. A stimulus is introduced in late diastole and scanned progressively earlier in 10- to 20-millisecond decrements until the stimulus fails to capture, defining the effective refractory period. The stimulus is then positioned later than the effective refractory period and a second extrastimulus is added late in diastole and scanned earlier. As the number of extrastimuli are increased, the likelihood of initiating ventricular fibrillation or "nonclinical arrhythmias" increases. Hence, most stimulation protocols proceed from a single-extrastimulus–scanning diastole during sinus rhythm or relatively slow ventricular pacing to two and then three or more extrastimuli during faster ventricular pacing.

Arrhythmias initiated by programmed stimulation can be classified according to duration and morphology (Table 23-3).[5] An arrhythmia is considered sustained if it lasts longer than 30 seconds (15 seconds in some laboratories) or requires earlier termination because of severe hemodynamic consequences, usually syncope. Some consider any arrhythmia that produces symptoms such as presyncope to be sustained. Sustained ventricular tachycardias can often be terminated by extrastimuli or rapid stimulus trains. Any tachycardia that produces syncope is immediately terminated with external direct current (DC) countershock.

Inducible Sustained Monomorphic Ventricular Tachycardia

Sustained monomorphic ventricular tachycardia (Fig. 23-1A) is the most specific response to programmed stimulation.[5] This arrhythmia is virtually never induced in a normal subject.[6-11] It is most commonly encountered in patients who have suffered a myocardial infarction weeks to years previously.

Patient With Sustained Monomorphic Ventricular Tachycardia After Myocardial Infarction

The most common mechanism of sustained monomorphic ventricular tachycardia late after myocardial infarction is reentry, involving the infarct scar. Programmed stimulation initiates sustained monomorphic ventricular tachycardia in more than 90% of patients who have suf-

TABLE 23-3. Inducible Arrhythmias

Sustained monomorphic VT—virtually never initiated in normal hearts. Predictive value for spontaneous VT occurrence varies with patient population

Nonsustained monomorphic VT—usually associated with structural heart disease, less specific than sustained VT

Sustained polymorphic VT—usually nonspecific*

Ventricular fibrillation—usually nonspecific

Nonsustained polymorphic VT—nonspecific

Repetitive ventricular responses—nonspecific

Nonspecific, arrhythmias with no or poor relation to spontaneous arrhythmia occurrence or sudden death.

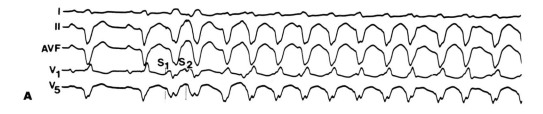

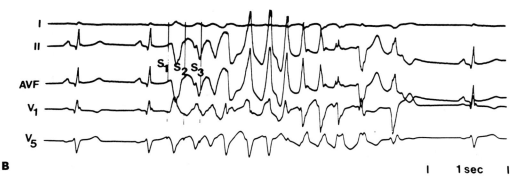

Figure 23-1. Two morphologically distinct ventricular tachycardias initiated by programmed electrical stimulation. From the top of each panel are surface electrocardiogram leads I, II, aV_f, V_1 and V_5. (**A**) Two extrastimuli (S_1, S_2) after a sinus beat initiate sustained monomorphic ventricular tachycardia. (**B**) Three extrastimuli (S_1, S_2, S_3) after a sinus beat initiate nonsustained polymorphic ventricular tachycardia.

fered spontaneous episodes of this arrhythmia in the absence of acute myocardial infarction (Fig. 23-2). Two extrastimuli are required in two thirds to three fourths of patients, and three extrastimuli are needed in a fourth of patients.[5,12-18] Increasing the pacing rate also facilitates tachycardia initiation. Use of a second right ventricular stimulation site, typically the right ventricular outflow tract, in addition to the right ventricular apex or a stimulus strength five to ten times greater than the late diastolic threshold current strength, increases the yield with two extrastimuli by 5% to 25%, achieving results similar to the use of three extrastimuli at the right ventricular apex alone.[10,12,13,15,19-21] Multiple repetitions without changing the coupling interval also increase the incidence of tachycardia induction with double extrastimuli.[22,23] Fast tachycardias (e.g., faster than 200 beats/minute) are more likely to require three or more extrastimuli for initiation.[12,24,25] Stimulation at a left ventricular site is required in fewer than 5% of patients.[12,13,26] Rapid burst pacing can also be used to initiate ventricular tachycardia but the precise timing and number of stimuli are critical and the response less reproducible than with extrastimuli.[27,28] Isoproterenol infusion is occasionally required, especially in patients with exercise- provokable ventricular tachycardia.[21,29-31] Although three or more extrastimuli reliably

initiate sustained monomorphic ventricular tachycardia in more than 90% of patients who present with this arrhythmia, the precise stimulus timing, number of stimuli, and pacing rate that initiates tachycardia vary from day to day in three fourths of patients.[32-35]

Repeated basic drive trains of stimuli at rates of 100 to 150 beats per minute, although typically only eight beats in duration and separated by a pause, can induce ischemia in some coronary artery disease patients.[36] Angina is rarely noted by the patient, although myocardial lactate production may occur. In occasional patients, ischemia may facilitate ventricular tachycardia initiation. This should be particularly suspected for inducible polymorphic ventricular tachycardia or ventricular fibrillation because some patients are rendered free of these inducible arrhythmias by coronary artery bypass surgery.[37] Sustained monomorphic ventricular tachycardia is rarely cured by coronary artery revascularization alone.[38]

In 80% of postmyocardial infarction patients with ventricular tachycardia, repeated programmed stimulation induces more than one morphology of ventricular tachycardia.[32,39-45] Multiple morphologies of ventricular tachycardia may be due to different exit points from the same arrhythmia focus, varied reentry circuit configurations arising in the same region, or multiple reentry circuits in

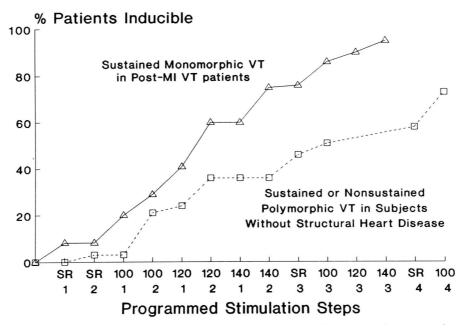

Figure 23-2. Cumulative incidence of initiating the most specific (sustained monomorphic ventricular tachycardia) and least specific (polymorphic ventricular tachycardia) types of ventricular tachycardia (*VT*) in two groups of patients. The ordinate is the cumulative percentage of patients with induced ventricular tachycardia. On the abscissa are steps in the stimulation protocol. The upper abscissa label is the basic drive, which was either sinus rhythm (*SR*) or ventricular pacing at the rates shown, progressing from 100 beats/minute to 140 beats/minute. The number of extrastimula are shown below the basic drive. The solid line depicts initiation of sustained monomorphic ventricular tachycardia in a group of patients who had suffered a spontaneous episode of this arrhythmia late after myocardial infarction (*MI*). The dashed line depicts initiation of polymorphic ventricular tachycardia (sustained or nonsustained) in patients who did not have structural heart disease or spontaneous ventricular arrhythmias. As the basic heart rate and number of extrastimuli increase, the incidence of both specific nonspecific arrhythmias increase. (Adapted from Wellens HJJ, Brugada P, Stevenson WG, et al: Programmed electrical stimulation: its role in the management of ventricular arrhythmias in coronary heart disease. Progress in Cardiovascular Disease 1986;29:165 and Stevenson WG, Brugada P, Waldecker B, Zhender M, Wellens HJJ: Can potentially significant polymorphic ventricular arrhythmias initiated by programmed ventricular stimulation be distinguished from those that are nonspecific? Am Heart J 1986; 112:1073.)

separate regions. Morphologies of inducible sustained ventricular tachycardia that have not previously occurred clinically may subsequently occur spontaneously in some patients but can be insignificant findings in others.[39]

Out-of-Hospital Ventricular Fibrillation Survivor

In up to 75% of patients resuscitated from cardiac arrest, ventricular fibrillation is the initial rhythm found by paramedics at the scene.[46] Of patients in whom evidence of acute myocardial infarction is absent after resuscitation, 27% to 55% have sustained monomorphic ventricular tachycardia inducible by programmed stimulation—almost all of whom have a ventricular scar from a prior

healed myocardial infarction.[47-54] Induced ventricular tachycardia is often faster than 200 beats per minute and commonly produces syncope, suggesting that ventricular tachycardia degenerating to ventricular fibrillation was the mechanism of the initial cardiac arrest.[48,55,56] Absence of inducible sustained ventricular tachycardia in a ventricular fibrillation survivor with coronary artery disease suggests acute ischemia as a likely cause of ventricular fibrillation.[46,47,53]

Syncope

Programmed stimulation initiates sustained monomorphic ventricular tachycardia in 4% to 33% of patients who have suffered undiagnosed episodes of syncope, suggesting that self-terminating ventricular tachycardia was the cause.[57–65] Patients with inducible tachycardia almost always have underlying structural heart disease, most commonly being healed myocardial infarction.

Risk Assessment in Patients Without Prior Sustained Ventricular Tachycardia

Programmed stimulation has been used to assess future arrhythmia risk in survivors of acute myocardial infarction who have not suffered spontaneous sustained ventricular tachycardia. Early after myocardial infarction, sustained monomorphic ventricular tachycardia can be initiated in 6% to 44% of patients.[66–78] The time from infarction importantly affects the incidence of inducible arrhythmias. Kuck and coworkers found inducible ventricular tachycardia in 11% of patients studied 5 days after infarction, increasing to 28% of patients studied 24 days after infarction.[72] Bhandari and associates found that about half of the patients with sustained ventricular tachycardia inducible 2 weeks after infarction do not have inducible ventricular tachycardia 5 months later.[69] Successful reperfusion during the acute phase of myocardial infarction reduces the incidence of inducible ventricular tachycardia.[71] Kersschot and colleagues found inducible sustained monomorphic ventricular tachycardia in 12% of patients who had successful reperfusion of the infarct artery, compared with 74% of patients in whom acute reperfusion was not achieved.[71] Left ventricular aneurysm and left ventricular ejection fraction less than 40% also increase the incidence of inducible ventricular tachycardia.[78, 79]

The rate of inducible sustained ventricular tachycardia may be an important indicator of potential clinical significance.[24, 72, 73] In patients studied 7 to 28 days after myocardial infarction, Denniss and coworkers found that the mean cycle length of inducible ventricular tachycardia was 248 ± 14 milliseconds in patients who subsequently suffered spontaneous sustained ventricular tachycardia or sudden death, compared with 209 ± 4 milliseconds in the patients who remained free of spontaneous sustained arrhythmias.[76] Inducible sustained monomorphic tachycardia with a cycle length shorter than 230 milliseconds (faster than 260 beats/minute) and inducible ventricular fibrillation do not confer an increased risk of sudden death during follow-up.[70, 76, 77] It appears that the faster reentry circuits are less likely to produce spontaneous arrhythmias.

Inducible ventricular tachycardia early after infarction is associated with an increased risk of spontaneous ventricular tachycyardia and sudden death. Bourke and associates performed programmed stimulation in 1209 survivors of acute myocardial infarction, excluding those requiring continued therapy for angina or more than 40 mg of furosemide daily for heart failure.[78] Programmed stimulation was performed before hospital discharge, a mean of 11 days after infarction. Sustained monomorphic ventricular tachycardia slower than 265 beats per minute was initiated in 6.2% of patients. During the first year of follow-up, 19% of patients with inducible tachycardia suffered sustained ventricular tachycardia or ventricular fibrillation, compared with 2.9% of the patients without inducible ventricular tachycardia.

Management of patients with inducible but not spontaneous tachycardia is controversial. In one study, antiarrhythmic drug treatment did not reduce the risk of sudden death.[80] The risks of antiarrhythmic therapy (especially as applied to the numerous patients who remain free of spontaneous arrhythmic events despite inducible tachycardia early after infarction) could offset any benefit.[81]

Programmed electric stimulation has also been used to assess the risk of sustained ventricular tachycardia in patients with spontaneous nonsustained ventricular tachycardia on ambulatory electrocardiogram monitoring. Sustained monomorphic ventricular tachycardia is initiated in 24% to 40% of those patients with coronary artery disease but is distinctly uncommon in patients with good left ventricular function and no prior myocardial infarction.[82–90] Absence of a late potential on the signal-averaged electrocardiogram is associated with a lower incidence of inducible tachycardia.[86, 87] Complex ventricular ectopy and nonsustained ventricular tachycardia is common in patients with dilated nonischemic cardiomyopathy but programmed stimulation initiates sustained monomorphic ventricular tachycardia in fewer than 5% of these patients if they have not suffered a spontaneous episode of sustained ventricular tachycardia.[91–93] Patients without inducible sustained ventricular tachycardia or whose arrhythmia is suppressed with antiarrhythmic drug therapy generally have a low risk of sudden death, except for those with severely depressed ventricular function, in whom sudden death risk remains substantial.[89, 91, 93] It is not known whether therapy guided by programmed stimulation is superior to no therapy. Programmed stimulation may be identifying patients who have a low or high risk of arrhythmic events, regardless of antiarrhythmic drug therapy, as described below.

Inducible Nonsustained Monomorphic Ventricular Tachycardia

Inducible nonsustained monomorphic ventricular tachycardia is uncommon in patients without structural heart disease but is observed in up to 24% of patients with prior myocardial infarction.[5] The prognostic significance of this induced arrhythmia is not clear.

Inducible Polymorphic Ventricular Arrhythmias

The most common causes of spontaneous sustained polymorphic ventricular tachycardia are acute myocardial ischemia and torsades de pointes associated with either congenital or acquired QT-interval prolongation. Torsade de pointes may be related to afterdepolarizations and is not inducible by programmed ventricular stimulation, at least as it is performed for other ventricular tachycardias.[94,95] Recurrent polymorphic ventricular tachycardia not occurring by one of these two causes is distinctly uncommon but programmed stimulation can initiate the tachycardia in some of these patients.[96] Sustained polymorphic ventricular tachycardia is often rapid and degenerates quickly to ventricular fibrillation.

Sustained polymorphic ventricular tachycardia or ventricular fibrillation can be initiated in normal subjects, usually by using more than two extrastimuli, and can be a nonspecific response to programmed stimulation.[5,8,9,97-102] Inducible ventricular fibrillation does not indicate an increased risk of sudden death in patients studied early after myocardial infarction or in patients with undiagnosed syncope.[58,61,76] It may be of more significance in patients with hypertrophic cardiomyopathy or those who have been resuscitated from ventricular fibrillation. Polymorphic ventricular tachycardia degenerating to ventricular fibrillation or ventricular fibrillation is initiated in 10% to 16% of patients who have been resuscitated from a cardiac arrest.[48-54] Although the clinical significance of inducible ventricular fibrillation is often not certain, it is usually considered evidence for the cause of cardiac arrest in ventricular fibrillation survivors if no other etiology is evident. Nonsustained polymorphic ventricular tachycardia (see Fig. 23-1B) is initiated in up to 38% of normal subjects subjected to up to three extrastimuli and is nonspecific.[5,8,9,98-102]

Because polymorphic ventricular tachycardia is usually nonspecific and often requires DC shock for termination, programmed stimulation protocols are designed to maximize initiation of monomorphic ventricular tachycardia while minimizing initiation of polymorphic ventricular tachycardia and ventricular fibrillation. Initiation of both polymorphic and monomorphic ventricular tachycardias increase as the number of extrastimuli are increased (see Fig. 23-2). Initiation of ventricular fibrillation is often preceded by prolongation of the time, "latency" between the stimulus, and local ventricular electrogram recorded from the proximal electrodes of the pacing catheter.[97] This is consistent with conduction slowing produced by propagation through relatively refractory tissue. Polymorphic arrhythmias are often initiated at shorter stimulus-coupling intervals than monomorphic ventricular tachycardia.[102] Initiation of ventricular fibrillation can probably be re-duced by performing stimulation with up to two extrastimuli at multiple pacing rates before using three or more extrastimuli. Limiting the shortest stimulus-coupling interval to 180 milliseconds and monitoring latency from the last stimulus have also been suggested.[97,102]

Repetitive Ventricular Responses

Short bursts of one to five ventricular beats initiated by programmed stimulation are commonly referred to as repetitive ventricular responses.[5] These may be due to intramyocardial reentry or macroreentry within the His-Purkinje system.[103] Multiple extrastimuli induce repetitive ventricular responses in virtually all patients with structural heart disease and in many normal subjects.[5,14] They are a nonspecific response to programmed stimulation.

ASSESSING ANTIARRHYTHMIC DRUG THERAPY WITH PROGRAMMED STIMULATION

Patients resuscitated from sustained ventricular tachycardia or ventricular fibrillation unrelated to acute myocardial infarction are at high risk for arrhythmia recurrence. Trappe and associates and Brugada and colleagues studied 108 survivors of sustained ventricular tachycardia or ventricular fibrillation who had coronary artery disease and were treated with antiarrhythmic drugs selected based on clinical judgment.[104,105] During a mean follow-up of 25 to 27 months, 19% of patients suffered a nonfatal arrhythmia recurrence and 7% died suddenly. Patients who initially presented with ventricular tachycardia were less likely to die suddenly (5%) but were more likely to suffer nonfatal arrhythmia recurrences (26%) than patients who presented with ventricular fibrillation, 6% of whom had nonfatal arrhythmia recurrences and 11% of whom died suddenly. In a multicenter study of 390 patients who survived an episode of sustained ventricular tachycardia or ventricular fibrillation remote from acute myocardial infarction and were treated predominantly with antiarrhythmic drugs, the actuarial 2-year risk of sudden death or fatal ventricular tachycardia was 19%.[106] Nonfatal arrhythmia recurrences were common, occurring in 49% of patients. Total mortality during follow-up is increased by the presence of cardiac arrest with the presenting arrhythmia, poor ventricular function with left ventricular ejection fraction below 30%, class III or IV heart failure, multiple prior infarctions, and initial arrhythmia occurrence less than 6 weeks after acute myocardial infarction (Table 23-4).[50,54,104,106-109] The time between arrhythmia recurrences is highly variable. Absence of spontaneous recur-

TABLE 23-4. Clinical Predictors of Mortality in Patients With Sustained Ventricular Tachycardia or Ventricular Fibrillation Remote From Acute Myocardial Infarction

Event	Relative Risk
Cardiac Arrest	1.7
Class III or IV heart failure	1.7–3.5
Multiple old myocardial infarctions	1.4–1.6
VT or VF 48 hours to 6 weeks after acute infarction	1.8

VF, ventricular fibrillation; VT, ventricular tachycardia.

Brugada P, Talajic M, Mulleneers R, Wellens HJJ: The value of the clinical history to assess prognosis of patients with ventricular tachycardia or ventricular fibrillation after myocardial infarction. Eur Heart J 1989;10:747.

rences during hospitalization for drug therapy does not reliably indicate long-term arrhythmia control. Suppression of ventricular ectopy on Holter-electrocardiogram recording and exercise treadmill testing is useful in some patients but limited by marked day-to-day variability in spontaneous ventricular ectopy and lack of spontaneous ventricular arrhythmias in others.[104, 105, 110–114]

Programmed electric stimulation supplies the "trigger" to induce the clinical arrhythmia in a controlled setting and has been used to guide therapy during serial testing of antiarrhythmic drugs.[112–137] Programmed ventricular stimulation is first performed in the drug-free state to define the inducible arrhythmia. An antiarrhythmic drug is then administered either orally or intravenously and programmed stimulation is repeated. Intravenous drug administration allows rapid assessment but is not uniformly predictive of the results during oral drug administration.[121–125, 134] If the first drug is deemed ineffective, a period for washout of this drug is allowed and a second drug is tested. The most desirable end point is inability to induce any sustained ventricular tachycardia. Marked variability in the precise step of the stimulation protocol that initiates ventricular tachycardia is common; therefore, a change in the mode of inducibility may not reliably predict drug efficacy.[32–35] If repeated drug trials are performed, drug suppression of inducible ventricular tachycardia can be achieved in 23% to 48% of patients.[47–54, 114, 126–136, 138] In the Electrophysiologic Study Versus Electrocardiographic Monitoring (ESVEM) trial, a standard protocol of drug testing was employed in 242 patients.[114] Inducible ventricular tachycardia was suppressed in 45% of patients. This required a mean of 3.2 drug trials per patient and a median hospital stay of 25 days. Suppression of inducible ventricular tachycardia is more often achieved in patients with left ventricular ejection fraction greater than 40% and in those who do not have

structural heart disease.[54, 129, 130, 135] Inducible ventricular tachycardia is suppressed in fewer than 25% of patients who have prior myocardial infarction with left ventricular ejection fraction less than 30%. If ventricular tachycardia can be suppressed by one antiarrhythmic drug, other drugs are also often effective.[121, 130] Waxman and coworkers found that 85% of inducible ventricular tachycardias suppressed by high-dose procainamide could also be suppressed by a second class I drug.[121] When high-dose procainamide was not successful, only 13% of tachycardias were suppressed by a different class I antiarrhythmic drug. The incidence of ventricular tachycardia suppression by antiarrhythmic drugs was examined in the ESVEM trial.[136] The class III drug sotalol had the greatest efficacy and was effective in 35% of drug trials, compared with 26% for procainamide, 16% for quinidine, 14% for propafenone, and 12% for Mexiletine. It is possible that the β-adrenergic blocking properties in addition to the potassium channel blocking properties of sotalol contribute to its efficacy but this also limits its usefulness in patients with congestive heart failure.

When antiarrhythmic drugs suppress inducible ventricular tachycardia, the risk of death from arrhythmia is 5% to 10% during the following year.[47–54, 108, 112, 113, 114, 127, 129, 131, 134] In the largest study, the risk of death from arrhythmia was 24% at 4 years.[114] The sudden-death risk is higher in patients with poor ventricular function.[50, 54, 108] Wilber and associates studied 166 survivors of out-of-hospital cardiac arrest and found that a left ventricular ejection fraction less than 30% and inducible ventricular tachycardia on drug therapy were independent predictors of sudden death.[50] One-year sudden-death–free survival was 95% when tachycardia was rendered noninducible, compared with 67% when tachycardia was inducible on antiarrhythmic drug therapy. Swerdlow and colleagues found that New York Heart Association functional classification and persistently inducible ventricular tachycardia on drug therapy were predictors of sudden death.[108] The better prognosis of patients with drug-suppressible ventricular tachycardia may be because of prevention of fatal arrhythmia recurrences. Alternatively, suppression with drug therapy may identify a group of patients who generally have better ventricular function and an inherently lower risk for sudden death.[137] Brugada and coworkers performed programmed electric stimulation during drug therapy of ventricular arrhythmias but did not alter therapy based on the results.[104, 105, 107, 137] Programmed-stimulation findings predicted the likelihood of ventricular tachycardia recurrences but not the risk of sudden death because many arrhythmia recurrences were not fatal. Drug-induced slowing of ventricular tachycardia may reduce the risk that an arrhythmia recurrence will be fatal, without preventing the arrhythmia.[105, 134, 138] Waller and associates found that a hemodynamically tolerated ventricular tachycardia, with cycle length prolonged by 100 milliseconds over that induced in the drug-free state, was associated with a 1-year sudden death risk similar to that of patients rendered free of inducible ventricular tachycardia on drug therapy.[131]

Amiodarone has often been used as a last-resort antiarrhythmic drug when other agents are not effective.[139–147] Several studies found a relatively low sudden death incidence when electrophysiologic testing was not performed or amiodarone was continued despite persistently inducible ventricular tachycardia.[143–147] Left ventricular function is the most important predictor of outcome.[139–142] Patients with severely depressed ventricular function (left ventricular ejection fraction less than 30% to 40%) have a greater risk of sudden death, regardless of the results of programmed stimulation. Amiodarone often slows the cycle length of inducible tachycardia, and this has been associated with a lower sudden death risk in some studies.[141–145] Persistently inducible ventricular tachycardia is associated with more arrhythmia recurrences than when ventricular tachycardia is not inducible during amiodarone therapy.

In summary, the severity of underlying heart disease and the clinical presentation are more important determinants of long-term prognosis and sudden death than the results of programmed stimulation, although programmed stimulation identifies groups at low and high risk for arrhythmia recurrences. Patients with well-perserved ventricular function can often be rendered free of inducible ventricular tachycardia with antiarrhythmic drugs and have a good prognosis. Patients with good left ventricular function whose ventricular arrhythmia occurred later than 6 weeks after myocardial infarction and did not result in cardiac arrest have a low risk of sudden death on antiarrhythmic drug therapy, although a third or more of patients with persistently inducible ventricular tachycardia suffer nonfatal arrhythmic recurrences. Patients with poor ventricular function and sustained ventricular tachycardia early after myocardial infarction have a 15% to 30% risk of sudden death while on antiarrhythmic drug therapy. Inducible ventricular tachycardia is also more difficult to suppress in patients with poor ventricular function. Implantable cardiovertor defibrillators or amiodarone are considered early in the management for this high-risk group.

MAPPING TO IDENTIFY THE VENTRICULAR TACHYCARDIA ORIGIN

Catheter and surgical ablation are important alternatives and adjuncts to therapy with antiarrhythmic drugs and implantable devices for ventricular tachycardia. Mapping to identify the arrhythmia origin is used to direct the ablation efforts. Surgical approaches are able to resect or damage relatively large regions. Methods of catheter ablation produce small lesions, and more precise localization of the arrhythmia focus or a critical site in a large reentry circuit is required.

Mapping in the catheterization laboratory is performed by exploring the ventricles with an endocardial electrode catheter. Access to the left ventricle is achieved either retrograde across the aortic valve or by a transatrial approach, puncturing the interatrial septum from the right atrium to reach the left atrium, then across the mitral valve to the left ventricle. Assessing catheter position in the ventricle requires fluoroscopic observation in a minimum of two projections, and precise localization is difficult. Transesophageal echocardiography allows more precise catheter positioning but requires additional experienced personnel and careful sedation and airway management.[148] A common mapping scheme divides the left ventricle into 12 sites, each having an estimated area of 5 to 10 cm^2.[149] In contrast, intraoperative mapping systems allow simultaneous recording from multiple sites, often with direct visual localization of the electrodes.

There are several approaches to locating the arrhythmia origin. These include analysis of electrograms during sinus rhythm and induced ventricular tachycardia, pacemapping, programmed electric stimulation during tachycardia, and application of radiofrequency current through the mapping catheter during ventricular tachycardia. The relative value of each technique in a given patient is determined by the suspected tachycardia mechanism, the ability to initiate tachycardia, and hemodynamic tolerance of the tachycardia. Many of these methods require hemodynamically stable ventricular tachycardia and are only applicable in selected patients. Catheter ablation for ventricular tachycardia is in its infancy and techniques are evolving. Tachycardias that arise from a small focus in a structurally normal heart are particularly susceptible to ablation. Myocardial infarction often creates large reentry circuits that are more difficult to localize with catheter techniques.

Technical Considerations in Recording Endocardial Electrograms for Mapping

Electrograms recorded with catheter techniques are typically analyzed with regard to timing, amplitude, and duration. These characteristics are importantly affected by the recording techniques (Table 23-5).[150] Recording amplifiers may be DC- or alternating current (AC)-coupled. In true DC amplifiers, the low-frequency response is 0.0 Hz. In AC-coupled amplifiers, commonly used for recording

TABLE 23-5. Factors Influencing Electrogram Characteristics

Recording technique
  Electrode size
  Interelectrode distance
    Unipolar
    Bipolar
  Electrode–tissue contact
  Amplification
  Filtering
Anatomic/Physiologic
  Direction of wavefront propagation
  Mass of excitable tissue
  Distance from recording electrode
  Fiber orientation
  Action potential
    Amplitude
    Upstroke
    Duration

the body-surface electrocardiogram, the lowest frequency response of near-DC filtering is 0.05 to 0.1 Hz. A small charge differential due to polarization at the catheter–electrode interface introduces a DC offset, which often fluctuates during true DC recordings.[151] High-pass filtering at 10 to 100 Hz is commonly employed in electrophysiology laboratories to remove baseline wandering and attenuate slow deflections produced by T waves and ST segments, which are not useful for identifying activation at the recording site. High-pass filtering differentiates the signal, so that the amplitude of the filtered signal is proportional to the rate of change of the input signal rather than to the amplitude of the input signal. In recordings from normal ventricular tissue, the electrogram height and duration diminish as the high-pass filter cut-off (corner frequency) is increased above 10 Hz.[152,153] Low-pass filtering has little effect on the appearance of normal ventricular electrograms unless the corner frequency is below 100 Hz, in which case electrogram amplitude diminishes. Because cardiac electrograms contain high-frequency components, low-pass–filter corner frequencies of 500 Hz or greater are recommended. For digital data-acquisition systems, sampling at rates of 1000 Hz (which allows acquisition of 500-Hz signals) or above are desirable.[154] Filtering alters electrogram morphology and hence the peaks and rapid deflections commonly used to determine local activation by visual inspection. In normal tissue, differences produced by changing the filter settings are usually less than 5 milliseconds.[152]

Recordings may be unipolar (with one electrode on the myocardium and the reference electrode distant from the heart) or bipolar (with both recording electrodes at the site of interest). In the catheterization laboratory, the reference electrode for unipolar recordings is most conveniently the Wilson central terminal or a cutaneous elec-

trode patch. Use of a catheter electrode positioned in the inferior vena cava is less subject to electric noise, however, allowing cleaner recordings without significantly altering electrogram amplitude.[153] Information about the direction of wavefront propagation can be derived from unfiltered unipolar recordings.[155–160] A positive deflection is recorded as the activation wavefront sweeps toward the electrode.[155] As the wavefront passes under the recording electrode, a sharp downward deflection (the intrinsicoid deflection) is inscribed, followed by a negative deflection as the wavefront propagates away from the recording electrode. With a small extracellular electrode positioned close to a myocardial fiber, the most rapid portion of the downstroke corresponds in time to the action potential upstroke of the underlying tissue.[156] When wavefronts are propagating through a tissue plane, collision of two wavefronts beneath the recording electrode produces a positive monophasic deflection. A dominant negative deflection is recorded at the site of earliest activation.[157–159] Other factors, however, complicate electrogram interpretation in vivo (see Table 23-5). At high amplification, considerable "far field" signals from depolarization of tissue remote from the exploring electrode are recorded.[161,162] The myocardium is composed of nonparallel sheets of muscle fibers, and conduction velocity is importantly influenced by the geometry of muscle cell bundles, relative to the wavefront direction.[158,163] Superimposition of potentials from adjacent muscle bundles, activated asynchronously, produces complex polyphasic waveforms. Hence, electrograms recorded by catheters in humans can be difficult to interpret, especially in and around regions of prior infarction.

Bipolar recordings are obtained by having both recording electrodes on the heart. The recorded signal is the sum of the unipolar signal at one electrode and the inverted unipolar signal at the other electrode.[160] Much of the far field electric activity is cancelled out, reducing the duration and amplitude of the recorded electrogram when compared with unipolar recordings.[155,160,162] The peak of the unfiltered bipolar recorded electrogram generally corresponds in time to the intrinsicoid deflection on the unipolar electrograms and therefore to local activation.[155] The direction of wavefront propagation cannot be inferred from a single bipolar recording. In contrast to unipolar recordings, the amplitude of a bipolar recording is influenced by the direction of wavefront propagation relative to the axis of the recording dipole. Theoretically, a wavefront moving perpendicular to this axis does not produce a signal. Interelectrode distance also affects bipolar electrogram amplitude and duration.[152] Interelectrode distances on intracardiac catheters commonly range from 1 mm to more than 1 cm. Close interelectrode spacing helps reduce far field signals, restricting the "field of view" to the tissue at the recording site.

Mapping Chronic Reentrant Ventricular Tachycardia Late After Myocardial Infarction

Pathophysiologic Considerations

Recurrent sustained ventricular tachycardia late after myocardial infarction is most commonly caused by reentry.[164–175] Histologic examination of chronic infarcts from patients with ventricular tachycardia reveals strands of surviving, often normal-appearing myocytes surrounded by fibrous scar.[163,165,172,176,177] Despite slow conduction through these regions, many cells have normal action potentials.[165,178,179] Conduction slowing is probably due to increased intercellular resistance that accompanies distortion of the intercellular architecture by interposition of fibrous tissue between cell bundles.[159,180] It is also possible that myofibril separation produces winding circuitous pathways, lengthening the microscopic routes for wavefront propagation and prolonging conduction time through the area from the macroscopic perspective.[171,172] Myocytes in infarct scars also demonstrate heterogeneity in action potential duration and refractoriness predisposing to reentry.[165,178,179]

The interplay between slow conduction and refractoriness is illustrated in Figure 23-3 for one mechanism of ventricular tachycardia initiation that has been studied in animal models.[181–185] A myocardial scar is present below and to the right of the thin dashed line. In Figure 23-3A a stimulus prematurely depolarizes a site (S) distant from the scar and the stimulated wavefronts (*solid arrows*) propagate toward the scar. On reaching the scar, the stimulated wavefront encounters tissue that has not yet recovered excitability.[185] Wavefronts propagate along both sides of the refractory tissue, forming an arc of conduction block (*hatched area*). In Figure 23-3B, the wavefronts continue, extending the arc of conduction block until they reach tissue that has recovered sufficiently to be excitable. The wavefront then propagates around both ends of the arc of block and proceeds back toward the center of the arc of block. In this animal model, conduction time through the central area is critical for reentry. If conduction is relatively fast, so that the wavefront reaches the central portion of the arc of block before it has recovered, block at that point

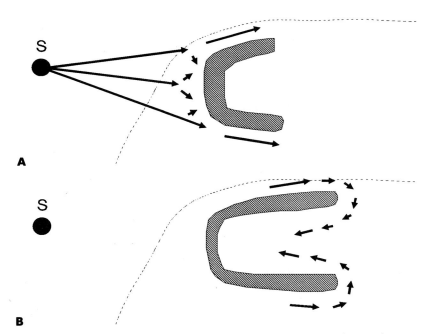

Figure 23-3. Initiation of reentry in a figure-eight reentry circuit is shown schematically. In all panels, an area of myocardial scar is present to the right and below the thin dashed line. *S* is a stimulation site in normal tissue. Propagating excitation wavefronts are shown as *solid arrows*. Areas through which wavefronts cannot propagate because of block or collision are shown as *hatched areas* or *solid lines*. (**A**) A premature stimulus captures site *S* and propagates toward the scar. Within the scar, the wavefronts encounters tissue that is not yet recovered after a previous depolarization. Excitation wavefronts propagate along both sides of the refractory tissue border, forming an arc of conduction block (*hatched area*). (**B**) The propagating wavefronts reach excitable tissue and turn in behind the arc of block. The two wavefronts merge, forming a common wavefront, which propagates toward the center of the arc of block. *(continued)*

extinguishes the wavefronts and reentry does not occur. If, however, conduction is sufficiently slow, allowing time for a portion of the arc of block to recover, the wavefront propagates through that area, reentering the tissue on the opposite side of the initial arc of block (Fig. 23-3C), producing the first reentrant beat. Wavefronts then propagate in clockwise and counterclockwise directions around the

remaining two arcs of block, forming a figure-eight type of reentry circuit, with wavefronts propagating around two arcs of block and sharing a central common pathway (Fig. 23-3D). The two apparent areas of block may be maintained by repetitive collision of wavefronts from the common central pathway and the wavefronts propagating around the outside of the arcs. The figure-eight model of

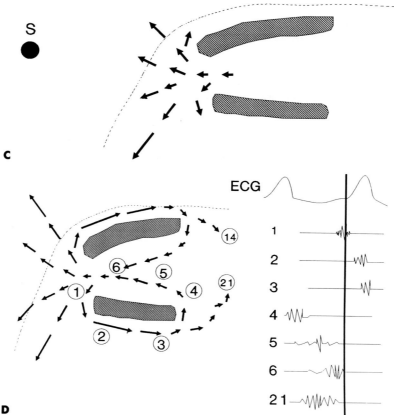

Figure 23-3 *(continued)* **(C)** The wavefront arrives at the center of the arc of block. Slow conduction through the scar has allowed sufficient time for tissue in this area to recover. The wavefront reenters tissue to the left of the initial arc of block and propagates out of the scar, generating the first tachycardia QRS complex. The common wavefront splits into two wavefronts, which propagate around the two remaining arcs of block. **(D)** The entire reentry circuit, with selected sites labeled. The two arcs of apparent conduction "block" may be maintained by continuous collision of wavefronts from the outer and central reentry paths. To the right is a schematic of the tachycardia surface electrocardiogram (*ECG*) and theoretical intracardiac electrograms, with timing derived from a computer simulation. A vertical line is drawn at the QRS onset. Wavefront propagation through the slow common central pathway from sites 4 to 6 generates only low-amplitude electrical activity which is not detectable on the surface ECG. The QRS onset occurs when the excitation wavefront propagates from the "exit" of the slow common pathway near site 1 to the surrounding myocardium. Presystolic electrical activity is recorded at sites 1, 5, and 21. Relatively rapid conduction around the arcs of block results in activation at the "entrance" to the slow common pathway near site 4 before inscription of the QRS complex is complete. Site 21 is within the scar adjacent to but not participating the reentry circuit. Slow conduction in this "bystander" region produces "diastolic" electrical activity that is unrelated to wavefront propagation in the circuit.

reentry has been observed in humans and extensively studied in canine models and is used to illustrate several important concepts for localizing reentry circuits.

In this model, reentry is ordered. The circulating wavefront follows a repeating path, and the revolution time through the circuit, which determines the tachycardia cycle length, is determined by the circuit length and conduction velocities. At each point in the circuit, the tissue must have time to recover before it is depolarized by the returning wavefront. The cycle length of the tachycardia, therefore, exceeds the longest recovery time of any point in the circuit. The time between recovery of the tissue and arrival of the next returning orthodromic wavefront is the "excitable gap" at that point in the circuit. An appropriately timed stimulus or excitation wavefront can prematurely depolarize a reentry circuit site during its excitable gap and reset, entrain, or terminate the tachycardia.

Reentry circuits may take any of a variety of geometric configurations.[165,168,171,174,175,183-189] In many cases, a region of slow conduction exists in or near the infarct scar and is a desirable target for ablation. Depolarization of these slowly conducting regions produces low-amplitude electric activity that is not detected in the standard body-surface electrocardiogram. The ventricular tachycardia QRS complex is produced when the excitation wavefront exits the slow conduction region and propagates across the ventricles. Microreentry theoretically may arise in a small segment of the infarct scar. A reentrant wavefront may propagate slowly through myocyte bundle crossing the scar, then exit from the scar and propagate through normal tissue around the border of the scar, reentering the scar some distance away from the exit. Alternatively, a macroreentrant wavefront may circulate around the border of the infarct scar. Multiple morphologies of sustained monomorphic ventricular tachycardia in a single patient are common.[32,39,40,41,190] These tachycardias can be due to different exits from the same reentry circuit; variations in the epicardial activation sequence, without a change in reentry circuit configuration; different reentry circuit configurations, involving the same slow conduction region; or anatomically separate reentry circuits.[42,44,168,190,191]

In canine models, coronary artery occlusion produces a layer of surviving cells in the subepicardium that can give produce reentrant arrhythmias.[163,182,184-186] In humans with ventricular tachycardia late after myocardial infarction, regions of abnormal conduction are most frequently located in left ventricular subendocardial regions.[165,171,176,177,192-205] In some patients, however, reentry circuits are in the subepicardium or intramurally or involve the right ventricle.[189,206,207]

Because chronic infarction is the substrate for postmyocardial infarction ventricular tachycardia, infarct location identified by abnormal ventricular wall motion is a useful guide to the region of interest. This is only a crude guide, however, because patients with ventricular tachycardia usually have large infarcted regions, with one or more reentry circuits that can be located anywhere in or around the infarct.

Standard 12-Lead Electrocardiogram

The QRS complex on the scalar electrocardiogram reflects the sequence of ventricular activation. For ventricular tachycardias that involve an area of slow conduction in an infarct scar (depolarization of which is not detectable in body-surface electrocardiogram), the QRS onset occurs after the excitation wavefront exits from the scar to propagate across the ventricles. The location of this exit is one determinant of the tachycardia QRS morphology.[208-213] A simplified summary of the QRS morphology as it relates to the likely exit location is shown in Table 23-6. Generally, postmyocardial infarction tachycardias with a left bundle branch configuration exit in or near the septum. A superiorly directed frontal plane axis often indicates early activation of the inferior wall or inferoseptum, whereas an inferior axis indicates a more superior location of earliest ventricular activation. A dominant R wave in V_4 and V_5 is consistent with early basal activation, whereas dominant S waves in these leads suggest early activation near the ventricular apex.

The QRS morphology is only a rough guide to the reentry circuit exit, however. The surface electrocardiogram QRS complex reflects predominantly the epicardial rather than the endocardial activation sequence. Slight differences in endocardial activation may sometimes produce dramatic changes in QRS configuration and substantial changes in epicardial activation and QRS morphology may occur without a change in endocardial activation.[168,209] The extent of the infarct scar, myocardial hyper-

TABLE 23-6. Relation of Ventricular Tachycardia QRS Morphology to Endocardial Site of Presystolic Electrograms

V_1	Frontal Plane Axis	V_4	LV Endocardial Location
LB	Left superior	S or qS	Apical septum
LB	Left superior	R	Basal septum
LB	Inferior	—	Anterior septum
RB	Left superior	R or rS	Inferobasal
RB	Left superior	S	Apical septum or apical inferior
RB	Right superior	S or rS	Apical inferior or apical septal
RB	Right superior	R	Inferobasal
RB	Inferior	S	Anterio-Apical
RB	Right inferior	R	Basal lateral

trophy, tachycardia rate, and the position of the heart in the chest also influence QRS morphology.[208, 210, 211, 214] The QRS morphology may also be misleading because exits from the infarct scar may be distant from other portions of the reentry circuit and therefor direct attention away from regions of interest. During rapid tachycardias or marked QRS prolongation due to antiarrhythmic drugs, superimposition of QRS and T waves hampers assessment of QRS morphology. The QRS morphology is a better guide to the origin of idiopathic ventricular tachycardias in structurally normal hearts than to tachycardias arising from infarct scars.

Sinus Rhythm Electrograms

The characteristics of left ventricular electrograms recorded during sinus rhythm from catheters with an interelectrode distance of 1 cm filtered at 30 to 500 Hz have been established by Cassidy and colleagues.[215] Normal ventricular electrograms have an amplitude greater than 3 mV and a duration of less than 70 milliseconds. In normal hearts, the earliest sinus rhythm (left ventricular) endocardial electrograms are recorded from the mid-septum, coincident with or immediately after the QRS onset in the surface electrocardiogram. The latest endocardial activation is recorded from the posterobasal left ventricle 50 milliseconds or less after the onset of the QRS in the surface electrocardiogram.

Slow conduction through myocardial scar produces delayed activation of tissue, even over relatively small areas. Endocardial electrograms from these areas have a prolonged duration, low amplitude, and multiple discrete rapid components that create a fractionated appearance (Fig. 23-4).[216-219] Fractionated electrograms often extend beyond the end of the QRS complex and are the likely source of late potentials detectable with high-gain low-noise recording techniques from the body surface. In a canine model, Gardner and coworkers showed that the multiple deflections seen in fractionated electrograms can be due to asynchronous depolarization of closely related muscle bundles.[220] It is important, however, to recognize that when recording at high amplification, fractionated electrograms can also be artifact.[221-223] Depolarizations occurring some distance from the recording site can sometimes create fractionated electrograms.[223] Interelectrode distance and filtering also influences whether an electrogram appears fractionated.[222]

Fractionated electrograms are generally recorded within or near akinetic or dyskinetic areas and are found over a larger area in patients with ventricular tachycardia than in those without this arrhythmia.[216, 217, 224-228] Wiener and associates recorded fractionated electrograms over a third to half of the aneurysm border zone in patients with ventricular tachycardia, as opposed to less than 20% of the border zone in patients without ventricular tachycardia.[228] Surgical endocardial resection of all areas with fractionated electrograms is associated with a high likelihood of cure.[226] Thus, it is likely that critical portions of reentry circuits are located somewhere within the areas that produce fractionated electrograms. Fractionated electrograms are often recorded over a relatively large region, however, and are not necessarily related to ventricular

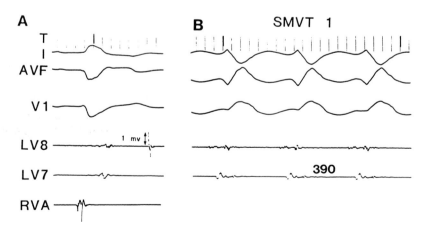

Figure 23-4. From the top of each panel are 50 millisecond surface electrocardiograms, leads I, aV$_f$, and V$_1$ and bipolar intracardiac electrograms filtered at 30–500 Hz from an area of left ventricular scar (LV$_8$ and LV$_7$) and the right ventricular apex (RVA). (**A**) A single sinus rhythm QRS complex. Compared with the RVA electrogram, electrograms at sites LV$_8$ and LV$_7$ are fractionated low-amplitude, with prolonged duration extending well beyond the end of the QRS complex. (**B**) Sustained monomorphic ventricular tachycardia at a cycle length of 390 millisecond is present. Fractionated electrograms at sites LV$_8$ and LV$_7$ precede the QRS onset.

tachycardia circuits. Some "bystander" areas generate abnormal electric activity but do not participate in a ventricular tachycardia circuit (see Fig. 23-3D).[229–232] Sinus rhythm mapping of endocardial activation may narrow the number of likely reentry circuit sites but does not establish whether a particular site is in the tachycardia circuit. At some sites, electrograms that are mildly abnormal during sinus rhythm become markedly fractionated at faster heart rates during pacing or ventricular tachycardia.[233]

Electrograms Recorded During Ventricular Tachycardia

Analysis of the sequence of ventricular electric activation during tachycardia (activation sequence mapping) is commonly used for mapping. During intraoperative mapping, electrograms from multiple epicardial sites can be simultaneously recorded using a mesh containing multiple electrodes pulled over the epicardium and a balloon covered with electrodes inserted into the left ventricle through the mitral valve or through an incision in a ventricular aneurysm.[165–168,175] With these methods, a complete reentry circuit can be delineated in only a few patients. In the remainder, it is likely that portions of the circuit are intramural, beyond range of the recording electrodes, or that activation of small amounts of tissue goes undetected by these recording techniques.[189] A common method of displaying these activation sequence maps is to draw lines through points having the same activation time, interpolating the activation time of the intervening tissue and creating an isochronal map. Limitations in this approach have been summarized and include difficulty in assessing the activation time in the presence of fractionated electrograms, typically present in areas of ventricular scar.[154,234]

During endocardial catheter mapping, only a limited number of sites can be simultaneously recorded. The timing of the endocardial electrograms is usually referenced to the onset of the surface electrocardiogram QRS complex.[235] If ventricular tachycardia is due to a small automatic focus surrounded by normal myocardium, the earliest ventricular electric activation immediately preceding the QRS onset is recorded at the tachycardia origin. With reentry tachycardias, some portion of the circuit is being activated throughout the cardiac cycle. A circuit in which the reentrant wavefront propagates around the border of an aneurysm, for example, is continuously depolarizing adjacent, more normal myocardium.[39,165,168,181] The surface electrocardiogram may reveal "ventricular flutter," with no definable onset or end to the QRS complex, especially if multiple electrocardiographic leads are simultaneously recorded. In circuits with an area of slow conduction through the scar that produces low-amplitude electric activity (see Fig. 23-4), the QRS onset occurs when the reentrant wavefront exits from the scar to depolarize

the more normal myocardium adjacent to the infarct scar. At or near the exit of the circuit (see Fig. 23-3D, site 1), electric activation immediately precedes the surface electrocardiogram QRS complex. The exit is commonly referred to as the site of origin. At other points in the circuit, the recorded electrograms may precede, follow, or coincide with the surface electrocardiogram QRS complex, depending on which part of the circuit is recorded (see Fig. 23-3D). If the reentry circuit is small, so that recording electrodes placed at the circuit record from the entire circuit, continuous electric activity spanning the cardiac cycle is recorded.[233,236,237]

Interpretation of electrograms is also complicated by the potential presence of bystander areas in the infarct region that are adjacent to but not actually participating in the reentry circuit (see Fig. 23-3D, site 21). These regions may generate fractionated electrograms, presystolic electric activity, and even continuous electric activity, which can often be dissociated from the tachycardia.[229–232] Electrograms may vanish and reemerge or display Wenckebacklike conduction behavior, with progressive delays followed by block despite there being no change in the ventricular tachycardia itself.[229,230] Ablation or cooling of a bystander area is unlikely to alter the tachycardia circuit.[164,231,232,238] In some cases, electrograms that suggest a bystander site are recording artifacts.

Electrogram timing has not been effective in guiding radiofrequency catheter ablation of postinfarct ventricular tachycardia, probably because of the limitations discussed above and the small lesions produced.[164,240] Some electrogram patterns do, however, indicate a high likelihood that the recording site is in a reentry circuit.[164,202,239] Fitzgerald and colleagues found that DC-shock catheter ablation at sites that displayed isolated mid- and early diastolic electric activity (Fig. 23-5) often abolished ventricular tachycardia.[202] To insure that these electrograms were not generated by bystander areas, these investigators excluded sites at which the electrograms could be dissociated from the tachycardia-QRS complexes during initiation and termination of tachycardia. In a study of radiofrequency catheter ablation involving 241 endocardial sites in 15 patients, isolated diastolic potentials were observed at only 5% of mapping sites but were associated with a fivefold increase in the likelihood of radiofrequency-current application at that site terminating ventricular tachycardia.[164]

Pace-Mapping

During ventricular pacing, the pacing-site location determines the ventricular activation sequence and hence the QRS morphology recorded in the 12-lead electrocardiogram.[208–211] Limitations of assessing endocardial activation from the QRS morphology also importantly influence pace-mapping. In some cases, pacing at closely adjacent

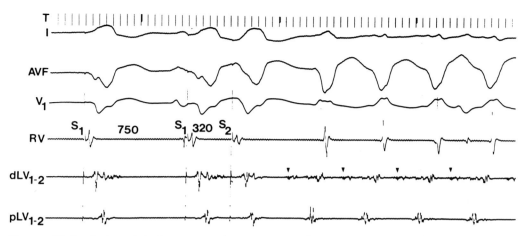

Figure 23-5. Endocardial electrograms during initiation of sustained monomorphic ventricular tachycardia. From the top are 50-millisecond time lines, surface electrocardiogram leads, I, aV₁ and V₁ and bipolar endocardial electrograms filtered at 30–500 Hz from the right ventricle (RV), and distal and proximal poles of a catheter positioned at the apical left ventricular septum (dLV₁₋₂ and pLV₁₋₂). A single extrastimulus (S₂) after a basic drive of 750 milliseconds (S₁) initiates monomorphic ventricular tachycardia. Electrograms at left ventricular site dLV₁₋₂ are markedly fractionated. A discrete mid-diastolic electrogram (arrows) is present before the first and all subsequent tachycardia beats, suggesting that this electrogram could arise from a portion of the tachycardia circuit.

sites produces dramatically different QRS complexes; in other cases, the same QRS morphology is observed during pacing at sites separated by centimeters. In patients with ventricular tachycardia, an endocardial site can often be identified at which pacing reproduces the ventricular tachycardia QRS morphology (Fig. 23-6).[200, 211, 240–243] This site often displays presystolic electrograms during ventricular tachycardia, suggesting that it is near the exit from the scar. At some reentry circuit sites, pace-mapping produces a QRS morphology markedly different from the tachycardia QRS.[44, 191, 241, 242] This is consistent with the relatively large size of some reentry circuits and the sometimes dramatic differences in QRS morphology that can occur with small changes in the initial site of endocardial activation.[165, 168, 209] The QRS morphology during pace-mapping has been a more reliable guide to tachycardia origin for idiopathic ventricular tachycardias than for post-infarct ventricular tachycardias.[240, 242, 244]

Pace-mapping can provide further evidence of slow ventricular conduction.[191, 241, 242, 245] At about half of the sites that have fractionated sinus rhythm electrograms, the QRS follows the stimulus by more than 40 milliseconds (see Fig. 23-6). This is consistent with slow conduction through abnormal myocardium surrounding the pacing site. The QRS is inscribed when the stimulated wavefront reaches the surrounding more normal myocardium. As is the case for sinus-rhythm mapping, evidence of slow conduction during pace-mapping does not confirm that the site is involved in a tachycardia circuit but facilitates identification of abnormal areas of interest for further evaluation.

Pacing at a rate close to that of the ventricular tachycar-dia is desirable for comparison of the paced and tachycardia QRS complexes. At some abnormal sites, relatively high pacing-current strengths are required for capture. Bipolar pacing has generally been used but introduces the possibility of local capture at the cathode, anode, or both electrodes simultaneously, depending on tissue contact, pacing current strength, and stimulus timing.[246–250] This concern can be obviated by unipolar pacing.

Programmed Stimulation During Tachycardia

ENTRAINMENT. If an excitable gap exists in a reentry circuit, appropriately timed excitation wavefronts from premature stimuli can depolarize a site in the reentry circuit in advance of the circulating tachycardia wavefront and advance or reset the circuit. A train of several stimuli may continuously reset the reentry circuit without terminating tachycardia. Waldo and coworkers and others define this response as entrainment (Fig. 23-7).[251–255] Entrainment is strong but not absolute evidence that reentry is the tachycardia mechanism.[251] Furthermore, entrainment can be used to identify the presence of slow conduction in the reentry circuit and to infer the location of pacing and recording sites relative to slow conduction in the circuit.[251–257] Entrainment can be demonstrated for most ventricular tachycardias arising in infarct scars if multiple pacing sites are explored.[164, 258–260]

During pacing, the presence of any one of four criteria is evidence that the tachycardia is entrained (Table 23-7). An example is shown in Figure 23-7. In Figure 23-7A, ventricular tachycardia with a cycle length of 570 milliseconds is present and the last four stimuli of a train at a cycle length of 470 milliseconds are shown. During pacing, the QRS complexes and all electrograms are accelerated to the pacing rate. After the last stimulus, the tachycardia con-

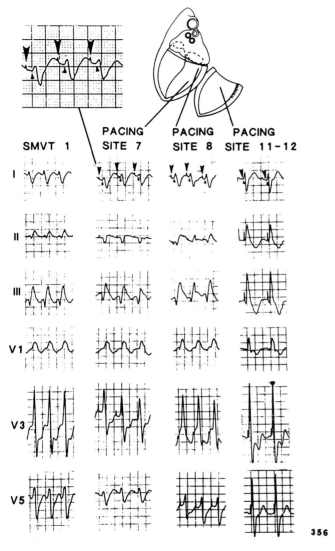

Figure 23-6. Six surface electrocardiogram leads, recorded during ventricular tachycardia (*SMVT-1*) and pacing at three left ventricular endocardial sites (7, 8, and 11–12). At each pacing site, the frontal and horizontal plane QRS axis is similar to that of the ventricular tachycardia. During pacing at sites 7 and 8, evidence for slow conduction is present, indicated by a delay of ≥ 80 milliseconds between the stimulus artifact (*large arrows* in lead I) and the QRS onset (*small arrows* in lead I) in all leads. During pacing at site 11, the stimulus to QRS interval is shorter than 20 milliseconds, consistent with rapid conduction away from the pacing site. Fractionated electrograms were recorded from sites 7 and 8 (not shown). An enlargement of lead I during pacing at site 7 is shown at the top left, and a schematic of the pacing site locations is at the top right. (Stevenson G, et al: Slow conduction in infarct scar: relevance to the occurance, detection, and ablation of ventricular re-entry circuits resulting from myocardial infarction. Am Heart J 1989; 117:457.)

tinues at its previous rate of 570 milliseconds. The mechanism of entrainment is shown schematically in Figure 23-7B, using the figure-eight reentry circuit model discussed above. The stimulation site is adjacent to the infarct scar. Each stimulated wavefront propagates into the area of slow conduction (toward site 5) and then toward the exit of the slow conduction area (site 1) and resets the tachycardia. All sites are accelerated to the pacing rate. Sites 5, 6, 1, 2, 3, RVS, and RVA are all activated orthodromically—by wavefronts traveling in the same direction as the tachycardia wavefronts.[256] Stimulation also produces antidromic wavefronts that propagate in the opposite direction in the circuit and wavefronts that propagate through myocardium outside the circuit in a different direction from the tachycardia wavefronts that exit the circuit. Electrograms from sites activated orthodromically have the same morphology during pacing as during tachycardia. In Figure 23-7A, electrograms at sites $LV_{6/8uni-2}$, RV_{ap}, and the right ventricular septum (*His*) have a similar morphology during pacing and tachycardia, consistent with depolarization from an orthodromic excitation wavefront. In Figure 23-7B, antidromic wavefronts depolarize sites 4 and 18 from a different direction than during tachycardia, altering electrogram morphology at these sites. In Figure 23-7A, the electrogram recorded from site $LV_{6/8p}$ is markedly different during pacing (compared with tachycardia), consistent with antidromic activation. During pacing, some of the ventricle distant from the circuit is activated by stimulated wavefronts that do not propagate through the circuit. This change in the sequence of ventricular activation alters the QRS morphology in the surface electrocardiogram. The antidromic wavefront collides with an orthodromic wavefront in myocardium distant from the circuit (see Fig. 23-7B, near site 18) producing fusion-QRS complexes. With continuous pacing, collision of the antidromic and orthodromic wavefronts occurs over a consistent zone;

TABLE 23-7. Criteria Indicating Entrainment of Ventricular Tachycardia*

1. Constant QRS fusion during pacing at a constant rate faster than the VT, which fails to terminate tachycardia, except for the last entrained beat, which with termination of pacing is not fused
2. Different degrees of constant QRS fusion during pacing at different rates, which fail to terminate VT
3. Localized conduction block during pacing at a rate that interrupts VT, indicated by failure of the stimulus to activate that site, followed by activation from the next stimulus with a shorter stimulus to electrogram interval
4. Electrogram equivalent of progressive fusion during pacing at two different rates that do not terminate tachycardia; the same site is activated from two different directions: from the wavefronts exiting the circuit (orthodromically) at the slower rate and from the stimulated wavefronts not propagating through the circuit (antidromically) at the faster rate

See references 239, 251–256.
VT, ventricular tachycardia.

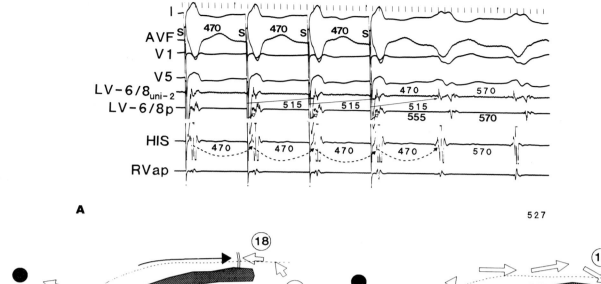

A

527

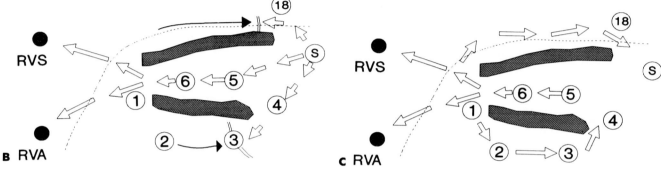

B RVA   **c** RVA

Figure 23-7. Entrainment of ventricular tachycardia. (**A**) From the top are 50-millisecond time lines, surface electrocardiogram leads, I, aV$_F$, V$_1$, V$_5$, and intracardiac electrograms recorded unipolar from electrode 2 at the left ventricular catheter (LV$_{6/8\,uni-2}$), bipolar from electrodes 3 and 4 of the left ventricular catheter (LV$_{6/8p}$), and bipolar right ventricular electrograms recorded from the His-bundle position (His) and apex (RV$_{ap}$). Sustained monomorphic ventricular tachycardia at a cycle length of 570 milliseconds was present. The last four stimuli (*S*) of a train at a cycle length of 470 milliseconds are shown. All electrograms are accelerated to the pacing cycle length. During pacing, QRS complexes have a constant morphology intermediate between completely paced and tachycardia QRS morphologies due to fusion. After the last stimulus, the subsequent QRS (515 milliseconds after the stimulus) occurs at the pacing cycle length (470 milliseconds) but has the same morphology as the unpaced tachycardia beats and is therefore not fused. During pacing electrogram in the His, RV$_{ap}$ and the sharp electrogram in the LV$_{6/8}$ uni-2 tracing, which occurs 515 milliseconds after the stimulus, are similar in morphology to those recorded during tachycardia in the absence of pacing, visible in the last electrograms at the right of the tracing. These sites appear to be depolarized by an orthodromic wavefront during entrainment. In contrast, electrograms at site LV$_{6/8p}$ are different during entrainment, as compared with tachycardia, consistent with depolarization of this site by an antidromic wavefront. (**B** and **C**) The likely mechanism, using the figure-eight reentry circuit model shown in Figure 22-3 *D*. The stimulus site (*S*) is adjacent to the reentry circuit near the entrance to the common pathway. Recording sites RVS and RVA are distant from the circuit, such as the His and RV$_{ap}$ recordings in *A*. Stimulated wavefronts are shown as open arrows, tachycardia wavefronts as *solid arrows*. (**B**) The first stimulus at site *S* produces orthodromic wavefronts that propagate through the circuit (e.g., to sites 5, 6) and an antidromic wavefront that collides (solid lines) near sites 18 and 3 with the returning tachycardia wavefront. Subsequent stimulated antidromic wavefronts collide at approximately the same site with returning stimulated orthodromic wavefronts. In panel *C*, the last stimulated orthodromic wavefront finds no antidromic wavefront with which to collide because (the antidromic wavefront from the last stimulus collided with the previous returning orthodromic wavefront). The QRS complex from the last stimulated orthodromic wavefront is therefore not fused. The last stimulated orthodromic wavefront reenters the common pathway, continuing the tachycardia.

thus, the degree of fusion and the QRS morphology are constant from beat to beat (see Fig. 23-7A, the first 4 beats). Constant fusion is the first criterion for entrainment. On termination of pacing (see Fig. 23-7C), the last stimulated orthodromic wavefront propagates through the circuit and exits from the slow pathway after a delay equal to the conduction time from the stimulus site to the exit from the circuit. This orthodromic wavefront finds no antidromic wavefront to collide with. Hence, in Figure 23-7A, the beat after the stimulus (indicated by the *last arrow*) occurs at the pacing rate (470 milliseconds) but the QRS is identical to the tachycardia QRS and is not fused—the second criterion that demonstrates entrainment.

The timing of electrograms after termination of pacing depends on the pacing- and recording-site locations relative to the tachycardia circuit. After the last stimulus, sites activated orthodromically by wavefronts that have propagated through the area of slow conduction (see Fig. 23-7A, ventricular electrograms labeled *His* and *RV$_{ap}$*; and Fig. 23-7B and C, sites *5*, *6*, *1*) are depolarized by the last paced orthodromic wavefront after a delay equal to the conduction time from the stimulus site through a portion of the reentry circuit to the exit that produces the QRS onset. Identifying the last electrogram that occurs at the pacing cycle length of 470 milliseconds at site LV$_{6/8uni-2}$ in Figure 23-7A (*arrow*), it becomes apparent that the electrogram immediately after each stimulus is actually produced by the stimulated orthodromic wavefront from the previous stimulus. In contrast to orthodromically activated sites, site LV$_{6/8p}$ in Figure 23-7A and sites 4 and 18 in Figure 23-7B and C are depolarized antidromically by a stimulated wavefront that arrives at the site from a different direction when compared with the tachycardia wavefronts. After termination of pacing, these sites are depolarized by a wavefront that propagates orthodromically through the circuit. The interval between the electrogram produced by antidromic capture of the site and depolarization of the site from the last stimulated orthodromic wavefront (see Fig. 23-7A, 555 milliseconds in LV$_{6/8p}$) is longer than the pacing-cycle length.

As the pacing rate is increased (not shown), there is evidence of progressive fusion. At a pacing rate slightly faster than the tachycardia cycle length, a relatively small amount of the ventricle is depolarized by the antidromic wavefront. At faster pacing rates, the antidromic wavefront propagates a greater distance before colliding with an orthodromic wavefront. The stimulated antidromic wavefront depolarizes a progressively greater proportion of the ventricle and the fusion QRS complexes more closely resemble a totally paced QRS morphology. Evidence of progressive fusion may also be detected in intracardiac recordings. Sites may be depolarized by orthodromic wavefronts at slow pacing rates and by antidromic wavefronts at faster rates. This is the electrogram equivalent of progressive fusion, the fourth criterion indicative of entrainment.[254]

At a critically rapid pacing rate, the orthodromic wavefront may block the circuit, terminating tachycardia. The orthodromic wavefront fails to depolarize sites distal to the block, which are then depolarized by a stimulated antidromic wavefront. Evidence of conduction block between the pacing and recording site, followed by depolarization of the site from a different direction (antidromically) accompanied by termination of tachycardia is the third criterion for entrainment. Presence of any one of these four criteria (see Table 23-7) indicates entrainment.

At rapid pacing rates or during pacing at sites close to the circuit exit, the stimulated antidromic wavefront may capture virtually all of the ventricle distant from the circuit while still continuously resetting the circuit. The QRS morphology appears totally paced, without fusion, yet entrainment can still be occurring and may be demonstrated if recordings are obtained from the circuit. This has been called "concealed entrainment."[255,257]

In these examples, the pacing site is located some distance from the reentry circuit; hence, the stimulated wavefront captures a portion of the ventricle antidromically (from a different direction relative to activation by the tachycardia wavefronts), producing a change in the QRS morphology, compared with the tachycardia-QRS complexes.

STIMULATION AT SITES IN AND ADJACENT TO REENTRY CIRCUITS. Programmed electric stimulation at some sites in or near ventricular reentry circuits can entrain or reset tachycardia but with a QRS morphology during pacing that is identical to that of the tachycardia QRS complexes (Figs. 23-8 and 23-9). QRS fusion is absent in the surface electrocardiogram.[261–271] This has been called entrainment with concealed fusion, exact entrainment, or another form of concealed entrainment.[43,44,164,191,203,207,244] Entrainment with concealed fusion can be observed with stimulus trains (see Fig. 23-9) or single stimuli (see Fig. 23-8). The mechanism is illustrated in Figure 23-8B for a theoretic figure-eight reentry circuit with a central slow-conduction zone. In this example, the stimulus site is in the common slow pathway. A capturing stimulus (during the excitable gap) produces excitation wavefronts that propagate in the orthodromic direction toward the exit from the slow common central pathway, and in the antidromic direction toward the entrance of the slow central pathway. The antidromic wavefront collides with a returning orthodromic wavefront within the circuit and does not reach tissue distant from the scar. The antidromic wavefront does not alter the sequence of ventricular activation distant from the scar and does not therefore alter the QRS morphology. The stimulated orthodromic wavefront propagates through the slow common pathway to its exit

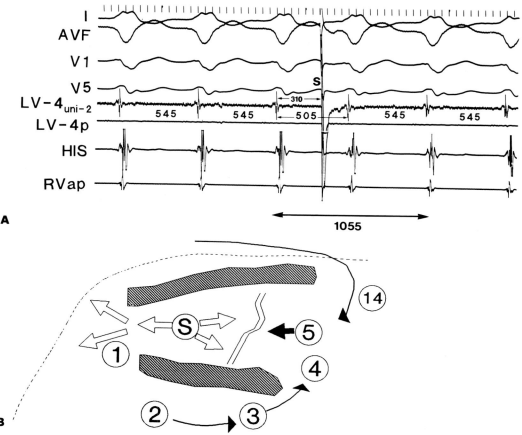

Figure 23-8. Resetting of ventricular tachycardia by a single stimulus at an area of slow conduction in the reentry circuit. (**A**) From the top are 50-millisecond time lines, surface electrocardiogram leads I, aV$_F$, V$_1$ and V$_5$, and intracardiac electrograms as follows: the unipolar recording from electrode 2 of the left ventricular catheter (*LV$_{4\ uni\ -2}$*); the bipolar recording from the proximal electrode pair of the left ventricular catheter (*L$_{V4p}$*); the bipolar recording from the His-bundle position (*His*); and the bipolar recording from the right ventricular apex (*RV$_{ap}$*). Sustained monomorphic ventricular tachycardia is from the same patient as in Figure 22-7 but has accelerated to a cycle length of 545 milliseconds. A single stimulus (*S*) at the distal LV electrode 310 milliseconds after the unipolar electrogram is shown. The stimulus advances the next QRS complex by 30 milliseconds (from 545 to 505 milliseconds) with no change in QRS morphology. The tachycardia is reset as indicated by the prematurity of the next QRS complex that occurs at 1055 milliseconds rather than at an interval of two cycle lengths (1090 milliseconds) after the QRS complex that precedes the stimulus. (**B**) The mechanism of this finding in the figure-eight reentry circuit model shown in Figure 22-3. A stimulus (*S*) in the common pathway produces orthodromic and antidromic wavefronts (*open arrows*). The antidromic wavefronts, moving from site *S* toward site 5, collide with returning tachycardia wavefronts (*solid arrows*) between the stimulus site and site 5 and are contained within the circuit. The stimulated orthodromic wavefront exits from the slow conduction pathways near site 1, initiating the early QRS complex and continues to propagate through the circuit, resetting the tachycardia. The QRS complex produced by the stimulated orthodromic wavefront has the same morphology as the tachycardia QRS because both the stimulated and tachycardia wavefronts exit the scar from the same site. In panel *A*, the relatively short delay (80 milliseconds) from stimulus to advanced QRS is consistent with a site in the distal portion of the common pathway.

and out into the surrounding myocardium, advancing the tachycardia. The interval between the stimulus and the premature QRS complex reflects the time required for the stimulated excitation wavefront to propagate from the pacing site to the exit. The premature QRS is similar in morphology to the tachycardia QRS complexes because the stimulated orthodromic wavefront exits the common slow pathway at the same site as the tachycardia wavefronts. Thus, the tachycardia is reset without altering the QRS morphology because the stimulated antidromic wavefronts are contained within or near the circuit. This can also be observed with a single stimulus. In some cases,

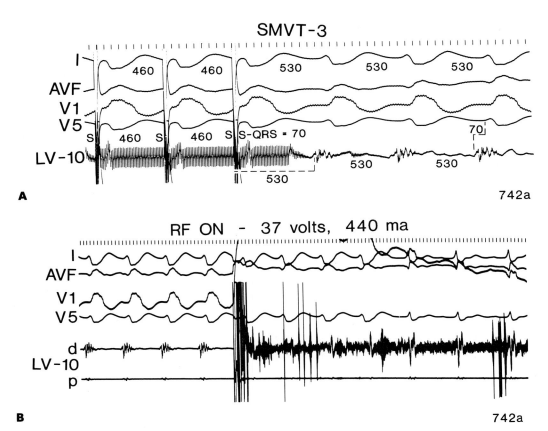

Figure 23-9. Programmed stimulation and application of radiofrequency current to a site near the exit of a reentry circuit. From the top of each tracing are 50-millisecond time lines, surface electrocardiogram leads I, aV$_f$, V$_1$ and V$_5$, and bipolar intracardiac recordings from the distal electrode pair of the mapping catheter at left ventricular site 10(LV$_{10}$). Sustained monomorphic ventricular tachycardia with a cycle length of 530 milliseconds is present. (**A**) The last three beats of stimulus train at a cycle length of 460 milliseconds. Pacing entrains tachycardia with concealed fusion. During pacing, there is considerable 60-Hz noise on the recording electrodes, which decays sufficiently to observe an electrogram occurring 530 milliseconds (*dashed line*) after the last stimulus at the pacing site. The postpacing interval matches the tachycardia cycle length of 530 milliseconds, consistent with a reentry circuit site. The stimulus-to-QRS interval (S-QRS) during entrainment is 70 milliseconds. The onset of the electrogram recorded from the pacing site during tachycardia is 70 milliseconds before the QRS complex. The S-QRS approximates the electrogram-to-QRS interval, consistent with a reentry circuit site. (**B**) Radiofrequency current is applied to this site during ventricular tachycardia. Tachycardia terminates after four beats, again suggesting that the site was in the reentry circuit. (Reproduced with permission from Stevenson WG, Khan H, Sager P, et al: Identification of reentry circuit sites during catheter mapping and radiofrequency ablation of ventricular tachycardia late after myocardial infarction. Circulation 1993;88[Pt1]:1647.)

stimuli produce only small changes in electrogram and QRS timing. Cursory observation may falsely suggest that the stimulus did not capture, and careful measurement may be required to demonstrate that the tachycardia has been reset in the manner described. Entrainment with concealed fusion is associated with a threefold increase likelihood that application of radiofrequency current at the site will terminate ventricular tachycardia (Table 23-8).[164]

Although entrainment with concealed fusion is consistent with stimulation at a reentry circuit site, it can also occur during pacing at some bystander sites adjacent to

the reentry circuit.[164, 244, 269] Methods to identify this possibility have been suggested.[164, 269] After the last paced stimulus at a reentry circuit site that entrains tachycardia, the next depolarization at the pacing site is due to arrival of the last stimulated orthodromic wavefront. This stimulated wavefront has made one revolution through the reentry circuit. Therefore, the interval from the last stimulus to the following electrogram (the postpacing interval) recorded at the pacing site approximates the revolution time through the circuit, which is the tachycardia cycle length, as shown in Figure 23-9A.[164] In contrast, when the stimulus

TABLE 23-8. Predictors of VT Termination by Radiofrequency Current Application

	Patients (n)	RF-Current Termination	%	Odds Ratio	95% CI
ECF					
Yes	86	15	17	3.4	1.4–8.3
No	155	9	6		
PPI–VTCL < 30 MS					
Yes	64	13	20	4.6	1.6–12.9
No	114	4	4		
DP OR CEA					
Yes	19	6	32	5.2	1.8–15.5
No	222	18	8		
S-QRS < 70% VTCL > 60 MS					
Yes	132	19	14	4.9	1.4–17.1
No	83	3	4		
ECF + PPI–VTCL <30 MS*					
Yes	40	10	25	5.3	2.0–13.8
No	168	11	7		
ECF + PPI + S-QRS < 70% > 60 MS*					
Yes	22	8	36	8.8	3.1–25.2
No	186	12	6		
ECF + DP OR CEA					
Yes	11	5	45	9.3	2.6–33.4
No	230	19	8		
ANY DP/CEA/PPI/ECF					
Yes	115	18	16	4.3	1.2–15.4
No	73	3	4		

CEA, continuous electrical activity; CI, confidence interval; DP, isolated diastolic potential; ECF, entrainment with concealed fusion; PPI, postpacing interval; RF, radiofrequency; S-QRS, stimulus to QRS interval during entrainment with concealed fusion; VT, ventricular tachycardia; VTCL, ventricular tachycardia cycle length.

*PPI-VTCL < 30 during ECF or entrainment with QRS fusion.

From Stevenson WG, Khan H, Sager P, et al: Identification of re-entry circuit sites during catheter mapping and radiofrequency ablation of ventricular tachycardia late after myocardial infarction. Circulation 1993;88(Pt1):1647.

site is not in the reentry circuit, stimulated wavefronts must propagate through tissue between the pacing site to reach the circuit. The interval from the last stimulus that entrains tachycardia to the next depolarization at the pacing site is the conduction time required for the last stimulated wavefront to propagate (1) from the pacing site, (2) to the reentry circuit, (3) through the reentry circuit, and (4) back to the pacing site. The postpacing interval exceeds the tachycardia cycle length (Fig. 23-10).

Analysis of the postpacing interval assumes that the electrogram recorded from the site reflects depolarization of the tissue captured by the pacing stimuli.[164,272] This is not always true. In some cases, far field electric activity may be recorded as discussed above. During bipolar pacing,

depolarization may occur at the cathode, anode, or both electrodes simultaneously. To eliminate this potential source of variability, unipolar pacing can be performed.[164] Validity of the postpacing interval as an indicator of pacing-site location relative to the reentry circuit assumes that the circuit and conduction velocities through the circuit are not altered by pacing. It cannot be applied if pacing alters the tachycardia morphology or cycle length.[149] Because alterations in conduction velocity or reentry circuit path are more likely at rapid pacing rates or with early premature stimuli, the postpacing interval should be assessed from pacing trains that are only slightly faster than the tachycardia or the latest single stimuli that capture. In one study, a postpacing interval within 30 milliseconds of the tachycardia cycle length during entrainment was associated with a 4.6-fold increase in the likelihood that radiofrequency current applied to the site would terminate ventricular tachycardia (see Table 23-8).[164]

During entrainment with concealed fusion, the S-QRS interval reflects the conduction time from the pacing site to the site at which the orthodromic wavefronts exit the scar to produce the QRS onset.[164,269] Pacing at a reentry circuit site, the S-QRS approximates the electrogram to QRS interval (see Fig. 23-9A). This is unlikely to occur during pacing at bystander regions (see Fig. 23-10). As with analysis of the postpacing interval, the slowest pacing rate that entrains tachycardia with concealed fusion or the latest single stimulus that captures should be used for this analysis. The S-QRS interval during entrainment with concealed fusion reflects the location of the pacing site relative to slow conduction in the circuit. Radiofrequency-current application terminates tachycardia more often at sites with S-QRS interval less than 70% of the tachycardia cycle length than when the S-QRS is longer, suggesting that sites proximal to regions of slow conduction are less desirable for ablation.[164]

A unique mode of tachycardia termination that is likely to indicate close proximity of the pacing site to the reentry circuit has been described in a few patients and in canine models.[183,262,266,273–275] Stimuli fail to elicit a premature QRS complex yet terminate the tachycardia (Fig. 23-11). Figure 21-11B illustrates a possible mechanism of this effect during stimulation in the common central pathway of slow conduction in a figure-eight reentry circuit.[276] The stimulated antidromic wavefront again collides with the returning orthodromic wavefronts near the entrance to the common pathway and is extinguished. The orthodromic wavefront encounters refractory tissue between the stimulation site and the exit from the common pathway and is blocked, terminating tachycardia. The stimulated orthodromic and antidromic wavefronts are not detectable in the electrocardiogram because they are confined in or near the circuit in scar tissue. An alternative explanation is prolongation of local refractoriness due to an electrotonic effect of a noncapturing stimulus.[274,276–278]

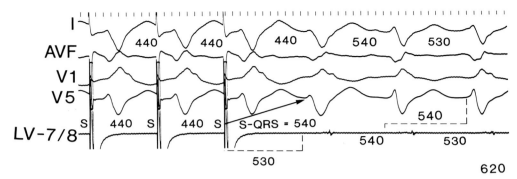

Figure 23-10. Entrainment with concealed fusion during pacing at a bystander site. From the top are 50-millisecond time lines, surface electrocardiogram leads I, aV$_f$, V$_1$, and V$_5$, and a bipolar recording from the distal electrode pair of the left ventricular mapping catheter at a site LV$_{7/8}$. Sustained monomorphic ventricular tachycardia with a cycle length of 520 to 540 milliseconds is present. The last three beats of a train of stimuli at a cycle length of 440 milliseconds at the mapping site are shown. Ventricular tachycardia is entrained, with minimal or no change in QRS morphology. At the mapping site, no electrograms are detectable 530 milliseconds (the tachycardia cycle length) after the last stimulus. The stimulus-to-QRS interval (*S-QRS*), measured to the last QRS entrained to the pacing cycle length, is quite long at 540 milliseconds. As shown by the *dashed line* from the last QRS, no electrograms are detectable at the mapping site 540 milliseconds preceding the QRS onset. These findings are consistent with a bystander area adjacent to the reentry circuit. Application of radiofrequency current to this site (not shown) failed to terminate ventricular tachycardia. (Reproduced with permission from Stevenson WG, Khan H, Sager P, et al: Identification of reentry circuit sites during catheter mapping and radiofrequency ablation of ventricular tachycardia late after myocardial infarction. Circulation 1993;88[Pt1]:1647.)

Application of Radiofrequency Current During Ventricular Tachycardia

Application of radiofrequency current to the mapping catheter heats the underlying myocardium, generally without eliciting propagated depolarizations. Heating impairs electric activity of the tissue. Hence, radiofrequency-current application can be used as a type of thermal mapping. Termination of ventricular tachycardia during radiofrequency-current application suggests that the ablation site is in the tachycardia circuit.[164] The relation of electrogram and programmed stimulation criteria discussed above to the likelihood that radiofrequency current will terminate ventricular tachycardia was investigated in 15 patients with 31 morphologies of monomorphic ventricular tachycardia late after myocardial infarction (see Table 23-8).[164] Entrainment with concealed fusion with a S-QRS interval less than 70% of the tachycardia cycle length, a minimum postpacing interval within 30 milliseconds of the tachycardia cycle length, and the presence of isolated diastolic potentials or continuous electric activity were predictors of likely reentry circuit sites.

Transcoronary Mapping and Chemical Ablation

Myocytes involved in producing ventricular tachycardia require a blood supply, as does all living cardiac tissue. In some patients, the coronary vessel supplying the arrhyth-

mogenic tissue can be identified and cannulated.[279, 280] Transient interruption of blood flow by catheter occlusion or saline injection terminates ventricular tachycardia. Sclerosis of the vessel with absolute ethanol has been successful in preventing inducible ventricular tachycardia in some patients. Potential complications of this experimental procedure include myocardial infarction and heart block from damage to septal vessels supplying the conduction system.

VENTRICULAR TACHYCARDIAS UNRELATED TO CORONARY ARTERY DISEASE

Bundle Branch Reentry Ventricular Tachycardia

Macroreentry within the bundle branches is commonly observed during programmed ventricular stimulation but usually terminates spontaneously within one or two beats.[103] Sustained macroreentry involving the bundle branches is an uncommon but important cause of ventricular tachycardia.[281, 282] When the tachycardia is initiated by right ventricular pacing, the circuit established tends to conduct retrograde over a portion of the left bundle branch system and antegrade over the right bundle. Tachy-

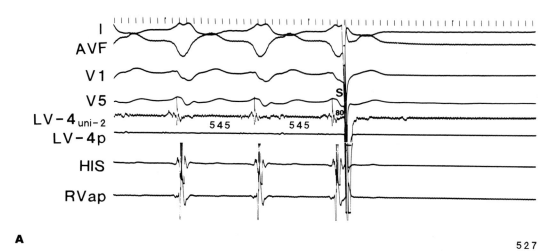

A

527

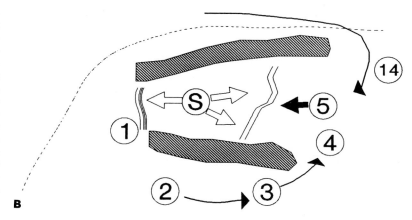

B

Figure 23-11. Termination of ventricular tachycardia by a nonpropagating stimulus is shown. (**A**) The same tachycardia and as in Figure 22-8. A single stimulus at LV site 4, 80 milliseconds after the local electrogram, fails to produce a detectable propagated response but terminates sustained monomorphic ventricular tachycardia. (**B**) One possible mechanism, using the figure-eight circuit shown in Figure 22-3. Stimulation is at a site in the slow common pathway (S) Late stimuli reset tachycardia, as shown in Figure 22-8. The antidromic wavefront from an early stimulus collides with the returning orthodromic wavefront and is extinguished. The stimulated orthodromic wavefront is blocked when it encounters refractory tissue, terminating tachycardia. All effects of the capturing stimuli are confined to the circuit.

cardias then have a left bundle branch block–QRS configuration. When tachycardia is initiated by left ventricular pacing, retrograde conduction typically is over the right bundle, with antegrade conduction and ventricular activation through the left bundle. Consequently, tachycardia displays a right bundle branch block–QRS morphology. A His-bundle deflection is present, preceding each QRS complex, usually by an interval exceeding the sinus rhythm His-bundle to ventricle (HV) interval. Bundle branch reentry is easily distinguished from supraventricular tachycardia with aberrancy by atrioventricular dissociation (absence of a one-to-one relation between the QRS complexes and atrial activity). Ventricular tachycardia with passive retrograde conduction through the His-Purkinje system can be excluded by careful analysis of His (and right bundle branch) activation. The His deflection cannot be dissociated from the tachycardia. Spontaneous changes in the His-bundle to His-bundle (H-H) interval are followed by a similar change in the ventricle to ventricle (V-V) interval. Tachycardia terminates if retrograde block occurs (His deflection absent after the last tachycardia QRS complex). Bundle branch macroreentry is occa-

sionally initiated by atrial programmed stimulation.[281] Initiation may be facilitated by use of long–short paced ventricular sequences, which tend to increase the disparity in refractoriness between the His-Purkinje system and ventricular myocardium.[283]

Bundle branch reentrant ventricular tachycardia comprised 6% of all ventricular tachycardias studied at a large referral center.[282] It should be particularly suspected when sustained ventricular tachycardia occurs in a patient with nonischemic dilated cardiomyopathy or valvular heart disease. The sinus rhythm electrocardiogram often displays a nonspecific intraventricular conduction delay. The HV interval during sinus rhythm is almost always prolonged.

Bundle branch reentry tachycardias tend to be rapid (mean cycle length, 280 milliseconds, ranging from 240 to 360 milliseconds) and can cause syncope and sudden death.[282] The right bundle is an obligate portion of the reentry circuit and can be easily located and ablated with an endocardial catheter, which is usually the treatment of choice.[284–287] In patients with prior myocardial infarction, bundle branch reentry may coexist with other ventricular tachycardias that require additional therapy.[286]

Ventricular Tachycardia in Nonischemic Dilated Cardiomyopathy

The electrophysiologic substrate responsible for ventricular tachycardia in patients with nonischemic causes of dilated cardiomyopathy has not been well-defined. Programmed stimulation can initiate ventricular tachycardia in most patients who have suffered a spontaneous episode of sustained ventricular tachycardia, again suggesting reentry or triggered automaticity as potential mechanisms.[288-291] In contrast to those of the postmyocardial infarction patients, fractionated endocardial electrograms are generally absent in nonischemic cardiomyopathy.[216] Examination of endomyocardial biopsies has shown a rough correlation of ventricular tachycardia with the extent of myocardial hypertrophy but not with the extent of fibrosis.[290] Biopsies are focal samplings, however, which may not include the portion of the ventricle generating the arrhythmia. Macroreentry within the bundle branches may cause a greater proportion of ventricular tachycardias in these patients than in postmyocardial infarction patients.

Right Ventricular Dysplasia

Right ventricular dysplasia is characterized by replacement of right ventricular myocardium by fatty and fibrous tissue.[292, 293] Involvement can be diffuse, with marked right ventricular enlargement or focal abnormalities producing discrete areas of akinesis or dyskinesis, typically located in the anterior infundibulum, right ventricular apex, or diaphragmatic aspect of the right ventricle. Occasionally, focal abnormalities of left ventricular wall motion are present.[294] Ventricular tachycardia may originate in any of the involved right ventricular areas and has a left bundle branch block–QRS configuration. Tachycardias originating in the right ventricular outflow tract have a frontal plane axis directed inferiorly between $+60°$ and $+135°$. Inferior and apical sites of origin produce tachycardias with a superiorly directed QRS axis, leftward of $-30°$. The sinus rhythm electrocardiogram often displays complete or incomplete right bundle branch block. In some patients, delayed right ventricular activation produces a slurred deflection after the QRS complex in the anterior precordial leads.[295] The signal-averaged electrocardiogram is usually abnormal, and epicardial intraoperative mapping confirms delayed ventricular activation at sites of right ventricular involvement.[295, 296]

At electrophysiology study, fractionated long-duration electrograms are recorded from areas of involvement. During pace-mapping, a long delay is present between the stimulus and the QRS onset (consistent with slow conduction) at some of these sites.[261, 295] Programmed electric stimulation initiates sustained monomorphic ventricular

tachycardia in more than 90% of patients who suffered this arrhythmia spontaneously.[293-299] Areas of slow conduction and the response to programmed stimulation are consistent with reentry. Multiple morphologies of tachycardia are common. Accelerated idioventricular rhythms may also arise from involved areas.[300] A history of exercise-provokable ventricular tachycardia is common and isoproterenol infusion facilitates tachycardia initiation in some patients.

Not all patients with right ventricular dysplasia suffer sustained ventricular arrhythmias. Programmed stimulation did not initiate sustained ventricular tachycardia in a series of 15 patients who had complex ventricular ectopy but no spontaneous or exercise-induced sustained ventricular tachycardia.[297]

Although sudden death and syncope occur, sudden death is relatively uncommon once the patient is under medical care and receiving therapy.[293, 299, 301] Class I and III antiarrhythmic drugs and β-adrenergic blockers can be effective in suppressing spontaneous arrhythmias. In one study, prognosis and risk of arrhythmia recurrence could not be predicted from electrophysiologic testing.[299] For patients with recurrent debilitating episodes of tachycardia, surgical ventriculotomy with or without cryoablation of arrhythmogenic foci and catheter ablation are alternatives.[302] Endocardial catheter ablation guided by activation mapping and pace-mapping have been successful in suppressing spontaneous sustained ventricular tachycardia in 40% to 70% of patients, although multiple sessions are often required.[303-305] It is likely that this approach will be supplanted by other ablation modalities. After surgery or catheter ablation, new arrhythmogenic foci develop with time in some patients.

Hypertrophic Cardiomyopathy

The incidence of sudden death in hypertrophic cardiomyopathy is 2% to 6% per year.[306] Young age at diagnosis, history of syncope, positive family history, and nonsustained ventricular tachycardia on ambulatory electrocardiogram recordings are associated with an increased risk of sudden death. Nonsustained ventricular tachycardia is present in a fourth of patients, however, and the positive predictive value for identifying future sudden death victims is poor. Spontaneous sustained monomorphic ventricular tachycardia is rare. Ventricular stimulation with up to two extrastimuli initiates sustained polymorphic ventricular tachycardia or ventricular flutter that rapidly degenerates to ventricular fibrillation in 18% to 45% of high-risk patients who have been resuscitated from cardiac arrest or who have a history of syncope or nonsustained ventricular tachycardia on ambulatory recordings.[307-310] Fananapazir and coworkers studied 155 patients referred because of syncope, cardiac arrest, nonsustained ventricular tachycardia, family history, or palpitations.[310] Programmed stimulation initiated sustained polymorphic ventricular tachycardia or ventricular fibrillation in 32% of patients and sustained monomorphic ventricular tachycardia with a mean cycle length of 266 ± 59 milliseconds in 10% of patients. Kuck and coworkers initiated sustained ventricular arrhythmias in 6 (14%) of 43 unselected patients who did not have a history of syncope or cardiac arrest.[308] In occasional patients, rapid atrial pacing or initiation of supraventricular arrhythmias precipitates ventricular fibrillation, an event that can also occur spontaneously.[311] During programmed stimulation, endocardial electrograms are frequently prolonged and multiphasic, suggesting slowed asynchronous myocardial activation that may facilitate reentry.[309] The prognostic significance of inducible arrhythmias or suppression of inducible arrhythmias in hypertrophic cardiomyopathy is not clear.

Ventricular Tachycardia in the Absence of Structural Heart Disease

Rare patients without identifiable structural heart disease suffer from sustained ventricular tachycardia.[312-320] In some cases, repetitive monomorphic ventricular tachycardia is incessant, with frequent ventricular tachycardia runs of three to 20 beats or longer present for more than 12 out of every 24 hours.[312,313,321,322]

The most common ventricular tachycardia in the absence of structural heart disease originates in the right ventricular outflow tract and has a left bundle branch block configuration and either a normal or rightward frontal plane axis.[313,314,316,317,323-326] Right ventricular wall motion abnormalities, an abnormal signal-averaged electrocardiogram, or other tachycardia morphologies strongly suggest right ventricular dysplasia rather than idiopathic tachycardia. Fibrosis on endomyocardial biopsy may indicate early right ventricular dysplasia despite apparently normal right ventricular wall motion.[327] Endocardial electrograms recorded during sinus rhythm appear normal, although at rapid heart rates, electrogram duration may prolong at the right ventricular outflow tract.[313,327] The predilection for right ventricular outflow tract origin is unexplained. Tachycardia is often exercise-induced and isoproterenol infusion is frequently required for initiation during electrophysiologic study. Some tachycardias are terminated by intravenous administration of adenosine, falsely suggesting a diagnosis of supraventricular tachycardia with aberrancy.[324] Although syncope and sudden death occur, sudden death is rare once the patient is receiving antiarrhythmic drug therapy, and the prognosis is good.[312] Therapy with β-adrenergic–blocking

drugs, and class I or III antiarrhythmic drugs has been effective, although not uniformly so.

Catheter ablation has been highly successful.[324,325,328-332] The absence of fractionated endocardial electrograms and the presence of normal ventricular function suggests that the arrhythmogenic focus is small. Pace-mapping often identifies a site where the paced QRS exactly matches the tachycardia in more than 10 of the 12 standard electrocardiogram leads. Endocardial activation at this site precedes the QRS complex by 10 to 40 milliseconds. Radiofrequency ablation eliminates tachycardia in more than 90% of patients, although follow-up longer than a few years is not yet available.

A second group of idiopathic ventricular tachycardias display right bundle branch block–QRS configurations.[312,319,333-338] The frontal plane QRS axis may be directed either superiorly or inferiorly. When the QRS frontal plane axis is directed superiorly, earliest endocardial activation has been recorded at the apical inferior left ventricle. When the frontal plane QRS axis is rightward or inferior, earliest endocardial activation has been recorded at the anterosuperior left ventricular apex. Endocardial electrograms are normal in appearance. An origin in or near the Purkinje fascicles of the left ventricle is suggested by the presence of a His-bundle potential 10 to 20 milliseconds after the earliest ventricular activation, consistent with early activation of the Purkinje system and rapid retrograde conduction to the His bundle.[320,333,335,337] Tachycardia is frequently provoked by exercise or isoproterenol infusion and terminated by intravenous verapamil and occasionally adenosine.[326,337] Tachycardia can often be entrained by pacing at the right ventricular outflow tract, suggesting reentry as the mechanism.[336]

Programmed stimulation initiates ventricular tachycardias in more than two thirds of patients, occasionally with rapid atrial pacing or atrial extrastimuli in addition to ventricular stimulation.[319,320,333-335] Ventricular tachycardia is often provokable by exercise and isoproterenol infusions. Therapy with β-adrenergic–blocking drugs, calcium channel blocking drugs, or class I or III antiarrhythmic drugs has been successful although not uniformly so. Radiofrequency catheter ablation has been attempted in only a few patients.[329,337] Nakagawa and coworkers eliminated ventricular tachycardia in seven of eight patients by targeting sites in the apical left ventricular septum, from which presystolic sharp potentials, possibly originating from Purkinje fibers, were recorded.[337]

References

1. Wellens HJJ, Schuilenberg RM, Durrer D: Electrical stimulation of the heart in patients with ventricular tachycardia. Circulation 1972;46:216.
2. Jazayeri MR, Van Whye G, Avitall B, McKinnie J, Tchou P,

Akhtar M: Isoproterenol reversal of antiarrhythmic effects in patients with inducible sustained ventricular tachyarrhythmias. J Am Coll Cardiol 1989;14:704.

3. Nattel S, Rinkenberger RL, Lehrman LL, Zipes DP: Therapeutic blood lidocaine concentrations after local anesthesia for cardiac electrophysiologyic studies. N Engl J Med 1979; 301:418.

4. Horowitz LN: Safety of electrophysiologic studies. Circulation 1986;73(Suppl II):28.

5. Wellens HJJ, Brugada P, Stevenson WG: Programmed electrical stimulation: its role in the management of ventricular arrhythmias in coronary heart disease. Prog Cardiovasc Dis 1986;29:165.

6. VandePol CJ, Farshidi A, Spielman SR, et al: Incidence and significance of induced ventricular tachycardia. Am J Cardiol 1980;45:725.

7. Livelli FD, Bigger JT, Reiffel JA: Response to programmed ventricular stimulation: sensitivity and relation to heart disease. Am J Cardiol 1982;50:452.

8. Brugada P, Green M, Abdollah H, et al: Significance of ventricular arrhythmias initiated by programmed ventricular stimulation: the importance of the type of ventricular arrhythmia induced and the number of preamature stimuli required. Circulation 1984;69:87.

9. Brugada P, Abdollah H, Heddle W, et al: Results of a ventricular stimluation protocol using a maximum of four premature stimuli in patients without documented or suspected ventricular arrhythmias. Am J Cardiol 1983;52:1214.

10. Mann DE, Luck JC, Griffin JE, et al: Induction of clinical ventricular tachycardia using programmed stimulation: value of third and fourth extrastimuli. Am J Cardiol 1983; 53:501.

11. Morady F, Shapiro W, Shen E, et al: Programmed ventricular stimulation in patients without spontaneous ventricular tachycardia. Am Heart J 1984;107:875.

12. Buxton AE, Waxman HL, Marchlinski FE, Untereker WJ, Waspe LE, Josephson ME: Role of triple extrastimuli during electrophysiologic study of patients with documented sustained ventricular tachyarrhythmias. Circulation 1984; 69:532.

13. Morady F, Dicarlo L, Winston S, Davis JC, Scheinman MM: A prospective comparison of triple extrastimuli and left ventricular stimulation in studies of ventricular tachycardia induction. Circulation 1984;79:52.

14. Zehender M, Brugada P, Giebel A, Waldecker B, Stevenson W, Wellens HJJ: Programmed electrical stimulation in healed myocardial infarction using a standardized ventricular stimulation protocol. Am J Cardiol 1987;59:578.

15. Herre JM, Mann DE, Luck JC, et al: Effect of increased current, multiple pacing sites and number of extrastimuli on induction of ventricular tachycardia. Am J Cardiol 1986; 57:102.

16. Estes NMA, Garan H, McGovern B, Ruskin JN: Influence of drive cycle length during programmed stimulation on induction of ventricular arrhythmias: analysis of 403 patients. Am J Cardiol 1986;57:108.

17. Summitt J, Rosenheck S, Kou WH, Schmaltz S, Kadish AH, Morady F: Effect of basic drive cycle length on the yield of ventricular tacycardia during programmed ventricular stimulation. Am J Cardiol 1990;65:49.

18. Breithardt G, Borggrefe M, Podczeck A, Budde T: Influence of the cycle length of basic drive on induction of sustained ventricular tachycardia associated with coronary artery disease. Am J Cardiol 1987;60:1306.

19. Doherty JU, Kienzle MG, Waxman HL, Buxton AE, Marchlinski FE, Josephson ME: Programmed ventricular stimulation at a second right ventricular site: an analysis of 100 patients, with special reference to sensitivity, specificity and characteristics of patients with induced ventricular tachycardia. Am J Cardiol 1983;52:1184.

20. Kudenchuk PJ, Kron J, Walance C, McAnulty JH: Limited value of programmed electrical stimulation from mutliple right ventricular pacing sites in clinically sustained ventricular fibrillation or ventricular tachycardia associated with coronary artery disease. Am J Cardiol 1988;61:303.

21. Brugada P, Wellens HJJ: A comparison in the same patient of 2 programmed ventricular stimulation protocols to induce ventricular tachycardia. Am J Cardiol 1985;55:380.

22. Belhassen B, Shapira I, Sheps D, Laniado S: Programmed ventricular stimulation using up to two extrastimuli and repetition of double extrastimulation for induction of ventricular tachycardia: a new highly sensitive and specific protocol. Am J Cardiol 1990;65:615.

23. Ho DSW, Cooper MJ, Richards DB, Uther JB, Yip ASB, Ross DL: Comparison of number of extrastimuli versus change in basic cycle length for induction of ventricular tachycardia by programmed ventricular stimulation. J Am Coll Cardiol 1993;22:1711.

24. Brugada P, Waldecker B, Kersschot Y, Zehender M, Wellens HJJ: Ventricular arrhythmias initiated by programmed stimulation in four groups of patients with healed myocardial infarction. J Am Coll Cardiol 1986;8:1035.

25. Doherty JU, Kienzle MG, Waxman HL, Buxton AE, Marchlinski FE, Josephson ME: Relation of mode of induction and cycle length of ventricular tachycardia: analysis of 104 patients. Am J Cardiol 1983;52:60.

26. Lin HT, Mann DE, Luck JC, et al: Prospective comparison of right and left ventricular stimulation for induction of sustained ventricular tachycardia. Am J Cardiol 1987;59:559.

27. El-Sherif N, Mehra R, Gough WB: Reentrant ventricular arrhythmias in the late myocardial infarction period. II. Burst pacing versus mutliple prematuer stimulation in the induction of reentry. J Am Coll Cardiol 1984;4:295.

28. Akhtar M: Clinical application of rapid ventricular burst pacing versus extrastimulation for induction of ventricular tachycardia. J Am Coll Cardiol 1984;4:305.

29. Olshansky B, Martins JB: Usefulness of isoproterenol facilitation of ventricular tachycardia induction during extrastimulus testing in predicting effective chronic therapy with beta-adrenergic blockade. Am J Cardiol 1987;59:573.

30. Freedman RA, Swerdlow CD, Echt DS, Winkle RA, Soderholm-Difatte V, Mason JW: Facilitation of ventriclular tachycardia induction by isoproterenol. Am J Cardiol 1984;54:765.

31. Reddy CP, Gettes LS: Use of isoproterenol as an aid to electric induction of chronic recurrent ventricular tachycardia. Am J Cardiol 1979;44:705.

32. Cooper MJ, Hunt LJ, Richards DA, Denniss AR, Uther JB, Ross DL: Effect of repitition of extrastimuli on sensitivity and reproducibility of modes of induction of ventricular tachy-

cardia by programmed stimulation. J Am Coll Cardiol 1988; 11:1260.

33. Cooper MJ, Hunt LJ, Palmer KJ, Denniss AR, Richard DA, Uther JB, Ross DL: Quantitation of day to day variability in mode of induction of ventricualr tachyarrhythmias by programmed stimulation. J Am Coll Cardiol 1988;11:101.

34. Beckman KJ, Velasco CE, Krafchek J, Lin HT, Magro SA, Wyndhan CRC: Significant variability in the mode of ventricular tachycardia induction and its implications for interpretation of acute drug testing. Am Heart J 1988;116:718.

35. McPherson CA, Rosenfeld LE, Batsford WP: Day-to-day reproducibility of responses to right ventricular programmed electrical stimulation: implications for serial drug testing. Am J Cardiol 1985;55:689.

36. Morady F, DiCarlo L, Krol RB, de Buitleir M, Nicklas JM, Annesley TM: Effect of programmed ventricular stimulation on myocardial lactate extraction in patients with and without coronary artery disease. Am Heart J 1986;111:252.

37. Kelly P, Ruskin JN, Vlahakes GJ, Buckley MJ, Freeman CS, Garan H: Surgical coronary revascularization in survivors of prehospital cardiac arrest: its effect on inducible ventricular arrhythmias and long-term survival. J Am Coll Cardiol 1990; 15:267.

38. Horowtiz LN, Harken AH, Josephson ME, Kastor JA: Surgical treatment of ventricular arrhythmias in coronary artery disease. Ann Intern Med 1981;95:88.

39. Miller JM, Kienzle MG, Harken AH, Josephson ME: Morphologically distinct sustained ventricular tachycardias in coronary artery disease: significance and surgical results. J Am Coll Cardiol 1984;6:1073.

40. Wilber DJ, Davis MJ, Rosenbaum M, Ruskin JN, Garan H: Incidence and determinants of multiple morphologically distince sustained ventricular tachycardias. J Am Coll Cardiol 1987;10:583.

41. Waspe LE, Brodman R, Kim SG, Matos JA, Johnston DR, Scavin GM: Activation mapping in patients with coronary artery disease with multiple ventricular tachycardia configurations: occurrence and therapeutic implications of widely separate apparent sites of origin. J Am Coll Cardiol 1985; 5:1075.

42. Josephson ME, Horowitz LN, Farshidi A: Recurrent sustained ventricular tachycardia. 4. Pleomorphism. Circulation 1979; 59:459.

43. Stevenson WG, et al: Slow conduction in infarct scar: relevance to the occurance, detection, and ablation of ventricular reentry circuits resulting from myocardial infarction. Am Heart J 1989;117:452.

44. Kuck KH, Schluter M, Kunze KP, Geiger M: Pleomorphic ventricular tachycardia: demonstration of conduction reversal within the reentry circuit. Pacing Clin Electrophysiol 1989;12:1055.

45. Mitrani RD, Biblo LA, Carlson MD, Gatzoylis KA, Henthorn RW, Waldo AL: Multiple monomorphic ventricular tachycardia configurations predict failure of antiarrhythmic drug therapy guided by electrophysiologic study. J Am Coll Cardiol 1993;22:1117.

46. Greene HL: Sudden arrhythmic cardiac death—mechanisms, resuscitation and classification: the Seattle perspective. Am J Cardiol 1990;65:4B.

47. Morady F, Schienman MM, Hess DS, et al: Electrophysiologic testing in the managment of survivors of out-of-hospital cardiac arrest. Am J Cardiol 1983;51:85.

48. Swerdlow CD, Bardy GH, McAnulty J, Kron J, Lee JT, Graham E, Peterson J, Greene HL: Determinants of induced sustained arrhythmias in survivors of out-of-hospital ventricular fibrillation. Circulation 1987;76:1053.

49. Eldar M, Sauve MJ, Scheinman MM: Electrophysiologic testing and follow-up of patients with aborted sudden death. J Am Coll Cardiol 1987;10:291.

50. Wilber DJ, Garan H, Finkelstein D, Kelly E, Newell J, McGovern B, Ruskin JN: Out-of-hospital cardiac arrest: use of electrophysiologic testing in the prediction of long-term outcome. N Engl J Med 1988;318:19.

51. Freedman RA, Swerdlow CD, Soderholm-Difatte V, Mason JW: Prognostic significance of arrhythmia inducibility or noninducibility at initial electrophysiologic study in survivors of cardiac arrest. Am J Cardiol 1988;61:578.

52. Roy D, Waxman HL, Kienzle MG, et al: Clinical characteristics and long-term follow up in 119 suriviors of cardiac arrest: relation to inducibility at electrophysiologic testing. Am J Cardiol 1983;52:969.

53. Kehoe R, Tommasco C, Zheutlier T, et al: Factors determining programmed stimulation responses and long-term arrhythmic outcome in survivors of ventricular fibrillation with ischemic heart disease. Am Heart J 1988;116:355.

54. Poole JE, Mathisen TL, Kudenchuk PJ, et al: Long-term outcome in patients who survive out of hospital ventricular fibrillation and undergo electrophysiologic studies: evaluation by electrophysiologic subgroups. J Am Coll Cardiol 1990;16:657.

55. Stevenson WG, Brugada P, Waldecker B, Zehender M, Wellens HJJ: Clinical, angiographic, and electrophysiologic findings in patients with aborted sudden death as compared with patients with sustained ventricular tachycardia after myocardial infarction. Circulation 1985;71:1146.

56. Adhar GC, Larson LW, Bardy GH, Greene HL: Sustained ventricular arrhythmia: differences between survivors of cardiac arrest and patients with recurrent sustained ventricular tachycardia. J Am Coll Cardiol 1988;12:159.

57. Doherty JU, Pembrook-Rogers D, Grogan EW, et al: Electrophysiologic evaluation and follow-up characteristics of patients with recurrent unexplained syncope and presyncope. Am J Cardiol 1985;55:703.

58. Morady F, Shen E, Schwartz A, et al: Long-term follow up of patients with recurrent unexplained syncope evaluated by electrophysiologic testing. J Am Coll Cardiol 1983;2:1053.

59. Morady F, Higgins J, Peters RW, et al: Electrophysiologic testing in bundle branch block and unexplained syncope. Am J Cardiol 1984;54:587.

60. Akhtar M, Shenasa M, Denker S, et al: Role of cardiac electrophysiologic studies in patients with unexplained recurrent syncope. Pacing Clin Electrophysiol 1983;6:192.

61. Krol RB, Morady F, Flaker GC, et al: Electrophysiologic testing in patients with unexplained syncope: clinical and noninvasive predictors of outcome. J Am Coll Cardiol 1987; 10:358.

62. Winters SL, Stewart D, Gomes A: Signal averaging of the surface QRS complex predicts inducibility of ventricular tachycardia in patients with syncope of unknown origin: a prospective study. J Am Coll Cardiol 1987;10:775.

63. Kuchar DL, Thorburn CW, Sammel NL: Signal-averaged electrocardiogram for evaluation of recurrent syncope. Am J Cardiol 1986;58:949.

64. Denes P, Uretz E, Ezri MD, Borbola J: Clinical predictors of electrophysiologic findings in patients with syncope of unknown origin. Arch Intern Med 1988;148;1922.

65. Gang ES, Peter T, Rosenthal ME, Mandel WJ, Lass Y: Detection of late potentials on the surface electrocardiogram in unexplained syncope. Am J Cardiol 1986;58:1014.

66. Roy D, Marchand E, Theroux P, Waters DD, Pelletier GB, Bourassa MG: Programmed ventricular stimulation in survivors of an acute myocardial infarction. Circulation 1985; 72:487.

67. Waspe LE, Seinfeld D, Ferrick A, Kim SG, Matos JA, Fisher JD: Prediction of sudden death and spontaneous ventricular tachycardia in survivors of complicated myocardial infarction: value of the repsonse to programmed stimulation using a maximum of three ventricular extrastimuli. J Am Coll Cardiol 1985;5:1292.

68. Bhandari AK, Rose JS, Koutlewski A, Rahomtoola SH, Wu D: Frequency and significance of induced sustained ventricular tachycardia or fibrillation two weeks after acute myocardial infarction. Am J Cardiol 1985;56:737.

69. Bhandari A, Au P, Rose JS, Kotlewski A, Blue S, Rahimtoola SH: Decline in inducibility of sustained ventricular tachycardia from two to twenty weeks after acute myocardial infarction. Am J Cardiol 1990;59:284.

70. Bhandari AK, Hong R, Kulick D, et al: Day to day reproducibility of electrically inducible ventricular arrhythmias in survivors of acute myocardial infarction. J Am Coll Cardiol 1990;15:1075.

71. Kersschot IE, Brugada P, Ramentol M, et al: Effects of early reperfusion in acute myocardial infarction on arrhythmias induced by programmed stimulation: a prospective randomized study. J Am Coll Cardiol 1986;7:1234.

72. Kuck KH, Costard A, Schulter M, Kunze KP: Significance of timing programmed electrical stimulation after acute myocardial infarction. J Am Coll Cardiol 1986;8:1279.

73. Marchlinski FE, Buxton AE, Waxman HL, Josephson ME: Identifying patients at risk of sudden death after myocardial infarction: value of the response of programmed stimulation, degree of ventricular ectopic activity and severity of left venticular dysfunction. Am J Cardiol 1983;52:1190.

74. Santarelli P, Bellocci F, Loperfido F, et al: Ventricular arrhythmia induced by programmed ventricular stimulation after acute myocardial infarction. Am J Cardiol 1985;55:391.

75. Cripps T, Bennett D, Camm J, Ward DE: Inducibility of sustained monomorphic ventricular tachycardia as a prognostic indicator in survivors of recent myocardial infarction: a prospective evaluation in relation to other prognostic variables. J Am Coll Cardiol 1989;14:289.

76. Denniss AR, Richards DA, Cody DV, et al: Prognostic significance of ventricular tachycardia and fibrillation induced at programmed stimulation and delayed potentials detected on signal-averaged electrocardiograms of survivors of acute myocardial infarction. Circulation 1986;74:731.

77. Breithardt G, Borggrefe, Haerten K: Role of programmed ventricular stimulation and noninvasice recording of ventricular late potentials for the identification of patients at risk of ventricular tachyarrhythmias after acute myocardial infarction. In: Zipes DP, Jalife J, eds. Cardiac electrophysiology and arrhythmias. New York: Grune & Stratton 1985:61.

78. Bourke JP, Richards DAB, Ross DL, Wallace EM, McGuire MA, Uther JB: Routine programmed electrical stimulation in survivors of acute myocardial infarction for prediction of spontaneous ventricular tachyarrhythmias during follow-up results, optimal stimulation protocol and cost-effective screening. J Am Coll Cardiol 1991;18:780.

79. Woelfel A, Foster JR, Rowe WW, Jain A, Gettes LS: Induction of ventricular tachycardia in patients with left ventricular aneurysms and no history of arrhythmia. Am J Cardiol 1988; 62:814.

80. Denniss AR, Ross DL, Russell PA, Young AA, Richards DA, Uther JB: Randomized controlled trial of prophylactic antiarrhythmic therapy in patients with inducible ventricular tachyarrhythmias after recent myocardial infarction. Eur Heart J 1988;9:746.

81. Ruskin JN, McGovern B, Garan H, DeMarco J, Kelly E: Antiarrhythmic drugs: a possible cause of out-of-hospital cardiac arrest. N Engl J Med 1983;309(21):1302.

82. Buxton AE, Marchlinski FE, Flores BT, Miller JM, Doherty JU, Josephson ME: Nonsustained ventricular tachycardia in patients with coronary artery disease: role of electrophysiologic study. Circulation 1987;75:1178.

83. Spielman SR, Greenspan AM, Kay HR, et al: Electrophysiologic testing in patients at high risk for sudden cardiac death. I. Nonsustained ventrifular tachycardia and abnormal ventricular function. J Am Coll Cardiol 1985;6:31.

84. Klein RC, Machell C: Use of electrophysiologic testing in patients with nonsustained ventricular tachycardia: prognostic and therapeutic implications. J Am Coll Cardiol 1989; 14:155.

85. Wilber DJ, Olshansky B, Moran JF, Scanlon PJ: Electrophysiological testing and nonsustained ventricular tachycardia: use and limitations in patients with coronary artery disease and impaired ventricular function. Circulation 1990;82:350.

86. Winters SL, Stewart D, Targonski A, Gomes JA: Role of signal averaging of the surface QRS complex in selecting patients with nonsustained ventricular tachycradia and high grade ventricular arrhythmias for programmed ventricular stimulation. J Am Coll Cardiol 1988;12:1481.

87. Turitto G, Fontaine JM, Ursell S, Caref EB, Bekheit S, El-Sherif N: Risk stratification and management of patients with organic heart disease and nonsustained ventricular tachycardia: role of programmed stimulation, left ventricular ejection fraction, and signal-averaged electrocardiogram. Am J Med 1990;88:35.

88. Kowey PR, Waxman HL, Greenspan A, et al: Value of electrophysiologic testing in patients with previous myocardial infarction and nonsustained ventricular tachycardia. Am J Cardiol 1990;65:594.

89. Gomes JAC, Hariman R, Kang PS, et al: Programmed electrical stimulation in patients with high grade ventricular ectopy: electrophysiologic findings and prognosis for survival. Circulation 1984;70:43.

90. Kharsa MH, Gold RL, Moore H, Yazaki Y, Haffajee CI, Alpert JS: Long-term outcome following programmed electrical stimulation in patients with high-grade ventricular ectopy. Pacing Clin Electrophysiol 1988;11:603.

91. Das SK, Morady F, DiCarlo L, et al: Prognostic usefulness of programmed ventricular stimulation in idiopathic dilated cardiomyopathy without symptomatic ventricular arrhythmias. Am J Cardiol 1986;58:998.

92. Meinertz T, Treese N, Kasper W, et al: Determinants of prognosis in idiopathic dilated cardiomyopathy as determined by programmed electrical stimulation. Am J Cardiol 1985;56:337.

93. Stevenson WG, Stevenson LW, Weiss J, Tillisch JH: Inducible ventricular arrhythmias and sudden death during vasodilator therapy of advanced heart failure. Am Heart J 1988; 116:1447.

94. Jackman WM, Friday KJ, Anderson JL, Aliot EM, Clark M, Lazzarra R: The long QT syndromes: a critical review, new clinical observation and a unifying hypothesis. Prog Cardiovasc Dis 1988;41:115.

95. Bhandari AK, Shapiro WA, Morady F, Shen EN, Mason J, Scheinman MM: Electrophysiologic testing in patients with the long QT syndrome. Circulation 1985;71:63.

96. Horowitz LN, Greenspan AM, Spielman SR, et al: Torsades de pointes: electrophysiologic studies in patients without transient pharmacologic or metabolic abnormalities. Circulation 1981;63:1120.

97. Avitall B, McKinnie J, Jazayeri M, Akhtar M, Anderson AJ, Tchou P: Induction of ventricular fibrillation versus monomorphic ventricular tachycardia during programmed stimulation. Role of premature beat conduction delay. Circulation 1992;85:1271.

98. Stevenson WG, Brugada P, Waldecker B, Zehender M, Wellens HJJ: Can potentially significant polymorphic ventricular arrhythmias initiated by programmed ventricular stimulation be distinguished from those that are nonspecific? Am Heart J 1986;112:1073.

99. Sager PT, Perlmutter RA, Rosenfeld LE, McPherson CA, Batsford WP: Rapid self-terminating ventricular tachycardia induced during electrophysiologic study: a prospective evaluation. J Am Coll Cardiol 1989;13:385.

100. Kou WH, de Buitleir M, Kadish AH, Morady F: Sequelae of nonsustained polymorphic ventricular tachycardia induced during programmed ventricular stimulation. Am J Cardiol 1989;64:1148.

101. Mahmud R, Denker S, Lehmann MH, Tchou P, Dongas J, Akhtar M: Incidence and clinical significance of ventricular fibrillation induced with single and double ventricular extrastimuli. 1986;58:75.

102. Morady F, DiCarlo LA, Baerman JM, de Buitleir M: Comparison of coupling intervals that induce clinical and nonclinical forms of ventricular tachycardia during programmed stimulation. Am J Cardiol 1986;57:1269.

103. Akhtar M, Damato AN, Batsford WP, et al: Demonstration of re-entry within the his-Purkinje system in man. Circulation 1974;50:1150.

104. Trappe HJ, Brugada P, Talajic M, et al: Prognosis of patients with ventricular tachycardia and ventricular fibrillation: role of underlying etiology. J Am Coll Cardiol 1988;12:166.

105. Brugada P, Talajic M, Della Bella P, Wellens HJJ: Treatment of patients with ventricular tachycardia or ventricular fibrillation. First lessions from the "PARALLEL" study. In: Brugada P, Wellens HJJ eds. Cardiac arrhythmias: where to go from here? Mount Kisco, NY: Futura Publishing, 1987;457.

106. Willems AR, Tijussen JG, Van Capelle FJL, et al: Determinants of prognosis in symptomatic ventricular tachycardia or ventricular fibrillation late after myocardial infarction. J Am Coll Cardiol 1990;16:521.

107. Brugada P, Talajic M, Mulleneers R, Wellens HJJ: The value of the clinical history to assess prognosis of patients with ventricular tachycardia or ventricular fibrillation after myocardial infarction. Eur Heart J 1989;10:747.

108. Swerdlow CD, Winkle RA, Mason JW: Determinants of survival in patients with ventricular tachyarrhythmias. N Engl J Med 1983;308:1436.

109. Furukawa T, Rozanski JJ, Nogami A, Moroe K, Gosselin AJ, Lister JW: Time-dependent risk of and predictors for cardiac arrest recurrence in survivors of out-of-hospital cardiac arrest with chronic coronary artery disease. Circulation 1989;80:599.

110. Horowitz LN: Ventricular arrhythmias: control of therapy by Holter monitoring. Eur Heart J 1989;10:53.

111. Saini V, Graboys T, Towne V, Lown B: Reproduciblity of exercise-induced ventricular arrhythmias in patients undergoing evaluation for malignant ventricular arrhythmia. Am J Cardiol 1989;63:697.

112. Mitchell LB, Duff HJ, Manyari DE, Wyse DG: A randomized clinical trial of the noninvasive and invasive approaches to drug therapy of ventricular tachycardia. N Engl J Med 1987; 317:1681.

113. Kim SG, Seiden SW, Felder SD, Waspe LE, Fisher JD: Is programmed stimulation of value in predicting the long-term success of antiarrhythmic therapy for ventricular tachycardias? N Engl J Med 1986;315:356.

114. Mason JW: A comparison of electrophysiologic testing with holter monitoring to predict antiarrhythmic-drug efficacy for ventricular tachyarrhythmia. N Engl J Med 1993;329:445.

115. Horowitz LN, Josephson ME, Farshidi A, Spielman SR, Michelson El: Recurrent sustained ventricular tachycardia. 3. Role of the electrophysiologic study in selection of antiarrhythmic regimens. Circulation 1978;58:986.

116. Mason JW, Winkle RA: Electrode-catheter arrhythmia induction in the selection and assessment of antiarrhythmic drug therapy for recurrent ventricular tachycardia. Circulation 1978;58:971.

117. Denes P, Wu D, Wyndham C, et al: Chronic longterm electrophysiologic study of paroxysmal ventricular tachycardia. Chest 1980;77:478.

118. Josephson MR, Horowitz LN: Electrophysiologic approach to therapy of recurrent sustained ventricular tachycardia. Am J Cardiol 1979;43 631.

119. Breithardt G, Borggrefe M, Seipel: Selection of optimal drug treatment of ventricular tachycardia by programmed electrical stimulation of the heart. Ann NY Acad Sci 1984;49.

120. Horowitz LN, Josephson ME, Kastor JA: Intracardiac electrophysiologic studies as a method for the optimization of drug therapy in chronic ventricular arrhythmia. Prog Cardiovasc Dis 1980;23:81.

121. Waxman HL, Buxton AE, Sadowski LM, Josephson ME: The response to procainamide during electrophysiologic study for sustained ventricular tachyarrhythmias predicts the response to other medications. Circulation 1983;67:30.

122. Swiryn S, Bauernfeind RA, Strasberg B, et al: Prediction of response to class I antiarrhythmic drugs during electro-

physiologic study of ventricular tachycardia. Am Heart J 1982;103:43.

123. Borggrefe M, Trampisch HJ, Breithardt G: Reappraisal of criteria for assessing drug efficacy in patients with ventricular tachyarrhythmias: complete versus partial suppression of inducible arrhythmias. J Am Coll Cardiol 1988;12;140.

124. Oseran DS, Gang ES, Rosenthal ME, Mandel WJ, Peter T: Electrophysiologic testing in sustained ventricular tachycardia associated with coronary artery disease: value of the response to intravenous procainamide in predicting the response to oral procainamide and oral quinidine treatment. Am J Cardiol 1985;56:883.

125. Marchlinski FE, Buxton AR, Vassallo JA, et al: Comparative electrophysiologic effects of intravenous and oral procainamide in patients with sustained ventricular arrhythmias. J Am Coll Cardiol 1984;4:1247.

126. Rae AP, Greenspan AM, Spielman SR, et al: Antiarrhythmic drug efficacy for ventricular tachyarrhythmias associated with coronary artery disease as assessed by electrophysiologic studies. Am J Cardiol 1985;55:1494.

127. Mason JW, Winkle RA: Accuracy of the ventricular tachycardia-induction study for predicting long-term efficacy and inefficacy of antiarrhythmic drugs. N Engl J Med 1980;303:1073.

128. Swerdlow CD, Winkle RA, Mason JW: Prognostic significance of the number of induced ventricular complexes during assessment of therapy for ventricular tachyarrhythmias. Circulation 1983;68:400.

129. Spielman SR, Schwartz JS, McCarthy DM, et al: Predictors of the success or failure of medical therapy in patients with chronic recurrent sustained ventricular tachycardia: a descriminant analysis. J Am Coll Cardiol 1983;1:401.

130. Kuchar DL, Rottman J, Berger E, Freeman CS, Garan H, Ruskin JN: Prediction of successful suppression of sustained ventricular tachyarrhythmias by serial drug testing from data derived at the initial electrophysiologic study. J Am Coll Cardiol 1988;12:982.

131. Waller TJ, Kay HR, Spielman SR, Kutalek SP, Greenspan AM, Horowitz LN: Reduction in sudden death and total mortality by antiarrhythmic therapy evaluated by electrophysiologic drug testing: criteria of efficacy in patients with sustained ventricular tachyarrhythmia. J Am Coll Cardiol 1987;10:83.

132. DiMarco JP, Garan H, Ruskin JN: Quinidine for ventricular arrhythmias: value of electrophysiologic testing. Am J Cardiol 1983;51:90.

133. Kuchar DL, Garan H, Vendeitti FJ, et al: Usefulness of sotalol in suppressing ventricular tachycardia or ventricular fibrillation in patients with healed myocardial infarcts. Am J Cardiol 1989;64:33.

134. Wynn J, Torres V, Flowers D, et al: Antiarrhythmic drug efficacy at electrophysiology testing: predictive effectiveness of procainamide and flecainide. Am Heart J 1986;111:632.

135. The ESVEM Investigators: Determinants of predicted efficacy of antiarrhythmic drugs in the electrophysiologic study versus electrocardiographic monitoring trial. Circulation 1993;87:323.

136. Mason JW: A comparison of seven antiarrhythmic drugs in patients with ventricular tachyarrhythmia. N Engl J Med 1993;329:452.

137. Brugada P, Wellens HJJ: Need and design of a prospective study to assess the value of different strategic approaches for management of ventricular tachycardia of fibrillation. Am J Cardiol 1986;57:1180.

138. Steinbeck G, Andresen D, Bach P, et al: A comparison of electrophysiologically guided antiarrhythmic drug therapy with beta-blocker therapy in patients with symptomatic, sustained ventricular tachyarrhythmias. N Engl J Med 1992; 327:987.

139. Herre JM, Sauve MJ, Malone P, et al: Long-term results of amiodarone therapy in patients with recurrent sustained ventricular tachycardia or ventricular fibrillation. J Am Coll Cardiol 1989;13:442.

140. Weinberg BA, Miles WM, Klein LS, et al: Five-year follow-up of 589 patients treated with amiodarone. Am Heart J 1993; 125:109.

141. Zhu J, Haines DE, Lerman BB, DiMarco JP: Predictors of efficacy of amiodarone and characteristics of recurrence of arrhythmia in patients with sustained ventricular tachycardia and coronary artery disease. Circulation 1987;76:802.

142. Olson PJ, Woelfel A, Simpson RJ, Foster JR: Stratification of sudden death risk in patients receiving long-term amiodarone treatment for sustained ventricular tachycardia or ventricular fibrillation. Am J Cardiol 1993;71:823.

143. Waxman HL, Groh WC, Marchlinski FE, et al: Amiodarone for control of sustained ventricular tachyarrhythmia: clinical and electrophysiologic effects in 51 patients. Am J Cardiol 1982;50:1066.

144. Horowitz LN, Greenspan AM, Spielman SR, et al: Usefulness of electrophysiologic testing in evaluation of amiodarone therapy for sustained ventricular tachyarrhythmias associated with coronary heart disease. Am J Cardiol 1985;55:367.

145. Kadish AH, Buxton AE, Waxman HL, Flores B, Josephson ME, Marchlinski FE: Usefulness of electrophysiologic study to determine the clinical tolerance of arrhythmia recurrences during amiodarone therapy. J Am Coll Cardiol 1987;10:90.

146. Greenspan AJ, Volosin KJ, Greenberg RM, Jefferies L, Rotmensch H: Amiodarone therapy: role of early and late electrophysiologic studies. J Am Coll Cardiol 1988;11:117.

147. Kadish AH, Marchlinski FE, Josephson ME, Buxton AE: Amiodarone: correlation of early and late electrophysiologic studies with outcome. Am Heart J 1986;112:1134.

148. Saxon LA, Stevenson WG, Fonorow GC, et al: Transesophageal echocardiography to guide energy delivery and catheter position during radiofrequency ablation of ventricular tachycardia. Am J Cardiol 1993;72:658.

149. Cassidy DM, Vassallo JA, Buxton AR, Doherty JU, Marchlinski FE, Josephson ME: The value of catheter mapping during sinus rhythm to localize site of origin of ventricular tachycardia. Circulation 1984;69:1103

150. Farre J, Grande A, Martinell J, Fraile J, Ramirez JA, Rabago G: Atrial unipolar waveform analysis during retrograde conduction over left-sided accessory atrioventriclular pathways. In: P Brugada, HJJ Wellens, eds. Cardiac arrhythmias: where to go from here? Mt. Kisco, NY: Futura Publishing, 1987:243.

151. Walton C, Gergley S, Economides AP: Platinum pacemaker electrodes: origins and effects of the electrode-tissue interface impedance. Pacing Clin Electrophysiol 1987;10:87.

152. Klitzner TS, Stevenson WG: Effects of filtering on right ventricular electrograms recorded from endocardial catheters in humans. Pacing Clin Electrophysiol 1990;13:69.

153. Kadish AH, Morady F, Rosenheck S, Summit J, Schmaltz S:

The effect of electrode configuration on the unipolar His-bundle electrogram. Pacing Clin Electrophysiol 1989;12:1445.

154. Ideker RE, Smith WM, Blanchard SM, et al: The assumptions of isochronal cardiac mapping. Pacing Clin Electrophysiol 1989;12:456.

155. Durrer D, van deer Tweel LH: Spread of activation in the left ventricular wall of the dog. Am Heart J 1953;46:683.

156. Spach MS, Barr RC, Serwer GA, Kootsey JM, Johnson EA: Extracellular potentials related to intracellular action potentials in the dog Purkinje system. Circ Res 1972;30:505.

157. Spach MS, Barr RC, Serwer GS, Johnson EA, Kootsey JM: Collision of excitation waves in the dog Purkinje system. Circ Res 1971;29:499.

158. Spach MS, Barr RC, Johnson EA, Kootsey JM: Cardiac extracellular potentials. Analysis of complex wave forms about the Purkinje networks in dogs. Circ Res 1973;33:465.

159. Spach MS, Miller WT, Geselowitz DB, Barr RC, Kootsey JM, Johnson EA: The discontinuous nature of propagation in normal canine cardiac muscle: evidence for recurrent discontinuities of intracellular resistance that effect the membrane currents. Circ Res 1981;48:39.

160. Gallagher JJ, Kasell J, Sealy WC, Pritchett EL, Wallace AG: Epicardial mapping in the Wolff-Parkinson-White syndrome. Circulation 1978;57:854.

161. Durrer D, Van Lier AAW, Builler J: Epicardial and intramural excitation in chronic myocardial infarction. Am Heart J 1964;68:765.

162. Damiano RJ, Blanchard SM, Asano T, Cox JL, Low JE: Effects of distant potentials on unipolar electrograms in an animal model utilizing the right ventricular isolation procedure. J Am Coll Cardiol 1988;11:1100.

163. Ursell PC, Gardner PI, Albala A, Fenoglio JJ, Wit AL: Structural and electrophysiologic changes in the epicardial border zone of canine myocardial infarcts during infarct healing. Circ Res 1985:56:436.

164. Stevenson WG, Khan H, Sager P, et al: Identification of reentry circuit sites during catheter mapping and radiofrequency ablation of ventricular tachycardia late after myocardial infarction. Circulation 1993;88(Pt 1):1647.

165. de Bakker JMT, Van Capelle FJL, Janse MJ, et al: Reentry as a cause of ventricular tachycardia in patients with chronic ischemic heart disease: electrophysiologic and anatomic correlation. Circulation 1988;77:589.

166. de Bakker JMT, Janse MJ, Van Capelle FJL, Durrer D: Endocardial mapping by simultaneous recording of endocardial electrograms during cardiac surgery for ventricular aneurysm. J Am Coll Cardiol 1983;2:947.

167. Krafchek J, Lawrie GM, Roberts R, Magro SA, Wyndham CRC: Surgical ablation of ventricular tachycardia: improved results with a map-directed regional approach. Circulation 1986;73:1239.

168. Harris L, Downar E, Mickleborough L, Shaikh N, Parson I: Activation sequence of ventricular tachycardia: endocardial and epicardial mapping studies in the human ventricle. J Am Coll Cardiol 1987;10:1040.

169. Wellens HJJ: Pathophysiology of ventricular tachycardia in man. Arch Intern Med 1975;135:473.

170. Josephson ME, Buxton AE, Marchlinski FE, et al: Sustained ventricular tachycardia in coronary artery disease-evidence for reentrant mechanism. In: Zipes DP, Jalife J, eds. Cardiac electrophysiology and arrhythmias. New York: Grune & Stratton, 1985;409.

171. de Bakker JMT, Coronel R, Tasseron S, et al: Ventricular tachycardia in the infarcted, Langendorf-perfused human heart: role of the arrangement of surviving cardiac fibers. J Am Coll Cardiol 1990:15:1594.

172. deBakker JMT, van Capelle FJL, Janse MJ, et al: Slow conduction in the infarcted human heart. 'Zigzag' course of activation. Circulation 1993;88:915.

173. Josephson ME, Horowitz LN, Farshidi A, Kastor JA: Recurrent sustained ventricular tachycardia. 1. Mechanisms. Circulation 1978;57:431.

174. Downar E, Harris L, Mickelborough LL, Shaikh NA, Parson ID: Endocardial mapping of ventricular tachycardia in the intact human ventricle: evidence for reentrant mechanisms. J Am Coll Cardiol 1988;11:783.

175. Kaltenbrunner W, Cardinal R, Dubuc M, et al: Epicardial and endocardial mapping of ventricular tachycardia in patients with myocardial infarction. Is the origin of the tachycardia always subendocardially localized? Circulation 1991;84:1058.

176. Fenoglio JJ, Pham TD, Harken AH, Horowitz LN, Josephson ME, Wit AL: Recurrent sustained ventricular tachycardia: structure and ultrastructure of subendocardial regions in which tachycardia originates. Circulation 1983;68:518

177. Bolick DR, Hackel DB, Reimer Ka, Ideker RE: Quantitative analysis of myocardial infarct structure in patients with ventricular tachycardia. Circulation 1986;74:1266.

178. Spear JF, Horowitz LN, Hodess AB, MacVaugh H, Moore EN: Cellular electrophysiology of human myocardial infarction. 1. Abnormalities of cellular activation. Circulation 1979;59:247.

179. Gilmour RF, Heger JJ, Prystowsky EN, Zipes DP: Cellular electrophysiologic abnormalities of diseased human ventricular myocardium. Am J Cardiol 1983;51:137.

180. Spear JF, Michelson EL, Moore EN: Reduced space constant in slowly conducting regions of chronically infarcted canine myocardium. Circ Res 1983;53:176.

181. Mehra R, Zeiler RH, Gough WB, El-Sherif N: Reentrant ventricular arrhythmias in the late myocardial infarction period. 9. Electrophysiologic-anatomic correlation of reentry circuits. Circulation 1983;67:11.

182. El-Sherif N, Mehra R, Gough WB, Zeiler RH: Reentrant ventricular arrhythmias in the late myocardial infarction period. Interruption of reentrant circuits by cryothermal techniques. Circulation 1983;68:644.

183. Garan H, Fallon JT, Rosenthal S, Ruskin JN: Endocardial, intramural, and epicardial activation patterns during sustained monomorphic ventricular tachycardia in late canine myocardial infarction. Circ Res 1987;60:879.

184. Cardinal R, Savard P, Carson L, Perry J, Page P: Mapping of ventricular tachycardia induced by programmed stimulation in canine preparations of myocardial infarction. Circulation 1984;70:136.

185. Gough WB, Mehra R, Restivo M, Zeiler RH, EL-Sherif N: Reentrant ventricular arrhythmias in the late myocardial infarction period in the dog. 13. Correlation of activation and refractory maps. Circ Res 1985;57:432.

186. Wit AL, Allessie MA, Bonke FIM, Lammers W, Smeets J, Fenolgio JJ: Electrophysiologic mapping to determine the

mechanism of experimental ventricular tachycardia initiated by premature impulses. Am J Cardiol 1982;49:166.

187. Mason JW, Stinson EB, Winkle RA, Oyer PE: Mechanisms of ventricular tachycardia: wide complex ignorance. Am Heart J 1981;102:1083.

188. Miller JM, Harken SH, Hargrove WC, Josephson ME: Patterns of endocardial activation during sustained ventricular tachycardia. J Am Coll Cardiol 1985;6:1280.

189. Pogwizd SM, Hoyt RH, Saffitz JE, Corr PB, Cox JL, Cain ME: Reentrant and focal mechanisms underlying ventricular tachycardia in the human heart. Circulation 1992;86:1872.

190. Kimber SK, Downar E, Harris L, et al: Mechanisms of spontaneous shift of surface electrocardiographic configuration during ventricular tachycardia. J Am Coll Cardiol 1992; 20:1397.

191. Stevenson WG, Weiss JN, Wiener I, Wohlgelernter D, Yeatman L: Localization of slow conduction in a ventricular tachycardia circuit by entrainment: implications for catheter ablation. Am Heart J 1987;114:1253.

192. Miller J, Kienzle M, Harken A, Josephson M: Subendocardial resection for ventricular tachycardia: predictors of surgical success. Circulation 1984;70:624.

193. Zee-cheng CS, Kouchoukos NT, Connors JP, Ruffy R: Treatment of life-threatening ventricular arrhythmias with nonguided surgery supported by electrophysiologic testing and drug therapy. J Am Coll Cardiol 1989;13:153.

194. Horowitz LN, Harken AH, Kastor JA, Josephson ME: Ventricular resection guided by epicardial and endocardial mapping for treatment of recurrent ventricular tachycardia. N Engl J Med 1980;302:589.

195. Garan H, Nguyen K, McGovern B, Buckley M, Ruskin JN: Perioperative and long-term results after electrophysiologically directed ventricular surgery for recurrent ventricular tachycardia. J Am Coll Cardiol 1986;8:201.

196. Mason JW, Stinson EB, Winkle RA, et al: Surgery for ventricular tachycardia: efficacy of left ventricular aneurysm resection compared with operation guided by electrical activation mapping. Circulation 1982;65:1148.

197. Lanymore RW, Gardner MA, McIntyre AJ, Barker RA: Surgical intervention for drug-resistant ventricular tachycardia. J Am Coll Cardiol 1990;16:37.

198. Moran JM, Kehoe RF, Loeb JM, Lichtenthal PR, Sanders JH, Michaelis LL: Extended endocardial resention for the treatment of ventricular tachycardia and ventricular fibrillation. Ann Thorac Surg 1982;34:538.

199. Haines DE, Lerman BB, Kron IL, DiMarco JP: Surgical ablation of ventricular tachycardia with sequential map-guided subendocardial resection: electrophysiologic assessment and long-term follow-up. Circulation 1988;77:131.

200. Morady F, Scheinman MM, Di Carlo L, et al: Catheter ablation of ventricular tachycardia with intracardiac shocks: results in 33 patients. Circulation 1987;75:1037.

201. Garan H, Steinhaus DM, Ruskin JN: Map-guided transcatheter electric ablation for recurrent ventricular tachycardia. In: Fontaine G, Scheinman MM, eds. Ablation in cardiac arrhythmias. Mt Kisco, NY: Futura Publishing, 1987:347.

202. Fitzgerald DM, Friday KJ, Wah JAYL, Lazzara R, Jackman WM: Electrogram patterns predicting successful catheter ablation of ventricular tachycardia. Circulation 1988;77:614.

203. Stevenson WG, Weiss JN, Wiener I, et al: Resetting of ventricular tachycardia: implications for localizing the area of slow conduction. J Am Coll Cardiol 1988;11:522.

204. Fontaine G, Tonet JL, Frank R, et al: Treatment of resistant ventricular tachycardia by endocavitary fulguration associated with antiarrhythmic therapy. In: Fontaine G, Scheinman MM eds. Ablation in cardiac arrhythmias. Mt Kisco, NY: Futura Publishing, 1987; 311.

205. Chouty F, Leclercq JF, Cauchemez V, Maison-Blanche P, Zimmerman M, Coumel P: Closed-chest catheter ablation for ventricular tachycardia: analysis of 16 proceedures in 11 patients. In: Fontaine G, Scheinman MM, eds. Ablation in cardiac arrhythmias. Mt Kisco, NY: Futura Publishing, 1987; 357.

206. Svenson RH, Gallagher JJ, Selle JG, Zimmern SH, Fedor JM, Robicsek F: Neodymium:YAG laser photocoagulation: a successful new map-guided technique for the intraoperative ablation of ventricular tachycardia. Circulation 1987;76:1319.

207. Littman L, Svenson RH, Gallagher JJ, et al: Functional role of the epicardium in post-infarction ventricular tachycardia. Observations derived from computerized epicardial activation mapping, entrainment, and epicardial laser photoablation. Circulation 1991;83:1577.

208. Waxman HL, Josephson ME: Ventricular activation during ventricular endocardial pacing: I. Electrocardiographic patterns related to the site of pacing. Am J Cardiol 1982;50:1.

209. Josephson ME, Waxman HL, Cain ME, Gardner MJ, Buxton AE: Ventricular activation during ventricular endocardial pacing. II. Role of pace-mapping to localize origin of ventricular tachycardia. Am J Cardiol 1982;50:11.

210. Holt PM, Smallpeice C, Deverall PB, Yates AK, Curry PVL: Ventricular arrhythmias. A guide to their localization. Br Heart J 1985;53:417.

211. Kuchar DL, Ruskin JN, Garan H: Electrocardiographic localization of the site of origin of ventricular tachycardia in patients with prior myocardial infarction. J Am Coll Cardiol 1989;13:893.

212. Josephson ME, Horowitz LN, Waxman HL, et al: Sustained ventricular tachycardia: role of the 12-lead electrocardiogram in localizing site of origin. Cirulation 1981;64:257.

213. Miller JM, Marchlinski FE, Buxton AE, Josephson ME: Relationship between the 12-lead electrocardiogram during ventricular tachycardia and endocardial site of origin in patients with coronary artery disease. Circulation 1988; 77:756.

214. Coumel P, Leclercq JF, Attuel P, Maisonblanche P: The QRS morphology in post-myocardial infarction ventricular tachycardia. A Study of 100 tracings compared with 70 cases of idiopathic ventricular tachycardia. Eur Heart J 1984;5:792.

215. Cassidy DM, Vassallo JA, Marchlinski FE, Buxton AE, Untereker WJ, Josephson ME: Endocardial mapping in humans in sinus rhythm with normal left ventricles: activation patterns and characteristics of electrograms. Circulation 1984;70:37.

216. Cassidy DM, Vassallo JA, Miller JM, et al: Endocardial catheter mapping in patients in sinus rhythm: relationship to underlying heart disease and ventricular arrhythmias. Circulation 1986;73:645.

217. Untereker WJ, Spielman SR, Waxman HL, Horowitz LN,

Josephson ME: Ventricular activation in normal sinus rhythm: abnormalities with recurrent sustained tachycardia and a history of myocardial infarction. Am J Cardiol 1985; 55:974.

218. Simson MB, Untereker WJ, Spielman SR, et al: Relation between late potentials on the body surface and directly recorded fragmented electrograms in patients with ventricular tachycardia. Am J Cardiol 1983;51:105.

219. Vassallo JA, Cassidy D, SImson MB, Buxton AE, Marchlinski FE, Josephson ME: Relation of late potentials to site of origin of ventricular tachycardia associated with coronary heart disease. Am J Cardiol 1985;55:985.

220. Gardner PI, Ursell PC, Fenoglio JJ, Wit AL: Electrophysiologic and anatomic basis for fractionated electrograms recorded from healed myocardial infarcts. Circulation 1985;72:596.

221. Gallagher JJ, Kasell JH, Cox JL, Smith WM, Ideker RE, Smith WM: Techniques of intraoperative electrophysiologic mapping. Am J Cardiol 1982;49:221.

222. Waxman HL, Sung RJ: Significance of fragmented ventricular electrograms observed using intracardiac recording techniques in man. Circulation 1980;62:1349.

223. Ideker RE, Lofland GK, Bardy GH, et al: Late fractionated potentials and continuous electrical activity caused by electrode motion. Pacing Clin Electrophysiol 1983;6:908.

224. Klein H, Karp RB, Kouchoukos NT, Zorn GL, James TN, Waldo AL: Intraoperative electrophysiologic mapping of the ventricles during sinus rhythm in patients with a previous myocardial infarction. Identification of the electrophysiologic substrate of ventricular arrhythmias. Circulation 1982; 66:847.

225. Kienzle MG, Miller J, Falcone RA, Harken A, Josephson ME: Intraoperative endocardial mapping during sinus rhythm: relationship to site of origin of ventricular tachycardia. Circulation 1984;70:957.

226. Wiener I, Mindich B, Pitchon R: Fragmented endocardial electrical activity in patients with ventricular tachycardia: a new guide to surgical therapy. Am Heart J 1984;107:86.

227. Wiener I, Mindich B, Pitchon R: Endocarrdial activation in patients with coronary artery disease: effects of regional contraction abnormalities. Am Heart J 1984;107:1146.

228. Wiener I, Mindich B, Pitchon R: Determinants of ventricular tachycardia in patients with ventricular aneurysms: results of intraoperative epicardial and endocardial mapping. Circulation 1982;65:856.

229. Brugada P, Abdollah H, Wellens HJJ: Continuous electrical activity during sustained monomorphic ventricular tachycardia. Observations on its dynamic behavior during the arrhythmia. Am J Cardiol 1985;55:402.

230. Miller JM, Vassallo JA, Hargrove WC, Josephson ME: Intermittent failure of local conduction during ventricular tachycardia. Circulation 1985;72:1286.

231. Gallagher JD, Del Rossi AJ, Fernandez J, et al: Cryothermal mapping of recurrent ventricular tachycardia in man. Circulation 1985;71:733.

232. Gessman LJ, Endo T, Egan J, Gallagher JD, Hastie R, Maroko PR: Dissociation of the site of origin from the site of cryotermination of ventricular tachycardia. Pacing Clin Electrophysiol 1983;6:1293.

233. Josephson ME, Horowitz LN, Farshidi A: Continuous local electrical activity. A mechanism of recurrent ventricular tachycardia. Circulation 1978;57:659.

234. Blanchard SM, Damiano RJ, Smith WM, Ideker RE, Lowe JE: Interpolating unipolar epicardial potantials from electrodes separated by increasing distances. Pacing Clin Electrophysiol 1989;12:1938.

235. Horowitz LN, Josephson ME, Harken AH: Epicardial and endocardial activation during sustained ventricular tachycardia in man. Circulation 1980;61:1227.

236. Kabell G, Scherlag BJ, Hope RR, Lazzara R: Patterns of interectopic activation recorded during plenomorphic ventricular tachycardia after myocardial infarction in the dog. Am J Cardiol 1982;49:56.

237. Brachmann J, Labell G, Scherlag B, Harrison L, Lazarra R: Analysis of interectopic activation patterns during sustained ventricular tachycardia. Circulation 1983;67:449.

238. Gessman LJ, Agrawal JB, Endo T, Helfant RH: Localization and mechanism of ventricular tachycardia by ice mapping 1 week after the onset of myocardial infarction in dogs. Circulation 1983;68:657.

239. Kay GN, Epstein AE, Plumb VJ: Region of slow conduction in sustained ventricular tachycardia: direct endocardial recordings and functional characterization in humans. J Am Coll Cardiol 1988;11:109.

240. Morady F, Harvey M, Kalbfleisch SJ, El-Atassi R, Calkins H, Langberg J: Radiofrequency catheter ablation of ventricular tachycardia in patients with coronary artery disease. Circulation 1993;87:363.

241. Kuck KH, Kentsch M, Geiger M: Pace-mapping in patients with ventricular tachycardia: different characteristics during pacing at the "site of origin." Circulation 1987;76(Suppl IV):413.

242. Stevenson WG, Sager P, Natterson PD, Saxon LA, Middlekauff HR, Wiener I: The QRS morphology does not predict ventricular tachycardia reentry circuit sites during pace-mapping. (Submitted) 1993.

243. Curry PVL, O'Keefe DB, Pitcher D, Sowton E, Deverall P, Yates AK: Localization of ventricular tachycardia by a new technique-pace-mapping. Circulation 1979;60(Suppl II):25A.

244. Morady F, Kadish A, Rosenheck S, et al: Concealed entrainment as a guide for catheter ablation of ventricular tachycardia in patients with prior myocardial infarction. J Am Coll Cardiol 1991;17:678.

245. Stevenson WG, Weiss JN, Weiner I, et al: Fractionated endocardial electrograms are associated with slow conduction in humans: evidence from pace mapping. J Am Coll Cardiol 1989;13:369.

246. Stevenson WG, Wiener I, Weiss JN: Contribution of the anode to ventricular excitation during bipolar programmed electrical stimulation. Am J Cardiol 1986;57:582.

247. Dam RTV, Strackee J, Tweeel HVD: The excitability cycle of the dogs left ventricle determined by anodal, cathodal and bipolar stimulation. Circ Res 1956;4:196.

248. Stevenson WG, Wiener I, Weiss JN: Comparison of bipolar and unipolar programmed electrical stimulation for the initiation of ventricular arrhythmias: significance of anodal excitation during bipolar stimulation. Circulation 1986; 73:693.

249. Van Gelder LM, El Gamal MIH, Tielen CHJ: Changes in

morphology of the paced QRS complex related to pacemaker output. Pacing Clin Electrophysiol 1989;12:1640.

250. Kadish AH, Childs K, Schmaltz S, Morady F: Differences in QRS configuration during unipolar pacing from adjacent sites: implications for the spatial resolution of pace-mapping. J Am Coll Cardiol 1991;17:143.

251. Waldo AL, Olshansky B, Okumura K, Henthorn RW: Current perspectives on entrainment of tachyarrhythmias. In: Brugada P, Wellens HJJ, eds. Cardiac arrhythmias: where to go from here. Mt Kisco, NY: Futura Publishing, 1987;171.

252. Waldo AL, Henthorn RW, Plumb VJ, MacLean WAH: Demonstration of the mechanism of transient entrainment and interruption of ventricular tachycardia with rapid atrial pacing. J Am Coll Cardiol 1984;3:422.

253. Okumura K, Olshansky B, Henthorn RW, Epstein AE, Plumb VJ, Waldo AL: Demonstration of the presence of slow conduction during sustained ventricular tachycardia in man: use of transient entrainment of the tachycardia. Circulation 1987;75:369.

254. Henthorn RW, Okumura K, Olshansky B, Plumb VJ, Hess PG, Waldo AL: A fourth criterion for transient entrainment: the electrogram equivalent of progressive fusion. Circulation 1988;77:1003.

255. Okumura K, Henthorn RW, Epstein AR, Plumb VJ, Waldo AL: Further observation on transient entrainment: importance of pacing site and properties of the components of the reentry circuit. Circulation 1985;72:1293.

256. Kay GN, Epstein AE, Plumb VJ: Resetting of ventricular tachycardia by single extrastimuli. Relation to slow conduction within the reentrant circuit. Circulation 1990;81:1507.

257. Almendral JM, Gottlieb CD, Rosenthal ME, et al: Entrainment of ventricular tachycardia: explaination for surface electrocardiographic phenomenon by analysis of electrograms recorded within the tachycardia circuit. Circulation 1988;77:569.

258. Mann DE, Lawrie GM, Luck JC, Griffin JC, Magro SA, Wyndham CRC: Importance of pacing site in entrainment of ventricular tachycardia. J Am Coll Cardiol 1985;5:781.

259. Anderson KP, Swerdlow CD, Mason JW: Entrainment of ventricular tachycardia. Am J Cardiol 1984;53:335.

260. Kay GN, Epstein AE, Plumb VJ: Incidence of reentry with an excitable gap in ventricular tachycardia: a prospective evaluation utilizing transient entrainment. J Am Coll Cardiol 1988;11:530.

261. Frank R, Tonet JL, Kounde S, Farenq G, Fontaine G: Localization of the area of slow conduction during ventricular tachycardia. In: Brugada P, Wellens HJJ, eds. Cardiac arrhythmias: where to go from here. Mt Kisco, NY: Futura Publishing, 1987:191.

262. Garan H, Ruskin JN: Reproducible termination of ventricular tachycardia by a single extrastimulus within the reentry circuit during the ventricular effective refractory period. Am Heart J 1988;116:546.

263. Ruffy R: Termination of ventricular tachycardia by nonpropagated local depolarization: further observations on entrainment of ventricular tachycardia from an area of slow conduction. Pacing Clin Electrophysiol 1990; 13:852.

264. Morady F, Frank R, Kou WH, et al: Identification and catheter ablation of a zone of slow conduction in the reentrant circuit

of ventricular tachycardia in humans. J Am Coll Cardiol 1988;11:775.

265. Fisher JD: Stimulation as a key to tachycardia localization and ablation. J Am Coll Cardiol 1988;11:889.

266. Podczeck A, Borgrefe M, Rubio A, Breithardt G, et al: Termination of re-entrant ventricular tachycardia by subthreshold stimulus applied to the zone of slow conduction. Eur Heart J 1988;9:1146.

267. El-Sherif N, Gough WB, Restivo M: Reentrant ventricular arrhythmias in the late myocardial infarction period: 14. mechanisms of resetting, entrainment, acceleration, or termination of reentrant tachycardia by programmed electrical stimulation. Pacing Clin Electrophysiol 1987;10:341.

268. Stevenson WG, Nademanee K, Weiss JN, et al: Programmed electrical stimulation at sites in ventricular reentry circuits: comparison of predictions from computer simulations with observations in humans. Circulation 1989;80:793.

269. Fontaine G, Frank R, Tonet J, Grosgogeat Y: Identification of a zone of slow conduction appropriate for ventricular tachycardia ablation: theoretical considerations. Pacing Clin Electrophysiol 1989;12:262.

270. Stevenson WG, Woo MA: Entrainment of ventricular tachycardia: relation of pacing site location within areas of slow conduction to antidromic wavefront distance. J Am Coll Cardiol 1990;15:253A.

271. Borggrefe M, Martinez-Rubio A, Karbenn U, Breithardt G: Pacing-interventions at the site of origins of VT: Improvement of results of catheter ablation. Ciruclation 1989;80 (Supp II):223.

272. Khan HH, Stevenson WG: Activation times in and adjacent to re-entry circuits during entrainment: implications for mapping ventricular tachycardia. Am Heart J 1994;127:833.

273. Ruffy R, Friday KJ, Southworth WF: Termination of ventricular tachycardia by single extrastimulation during the ventricular effective refractory period. Circulation 1983;67:457.

274. Shenasa M, Cardinal R, Kus T, et al: Termination of sustained ventricular tachycardia by ultrarapid subthreshold stimulation in humans. Circulation 1988;78:1135.

275. Stevenson W, Sager P, Nademanee K, Hassan H, Middlekauff HG: Identifying sites for catheter ablation of ventricular tachycardia. Herz 1992;17:158.

276. Malik M, Camm AJ: Termination of macro-reentrant tachycardia by a single extrastimulus delivered during the effective refractory period: a computer modeled case report. Pacing Clin Electrophysiol 1990:13:103.

277. Antzelevitch C, Moe GK: Electrotonic inhibition and summation of impulse conduction in mammalian purkinje fibers. Am J Physiol 1983;245:1442.

278. Ruffy R: Subthreshold stimulation of the heart: small but important. Pacing Clin Electrophysiol 1990;13:110.

279. Brugada P, de Swart H, Smeets JLRM, Wellens HJJ: Transcoronary termination and ablation of ventricular tachycardia. Circulation 1989;79:475.

280. Kay GN, Epstein AE, Bubien RS, Anderson PG, Dailey SM, Plumb VJ: Intracoronary ethanol ablation for the treatment of recurrent sustained ventricular tachycardia. J Am Coll Cardiol 1992;19:159.

281. Touboul P, Kirkorian G, Atallah G, Moleur P: Bundle branch

reentry: a possible mechanism of ventricular tachycardia. Circulation 1983;67:674.

282. Cacceres J, Jazayeri M, McKinnie J, et al: Sustained bundle branch reentry as a mechanism of clinical tachycardia. Circulation 1989;79:256.

283. Denker S, Lehmann M, Mahmud R, Gilbert C, Akhtar M: Facilitation of ventricular tachycardia induction with abrupt changes in ventricular cycle length. Am J Cardiol 1984; 53:508.

284. Touboul P, Kirkorian G, Attalah G, et al: Bundle branch reentrant tachycardia treated by electrical ablation of the right bundle branch. J Am Coll Cardiol 1986;7:1404.

285. Tchou P, Jazayeri M, Denker S, Dongas J, Caceres J, Akhtar M: Transcatheter electrical ablation of right bundle branch: a method of treating macroreentrant ventricular tachycardia attributed to bundle brach reentry. Circulation 1988;78:246.

286. Cohen T, Chien W, Lurie K, et al: Radiofrequency catheter ablation for treatment of bundle branch reentrant ventricular tachycardia: results and long-term follow-up. J Am Coll Cardiol 1991;18:1767.

287. Blanck Z, Dhala A, Deshpande S, Sra J, Jazayeri M, Akhtar M: Bundle branch reentrant ventricular tachycardia: cumulative experience in 48 patients. J Cardiovasc Electrophysiol 1993;4:253.

288. Poll DS, Marchlinski FE, Buxton AE, Doherty JU, Waxman HL, Josephson ME: Sustained ventricular tachycardia in patients with idiopathic dilated cardiomyopathy: electrophysiologic testing and lack of response to antiarrhythmic drug therapy. Circulation 1984;70:451.

289. Liem LB, Swerdlow CD: Value of electropharmacologic testing in idiopathic dilated cardiomyopathy and sustained ventricular tachyarrhythmias. Am J Cardiol 1988;62:611.

290. Lo YSA, Billingham M, Rowan RA, Lee HC, Liem LB, Swerdlow CD: Histopathologic and electrophysiologic correlations in idiopathic dilated cardiomyopathy and sustained ventricular tachyarrhythmia. Am J Cardiol 1989;64:1063.

291. Rae AP: Apielman SR, Kutalek SP, Kay HR, Horowitz LN: Electrophysiologic assessment of antiarrhythmic drug efficacy for ventricular tachyarrhythmias associated with dilated cardiomyopathy. Am J Cardiol 1987;59:291.

292. Fontaine G, Guiraudon G, Frank R, et al: Stimulation studies and epicardial mapping in ventricular tachycardia: study of mechanisms and selection for surgery. In: Kulbertus H, ed. Reentrant arrhythmias. Lancaster, PA: MTP Publishing, 1977:334.

293. Marcus FI, Fontaine GH, Guiraudon G, et al: Right ventricular dysplasia: a report of 24 adult cases. Circulation 1982; 65:384.

294. Blomstrom-Lundqvist C, Selin K, Jonsson R, Johansson SR, Schlossman D, Olsson SB: Cardioangiographic findings in patients with arrhythmogenic right ventricular dysplasia. Br Heart J 1988;59:556.

295. Fontaine G, Guiraudon G, Frank R: Intramyocardial conduction defects in patients prone to ventricular tachycardia. III. A dynamic study of the post-excitation syndrome. In: Sandoe E, Julian DG, Bell JW, eds. Management of ventricular tachycardia: role of mexiletine. Amsterdam: Excerpta Medica 1978:56.

296. Blomstrom-Lundqvist C, Olsson SB, Edvardsson N: Follow-up by repeated signal-averaged surface QRS in patients with the syndrome of arrhythmogenic right ventricular dysplasia. Eur Heart J 1989;10:54.

297. Di Biase M, Favale S, Massari V, Amodio G, Chiddo A, Risson P: Programmed stimulation in patients with minor forms of right ventricular dysplasia. Eur Heart J 1989;10:49.

298. Foale RA, Nihoyannopoulos R, Ribeiro P, et al: Right ventricular abnormalities in ventricular tachycardia of right ventricular origin: relation to electrophysiological abnormalities. Br Heart J 1986;56:45.

299. Lemery R, Brugada P, Janssen J, Cheriex E, Dugernier T, Wellens HJJ: Nonischemic sustained ventricular tachycardia: clinical outcome in 12 patients with arrhythmogenic right ventricular dysplasia. J Am Coll Cardiol 1989;14:96.

300. Martini B, Nava A, Thine G, et al: Accelerated idioventricular rhythm of infundibular origin in patients with a concealed form of arrhythmogenic right ventricular dysplasia. Br Heart J 1989;59:564.

301. Blomstrom-Lundqvist C, Sabel KG, Olsson SB: A long term follow up of 15 patients with arrhythmogenic right ventricular dysplasia. Br Heart J 1987;58:477.

302. Guiraudon G, Fontaine G, Frank R, Leandri R, Barra J, Cabrol C: Surgical treatment of ventricular tachycardia guided by ventricular mapping in 23 patients without coronary artery disease. Ann Thorac Surg 1981;32:439.

303. Leclercq JF, Chouty F, Couchemez B, Leenhardt A, Coumel P, Slama R: Results of electrical fulguration in arrhythmogenic right ventricular disease. Am J Cardiol 1988;62:220.

304. Hauer RN, de Medina EOR, Kuijer PJ, Westerhof PW: Electrode catheter ablation for ventricular tachycardia: efficacy of a single cathodal shock. Br Heart J 1989;61:38.

305. Borgreffe M, Breithardt G, Podczeck A, Rohner D, Budde T, Martinez-Rubio A: Catheter ablation of ventricular tachycardia using defibrillator pulses: electrophysiological findings and long-term results. Eur Heart J 1989;10:591.

306. McKenna WJ: Sudden death in hypertrophic cardiomyopathy: assessment of patients at high risk. Circulation 1989; 80:1489.

307. Kowey PR, Eisenberg R, Engel TR: Sustained arrhythmias in hypertrophic obstructive cardiomyopathy. N Engl J Med 1984;310:1566.

308. Kuck KH, Kunze KP, Geiger M, Costard A, Schluter M: Programmed electrical stimulation in patients with hypertrophic cardiomyopathy: results in patients with and without cardiac arrest or syncope. In: Brugada P, Wellens HJJ, eds. Cardiac arrhythmias: where to go from here? Mount Kisco, NY: Futura Publishing, 1987:367.

309. Watson RM, Schwartz JL, Maron BJ, Tucker E, Rosing DR, Josephson ME: Inducible polymorphic ventricular tachycardia and ventricular fibrillation in a subgroup of patients with hypertrophic cardiomyopathy at high risk for sudden death. J Am Coll Cardiol 1987;10:761.

310. Fananapazir L, Tracy CM, Leon MB, et al: Electrophysiologic abnormalities in patients with hypertrophic cardiomyopathy. a consecutive analysis in 155 patients. Circulation 1989; 80:1259.

311. Nicod P, Polikar R, Peterson KL: Hypertrophic cardiomyopathy and sudden death. N Engl J Med 1988;318:1255.

312. Lemery R, Brugada P, Della Bella P, Dugernier T, van den

Dool A, Wellens HJJ: Nonischemic ventricular tachycardia: clinical course and long-term follow-up in patients without clinically overt heart disease. Circulation 1989;79:990.

313. Buxton AE, Waxman AL, Marchlinski FE, Simson MB, Cassidy D, Josephson ME: Right ventricular tachycardia: clinical and electrophysiologic characteristics. Circulation 1983;68:917.

314. Palileo EV, Ashley WW, Swiryn S, et al: Exercise provocable right ventricular outflow tract tachycardia. Am Heart J 1982; 104:185.

315. Coumel P, Leclerq JF, Slama R: Repetitive monomorphic idiopathic ventricular tachycardia, In: Zipes DP, Jalife G, eds. Cardiac electrophysiology and arrhythmias. New York: Grune & Stratton, 1985:457.

316. Pietras RJ, Lam W, Bauernfeind R, et al: Chronic recurrent right ventricular tachycardia in patients without ischemic heart disease: clinical, hemodynamic, and angiographic findings. Am Heart J 1983;105:357.

317. Reiter MJ, Smith WM, Gallagher JJ: Clinical spectrum of ventricular tachycardia with left bundle branch morphology. Am J Cardiol 1983;51:112.

318. Sung Ruey J, Shen EN, Morady F, Scheinman MM, Hess D, Botvinick EH: Electrophysiologic mechanism of exercise-induced sustained ventricular tachycardia. Am J Cardiol 1983;51:525.

319. Lin FC, Finley D, Rahimtoola SH, Wu D: Idiopathic paroxysmal ventricular tachycardia with a QRS pattern of right bundle branch block and left axis deviation: a unique clinical entity with specific properties. Am J Cardiol 1983;52:97.

320. German LD, Packer DL, Bardy GH, Gallagher JJ: Ventricular tachycardia induced by atrial stimulation in patients without symptomatic cardiac disease. Am J Cardiol 1983;52:1202.

321. Rahilly GM, Prystowsky EN, Zipes DP, Naccarelli GV, Jackman WM, Heger JJ: Clinical and electrophysiologic findings in patients with repetitive monomorphic ventricular tachycardia and otherwise normal electrocardiogram. Am J Cardiol 1982;50:459.

322. Zimmermann MA, Maisonblanche R, Cauchemez B, Leclerq JF, Coumel P: Determinants of spontaneous ectopic acitvity in repetitive monomorphic idiopathic ventricular tachycardia. J Am Coll Cardiol 1986;6:1219.

323. Wilber DJ, Blakeman BM, Pifarre R, Schlon PJ: Catecholamine sensitive right ventricular outflow tract tachycardia: intraoperative mapping and ablation of a free-wall focus. Pacing Clin Electrophysiol 1989;12:1851.

324. Wilber DJ, Baerman J, Olshansky B, Kall J, Kopp D: Adenosine-sensitive ventricular tachycardia: Clinical characteristics and response to catheter ablation. Circulation 1993; 87:126.

325. Klein LS, Shih HT, Hackett FK, Zipes DP, Miles WM: Radiofrequency catheter ablation of ventricular tachycardia in patients without structural heart disease. Circulation 1992; 85:1666.

326. Lerman BB: Response of nonreentrant catecholamine-mediated ventricular tachycardia to endogenous adenosine and acetyl-choline: evidence for myocardial receptor-mediated effects. Circulation 1993;87:382.

327. Mehta D, McKenna W, Ward DE, Davies M, Camm AJ: Significance of signal-averaged electrocardiography in relation to endomyocardial biopsy and ventricular stimulation studies in patients with ventricular tachycardia without clinically apparent heart disease. J Am Coll Cardiol 1989;14:372.

328. Hartzler GO: Electrode catheter ablation of refractory focal ventricular tachycardia. J Am Coll Cardiol 1983;2:1107.

329. Calkins H, Kalbfleisch SJ, El-Atassi R, Langberg JJ, Morady F: Relation between efficacy of radiofrequency catheter ablation and site of origin of idiopathic ventricular tachycardia. Am J Cardiol 1993;71:827.

330. Stevenson WG, Nademanee K, Weiss JN, Wiener I: Treatment of catecholamine-sensitive right ventricular tachycardia by endocardial catheter ablation. J Am Coll Cardiol 1990;16:752.

331. Jordeans L, Roelandt R, Palmer A, van Wassenhove E, Clement D: Ablation of ventricular tachycardia of right ventricular origin with low energy shocks. Pacing Clin Electrophysiol 1989;12:911.

332. Morady G, Kadish AH, DiCarlo L, et al: Long-term results of catheter ablation of idiopathic right ventricular tachycardia. Circulation 1990;82:2093.

333. Zipes DP, Foster PR, Troup PJ, Pedersen DH: Atrial induction of ventricular tachycardia: reentry versus triggered automaticity. Am J Cardiol 1979;44:1.

334. Morgera T, Slavi A, Alberti E, Silvestri F, Camerini F: Morphological findings in apparently idiopathic ventricular tachycardia. An echocardiographic haemodynamic and histologic study. Eur Heart J 1985;6:323.

335. Ohe T, Shimomura K, Ahara N, et al: Idiopathic sustained left ventricular tachycardia: clinical and electrophysiologic conditions. Circulation 1988;77:560.

336. Okumura K, Matsuyama K, Miyagi H, Tsuchiya T, Yasue H: Entrainment of idiopathic ventricular tachycardia of left ventricular origin with evidence for reentry with an arc of slow conduction and effect of verapamil. Am J Cardiol 1988; 62:727.

337. Nakagawa H, Beckman KJ, McClelland JH, et al: Radiofrequency catheter ablation of idiopathic left ventricular tachycardia guided by a Purkinje potential. Circulation 1993; 88:2607.

338. Wu D, Kou HC, Hung JS: Exercise-triggered paroxysmal ventricular tachycardia. Ann Intern Med 1981;85:410.

Cardiac Arrhythmias, 3rd edition, edited by William J. Mandel.
J. B. Lippincott Company, Philadelphia © 1995.

24

Antoni Martínez-Rubio • Martin Borggrefe • Thomas Fetsch
Lutz Reinhardt • Markku Mäkijärvi • Günter Breithardt

Ventricular Late Potentials: Mechanisms, Methodology, Prevalence and Clinical Significance*

Experimental and clinical studies have provided convincing evidence that the reentry mechanism plays a major role in the genesis of malignant ventricular arrhythmias.[1–5] The prerequisites for reentry are unidirectional block, slow conduction, and recovery of the tissue ahead of the wavefront of excitation.[1–5] In this context, one of the most compelling findings attributed to slow conduction is the detection of delayed fractionated electric activity during diastole in regions of experimental infarction.[3–5] These potentials occurring in or after the end of the QRS complex have been called "ventricular late potentials."[6,7] They are characterized by multiple low-amplitude spikes, sometimes separated by isoelectric intervals. The presence of such electrograms during sinus rhythm may indicate sites for potential reentrant circuits. Delayed and fractionated potentials have been observed during intraoperative epicardial and endocardial mapping and in endocardial catheter mapping in patients having ventricular tachycardia (Fig. 24-1).[6–12]

Ventricular late potentials have been recorded noninvasively, using appropriate recording and filtering techniques.[7,13–21] In this chapter, the recording technologies and the available clinical results in patients with or without documented ventricular tachyarrhythmias after myocardial infarction in addition to the results of interventions are presented. The European Society of Cardiology, the American College of Cardiology, and the American Heart Association developed the guidelines for recording and analysis of ventricular late potentials using high-resolution or signal-averaged electrocardiography.[22]

ELECTROPHYSIOLOGIC AND ANATOMIC BASIS OF VENTRICULAR LATE POTENTIALS

In experimental myocardial infarction, continuous electric activity that regularly and predictably bridged the entire diastolic interval between the initiating beat and the reentrant beats as well as between consecutive reentrant beats was demonstrated by El-Sherif and colleagues, using a specially designed composite electrode (Fig. 24-2).[3] The

*Partly supported by the Deutsche Forschungsgemeinschaft, Bonn-Bad Godesberg, Germany (DFG Project Nr. Br 759/2-1) Bonn, Germany

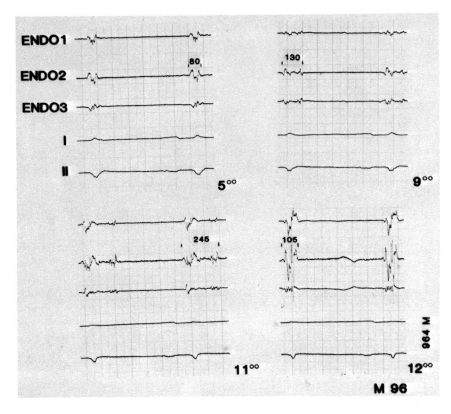

Figure 24-1. Intraoperative recording of fractionated activity in a patient with documented ventricular tachycardia, using endocardial bipolar mapping techniques. The site of recording is in the border zone of an aneurysm. The fractionated activity starts before the end of the QRS complex in the surface electrocardiogram and extends into the ST segment.

ventricular late potentials originate from areas of previous myocardial infarction, which may leave a zone of electrically abnormal ventricular myocardium as a potential site of origin for ventricular tachycardia.[6-11] This tissue is normally located at the border zone of the previous infarction and is characterized by islands of relatively viable muscle alternating with areas of necrosis and later, fibrosis. Such tissue may result in fragmentation of the propagating electromotive forces because of slow asynchronous conduction, with the consequent development of high-frequency components that can be recorded directly from these areas.[3,4,5,23-28] Gardner and associates demonstrated that (1) slow conduction caused by depressed resting potential, and (2) action potential upstroke velocity, with elevated potassium concentration in the superfusion solution, were associated with a reduced electrogram amplitude and increased duration but did not cause fragmented activity.[29] Therefore, slow conduction alone does not cause fragmented activity. Highly fractionated electrograms only occurred in preparations from chronic infarcts in which interstitial fibrosis formed insulating boundaries between muscle bundles. Therefore, the individual components of fragmented electrograms most likely represent asynchronous electric activity in each of the separate bundles of surviving muscle under the electrode. The intrinsic asymmetry of cardiac activation due to fiber orientation is accentuated by infarction and may predispose to reentry.[25,29] The transmembrane potentials of muscle fibers in

areas of fractionated activity in the epicardial border zone of healed canine infarcts were not depressed.[29] Instead, slow conduction in these areas was attributed to diminished intercellular connections between muscle fibers. The low amplitude of the electrograms probably resulted from the paucity of surviving muscle fibers under the electrode because of the large amounts of connective tissue and not because the action potentials were depressed. Prolonged fractionated electrograms recorded in these regions reflect a slow, dissociated conduction, which may cause an increase in the duration of the local electrogram. The intrinsic activation time of the local electrogram may be normal because the time required for an impulse to conduct through the remaining myocardium to that site may not be altered. The prolonged duration of the local electrogram depends on the impulse traversing the immediate field of view of a local recording electrode and thus reflects local conduction characteristics.[27-29] Therefore, the anatomic substrate for reentry seems to be present in regions where fragmented electrograms can be recorded, indicating slow inhomogenous conduction. Fragmented electrograms are probably found wherever myocardial fibers are separated by connective tissue, even if reentry does not occur in the region.[30,31] Richards and colleagues showed that sustained reentry may occur in areas of the epicardium showing fractionated electrograms as small as 5 cm.[3,25]

A close correlation between the presence of con-

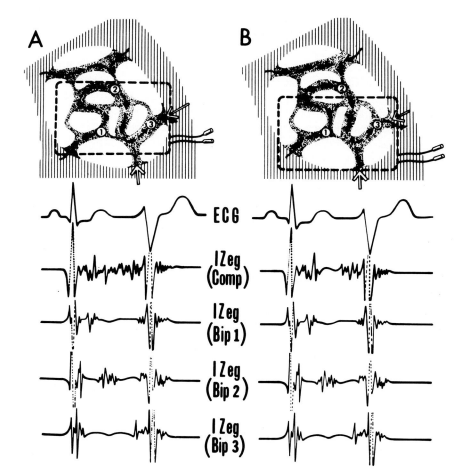

Figure 24-2. Schematic representation of the conduction disorder in the zone of experimental infarction leading to reentry. Tracings from top to bottom represent a standard electrocardiographic lead, a composite electrode recording (*Comp*) with an electrogram from the ischemic zone (*IZeg*), and three close bipolar recordings (*IZeg [Bip] 1* to *3*). (**B**) The composite electrode (*dotted line*) does not cover the entire reentrant pathway, which explains failure of the *IZeg* (*Comp*) to depict a continuous series of multiple asynchronous spikes. (El-Sherif N, Scherlag BJ, Lazzara R, Hope RR: Reentrant ventricular arrhythmias in the late myocardial infarction period. I. Conduction characteristics in the infarction zone. Circulation 1977;55:686.)

tinuous fractionated electric activity and perpetuation of ventricular tachycardia was demonstrated by Garan and colleagues.[32] In these studies, ventricular pacing that captured the ventricles without affecting continuous electric activity never terminated the tachycardia. Transformation of continuous electric activity into abbreviated discrete electrograms by rapid pacing terminated ventricular tachycardia, however. Interruption of continuous electric activity by a single ventricular stimulus, without capture of the ventricles during ventricular tachycardia, also terminated ventricular tachycardia. Surgical ablation of the site of continuous electric activity abolished inducible ventricular tachycardia. This has also been reported in patients with previous ventricular tachycardia, in whom the propensity to this arrhythmia had been successfully abolished by surgical intervention.[33,34] These studies elegantly show the pathogenetic significance of these areas for the perpetuation of ventricular tachycardia. Thus, the areas from which ventricular late potentials can be recorded have been considered as the arrhythmogenic electrophysiologic substrate for reentrant ventricular tachycardia. The presence of an arrhythmogenic electrophysiologic substrate in the form of regional slow ventricular activa-

tion is not sufficient to develop ventricular tachycardia, however. Instead, an additional factor (such as ventricular ectopic beats) is necessary to initiate reentrant ventricular tachycardia by triggering the arrhythmogenic substrate. Once initiated, reentrant tachycardia may perpetuate itself within the reentrant circuit if the conditions are adequate.

A zone with arrhythmogenic properties may arise acutely (and be present only transiently) or it may exist chronically in the form of myocardium interspersed with fibrosis after a previous myocardial infarction. The classic example of an acutely developing arrhythmogenic tissue that leads to ventricular tachyarrhythmias is acute myocardial infarction, which is frequently accompanied by ventricular fibrillation. The changes that occur in this situation are frequently transient in nature and may subside as soon as the tissue is completely necrotic. In contrast, strands of surviving myocardial fibers surrounded by fibrous tissue may develop during the healing phase of myocardial infarction and may persist chronically, even for many years, as the basis for ventricular late potentials.[28]

A more detailed discussion of the pathophysiologic mechanisms of ventricular late potentials has previously been presented.[12,35]

METHODOLOGICAL ASPECTS OF NONINVASIVE RECORDING OF VENTRICULAR LATE POTENTIALS

The amplitude of ventricular late potentials is in the low millivolt range, even when direct recordings are used. Using conventional methods of electrocardiographic recording, these signals can rarely be recovered from the body surface.[13,36] These signals can be recorded from the body surface by using high-gain amplification and computer-averaging techniques, however, as has been shown for the first time by Berbari and colleagues in the experimental animal and by Fontaine and colleagues in patients having idiopathic ventricular tachycardia.[7,13] This is confirmed by many other reports.[14–18,20,21,37,38] These different types of recording are termed "high-resolution electrocardiography."

In principle, three different approaches of high-resolution electrocardiography have been used for detection of ventricular late potentials. First, signal-averaging in the time domain. Second, spatial-averaging on a beat-to-beat basis. Third, signal-averaging in the frequency domain.

Signal-averaging in the time domain is based on high-gain amplification, band-pass filtering, and signal-averaging of a given number of identical beats to eliminate the random noise and to improve the signal-to-noise ratio (Fig. 24-3).[8,22,39–41]

A major problem with high-gain amplification is the level of noise that is generated by several sources (Table 24-1), making some method of noise reduction necessary. The amplitude of these signals is usually smaller than the electric noise produced by the various sources. In addition to careful shielding of all cables and the use of preamplifiers with a high signal-to-noise ratio, signal-averaging is used to eliminate the remaining random noise. With increasing repetition of the averaging process, randomly occurring noise is cancelled, whereas the amplitude of the repetitively occurring true signal stabilizes, thus increasing the signal-to-noise ratio (see Fig. 24-3). This technique is applicable only to repetitive electrocardiographic signals and cannot detect moment-to-moment dynamic changes in the signal.

The necessary sampling rate of the averaging system is determined by the frequency content of the signal. To recover a signal with good fidelity, the frequency response of the instrumentation must be commensurate with the frequency components of the signal. Ideally, there should be no frequency components of the input signal (including noise) that are higher in frequency than the sampling frequency. Higher input frequencies cause aliasing, which means that frequencies appear the same number of hertz below half the sampling frequency as the input component is above it. In our own system, aliasing was no problem because the signals were filtered with a low-pass cutoff of 300 Hz and the sampling frequency was 10 kHz.[18]

For better identification of late potentials, elimination of low-frequency components of the signal is mandatory.[22] This prevents the ST segment from saturating at extremely high amplifications and excludes respiratory movements. Depending on the characteristics of the filters, high-pass cutoff points between 25 and 100 Hz are suggested.[18,22,40–43] One problem with high-gain amplification of biologic signals is filter-ringing, especially if sharp high-pass filters are used. This may occur at a point of rapid transition of a high-amplitude signal to baseline. Conventional filtering of the highly amplified QRS complex distorts the end of the signal. The degree of filter-ringing increases with elevation of the high-pass cutoff. Thus, in any study, the characteristics of the filters used should be stated. Multiple-ringing lasting for a significant time after the end of the QRS complex occurs with some filters.[20] To prevent filter-ringing, either filters with flat characteristics should be used or the signal should be analyzed retrogradely, as suggested by Simson.[20] In the latter approach, a bidirectional filter is used that first processes forward in time until 40 milliseconds into the QRS complex and then processes backward in that time up to the same point within the QRS complex.

One of the prerequesites for signal-averaging is that the timing and morphology of late potentials is identical for beats of similar QRS morphology. Whether this is correct is still unsettled. Variation of the timing and configuration of ventricular late potentials may occur on a beat-to-beat basis and may thus cause progressive attenuation during the averaging process. Therefore, premature ventricular beats should be excluded. This can either be done simply by rejecting all beats of a given prematurity or by passing all electrocardiographic signals through a template-recognition program to reject ectopic beats and grossly noisy signals.[18,20] In the latter approach, an initial eight-beat template is accepted if the mean standard deviation of the signals is less than 10 μV. All subsequent beats are tested against this template and accepted if the deviation from the template is less than twice the template standard deviation. The template is updated every fourth beat.

Instability (jitter) of the trigger point for the QRS complex may attenuate the signals and act as a low-pass filter. This is not only a limitation of signal-averaging in the time domain but also in the frequency domain. In pre-

TABLE 24-1. Causes of Noise During High-Gain Recordings of the Electrocardiogram

Environmental noise
Noise generated from the skin–electrode interface
Myotonic noise
Amplifier noise

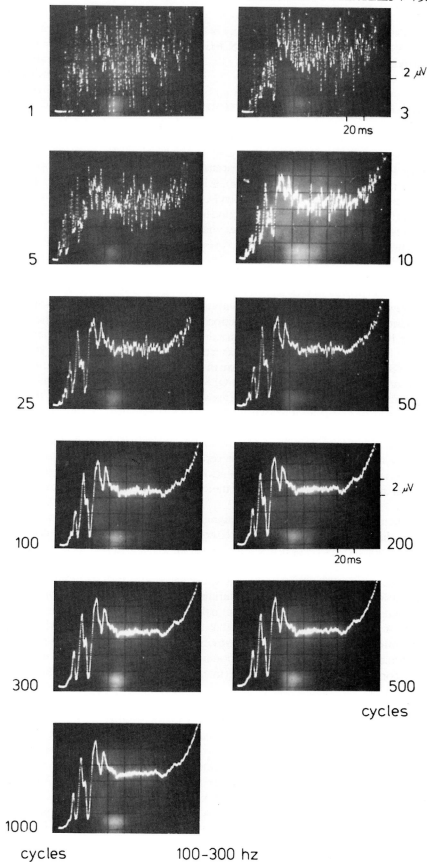

Figure 24-3. Progress of the averaging process with evolution of the final signal depending on the number of cycles, which ranged from 1 to 1000 in a patient with left ventricular aneurysm. A circumscribed high-frequency activity represents a late potential shortly after the QRS complex in this patient with ventricular tachycardia.

vious studies, values for the instability of the trigger point of QRS between 0.5 to 2.0 milliseconds have been reported.[13, 14, 18, 21, 22, 40, 44–46]

End Point of Noise Reduction

Prior studies used a fixed number of QRS complexes for performing signal-averaging. Because the background noise level in individual patients is variable, Steinberg and Bigger analyzed whether variable noise levels after signal processing interfered with the detection of late potentials.[47] They performed signal-averaging for each patient of their study to two prespecified noise end points. The first end point was 1.0 μV, which was also used in other studies as a minimal residual noise level. The second was 0.3 μV, a low level that generally can be attained in less than 450 beats. The prevalence of late potentials was significantly greater with the 0.3-μV level than with the 1.0-μV level in patients with prior myocardial infarction. In normal volunteers, however, the prevalence did not depend on the final noise level achieved. The greater detection of late potentials with the 0.3-μV level was because of improved resolution of the terminal low-amplitude QRS segment. Therefore, using a lower noise level increased the sensitivity of detection of late potentials without a loss of specificity, whereas relatively high noise levels may obscure the presence of late potentials and yield an incorrect prevalence of late potentials. This may alter the reproducibility of a study. Based on these results, it is advisable to perform signal-averaging to this prespecified low-noise end point.[22]

Reproducibility of signal-averaging in the time domain depends on interobserver and day-to-day variability. The major factors responsible for this variability are (1) electrode position, (2) level of noise, (3) stability of the triggering of QRS, (4) stability of the cardiac status and medication, (5) use of identical criteria to judge the onset and offset of QRS, and (6) the terminal low-voltage portion. Available evidence suggests that day-to-day reproducibility is high, with a large percentage of patients (more than 90%) still having late potentials detectable at a second recording if no change in the clinical status occurs.[18, 20, 39, 40, 48]

The basic equipment for the temporal signal-averaging technique consists of a preamplifier, an analog–digital (AD) converter, a signal-averager, and a method for data presentation and storage. In addition, a trigger signal must be derived from either the same electrocardiographic source or another lead. This trigger signal is used to initiate the averaging process at a given point within each QRS complex. To record portions of the signal before the trigger point, a transient recording device may be interposed. Abnormal QRS complexes should be excluded from the averaging process, as described above.

Some major technical differences between the various systems in use in several laboratories are due to lead positioning for recording, filter characteristics, and type of data presentation, storage, and evaluation. A short description of some techniques follows.

In our first signal-averaging system, four bipolar electrodes were connected to a high-gain low-noise battery powered preamplifier (model 113, Princeton Applied Research), using shielded leads.[18] Band-pass filter settings (single-pole analog filters, 6 dB/octave) were from 100 to 300 Hz. The high-pass cutoff of 100 Hz was necessary to eliminate respiratory baseline drifts and to flatten the ST segment, which otherwise would have had a steep upstroke at the gain used. The low-pass cutoff of 300 Hz was chosen to eliminate noise originating from muscular activity. The preamplified signal was connected to a dual-channel signal-averager (model 4202, Princeton Applied Research). Both channels were combined to a single 2048-word memory. The averager was externally triggered from the QRS complex of an additional bipolar lead that was selected to yield a high-amplitude monophasic QRS signal. The threshold was adjusted for consistent triggering at the time of averaging. The jitter for triggering was ±1.5 milliseconds. The trigger signal initiated a sweep that at the selected positions lasted 204.8 milliseconds (consisting of 2048 consecutive dwell time intervals, each lasting 100 μs). In this mode of operation, the signal was digitized at a sampling rate of 10 kHz. The signal-averager allowed continuous monitoring of the progress of the averaging process on a storage oscilloscope. In most cases, the number of cardiac cycles averaged varied between 150 to 200. Care was taken not to include premature ventricular beats. For this purpose, a special circuit was included that automatically measured the RR intervals on a beat-to-beat basis. Premature complexes were thus eliminated from being triggered. The averaged signals were photographed with a Polaroid camera.

We have also been using the system developed by Simson and modified by Karbenn and colleagues,[m] which uses the three bipolar orthogonal leads X, Y, and Z.[20, 43] The high-resolution electrocardiogram (ECG) is amplified 1000- to 5000-fold and prefiltered at a band width of 0.05 to 300 Hz. The signal from each lead is then passed through four-pole 250-Hz low-pass filters and then AD-converted to 12-bit accuracy at 1000 samples per second. The digital information is stored on floppy disks by a Hewlett-Packard 9826 desktop computer. Each lead is sequentially recorded for 133 seconds. Only those complexes identified as normal by a template-recognition program are averaged for each lead separately. To reject the low frequencies in the ECG, a bidirectional digital filter of 25 Hz (four-pole high-pass Butterworth design) is used. The filter processes forward until 40 milliseconds into the QRS complex and then processes retrogradely, beginning in the ST segment to avoid filter-ringing.[20] The filtered signals for the three leads are then combined into a vector magnitude (root square of $X^2 + Y^2 + Z^2$), referred to as "filtered QRS complex." The onset and the end of the total signal are automatically defined as the points where the mean amplitude within a portion of the ST segment exceeds a given proportion of the voltage of the random noise. The onset and end of the total filtered QRS complex and the mean voltage of the total signal are calculated. Furthermore, the mean H voltage of the last 40 milliseconds of the signal is measured.[20]

Some authors suggest the use of more than three leads for improving the detection of delayed depolarization by signal-averaging.[12, 49–51]

Because the temporal signal-averaging technique can only detect repetitive electrocardiographic signals, dynamic changes that occur on a beat-to-beat basis cannot be detected. For the latter condition, El-Sherif and associates designed the technique of spatial-averaging.[52] In this technique, electronic summation of potentials recorded from 16 pairs of electrodes is performed, using a specially designed volume-conductor electrode that reduces the noise to 1 to 1.4 μV. It is assumed that the electrocardiographic signal between any pair of electrodes is almost identical, whereas the noise from electromyographic sources, electrode-tissue interface, and the amplifier are not completely correlated. With spatial-averaging, one expects to reinforce the identical signal and to reduce the noise. Although the electrode-tissue interface and amplifier noise can be considered as completely random, electromyographic potentials are not completely incoherent.[53] The greater the distance between the electrodes, the smaller the coherence function of the electromyographic signal. This also reduces the coherence function of the electrocardiographic signal.

The volume conductor electrode improves the ratio of electrocardiographic-to-electromyographic signal because the bioelectric source of the electromyographic potentials is immediately underneath the skin and the cardiac source is more distant.[52] Both the electromyographic and electrocardiographic potentials undergo an approximate inverse square attenuation. Because the electromyographic source is closer, it undergoes greater attenuation. Others have used specially shielded rooms to reduce interference from external sources (mainly alternating current).[39, 42]

Signal-Averaging From Holter-Monitor Tapes

Despite inherent obstacles, it is technically feasible to perform signal-averaging and detect late potentials from conventionally recorded Holter-monitor tapes.[54–56] This approach may provide a method to obtain information on spontaneous ventricular arrhythmias and the underlying arrhythmogenic substrate from the same recording. It may also provide insight into the spontaneous variability of late potentials. Kelen and coworkers obtained signal-averaged ECGs from three-channel Holter-monitor recordings that were compared, using the same skin electrodes, with signal-averaged real-time recordings in 32 subjects.[55] The numeric late potential parameters and morphologic appearances correlated closely between the two methods. The restricted high-frequency response of Holter-monitor systems appears not to militate against clinically useful late potential analysis from Holter-monitor tapes. This study suggests that diagnostic accuracy, using real-time 25- to 250-Hz criteria, is acceptable for clinical use until criteria derived specifically for Holter-monitor applications become available. The authors concluded that Holter-monitor analysis may confer significant benefits, resulting from an ability to perform late-potential analysis on the same tape used for conventional arrhythmia analysis, and may allow further studies of possible dynamic changes of late potentials in relation to transit ischemia and spontaneous ventricular tachyarrhythmias. These results were confirmed by Fetsch and associates.[56]

In addition to signal-averaging in the time domain, signal-averaging in the frequency domain using fast Fourier transform analysis (FFTA) has been suggested as an alternative approach by Cain and colleagues to circumvent the limitations of signal-averaging in the time domain (e.g., filter-ringing or attenuation of the signal by filtering).[18, 20, 21, 40, 41, 44, 48, 57] This technique is based on the assumption that late potentials have different frequency characteristics when compared with the QRS complex and the ST segment. Signals are processed for their frequency content (frequency domain) by analyzing all signals for higher sinusoidal components (harmonics) in relation to the sinusoidal component with the lowest frequency. All harmonics have frequencies that are integer multiples of the fundamental frequencies. Fast Fourier transform analysis for a discrete sample of a periodic waveform, such as the terminal portion of the QRS complex, is based on the assumption that the signal is a repetitive function and that the initial and final sample points are at a potential of zero. If this is not the case, a sharp-edged discontinuity would be introduced between the end of one cycle and the beginning of the next that would artifactually add both high and low frequencies to the original signal. To eliminate this source of harmonic error, time-domain samples are multiplied by a window function (e.g., the four-term Blackman-Harris window) that smooths the initial and final sampling points to zero at the boundaries, allowing periodic extension of the finite signal.[44] This window function reduces spectral leakage by edge discontinuities associated with analysis of a discrete subset of the complex periodic waveform. The major problem of FFTA of the ECG is the selection of the interval of interest. According to the fixed data-acquisition sampling rate, time series of different lengths yield different spectral resolutions. For example, if a waveform sampled at 1.000 Hz is analyzed during a 50-millisecond period, 50 samples are used for the FFT spaced between 0 and 1.000 Hz; the resulting frequency resolution is 20 Hz. The longer the time period, the higher the frequency resolution. Conversely, if signals with changing frequency characteristics are analyzed in a long time window, the resulting frequency curve is an average of all frequency spectra within the observed interval. Transient frequency components are difficult to detect because of their small contribution to the total spectrum. Therefore, the actual length of a timeframe used for FFTA is always a compromise between the maximum frequency resolution and the ability to detect dynamic changes in time.

Haberl and colleagues reported on the use of FFTA to perform a single-beat analysis of the total and terminal QRS and ST segment after high-gain low-noise amplification (0 to 300 Hz).[58] In addition, they suggest performing spectral mapping with FFTA of multiple segments of the surface ECG during sinus rhythm after signal-averaging.[59] The ST segment was divided into 25 segments: the first segment started 50 milliseconds after the end of QRS (segment size, 80 milliseconds), the subsequent segments started progressively earlier in the ST segment in steps of 3 milliseconds. Thus, the 25th segment started 25 milliseconds inside the QRS complex. The frequency components of each segment were calculated with FFTA. The segments were multiplied point by point, with a Hanning window to avoid edge discontinuities. The 25 frequency spectra were combined into a three-dimensional plot. The frequency spectrum of segment 1 (which started far outside the QRS) was defined as a reference spectrum; the spectra of segments 2 to 25 were compared with this reference spectrum by cross-correlation in the frequency range of 40 to 150 Hz. The similarity of spectra was indicated by the correlation coefficient: the correlation coefficient was 0 if two spectra showed no similarity and was 1 if two spectra were identical. A "factor of normality" was then calculated. The mean of the correlation coefficients of segments 20 to 25 was divided by the mean of the correlation coefficients of spectra 1 to 5 multiplied by 100. High frequency content at the end of QRS that is absent far outside QRS causes the factor of normality to be low. The factor of normality may range between 0% and 100% (0% = strong evidence of late potentials; 100% = no evidence of late potentials). A factor of normality below 30% was considered abnormal.

Haberl and colleagues suggest that the advantage of the spectral mapping of the ST segment is that it does not require an exact definition of the onset and end of QRS, which often is difficult to determine.[59] Furthermore, a distinction between normal and abnormal is simpler and does not require criteria that are more or less arbitrary because the factor of normality is calculated as a single parameter. Complex high-pass filtering is not necessary and a discussion about filter artifacts, signal-distortion, and the choice of adequate cutoff frequencies is not necessary.[35, 60] Finally, spectral mapping allows discrimination between late potentials and noise, which both have a typical spectral representation. Noise can easily be identified by spectral peaks that are present in all segments. Late potentials generate spectral peaks only in segments at the end of the QRS but not far outside the QRS-complex. In contrast, the definitions of Simson's approach depend directly on the noise level, which thus represent a possible source of error.[20]

In 1991, Kelen and coworkers proposed a new technique of spectral analysis. Because the arrhythmogenic substrate causes electric inhomogeneities that occur at a time when normal parts of the ventricle still undergo depolarization, the uniform activation is superimposed by the inhomogenous activation of the arrhythmogenic substrate. This may cause changes in the frequency content of the QRS complex, assumed to be detectable by the spectral turbulence analysis technique. To analyze dynamic changes in the frequency content of a signal, short windows are necessary, resulting in a poor frequency resolution. The use of the first derivative of the ECG raw data for FFTA calculation yields to a shift of the frequency spectrum into a higher range. This results in a compromise between optimal frequency resolution and the possibility of detecting dynamic processes. Kelen and coworkers used a 24-millisecond window, starting 25 milliseconds before the onset of QRS and shifting progressively in steps of 2 milliseconds into QRS, terminating 125 milliseconds after the end of the QRS complex.[60a] Fast Fourier transform analysis curves were calculated at each step and plotted in a three-dimensional graph. The mean correlation of each time slice to its neighbor and the average discordance of each slice with an imaginary average slice were calculated. The results indicate a total predictive accuracy of 94% for the spectral turbulence analysis, compared with 73% for the time-domain analysis discriminating patients after myocardial infarction and with inducible sustained ventricular tachycardia from those without inducible ventricular tachycardia and from healthy volunteers. Validation of this technique using larger populations is needed to estimate its clinical value, however.

EXAMPLES OF LATE POTENTIALS RECORDED USING VARIOUS TECHNIQUES

The progression of the averaging process, with improvement in signal quality using our early approach, is shown in Figure 24-3.[18] A typical averaged recording in a normal subject exhibiting the terminal portion of the QRS complex and a part of the ST segment immediately after the QRS complex is shown in Figure 24-4. Two repeated averaging processes were assembled on the same picture by dual exposure to demonstrate the reproducibility. There was a smooth transition from the high-gain QRS complex to the ST segment, which does not show any low-amplitude high-frequency signal. The small fluctuations of the baseline are due to remaining noise, the level of which is less than 1 μV. There was no filter-ringing. A typical late potential in a patient after myocardial infarction is demonstrated in Figure 24-5.

The results of signal processing, using the system described by Simson in a normal subject, are presented in Figure 24-6.[20] The QRS duration was normal (86 milliseconds); there was no low-amplitude tail at the end of the high-gain filtered QRS complex (high-pass cutoff, 25 Hz); the mean voltage in the terminal 40 milliseconds of the QRS complex was high (V, 128.52 μV), indicating the absence of low-amplitude activity. The end of the high-amplitude filtered QRS complex in the top tracing corresponds to the end in the standard surface leads X, Y, and Z (*bottom*). In contrast, a low-amplitude tail appears at the end of the high-voltage part of the QRS complex in a patient with documented sustained ventricular tachycardia after myocardial infarction (Fig. 24-7). The duration of the total filtered QRS complex was 134 milliseconds; the voltage in the terminal 40 milliseconds of the filtered QRS complex was low (V, 3.57 μV). In Figure 24-8, the low-amplitude signal extended far into the ST segment. Using automated signal analysis (Fig. 24-9), the program identi-

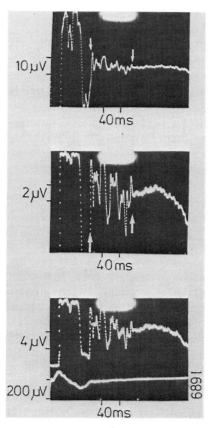

Figure 24-5. Visual identification of a late potential at different degree of amplification in a patient after myocardial infarction. (*Upper panel*) At low amplification (10 μV/division), a low-amplitude signal (between *arrows*) is apparent after the steep downstroke of the high-amplitude part of the QRS complex. (*Middle panel*) After rough visual identification of a late potential, a higher magnification is used (2 μV/division) to define more carefully the onset and end of the late potential. The median amplitude of the late potential is estimated from that part of the signal that has been identified at lower amplification (*upper panel*). *Onset and end of the late potential are marked by arrows.* (*Lower panel*) Dual-channel recording from the same patient, showing the late potential (*upper tracing*) at 4 μV/division and the unfiltered terminal part of the surface electrocardiogram to demonstrate that the late potential appears within the ST segment.

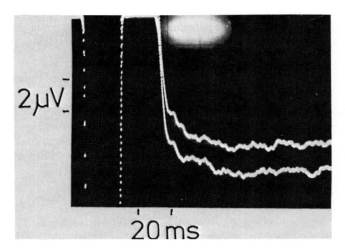

Figure 24-4. Averaged recording of 200 cardiac cycles, showing the terminal portion of the QRS complex and a part of the ST segment in a normal subject. There were no late potentials during the terminal portion of the QRS complex and ST segment. The rapid downstroke of the QRS complex showed a smooth transition to the ST segment. To demonstrate reproducibility, the signal was recorded twice.

fied true QRS, total QRS, and late potentials with a duration of 73 milliseconds.[43] Similarly, a terminal low-amplitude signal of 55 milliseconds duration in Figure 24-7 and of 138 milliseconds duration in Figure 24-8 were also automatically identified.

Figures 24-10 and 24-11A present the signal-averaged recordings from a normal subject and from a patient with documented ventricular tachycardia with time-domain and frequency-domain analysis. Spectral mapping from leads X, Y, and Z is also presented. Figure 24-11B and C present an example of FFTA and of spectral turbulence

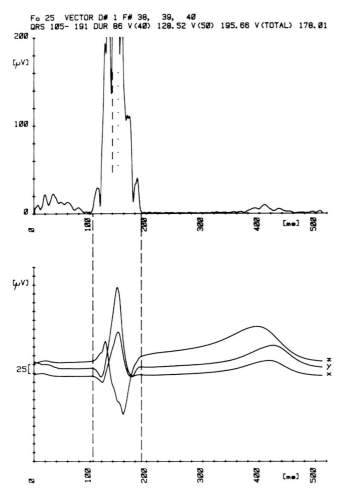

Figure 24-6. Original recording, using the system developed by M Simson[20] in a patient with normal left ventricular function and no history of ventricular tachycardia. (*Top*) Signal-averaged and filtered beats (high-pass cutoff, 25 Hz) from the body surface (leads *X, Y, Z*), showing the vector magnitude. There is no low-amplitude signal at the end of the filtered QRS complex. (*Bottom*) Signal-averaged leads from the body surface at a lower magnification.

analysis of patients with and without ventricular late potentials.

DEFINITION OF VENTRICULAR LATE POTENTIALS IN SURFACE ELECTROCARDIOGRAPHIC AVERAGED RECORDINGS

A schematic representation of the various parameters that are usually analyzed in time domain is presented in Figure 24-12.

Generally, ventricular late potentials may be defined

as low-amplitude fractionated activity appearing at the end of the QRS complex and extending into the ST segment. No universally accepted criteria for definition of late potentials exist.[22] One of the issues is whether only those potentials appearing after the end of the QRS complex should be considered or whether any low-amplitude activity, even when appearing before the end of the surface ECG, should be termed ventricular late potential. In this context, it is apparent that a definition of the end of QRS is not easy because it depends on the degree of amplification and filtering. We and others did not factor the end of the QRS complex in the surface ECG, whereas others consider low-amplitude activity to represent a late potential only if it extends for a certain period beyond the end of the QRS complex (see Fig. 24-8).[18, 20, 46, 61] The former approach is based on findings during intraoperative mapping that demonstrate that fractionated low-amplitude activity, mostly in the border zone of an aneurysm, started within the QRS complex. This is confirmed by Simson and co-workers.[62] Therefore, in some cases, the terminal part of the QRS complex in the standard surface ECG is already constituted by low-amplitude activity. That is the reason that after successful exclusion of an arrhythmogenic area after intraoperative mapping and application of semicircular subendocardial ventriculotomy or subendocardial resection these potentials may no longer be recorded at the end of the QRS complex, which, at the same time, becomes shorter.[33, 34, 63, 64]

Simson considered delayed depolarization (late potential) to be present when the vector magnitude during the last 40 milliseconds of the filtered and averaged QRS complex was less than 25 μV (see Figs. 24-7, 24-8, and 24-12).[20] This is a more objective approach because the measurement of amplitude in the terminal portion of the high-gain QRS complex is performed by computer software. It represents the most widely used criterion to identify late potentials. In addition, Simson defined as abnormal any prolongation of the highly amplified and filtered QRS complex of 120 or more milliseconds in the absence of classic bundle branch block (see Fig. 24-12).[20]

Denes and colleagues suggest identifying the point where the downstroke of the QRS complex falls short of 40 μV (see Fig. 24-12).[40] The distance between this point and the end of the high-gain filtered and averaged QRS complex represents the late potential, as estimated by the software developed by Simson.[20]

In addition to the original computer program designed by Simson, we developed an algorithm for automated recognition of the late potential (see Fig. 24-9) that recognizes the transition point between the true QRS complex and late potentials if they exists.[20, 43] This approach analyses both the voltage and the morphology of the terminal QRS complex.

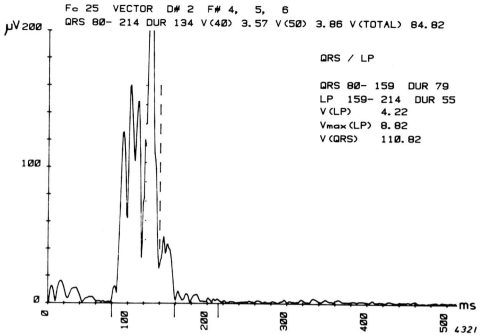

Figure 24-7. Signal-averaged and filtered recording of leads X, Y, Z (vector magnitude) in a patient with ventricular tachycardia. QRS duration was 134 milliseconds. The program automatically identified the end of the total QRS complex at 214 milliseconds on the horizontal axis. The amplitude in the terminal 40 milliseconds was low (V[40], 3.57 μV), which was automatically measured by the program described in the text.[20,43] Additionally, the onset of low-amplitude activity was automatically identified at 159 milliseconds on the horizontal axis by the automated recognition program. The latter program additionally measured the mean voltage of the late potential (V [LP]), the maximal voltage of the late potential (V_max), and the mean voltage of the true QRS complex (V [QRS]).

In comparison with visual analysis, the automated evaluation of the high-amplitude signal-averaged recordings is independent of the bias of observers, does not depend on personal experience, and is reproducible. Nevertheless, the results of automated analysis should not be accepted blindly, and some visual control may still be necessary.

In most studies, patients with bundle branch block were excluded because it was assumed that delayed conduction associated with these abnormalities would interfere with the detection of late potentials. Conduction defects are known to delay and fragment the ECG signal and may be expected to cause changes of the signal-averaged ECG that may mimic late potentials. Because patients with bifascicular block are at high risk of sudden cardiac death, it is in this group of patients that signal-averaging may be of special importance. Only a few studies have examined the effect of conduction defects on the signal-averaged ECG.[65–67] The new techniques of analysis using frequency domain signal-averaging (e.g., spectral turbulence analysis) may be of use for risk stratification of patients with bundle branch block, using noninvasive methods.

It is difficult to make firm recommendations of the criteria to use to diagnose late potentials in the presence of conduction defects. These criteria must be changed when cardiac conduction defects are seen. Therefore, a 12-lead ECG has to be performed at the time of the signal-averaged ECG recording to detect conduction defects.

Selection of Criteria of Late Potentials

The ultimate selection of criteria for clinical use is governed by the intended use of the diagnostic test and the patient population to which it is applied. For example, if signal-averaged ECGs were being used to screen a low-risk population, with subsequent assignment of late potential–positive patients to a treatment having some risk (i.e., antiarrhythmic drugs), the criteria could be adjusted to provide a high specificity. Alternatively, in a high-risk population (e.g., patients with recurrent syncope of unknown cause in the setting of structural heart disease) being considered for further diagnostic procedures (i.e., invasive electrophysiologic studies) before assignment to

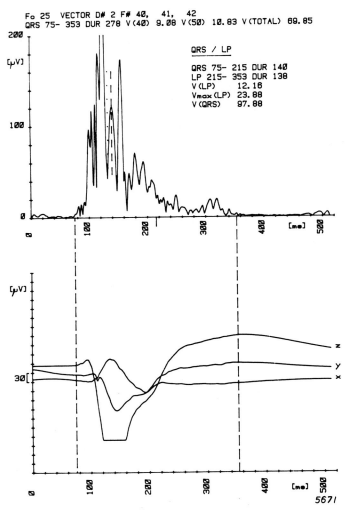

Figure 24-8. An example that shows the filtered-surface electrocardiogram. In this patient, who also has sustained ventricular tachycardia and left ventricular aneurysm, a very large low-amplitude tail was identified, extending into the ST segment. Some fluctuation was also seen in the surface electrocardiogram recordings.

treatment, these criteria could be adjusted to provide high sensitivity.

COMPARISON OF VARIOUS METHODS FOR RECORDING LATE POTENTIALS

To evaluate the methodological problems of noninvasive registration of ventricular late potentials, a comparative multicenter study was performed.[68] The results were obtained with (1) a Princeton 4202 signal-averager (methods A and B), (2) the Marquette MAC I signal-averager (method

C), and (3) the software-averaging system developed by Simson (method D) were compared in the same group of 109 patients (80 having coronary artery disease, 29 having dilated cardiomyopathy).[16,18,20,21,61] In each patient, all registrations were done within 2 hours. The main difference between methods A and B is that in method A, only low-amplitude signals appearing *after* the end of the QRS complex in the standard surface leads were evaluated.

Ventricular late potentials were recorded in 12% of patients using method A, in 21% using method B, in 14% using method C, and in 20% using method D. Corresponding positive results were obtained in 6% and corresponding negative results in 69%. Differences in comparison with the other three methods were seen 12 times for method D, five times for method B, and two times for method A. In 10% of the patients, two methods showed

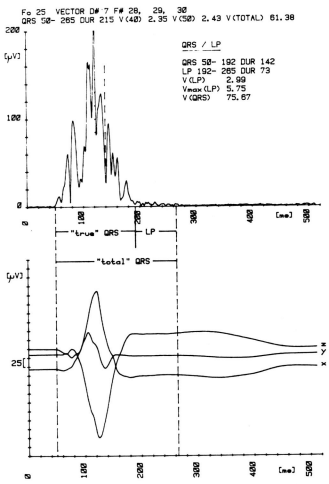

Figure 24-9. Definition of "true" QRS, "total" QRS, and "late potential," as used for automated identification of late potentials with the software program designed by Karbenn and colleagues.[43]

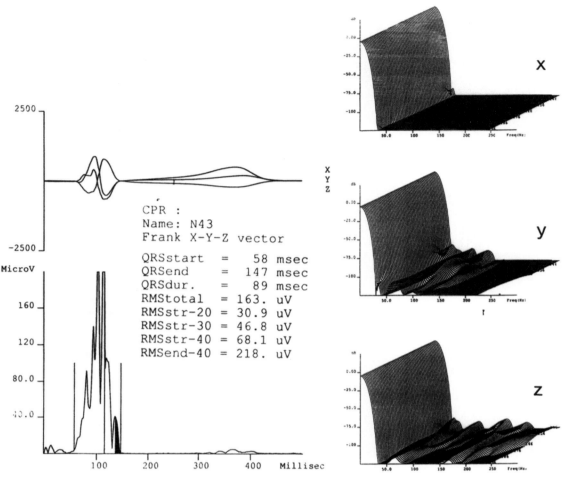

Figure 24-10. The signal-averaged electrocardiogram from a patient without late potentials. The QRS duration is 89 milliseconds, the root mean square of the voltage in the last 40 milliseconds is 218 μV. There is abrupt termination of the QRS-complex. In the *right panel*, spectral mappings of the leads *x*, *y*, and *z* are presented. The "undulations" observable in leads Y and Z during the ST segment correspond to registered noise. For further explanation, see text; for comparison with a patient with late potentials, see Figure 24-11.

the same results. Despite these differences between the various methods, detailed analysis of the tracings of patients who had controversial results revealed that the differences (mainly using methods A, B, and C) were due to differences in visual interpretation. Methods that did not factor the QRS width (methods B and D) showed a greater number of positive results than the methods that did (methods A and C). Further prospective studies must show whether delayed depolarizations occurring in the terminal portion of the QRS complex or only those occurring after the end of the QRS complex are of prognostic significance.

We performed a comparative study between the Arrhythmia Research Technology (ART) signal-averager

(based on Simson's algorithm)[20] and the LP-3000 signal-averager from Fidelity Medicals. Thirty-seven patients were included in the study (19 patients had documented sustained ventricular tachyarrhythmias). With both signal-averagers, late potentials were considered to be present when the root mean square (RMS) of the voltage during the last 40 milliseconds of the averaged and filtered QRS (V40) was less than 25 μV using the same filtering, number of averaging cycles, and electrode position in a randomized sequence. Nonsignificant differences were observed in the QRS duration (121 ± 32 milliseconds versus 124 ± 30 milliseconds); in the time of QRS with a voltage below 40 μV (34 ± 20 milliseconds versus 33 ± 19 milliseconds); or in the V40 (41 ± 41 μV versus 41 ± 31 μV). With

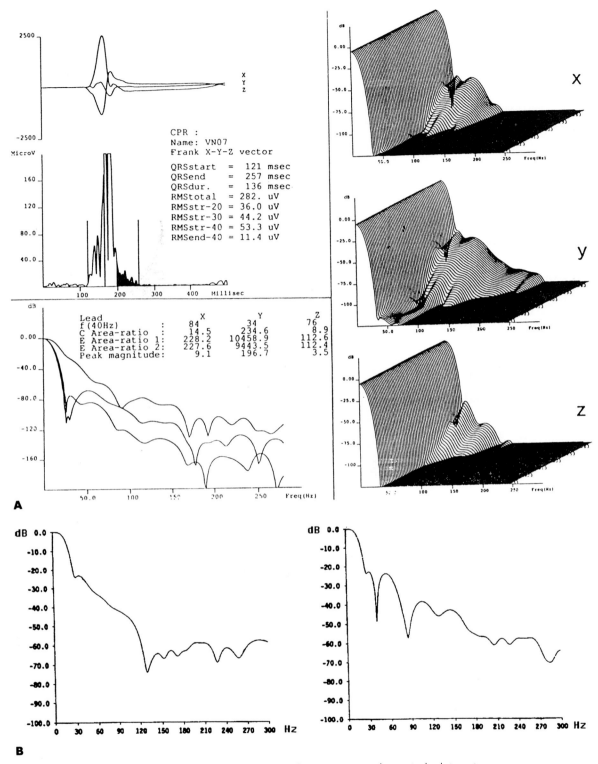

Figure 24-11. (**A**) Signal-averaged electrocardiogram from a patient with ventricular late potentials. The QRS duration was 136 milliseconds and the root mean square of the voltage during the last 40 milliseconds was 11.4 μV. (**B**) The frequency contents of leads *X*, *Y*, and *Z* are presented with Cain algorithm (*C*) and with El-Sherif (*E*) algorithms (left side, *bottom*). (*continued*)

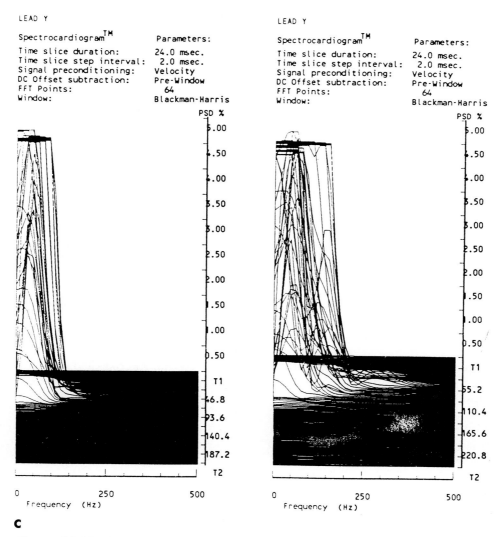

C

Figure 24-11. *(continued)* (**C**) Spectral mappings of the frequency content of leads *X*, *Y* and *Z* are presented on the right side of the figure. In the FFT curve, multiple significant frequency peaks in a range of 30 to 150 Hz are visible at a high level of amplitude (> −50 dB) (**B**). These high-frequency components of the FFT curve represent the ventricular late potentials. Spectral turbulence analysis (STA) of the signal-averaged electrocardiogram of a 62-year-old female patient after myocardial infarction with inducible sustained ventricular tachycardia. All FFT curves of the shifting window are plotted in a three-dimensional graph, with the frequency (Hz) on the x axis, the power spectrum density (%) on the y axis, and the time (ms) on the z axis (DELMAR/Avionics, 850). Markedly inhomogenous FFT spectra inside the QRS complex are visible.

the ART signal-averager and the Fidelity Medicals signal-averager, 11 and 12 patients (respectively) of the 19 patients with documented ventricular tachyarrhythmias had late potentials. In addition, the ART signal-averager and the Hipec Analyzer HA-100 were compared based on the approach by Abboud and colleagues.[69] Ten patients with documented ventricular tachycardia were included. The second system used a filter setting of 30 to 250 Hz, a cross-correlation function for triggering, and allowed analysis of

different windows of the ST segment. With both systems, the same leads and definitions of late potentials were used (V40 less than 25 μV). Different windows of 75, 100, 125, and 150 milliseconds duration after the visual end of the QRS were analyzed for their noise content. The window of analysis influenced the results because it yielded different noise levels, which were used to define the end of QRS. The maximal concordance of the presence or absence of late potentials with both systems was found with the use of

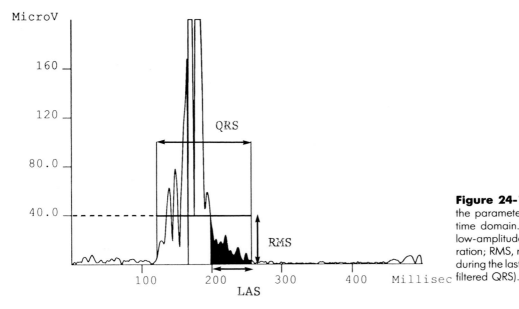

Figure 24-12. Schematic presentation of the parameters that are usually analyzed in time domain. (LAS, duration of the terminal low-amplitude [<40 µV] signal. QRS, QRS duration; RMS, root mean square of the voltage during the last 40 milliseconds of the averaged filtered QRS).

a window of 150 milliseconds (Martínez-Rubio, unpublished data.

Thus, different recording systems and interpretation may lead to different results. The differences between groups may be explained by the use of different leads, amplification, number of averaged cycles, filter setting, stability of trigger point, noise level, window of analysis, and definitions of late potentials. Thus, there is an urgent need for standardization to allow reliable comparison between different studies and different methods of analysis.[22]

DURATION OF LATE POTENTIALS

In early reports, we demonstrated that the duration of late potentials may vary between 50 milliseconds and 180 milliseconds.[18,46,70] The median duration of late potentials in patients with one (40 milliseconds) or more than one episode of ventricular tachycardia (35 milliseconds) was longer than in those with previous ventricular fibrillation (16 milliseconds). Kertes and colleagues report a mean value for the duration of late potentials of 35 milliseconds (range, 15 to 70 milliseconds) in 12 of 15 patients having ventricular tachycardia.[71] Gomes and colleagues found "very late" potentials (ending 69 ± 23 milliseconds after the end of the QRS complex) in 35% of the patients having ventricular tachycardia after myocardial infarction.[72]

The factors that govern the duration of late potentials have not been studied sufficiently. It may depend on heart rate and the conduction velocity and the size of a potential reentrant circuit.

The effect of spontaneous or pacing-induced changes in ventricular rate on ventricular late potentials needs

further evaluation. Studies by El-Sherif and colleagues show that conduction in a reentrant pathway is markedly rate-dependent.[3,5] Berbari and colleagues, in preliminary experimental studies, reported that the duration of fractionated activity increased with increasing rates of atrial pacing.[13] In a subsequent preliminary clinical report, however, the same authors suggest that an increase in atrial rate does not exert any influence on the duration of a late potential, whereas the high-frequency components of the signal change.[73] In contrast, Landreneau and associates reported a decrease in duration of late potentials in dogs having 2- to 10-day-old myocardial infarction during atrial pacing.[74] This response was attributed to the creation of block in the region of slow conduction. This was the opposite of ventricular pacing, which caused a significant increase in the duration of late potentials when compared with sinus rhythm.[74] Stimulation of the ventricles during the vulnerable period, using either single pulses or a train, showed marked fragmentation in electrograms recorded within 2 mm of the stimulation site. With stimulus intensities that evoked multiple ventricular extrasystoles or ventricular fibrillation, the fragmented ventricular activity became continuous and bridged the diastolic interval between successive ectopic beats.[75]

A short duration of a late potential may be due to a small area with slow fractionated conduction or to more rapid conduction in a larger area. Because the wavefront of excitation probably travels along multiple pathways and in various directions, no calculations of conduction velocity or of wave length can be performed. In experimental studies, the amplitude and duration of electrograms in dogs with inducible ventricular fibrillation were more normal than those recorded in animals with inducible ventricular tachycardia, thus exhibiting an inverse relation between cycle length of ventricular tachycardia and duration of late potentials.[25] A similar trend was also demonstrated in patients with sustained ventricular tachycardia.[70, 76]

This inverse relation between the rate of ventricular tachycardia and the duration of late potentials points to one of the limitations of this technique.[76] Particularly in those patients at highest risk of sudden cardiac death (i.e., those with a propensity to rapid rates of ventricular tachycardia), ventricular late potentials may be too short to be detected because they may not extend beyond the end of the QRS complex on the body surface. Therefore, techniques that exert a stress—causing a prolongation and thus appearance of hidden late potentials—would be desirable.

LATE POTENTIALS IN PATIENTS WITH VENTRICULAR TACHYCARDIA

Ventricular late potentials have rarely been detected in subjects with normal ventricular function.[16, 18, 20, 21, 46, 61, 69, 71, 77, 78] This is in contrast to patients with previously documented sustained ventricular tachycardia or fibrillation (outside the acute phase of myocardial infarction), in whom there is a high incidence of ventricular late potentials.[18, 20, 21, 46, 71, 76, 79–81] We previously reported that 45 out of 63 patients (71%) having documented sustained ventricular tachycardia or fibrillation had ventricular late potentials of any duration. The proportion of patients with late potentials increased to 37 of 47 patients (79%) when only patients with coronary artery disease were considered.[46] Simson reports that patients with sustained ventricular tachycardia had a low-amplitude signal in the last 40 milliseconds of the filtered QRS complex that was not detectable in the filtered output from patients without ventricular tachycardia.[20] The V40 discriminated well between patients with and those without ventricular tachycardia. Patients with ventricular tachycardia had 15 ± 14.4 μV of high-frequency signal in this segment; in contrast, patients without ventricular tachycardia had 74 ± 77.7 μV ($p < .0001$). Twenty-five microvolts was the best threshold to discriminate between patients with and those without ventricular tachycardia.[20] In only three of 39 patients (8%) with ventricular tachycardia, it exceeded 25 μV. The filtered QRS voltage tended to be lower in patients with ventricular tachycardia than in those without (103 ± 30 versus 127 ± 43 μV; nonsignificant). The QRS duration was longer in patients with ventricular tachycardia (139 ± 26 versus 95 ± 10 milliseconds; $p < .0001$). Therefore, Simson suggests as a criterion for late potentials either (1) a low-amplitude signal in the terminal 40 milliseconds below 25 μV, or (2) a QRS duration of 120 or more

milliseconds.[20] Freedman and colleagues, using a similar methodology, found late potentials in 33 of 53 patients (62%) having ventricular tachycardia.[79] Kanovsky and colleagues studied 174 patients after myocardial infarction.[81] Eighty-nine of these patients had recurrent sustained ventricular tachycardia. By multivariate logistic regression analysis, the signal-averaged ECG, peak premature ventricular contractions of more than 100 per hour, and the presence of a left ventricular aneurysm were found to be independently significant. Patients with nonsustained ventricular tachycardia, in whom sustained ventricular tachycardia can be induced by programmed ventricular stimulation, also have a significantly higher incidence of late potentials (67%) than patients without inducible sustained ventricular tachycardia (25%).[82] The filtered QRS duration was also longer (127 versus 100 milliseconds).[82] Similar to patients with ventricular tachycardia after myocardial infarction, patients with congestive cardiomyopathy and a history of sustained ventricular tachycardia had a significantly greater incidence of late potentials and a longer QRS duration than those without ventricular tachycardia.[83, 84]

Zimmermann and colleagues compared the high-resolution ECG on a beat-to-beat basis and signal-averaging in 31 normal subjects, 28 patients with coronary artery disease without ventricular tachycardia, and 21 patients with coronary artery disease and documented ventricular tachycardia.[85] They found concordant results using both techniques in 46 of 49 patients (94%, 32 positive and 14 negative results).

Using FFTA, patients with sustained ventricular tachycardia have a higher frequency content in their terminal QRS complex when compared with normal patients.[44, 57, 58] Cain and colleagues demonstrated an increase in the amplitude of high-frequency components in the terminal QRS in 88% of patients with sustained ventricular tachycardia, in contrast to 15% in patients without ventricular tachycardia.[44] In a subsequent report, these authors studied 87 patients (23 patients with and 53 patients without ventricular tachycardia after myocardial infarction in addition to 11 normal subjects) in whom the terminal 40 milliseconds of the QRS complex and the ST segment were analyzed as a single unit to enhance the frequency resolution.[57] The terminal QRS and ST segment from patients with sustained ventricular tachycardia contained 10- to 100-fold greater amplitudes of components in the 20- to 50-Hz range, compared with corresponding electrocardiographic segments in patients without sustained ventricular tachycardia. There were no significant differences in the peak frequencies among the patient groups. The relative contribution of the magnitudes of these peak frequencies to the overall magnitude of the spectral plot differed significantly, however. No frequencies above 50 Hz contributed substantially to the energy spectra of the terminal QRS and ST segments in any group. Haberl and colleagues found an increased spectral area in the range of 60 to 120 Hz and spectral peaks of more than 10 dB in 21 of 30 patients with ventricular tachycardia.[86] In contrast, of 15 patients without ventricular tachycardia, only one demonstrated abnormal frequency spectra; none of 15 healthy subjects manifested abnormal findings. The choice of an appropriate ST segment was crucial; if the segment was too long in comparison with the duration of late potentials and if it extended too far into the QRS complex, FFTA yielded random results.

In another report, Haberl and colleagues presented the results of spectral analysis.[59] They studied 32 patients having sustained ventricular tachycardia after myocardial infarction in addition to 19 patients after myocardial infarction without ventricular tachycardia and 17 healthy subjects. A total of 18 patients had bundle branch block. Twenty-four of 32 patients after myocardial infarction with ventricular tachycardia had a factor of normality below 30%, whereas this parameter was below 30% in only two of 19 postmyocardial infarction patients without ventricular arrhythmias and in only one of 17 healthy subjects. The differences between the first group and the last two groups were highly significant ($p < .001$). Comparison with the method by Simson[20] was made only in those patients who had no bundle branch block. This comparison showed that 13 of 19 patients (68%) with ventricular tachycardia after myocardial infarction had a factor of normality below 30% (abnormal), whereas using Simson's method (high-pass filter of 25 Hz, QRS duration more than 120 milliseconds, or RMS voltage less than 25 μV), 10 of 19 patients (53%) were classified as abnormal. In the remaining 13 patients with bundle branch block, the factor of normality was below 30% in 11 patients. In those 19 patients with a previous myocardial infarction without a history of ventricular tachycardia, only two of 15 patients without bundle branch block (13%) had a factor of normality below 30%, whereas Simson's approach classified five of these patients (33%) as abnormal. In 17 healthy subjects, one patient had bundle branch block. In the remaining 16, one patient (6%) had a factor of normality below 30%, whereas Simson's method classified three of 16 subjects (19%) as abnormal.

It remains unclear whether FFTA is superior to signal-averaging in the time domain. To address this issue, some preliminary studies were performed.[86–92] Both methods were assessed in 54 subjects (26 patients with sustained ventricular tachycardia, 18 control patients with organic heart disease but without sustained ventricular tachycardia and 10 normal volunteers).[87] Time-domain analysis was performed with high-pass filtering of 25, 40, and 80 Hz and low-pass filtering of 250 Hz. Frequency-domain analysis was performed on the terminal 40 milliseconds of the QRS complex, either alone or with 216 or 150 milliseconds of the ST segment. Absolute summed energies of discrete frequency bands and band-energy ratios were calculated. Frequency-domain analysis was not considered as an improvement over time-domain analysis in differentiating patients with ventricular tachycardia from those without; Worley and colleagues presented similar results.[88] The major problem of the FFTA technique detected by both groups was the variation of results, depending on time-varying frequency spectra.[87,88] In contrast, Haberl and colleagues claimed superiority of frequency-domain analysis over time-domain analysis.[86] This different estimation of the value of these two methods largely was due to exclusion of patients with bundle branch block from time-domain analysis; those patients underwent frequency-domain analysis. Thus, these differences may be due to different methodology and may need further evaluation. Malik and associates, Kulakowski and coworkers, and Odemuyiwa and colleagues examined the reproducibility of frequency- versus time-domain analysis of signal-averaged ECG, the predictive accuracy in identification of patients with ventricular tachycardia, and the detection of patients at risk of arrhythmic events.[90–92] The results of their studies provide the following conclusions: (1) compared with different methods of frequency-domain analysis, time-domain analysis had the highest reproducibility of the results; (2) frequency-domain analysis and spectral temporal mapping did not increase the sensitivity of the signal-averaged ECG in identification of patients with ventricular tachycardia nor detection of arrhythmic events in postinfarction patients.

DIFFERENCES BETWEEN PATIENTS WITH VENTRICULAR TACHYCARDIA VERSUS VENTRICULAR FIBRILLATION

The type of documented ventricular tachyarrhythmia has some influence on the incidence and duration of ventricular late potentials. Among patients with chronic recurrent sustained ventricular tachycardia, 46 of 62 patients (74%) had late potentials, which was almost similar to the percentage of patients with only one documented episode of ventricular tachycardia (21 of 26 patients; 81%). In contrast, patients with a history of ventricular fibrillation outside acute myocardial infarction with no previous documentation of sustained ventricular tachycardia had late potentials in only eight of 15 patients (53%), in six of 27 patients (22%), and in one of 14 patients (7%).[70,71,79] Vaitkus and coworkers report differences in the electrophysiologic substrate of those patients with coronary artery disease presenting with hemodynamically well-tolerated ventricular tachycardia and those presenting with cardiac arrest (ventricular fibrillation).[93] Longer mean–filtered QRS duration and lower RMS of the voltage uring the last 40 milliseconds were found in patients with entricular tachycardia ($p < .01$). In addition, 63% of patients with ventricular fibrillation and 87% of patients with entricular tachycardia presented abnormal signal-averaged ECGs ($p = .001$). Patients with ventricular tachycardia had more extensive endocardial substrate than patients with ventricular fibrillation, which translates into greater and more frequent signal-averaged ECG abnormalities. Denniss and colleagues detected late potentials in only 32% of patients with previous ventricular fibrillation, in 58% of those with sustained ventricular tachycardia with rates greater than 270 beats per minute, and in 95% of those with rates of 270 beats per minute or less.[94] Late potentials were significantly more frequent in those patients in whom the cycle length of induced ventricular tachycardia was greater than 250 milliseconds (90%), compared with those with cycle lengths less than 250 milliseconds (40%).[79] A similar relation was reported by Spielman and coworkers and Martínez-Rubio and colleagues.[76, 95] Thus, patients with inducible ventricular fibrillation or with inducible rapid ventricular tachycardia have less extensive areas of slow conduction.

During programmed ventricular stimulation, longer coupling intervals are sufficient for the induction of ventricular tachycardia, compared with those necessary for the induction of ventricular fibrillation.[76, 96] This suggests a greater propensity of the arrhythmogenic substrate to reentry in cases of inducible ventricular tachycardia than in cases of ventricular fibrillation. Furthermore, with the use of faster drive-cycle lengths and shorter coupling intervals, more dispersion of regional activation and of refractoriness may be achieved, facilitating the induction of reentrant tachycardias. These data suggest that the ease of induction of ventricular tachycardia versus fibrillation represents the inherent properties of the reentrant circuit. Kus and associates demonstrated the correlation between dispersion of ventricular refractoriness and the ability to induce ventricular tachycardia in patients with prior myocardial infarction.[97] Thus, if ventricular late potentials indicate the degree of preexisting conduction impairment, they should correlate to the ease of induction of ventricular tachyarrhythmias. Compared with patients with inducible ventricular fibrillation, patients with inducible sustained ventricular tachycardia had longer QRS duration, longer terminal low-amplitude signals, and lower RMS of the voltage during the last 40 milliseconds.[76] The incidence of ventricular late potentials was higher in patients with inducible ventricular tachycardia than in patients with inducible ventricular fibrillation ($p < .007$).[76] In addition, for arrhythmia induction, significantly shorter coupling intervals were necessary in those patients without late potentials than those with.[76]

LATE POTENTIALS IN PATIENTS WITH SYNCOPE

Syncope may result from many conditions and has a variable prognosis.[98, 99] Analysis of the high-frequency components of the terminal QRS complex using signal-averaged electrocardiography is a means to identify patients with a propensity to ventricular tachycardia after myocardial infarction, especially in the presence of a left ventricular aneurysm and in patients with arrhythmogenic right ventricular disease.[6, 100–102] Therefore, signal-averaging also may be useful to identify those patients with recurrent syncope in whom a ventricular tachyarrhythmia may be the underlying mechanism.

Gang and colleagues assessed the usefulness of signal-averaging for detecting hitherto undocumented ventricular tachycardia in 24 patients with unexplained syncope.[101] Sustained ventricular tachycardia was documented in nine patients (eight with inducible ventricular tachycardia and one with a spontaneous episode). The signal-averaged ECG contained late potentials and a filtered QRS complex longer than 120 milliseconds in eight of these nine patients (sensitivity, 89%). None of the remaining 15 patients had these electrocardiographic abnormalities.

We studied 40 patients (mean age, 54 years) with syncope of unknown origin even after thorough medical and neurologic evaluation.[100] Twenty-two patients had late potentials (mean duration, 34 ± 10.2 milliseconds). In 18 of these 22 patients with late potentials, sustained ventricular tachycardia or fibrillation was inducible, whereas only eight of 18 patients without late potentials had inducible sustained ventricular tachycardia ($p < .05$).

A larger group of 150 consecutive patients presenting with syncope was studied by Kuchar and colleagues.[102] Twenty-nine patients had late potentials, 107 had a normal signal-averaged ECG, and 14 patients had bundle branch block on the 12-lead ECG. The signal-averaged ECG (1) identified late potentials in 16 of 22 patients having ventricular tachycardia, (2) was normal in 101 of 114 patients in whom syncope was attributed to causes other than ventricular tachycardia or remained unexplained (sensitivity, 73%; specificity, 89%; predictive accuracy, 54%). Absence of late potentials identified a group of patients with a low incidence of ventricular tachycardia. During follow-up of 1 to 20 months (mean, 11 months), 15 patients (10%) died, six of whom died suddenly. There was no significant difference in survival or recurrence of syncope between patients with or without late potentials.

These results suggest that signal-averaging of the surface ECG may be a noninvasive test for detecting a high-risk subset of patients prone to lethal tachyarrhythmias. Further studies are needed, however.

LATE POTENTIALS AND LEFT VENTRICULAR FUNCTION

In patients with documented ventricular tachycardia, the highest incidence of late potentials has been found in those with left ventricular aneurysms due to coronary artery disease. Similarly, there is a close correlation between the detection of late potentials and left ventricular function in patients without previously documented ventricular tachycardia or fibrillation (Table 24-2).[46] Conversely, the degree and extent of coronary artery involvement did not influence the prevalence of late potentials in patients with ventricular tachycardia or fibrillation, unless indirectly by causing left ventricular contraction abnormalities.

These correlations between the presence of late potentials and left ventricular function were confirmed in a larger group of 404 prospectively studied patients without documented complex ventricular arrhythmias (Fig. 24-13). In this group, late potentials of long duration (40 or more milliseconds) were almost exclusively found in patients with hypokinesia, akinesia, or aneurysms. Moreover, about 20% of late potentials appeared in patients with left ventricles that seemed angiographically normal (see Fig. 24-13). Despite normal findings during left ventricular angiography, many of these patients were not considered to have true normal left ventricular function. Most of them complained of atypical angina pectoris; a great variety of abnormal findings existed such as ST-segment depression during exercise despite normal coronary arteries, an abnormal increase in pulmonary artery pressure during exercise, and perfusion defects during thallium scintigraphy.

That late potentials are found more frequently in patients with regional or diffuse ventricular contraction abnormalities suggests that the anatomic substrate for late potentials is diseased tissue. A transmural infarction may show no abnormal activation pattern because such tissue is electrically silent. In contrast, tissue immediately adjacent to the infarction contains viable myocardium interspersed with fibrotic tissue.[103] Such tissue may result in fragmentation of the propagating electromotive surface, with the consequent development of high-frequency components.[24, 103, 104] The border zone of old myocardial infarcts was identified as the site of origin for delayed ventricular potentials by comparing precordial recordings using the averaging technique and intraoperative mapping techniques.[62] Because late potentials are abolished by subendocardial partial or complete encircling ventriculotomy in patients with documented ventricular tachycardia, it is probable that they are related to the propensity to ventricular tachycardia and that they probably originate in the border zone between myocardial scars and normal myocardium (Fig. 24-14).[34, 63, 64, 105]

LATE POTENTIALS AND SPONTANEOUS VENTRICULAR ARRHYTHMIAS DURING HOLTER-MONITOR RECORDING

In 170 patients, the results of 24-hour long-term electrocardiographic recordings and of signal-averaging were compared (Fig. 24-15). Although there was a significant increase in the prevalence of late potentials with increasing numbers of ventricular extrasystoles, it was also apparent that late potentials of long duration (40 or more milliseconds) were not significantly correlated to spontaneous arrhythmias. They occurred in patients with either no extrasystoles or with less than 30 per hour, as they did in those with more frequent extrasystoles or with couplets or salvoes. Thus, spontaneous ventricular extrasystoles were independent of the presence or absence of fractionated activity (Breithardt and coworkers, unpublished data).

Preliminary data suggest that heart rate variability measured in the time and frequency domains is a powerful noninvasive marker of risk of developing spontaneous arrhythmic events (sustained ventricular tachyarrhythmias or sudden cardiac death) after myocardial infarction.[106] In combination with parameters from the signal-averaged ECG, it was even possible to improve the predictive power of risk stratification of these patients.

LATE POTENTIALS AND INDUCIBILITY OF VENTRICULAR TACHYARRHYTHMIAS

To get more insight into the mechanisms and potential prognostic value of late potentials, 110 male patients without previously documented ventricular tachycardia or

TABLE 24-2. Correlation Between Detection of Late Potentials and Angiograpic Findings

	Patients Without VT/VF	Patients With VT/VF
Normal subjects	0/12	
Normal coronary arteries, normal LV	0/15	1/3
CAD, normal LV	3/17	
COCM	3/9	4/7
Diffuse hypokinesia, CAD	3/15	5/8
Regional hypokinesia, CAD	8/36	3/3
Akinesia, CAD	14/26	4/6
Aneurysm, CAD	18/43	25/30
Various findings		3/6
Mean potential duration (msec)	31 ± 15.3	51 ± 31.5

VT, ventricular tachycardia; VF, ventricular fibrillation; LV, left ventricle. CAD, coronary artery disease; COCM, congestive cardiomyopathy.

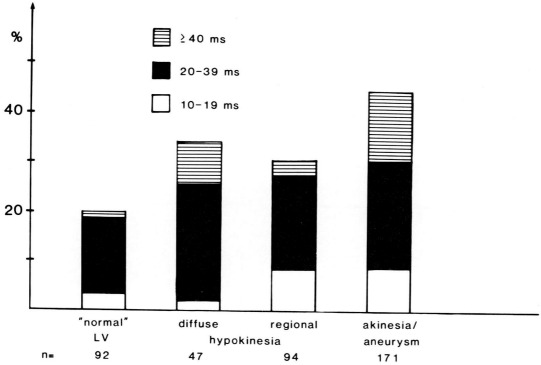

Figure 24-13. Correlation between the presence and duration of late potentials and various types of left ventricular contraction abnormalities, as estimated by left ventricular angiography.

fibrillation and without a history of resuscitation or syncope were studied.[107] In addition to recording late potentials, an electrophysiologic study was performed, using single and double ventricular extrastimuli during sinus rhythm and paced ventricular rhythms at rates of 120, 140, 160, and 180 beats per minute. Because the patients studied did not have documented ventricular tachycardia, programmed ventricular stimulation was stopped as soon as nonsustained or sustained ventricular tachycardia (defined as four or more consecutive ventricular beats) was induced. Based on the results of a previous study, this response was considered abnormal.[108] There was a significant correlation between the absence of ventricular late potentials and programmed ventricular stimulation.[107] In 70 patients in whom no late potentials were detected on the body surface, four or more ventricular echo beats were induced less frequently than in those patients with late potentials. The incidence of abnormal responses increased in relation to the duration of late potentials (chi square, 20.97; $p < .001$). Of note, 11 of 12 patients (92%) with late potentials of duration of 40 or more milliseconds had an abnormal finding. Similar correlations between the results of programmed ventricular stimulation and FFTA have been reported by Lindsay and colleagues.[109]

Our group demonstrated that the combined use of the signal-averaged ECG and programmed ventricular stimulation helps to identify those at risk of ventricular

tachycardia and sudden death in patients with coronary artery disease without a history of ventricular tachycardia or fibrillation.[110] Winters and colleagues suggest using signal-averaging to select patients with myocardial infarction who have left ventricular dysfunction and complex ventricular ectopy for programmed ventricular stimulation.[111] They found late potentials are stronger predictors of ventricular tachycardia than left ventricular ejection fraction. Although late potentials were moderately specific (50%), they were sensitive (88%) in detecting patients with inducible ventricular tachycardia. Pagé and colleagues found signal-averaging to be superior to left ventricular ejection fraction in predicting inducible ventricular tachycardia.[112] Those patients with noninducible sustained ventricular tachycardia had a low risk for suffering ventricular tachycardia or sudden death. Fananapazir and colleagues report that the signal-averaged ECG is also useful to predict inducibility of ventricular tachycardia in patients with hypertrophic cardiomyopathy.[113]

Late potentials can therefore be considered as indicators of increased ventricular vulnerability. Patients with late potentials had more vulnerable myocardium than did those without late potentials. Statistical analyses revealed left ventricular function as the predominant factor, with late potentials and the induced ventricular responses being highly significantly correlated with it.[107] Late potentials and induced ventricular responses were less closely asso-

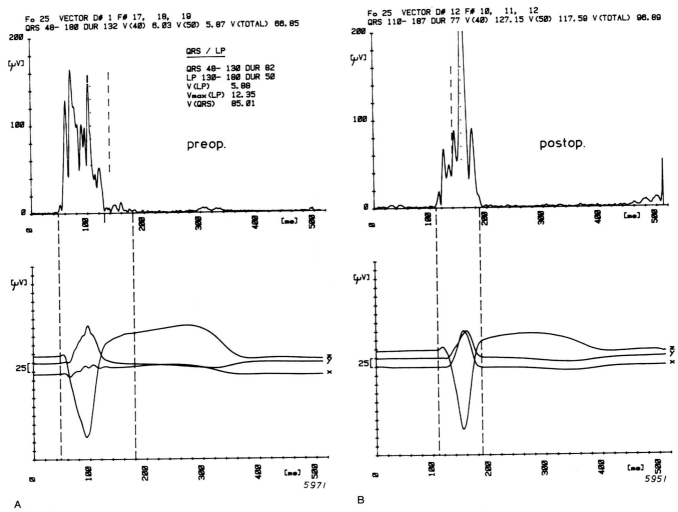

Figure 24-14. Preoperative (**A**) and postoperative (**B**) signal-averaged recording in a patient with recurrent sustained ventricular tachycardia. Before surgery (**A**), the amplitude in the terminal 40 milliseconds of the filtered (total) QRS complex was low (V [40], 6.03 μV); a late potential of 50-milliseconds duration was automatically identified. After map-guided surgery (**B**), the amplitude in the terminal 40 milliseconds of the QRS complex was normal (V [40], 127.15 μV); there was no longer any low-amplitude tail at the end of QRS. Postoperatively, the patient was free of inducible and spontaneous ventricular tachycardia.

ciated. Late potentials of 40 milliseconds duration or more predicted the inducibility of nonsustained or sustained ventricular tachycardia with high sensitivity. Nevertheless, even in the absence of late potentials, ventricular tachycardia was induced in 9% of patients.[107] This apparent discrepancy may be explained in different ways. First, induced ventricular tachycardia may not be related to regional slow conduction but to some other mechanism such as triggered automaticity.[114,115] Although this cannot be excluded, another explanation seems more likely. Depending on the arrival of excitation, a given area of slow conduction may still be activated so early that it is completely hidden within the QRS complex (Fig. 24-16).[62] In

these cases, slow conduction may only extend far enough into diastole if some stress such as premature stimulation is exerted. In other patients, abnormal ventricular responses were not inducible despite the presence of late potentials. This may be due to the fact that only one site of stimulation was used. Using more than one site or more than two premature stimuli may increase the number of abnormal findings. An extensive stimulation protocol, using five different cycle lengths of basic rhythm, was applied. It is also conceivable that in these patients, the presence of late potentials is an unspecific finding related to the presence of scarred tissue that has no propensity to ventricular tachycardia.

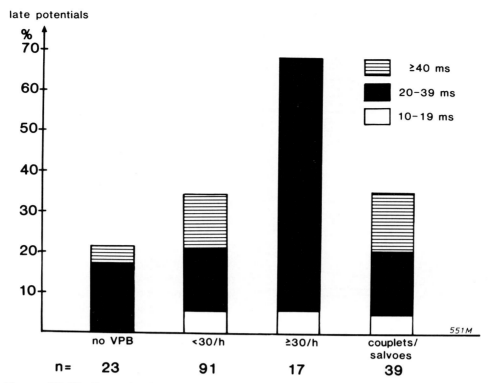

Figure 24-15. Twenty-four-hour long-term electrocardiographic findings correlated to the results of signal averaging in 170 patients without documented ventricular tachycardia or fibrillation who were studied prospectively. The prevalence of late potentials and their duration are shown.

SENSITIVITY AND SPECIFICITY OF LATE POTENTIALS

Not all patients with documented ventricular tachycardia or fibrillation have late potentials detectable in their body surface recordings. One explanation may be that their ventricular tachycardia is not of the reentry type but instead may be due to some form of triggered automaticity. In the latter case, no regional slow conduction can be anticipated. How frequently this is the case has not been determined. There are several other reasons why late potentials may not be detectable on the body surface.

First, the amount of tissue with regional slow conduction and thus late activation may be too small. We compared the results of signal-averaging and of intraoperative endocardial mapping.[116,117] The extent of regional slow conduction during intraoperative mapping (i.e., the duration of local activation) did not correlate to the duration of late potentials on the body surface. The greater the number of sites with abnormal slow activation during endocardial mapping, however, the greater the chance of recording ventricular late potentials on the body surface. Thus, a given amount of abnormal slow activation probably was necessary to be detected from the body surface.

Second, fragmented activation of an area of the myocardium may occur so early that it takes place at the time of activation of the remaining normal myocardium. Therefore, its activity is hidden within the QRS complex.[62] The finding that various left ventricular sites are activated at different times may also be important.[70] The infero-posterobasal areas of the left ventricle are activated later than the other areas. Thus, an electrogram of a given duration from an inferoposterobasal area may clearly extend beyond the QRS complex because this area is activated later than (for instance) the anterior wall of the left ventricle.

Third, the signals may be too short and may occur immediately at the end of QRS at a time when filter-ringing occurs. This may be a problem if filters with steep characteristics are used. As a solution to this problem, Simson suggests analyzing the QRS complex retrogradely, starting within the ST segment.[20] To avoid filter-ringing, we used single-pole filters with flat characteristics in our initial system, which showed a negligible degree of filter-ringing.[18]

Fourth, unstable triggering of the QRS complex (jitter) may prevent the recording of late potentials, which may be cancelled by the always changing timing in rela-

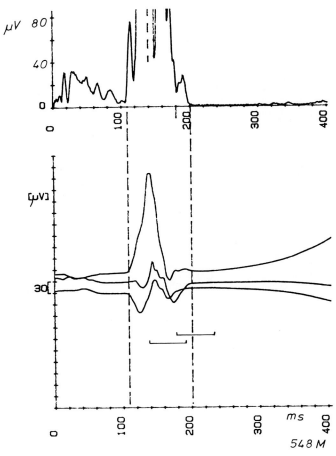

Figure 24-16. Signal-averaged recording, with schematic representation of fragmented low-amplitude activity (*horizontal bars*) that starts at different times during ventricular excitation. A signal from an area, that is activated early may be hidden within the QRS complex.

tion to the trigger point. This seems to be of minor importance because the jitter for triggering is relative small in available systems. There may be beat-to-beat variations in the configuration and timing of late potentials, however, which may lead to cancellation during the averaging process. This may cause some attenuation in the high-frequency components, thus acting as a low-pass filter.

Fifth, the level of baseline noise originating from muscular activity or from interference of alternating current may hide ventricular late potentials if it is too high.[47]

The signal-averaged ECG proved to be specific because it did not detect late ventricular activity in patients in whom there was no delayed activity during intraoperative mapping.[118] It may miss delayed activity on the body surface in patients in whom it can be demonstrated by epicardial mapping. These studies show that the mean number of epicardial sites with a delayed activity is greater in patients with concordant results than in patients with

discordant results. Total ventricular activation time in the concordant groups with delayed activity was 199 ± 16 milliseconds at mapping and 167 ± 17 milliseconds on the signal-averaged ECG.[118]

Although comparison of signal-averaging of the ECG with intraoperative or catheter mapping shows the specificity of the signal-averaging technique for the detection of late potentials, comparative studies of patients with and without a history of ventricular tachycardia show that even those without a history of ventricular tachycardia may exhibit late potentials.[46] The detection of late potentials in patients without a history of sustained ventricular tachycardia may be explained in two different ways. First, this may be a true false-positive finding due to some methodological inadequacy of the technique. Second, the presence of late potentials in a patient free of sustained ventricular tachycardia may herald the propensity to ventricular tachycardia although is not manifest. To address this question, we prospectively studied 110 patients without a history of sustained ventricular tachycardia in whom programmed ventricular stimulation was performed.[107] There was a significant correlation (1) between left ventricular function and presence and duration of late potentials, and (2) between left ventricular function and the results of programed ventricular stimulation. Thus, in these patients, late potentials indicated an increase in the propensity to ventricular tachycardia in those who had been free of symptomatic tachyarrhythmias up to the time of the study. Late potentials may therefore be considered as an indicator of the presence of an arrhythmogenic substrate. Subsequent follow-up studies of larger groups of patients show that a significant proportion of these patients developed a spontaneous episode of ventricular tachycardia or died suddenly.

EFFECTS OF NONPHARMACOLOGIC APPROACHES ON LATE POTENTIALS

Antitachycardia Surgery

Map-guided cardiac surgery is an effective measure in the treatment of drug-resistant ventricular tachycardia. The aim of this approach is to identify the site of origin of ventricular tachycardia and to take appropriate measures of ablation, such as partial or complete endomyocardial ventriculotomy, endomyocardial resection, or cryosurgery. Because late fractionated electric activity can often be found during sinus rhythm at the site of origin of ventricular tachycardia, one may expect that successful abolition of the propensity to ventricular tachycardia would be accompanied by loss of ventricular late potentials (see Fig. 24-14).

Early reports included only a few patients. Uther and colleagues report that in two of three patients who had surgery for their ventricular tachycardia with excision of diseased myocardium, ventricular tachycardia could no longer be induced and late potentials were no longer detectable.[14] In the third patient, ventricular tachycardia could still be induced and late potentials were still present. Rozanski and colleagues report the data of four patients in whom ventricular late potentials were abolished by aneurysmectomy.[21]

In a series of 19 patients, we were able to confirm these results.[34] All patients underwent surgery for recurrent sustained ventricular tachycardia, using a map-guided approach. During the postoperative electrophysiologic study, sustained ventricular tachycardia was no longer inducible in 12 of 13 cases (92%) in whom late potentials disappeared after surgery, compared with four of six patients (67%) in whom late potentials were still present. Noninducibility of ventricular tachycardia and absence of late potentials after surgery correlated with a favorable long-term prognosis. Similar data were reported by Marcus and colleagues in 37 patients in whom endocardial resection for ventricular tachycardia was performed.[119] In 24 patients in whom ventricular tachycardia became noninducible after surgery, QRS duration decreased and the voltage in the terminal 40 milliseconds of the averaged and filtered QRS complex increased, indicating that low-amplitude electric activity had been removed. The presence of late potentials decreased from 71% to 33%. In contrast, in 13 patients in whom ventricular tachycardia was still inducible, there was no significant change in either QRS duration or V40. Late potentials were still present in 85% of these cases.

We reviewed our pre- and postoperative recordings of the signal-averaged ECG using the same algorithm as reported by Simson and colleagues.[20, 119, 120] The aims of the study were to gain some insight into whether the absence or presence of late potentials before surgery predicts outcome after surgical ablation of ventricular tachycardia and to assess whether changes in these noninvasive recordings predict surgical outcome. Eighty-six patients underwent direct map-guided antitachycardia surgery. Postoperatively, 41 patients were rendered noninducible (48%); in 26 patients (30%), only nonsustained tachyarrhythmias were induced, whereas sustained ventricular tachycardia was still inducible in 19 patients (22%). These ventricular tachycardias were mostly nonclinical forms. Most of the latter patients were controlled by previously ineffective antiarrhythmic agents. Thus, the overall surgical efficacy rate was 78%. Of these 86 patients, 40 (46%) did not have late potentials before surgery. Thus, in only 46 patients (53%), this noninvasive test was used to assess surgical efficacy. The presence or absence of late potentials before surgery did not predict surgical outcome

because 34 of 67 patients (51%) who were treated successfully did not have late potentials before surgery, compared with six of 19 patients (31%) with still inducible ventricular tachycardia up to the time of surgery. These differences were not significantly different. Patients with noninducible ventricular tachycardia after surgery showed a significant increase in V40 of the signal-averaged QRS complex ($p < 0.03$), whereas this parameter remained unchanged in patients with inducible sustained and nonsustained ventricular tachycardia postoperatively. Overall, the presence or absence of late potentials after antitachycardia surgery can be used in assessing noninvasively the efficacy of this procedure. The sensitivity of this noninvasive technique was 36%, the specificity 69%, and the predictive accuracy 46%, respectively.

Based on these results, subgroups of patients can be identified after antitachycardia surgery in whom the outcome can be predicted. For the individual case, however, postoperative programmed stimulation is mandatory to assure postoperative noninducibility because the sensitivity and specificity of noninvasive recording of late potentials are too low. Despite these limitations, the changes of the signal-averaged QRS complex after direct surgery have given more insight into the pathophysiologic mechanisms underlying late potentials.

The mechanisms by which the various techniques lead to a cure of ventricular tachycardia have not been clearly established. In the encircling endocardial ventriculotomy approach, which has been mainly used by our group, the arrhythmogenic tissue is theoretically isolated from the pumping ventricular chamber. Thus, the reentrant circuit is prevented from engaging the normal portion of the ventricle. According to this concept, one may therefore expect that late potentials do persist postoperatively. This was not the case, however, in many of the patients. One explanation may be that by the combined surgical procedure (subendocardial encircling ventriculotomy and aneurysmectomy) used, the arrhythmogenic zone is not only isolated but also devitalized. Another explanation may be that in this zone, electric activity still persists but is no longer synchronized to the normal heart beat by entrance and exit block and thus goes undetected during signal-averaging. Conversely, the endocardial excision approach of controlling ventricular tachyarrhythmias theoretically either damages or completely excises the reentrant circuit; thus, in patients successfully treated, late potentials should not exist postoperatively. Even if late potentials still persist after surgery, ventricular tachycardia is not inducible in all patients. This may be explained by the observation that low-amplitude fractionated activity during endocardial mapping can be found also in regions of the left ventricle that are at some distance from the site of origin of ventricular tachycardia and that probably do not participate in the reentrant circuit. Removal of the arrhythmogenic tissue at the site of origin of ventricular tachycardia can therefore not be expected to lead to a loss of ventricular late potentials on the body surface if abnormal electric activity at a distant site persists.

Catheter Ablation

Catheter ablation is a new nonpharmacologic approach to control drug-refractory ventricular tachycardias.[121] Its effects on the signal-averaged QRS complex are unknown. Because the overall clinical efficacy of this new approach is reported to range between 60% to 80%, one may expect that recording of late potentials may be useful in assessing acute and long-term outcome of patients after catheter ablation. We analyzed 12 patients who underwent catheter ablation and in whom (before and after ablation) signal-averaging was performed. Overall, the QRS duration and the V40 did not reveal any significant changes after ablation.[122] Furthermore, analysis of successful and ineffective ablation attempts did not show any differences in measured parameters of the filtered QRS complex. Although the number of patients studied is relatively small, the results indicate that recording of late potentials seems not to be helpful in assessing acute and long-term outcome of patients undergoing catheter ablation. The underlying mechanisms are not understood. Probably, the area of damage created by catheter ablation is too small to have any effect on low-amplitude fragmented endocardial activation. Previous studies show that many endocardial sites outside the area of origin of ventricular tachycardia display low fragmented endocardial activation. Thus, one cannot expect catheter ablation to eliminate these areas completely. Probably the critical part of the reentrant circuit (i.e., the area of slow conduction) is sufficiently altered without an effect on areas of slow myocardial activation that function as bystanders. Further studies are needed to elucidate the underlying mechanisms.

EFFECTS OF ANTIARRHYTHMIC DRUGS ON LATE POTENTIALS

One would expect that antiarrhythmic drugs that prolong ventricular conduction time produce prolongation of activation time in those regions with ischemia and in the border zone of infarcted areas. Similarly, these areas of slow conduction and delayed activation may be more sensitive to increments in heart rate than normally activated areas. It would therefore be desirable to find methods to improve the sensitivity of signal-averaged ECG and predict efficacy of antiarrhythmic agents. Several authors report on the use of signal-averaging for predicting

the antiarrhythmic effects of different drugs.[21, 123–136] Most analyzed the effects of class I and II agents and found that the changes detected on signal-averaged ECG variables did not correlate with drug effectiveness against ventricular tachycardia induction.[21, 124–126, 128–131, 134]

Denniss and colleagues studied whether the timing of ventricular late potentials was modified by antiarrhythmic agents and whether any such changes correlated with suppression of clinical and inducible ventricular tachycardia in 32 patients.[127] There was no consistent effect of quinidine, mexiletine, and metoprolol on the timing of late potentials. Late potentials were abolished in five of 53 trials of antiarrhythmic agents (9.4%), whereas ventricular tachycardia was not inducible after antiarrhythmic agents in seven trials (13.2%). Both late potentials and inducibility of ventricular tachycardia were abolished in only one trial. During long-term follow-up (mean, 6 months), ventricular tachycardia recurred in four of nine patients in whom it was still inducible using these antiarrhythmic agents and in one of seven patients in whom it was no longer inducible. These five patients with a recurrence of ventricular tachycardia had persistent late potentials on antiarrhythmic agents.

Cain and colleagues characterized the effects of antiarrhythmic drugs on ventricular late potentials by frequency analysis of signal-averaged ECGs.[135] Squared fast Fourier–transformed data of signal-averaged orthogonal ECGs were compared in 14 patients having ventricular tachycardia before and during treatment with antiarrhythmic drugs. A total of 20 trials were performed. The ratio of the amplitudes of 20- to 50-Hz components to the total spectral amplitudes decreased substantially (81 ± 19%) in eight of 10 successful trials when compared with control values but in only one of 10 unsuccessful trials ($p < .001$). Thus, effective drugs were associated with a significant decrease in the proportion of relatively high-frequency components in the terminal QRS and ST segment. In contrast, Simson and colleagues found no correlation between changes in the high-frequency content of the signal-averaged ECG and successful control of antiarrhythmic drug therapy in ventricular tachycardia.[136] They studied 49 patients having sustained ventricular tachycardia after myocardial infarction. For all trials, the drugs (1) prolonged the filtered QRS complex by 7.4%, (2) decreased the high-frequency content in the first 80 milliseconds of the QRS-complex by 7.8% and in the last 40 milliseconds by 9.6%, and (3) extended the duration that the high-frequency content stayed under 40 μV at the end of the QRS. No differences were found in the four measured parameters between 21 successful and 49 unsuccessful trials. Other authors, using new recording devices and analysis techniques, found that the response to antiarrhythmic drugs (classes IA and III) may be predicted by signal-averaging variables.[131–133] Thus, this noninvasive method may prove to be useful in guiding antiarrhythmic drug therapy. These preliminary results need further prospective evaluation, however.

PROGNOSTIC SIGNIFICANCE OF LATE POTENTIALS

Several studies have addressed the prognostic value of ventricular late potentials (Table 24-3). Our own experience is primarily based on two studies, both using signal-averaging in the time domain. The first prospective trial was initiated at Düsseldorf University in 1980; it used the methodology for signal-averaging that was developed in our department between 1978 und 1979. This system was based on a hard-wired signal-averager, which has subsequently been used by other groups.[18,46,68,107,129,137,138] The second study (PILP; Post-Infarction Late Potential study) began in January 1983. It was completed after inclusion of 777 patients.[139,140]

The results of the first prospective pilot study in 160 patients was reported in 1983.[137] Subsequently, another 628 patients without a history of sustained ventricular tachycardia or fibrillation outside the acute phase of myocardial infarction were studied. Mean duration of follow-up was 39 ± 15.0 months. A major arrhythmic event occurred in 35 patients (21 sudden deaths, 14 episodes of symptomatic spontaneous sustained ventricular tachycardia). The risk of major arrhythmic complications was 2.8 times greater in patients with late potentials of less than 40 milliseconds duration when compared with those without and 9.3 times greater in those with a duration of 40 milliseconds or more. The chance of sudden cardiac death within 1 hour was 3.3 and 5.4 times greater, respectively, whereas the chance for symptomatic sustained ventricular tachycardia was 2.0 and 17.4 times greater, respectively, depending on the duration of late potentials (less or greater than 40 milliseconds). The chance of major arrhythmic complications such as sudden cardiac death or sustained symptomatic ventricular tachycardia was greatest in those patients who were studied within the first 4 to 8 weeks after their qualifying myocardial infarction. In the second study (PILP[139,140]), we included a total of 777 patients during the second or third week after myocardial infarction. Signal-averaging was performed using the software by Simson.[20] In patients with late potentials (RMS of the V40 less than 25 μV or filtered QRS duration 120 or more milliseconds), serious arrhythmic events (symptomatic sustained ventricular tachycardia or sudden cardiac death) occurred in 5.91% of cases but only in 2.15% if there were no late potentials ($p = .01$).

These data are supported by other studies that also used signal-averaging in the time domain. Denniss and colleagues studied 110 patients 7 to 28 days after acute myocardial infarction.[141] Follow-up of these patients ranged between 2 to 12 months (mean, 5 months). There was a significant difference in the subsequent occurrence of symptomatic sustained ventricular tachycardia during follow-up in patients without late potentials (1.1%), compared with those with late potentials (17.4%). The incidence of sudden cardiac death was not reported in this study. In a newer report, the same group presented the results of long-term observation in 403 clinically well survivors of transmural infarction who were 65 years old or younger.[142] Twenty-six percent of the patients had late potentials. At 2 years follow-up, the probability of remaining free from cardiac death or nonfatal ventricular tachycardia or fibrillation was 0.73 for patients with late potentials and 0.95 for patients without. For patients with late potentials, the probability of remaining free from instantaneous death or nonfatal ventricular tachycardia or fibrillation was 0.85 at 1 year and 0.79 at 2 years, lower than the corresponding figures of 0.98 ($p < .001$) and 0.96 ($p < .001$) for patients without late potentials.[142] Within the group of patients with late potentials, the patients who either died instantaneously or had nonfatal ventricular tachycardia or fibrillation had a longer mean ventricular activation time, a lower mean left ventricular ejection fraction, and a higher incidence of left ventricular aneurysms than patients who were event-free.

Kacet and colleagues (personal communication) studied a population of 104 patients who were followed-up for 8.5 ± 4 months. The incidence of subsequent symptomatic sustained ventricular tachycardia in patients without late potentials was 4.5%, compared with 28.9% in patients with late potentials. None of the patients without late potentials died suddenly, compared with 13% of patients with late potentials. Kuchar and colleagues report the results of follow-up (3 to 12 months) of 123 patients who were studied 10 days (mean) after acute myocardial infarction.[143,144] The incidence of major arrhythmic complications such as sudden death or symptomatic ventricular tachycardia was only 1.4% in patients without late potentials, compared with 20.5% in patients with late potentials. In a study by Höpp and colleagues, 50 patients were studied in the early postinfarction period.[145] These patients were followed-up for 24 ± 5 months. Twelve of 30 patients who had late potentials (40%) died suddenly. On the contrary, none of the 20 patients without late potentials died suddenly. The same authors studied another group of 200 patients who had chronic stable coronary artery disease.[145] Mean follow-up was 20 ± 5 months. One hundred eight of 200 patients had ventricular late potentials. Fifteen of these patients (13.9%) died suddenly, compared with four of 92 patients (4.3%) without late potentials ($p < .001$). Von Leitner and colleagues followed-up 518 patients who took part in a rehabilitation program after

TABLE 24-3. Prognostic Significance of Signal-Averaging

Study	Patients (n)	Interval After MI	Follow-up Duration	Definition	Prognostic Value of Late Potentials		
					Cardiac mortality	Sudden death or Symptomatic VT or V/F	Sustained VT or VF
Breithardt, et al	628	<1 mo; n, 258 2 mo; n, 52 3–12 mo; n, 60 >12 mo; n, 99 no MI; n, 159	39±15 months (mean, ±SD)	No LP <40 ms >40 ms	4.5% 7.3% 12.1%	1.6% 5.2% 8.6%	0.8% 1.6% 13.8%
Von Leitner, et al (146)	518	6–8 weeks	10 months (mean)	LP absent LP present	1.5% 7.3%	0.9% 3.6%	No event
Denniss et al (141)	110	7–28 days (mean, 11)	2–12 months (mean, 5)	LP absent LP present	NA		1.1% 17.4%
Kuchar, et al (143, 144)	123	10 d	3–12 mo	LP absent LP present		1.4% 20.5%	
Höpp, et al (165)	50	<4 wks	24±5 mo	LP absent LP present	0% 40%		
Höpp, et al (145)	200	Chronic CAD	20±5 mo	LP absent LP present		4.3% 13.9%	
Denniss, et al (142)	403	11–12 d	2 y	LP absent LP present		At 1 year: 2%, 15%; at 2 years: 4%, 21%	
Eldar, et al (147)	121	Until 48 h	2–10 d	QRS<110 ms QRS>110 ms RMS 40 ms>8.3 µV RMS 40 ms<8.3 µV		4.1% 29.2% 6.9% 19%	
Hong, et al (154)	240	3±2 d	1–10 d	LP absent LP present			23% 65%

MI, myocardial infarction; VF, ventricular fibrillation; VT, ventricular tachycardia. Data not available if not indicated.

myocardial infarction.[146] These patients were studied 6 to 8 weeks after onset of infarction. During a mean follow-up period of 10 months, cardiac mortality was 1.5% in patients without late potentials, compared with 7.3% in patients with ventricular late potentials. Sudden cardiac death occurred in 0.9% of patients without late potentials, compared with 3.6% of patients with late potentials. In none of these patients was symptomatic sustained ventricular tachycardia reported.

Eldar and colleagues demonstrated the use of the signal-averaged ECG in detecting an increased mortality risk in the early postinfarction period.[147] Denniss and colleagues performed exercise testing and signal-averaged ECG in 250 patients within 2 months after myocardial infarction.[148] The odds ratio for presence or absence of late potentials was 7.4 in patients who died or suffered sustained ventricular tachyarrhythmias, compared with those free of serious arrhythmic events. In contrast, the odds ratio was 1.5 in patients with abnormal exercise testing compared with patients without abnormal exercise testing. Similar results were reported by Cripps and associates.[149] Using multivariate analysis, the only independent variable in predicting ischemic events was exercise testing. Arrhythmic events, however, were independent of exercise test results. They were best predicted by the values of (1) size of myocardial infarction, such as Killip class on admission; (2) presence of late potentials; (3) previous infarction; (4) occurrence of in-hospital complications; and (5) non–Q-wave infarction, which were independently associated with arrhythmic events. The independent variables predicting any event (reinfarction, symptomatic ventricular tachycardia, sudden death, or coronary artery bypass grafting) included (in order of importance) Killip class, exercise test result, presence of late potentials, and non–Q-wave infarction. They reported, however, that only about one of five patients with late potentials suffer an arrhythmic event.[149] Therefore, they suggest the addition of clinical observations and the results of exercise testing for enhancing the predictive accuracy of signal-averaging. Patients having negative results of exercise testing and signal-averaging and absence of complications during the acute phase of myocardial infarction were at low risk of suffering arrhythmic events. A good outcome with no arrhythmic or ischemic events could be predicted with a certainty of 99% by using combinations of these parameters. In addition, other authors have demonstrated that the combination of noninvasive algorithms (i.e., signal-averaged ECG, Holter-monitoring, and left ventricular ejection fraction) is useful for screening the population at high risk of suffering arrhythmic events after myocardial infarction.[106, 144, 148–152]

Ursell and colleagues report that the incidence of an abnormal signal-averaged ECG is highest at 6 to 30 days after myocardial infarction and that the recordings at this time have the best sensitivity and predictive accuracy for sudden death or sustained ventricular tachycardia (sensitivity, 75%; specificity, 79%; predictive accuracy, 23%).[153] A transiently abnormal signal-averaged ECG up to 5 days after myocardial infarction and the late appearance of an abnormal signal-averaged ECG (31 to 60 days after myocardial infarction) were not associated with serious arrhythmic events. Hong and colleagues found that the presence of ventricular tachycardia or fibrillation in the prehospital and early in-hospital phase (fewer than 10 days) after acute myocardial infarction was associated with a high incidence of late potentials.[154] The presence of late potentials in this setting was independent of infarct size.

Large multicenter studies demonstrate that early thrombolytic therapy reduces the incidence of late potentials after myocardial infarction.[155–158] This reduced incidence is not related to global left ventricular function but appears to depend on the patency of the infarct-related artery.[155–158] This may reduce the propensity to ventricular tachyarrhythmias. The sensitivity and specificity of signal-averaging are not sufficient to allow reliable monitoring of coronary reperfusion at the bedside.[157]

In contrast to this extensive information on the prognostic significance of signal-averaging in the time domain, there are no prospective large-scale studies using signal-averaging in the frequency-domain.

CLINICAL APPROACH TO THE EVALUATION OF POSTMYOCARDIAL INFARCTION PATIENTS

From the clinical point of view, noninvasive procedures are desirable for screening purposes, although it would be acceptable to use more aggressive invasive techniques in certain subsets of patients. A stepwise approach, using noninvasive recording of late ventricular potentials as the initial step, would allow preselection of patients for further evaluation by invasive electrophysiologic techniques. Feasibility of this approach was tested in 132 postmyocardial infarction patients studied prospectively.[138, 159] The combined use of signal-averaging and programmed ventricular stimulation helped to identify subgroups of patients at markedly different risk of developing spontaneous symptomatic sustained ventricular tachycardia (Fig. 24-17). Patients with late potentials, irrespective of duration, had a 4.4 times greater risk of developing symptomatic sustained ventricular tachycardia (seven of 59 patients; 11.9%) than those without (two of 73 patients; 2.7%). A further increase in the risk of ventricular tachycardia was observed in those patients having late potentials, in whom an abnormal response to ventricular stimulation was observed. Ventricular tachycardia supervened in seven of 35

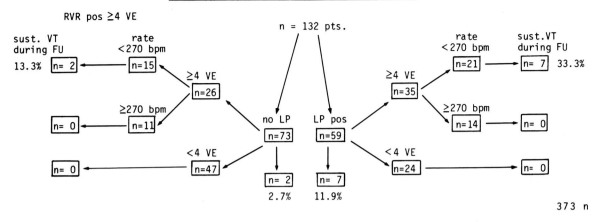

LP and VE early after MI (≤ 1.5 mo.)

Figure 24-17. Value of late potentials and programmed ventricular stimulation in 132 patients after recent myocardial infarction for prediction of spontaneous occurrence of sustained ventricular tachycardia. (*VE*, ventricular echo beat; *LP*, late potential; *sust. VT during FU*, sustained ventricular tachycardia during follow-up study).

patients (20%) having an abnormal response to ventricular stimulation, compared with none of 24 patients who had a normal response. A further important criterion was the rate of the induced ventricular arrhythmia. Only if the rate was less than 270 beats per minute were there any spontaneous episodes of ventricular tachycardia. Thus, the induction of ventricular flutter or fibrillation (rate, 270 or more beats per minute) was of no clinical significance, compared with the induction of a monomorphic and relatively slow tachyarrhythmia.

Patients at highest risk of developing symptomatic sustained ventricular tachycardia after myocardial infarction were characterized by an abnormal result of programmed ventricular stimulation and a rate of the induced ventricular arrhythmia of fewer than 270 beats per minute (see Fig. 24-17). With regard to establishing antiarrhythmic therapy, this may be a subgroup of postmyocardial infarction patients that would benefit most.

If these data are confirmed by future studies, it must still be determined which type of antiarrhythmic therapy should be initiated and how its effect should be controlled. Previous experience in patients with documented sustained ventricular tachycardia suggests that serial electrophysiologic testing may be an appropriate approach.[160-162] This is especially the case if patients present with a low level and grade of spontaneous ventricular ectopy between attacks. In those with frequent and complex ventricular ectopy, preliminary data suggest that the use of antiarrhythmic drugs to suppress these spontaneous arrhythmias improves the prognosis.[163,164] The results of the Cardiac Arrhythmia Suppression Trial study have generated severe doubts that suppression of spontaneous ventricular ectopic beats is helpful in improving prognosis,

at least with the two drugs used (i.e., flecainide and encainide).[165]

SIGNIFICANCE OF LATE POTENTIALS TO PREDICT REJECTION AFTER HEART TRANSPLANTATION AND IN PATIENTS WITH NON–CORONARY ARTERY DISEASE

Haberl and colleagues report the use of frequency analysis of low-noise electrocardiographic recordings as a new noninvasive approach to detect early rejection after cardiac transplantation.[166,167] Thirty-six acute rejection crises that required treatment in heart-transplantation patients were diagnosed by cytoimmunologic monitoring and endomyocardial biopsy. In 33 of 36 cases (91.7%), a significant increase in the frequency content of the QRS complex between 70 and 110 Hz was observed on the days of rejection. The frequency content of the ST segment in a 300-millisecond window was found to be decreased between 10 and 30 Hz. These changes in the frequency content were reversible within 1 to 2 weeks in most patients after successful treatment. They found only two false-positive results (two patients with acute mediastinitis). The mechanism of these changes and the potential use of this method for the evaluation of acute and chronic rejection after orthotopic heart transplantation seems to be a promising new approach that still needs further evaluation.

Thus, actual data suggest that the signal-averaged ECG is an useful noninvasive method for detection of early rejection after cardiac transplantation and for identifying patients with ventricular tachycardia after surgery of tetralogy of Fallot.[166-170] In patients with arrhythmogenic right ventricular disease, a good correlation between the extent of right ventricular involvement, history of sustained ventricular tachycardia, presence of ventricular late potentials, and inducibility of ventricular tachycardia during programmed ventricular stimulation has been reported.[171-174] The role of this technique in patients with nonischemic dilated cardiomyopathy is not established.[175] It may be helpful to detect a propensity to spontaneous ventricular tachycardia but the correlation between an abnormal signal-averaged ECG and the results of programmed ventricular stimulation is poor.[84, 176-178] Furthermore, the role of signal-averaging in patients with hypertrophic cardiomyopathy and in patients with mitral valve prolapse remains unclear.[179-183] Thus, the role of noninvasive recovery of late potentials in patients with nonischemic cardiac disease needs further examination.

CONCLUSIONS

With respect to available information, signal-averaging for the detection of late ventricular potentials seems to be a promising new technique for the identification of patients at risk of ventricular tachyarrhythmias. The relative value of this technique for the prediction of ventricular tachycardias in comparison with sudden cardiac death demands future studies. Which of the various characteristics of low-amplitude fractionated activity (duration, voltage, frequency content) is the most appropriate to predict prognosis in patients after myocardial infarctions needs further evaluation. With regard to the numerous false-positive results (which is not only the case with signal-averaging but also with long-term electrocardiographic recording, as an example), it seems unjustified to expect any single method to be able to identify a given patient at risk of sustained ventricular tachycardia or sudden death with sufficient accuracy. Instead, a combined approach is necessary. In this context, long-term electrocardiographic recording and signal-averaging may prove useful as screening methods, whereas programmed ventricular stimulation may serve for further categorization of risk.

References

1. Williams DO, Scherlag BJ, Hope RR, et al: The pathophysiology of malignant ventricular arrhythmias during acute myocardial ischemia. Circulation 1974;50:1163.
2. Zipes DP: Electrophysiological mechanisms involved in ventricular fibrillation. Circulation 1975;52(Suppl III):120.
3. El-Sherif N, Scherlag BJ, Lazzara R, Hope RR: Reentrant ventricular arrhythmias in the late myocardial infarction period. I. Conduction characteristics in the infarction zone. Circulation 1977;55:686.
4. El-Sherif N, Scherlag BJ, Lazzara R, Hope RR: Reentrant ventricular arrhythmias in the late myocardial infarction period. II. Patterns of initiation and termination of reentry. Circulation 1977;55:702.
5. El-Sherif N, Lazzara R, Hope RR, Scherlag BJ: Reentrant arrhythmias in the late myocardial infarction period. III. Manifest and concealed extra-systolic grouping. Circulation 1977;56:225.
6. Fontaine G, Guiraudon G, Frank R: Intramyocardial conduction defects in patients prone to ventricular tachycardia. III. The post-excitation syndrome in ventricular tachycardia. In: Sandoe E, Julian DG, Bell JW, eds. Management of ventricular tachycardia—role of mexiletine. Amsterdam: Excerpta Medica, 1978:67.
7. Fontaine G, Frank R, Gallais-Hamonnno F, Allali I, Phan-Thuc H, Grosgogeat Y: Electrocardiographie des potentiels tardifs du syndrome de post-excitation. Arch Mal Coeur 1978;71:854.
8. Ostermeyer J, Breithardt G, Kolvenbach R, et al: Intraoperative electrophysiologic mapping during cardiac surgery. Thorac Cardiovasc Surg 1979;27:260.
9. Klein H, Karp RB, Kouchoukos NT, Zorn GL, James TN, Waldo AL: Intraoperative electrophysiologic mapping of the ventricles during sinus rhythm in patients with previous myocardial infarction. Identification of the electrophysiologic substrate of ventricular arrhythmias Circulation 1982;66:847.
10. Josephson ME, Horowitz LN, Farshidi A, Spielman SR, Michelson EL, Greenspan AM: Sustained ventricular tachycardia: evidence for protected localized reentry. Am J Cardiol 1978;42:416.
11. Spielman SR, Untereker WJ, Horowitz LN, et al: Fragmented electrical activity—relationship to ventricular tachycardia. Am J Cardiol 1981;47:448. Abstract.
12. Shenasa M, Borggrefe M, Breithardt G: Cardiac mapping. Mt Kisco, NY: Futura Publishing, 1993.
13. Berbari EJ, Scherlag BJ, Hope RR, Lazzara R: Recording from the body surface of arrhythmogenic ventricular activity during the ST-segment. Am J Cardiol 1978;41:697.
14. Uther JB, Dennett CJ, Tan A: The detection of delayed activation signals of low amplitude in the vectorcardiogram of patients with recurrent ventricular tachycardia by signal averaging. In: Sando AE, Julian DG, Bell JW, eds. Management of ventricular tachycardia—role of mexiletine. Amsterdam: Excerpta Medica, 1978:80.
15. Breithardt G, Becker R, Seipel L: Non-invasive recording of late ventricular activation in man. Circulation 1982;62 (Suppl):III.
16. Hombach V, Höpp HW, Braun V, Behrenbeck DW, Tauchert M, Hilger HH: Die Bedeutung von Nachpotentialen innerhalb des ST-Segmentes im Oberflächen-EKG bei Patienten mit koronarer Herzkrankheit. Dtsch Med Wochenschr 1980;105:1457.
17. Simson M, Horowitz L, Josephson M, et al: A marker for ventricular tachycardia after myocardial infarction. Circulation 1980;62(Suppl):III.
18. Breithardt G, Becker R, Seipel L, Abendroth RR, Ostermeyer

J: Non-invasive detection of late potentials in man—a new marker for ventricular tachycardia. Eur Heart J 1981;2:1.

19. Simson MB: Identification of patients with ventricular tachycardia after myocardial infarction from signals in the terminal QRS complex. Circulation 1981;64:235.

20. Simson MB: Use of signals in the terminal QRS-complex to identify patients with ventricular tachycardia after myocardial infarction. Circulation 1981;64:235.

21. Rozanski JJ, Mortara D, Myerburg RJ, Castellanos A: Body surface detection of delayed depolarizations in patients with recurrent ventricular tachycardia and left ventricular aneurysm. Circulation 1981;63:1172.

22. Breithardt G, Cain ME, El-Sherif N, et al: Standards for analysis of ventricular late potentials using high resolution or signal-averaged electrocardiography. Eur Heart J 1991; 12:473.

23. Durrer D, Formaijne P, Van Dam R, Buller J, Van Lier A, Meyler F: Electrogram in normal and some abnormal conditions. Am Heart J 1961;61:303.

24. Flowers NC, Horan LG, Thomas JR, Tolleson WJ: The anatomic basis for high frequency components in the electrocardiogram. Circulation 1969;39:531.

25. Richards DA, Blake GJ, Spear JF, Moore EN: Electrophysiologic substrate for ventricular tachycardia: correlation of properties in vivo and in vitro. Circulation 1984;69:369.

26. Gardner PI, Ursell PC, Fenoglio JJ, Wit AL: Electrophysiologic and anatomic basis for fractionated electrograms recorded from healed myocardial infarcts. Circulation 1985;72:596.

27. Gardner PI, Ursell PC, Pham TD, Fenoglio JJ, Wit AL: Experimental chronic ventricular tachycardia: anatomic and electrophysiologic substrates. In: Josephson ME, Wellens HJJ, eds. Tachycardias: mechanisms, diagnosis, treatment. Philadelphia: Lea & Febiger, 1984:29.

28. Hanich RF, de Langen CDJ, Kadish AH, et al: Inducible sustained ventricular tachycardia 4 years after experimental canine myocardial infarction: electrophysiologic and anatomic comparisons with early healed infarcts. Circulation 1988;77:445.

29. Gardner PI, Ursell PC, Fenoglio JJ Jr, Wit AL: Anatomical and electrophysiological basis for electrograms showing fractionated activity. Circulation 1982;66(Suppl II):78.

30. Kienzle MG, Miller J, Falcone R, Harken A, Josephson ME: Intraoperative endocardial mapping during sinus rhythm: relationship to site of origin of ventricular tachycardia. Circulation 1984;70:957.

31. Hood MA, Pogwizd SM, Peirick J, Cain ME: Contribution of myocardium responsible for ventricular tachycardia to abnormalities detected by signal-averaged ECG. Circulation 1992;86:1888.

32. Garan H, Ruskin JN: Association of continuous electrical activity and localized reentry: proposed criteria for causal relationship. Circulation 1982;66(Suppl II):79.

33. Simson MB, Spielman SR, Horowitz LN, et al: Effects of surgery for control of ventricular tachycardia on late potentials. Circulation 1981;64(Suppl):IV.

34. Breithardt G, Seipel L, Ostermeyer J, et al: Effects of antiarrhythmic surgery on late ventricular potentials recorded by precordial signal averaging in patients with ventricular tachycardia. Am Heart J 1983;104:966.

35. Breithardt G, Borggrefe M: Pathophysiological mechanisms

and clinical significance of ventricular late potentials. Eur Heart J 1986;7:364.

36. Fontaine G, Guiraudon G, Frank R, et al: Stimulation studies and epicardial mapping in ventricular tachycardia: study of mechanisms and selection for surgery. In: Kulbertus HE, ed. Reentrant arrhythmias, mechanisms and treatment. Lancaster: MTP Press, 1977:333.

37. Höpp HW, Hombach V, Braun V, et al: Kammerarrhythmien und ventrikuläre Spätdepolarisationen bei akutem Myokardinfarkt. Z Kardiol 1981;70:319. Abstract.

38. Simson M, Spielman S, Horowitz L, et al: Slow ventricular activation detected on the body surface in patients with ventricular tachycardia after myocardial infarction. Am J Cardiol 1981;47:498. Abstract.

39. Hombach V, Kebbel V, Höpp HW, et al: Fortlaufende Registrierung von Mikropotentialen des menschlichen Herzens. Dtsch Med Wochenschr 1982;107:1951.

40. Denes P, Santarelli P, Hauser RG, Uretz EF: Quantitative analysis of the high frequency components of the terminal portion of the body surface QRS in normal subjects and in patients with ventricular tachycardia. Circulation 1983; 67:1129.

41. Hombach V, Kebbel V, Höpp HW, Winter V, Hirche H: Noninvasive beat-by-beat registration of ventricular late potentials using high resolution electrocardiography. Int J Cardiol 1984;6:167.

42. Oeff M, von Leitner ER, Erne SN, Lehmann HP, Fenici RR: Failure of signal-averaging technique to record arrhythmogenic diastolic potentials: advantage of non-invasive beat for beat recording. Circulation 1983;68:III.

43. Karbenn U, Breithardt G, Borggrefe M, Simson MB: Automatic identification of late potentials. J Electrocardiol 1985; 18:123.

44. Cain ME, Ambos D, Witkowski FX, Sobel BE: Fast-Fourier Transform analysis of signal-averaged electrocardiograms for identification of patients prone to sustained ventricular tachycardia. Circulation 1984;69:711.

45. Simson MB, Euler D, Mickelson EL, Falcone RA, Spear JF, Moore EN: Detection of delayed ventricular activation on the body surface in dogs. Heart Circ Physiol 1981;241:10 H363.

46. Breithardt G, Borggrefe M, Karbenn U, Abendroth RR, Yeh HL, Seipel L: Prevalence of late potentials in patients with and without ventricular tachycardia: correlation to angiographic findings. Am J Cardiol 1982;49:1932.

47. Steinberg JS, Bigger JT Jr: Importance of the endpoint of noise reduction in analysis of the signal-averaged electrocardiogram. Am J Cardiol 1989;63:556.

48. Goedel-Meinen L, Hofmann M, Schmidt G, Höglsperger H, Jahns G, Baedecker W, Blömer H: Reproducibility of data of the signal-averaged electrocardiogram. Circulation 1987; 76(Suppl IV):124. Abstract.

49. Denniss AR, Cooper MJ, Ross DL, Wallace E, Uther JB, Richards DA: Improved detection of delayed potentials by signal averaging of 28 body surface ECG leads. Circulation 1988; 78(Suppl II):137.

50. Faugère G, Savard P, Nadeau RA, et al: Characterization of the spatial distribution of late ventricular potentials by body surface potential mapping in patients with ventricular tachycardia. Circulation 1986;74:1323.

51. Berbari BJ, Friday LJ, Jackman WM, et al: Precordial mapping

of signal averaged late potentials compared to XYZ leads. J Am Coll Cardiol 1986;7:127.

52. El-Sherif N, Mehra R, Gomes JAC, Kelen G: Appraisal of a low noise electrocardiogram. J Am Coll Cardiol 1983;1:456.

53. Santipetro RF: The origin characterisation of the primary signal, noise and interface sources in the high frequency electrocardiogram. IEEE Trans Biomed Eng 1977;65:707.

54. Steinberg JS, Lander P, Bigger T, Berbari EJ: Signal averaging directly from Holter tapes—results of a new technique. Circulation 1988;78(Suppl II):50.

55. Kelen G, Henkin R, Lannon M, Bloomfield D, El-Sherif N: Correlation between the signal-averaged electrocardiogram from Holter-tapes and from real-time-recordings. Am J Cardiol 1989;63:1321.

56. Fetsch T, Pietersen AH, Karbenn U, Borggrefe M, Breithardt G: Analysis of late potentials from Holter tapes—a comparison of Holter recorded and real-time signal averaged ECG. Pace 1994. (In press).

57. Cain ME, Ambos HD, Markham J, Fischer AE, Sobel BE: Quantification of differences in frequency content of signal-averaged electrocardiograms in patients with compared to those without sustained ventricular tachycardia. Am J Cardiol 1985;55:1500.

58. Haberl R, Hengstenberg E, Pulter R, Steinbeck G: Frequenz-analyse des Einzelschlag-Elektrokardiogrammes zur Diagnostik von Kammertachykardien. Z Kardiol 1986;75:659.

59. Haberl R, Jilge G, Pulter R, Steinbeck G: Spectral mapping of the electrocardiogram with Fourier transform for identification of patients with sustained ventricular tachycardia and coronary artery disease. Eur Heart J 1989;10:316.

60. Rabiner LR, Gold B: Theory and application of digital signal-processing. Englewood Cliffs, NJ: Prentice-Hall, 1975: 356.

60a. Kelen GJ, Henkin R, Starr AM, Caref EB, Bloomfield D, El-Sherif N: Spectral turbulence analysis of the signal-averaged electrocardiogram and its predictive accuracy for reducible sustained monomorphic ventricular tachycardia. Am J Cardiol 1991;67:965.

61. Oeff M, von Leitner ER, Brüggemann T, Andresen D, Sthapit R, Schrüder R: Methodische Probleme bei der Registrierung ventrikulärer Spätpotentiale (Abstract.). Z Kardiol 1982; 71:204.

62. Simson MB, Untereker WJ, Spielman SR, et al: Relation between late potentials on the body surface an directly recorded fragmented electrocardiograms in patients with ventricular tachycardia. Am J Cardiol 1983;51:105.

63. Breithardt G, Borggrefe M, Karbenn U, et al: Verhalten ventrikulärer Spätpotentiale nach operativer Therapie ventrikulärer Tachykardien. Z Kardiol 1982;71:381.

64. Borggrefe M, Breithardt G, Ostermeyer J, Bircks W: Long-term efficacy of endocardial encircling ventriculotomy for ventricular tachycardia: Complete vs partial incision. Circulation 1983;68(Suppl):III.

65. Oeff M, von Leitner ER, Schwarz W, Schröder R: Nichtinvasive Registrierung ventrikulärer Spätpotentiale bei Herzgesunden und bei Patienten mit intraventrikulären Reizleitungsstörungen—Methode und Ergebnisse der Signalmittelungstechnik. Z Kardiol 1986;75:666.

66. Zimmermann M, Friedli B, Adamec R, Oberhänsli I: Frequency of ventricular late potentials and fractionated right ventricular electrograms after operative repair of tetralogy of Fallot. Am J Cardiol 1987;59:448.

67. Buckingham TA, Thessen CC, Stevens LL, Redd RM, Kennedy HL: Effect of conduction defects on the signal-averaged electrocardiographic determination of late potentials. Am J Cardiol 1988;61:1265.

68. Oeff M, von Leitner ER, Sthapit R, et al: Methods for non-invasive detection of ventricular late potentials—a comparative multicenter study. Eur Heart J 1986;7:25.

69. Abboud S, Belhassen B, Laniado S, Sadeh D: Non-invasive recording of late ventricular activity using an advanced method in patients with a damaged mass of ventricular tissue. J Electrocardiol 1983;16:245.

70. Borggrefe M, Karbenn U, Breithardt G: Spätpotentiale und elektrophysiologische Befunde bei ventrikulären Tachykardien. Z Kardiol 1982;71:627. Abstract.

71. Kertes PJ, Glaubus M, Murray A, Julian DG, Campbell RWF: Delayed ventricular depolarization-correlation with ventricular activation and relevance to ventricular fibrillation in acute myocardial infarction. Eur Heart J 1984;5:974.

72. Gomes J, Winters S, Stewart D: "Late" late potentials on the signal-averaged ECG: incidence, characteristics and significance. Circulation 1988;78(Suppl II):52.

73. Berbari EJ, Friday KJ, Jackmann WM, Beck B, Scherlag BJ, Lazzara R: Effects of atrial pacing on surface recorded late potentials in patients with ventricular tachycardia. Circulation 1984;70(Suppl II):II.

74. Landreneau JW, Arenburg JH, Hanley HG, Reddy CP: Effect of atrial and ventricular pacing on the incidence and duration of signal averaged ECG late potentials in canine myocardial infarction. Circulation 1985;72(Suppl III):162.

75. Euler DE, Moore EN: Continuous fractionated electrical activity after stimulation of the ventricles during the vulnerable period: evidence for local reentry. Am J Cardiol 1980; 46:783.

76. Martínez-Rubio A, Shenasa M, Borggrefe M, Chen X, Benning F, Breithardt G: Electrophysiologic parameters characterizing the induction of ventricular tachycardia versus ventricular fibrillation after myocardial infarction: relation between ventricular late potentials and coupling intervals for the induction of sustained ventricular tachyarrhythmias. J Am Coll Cardiol 1993;21:1624.

77. Klempt HW, Wulschner W: Die Analyse des QRS-Komplexes sowie des ST-Abschnittes mit der Signalmittelungstechnik bei Herzgesunden. Z Kardiol 1983;72:369.

78. Wilner J, Mindlich B: Fragmented endocardial eljgectrical activity in patients with ventricular tachycardia: a guide to surgical therapy. Am J Cardiol 1982;49:946.

79. Freedman RA, Gillis AM, Keren A, Soderholm-Difatte V, Mason JW: Signal-averaged ECG late potentials correlate with clinical arrhythmia and electrophysiology study in patients with ventricular tachycardia or fibrillation. Circulation 1984;70:II.

80. Höpp HW, Hombach V, Deutsch HJ, Osterspey A, Winter U, Hilger HH: Assessment of ventricular vulnerability by Holter ECG, programmed ventricular stimulation and recording of ventricular late potentials. In: Steinbach D, Glogan D, Caszkovics A, Scheibelhofer W, Weber H, eds. Cardiac pacing. Darmstadt: Steinkopff Verlag, 1983:625.

81. Kanovsky MS, Falcone RA, Dresden CA, Josephson ME, Sim-

son ME: Identification of patients with ventricular tachycardia after myocardial infarction: signal-averaged electrocardiogram, Holter monitoring, and cardiac catheterization. Circulation 1984;70:264.

82. Buxton AE, Simson MB, Falcone R, et al: Signal averaged ECG in patients with nonsustained ventricular tachycardia: identification of patients with potential for sustained ventricular arrhythmias. J Am Coll Cardiol 1984;3:495. Abstract.

83. Poll DS, Marchlinski FE, Falcone RA, Simson MB: Abnormal signal averaged ECG in nonischemic congestive cardiomyopathy: relationship to sustained ventricular tachyarrhythmias. Circulation 1984;70:II.

84. Poll DS, Marchlinski FE, Falcone RA, Simson MB: Abnormal signal-averaged ECG in nonischemic congestive cardiomyopathy: relationship to sustained ventricular tachyarrhythmias. Circulation 1986;72:1308.

85. Zimmermann M, Adamec R, Simonin P, Richez J: Beat to beat detection of ventricular late potentials using high-resolution ECG and comparison with signal averaging. Circulation 1988;78(Suppl II):139.

86. Haberl R, Jilge G, Pulter R, Steinbeck G: Comparison of frequency and time domain analysis of the signal-averaged electrocardiogram in patients with ventricular tachycardia and coronary artery disease: methodologic validation and clinical relevance. J Am Coll Cardiol 1988;12:150.

87. Machac J, Weiss A, Winters SL, Baricca P, Gomez JA: A comparative study of frequency-domain and time-domain analysis of signal averaged electrocardiograms in patients with ventricular tachycardia. J Am Coll Cardiol 1988;11:284.

88. Worley SJ, Mark DB, Smith WM, et al: Comparison of time domain and frequency domain variables from the signal-averaged electrocardiogram: a multivariable analysis. J Am Coll Cardiol 1988;11:1041.

89. Buckingham TA, Thessen CM, Hertweck D, Janosik DL, Kennedy HL: Signal-averaged electrocardiography in the time and frequency domains. Am J Cardiol 1989;63:820.

90. Malik M, Kulakowski P, Poloniecki J, et al: Frequency versus time domain analysis of signal-averaged electrocardiograms. I. Reproducibility of the results. J Am Coll Cardiol 1992;20:127.

91. Kulakowski P, Malik M, Poloniecki J, et al: Frequency versus time domain analysis of signal-averaged electrocardiograms. II. Identification of patients with ventricular tachycardia after myocardial infarction. J Am Coll Cardiol 1992;20:135.

92. Odemuyiwa O, Malik M, Poloniecki J, et al: Frequency versus time domain analysis of signal-averaged electrocardiograms. III. Stratification of postinfarction patients for arrhythmic events. J Am Coll Cardiol 1992;20:144.

93. Vaitkus PT, Kindwall KE, Marchlinski FE, Miller JM, Buxton AE, Josephson ME: Differences in electrophysiological substrate in patients with coronary artery disease and cardiac arrest or ventricular tachycardia. Insights from endocardial mapping and signal-averaged electrocardiography. Circulation 1991;84:672.

94. Denniss AR, Holley LK, Cody DV, et al: Ventricular tachycardia and fibrillation: differences in ventricular activation times and ventricular function. J Am Coll Cardiol 1983;1:606. Abstract.

95. Spielman SR, Horowitz LN, Greenspan AM, et al: Activation mapping in sinus rhythm in patients with ventricular tachycardia—relationship to cycle length and site of origin. Am J Cardiol 1981;47:497. Abstract.

96. Morady F, Di Carlo LA, Baerman JM, Buitleir M: Comparison of coupling intervals that induce clinical and nonclinical forms of ventricular tachycardia during programmed stimulation. Am J Cardiol 1986;57:1269.

97. Kus T, Fromer M, Dubuc M, Shenasa M: Dispersion of refractoriness in ventricular tachycardia induction from the right ventricle. J Electrophysiol 1989;3:117.

98. Wright KE, McIntosch HD: Syncope: a review of pathophysiologic mechanisms. Progr Cardiovasc Dis 1971;13:580.

99. Silverstein MB, Singer DE, Mulley AG, Thibault GE, Barnett GO: Patients with syncope admitted to medical intensive units. JAMA 1982;248:1185.

100. Borggrefe M, Karbenn U, Breithardt G: Usefulness of Holter monitoring and non-invasive recording of late potentials in selection of patients for programmed ventricular stimulation. Circulation 1986;74(Suppl II):745. Abstract.

101. Gang ES, Peter TH, Rosenthal ME, Mandel WJ, Lass Y: Detection of late potentials on the surface electrocardiogram in unexplained syncope. Am J Cardiol 1986;58:1014.

102. Kuchar Dl, Thorburn CW, Sammel NL: Signal-averaged electrocardiogram for evaluation of recurrent syncope. Am J Cardiol 1986;58:949.

103. Daniel T, Boineau J, Sabiston D: Comparison of human ventricular activation with canine model in chronic myocardial infarction. Circulation 1971;44:74.

104. Langner PH Jr, Greselowitz DB, Briller SA: Wide band recording of the electrocardiogram and coronary heart disease. Am Heart J 1973;86:308.

105. Guiraudon G, Fontaine G, Frank R, et al: Encircling endocardial ventriculotomy. A new surgical treatment for life-threatening ventricular tachycardias resistant to medical treatment following myocardial infarction. Ann Thorac Surg 1978;26:438.

106. Reinhardt L, Mäkijärvi M, Fetsch T, et al: The prognostic significance of heart rate variability after acute myocardial infarction. Experience from the Post-Infarction Late Potential Study. Submitted.

107. Breithardt G, Borggrefe M, Quantius B, Karbenn U, Seipel L: Ventricular vulnerability assessed by programmed ventricular stimulation in patients with and without late potentials. Circulation 1983;68:275.

108. Breithardt G, Seipel L, Meyer T, Abendroth RR: Prognostic significance of repetitive ventricular response during programmed ventricular stimulation. Am J Cardiol 1982;49:693.

109. Lindsay BD, Ambos D, Schechtman KB, Cain ME: Improved selection of patients for programmed ventricular stimulation by frequency analysis of signal-averaged electrocardiograms. Circulation 1986;73:675.

110. Breithardt G, Borggrefe M, Haerten K: Ventricular late potentials and inducible ventricular tachyarrhythmias as a marker for ventricular tachycardia after myocardial infarction. Eur Heart J 1986;7(Suppl A):127.

111. Winters S, Stewart D, Targonski A, Squire A, Gomes J: Late potentials identiy patients post myocardial infarction with left ventricular dysfunction and complex ventricular ectopy

who have inducible ventricular tachycardia. Circulation 1988;78(Suppl II):578.

112. Pagé RL, Smith PN, Irwin JM, Wharton M, Prystowsky EN: Noninvasive predictors of sustained ventricular tachycardia induction in patients with asymptomatic nonsustained ventricular tachycardia. Circulation 1988;78(Suppl II):629.

113. Fananapazir L, Barbour DJ, Winkler JB: Signal-averaged electrocardiographic identification of patients with inducible ventricular tachycardia with hypertrophic cardiomyopathy. Circulation 1988;78(Suppl II):51.

114. Rosen M, Fisch C, Hoffmann B, Knoebel S: Delayed afterdepolarisations as a mechanism for accelerated junctional escape rhythm. Circulation 1979;60(Suppl):II.

115. Moak JP, Rosen MR: Induction and termination of triggered activity by pacing in isolated canine Purkinje fibers. Circulation 1984;69:149.

116. Schwarzmaier J, Karbenn U, Borggrefe M, Ostermeyer J, Breithardt G: Quantitative relation between intraoperative registration of late endocardial activation and late potentials in signal-averaged electrocardiogram. Circulation 1987;76 (Suppl IV):1363. Abstract.

117. Schwarzmaier HJ, Karbenn U, Borggrefe M, Ostermeyer J, Breithardt G: Relation between ventricular late endocardial activity during intraoperative endocardial mapping and low-amplitude signals within the terminal QRS complex on the signal-averaged surface electrocardiogram. Am J Cardiol 1990;66:308.

118. Denniss AR, Ross DL, Johnson DC, Nunn G, Uther JB: Comparison of ventricular activation times obtained by signal averaged ECG and epicardial mapping. (Abstr.). J Am Coll Cardiol 1984;3:623. Abstract.

119. Marcus NH, Falcone RA, Harken AH, Josephson ME, Simson MB: Body surface late potentials: effects of endocardial resection in patients with ventricular tachycardia. Circulation 1984;70:632.

120. Borggrefe M, Karbenn U, Podczeck A, Martinez-Rubio A, Schwarzmaier J, Breithardt G: Effects of nonpharmacological intervention on ventricular late potentials. Herz 1988;13:197.

121. Breithardt G, Borggrefe M, Zipes D: Non-pharmacological therapy of tachyarrhythmias. Mt. Kisco, NY: Futura Publishing, 1987.

122. Seifert T, Borggrefe M, Karbenn U, Martinez-Rubio A, Breithardt G: Verhalten ventrikulärer Spätpotentiale nach Katheterablation ventrikulärer Tachykardien. Z Kardiol 1989;78:647.

123. El-Sherif N, Scherlag BJ, Lazzara R, Hope RR: Reentrant ventricular arrhythmias in the late myocardial infarction period. 4. Mechanisms of action of lidocaine. Circulation 1987;56:395.

124. Simson MB, Waxman HL, Falcone R, Marcus NH, Josephson ME: Effects of antiarrhythmic drugs on noninvasively recorded late potentials. In: Breithardt G, Loogen F, eds. New aspects in the medical treatment of tachyarrhythmias. München, 1987:80.

125. Breithardt G, Borggrefe M, Karbenn U, Schwarzmaier HJ: Effects of pharmacological and non-pharmacological interventions on ventricular late potentials. Eur Heart J 1987; 8(Suppl A):97.

126. Lombardi F, Finocchiaro ML, Dalla Vecchia L, et al: Effects of mexiletine, propafenone and flecainide on signal-averaged electrocardiogram. Eur Heart J 1992;13:517.

127. Denniss AR, Ross DL, Cody DV, Ho B, Russell PA, Young AA: Effect of antiarrhythmic therapy on delayed potentials in patients with ventricular tachycardia. J Am Coll Cardiol 1984;3:495. Abstract.

128. Höpp HW, Deutsch H, Hombach V, Braun V, Hilger HH: Medikamentöse Beeinflussbarkeit ventrikulärer Spätpotentials. Z Kardiol 1982;71:206.

129. Jauernig RA, Senges J, Langfelder W, et al: Effect of antiarrhythmic drugs on ventricular late potentials at sinus rhythm and at constant heart rate. In: Steinbach D, Glogar D, Laszkovics A, Scheibelhofer W, Weber H, eds. Cardiac pacing. Darmstadt: Steinkopff Verlag, 1983:767.

130. Shenasa M, Fetsch T, Shenasa J, et al: The effect of antiarrhythmic drugs on the signal-averaged ECG. Does it predict response to therapy?. In: Gomes JA, ed. Signal averaged electrocardiography. Dordrecht: Kluwer Publishing, 1993;527.

131. Freedman RA, Steinberg JS: Selective prolongation of QRS late potentials by sodium channel blocking antiarrhythmic drugs: relation to slowing of VT. J Am Coll Cardiol 1991; 17:1017.

132. Fetsch T, Reinhardt L, Shenasa M, et al: Is the efficacy of sotalol treatment predictable by the analysis of spectral turbulences (STA) from the signal averaged ECG?. Circulation 1993;88:413. Abstract.

133. Hopson JR, Kienzle MG, Aschoff AM, Shirkey DR: Noninvasive prediction of efficacy of type IA antiarrhythmic drugs by the signal-averaged electrocardiogram in patients with coronary artery disease and sustained ventricular tachycardia. Am J Cardiol 1993;72:288.

134. Gessman L, Gallagher J, Del Rossi A, Fernandez J, Strong M, Maranhao V: Prolongation of late potentials by type I antiarrhythmic drugs coincident with inducibility of ventricular tachycardia. Circulation 1983;68(Suppl III):173.

135. Cain ME, Ambos HD, Fischer AE, Markham J, Schechtman KB: Noninvasive prediction of antiarrhythmic drug efficacy in patients with sustaine ventricular tachycardia from frequency analysis of signal average ECGs. Circulation 1984; 70(Suppl II):252.

136. Simson MB, Falcone R, Kindwall E: The signal averaged electrocardiogram does not predict antiarrhythmic drug success. Circulation 1985;72(Suppl III):7.

137. Breithardt G, Schwarzmaier J, Borggrefe M, Haerten K, Seipel L: Prognostic significance of ventricular late potentials after acute myocardial infarction. Eur Heart J 1983; 4:487.

138. Breithardt G, Borggrefe M, Haerten K: Role of programmed ventricular stimulation and noninvasive recording of ventricular late potentials for the identification of patients at risk of ventricular tachyarrhythmias after acute myocardial infarction. In: Zipes DP, Jaliffe J, eds. Cardiac electrophysiology and arrhythmias. Orlando, FL: Grune & Stratton, 1985:553.

139. Breithardt G, Borggrefe M: Post-Infarction Late Potential Study. In preparation.

140. Mäkijärvi M, Fetsch T, Reinhardt L, Borggrefe M, Breithardt G: Noninvasive risk assessment after acute myocardial infar-

ction in the thrombolytic era. The results of the Post-Infarction Late Potential Study. Submitted.

141. Denniss AR, Cody DV, Fenton SM, et al: Significance of delayed activation potentials in survivors of myocardial infarction. (Abstr.) J Am Coll Cardiol 1983;1:582.

142. Denniss AR, Richards DA, Cody DV, et al: Prognostic significance of ventricular tachycardia and fibrillation induced at programmed stimulation and delayed potentials detected on the signal-averaged electrocardiogram of survivors of acute myocardial infarction. Circulation 1986;74:731.

143. Kuchar D, Thorburn C, Sammel N: Natural history and clinical significance of late potentials after myocardial infarction. Circulation 1985;72:III.

144. Kuchar DL, Thorburn CW, Sammel NL: Late potentials detected after myocardial infarction: natural history and prognostic significance. Circulation 1987;74:1280.

145. Höpp HW, Hombach V, Osterspey A, et al: Clinical and prognostic significance of ventricular arrhythmias and ventricular late potentials in patients with coronary heart disease. In: Hombach V, Hilger HH, eds. Holter monitoring technique. Technical aspects and clinical applications. Stuttgart-New York, 1985:297.

146. von Leitner ER, Oeff M, Loock D, Jahns B, Schröder R: Value of non invasively detected delayed ventricular depolarizations to predict prognosis in post myocardial infarction patients. Circulation 1983;68:III.

147. Eldar M, Leor J, Rotstein Z, Hod H, Truman S, Abboud S: Signal averaging identifies increased mortality risk at early post-infarction period. Circulation 1988;78(Suppl II):51.

148. Dennis AR, Cody DV, Richards DA, et al: Signal-averaged electrocardiogram is superior to exercise testing in predicting death and arrhythmias after myocardial infarction. Circulation 1988;78(Suppl II):578.

149. Cripps T, Bennet D, Camm J, Ward D: Prospective evaluation of clinical assessment, exercise testing and signal-averaged electrocardiogram in predicting outcome after acute myocardial infarction. Am J Cardiol 1988;62:995.

150. El-Sherif N, Ursell SN, Bekheit S, et al: Prognostic significance of the signal-averaged electrocardiogram depends on the time of recording in the post-infarction period. Am Heart J 1989;118:256.

151. Gomes JA, Winters SL, Stewart D, et al: A new noninvasive index to predict sustained ventricular tachycardia and sudden death in the first year after myocardial infarction: based on signal-averaged electrocardiogram, radionuclide ejection fraction and Holter monitoring. J Am Coll Cardiol 1987; 10:349.

152. Gomes JA, Winters SL, Ip J: Signal averaging of the surface QRS complex: practical applications. J Cardiovasc Electrophysiol 1991;2:316.

153. Ursell S, Bekheit S, Ibrahim B, et al: The predictive accuracy of the signal averaged ECG in the post-infarction patient depends on the time of recording. Circulation 1988;78(Suppl II):302.

154. Hong M, Gang ES, Wang FZ, Siebert C, Xu YX, Simonson J, Peter T: Ventricular late potentials are associated with ventricular tachyarrhythmias in the early phase of myocardial infarction. Circulation 1988;78(Suppl II):302.

155. Gang ES, Leur AS, Hong M, Wang FZ, Siebert CA, Peter TH:

Decreased incidence of ventricular late potentials after successful thrombolytic therapy for acute myocardial infarction. N Engl J Med 1989;321:712.

156. Breithardt G, Borggrefe M, Karbenn U: Late potentials as predictors of risk after thrombolytic therapy? Br Heart J 1990;64:174.

157. Tranchesi B Jr, Verstraete M, Van de Werf F, et al: Usefulness of high-frequency analysis of signal-averaged surface electrocardiograms in acute myocardial infarction before and after coronary thrombolysis for assessing coronary perfusion. Am J Cardiol 1990;66:1196.

158. Zimmermann M, Adamec R, Ciaroni S: Reduction in the frequency of ventricular late potentials after acute myocardial infarction by early thrombolytic therapy. Am J Cardiol 1991;67:697.

159. Breithardt G, Borggrefe M, Haerten K, Trampisch HJ: Value of late potentials and programmed ventricular stimulation in predicting long-term arrhythmic complications in patients with coronary artery disease. Circulation 78(Suppl):301.

160. Breithardt G, Seipel L, Abendroth RR, Loogen F: Serial electrophysiological testing of antiarrhythmic drug efficacy in patients with recurrent ventricular tachycardia. Eur Heart J 1980;1:11.

161. Horowitz LN, Josephson ME, Kastor JA: Intracardiac electrophysiologic studies as a method for the optimization of drug therapy in chronic ventricular arrhythmia. Prog Cardiovasc Dis 1980;23:81.

162. Breithardt G, Borggrefe M, Seipel L: Present status of serial electrophysiologic testing for predicting antiarrhythmic drug-efficacy in patients with ventricular tachycardia. In: Breithardt G, Loogen F, eds. New aspects in the medical treatment of tachyarrhythmias. Role of amiodarone. Baltimore: Urban & Schwarzenberg, 1983:112.

163. Graboys TB, Lown B, Podrid PJ, de Silva R: Long-term survival of patients with malignant ventricular arrhythmia treated with antiarrhythmic drugs. Am J Cardiol 1982;50: 437.

164. Hoffmann A, Schütz E, White R, Follath F, Burckhardt D: Suppression of high-grade ventricular ectopic activity by antiarrhythmic drug treatment as a marker for survival in patients with chronic coronary artery disease. Am Heart J 1984;107:1103.

165. Rogers WJ, Epstein AE, Arciniegas JG, et al. Cardiac Arrhythmia Suppression Trial (CAST) Investigators: preliminary report: effect of encainide and flecainide on mortality in a randomized trial of arrhythmias suppression after myocardial infarction. N Engl J Med 1989;321:406.

166. Haberl R, Weber M, Kemkes B, Steinbeck G: Frequency analysis of the QRS-complex and ST-segment for noninvasive detection of acute rejection after orthotopic heart transplantation. Circulation 1987;76(Suppl IV):204. Abstract.

167. Haberl R, Weber M, Reichenspurner H, et al: Frequency analysis of the surface electrocardiogram for recognition of acute rejection after orthotopic cardiac transplantation. Circulation 1987;76:101.

168. Keren A, Gillis AM, Freedman RA: Heart transplant rejection monitored by signal-averaged electrocardiography in patients receiving cyclosporine. Circulation 1984;70(Suppl I):124.

169. Lacroix D, Kacet S, Savard P, et al: Signal-averaged electro-

cardiography and detection of heart transplant rejection: comparison of time and frequency domain analysis. J Am Coll Cardiol 1992:19:553.

170. Danford DA, Garson A Jr: Abnormal conduction related to ventricular dysrhythmias by signal averaged electrocardiography in postoperative tetralogy of Fallot. Circulation 1984;70(Suppl II):207. Abstract.

171. Blomström-Lundqvist C, Hirsch I, Olsson SB, Edvardsson N: Quantitative analysis of the signal-averaged QRS in patients with arrhythmogenic right ventricular dysplasia. Eur Heart J 1988;9:301.

172. Wichter T, Martínez-Rubio A, Borggrefe M, Breithardt G: Clinical value of the signal-averaged ECG in patients with arrhythmogenic right ventricular disease. Eur Heart J 1992; 13(Suppl):378.

173. Wichter T, Martínez-Rubio A: Value of the signal-averaged ECG in patients with arrhythmogenic right ventricular disease. Circulation 1992;86(Suppl I):319.

174. Kinoshita O, Kamakura S, Ohe T, et al: Frequency analysis of signal-averaged electrocardiogram in patients with right ventricular tachycardia. J Am Coll Cardiol 1992;20:1230.

175. Winters SL, Goldman DS, Banas JS Jr: Prognostic impact of late potentials in nonischemic dilated cardiomyopathy. Circulation 1993;87:1405.

176. Denereaz D, Zimmermann M, Adamec R: Significance of ventricular late potentials in non-ischaemic dilated cardiomyopathy. Eur Heart J 1992;13:895.

177. Mancini DM, Wong KL, Simson MB: Prognostic value of an abnormal signal-averaged electrocardiogram in patients with nonischemic congestive cardiomyopathy. Circulation 1993;87:1083.

178. Martínez-Rubio A, Borggrefe M, Budde T, Chen X, Breithardt G: Signal-averaging and programmed ventricular stimulation in patients with dilated cardiomyopathy. Eur Heart J 1989;10(Suppl):232.

179. Crips TR, Counihan PJ, Frenneaux MP, Ward DE, Camm AJ, McKenna WJ: Signal-averaged electrocardiography in hypertrophic cardiomyopathy. J Am Coll Cardiol 1990;15:956.

180. Fleischmann C, Gonska BD, Brune S, Kreuzer H: Ventrikuläre Rhythmusstörungen und Spätpotentiale bei Patienten mit hypertropher Kardiomyopathie. Z Kardiol 1990;79:113.

181. Kulakowski P, Counihan PJ, Camm AJ, McKenna WJ: The value of time and frequency domain, and spectral temporal mapping analysis of the signal-averaged electrocardiogram in identification of patients with hypertrophic cardiomyopathy at increased risk of sudden death. Eur Heart J 1993;14:941.

182. Newton G, Sochowski RA, Tang ASL: Late potentials in patients with mitral valve prolapse do not contain abnormal high frequency. Circulation 1992;86(Suppl I):319.

183. Jabi H, Burger AJ, Orawiec B, Touchon RC: Late potentials in mitral valve prolapse. Am Heart J 1991;122:1340.

Cardiac Arrhythmias, 3rd edition, edited by William J. Mandel.
J. B. Lippincott Company, Philadelphia © 1995.

25

S. Bertil Olsson • Shiwen Yuan

Technique and Use of Monophasic Action Potential Recordings

Knowledge of the electrophysiologic behavior of the heart depends largely on the findings obtained using intracellular microelectrode technique, developed in 1949.[1] As long ago as 1936, however, Schütz described how monophasic signals could be recorded from the beating heart with the aid of a suction electrode device.[2] The signal recorded in this way has been named the monophasic action potential (MAP), which distinguishes it from the signal recorded by the intracellular microelectrode, the transmembrane action potential (AP). Monophasic action potential recordings from the intact human heart were initially obtained using the suction catheter technique.[3–5] Today, the recording of MAPs is performed with the contact catheter technique.[6–8]

The MAP reproduces the repolarization time (RT) course of AP of the myocardial cells with high accuracy and provides precise information on the local activation time (AT).[9–11] With the advantage of in vivo applicability and the realization that specific cardiac arrhythmias cannot be mimicked in isolated animal preparations but are best studied in patients, MAP recordings have been widely used in the last decade.[12] They are believed to be the method of choice for evaluating myocardial repolarization changes.

This chapter aims to provide information on practical use of MAP recordings, with emphasis on clinical applications.

GENESIS OF MONOPHASIC ACTION POTENTIAL

Although the electric origin of the MAP has been extensively discussed, the actual mechanism of the genesis of the MAP is still limited to theoretic considerations.[7,9,12,13] It is commonly accepted that the MAPs are recorded between an area of injury or local depolarization and an indifferent electrode.[12] The injured or depolarized area, which is the prerequisite for recording MAPs, can be produced by applying a suction, mechanical pressure or even thermal and chemical factors onto the endo- or epicardium.[5,14,15] Thus, the cells immediately subjacent to the tip electrode are depolarized and electrically inactivated, whereas the adjacent cells surrounding these depolarized cells are unaffected. An electric gradient develops between the inexcitable and adjacent normal cells. During the electric diastole, a source current emerges from the normal cells and a sink current descends into the depolarized cells. Under the volume-conductor condition, the sink current results in a negative electric field. During electric systole, the former current sink reverses to a current source, producing an electric field of opposite polarity. According to this hypothesis, the MAPs reflect the voltage time-course of the normal cells surrounding the injured cells. Both the injured and normal cells contribute equally to the genesis of the boundary current, which produces the MAP field potential.[12] A modeling study performed by Hirsch and coworkers provides theoretic support for this hypothesis.[16]

It should be stressed that the intentionally produced cellular injury is reversible, provided that the tissue damage is spatially and temporally limited.[14] The contact electrode catheters used for MAP recordings do not differ in this respect from conventionally used intracardiac electrode catheters for the recording of intracardiac electrograms.

Relation Between Monophasic Action Potential and Transmembrane Action Potential

The MAP has a gross configuration that is similar to that of an AP.[9–11,13] When a MAP and an AP are recorded from closely adjacent areas, the onset of depolarization of these two signals occurs simultaneously. Furthermore, the repolarization courses are almost completely superimposable if the MAP amplitude is normalized to the same level of the AP (Fig. 25-1).[10]

Important differences do exist between the MAP and AP recordings, however: (1) the MAP always has a lower amplitude and consequently a slower upstroke velocity than the AP because it reflects a summation of the electric activity from hundreds of cells that depolarize sequentially with time; (2) the relation of a resting membrane potential level to the AP amplitude and overshoot is not reproduced in the MAP recording (the MAP has a proportionally higher overshoot; Fig. 25-2); and (3) the upstroke of the MAP is always slower than that of the AP and in addition, it is commonly contaminated by a rapid biphasic deflection (i.e., the remnant of the intrinsic deflection; see Fig. 25-1).[12,17] Moreover, mechanically induced artifacts may highly influence the similarity between the MAP and the AP. Generally, MAPs can provide important information on myocardial repolarization and activation, as does the AP, whereas they have the advantage of in vivo applicability in human subjects, which bridges the gap between basic and clinical electrophysiology.[18]

Relation Between Monophasic Action Potential and the Surface Electrocardiogram

The surface electrocardiogram (ECG) is the most readily available method for evaluating cardiac activation and repolarization. Compared with the ECG, MAPs provide more precise and representative local information because they derive from a limited area not more than 5 mm in diameter, whereas the ECG reflects the electric activity of the whole heart.[10,12] Thus, the local activation is accurately measured on MAP recordings by the AT and the local repolarization by MAP duration (MAPd). The atrial repolarization, which is almost undetectable by ECG, can also be well evaluated by recording the atrial MAP.

The QT interval has been frequently used in clinical settings to study the repolarization disturbances and the

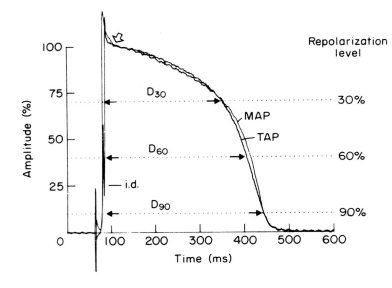

Figure 25-1. Comparison between the monophasic action potential (*MAP*) recorded with a contact electrode and the transmembrane action potential (*TAP*) recorded with a microelectrode. The plateau amplitude (*open arrow*) of the signals are scaled to the same level to facilitate comparison. Note the similarities between the repolarization courses of these two signals and the remnant of the intrinsic deflection (*i.d.*) on the upstroke of the MAP (Reproduced with permission from Franz MR, Burkhoff D, Spurgeon H, Weisfeldt ML, Lakatta EG: In vitro validation of a new cardiac catheter technique for recording monophasic action potentials. Eur Heart J 1986;7:34–41.)

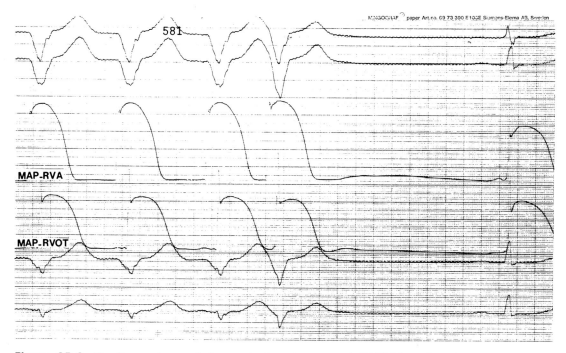

Figure 25-2. Simultaneously recorded monophasic action potentials (MAPs) from the right ventricular apex (*MAP-RVA*) and outflow tract (*MAP-RVOT*), using a MAP-pacing combination catheter during programmed stimulation in a patient with ischemic heart disease. The repolarization phase of the MAPs is smooth at both recording sites. A pacing artifact can be seen on the RVA channel and does not influence the MAP measurement. Note that the overshoot of the upstrokes are relatively high, as compared with those of the transmembrane action potentials. A small notch is recorded just before the upstroke of the MAP-RVOT.

effect of antiarrhythmic drugs; a gross relation between the QT interval and ventricular MAPd has been observed.[19-22] Monophasic action potential recordings, however, have been verified to be more sensitive and reliable than the QT interval in detecting early ischemia, the effects of antiarrhythmic drugs, and the mechanoelectric feedback phenomenon.[6, 22-26] During ventricular pacing or programmed stimulation, the aberrant T waves make it difficult to measure the QT interval. In contrast, the MAP signal represents local myocardial activity that is little influenced by the ventricular activation sequence. Conversely, normal MAPs can be recorded even when the ST-T are markedly changed on the surface ECG if the myocardial cells at the recording site are normal.

TECHNICAL ASPECTS

Monophasic action potentials can easily be recorded from the endocardium, using the contact catheter technique during the electrophysiologic study, and from the epicardium, using the contact electrode probe during openheart surgery. To assure good quality MAP recordings, the following technical aspects must be considered in addition to the demands of conventional electrophysiology.

Catheters

The contact electrode catheter is generally adopted for endocardial MAP recordings because of its simplicity, safety, and stability over time, although the suction catheter is still used in some animal experiments and clinical studies.[7, 27, 28] The Franz contact catheter is designed with a hemispheric electrode of 1.5 mm in diameter at the tip and a reference electrode of 1 mm in diameter, 5 mm proximal to the tip.[7, 12] It contains an intraluminal stylet, which gives the distal catheter shaft sufficient elasticity and resilience, allowing the catheter to follow the myocardial wall movement without losing its contact pressure or being dislodged. The electrodes are made of nonpolarizable material (Ag-AgCl) to allow true direct current (DC) amplification and minimize the polarization phenomena in the interface between electrode and tissue. The catheter size is usually 6 to 7 French. A MAP-pacing combination catheter (EP technologies, Mountain View, CA) allows both MAPd and effective refractory period (ERP) to be measured at the same endocardial site.[12, 29, 30] The diametrically mounted pacing electrodes of this combination catheter provide unusually low and stable pacing threshold and consequently, a tiny or invisible pacing spike on the MAP recording, which facilitates high-fidelity measurements without interference from the pacing spike (see Fig. 25-2). We found also that the combination catheter is well sheltered because 50-Hz noise is seldom collected by this catheter. A MAP catheter with a steerable tip is also commercially available (EP Technologies) that facilitates catheter placement and allows stable long-term recording. Several contact electrode probes have also been developed for recording epicardial MAPs in man and in animal experiments.[12, 24, 31–33]

Catheter Manipulation

The catheter is advanced into the right or left ventricle percutaneously through the femoral vein or artery using the Seldinger procedure. The right access is more frequently used than the left in the clinical setting. The apex or outflow tract of the right ventricle is the most common recording position. For atrial MAP recordings, the high lateral free wall of the right atrium is usually chosen. One catheter is frequently used, although the use of two catheters to record MAPs simultaneously from one or both sides of the ventricles has also been reported.[34–38] Multiple-site recording permits the evaluation of the dispersion of myocardial repolarization.[34–39]

The objective of the contact technique is to keep the tip electrode in close apposition with the endocardium under as stable a contact pressure as possible throughout the cardiac cycle. The trabecularization of the ventricular endocardium usually aids in keeping the spring-loaded catheter tip in its desired location. Care should be taken to keep the contact pressure against the endocardial surface strong enough to produce the appropriate amount of local myocardial depolarization and at the same time gentle enough to avoid damaging the endocardium or causing other complications. Suitable contact pressures range between 10 and 30 g/mm^2.[12] Using an introducer with rubber valves and leaving it in the vessel during MAP recording can help to avoid loss of the contact pressure and dislocation of the catheter. When the indifferent electrode is in contact with the endocardium, distorted MAP signals may be recorded. We recorded a simultaneous unipolar electrogram through the indifferent electrode, with a bandwidth from 0.1 to 500 Hz, to avoid this problem.[14] An ST elevation in the unipolar electrogram usually suggests that the contact pressure is too strong, which can be avoided by slightly withdrawing the catheter or better positioning.[14] For epicardial MAP recording, the tip electrode of the probe should be held firmly and perpendicularly against

the epicardium. The mapping of the entire ventricular endo- or epicardial surface can be completed within a few minutes using one-catheter technique.[31–33, 40, 41] It should be noted that MAPs cannot be recorded in areas covered by fatty tissue or from nonviable tissue such as a myocardial scar.

Amplifiers and Recorder

The technique for recording MAPs is different from that for recording conventional intracardiac electrograms. Thus, a DC-coupled differential amplifier is mandatory for amplification of the signal and elimination of the alternating current (AC) or high-frequency noise.[14] The conventional amplifiers of electrocardiographic recorders are AC-coupled and tend to move the recorded diastolic potential upward, mimicking spontaneous phase 4 depolarization, and are therefore not suitable for MAP recordings.[12, 39] Gould universal amplifiers (11G4133, Gould Inc., Cleveland, OH) are used in our laboratory. The distal electrode of the MAP catheter is connected to the positive input and the proximal electrode is connected to the negative input of the amplifier. The frequency response of the recording system should cover the range from DC to more than 1000 Hz to properly reproduce the MAP signal. Franz suggests a bandwidth from DC to at least 5000 Hz.[12] Using the Gould amplifier, we set the filter from DC to 3000 Hz and obtain satisfactory recordings. The amplified MAP signals can be recorded by a multichannel recorder on paper (with a speed from 100 to 200 mm per second), on tapes, or digitized on computer disks for detailed analysis.

Safety

Transvenous MAP recording has proved safe.[7, 15] The recording of an endocardial MAP, however, necessitates a contact pressure of the catheter against the endocardium and consequently, there is a theoretic possibility that a MAP catheter may perforate the myocardial wall. The catheter used for MAP recordings is usually less flexible than the conventional electrode catheter of the same diameter. It is therefore advisable to abstain from a catheter manipulation that may be associated with increased risk of perforation for other reasons—for instance, in connection with DC-conversion of cardiac arrhythmias.

In our series, extended to 635 cases of endocardial right ventricular or atrial MAP recordings, pericardial tamponade occurred in one case and was uneventfully treated. It was unclear whether the perforation was caused by the suction MAP catheter or a quadripolar 5F right ventricular apical catheter.[15]

NORMAL FINDINGS

Typical ventricular MAPs are almost identical in configuration to APs recorded from closely adjacent sites when normalized in amplitude (see Fig. 25-1).[10,12] They should have a stable, negative diastolic baseline (phase 4); a sharp positive overshooting phase during early depolarization (phase 0), followed by a short downward deflection (phase 1); a plateau (phase 2); and a downward repolarization (phase 3) returning to the baseline (see Figs. 25-1 and 25-2).

Small negative deflections, or notches, can sometimes be seen just before or during the upstroke of the MAP (see Fig. 25-2). They reflect relatively remote electric activity, the intracardiac QRS complex, or the intrinsic deflection of the nearby endocardial electrogram. A sufficiently large MAP signal may provide a more favorable ratio between the MAP signal and remote potentials and thereby minimize the influence of this artifact on MAP measurement.[12] The upstroke phase of the MAP often contains a rapid biphasic deflection, appearing as a notch or spike in high-frequency recordings, which represents the remnant of the intrinsic deflection and usually has little influence on MAP measurements (see Fig. 25-1).[12,15]

Criteria for Acceptable Monophasic Action Potentials

Monophasic action potentials of perfect quality are not always obtainable, especially in the clinical setting, because of time limitations or electric or movement artifacts (Fig. 25-3).[12,15,17] The criteria for acceptable quality of MAP recordings have not been well established.[15,42] In 1985, Olsson proposed criteria as follows: (1) MAPs should have a level of undisturbed baseline that coincides in time with phase 4 of an AP recording and the requirement must be fulfilled at heart rates below 100 per minute; (2) the right atrial MAP amplitude should exceed 3 mV in all rhythms but atrial fibrillation and the right ventricular MAP amplitude should exceed 15 mV; (3) if any pre- and afterpotential exist that coincides in time with atrial or ventricular

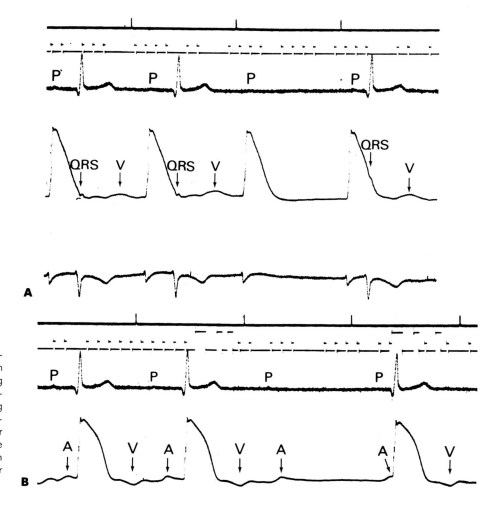

Figure 25-3. Example of mechanical disturbances in monophasic action potential (MAP) recordings, showing the effect of mechanical ventricular activity (*V*) in the atrial MAP recording (*upper*) and the effect of the mechanical atrial activity (A) in the ventricular MAP recording (lower). Note that the ventricular mechanical activity (*V*) can also be recorded on the ventricular MAP recordings.

mechanical activity, its amplitude should not exceed 10% of the total amplitude of the MAP.[15]

Monophasic Action Potential Measurements

Three main time intervals are usually measured (Fig. 25-4):[31, 43]

1. AT—Defined as the interval from the earliest onset of the QRS complexes or the stimulus artifact during pacing on the surface ECG to the take-off point of the MAP upstroke or the point where the MAP upstroke reaches the 10% depolarization level, it represents

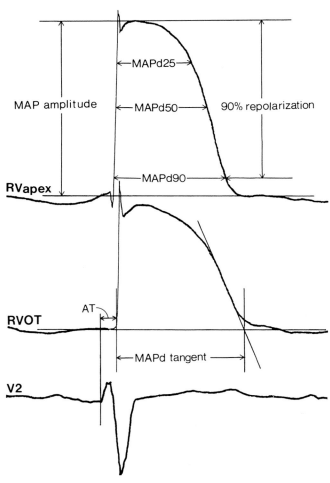

Figure 25-4. Measurements of monophasic action potential (MAP) duration at different levels of repolarization (*MAPd25, MAPd50, MAPd90* and *MAPd$_{tangent}$*), activation time (AT), and MAP amplitude. The MAP upstroke has been redrawn for clear reproduction (*RVapex*, right ventricular apex; *RVOT*, right ventricular outflow tract.)

the conduction time from the start of ventricular activation to the activation at the recording site.

2. MAPd—Usually measured at a repolarization of 90% of the total amplitude from the diastolic baseline to the crest of the plateau (MAPd90) because the asymptotic end of repolarization makes precise measurement of total MAPd difficult; the intersection between the baseline and a tangent on the maximal negative slope in phase 3 (MAPd$_{tangent}$) is also used to represent the end of repolarization (see Fig. 25-4).[44, 45] Monophasic action potential duration at earlier levels such as 20% or 25%, and 50% of repolarization (MAPd20, MAPd25, MAPd50, respectively) is also measured, which may help to detect the configuration changes of MAPs.[37, 46]

3. RT—Measured from the earliest onset of the QRS complexes or the stimulus artifact during pacing to the end point of 90% repolarization (equal to AT plus MAPd90), it represents the total time of repolarization.

In early premature beats, if the depolarization began before 90% repolarization of the preceding beat, an extrapolative line along the maximal slope of MAP upstroke (V$_{max}$) down to the baseline can be drawn and MAPd90 and MAPd$_{tangent}$ can be estimated from this line. Similarly, MAPd90 of the preceding beat can be estimated using the above-mentioned tangent line for MAPd$_{tangent}$ measurement.[44, 45]

The V$_{max}$ and rising time of MAP upstroke are measured; their changes are reported to be a highly sensitive marker of myocardial ischemia and drug effects.[24, 47, 48] To eliminate the influence of MAP amplitude variation on the velocity, a relative velocity of the upstroke (V$_{max}$%) can be derived by dividing the maximal velocity by the total amplitude of the MAP.[45] Similarly, the relative slope of the repolarization phase (R$_{max}$%) is calculated and its relation with the change of MAPd has been found.[43, 45]

The amplitude of MAPs differs greatly from that of APs and varies, depending on the type of tissue, the contact pressure, the angle between the catheter and the myocardial surface, and the electrophysiologic properties of the myocardial cells underlying the recording electrode.[49, 50] The MAPs therefore do not reproduce the diastolic- and action-potential amplitude of the AP. The relative changes of MAP amplitude can be assessed, however, and may provide information on changes of extracellular ion concentration and myocardial ischemia, for example.[10, 24, 51–54] The plateau amplitude was taken as the amplitude of MAPs because the amplitude of the upstroke is contaminated by the intrinsic deflection of the electrogram.[7] The amplitude of atrial MAPs is lower than that of ventricular MAPs. This may partly be explained by the subendocardial connective tissue layer being thicker in the atrium than in the ventricle.[14] The thin myocardial layer of the atrial wall may also contribute to the low amplitude of the atrial MAP, an explanation that is supported by the modeling study of Hirsch and coworkers.[16] In fact, the atrial myocardial AP is of lower amplitude than that of the ventricle.[55]

Reference Values for Monophasic Action Potential Measurements

The normal ranges of MAP parameters have not been well established in man because of difficulties in getting MAPs from large series of healthy subjects. Brorson and co-workers reported a set of reference values for atrial MAP measurements in 1975 based on right atrial MAP recordings in 40 healthy men (Table 25-1).[49,56–58] In 1984, Edvardsson and colleagues reported reference values for right ventricular MAPs based on recordings during pacing with a cycle length of 500 milliseconds in 48 healthy young men (see Table 25-1).[50] Franz and coworkers recorded MAPs from the right ventricular endocardium using contact-catheter technique during right ventricular pacing with cycle lengths of 600 milliseconds and 400 milliseconds in 25 patients with normal right ventricle; they reported a set of reference values that are in concordance with those obtained using suction-catheter technique.[30,50]

INFLUENCE OF RATE AND RHYTHM ON MONOPHASIC ACTION POTENTIAL DURATION

The influence of heart rate and rhythm on MAPd has been extensively studied using MAP recordings. A number of experimental studies show that heart rate and rhythm

modify the MAPd in two ways.[21,59–62] The first is known as the electric restitution, which manifests as a smooth increase in MAPd when pacing at a given steady rate and delivering extrastimulation at progressively increasing coupling intervals, with the MAPd increase being more rapid at earlier phase near the ERP (Fig. 25-5). This is an intrinsic electrophysiologic feature of the myocardium and can also be observed during functional variation of the heart rate and during arrhythmias.[14,43,63] Olsson found that the changes of MAPd in beats with different prematurity are not equal in all phases of repolarization but the earlier extra beats are terminated by a shorter MAPd with an unchanged repolarization rate of phase 3 and later extra beats by a relatively longer MAPd and decreased repolarization rate of phase 3.[14] The electric restitution is believed to be due to incomplete recovery of the plateau currents and contribution from electrogenic pump currents between one action potential and the next.[60,64,65]

The second way by which the heart rate influences the MAPd is related to a sudden change of the heart rate. Previous studies show that in the event of a sudden increase in heart rate (e.g., the introduction of pacing to sinus rhythm or rate change during pacing with a constant cycle length), a sharp drop of the MAPd occurs in the first few beats, followed by a slow progressive shortening until a steady state is reached over a period of several minutes (Fig. 25-6).[14,43,60,66,67] If the electric restitution curve is redefined at this new steady-state MAPd, a new curve with a shorter MAPd at all RR intervals will be obtained. The sharp drop of the MAPd in the first few beats is covered by the electric restitution, whereas the slow change is due to the accumulation of an ion or metabolite or to changes in activity of the Na^+-K^+ pump through an increase in outward background current.[60]

The electric restitution has been identified in man

TABLE 25-1. Measurements From Right Atrial and Ventricular Monophasic Action Potentials In Healthy Men or Patients With Relatively Normal Right Ventricle

Site, Rhythm	Patients (n)	MAPd90 (ms)	Amplitude (mV)	AT (ms)	ERP (ms)	VERP/MAPd
Atrial[49,56–58]						
Sinus	40	271 ± 38.5	6.2 ± 2.6	19 ± 9	—	—
Pacing, CL = 500 ms	25	251 ± 34.8	—	51 ± 31	253 ± 36.8*	—
Ventricular[30,50]						
Pacing, CL = 600 ms	25	244 ± 32	—	—	220 ± 35	0.90 ± 0.04
Pacing, CL = 500 ms	48	243 ± 18	27 ± 10	—	236 ± 14	0.96 ± 0.09
Pacing, CL = 400 ms	25	225 ± 38	—	—	220 ± 42	0.88 ± 0.05

Values are presented as M ± SD. MAPd90, monophasic action potential duration at 90% repolarization; AT, activation time; ERP, effective refractory period; VERP/MAPd, the ratio between ventricular ERP and MAPd90; CL, cycle length; *, measured during right atrial pacing at a driving cycle length of 800 ms; —, data note available.

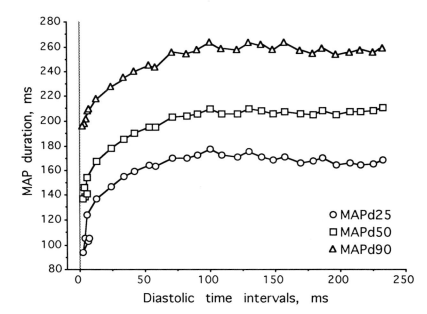

Figure 25-5. Electrical restitution curve of monophasic action potential (MAP) duration, measured from right ventricular apex at a driving cycle length of 500 milliseconds, with extrastimuli delivered from 1 to 280 milliseconds longer than the ventricular effective refractory period. Note the shifting of MAP duration at three levels of repolarization along the restitution curve plateau toward the shoulder and the sharp descent of the curve at the earlier phase of the diastolic time intervals. (MAPd25, 50 and 90, MAP duration at 25%, 50%, and 90% repolarization, respectively.) (Reproduced by permission from Yuan S, Blomström-Lundquist C, Olsson SB: Monophasic action potentials: concept of practical application. J Cardiovasc Electrophysiol 1994;5:287.)

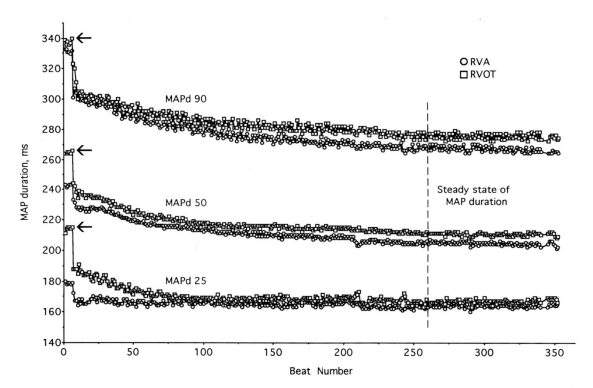

Figure 25-6. Monophasic action potential (MAP) duration, measured from the right ventricular apex (*RVA*) and outflow tract (*RVOT*) during RVA pacing at a cycle length of 500 milliseconds. When the pacing started suddenly during sinus rhythm with a mean RR interval of 690 milliseconds (*arrows*), the MAP duration dropped immediately by 25 to 40 milliseconds in the first few beats and then shortened progressively until it reached a steady state (after the *vertical dashed line*) over a period of 2.2 minutes. Note that the changes in MAP duration at three levels of repolarization at both recording sites followed a similar pattern. (MAPd25, 50 and 90, MAP duration at 25%, 50% and 90% repolarization, respectively.) (Reproduced by permission from Yuan S, Blomström-Lundquist C, Olsson SB: Monophasic action potentials: concept of practical application. J Cardiovasc Electrophysiol 1994;5:287.)

in several studies using MAP recordings.[14, 28, 63, 64, 67-69] In 1971, Olsson and associates reported the effects of abrupt changes of cycle length on MAPd in man and found that a shorter cycle length was terminated by a shorter MAPd and vice versa.[14, 63] In some clinical studies, a hump on the restitution curve was observed, as in an experimental study in rabbits.[28, 64, 69, 70] Seed and colleagues, however, did not observe such a hump but found a restitution curve similar to that established in experiments in cats and dogs.[59, 67] The rate-dependence of MAPd and ventricular ERP (VERP) has been demonstrated to be parallel and it was reported that the value of VERP minus MAPd in 24 patients with suspected ventricular tachycardia was almost constant (range, -12 to -15 milliseconds) at all cycle lengths.[68, 71-73]

One of the clinical implications of these findings is that they argue against the widely used Bazett's correction of the QT interval (QTc) for physiologic variation in heart rate. Seed and coworkers studied 14 patients by correlating the MAPd (and QT interval) with the cycle length and found that after one beat at a different interval, it took up to 10 beats for a steady state to be regained; after a switch from one sustained rate to another faster sustained rate, it took at least 3 minutes for a new steady state to be reached.[67] Based on the finding that the relation between heart rate and MAPd (and QT intervals) is not constant, they concluded that the use of the rate-corrected QT interval is not valid and suggest the use of QT obtained during pacing with constant cycle length for at least 3 minutes instead of the QTc.

The findings also raise questions about the routine protocol of programmed stimulation for clinical electrophysiologic studies. Kanaan and associates studied the changes of MAPd during programmed stimulation and the difference between MAPd during pacing with constant cycle length and that with an intertrain pause.[61] They found that with a sudden acceleration in pacing rate, MAPd decreased exponentially. During constant rate pacing, MAPd was always shorter than during pacing with an intertrain pause. With the intertrain pause shorter than 16 seconds, there was a decremental shortening in MAPd in successive drivetrains until about 50 to 56 seconds. They concluded that when performing programmed stimulation using a pause, a conditioning period of at least 2 minutes should be used before diastole scanning to allow MAPd to reach the steady state. We have similar findings in our patients.[45] From a practical point of view, however, we believe that if the protocol takes more than 2 minutes before the final step of the diastole scanning by which the ERP is determined, it is still valid for clinical use of ERP testing.

Thus, the electric restitution studied by MAP technique in intact human heart resembles that in cellular preparations.[69] Characterization of the rate-dependent changes of MAPd in patients with arrhythmias may give insight into the contribution of cellular mechanisms to the arrhythmogenic substrate.[36-38]

EVALUATION OF ANTIARRHYTHMIC DRUGS

Monophasic action potentials allow quantification of myocardial repolarization (offering a unique opportunity to assess the drug action during electrophysiologic study in vivo) and have been extensively used to evaluate the effects of antiarrhythmic drugs in animals and in man.[74, 75]

Drug Effects on Myocardial Repolarization and Refractoriness

Because the prolongation of MAPd and VERP is a property of many antiarrhythmic drugs and is considered a prerequisite for their efficacy, confirmation and quantification of the drug effects on MAPd and VERP in animals and in man has long been the main focus of interest in this area. The VERP to MAPd ratio is also a useful parameter because antiarrhythmic drugs may have disparate effects on MAPd and VERP. An increase of the VERP to MAPd ratio was believed to be important for antiarrhythmic drug efficacy and was found to reflect a use-dependent sodium channel blockade that is quantitatively similar to V_{max}.[76]

Class Ia drugs (Vaughan-Williams classification) usually prolong myocardial repolarization and refractoriness, which manifest as prolongation of MAPd and ERP. Quinidine prolongs both right atrial and ventricular MAPd.[22, 72, 77] Gavrilescu and colleagues found that quinidine lengthened right atrial MAPd to a greater degree in atrial premature beats than in sinus beats, which may explain why quinidine can prevent atrial arrhythmias in doses that do not influence sinus rhythm.[78] Edvardsson and coworkers, using a relatively low dose of procainamide (500 mg, intravenously) in eight healthy volunteers found only a prolongation of VERP, with no change in MAPd, whereas Platia and associates, using a higher dose of 20 to 25 mg/kg, noted prolongation of both parameters.[22, 79] Endresen and colleagues documented that disopyramide prolonged MAPd and VERP with an increased VERP to MAPd ratio.[80] Platia and coworkers reported similar effects of quinidine and procainamide and found that the plasma drug level correlated more closely with MAPd than with QT interval, QRS duration, or VERP.[22]

Class Ib drugs tend to shorten the time course of repolarization. Edvardsson and associates found that a bolus injection of lidocaine (75 mg) shortened MAPd but had no effect on VERP, whereas Endresen and Amlie reported that lidocaine (100 mg, intravenously) shortened both MAPd and VERP.[50,81] After giving 2 mg/kg of mexiletine to nine healthy volunteers, Olsson and Harper found a slight, nonsignificant shortening of MAPd and VERP.[82,83]

The effect of class Ic agents on repolarization and refractoriness in human subjects has rarely been reported. Olsson and Edvardsson gave a single intravenous dose of flecainide (2 mg/kg) to nine healthy men and found a significant prolongation of MAPd and VERP that was even enhanced in early premature beats.[84] Interestingly, a new class I drug, pentisomide, has been verified in a clinical study to possess class Ic, Ia, and Ib effects, so that it is difficult to further classify this drug into subgroups according to the Vaughan-Williams's definition.[20]

Clinical evaluation of the influence of β-blockers on repolarization and refractoriness is somewhat difficult and available data are conflicting. This is partly because of the variability of the baseline sympathetic tone. Edvardsson and Olsson tested acute and chronic effects of metoprolol on ventricular repolarization in healthy volunteers and found that 15 mg, intravenously, had no statistically signifi-

cant effect on VERP, MAPd, or QT interval, whereas 400 mg daily for 5 weeks resulted in significant prolongation of all three parameters.[85] The effect of propranolol on repolarization has been studied in patients and—differing from an earlier experimental study—a shortening of MAPd was found, whereas VERP not changed.[86-88]

Many class III drugs have been tested in human subjects concerning their electrophysiologic effects on repolarization, and the prolongations of MAPd and ERP were documented.[75] Olsson and associates found a 30% prolongation of right atrial MAPd after chronic administration of amiodarone for 4 or more weeks.[89] After intravenous injection of amiodarone (5 mg/kg), Blomström and colleagues observed a significant prolongation of both MAPd and VERP.[90] Sotalol was also repeatedly demonstrated to prolong both the atrial and ventricular MAPd and ERP.[86,91] A similar class III drug action of melperone and bunaphtine has also been documented in human subjects.[92,93] Dofetilide, a new class III drug, prolonged MAPd (Fig. 25-7) and VERP in a parallel fashion in patients with ventricular tachycardia but did not affect AT, which verifies the highly selective class III effect of this drug.[37,94,95]

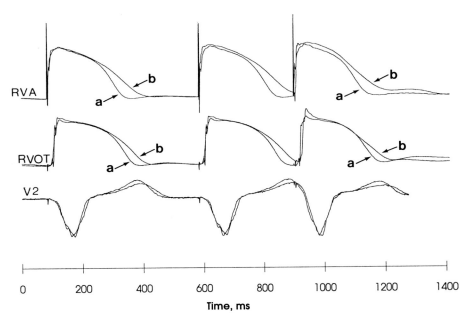

Figure 25-7. Superimposed monophasic action potentials (MAPS) before (*a*) and after (*b*) dofetilide infusion during right ventricular (RV) extrastimulation at a driving cycle length of 500 milliseconds reproduced from the digitized MAP recordings at the RV apex (*RVA*) and the outflow tract (*RVOT*) in a patient with ventricular tachycardia. The amplitudes of the MAPs were normalized to the same level to facilitate comparison. The MAP duration of both the drive-train beats and the premature beats was markedly prolonged after dofetilide at both recording sites. Note that the prolongation of the MAP duration was more pronounced in the later than in the earlier phase of repolarization. (Reproduced by permission from Yuan S, Rasmussen HS, Olsson SB, Blomström-Lundquist C: Effect of dofetilide on cardiac repolarization in patients with ventricular tachycardia. A study using simultaneous monophasic action potential recording from two sites in the right ventricle. Eur Heart J 1994;15:514.)

The effects of calcium channel blockade on repolarization in humans have rarely been reported. Edvardsson and coworkers gave a single intravenous dose of verapamil (0.15 mg/kg) to 10 patients with supraventricular tachycardia and found that the atrial MAPd was unexpectedly shortened, whereas the ventricular MAPd and ERP were not affected.[96]

The influence of cardiac glycosides on repolarization includes direct effects and those mediated by the autonomic nervous system. Edvardsson and associates gave a bolus dose of digoxin (0.75 mg, intravenously) to eight healthy men and observed a significant prolongation of VERP in the right outflow tract but no change of MAPd was found.[79] This result was attributed to a vagal effect because the opposite result had previously been obtained after administration of digoxin under autonomic blockade in dogs, in which a shortening of both VERP and MAPd with an increase of the VERP to MAPd ratio was observed.[97] This

hypothesis was further supported by the effect of atropine, which caused a significant decrease in VERP.[79]

Table 25-2 summarizes the effects of these antiarrhythmic drugs on MAPd and ERP in human subjects.

Use-Dependency of Antiarrhythmic Drugs

Measuring the steady-state MAPd during pacing at different cycle lengths may provide information on the use-dependency of antiarrhythmic drugs. The use dependency of drugs can also be evaluated by constructing the restitution curve of MAPd. In a study in patients with angina pectoris, Sedgwick and colleagues measured the MAPd during pacing at four cycle lengths and found a similar MAPd increase after dofetilide infusion at all the cycle lengths.[94] Morgan and coworkers obtained a similar result in patients with

TABLE 25-2. Effect of Antiarrhythmic Drugs on Human Myocardial Repolarization and Refractoriness

Class	Drugs	Site	Patients (n)	MAPd90	VERP	VERP/MAPd
Ia	Quinidine[78]	RA†	11	‡	—	—
	Quinidine[22,72]	RV†	15	‡	‡	NS
	Procainamide[22,73,79]	RV†*	34	‡	‡	NS
	Disopyramide[80]	RV†	10	‡	‡	‡
Ib	Lidocaine[79,81]	RV†*	18	§	§	NS
	Mexiletine[83]	RV*	9	NS	NS	NS
Ic	Flecainide[84]	RV†*	9	‡	‡	NS
I	Pentisomide[20]	RV†	17	§	§	‡
II	Metoprolol (acute)[85]	RV*	16	NS	NS	NS
	Metoprolol (chronic)[85]	RV*	8	‡	‡	NS
	Propranolol[87,88]	RV†	20	§	NS	‡
III	Amiodarone (chronic)[89]	RA†	8	‡	—	—
	Amiodarone (acute)[90]	RV†	13	‡	‡	NS
	Sotalol[86,91,161]	RV†	38	‡	‡	NS
	Sotalol[86]	RA†	9	‡	‡	—
	Melperone[92]	RA†*	8	‡	—	—
	Bunaphtine[162]	RA, RV†	13	‡	‡	NS
	Dofetilide[94,95]	RV†	28	‡	‡	NS
IV	Verapamil[96]	RA†	10	§	NS	‡
		RV†	10	NS	NS	NS
Other	Digoxin[79]	RV*	8	NS	‡	NS
	Atropine[79]	RV*	8	NS	§	NS

RA and RV, Right atrial and ventricular endocardium, respectively. See Table 25-1 for other abbreviations.
*In healthy volunteers.
†In patients with ischemic heart disease and/or arrhythmias.
‡Duration prolonged or ratio increased.
§Duration shortened.
NS, no statistically significant changes observed; — data not available.

supraventricular tachycardia.[98] Yuan and associates found that dofetilide has a relatively marked effect of prolongation of MAPd at shorter rather than at longer diastolic time intervals.[37,95] These findings suggest that the effect of dofetilide is not reverse–use-dependent in humans, which differs from the other class III drugs.

Drug Effects on Conduction

The accurate measurement of local AT from MAP recordings can be used to study the influence of antiarrhythmic drugs on intraventricular conduction velocity, although it is not as widely used as MAPd. Olsson and Harper demonstrated subnormal and supernormal conductions by measuring AT of the premature beats during ventricular programmed stimulation in healthy young men.[82,99] They found an increased period of subnormal conduction with the abolition of the supernormal conduction period after the administration of mexiletine (2 mg/kg, intravenously; Fig. 25-8).

Thus, the use of MAP recording in antiarrhythmic drug studies bridges clinical and cellular electrophar-macology, allowing the findings of the cellular electro-pharmacology in vitro to be explored in a clinical setting in vivo.

AFTERDEPOLARIZATIONS AND TRIGGERED ARRHYTHMIA

Triggered activity is a transient membrane oscillation triggered by cardiac depolarization.[100] When this occurs early, before repolarization is complete, it is called early after-depolarization (EAD), whereas when it occurs after the completion of repolarization it is called delayed after-depolarization. These afterdepolarizations are relatively slow waveforms that interrupt or follow myocardial repolarization. They cannot be detected by conventional intracardiac recordings or surface ECG but can be demonstrated by MAP recording in both animals and in man.[34,101–106] On MAP recordings, the EAD manifests as a deviation from the smooth repolarization in phase 3 (Fig. 25-9). The amplitude of EAD is defined as the distance between phase 4 and the first deviation from the smooth repolarization in

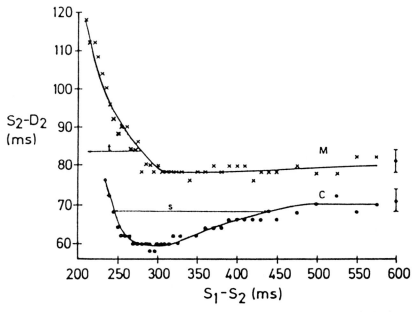

Figure 25-8. Intraventricular conduction curves during ventricular programmed stimulation in a healthy young man, constructed using the intervals of the stimulus artifact to the onset of the menophasic actions potential upstroke (S_2-D_2) in the extra beats against the coupling intervals(S_1-S_2). In the control recording (C), a phase of supernormal conduction(s) is clearly visible. After the administration of mexiletine (M), there is no obvious supernormal conduction phase but a substantial delay of the conduction in the earlier extra beats (i.e., a phase of subnormal conduction (t); reproduced by permission from Harper RW, Olsson SB: Effect of mexiletine on conduction of premature ventricular beats in man: a study using monophasic action potential recordings from the right ventricle. Cardiovasc Res 1979;13(6):311–9.)

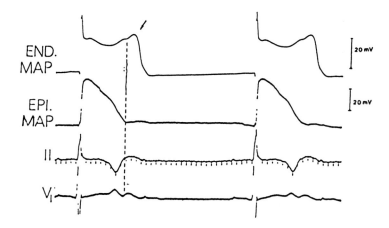

From N El-Sherif et al, 1988 (Circ Res)

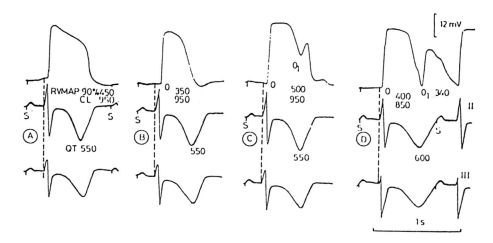

From Gavrilescu et al, 1978 (Brit H Journal)

Figure 25-9. (Upper panel) Endocardial (*END*) and epicardial (*EPI*) monophasic action potentials (*MAPs*) recorded from a dog with experimentally induced QTU prolongation and polymorphic ventricular arrhythmias. Note the marked repolarization disturbance i.e., early after depolarization (EAD) on the endocardial MAP (*arrow*), whereas the epicardia MAP is normal. **(Lower panel)** MAP recordings in a patient with long QT syndrome, showing the EAD is significantly evident in MAP recordings *C* and *D*. Note that the EADs coincide with the repolarization abnormalities on the surface electrocardiogram (Reproduced with permission from El-Sherif N, Zeiler RH, Craelius W, Gough WB, Henkin R: QTU prolongation and polymorphic ventricular tachyarrhythmias due to bradycardia-dependent early afterdepolarizations. Afterdepolarizations and ventricular arrhythmias. Circ Res 1988;63(2):286–305, and Gavrilescu S, Luca C: Right ventricular monophasic action potentials in patients with long QT syndrome. Br Heart J 1978;40(9):1014–8.)

phase 3 and is expressed as a percentage of the total MAP amplitude because the latter is variable, depending on the recording position and contact pressure.[100]

The manifestation of EAD-induced activity requires the following steps: (1) critical prolongation of the repolarization phase, (2) a net depolarizing current carrying the charge for EAD, and (3) propagation of EADs, which are locally generated to capture the entire heart, resulting in one or more extrasystoles.[107]

There is growing evidence that the EAD and EAD-triggered activity play an important role in the development of triggered arrhythmias, such as torsades de points.[101, 103] In canine models, Levine and colleagues recorded MAPs with cesium chloride–induced phase 3 EAD, which preceded the onset of the tachyarrhythmias, and observed coupling intervals identical to the ventricular premature beats.[101] Both EAD and ventricular arrhythmias resolved concurrently during overdrive pacing. This study established the validity of using MAP recordings to identify the presence of EADs and triggered activity in vivo, which was further supported by later studies.[102-104] Although the experimentally induced EADs were neither uniform nor stable, they coincided with repolarization abnormalities of the surface ECG (see Fig. 25-9).

In clinical studies, the presence or inducibility of EAD on MAP recordings, concurrent with deformations of the final portion of the T wave, and their relation with torsades de pointes in patients with long QT syndrome have repeatedly been reported.[93, 105, 106, 108-111] Bonatti and coworkers recorded right ventricular MAPs in 10 patients with long QT syndrome and found marked repolarization abnormalities, with humps preceding the completion of repolarization.[112] Although we believe that some of the humps may possibly be induced by mechanical atrial activity, humps consistent with EAD existed before the author indicated humps in the same recording.[15, 17, 112] El-Sherif and colleagues recorded MAPs from the right ventricle in a patient with quinidine-induced long QT interval and torsades de pointes and found a distinct hump on phase 3 repolarization characteristic of EAD, which was synchronous with the U wave and its amplitude correlated to that of the U wave.[105] Ventricular ectopic beats arose close to the peak of EADs after long cycle lengths. With rapid ventricular pacing, the EADs and U waves were suppressed together with the ventricular ectopic beats. Habbab and coworkers reported a case of procainamide-induced torsades de pointes with simultaneous MAP recordings from the right and left ventricular endocardial sites.[34] They found a markedly prolonged MAPd and a "hump" deflection on the repolarization phase compatible with EAD from the right ventricle. Shimizu and associates reported that EAD was induced by isoprenaline infusion in congenital long-QT patients but not in the control patients, with significant prolongation of MAPd in the long-QT patients when compared with shortening of MAPd in the control patients.[39] This study further confirms the existence of primary repolarization abnormalities in patients with congenital long-QT syndrome and suggests an important role of sympathetic activity in the exaggeration of the repolarization abnormalities.

The above evidences support for the lengthened RT and ventricular tachyarrhythmias found in patients with acquired or idiopathic long-QT syndromes. Further studies in these patients and in patients with other triggered arrhythmias using MAPs are needed and care should be taken to eliminate mechanical artifacts that may mimic EAD on MAP recordings.[15, 17, 113] The application of MAP recordings in this area may be extended to evaluation of effects of antiarrhythmic drugs because the disappearance or decrease in amplitude of the EAD is a good parameter.[114]

MEASUREMENT OF DISPERSION OF REPOLARIZATION

Reentrant activity is considered a major underlying mechanism for ventricular arrhythmias, and the presence of increased dispersion of repolarization may create the electrophysiologic environment that favors reentry.[115-117] Monophasic action potentials reliably represent the local repolarization at the recording site. The spatial time differences of MAPd, RT, and AT measured at multiple sites and their changes after electric or pharmacologic interventions are unique for evaluating dispersions of repolarization in vivo.

Dispersion of RT is defined as the time difference between the ends of simultaneously recorded MAPs. It measures the disparity of the termination of repolarization, which is influenced by the dispersion of both AT and MAPd. For accurate determination and practical convenience in manual and computerized measurements, we take the point of 90% repolarization as the end of a MAP.[38] Kuo and colleagues used this measurement in their series of experimental studies and established the links between the dispersion of repolarization and the genesis of ventricular arrhythmias.[115, 118-120] The dispersion of RT is commonly used in clinical studies.[27, 31, 41, 94]

Dispersion of MAPd is defined as the time difference of the MAPd90 between simultaneously recorded MAPs. This measurement eliminates the contribution of the disparity of AT to the dispersion of RT and thereby reflects the pure disparity of the local repolarizations. It is used in the clinical studies as a main parameter or together with other parameters in evaluation of the dispersion.[27, 31, 36, 39, 41, 94]

Dispersion of AT is defined as the time difference of AT between simultaneously recorded MAPs, which represents the disparity of the local conduction delay.[27, 31, 34, 41, 115]

Premature dispersion is that measured during programmed extrastimulation, which is usually more pronounced than that measured during sinus rhythm or pacing.[36, 115] The maximal premature dispersion is often seen in the extra beats at coupling intervals within 30 milliseconds, close to the VERP but usually not in the earliest extra beat because the latter tends to be associated with the slowest conduction and the greatest MAPd shortening.[118] The premature dispersion at the time of induction of ventricular arrhythmias is also measured and termed critical dispersion.[119]

Adjacent dispersion is that measured between two adjacent sites with the same AT during ventricular pacing, which helps to remove the contribution of AT to the dispersion of repolarization. In one study, Morgan and coworkers found that the adjacent dispersion in patients with ventricular tachycardia was not different from the control during steady-state but was significantly exaggerated after programmed extrastimulation.[36]

We are of the opinion that the dispersion should be measured in all the three parameters (i.e., dispersions of RT, MAPd and AT). This is especially helpful in specifying either the disparity of local repolarization, conduction delay, or both being responsible for the genesis of ventricular arrhythmias in patients with different pathophysiologic substrates.[121] In the clinical setting, extensive endocardial mapping is often not practically possible. The MAPs are usually recorded using one catheter at one site at a time or two catheters at selected sites, which limits the extensive use of this method in practice.[31,36-38,94]

The normal reference values for evaluating dispersion of repolarization have not been well established in man. In patients with coronary artery or valvular diseases, Franz and associates recorded left ventricular endocardial MAPs and reported that the dispersion of MAPd ranged from 21 to 64 milliseconds (Table 25-3).[31] In patients undergoing coronary bypass or aortic valve replacement, Cowan and colleagues recorded left ventricular epicardial MAPs and found that the dispersion of MAPd ranged from 21 to 89 milliseconds (see Table 25-3).[41] Morgan and coworkers report that in patients with supraventricular tachycardia or sinus node disease, the geographic dispersion of MAPd in right ventricular endocardium ranged from 20 to 45 milliseconds and from 25 to 60 milliseconds during right ventricular pacing at cycle lengths of 430 and 600 milliseconds, respectively (see Table 25-3).[36] These reported data were obtained from multiple myocardial sites and in patients with relatively normal ventricles and therefore can be used as references in evaluating the dispersion of

repolarization. It is also important to measure the dynamic changes of dispersion during programmed stimulation, sympathetic stimulation, or pharmacologic intervention, which may possess more clinical relevance than the absolute values (Fig. 25-10).

Experimental evidence links a marked increase in dispersion of repolarization to the induction of ventricular arrhythmias.[27,115,118-120] By recording six MAPs simultaneously from the epicardium of the modified canine thermal-lesion model, Kuo and associates found that when the premature dispersion of repolarization increased up to 111 ± 16 milliseconds, ventricular arrhythmias could be induced by programmed stimulation in all dogs.[118,119] Gotoh recorded four MAPs simultaneously from the surface of the right and left ventricles in dogs and found that the increased dispersion of ventricular repolarization played an important role in the induction of ventricular fibrillation.[27]

In the clinical setting, an increased dispersion of repolarization was found in patients with long-QT syndrome and believed responsible for the polymorphic ventricular tachycardia or torsades de pointes.[34,35,39,93,110,122] Habbab and El-Sherif recorded two MAPs simultaneously from both ventricles in a case of procainamide-induced torsades de pointes and found marked dispersion of MAPd, ranging from 180 to 280 milliseconds, and marked dispersion of local AT between right and left ventricular recording sites during torsades de pointes.[34] Nonsustained runs of torsades de pointes in this case consistently arose from the right ventricular site when the left ventricular site had already completed repolarization. It was believed that the persistent dispersion of repolarization in subsequent short cycles could create the electrophysiologic prerequisites for the torsades de pointes.

Shimizu and colleagues found that dispersion of MAPd90 between the left and right ventricular endocar-

TABLE 25-3. The Dispersion of Ventricular Activation Time, Monophasic Acting Potential Duration, and Repolarization Time in Patients With Relatively Normal Ventricles

Site	Rhythm	Patients (n)	Sites (n)	AT	MAPd90	RT
Left endocardial[31]	Sinus or RA pacing*	7	5–11	24.9 ± 6.1 (13–32)	41.4 ± 14.6 (21–64)	26.4 ± 12.0 (10–46)
Left epicardial[41]	RA pacing†	10	8–10	27.1 ± 7.0 (16–34)	39.7 ± 19.4 (21–89)	26.7 ± 11.4 (15–55)
Right endocardial[36]	RV pacing, CL = 430, CL = 600	10	9–12 8–15	— —	30‡ (20–45) 40‡ (25–60)	— —

RT, repolarization time; RV, right ventricle.
Data not available; See Table 25-1 for other abbreviations.
*If sinus rate varied more than 5 beats/min, pacing with the lowest rate to overdrive the spontaneous rhythm; † RA pacing at rate 10-20 beat/min above the spontaneous rate; ‡ Median.

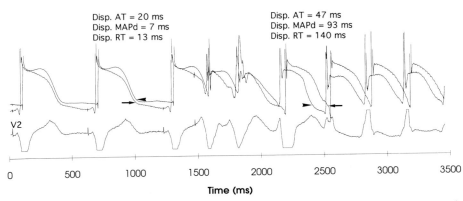

Figure 25-10. Monophasic action potential recordings from the right ventricular apex (*arrow*) and outflow tract (*arrow head*) during ventricular programmed stimulation in a patient with ischemic heart disease, showing that a sustained ventricular tachycardia (VT) was induced when the dispersion of repolarization time (*RT*) increased from 13 milliseconds in the drive-train beat to 140 milliseconds in the premature beat immediately before the initiation of the VT. Note that the sequence of activation between these two sites changed in the premature beat immediately before the VT initiation. The dispersion of RT during the VT was constant and less pronounced than in the premature beat.

dium was increased by isoprenaline infusion in long-QT patients, whereas it was not changed in the control patients.[39] This result suggests that sympathetic stimulation plays an important role in the exaggeration of the repolarization abnormalities and may be, together with the occurrence of EAD, responsible for the ventricular arrhythmias in these patients. Linker and coworkers performed right ventricular endocardial mapping of four to six sites in two patients with congenital long-QT syndrome and demonstrated a significant dispersion of repolarization, up to 50 and 65 milliseconds, which was excessive compared with the reference values.[35, 36]

The role of dispersion in the genesis of sustained monomorphic ventricular tachycardia has not been well clarified, however. Morgan and associates report that the geographic dispersion of MAPd in their 22 patients with ventricular tachycardia was not significantly different from the control patients.[36] The adjacent dispersion during programmed ventricular stimulation, however, was significantly higher in patients with right or left ventricular dysplasia or both than in patients with ischemic heart disease or control patients. The dispersion of AT and that of RT were not evaluated in this study but evidence that the dispersion of AT is more evident than that of refractory period in patients with monomorphic ventricular tachycardia has been obtained in another study.[121] We recorded MAPs simultaneously from two sites in the right ventricle in 24 patients with documented monomorphic ventricular tachycardia and found that dispersion of repolarization is linked to the inducibility of the ventricular tachycardia and that dispersion of both AT and MAPd contributed to the dispersion of RT in these patients. Our result suggests that the increased dispersion of repolarization plays an impor-

tant role in the genesis of a monomorphic ventricular tachycardia.[38]

Monophasic action potential recordings provide a valuable tool for evaluating the dispersion of ventricular repolarization; however, the clinical difficulties entailed in recording MAPs simultaneously from multiple sites limit their use.

DETECTION OF MYOCARDIAL ISCHEMIA

Early ionic and electric changes that occur during myocardial ischemia are involved in the development of ventricular arrhythmias and abnormalities of myocardial contractility.[6] These changes can provide important information needed for clinical use and research. The initial change, however, is confined to a small region of the endocardium; the surface ECG is usually not able to reveal it. Even in the later settings of myocardial ischemia, surface ECG changes reflect the electric activity of the whole heart; therefore, no information of local cellular electrophysiology can be obtained. Floating microelectrodes and unipolar electrograms have been used in attempt to study these changes. Various factors limit the value of these methods for clinical applications, however.[25] Compared with the above-mentioned methods, MAP recordings in vivo provide the closest assessment of the cellular electrophysiologic changes that occur during ischemia.

Cellular electrophysiologic studies show that in severely ischemic tissue, the action potential is characterized by a greatly diminished upstroke velocity and a smaller amplitude. The action potential duration increased initially, followed by reduction and changes of the time course of recovery of excitability. Consequently, conduction in the ischemic myocardium is affected. These electric changes are believed to have important consequences for the development of ischemia-induced arrhythmias and are sensitive and reliable parameters for localizing ischemic and infarcted area in experimental studies.[24, 51–54, 123, 124]

Monophasic action potential recordings have also been used in the clinical setting to detect myocardial ischemia. Donaldson and colleagues recorded MAPs during pacing stress tests in 10 patients with reversible myocardial ischemia and found a decrease in MAP amplitude and duration in the ischemic zone but no changes in the normal zone.[125] The MAP changes occurred before the clinical symptoms and ECG abnormalities of ischemia. Within 30 seconds after nitroglycerin administration and cessation of angina, the MAP changes rapidly reversed, preceding the reversal of ECG changes. The investigators believed that a decrease of MAPd by more than 5% may indicate early ischemia. Similar evidence that MAP recordings are more sensitive and are an earlier indicator of myocardial ischemia than the surface ECG has been obtained in other studies.[23, 25]

Taggart and coworkers recorded epicardial MAPs from eight patients undergoing coronary bypass surgery and found a significant decrease of MAP amplitude and shortening of MAPd in addition to loss of diastolic potential during the graft occlusion of 90 seconds.[40] These changes reversed on reperfusion. The same group recorded MAPs from the right ventricular septum in 20 patients undergoing balloon angioplasty and found that of a total 25 occlusions of the left anterior descending coronary artery during balloon inflation, 19 showed less than 5% shortening of MAPd, five showed between 5% and 10%, and one showed 16.4%.[26] The shortening of the MAPd occurred concomitantly with an ST-segment shift (Fig. 25-11).[26]

John and associates recorded endocardial MAPs from normal and ischemic areas that were identified by the simultaneous use of a radionuclide tracer in 26 patients with ischemic heart disease.[126] They found that during atrial pacing, the shortening of MAPd90 was significantly greater in the ischemic areas (33.8 ± 9.7 milliseconds) than in the normal areas (22.0 ± 4.8 milliseconds). This confirmed the effect of local myocardial ischemia on the MAPd with strong clinical evidence and validates the applicability of the endocardial MAPs for the detection of ischemia. The method may be further used in assessing therapeutic interventions aimed at the early phase of ischemia.

A limitation of MAP recordings in detection of myocardial ischemia is that the upstroke velocity and the amplitude of the MAP are influenced by the contact pressure of the MAP catheter on the myocardium. Therefore, the change in myocardial wall tension caused by ischemia may underlie the MAP changes by the intracellular ionic alterations. This complicates the interpretation of the MAP changes during ischemia. The available MAP catheter with

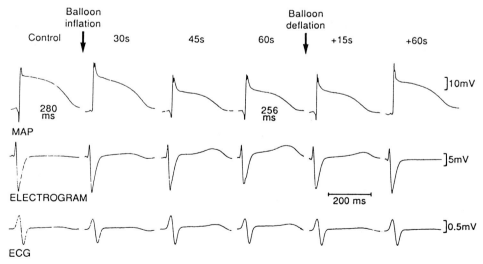

Figure 25-11. Right ventricular monophasic action potential (MAP), intracardiac electrogram, and electrocardiogram (V5) recorded during balloon angioplasty of the left anterior descending coronary artery in a patient. Note that during the 60 seconds of balloon inflation, the MAP duration decreased concomitant with the ST elevation in the intracardiac electrogram, whereas no marked change can be seen in the electrocardiogram. (Reproduced with permission from Taggart P, Sutton P, John R, Hayward R, Swanton H. The epicardial electrogram: a quantitative assessment during balloon angioplasty incorporating monophasic action potential recordings. Br Heart J 1989;62(5):342–52.)

an intraluminal stylet is more elastic and resilient, making the MAP more sensitive to electrophysiologic than to mechanical changes.[7] With improvement of the technology, MAP recordings can provide more information of theoretic and practical significance in this area.

LOCAL ACTIVATION AND THE GENESIS OF T WAVE

In conventional recordings of epicardial or endocardial electrograms, the local AT is usually determined at the maximal slope, maximal amplitude or onset of the bipolar electrogram, and the intrinsic deflection of the unipolar electrogram. In practice, the determination of AT from these multiphasic deflections is sometimes difficult.[127, 128] The upstroke of MAP is sharp, unambiguous, and precisely represents the local AT, however.[10, 12, 129] Thus, not only repolarization but also activation can be studied better on MAP recordings than on the conventional electrograms, which has greatly facilitated study on the development of the T wave in surface ECGs, both experimentally and clinically.[31, 33, 41, 84, 130, 131]

In the normal ECG, the T wave has the same polarity as the QRS complex in almost all leads. This paradox of T-wave concordance has been explained by assuming that the repolarization wave travels in the direction opposite that of depolarization. This hypothesis was first verified in man by Olsson using MAP recording technique.[14] Thus, MAPs were recorded from different sites in the right ventricular endocardium and a shorter AT was found to be associated with a longer MAPd and vice versa, with the MAPs at the basal part having a significantly shorter duration than those close to the apex. Findings by Franz and coworkers further supported the hypothesis.[31] They performed MAP mapping in five to 11 endocardial sites in seven patients and in five to eight epicardial sites in three patients and found a close inverse relation between MAPd and AT, independent of the recording site, so that progressively later activation was associated with progressively earlier repolarization. These data suggest a transmural gradient of repolarization, with earlier repolarization occurring at the epicardium.

Cowan and associates studied epicardial activation and repolarization sequences in patients with upright or inverted T waves.[41] They found an inverse relation between the MAPd and AT in patients with upright T waves. As a consequence, activation and repolarization proceeded in opposite directions, and the dispersion of MAPd was less than the dispersion of AT. In patients with T-wave inversion, there was no relation between MAPd and AT; the repolarization sequence resembled the activation sequence and the dispersion of MAPd was greater than that of AT. Thus, the epicardial repolarization gradients are related to the configuration of the T wave. Chen and colleagues studied the patterns of epicardial activation and repolarization in patients with right ventricular hypertrophy, using MAPs recorded by a computer mapping system.[132] They found that the right ventricle completed activation and repolarization later than the left and that the distribution of T wave morphologies is nonuniform, with predominantly positive T waves over the left ventricle and negative or biphasic T waves over the right ventricle. These findings further support the above-mentioned hypothesis on the development of the T wave.

With the increasing knowledge obtained from MAP recordings and other electrophysiologic studies, the development of the T wave, that of the U wave, and their clinical relevance will be further clarified.[103, 105, 107]

MONOPHASIC ACTION POTENTIAL AND MECHANOELECTRIC FEEDBACK

Most studies of ventricular arrhythmias have concerned the abnormal electric behavior of the heart. The evidence that mechanical changes can initiate electrophysiologic changes, however, made the mechanoelectric feedback, or contraction–excitation recoupling, another possible mechanism underlying the occurrence of ventricular arrhythmias.[133–138] In vitro studies demonstrate that mechanical changes are capable of influencing the AP duration, excitability, and ERP and of inducing apparently abnormal depolarization to produce ventricular arrhythmia.[137] Monophasic action potential recordings have played a definitive role in verifying this hypothesis in vivo.

Lab and coworkers and many others have demonstrated that mechanical or pharmacologic reduction of the load is followed by prolongation of the MAPd and vice versa.[46, 134, 135, 137] Franz and associates found also that the increases of the left ventricular volume and pressure in canine models resulted in linear decreases in MAP amplitude, MAPd20, and the appearance of the EADs.[46] These loading-induced changes were associated with occurrence of ectopic ventricular beats.

In patients undergoing balloon pulmonary valvuloplasty, Levine and colleagues found that MAPd was significantly shortened and EAD developed during acute right ventricular outflow tract obstruction, whereas the MAPd was prolonged after successful valvuloplasty.[139] In patients undergoing cardiopulmonary bypass, Taggart and colleagues found that when the systolic pressure increased, the left ventricular epicardial MAPd was shortened and a strong correlation between the absolute MAPd and systolic pressure was obtained.[140] This was later confirmed in conscious man.[141]

Controversy also exists in this area. Calkins and coworkers applied an increased end-diastolic volume to 14 isolated canine ventricles and found no or little effect on MAPd and MAP contour under ejecting or isovolumic conditions.[142] The same group found also that two- to three-fold increases in left ventricular wall stress (induced by transient proximal aortic occlusion in dogs) resulted in less than 5% MAPd shortening.[143] Early afterdepolarizations were observed in less than 10% of the occlusions and were not correlated to the magnitude or rate of the loading change. Based on these findings, they believe that alterations in volume load are of little electrophysiologic or arrhythmogenic importance, whereas load-induced ventricular ectopy is due to stretch-induced automaticity rather than to triggered activity or reentry.

The effect of mechanoelectric feedback on repolarization and its clinical relevance are still uncertain, and further study using MAP recordings and other electrophysiologic methods is needed. Based on the present data, it is commonly believed that even if mechanically induced changes are not central to causes of arrhythmogenesis, they at least contribute to the genesis of arrhythmia in the altered electrophysiologic milieu of regional ischemia and heart failure.[137]

OTHER APPLICATIONS

Atrial Monophasic Action Potential Recordings

Monophasic action potentials are most frequently recorded from the ventricles and are extensively used in the study of ventricular arrhythmias. In contrast, the atrial MAP recordings have been shown to be important in the study of atrial arrhythmias by Olsson and associates and Gavrilescu and colleagues.[77, 144–148]

Monophasic Action Potential Recordings in Electrolyte Disorders

Human atrial or ventricular MAPs have been recorded at different concentrations of serum calcium and potassium. The observed changes are similar to those in corresponding in vitro experiments (i.e., high serum potassium markedly shortens the MAPd, whereas low calcium results in a marked prolongation of repolarization).[4, 149]

Monophasic Action Potential Recordings in Thyroid Disorders

Monophasic action potential recordings have been performed in patients with hyper- and hypothyroid functions.[77, 150, 151] Significant prolongations of atrial and

ventricular MAP were observed in patients with hypothyroidism. Thyroid hormone substitution resulted in normalization of atrial and ventricular MAPd. The findings are in agreement with the results of the earlier experimental studies, in which accelerated repolarization was observed as a consequence of hyperthyroid activity and delayed repolarization was found during decreased thyroid function.[152]

Monitoring the Effect of Radiofrequency Ablation

Franz and coworkers used an ablation-MAP combination catheter, which has a small MAP electrode imbedded into the tip of the distal ablation electrode, to record MAPs at the ablation site during the delivery of radiofrequency energy in dogs.[153] They found that after ablation, the reduction of the MAP amplitude to less than 20% of the baseline value was associated with a large and permanent myocardial lesion and the reduction to 35% to 65% of the baseline was associated with smaller and temporary lesions. Thus, the MAP may serve as an instantaneous feedback about the magnitude and permanence of the myocardial destruction.

COMPUTERIZED MONOPHASIC ACTION POTENTIAL MEASUREMENT

The MAP measurements are traditionally made by manual methods on paper recordings, which is time-consuming, especially if detailed measurement in a long-term recording is needed. It is almost impossible to measure beat by beat manually, and the result obtained by selected measurement may lose important information. In addition, visual judgment of repolarization levels may not be accurate when the amplitude of the MAP is low and the same applies to MAPd measurements. Computerized MAP measurement has consequently been developed, which is reported to be quick and accurate, with 1-millisecond resolution at a sampling rate of 1 kHz.[44, 47, 154–157]

Hirsch and associates reported the first application of computer-based analysis of MAP recordings in man.[155, 158] Their system featured off-line data acquisition from tape-recorded MAPs at a sampling rate of 1 kHz by a minicomputer. It allowed user-controlled automatic measurements of MAPd90, MAPd50, V_{max}, and AT as well as MAP amplitude.

Kanaan and colleagues report a microcomputer system that allows off-line data acquisition of MAP signals, with a sampling rate of 1 kHz and automatic measurement of AT and MAPd.[44, 61] This system also provides a new algorithm for detecting the end of the repolarization phase, using the intersection of the baseline and the tangent of the peak negative slope (dV/dT) during repolarization (MAPd$_{tangent}$). The algorithm allows estimation of MAPd90 even if a subsequent premature beat comes before the completion of 90% repolarization. This system was further used to reevaluate the clinically used protocol for determination of VERP and induction of tachyarrhythmias in an experimental study.[61]

A similar computerized system has been clinically used in our laboratory since 1991.[45] It features on-line acquisition of multichannel MAP signals and one-channel ECG and on-screen–monitored automatic measurement of AT, MAPd (at three different levels of repolarization), RT, MAPd$_{tangent}$, MAP amplitude, V$_{max}$, rising time, R$_{max}$, V$_{max}$%, and R$_{max}$%, with the capability of manual corrections. The MAPd90 and MAPd$_{tangent}$ in early extra beats can be estimated from an extrapolated line along the V$_{max}$, as mentioned earlier. A digital filter is equipped to minimize 50-Hz noise, which exists in our early recordings. The resulting values can be exported to any database or graphics program for further analysis. Using this computer system, it is possible to measure every beat of a recording with two channels of MAPs and more than 300 consecutive beats in a few minutes. This allows determination of steady-state MAPd individually (see Fig. 25-6) and more detailed analyses of the rate-dependent variation of the MAPd, the restitution curve (see Fig. 25-5), and the relation between conduction and refractoriness. In addition to the advantage in speed, information with potential theoretic and clinical significance may also be obtained from the computerized measurement.[45]

Computerized MAP measurement is reliable, quick, and accurate. With the rapid development of computer technique and lower computer cost, it will not be surprising to see computerized measurement replace the manual method in the near future.

LIMITATIONS OF THE MONOPHASIC ACTION POTENTIAL TECHNIQUE

Compared with AP, the main limitation of MAPs is their inability to provide information on absolute voltage of resting and action-potential amplitude or on absolute upstroke velocity. The amplitude and upstroke velocity of MAP are related to the contact pressure of the catheter against the myocardium. Any change that influences the contact pressure, such as the changes in myocardial wall tension, may change the upstroke velocity and the amplitude of the MAP. This can be minimized or abolished by using highly elastic catheters and careful catheter positioning, which helps in maintaining a steady contact pressure.[12] Moreover, the MAP upstroke is commonly contaminated by the intrinsic deflection, as mentioned above.

These phenomena have markedly hampered the interpretation on the depolarization phase of MAPs. To eliminate the influence of MAP amplitude and obtain more representative information from the depolarization phase, we use a relative slope of the upstroke (V$_{max}$%), which is the depolarizing velocity divided by the MAP amplitude.[45]

Further limitations of MAP recordings are caused by the mechanical activity of the heart. A distorted MAP may be recorded because of the change of the contact pressure caused by irregular contractions, such as a premature beat or programmed stimulation, and even by the rhythmic movement of a beating heart. A ventricular MAP recording can be influenced by the mechanical activity of the atrium and the ventricle per se. Similarly, an atrial MAP recording is affected by the ventricular mechanical activity as well as that of the atrium (see Fig. 25-3). The mechanical artifacts of ventricular or atrial origin limit the interpretation of possible true pathoelectrophysiologic phenomena concomitant with mechanical cardiac activity. For instance, the atrial-movement artifacts in ventricular MAP recordings may mimic afterdepolarization in patients with long-QT syndrome.[9,17] Although signal stability and reproducibility at multiple recording sites are used as indicators of true electrophysiologic findings, making a reliable distinction between true and false mechanical changes is still one of the greatest challenges of the MAP method.[12,17,159]

Although long-term recording (up to 3 hours) of MAPs from the same endocardial site without further manipulation of the catheter have been reported, a gradual decrease of MAP amplitude is often seen in our practice when the recording time is longer than 30 minutes.[7,160] This may be due to the loss of contact pressure and can be solved by sending the catheter a few millimeters forward. Sometimes, MAP amplitude cannot resume to the level of more than 15 mV, despite catheter manipulation. This may indicate injury of the myocardial cells underneath the electrode and requires repositioning of the catheter. In practice, however, keeping the catheter at the same recording site is often a prerequisite for the comparison of MAP change between interventions. Thus, more careful catheter manipulation and positioning and a high elastic tip on the MAP catheter are required to ensure reliable long-term recording of MAPs.

SUMMARY

Monophasic action potential recordings provide precise information on local myocardial repolarization and activation. With the advantage of in vivo application, MAPs have been widely used in the last decade. Monophasic action potential recording is considered the method of choice for evaluating myocardial repolarization changes.

In the clinical setting, MAPs can be recorded without special difficulties from the endocardium with the contact-catheter technique in the electrophysiology laboratory and from the epicardium with electrode probes during cardiac surgery. Although the normal values of MAP parameters have not been well established in man, several sets of references are available. Using MAP recordings, rate dependence of myocardial repolarization and excitability and its clinical relevance have been well elucidated and the effects of antiarrhythmic drugs on repolarization have been thoroughly tested. Studies on EADs and dispersion of repolarization have provided more evidence concerning their relation to triggered arrhythmias in patients with long-QT syndrome. Links between dispersion of repolarization and the induction of monomorphic ventricular tachycardia have also been found. Attempts to detect early myocardial ischemia using MAP recordings yielded favorable results. Monophasic action potential recordings have also been helpful in the analysis of intracardiac conduction and in the assessment of the development of the T wave. On the controversial subject of mechanoelectric feedback, MAP recordings are the best available technique for verifying its arrhythmogenic effect. The development of computerized MAP recording and measurement may add new capabilities of clinical or theoretic significance to the MAP technique.

With further improvement of the technique and with limitations in mind, MAP recordings can provide more useful information in clinical electrophysiologic studies.

References

1. Ling G, Gerard RW: The normal membrane potential of frog sartorius fibers. J Cell Comp Physiol 1949;34:383.
2. Schütz E: Elektrophysiologie des Herzens bei einphasischer Ableitung. Ergebnisse der Physiologie 1936;38:493.
3. Korsgren M, Leskinen E, Sjostrand U, Varnauskas E: Intracardiac recording of monophasic action potentials in the human heart. Scand J Clin Lab Invest 1966;18:561.
4. Shabetai R, Surawicz B, Hammill W: Monophasic action potentials in man. Circulation 1968;38:341.
5. Olsson SB, Varnauskas E, Korsgren M: Further improved method for measuring monophasic action potentials of the intact human heart. J Electrocardiol 1971;4:19.
6. Donaldson RM, Taggart P, Swanton H, Fox K, Noble D, Richards AF: Intracardiac electrode detection of early ischaemia in man. Br Heart J 1983;50(3):213.
7. Franz MR: Long-term recording of monophasic action potentials from human endocardium. Am J Cardiol 1983;51(10):1629.
8. Olsson SB, Edvardsson N, Hirsch I, Blomström P: Methodological aspects on invasive evaluation of myocardial repolarization. In: Butrous GS, Schwartz PJ, eds. Clinical aspects of ventricular repolarization. London: Farrand Press, 1989:67.
9. Hoffman BF, Cranefield PF, Lepeschkin E, Surawicz B, Herrlich HC: Comparison of cardiac monophasic action potentials recorded by intracellular and suction electrodes. Am J Physiol 1959;196:1297.
10. Franz MR, Burkhoff D, Spurgeon H, Weisfeldt ML, Lakatta EG: In vitro validation of a new cardiac catheter technique for recording monophasic action potentials. Eur Heart J 1986;7:34.
11. Ino T, Karagueuzian HS, Hong K, Meesmann M, Mandel WJ, Peter T: Relation of monophasic action potential recorded with contact electrode to underlying transmembrane action potential properties in isolated cardiac tissues: a systematic microelectrode validation study. Cardiovasc Res 1988;22(4):255.
12. Franz MR: Method and theory of monophasic action potential recording. Prog Cardiovasc Dis 1991;33(6):347.
13. Churney L, Ohshima H: An improved suction electrode for recovery from the dog heart in situ. J Appl Physiol 1964;196:1297.
14. Olsson SB: Monophasic action potentials of right heart. Suction electrode method in clinical investigations. Göteborg: Elanders Boktryckeri AB, 1971. Thesis.
15. Olsson SB: Estimation of ventricular repolarization in man by monophasic action potential recording technique. Eur Heart J 1985;6(Suppl D):71.
16. Hirsch I, Edvardsson N, Olsson SB, Broman H: Cardiac monophasic action potentials related to intracellular action potentials. A modeling study. In: Hirsch I, ed. On the generation, analysis and clinical use of cardiac monophasic action potentials. Göteborg: Vasastadens Bokbinderi, 1984:(I)1. Thesis.
17. Olsson SB, Blomström P, Blomström-Lundqvist C, Wohlfart B: Endocardial monophasic action potentials. Correlations with intracellular electrical activity. Ann NY Acad Sci 1990;601:119.
18. Franz MR: Monophasic action potential symposium. I. Introduction. Prog Cardiovasc Dis 1991;33(6):345.
19. Surawicz B: Mechanisms of QT prolongation and arrhythmias. In: Butrous GS, Schwartz PJ, eds. Clinical aspects of ventricular repolarization. London: Farrand Press, 1988:227.
20. Olsson SB, Edvardsson N, Newell PA, Yuan S, Zeng Z: Effect of pentisomide (CM 7857) on myocardial excitation, conduction, repolarization, and refractoriness. An electrophysiological study in humans. J Cardiovasc Pharmacol 1991;18(6):849.
21. Zaza A, Malfatto G, Schwartz PJ: Sympathetic modulation of the relation between ventricular repolarization and cycle length. Circ Res 1991;68(5):1191.
22. Platia EV, Weisfeldt ML, Franz MR: Immediate quantitation of antiarrhythmic drug effect by monophasic action potential recording in coronary artery disease. Am J Cardiol 1988;61(15):1284.
23. Donaldson RM, Taggart P, Swanton H, Fox K, Rickards AF, Noble D: Effect of nitroglycerin on the electrical changes of early or subendocardial ischaemia evaluated by monophasic action potential recordings. Cardiovasc Res 1984;18(1):7.
24. Franz MR, Flaherty JT, Platia EV, Bulkley BH, Weisfeldt ML: Localization of regional myocardial ischemia by record-

ing of monophasic action potentials. Circulation 1984; 69(3):593.

25. Mohabir R, Franz MR, Clusin WT: In vivo electrophysiological detection of myocardial ischemia through monophasic action potential recording. Prog Cardiovasc Dis 1991; 34(1):15.

26. Taggart P, Sutton P, John R, Hayward R, Swanton H: The epicardial electrogram: a quantitative assessment during balloon angioplasty incorporating monophasic action potential recordings. Br Heart J 1989;62(5):342.

27. Gotoh M: A study on the role of the dispersion of repolarization in the induction of ventricular fibrillation using the suction electrode technique. Nippon Ika Daigaku Zasshi 1989;56(4):349.

28. Endresen K, Amlie JP: Electrical restitution and conduction intervals of ventricular premature beats in man: influence of heart rate. Pacing Clin Electrophysiol 1989;12(8):1347.

29. Franz MR, Chin MC, Sharkey HR, Griffin JC, Scheinman MM: A new single catheter technique for simultaneous measurement of action potential duration and refractory period in vivo. J Am Coll Cardiol 1990;16(4):878.

30. Franz MR, Cohen T, Lee R, Lee M, Griffin JC, Scheinman MM: Correlation between action potential duration and effective refractory period in vivo: results from 25 patients with normal right ventricular myocardium. Pacing Clin Electrophysiol 1991;14:703. Abstract.

31. Franz MR, Bargheer K, Rafflenbeul W, Haverich A, Lichtlen PR: Monophasic action potential mapping in human subjects with normal electrocardiograms: direct evidence for the genesis of the T wave. Circulation 1987;75(2):379.

32. Cowan JC, Griffiths CJ, Hilton CJ, et al: Epicardial repolarization mapping in man. Eur Heart J 1987;8(9):952.

33. Runnalls ME, Sutton PM, Taggart P, Treasure T: Modifications of electrode design for recording monophasic action potentials in animals and humans. Am J Physiol 1987;253(5Pt 2):H1315.

34. Habbab MA, El-Sherif N: Drug-induced de pointes: role of early afterdepolarizations and dispersion of repolarization. Am J Med 1990;89:241.

35. Linker NJ, Camm AJ, Ward DE: Dynamics of ventricular repolarisation in the congenital long QT syndromes. Br Heart J 1991;66(3):230.

36. Morgan JM, Cunningham D, Rowland E: Dispersion of monophasic action potential duration: demonstrable in humans after premature ventricular extrastimulation but not in steady state. J Am Coll Cardiol 1992;19(6):1244.

37. Yuan S, Wholfart B, Rasumussen HS, Olsson SB, B-Lundqvist C: Effect of dofetilide on cardiac repolarization in patients with ventricular tachycardia. A study using simultaneous monophasic action potential recordings from two sites in the right ventricle. Eur Heart J 1994;15:514.

38. Yuan S, Wholfart B, Olsson SB, B-Lundqvist C: Dispersion of repolarization in patients with ventricular tachycardia. A study using simultaneous monophasic action potential recordings from two sites in the right ventricle. 1993. Submitted.

39. Shimizu W, Ohe T, Kurita T, et al: Early afterdepolarizations induced by isoproterenol in patients with congenital long QT syndrome. Circulation 1991;84(5):1915.

40. Taggart P, Sutton P, Runnalls M, et al: Use of monophasic action potential recordings during routine coronary-artery bypass surgery as an index of localised myocardial ischaemia. Lancet 1986;1(8496):1462.

41. Cowan JC, Hilton CJ, Griffiths CJ, et al: Sequence of epicardial repolarisation and configuration of the T wave. Br Heart J 1988;60(5):424.

42. Kuo CS, Surawicz B: Ventricular monophasic action potential changes associated with neurogenic T wave abnormalities and isoproterenol administration in dogs. Am J Cardiol 1976;38(2):170.

43. Olsson SB: Right ventricular monophasic action potentials during regular rhythm. A heart catheterization study in man. Acta Med Scand 1972;191(3):145.

44. Kanaan N, Jenkins J, Kadish A: An automatic microcomputer system for analysis of monophasic action potentials. Pacing Clin Electrophysiol 1990;13(2):196.

45. Yuan S, B-Lundqvist C, Olsson SB, Wholfart B: Clinical application of a computer system for recording and measuring monophasic action potentials. 1994. Submitted.

46. Franz MR, Burkhoff D, Yue DT, Sagawa K: Mechanically induced action potential changes and arrhythmia in isolated and in situ canine hearts. Cardiovasc Res 1989;23(3):213.

47. Duker G, Almgren O, Axenborg J: Computerized evaluation of drug-induced changes in guinea-pig epicardial monophasic action potentials. Pharmacol Toxicol 1988;63(2):85.

48. Duker DG: Frequency dependent effects of tocainide, quinidine, and flecainide on conduction as reflected in the rise time of the monophasic action potential in the isolated guinea pig heart. Cardiovasc Res 1991;25(3):217.

49. Brorson L, Olsson SB: Atrial repolarization in healthy males. Studies with programmed stimulation and monophasic action potential recordings. Acta Med Scand 1976;199(6):447.

50. Edvardsson N, Hirsh I, Olsson SB: Right ventricular monophasic action potentials in healty young men. Pacing Clin Electrophysiol 1984;7(5):813.

51. Kingaby RO, Lab MJ, Cole AW, Palmer TN: Relation between monophasic action potential duration, ST segment elevation, and regional myocardial blood flow after coronary occulusion in the pig. Cardiovasc Res 1986;20(10):740.

52. Dilly SG, Lab MJ: Changes in monophasic action potential duration during the first hour of regional myocardial ischaemia in the anaesthetised pig. Cardiovasc Res 1987;21(12):908.

53. Blake K, Clusin WT, Franz MR, Smith NA: Mechanism of depolarization in the ischaemic dog heart: discrepancy between T-Q potentials and potassium accumulation. J Physiol (Lond) 1988;397:307.

54. Dilly SG, Lab MJ: Electrophysiological alternans and restitution during acute regional ischaemia in myocardium of anaesthetized pig. J Physiol (Lond) 1988;402:315.

55. Hoffman BF, Cranefield PF: Electrophysiology of the heart. New York: McGraw-Hill, 1960.

56. Brorson L, Olsson SB: Right atrial monophasic action potential in healthy males. Studies during spontaneous sinus rhythm and atrial pacing. Acta Med Scand 1976;199(6):433.

57. Brorson L, Olsson SB: Human atrial conduction with reference to heart rate and refractory periods. Acta Med Scand 1977;201(1–2):111.

58. Brorson L, Conradson TB, Olsson B, Varnauskas E: Right atrial monophasic action potential and effective refractory periods in relation to physical training and maximal heart rate. Cardiovasc Res 1976;10(2):160.

59. Boyett MR, Jewell BR: A study of the factors responsible for rate-dependent shortening of the action potential in mammalian ventricular muscles. J Physiol (Lond) 1978;285:359.

60. Boyett M, Fedida D: Changes in the electrical activity of dog cardiac Purkinje fibres at high heart rates. J Physiol (Lond) 1984;35:361.

61. Kanaan N, Jenkins J, Childs K, Ge YZ, Kadish A: Monophasic action potential duration during programmed electrical stimulation. Pacing Clin Electrophysiol 1991;14(6):1049.

62. Rosenbaum DS, Kaplan DT, Kanai A, et al: Repolarization inhomogeneities in ventricular myocardium change dynamically with abrupt cycle length shortening. Circulation 1991;84(3):1333.

63. Olsson SB, Varnauskas E: Right ventricular monophasic action potentials in man. Effect of abrupt changes of cycle length and of atrial fibrillation. Acta Med Scand 1972;191(3):159.

64. Franz MR, Schaefer J, Schoettler M, Seed WA, Noble MIM: Electrical and mechanical restitution of the human heart at different rates of stimulation. Circ Res 1983;53:815.

65. Litovsky SL, Antzelevitch C: Rate dependence of action potential duration and refractoriness in canine ventricular endocardium differs from that of epicardium: role of the transient outward current. J Am Coll Cardiol 1989;14(4):1053.

66. Franz M, Schöttler M, Schaefer J, Seed WA: Simultaneous recording of monophasic action potentials and contractile force from the human heart. Klin Wochenschr 1980;58(24):1357.

67. Seed WA, Noble MI, Oldershaw P, et al: Relation of human cardiac action potential duration to the interval between beats: implications for the validity of rate corrected QT interval (QTc). Br Heart J 1987;57(1):32.

68. Morgan JM, Cunningham AD, Rowland E: Relationship of the effective refractory period and monophasic action potential duration after a step increase in pacing frequency. Pacing Clin Electrophysiol 1990;13(8):1002.

69. Morgan JM, Cunningham D, Rowland E: Electrical restitution in the endocardium of the intact human right ventricle. Br Heart J 1992;67(1):42.

70. Wohlfart B: Relationships between peak forfe, action potential duration, and stimulus interval in rabbit myocardium. Acta Physiol Scand 1979;196:1297.

71. Franz MR, Swerdlow CD, Liem LB, Schaefer J: Cycle length dependence of human action potential duration in vivo. Effects of single extrastimuli, sudden sustained rate acceleration and deceleration, and different steady-state frequencies. J Clin Invest 1988;82(3):972.

72. Nademanee K, Stevenson WG, Weiss JN, et al: Frequency-dependent effects of quinidine on the ventricular action potential and QRS duration in humans. Circulation 1990;81(3):790.

73. Lee RJ, Liem LB, Cohen TJ, Franz MR: Relation between repolarization and refractoriness in the human ventricle: cycle length dependence and effect of procainamide. J Am Coll Cardiol 1992;19:614.

74. O'Donoghue S, Platia EV: Monophasic action potential recordings: evaluation of antiarrhythmic drugs. Prog Cardiovasc Dis 1991;34:1.

75. Olsson SB: Class III antiarrhythmic action. In: Vaughan Williams EM, ed. Antiarrhythmic drugs. Berlin & Heidelberg: Springer-Verlag, 1989:323.

76. Franz MR, Costard A: Frequency-dependent effects on quinidine on the relationship between action potential duration and refractoriness in the canine heart in situ. Circulation 1988;77(5):1177.

77. Gavrilescu S, Luca C, Streian C, Lungu G, Deutsch G: Monophasic action potentials of right atrium and electrophysiological properties of AV conducting system in patients with hypothyroidism. Br Heart J 1976;38(12):1350.

78. Gavrilescu S, Dragulescu SI, Luca C, Streian C, Comsulea L, Popovici V: The effects of quinidine on the monophasic action potential of the right atrium in patients with atrial fibrillation. Agressologie 1976;17(2):111.

79. Edvardsson N, Hirsch I, Olsson SB: Acute effects of lignocaine, procainamide, metoprolol, digoxin and atropine on human myocardial refractoriness. Cardiovasc Res 1984;18(8):463.

80. Endresen K, Amlie JP, Forfang K: Effects of disopyramide on repolarisation and intraventricular conduction in man. Eur J Clin Pharmacol 1988;35(5):467.

81. Endresen K, Amlie JP: Acute effects of lidocaine on repolarization and conduction in patients with coronary artery disease. Clin Pharmacol Ther 1989;45(4):387.

82. Olsson SB, Harper RW: Mexiletine effect on monophasic action potential (MAP) of right ventricle in man. Acta Med Scand 1978;615:93.

83. Harper RW, Olsson SB, Varnauskas E: Effect of mexiletine on monophasic action potentials recorded from the right ventricle in man. Cardiovasc Res 1979;13(6):303.

84. Olsson SB, Edvardsson N: Clinical electrophysiologic study of antiarrhythmic properties of flecainide: acute intraventricular delayed conduction and prolonged repolarization in regular paced and premature beats using intracardiac monophasic action potentials with programmed stimulation. Am Heart J 1981;102(5):864.

85. Edvardsson N, Olsson SB: Effects of acute and chronic beta-receptor blockade on ventricular repolarisation in man. Br Heart J 1981;45(6):628.

86. Echt DS, Berte LE, Clusin WT, Samuelsson RG, Harrison DC, Mason JW: Prolongation of the human cardiac monophasic action potential by sotalol. Am J Cardiol 1982;50(5):1082.

87. Duff HJ, Roden DM, Brorson L, et al: Electrophysiologic actions of high plasma concentrations of propranolol in human subjects. J Am Coll Cardiol 1983;2(6):1134.

88. Endresen K, Amlie JP: Effects of propranolol on ventricular repolarization in man. Eur J Clin Pharmacol 1990;39(2):123.

89. Olsson SB, Brorson L, Varnauskas E: Class 3 antiarrhythmic action in man. Observations from monophasic action potential recordings and amiodarone treatment. Br Heart J 1973;35(12):1255.

90. Blomström P, Bodnar J, Edvardsson N, B-Lundqvist C, Olsson SB: Acute effect of intravenous amiodarone on ventricular refractoriness and repolarization. Pacing Clin Electrophysiol 1987;10(40:II):1004.

91. Edvardsson N, Hirsch I, Emanuelsson H, Pontén J, Olsson SB: Sotalol-induced delayed ventricular repolarization in man. Eur Heart J 1980;1:335.

92. Edvardsson N, Olsson SB: Effect of intravenous melperone on atrial repolarization in man. Scand J Clin Lab Invest 1981;41(1):87.

93. Bonatti V, Rolli A, Botti G: Recording of monophasic action potentials of the right ventricle in long QT syndromes complicated by severe ventricular arrhythmias. Eur Heart J 1983;4(3):168.

94. Sedgwick ML, Rasmussen HS, Cobbe SM: Effects of the class III antiarrhythmic drug dofetilide on ventricular monophasic action potential duration and QT interval dispersion in stable angina pectoris. Am J Cardiol 1992;70(18):1432.

95. Yuan S, Wohlfart B, Rasmussen HS, Olsson B, B-Lundqvist C: Effect of dofetilide on cardiac repolarization in patients with ventricular tachycardia. Cardiovasc Drugs Ther 1993;7 (Suppl 2):399. Abstract.

96. Edvardsson N, Talwar KK, Hirsch I, Olsson SB: Acute effects of verapamil on the human right atrium and ventricle. Procedings of the International symposium on Cardiovascular Pharmacotherapy. Geneva, 1985;276.

97. Amlie JP: The modifying effect of autonomic blockade on digitoxin-induced changes in monophasic action potential and refractoriness of the right ventricle of the dog heart. Acta Pharmacol Toxicol (Copenh) 1980;47(2):112.

98. Morgan J, Cunningham D, Connelly DT, Rowland E: Effect of dofetilide (UK-68,798) on electrical restitution in the intact human heart. Pacing Clin Electrophysiol 1992;15(4-II):552. Abstract.

99. Harper RW, Olsson SB: Effect of mexiletine on conduction of premature ventricular beats in man: a study using monophasic action potential recordings from the right ventricle. Cardiovasc Res 1979;13(6):311.

100. Zipes DP: Monophasic action potentials in the diagnosis of triggered arrhythmias. Prog Cardiovasc Dis 1991;33(6):385.

101. Levine JH, Spear JF, Guarnieri T, et al: Cesium chloride-induced long QT syndrome: demonstration of afterdepolarizations and triggered activity in vivo. Circulation 1985;72(5):1092.

102. Bailie DS, Inoue H, Kaseda S, Ben DJ, Zipes DP: Magnesium suppression of early afterdepolarizations and ventricular tachyarrhythmias induced by cesium in dogs. Circulation 1988;77(6):1395.

103. El-Sherif N, Zeiler RH, Craelius W, Gough WB, Henkin R: QTU prolongation and polymorphic ventricular tachyarrhythmias due to bradycardia-dependent early afterdepolarizations. Afterdepolarizations and ventricular arrhythmias. Circ Res 1988;63(2):286.

104. Ben-David J, Zipes DP: Differential response to right and left ansae subclaviae stimulation of early afterdepolarizations and ventricular tachycardia induced by cesium in dogs. Circulation 1988;78(5Pt 1):1241.

105. El-Sherif N, Bekheit SS, Henkin R: Quinidine-induced long QTU interval and torsade de pointes: role of bradycardia-dependent early afterdepolarizations. J Am Coll Cardiol 1989;14(1):252.

106. Shimizu W, Tanaka K, Suenaga K, Wakamoto A: Bradycardia-dependent early afterdepolarizations in a patient with QTU prolongation and torsade de pointes in association with marked bradycardia and hypokalemia. Pacing Clin Electrophysiol 1991;14(7):1105.

107. El-Sherif N: Early afterdepolarizations and arrhythmogenesis. Experimental and clinical aspects. Arch Mal Coeur Vaiss 1991;84(2):227.

108. Luca C: Right ventricular monophasic action potential during quinidine induce marked T and U waves abnormalities. Acta Cardiol 1977;32(4):305.

109. Gavrilescu S, Luca C: Right ventricular monophasic action potentials in patients with long QT syndrome. Br Heart J 1978;40(9):1014.

110. Ohe T, Kurita T, Aihara N, Kamakura S, Matsuhisa M, Shimomura K: Electrocardiographic and electrophysiologic studies in patients with torsades de pointe—role of monophasic action potentials. Jpn Circ J 1990;54(10):1323.

111. Sakurada H, Tejima T, Hiyoshi Y, Motomiya T, Hiraoka M: Association of humps on monophasic action potentials and ST-T alternans in a patient with Romano-Ward syndrome. Pacing Clin Electrophysiol 1991;14(10):1485.

112. Bonatti V, Rolli A, Botti G: Monophasic action potential studies in human subjects with prolonged ventricular repolarization and long QT syndromes. Am Heart J 1985;6 (Suppl D):131.

113. Gough WB, Henkin R: The early afterdepolarization as recorded by the monophasic action potential technique: fact or artifact. Circulation 1989;80:II 130. Abstract.

114. Graham B, Gilmour RF, Stanto MS: OPC88117 suppresses early afterdepolarizations and arrhythmias induced by cesium, 4-aminopyridine and digitalis in canine Purkinje fibers and in the canine heart in situ. Am Heart J 1989;118:708.

115. Kuo CS, Reddy CP, Munakata K, Surawicz B: Mechanism of ventricular arrhythmias caused by increased dispersion of repolarization. Eur Heart J 1985;6(Suppl D):63.

116. Mitchell L, Wyse D, Duff H: Programmed electrical stimulation for ventricular tachycardia induction in humans. I. The role of ventricular functional refractoriness in tachycardia induction. J Am Coll Cardiol 1986;8:567.

117. Downar E, Harris L, Mickelborough L, Shaikh N, Parson I: Endocardial mapping of ventricular tachycardia in the intact human ventricle: evidence for reentrant mechanisms. J Am Coll Cardiol 1988;11:783.

118. Kuo CS, Amlie JP, Munakata K, Reddy CP, Surawicz B: Dispersion of monophasic action potential durations and activation times during atrial pacing, ventricular pacing, and ventricular premature stimulation in canine ventricles. Cardiovasc Res 1983;17(3):152.

119. Kuo CS, Munakata K, Reddy CP, Surawicz B: Characteristics and possible mechanism of ventricular arrhythmia dependent on the dispersion of action potential durations. Circulation 1983;67(6):1356.

120. Kuo CS, Atarashi H, Reddy CP, Surawicz B: Dispersion of ventricular repolarization and arrhythmia: study of two consecutive ventricular premature complexes. Circulation 1985;72(2):370.

121. Vassallo JA, Cassidy DM, Kindwall MFE, Josephson ME: Non-uniform recovery of excitability in the left ventricle. Circulation 1988;78:1365.

122. Habbab MA, El SN: TU alternans, long QTU, and torsade de

pointes: clinical and experimental observations. Pacing Clin Electrophysiol 1992;15(6):916.

123. Downar E, Janse MJ, Durrer D: The effect of acute coronary artery occlusion on subepicardial transmembrane potentials in the intact porcine heart. Circulation 1977;56(2):217.

124. Janse MJ, Kléber AG: Electrophysiological changes and ventricular arrhythmias in the early phase of regional ischemia. Circ Res 1981;49:1069.

125. Donaldson RM, Taggart P, Swanton H, Fox K, Noble D, Richards AF: Intracardiac electrode detection of early ischaemia in man. Br Heart J 1983;50:213.

126. John RM, Taggart PI, Sutton PM, Costa DC, Ell PJ, Swanton H: Endocardial monophasic action potential recordings for the detection of myocardial ischemia in man: a study using atrial pacing stress and myocardial perfusion scintigraphy. Am Heart J 1991;122(6):1599.

127. Paul T, Moak JP, Morris C, Garson A: Epicardial mapping: how to measure local activation? Pacing Clin Electrophysiol 1990;13:285.

128. Olsson SB, Zeng ZR, Blomström P, et al: Determination of local activation times from bipolar electrograms of epicardial mapping. A comparative study of three manual methods and a computerised timer. New Tren Arrhyth 1992;8:193.

129. Levine JH, Moore EN, Kadish AH, Guarnieri T, Spear JF: The monophasic action potential upstroke: a means of characterizing local conduction. Circulation 1986;74(5):1147.

130. Endresen K, Amlie JP, Forfang K, Simonsen S, Jensen O: Monophasic action potentials in patients with coronary artery disease: reproducibility and electrical restitution and conduction at different stimulation rates. Cardiovasc Res 1987;21(9):696.

131. Autenrieth G, Surawicz B, Kuo CS, Arita M: Primary T wave abnormalities caused by uniform and regional shortening of ventricular monophasic action potential in dog. Circulation 1975;51(4):668.

132. Chen PS, Moser KM, Dembitsky WP, et al: Epicardial activation and repolarization patterns in patients with right ventricular hypertrophy. Circulation 1991;83(1):104.

133. Lab MJ: Contribution of mechano-electric coupling to ventricular arrhythmias during reduced perfusion. Int J Microcirc Clin Exp 1989;8(4):433.

134. Lab MJ, Woollard KV: Monophasic action potentials, electrocardiograms and mechanical performance in normal and ischaemic epicardial segments of the pig ventricle in situ. Cardiovasc Res 1978;12(9):555.

135. Lab MJ: Mechanically dependent changes in action potentials recorded from the intact frog ventricle. Circ Res 1978; 42(4):519.

136. Lab MJ, Yardley J: A simple device for simultaneously monitoring monophasic action potentials from epicardium and endocardium in the intact ventricle of the pig. proceedings. J Physiol (Lond) 1979;289:12p.

137. Lab MJ: Monophasic action potentials and the detection and significance of mechanoelectric feedback in vivo. Prog Cardiovasc Dis 1991;34(1):29.

138. Dean JW, Lab MJ: Effect of changes in load on monophasic action potential and segment length of pig heart in situ. Cardiovasc Res 1989;23(10):887.

139. Levine JH, Guarnieri T, Kadish AH, White RI, Calkins H, Kan JS: Changes in myocardial repolarization in patients undergoing balloon valvuloplasty for congenital pulmonary stenosis: evidence for contraction-excitation feedback in humans. Circulation 1988;77(1):70.

140. Taggart P, Sutton PM, Treasure T, et al: Monophasic action potentials at discontinuation of cardiopulmonary bypass: evidence for contraction-excitation feedback in man. Circulation 1988;77(6):1266.

141. Taggart P, Sutton PMI, John R: Evidence for contraction excitation feedback in conscious man. J Physiol 1990;426:9P. Abstract.

142. Calkins H, Maughan WL, Kass DA, Sagawa K, Levine JH: Electrophysiological effect of volume load in isolated canine hearts. Am J Physiol 1989;256(6Pt 2):H1697.

143. Calkins H, Levine JH, Kass DA: Electrophysiological effect of varied rate and extent of acute in vivo left ventricular load increase. Cardiovasc Res 1991;25(8):637.

144. Olsson SB: Recording of monophasic action potentials in the study of atrial dysrhythmias. G Ital Cardiol 1972;2 (4):536.

145. Olsson SB, Cai N, Edvardsson N, Talwar KK: Prediction of terminal atrial myocardial repolarisation from incomplete phase 3 data. Cardiovasc Res 1989;23(1):53.

146. Gavrilescu S, Luca C: Right atrium monophasic action potentials during atrial flutter and fibrillation in man. Am Heart J 1975;90(2):199.

147. Gavrilescu S, Cotoi S, Pop T: Monophasic action potential of the right atrium in paroxysmal atrial flutter and fibrillation. Br Heart J 1973;35(6):585.

148. Gavrilescu S, Cotoi S: Monophasic action potential of right human atrium during atrial flutter and after conversion to sinus rhythm. Argument for re-entry theory. Br Heart J 1972;34(4):396.

149. Gavrilescu S, Streian C, Comsulea L, Luca C: Refractoriness of the right atrium and AV conducting system. Influence of practocol, chronic hypoxia and uremia. Rev Roum Med 1974;12:255.

150. Cotoi S, Constantinescu L, Gavrilescu S: The effect of thyroid state on monophasic action potential in human heart. Experientia 1972;28(7):797.

151. Fredlund B-O, Olsson SB: Long QT interval and ventricular tachycardia of "torsade de pointe" type in hypothyroidism. Acta Med Scand 1983;213:231.

152. Freedberg AS, Papp JG, Vaughan Williams EM: The effect of altered thyroid state on atrial intracellular potentials. J Physiol 1970;207:357.

153. Franz MR, Chin MC, Wang D, Stern R, Scheinman MM: Monitoring of radiofrequency ablation effect by simultaneously monophasic action potential recording. Pacing Clin Electrophysiol 1991;14:703. Abstract.

154. Leblanc AR, Senecal L, Guimond C, Nadeau RA: Computer processing of intracardiac electrograms for conduction studies. Comput Programs Biomed 1979;10(2):151.

155. Hirsch I, Edvardsson N, Olsson SB: Computer based analysis of monophasic action potentials in man. In: Hirsch I, ed. On the generation, analysis and clinical use of cardiac monophasic action potentials. Göteborg: Vasastadens Bokbinderi, 1984:(II)1. Thesis.

156. Cole PG, Dilly S, Lab M: A computerized method of cardiac

action-potential duration analysis. J Physiol (Lond) 1985; 366:118P. Abstract.

157. Kanaan N, Kadish A, Jenkins J, Childs K, MacDonald R: Automated detection and analysis of monophasic action potentials in vivo. J Electrocardiol 1989;22(Suppl):127.

158. Hirsch I, Edvardsson N: Computerized analysis of monophasic action potentials recorded from the intact human heart. Proceeding of the 5th Nordic meeting on medical and biological engineering. Linköping, Sweden, 1981:85.

159. Butrous GS, Schwartz PJ: Clinical aspects of ventricular repolarization. London: Farrand Press, 1989:67.

160. Franz MR, Burkhoff D, Lakatta EG: Monophasic action poten-

tial recording by contact electrode technique: in vitro validation and clinical applications. In: Butrous GS, Schwartz PJ, ed. Clinical aspects of ventricular repolarization. London: Farrand, 1989:81.

161. Schmitt C, Brachmann J, Karch M, et al: Reverse use-dependent effects of sotalol demonstrated by recording monophasic action potentials of the right ventricle. Am J Cardiol 1991;68(11):1183.

162. Bonatti V, Finardi A, Cabasson J, Botti G: A study of the mechanism of the action of Bunaphtine recording the myocardial monophasic action potentials in man. Conclusive report. G Ital Cardiol 1976;6(8):1378.

Cardiac Arrhythmias, 3rd edition, edited by William J. Mandel.
J. B. Lippincott Company, Philadelphia © 1995.

26

William J. Mandel • C. Thomas Peter • Selvyn B. Bleifer

Holter-Monitor Recording

Holter-monitor recording means the recording of all cardiac cycles for periods up to or more than 24 hours. The fundamental concept of this method of electrocardiographic monitoring differs from other methods of intermittent surveillance using the electrocardiogram (ECG) in which only a segment of cardiac electric activity is recorded; therefore, these other methods cannot be considered true Holter-monitor recordings.

The ability to transmit the ECG by means of radio frequencies was first demonstrated by Holter and Gengerelli as early as 1949 (Fig. 26-1).[1] Further development by Holter and colleagues led to the introduction of the first magnetic tape recording unit.[2-4] Subsequently, over the next two decades, a large body of investigators demonstrated the usefulness of this technique.[5-34]

The initial electronic design characteristics of the Holter monitor allowed small recorder size and the ability to obtain electrocardiographic data over 8 hours using a rechargeable direct current power source. Because of significant advances in electronic component design, the quality and fidelity of recordings have been improved and the size and weight of the recorders have been scaled downward. In addition, multichannel devices have become available, enabling the simultaneous recording of two or more leads with the added possibility of an additional channel for timing calibration.

Most contemporary Holter-monitor systems do not absolutely meet the standards of the American Heart Association of electrocardiography frequency response (i.e., 0.05 to 100 Hz).[31] Assuming proper hookup techniques, the recordings appear to reproduce accurate rate and ST-segment abnormalities. The entire system must be evaluated, including both the recorder and the playback system.[35,36]

HOLTER-MONITOR EQUIPMENT

The Holter-monitor recorders are small and battery-operated (using either disposable or rechargeable batteries) and use standard-size cassettes or reel-to-reel tape. Recorder size varies, with small models measuring about $3\frac{1}{2}$ by 5 by $1\frac{1}{2}$ inches and several models being just slightly larger; the weight varies, with most models weighing just more than one pound (Fig. 26-2*A* and *B*). This small size

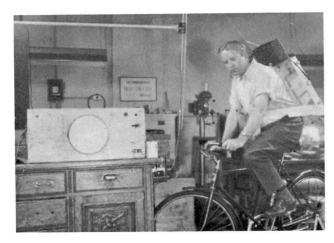

Figure 26-1. Photograph from Holter's laboratory, showing the original electrocardiographic telemetry unit. (Courtesy Hoechst Pharmaceuticals)

and weight enable the patient to carry the recorder comfortably as a harness or purse over the shoulder or attached to a belt. Most recorders have both an event marker (which the patient can activate in case of symptoms) and a continuous digital time display (which allows the patient to record, in a diary, the exact time of any symptom). Furthermore, time-marking channels are available in some units, enabling accurate time definition.

ALTERNATIVE DEVICES

Many small ambulatory devices have been developed and marketed that record or transmit the ECG. These ambulatory devices may be grouped into (1) automatic, (2) patient-activated, and (3) telephone transmitters.

The cardiac event recorder has been available for several years. It contains a preprocessor that initiates the electrocardiographic recording when certain predetermined characteristics—based on rate, QRS change, or arrhythmia, as defined by the program—occur. In addition to the automatic recording, the patient may initiate a recording sequence if symptoms occur. Furthermore, the instrument is programmed to automatically obtain brief recordings at regular intervals. This format includes the following limitations: (1) the recording cassette is small, and the tape may be completed before more important asymptomatic or symptomatic events occur; and (2) the reliability of the preprocessor in detecting the enormous spectrum of electrocardiographic changes remains uncertain. Difficulties encountered with computer analysis of arrhythmias in conventional electrocardiography and in Holter-monitor electrocardiography have shown this to be a far more difficult task than was originally anticipated.

Another alternative approach uses patient- or symptom-activated recording. The patient is monitored by an ambulatory tape recorder, in which each recording sequence is triggered by the patient in response to symptoms or to specific instructions. There are several limitations to this approach, however (e.g., due to syncope, altered mental state, or slow response time, the patient may be unable to initiate the recording). Therefore, the diagnostic changes may be missed, particularly the rhythm present just before symptoms appear.

Both the automatic and symptom-activated recorders fail to provide an essential characteristic of Holter-monitor recording—namely, the recording of every cardiac cycle. It is well documented that informative or diagnostic changes commonly occur without symptoms, and these changes are best detected by continuous recordings. Additionally, access to quantitative data (particularly for ventricular premature complexes) requires that all such complexes be recorded. Other quantitative data such as trend records and ST-segment shifts also require uninterrupted recording.

A third type of ambulatory device employs telephone transmission of the electrocardiographic signal. This device differs from Holter-monitor electrocardiography and from the two other types of devices described above because an ambulatory tape recording of the ECG is not made. An electrocardiographic signal is transmitted by telephone and reproduced directly through a strip-chart recorder, with or without tape recording at the receiving end. The patient generally transmits his ECG because of symptoms or because a signal from the device tells him that a change has occurred. This approach has not found wide acceptance because of the following logistic difficulties: (1) there must be immediate access to a telephone for the system to operate, (2) the receiving station should provide 24-hour availability to both receive the signal and provide instructions to the patient, and (3) the patient may become anxious if he is not near a telephone or if his transmission cannot be received in a clinically effective fashion. (The method is in contrast to the scheduled telephone transmission of pacemaker signals, which has wide acceptance and provides reassurance to the patient with a pacemaker.)

Newer devices allow the patient to record the index event with the unit and then use telephone transmission at his leisure (see Fig. 26-2).

TECHNICAL ASPECTS

Essential to the recording technique is adequate hookup of the recorder by the technician. Skin preparation, satisfactory electrodes (preferably silver or silver chloride),

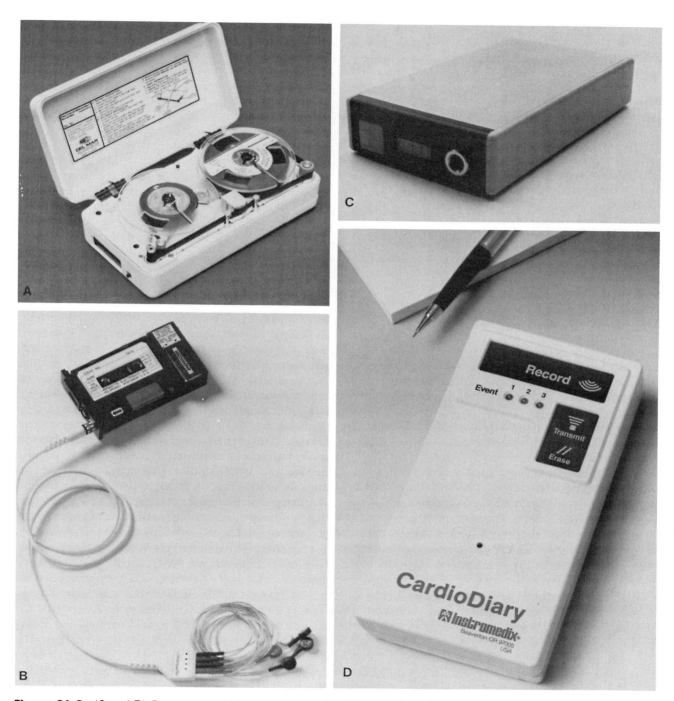

Figure 26-2. (**A** and **B**) Contemporary Holter-monitor recorder (**A**) A two-channel reel-to-reel tape recorder with a digital timing tract. (**B**) A cassette recorder with three channels of electrocardiographic data plus a time channel. (**C**) A unit that allows real-time preprocessing of electrocardiographic data. This unit is used with the analysis system shown in Figure 26-4C. (**D**) A pocket recorder capable of recording three separate 30-second events initiated at the patient's command. The data can later be played back by transtelephonic transmission.

and secure taping of the electrodes to the chest ensure technically adequate 24-hour recordings (Fig. 26-3).

The tape scanners or analyzers vary considerably in concept and function (Fig. 26-4). The fundamental principle of tape review and documentation is the ability to perform high-speed analysis and still detect every abnormality. The typical 24-hour recording contains more than 100,000 cardiac cycles. Primary interest is directed to those episodes in the recording that contain abnormalities, such as premature complexes, atrioventricular (AV) block, and paroxysmal tachycardia. Originally, visual scanning was accomplished by superimposing each P-QRS-T complex, so that a uniform, stationary image results if identical complexes are present (i.e., sinus rhythm). If a complex differs from the preceding one (e.g., a ventricular premature complex), the mismatched complex can readily be detected by visual inspection. The speed of playback is variable but is usually 60 to 120 times the real time of the recording. The trained observer is able to detect electrocardiographic changes, which can then be documented by recording them at real time.

In some analyzer systems, an audio signal (i.e., a constant hum) is provided in addition to the video display, the tone of which depends on the heart rate. The faster the heart rate, the higher the pitch. A sudden tachycardia is signaled by a dramatic change in pitch and even a single ectopic beat interrupts the constant hum. Therefore, any change in heart rate or in the morphology of the electrocardiographic complex can be detected.

"Full disclosure" systems have been introduced to allow more rapid scanning, even by technicians of limited experience. This system permits playback of all taped data at 120 times the recorded speed and produces a report with time coordinates (Fig. 26-5). This report allows review of all data, albeit compressed, with ability to (1) review the quality of the recording, (2) check on technician accuracy, and (3) physically count all premature complexes. The system also allows expansion of the compressed data to permit a real-time report of selected data. The visual scanning system has been updated by the addition of microprocessors that can create templates of QRS waveforms, allowing the operator to select with greater accuracy those normal, artifact, and abnormal QRS waveforms.

These systems have been further improved with semiautomated modes of data processing. Some of these systems have central microcomputers with hard disk. These systems filter the original ECG to eliminate voltage or frequency artifacts. Analog-to-digital conversion is then performed, with storage on hard disk. Sophisticated algorithms are used to analyze the digitalized QRS data in a second pass-through core memory.

Real-time analyzers have been developed that are digitally based and microprocessor driven. These units automatically detect arrhythmias while the patient wears them. They do not, however, analyze the P wave and may have some difficulty with ST-segment analysis. These units have potential disadvantages, including reduced frequency response, higher unit cost, and inability to validate data. Processing is simple and rapid, however.

Sampling recorders are available in which electrocardiographic data are obtained on a prescheduled time format as well as when activated by the patient. The data is then replayed in real time on hard copy for analysis. This offers some advantages in patients with infrequent events who may also have silent episodes.

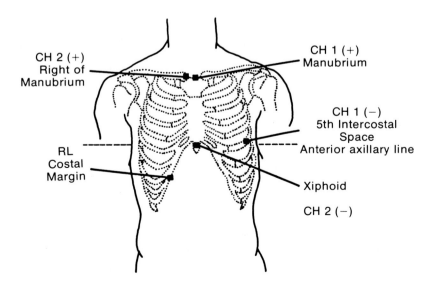

Figure 26-3. Diagram of the typical hookup used for standard Holter-monitor recording with a five-electrode combination. Two bipolar electrode pairs are used as well as a ground electrode, seen at the right lower (*RL*) costal margin. (*CH*, channel)

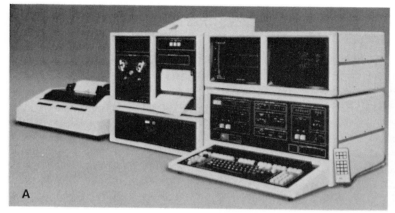

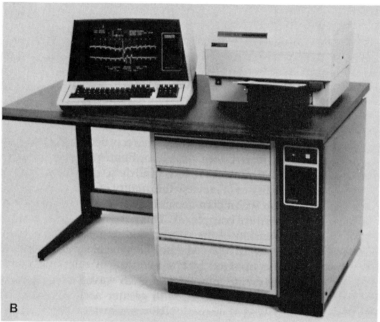

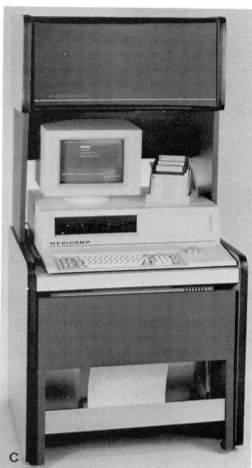

Figure 26-4. Three contemporary analysis systems. (**A**) A reel-to-reel analysis system with computer-assisted hardware. (**B**) A cassette analysis system with a central computer with hard disk drive that allows semiautomated analysis. (**C**) A central processing unit for a system using a preprocessing device, as shown in Figure 26-2C.

INDICATIONS

The clinical indications for Holter monitoring are numerous. In the context of this text, however, Holter-monitor recordings are useful for documenting the presence of arrhythmias and evaluating their frequency, identifying the types of arrhythmia, relating pharmacologic therapy to effectiveness, identifying the possible mechanism of arrhythmias, identifying the arrhythmic etiology of clinical symptoms, and evaluating pacemaker function (Table 26-1).

Evaluation of Atrial Arrhythmias

Holter monitoring offers significant advantages in evaluating patients with suspected or documented episodes of atrial arrhythmias. The patient who presents with a history of recurrent palpitations and a normal resting ECG may require investigation by Holter monitoring; the presence of atrial premature complexes, although usually considered innocuous, may indeed identify the source of the patient's clinical symptoms. The documentation by Holter monitoring of infrequent atrial premature complexes can

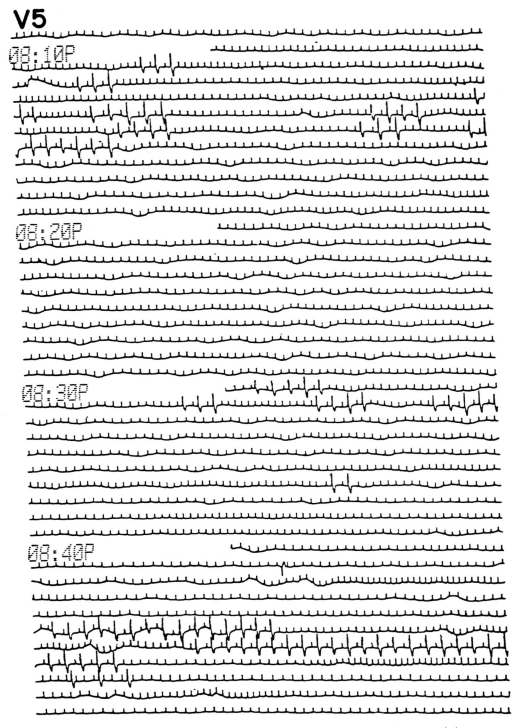

Figure 26-5. A printout of 40 minutes of a typical patient record, using a compressed-data system. This system allows recording at very slow paper speed, so that the entire 24-hour record can be printed out in 12 minutes at 120 times real time and compressed, as shown here. Time marks are available for continuous analysis of data from a time-point reference system. Even though the data is highly compressed, it is easy to identify and count the ventricular premature complex activity. In addition, rate can be assessed by using an overlay to give accurate rate changes.

TABLE 26-1. Indications for Holter Monitoring

Possible cardiac symptoms
  Palpitations
  Syncope
  Chest pain
  Transient central nervous system events
High-risk patients
  Conduction system disease
  Sick sinus syndrome
  Prolonged QT syndromes
  Wolff-Parkinson-White syndrome
  Ischemic heart disease
  Postmyocardial infarction
  Cardiomyopathy
  Mitral valve prolapse
  Sudden-death survivors
  Possible pacemaker malfunction
Antiarrhythmic drug evaluation

be reassuring. If frequent atrial premature complexes are noted or if unusual characteristics of the atrial premature complexes are identified, more detailed investigation may be indicated (e.g., studies of thyroid function or echocardiographic evaluation). Furthermore, atrial premature complexes may be a precursor of more sustained atrial arrhythmias or may identify the earliest features of sinus node dysfunction. Of additional importance are the clinical symptoms associated with atrial premature complexes, which may actually not be due to the irregularity of the rhythm but to episodic pronounced slowing of the heart rate because of nonconducted atrial premature complexes. Moreover, the documentation of atrial premature complexes allows a clearer understanding of various features of atrial electrophysiology and an understanding of the AV-conduction characteristics in a particular patient. That a single Holter-monitor recording can identify the many facets described above is clearly shown in Figure 26-6.

More sustained atrial arrhythmias cannot be clearly distinguished from frequent atrial premature complexes by a detailed history. That the Holter monitor may be critical in documenting recurrent sustained atrial arrhythmias is exemplified in Figure 26-7. Although controversy exists on the relation between atrial premature complexes, their coupling interval, and the onset of atrial fibrillation, innumerable tracings are available from all large Holter-monitoring centers, demonstrating the relation between atrial premature complexes and the initiation of atrial fibrillation. Nevertheless, these tracings do not identify the etiology, which must be more clearly evaluated by the physician (e.g., catecholamine excess, hyperthyroidism, drug-related arrhythmias, valvular dysfunction).

The onset of atrial fibrillation is usually related to atrial premature complexes in most instances observed on a Holter-monitor recording (see Fig. 26-7 and Fig. 26-8).

Atrial premature complexes are frequently noted to have short coupling intervals and may relate to initiation of atrial fibrillation by impinging on the atrial "vulnerable period." Additional information other than the mode of onset may be obtained from records obtained from patients who have had repeated bouts of atrial fibrillation during the course of monitoring. Dramatic alterations in rate, rhythm, and QRS morphology during such monitor recordings may frequently be observed (see Fig. 26-8). It is clear from such records and associated clinical histories that patients are occasionally unaware of dramatic changes in rhythm disturbance and may report that they have sustained palpitations throughout the day with no clear-cut relation to rate or shift in rhythm. These phenomena may be precursors of a variant of sinus node dysfunction (i.e., bradycardia–tachycardia syndrome).

In some patients, regulation of the ventricular rate in atrial fibrillation may be a significant clinical problem. During Holter-monitor recordings, however, many patients with sustained atrial fibrillation may have marked variations in the ventricular response to atrial fibrillation that is related to changes in activity or time of day. This can result in significant difficulties in regard to developing an appropriate maintenance dose of digitalis or the use of associated AV-conduction–blocking agents such as beta blockers. A typical example of such a patient is illustrated in Figure 26-9.

Atrial flutter on a sustained basis is a less common atrial arrhythmia. Nevertheless, its behavior mimics to some degree the phenomena described above in patients who have paroxysmal or sustained atrial fibrillation. Dramatic swings in the ventricular rate with atrial flutter appear to be less common than in those seen with atrial fibrillation. Nevertheless, such events occur and may produce dramatic clinical symptoms. This is clearly illustrated in Figure 26-10.

In many instances, the onset of atrial flutter, like the onset of atrial fibrillation, appears to be related to the presence (and prematurity) of atrial premature complexes. In patients with recurrent palpitations, intermittent atrial flutter should be considered among the differential diagnoses. The presence of palpitations associated with dizziness suggests that the ventricular rate may be rapid. On rare occasions, rapid ventricular rates are noted with the onset of atrial flutter (Fig. 26-11).

Atrial flutter may be a sustained arrhythmia and generally requires larger maintenance doses of digitalis than does atrial fibrillation, sometimes with the additional use of ancillary agents to depress AV conduction. The use of higher doses of digitalis, with or without adjuvant agents, may depress AV conduction more than necessary for clinical effectiveness. This phenomenon is exemplified in Figure 26-12.

Text continues on p. 820

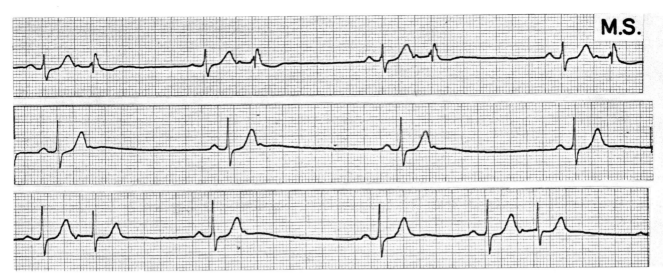

Figure 26-6. Three Holter-monitor strips obtained from a patient complaining of palpitations. The *top recording* reveals atrial premature complexes that occur in a bigeminal fashion and conduct with aberration (i.e., long–short cycle lengths), consistent with phase 3 aberration or Ashman's phenomenon. In the *middle strip*, similar atrial premature complexes are noted to occur; however, they are nonconducted and lead to a dramatic slowing of the heart rate. In the *bottom strip*, atrial premature complexes occur, with even later coupling intervals on occasion, which allow conduction with normal QRS configuration. Blocked atrial premature complexes are also noted.

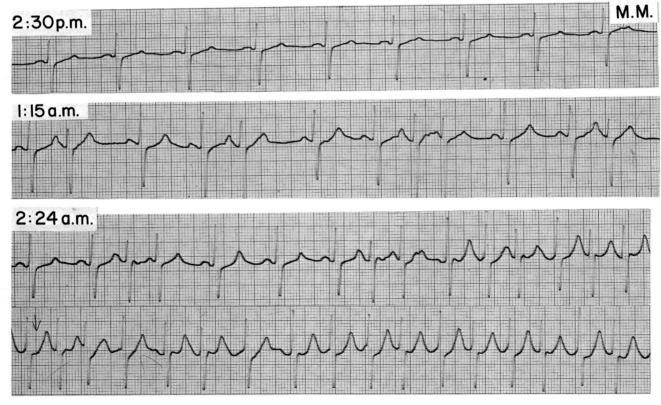

Figure 26-7. Three representative periods during a Holter-monitor recording from a patient complaining of recurrent palpitations. In the *top panel*, sinus rhythm is seen. In the *middle panel*, atrial premature complexes occur singly and in couplets. In the *bottom panel*, atrial premature complexes occur in couplets. In the later part of the *bottom strip*, three atrial premature complexes occur in a row. The last complex occurs quite early and initiates an episode of atrial fibrillation, with a moderately rapid ventricular response.

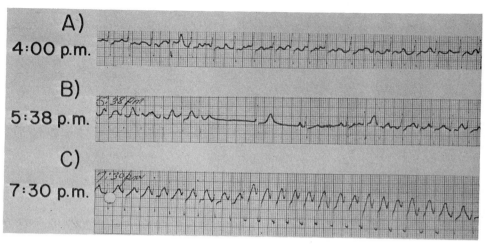

Figure 26-8. Three representative strips from a patient with recurrent palpitations. (**A**) Atrial fibrillation with a moderately rapid ventricular rate is noted. (**B**) Atrial fibrillation terminates spontaneously with a junctional escape complex followed by sinus rhythm. After the second sinus complex, an atrial premature complex initiates another episode of atrial fibrillation. (**C**) Atrial fibrillation with a much more rapid ventricular response is noted and intermittent ventricular aberration is seen.

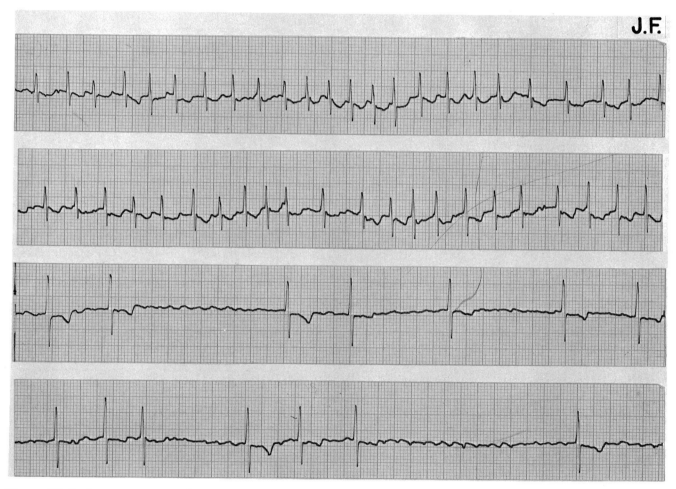

Figure 26-9. Representative recordings taken from a patient with sustained long-standing atrial fibrillation. In the *top two panels*, atrial fibrillation is seen, with ventricular rates generally in excess of 150 beats/min. The *bottom two panels*, from the same patient at a different time, show atrial fibrillation with pronounced slowing of the ventricular rate, with pauses exceeding 2 seconds on two occasions.

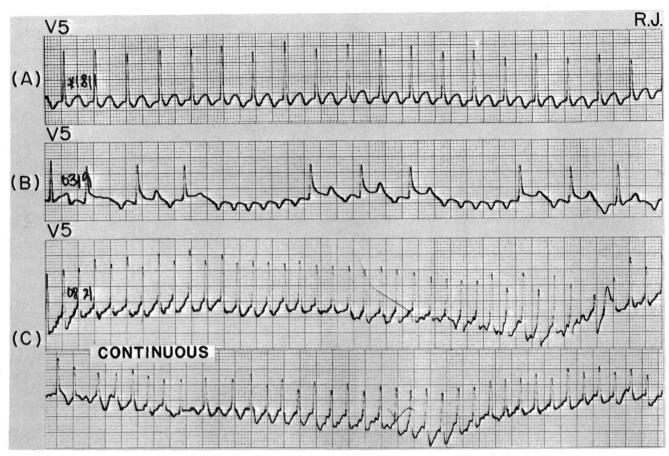

Figure 26-10. Three representative periods obtained from a Holter-monitor recording from a patient with atrial flutter. (**A**) Atrial flutter is seen with a 2:1 ventricular response. (**B**) Later, the patient is in atrial flutter with a controlled ventricular rate, in which long pauses are seen. (**C**) During an episode of sustained dizziness, the patient is in atrial flutter but with 1:1 conduction, with ventricular response of approximately 300 beats/min.

Episodic tachyarrhythmias, palpitations, or both may be documented by a Holter-monitor recording and yet may not fit into the classic categories of atrial arrhythmias (Fig. 26-13). Once these unusual atrial arrhythmias (e.g., paroxysmal atrial tachycardia with block, multifocal atrial tachycardia, ectopic atrial tachycardia) are documented, they may explain the difficulty in managing such patients with routine therapeutic agents.

Recurrent supraventricular tachycardias such as those described above may occasionally be associated with alternating periods of bradyarrhythmias. If ventricular rates are not dramatically different from those observed during

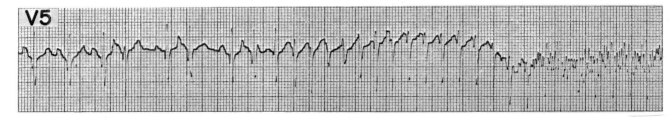

Figure 26-11. Onset of atrial flutter in a patient with a history of recurrent palpitations. The beginning of the strip shows premature complexes as isolated events. The third atrial premature complex initiates a sustained episode of atrial flutter with a 1:1 ventricular response and with a ventricular rate of approximately 300 beats/min.

R.G.

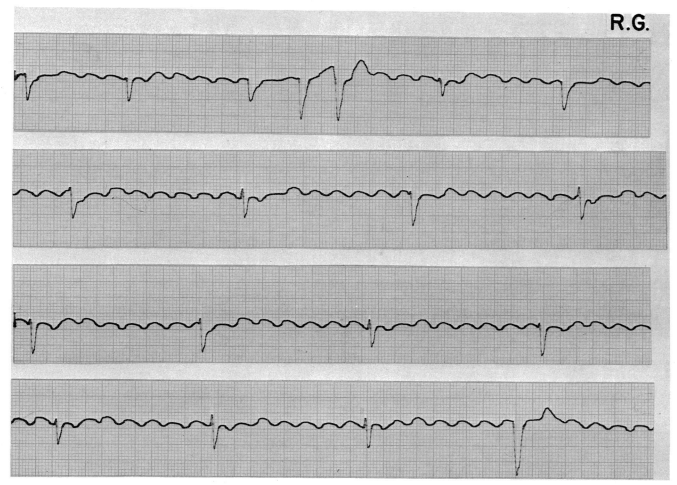

Figure 26-12. Strips obtained from a Holter-monitor recording in a patient with sustained atrial flutter. Throughout the recording, the patient demonstrates atrial flutter with a profound degree of atrioventricular conduction disturbance. Ventricular premature complexes are seen, and a possible ventricular escape complex is also noted in the last strip.

sinus rhythm, limited or no symptoms may be recounted by the patient. Nevertheless, these arrhythmias may be dramatic and may be precursors of more pronounced degrees of supraventricular arrhythmias. Exaggerated versions of the alternation of tachycardia and bradycardia may be associated with clinical symptoms of cerebral hypoperfusion. Figures 26-14 and 26-15 offer dramatic examples of such instances.

Palpitations may be reported as clinical symptoms of minor magnitude or of major clinical significance. Holter-monitor recordings can identify clinically insignificant episodes or episodes associated with major clinical problems. Furthermore, these recordings can offer some significant insight into the mechanism of the tachyarrhythmias as well as insight into the function of the sinus and AV nodes. These features are illustrated in Figures 23-16 and 23-17.

Detection and Quantitation of Ventricular Arrhythmias

Holter monitoring has been a mainstay in the detection and quantitation of ventricular arrhythmias, especially ventricular premature complexes. Extensive studies emphasize clearly that spontaneously occurring fluctuations in the ventricular premature complex frequency are such that brief periods of recording may give an extremely erroneous impression of the frequency of arrhythmias and the success or failure of antiarrhythmic drug therapy. Multiple studies adequately emphasize the importance of longer-duration recordings.[37-46] Spontaneous variability in the ventricular premature complex frequency is so great that it mimics the effects of antiarrhythmic drug therapy (Fig. 26-18). Furthermore, these studies emphasize that the spontaneous incidence of ventricular arrhyth-

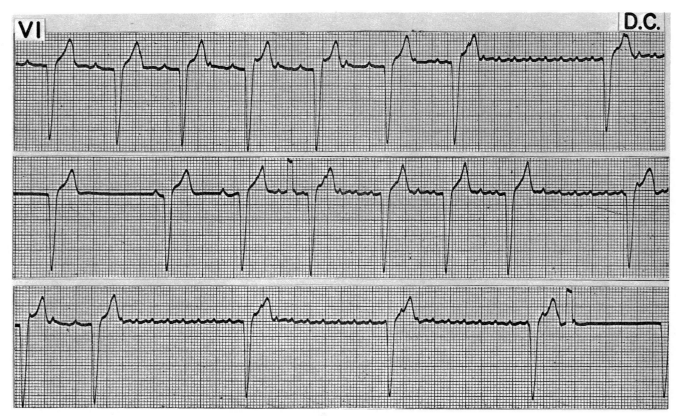

Figure 26-13. An unusual recording obtained from a patient complaining of recurrent palpitations. In these representative Holter-monitor strips, several unusual arrhythmias are noted. In the *top strip*, atrial tachycardia with variable conduction delay is initiated by an atrial premature complex. The atrial tachycardia suddenly converts into an episode of apparent atrial flutter, with peculiar flutter waves and with an atrial flutter rate of approximately 300 beats/min. The flutter terminates spontaneously, with resultant junctional escape complex and then restoration of sinus rhythm. In the *middle strip*, after restoration of sinus rhythm, the atypical atrial flutter is initiated again and ultimately results in termination and restoration of junctional escape rhythm in the last complex of the *bottom strip*.

mias may largely depend on daytime or nighttime recordings, so that during sleep, the ventricular arrhythmias may be nearly abolished (Fig. 26-19). Finally, the spontaneous day-to-day variability is such that on three different days, the number of ventricular premature complexes may vary from as few as 70 to as many as 700 per hour (Fig. 26-20). This variability may greatly inhibit accurate evaluation of antiarrhythmic drug therapy and may be a critical point with regard to the long-term management of patients with ventricular arrhythmias. These authors emphasize clearly that statistically significant reductions in ventricular premature complex activity cannot be observed at the 5% confidence limit unless there is a 90% reduction in ventricular premature complex activity over 24 hours. Longer periods allow statistical comparison, with less of a reduction in ventricular premature complex activity.[37–46] The random ECG may identify the presence of ventricular premature complexes and may clarify the mechanism of

patient-related symptoms (i.e., the sensation of palpitation). Albeit controversial, the use of grading systems for evaluating the nature of ventricular arrhythmias suggests that a more detailed evaluation of the frequency and nature of the ventricular premature complex activity be obtained. This necessitates more protracted periods of electrocardiographic observation. During such observation, it is common to determine episodic complex ventricular arrhythmia activity without sustained ventricular tachycardia, as exemplified in Figure 26-21. (In this regard, it is necessary to point out the importance of two-channel recordings. The nature of the premature complex may not be obvious without two separate ECG channels; Fig. 26-22.)

Studies by Pratt and coworkers reveal that the variability of complex ventricular arrhythmias is significantly higher in patients with (rather than without) coronary artery disease.[40,47] This is especially true in patients with

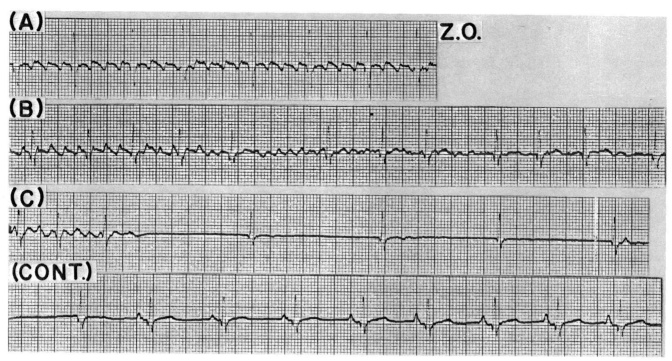

Figure 26-14. Representative Holter-monitor strips from a recording in a patient with recurrent tachycardia alternating with bradycardia. (**A**) Atrial flutter is seen, with typical flutter waves both in rate and in configuration. The ventricular response is controlled. (**B**) The flutter waves change in configuration in the early portion of the record and then convert into atrial fibrillation with a controlled ventricular response. (**C**) (Continuous strip) atrial fibrillation terminates and is followed by junctional bradycardia. Subsequently, sinus rhythm is restored, with normal heart rate and normal atrioventricular conduction seen in the later portion of **C**.

runs of ventricular tachycardia. The importance of variability has been further emphasized in studies by Kennedy and colleagues in asymptomatic healthy subjects having frequent and complex ectopy.[48] This study found that the long-term prognosis in this group is similar to that in a cohort of healthy patients and that no increased incidence of death should be anticipated.

Age may predispose to cardiac arrhythmias. Fleg and Kennedy studied an elderly (60 to 85 years of age) population without clinical cardiac disease.[49] These patients demonstrated a significant prevalence of supraventricular and ventricular premature complexes, isolated and complex. Marked bradycardia, sinus arrest, or high degrees of AV block were not noted, however.

More sustained episodes of ventricular arrhythmias may occur but may be unrelated to clinical symptoms. Accelerated idioventricular rhythm (AIVR) may occur in patients without obvious clinical evidence of heart disease: AIVR may be of brief duration associated with sinus arrhythmia (Fig. 26-23) or it may occur on a more sustained basis, usually in patients with significant organic heart disease (Fig. 26-24). The ventricular rate seen during

AIVR is by definition less than 100 beats per minute. This largely explains the general lack of symptoms associated with the presence of intermittent short-lived or even sustained episodes of AIVR.

Symptomatic ventricular arrhythmias can occur in patients without overt cardiovascular disease but in most instances, organic cardiovascular disease is present. In clinical practice, the most common background for the development of ventricular arrhythmias is ischemic heart disease. The presence of intermittent ischemia may play a substantive role in the development of short or more sustained episodes of ventricular tachycardia. This is exemplified by the findings in Figure 26-25, showing that the development of ST-segment depression associated with clinically important ischemia was associated with the development of ventricular tachycardia.

Sustained episodes of ventricular tachycardia generally are associated with clinical symptoms such as palpitations, lightheadedness, dizziness, or frank syncope. The development of sustained ventricular tachycardia may occur at rates below 150 beats per minute, however, and may be associated only with the sensation of mild palpitations

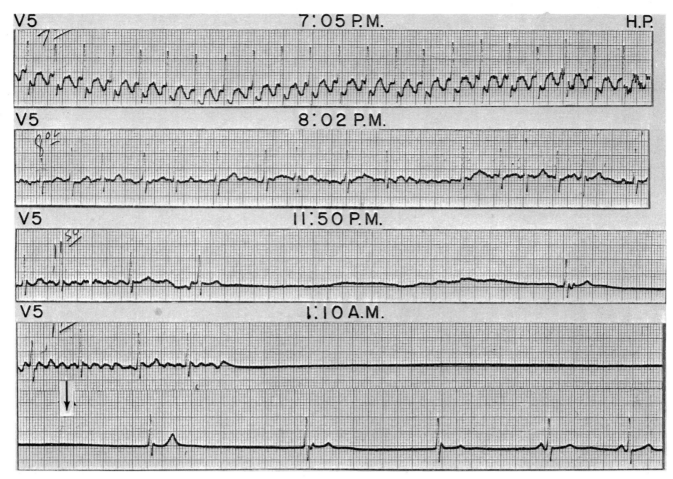

Figure 26-15. Representative Holter-monitor strips from a patient with recurrent tachycardia and bradycardia. In the first strip (at 7:05 PM), atrial flutter with 2:1 ventricular response is noted. Approximately 1 hour later (the second strip, at 8:02 PM), atrial flutter has converted to atrial fibrillation with a moderately rapid ventricular response. In the third strip (at 11:50 PM), atrial fibrillation terminates spontaneously with a profound sinus arrest terminated by a junctional escape complex. In the final strips (at 1:10 AM), atrial flutter/fibrillation terminates spontaneously with a dramatic sinus arrest terminated by three junctional escape complexes, followed by restoration of sinus rhythm.

(Fig. 26-26). Ventricular tachycardia occurring at slow rates in the presence of organic heart disease is usually clinically evident. In the setting of relatively normal ventricular function, the presence of ventricular tachycardia at rates below 150 beats per minute should not lead to significant hemodynamic compromise and therefore may not be clinically evident by review of the patient's history. In contrast to the findings listed above, more rapid ventricular rates in patients with impaired hemodynamic function invariably lead to significant hemodynamic compromise (Fig. 26-27).

Therapy with antiarrhythmic agents is used in many instances in patients with significant ventricular arrhythmias but the initiation of therapy with antiarrhythmic agents may precipitate rather than prevent ventricular arrhythmias. This is particularly true with quinidine. During the early stages of therapy with quinidine, QT-interval prolongation may occur without suppression of ventricular arrhythmias and may lead to enhanced vulnerability and to the development of sustained ventricular arrhythmias (quinidine syncope). An example is demonstrated in Figure 26-28.

Other conditions also predispose to the development of sustained ventricular arrhythmias. If these conditions are not readily recognized, historical features of syncope may be associated with Holter-monitor–documented severe ventricular arrhythmias. This is most clearly demonstrated in hereditary QT-interval prolongation syndromes, in which syncope and near syncope are associated with the presence of sustained ventricular arrhythmias and even episodic ventricular fibrillation. A typical example is shown in Figure 26-29.

Multiple studies have evaluated Holter-monitoring

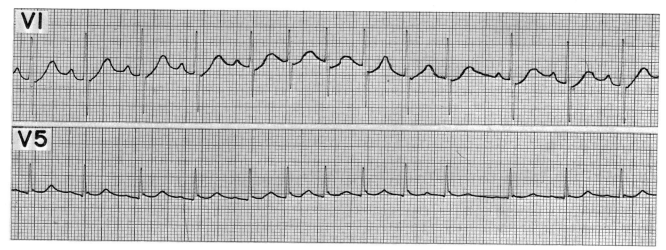

Figure 26-16. Representative two-channel Holter-monitor strips from a patient with a recurrent history of palpitations. In the *middle portion* of this recording, a short burst of supraventricular tachycardia lasting for five complexes is seen with a ventricular rate of approximately 130 beats/min. After the burst of tachycardia, sinus rhythm is restored with a normal sinus node recovery time. Throughout the 24-hour period of this recording, the patient had repeated short bursts of supraventricular tachycardia. Documentation by electrocardiography had never been made in previous examinations.

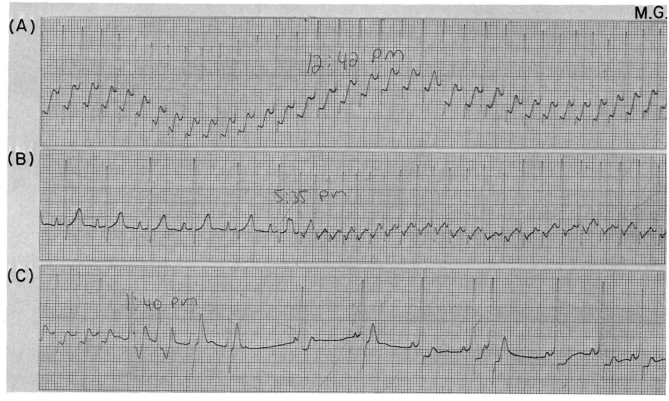

Figure 26-17. Representative Holter-monitor strips from a patient with recurrent paroxysmal supraventricular tachycardia. (**A**) At 12:42 AM, the patient had a sustained episode of supraventricular tachycardia with a ventricular rate in excess of 220 beats/min. Atrial activity after the QRS appears to be present. (**B**) At 5:35 PM, the onset of supraventricular tachycardia is observed in the same patient. The tachycardia is initiated by an atrial premature complex with modest prolongation of the PR interval, followed by atrial activation after the QRS complex. (**C**) At 1:40 PM, an episode of supraventricular tachycardia terminates, with bizarre complex activity, possibly ventricular in origin, seen just before termination.

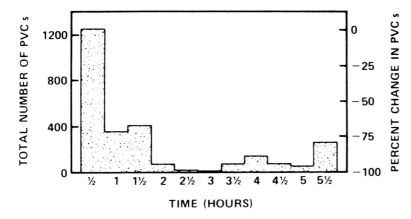

Figure 26-18. Graph demonstrating the highly variable nature of ventricular premature complex activity seen in one patient's Holter-monitor recording over a 5½-hour time span. The patient was not receiving antiarrhythmic drugs at the time of the Holter-monitor recording. (Winkle RA: Antiarrhythmic drug effect mimicked by spontaneous variability of ventricular ectopy. Circulation 1978;57:1116. By permission of the American Heart Association.)

data in postmyocardial infarction patients.[50–65] The major problem with these studies has been the inability to compare data because of striking differences in study design (e.g., the number of hours of recording time after the index event, duration of follow-up). The data, as reviewed by DiMarco and Philbrick, indicate that prognostic information could be obtained from the standpoint of mortality (all causes), sudden death, and total cardiac mortality.[34] The major negative variables included (1) ventricular tachycardia, (2) more than 10 premature ventricular complexes (PVCs) per hour, and (3) complex ventricular arrhythmias. It is important to note, however, that arrhythmia variables (Holter-monitor data) were not as good a

predictive force as some clinical variables (e.g., left ventricular ejection fraction, presence of late potentials). It therefore remains unclear whether routine use of Holter monitoring in postmyocardial infarction is an appropriate clinical tool.

Holter-monitoring studies in patients with ischemic heart disease monitored at a time not related to myocardial infarction are a parallel to the above. Data are limited but do not support the routine use of Holter monitoring as a screening procedure for prognostic purposes.[66–69]

Other Holter-monitor screening studies have been performed in patients having congestive heart failure of a variety of etiologies, complex ventricular arrhythmias and

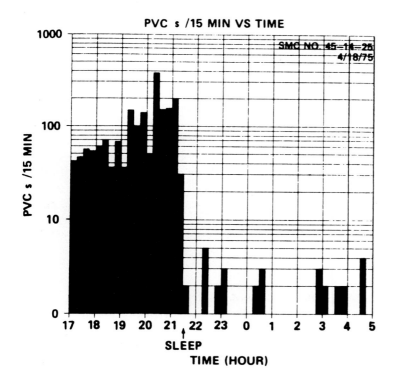

Figure 26-19. The horizontal axis shows the time during a 24-hour span, and the vertical axis shows the number of premature ventricular contractions (PVCs) per 15 minutes. Note the dramatic reduction in PVC frequency when the patient falls asleep. (Winkle RA: Antiarrhythmic drug effect mimicked by spontaneous variability of ventricular ectopy. Circulation 1978;57:1116. By permission of the American Heart Association.)

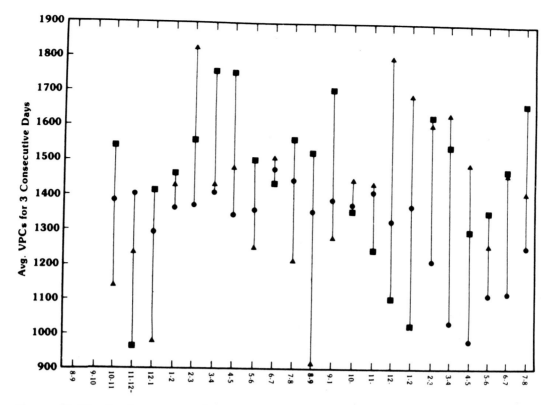

Figure 26-20. One-hour time periods are plotted on the horizontal axis, and the average numbers of premature ventricular contracts (PVCs) seen on three consecutive days are shown on the vertical axis. Note the dramatic swings in PVC frequency relative to the days the Holter-monitor recording was taken. (Morganroth J, Michelson EL, Horowitz LN, et al: Limitations of routine long-term electrocardiographic monitoring to assess ventricular ectopic frequency. Circulation 1978;58:408. By permission of the American Heart Association.)

no apparent heart disease, and chronic pulmonary disease.[70–74] All studies suggest that the Holter-monitor data cannot be used prognostically.

Monitoring the effectiveness of therapy in patients judged in need of antiarrhythmic drug treatment has been routinely performed with Holter-monitoring recording. This evaluation procedure is based on the hypothesis that mortality can be reduced by reducing the number and quality of ventricular premature complexes.[75] Studies using Holter-monitor data have been flawed but some have been completed with randomized controlled trials and a comparable control group.[76–84] These studies have been partially flawed because no systematic protocol was in place nor were alternative drugs available. No clear decrease in mortality was seen, however. The CAPS trial (*C*ardiac *A*rrhythmias *P*ilot *S*tudy) used multiple agents in the same patient.[85] This was followed by the CAST study (*C*ardiac *A*rrhythmias *S*uppression *T*rial), which has shown some disquieting negative effects of antiarrhythmic drugs (e.g., encainide and flecainide).[86] An overview

therefore indicates that there are no convincing data available that validate the reduction or elimination of ventricular premature complexes as a guide to reduction in mortality.

Another iatrogenic cause of sustained ventricular arrhythmias has been noted in patients who have developed a QT-interval prolongation associated with the use of liquid protein mixtures for weight loss. Serious and even life-threatening arrhythmias associated with a significant QT-interval prolongation have been documented in such patients. These patients frequently demonstrated torsades de pointes and even episodes of ventricular flutter or fibrillation (Fig. 26-30).

Sudden Cardiac Death

Holter monitoring has been useful in identifying the arrhythmic mechanism or mechanisms of sudden cardiac death. The original documentation of sudden death dur-

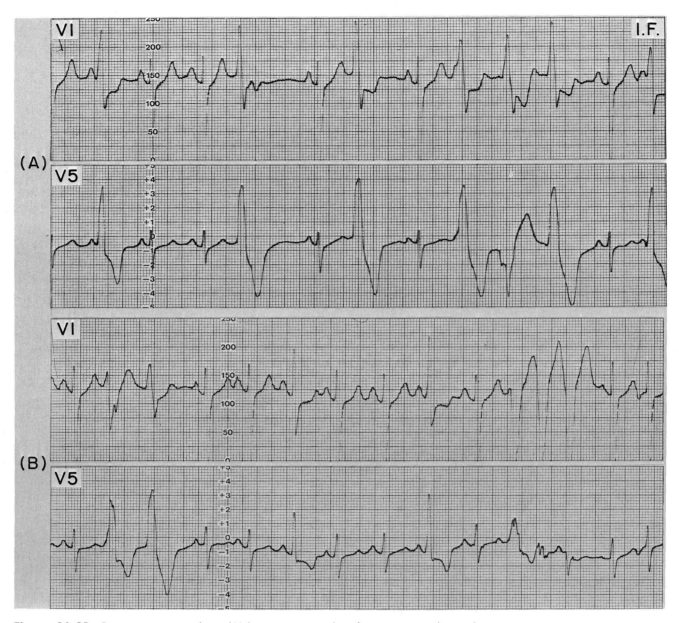

Figure 26-21. Representative two-channel Holter-monitor recordings from a patient with a cardio-myopathy and a history of palpitations. Multiform frequent ventricular premature complexes are noted occurring (**A**) as isolated events and (**B**) in groups of up to three premature ventricular contractions in a row.

ing Holter monitoring by Bleifer and colleagues has been followed-up by observation from multiple centers.[14,87–92]

Denes and associates, in their observations on five patients, identified an increase in the QT_c that is possibly related to quinidine as a cause of the events.[93] Detailed analysis of premonitory data in other reports has further aided understanding of the premorbid changes in ventricular arrhythmias that may herald sudden death. Nikolie and coworkers identified complex ventricular arrhythmias, variations of cycle length, and the R-on-T phenomenon as major events in six patients.[94] In 12 patients, Lewis and coworkers further confirmed (1) an increase in premature complexes or complexity preceding the terminal event, (2) R-on-T phenomenon, and (3) repolarization abnormality for several hours before the termination event.[95] They did not find changes in cycle length to be an

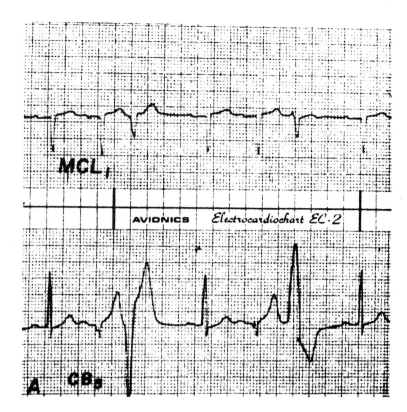

Figure 26-22. Two-channel Holter-monitor recording, demonstrating the importance of a two-channel recording system to define the nature of premature complexes. In the *top strip*, using only the upper channel, premature complexes are noted, but the exact nature is uncertain. In the *bottom strip*, a simultaneous record demonstrates multiform configurations of the premature ventricular complexes.

important factor. Finally, Pratt and coworkers, in their study of 15 patients with ventricular fibrillation confirmed that this arrhythmia was preceded by an increase in ventricular premature complexes (number and complexity) followed by ventricular tachycardia in all patients.[96] R-on-T phenomenon and QT-interval prolongation were not significant factors. In contrast, Roelandt and colleagues found

that no specific arrhythmic pattern predicted sudden cardiac death.[97]

Subsequently, other investigators have accumulated larger series of Holter-monitor recordings at the time of sudden cardiac death.[98–100] These studies analyze data from groups of 61, 69, and 157 patients. Repetitive ven-

Text continues on p. 832

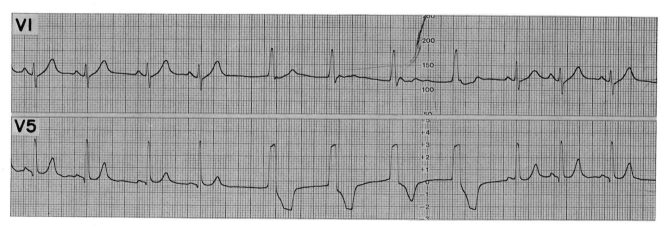

Figure 26-23. Two-channel Holter-monitor recordings obtained from a patient without clinical symptoms. In the *middle* of the recordings, note that the significant sinus arrhythmia was terminated by the appearance of accelerated idioventricular rhythm lasting four complexes. Subsequently, sinus rhythm is restored.

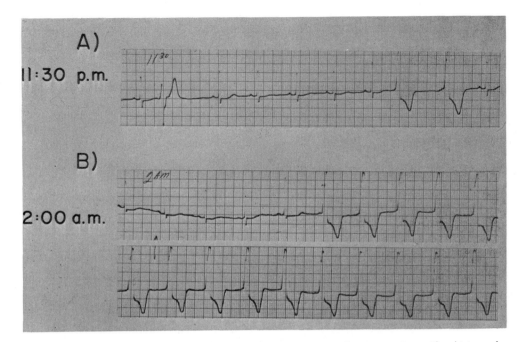

Figure 26-24. Representative strips from a Holter-monitor recording in a patient with a history of vague chest distress. (**A**) Premature ventricular complexes are seen with varying configurations. The latter portion of the record demonstrates two premature ventricular complexes in a row. (**B**) A sustained episode of accelerated idioventricular rhythm at a rate of approximately 70 beats/min is noted. The patient had no clinically apparent symptoms during this latter portion of the record.

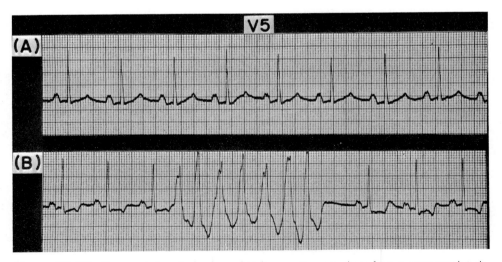

Figure 26-25. Representative single-channel Holter-monitor recordings from a patient with ischemic heart disease and a history of palpitations. (**A**) During a time when the patient was free from pain, normal ST segments are noted and the patient has no ventricular arrhythmias. (**B**) During an episode of significant angina, the patient complained of palpitations. ST-segment depression of significant degree is noted, associated with a short run of ventricular tachycardia lasting seven complexes.

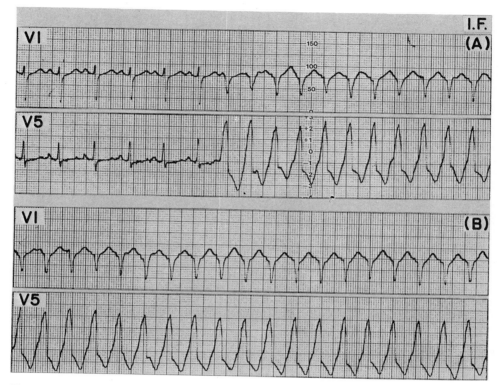

Figure 26-26. Paroxysms of ventricular tachycardia are not always recognized by the patient, even though the ventricular rates during such tachycardia episodes are over 100 beats/min. This is illustrated by the recordings shown in this figure. (**A**) The onset of ventricular tachycardia at a rate of approximately 140 beats/min is noted. (**B**) A sustained episode of the ventricular tachycardia is observed. The patient had a history of palpitations but was unaware of this episode despite the relatively rapid rate.

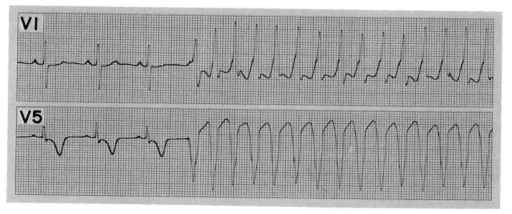

Figure 26-27. Two-channel Holter-monitor recordings obtained from a patient with recurrent palpitations and near-syncopal episodes. The onset of ventricular tachycardia is clearly observed. The ventricular tachycardia rate is approximately 170 beats/min. After the tachycardia began, the patient was clinically symptomatic and had a near-syncopal episode.

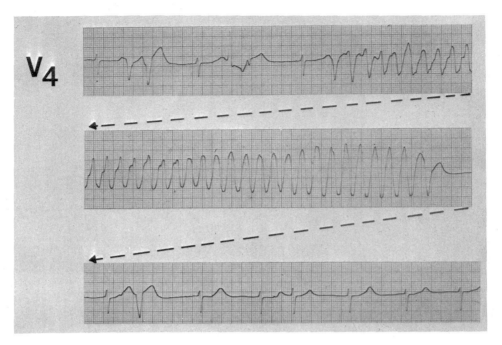

Figure 26-28. Recordings obtained from a patient with recurrent near-syncopal episodes after institution of quinidine therapy. Note that multiform premature ventricular complexes are present at the beginning of the *top strip*. A sustained burst of ventricular tachycardia is observed, initiated by a ventricular premature complex that interrupts the T wave in a complex with a markedly prolonged QT interval. The ventricular tachycardia/flutter terminates spontaneously with restoration of sinus rhythm.

tricular arrhythmias were found in more than 75% of patients in the hours before death. Monomorphic ventricular tachycardia was found in nearly 50% of the patients before the terminal event. Complex ectopy increased significantly in the hour before death but R-on-T events were uncommon.

Vlay and colleagues found that Holter monitoring 1 month after the index event in patients who survive sudden cardiac death has important prognostic value.[101] If ventricular tachycardia (asymptomatic) were present (three or more beats, 120 or more beats/minute) at that time, 42% of the patients had syncope or sudden death within 700 days of the follow-up study.

In the patient who is considered at high risk for development of ventricular tachycardia or sudden death, studies have been designed to compare electrophysiologic testing with Holter monitoring.[102–108] A cooperative study has been designed by the National Institutes of Health to evaluate this point (the ESVEM trial—endocardial *s*timulation *v*ersus *e*lectrocardiographic *m*onitoring).[109] This study was initiated in 1985 and is expected to randomize about 500 patients. It examines the antiarrhythmic effects of six drugs: mexiletine, quinidine, procainamide, sotalol, propafenone, and pirmenol.

The results of this study have been reported, detailing the evaluation of 486 patients.[109a, 109b] Invasive electrophysiologic studies were efficacious in 45% of patients, whereas Holter monitoring was efficacious in 77% of patients. There were no significant differences between the two groups, however, in actuarial probabilities of the arrhythmic deaths (34 patients; i.e., no significant difference in the success of drug therapy, as selected by these two methods). These data have been subjected to some scrutiny and the final outcome has not been published.

Diagnosis of Atrioventricular Block

In clinical practice, the electrocardiographic diagnosis of AV block seldom requires the additional use of Holter-monitor recording. Moreover, Holter-monitor recordings generally play only a limited role in the clinical management of asymptomatic patients having first-degree AV block. Generally, second-degree AV block of the type II (Mobitz) variety also should be managed with permanent pacing without the need for Holter-monitor recordings. In the setting of second-degree AV block of the type I (Wenckebach) variety, however, Holter-monitor record-

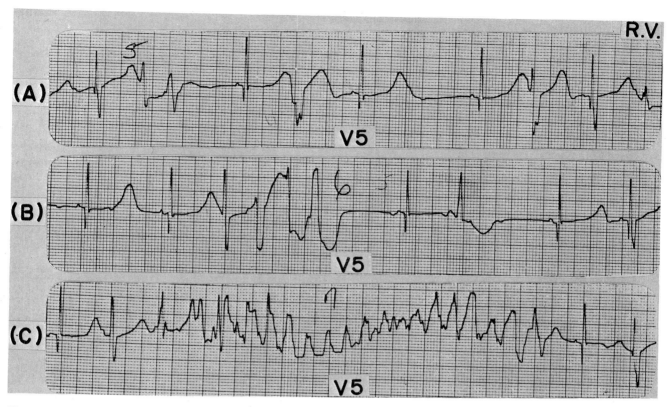

Figure 26-29. Holter-monitor strips obtained from a girl aged 7 years with recurrent syncopal episodes. (**A** and **B**) The patient demonstrates multiform premature ventricular complexes, sometimes occurring in short bursts. (**C**) A ventricular premature complex initiates a burst of ventricular tachycardia with features suggestive of torsade de pointes. This patient had a hereditary long QT-prolongation syndrome.

ings may give the clinician needed data. This is especially the case in asymptomatic patients without evidence of acute or chronic cardiac disease who are not receiving cardioactive drugs. Data have been accumulated that identify a category of younger patients (under 40 years of age) having second-degree AV block with no evidence of underlying heart disease or central nervous system symptoms.[110] Conduction studies in these patients identify AV nodal dysfunction secondary to altered response to parasympathetic tone as being the apparent pathophysiologic basis. In these patients, exercise and atropine reduced or eliminated second- and first-degree AV block. Figure 26-31A shows an episode of second-degree AV block of the Wenckebach type that is followed (Fig. 26-31B) by sinus tachycardia, with a normal PR interval. This recording was obtained from a man aged 30 years without symptoms who at rest had persistent second-degree AV block (type I). Conduction studies identified the site of block at the AV nodal level. Atropine administration and exercise abolished the block. Although the long-term prognosis of these patients is uncertain, repeated Holter-monitor re-

cordings appear to be necessary to follow-up their clinical status.

In patients with a history of intermittent syncope or near syncope, Holter-monitor recordings can be invaluable. The documentation of paroxysmal advanced AV block in patients with intermittent central nervous system symptoms may prove lifesaving. Nevertheless, persistence on the part of the clinician may be of paramount importance, especially in the patient with infrequent symptoms. An example of this clinical problem is shown in Figure 26-32. The record in this figure was obtained from a woman aged 50 years, with a 5-year history of seizures of the grand mal type. The patient had previously been investigated by three neurologists, who had been unsuccessful in eliminating her seizures despite extensive neurologic evaluation and pharmacologic therapy. The patient was hospitalized by her physician for further studies, during which time she was noted to have an ECG with right bundle branch block, left anterior superior fascicular block, and first-degree AV block. The patient was to undergo conduction studies but had a Holter-monitor re-

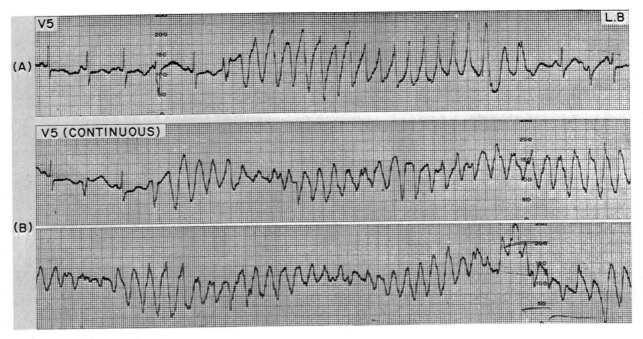

Figure 26-30. Two representative strips from a patient who had been taking a liquid protein mixture without medical supervision to lose weight. (**A**) A burst of ventricular tachycardia is noted with characteristic features of torsade de pointes. (**B**) A continuous episode of ventricular tachycardia/flutter/fibrillation is observed.

cording before the catheterization. The Holter-monitor recording shown in Figure 26-32 was obtained during this study and shows an episode of paroxysmal AV block during a seizure episode. The patient subsequently had a permanent pacemaker implanted, with complete cure of her seizure disorder.

These examples, albeit unusual, point out the benefits of Holter-monitor recording in patients with onset of suspected paroxysmal AV block. Pacemaker therapy may be justifiably withheld or urgently implemented based on the results of such studies.

Unexplained Symptoms

Holter monitoring is routinely used to evaluate patients with recurrent palpitations, dizziness, or syncope. Studies document potentially causative arrhythmias in from 10% to 64% of patients evaluated.[111–121] Importantly, 4% to 30% of patients *without* symptoms had significant arrhythmias documented. The importance of such studies may frequently be to give evidence that the patient's symptoms were *not* due to arrhythmias. These studies, however, were only done with 12 to 24 hours of monitoring. A study by Bass and colleagues indicates that the yield in patients with unexplained syncope may be increased significantly by a second 24-hour period of recording (positive

yield, 15% with 24 hours and 36% with 48 hours of recording).[122]

Hypertrophic Cardiomyopathy

Patients with hypertrophic cardiomyopathy are noted to have a significant incidence of syncope and sudden death. Holter monitoring has been used as a tool to assess the incidence and complexity of ventricular arrhythmias in this patient population. Maron and colleagues determined that 66% of a cohort of 99 patients had high-grade ventricular arrhythmias, including 19% with asymptomatic ventricular tachycardia.[123] This latter group appears to identify a subset of patients who are at high risk for sudden death. McKenna and coworkers confirm these observations.[124]

Digitalis-Induced Arrhythmias

The relation between digitalis administration, serum digoxin levels, and the incidence of arrhythmias considered to represent digitalis intoxication was studied in a prospective manner by Goren and Denes.[125] These authors noted that digitalis-provoked arrhythmias were demon-

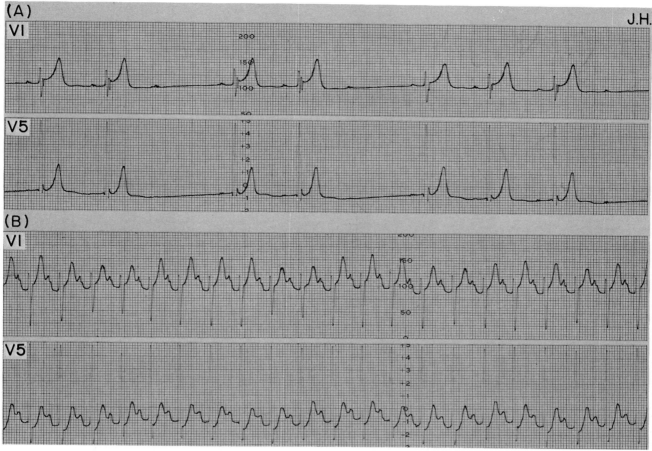

Figure 26-31. Representative Holter-monitor two-channel recordings from a patient with episodic second-degree atrioventricular (AV) block. (**A**) Typical group-beating episodes are seen with characteristic features suggestive of AV nodal Wenckebach phenomenon. (**B**) During an episode of vigorous activity. 1:1 AV conduction is noted with a PR interval that is within the normal range.

strated in 10 of 69 patients undergoing Holter monitoring. There was *no* relation between these arrhythmias and the digoxin level. It was concluded that rhythm disorders considered typical for digitalis intoxication do not always reflect clinically evident toxicity.

Cardiac Surgery

Patients subjected to cardiac surgery are frequently noted to have atrial and ventricular arrhythmias in the perioperative period. Dewar and associates reported on a detailed preoperative, intraoperative, and postoperative Holter-monitoring study in 52 adult patients undergoing cardiac surgery.[126] Their investigations identified (1) a high incidence of arrhythmias associated with anesthesia induction and thoracotomy, (2) a lack of correlation between peak creatinine kinase and arrhythmias, and (3) a higher incidence of arrhythmias in valve replacements.

In children undergoing cardiac surgery, arrhythmias have been well documented, especially in patients who have undergone repair of an atrial septal defect or a Mustard procedure. Potentially more important is the group that includes patients having repair for tetralogy of Fallot, in whom ventricular arrhythmias and sudden death have been documented. In a prospective study, Ringel and colleagues evaluated 65 patients with Holter-monitor recordings preoperatively and early (1 to 10 days) and late (3 to 12 months) postoperatively.[127] The preoperative data indicate a 25% incidence of supraventricular and a 39% incidence of ventricular arrhythmias. These percentages increased dramatically in the early postoperative state and were still above preoperative values in the later postoperative period.

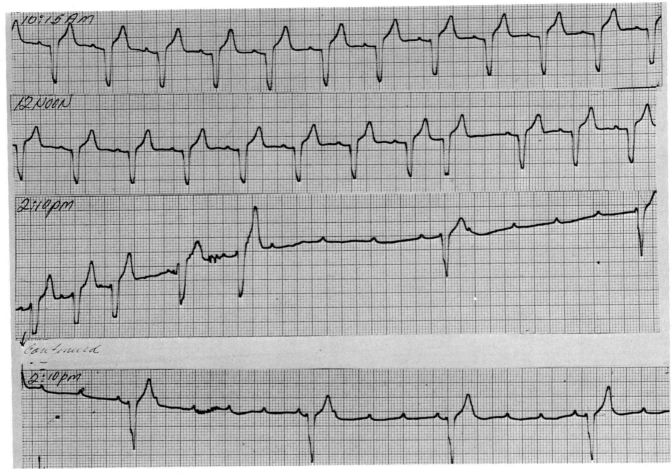

Figure 26-32. Holter-monitor strips obtained from a patient with recurrent epileptic "seizures" who had, on a standard electrocardiogram, right bundle branch block with anterior superior fascicular block and first-degree AV block. The *two lower strips* demonstrate the features seen during a typical "seizure," in which paroxysmal atrioventricular block occurred.

Pacemaker Evaluation

Implantations of permanent pacemakers have increased at a dramatic rate since their introduction. Over the past two decades, electronic circuitry and design have improved at a spectacular rate, allowing pacemaker manufacturers to develop smaller and more reliable units. These developments have been paralleled by the development of new power sources, which has increased the longevity of the devices. Moreover, new units have been developed that allow the addition of new pacemaker functions, making the implanted unit an even more highly specialized electronic instrument. External programmability of (1) multiple parameters, (2) sensing and pacing of multiple chambers, (3) multiple pacing modes for the same unit, and (4) especially the DDD pacemaker has introduced a complexity into the evaluation of unit function that requires spe-

cialized knowledge. The use of pacemakers has necessitated a sophisticated system of follow-up study of the functional integrity of the entire system (generator, power source, electrodes). In many cardiologic centers, the development of pacemaker-evaluation units designed solely to analyze pacemaker function has proved invaluable in the long-term follow-up study of pacemaker patients. Critical rate analysis, rhythm-strip interpretation, and waveform analysis are inherent in the evaluation of these patients. Nevertheless, some patients have intermittent pacemaker malfunction that escapes detection, even with sophisticated analysis. The electrocardiographic surveillance used in most pacemaker clinics requires the recording of a short (30-second to 2-minute) rhythm strip directly or transtelephonically. This limited database may fail to reveal any significant intermittent malfunctions, which may also not be detected by rate or waveform analysis.

Holter-monitor recordings are invaluable in evaluating intermittent pacemaker malfunction in symptomatic patients. In addition, Holter-monitor recordings may prove to be invaluable in the detection of pacemaker malfunction that is not yet significant enough to be associated with clinical complaints.

Holter monitoring is not suggested as a replacement for the present mode of pacemaker evaluation but is suggested for use as an important ancillary tool to evaluate pacemaker patients. In this regard, this chapter demonstrates the usefulness of Holter-monitor recording by illus-

trating a variety of examples of intermittent pacemaker failure. Figure 26-33 is a 24-hour Holter-monitor record from a patient with a permanent ventricular demand pacemaker who complained of the recent onset of palpitations. Rhythm-strip analysis at the time of follow-up study revealed rare PVCs that were appropriately sensed and suppressed by the pacemaker unit. During the course of the 24-hour recording, however, numerous examples of both failure to pace and failure to sense were recorded, which resulted in the replacement of the unit. The observations in such patients have led Kelen and colleagues to develop a

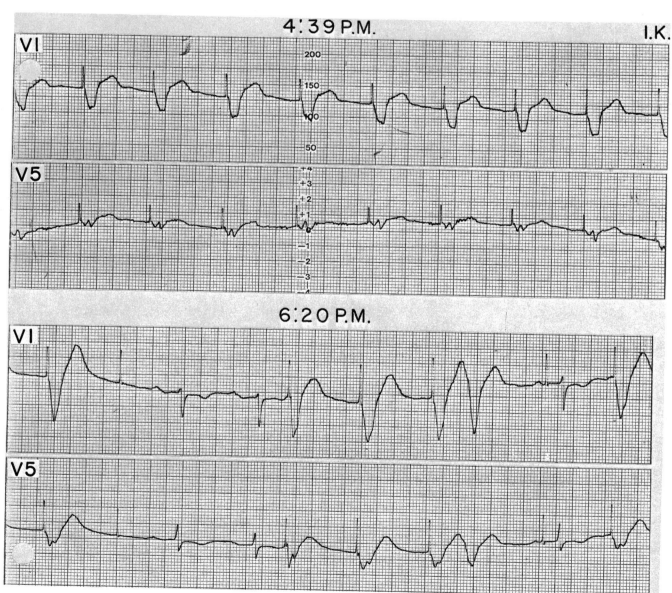

Figure 26-33. Representative two-channel Holter-monitor recordings from a patient with a history of palpitations after pacemaker implantation. (*Top panel*) 1:1 Ventricular capture from the ventricular pacemaker is seen. (*Bottom panel*) Episodes of failure to capture and to sense are observed.

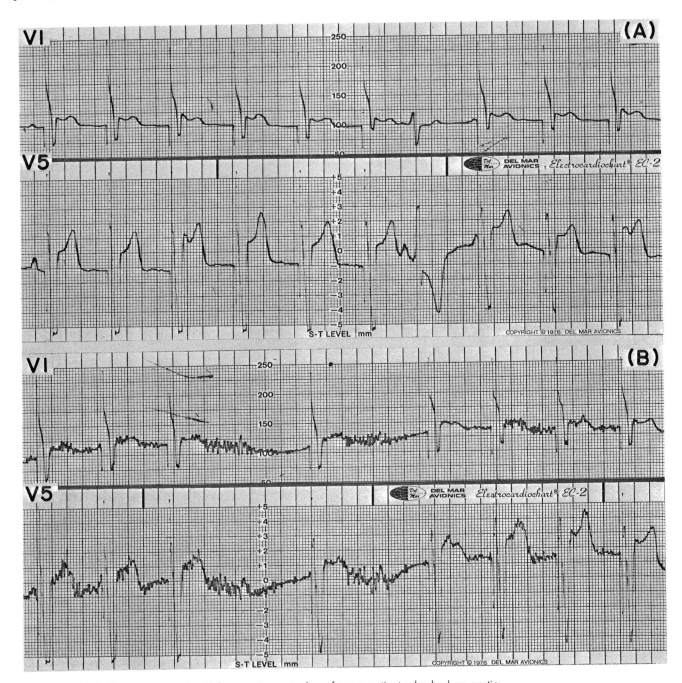

Figure 26-34. Two representative Holter-monitor recordings from a patient who had an aortic valve replacement and an implanted permanent ventricular demand pacemaker. The patient complained of a recent onset of near-syncopal episodes. (**A**) A premature complex is sensed by the pacemaker. (**B**) Irregular firing of the ventricular pacemaker is noted without premature complexes being observed. The artifacts seen on the electrocardiogram represent somatic muscle noise. The original interpretation of this tracing was that concealed ventricular premature complexes were producing recycling of the pacemaker. On further examination, when the patient voluntarily produced pectoralis muscle activity, the pacemaker was suppressed, indicating myopotential sensing by the unipolar pacemaker. The pacemaker was converted to a bipolar mode and no more syncopal or near-syncopal episodes occurred.

Holter-monitor scanning system that enables the technician to evaluate even rare episodes of failure to sense or capture.[128] Their circuitry allows the isolation of pacemaker artifact from the QRS waveform, with quantification of waveforms, analog display, and statistical presentation. This system enables the Holter monitor to serve as a tool in evaluating potential pacemaker malfunction.

The pacemaker patient with recurrent dizzy episodes postimplantation may be a frustrating clinical problem. Noncardiac causes must be evaluated in detail but pacemaker malfunction must also be considered. Detailed pacemaker function analysis may fail to identify any significant abnormality. Figure 26-34 was recorded from a patient with recent onset of recurrent near-syncopal episodes. The 24-hour Holter-monitor recording did not demonstrate prolonged pauses but did show occasional isolated PVCs (see Fig. 26-34A) that were sensed ap-

propriately. Occasional irregular firing was noted, however (see Fig. 26-34B). The initial impression was of concealed PVCs that were being sensed, resulting in recycling of the pacemaker, but antiarrhythmic therapy failed to suppress these pauses. In this patient with a unipolar unit, significant pectoralis muscle exercise produced total suppression of the device and thereby duplicated the patient's symptoms. In retrospect, Figure 26-34B was an example of muscle artifact that was sensed by the unit, resulting in partial suppression. The unipolar device was converted to a bipolar unit, with total elimination of the patient's symptoms.

A somewhat similar clinical situation is illustrated in Figure 26-35, which shows the Holter-monitor recordings from a patient with sick sinus syndrome and a permanent atrial pacemaker. This patient also complained of recurrent dizzy episodes postimplantation; however, pace-

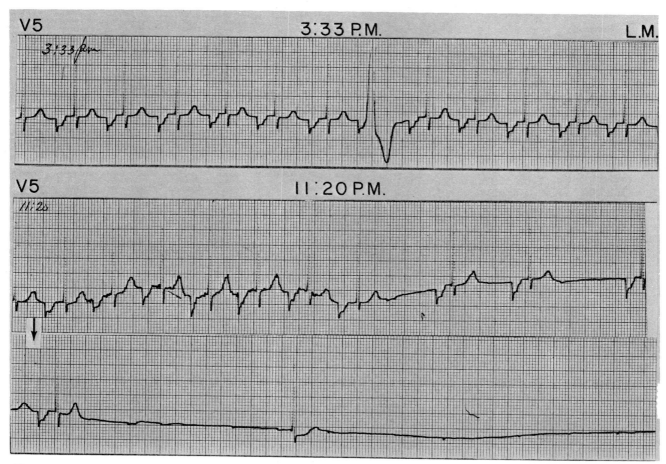

Figure 26-35. Two representative strips obtained from a Holter-monitor recording in a patient with an atrial pacemaker who complained about recurrent syncopal episodes. In the *upper panel*, atrial pacing was noted, with one ventricular premature complex seen. In the *lower strip*, when the patient turned abruptly onto her left side, the atrial pacemaker became irregular and finally ceased to fire. Further detailed evaluation revealed that the patient had a fractured lead wire. The pacemaker functioned appropriately once the lead was replaced.

maker clinic evaluation was normal. A 24-hour Holter-monitor recording was performed, showing multiple episodes of pacemaker failure during the dizzy spells. In retrospect, the patient revealed that she only had symptoms while in certain positions. Subsequent evaluation revealed a partial lead fracture in this patient. Implantation of a new lead restored normal pacemaker function.

Holter-monitor recording is not only useful for evaluation of pacemaker malfunction but can also identify unusual causes of pacemaker-associated problems. A 24-hour Holter-monitor recording was obtained from a patient with a newly implanted ventricular demand unit who had noted recurrent dizzy episodes (Fig. 26-36). Routine pacemaker-clinic evaluation failed to demonstrate any abnormalities, and the Holter-monitor recording was obtained as part of the patient workup. Recurrent episodes of paroxysmal supraventricular tachycardia were demonstrated during this 24-hour recording. Atrioventricular dissociation was present and with an appropriately timed P wave, sinus capture occurred. If the P waves were appropriately positioned, significant anterograde delay occurred, allowing sustained AV nodal reciprocating tachycardia to develop. This patient was treated with both a

change in his pacemaker rate and digoxin, with complete elimination of the episodes of dizziness and paroxysmal supraventricular tachycardia.

Heart Rate Variability

Sudden death after myocardial infarction continues to be a major concern to the cardiologist because up to 50% of these deaths occur without warning.[129-132] Ventricular arrhythmias are an independent predictor of total cardiac mortality and sudden cardiac deaths.[133-137]

Sudden cardiac death appears to be due to structural and functional events that interact, leading to fatal arrhythmias.[138] Data both from experimental and clinical sources support the importance of alterations of autonomic tone as a major force in the development of sudden death.[139-144]

The sinus node is richly innervated by parasympathetic fibers. The right sympathetic nerve has more influence on sinus function than does the left sympathetic nerve, with nerve distribution being mostly epicardial by superficial epicardial coronary artery.[145] The sinus node responds more rapidly to changes in vagal tone because

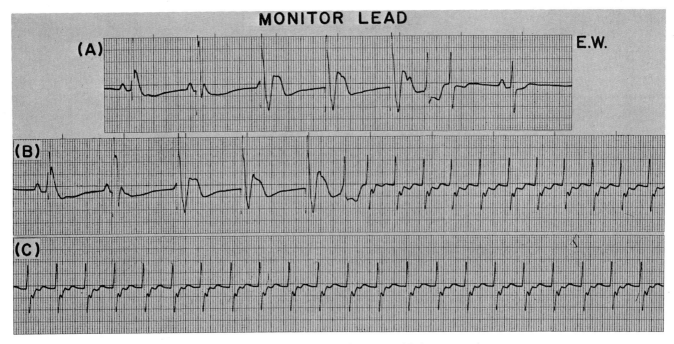

Figure 26-36. Representative records from a Holter-monitor recording in an elderly patient who had a permanent ventricular demand pacemaker implanted because of bradycardia associated with near syncope. After implantation of the pacemaker, the patient continued to have syncopal episodes. (**A**) The Holter-monitor record demonstrates the presence of atrioventricular (AV) dissociation and supraventricular captures. (**B**) AV dissociation is again noted, with a sinus complex occurring at a time that allows for capture of the ventricle but with an extremely long PR interval. Supraventricular tachycardia is then initiated, resulting in sustained reentrant tachycardia associated with severe central nervous system symptomatology in this elderly patient with diminished cardiovascular reserve.

there is a shorter latency between release and effect of acetylcholine.[146] Vagal fibers in the myocardium are located predominantly on the endocardial surface.[147]

Myocardial ischemia and infarction can produce a significant alteration in cardiac autonomic tone by directly affecting neural fibers and altering afferent autonomic action.[148-150] The exact mechanism or mechanisms by which specific alterations are noted is not clear, however. Nevertheless, myocardial infarction can affect autonomic tone, as measured by altered heart rate variability.[140]

Heart rate variability is a measure of autonomic tone, predominantly reflecting parasympathetic activity but multiple control mechanisms are operative (Fig. 26-37). Heart rate variability is decreased in patients postmyocardial infarction and may be a marker for those patients at risk for sudden cardiac death.[151,152]

Heart rate variability generally is measured using Holter-monitor recordings. Data have been obtained using time-domain or nonspectral analysis but frequency-domain or spectral analysis may be more sensitive.

Nonspectral measurements appear to reflect predominantly parasympathetic tone. Multiple measurement formats have been used to obtain the data.[143,153-156] Nonspectral analysis is performed on the entire 24-hour recording, whereas frequency-domain analysis is generally performed on 256 successive beats. Spectral analysis is performed using fast Fourier transform methods to translate RR intervals into different frequency domains. This data generally is expressed as three peaks: (1) very-low-frequency band–sympathetic, parasympathetic, and renin–angiotensin activity (0.02 to 0.09 Hz); (2) low-frequency band–baroreceptor reflex and blood pressure

regulation (0.09 to 0.15 Hz); and (3) high-frequency band–respiratory driven parasympathetic activity (0.15 to 0.40 Hz; Fig. 26-38),.[157-161]

Heart rate variability in normal subjects appears to be stable in any individual (over at least several weeks) having higher variability at night with a peak in early morning hours.[162] Variability decreases with age and is higher in physically well-trained individuals.[163]

Heart rate variability has been described as decreasing after myocardial infarction, as first observed by Schneider and Costiloe.[164] In 1987, the Multicenter Infarction Group demonstrated in a 31-month follow-up of acute myocardial infarction patients that 34% of 125 patients with a heart rate variability of less than 50 milliseconds died, whereas only 12% of 683 patients with a value of more than 50 milliseconds died. This variable was found to be an independent predictor of mortality, with the vulnerable group having a 5.3% greater relative risk of dying than the normal group.[165]

A subsequent study of 487 patients used heart rate variability, Holter-monitor data, signal-averaged ECGs, and left ventricular ejection fraction to predict both arrhythmic and all-cause cardiac death for a 20-month follow-up.[139] There were 24 arrhythmic deaths, and this group had a markedly reduced heart rate variability. In combination with an abnormal signal-averaged ECG, there was a sensitivity of 58%, a positive predicted accuracy of 33%, and a relative risk of 18.

Heart rate variability can be modified by a variety of interventions. Physical endurance training increases vagal tone and heart rate variability. Interestingly, biofeedback training appears potentially to alter heart rate

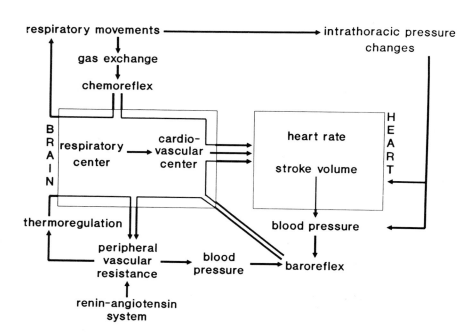

Figure 26-37. (**A**) Cardiovascular control mechanisms for heart-rate adjustment. (van Ravenswaaij-Arts MA, Kollee LAA, Hopman JCW, Stoelinga GBA, van Geijn HP: Heart rate variability. Ann Intern Med 1993;118:436.)

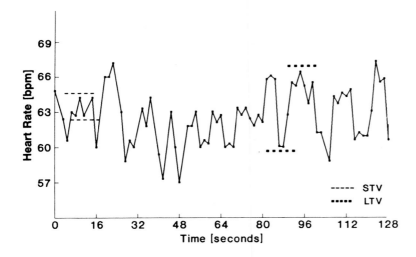

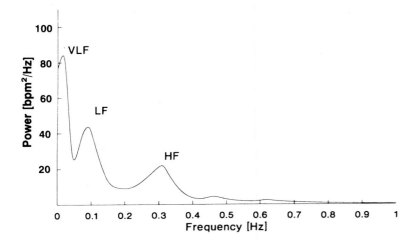

Figure 26-38. (**A**) The *top panel* shows beat-to-beat short-term variability (*STV*) and long-term variability (*LTV*). The *bottom panel* shows a power spectrum plot of the heart-rate tracing shown in the top panel. The three main peaks are very low frequency (*VLF*; 0.05 Hz) fluctuations; low-frequency (*LF*; 0.1 Hz) fluctuations; and high-frequency (*HF*; 0.32 Hz) fluctuations. The area under each peak corresponds to the amount of each fluctuation presented in the top heart rate plot. (van Ravenswaaij-Arts MA, Kollee LAA, Hopman JCW, Stoelinga GBA, van Geijn HP: Heart rate variability. Ann Intern Med 1993;118:436.)

variability.[166,167] β-Adrenergic–blocking therapy reduces mortality in the postmyocardial infarction patient. This may be partly due to a reduction in heart rate variability related to augmented vagal tone and possibly to central vagal tonic effects.[139,168] Parasympathetic tone may also be altered pharmacologically and therefore increase heart rate variability. Drugs such as transdermal scopolamine have been used to increase heart rate variability in normal patients.[169]

The effect of antiarrhythmic drugs on heart rate variability has also been studied in light of the CAST trial results.[99,170,171] In one study, amiodarone produced no significant change, whereas flecainide and propafenone decreased heart rate variability.[99]

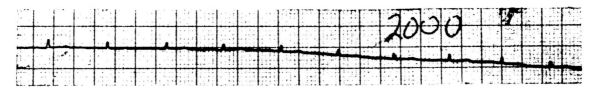

Figure 26-39. This record demonstrates the influence of partial battery failure on Holter-monitor recordings. Note the predominant voltage reduction. (Krasnow AZ, Bloomfield DK: Artifacts in portable electrocardiographic monitoring. Am Heart J 1976;91:349.)

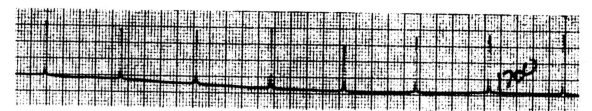

Figure 26-40. Example of pseudojunctional rhythm seen in a Holter-monitor record, during which the low-frequency cut-off is abnormal, resulting in lack of atrial activity and loss of repolarization. (Krasnow AZ, Bloomfield DK: Artifacts in portable electrocardiographic monitoring. Am Heart J 1976;91:349.)

ARTIFACTS IN HOLTER MONITORING

The previous sections discussed the use of Holter-monitor recordings in the evaluation and management of cardiovascular patients. It is essential, however, that both the technician and the physician be aware of the many pitfalls that may occur with the use of 24-hour recorders and playback units.[172,173] It is critical to the patient's well-being that inappropriate interpretation of inaccurate data be prevented from influencing the patient's medical management. Although the Holter-monitor recording may be invaluable in the clinical care of many patients, errors in evaluation may be equally costly. This section identifies many of the technical problems that—when recognized— clarify the appropriate clinical decision-making process.

Technical problems with the recorders, playback amplifier, or stylus may become manifest in a variety of ways, which may result in inability to evaluate the electrocardiographic events. Excessive damping, inappropriate calibration, saturation of the amplifier, and poorly adjusted stylus are just a few of many potential examples that may render the final report worthless for interpretation (Figs. 26-39 and 26-40).

Vacillation in QRS- or T-wave morphology may frequently be noted in relation to change in respiration or body position. Recognition of these frequently observed variations is essential for proper interpretation of Holter-monitor recordings, especially in patients with suspected ischemic heart disease (Fig. 26-41).

Inappropriate display or inappropriate mounting of the tape during playback leads to misdiagnosis if not recognized, with significant associated clinical implications. In Figure 26-42, the electrocardiographic signal has been displayed in an inverted fashion, resulting in an electrocardiographic record with an inverted P wave, a prominent Q wave, and an inverted T wave. Because of this inversion, the inappropriate diagnosis of ectopic atrial or junctional rhythm and repolarization abnormalities could clearly have been made.

In Figure 26-43, the initial impression of this record may be of first-degree AV block with short QT interval (see Fig. 26-43A and B) and ST-segment elevation with a PVC during a tachycardia of possible supraventricular origin (see Figure 26-43C). More careful analysis of the tracing reveals that the tape has been analyzed in a reverse fashion, with the resultant ECG displaying T, QRS, and P; the ST-segment elevation is actually ST-segment depression.

The use of two-channel recorders has previously been emphasized (see Fig. 26-22) with regard to documenting the potential origin of premature complexes. Of equal importance is the significance of two-channel recordings in evaluating artifacts, which may lead to erroneous clinical decisions if only single-channel data are available. In Figure 26-44, lead V₅ identifies a sudden pause

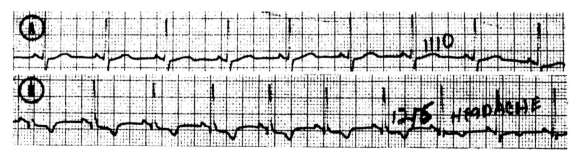

Figure 26-41. Positional changes in the ST-T wave and the QRS seen in this tracing are commonly noted in Holter-monitor recordings in patients without significant cardiac disease. (Krasnow AZ, Bloomfield DK: Artifacts in portable electrocardiographic monitoring. Am Heart J 1976;91:349.)

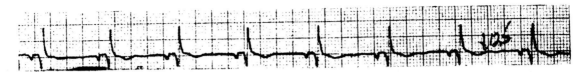

Figure 26-42. Recording in which reversed polarity is obtained, with inversion of the P, QRS, and T waves because of improper lead placement. (Krasnow AZ, Bloomfield, DK: Artifacts in portable electrocardiographic monitoring. AM Heart J 1976;91:349.)

that is a multiple of the sinus rate, suggesting 2:1 sinoatrial block. In lead V_1, however, the absent sinus complex was clearly recorded, thereby identifying the sinoatrial block as a lead artifact.

More protracted technical artifacts may lead to the clinical decision for urgent permanent pacing, even if the patient remains asymptomatic. In Figure 26-45, such an example is seen in which transient recording failure has produced a short pause (MV_1) followed by a long pause, despite the use of a two-channel Holter-monitor. The clue to the artifactual nature of this record is the absence of the pause in the first portion of the record (MV_5) and the irregular nature of the second and longer pause in MV_1 and MV_5.

In Figures 26-44 and 26-45, sudden pauses are apparent that are multiples of the basic sinus cycle length. These technical artifacts are due to lead electrode artifacts or electronic artifacts. Another form of artifact, however, may result in dramatic rate changes that can be misinterpreted as sinus arrest, with a resultant clinical decision for urgent

pacemaker therapy. This artifact is dramatically illustrated in Figure 26-46. In this recording, marked sinus arrest and sinus slowing are noted. Closer inspection of the record reveals that PR-, QRS-, and QT-interval prolongation of varying degrees can be identified before, during, and after the pauses. This record is properly identified as artifact secondary to stretching of the tape and subsequent distortion of the analog waveforms and associated PP intervals.

Pseudoarrhythmias may also occur secondary to technical artifact. In a minor fashion, their misinterpretation may not lead to clinical changes but recurrent arrhythmias may result in serious errors in clinical management. In Figure 26-47A, an example of pseudoatrial premature complexes is seen. These premature complexes occur because of sudden momentary changes in tape transport speed. In Figure 26-47B, an example of a junctional rhythm with supraventricular premature complexes is seen. This also is artifact and results from a combination of amplifier artifact (see Fig. 26-40) and tape transport distortion.

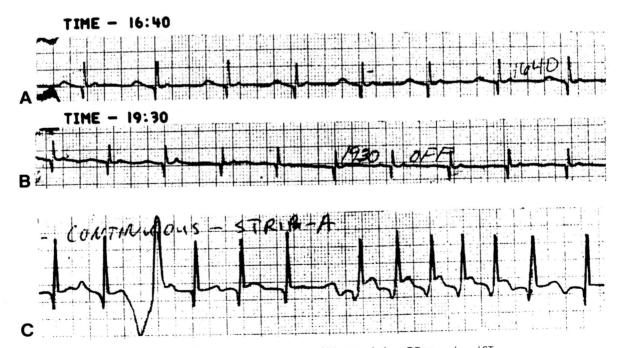

Figure 26-43. Strips in this recording demonstrate prolonged PR interval, short QT interval, and ST-segment elevation. In reality, these strips represent a mirror image sequence in which the tape has been run in reverse. (Krasnow AZ, Bloomfield DK: Artifacts in portable electrocardiographic monitoring. Am Heart J 1976;91:349.)

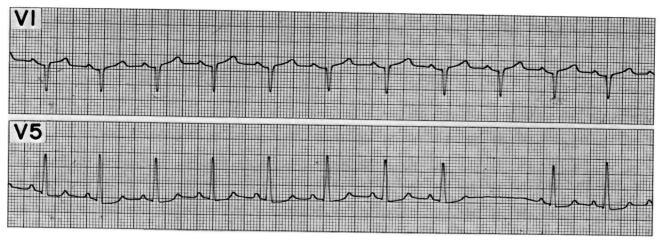

Figure 26-44. The advantages of a two-channel system are clearly demonstrated by looking at the simultaneously obtained lead V₁ and lead V₅ recordings. In lead V₅, an episode of what appears to be 2:1 sinoatrial block is actually loss of signal on the V₅ electrode during a time at which the patient was clearly in sinus rhythm.

Artifact outside of the recorder-playback system may also result in an inappropriate rhythm diagnosis. Figure 26-48A shows an apparent episode of atrial flutter with a controlled ventricular rate. On closer inspection, in Figure 26-48B, the initial portion of the record shows atrial flutter that disappears as the baseline changes. This is an example of sinus rhythm with extraneous surface electrode noise mimicking a paroxysmal episode of atrial flutter.

Episodes of paroxysmal tachycardia also can be a manifestation of technical artifact. Variations in the degree of artifact can produce subtle or overt manifestations of this event. Figure 26-49A shows sinus rhythm with narrow PR, QRS, and QT intervals. In Figure 26-49B, at a time when the battery was near depletion, there is an apparent sinus tachycardia. Closer inspection reveals that there is not only an increase in heart rate but also a decrease in the

PR, QRS, and QT intervals, indicating a significant change in tape transport speed. A more dramatic example of this phenomenon is illustrated in Figure 26-50. In the upper panel, intermittent decrease in battery output results in sudden acceleration of heart rate; this phenomenon is both more sustained and increased in rate in the lower panel. The heart rate of about 300 beats per minute in the lower panel mimics atrial flutter with 1:1 conduction but is clearly artifact for the reasons outlined above.

Artifacts can also mimic ventricular arrhythmias; this has important clinical implications if they are misinterpreted by the reviewing physician. This is dramatically illustrated by the Holter-monitor strips shown in Figure 26-51. In Figure 26-51A, sinus rhythm is seen with normal PR, QRS, and QT intervals. Moments later, as depicted in Figure 26-51B, the recording shows a marked increase in

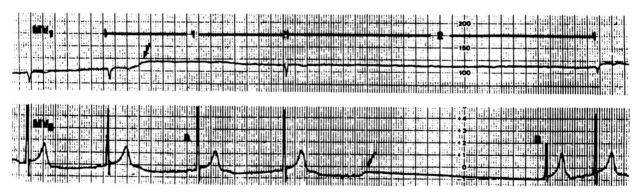

Figure 26-45. A more dramatic example of the events illustrated in Figure 26-44. This two-channel recording identifies repeated loss of signal in the *upper strip* and intermittent loss of signal in the *lower strip*. The data suggest marked sinus node dysfunction but in reality are artifactual secondary to signal loss. (Gardin JM, Belic N, Singer DH: Pseudoarrhythmias in ambulatory ECG monitoring. Arch Intern Med 1979;139:809.)

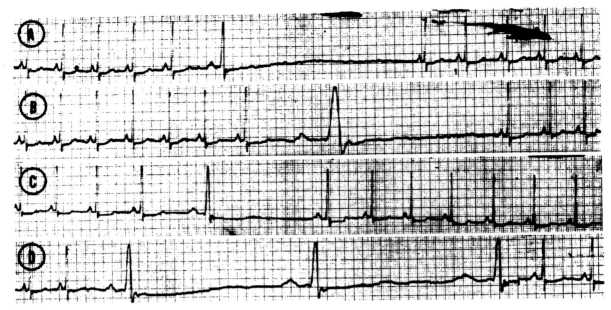

Figure 26-46. Episodes suggestive of pseudosinus arrest that are actually due to marked alterations in tape speed or tape stretching or both. The patient had no demonstratable abnormalities of sinus function. Note the marked prolongation of the PR interval and QRS interval, especially well-seen in **B** and **D**. (Krasnow AZ, Bloomfield DK: Artifacts in portable electrocardiographic monitoring. Am Heart J 1976;91:349.)

heart rate associated with a wide QRS complex. On close inspection, a regular QRS can be discerned among the bizarre QRS complexes at a rate of about 120 beats per minute. This recording represents electrode artifact during exercise in a patient with sinus tachycardia.

Conduction defects can also be simulated by artifacts. These defects in conduction may have minor clinical im-

plications or may result in significant but inappropriate clinical decisions with regard to permanent pacing. A dramatic example with substantial clinical implications is evident in the tracings shown in Figure 26-52. Episodic second-degree AV block (Mobitz type II) appears to be present in Figure 26-52*A*, which progresses to a more advanced degree of AV block in Figure 26-52*B*. More care-

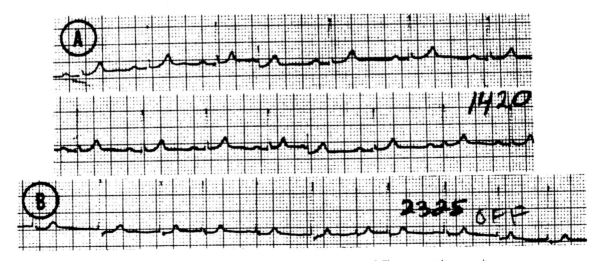

Figure 26-47. Pseudoextrasystoles due to tape sticking are demonstrated. This tape sticking results in "premature complexes" with extremely short PR and QRS duration. (Krasnow AZ, Bloomfield DK: Artifacts in portable electrocardiographic monitoring. Am Heart J 1976;91:349.)

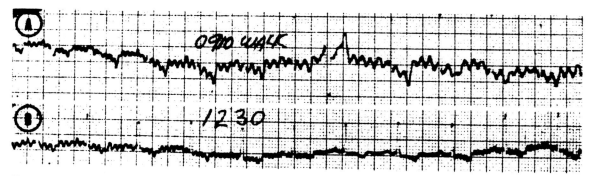

Figure 26-48. (**A**) Pseudoatrial fibrillation/flutter. (**B**) Clear-cut sinus rhythm which, in retrospect, is the circumstance seen in **A**. This patient's records showing pseudoatrial fibrillation/flutter are due to electrode noise and are not associated with patient tremor or atrial flutter. (Krasnow AZ, Bloomfield DK: Artifacts in portable electrocardiographic monitoring. Am Heart J 1976;91:349.)

ful inspection of the records reveals that the nonconducted P waves represent distorted QRS complexes secondary to amplifier artifact.

Decisions to implant permanent pacemakers based on inadequate data or misinterpretation must be avoided. Occasionally, the Holter-monitor recording may demonstrate evidence of normal pacemaker function in the absence of any pacemaker, temporary or permanent. This is graphically illustrated in Figure 26-53. In the lower strip, this continuous record shows a rapid artifact similar to a pacemaker spike. This actually represents electrode motion artifact in a patient in whom there is neither a temporary nor a permanent pacemaker.

The ultimate artifactual arrhythmia is illustrated in Figure 26-54. In this case, two distinct QRS types suggest two independent supraventricular sites of origin (e.g., sinus and junctional parasystole). The true explanation of this most unusual rhythm is readily apparent when one discovers that this tracing was obtained from a tape that had previously been used for another Holter-monitor recording. This resulted in the recording of the present patient's ECG (small QRS) superimposed on the previous patient's ECG (large QRS). This has been described as the "siamese-twin" effect.

MISCELLANEOUS

There are a variety of uncategorized areas in which Holter monitoring can be invaluable in the evaluation and management of cardiac patients. This section illustrates some aspects of a potpourri of clinical situations in which long-term electrocardiographic monitoring may be useful.

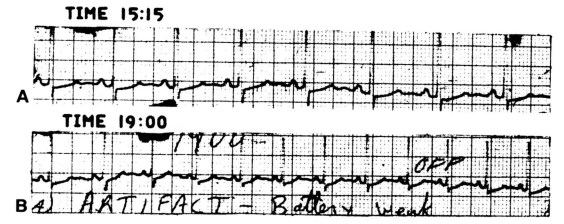

Figure 26-49. Paroxysmal pseudosinus tachycardia. (**B**) Increase in the heart rate, suggestive of sinus tachycardia seen in B with shortening of the PR, QRS, and QT intervals, consistent with early battery failure. (Krasnow AZ, Bloomfield DK: Artifacts in portable electrocardiographic monitoring. Am Heart J 1976;91:349.)

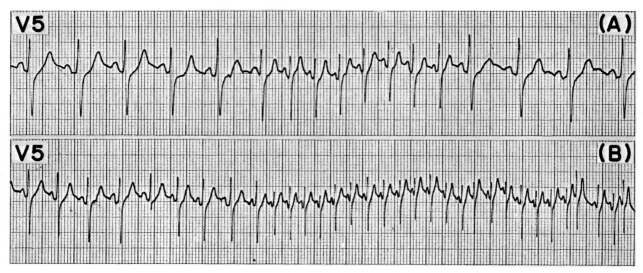

Figure 26-50. Two representative strips from a patient's Holter-monitor recording, during which time battery failure occurred. (**A**) A short period of diminished battery output apparently accelerates the heart rate. (**B**) More prominent battery failure results in apparent supraventricular "tachycardia" at rates of nearly 300 beats/min.

In Figure 26-55, a record obtained from a patient with a history of recurrent tachycardias is shown. The upper panel shows sinus rhythm with first-degree AV block, yet in the lower panel, with a decrease in the sinus rate, the PR interval shortens and QRS complexes with initial slurring of the upstroke appear. These latter complexes only appeared at slow sinus rates, with a fixed PR associated with a uniform bizarre QRS during such times. Therefore, the Holter-monitor recording indicated that this patient had ventricular preexcitation with a long bypass refractory period. His tachyarrhythmias could thus be explained, and a more critical formulation of antiarrhythmic therapy could be designed. (Prior studies in patients with Wolff-Parkinson-White syndrome document tachyarrhythmias without symptoms and symptoms without tachyarrhythmias.)[174, 175]

On many occasions, patients with ischemic heart disease have a prominent variability in clinical symptoms. Nevertheless, there are times when patients may not manifest clinical complaints but have electrocardiographic evidence of ischemia with a potential for significant ventricular arrhythmias. This vacillation in the electrocardiographic manifestations of ischemia (i.e., ST-segment depression) is clearly illustrated by the records obtained over a 24-hour period in a patient with intermittent angina (Fig. 26-56). That ST-segment depression can occur during sleep, unassociated with clinical symptoms, is clearly illustrated (see also Fig. 26-25).

An equally important use of Holter monitoring may be in the patient with clinically atypical but angina-like chest pain. These patients may represent variant angina, and electrocardiographic recordings during episodes of chest pain may be crucial to their diagnosis and management. The patients may present not only with histories of chest distress but also with a history of palpitations. The Holter-monitor recordings allow clear documentation of the basis for these symptoms. The spectrum of such a clinical situation is illustrated in Figures 26-57 to 26-58, obtained from a woman aged 48 years with burning epigastric pain of recent onset occurring at rest and unrelated to food intake. Her internist could not control the episodes of pain (more than 15 per day) with routine antacid therapy. A gallbladder series was negative and an upper gastrointestinal series demonstrated a small hiatus hernia. The patient was referred to a gastroenterologist for further workup. His evaluation was inconclusive but he felt the pain was not gastrointestinal in origin. A Holter monitoring was ordered because the patient also admitted that she experienced palpitations during some of those episodes of pain. In Figure 26-57, obtained during an episode of pain, dramatic ST-segment elevation is seen in lead V₅. These electrocardiographic events were repeatedly documented during all episodes of pain that the patient experienced during the 24-hour recording. On several occasions, the patient complained of palpitations and in Figure 26-58, a recording shows repetitive short bursts of probable ventricular tachycardia that were documented on multiple occasions, associated with clinical complaints of chest pain and palpitations. These, however, were not the only events documented during such periods of chest pain

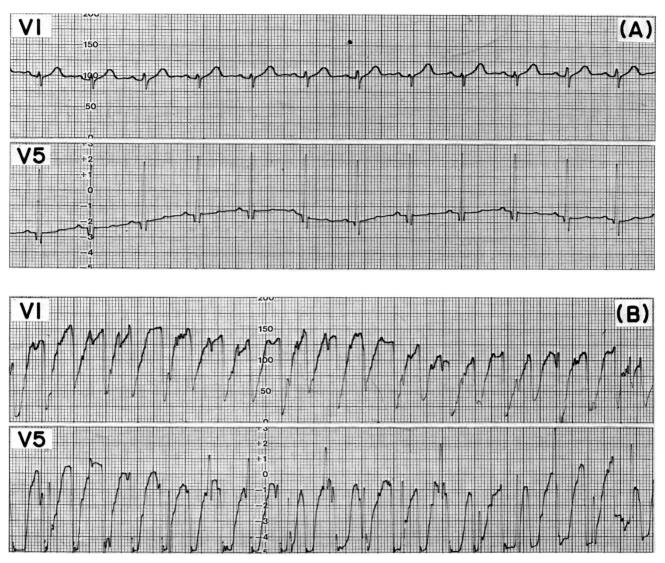

Figure 26-51. Pseudoventricular tachycardia is illustrated in this record obtained from a patient without significant palpitations. **(A)** Sinus rhythm is demonstrated. **(B)** Bizarre regular activity is noted in both V₁ and V₅ electrode leads. More careful inspection of the record demonstrates sinus tachycardia, with narrow QRS complexes interspersed between the bizarre waveforms. Marked electrode artifact is demonstrated.

and palpitations. On several other occasions, the patient had recordings during which paroxysmal AV block occurred during complaints of chest pain and palpitations (see Fig. 26-59). Therefore, in this patient, the gamut of phasic ST-segment elevation, ventricular arrhythmias, and AV block were all recorded during episodes of chest pain. The diagnosis of variant angina was established and appropriate medical therapy was initiated. Therefore, Holter-monitor recordings such as those shown in these figures may be an invaluable tool in evaluating patients with suspected or documented ischemic heart disease.

Ideally, in many patients with cardiac arrhythmias, magnification of atrial activity would offer significant diagnostic (and potentially therapeutic) advantages. The use of various lead placement changes can occasionally enhance atrial activity on the surface ECG (i.e., Lewis lead). Nevertheless, even with the use of dual-channel systems and novel lead placements, Holter-monitor recordings may not always allow accurate rhythm interpretation.

Jenkins and coworkers demonstrated that a bipolar electrode can be introduced per os for continuous re-

Text continues on p. 854

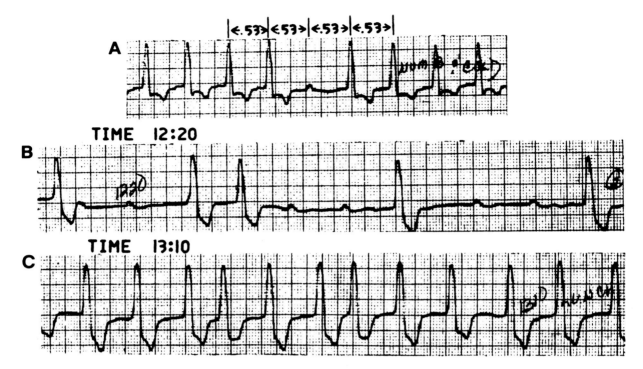

Figure 26-52. Pseudoatrioventricular block is illustrated in this record obtained from a patient without a history of syncope but with an intraventricular conduction defect of the left bundle branch block type. Episodes of apparent second-degree atrioventricular block with nonconducted sinus complexes are seen in **A** and **B**. The small complexes initially interpreted as atrial activity are actually normal QRS complexes that are damped by amplifier artifact. (Krasnow AZ, Bloomfield DK: Artifacts in portable electrocardiographic monitoring. Am Heart J 1976;91:349.)

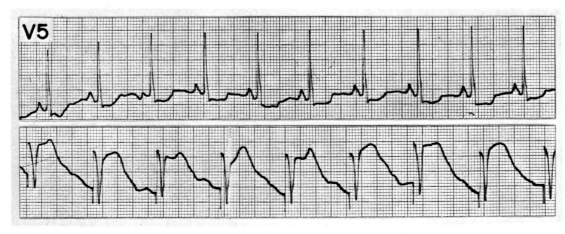

Figure 26-53. Pseudopacemaker activity in a continuous record from a single-channel recording. Marked amplifier and electrode artifact mimics the presence of a demand pacemaker.

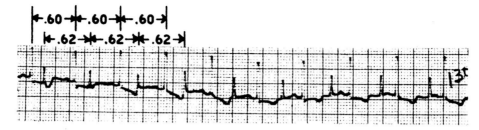

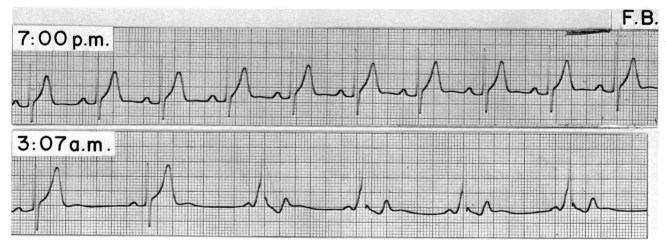

Figure 26-54. Pseudoelectric alternans due to the presence of a "siamese-twin" effect. This record illustrates the ultimate complex arrhythmia in Holter-monitor recording. The electrocardiograms of two patients have been recorded on the same tape, explaining the bizarre arrhythmia seen in this tracing. (Krasnow AZ, Bloomfield DK: Artifacts in portable electrocardiographic monitoring. Am Heart J 1976;91:349.)

Figure 26-55. Two representative strips from a patient with a history of tachycardia. In the *top strip*, sinus rhythm with normal atrioventricular conduction is noted. In the *bottom strip*, during the sinus bradycardia, ventricular preexcitation is now noted.

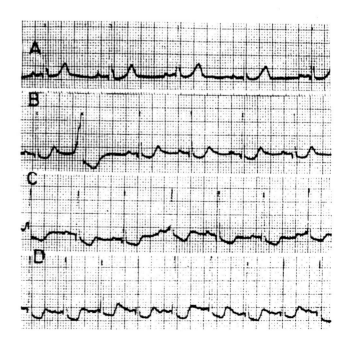

Figure 26-56. Significant ST-segment changes at various times of the day but unassociated with significant clinical symptomatology in a patient with coronary artery disease. (Stern S, Tzivoni D: The dynamic nature of ST-T segment in ischemic heart disease. Am Heart J 1976;91:820.)

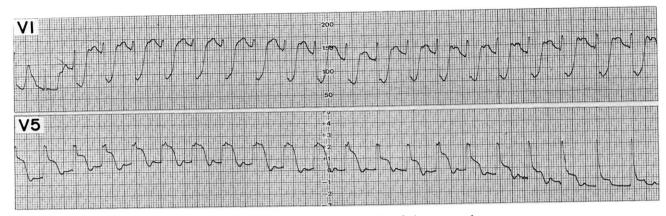

Figure 26-57. Recording obtained from a patient with recurrent episodes of chest pain of an atypical variety but suggestive of reflux esophagitis. During an episode of chest pain, marked ST-segment elevation is seen in lead V₅, consistent with Prinzmetal's variant angina.

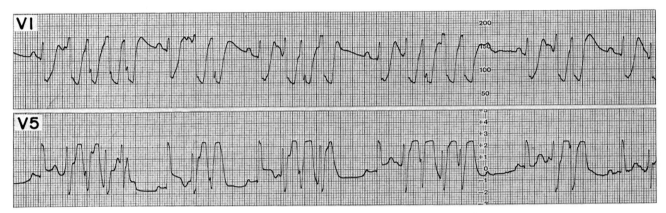

Figure 26-58. Another portion of the recording from the same patient as in Figure 25-55. This portion of the recording was obtained during a period when the patient had both palpitations and chest pain. Note the prominent ST-segment elevation and the burst of ventricular premature complexes.

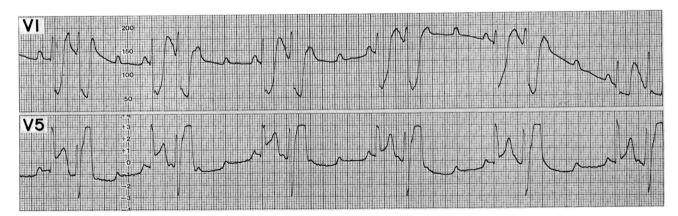

Figure 26-59. Another portion of the Holter-monitor recording obtained from the same patient as in Figures 26-57 and 26-58, illustrating another period during which the patient complained of palpitations and chest pain. Note the presence of marked ST-segment elevation, atrioventricular block, and ventricular premature complexes.

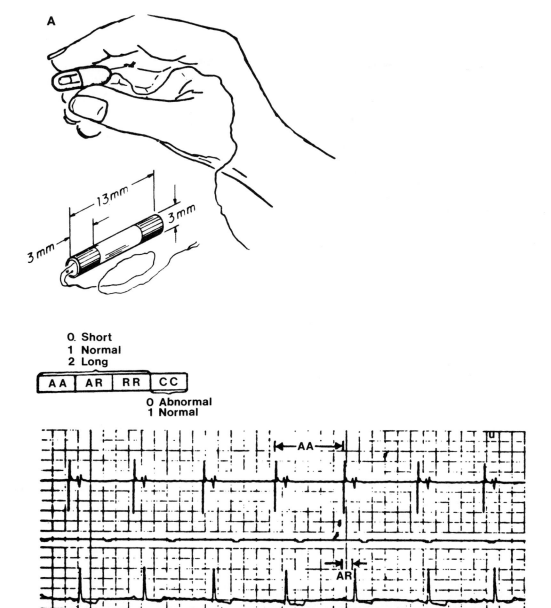

Figure 26-60. (**A**) The swallowable bipolar electrode that may be used for recording an atrial electrogram in an ambulatory patient during Holter-monitor recording. (**B**) The atrial electrogram is seen in the *upper channel*, and the surface electrocardiogram is seen in the *lower channel*. (Jenkins JM, Wu D, Arzbaecher RL: Computer diagnosis of supraventricular and ventricular arrhythmias. A new esophageal technique. Circulation 1979;60:977. By permission of the American Heart Association.)

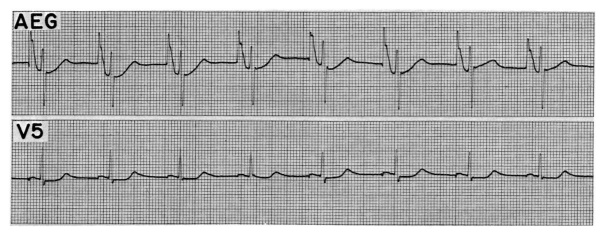

Figure 26-61. Atrial electrodes implanted at cardiac surgery were used to obtain an atrial electrogram during recording with the two-channel Holter-monitor. In the *top strip*, the atrial electrogram was recorded with a prominent atrial spike and a QRS spike. The surface electrocardiogram in the *bottom strip* was obtained during sinus rhythm.

cording of an atrial electrogram on one channel of a dual-channel recorder (Fig. 26-60A).[176] This swallowable bipolar esophageal electrode gives an adequate atrial recording that is satisfactory for the use of computerized techniques for arrhythmia analysis (see Fig. 26-60B).

In studies from our institution, we found that a similar quality atrial recording can be obtained over 24-hour periods with the use of atrial wires implanted at cardiac surgery (Fig. 26-61). Adequate atrial signals can be continuously recorded on one of the two channels of the Holter-monitor recorder, allowing accurate evaluation of many transient or more persistent arrhythmias. Atrial arrhythmias, such as isolated atrial premature complexes or atrial

flutter, can be clearly documented (Fig. 26-62 and 26-63). Atrioventricular dissociation, PVCs, and ventricular tachycardia also can readily be diagnosed (Figs. 23-64 through 23-66). The techniques described above can be anticipated to extend significantly the usefulness of Holter-monitor recording devices.

Conclusion

This chapter and the position papers sponsored by the American College of Physicians,[34] the joint report by the American Heart Association, and the American College of

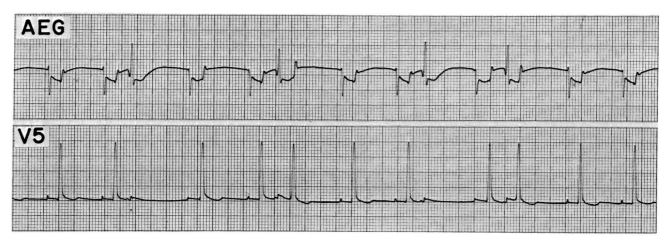

Figure 26-62. Using the technique discussed in Figure 26-61, a record is obtained during standard Holter-monitor recording in a postoperative cardiac surgical patient. The *top strip* demonstrates the atrial electrogram, and the *bottom strip* demonstrates a surface electrocardiogram. Note the presence of premature complexes that are clearly atrial in origin, as demonstrated by the prominent P waves seen both during the nonconducted complexes and during the conducted complexes.

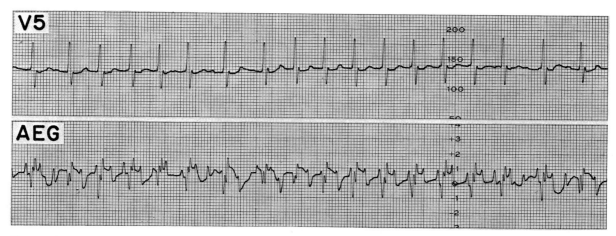

Figure 26-63. A representative recording from a patient after cardiac surgery, during which time recurrent supraventricular tachycardia was noted on Holter monitoring. The *bottom strip* shows the atrial electrogram, which clearly identifies the presence of two atrial complexes for each QRS complex (i.e., atrial flutter with 2:1 ventricular response).

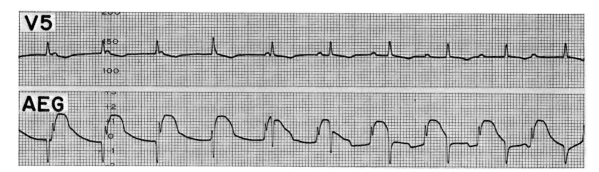

Figure 26-64. A two-lead Holter-monitor recording from a patient after cardiac surgery; during the recording, the lower channel was used to record the atrial electrogram. Note the presence of atrioventricular dissociation, clearly seen in the atrial electrogram, with varying QRS and P wave rates.

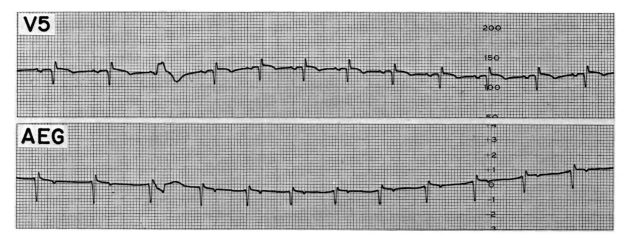

Figure 26-65. A two-lead Holter-monitor recording, during which one channel was used to record an atrial electrogram in a patient after cardiac surgery. Note the presence of the premature complex unassociated with a change in sinus rate (suggesting ventricular origin).

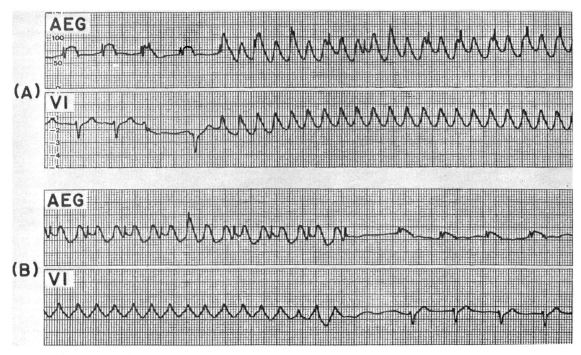

Figure 26-66. A two-channel Holter-monitor recording obtained from a postoperative cardiac surgical patient during an episode of tachycardia. The upper tracing in both **A** and **B** is an atrial electrogram. The lower tracings are lead V₁ surface electrocardiograms. (**A**) The onset of a wide QRS rapid tachycardia is noted. Inspection of the atrial electrogram recordings clearly demonstrates atrioventricular dissociation, indicating a very high likelihood of ventricular origin of the tachycardia.

Cardiology[33] will serve as a resource guide to the clinician with an interest in Holter-monitor electrocardiography.

References

1. Holter NJ, Gengerelli JA: Remote recording of physiologic data by radio. Rocky Mt Med J 1949;46:79.

2. Holter NJ: Radioelectrocardiography: new technique for cardiovascular studies. Ann NY Acad Sci 1957;65:913.

3. Holter NJ: New method for heart studies. Science 1961; 134:1214.

4. Gilson JS, Holter NJ, Glascock WR: Continuous ambulant electrocardiograms and their analysis—clinical observations using the electrocardiocorder and a Vsep analyzer. Circulation 1961;24:940.

5. Gilson JS, Holter NJ, Glascock WR: Clinical observations using electrocardiocorder and A Vsep continuous electrocardiographic system. Am J Cardiol 1964;14:204.

6. Sanders JS, Martt JM: Dynamic electrocardiography at high altitude. Am J Cardiol 1964;14:287.

7. Corday E, Bazika V, Lang T-W, et al: Detection of phantom arrhythmias and evanescent electrocardiographic abnormalities. JAMA 1965;193:417.

8. Hinkle LE, Meyer J, Stevens M, et al: Tape recording of the ECG of active men: limitations and advantages of the Holter-Avionics instruments. Circulation 1967;36:752.

9. Walter PF, Reid SJ Jr, Wenger NK: Transient cerebral ischemia due to arrhythmias. Ann Intern Med 1970;72:471.

10. Karpman HL, Bleifer SB, Bleifer DF: Clinical applications of dynamic electrocardiography. Chest 1970;58:283.

11. Crook BRM, Cashman PMM, Stott FD, et al: Tape monitoring of the electrocardiogram in ambulant patients with sino-atrial disease. Br Heart J 1973;35:1009.

12. Crawford M, O'Rourke R, Ramakrishna N, et al: Comparative effectiveness of exercise testing and continuous monitoring for detecting arrhythmias in patients with previous myocardial infarction. Circulation 1974;50:301.

13. Kleiger RE, Senior RM: Long-term electrocardiographic monitoring of ambulatory patients with chronic airway obstruction. Chest 1974;65:483.

14. Bleifer SB, Bleifer DJ, Hausmann DR, et al: Diagnosis of occult arrhythmias by Holter electrocardiography. Prog Cardiovasc Dis 1974;16:569.

15. Stein IM: Ambulatory long-term electrocardiography—the "LCG." Am Heart J 1974;88:37.

16. Ryan M, Lown B, Horn H: Comparison of ventricular ectopic activity during 24-hour monitoring and exercise testing in patients with coronary heart disease. N Engl J Med 1974; 292:224.

17. Winkle RA, Lopes MG, Fitzgerald JW, et al: Arrhythmias in patients with mitral valve prolapse. Circulation 1975;52:73.

18. Coumel P: Continuous electrocardiographic recording. Clinical, diagnostic and therapeutic value. Arch Mal Coeur 1975;68:941.

19. Harrison DC, Fitzgerald JW, Winkle RA: Ambulatory electrocardiography for diagnosis and treatment of cardiac arrhythmias. N Engl J Med 1976;294:373.

20. Vismara LA, Pratt C, Miller RR, et al: Correlation of standard electrocardiogram and continuous ambulatory monitoring in detection of ventricular arrhythmias in coronary patients. Circulation 1976;53:27.

21. Stern S, Tzivoni D: The dynamic nature of the ST-T segment in ischemic heart disease. Am Heart J 1976;91:820.

22. Schroeder JS: Ambulatory electrocardiographic monitoring—technique and clinical indications. JAMA 1976;236:494.

23. Romero CA: Holter monitoring in diagnosis and management of cardiac rhythm disturbances. Med Clin North Am 1976;60:299.

24. Johansson BW: Long term ECG in ambulatory clinical practice. Analysis and two year follow-up of 100 patients studied with a portable ECG tape recorder. Eur J Cardiol 1977;5:39.

25. Brodsky M, Wu D, Denes P, et al: Arrhythmias documented by 24 hour continuous electrocardiograph monitoring in 50 male medical students without apparent heart disease. Am J Cardiol 1977;39:390.

26. Kennedy HL: Ambulatory electrocardiography. Ann Intern Med 1977;87:729.

27. Fletcher GF, Cantwell JD: Continuous ambulatory electrocardiographic monitoring. Use in cardiac exercise programs. Chest 1977;71:27.

28. McLeod AA, Jewitt DE: Role of 24 hour ambulatory electrocardiographic monitoring in a general hospital. Br Med J 1978;1:1197.

29. Michelson EL, Morganroth J, MacVaugh H III: Postoperative arrhythmias after coronary artery and cardiac valvular surgery detected by long-term electrocardiographic monitoring. Am Heart J 1979;97:442.

30. Gradman AH, Bell PA, DeBusk RF: Sudden death during ambulatory monitoring. Circulation 1977;55:210.

31. Morganroth J: Ambulatory Holter electrocardiography: choice of technologies and clinical uses. Ann Intern Med 1985;102:73.

32. Pratt CM Eaton T, Francis M, Pacifico A: Ambulatory electrocardiographic recordings: the Holter monitor. Curr Probl Cardiol 1988;13:521.

33. Fisch C, DeSanctis RW, Dodge HT, Reeves TJ, Weinberg SL: Guidelines for ambulatory electrocardiography: a report of the American College of Cardiology/American Heart Association Task Force on Assessment of Diagnostic and Therapeutic Cardiovascular Procedures (Subcommittee on Ambulatory Electrocardiography). J Am Coll Cardiol 1989; 13:249.

34. DiMarco JP, Philbrick JT: Use of ambulatory electrocardiographic (Holter) monitoring. Ann Intern Med 1990; 113:53.

35. Winkle RA, Rodriguez I, Bragg-Remschel DA: Technological status and problems of ambulatory electrocardiographic monitoring. Ann NY Acad Sci 1984;432:108.

36. Sheffield L, Berson A, Bragg-Remschel D, et al: Recommendations for standards of instrumentation and practice in the use of ambulatory electrocardiography. Circulation 1985; 71:626A.

37. Morganroth J, Michelson EL, Horowitz LN, et al: Limitations of routine long-term electrocardiographic monitoring to assess ventricular ectopic frequency. Circulation 1978; 58:408.

38. Winkle RA: Antiarrhythmic drug effect mimicked by spontaneous variability of ventricular ectopy. Circulation 1978; 57:1116.

39. Winkle RA, Peters F, Hall R: Characterization of ventricular tachyarrhythmias on ambulatory ECG recordings in postmyocardial infarction patients: arrhythmia detection and duration of recording, relationship between arrhythmia frequency and complexity, and day-to-day reproducibility. Am Heart J 1981;102:162.

40. Pratt CM, Theroux P, Slymen D, et al: Spontaneous variability of ventricular arrhythmias in patients at increased risk for sudden death after acute myocardial infarction: consecutive ambulatory electrocardiographic recordings of 88 patients. Am J Cardiol 1987;59:278.

41. The Cardiac Arrhythmia Pilot Study (CAPS) Investigators: Effects of encainide, flecainide, imipramine and moricizine on ventricular arrhythmias during the year after acute myocardial infarction: the CAPS. Am J Cardiol 1988;61:501.

42. Mulrow JP, Healy MJ, McKenna WJ: Variability of ventricular arrhythmias in hypertrophic cardiomyopathy and implications for treatment. Am J Cardiol 1986;58:615.

43. Raeder EA, Hohnloser SH, Graboys TB, Podrid PJ, Lampert S, Lown B: Spontaneous variability and circadian distribution of ectopic activity in patients with malignant ventricular arrhythmia. J Am Coll Cardiol 1988;12:656.

44. Toivonen L: Spontaneous variability in the frequency of ventricular premature complexes over prolonged intervals and implications for antiarrhythmic treatment. Am J Cardiol 1987;60:608.

45. Schmidt G, Ulm K, Barthel P, Goedel-Meinen L, Jahns G, Baedeker W: Spontaneously variability of simple and complex ventricular premature contractions during longtime intervals in patients with severe organic heart disease Circulation 1988;78:296.

46. Anastasiou-Nana MI, Menlove RL, Nanas JN, Anderson JL: Changes in spontaneous variability of ventricular ectopic activity as a function of time in patients with chronic arrhythmias. Circulation 1988;78:286.

47. Pratt CM, Slymen DJ, Wierman AM, et al: Analysis of the spontaneous variability of ventricular arrhythmias: consecutive ambulatory electrocardiographic recordings of ventricular tachycardia. Am J Cardiol 1985;56:67.

48. Kennedy HL, Whitlock JA, Sprague MK, et al: Long-term follow-up of asymptomatic healthy subjects with frequent and complex ventricular ectopy. N Engl J Med 1985;312:193.

49. Fleg JL, Kennedy HL: Cardiac arrhythmias in a healthy elderly population. Chest 1982;81:3 302.

50. Cleempoel H, Vainsel H, Bernard R, et al: Predictors of early death after acute myocardial infarction: two months follow-up. Eur Heart J 1986;7:305.

51. Hakki AH, Nestico PF, Heo J, Unwala AA, Iskandrian AS: Relative prognostic value of rest thallium-201 imaging, radionuclide ventriculography and 24 hour ambulatory electrocardiographic monitoring after acute myocardial infarction. J Am Coll Cardiol 1987;10:25.

52. Rapaport E, Remedios P: The high risk patient after recovery from myocardial infarction: recognition and management. J Am Coll Cardiol 1983;1:391.

53. Gomes JA, Winters SL, Stewart D, Horowitz S, Milner M, Barreca P: A new noninvasive index to predict sustained ventricular tachycardia and sudden death in the first year after myocardial infarction: based on signal-averaged electrocardiogram, radionuclide ejection fraction and Holter monitoring. J Am Coll Cardiol 1987;10:349.

54. Gomes JA, Winters SL, Martinson M, Machac J, Stewart D, Targonski A: The prognostic significance of quantitative signal-averaged variables relative to clinical variables, site of myocardial infarction, ejection fraction and ventricular premature beats: a prospective study. J Am Coll Cardiol 1989; 13:377.

55. Kuchar DL, Thorburn CW, Sammel NL: Prediction of serious arrhythmic events after myocardial infarction: signal-averaged electrocardiogram, Holter monitoring and radionuclide ventriculography. J Am Coll Cardiol 1987;9:531.

56. Mukharji J, Rude RE, Poole WK, et al: Risk factors for sudden death after acute myocardial infarction: two-year follow-up. Am J Cardiol 1984;54:31.

57. The Multicenter Postinfarction Research Group: Risk stratification and survival after myocardial infarction. N Engl J Med 1983;309:331.

58. Bigger JT Jr, Fleiss JL, Kleiger R, Miller JP, Rolnitzky LM: The relationships among ventricular arrhythmias, left ventricular dysfunction, and mortality in the 2 years after myocardial infarction. Circulation 1984;69:250.

59. DeBusk RF, Davidson DM, Houston N, Fitzgerald J: Serial ambulatory electrocardiography and treadmill exercise testing after uncomplicated myocardial infarction. Am J Cardiol 1980;45:547.

60. Kostis JB, Byington R, Friedman LM, Goldstein S, Furberg C: Prognostic significance of ventricular ectopic activity in survivors of acute myocardial infarction. J Am Coll Cardiol 1987;10:231.

61. Kostis JB, Wilson AC, Sanders MR, Byington RP: Prognostic significance of ventricular ectopic activity in survivors of acute myocardial infarction who receive propranolol. Am J Cardiol 1988;61:975.

62. Bigger JT Jr, Weld FM, Rolnitzky LM: Prevalence, characteristics and significance of ventricular tachycardia (three or more complexes) detected with ambulatory electrocardiographic recording in the late hospital phase of acute myocardial infarction. Am J Cardiol 1981;48:815.

63. Kleiger RE, Miller JP, Bigger JT Jr, Moss AJ: Decreased heart rate variability and its association with increased mortality after acute myocardial infarction. Am J Cardiol 1987;59:256.

64. Davis HT, DeCamilla J, Bayer LW, Moss AJ: Survivorship patterns in the posthospital phase of myocardial infarction. Circulation 1979;60:1252.

65. Ruberman W, Weinblatt E, Frank CW, Goldberg JD, Shapiro S: Repeated 1 hour electrocardiographic monitoring of survivors of myocardial infarction at 6 month intervals: arrhythmia detection and relation to prognosis. Am J Cardiol 1981; 47:1197.

66. Rubin DA, Nieminski KE, Monteferrante JC, Magee T, Reed GE, Herman MV: Ventricular arrhythmias after coronary artery bypass graft surgery: incidence, risk factors and long-term prognosis. J Am Coll Cardiol 1985;6:307.

67. Ruberman W, Weinblatt E, Goldberg JD, Frank CW, Shapiro S, Chaudhary BS: Ventricular premature complexes in prognosis of angina. Circulation 1980;61:1172.

68. Califf RM, McKinnis RA, Burks J, et al: Prognostic implications of ventricular arrhythmias during 24 hour ambulatory monitoring in patients undergoing cardiac catheterization for coronary artery disease. Am J Cardiol 1982;50:23.

69. Batchelor AJ, Kruyer WB, Hickman JR Jr: Ventricular ectopy in totally symptom-free subjects with defined coronary artery anatomy. Am Heart J 1989;117:1265.

70. Wilson JR, Schwartz JS, Sutton MS, et al: Prognosis in severe heart failure: relation to hemodynamic measurements and ventricular ectopic activity. J Am Coll Cardiol 1983;2:403.

71. Huang SK, Messer JV, Denes P: Significance of ventricular tachycardia in idiopathic dilated cardiomyopathy: observations in 35 patients. Am J Cardiol 1983;51:507.

72. Kron J, Hart M, Schual-Berke S, Niles NR, Hosenpud JD, McAnulty JH: Idiopathic dilated cardiomyopathy. Role of programmed electrical stimulation and Holter monitoring in predicting those at risk of sudden death. Chest 1988; 93:85.

73. Kennedy HL, Whitlock JA, Sprague MK, Kennedy LJ, Buckingham TA, Goldberg RJ: Long-term follow-up of asymptomatic healthy subjects with frequent and complex ventricular ectopy. N Engl J Med 1985;312:193.

74. Shih HT, Webb CR, Conway WA, Peterson E, Tilley B, Goldstein S: Frequency and significance of cardiac arrhythmias in chronic obstructive lung disease. Chest 1988;94:44.

75. Lown B, Wolf M: Approaches to sudden death from coronary heart disease. Circulation 1971;44:130.

76. Lovell RR, Mitchell ME, Prineas RJ, et al: Phenytoin after recovery from myocardial infarction. Controlled trial in 568 patients. Lancet 1971;2:1055.

77. Peter T, Ross D, Duffield A, et al: Effect on survival after myocardial infarction of long-term treatment with phenytoin. Br Heart J 1978;40:1356.

78. Ryden L, Arnman K, Conradson TB, Hofvendahl S, Mortensen O, Smedgard P: Prophylaxis of ventricular tachyarrhythmias with intravenous and oral tocainide in patients with and recovering from acute myocardial infarction. Am Heart J 1980;100:1006.

79. Chamberlain DA, Jewitt DE, Julian DG, Campbell RW, Boyle DM, Shanks RG: Oral mexiletine in high-risk patients after myocardial infarction. Lancet 1980;2:1324.

80. Hugenholtz PG, Hagemeijer F, Lubsen J, Glazer B, Van Durme JP, Bogaert MG: One year follow-up in patients with persistent ventricular dysrhythmias after myocardial infarction treated with aprindine or placebo. In: Sandoe E, Julian DG, Pell JW, eds. Management of ventricular tachycardia: role of mexiletine. Amsterdam: Excerpta Medica, 1978:572.

81. Impact Research Group: International mexiletine and placebo antiarrhythmic coronary trial: I. Report on arrhythmia and other findings. J Am Coll Cardiol 1984;4:1148.

82. Julian DG, Prescott RJ, Jackson FS, Szekely P: Controlled trial of sotalol for one year after myocardial infarction. Lancet 1982;1:1142.

83. Gottlieb SH, Achuff SC, Mellits ED, et al: Prophylactic antiarrhythmic therapy of high-risk survivors of myocardial infarction: lower mortality at 1 month but not at 1 year. Circulation 1987;75:792.

84. Hockings BE, George T, Mahrous F, Taylor RR, Hajar HA: Effectiveness of amiodarone on ventricular arrhythmias during and after acute myocardial infarction. Am J Cardiol 1987;60:967.

85. The CAPS Investigators: The Cardiac Arrhythmia Pilot Study. Am J Cardiol 1986;57:91.

86. The CAST Investigators: Preliminary report: effect of encainide and flecainide on mortality in a randomized trial of arrhythmia suppression after myocardial infarction. N Engl J Med 1989;321:406.

87. Hinkle LE, Argyros DC, Hayes JC, et al: Pathogenesis of an unexpected sudden death: role of early cycle ventricular premature contractions. Am J Cardiol 1977;39:873.

88. Gradman AH, Bell PA, DeBusk RF: Sudden death during ambulatory monitoring. Circulation 1977;55:210.

89. Pool I, Kunst K, Van Wermeskerken J: Two monitored cases of sudden death outside hospital. Br Heart J 1978;40:627.

90. Lahiri A, Balasubramanian V, Raferty EB: Sudden death during ambulatory monitoring. Br Med J 1979;1:1676.

91. Bissett JK, Watson JW, Scovil JA, et al: Sudden death in cardiomyopathy: role of bradycardia-dependent repolarization changes. Am Heart J 1980;99:625.

92. Salerno D, Hodges M, Graham E, et al: Fatal cardiac arrest during continuous ambulatory monitoring. N Engl J Med 1981;305:700.

93. Denes P, Gabster A, Huang SK: Clinical, electrocardiographic and follow-up observations in patients having ventricular fibrillation during Holter monitoring: role of quinidine therapy. J Am Coll Cardiol 1981;48:9.

94. Nikolie G, Bishop RL, Singh JB: Sudden death recorded during Holter monitoring. Circulation 1982;66:218.

95. Lewis BH, Antman EM, Graboys TB: Detailed analysis of 24 hour ambulatory electrocardiographic recordings during ventricular fibrillation or torsade de pointes. J Am Coll Cardiol 1983;2:426.

96. Pratt CM, Francis MJ, Luck JC, et al: Analysis of ambulatory electrocardiograms in 15 patients during spontaneous ventricular fibrillation with special reference to preceding arrhythmic events. J Am Coll Cardiol 1983;2:789.

97. Roelandt J, Klootwijk P, Lubsen J, Jansen MJ: Sudden death during longterm ambulatory monitoring. Eur Heart J 1984;5:7.

98. Olshausen KV, Witt T, Pop T, Treese N, Bethge K-P, Meyer J: Sudden cardiac death while wearing a Holter monitor. Am J Cardiol 1991;67:381.

99. Leclercq JF, Coumel P, Maison-Blache P, et al: The mechanism of sudden death: a cooperative study of 69 cases recorded by the Holter method. Arch Mal Coeur 1986; 79:1024.

100. Bayes de Luna A, Coumel P, Leclercq JF: Ambulatory sudden cardiac death: mechanisms of production of fatal arrhythma on the basis of data from 157 cases. Am Heart J 1989;117:151.

101. Vlay SC, Kallman CH, Reid PR: Prognostic assessment of survivors of ventricular tachycardia and ventricular fibrillation with ambulatory monitoring. Am J Cardiol 1984;54:87.

102. Platia EV, Reid PR: Comparison of programmed electrical stimulation and ambulatory electrocardiographic (Holter) monitoring in the management of ventricular tachycardia and ventricular fibrillation. J Am Coll Cardiol 1984;4:493.

103. Swerdlow CD, Peterson J: Prospective comparison of Holter monitoring and electrophysiologic study in patients with coronary artery disease and sustained ventricular tachyarrhythmias. Am J Cardiol 1985;56:577.

104. Ezri MD, Huang SK, Denes P: The role of Holter monitoring in patients with recurrent sustained ventricular tachycardia: an electrophysiologic correlation. Am Heart J 1986;108:1229.

105. Skale BT, Miles WM, Heger JJ, Zipes DP, Prystowsky EN: Survivors of cardiac arrest: prevention of recurrence by drug therapy as predicted by electrophysiologic testing or electrocardiographic monitoring. Am J Cardiol 1986; 57:113.

106. Mitchell LB, Duff HJ, Manyari DE, Wyse DG: A randomized clinical trial of the noninvasive and invasive approaches to drug therapy of ventricular tachycardia. N Engl J Med 1987; 317:1681.

107. Wilber DJ, Garan H, Finkelstein D, et al: Out-of-hospital cardiac arrest. Use of electrophysiologic testing in the prediction of long-term outcome. N Engl J Med 1988;318:19.

108. Marchlinski FE: Treatment of sustained ventricular arrhythmias: which therapy to use? Ann Intern Med 1988;109:522.

109. The ESVEM Investigators: The ESVEM trial. Circulation 1989;79:1354.

109a. The ESVEM Investigators: Determinants of predicted efficacy of antiarrhythmic drugs in the electrophysiologic study versus electrocardiographic monitoring trial. Circulation 1993:87:323.

109b. Mason JW, for the Electrophysiologic Study Versus Electrocardiographic Monitoring investigators. A comparison of electrophysiologic testing with holter monitoring to predict antiarrhythmic-drug efficacy for ventricular tachyarrhythmias. N Engl Med 1993;329:445.

110. Lightfoot PR, Sasse L, Mandel WJ, et al: His bundle electrograms in healthy adolescents with persistent second degree AV block. Chest 1973;63:358.

111. Jonas S, Klein I, Dimant J: Importance of Holter monitoring in patients with periodic cerebral symptoms. Ann Neurol 1977;1:470.

112. Boudoulas H, Schaal SF, Lewis RP, Robinson JL: Superiority of 24-hour outpatient monitoring over multi-stage exercise testing for the evaluation of syncope. J Electrocardiol 1979; 12:103.

113. Zeldis SM, Levine BJ, Michelson EL, Morganroth J: Cardiovascular complaints. Correlation with cardiac arrhythmias on 24-hour electrocardiographic monitoring. Chest 1980; 78:456.

114. Clark PI, Glasser SP, Spoto E Jr: Arrhythmias detected by ambulatory monitoring. Lack of correlation with symptoms of dizziness and syncope. Chest 1980;77:722.

115. Klein GJ, Gulamhusein SS: Undiagnosed syncope: search for an arrhythmic etiology. Stroke 1982;13:746.

116. Kala R, Viitasalo MT, Toivonen L, Eisalo A: Ambulatory ECG recording in patients referred because of syncope or dizziness. Acta Med Scand 1982;688(Suppl):13.

117. Abdon NJ, Johansson BW, Lessem J: Predictive use of routine 24-hour electrocardiography in suspected Adams-Stokes syndrome: comparison with cardiac rhythm during symptoms. Br Heart J 1982;47:553.

118. Kapoor WN, Karpf M, Wieand S, Peterson JR, Levey GS:

A prospective evaluation and follow-up of patients with syncope. N Engl J Med 1983;309:197.

119. Diamond TH, Smith R, Myburgh DP: Holter monitoring—a necessity for the evaluation of palpitations. S Afr Med J 1983;63:5.

120. Gibson TC, Heitzman MR: Diagnostic efficacy of 24-hour electrocardiographic monitoring for syncope. Am J Cardiol 1984;53:1013.

121. Kapoor WN, Cha R, Peterson JR, Wieand HS, Karpf M: Prolonged electrocardiographic monitoring in patients with syncope: importance of frequent or repetitive ventricular ectopy. Am J Med 1987;82:20.

122. Bass EB, Curtiss EI, Arena VC, et al: The duration of Holter monitoring in patients with syncope. Arch Intern Med 1990;150:1073.

123. Maron BJ, Savage DD, Wolfson JK, Epstein SE: Prognostic significance of 24 hour ambulatory electrocardiographic monitoring in patients with hypertrophic cardiomyopathy: A prospective study. J Am Coll Cardiol 1981;48:252.

124. McKenna WJ, England D, Doi YL, Deanfield JE, Oakley C, Goodwin JF: Arrhythmia in hypertrophic cardiomyopathy. I: Influence on prognosis. Br Heart J 1981;46:168.

125. Goren C, Denes P: The role of Holter monitoring in detecting digitalis-provoked arrhythmias. Chest 1981;79:555.

126. Dewar ML, Rosengarten MD, Bundell PE, Chiu RCJ: Perioperative Holter monitoring and computer analysis of dysrhythmias in cardiac surgery. Chest 1985;87:593.

127. Ringel RE, Kennedy HL, Brenner JI, et al: Detection of cardiac dysrhythmias by continuous electrocardiographic recording in children undergoing cardiac surgery. J Electrocardiol 1984;17:1.

128. Kelen G, Bloomfield D, Hardage M: Holter monitoring the patient with an artificial pacemaker—a new approach. Amb Electrocardiol 1978;1:1.

129. Beta-blocker Heart Attack Trial Research Group: A randomized trial of propranolol in patients with acute myocardial infarction. 1. Mortality results. JAMA 1982;247:1707.

130. Bigger JT Jr, Heller CA, Wenger TL, et al: Risk stratification after acute myocardial infarction. Am J Cardiol 1978;42:202.

131. Moss AJ, DeCamilla J, Davis H: Cardiac death in the first 6 months after myocardial infarction: potential for mortality reduction in the early posthospital period. Am J Cardiol 1977;39:816.

132. The Norwegian Multicenter Study Group: Timolol-induced reduction in mortality and reinfarction in patients surviving acute myocardial infarction. N Engl J Med 1981;304:801.

133. Ruberman W, Weinblatt E, Goldberg JD, et al: Ventricular premature beats and mortality after acute myocardial infarction. N Engl J Med 1977;297:750.

134. Moss AJ, Davis HT, DeCamilla J, Bayer LW: Ventricular ectopic beats and their relation to sudden and nonsudden cardiac death after myocardial infarction. Circulation 1979;60:998.

135. Mukharji J, Rude RE, Poole WK, et al: Risk factors for sudden death after myocardial infarction: two year follow up. Am J Cardiol 1984;54:31.

136. Bigger JT Jr, Fleiss JL, Kleiger K, et al: The Multicenter Postinfarction Research Group. The relationship between ventricular arrhythmias, left ventricular dysfunction and mortality in the two years after myocardial infarction. Circulation 1984;69:250.

137. Kostis JB, Byington R, Friedman LM, et al: Prognostic significance of ventricular ectopic activity in survivors of acute myocardial infarction. J Am Coll Cardiol 1987;10:231.

138. Myerburg RJ, Kessler KM, Bassett AL, Castellanos A: A biological approach to sudden cardiac death: structure, function and cause. Am J Cardiol 1989;63:1512.

139. Farell TG, Bashir Y, Cripps T, et al: Risk stratification for arrhythmic events in postinfarction patients based on heart rate variability, ambulatory electrocardiographic variables and the signal-averaged electrocardiogram. J Am Coll Cardiol 1991;18:687

140. Hull SS Jr, Evans AR, Vanoli E, et al: Heart rate variability before and after myocardial infarction in conscious dogs at high and low risk of sudden death. J Am Coll Cardiol 1990;16:978.

141. Billman GE, Hoskins RS: Time series analysis of heart rate variability during submaximal exercise. Evidence for reduced cardiac vagal tone in animals susceptible to ventricular fibrillation. Circulation 1989;80:146.

142. Schwartz PJ, Vanoli E, Stamba-Badiale M, De Ferrari GM, Billman GE, Foreman RD: Autonomic mechanisms and sudden death. New insights from analysis of baroreceptor reflexes in conscious dogs with and without a myocardial infarction. Circulation 1988;78:969.

143. Kleiger RE, Miller JP, Bigger JT Jr, Moss AJ, the Multicenter Post-Infarction Research Group: Decreased heart rate variability and its association with increased mortality after acute myocardial infarction. Am J Cardiol 1987;59:256.

144. Martin GJ, Magid NM, Myers G, et al: Heart rate variability and sudden death secondary to coronary artery disease during ambulatory electrocardiographic monitoring. Am J Cardiol 1987;60:86.

145. Randall WC, Szentivanya M, Pace JB, Wechsler JS, Kaye MP: Patterns of sympathetic nerve projections onto the canine heart. Circ Res 1968;22:315.

146. Löffelholz K, Pappano AJ: The parasympathetic neuroeffector junction of the heart. Pharmacol Rev 1985;37:1.

147. Takahashi N, Barber MJ, Zipes DP: Efferent vagal innervation of the canine left ventricle. Am J Physiol 1985;248(Heart Circ Physiol 17):H89.

148. Barber MJ, Mueller TM, Henry DP, Felten SY, Zipes DP: Transmural myocardial infarction in the dog produces sympathectomy in noninfarcted myocardium. Circulation 1983;67:787.

149. Malliani A, Recordati G, Schwartz PJ: Nervous activity of afferent cardiac sympathetic fibres with atrial and ventricular endings. J Physiol (Lond) 1973;229:457.

150. van Ravenswaaij-Arts CMA, Kollee LAA, Hopman JCW, Stoelinga GBA, van Geijn HP: Heart rate variability. Ann Intern Med 1993;118:436.

151. Hull SS Jr, Evans AR, Vanoli E, et al: Heart rate variability before and after myocardial infarction in conscious dogs at high and low risk of sudden death. J Am Coll Cardiol 1990;16:978.

152. Osculati G, Grassi G, Giannattasio C, et al: Early alterations of the baroreceptor control of heart rate in patients with acute myocardial infarction. Circulation 1990;81:939.

153. Magid NM, Martin GJ, Kehoe RF, et al: Diminished heart rate variability in sudden cardiac death. Circulation 1985;72(Suppl III):241. Abstract.

154. Kleiger RE, Miller JP, Bigger JT Jr, et al: Heart rate variability: a variable predicting mortality following acute myocardial infarction. J Am Coll Cardiol 1984;3:547. Abstract.

155. Ewing DJ, Neilson JM, Travis P. New method for assessing cardiac parasympathetic activity using 24 hour electrocardiograms. Br Heart J 1984;52:396.

156. Malik M, Farell T, Cripps TR, Camm AJ: Heart rate variability in relation to prognosis after myocardial infarction: selection of optimal processing techniques. Eur Heart J 1989; 10:1060.

157. Akselrod S, Gordon D, Ubel FA, et al: Power spectrum analysis of heart rate fluctuation: a quantative probe of beat to beat cardiovascular control. Science 1981;213:220.

158. Pagani M, Lombardi F, Guzzette S, et al: Power spectral analysis of heart rate and arterial pressure variabilities as a marker of sympatho-vagal interaction in man and conscious dog. Circ Res 1986;59:178.

159. Pomeranz B, Macaulay JB, Caudill MA, et al: Assessment of autonomic function in humans by heart rate spectral analysis. Am J Physiol 1985;248:H151.

160. Eckberg DL, Kifle YT, Roberts VL: Phase relationship between human respiration and baroreflex responsiveness. J Physiol 1980;304:489.

161. Katona PG, Jih F: Respiratory sinus arrhythmia: noninvasive measure of parasympathetic cardiac control. J Appl Physiol 1975;39:801.

162. Kleiger RE, Bigger JT, Bosner MS, et al: Stability over time of variables measuring heart rate variability in normal subjects. Am J Cardiol 1991;68:626.

163. Mölgaard H, Sörensen KE, Bjerregaard P: Circadian variation and influence of risk factors on heart rate variability in healthy subjects. Am J Cardiol 1991;68:777.

164. Schneider RA, Costiloe JP: Relationship of sinus arrhythmia to age and its prognostic significance in ischemic heart disease. Clin Res 1965;13:219.

165. Wolf MM, Varigos GA, Hunt D, Sloman JG: Sinus arrhythmia in acute myocardial infarction. Med J Aust 1978;2:52.

166. Seals DR, Chase PB: Influence of physical training on heart rate variability and baroreflex circulatory control. J Appl Physiol 1989;66:1886.

167. Cowan MJ, Kogan H, Burr R, Hendershot S, Buchanan L: Power spectral analysis of heart rate variability after biofeedback training. J Electrocardiol 1990;23(Suppl):85.

168. Bittiner SB, Smith SE: Beta-adrenoceptor antagonists increase sinus arrhythmia, a vagotonic effect. Br J Clin Pharmacol 1986;22:691.

169. Vybiral T, Bryg RJ, Maddens ME, et al: Effects of transdermal scopolamine on heart rate variability in normal subjects. Am J Cardiol 1990;65:604.

170. Echt DS, Liebson PR, Mitchell LB, et al: Mortality and morbidity in patients receiving encainide, flecainide, or placebo. The Cardiac Arrhythmia Suppression Trial. N Engl J Med 1991;324:781.

171. Zuanetti G, Latini R, Neilson JMM, Schwartz PJ, Ewing DJ, The Antiarrhythmic drug Evaluation Group: Heart rate variability in patients with ventricular arrhythmias: effect of antiarrhythmic drugs. J Am Coll Cardiol 1991;17:604.

172. Krasnow AZ, Bloomfield DK: Artifacts in portable electrocardiographic monitoring. Am Heart J 1976;91:349.

173. Gardin JM, Belic N, Singer DH: Pseudoarrhythmias in ambulatory ECG monitoring. Arch Intern Med 1979;139:809.

174. Isaeff DM, Harrison DC: Tachyarrhythmias in patients with Wolff-Parkinson-White syndrome in long-term Holter monitoring. Chest 1970;58:282.

175. Hindman MC, Last JH, Rosen KM: Wolff-Parkinson-White syndrome observed by portable monitoring. Ann Intern Med 1973;79:654.

176. Jenkins JM, Wu D, Arzbaecher RL: Computer diagnosis of supraventricular and ventricular arrhythmias. A new esophogeal technique. Circulation 1979;60:977.

Cardiac Arrhythmias, 3rd edition, edited by William J. Mandel.
J. B. Lippincott Company, Philadelphia © 1995.

27

Fred Morady

Electrophysiologic Testing in the Management of Patients With Unexplained Syncope

Syncope, defined as transient loss of consciousness with spontaneous recovery, can be caused by a variety of metabolic, neurologic, and cardiac causes. In some patients, for example the patient who has a "fainting spell" during phlebotomy, syncope is a benign condition of little or no prognostic significance. In other patients, if syncope is caused by ventricular tachycardia, it may be a harbinger of sudden death. It is, therefore, important to establish the cause of syncope.

The most common causes of syncope are listed in Table 27-1. The patient who experiences syncope should be evaluated initially with a thorough history, physical examination, and electrocardiogram. Several potential causes of syncope can be diagnosed based on this initial evaluation, for example, classic vasodepressor syncope, orthostatic hypotension, carotid sinus hypersensitivity, obstructive cardiac lesions, and high-degree atrioventricular (AV) block. Depending on clues obtained from the history, physical examination, and electrocardiogram, it may be appropriate for the patient to have a thorough neurologic evaluation, echocardiogram, exercise treadmill test, or cardiac catheterization. Unless the cause of syncope is apparent, the evaluation should always include electrocardiographic monitoring, preferably on a prolonged, contin-

uous, ambulatory basis, to look for potential arrhythmic causes of syncope. Passive upright tilting may be helpful in reproducing symptomatic bradycardia or hypotension in patients who have had vasodepressor syncope.[1]

The cause of syncope can reportedly be determined by history, physical examination, or noninvasive evaluation in 52% to 87% of unselected patients who are hospitalized with syncope.[2,3] However, in a significant proportion of patients, the cause of syncope is unclear despite a thorough metabolic, neurologic, and noninvasive cardiac evaluation. In these patients, the sporadic and infrequent nature of the syncopal episodes may make it difficult to establish arrhythmia as the cause of syncope. Although ambulatory electrocardiographic monitoring may demonstrate an arrhythmic cause of syncope, experience indicates that it is uncommon for syncope to occur while the patient is undergoing ambulatory monitoring. Gibson and Heitzman found that, among 1512 patients who underwent ambulatory electrocardiographic monitoring because of syncope, only 15 patients (1%) had syncope during the monitoring period.[4] It is more often the case that ambulatory monitoring demonstrates arrhythmias, such as short episodes of nonsustained ventricular tachycardia or a sinus pause, that are not associated with cere-

TABLE 27-1. Common Causes of Syncope

Metabolic
  Hypoxemia
  Hypoglycemia
  Hypocapnia, alkalosis
Neuropsychiatric
  Syncopal migraine
  Akinetic temporal lobe seizure
  Partial complex seizure
  Posterior circulation transient ischemic attack
Cardiovascular
  Vagally mediated (cardioinhibitory or vasodepressor)
    Common faint
    Carotid sinus hypersensitivity
    Postmicturition syncope
    Swallow syncope
    Cough syncope
  Orthostatic hypotension
    Drug induced
    Hypovolemia
    Idiopathic
  Obstructive lesions
    Aortic stenosis
    Hypertrophic obstructive cardiomyopathy
    Atrial myxoma
    Pulmonary vascular disease
  Arrhythmias
    Sick sinus syndrome
    Atrioventricular block
    Supraventricular tachycardia
    Ventricular tachycardia

bral symptoms. In these patients, it cannot be assumed that the observed asymptomatic arrhythmia is the cause of syncope.

This chapter reviews the usefulness of electrophysiologic testing in establishing the cause of syncope in patients with unexplained syncope. Electrophysiologic testing may be helpful in uncovering the following potential arrhythmic causes of syncope: sinus node dysfunction, supraventricular tachycardia, AV block, and ventricular tachycardia.

INDICATIONS FOR ELECTROPHYSIOLOGIC STUDY

Syncope does not recur in a significant proportion of patients who experience an episode.[5,6] Electrophysiologic testing should, therefore, generally be considered only for patients in whom syncope is a recurrent unexplained problem. However, in some patients, it may be appropriate to perform electrophysiologic testing after only one episode of unexplained syncope. For example, if a patient suffers a severe injury as a result of a syncopal episode, a thorough evaluation including electrophysiologic testing may be indicated to minimize the possibility of additional injury. An electrophysiologic study should be considered in patients with one episode of unexplained syncope who are at risk of sudden death, for instance, patients with a cardiomyopathy or coronary artery disease and a history of myocardial infarction who have asymptomatic complex ventricular ectopic activity; in these patients, one must consider the possibility that the syncope was caused by ventricular tachycardia and that the next episode might be fatal.[7–9]

In patients with syncope who are found to have carotid hypersensitivity, electrophysiologic testing may be indicated if the patient has structural heart disease. Nelson and coworkers demonstrated that one third of patients presumed to have carotid sinus syndrome and who had structural heart disease had unimorphic ventricular tachycardia induced during electrophysiologic testing, raising the possibility that ventricular tachycardia was the cause of syncope.[10] Therefore, an electrophysiologic test is needed to eliminate ventricular tachycardia as a cause of syncope in patients with carotid hypersensitivity and structural heart disease.

EVALUATION OF SINUS NODE FUNCTION

Sinus node function is evaluated during electrophysiologic testing by determining the sinus node recovery time (SNRT), sinoatrial conduction time, and sinus node refractory period.[11–15] SNRT is determined by pacing the right atrium at various cycle lengths (e.g., 600 to 300 milliseconds in 50-millisecond decrements) for 30 to 60 seconds. The SNRT is defined as the interval between the last paced atrial depolarization and the first spontaneous atrial depolarization resulting from sinus node discharge. The SNRT is corrected for the patient's spontaneous cycle length by subtracting the spontaneous cycle length from the SNRT. The upper limits of normal of the corrected SNRT is approximately 550 milliseconds. The normal response after the first sinus recovery beat is a gradual return to the baseline spontaneous cycle length after three to four beats. A secondary pause has been defined as an inappropriately long cycle length among the nine beats that follow the first sinus recovery beat after atrial overdrive pacing.[16] Evaluation of secondary pauses increases the sensitivity of the SNRT in the detection of sinus node dysfunction.[17]

The sinoatrial conduction time can be measured indirectly by the extrastimulus or the overdrive technique.[13,14] Reiffel and coworkers have described a catheter technique for recording the sinus node electrogram in humans, allowing direct measurements of the sinoatrial conduction time.[18]

Sinus node refractoriness can be determined in humans with an extrastimulus technique and has been reported to more clearly differentiate patients with and without sinus node dysfunction than does the SNRT or sinoatrial conduction time.[15]

Most patients with sick sinus syndrome demonstrate evidence of sinus node dysfunction during prolonged, continuous, ambulatory electrocardiographic recordings.[19,20] Patients with unexplained syncope have been screened for evidence of sinus node dysfunction during ambulatory electrocardiographic monitoring, and sinus node dysfunction has been an infrequent finding. DiMarco and coworkers found a prolonged SNRT in only one of 25 patients with recurrent unexplained syncope who underwent electrophysiologic testing.[21] Akhtar and coworkers found that four of 30 patients with recurrent unexplained syncope had a corrected SNRT greater than 800 milliseconds.[22] Morady and coworkers reported that only two of 53 patients with recurrent unexplained syncope had evidence of sinus node dysfunction—a prolonged SNRT in one patient and an abnormal sinoatrial conduction time in another.[23] Therefore, among a total of 108 patients with recurrent unexplained syncope who did not have evidence of sinus node dysfunction during ambulatory monitoring and who underwent complete electrophysiologic testing, only seven patients (6%) were found to have sinus node dysfunction as the potential cause of syncope.

Because sinus node dysfunction may, in some patients, be an incidental finding unrelated to syncope, demonstration of an abnormal SNRT or sinoatrial conduction time during electrophysiologic testing does not guarantee that syncope will resolve after a permanent pacemaker is implanted. For example, Akhtar and coworkers reported that syncope recurred in two of four patients with unex-

plained syncope who were found to have a prolonged SNRT.[22] The clinical significance of a prolonged SNRT appears to be partly related to the degree of prolongation. Symptoms are most likely to resolve with pacemaker implantation when the SNRT is greater than 2 seconds (Fig. 27-1).[24] Reproduction of the patient's symptoms during a postpacing pause may indicate that the cause of the patient's symptoms has been identified. However, the significance of a mildly prolonged SNRT in a patient with unexplained syncope and no evidence of sinus node dysfunction during ambulatory electrocardiographic monitoring is unclear. The decision to implant a permanent pacemaker in such patients is a matter of clinical judgment.

In elderly patients with cerebral symptoms, ambulatory electrocardiographic recordings frequently demonstrate asymptomatic sinus bradycardia. In these patients, symptoms cannot be assumed to be related to the sick sinus syndrome unless there is documentation that the symptoms are related to the bradyarrhythmia. Electrophysiologic testing may be helpful in evaluating these patients. Gann and coworkers reported that an abnormal SNRT was useful in selecting patients with chronic sinus bradycardia and dizziness or syncope for pacemaker therapy.[25] Among a group of 36 patients with a history of syncope and sinus bradycardia, 16 of 18 patients who had an abnormal SNRT had a permanent pacemaker implanted, and all subsequently remained asymptomatic; the two patients with an abnormal SNRT who refused pacemaker implantation remained symptomatic. Among the remaining 18 patients who had a normal SNRT, nine of 10 without pacemakers became asymptomatic, and two of eight who underwent pacemaker implantation continued to have syncope. Therefore, a prolonged SNRT appeared to predict a response to pacemaker implantation. How-

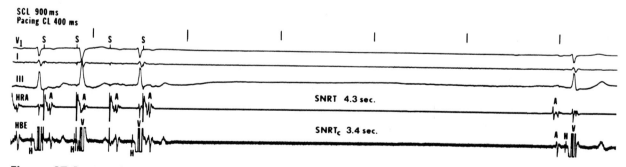

Figure 27-1. A markedly prolonged sinus node recovery time (SNRT) in a patient with recurrent, unexplained syncope. From top to bottom are electrocardiographic leads V_1, I, and III, a high right atrial (HRA) electrogram, and the His bundle electrogram (HBE). Upon cessation of atrial pacing at a cycle length (CL) of 400 milliseconds there is a 4.3-second pause between the last paced atrial depolarization and the first spontaneous atrial depolarization resulting from sinus node discharge. Subtracting the spontaneous cycle length (SCL) of 900 milliseconds yields a corrected sinus node discharge. Syncope did not recur after a permanent pacemaker was implanted. Time lines in this and subsequent figures represent 1-second intervals. A, atrial depolarization; H, His bundle depolarization; S, pacing stimulus; V, ventricular depolarization.

ever, Gann and coworkers did not consider the degree of prolongation of the SNRT. The same considerations regarding the clinical significance of a prolonged SNRT apply in patients with syncope and chronic sinus bradycardia as apply in patients with syncope and no evidence of sinus node dysfunction during ambulatory monitoring. The clinical significance of a mildly prolonged SNRT should be interpreted with caution.

Although the sinoatrial conduction time is a sensitive indicator of sinus node disease, it lacks a high degree of specificity and has been of limited value in evaluating the need for a permanent pacemaker.[26] For example, Morady and coworkers reported that a patient with recurrent unexplained syncope, an abnormal sinoatrial conduction time, and no other abnormalities during electrophysiologic testing had recurrent syncope despite implantation of a permanent pacemaker.[23]

Measurement of sinus node refractoriness using an extrastimulus technique has been found to increase the sensitivity of diagnosis of patients with sinus node dysfunction when compared to the SNRT and sinoatrial conduction time.[15] However, the usefulness of this measure of sinus node function in selecting patients with unexplained syncope for pacemaker implantation has not been assessed.

SUPRAVENTRICULAR TACHYCARDIA

It is uncommon for supraventricular tachycardia to cause syncope, unless the patient has underlying heart disease or the rate of the tachycardia is extremely rapid. In many patients, syncope or near-syncope may occur at the onset of an episode of supraventricular tachycardia because of an initial drop in blood pressure, especially if the patient is standing. Compensatory mechanisms, that is, peripheral vasoconstriction, and assumption of a supine position then result in an increase in blood pressure and cerebral perfusion, and the patient often regains consciousness although the tachycardia persists. Many patients with syncope caused by supraventricular tachycardia do not experience syncope with every episode of tachycardia. For these reasons, patients who have syncope caused by supraventricular tachycardia often do not present a diagnostic problem. However, an occasional patient with supraventricular tachycardia may have sporadic episodes of syncope as the only manifestation of the tachycardia. Repeated ambulatory electrocardiographic recordings may be unrevealing unless the patient has an episode of syncope during the monitoring period. Electrophysiologic testing may be helpful in demonstrating the cause of syncope in these patients.

Electrophysiologic testing in patients with unexplained syncope should include incremental atrial and ventricular pacing and programmed atrial and ventricular stimulation with one extrastimulus to uncover the presence of an accessory pathway, dual AV nodal pathways, and enhanced AV nodal conduction.[27-32] Attempts should be made to induce AV nodal reentrant tachycardia, AV reciprocating tachycardia using an overt or concealed accessory pathway, atrial tachycardia, and atrial fibrillation/flutter.[33] The aggressiveness of the stimulation protocol used to induce these tachycardias should be guided by the clinical picture. In patients with recurrent unexplained syncope who have repeated ambulatory electrocardiographic recordings that do not reveal symptomatic or asymptomatic supraventricular tachycardia, it is unlikely that electrophysiologic testing will demonstrate supraventricular tachycardia as the potential cause of syncope. Accordingly, among 108 patients with recurrent unexplained syncope and negative ambulatory electrocardiographic recordings who underwent electrophysiologic testing, only one patient was found to have a supraventricular tachycardia felt to be the cause of syncope (atrial flutter with a ventricular rate of 205 beats per minute).[21-23] However, if the patient is an otherwise healthy person who describes a prodrome of rapid palpitations in association with syncope or if ambulatory electrocardiographic recordings demonstrate short runs of supraventricular tachycardia, then supraventricular tachycardia is more likely to be the cause of syncope and the electrophysiologic study should include vigorous attempts to induce the tachycardias described (Fig. 27-2). If supraventricular tachycardia cannot be induced in the baseline state, atrial and ventricular stimulation repeated during an infusion of isoproterenol may induce a symptomatic supraventricular tachycardia (Fig. 27-3).[34,35]

In patients with Wolff-Parkinson-White syndrome, the arrhythmias most likely to cause syncope are atrial fibrillation or flutter with a rapid ventricular response or AV reciprocating tachycardia. However, if these arrhythmias are not inducible during electrophysiologic testing or if they are not rapid and associated with hypotension, a complete evaluation should be performed to look for other causes of syncope. Lloyd and coworkers reported on five patients with ventricular preexcitation and syncope who, based on the results of electrophysiologic testing, were found to have ventricular tachycardia rather than supraventricular tachycardia as the cause of syncope.[36]

Supraventricular tachycardia may, at times, be inducible during electrophysiologic testing in patients who have never had spontaneous episodes of supraventricular tachycardia. An induced tachycardia is unlikely to be the cause of syncope unless it is rapid and associated with a significant fall in blood pressure. In patients who have had syncope in association with supraventricular tachycardia, syncope usually does not occur when the supraventricular tachycardia is induced during electrophysiologic testing in the supine position; however, the patient often experiences dizziness or near-syncope. Supraventricular tachy-

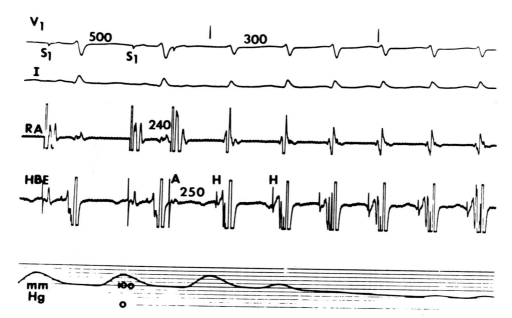

Figure 27-2. Supraventricular tachycardia induced during electrophysiologic testing in a woman aged 36 years with a several-year history of paroxysmal palpitations, on one occasion associated with syncope. From top to bottom are electrocardiographic leads V_1 and I, a right atrial (RA) electrogram, the His bundle electrogram (HBE), and recording of arterial blood pressure on a scale of 200 mm Hg. Right atrial programmed stimulation at a drive cycle length (S_1-S_1) of 500 milliseconds with a single atrial extrastimulus (coupling interval 240 milliseconds) induced atrioventricular nodal reentrant tachycardia, cycle length 300 milliseconds. The systolic blood pressure fell rapidly from 160 to 70 mm Hg, and the patient experienced rapid palpitations and lightheadedness, similar to the symptoms she experienced before her episode of syncope. Propranolol was effective in suppressing the induction of this tachycardia, and no further episodes of palpitations or syncope occurred while the drug was given.

cardia is probably not the cause of syncope if it is not associated with a fall in blood pressure or cerebral symptoms when induced in the electrophysiology laboratory. For example, Akhtar and coworkers found that AV nodal reentrant tachycardia could be initiated in three of 30 patients with recurrent unexplained syncope who underwent electrophysiologic testing.[22] The rate of the tachycardia was 146 to 158 beats per minute, and in none of the patients was the tachycardia associated with a significant fall in blood pressure or symptoms of dizziness. Despite treatment aimed at preventing the supraventricular tachycardia, these three patients continued to have syncope during the follow-up period, indicating that the supraventricular tachycardia was most likely an incidental finding.

ATRIOVENTRICULAR BLOCK

Some patients with syncope caused by intermittent high-degree AV block may have normal AV conduction between episodes of AV block. Because syncope may be infrequent and unpredictable in these patients, it may not be possible to demonstrate the intermittent high-degree AV block de-

spite repeated ambulatory electrocardiographic recordings. Electrophysiologic testing may be helpful in evaluating these patients.

Evaluation of AV conduction during electrophysiologic testing includes determining the baseline AV nodal to His bundle conduction time (AH interval) and the His bundle to ventricular conduction time (HV interval). AV conduction is assessed by incremental atrial pacing, and AV nodal and His–Purkinje refractory periods are determined by the extrastimulus technique.[37]

Because it is uncommon for AV nodal block to be associated with severe bradycardia or syncope, the finding of a prolonged AV nodal refractory period may not be clinically significant. A complete evaluation for other potential causes of syncope should be performed before attributing the patient's syncope to intermittent second or third degree AV nodal block. If the only abnormality found during electrophysiologic testing in a patient with unexplained syncope is prolongation of AV nodal refractoriness, then implantation of a permanent pacemaker is usually not indicated unless a symptomatic bradyarrhythmia is documented during repeated ambulatory electrocardiographic recordings.

The clinical usefulness of the HV interval in patients with unexplained syncope is controversial. Because pa-

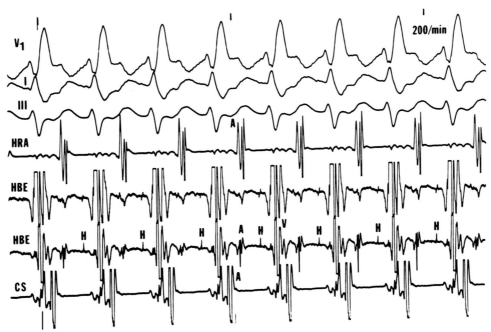

Figure 27-3. Orthodromic reciprocating tachycardia induced during an infusion of isoproterenol. From top to bottom are leads V₁, I, and III, high right atrial (HRA) electrogram, two His bundle electrograms (HBE), and a distal coronary sinus (CS) electrogram. The patient had a concealed left-sided accessory pathway. Before the infusion of isoproterenol, only single echo beats were induced by atrial programmed stimulation. During infusion of isoproterenol, 2 μg/per minute sustained orthodromic reciprocating tachycardia (rate 200 beats per minute) was induced. Note the eccentric pattern of atrial activation, with earliest activation recorded in the distal coronary sinus, consistent with retrograde conduction over a left-sided accessory pathway. (See Fig. 26-1 for key to abbreviations.)

tients with bundle branch block are more likely to have a prolonged HV interval than patients without bundle branch block, most published studies on the clinical significance of a prolonged HV interval have been conducted with patients with bundle branch block.

Dhingra and coworkers evaluated the clinical significance of the HV interval in a prospective study of 517 patients with bundle branch block, most of whom did not have syncope.[38] The HV interval was normal in 319 patients and prolonged (>55 milliseconds) in 198 patients. The cumulative 7-year incidence of high-degree AV block was 3% in the patients with a normal HV interval and 12% in the patients with a prolonged HV interval. The authors concluded that the HV interval is useful for evaluating patients with bundle branch block and that a prolonged HV interval in patients with bundle branch block and syncope implicates intermittent high-degree AV block as the cause of symptoms.

McAnulty and coworkers also conducted a prospective study of patients with bundle branch block, most of whom did not have syncope.[39] The HV interval was normal in 161 patients and prolonged in 190 patients. The mean followup period was 42 ± 8 months (± SD). In contrast to the findings of Dhingra and colleagues, these authors found that patients with a prolonged HV interval did not have a statistically increased risk of high-degree AV block as compared with patients with a normal HV interval (4.9% versus 1.9% $P > 0.05$). McAnulty and coworkers concluded that the HV interval cannot be used to determine which patients with bundle branch block are at increased risk of developing AV block.

In the studies of Dhingra and coworkers and of McAnulty and associates, patients with a prolonged HV interval were not categorized according to the degree of HV prolongation.[38,39] Scheinman and coworkers performed a prospective study of 313 patients with bundle branch block (60% of whom did not have syncope) in which patients with a prolonged HV interval were categorized according to the degree of HV interval prolongation: normal in 97 patients, 55 to 69 milliseconds in 99 patients, and at least 70 milliseconds in 117 patients.[40] The mean follow-up period was approximately 3 years. The progression to high-degree AV block was greater in the group with an HV interval greater than or equal to 70 milliseconds (12%) than in the other groups (2% to 4%). High-degree AV block occurred in four of 17 patients (24%) with an HV interval of at least 100 milliseconds. Scheinman and associates concluded that an HV interval of at least 70 milliseconds is an independent risk factor for progression to high-degree AV block and that an HV interval of at least 100 milliseconds identifies a subgroup at particularly high risk.[40] These authors recommended pacemaker implantation in patients with bundle branch block and unexplained transient neurologic symptoms who have an HV interval of at least 70 milliseconds, particularly if the HV interval is greater than or equal to 100 milliseconds.

There is a significant limitation in applying the results of the large-scale studies cited above to the management of patients who undergo electrophysiologic testing because of unexplained syncope; that is, both symptomatic and asymptomatic patients with bundle branch block were included in these studies and most patients did not have a history of syncope. In the studies summarized above, the prognostic significance of HV interval prolongation was not analyzed in the subgroup of patients who had syncope. It cannot be assumed that the results obtained by analyzing all patients with bundle branch block can be applied to patients with bundle branch block who have had syncope.

A study by Altschuler and coworkers assessed the significance of HV interval prolongation in a group of patients who all had either dizziness or syncope.[41] Eighteen patients who had a normal HV interval (<55 milliseconds) did not undergo pacemaker implantation. Among 35 patients with HV interval prolongation (≥60 milliseconds), 18 underwent pacemaker implantation and 17 did not. The decision to implant a pacemaker was left to the referring physician. Over a mean follow-up period of 22 ± 17 months, none of the patients with a normal HV interval died or developed AV block. Among the 17 patients with prolonged HV interval who did not receive a pacemaker, after a mean follow-up period of 6 ± 5 months, three

patients died suddenly, three progressed to high-degree AV block and required a pacemaker, and nine remained symptomatic. In contrast, among the 18 patients who received a pacemaker, after a mean follow-up period of 23 ± 13 months, none of the patients died suddenly and only two remained symptomatic with syncope or dizziness. These results suggested that symptomatic patients with a prolonged HV interval were at increased risk of dying suddenly and that the incidence of both sudden death and symptoms could be diminished by pacemaker implantation. Altschuler and coworkers concluded that patients with unexplained transient neurologic symptoms whose HV interval is greater than or equal to 60 milliseconds should receive a permanent pacemaker.[41]

The principal limitations of this study are the relatively small number of patients in the various subgroups and the nonrandom fashion in which pacemakers were implanted in the patients with a prolonged HV interval. Although the study of Altschuler and coworkers does not prove that patients with HV interval prolongation and syncope have an improved outcome with pacing, their results do suggest that pacemaker implantation should be considered for patients with recurrent unexplained syncope whose only abnormality during electrophysiologic testing is a prolonged HV interval.[41] The findings of Scheinman and coworkers suggest that a permanent pacemaker would be appropriate in patients with unexplained syncope who have a markedly prolonged HV interval (≥100 milliseconds) (Fig. 27-4).[40] However, although there is a correlation between the degree of HV interval prolongation and the risk of high-degree AV block, a normal or mildly prolonged HV interval does not exclude the possibility of intermittent high-degree AV block in a patient with unexplained syncope (Fig. 27-5).

A helpful but uncommon finding in patients with

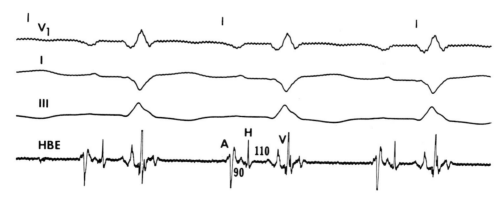

Figure 27-4. A markedly prolonged HV interval. From top to bottom are electrocardiographic leads V₁, I, and III and a His bundle electrogram (HBE). This patient with recurrent, unexplained syncope had a right bundle branch block, a normal AH interval of 90 milliseconds, and a markedly prolonged HV interval of 110 milliseconds (upper limits of normal = 55 milliseconds). Ventricular tachycardia was not inducible. The patient had further syncope after a permanent pacemaker was implanted. (See Fig. 26-1 for key to abbreviations.)

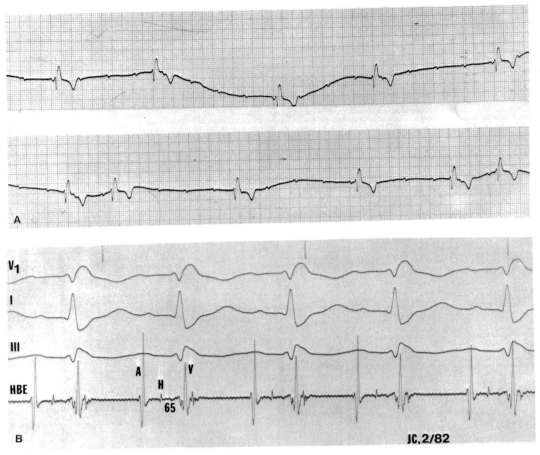

Figure 27-5. An example of high-degree atrioventricular block in a patient with an HV interval that was only mildly prolonged. (**A**) The patient had a history of recurrent syncope. During a syncopal episode that occurred during hospitalization, an electrocardiogram demonstrated high-degree atrioventricular block with an average ventricular rate of 30 beats per minute. Shown is a continuous recording of lead V_1. (**B**) A His bundle electrogram (HBE) recorded at permanent pacemaker implantation, when there was 1:1 atrioventricular conduction, demonstrated an HV interval of 65 milliseconds. This example shows that a mildly prolonged HV interval does not rule out the possibility that syncope is due to intermittent high-degree atrioventricular block.

bundle branch block is infranodal block during atrial pacing. However, "pathologic" infranodal block must be distinguished from "functional" infranodal block.[42] Pathologic infranodal block during atrial pacing occurs when AV nodal conduction is intact (Fig. 27-6). Functional infranodal block during atrial pacing occurs when there is AV nodal Wenckebach; that is, failure of impulse propagation in the AV node results in a pause that lengthens refractoriness in the His–Purkinje system such that the second beat in the next Wenckebach cycle blocks in or distal to the His bundle ("long–short" phenomenon, Fig. 27-7). Dhingra and coworkers reported that patients with functional infranodal block had a benign prognosis when left untreated, whereas, among 15 patients with pacing-induced infranodal AV block during intact AV nodal conduction, eight patients developed AV block over a mean follow-up period of 3.4 years.[42] The electrophysiologic evaluation of patients with unexplained syncope should, therefore, include an assessment of the response to atrial pacing. Because of the high risk of AV block in patients with pathologic infranodal block induced by atrial pacing, pacemaker implantation is indicated in patients in whom no other apparent cause of syncope is found.

In patients who develop AV nodal Wenckebach block during atrial pacing at a long cycle length ($\geq$450 milliseconds), it may not be possible to assess conduction adequately within the His–Purkinje system. In these patients, it may be helpful to perform incremental atrial pacing after

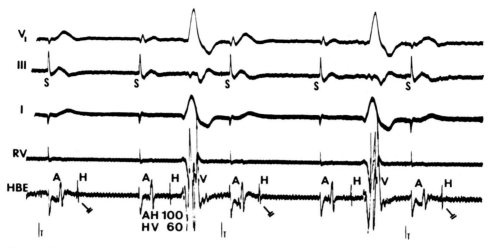

Figure 27-6. Pathologic infranodal atrioventricular block during atrial pacing. From top to bottom are leads V₁, III, and I, a right ventricular (RV) electrogram, and a His bundle electrogram (HBE). The atrial pacing cycle length is 500 milliseconds. There is intact atrioventricular nodal conduction, with an AH interval of 100 milliseconds. Two-to-one infra-Hisian block is seen. This abnormality is associated with a high risk of high-degree atrioventricular block. (See Fig 26-1 for key to abbreviations.)

the administration of atropine (0.5 to 1 mg intravenously). By shortening the cycle length at which AV nodal Wenckebach periodicity occurs, the His–Purkinje system is subjected to greater stress and infranodal block may be uncovered. However, if infranodal block occurs only at a very short atrial pacing cycle length (<300 milliseconds), this may not be an abnormal response and is not necessarily an indication for pacemaker implantation in the patient with unexplained syncope.

VENTRICULAR TACHYCARDIA

Several studies have demonstrated that the most common abnormality in patients with recurrent unexplained syncope who undergo electrophysiologic testing is ventricular tachycardia.[21-23] The prevalence of inducible ventricular tachycardia in patients with recurrent unexplained syncope ranges from 36% to 53%.[21-23] However, it cannot be assumed that ventricular tachycardia is always the cause

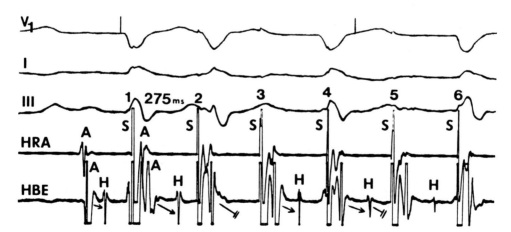

Figure 27-7. Functional infranodal atrioventricular block during atrial pacing. From top to bottom are leads V₁, I, and III, a high right atrial (HRA) electrogram, and a His bundle electrogram (HBE). The atrial pacing cycle length is 275 milliseconds. There is atrioventricular nodal Wenckebach block, with atrioventricular nodal block following stimulus number 2. The HH interval preceding stimulus number 4 is therefore lengthened, prolonging refractoriness in the His-Purkinje system. This accounts for the infra-Hisian block following stimulus number 4. This type of functional infranodal block is not associated with an increased risk of high-degree atrioventricular block (See Fig. 26-1 for key to abbreviations.)

of syncope in these patients. Programmed ventricular stimulation is helpful in evaluating patients with unexplained syncope only in that it results in the induction of clinical forms of ventricular tachycardia, that is, spontaneous ventricular tachycardia. Because programmed ventricular stimulation may result in the induction of nonclinical forms of ventricular tachycardia and because the "clinical" ventricular tachycardia (if there is one) in a patient with unexplained syncope has not been documented, it may be unclear whether an induced episode of ventricular tachycardia is clinically significant. A judgment on the clinical significance of induced ventricular tachycardia in a patient with unexplained syncope must be based on knowledge of the sensitivity and specificity of the particular stimulation protocol being used, the type of ventricular tachycardia induced, and the results of therapy reported in published studies.

Nonclinical forms of ventricular tachycardia are induced infrequently when the stimulation protocol includes only single and double extrastimuli.[43, 44] However, recent studies have demonstrated that triple extrastimuli are often required to induce the clinical form of ventricular tachycardia in patients with documented ventricular tachycardia.[45, 46] Although the sensitivity of programmed ventricular stimulation increases when triple extrastimuli are used, the specificity decreases. When the ventricular stimulation protocol includes triple extrastimuli, ventricular tachycardia can be induced in 37% to 45% of patients who have no documented or suspected history of ventricular tachycardia.[46–49] The nonclinical episodes of ventricular tachycardia induced in these patients are usually polymorphic, rapid (cycle length < 230 milliseconds), and unsustained and are more commonly induced in patients who have structural heart disease than in those who do not.[46–49] In contrast, sustained, unimorphic ventricular tachycardia is rarely inducible in patients who have not had spontaneous ventricular tachycardia.[46–49]

Based on studies that have assessed the specificity of ventricular stimulation protocols, it can be predicted that, in patients with unexplained syncope, sustained unimorphic ventricular tachycardia induced during electrophysiologic testing is more likely to be clinically significant than is polymorphic nonsustained ventricular tachycardia. This is supported by the results of a study by Morady and coworkers in which 53 patients with unexplained, recurrent syncope underwent electrophysiologic testing, including ventricular stimulation with as much as triple extrastimuli.[23] Nonsustained ventricular tachycardia (usually polymorphic) was induced in 15 patients (28%), sustained ventricular tachycardia (usually unimorphic) was induced in nine (17%), and ventricular fibrillation was induced in four (8%). In the majority of patients, sustained ventricular tachycardia, nonsustained ventricular tachycardia, and ventricular fibrillation were induced by triple

extrastimuli. These patients were treated with antiarrhythmic drugs selected on the basis of the results of electropharmacologic testing. The recurrence rate of syncope was 40% over 22 ± 6 months of follow-up study in patients with inducible nonsustained ventricular tachycardia, 0% over 30 ± 12 months of follow-up study in patients with inducible sustained ventricular tachycardia, and 25% over 21 ± 10 months of follow-up study in patients with inducible ventricular fibrillation. The excellent response rate in patients treated for sustained ventricular tachycardia implies that the cause of syncope was correctly identified and treated (Fig. 27-8). However, the 25% to 40% recurrence rate in the patients with induced polymorphic unsustained ventricular tachycardia or ventricular fibrillation suggests that, at least in some patients, the induced arrhythmia may have been a nonspecific response to an aggressive stimulation protocol unrelated to syncope (Fig. 27-9).

Because of the uncertainty that may arise regarding the clinical significance of ventricular tachycardia induced during electrophysiologic testing in patients with unexplained syncope, it is important to use a stimulation protocol that is sensitive in detecting ventricular tachycardia but that has maximum specificity. Multiple variables exist in a stimulation protocol (e.g., stimulus strength, number of extrastimuli, number of basic drive rates, number of right ventricular stimulation sites, and the use of left ventricular stimulation). The ideal stimulation protocol, taking into account all these variables, has yet to be determined. However, based on available data, it seems prudent to use a relatively low current strength (between twice diastolic threshold and 5 mA), at least two right ventricular stimulation sites, at least two basic drive rates, and left ventricular stimulation only if ventricular tachycardia is not induced by right ventricular stimulation and if the patient has structural heart disease. The latter recommendation is based on the observation that the yield of inducible ventricular tachycardia in patients with unexplained syncope who do not have structural heart disease is exceedingly small; the additional time and potential morbidity involved in performing left ventricular stimulation does not seem warranted in these patients.[21–23]

Coupling intervals of less than 200 milliseconds are rarely required to induce unimorphic ventricular tachycardia during programmed stimulation, whereas more than 50% of nonclinical polymorphic ventricular tachycardias are induced with coupling intervals less than 200 milliseconds. Therefore, specificity can be improved without impairing sensitivity if the extrastimulus coupling intervals are limited to 200 milliseconds.[50]

Ventricular stimulation during an isoproterenol infusion increases the sensitivity of electrophysiologic testing.[51] The use of single and double extrastimuli during an infusion of isoproterenol has a sensitivity equiv-

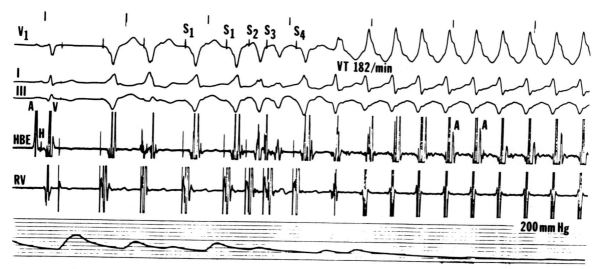

Figure 27-8. Sustained unimorphic ventricular tachycardia (VT) induced in a patient with recurrent, unexplained syncope who had coronary artery disease, a history of myocardial infarction, and occasional ventricular premature depolarizations during prolonged ambulatory electrocardiographic monitoring. From top to bottom are leads V_1, I, and III, a His bundle electrogram (HBE), a right ventricular (RV) electrogram, and a recording of arterial blood pressure on a scale of 200 mm Hg. Triple extrastimuli (S_2, S_3, S_4) introduced during ventricular drive (S_1, S_1) induced VT, rate 182 beats per minute. Systolic blood pressure fell rapidly from 120 to 0 mm Hg. The patient lost consciousness, and the VT was terminated by direct current countershock. Based on the results of electropharmacologic testing, the patient was treated with procainamide and has no further episodes of syncope. Sustained unimorphic VT has high diagnostic value when induced in a patient with unexplained syncope. (See Fig. 26-1 for key to abbreviations.)

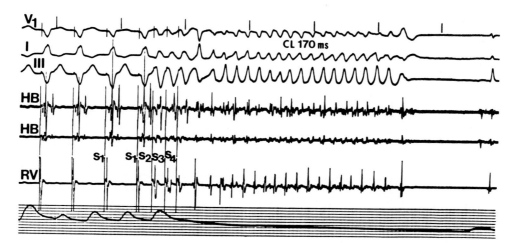

Figure 27-9. Polymorphic, unsustained ventricular tachycardia, cycle length 170 milliseconds, induced by triple extrastimuli (S_2, S_3, S_4) in a patient who had mitral valve prolapse and recurrent, unexplained syncope. From top to bottom are leads V_1, I, and III, two His bundle electrograms (HBE), a right ventricular (RV) electrogram, and an arterial blood pressure recording on a scale of 200 mm Hg. The patient was monitored and was documented to be in sinus rhythm during a typical episode of syncope that occured after the electrophysiologic study. The VT induced in this patient was, therefore, most likely a laboratory artifact unrelated to syncope. This type of polymorphic, unsustained VT is often a nonspecific response to programmed stimulation with triple extrastimuli.

alent to that of triple extrastimuli and has a greater degree of specificity.[52] Isoproterenol should be used as an additional provocative maneuver particularly in patients in whom syncope occurred in the setting of elevated catecholamine levels (e.g., during or immediately after exercise).

Because single and double extrastimuli induce non-clinical forms of ventricular tachycardia less often than do triple extrastimuli, it seems prudent to perform ventricular stimulation at two or more sites with single and double extrastimuli, reserving the use of triple extrastimuli for patients who do not have inducible ventricular tachycardia with fewer extrastimuli. This type of stimulation protocol minimizes the yield of nonclinical forms of ventricular tachycardia and maximizes the yield of clinical forms of ventricular tachycardia.[53]

Although unimorphic ventricular tachycardia is more likely than polymorphic ventricular tachycardia to be a clinically significant arrhythmia when induced in a patient with unexplained syncope, the clinical significance of polymorphic ventricular tachycardia in a given patient may be difficult to assess. In some patients, polymorphic ventricular tachycardia is a laboratory artifact, while in others it is the cause of syncope; the dilemma is how to distinguish the two (Fig. 27-10). Based on available data regarding the specificity of ventricular tachycardia induction protocols, the probability that polymorphic ventricular tachycardia is the cause of syncope appears to be inversely related to the number of extrastimuli needed to induce the ventricular tachycardia; that is, the greater the number of extrastimuli needed to induce the polymorphic ventricular tachycardia, the less likely it is to be the cause of syncope. If no other potential cause for syncope is found, a clinical trial of antiarrhythmic drug therapy aimed at suppressing polymorphic ventricular tachycardia may be indicated. If syncope recurs despite antiarrhythmic drug therapy predicted to be efficacious on the basis of electro-pharmacologic testing, polymorphic ventricular tachycardia may not be the cause of syncope.

In patients with bundle branch block and unexplained syncope, Ezri and coworkers found that ventricular tachycardia was inducible in four of 13 patients.[54] In a group of 32 patients with bundle branch block and unexplained syncope, Morady and coworkers reported that unimorphic ventricular tachycardia was inducible in nine (28%); one of these patients (who was noncompliant) died suddenly, and the other eight patients, who were treated with antiarrhythmic drugs directed at suppressing ventricular tachycardia, did not have recurrent syncope.[55] Four of the nine patients had an HV interval greater than or equal to 70 milliseconds, indicating a second potential cause of syncope, namely, intermittent AV block. These results demonstrate that patients with bundle branch block and unexplained syncope should undergo programmed ventricular stimulation even when a prolonged HV interval indicates that AV block may be a cause of syncope. Some patients with bundle branch block may be found to have two potential causes of syncope and may require more than one form of therapy (i.e., a pacemaker plus antiarrhythmic drugs).

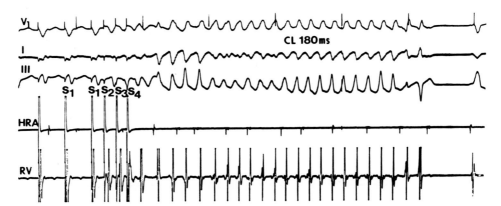

Figure 27-10. Polymorphic, unsustained ventricular tachycardia, cycle length (CL) 180 milliseconds induced by triple extrastimuli (S_2, S_3, S_4) in a patient with a congestive cardiomyopathy and recurrent syncope and presyncope. Ambulatory electrocardiographic recordings demonstrated bursts of rapid, polymorphic ventricular tachycardia, CL200 milliseconds, associated with presyncope. From top to bottom are leads V_1, I, and III, a high right atrial (HRA) electrogram, and a right ventricular (RV) electrogram. In this patient, polymorphic, unsustained ventricular tachycardia induced by triple extrastimuli appeared to be a clinically significant arrhythmia. However, if the patient had not been found to have similar episodes of ventricular tachycardia during ambulatory monitoring, the polymorphic, unsustained tachycardia might have mistakenly been thought to be a nonspecific response to an aggressive stimulation protocol, as was the case in the example presented in Figure 26-9.

PATIENTS MOST LIKELY TO HAVE A POSITIVE ELECTROPHYSIOLOGIC STUDY

An analysis of clinical variables may be helpful in selecting the patients with unexplained syncope who are the most likely to have a clinically significant abnormality during electrophysiologic testing. In a group of 104 patients with unexplained syncope who underwent an electrophysiologic test, Krol and coworkers demonstrated that the most powerful predictor of a positive electrophysiologic study is a left ventricular ejection fraction of less than or equal to 0.40, followed by the presence of bundle branch block, coronary artery disease, remote myocardial infarction, injury related to loss of consciousness, and male sex.[56] A negative electrophysiologic study was associated with an ejection fraction of more than 0.40, the absence of structural heart disease, a normal electrocardiogram, and normal ambulatory electrocardiographic monitoring. The probability of a negative study increased as the number and duration of syncopal episodes increased. Therefore, based on clinical variables, it is possible to stratify patients with unexplained syncope into subgroups with high and low probability of having a positive electrophysiologic study.

A noninvasive technique for identifying patients with unexplained syncope who are likely to have inducible ventricular tachycardia is the signal-averaged electrocardiogram. This technique has a sensitivity of 73% to 82% and a specificity of approximately 90% in detecting patients with unexplained syncope who have inducible ventricular tachycardia during electrophysiologic testing.[57–59]

IMPLICATIONS OF A NEGATIVE ELECTROPHYSIOLOGIC STUDY

In a group of 34 patients without organic heart disease who had unexplained syncope or presyncope, Gulamhusein and coworkers reported that 15 of 28 patients (44%) who had a normal electrophysiologic study had no recurrence of syncope over a mean of 15 months of follow-up study (range, 2 to 44 months).[60] Morady and coworkers also found a high spontaneous remission rate in patients with a normal electrophysiologic study; 7 of 10 patients (70%) who received no therapy had no recurrence of syncope over 31 ± 10 months of follow-up study.[23] In a group of 32 patients with bundle branch block and unexplained syncope, no diagnostic abnormalities were found during electrophysiologic testing in eight patients; only one of these eight patients had a recurrence of syncope over a mean of 18 months follow-up study (range, 6 to 41 months).[55] Therefore, it appears that patients with unexplained syncope who have a negative electrophysiologic study may have a low incidence of recurrent syncope.

The reason for the high spontaneous remission rate among patients who have a negative electrophysiologic study is unclear. The apparent remission may be due to spontaneous fluctuations in frequency; syncope may eventually recur with longer follow-up study. Some of these patients may have a psychiatric or hysterical basis for syncope and benefit from a placebo effect associated with undergoing an electrophysiologic study.

A normal electrophysiologic study does not eliminate the possibility of an arrhythmic cause for a patient's syncope. Patients with bundle branch block and intermittent high-degree infranodal AV block may, at times, have a normal HV interval between episodes of AV block.[61, 62] If syncope is caused by ventricular tachycardia that is caused by abnormal automaticity rather than reentry, the ventricular tachycardia is usually not inducible by programmed ventricular stimulation and may not be provoked by isoproterenol either. In some patients with coronary artery disease, syncope caused by ventricular tachycardia may occur only in the setting of myocardial ischemia; these patients may not have inducible ventricular tachycardia if ischemia is not present during electrophysiologic testing. Therefore, although a normal electrophysiologic study decreases the likelihood that syncope is caused by an arrhythmia, it does not eliminate the possibility.

Also, a benign prognosis is not guaranteed by an electrophysiologic study that does not demonstrate any diagnostic abnormalities. Among 12 patients with unexplained syncope and a negative electrophysiologic study who were treated empirically with an antiarrhythmic drug because of ventricular premature depolarizations, two patients (both of whom had coronary artery disease) died suddenly.[23] The mechanism of sudden death and whether antiarrhythmic drug therapy was a contributor is unclear.

What is the most appropriate management of the patient with unexplained syncope who has frequent ventricular premature depolarizations or nonsustained ventricular tachycardia without associated symptoms during ambulatory electrocardiographic monitoring and a normal electrophysiologic study? The asymptomatic ventricular ectopy may be an incidental finding, or the ventricular ectopy may be a clue that the patient's syncope is caused by ventricular tachycardia that is not inducible by programmed stimulation. Although no definitive recommendations can be made, it seems reasonable to suppress the ectopy with antiarrhythmic drugs in patients who, regardless of their syncope, may be at increased risk of sudden death, for example, patients with coronary artery disease or dilated cardiomyopathy who have complex forms of ventricular ectopy.[7–9] In patients with unexplained syncope, complex but asymptomatic ventricular arrhythmias, and a normal electrophysiologic study and who do not fall into a "high-risk" subgroup, for example, patients without identifiable structural heart disease, an empiric trial of antiarrhythmic drug therapy becomes a matter of clinical judgment. The potential toxicity and expense of chronic antiarrhythmic drug treatment must be weighed against the risk of symptomatic ventricular tachycardia or sudden death; the latter risk appears to be small in patients without identifiable heart disease.[63]

Is there a role for empiric pacemaker implantation in the patient with recurrent unexplained syncope who has a normal electrophysiologic study? Gulamhusein and co-workers reported that there was no recurrence of syncope in seven patients with syncope or presyncope who had a normal electrophysiologic study and underwent pacemaker implantation.[60] However, these authors also found a high remission rate in patients with a normal electrophysiologic study who received no therapy. Morady and co-workers found that syncope recurred in two of three patients with recurrent syncope and a normal electrophysiologic study who received a permanent pacemaker.[23] It seems that there is little or no role for pacemaker implantation in patients with unexplained syncope who have no abnormalities demonstrated by electrocardiographic monitoring or electrophysiologic testing. However, it may be appropriate to institute an empiric trial of permanent pacing in the patient who has recurrent unexplained syncope that causes injury and who is found to have a borderline abnormal but asymptomatic bradyarrhythmia during electrocardiographic monitoring (e.g., a 1.7-second sinus pause).

CONCLUSION

Electrophysiologic testing in the evaluation of patients with unexplained syncope is associated with several limitations. Diagnosis of the cause of syncope based on the results of electrophysiologic testing is inferential. Electrophysiologic testing may demonstrate abnormalities that are not related to the patient's syncope. A normal electrophysiologic study does not rule out an arrhythmic cause of syncope. These limitations must be kept in mind when selecting patients to undergo electrophysiologic testing and when interpreting the results.

Among patients with unexplained syncope who do not have organic heart disease, an arrhythmic cause of syncope is unlikely; therefore, the diagnostic yield of electrophysiologic testing is low. Unless there is a specific reason to suspect an arrhythmic cause of syncope (e.g., abrupt onset of rapid palpitations before syncope), electrophysiologic testing is unlikely to be of value in these patients.

On the other hand, electrophysiologic testing can uncover an abnormality that is likely to be the cause of syncope in a significant percentage of patients with or-

ganic heart disease. Probably the most significant contribution of electrophysiologic testing in the evaluation of patients with organic heart disease and unexplained syncope is to demonstrate whether ventricular tachycardia may be the cause of syncope. Electrophysiologic testing is, therefore, particularly appropriate in patients who belong to subgroups demonstrated to be at increased risk of sudden death.

The following abnormalities have the highest diagnostic value: inducible unimorphic ventricular tachycardia, a markedly prolonged SNRT (>2 to 3 seconds), inducible supraventricular tachycardia that is rapid and causes hypotension, a markedly prolonged HV interval (≥ 100 milliseconds), and pacing-induced infranodal AV block during intact AV nodal conduction. The diagnostic value of these abnormalities is enhanced if the induced arrhythmia reproduces the patient's symptoms.

A mildly prolonged SNRT, an abnormal sinoatrial conduction time, a moderately prolonged HV interval (70 to 100 milliseconds), and inducible polymorphic ventricular tachycardia or ventricular fibrillation may be related to the cause of syncope in some patients; however, in many patients these may be incidental findings or laboratory artifacts unrelated to syncope.

Despite its limitations, electrophysiologic testing can make an important contribution to the diagnosis and treatment of selected patients with unexplained syncope.

References

1. Milstein S, Reyes WJ, Benditt DG: Upright body tilt for evaluation of patients with recurrent, unexplained syncope. PACE 1989;12:117.
2. Day SC, Cook EF, Funkenstein H, Goldman L: Evaluation and outcome of emergency room patients with transient loss of consciousness. Am J Med 1982;73:15.
3. Kapoor WN, Karpf M, Wieand S, et al: A prospective evaluation and follow-up of patients with syncope. N Engl J Med 1983;309:197.
4. Gibson TC, Heitzman MR: Diagnostic efficacy of 24-hour electrocardiographic monitoring for syncope. Am J Cardiol 1984;53:1013.
5. Dhingra RC, Denes P, Wu D, et al: Syncope in patients with chronic bifascicular block. Significance, causative mechanisms, and clinical implications. Ann Intern Med 1974; 81:302.
6. Peters RW, Scheinman MM, Modin G, et al: Prophylactic permanent pacemaker for patients with chronic bundle branch block. Am J Med 1979;66:978.
7. Meinertz T, Hofmann T, Wolfgang K, et al: Significance of ventricular arrhythmias in idiopathic dilated cardiomyopathy. Am J Cardiol 1984;53:902.
8. Ruberman W, Weinblatt E, Goldberg JD, et al: Ventricular premature complexes and sudden death after myocardial infarction. Circulation 1981;64:297.
9. Bigger JT Jr, Fleiss JL, Kleiger R, et al: The relationships

among ventricular arrhythmias, left ventricular dysfunction, and mortality in the 2 years after myocardial infarction. Circulation 1984;69:250.

10. Nelson SD, Kou WH, DeBuitleir M, DiCarlo LA, Morady F: Value of programmed ventricular stimulation in presumed carotid sinus syndrome. Am J Cardiol 1987;60:1073.

11. Mandel WJ, Hayakawa H, Danzig R, Marcus HS: Evaluation of sinoatrial node function in man by overdrive suppression. Circulation 1971;44:59.

12. Narula OS, Samet P, Javier RP: Significance of the sinus node recovery time. Circulation 1972;45:140.

13. Strauss HC, Saroff AL, Bigger JT, Giardina EGV: Premature atrial stimulation as a key to the understanding of sinoatrial conduction in man. Presentation of data and critical review of the literature. Circulation 1973;47:86.

14. Narula OS, Shantha N, Vasquez M, et al: A new method for measurement of sinoatrial conduction time. Circulation 1978;58:706.

15. Kerr CR, Strauss HC: The measurement of sinus node refractoriness in man. Circulation 1983;68:1231.

16. Benditt DG, Strauss HC, Scheinman M, et al: Analysis of secondary pauses following termination of rapid atrial pacing in man. Circulation 1976;54:436.

17. Scheinman MM, Strauss HC, Abbott JA, et al: Electrophysiologic testing in patients with sinus pauses and/or sinoatrial exit block. Eur J Cardiol 1978;8:51.

18. Reiffel JA, Gang E, Gliklich J, et al: The human sinus node electrogram: A transvenous catheter technique and a comparison of directly measured and indirectly estimated sinoatrial conduction time in adults. Circulation 1980;62:1324.

19. Moss AJ, Davis RJ: Brady-tachy syndrome. Prog Cardiovasc Dis 1974;16:439.

20. Scheinman MM, Peters R, Hirschfeld DS, et al: The sick sinus ailing atrium. West J Med 1974;121:473.

21. DiMarco JP, Garan H, Harthorne JW, Ruskin JN: Intracardiac electrophysiologic techniques in recurrent syncope of unknown cause. Ann Intern Med 1981;95:542.

22. Akhtar M, Shenasa M, Denker S, et al: Role of cardiac electrophysiologic studies in patients with unexplained recurrent syncope. PACE 1983;6:192.

23. Morady F, Shen E, Schwartz A, et al: Long-term follow-up of patients with recurrent unexplained syncope evaluated by electrophysiologic testing. J Am Coll Cardiol 1983;2:1053.

24. Scheinman MM, Strauss HC, Abbott JA: Electrophysiologic testing for patients with sinus node dysfunction. J Electrocardiol 1979;12:211.

25. Gann D, Tolentino A, Samet P: Electrophysiologic evaluation of elderly patients with sinus bradycardia. A long-term follow-up study. Ann Intern Med 1979;90:24.

26. Dhingra RC, Amat-Y-Leon F, Wyndham C, et al: Clinical significance of prolonged sinoatrial conduction time. Circulation 1977;55:8.

27. Durrer D, Schoo L, Schuilenburg RM, Wellens HJJ: The role of premature beats in the initiation and the termination of supraventricular tachycardia in the Wolff-Parkinson-White syndrome. Circulation 1967;36:644.

28. Sung RJ, Castellanos A, Mallon SM, et al: Mode of initiation of reciprocating tachycardia during programmed ventricular stimulation in the Wolff-Parkinson-White syndrome: With reference to various patterns of ventriculoatrial conduction. Am J Cardiol 1977;40:24.

29. Denes P, Wu D, Dhingra RC, et al: Demonstration of dual A-V nodal pathways in patients with paroxysmal supraventricular tachycardia. Circulation 1973;48:549.

30. Rosen KM, Mehta A, Miller RA: Demonstration of dual atrioventricular nodal pathways in man. Am J Cardiol 1974; 33:291.

31. Benditt DG, Pritchett EL, Smith WM, et al: Characteristics of atrioventricular conduction and the spectrum of arrhythmias in Lown-Ganong-Levine syndrome. Circulation 1978; 57:454.

32. Moleiro F, Mendoza IJ, Medina-Ravell V, et al: One to one atrioventricular conduction during atrial pacing at rates of 300/minute in absence of Wolff-Parkinson-White syndrome. Am J Cardiol 1981;48:789.

33. Farshidi A, Josephson ME, Horowitz LN: Electrophysiologic characteristics of concealed bypass tracts: Clinical and electrocardiographic correlates. Am J Cardiol 1978;41:1052.

34. Przybylski J, Chiale PA, Halpern MS, et al: Unmasking of ventricular preexcitation by vagal stimulation or isoproterenol administration. Circulation 1980;61:1030.

35. Hariman RJ, Gomes JAC, El-Sherif N: Catecholamine-dependent atrioventricular nodal reentrant tachycardia. Circulation 1983;67:681.

36. Lloyd EA, Hauer RN, Zipes DP, et al: Syncope and ventricular tachycardia in patients with ventricular preexcitation. Am J Cardiol 1983;52:79.

37. Josephson ME, Seides SF: Clinical cardiac electrophysiology: Techniques and interpretations. Philadelphia: Lea & Febiger, 1979:23.

38. Dhingra RC, Palileo E, Strasberg B, et al: Significance of the HV interval in 517 patients with chronic bifascicular block. Circulation 1981;64:1265.

39. McAnulty JH, Rahimtoola SH, Murphy E, et al: Natural history of "high-risk" bundle-branch block. Final report of a prospective study. N Engl J Med 1982;307:137.

40. Scheinman MM, Peters RW, Sauve MJ, et al: Value of the H-Q interval in patients with bundle branch block and the role of prophylactic permanent pacing. Am J Cardiol 1982;50:1316.

41. Altschuler H, Fisher JD, Furman S: Significance of isolated H-V interval prolongation in symptomatic patients without documented heart block. Am Heart J 1979;97:19.

42. Dhingra RC, Wyndham C, Bauernfeind R, et al: Significance of block distal to the His bundle induced by atrial pacing in patients with chronic bifascicular block. Circulation 1979; 60:1455.

43. Vandepol CJ, Farshidi A, Spielman SR, et al: Incidence and clinical significance of induced ventricular tachycardia. Am J Cardiol 1980;45:725.

44. Livelli FD Jr, Bigger JT Jr, Reiffel JA, et al: Response to programmed ventricular stimulation: sensitivity, specificity and relation to heart disease. Am J Cardiol 1982;50:452.

45. Mann DE, Luck JC, Griffin JC, et al: Induction of clinical ventricular tachycardia using programmed stimulation: Value of third and fourth extrastimuli. Am J Cardiol 1983; 52:501.

46. Buxton AE, Waxman HL, Marchlinski FE, et al: Role of triple extrastimuli during electrophysiologic study of patients

with documented sustained ventricular tachyarrhythmias. Circulation 1984;69:532.

47. Brugada P, Abdollah H, Heddle B, Wellens HJJ: Results of a ventricular stimulation protocol using a maximum of 4 premature stimuli in patients without documented or suspected ventricular arrhythmias. Am J Cardiol 1983;52:1214.

48. Brugada P, Green M, Abdollah H, Wellens HJJ: Significance of ventricular arrhythmias initiated by programmed ventricular stimulation: The importance of the type of ventricular arrhythmia induced and the number of premature stimuli required. Circulation 1984;69:87.

49. Morady F, Shapiro W, Shen E, et al: Programmed ventricular stimulation in patients without spontaneous ventricular tachycardia. Am Heart J 1984;107:875.

50. Morady F, DiCarlo LA, Baerman JM, DeBuitleir M: Comparison of coupling intervals that induce clinical and nonclinical forms of ventricular tachycardia during programmed stimulation. Am J Cardiol 1987;57:1269.

51. Reddy CP, Gettes LS: Use of isoproterenol as an aid to electric induction of chronic recurrent ventricular tachycardia. Am J Cardiol 1979;44:705.

52. Baerman JM, Morady F, DeBuitleir M, DiCarlo LA, Kou WH, Nelson SD: A prospective comparison of programmed ventricular stimulation with triple extrastimuli versus single and double extrastimuli during infusion of isoproterenol. Am Heart J 1989;117:342.

53. Morady F, DiCarlo L, Winston S, et al: A prospective comparison of triple extrastimuli and left ventricular stimulation in ventricular tachycardia induction studies. Circulation 1984;70:52.

54. Ezri M, Lerman BB, Marchlinski FE, et al: Electrophysiologic

55. Morady F, Higgins J, Peters RW, et al: Results of electrophysiologic testing in patients with bundle branch block and unexplained syncope. Am J Cardiol 1984;54:587.

56. Krol RB, Morady F, Flaker GC, et al: Electrophysiologic testing in patients with unexplained syncope: Clinical and noninvasive predictors of outcome. J Am Coll Cardiol 1987;10:358.

57. Winters SL, Stewart D, Gomes JA: Signal averaging of the surface QRS complex predicts inducibility of ventricular tachycardia in patients with syncope of unknown origin: A prospective study. J Am Coll Cardiol 1987;10:775.

58. Kuchar DL, Thorburn CW, Sammel NL: Signal-averaged electrocardiogram for evaluation of recurrent syncope. Am J Cardiol 1986;58:949.

59. Gang ES, Peter T, Rosenthal ME, Mandel WJ, Lass Y: Detection of late potentials on the surface electrocardiogram in unexplained syncope. Am J Cardiol 1986;58:1014.

60. Gulamhusein S, Naccarelli GV, Ko PT, et al: Value and limitations of clinical electrophysiologic study in assessment of patients with unexplained syncope. Am J Med 1982;73:700.

61. DeJoseph RL, Zipes DP: Normal HV time in a patient with right bundle branch block, left anterior hemiblock and intermittent complete distal His block. Chest 1973;63:564.

62. McKenna WJ, Rowland E, Davies J, Krikler DM: Failure to predict development of atrioventricular block with electrophysiological testing supplemented by ajrnaline. PACE 1980;3:666.

63. Montague TJ, McPherson DD, MacKenzie BR, et al: Frequent ventricular ectopic activity without underlying cardiac disease: Analysis of 45 subjects. Am J Cardiol 1983;52:980.

evaluation of syncope in patients with bifascicular block. Am Heart J 1983;106:693.

Cardiac Arrhythmias, 3rd edition, edited by William J. Mandel.
J. B. Lippincott Company, Philadelphia © 1995.

28

David G. Benditt • MaryAnn Goldstein* • Stuart Adler
Scott Sakaguchi* • Keith Lurie

Neurally Mediated Syncopal Syndromes: Pathophysiology and Clinical Evaluation

Apart from the burden imposed by gravity during upright posture, numerous other daily stresses test the boundaries of human vasomotor stability. Physical exercise, emotional upset, metabolic disturbances, disease, and myriad other demands are mostly dealt with promptly and successfully by a complex interaction of neurologic, cardiac, and vascular compensatory mechanisms. Although many individuals occasionally encounter transient disturbances of circulatory homeostasis (e.g., symptoms accompanying rapid movement to the upright posture), it is remarkable that the cardiovascular adjustments needed to prevent transient cerebral ischemia are not subject to frequent dramatic symptomatic failures.

Under normal conditions, total cerebral blood flow averages 50 to 60 mL/100 g tissue, a range maintained primarily by the autoregulatory features of the cerebral vascular bed.[1] As a consequence, in the absence of clinically significant obstructive cerebrovascular disease, adequate cerebral perfusion can typically be assured as long as the mean arterial pressure is more than 80 mmHg (Fig.

28-1). Lesser flow levels lasting for 10 seconds or longer may be expected to be accompanied by loss of both consciousness and postural tone, whereas briefer periods of diminished flow may initiate a transient premonitory sensation of imminent loss of consciousness.[2] The former condition is usually termed syncope, whereas the latter has become characterized as presyncope (although in the absence of a subsequent syncopal event, this usage is obviously imprecise). In either case, the clinical event must be carefully distinguished from other states, such as seizure disorders and sleep.

A wide array of clinical conditions may be responsible for or closely associated with occurrence of spontaneous syncopal episodes.[3–7] These conditions are often divided into two principal subgroups based on the presence or absence of identifiable organic cardiovascular disease. The use of this approach, however, is limited for several reasons. First, most syncopal episodes fall into the cardiovascular class. Second, the pathophysiology of syncope crosses these classification boundaries. For example, syncope associated with valvular aortic stenosis is not solely due to failure of forward blood flow but is importantly contributed to by neurally mediated vasodilation.[8,9] Similarly, syncope accompanying certain tachyarrhythmias appears to exhibit a neurally mediated component.[10] Finally,

---

*Dr. Goldstein and Dr. Sakaguchi were recipients of postgraduate fellowships from the North American Society for Pacing and Electrophysiology (NASPE).

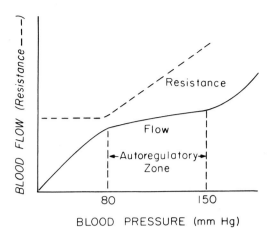

Figure 28-1. "Autoregulation" of blood flow in the cerebrovascular bed. Blood flow (*solid line*) and vascular resistance (*hatched line*) are shown on the ordinate, and systemic blood pressure (mmHg) is indicated in the abscissa. In the "autoregulatory range" changes in blood flow are less influenced by changes in arterial pressure than outside the autoregulatory range. Humans exhibit approximately a 6%–7% decrease in cerebral blood flow for every 10 mmHg reduction of arterial blood pressure in this zone. (Rowell LB: Human Circulation. Regulation during physical stress. New York: Oxford University Press, 1986:16. Reproduced with permission.)

the prognosis associated with similar mechanisms may be different. For instance, syncope in patients with aortic stenosis is accorded a worse prognosis than that of other neurally mediated syncopal syndromes. Given these limitations, we proposed an alternative classification of the causes of syncope that more evenly separates etiologies and their associated prognoses.[11]

Despite the difficulties associated with the classic cardiovascular and noncardiovascular division, it is important to remember that syncope associated with structural cardiovascular disease has a relatively grave prognosis, with the symptoms presumed to be both the direct result of the coexisting cardiac or cardiovascular disturbance and reflective of its severity.[12–14] Conversely, the prognosis of patients with symptoms unassociated with organic cardiovascular disease is generally considered less severe, although mortality has been reported and recurrences of syncope may be distressing (to both patients and their families) and the cause of considerable morbidity.[13,14] In this latter subgroup of patients, it is always important to consider metabolic, pulmonary, or organic neurologic disturbances. Nonetheless, most patients appear to be those susceptible to unexpected and inappropriate neurally mediated reflex activity, which results in various combinations of inadequate venous return, excessive peripheral vascular capacity, and paradoxical chronotropic, dromotropic, and possible inotropic responses. It is the understanding and clinical evaluation of this large subset of

neurally mediated (sometimes referred to as cardioneurogenic) syncopal and presyncopal conditions that form the focus of this chapter.

NEURALLY MEDIATED SYNCOPAL SYNDROMES

Among all causes of syncope, the neurally mediated reflex syncopal syndromes (Table 28-1) are believed to be the most common. Only the emotional or vasovagal faint occurs frequently, however. Some other syndromes may be considered to be infrequent (e.g., carotid sinus syndrome, postmicturition syncope), whereas yet others are rare

TABLE 28-1. Neurally Mediated Reflex Syncopal Syndromes

Syndrome	Suspected "Trigger" receptors
Vasovagal (emotional, common) faint	CNS higher centers, central C-P receptors
Carotid sinus syncope	Carotid artery baroreceptors
Increased intrathoracic pressure Cough syncope Sneeze syncope Trumpet playing Weight lifting "Mess trick" Valsalva-induced	Central C-P receptors
Postmicturition syncope	Bladder mechanoreceptors
GI stimulation Rectal examination Defecation syncope GI instrumentation	GI mechanoreceptors + C-P mechanoreceptors, due to straining
Esophageal-nasopharyngeal Swallowing syncope Glossopharyngeal neuralgia Oropharyngeal esophageal	Glossopharyngeal neural afferents ± carotid baroreceptor stimulation
Airway stimulation	Tracheal vagal afferent stimulation
"Diving" reflex	Cutaneous trigeminal nerve afferents
Drug-induced Nitroglycerin Isoproterenol Sympatholytic agents (e.g., bretylium, guanethidine)	Direct reduction of CO and arterial pressure, reflex actions by central C-P mechanoreceptors
Head-up tilt/gravitational	Central C-P mechanoreceptors
Second stage of hemorrhage	Carotid baroreceptor and central C-P mechanoreceptors ± CNS opiod receptors

CNS, central nervous system; C-P, cardiopulmonary; CO, cardiac output; GI, gastrointestinal.

(e.g., cough syncope). As understood, the principal features distinguishing each of these syndromes appears to be the nature and site of the initiating stimulus. Thus, the afferent limb (i.e., signals transmitted to the central nervous system [CNS]) of the culpable neural reflex arc differs among the syndromes. In contrast, although our understanding is incomplete, it appears that the efferent limbs, which result in the development of varying degrees (from patient to patient and within patients at various times) of symptomatic hypotension or bradycardia, are more or less common to all the syndromes.

Emotional or Vasovagal Faint

The term vasovagal (vasodepressor) syncope, although employed initially by Gowers for a different purpose, can be reasonably credited to Lewis, who first used it to describe the emotional or "common" faint.[15,16] Critical to Thomas' description was the recognition that hypotension and bradycardia were independent of each other in most instances. Thus, he indicated that atropine, while raising the pulse rate leaves the blood pressure below normal and the patient still pale and not fully conscious.[16] Further, Lewis clearly pointed out a concept often forgotten today; namely, that the main cause of the fall of blood pressure and the enfeeblement or loss of pulse is independent of the vagus and lies in the blood vessels. He recognized that the bradycardia associated with spontaneous and induced vasovagal faints may be impressive and contribute importantly to syncopal symptoms; however, it was not essential for development of hypotension:

> . . . from the beginning of the attack, the blood pressure falls progressively and is almost always accompanied by a steep fall of heart rate, the pulse often becomes imperceptible and the rate falling . . .[17]

Numerous factors are associated with triggering emotional or vasovagal faints in susceptible individuals, including noxious or unpleasant sights (e.g., blood), unanticipated pain, abrupt movement to the upright posture or prolonged exposure to upright posture, heat, dehydration, physical exercise, and venipuncture. As a rule, the temporal sequence of events documented in both spontaneous and tilt-table–induced episodes reveals an initial period of hypotension preceding onset of marked bradycardia.[18–20] The latter may be expected to markedly exacerbate the degree of hypotension.

Both venous and arteriolar dilation contribute to development of symptomatic hypotension in patients having vasovagal episodes. The former directly impairs stroke volume and cardiac output, both of which drop substantially despite reduced resistance to ejection. The latter

compounds the problem and probably reduces the time during which the cerebrovascular bed remains in its autoregulatory range. A negative cardiac inotropic effect has also been implicated but has not been clearly substantiated.[21] Indeed, a sizable negative inotropic component would be surprising given concepts regarding the probable contributory role played by central mechanoreceptors triggering or facilitating the event.[22–27]

Potentially, the initial reduction in systemic pressure may be an efferent neural response, resulting in both diminished vasoconstriction and a direct vasodilatory action, comparable with effects reported to occur in association with mental or emotional stress.[28] The efferent nerves may be sympathetic cholinergic fibers, resulting in muscle vasodilation, but the usual ineffectiveness of atropine for reversing the hypotension likely excludes a predominant muscarinic neurotransmitter.[29] Withdrawal of sympathetic vasoconstrictor tone remains the most likely basis for the vasodilation. Subsequently, active venous dilation may contribute directly by reducing venous return to the heart, whereas an unbalanced β-adrenergic–agonist action of elevated circulating epinephrine levels may play a contributory vasodilatory role in the systemic circulation.[29]

Although the vascular phenomena remain the more intriguing from both pathophysiologic and therapeutic perspectives, it is the heart rate slowing that usually accompanies vasovagal spells that tends to draw the greatest clinical attention. The latter may be because techniques are more readily available to document bradycardia in the free-living subject, whereas substantiating changes in blood pressure is far more difficult. Consequently, on those relatively rare occasions when prolonged asystolic pauses are fortuitously recorded, they tend to become a source of considerable medical concern. It is likely, however, that asystolic periods of 10 to 20 seconds (and perhaps longer) are common in the various forms of spontaneous neurally mediated syncope but are poorly appreciated because of the relative infrequency with which these events are documented. In support of this contention, a relatively early study in which vasovagal spells were induced by exposing a susceptible subject to a noxious stimulus demonstrated asystolic periods of 11 seconds and longer.[30] Fitzpatrick and Sutton, in a study comprising 40 patients having primarily cardioinhibitory vasovagal syncope, noted that five patients had pauses of more than 10 seconds.[31] Additionally, Yerg and coworkers observed a 22-second ventricular asystolic arrest, resulting in a vasovagal faint, in an endurance athlete before exercise.[32] Incidentally, periods of comparably severe bradycardia are commonly reported in related neurally mediated syndromes.[33–36] There is no evidence to suggest any additional risk associated with long versus short asystolic periods. Detailed follow-up studies of such patients are needed.

Carotid Sinus Syncope

The carotid sinus baroreceptors are the best known of the numerous cardiac and central vascular mechanoreceptors; stimulation of any of these receptors can result in various degrees of sinus bradycardia or pauses, paroxysmal atrioventricular (AV) block, and vasodilation with hypotension (Fig. 28-2). Anatomically, the carotid sinus baroreceptors are located in the adventitia of an enlarged segment of the carotid artery near its bifurcation. Mechanical deformation of the receptor tissue, particularly that due to steady repeated changes in vessel length, results in afferent impulses within the carotid sinus nerve, which travels primarily but not exclusively within the glossopharyngeal nerve. These impulses are thereby transmitted to the nucleus solitarius in the medulla, which is closely connected to the dorsal and ambiguous nuclei of the vagus nerve.[37]

An apparent relation between mechanical stimulation of the region known to incorporate the carotid sinus baroreceptors and resultant slowing of heart rate has been recognized for at least two centuries.[38] The true mechanism of the effect remained uncertain until clarified by Hering.[39] Indeed, as pointed out by Burchell, as prominent a physiologist as A. V. Waller argued strongly that the symptoms produced by his pressure on the carotid arteries were related to the pressure on the vagal nerves and not on the carotid arteries.[40,41]

The potential role of carotid sinus hypersensitivity as a cause of syncope was not widely appreciated until the comprehensive studies reported by Weiss and Baker.[33] It was these investigators who clearly distinguished the cardioinhibitory and vasodepressor elements associated with carotid sinus stimulation, although they also characterized a third condition that was classed as the central or cerebral type. The latter has since been discarded as probably having been due to carotid artery obstruction, with consequent cerebral ischemia. Overall, most patients exhibit a combination of both cardioinhibitory and vasodepressor elements in association with carotid sinus stim-

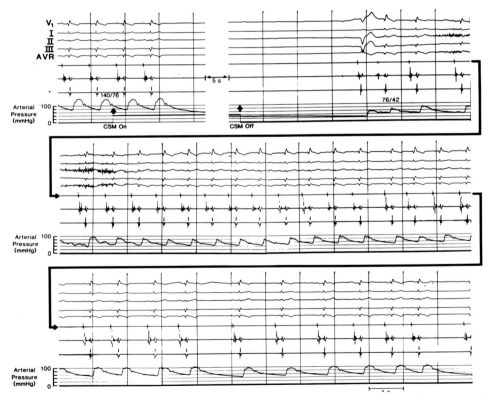

Figure 28-2. Electrocardiographic (ECG) and arterial pressure recordings obtained during carotid sinus massage. From top to bottom, the recordings in each panel are ECG leads V_1, I, II, III, and AVR, and intracardiac electrograms from the right atrium, His-bundle recording site, and right ventricular apex. The arterial pressure tracing was obtained from a cannula within the femoral artery. The onset and offset of carotid sinus massage (*CSM*) are indicated. Carotid sinus massage produced a 10.2-second period of atrial and ventricular asystole. Cardiac rhythm was restored by a ventricular escape beat and sinus bradycardia ensued. Systolic arterial pressure declined by 64 mmHg and did not return to control for 60 seconds (not shown). Time lines indicate one-second intervals. Recording speed was 50 mm/second. (Almquist A, et al: Carotid sinus hypersensitivity: evaluation of the vasodepressor component. Circulation 1985;71:927. Reproduced with permission of the American Heart Association.)

ulation, with only rare individuals exhibiting a pure form of either (Fig. 28-3).[42] Additionally, in contrast to the bradycardic response, which is nearly always immediate in onset after carotid sinus stimulation, the timing of the vasodepressor component is varied. In our experience, the nadir of the hypotensive response generally occurred within 10 to 15 seconds of the initiation of the stimulus (carotid sinus massage) and was sustained for a variable period (range, 6 to 84 seconds).[42] Further, neither muscarinic blockade alone (atropine) nor combined muscarinic and β-adrenergic blockade (atropine plus propranolol) prevented hypotension.

The frequency with which carotid sinus hypersensitivity is responsible for syncopal symptoms is uncertain. This uncertainty may be partly due to the frequency with which individuals (particularly older patients) exhibit marked bradycardia with carotid sinus stimulation and partly be due to the difficulty establishing an unequivocal relation between spontaneous syncope and demonstrable carotid sinus hypersensitivity.[43–50] Estimates suggest that only 5% to 20% of patients exhibiting carotid sinus hypersensitivity actually have syncope of carotid sinus origin.[44, 46, 51] Clinically, the diagnosis is suspected if the attack is triggered by or associated with turning or extending the neck, tight collars or ties, physical exertion, or previous neck surgery or irradiation. Hyperactivity of the reflex is more frequent in older individuals and has been reported to be closely correlated to the presence of atherosclerotic disease.[52]

Syncope Associated With Increased Intrathoracic Pressure

A variety of syncopal syndromes are associated with increased intrathoracic pressure, including cough and sneeze syncope (Fig. 28-4); syncope associated with playing certain musical instruments (e.g., trumpet players) or lifting heavy objects; straining during bowel movement; and Valsalva's maneuver, with or without concomitant ex-

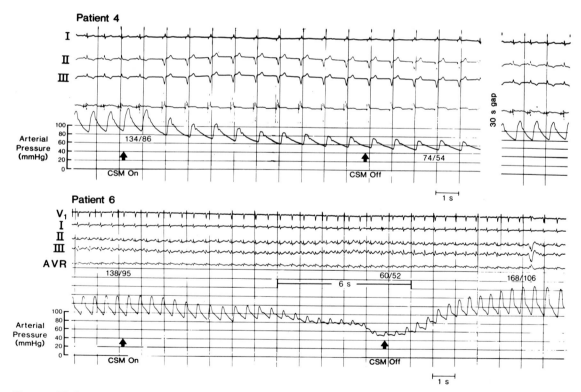

Figure 28-3. Recordings illustrating the temporal response of arterial hypotension induced by carotid sinus massage (*CSM*) in two patients. Traces from top to bottom are surface electrogram leads, as indicated; an intercardiac electrogram; and systemic arterial pressure. In patient 4 (*top panel*), hypotension occurred during CSM despite cardiac pacing, and the recovery period after CSM was prolonged. In patient 6 (*lower panel*), carotid sinus massage was associated with an almost pure vasodepressor response, and blood pressure recovered quickly with some overshoot in the post-CSM period. (Almquist A, et al: Carotid sinus hypersensitivity: evaluation of the vasodepressor component. Circulation 1985;71:927. Reproduced with permission of the American Heart Association.)

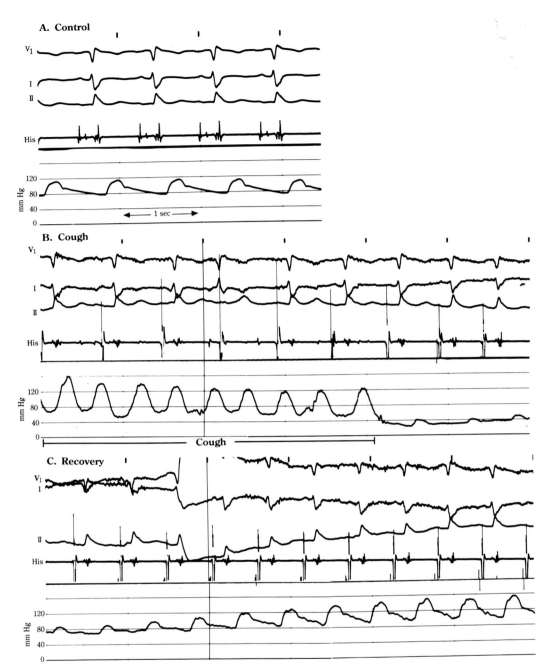

Figure 28-4. Electrocardiographic, intracardiac, and blood pressure traces illustrating findings in a patient with cough syncope. In each panel, the recordings from top to bottom are electrocardiogram leads V₁, I, II, an electrogram from the region of the His bundle, and an intraarterial pressure recording. (**A**) Baseline heart rate and blood pressure prior to cough. (**B**) Recorded during a period of coughing (duration of cough is indicated at the bottom of this panel). After the coughing episode (also revealed by the erratic blood pressure changes), the systemic pressure was markedly diminished (mean pressure, about 40 mmHg). (**C**) The slow recovery of systemic pressure in the post-cough period. Panel **C** is continuous with panel **B**. (Recordings provided through the courtesy of Charles C. Gornick, MD, Veterans Administration Medical Center, Minneapolis, Minnesota.)

ternal chest compression (the mess trick in which both a Valsalva is performed while a second individual compresses the subject's chest).[53-56] The basis for these forms of syncope is believed to be primarily related to a critical diminution of systemic venous return, with consequent reduction of cardiac output and cerebral blood flow. Other factors may facilitate the faint, however. First, as in the case of Valsalva's maneuver, circulatory attempts to overcome the impact of diminished stroke volume (e.g., increased inotropic activity, presumably partly due to carotid baroreceptor activation) may be inadequate, thereby aggravating empty ventricle activation of myocardial mechanoreceptors. The net result could be neurally mediated reflex hypotension and bradycardia comparable in mechanism with that associated with the vasovagal or emotional faint. Second, especially in the case of cough or sneeze syncope, a concussive effect may directly activate vascular mechanoreceptors, resulting in more prolonged periods of hypotension than would seem likely if diminished venous return were the sole cause. The latter mechanism seems plausible, given evidence suggesting that vigorous cough can increase intrathoracic pressure 100 mmHg or more.[56] Finally, vigorous coughing may result in substantial pressure transmission to the subarachnoid space, which may reduce cerebral blood flow.[37,57]

Postmicturition Syncope

This form of neurally mediated syncope is typically thought to be most frequent in young males, in whom it occurs as an isolated event in the absence of other significant disease, although older males and occasionally females may manifest the disorder.[58] The event tends to be closely associated with arising from sleep to empty the bladder and syncope occurs a few moments after the bladder emptying is completed. It is believed that marked bladder distention results in systemic vasoconstriction induced by a spinal cord reflex, which triggers widespread sympathetic discharge.[59,60] The latter is compensated in most cases by baroreceptor diminution of sympathetic activity, thereby normally preventing the hypertension that has been documented with bladder distention in patients with spinal cord transections.[60] As noted by Johnson and associates and Lukash and colleagues, if baroreceptor activation is not terminated promptly when the bladder contraction stimulus ends, both bradycardia and hypotension can result.[61,62] Fortunately, this rarely results in syncope. If the bladder is markedly distended and the patient dehydrated and vasodilated, symptoms can occur. The latter scenario appears to be facilitated by having just awakened from sleep and having been a recent consumer of at least a moderate amount of alcohol.[63]

Syncope Associated With Defecation and Other Forms of Pelvic Stimulation

Vagal afferents from the gut transmit impulses from gut wall tension receptors, with the frequency of the signals being related to the rapidity of the distention or contraction.[64] As a result, afferent neural signals may induce hypotensive and bradycardia episodes with syncope, comparable with the mechanism proposed for the vasovagal or emotional faint. According to Pathy, defecation syncope occurs more commonly in the morning and is most frequent in constipated individuals using laxatives or in association with the evacuation of large quantity of stool.[65]

Syncope is also known to occur in association with rectal and pelvic examinations and during sigmoidoscopic study. Again, marked bradycardia presumably associated with a vasodepressor component has been implicated.[66,67] The possibility of ventricular tachyarrhythmias should not be disregarded, however.[65]

Syncope Associated With Swallowing, Glossopharyngeal Neuralgia, and the Postprandial State

Syncope associated with swallowing is rare and usually associated with esophageal or other pharyngeal abnormalities.[37,45,68-72] Esophageal spasm may contribute to triggering the neural signals. Syncope tends to occur during or immediately after swallowing food, although severe bradycardia during passage of a gastroscope or feeding tube is likely a comparable condition. Syncope associated with swallowing a cold drink is probably also related, as is the development of presumed vagally mediated atrial tachyarrhythmias (fibrillation or flutter) in rare cases.[61] In all these situations, afferent neural impulses arise in territories subserved by the glossopharyngeal or vagus nerves. Transmission to the CNS is thereafter probably comparable with that of impulses generated by carotid sinus stimulation. Subsequently, efferent neural signals produce both bradycardia by a vagal mechanism and a vasodepressor action by mechanisms common to all the neurally mediated hypotension and bradycardia syndromes.

The glossopharyngeal nerve (ninth cranial nerve) incorporates afferents from the carotid sinus and the posterior pharyngeal wall.[37] Pain associated with glossopharyngeal neuralgia may initiate afferent impulses, which can trigger a hypotension and bradycardia episode.[73-77] Glossopharyngeal neuralgia may be the result of lesions of the cerebellopontine angle, base of the skull, or carotid artery. Often, however, no evident structural abnormality is present and no specific therapy is available. Although cardiac pacing has been used in some instances to counteract symptomatic bradycardia, prevention of syncope or dizziness would clearly be most effective if adequate prophylaxis against the painful trigger could be reliably achieved.[74,77,78]

Syncope Associated With Airway Stimulation

Airway stimulation, such as may occur during endotracheal intubation, has been associated with development of marked bradycardia by a vagal afferent or vagal efferent mechanism. These cases may exhibit substantial vasopressor action, however, and as illustrated in the case reported by Frankel and coworkers, the vasodepressor effect may be manifest even in the presence of apparent complete cervical cord transection.[79] Consequently, the efferent limb of the circuit is probably complex and may involve elements not solely restricted to the spinal column.

It is suggested that abrupt exposure of the airways to cold (e.g., cold water) can elicit a hypotensive and bradycardic response.[61] Although this probably can occur, it may be difficult to distinguish from the so-called diving reflex. The diving reflex appears to be triggered primarily by cutaneous receptors in the trigeminal nerve distribution and is characterized by apnea, bradycardia, and vasoconstriction. A vagal efferent mechanism, initially elicited from the trigeminal receptors and subsequently maintained by asphyxia-mediated carotid body afferent signals, has been observed in a variety of species, including some humans. The vasoconstriction is associated with a major shift of systemic blood flow away from viscera and toward working skeletal muscle.[80] Potentially, as in the case of postmicturition syncope, it may be speculated that after initial vasoconstriction, an excessive or unrelieved baroceptor reflex response may induce paradoxical vasodilation in conjunction with marked bradycardia. Such an outcome could be sufficiently catastrophic to explain several swimming- or diving-related fatalities due to asystolic cardiovascular collapse.[26,81]

Drug-Induced Reflex Syncope

Although nitrates in moderate doses induce arterial dilation, their principal effect is marked venous dilation, with a consequent decrease in the volume of blood returning to the heart in the upright patient. The resulting diminished cardiac output and systemic pressure usually elicit a compensatory carotid baroreceptor response, with initial parasympathetic withdrawal and increasing sympathetic drive. The result is tachycardia accompanied by an enhanced cardiac inotropic state. In certain susceptible individuals (perhaps facilitated by dehydration and the

upright posture), it is speculated that the resulting accentuation of central cardiopulmonary mechanoreceptor afferent activity may trigger an episode of symptomatic neurally mediated hypotension and bradycardia.[34,82,83] The potential importance of the noncardiac mechanoreceptors in this syndrome can be inferred from the report by Scherrer and associates, who describe induction of a vasovagal episode by the administration of a vasodilator to a heart-transplant recipient.[84] Presumably, the ventricular mechanoreceptors were isolated in this patient (i.e., absence of neural afferents) and could not participate in the neural reflex events.

Weiss and coworkers assessed the ability of nitrates to induce the equivalent of a vasovagal faint more than 55 years ago.[85] Subsequently, Weissler and colleagues, using nitrates and 60° upright tilt to induce syncope, determined that cardiac output failed to rise appropriately in the presence of diminished peripheral vascular resistance.[86] The latter is presumably due to inadequate venous return because it can be reversed by use of antigravity suits. Similar observations have been made with nitroglycerin.[83] The tendency for isoproterenol to induce hypotension and bradycardia episodes in susceptible individuals is probably comparable but additionally may relate to a direct drug effect on myocardial inotropic state and thereby on central cardiopulmonary mechanoreceptor afferent activity as well as by eliciting enhancement of receptor sensitivity.[24,87]

Head-Up Tilt-Induced and Hemorrhage-Induced Hypotension and Bradycardia

Under normal conditions, head-up tilt is associated with reduced venous return to the heart and a consequent diminution of stroke volume and cardiac output. Concomitant dehydration or inefficient dependent venoconstriction (e.g., patients subjected to prolonged bed rest, afflicted with certain neuropathies, or exposed to weightlessness) would be expected to exacerbate sensitivity to development of such a reaction with assumption of upright posture.[1,88]

The basis for development of hypotension and bradycardia with upright posture appears to be best explained by neurally mediated reflex activity initiated from the central circulation. In susceptible individuals, the impact of central volume changes and the resulting compensatory increase in cardiac inotropic state may induce a paradoxical hypotension and bradycardia secondary to afferent signals generated by both the carotid sinus baroreceptor and the central cardiopulmonary mechanoreceptors. A similar scenario occurs during abrupt hemorrhage and is presumed to initiate the second stage response, in which marked bradycardia and vasodilation develop.[89–94]

Reflex Hypotension and Bradycardia Associated With Exercise

The occurrence of neurally mediated hypotension and bradycardia in association with exercise may occur in individuals without apparent structural heart disease, although infrequently (Fig. 28-5).[26, 95-104] As an example, Fleg and Asante describe an 11-second asystolic pause with a prolonged syncopal event after completion of a maximal treadmill exercise test in a 52-year-old male.[95] This patient had apparently experienced a comparable event after treadmill exercise 4 years earlier. Kapoor describes a similar series of events in a 34-year-old jogger, in whom ambulatory electrocardiographic recording during usual exercise ultimately detected symptoms in conjunction with a rapid change from sinus tachycardia to sinus bradycardia, followed by multiple sinus and ventricular pauses, with longest pauses of 6.8 seconds.[99] Additionally, we describe findings in several patients presenting with what appeared to be severe cardiovascular collapse due to cardiac asystole. In several of these patients, spontaneous symptoms developed in association with physical exertion.[26, 104] Finally, Tamura and coworkers also note the abrupt development of cardiac slowing immediately after treadmill exercise in a 45-year-old male who had had a history of recurrent syncopal attacks after strenuous exercise.[100] In this case, atrial asystole of 30 seconds duration occurred, and temporary pacing was instituted because of the prolonged bradycardia.

Although orthostatic hypotension has been reported after heavy exertion, the development of both hypotension and bradycardia in otherwise healthy individuals in close association with exercise is compatible with a neurally mediated reflex phenomenon.[26, 101, 102, 104] In this case, the increased catecholamines associated with exercise may both sensitize the cardiopulmonary mechanoreceptors and increase the inotropic force applied to them. Additionally, at termination of exercise, the central circulation may be faced with both an abrupt diminution of venous return and a general reduction in circulating volume due to dehydration and shifts of flow to facilitate heat dissipation. The net result of these physiologic events is enhanced susceptibility to neurally mediated vasovagal events through mechanisms.

PATHOPHYSIOLOGY OF NEURALLY MEDIATED SYNCOPAL SYNDROMES

Afferent and Efferent Neural Pathways

The precise origins of the various neurally mediated syncopal syndromes are incompletely understood. Despite evident important clinical and pathophysiologic differences among the syndromes (some of which have already been noted), their many characteristics in common suggest that it is reasonable to consider them as being a group of closely related disorders. For practical purposes, the major distinguishing feature among the syndromes appears to be the site or nature of the factor or factors that triggers the episode and consequently the route of the initial afferent neural impulses (Fig. 28-6). Nonetheless, there is already evidence indicating that there are differences in the manner in which the CNS processes the afferent impulses. For example, the temporal relation of induced hypotension and bradycardia are different in carotid sinus stimulation when compared with tilt-induced vasovagal syncope.[20, 42] Most of the differences in the manner in which the CNS responds to afferent impulses lie beyond the resolution of available clinical investigational techniques. Potentially, future studies will profitably address this issue.

Carotid sinus hypersensitivity and the vasovagal faint have been the most thoroughly studied of the neurally mediated syncopal syndromes, and hypotheses regarding mechanisms of spontaneous hypotension and bradycardia are mostly based on clinical and experimental observations in these conditions. Essentially, the origin of the afferent signals in each of these conditions appears to be receptors that respond to mechanical stimuli (e.g., increased or decreased wall stress); pain; or less commonly, temperature change. In the most common of the neurally mediated syncopal syndromes, mechanoreceptors located in any of various organ systems provide the trigger. In the case of the carotid artery and aortic arch mechanoreceptors (baroreceptors), the afferent traffic in both myelinated and unmyelinated nerves is enhanced by activation resulting from increased systemic blood pressure (or the receptors are otherwise stimulated, such as by carotid sinus massage). The carotid sinus nerve joins the glossopharyngeal nerve, whereas the nerves from the aortic arch become afferent elements within the vagus nerve. Under normal conditions, an increase in afferent nerve traffic from these receptors results in bradycardia and reduced systemic vascular resistance, thereby providing a means of short-term modulation of systemic pressure changes.[61, 105]

Mechanoreceptors similar to those of the carotid arteries and aortic arch are also found elsewhere in the cardiopulmonary system. For example, the atrial and ventricular myocardium is networked by mechanoreceptors with afferent connections to the CNS by both myelinated and unmyelinated fibers (so-called C fibers), which travel predominantly in the vagus nerve (tenth cranial nerve).[105-109] The atrial afferents (predominantly myelinated) are derived from several types of receptors located primarily in the region of the atrial junctions with the vena cavae and the pulmonary veins. These receptors appear to be particularly sensitive to central volume changes and relatively

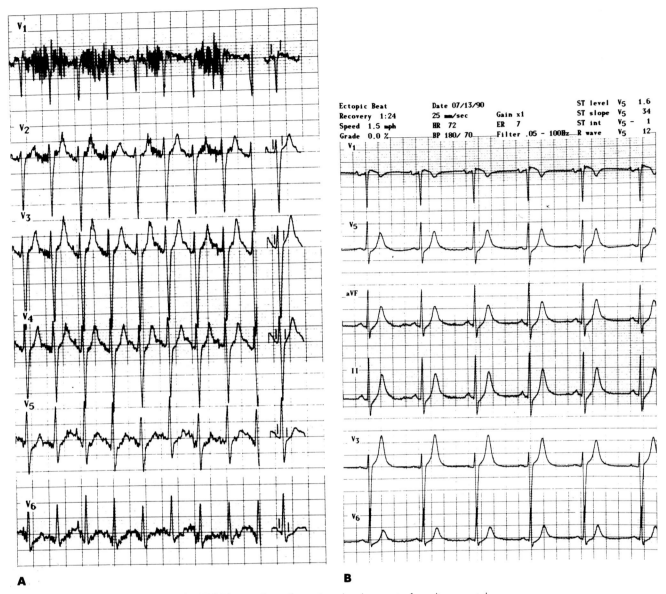

Figure 28-5. Electrocardiographic (ECG) recordings illustrating development of cardiac asystole after vigorous exercise in a 32-year-old male (ECG leads as indicated). (**A**) An ECG recording obtained at peak exercise during a Bruce treadmill exercise protocol. The maximum heart rate was about 170 beats/min, with a corresponding blood pressure of 170/65 mmHg. (**B**) A recording obtained at 1-minute 24 seconds into the recovery period. A moderate but premature bradycardia has begun to emerge. *(continued)*

insensitive to changes in myocardial contractile state.[105] Atrial receptor distension increases heart rate and urinary output (the latter by both enhanced vasopressin release and by atrial peptides). Afferents from ventricular receptors are predominantly unmyelinated C fibers from both chemical-sensitive (e.g., veratidine, nicotine) and mechanically sensitive sites. The frequency of impulses generated by the mechanically sensitive receptors is directly related to contractile state and end-diastolic pressure. Thus, in-

creased wall stress by excessive wall distension or due to marked increases in inotropic state may result in an increased frequency of afferent neural signals, which ultimately trigger development of vasodilation and bradycardia.[109] Thus, positive inotropic agents enhance ventricular mechanoreceptor discharge, whereas negative inotropes reduce the intensity of afferent signals.[107,110,111] Perhaps the occurrence of vasodilation and bradycardia in the presence of increased wall stress can be thought of as

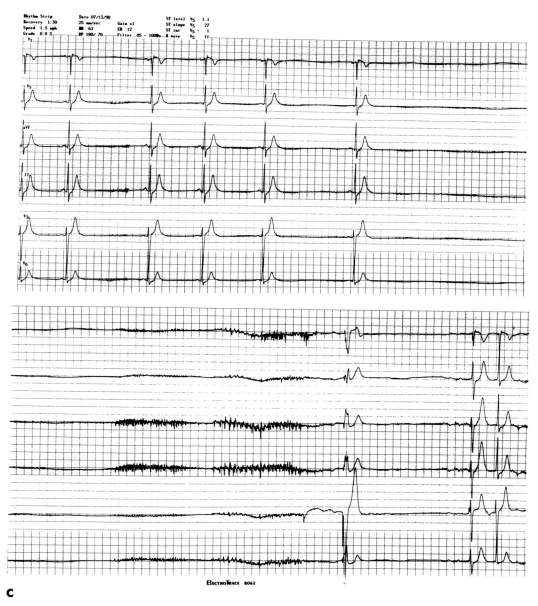

Figure 28-5. *(continued)* (**C**) At 1-minute 30 seconds into the recovery phase, while the patient was walking slowly on the treadmill, an abrupt asystolic pause developed. The maximum asystolic pause was approximately 11 seconds duration with development of seizure-like activity. The initial asystolic pause was terminated by a ventricular escape beat after which marked bradycardia persisted until sinus rhythm resumed as the patient recovered in the supine position. (Electrocardiographic tracings provided courtesy of the cardiopulmonary exercise laboratory at University of Minnesota Hospital.)

being a cardioprotective device, although at times it appears to be disadvantageous to other elements of the circulation.[24, 25]

The relation between myelinated and unmyelinated afferent activity on ultimate heart rate and vascular control is complex and incompletely understood. Nonetheless, it appears that cardiac afferent activity does participate in establishing the level of tonic sympathetic neural outflow

to the renal and splanchnic beds in particular, with a smaller impact on skeletal muscle blood flow.[105–112] Additionally, these afferent signals also importantly influence renin secretion and contribute to control of vasopressin release from hypothalamic sites.[105, 113–115]

Hypotension elicited by reflex, based on central mechanoreceptor stimulation, is thought to be due primarily to diminished sympathetic vasoconstrictor tone.[18, 116–118]

NEURALLY-MEDIATED SYNCOPAL SYNDROMES

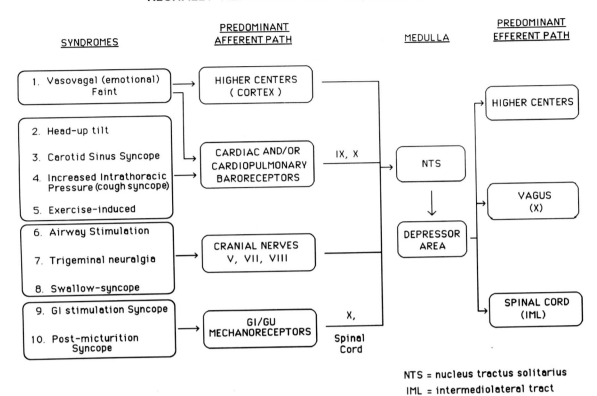

Figure 28-6. Relation among various neurally mediated syncopal syndromes, their predominant afferent neural pathways, and their predominant efferent neural connections.

Microneurographic recordings offer the most specific view of sympathetic neural activity, although the selected nature of available recording sites is a major limitation of the technique. Nonetheless, reported neural recordings in two patients with vasovagal syncope and in one patient with syncope associated with glossopharyngeal neuralgia revealed diminished sympathetic neural activity in close temporal association with documented hypotension and bradycardia (Fig. 28-8).[18,76] In the former report, the authors noted that sympathetic neural activity was increased before syncope. Careful inspection of Figure 28-7, however, (see Fig. 28-1 from reference 18) reveals that the onset of hypotension substantially preceded the abrupt reduction in recorded sympathetic neural traffic. Further clarification of the temporal relation between alterations of neural activity and hemodynamic changes remains essential.

Measurement of circulating catecholamine concentrations before and during induced faints provides an alternative although indirect assessment of sympathetic neural state. With this technique, there appears to be some discrepancy between the sympathetic neural withdrawal hypothesis and reported norepinephrine levels (the best

readily available marker for the general state of sympathetic neural activity in patients with neurally mediated syncope).[119] Sander-Jensen and colleagues and Fitzpatrick and associates noted no evident diminution of circulating norepinephrine levels (see Fig. 28-8).[120,121] Norepinephrine actually increased, as has been observed in normal individuals subjected to upright posture. Goldstein and colleagues, in a case report illustrating findings in a young woman with easily inducible syncopal episodes, similarly failed to detect a significant fall in circulating norepinephrine.[19] Our experience has been comparable. Conversely, Ziegler and coworkers observed lesser circulating plasma norepinephrine levels in vasodepressor-susceptible patients on arising, compared with increases noted in individuals who were apparently not susceptible.[117] In our experience, when one attempts to factor out adrenal contribution to circulating norepinephrine, there does appear to be a less prominent rise in norepinephrine levels in fainters than in nonfainters during head-up tilt-table testing. The stress of the syncopal episode may induce simultaneous release of both adrenal-origin epinephrine and norepinephrine, whereas norepinephrine of neural-origin is diminished.[120] Such a combination of

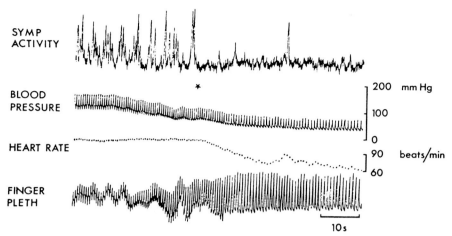

Figure 28-7. Changes in muscle sympathetic activity, systemic arterial blood pressure, heart rate, and finger pulse plethysmographic recordings during spontaneous vasovagal syncope. The *asterisk* indicates the time of syncope in this patient. Note the syncope was temporally closely associated with a marked diminution of sympathetic neural activity. Further, heart-rate decline was closely associated with the onset of syncope and with the reduction in neural sympathetic activity. It should be noted, however, that systemic blood pressure began to decline considerably before either reduction of neural sympathetic activity or fall in heart rate. Similarly, the plethysmographic recording appears to show an increase in the vascular bed before diminution of evident sympathetic neural activity. (Wallin BG, Sundlof G: Sympathetic outflow to muscles during vasovagal syncope. J Auton Nerv Syst 1982;6:287. Reproduced with permission.)

events could explain the reported relatively stable levels of circulating norepinephrine despite reduced sympathetic neural activity.[120, 121]

Central Nervous System Connections and Sympathetic and Nonsympathetic Efferent Neural Control

The medulla is the principal site of CNS connections subserving the reflexes of interest. The nucleus tractus solitarius (NTS) provides the most important region, integrating afferent impulses from most cardiovascular baro- and chemoreceptors arriving in the vagus and glossopharyngeal nerves. It also receives afferent impulses from other cranial nerves, the hypothalamus, the spinal cord and brainstem. Nucleus tractus solitarius may also be influenced by circulating humoral factors because of its close vascular and neural relation to the area postrema, which lacks a blood–brain barrier. Efferent signals from the NTS stimulate vagal preganglionic nuclei in the medulla, sympathetic preganglionic nuclei in the intermediolateral nuclei of the spinal cord, and other brainstem nuclei and higher CNS centers.[37, 105]

The hypothalamus also appears to be capable of eliciting both pressor and depressor responses. Both sympathetic and parasympathetic responses are affected, with the pressor response being initiated by stimulation of the supraoptic region, whereas depressor responses originate in a more rostral region. When stimulated, the latter produces a bradycardia and vasodepressor response comparable with that associated with baroreceptor stimulation.[122] Potentially, in the neurally mediated syncopal syndromes, the reported diminution in sympathetic nerve activity, which presumably contributes to the negative chronotropic and vasodepressor responses, may partly be the result of occupation of CNS delta-opiode receptor sites.[18, 76] The latter is consistent with the increase in β-endorphin levels reported in both vasovagal syncope and the analogous second stage of hemorrhagic shock.[123–126] In the latter condition, the administration of the opiod-receptor–blocker naloxone is far more effective in preventing hypotension when administered intracisternally than when administered intravenously.[127] There has also been interest in the role played by serotonin in modulating CNS sympathetic outflow. Clinical observations suggest that serotonin re-uptake blockers may diminish susceptibility to certain neurally mediated syncopal events, a finding compatible with the notion that increased CNS serotonin diminishes efferent adrenergic nerve traffic.[128] Finally, certain vasoactive peptides (e.g., vasoactive intestinal peptide, calcitonin gene-related peptide) and purinergic agonists (e.g., adenosine) released from perivascular nerves may decrease norepinephrine

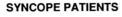

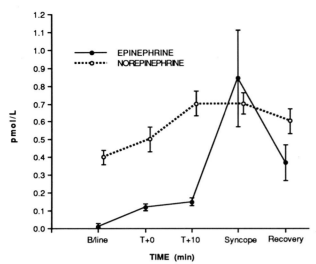

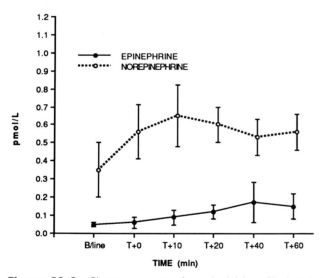

Figure 28-8. Changes in epinephrine (*solid line, filled circles*) and norepinephrine (*dotted line, empty circles*) during head-uptilt testing in patients in whom syncope developed (*top panel*) and in nonsyncope patients (*bottom panel*). In each panel, the catecholamine concentration is indicated in pmol/L on the ordinate and time is indicated on the abscissa. The baseline control values are indicated by the abbreviation *B/line*. In syncope patients, there was a marked increase in circulating epinephrine levels just before occurrence of syncope, compared with findings in nonsyncope patients. Norepinephrine concentrations were comparable in both groups of patients. It is noted that baseline epinephrine levels tended to be lower in syncope patients than in nonsyncope patients. (Data for graphical presentation provided through the courtesy of Drs. A. Fitzpatrick and R. Sutton, London, England.)

release and contribute directly to vasodilation.[129–132] The role of cholinergic vasodilator mechanisms in eliciting the vasodepressor response remains controversial.[1, 130] Based on failure of muscarinic blockade with atropine to substantially affect hypotension in most patients, it is difficult to assign this mechanism a crucial role. A cholinergic vasodilator mechanism may be clinically relevant in a subset of individuals (about 10% of those with hypotension and bradycardia syndromes) in whom atropine does prove effective. In contrast, the specificity of atropine as a pure muscarinic blocker differs in various vascular beds.[131] For example, atropine is reported to antagonize serotoninergic and α-adrenergic receptors in some tissues.[133, 134] Consequently, a cholinergic vasodilator mechanism may yet play a role in the development of hypotension during neurally mediated syncopal events but further studies are required to substantiate its contribution.

Higher Cerebral Centers

It is evident clinically that higher CNS centers are frequently involved in initiating spontaneous syncopal episodes. They probably also play an important role in facilitating development of symptoms in susceptible patients, thereby perhaps partially explaining the variability in occurrence of syncopal events. Clearly, fear, pain, and unpleasant experiences or smells can instigate hypotension and bradycardia episodes. As reviewed by Abboud and Thames, stimulation of certain cortical and subcortical regions can elicit vasodepressor responses in addition to bradycardia and apnea, whereas other cortical regions are associated with suppression of baroreceptor-induced bradycardia and hypotension.[105] Satisfactory tests evaluating the role of higher cerebral inputs are not available, precluding clinical assessment of their role in individual patients.

Overview of the Pathophysiology of Neurally Mediated Syncopal Syndromes

The neural and hemodynamic events culminating in a neurally mediated syncopal episode are complex and only incompletely characterized. Although many elements of the puzzle remain to be defined, three appear to be relatively well substantiated: (1) effects of posture or loss of central blood volume; (2) neuroendocrine activation initiated by peripheral (i.e., non-CNS) receptors or cortical sites; and (3) a factor that can perhaps best be categorized as susceptibility (i.e., the tendency for certain individuals to be more frequently troubled by neurally mediated syncopal syndromes despite the probable universal presence of the reflex arcs in humans).

Typically, neurally mediated syncopal syndromes are associated with the upright posture, in which circulating volume is displaced from intrathoracic to more dependent vascular spaces. Central venous pressure, stroke volume, and systemic arterial pressure tend to fall, activating arterial and central cardiopulmonary baroreceptors. Normally, afferent neural signals to the various medullary centers ultimately result in efferent accentuation of sympathetic neural output, with relative diminution of parasympathetic activity and activation of the renin–angiotensin aldosterone and vasopressin systems. Similar responses may be elicited with modest hemorrhage or dehydration. Thus, usually a compensatory series of events occur, resulting in vasoconstriction, increased heart rate, enhanced inotropic state, and ultimately, salt and water retention. The result is typically a modest tachycardia, a small drop in systolic pressure, and a slight increase in diastolic pressure. Under certain circumstances, a different outcome may transpire. Rapid loss of central volume, such as may occur with hemorrhage, administration of nitroglycerin or amyl nitrite, and probably the abrupt assumption of upright posture alone can result in a relatively empty ventricle with a vigorous left ventricular contraction.[34, 83, 89, 90, 93, 135] The latter effect, perhaps amplified by increased circulating catecholamines of adrenal origin, may result in exaggerated afferent neural activity (a positive feedback effect), with consequent efferent neural signals calling for bradycardia and vasodilation.[120, 121] Observations by Doppler ultrasound support the view that a strong ventricular contraction is associated with and may be an initiating factor in development of hypotension and bradycardia episodes. Under these circumstances, the induced hypotension and bradycardia may be interpreted as a myocardial protective mechanism.

The concept of susceptibility to neurally mediated hypotension and bradycardia has not been well established scientifically, although it appears to be a real phenomenon clinically. Perhaps the baseline neuroendocrine state of the individual is a marker. Previous studies in patients with inducible vasovagal reactions note heart rate and blood pressure increases preceding loss of consciousness, whereas others suggest a transient premonitory increase in sympathetic neural and adrenal activity.[18, 21, 81, 136–138] Findings suggest that the level of heart rate and circulating epinephrine increment during onset of upright tilt testing appear to predict susceptibility to a positive test.[121] Additionally, the hyperparasympathetic state may be a marker of increased susceptibility. The latter, perhaps compounded by dehydration, upright posture, and rising catecholamines, may partly contribute to occurrence of syncopal events in close association with exercise, especially in well-trained athletes.[26, 32, 95, 97, 100, 103, 139] Conversely, susceptibility to one form of the neurally mediated syncopal syndromes does not necessarily confer susceptibility to other mechanoreceptor-mediated hypotension and bradycardia events. Thus, for example, coincidence of marked carotid sinus hypersensitivity in patients with tilt-table proved neurally mediated vasovagal reactions has been the exception rather than the rule in our experience. Additional studies of correspondences such as these are certainly warranted.

CLINICAL LABORATORY TECHNIQUES FOR EVALUATION OF NEURALLY MEDIATED SYNCOPAL SYNDROMES

Head-up tilt-table testing in conjunction with other tests of autonomic neural control such as carotid sinus stimulation and Valsalva's maneuver are the most commonly employed techniques for evaluation of susceptibility to neurally mediated syncopal syndromes. Assessment of observed intrinsic heart rate may also be used to evaluate the relative predominance of parasympathetic and sympathetic control on sinus node and AV node electrophysiologic properties.[140] Additionally, estimation of circulating blood volume and its distribution has been advocated in some studies, although its clinical use has been questioned.[141] In the future, measurement of heart rate and blood pressure variability and response to lower-body negative pressure may also contribute to the examination of patients.[135] For purposes of this review, only those techniques in common clinical use for assessment of patients with suspected neurally mediated syncope are discussed (i.e., head-up tilt, carotid sinus massage, and Valsalva's maneuver).

Head-up Tilt-Table Testing

The physiologic responses to upright posture during tilt-table testing have been the subject of study for some time.[86, 142–148] In particular, the understanding of circulatory adjustments to gravitational stress in health and disease has been of considerable interest in aviation and aerospace environments.[149–152] Only recently, however, has the role of upright posture been seriously considered in evaluation of individuals with symptomatic arrhythmias. As a result, it is recommended that the clinical significance of induced arrhythmias during electrophysiologic testing be assessed during upright tilt.[153] This concept makes sense, given the clinical observation that symptoms associated with clinical arrhythmias are usually most apparent when patients are upright, presumably due to inadequacy of the circulatory compensation to gravitational stress given the limitation imposed by a concomitant rhythm disturbance. Furthermore, cardiac electrophysiologic characteristics are affected by the neuroendocrine responses to postural change and consequently, it should not be surprising that both arrhythmia susceptibility and characteristics (i.e., rate, frequency of occurrence) may be sensitive to postural changes.[154,155]

The head-up tilt-table testing technique has generated widespread interest as a tool for assessing susceptibility to spontaneous neurally mediated reflex syncopal syndromes.[20,24,26,87,156–165] The potential use of upright tilt testing in this setting may be evident from the preceding discussion of the physiologic effects of upright posture and its role in eliciting the neural reflex activity believed critical to initiating hypotension and bradycardia. Beyond these hypothetical considerations, however, several clinical and laboratory observations lend support to the notion that tilt-table testing is capable of reproducing the neurally mediated vasovagal syncopal syndrome in susceptible individuals:

1. There is a close clinical similarity between tilt-induced syncopal events and spontaneous vasovagal episodes, as evidenced by comparable premonitory symptoms (e.g., nausea, hearing and visual loss, diaphoresis) and signs (e.g., marked pallor, variable respiratory movements, loss of postural tone, bradycardia, and occasionally extreme asystole and seizure-like musculoskeletal activity).

2. The hemodynamic and electrocardiographic parallels are striking. For example, studies from this laboratory assessed the temporal sequence of blood pressure and heart rate changes during tilt-induced syncopal spells to compare them with those reported for spontaneous syncopal episodes.[20] Findings in nine syncope patients having positive tilt tests (i.e., induced hypotension and bradycardia) and five syncope patients having negative tilt tests were reported. Briefly, the tilt-test–positive patients manifested progressive RR-interval and prolongation, with marked systolic and diastolic hypotension (Fig. 28-9). Conversely, tilt-

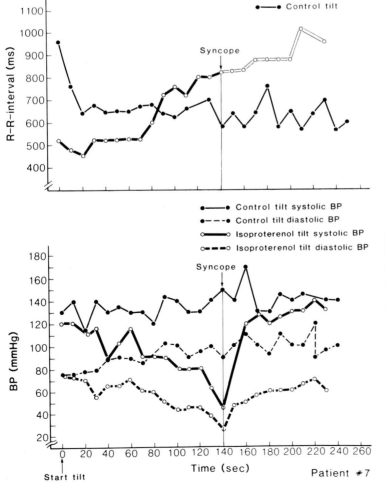

Figure 28-9. RR interval (*top panel*) and blood pressure (*bottom panel*) responses during a control head-up tilt in the absence of isoproterenol and during upright tilt in the presence of isoproterenol (2 µg/min). During the control tilt, the RR-interval shortening was not associated with significant changes in systolic pressure. The slight increase in diastolic pressure is considered a normal response. During combined head-up tilt and isoproterenol infusion, measurable RR-interval prolongation and blood pressure decline started at 70 and 60 seconds after tilt, respectively. Syncope occurred in close temporal proximity to the nadir of the blood pressure response and approximately 70 seconds before maximal RR-interval prolongation occurred. The patient was returned to the supine position immediately upon development of syncope, with consequent restoration of systemic pressure. Nonetheless, RR-interval prolongation continued. (Chen MY, et al: Cardiac electrophysiologic and hemodynamic correlates of neurally mediated syncope. Am J Cardiol 1989;63:66. Reproduced with permission.)

test–negative patients exhibited RR-interval shortening, with only a minimal fall in systemic blood pressure, consistent with the upright posture. Of note, in the tilt-test–positive patients, onset of hypotension invariably preceded onset of bradycardia, and the timing of maximum systemic hypotension both closely paralleled development of syncope and preceded maximum RR-interval prolongation. In essence, the observed temporal sequence of events correlates well with the findings of Epstein and associates in patients with vasovagal episodes induced by upright tilt alone and those of Wallin and Sundlof and Goldstein and colleagues in pure spontaneous vasovagal episodes.[18, 19, 166]

3. Plasma catecholamines measured before and during spontaneous and tilt-induced syncope exhibit important similarities. First, as noted earlier, premonitory increases in circulating catecholamines appear to characterize the spontaneous vasovagal faint.[19, 138, 139] Chosy and Graham observed about 30% greater urinary epinephrine and norepinephrine concentrations in fainters before spontaneous vasovagal syncopal episodes when compared with control subjects.[137] Furthermore, Vingerhoets reported an increase of 60% or more in plasma epinephrine and norepinephrine concentrations in two patients just before a vasovagal faint, compared with control (sitting) values.[138] Similar findings are reported in tilt-induced syncope, with the increased catecholamine being primarily epinephrine. For instance, during 60° head-up tilt-table testing, Fitzpatrick and coworkers observed both a more abrupt increase and higher overall levels of circulating epinephrine in 14 patients in whom syncope occurred when compared with control subjects (see Fig. 28-8).[121] Sander-Jensen and associates similarly observed a doubling of epinephrine levels in fainters when the episode was induced during 60° head-up tilt yet reported no substantial change in norepinephrine levels.[120] The latter is also consistent with findings reported by Abi-Samra and colleagues.[158] In our laboratory, circulating epinephrine and norepinephrine concentrations have also been studied during head-up tilt procedures. Generally, the most evident change is a marked increase in circulating epinephrine concentration. Furthermore, this increase antedates evident changes of heart rate or blood pressure, suggesting that it is *not* simply reactive but may be part of the trigger mechanism.[167]

4. Pancreatic polypeptide and vasopressin are both noted to increase in association with spontaneous and tilt-induced syncope.[120, 121, 168] Pancreatic polypeptide is closely associated with and often considered a marker of parasympathetic efferent neural activity.[168] In contrast, vasopressin release (Fig. 28-10) is attributable to neural connections from the NTS, which are

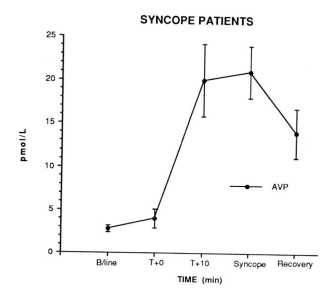

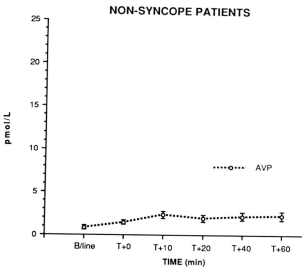

Figure 28-10. Changes in arginine vasopressin (AVP) plasma concentrations during head-up tilt testing in patients developing syncope and in nonsyncope control patients. In each panel, the AVP concentration is indicated on the ordinate in pmol/L. Time is indicated on the abscissa. In syncope patients, a marked increase of AVP concentrations was observed before development of syncope. Nonsyncope control patients did not exhibit significant changes of AVP concentrations despite tilt-table testing of up to 60 minutes duration. (Data for graphical presentation provided through the courtesy of Drs. A. Fitzpatrick and R. Sutton, London, England.)

presumably triggered by the afferent neural impulses from peripheral receptors.

Protocols for Head-Up Tilt-Table Testing

Based on the apparent similarities between their clinical and neuroendocrine features, it seems reasonable to conclude that the combined hypotension and bradycardia that is induced by head-up tilt provides a model of spontaneous neurally mediated vasovagal syndromes. The neural reflexes believed responsible for these syndromes are probably universally present in humans. Consequently, the manner in which tilt-table testing is conducted determines the sensitivity and specificity of head-up tilt-table testing as a diagnostic tool in patients undergoing evaluation for syncope.[169,170] Several factors must be considered: (1) design of the tilt table, (2) tilt angle, (3) duration of exposure to upright posture, (4) associated procedures and instrumentation, and (5) concomitant administration of pharmacologic agents.

TILT TABLE DESIGN. Both saddle-support and foot-board support techniques are feasible. The former, however (probably because of excessive compression of leg and pelvic veins), is associated with a high incidence of positive tests in control subjects (8 of 12, 67%[161,171]). Conversely, the foot-board support technique is reported to result in only a 2% to 11% false-positive rate (i.e., a positive test in an asymptomatic control subject) and at the same time provides a reasonable level of sensitivity (Table 28-2).[24,161,171] Therefore, although the foot-board support may be susceptible to the confounding effect of greater leg muscle–pump activity during upright tilt, it appears to be the preferable method for diagnostic testing.

TILT ANGLE. The physiologic effects of upright posture appear to be comparable for tilt angles of 60° or greater. As a result, from the perspective of orthostatic stress, tilt-table testing protocols employing angles of 60° or more are

probably similar. Lesser angles—specifically, those in the range of 30° to 45°—do not seem to exert sufficient gravitational stress and provide a lower yield of positive tests in syncope patients than do steeper tilt angles (3 of 10 [30%] versus 53 of 71 [75%]).[161,171] Consequently, the 60° to 80° tilt angle has become the most widely used. Lower angles are used in some laboratories as an intermediate step in the test protocol before proceeding to steeper values.[158,172,173] The added benefit of intermediate steps is uncertain, however, and consequently, a one-step procedure employing angles in the range of 60° to 80° provides a clinically practicable approach.

DURATION OF HEAD-UP TILT. The duration of exposure to 60° or greater upright posture is probably crucial in determining the sensitivity and specificity of the test, and the optimal value of test duration has yet to be agreed on.[11,169,170,174] Test durations of 10 to 60 minutes have been advocated by various laboratories.[24,156,158,175,176] There is a trend, however, for proponents of the shorter procedures to lengthen the protocol to 45 minutes, whereas those who initially favored 60-minute tilts have gravitated toward 45 minutes also.[11] The 45-minute test is largely based on a determination of the mean time to syncope plus two standard deviations of the mean in 53 patients.[161] We use a 45-minute 80° upright tilt in the absence of pharmacologic intervention, followed if necessary (i.e., nondiagnostic baseline tilt) by 10-minute 80° upright tilts in conjunction with isoproterenol infusion.[11,20,24,177] If pharmacologic provocation is not planned, the 60-minute tilt duration is probably essential.

TABLE 28-2. Frequency of Induced Symptomatic Hypotension/Bradycardia With Head-Up Tilt-Table Testing

Study	Controls	Suspected NMS	Time to Syncope (min)
1) Westminister Hosp London, England[161]	2/27 (7%)	53/71 (75%)	24.5 + 10
2) Cleveland, Clinic Cleveland, Ohio[158]	0/15 (0)	62/151 (42%)	11.7 + 6.1 (total time, about 14 min)*
3) Ospedale Umberto I Mestra-Venezia, Italy[159,160]	0/11 (0%)	15/30 (50%)	24.9 + 17.3
4) Children's Memorial Hospital Chicago, Illinois[178]	Not reported	4/20 (20%)	Not reported
5) University of Minnesota	0/18 (0%) 2/18 (11%)	4/15 (27%) 13/15 (87%)†	Not reported

*The graded tilt protocol used by Abi-Samra and coworkers[158] included a 2-minute interval at 30° before proceeding to 60. This 2-minute period was not included in the mean time to syncope reported by the authors.
†The lower yield with tilt alone (*top line*) may have been due to the relatively short tilt duration (10–15 min). The daggered (†) values refer to findings with combined tilt plus isoproternol infusion.
NMS, neurally mediated syncope.

ASSOCIATED PROCEDURES. The diagnostic use of tilt-table testing may be influenced by anxiety, pain, time of day, or volume loss associated with the conduct of concomitant procedures. Thus, results of testing may be biased by (1) apprehension reasonably associated with first exposure to a cardiac catheterization laboratory, (2) the patient having been instrumented (intravenous or arterial lines) in close temporal proximity to the tilt test, or (3) the patient having undergone a prolonged electrophysiologic procedure on the same day and thereby being perhaps both fatigued and relatively volume depleted. Chronobiologic factors may also play an important role, especially if reproducibility is crucial to assess therapeutic interventions. Consideration should be accorded each of these factors when establishing a laboratory protocol.

PHARMACOLOGIC INTERVENTIONS. Certain laboratories, including our own, have found the administration of isoproterenol to be useful in facilitating recognition of patients with susceptibility to neurally mediated syncope.[24,87,164,178] Our preference has been to administer the drug in graded infusions during sequential 10-minute tilt-table test procedures, although bolus administration is also effective.[87]

The use of isoproterenol as an adjunct to head-up tilt testing is controversial.[163,176] Nonetheless, this provocative measure is based on the well-documented increase in circulating epinephrine associated with spontaneous symptomatic episodes. Conceivably, variability in the magnitude of the increase of circulating epinephrine (in addition to other hemodynamic and neurohumoral factors) may contribute to the unpredictable nature of neurally mediated syncopal events. Thus, administration of exogenous catecholamine may facilitate recognition of susceptible patients in cases where tilt-table testing alone fails to elicit a syncopal event. Additionally, in our experience, use of isoproterenol infusion technique shortens overall study duration, without apparent adverse effect on test specificity.[11]

Several other provocative agents have been evaluated for use during tilt-table testing. Edrophonium is the most thoroughly studied of these, although adenosine triphosphate (ATP) is favored by some European investigators.[11,165]

Findings During Head-Up Tilt-Table Testing in Control Subjects and Patients With Unexplained Syncope

Control Subjects

Because the reflexes thought to be responsible for neurally mediated syncopal syndromes are probably universally present in humans, it is reasonable to assume that upright tilt-table testing induces syncopal symptoms among some asymptomatic individuals subjected to the procedure. Such false-positive test results occur only infrequently (see Table 28-2). For example, Shvartz reported only one syncopal episode and one episode of dizziness among 18 apparently healthy males, whereas Shvartz and Meyerstein noted only two syncopal episodes (at 10 and 12 minutes tilt duration) among 36 other young men and women undergoing 70° upright tilt for 20 minutes duration.[140,151] Similarly, Vogt observed only two syncopal events during 64 trials of 70° upright tilt in nine subjects, whereas in our own laboratory, 80° upright tilt for 10 to 15 minutes duration was unassociated with syncope among 18 control subjects.[20,150] Finally, Fitzpatrick and Sutton indicate that prolonged (45 minutes) 60° upright tilt-table testing was accompanied by development of syncope in only 7% of 27 control subjects (mean time to syncope, 35 ± 5 minutes).[161,175,176] Consequently, the commonly used head-up tilt-table test protocols appear to exhibit a predictable and relatively low (but not zero) false-positive rate among asymptomatic control subjects.

Vardas and coworkers extended the tilt table experience in asymptomatic individuals by examining responses to 60° upright tilt (45 minutes duration) in patients with marked sinus bradycardia but without a history of syncope.[179] Among the 28 patients evaluated (19 males, nine females; age range, 38 to 72 years), only two (7%) developed syncopal symptoms (time to syncope, 15 and 20 minutes, respectively). Thus, even in patients with asymptomatic sinus bradycardia, head-up tilt-table testing appears to be relatively free of an excessive number of false-positive outcomes.

Patients With Syncope of Unknown Origin

Syncope has many potential causes, of which cardiac rhythm disturbances and neurally mediated vasovagal syndromes probably comprise most.[4,5,7,11,12,180] Unfortunately, the transient and unpredictable nature of syncopal symptoms usually preclude substantiation of symptom-related cardiac arrhythmias by conventional ambulatory electrocardiographic monitoring technique. Furthermore, in the case of neurally mediated syncopal syndromes, the vasodepressor component may overshadow the bradyarrhythmia, thereby further diminishing the value of electrocardiographic monitoring alone.

Conventional programmed electrical stimulation (PES) of the heart during cardiac electrophysiologic testing has proved useful for defining probable arrhythmic causes of syncope in many patients. Programmed electric stimulation is generally most helpful in individuals with underlying structural heart disease (including congenital anomalies such as accessory connections). In contrast, it has been far less successful among patients without evident structural substrate for arrhythmia.[181–185] In particular, conventional PES techniques do not address the pathophysiology of the hypotension and bradycardia associated with the neurally mediated syncopal syndromes, which are often the cause of syncope in patients without evident structural cardiac disease.

In most published studies examining the effectiveness of head-up tilt-table testing for assessment of unexplained syncope, the preceding diagnostic evaluation in each patient included a detailed medical history and physical examination, hematologic and biochemical assessment, 12-lead electrocardiogram, ambulatory electrocardiographic recordings, and conventional PES studies. In addition, in earlier studies, neurologic consultation was usually obtained and an electroencephalogram or computed axial tomography obtained if the neurology consultant thought it appropriate. Patients in whom these studies are nondiagnostic may be termed "PES-negative." Many of these patients are suspected of experiencing symptoms due to neurally mediated syncope. Patients in whom the conventional diagnostic tests provided a presumed cause of syncope may be termed "PES-positive." These latter patients probably do not experience symptoms due to neurally mediated syncope but nonetheless, the response to tilt-table testing must be examined in these cases to assess the overall clinical use of the technique.

The response to upright tilt-table testing in patients with suspected neurally mediated syncope is different than that observed in asymptomatic control subjects or in PES-positive patients (see Table 28-2; Fig. 28-11). The following published examples illustrate this point. Among 104 patients subjected to 60° upright tilt-table testing by Hammill and associates, only the six patients with histories most compatible with vasovagal syncope developed hypotension- and bradycardia-related syncopal symptoms.[153] Similarly, among 28 young patients with recurrent syncope reported by Ross, symptoms resulting from induced hypotension and bradycardia were reproduced in 14 (50%) within 5 minutes of tilt onset.[186] Abi-Samra and coworkers, using the graded uptight tilt-table protocol above, found tilt-table testing effective for reproducing symptoms in 27 of 34 (79%) patients with previously unexplained symptoms.[158] Furthermore, among 71 patients with recurrent unexplained syncope, Fitzpatrick and Sutton found that 60° upright tilt-table testing reproduced symptoms in 53 (75%), of whom 40 exhibited both hypotension and bradycardia, whereas in 13, the symptoms were primarily due to vasodepression.[31] In an update from this same group, a total of 53 positive tilt-table tests (75%) have been observed among 71 patients with unexplained syncope.[161] Finally, our own laboratory reported that short duration (10 minutes) 80° upright tilt (using isoproterenol infusion as an adjunctive provocative measure when necessary [Fig. 28-12]) reproduced symptoms

in 9 of 11 patients with suspected neurally mediated syncope (sensitivity, about 82%).[24] Conversely, among nine PES-positive syncope patients, only two (22%) developed symptoms during tilt-table testing (Fig. 28-13). Pongiglione and associates confirmed the use of adding isoproterenol to the tilt-test protocol (see Table 28-2).[178]

In addition to its diagnostic use, preliminary reports suggest that the intrapatient reproducibility of tilt-table testing is excellent.[161, 162, 164, 177] In this regard, it should be noted that the response of cardiopulmonary mechanoreceptors does fatigue. Consequently, although Chen and colleagues from our laboratory reported high reproducibility levels for tests repeated within 30 minutes on the same day, multiple repetitions might not be expected to yield the same outcome.[177] Testing at the same time on subsequent days might prove more useful in the future to assess treatment efficacy.[27, 187, 188]

Carotid Sinus Stimulation and Valsalva's Maneuver

Carotid sinus stimulation provides a means of directly initiating afferent neural activity from at least one set of mechanoreceptors known to be capable of inducing neurally mediated hypotension and bradycardia.[33, 42, 45, 46, 66] The potential role that paroxysmal bradyarrhythmias of carotid sinus origin may play in the initiation of syncopal syndromes has been discussed. It should be stressed, however, that stimulation of one or other carotid sinus may induce marked bradycardia or hypotension in many asymptomatic individuals, especially among older men and individuals with coronary artery disease; this finding is more appropriately termed carotid sinus hypersensitivity.[52, 189] In contrast, carotid sinus syncope is a less frequent phenomenon, and its diagnosis depends on both the presence of a hypersensitive carotid sinus and a medical history compatible with spontaneous carotid baroreceptor stimulation (e.g., stiff collar, previous neck surgery or irradiation).

The diagnostic value of carotid sinus stimulation as a means of assessing susceptibility to the broad range of neurally mediated syncopal syndromes is uncertain. In our experience, only infrequently have patients with positive tilt-table responses also exhibited carotid sinus hypersensitivity. Conversely, Fitzpatrick and Sutton observed the development of syncope during upright tilt in 6 of 12 (50%) patients with demonstrable carotid sinus hypersensitivity.[161] Conceivably, the latter patients may have been older than our patients, thereby explaining the discrepancy. It is more intriguing, however, to postulate that tilt-table testing may elicit a particular susceptibility in the CNS or efferent neural reflex arc in a segment of the population of individuals manifesting carotid sinus hyper-

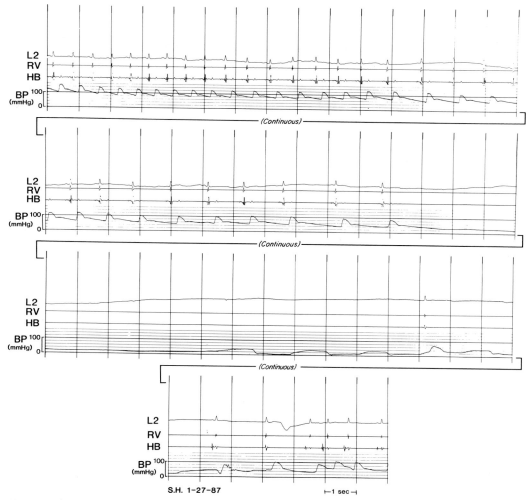

Figure 28-11. Continuous electrocardiographic and intraarterial blood pressure recording during an induced asystolic event in a young male with a history of recurrent syncope. At 2 minutes of 80° head-up tilt testing, the arterial blood pressure was 140/100 mmHg and the heart rate was 94 beats/min. Subsequently, there was a progressive decrease in arterial blood pressure to 120/80 mmHg, with the heart rate at approximately 83 beats/min (*top panel*). Thereafter (*second panel*), a steady decrease in arterial pressure was observed. The heart rate slowed markedly at a time when the arterial pressure had already fallen to 80/40 mmHg and the patient became asystolic. Asystole lasted for 16 seconds, during which the patient was returned to the supine position. After a few seconds in the supine position, there was a junction escape beat and subsequently, a further pause of 4 seconds before sinus rhythm resumed. HB, His-bundle electrogram; L_2, lead II of the electrocardiogram; RV, right ventricular electrogram. (Milstein, et al: Cardiac asystole: manifestation of neurally mediated hypotension-bradycardia. J Am Coll Cardiol 1989;14:1626. Reproduced with permission.)

sensitivity. In contrast, because carotid sinus stimulation does not appear to elicit a comparable finding in tilt-positive patients, one may infer that their susceptibility resides in the afferent aspects of the reflex arc. Clearly, such inferences are premature but potentially open avenues for future research.

As discussed earlier, Valsalva's maneuver contributes directly to rare forms of neurally mediated syncope such as the mess trick.[37] The predictive value of this maneuver for detecting susceptibility to neurally mediated syncopal syndromes has not yet been the subject of sufficient study. Lagi and coworkers report results of Valsalva's maneuver—testing in 24 young patients (age, 17 to 40 years) with suspected vasodepressor syncope and seven apparently healthy control subjects.[190] Baseline variables appeared to be similar in the two groups. During the maneuver, how-

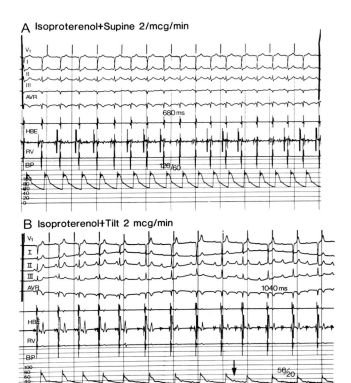

Figure 28-12. Electrocardiographic, intracardiac, and blood pressure recordings during 80° head-up tilt testing in a patient with recurrent syncope and nondiagnostic neurologic and conventional electrophysiologic testing. (**A**) Recordings were obtained with the patient in the supine posture during isoproterenol infusion at 2 μg/min. The cardiac cycle length was 680 milliseconds and the blood pressure was 128/60 mmHg. (**B**) Recordings obtained during 80° head-up tilt testing revealed onset of a relative sinus bradycardia (cycle length, 1040 milliseconds) and marked hypotension (blood pressure, 56/20 mmHg) associated with syncope. The patient was returned to the supine position (*arrow*) and recovered promptly.

ever, the syncope patients manifested both lower systolic and diastolic blood pressure nadirs and a substantially longer time to blood pressure recovery (mean values: patients, 2720 milliseconds; controls, 1560 milliseconds). Perhaps if further experience with Valsalva's maneuver in this clinical setting confirms these findings, it may yet prove helpful in identifying individuals in whom neurally mediated reflex responses are responsible for spontaneous symptoms.

CONCLUSION

The Framingham study, based on a survey of more than 5200 subjects, suggested that during a 26-year follow-up, at least one syncopal episode may be anticipated in 3% of

men and 3.5% of women.[6] Earlier estimates indicated that about 20% of adults experience a syncopal episode by age 75 years, whereas others reported that up to 50% of young adults have experienced a syncopal spell.[3,7,180] In numeric terms, these estimates imply a substantial patient population, although in most cases a single symptomatic episode only rarely occasions referral for evaluation. Conversely, recurrent events may be expected in about a third of such patients and certainly warrant thorough assessment.

Despite availability of a broad range of diagnostic techniques, the assessment of patients with recurrent syncopal spells remains suboptimal.[185,191,192] Indeed, substantiating a basis for syncopal symptoms with sufficient certainty to permit an assessment of prognosis and direct therapy was previously achieved in only 30% to 60% of cases. Moreover, establishing a diagnosis of neurally mediated vasovagal syncope with a reasonable level of certainty was rarely possible. At best, until the advent of tilt-table testing, this latter diagnosis relied solely on clinical suspicion based on a thorough medical history.

The neurally mediated syncopal syndromes comprise a broad range of clinical conditions, of which the common or vasovagal faint is by far the most common. Furthermore, these syndromes are almost certainly the most frequent causes of syncope or dizziness, especially among individuals without evidence of structural heart disease. At this time, we have only an imperfect understanding of the contributing neural reflex arcs, the elements that modulate individual susceptibility to neurally mediated hypotension and bradycardia episodes, and the factors that permit symptoms to become manifest periodically. Newer concepts suggest that the CNS connections and the efferent neural limb of the circuit may be a common thread. In contrast, the afferent limb seems variable and in clinical terms denotes the particular syndrome (e.g., carotid sinus syndrome, micturition syncope, cough syncope).

Attempting to substantiate a diagnosis of suspected neurally mediated syncope previously has been time-consuming, expensive, and often unrewarding. Availability of head-up tilt-table testing has markedly altered this picture. Although its role in the assessment of susceptibility to some of the less common forms of neurally mediated syncope (e.g., postmicturition syncope, cough syncope) remains to be clarified, head-up tilt-table testing provides a readily available technique for inducing certain of the physiologic stresses typically associated with the most common forms of spontaneous neurally mediated syncope (e.g., upright posture, sympathetic-adrenal activation). Additionally, head-up tilt-table testing has already opened the door to innovative approaches to the treatment of severely symptomatic patients, including the use of β-adrenergic blockade, disopyramide, belladonna alkaloids, and serotonin re-uptake inhibitors.[123,128,158,187,188]

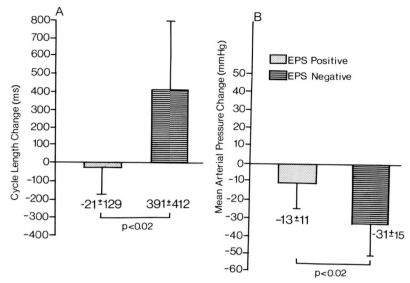

Figure 28-13. The response to 80° head-up tilt testing in two groups of patients with recurrent syncope. Patients with syncope in whom conventional electrophysiologic testing appeared to provide a basis for symptoms were categorized as PES-positive (*stippled bars*). Patients in whom conventional electrophysiologic testing failed to provide a reasonable basis for recurrent syncope are indicated as PES-negative (*hatched bars*). (**A**) Maximum changes in cardiac cycle length (RR interval) during head-up tilt testing are indicated. In PES-positive patients, there was a small decrease in cardiac cycle length (i.e., increased heart rate), resulting from a physiologic response to upright posture. Conversely, as a group, PES-negative patients exhibited marked cycle length prolongation (heart rate slowing) during the head-up tilt testing procedure. (**B**) Maximum changes of mean arterial blood pressure during head-up tilt testing are indicated for the two patients groups. PES-positive patients exhibited a small decrease in mean arterial blood pressure consistent with a physiologic response to head-up tilt testing. In contract, PES-negative patients tended to exhibit a much more marked fall of mean arterial blood pressure, compatible with neurally-mediated hypotension-bradycardia syndrome. (Findings adapted from Almquist A, et al: Provocation of bradycardia and hypotension by isoproterenol and upright posture in patients with unexplained syncope. N Engl J Med 1989;320:346.)

Furthermore, although their predictive value requires more study, provocative upright tilt-testing appears to permit direct assessment of treatment efficacy within patients and provide an opportunity to undertake double-blind controlled testing of therapeutic alternatives.[188] Consequently, based on a rapidly expanding body of published evidence, it seems evident that head-up tilt-table testing offers the most effective available means for identifying susceptibility to vasovagal episodes, studying the mechanisms of the phenomena, and defining appropriate treatments.

Acknowledgment

The authors would like to thank Charles C. Gornick, MD, for providing Figure 28-4, Barry L.S. Detloff for valuable technical assistance, and Wendy Braatz for preparing the manuscript.

References

1. Rowell LB: Human Circulation. Regulation during physical stress. New York: Oxford University Press, 1986.
2. Wood E: Hydrostatic homeostatic effects during changing force environments. Aviat Space Environ Med 1990;61:366.
3. Stults BM, Gandolfi RJ: Diagnostic evaluation of syncope. Western Med J 1936;144:234.
4. Wayne HH: Syncope: physiological considerations and an analysis of the clinical characteristics in 510 patients. Am J Med 1961;30:418.
5. Ruetz PP, Johnson SA, Callahan R, Meade RC, Smith JJ: Fainting: a review of its mechanisms and a study in blood donors. Medicine (Baltimore) 1967;46:363.
6. Savage DD, Corwin L, McGee DL, Kannell WB, Wolf PA: Epidemiologic features of isolated syncope: The Framingham study. Stroke 1985;16:626.
7. Kudenchuk PJ, McAnulty JH: Syncope: evaluation and treatment. Mod Conc Cardiovasc Dis 1985;54:25.

8. Atwood JE, Kawanishi S, Meyers J, Froelicher VF: Exercise testing in patients with aortic stenosis. Chest 1988;93:1083.

9. Johnson AM: Aortic stenosis, sudden death; and the left ventricular baroreceptors. Br Heart J 1971;33:1.

10. Leitch JW, Klein GJ, Yee R, Leather RA, Kim YH: Syncope associated with supraventricular tachycardia: an expression of tachycardia or vasomotor response. Circulation 1992; 85:1064.

11. Benditt DG, Sakaguchi S, Schultz JJ, Remole S, Adler S, Lurie KG: Syncope. Diagnostic considerations and the role of tilt table testing. Cardiol Rev 1993;1:146.

12. Kapoor WN, Karpf M, Wieand S, Peterson JR, Levey GS: A prospective evaluation and follow-up of patients with syncope. N Engl J Med 1983;309:197.

13. Kapoor WN, Peterson J, Wieand HS, Karpf M: Diagnostic and prognostic implications of recurrences in patients with syncope. Am J Med 1987;83:700.

14. Bass EB, Elson JJ, Fogoros RN, Peterson J, Arena VC, Kapoor WN: Long-term prognosis of patients undergoing electrophysiologic studies for syncope of unknown origin. Am J Cardiol 1988;62:1186.

15. Gowers WR: A lecture on vagal and vaso-vagal attacks. Lancet 1907;173:1551.

16. Lewis T: Vasovagal syncope and the carotid sinus mechanism. With comments on Gower's and Nothnagel's syndrome. Br Med J 1932;1:873.

17. Lewis T: Diseases of the heart. Described for practitioners and students. New York: McMillan, 1933:96.

18. Wallin BG, Sundlof G: Sympathetic outflow in muscles during vasovagal syncope, J Auton Nerv Syst 1982;6:287.

19. Goldstein DS, Spanarkel M, Pitterman A, et al: Circulatory control mechanisms in vasodepressor syncope. Am Heart J 1982;104:1071.

20. Chen M-Y, Goldenberg IF, Milstein S, et al: Cardiac electrophysiologic and hemodynamic correlates of neurally-mediated syncope. Am J Cardiol 1989;63:66.

21. Glick G, Yu PN: Hemodynamic changes during spontaneous vasovagal reactions. Am J Med 1963;34:42.

22. Sharpey-Schafer EP: The mechanism of syncope after coughing. Br Med J 1953;2:860.

23. Sharpey-Schafer EP, Hayter CJ, Barlow ED: Mechanism of acute hypotension from fear and nausea. Br Med J 1958; 2:878.

24. Almquist A, Goldenberg IF, Milstein S, et al: Provocation of bradycardia and hypotension by isoproterenol and upright posture in patients with unexplained syncope. N Engl J Med 1989;320:346.

25. Abboud FM: Ventricular syncope. Is the heart a sensory organ? Editorial. N Engl J Med 1989;320:390.

26. Milstein S, Buetikofer J, Lesser J, et al: Cardiac asystole: a manifestation of neurally mediated hypotension-bradycardia. J Am Coll Cardiol 1989;14:1626.

27. Milstein S, Buetikofer J, Lesser J, et al: Usefulness of disopyramide for prevention of upright tilt induced hypotension bradycardia. Am J Card 1990;65:1339.

28. Roddie IC, Shepherd JT: Nervous control of the circulation in skeletal muscle. Br Med Bull 1963;19:115.

29. Shepherd JT: Physiology of the circulation in human limbs in health and disease. Philadelphia: WB Saunders, 1963.

30. Greenfield ADM: An emotional faint. Lancet 1951;1:1302.

31. Fitzpatrick A, Sutton R: Tilting towards a diagnosis in unexplained syncope. Lancet 1989;1:658.

32. Yerg JE, Seals DR, Hagberg JM, Ehsani AA: Syncope secondary to ventricular asystole in an endurance athlete. Clin Cardiol 1986;9:220.

33. Weiss S, Baker JP: The carotid sinus reflex in health and disease. Its role in the causation of fainting and convulsions. Medicine 1933;12:297.

34. Rosoff MH, Cohen MV: Profound bradycardia after amyl nitrite in patients with a tendency to vasovagal episodes. Br Heart J 1986;55:97.

35. Maloney JD, Jaeger FJ, Fouad-Tarazi F, Morris HH: Malignant vasovagal syncope: prolonged asystole provoked by head-up tilt. Cleve Clin J Med 1988;55:543.

36. Strasberg B, Lam W, Swiryn S, et al: Symptomatic spontaneous paroxysmal AV nodal block due to localized hyperresponsiveness of the AV node to vagatonic reflexes. Am Heart J 1982;103:795.

37. Ross RT: Syncope. London: WB Saunders, 1988.

38. Parry CH: An inquiry into the symptoms and causes of the syncope anginosa. Bath: R Cuttwell, 1799:102.

39. Hering HE: Die Karotidssinusreflexe auf Herz und Gefasse, Dresden und Liepzig: Th Steinkopff, 1927.

40. Burchell HB: A. V. Waller (1816–1870) and "Vagus" pressure. Pacing Clin Electrophysiol 1988;11:1499.

41. Waller AV: On the effects of compression of the vagus nerve in the cure and relief of various nervous affections. Practitioner 1870;4:193.

42. Almquist A, Gornick CC, Benson DW Jr, Dunnigan A, Benditt DG: Carotid sinus hypersensitivity: evaluation of the vasodepressor component. Circulation 1985;67:927.

43. Heidorn GH, McNamara AP: Effect of carotid sinus stimulation on the electrocardiograms of clinically normal individuals. Circulation 1956;14:1104.

44. Nathanson MH: Hyperactive cardioinhibitory carotid sinus reflex. Arch Intern Med 1946;77:491.

45. Lown B, Levine JA: The carotid sinus. Clinical value of its stimulation. Circulation 1961;23:766.

46. Thomas JE: Hyperactive carotid sinus reflex and carotid sinus syncope. Mayo Clin Proc 1969;44:127.

47. Davies AB, Stephens MR, Davies AG: Carotid sinus hypersensitivity in patients presenting with syncope. Br Heart J 1979; 42:583.

48. Leatham A: Carotid sinus syncope. Br Heart J 1982;47: 409.

49. Sugrue DD, Wood DL, McGoon MD: Carotid sinus hypersensitivity and syncope. Mayo Clin Proc 1984;59:637.

50. Strasberg B, Pinchas A, Lewin RF, Sclarovsky S, Arditti A, Agmon J: Carotid sinus syndrome: an overlooked cause of syncope. Isr J Med Sci 1985;21:430.

51. Strasberg B, Sagie A, Erdman S, Kusniec J, Sclarovsky S, Agmon J: Carotid sinus hypersensitivity and the carotid sinus syndrome. Prog Cardiovasc Dis 1989;31:379.

52. Brown KA, Maloney JD, Smith HC, Hartzler GO, Ilstrup DM: Carotid sinus reflex in patients undergoing coronary angiography: relationship of degree and location of coronary artery disease to response to carotid sinus massage. Circulation 1980;62:697.

53. Charcot JM: Discussion on a paper by M. Levan. Gaz Med Paris 1876;5:588.

54. Faulkner M, Sharpey-Schafer EP: Circulatory effects of trumpet playing. Br Med J 1959;1:685.

55. Klein LJ, Saltzman AJ, Heyman A, Sieker HO: Syncope induced by the valsalva maneuver. Am J Med 1964;37:263.

56. Skolnick JL, Dines DE: Tussive syncope. Minn Med 1969;52:1609.

57. Williams B: Cerebrospinal fluid pressure changes in response to coughing. Brain 1976;99:331.

58. Kapoor WN, Peterson JR, Karpf M: Micturition syncope: a reappraisal. JAMA 1985;253:796.

59. Guttman L, Whitteridge D: Effects of bladder distention on autonomic mechanisms after spinal cord injuries. Brain 1947;70:361.

60. Mathias CJ, Christensen NJ, Corbett JL, Frankel HL, Spalding JMK: Plasma catecholamines during paroxysmal neurogenic hypertension in quadriplegic man. Circ Res 1976;39:204.

61. Johnson RH, Lambie DG, Spalding JMK: Neurocardiology. The interrelationships between dysfunction in the nervous and cardiovascular systems. London: WB Saunders, 1984.

62. Lukash WM, Sawyer GT, Davies JE: Micturition syncope produced by orthostasis and bladder distention. N Engl J Med 1964;270:341.

63. Lyle CB, Monroe JT, Flinn DE, Lamb LE: Micturition syncope. Report of 24 cases. N Engl J Med 1961;265:982.

64. Iggo A: Gastrointestinal tension receptors with unmyelinated afferent fibres in the vagus of the cat. Q J Exp Physiol 1957;42:130.

65. Pathy MS: Defecation syncope. Age Ageing 1978;7:233.

66. Bilbro RH: Syncope after prostatic massage. N Engl J Med 1970;282:167. Letter.

67. Menzies DN: Syncope on pelvic examination. Br Med J 1970;716:221. Letter.

68. Levin B, Posner JB: Swallow syncope-report of a case and review of the literature. Neurology (Minneapolis) 1972;22:1086.

69. Palmer ED: The abnormal upper gastrointestinal vasovagal reflexes that affect the heart. Am J Gastroenterol 1976;66:513.

70. Bortolotti M, Cirignotta F, Labo G: Atrioventricular block induced by swallowing with documentation by His bundle recordings. JAMA 1982;248:2297.

71. Armstrong PW, McMillan DG, Simon JB: Swallow syncope. Can Med Assoc J 1985;132:1281.

72. Garretson HD, Elvidge AR: Glossopharyngeal neuralgia with asystole and seizures. Arch Neurol 1963;8:26.

73. Kjellin K, Muller R, Widen L: Glossopharyngeal neuralgia associated with cardiac arrest and hypersecretion from the ipsilateral parotid gland. Neurology 1959;9:527.

74. Khero BA, Mullins CB: Cardiac syncope due to glossopharyngeal neuralgia. Treatment with a transvenous pacemaker. Arch Intern Med 1971;128:806.

75. Dykman TR, Montgomery EB Jr, Gerstenberger PD, Ziegier HE, Clutter WE, Cryer PE: Glossopharyngeal neuralgia with syncope secondary to tumour. Am J Med 1981;71:165.

72. Elam MP, Laird JR, Johnson S, Stratton JR: Swallow syncope associated with complete atrioventricular block: a case report and review of the literature. Mil Med 1989;154:465.

76. Wallin BG, Westerberg C-E, Sundlof G: Syncope induced by glossopharyngeal neuralgia sympathetic outflow to muscle. Neurology 1984;34:522.

77. Jamshidi A, Masroor MA: Glossopharyngeal neuralgia with cardiac syncope. Treatment with a permanent pacemaker and carbamazepine. Arch Intern Med 1976;136:842.

78. Taylor PH, Gray K, Bicknell PG, Rees JR: Glossopharyngeal neuralgia with syncope. J Laryngol Otolaryngol 1977;91:859.

79. Frankel HL, Mathias CJ, Spalding JMK: Mechanisms of reflex cardiac arrest in tetraplegic patients. Lancet 1975;II:1183.

80. Rowell LB: Reflex control of regional circulations in humans. J Auton Nerv Syst 1984;11:101.

81. Engel GL: Psychologic stress, vasodepressor (vasovagal) syncope and sudden death. Ann Intern Med 1978;89:403.

82. Prodger SH, Ayman D: Harmful effects of nitroglycerin with special reference to coronary thrombus. Am J Med Sci 1932;184:480.

83. Come PC, Pitt B: Nitroglycerin-induced severe hypotension and bradycardia in patients with acute myocardial infarction. Circulation 1976;54:624628.

84. Scherrer U, Vissing S, Morgan BJ, Hanson P, Victor RG: Vasovagal syncope after infusion of a vasodilator in a heart-transplant recipient. N Engl J Med 1990;322:602.

85. Weiss S, Wilkins RW, Haynes FW: The nature of circulatory collapse induced by sodium nitrite. J Clin Invest 1937;16:73.

86. Weissler AM, Warren JV, Estes EH Jr, McIntosh HD, Leonard JJ: Vasodepressor syncope. Factors influencing cardiac output. Circulation 1957;15:875.

87. Waxman MB, Yao L, Cameron DA, Wald RW, Roseman J: Isoproterenol induction of vasodepressor-type reaction in vasodepressor-prone persons. Am J Cardiol 1989;63:58.

88. Katuntsev VP, Katkov VE, Baranov VM, Vil-Vilyams IF, Genin AM: Cardiorespiratory responses to lower body negative pressure and tilt tests after exposure to simulated weightlessness. Physiologist 1985;28(Suppl):40.

89. Barcroft H, Edholm OG, McMichael J, Sharpey-Shafer EP: Posthaemorrhagic fainting. Lancet 1944;I:489.

90. Barcroft H, Edholm OG: On the vasodilatation in human skeletal muscle during posthemorrhagic fainting. J Physiol (Lond) 1945:104:161.

91. Oberg B, White S: The role of vagal cardiac nerves and arterial baroreceptors in the circulatory adjustments to hemorrhage in the cat. Acta Physiol Scand 1970;80:395.

92. Oberg B, Thoren P: Increased activity in vagal cardiac afferents correlated to the appearance of reflex bradycardia during severe hemorrhage in cats. Acta Physiol Scand 1970;80:22A.

93. Oberg B, Thoren P: Increased activity in left ventricular receptors during hemorrhage or occlusion of caval veins in the cat. A possible cause of the vaso-vagal reaction. Acta Physiol Scand 1972;85:164.

94. Secher NH, Sander-Jensen K, Werner C, Warberg J, Bie P: Bradycardia, a severe but reversible hypovolemic shock in man. Circ Shock 1984;14:267.

95. Fleg JL, Asante AVK: Asystole following treadmill exercise in a man wthout organic heart disease. Arch Intern Med 1983;143:1821.

96. Hirata T, Yano K, Okui T, Mitsuoka T, Hashiba K: Aystole with

syncope following strenuous exercise in a man without organic heart disease. J Electrocardiol 1987;20:280.

97. Huycke EC, Card HG, Sobol SM, Nguyen NX, Sung RJ: Post-exertional cardiac asystole in a young man without organic heart disease. Ann Intern Med 1987;106:844.

98. Pedersen WR, Janosik DL, Goldenberg IF, Stevens LL, Redd RM: Post-exercise asystolic arrest in a young man without organic heart disease. Utility of head-up tilt testing in guiding therapy. Am Heart J 1989;118:410.

99. Kapoor WN: Syncope with abrupt termination of exercise. Am J Med 1989;87:597.

100. Tamura Y, Onodera O, Kodera K, et al: Atrial standstill after treadmill exercise test and unique response to isoproterenol infusion in recurrent postexercise syncope. Am J Cardiol 1990;65:533.

101. Brogdon E, Hellebrandt FA: Post-exercise orthostatic collapse. Am J Physiol 1940;129:P318.

102. Eichna LW, Bean WB: Orthostatic hypotension in normal young men following physical exertion, environmental thermal loads, or both. J Clin Invest 1944;23:942. Abstract.

103. Eichna LW, Horvath SM, Bean WB: Cardiac asystole in a normal young man following physical effort. Am Heart J 1947;33:354.

104. Sakaguchi S, Shultz JJ, Remole SC, Adler SW, Lurie KG, Benditt DG: Syncope accompanying vigorous exercise in young patients without overt heart disease: a manifestation of neurally-mediated syncope. Pacing Clin Electrophysiol 1993;16:893. Abstract.

105. Abboud FM, Thames MD: Interaction of cardiovascular reflexes in circulatory control. In: Shepherd JT, Abboud FM, eds. Handbook of physiology. The cardiovascular system. Peripheral circulation and organ blood flow. Bethesda, MD: American Physiological Society, 1983:675.

106. Pelletier CL, Shepherd JT: Circulatory reflexes from mechanoreceptors in the cardio-aortic area. Circ Res 1973;33:131.

107. Thoren P: Characteristics of left ventricular receptors with nonmedullated vagal afferents in cats. Circ Res 1977;40:415.

108. Donald DE, Shepherd JT: Reflexes from the heart and lungs: physiological curiosities or important regulatory mechanisms. Cardiovasc Res 1978;12:449.

109. Thoren P: Role of cardiac vagal C-fibres in cardiovascular control. Rev Physiol Biochem Pharmacol 1979;86:1.

110. Sleight P, Widdicombe JG: Action potentials in fibres from receptors in the epicardium and myocardium of the dog's ventricle. J Physiol (Lond) 1965;181:235.

111. Thames MD: Effect of d- and l-propranolol on the discharge of cardiac vagal C-fibers. Am J Physiol 1980;238:H465.

112. Mancia G, Donald DE: Demonstration that atria, ventricles, and lung each are responsible for a tonic inhibition of the vasomotor center in the dog. Circ Res 1975;36:310.

113. Share L: Role of cardiovascular receptors in the control of ADH release. Cardiology 1976;61(Suppl 1):51.

114. Jarecki M, Thoren PN, Donald DE: Release of renin by the carotid baroreflex in anesthetized dogs: role of cardiopulmonary vagal afferents and renal arterial pressure. Circ Res 1978;42:614.

115. Schrier RW, Bichet DG: Osmotic and nonosmotic control of vasopressin release and the pathogenesis of impaired water

116. excretion in adrenal, thyroid, and edematous disorders. J Lab Clin Med 1981;98:1.

116. Beiser GD, Zelis R, Epstein SE, Mason DT, Braunwald E: The role of skin and muscle resistance vessels in reflexes mediated by the baroreceptor system. J Clin Invest 1970;49:225.

117. Ziegler MG, Echon C, Wilner KD, Specho P, Lake CR, McCutchen JA: Sympathetic nervous withdrawal in the vasodepressor (vasovagal) reaction. J Auton Nerv Syst 1986;17:273.

118. Kellogg DL, Johnson JM, Kosiba WA: Baroreflex control of the cutaneous active vasodilator system in humans. Circ Res 1990;66:1420.

119. Goldstein DS, McCarty R, Polinsky RJ, Kopin IJ: Relationship between plasma norepinephrine and sympathetic neural activity. Hypertension 1983;5:552.

120. Sander-Jensen K, Secher NH, Astrup A, et al: Hypotension induced by passive head-up tilt: endocrine and circulatory mechanisms. Am J Physiol 1986;251:R742.

121. Fitzpatrick A, Williams T, Jeffrey C, Lightman S, Sutton R: Pathogenic role for arginine vasopressin (AVP) and catecholamines (EP & NEP) in vasovagal syncope. J Am Coll Cardiol 1990;15:98. Abstract.

122. Hilton SM, Spyer KM: Participation of the anterior hypothalamus in the baroreceptor reflex. J Physiol (Lond) 1971;218:271.

123. Perna GP, Ficola U, Salvatori MP, et al: Increase of plasma beta endorphins in vasodepressor syncope. Am J Cardiol 1990;65:929.

124. Faden AI, Jacobs TP, Holaday JW: Opiate antagonist improves neurologic recovery after spinal injury. Science 1981;211:493.

125. Rutter PC, Potocnik SJ, Ludbrook J: Sympathoadrenal mechanisms in cardiovascular responses to naloxone after hemorrhage. Am J Physiol 1987;252:H40.

126. Morita H, Nishida Y, Motochigawa H, Uemura H, Hosomi, H, Vatner SF: Opiate receptormediated decrease in renal nerve activity during hypotensive hemorrhage in conscious rabbits. Circ Res 1988;63:165.

127. Evans RG, Ludbrook J, Potocnik SJ: Intracisternal naloxone and cardiac nerve blockade prevent vasodilation during simulated hemorrhage in awake rabbits. J Physiol (Lond) 1989;409:1.

128. Kosinski D, Grubb BP: Role of serotonin in neurocardiogenic syncope. J Serotonin Res 1994;1:85.

129. Burnstock G: Purinergic nerves. Pharmacol Rev 1972;24:509.

130. Brody MJ: Histaminergic and cholinergic vasodilator systems. In: Vanhoutte PM, Leusen I, eds. Mechanisms of vasodilatation. Basel: Karger AG, 1978:266.

131. Bevan JA, Brayden JE: Nonadrenergic neural vasodilator mechanisms. Circ Res 1987;60:309326.

132. Warner MR, Levy MN: Inhibition of cardiac vagal effects by neurally released and exogenous neuropeptide Y. Circ Res 1989;65:1536.

133. Abraham S, Cantor EH, Spector S: Atropine lowers blood pressure in normotensive rats through blockade of alpha-adrenergic receptors. Life Sci 1981;28:315.

134. Tayo FM: Effect of atropine on the rat anococcygeus muscle. J Pharm Pharmacol 1982;34:202.

135. Sjostrand T: Circulatory control via vagal afferents VI: the

bleeding bradycardia in the rat, its elicitation and relation to the release of vasopressin. Acta Physiol Scand 1973;89:39.

136. Graham DT, Kabler JD, Lunsford L Jr: Vasovagal fainting: a diphasic response. Psychsom Med 1961;23:493.

137. Chosy JJ, Graham DT: Catecholamines in vasovagal fainting. J Psychosom Res 1965;9:189.

138. Vingerhoets AJJM: Biochemical changes in two subjects succumbing to syncope. Psychosom Med 1984;46:95.

139. Schlesinger Z: Life-threatening "vagal reaction" to physical fitness test. JAMA 1973;226:1119.

140. Benditt DG, Sakaguchi S, Goldstein MA, Lurie KG, Gornick CC, Adler SW: Sinus node dysfunction: Pathophysiology, clinical features, evaluation and treatment. In: Zipes DP, Jalife J, eds. Cardiac electrophysiology: from cell to bedside. Philadelphia: WB Saunders 1994. In Press.

141. Jaegar F, Fouad-Tarazi F, Maloney J: Vasovagal syncope: lack of relationship between baseline blood volume and presyncopal chronotropic orthostatic response. Revue Europeene de Technologie Biomedicale 1990;12:92. Abstract.

142. Lipsitz LA, Mietus J, Moody GB, Goldberger A: Spectral characteristics of heart rate variability before and during postural tilt. Relations to aging and risk of syncope. Circulation 1990;81:1803.

143. Barach JH, Marks WL: Effect of change of posture without active muscular exertion on the arterial and venous pressures. Arch Intern Med 1913;11:485.

144. Nielsen M, Herrington LP, Winslow A: The effect of posture upon peripheral circulation. Am J Physiol 1939;147:573.

145. Asmussen E, Christensen EH, Neilsen M: The regulation of circulation in different postures. Surgery 1940;8:604.

146. Stead EA, Warren JV, Merril AJ, Brannan ES: The cardiac output in male subjects as measured by the technique of right arterial catheterization. Normal values with observations on the effect of anxiety and tilting. J Clin Invest 1945;24:326.

147. Lagerlof H, Eliasch H, Werdo L, Berglund E: Orthostatic changes of the pulmonary and peripheral circulation in man. A preliminary report. Scand J Clin Lab Invest 1951;3:85.

148. Weissler AM, Warren JV: Vasodepressor syncope. Am Heart J 1959;57:786.

149. Shvartz E: Reliability of quantitatible tilt table data. Aerospace Med 1968;39:1094.

150. Vogt FB: Tilt table and plasma volume changes with short term deconditioning experiments. Aerospace Med 1967;38:564.

151. Shvartz E, Meyerstein N: Tilt tolerance of young men and women. Aerospace Med 1970;41:253.

152. Wood EH: Contributions of aeromedical research to flight and biomedical science. Cause and prevention of GLOC. Aviat Space Environ Med 1986;57:A13.

153. Hammill SC, Holmes DR, Wood DL, et al: Electrophysiologic testing in the upright position: improved evaluation of patients with rhythm disturbances using a tilt table. J Am Coll Cardiol 1984;4:65.

154. Hermiller JB, Wallcer SS, Binkley PF, et al: The electrophysiologic effects of upright posure. Am Heart J 1984;108:1250.

155. Mann DE, Sensecqua JE, Easley AR, Reiter MJ: Effects of upright posture on antegrade and retrograde atrioventricular conduction in patients with coronary artery disease, mitral prolapse, or no structural heart disease. Am J Cardiol 1987;60:625.

156. Kenny RA, Ingram A, Bayliss J, Sutton R: Head-up tilt: a useful test for investigating unexplained syncope. Lancet 1986;1:1351.

157. Kenny RA, Ingram I, Vardas P, Sutton R: Unexplained cardiac syncope: the role of the vasovagal syndrome. In: Belhassen B, Feldman S, Copperman Y, eds. Cardiac pacing and electrophysiology. Proceedings of the VIIIth World Symposium on Cardiac Pacing and Electrophysiology. Tel Aviv: R & L Creative Communications, 1987:233.

158. Abi-Samra F, Maloney JD, Fouad-Tarazi FM, Castle L: The usefulness of head-up tilt testing and hemodynamic investigations in the workup of syncope of unknown origin. Pacing Clin Electrophysiol 1988;11:1202.

159. Raviele A, Gasparini G, Di Pede F, Delise P, Bonso A, Piccolo E: Sincopi di natura indeterminata dopo studio elettrofisiologico. Utilita dell'head-up tilt test nella diagnosi di origine vaso-vagale e nella scelta della terapia. G Ital Cardiol 1990;20:185.

160. Raviele A, Gasparini G, Di Pede F, Delise P, Bonso A, Piccolo E: Usefulness of head-up tilt test in evaluating patients with syncope of unknown origin and negative electrophysiologic study. Am J Cardiol 1990;65:1322.

161. Fitzpatrick A, Theodroakis G, Vardas P, Sutton R: Methodology of head-up tilt testing in patients with unexplained syncope. J Am Coll Cardiol 1991;17:125.

162. Grubb BP, Wolf W, Temesy-Aromos P, Hahn H, Elliot L: Reproducibility of head-up tilt table test results in patients with syncope. Pacing Clin Electrophysiol 1992;15:1477.

163. Kapoor WN, Brant N: Evaluation of syncope by upright tilt testing with isoproterenol. A nonspecific test. Ann Intern Med 1992;116:358.

164. Sheldon R, Splawinski J, Killam S: Reproducibility of upright tilt-table tests in patients with syncope. Am J Cardiol 1992;69:1300.

165. Lurie KG, Dutton J, Mangat R, Newman D, Eisenberg S, Scheinman MM: Evaluation of edrophonium as a provocative agent for vasovagal syncope during head-up tilt table testing. Am J Cardiol 1993;72:1286.

166. Epstein SE, Stampfer M, Beiser GD: Role of the capacitance and resistance vessels in vasovagal syncope. Circulation 1968;37:524.

167. Remole SC, Neustel M, Bailin S, Chen M-Y, Milstein S, Benditt DG: Adrenal effluent may account for increased norepinephrine levels during tilt-induced syncope. Circulation 1991;84(Suppl II):233. Abstract.

168. Sander-Jensen K, Garne S, Schwartz TW: Pancreatic polypeptide release during emotionally induced vasovagal syncope. Lancet 1985;II:1132.

169. Benditt DG, Remole SC, Bailin S, Dunnigan, Asso A, Milstein S: Tilt table testing for evaluation of neurally-mediated (cardioneurogenic) syncope: rationale and proposed protocols. Pacing Clin Electrophysiol 1991;14:1.

170. Benditt DG, Lurie K, Adler S, Sakaguchi S: Rationale and methodology of head-up tilt table testing for evaluation of neurally-mediated (cardioneurogenic) syncope. In: Zipes

DP, Jalife J, eds. Cardiac electrophysiology. From cell to bedside. 2nd ed. Philadelphia: WB Saunders, 1994. In Press.

171. Fitzpatrick A, Theodorakis G, Ahmed R, Marriott R, Sutton R: Methodology of head-up tilt testing in the investigation of unexplained syncope (Abstract). Pacing Clin Electrophysiol 1990;13:561.

172. Fouad FM, Tarazi RC, Bravo EL: Dihydroergotamine in idiopathic orthostatic hypotension: short-term intramuscular and long-term oral therapy. Clin Pharmacol Ther 1981; 30:782.

173. Tarazi RC, Fouad FM: Circulatory dynamics in progressive autonomic failure. In: Bannister R, ed. Autonomic failure, a textbook of clinical disorders of the autonomic nervous system. Oxford: Oxford University Press, 1983:96.

174. Gasparini G, Raviele A, DePede F, Piccolo E: Terapia delle sincopi vasovagali. Qual'E l'importanza del tilting test seriati? In: Piccolo E, Raviele A, eds. Aritmie cardiache. Third International Workshop. Torino: Centro Scientifico Editore, 1993:442.

175. Fitzpatrick A, Theodorakis G, Ahmed R, Sutton R: Clinical features of patients with unexplained syncope. Revue Europeene de Technologie Biomedicale 1990;12:91. Abstract.

176. Fitzpatrick AP, Sutton R: Tilt-induced syncope. N Engl J Med 1989;321:331.

177. Chen XC, Chen M-Y, Remole S, et al: Reproducibility of head-up tilt table testing for eliciting susceptibility to neurally-mediated syncope in patients without structural heart disease. Am J Cardiol 1992;69:766.

178. Pongiglione G, Fish F, Strasburger JF, Benson DW Jr: Heart rate and blood pressure response to upright tilt in young patients with unexplained syncope. J Am Coll Cardiol 1990; 16:165.

179. Vardas P, Vemmos C, Vrouchos G, Moulopoulos S: The tilting test in asymptomatic individuals with severe and unexplained sinus bradycardia (Abstract). Revue Europeene de Technologie Biomedicale 1990;12:91. Abstract

180. Lipsitz LA, Wei JY, Rowe JW: Syncope in an elderly, institutionalized population: prevalence, incidence, and associated risk. Q J Med 1985;55:45.

181. DiMarco JP, Garan H, Harthorne NW, Ruskin JN: Intracardiac electrophysiologic techniques in recurrent syncope of unknown cause. Ann Intern Med 1981;95:542.

182. Gulamhusein S, Naccarelli GV, Ko PT, et al: Value and limitations of clinical electrophysiologic study in assessment of patients with unexplained syncope. Am J Med 1983;73:700.

183. Morady F, Shen E, Schwartz A, et al: Long-term follow-up of patients with recurrent unexplained syncope evaluated by electrophysiologic testing. J Am Coll Cardiol 1983;2:1053.

184. Akhtar M, Shenasa M, Denker S, Gilbert CJ, Rizwi N: Role of cardiac electrophysiologic studies in patients with unexplained recurrent syncope. Pacing Clin Electrophysiol 1983;6:192.

185. Kapoor WN, Hammill SC, Gersh BJ: Diagnosis and natural history of syncope and the role of invasive electrophysiologic testing. Am J Cardiol 1989;62:730.

186. Ross BA: Evaluation and treatment of syncope in children. Learning center highlights. Am Coll Cardiol 1990:7.

187. Goldenberg IF, Almquist A, Dunbar D, Milstein S, Pritzker MR, Benditt DG: Prevention of neurally-mediated syncope by selective beta-1 adrenoreceptor blockade. Circulation 1987;76(Suppl IV):133. Abstract.

188. Fitzpatrick A, Williams S, Ahmed R, Travill C, Sutton R: A randomised trial of medical therapy for vasodepressor vasovagal syncope. J Am Coll Cardiol 1990;15:97. Abstract.

189. Mankikar GD, Clark ANG: Cardiac effects of carotid sinus massage in old age. Age Ageing 1975;4:86.

190. Lagi A, Arnetoli G, Vannucchi PL, et al: The Valsalva maneuver in vasodepressor syncope. Angiology 1989;40:958.

191. Haissaguerre M, Commenyes D, Mathio JL, Lemetayer PH, Salamon R, Warin JF: Etude electrophysiologique des syncopes. Prevision du resultat. Le Presse Medicale 1989;18:212.

192. Fujimura O, Yee R, Klein GJ, Sharma AD, Boahene KA: The diagnostic sensitivity of electrophysiologic testing in patients with syncope caused by transient bradycardia. N Engl J Med 1989;321:1703.

Cardiac Arrhythmias, 3rd edition, edited by William J. Mandel.
J. B. Lippincott Company, Philadelphia © 1995.

29

Alan B. Wagshal • Shoei K. Stephen Huang

The Use of Radiofrequency Current as an Energy Source for Catheter Ablation Therapy

Successful catheter ablation depends on two distinct aspects—successful identification and mapping of the critical portion of the arrhythmia being treated, and adequate lesion formation at that site. In this chapter we will discuss radiofrequency (RF) energy as an energy source for catheter ablation, paying particular attention to the mechanism of lesion formation with RF energy, the histopathologic effects of RF ablation on normal and abnormal tissues, and the results of clinical studies. We will also compare RF energy to direct current (DC) energy, which was the first form of energy used for catheter ablation, and discuss the advantages of RF energy compared with DC energy. Finally, we will briefly review the various arrhythmias for which RF ablation has been applied, as well as the uses and limitations of RF energy for catheter ablation of these various arrhythmias. Hopefully, by the end of this chapter it will be clear why the introduction of RF energy has revolutionized the field of catheter ablation and electrophysiology as a whole.

HISTORIC ASPECTS

RF current is not new to medicine, having been used in electrosurgery for over 50 years (Table 29-1). D'Arsonval in 1891 first applied the principle of using alternating current to avoid the undesirable effect of neuromuscular stimulation during surgical procedures.[1] In 1928, W.T. Bovie, together with the famous neurosurgeon Dr. Harvey Cushing, introduced the prototype electrosurgical unit for surgical cutting and coagulation that still is referred to by his name today.[2] RF current has gained wide usage in many areas of medicine, particularly because of its ability to produce discrete lesions in the central and peripheral nervous system.[3,4] RF energy has also been used in a variety of dermatologic and other malignancies[5] and for the control of chronic pain syndromes.[6]

RF energy was first used in the experimental treatment of cardiac arrhythmias in animal models in the mid 1980s by Huang and colleagues and was shown to be able to safely produce lesions in the atrioventricular (AV) node as well as the atrial and ventricular myocardium.[7-11] The first application of radiofrequency energy for catheter ablation in humans was the creation of complete AV block.[12,13] Subsequently, the use of radiofrequency energy has spread to include selective AV node modification,[14-17] ablation of accessory atrioventricular connections,[18,19] and, more recently, ablation of ventricular tachycardia, including ventricular tachycardia related to coronary artery disease[20] as well as idiopathic left and right ventricular tachycardia.[21]

907

TABLE 29-1. History of Use of Radiofrequency (RF) Energy for Therapeutic Lesion Formation

- Beginning of twentieth century: Ham radio operators, while experimenting with radio waves, burn fingers, thereby discovering accidentally potential for radio waves to generate localized heating.
- 1920s: Dr. Harvey Cushing and his technician, W.T. Bovie, used RF currents for electrocoagulation in neural tissue.
- 1920s: Horsely and Clarke in England use DC lesions for tissue destruction, particularly in the brain.
- 1950: Drs. Aranow and Mark showed that RF energy produced much more reproducible and controllable neural lesions than DC energy.
- Late 1950s: Drs. Aranow and Cosman develop first commercially available RF lesion generators for neurosurgery at Massachusetts General Hospital.
- 1960s to the present: RF lesion generators find growing applications, including dermatology, central and peripheral nervous system.
- Mid 1980s: Dr. Huang and coworkers introduce RF energy for cardiac lesion formation for control of arrhythmias.

BIOPHYSICS OF RADIOFREQUENCY ENERGY: SIMILARITIES AND DIFFERENCES FROM DIRECT CURRENT SHOCKS

RF current is an alternating current that occupies the lowest frequencies of the electromagnetic spectrum and extends up to microwave energy, which begins at a frequency of around 10^9 Hz. Medical and other commercial uses of RF energy use primarily the frequencies between 100 kHz and 1.5 MHz (between 10^5 and 1.5×10^7 cycles per second). For comparison, regular alternating household current, which is in the lowest frequency range of RF energy, has a frequency of 60 Hz, whereas visible light has a frequency of 10^{14} to 10^{15} Hz (Fig. 29-1). It is particularly important for RF energy in medical use to avoid the lower frequencies (<10,000 Hz, including 60-Hz alternating household current), because energy at this frequency has the capability of repetitively depolarizing muscle, including cardiac tissue, thereby potentially inducing ventricular fibrillation.[22]

The radiofrequency energy used for catheter ablation is applied in such a fashion as to selectively produce tissue desiccation (Fig. 29-2). Most generators for catheter ablation deliver a continuous unmodulated sine wave current between 300,000 and 750,000 Hz at an output in the range of 40 to 60 V (Fig. 29-3). In contrast, electrosurgical units use RF energy with much higher voltages that is applied as a series of short pulses to create cutting and coagulation. To selectively achieve tissue desiccation, the RF energy source must be in direct contact with the tissue, and the energy must be delivered at a steady rate directly from the energy source into the low-resistance tissue. Because of this, tissue contact is an important variable in the successful use of RF energy for catheter ablation. This fact explains both the safety of RF energy (i.e., unlike DC shocks, because direct tissue contact is needed for energy transfer during RF ablation, there are no significant "far-field" effects on cardiac tissue away from the catheter) and some of its potential limitations. For example, because of this dependence on direct tissue contact, the size of the lesion

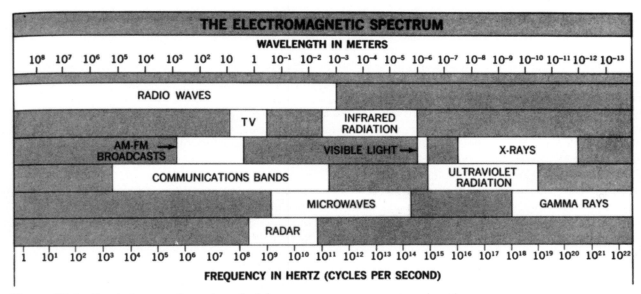

Figure 29-1. The electromagnetic spectrum. Radiofrequency energy encompasses a broad range of frequencies, between 1 and 10^{11} H. (Encyclopedia Americana, Vol 10. Danbury, CT, Grolier Publishing, 1989:157.)

DESICCATION

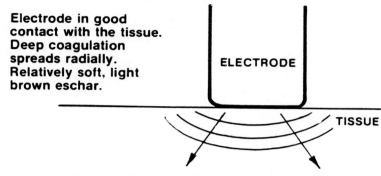

Electrode in good contact with the tissue. Deep coagulation spreads radially. Relatively soft, light brown eschar.

ELECTRODE

TISSUE

A   TYPICAL CURRENT = 0.5 AMP RMS

ELECTROSURGICAL CUTTING

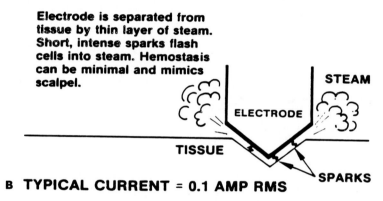

Electrode is separated from tissue by thin layer of steam. Short, intense sparks flash cells into steam. Hemostasis can be minimal and mimics scalpel.

STEAM

ELECTRODE

TISSUE

SPARKS

B TYPICAL CURRENT = 0.1 AMP RMS

FULGURATION

Electrode free from tissue. Long sparks to tissue result in superficial coagulation first, then deeper necrosis as fulguration continues. Eschar is hard and black.

ELECTRODE

SPARKS

TISSUE

Figure 29-2. (**A**) Schematic illustration of the effect of electrosurgical desiccation on tissue, as compared to electrosurgical cutting and fulguration (**B** and **C**). (Force 4 Instruction Manual, Valleylab, Inc., Boulder, Colorado.)

C   TYPICAL CURRENT = 0.1 AMP RMS

tends to be small; thus, RF energy may be inadequate where larger lesions may be needed (such as in some patients with ventricular tachycardia associated with coronary disease).

In contrast, DC energy produces its effects by very different mechanisms (Table 29-2). The delivered shock results in an initial explosion at the catheter tip accompanied by extremely high temperatures, which damages the myocardium by the passage of electrical current as well as by the release of heat and barotrauma.[23,24] The lesion size is large and inhomogeneous with irregular wide margins. Because of widespread muscular activation by the electrical current, the process is quite painful, and general anesthesia is required. The myocardial damage is

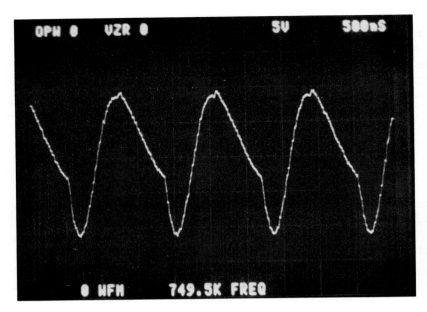

Figure 29-3. Oscilloscope recording of a typical radiofrequency waveform used for cardiac catheter ablation (750 kHz continuous unmodulated sinusoidal waveform). (Huang SKS: Use of radiofrequency energy for catheter ablation of the endomyocardium: prospective energy source. J Electrophysiol 1987; 1:78.)

felt to be the result of the direct electrical effects plus, to a lesser extent, thermal and barotrauma effects.[25] These effects do make DC energy a powerful ablation source, so that by positioning the catheter electrode directly on the endocardial surface, selective ablation of a relatively large area (1 to 3 cm³) of myocardium can be achieved, which obviates the need for pinpoint localization of the structure to be ablated, which is required in RF ablation. DC ablation is also easy to perform, using standard catheters and using the energy directly from an external defibrillator. It is the barotrauma (i.e., tissue damage from exploding vapor pockets) that can create unpredictable and potentially serious side effects; this is the major limitation to DC ablation in clinical use. Thus, such adverse effects as rupture of the coronary sinus, myocardial dysfunction, cardiac tamponade, ventricular arrhythmia, and sudden death following DC ablation have all been reported.[24-31]

Another advantage of RF compared to DC energy is that because RF energy in the frequencies used for catheter ablation does not cause cellular depolarization, it does not result in cardiac muscle contraction or nervous tissue stimulation. Therefore, its use is almost painless (even for the conscious patient) and free of the risk of ventricular fibrillation.[32] Thus, general anesthesia during energy delivery is not required.

The mechanism of heating by RF catheter ablation is

TABLE 29-2. Comparison of Direct Current (DC) Versus Radiofrequency (RF) Current for Catheter Ablation

	Direct Current	**RF Current**
Waveform	Monophasic damped sinusoid	Continuous unmodulated sinusoid
Peak voltage	2,000–4,000 V	<100 V
Barotrauma	Yes	No
Sparking	Yes	No
General anesthesia	Yes	No
Arrhythmogenicity	High	Low
Depression of left ventricular function	Yes	No
Catheter damage	Frequent	Infrequent
Energy control	Less possible	Possible
Lesion necrosis	Inhomogeneous with an irregular and wide margin	Homogeneous with a sharp and narrow margin
Lesion size	Larger	Smaller

identical to that used by a wide variety of household appliances, which all have in common the basic mechanism of passing electrical energy through an area of high resistance to generate heat, whether it be a toaster, electric heater, hair dryer, and so forth. This mechanism of heating is called resistive heating. When a current I passes through a resistor with a resistance R, the amount of electrical power converted into heat can be calculated according to the following equation:

$$P = I^2R$$

For a circuit with a given resistance, a fixed amount of resistive heating can be produced by either delivering a certain power to the element or creating a certain voltage drop across it, because the resistance is also related to the voltage V by Ohm's law:

$$V = IR$$

For a typical RF ablation with a resistance of 100 Ω and an applied voltage of 50 V, the resulting current passing through the electrode into the heart would be 50 V/100 Ω or 0.5 A, corresponding to a power (from equation 1) of $0.25 \times 100 = 25$ W; with a higher impedance of 150 Ω in order to deliver the same power of 25 W would require 60 V.

During catheter ablation, the radiofrequency energy is delivered in a unipolar fashion from the catheter tip to an indifferent skin electrode. The circuit created during radiofrequency ablation consists of the radiofrequency generator, the connecting wire to the electrode catheter that is in contact with the endocardium, the skin patch, and the wire connecting back to the RF generator. The circuit is completed by the myocardium and the tissue between the heart and the body surface, taking advantage of the fact that the body tissues are a conductive electrolytic medium (Fig. 29-4). Within this circuit, resistive heating will occur in an area with both a high current density and a high electrical resistance. In the ablation circuit outlined above, current density and electrical resistance are both highest at the interface between the electrode and the endocardium, and it is at this interface that essentially all of the RF energy–induced heating is produced.

The relatively small surface area of the ablation electrode results in a high current density at the electrode–tissue interface. The much larger area of contact between the skin and the indifferent electrode results in only minimal current density and heat production to the skin. The location of this skin patch is irrelevant, but care must be taken to apply it firmly to the skin so that the energy is spread out over the entire patch and not localized to a small area that could produce a skin burn. Compared with the electrode–tissue interface, the resist-

ance of the generator and connecting wires is usually minor. However, one must be sure that all connections are tight and that the wires are all intact and not excessively long.

A characteristic of resistive heating is that only the thin rim of tissue in immediate contact with the RF electrode is directly heated. Current density, J, falls off as the square of the distance from the current source, according to the following equation:

$$J = 1/4\pi r^2$$

where r represents the distance from the electrode tip. Because the actual tissue heating that results is proportional to the power density in the tissue, which in turn is proportional to the square of the current density (see equation 1 above), the actual tissue heating that results from a unipolar delivery of RF energy will fall off with the

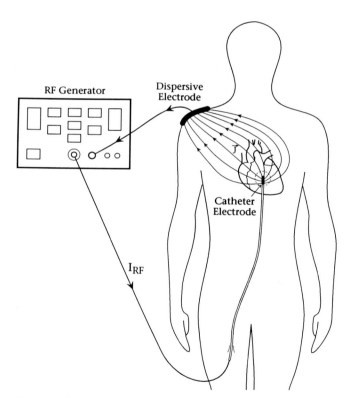

Figure 29-4. Diagram of the radiofrequency current circuit. While there is continuous current flow throughout the patient between the catheter electrode ("active" electrode) and the skin patch ("dispersive" electrode), current density and resistance are highest at the electrode tip, so essentially all of the heating is generated at the tip–tissue interface (*dotted circle*). This figure makes the important point that the patient's tissues themselves are an essential part of the radiofrequency circuit. I_{RF} radiofrequency current carried through connecting wires; J, resulting radiofrequency current density in the tissue between the active and dispersive electrodes.

fourth power of the distance from the electrode tip, according to the following equation:

$$h = R/16\pi^2 r^4$$

where h is the heat production in a unit volume of tissue of resistivity at a distance r from the electrode center.[33] As a result of this inverse r^4 factor, the area of tissue directly affected by the resistive heating is quite shallow. The heat that is generated within this small margin of tissue is then transferred by conduction and convection to deeper tissue layers through the fluid components of the cells and the extracellular fluid. This, of course, is a much slower process and must compete with the dissipation of heat through blood vessels.

These theoretic calculations have been validated by Haines and colleagues in isolated perfused heart muscle strips.[33] The fact that the effects of RF energy on cardiac tissues are often visualized within a second or so of delivery (e.g., by resulting in loss of delta waves in patients with accessory pathways) demonstrates the close proximity of the catheter to the tissue being targeted by the ablation. In a series of 195 patients undergoing ablation of accessory pathways, the mean time to initial accessory pathway block was only 2.9 ± 3.4 seconds.[34] If more time is required to produce an effect, this suggests that the target tissue is deeper or otherwise farther from the catheter tip, in which case it does not undergo direct resistive heating but instead depends on these other mechanisms of heat transfer. Because these not only are slower processes but also generate lower degrees of heating, these patients are more susceptible to recurrence of their underlying arrhythmia (see later discussion). On the other hand, when the target arrhythmia is more deep-seated, a longer duration of energy pulses may be able, at least to some extent, to overcome this handicap by allowing for greater energy to the tissue.[33,35,36] Longer pulse durations may also have some benefit in cases in which the ablation is limited by poor tissue contact. However, there is no increase in lesion size for RF applications longer than approximately 50 to 60 seconds because by that time the rate of heat loss via the bloodstream at the lesion edge is equal to the incoming conductive and convective spread of heat from the electrode catheter.[35] This discussion by no means denies the crucial role of adequate catheter–tissue contact, and the fact that RF energy is clearly more effective in ablating surface foci rather than deeply seated foci.

The extent of tissue heating and thereby the amount of myocardium that will be coagulated during RF current application depends on multiple variables, which are summarized in Table 29-3. Although *in vitro* studies have shown a good correlation between lesion size and applied power or voltage, this has not been the case for *in vivo* lesions.[7,36] This is undoubtedly due to the importance of

TABLE 29-3. *In vivo* Determinants of Lesion Size in Radiofrequency Ablation

1. Applied power (Refs. 8, 41)
2. Duration of energy delivery (Refs. 8, 35, 36, 41)
3. Electrode size and contact surface area (Refs. 13, 52, 54, 55)
4. Impedance of the tissues and the electrode catheter system (Refs. 8, 65)
5. Contact pressure and catheter tip angle of contact with the heart (Refs. 8, 36, 38, 65, 103)
6. Convective heat loss via intracavitary blood flow (Refs. 35, 69)
7. Electrode–tissue interface temperature, in turn based on delivered power or voltage, pulse duration, and contact pressure, as well as the impedance at the tissue–electrode interface (Refs. 33, 37, 38, 52, 67–69, 71)

variables that are difficult to control in the beating heart, such as electrode tissue coupling and contact pressure, and the amount of convective heat loss due to local blood flow. Irreversible myocardial injury, as demonstrated by histochemical staining, has been reported to occur at a temperature of 52°C to 55°C in an *in vitro* model of radiofrequency ablation.[37,38] The effects of such levels of hyperthermia on cells have been studied and shown to involve profound effects on cell membranes, the cytoskeleton, and the nucleus, all of which can produce cell death with only a brief exposure to heat (from less than a second to a few seconds, depending on the exact temperature reached).[39,40]

HISTOPATHOLOGY OF RADIOFREQUENCY ENERGY–INDUCED LESIONS AND ANIMAL EXPERIMENTS

Catheter-delivered radiofrequency current usually induces well-demarcated coagulation necrosis of the myocardium without destruction of the surrounding normal tissue. With a regular 2 mm–tipped electrode, the size of surface necrosis is usually 5 to 8 mm in diameter. The shape of the lesion is usually spherical or oval as a result of the radial flow of current from the electrode to the tissue (Figs. 29-5 and 29-6).[7,9,11,41] Huang and colleagues performed a detailed histologic analysis in dogs sacrificed at various times following radiofrequency ablation.[9] At the subacute stage (4 to 14 days) there was a central pit surrounded by a discrete area of homogeneous coagulation necrosis (see Fig. 29-6). Surrounding the necrotic area was a narrow zone (0.1 to 0.3 mm) of hemorrhage and granulation tissue with proliferating capillaries, fibroblasts, and inflammatory cells (mononuclear cells and neutrophils). This rim of granulation tissue was sharply demarcated from the surrounding normal tissue,

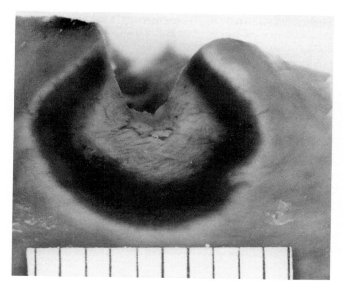

Figure 29-5. A cross-sectional view of a spherical lesion induced by radiofrequency catheter ablation (14.2 W for 30 seconds) of the canine left ventricular myocardium. The dog was killed 4 days after ablation. The sharply circumscribed coagulation necrosis was separated from the normal myocardium by a hemorrhagic zone and a rim of mononuclear cell infiltration. The top center of the necrotic lesion is the endocardial surface of a pit in the left ventricle. (Huang SKS: Radiofrequency catheter ablation of cardiac arrhythmias: appraisal of an evolving therapeutic modality. Am Heart J 1989;118:1317.)

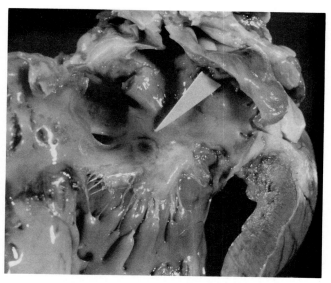

Figure 29-6. Right atrial and right ventricular view of a canine heart showing the effect of RF catheter ablation at the AV nodal area. Arrow points to a well-demarcated circular lesion at the AV junction. The dog was killed 7 days after ablation. Complete AV block was achieved after three applications of RF current to the distal electrode of a regular 7F tripolar catheter. (Huang SKS: Radiofrequency catheter ablation of cardiac arrhythmias: appraisal of an evolving therapeutic modality. Am Heart J 1989;118:1317.)

which revealed no fiber changes or vacuolization. The chronic (>2 months) lesions demonstrated localized whitish, thickened scar with fibrosis, granulation tissue, and infiltration with fat and chronic inflammatory cells (Figs. 29-7 and 29-8).

Extensive animal studies with RF catheter ablation have been reported using a variety of tissues. Acute and persistent complete heart block was reliably produced at a fairly low power output of 5 to 15 W at a pulse duration of 10 to 20 seconds. On pathologic examination, an area of well-demarcated coagulation necrosis was found at the AV junction (see Figs. 29-6 and 29-7), and most of the lesions involved the AV node, the approaches to the AV node, and the penetrating His bundle (see Fig. 29-8).[7,9]

The feasibility of ablating left-sided and right-sided accessory pathways with RF current was demonstrated in several animal experiments.[11,42–44] Huang and associates[11] and Langberg and colleagues[43] produced discrete lesions in the coronary sinus, extending to the left atrial and left ventricular myocardium (Fig. 29-9). RF catheter ablation directly in the coronary sinus was shown to be capable of producing lesions large enough to ablate left-sided accessory pathways, without coronary sinus thrombosis or rupture or occlusion of the nearby coronary artery. Similarly effective abilities to induce lesions along the tricuspid annulus have also been shown.[45,46]

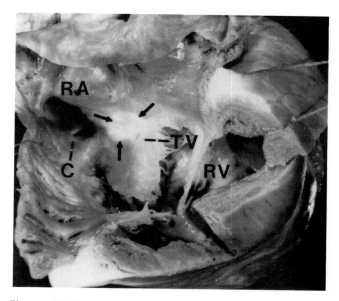

Figure 29-7. Right atrial and right ventricular view of a canine heart showing the chronic changes at the AV junction 2 months after ablation with radiofrequency current. The arrows point to the thickened whitish plaque between the coronary sinus and the medial leaflet of the tricuspid valve. C, coronary sinus; RA, right atrium; RV, right ventricle; TV, tricuspid valve. (Huang SKS, Bharati S, Graham AR, et al: Chronic incomplete atrioventricular block induced by radiofrequency catheter ablation. Circulation 1989;80:951.)

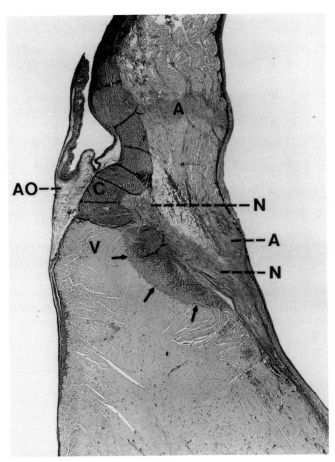

Figure 29-8. Photomicrograph of longitudinal sectioning of AV nodal area in a canine heart showing the chronic effect (2 months) of radiofrequency ablation at the AV junction. Note that the AV node (*N*) and the immediate approaches (*A*) and the right side of the summit of the ventricular septum (*arrows*) were completely within the discrete necrotic lesion and were replaced by granulation tissue. Note also fatty infiltration separating the superior approaches from the AV node. *AO*, aortic valve; *C*, central fibrous body; *V*, summit of the ventricular septum (Weigert–van Gieson stain ×17.25). (Huang SKS, Bharati S, Lev M, et al: Electrophysiologic and histologic observations of chronic atrioventricular block induced by closed-chest catheter desiccation with radiofrequency energy. Pacing Clin Electrophysiol 1987;10:805.)

The use of RF current to produce discrete lesions in the atrial or ventricular myocardium has been shown to be safe.[10,11,35,44,47,48] Serious arrhythmias did not occur during or after ablation (unlike DC energy, to which canines and other laboratory animals are particularly sensitive—they frequently develop ventricular tachycardia or fibrillation). Transmural lesions without perforation were occasionally found when RF ablation was delivered to the thin right atrial or right ventricular wall. Occasionally, mural thrombi were found on the acute atrial or ventricular lesions. Visible lesions were less consistently found in the left ventricle after a single pulsed delivery of RF energy, presumably because of poor control of the elec-

trode–tissue contact in the contractile left ventricle, and the presence of trabeculae and pits in the endocardial surface.

Huang and colleagues compared the electrophysiologic and histologic effects of DC and radiofrequency energy in dogs.[49] DC shocks were associated with induction of sustained ventricular tachycardia, and, in one dog, intractable ventricular fibrillation. The induced lesions were larger and poorly circumscribed with inhomogeneous margins of necrosis, in comparison to the much smaller and discrete radiofrequency-induced lesions. Other investigators have also noted the arrhythmogenicity of DC lesions in canines and have speculated as to its mechanism.[50,51]

Animal experiments have been particularly valuable in studying the effects of various parameters on RF energy–induced lesion size, particularly in an effort to combine the safety and predictability of RF lesions with a technique to generate larger lesion size. For example, a number of animal studies have investigated the influence of varying electrode size on local current density and thus on lesion size in an attempt to identify the ideal electrode size.[36,52–54] In an animal study by Langberg and associates,[54] increasing electrode length from 2 to 4 mm more than doubled the mean lesion volume from 143 to 326 mm^3 at the same applied power, whereas further increases in electrode length beyond 4 mm produced progressively smaller lesions, either because of a lower power

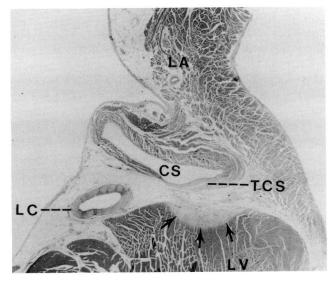

Figure 29-9. Photomicrograph of the coronary sinus showing the effect of RF ablation in a canine heart. A discrete area of fibrosis (*arrows*) of the left ventricle (*LV*) was produced by RF catheter ablation of the coronary sinus (*CS*). *LA* left atrium; *LC*, left circumflex coronary artery; *TCS*, fibrosis of part of the wall of the coronary sinus (hematoxylin and eosin stain, ×7.5). (Huang SKS, Bharati S, Graham AR, et al: Short and long-term effects of transcatheter ablation of the coronary sinus by radiofrequency energy. Circulation 1988;78:416.)

density or as the result of loss of contact between portions of the electrode surface and the tissue. A subsequent study from the same author, however, showed that if the RF energy was applied to achieve a preset temperature rather than delivering a set amount of power, the use of longer electrode tips (8 or 12 mm long) required a significantly higher radiofrequency power output to achieve the desired temperature, but this in turn was able to produce larger lesions up to 1 cm in diameter. However, ablation with these larger electrodes was associated with a drop in arterial pressure and with ventricular ectopy in the dogs used in the study, and the lesions were sometimes associated with charring and crater formation.[55]

As a direct result of these animal studies, clinical studies have been performed to prove that the optimum electrode tip length is at least 4 mm, and this is now the standard size of all ablation catheters. For example, Jackman and colleagues compared standard electrodes with a 1.25-mm tip to a 4-mm tip electrode in 17 patients undergoing complete AV node ablation.[13] Compared with the standard tip, the larger electrode allowed a significant increase in power delivery and a decreased incidence of impedance rise, resulting in marked improvement in ease of achieving AV block.

Other novel efforts to increase lesion size have also been made. Cooling of the distal electrode with saline infusion via a central lumen has been proposed as a means to control the electrode–tissue interface temperature and prevent coagulum formation and impedance rise, allowing greater power to be delivered for maximal lesion size.[56, 57] Other examples of altering RF energy delivery to increase lesion size include multiple sequential applications[58] and use of an orthogonal catheter array.[59] Another research effort, although beyond the scope of this chapter to discuss in detail, has been the use of microwave energy as an alternative to RF energy to increase lesion size. The rationale behind these efforts is that microwave energy, unlike RF energy, is not dependent on direct flow of energy from catheter to tissue. Instead, microwave energy has the capacity to deliver energy to tissue by generating a local electromagnetic field; this field in turn heats the surrounding tissue by molecular friction. This technique may prove valuable in circumstances where good catheter–tissue contact cannot be achieved or a larger lesion size is desired.[60–63]

LESION FORMATION WITH RF ENERGY AND USE OF TEMPERATURE TO GUIDE RADIOFREQUENCY ABLATION

A typical radiofrequency current generator allows continuous monitoring and adjustment of impedance, output power in watts, volts, current, and (in some models) catheter tip temperature. Other requirements for the generator are electrical isolation to prevent current leakage to the heart, similar to all other equipment used in electrophysiologic testing, as well as appropriate filtering to allow continuous monitoring of the surface and intracardiac electrograms during energy application.

The impedance calculated from current and voltage measurements during radiofrequency catheter ablation in the normal heart usually ranges from 100 to 150 Ω. If the initial or baseline impedance is significantly higher than this, the most likely reason is that the electrical circuit is not properly closed (poor wire connections or disruption of a wire or the catheter). However, if the initial impedance is normal but then rises abruptly during energy application, the most likely cause is coagulum formation on the tip electrode (see discussion later). The specific resistance varies for different types of tissues. For example, *in vitro* studies have shown that for muscle tissue the specific resistance ranges approximately between 100 and 230 Ω, whereas for fatty tissue the specific resistance ranges from 1600 to 2300 Ω.[33] The specific resistance for blood is in the same range as that for muscle[33]; thus, it is difficult to differentiate between current applications to blood and to myocardial tissues from the impedance measurements alone.

Because of its low resistance, no direct heating of the catheter electrode itself occurs. However, the temperature of the electrode tip in close contact with the tissue rises during current application because of the heat that is reflected from the tissue surface. This allows one to monitor the heat generated in the directly surrounding tissue by the use of a thermistor or thermocouple in the tip electrode of the catheter. As will be discussed shortly, the ability to measure directly the temperature at the electrode–tissue interface allows the operator the best control over the ablation process and the size of the induced lesion. Because the catheter tip itself is not heated directly but is only indirectly heated from the nearby tissue, special care is required to ensure accurate temperatures. Blouin and associates directly compared two thermistor probes, one directly centered over the area to be heated and protruding from, and thermally isolated from, the electrode, and the second bonded to the inner surface of the electrode at the tip. The second thermistor consistently underestimated the tissue temperature compared with the first thermistor (between 1.8°C at 46°C and between 8.3°C at 75°C.).[64] They concluded that for accurate temperature monitoring, the thermistor must be directly in contact with the tissue and thermally isolated from the delivery electrode.

Because the mechanism of lesion formation in RF ablation is heat-induced necrosis (desiccation), it is logical to assume that temperature monitoring may provide the best way to control and monitor radiofrequency ablation. Whereas the contact pressure and the amount of heat loss by local blood flow cannot be determined *in vivo* or by measuring power or voltage output, demonstration of prompt and adequate temperature rise at the electrode–tissue interface can ensure adequate energy delivery to the tissue. As discussed above, because muscle and blood have a similar effective tissue impedance, it is impossible to distinguish between energy delivery to the blood or to the myocardium from measurements of current, voltage, or calculated impedance; only with tissue contact would there be a significant temperature rise. As a result of these limitations, several ablation catheters capable of monitoring tip temperature are undergoing clinical trials.

Another significant advantage of temperature monitoring is the ability to prevent impedance rises at the catheter tip–tissue interface. Although theoretically one might think that an unlimited amount of electrical energy could be supplied to the tissue, creating an unlimited amount of heat energy and very large lesion sizes, in reality, lesion size is limited by the fact that the temperature of the tissue immediately apposed to the catheter tip can rise no higher than 100°C. This is because higher temperatures result in coagulum formation at the catheter tip. This in turn coats the catheter tip and insulates the electrode, causing an abrupt increase in impedance in the delivery system and preventing any further current flow into the tissue.

The mechanism of coagulum formation has been studied by Haines and colleagues.[65] Using both *in vitro* and *in vivo* models, they showed that coagulum formation was related to raising the tissue temperature directly apposed to the electrode to 100°C, with the resultant boiling of plasma and adherence of denatured plasma proteins to the electrode. Impedance rises were associated with sudden boiling and audible popping. In the *in vivo* preparations in which electrode–tissue heating to 100°C or greater had occurred, there was charring and coagulum or clot adherent to the electrodes (as well as a small amount of adherent tissue). In more than 50% of such cases, fibrin or clot was adherent to the surface of the lesion as well. Neither delivered current, voltage, nor power could be used to reliably predict the occurrence of an impedance rise, which correlated only with tissue temperature achieved.[65] Ring and colleagues compared the histology of lesions created with radiofrequency energy associated with or without an impedance rise.[53] Rises in impedance were associated with lesions demonstrating marked and extensive endocardial disruption and coagulum formation. In addition, ablations associated with an impedance rise have been shown to cause catheter disruption.[66] Thus, temperature monitoring is important to ensure a successful delivery of radiofrequency energy to the tissue and to potentially decrease adverse effects of the ablation procedure resulting from impedance rises, such as the risk of thrombus formation at the ablation site.

The ability of temperature monitoring to predict lesion size and ablation efficacy has been verified by both *in vitro*[33,38,52,67,68] and *in vivo* studies.[69–71] The first measurements of catheter tip temperature during radiofrequency application to the intact heart were performed by Hindricks and colleagues using Ni-Cr/Ni thermo-elements that were built in to the active electrode.[38] From this study it became clear that catheter tip temperature is highly predictive of lesion size when radiofrequency currents are applied to intact hearts. The rate and amount of temperature increase provide a rough estimate of the adequacy of tissue–electrode contact. These results were further quantified and a theoretic model was verified by Haines and associates.[68]

Langberg and colleagues presented a series of 20 patients undergoing ablation of accessory pathways with a temperature-guided catheter fitted with a thermistor embedded in the distal electrode.[69] Ablation of left-sided accessory pathways, with the catheter wedged on the left ventricle against the mitral annulus, was associated with higher temperatures than right-sided ablation performed from the atrial aspect of the tricuspid valve, presumed secondary to the greater contact pressure and lesser competing blood flow associated with the left-sided location. Temperature at the electrode–tissue interface rose to its steady-state level within a few seconds. Applications of radiofrequency energy that caused transient accessory pathway block were associated with a mean temperature of 50°C ± 8°C (presumably causing reversible tissue injury rather than complete necrosis), whereas those that permanently eliminated accessory pathway function were associated with a temperature of 62°C ± 15°C. They also confirmed that impedance rise was associated only with applications creating a temperature of 95°C to 100°C. In addition, they showed that at a power output of 20 or 30 W, a typical power for performing radiofrequency ablation, a majority of sites had sufficiently poor coupling between the ablating electrode and adjacent tissue to prevent temperatures from exceeding 48°C, the minimum temperature associated with permanent accessory pathway block. Similar results were shown by Calkins and colleagues[70] and Chen and associates.[71]

In summary, temperature at the electrode–tissue interface is an ideal parameter to be monitored during radiofrequency ablation. If the thermistor is properly located in the electrode tip and the temperature is accurately measured, it is by far the best way to prevent an impedance rise, it ensures adequate tissue contact and delivery of energy to the tissue, and it is the best correlate with lesion size. Until temperature monitoring catheters are clinically available, however, one should monitor impedance to ensure good tissue contact and to stop energy delivery at the first sign of an impedance rise, and use incremental power output while monitoring clinical effect in an attempt to avoid an impedance rise, usually adjusting the power to produce no more than 65 to 70 V (approximately 35 to 40 W at an average tissue impedance of 110 to 120 Ω).

RECURRENCE AND "DELAYED CURE" FOLLOWING ABLATION

The above histologic and biophysical aspects of RF ablation may be helpful in understanding such phenomena as recurrence and delayed cure following ablation. A recurrence rate of 8% to 12% following radiofrequency ablation of accessory pathways has been reported.[34, 72] Interestingly enough, there was a statistically significant greater incidence of recurrence in right-sided or posteroseptal pathways, suggesting that the lower temperature associated with ablation in these locations (see discussion above)[69] may be the cause, in that the pathways were damaged but true necrosis was not produced. Leitch and colleagues observed several patients undergoing seemingly unsuccessful ablation who subsequently exhibited delayed loss of pre-excitation 3 to 5 days after ablation.[73] However, the success was not permanent, because all patients regained pre-excitation between 3 and 5 months later. It is quite reasonable to hypothesize that these patients' accessory pathways were located not in the area of necrosis but in the surrounding area of inflammation. Thus, between 3 and 5 days later, when the inflammatory response would be expected to be at its height, there could be loss of accessory pathway function, followed by recurrence of this function after healing had occurred. Wagshal and colleagues presented a group of patients undergoing initially successful RF ablation of accessory pathways who developed transient recurrence of accessory pathway function but were shown to have delayed cure during follow-up electrophysiologic testing and long-term clinical observation. This suggested that these patients' accessory pathways were also on the edge of the original necrotic lesion such that complete necrosis did not occur immediately but several days later.[74] Because these patients demonstrated immediate loss of pre-excitation, presumably the accessory pathways of these patients were closer to the central zone of necrosis than those reported by Leitch and associates. Reports of similar patients have also been published by other investigators.[75–77] The important lesson to be learned from these reports is that there can be considerable evolution of the ablation lesion over the first few days following ablation, which can lead to either recurrent accessory pathway conduction or a long-lasting complete cure. Accordingly, we feel it is appropriate to observe the patients for several days before making a decision as to whether or not a repeat ablation procedure is required, and then to obtain full electrophysiologic evaluation of the residual accessory pathway characteristics before actually undertaking repeat RF energy deliveries.

As to the mechanism of these findings, one possibility was suggested by Nath and colleagues.[78] These authors have shown that the zone of tissue injury extending beyond the edge of the actual area of immediate necrosis is characterized by a marked reduction in microvascular blood flow and is associated with histologic findings of microvascular endothelial injury. Progression or resolution of this area of potential ischemia could account for either the late progression or the resolution of the RF-induced tissue injury. This phenomenon may be the explanation for the "forward creep" observed in several patients undergoing radiofrequency ablation for ventricular tachycardia in whom the full effect of the ablation was not seen until several hours later.[21, 79]

COMPLICATIONS OF CATHETER ABLATION WITH USE OF RADIOFREQUENCY ENERGY

Undoubtedly because of the controlled and small, well-circumscribed lesions produced by radiofrequency ablation, the incidence of complications reported has been quite low, and most of the complications have been related to either arterial or venous cannulation or intracardiac catheter manipulation.[80, 81] DC energy, however, which produces significant barotrauma and larger lesions, has been associated with more complications (see introduction and next section). Of the 106 patients treated with radiofrequency ablation by Calkins and associates,[18] one patient suffered a myocardial infarction as a result of occlusion of the left circumflex coronary artery, and one developed complete AV block. Jackman and associates reported one incidence of complete AV block, one episode of cardiac tamponade from radiofrequency current delivery into a small branch of the coronary sinus, and one case of pericarditis out of 166 patients.[19] Olgin and Scheinman followed 54 patients undergoing complete AV junction ablation with radiofrequency energy for a mean of 24 months; one patient suffered a pulmonary embolus shortly after the procedure, and two patients died suddenly 7 and 11 months later.[82] A third patient was successfully resuscitated from an episode of ventricular fibrillation 20 months later. However, two of these three patients had significant underlying coronary artery disease, so we cannot be certain that these events were related to their earlier ablation procedure. So far, this is the only report in the literature of late sudden death possibly related to prior RF complete AV junction ablation. A significantly higher incidence of serious arrhythmias and sudden deaths has been reported following DC ablation (see discussion at the beginning of this chapter).

Several studies have looked at the potential arrhythmogenicity of radiofrequency energy–induced lesions. Chiang and coworkers performed 24-hour Holter monitoring, signal-averaged electrocardiograms, treadmill exercise testing, and programmed electrical stimulation before and serially after both DC and RF energy ablation of accessory pathways or of the AV node.[83] They noted a significant increase in the number of premature ventricular beats and short runs of nonsustained ventricular tachycardia in the first week after ablation in both groups, although the findings were more persistent and more frequent in those patients undergoing DC ablation. No patient, however, developed inducible ventricular tachycardia. Twidale and colleagues also showed no inducible ventricular tachycardia on programmed stimulation after radiofrequency ablation of accessory pathways.[84]

An interesting report by Mittleman and associates documented the presence of new inducible atrial tachycardia in a group of six patients following RF catheter ablation of the slow AV nodal pathway.[85] The tachycardia origin was from the low right atrium and appeared to be the result of the RF lesions created at the site of the ablation attempts. Correspondingly, this arrhythmia was more frequently demonstrated in patients receiving a larger number of ablation lesions during the ablation session.

The acute electrophysiologic effects of hyperthermia on isolated guinea pig papillary muscle were studied *in vitro* by Nath and associates.[86] In muscle strips warmed to >50°C, depolarization of the resting membrane potential was observed with a decrease in the action potential duration and loss of excitability. Spontaneous automaticity was also observed at this temperature; thus, this may be a marker for the frequent occurrence of short flurries of junctional tachycardias in patients undergoing modification or complete ablation of the AV node.[87–89] Ge and colleagues analyzed the effects of RF and DC ablations applied to isolated myocardial strips on the action potential of the surrounding myocardial cells.[90] Significantly greater alterations of the action potential were seen with DC ablation compared with RF ablation; this may explain the low incidence of proarrhythmia and perhaps explain as well the lower incidence of late sudden death associated with RF ablation.

Several studies performed echocardiograms routinely after RF ablation; no pericardial effusion (except in clinically overt pericardial tamponade from catheter perforation), intracardiac thrombus, or valve disruption was detected.[91,92] Two studies have specifically addressed the issue of possible effects on the nearby coronary artery after radiofrequency ablation of accessory pathways located along either the tricuspid or mitral annulus.[93,94] In both studies no effects were seen. In the series of 100 patients undergoing RF ablation of a left anterolateral accessory pathway described by Lesh and colleagues, one patient developed chest pain and transient ST segment elevation during application of RF energy.[91] Coronary spasm was suspected, but results of coronary angiography were normal. This demonstrated lack of effect of RF ablation on coronary arteries is not unexpected given the small size of the RF lesion produced during ablation as well as the fact that the rapid blood flow through the coronary arteries would prevent any local heat build-up.

It must be realized, however, that experience with radiofrequency catheter ablation is too short-lived to fully evaluate possible late side effects. This point was made by Brodman in a recent editorial describing some of the ecchymoses, induration, and scarring seen at surgery after failed radiofrequency ablation.[95] Another source of possible late side effects is the substantial fluoroscopic exposure to the patient undergoing lengthy ablation procedures.[96,97]

APPLICATION OF RADIOFREQUENCY ENERGY TO TREAT SPECIFIC ARRHYTHMIAS

Arrhythmias Associated With Accessory Atrioventricular Connections

For many reasons, accessory pathways have been the most successful and well-studied targets for RF ablation. Among these are the fact that in most cases accessory pathways result in pre-excitation on the surface ECG, allowing relatively easy diagnosis of their potential role in cardiac arrhythmias. The accessory pathways run in well-defined anatomic sites in the AV grooves, where their exact location can be easily mapped (particularly left-sided pathways, which run close to the coronary sinus). They result in arrhythmias that in addition to being clinically bothersome can also be associated with sudden cardiac death (particularly from degeneration of rapid atrial fibrillation over the bypass tract into ventricular fibrillation), and the success (or recurrence after initially successful ablation) can be easily gauged by the surface EKG. Over the past few years, several large centers have accumulated and published experience in hundreds of patients.[19,98–100]

Anatomically, accessory pathways can be divided into four groups—left free wall (along the mitral annulus), posteroseptal (in the fairly large space between and posterior to the mitral and tricuspid rings), right free wall (along the tricuspid annulus), and anteroseptal and midseptal (in the anterior space near the His bundle region) pathways (Fig. 29-10). Once the accessory pathway has been located to a particular region in the heart, more pinpoint mapping is required, which is usually performed directly from the ablation catheter itself because of the restricted size of the radiofrequency lesion. Several studies have addressed the electrogram characteristics that identify successful ablation

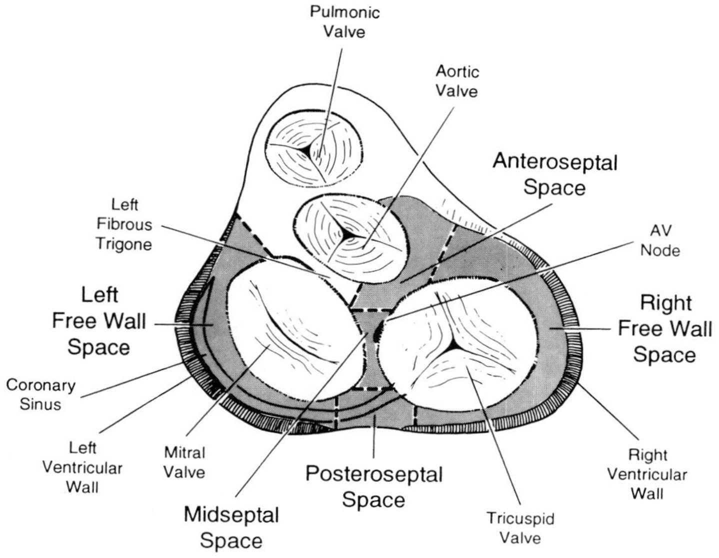

Figure 29-10. Diagram of a cross section of the human heart at the level of the atrioventricular groove with the atria cut away, showing the distribution of the five anatomic spaces (*stippled area*) through which accessory pathways traverse the AV groove. These regions are the left free wall, right free wall, posteroseptal, midseptal, and anteroseptal spaces. Accessory pathways are not found in the far anterior portion of the mitral annulus where the left fibrous trigone connects the mitral valve and aortic valve apparatus. The extreme anterior right free wall space can contain accessory pathways because there is no similar tricuspid valve–aortic valve continuity, and this area merges into the anteroseptal space. The midseptal space runs from just anterior to the coronary sinus os to the level of the AV node.

sites.[101,102] Calkins and colleagues found the following criteria to be independent predictors of success.[103] For pathways with manifest pre-excitation:

1. A short AV interval (measured from the peak of the atrial electrogram to the peak of the ventricular electrogram, and ideally <30 msec) or the onset of the local ventricular electrogram occurring prior to the surface QRS complex

2. The presence of an accessory pathway potential

3. Electrogram stability as assessed by a constant (<10% variation) electrogram morphology for three to five consecutive beats immediately before ablation.

The corresponding criteria for concealed accessory pathways were:

1. Continuous electrical activity between the ventricular and atrial electrograms during either ventricular pacing or orthodromic AV reciprocating tachycardia

2. The presence of an accessory pathway potential

3. Electrogram stability.

Accessory pathway potentials were previously described and proved to represent rapid conduction through the accessory pathway itself.[104,105] A typical example is shown in Figure 29-11. The requirement of electrogram stability is presumably a reflection of firm catheter––tissue contact, a prerequisite for adequate transfer of RF energy from the catheter to the tissue to produce adequate heating and lesion formation at the target site. In our experience, at ablation sites where we ultimately achieve long-term success, the accessory pathway conduction is usually lost quite rapidly (within 1 or 2 seconds), presumably reflecting nearly direct contact between the accessory

pathway and the ablation catheter. Although we regularly use the criteria of Calkins and colleagues and have confirmed their validity, we have found a significant subset of patients with comparably slow retrograde conduction through their accessory pathway and have found that a much more reliable predictor of successful ablation sites in patients with concealed accessory pathways is the earliest retrograde atrial activation during orthodromic AVRT (Fig. 29-12).

Left free wall pathways can be approached either from the left ventricular aspect of the mitral valve, usually by passing the catheter across the aortic valve and positioning it under the mitral annulus, or by way of the atrial aspect, usually performed via a transseptal approach. In general, either of these two techniques can be used, depending on the operator's preference, although occasionally only one or the other will be successful in a particular patient, so the ability to use both techniques is desirable. The transseptal technique is also preferred in children, the elderly, and those with arterial disease or left ventricular hypertrophy.[106–108] A third, less frequently used approach is via the coronary sinus, which runs posteriorly along the left atrioventricular groove in close proximity to most left free wall pathways (Fig. 29-13). Although most pathways can be approached from either the atrial or ventricular aspects, occasionally one encounters pathways that run more subepicardially and can be approached only from the coronary sinus. A coronary sinus approach is also required for those pathways associated with a coronary sinus diverticulum, and these pathways can often be ablated by applying RF energy to the neck of the diverticulum.[109,110] In one series of 51 consecutive patients with left free wall pathways, five patients could be ablated only from within the coronary sinus.[111] In all cases, a large accessory pathway

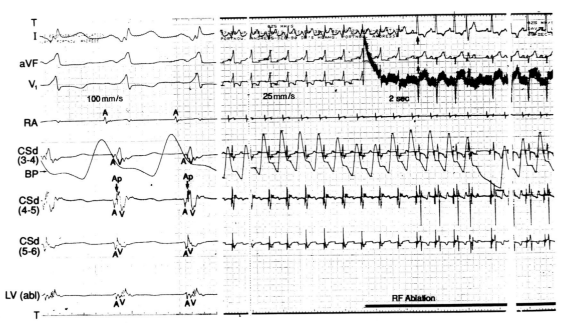

Figure 29-11. Example of an accessory pathway potential recorded in a patient undergoing RF catheter ablation of a left free wall accessory pathway. A large sharp deflection (indicated by the arrows labeled Ap) separating the closely spaced atrial and ventricular electrograms from the coronary sinus recording (poles 4 and 5) was present. The ablation catheter was maneuvered against the mitral annulus directly opposite these poles of the coronary sinus catheter, where there was also a smaller accessory pathway potential recorded between the closely spaced atrial and ventricular electrograms. Within approximately 2 seconds of energy delivery at this site, pre-excitation was permanently lost (right-hand panel), as marked by the arrows in the ECG. The first half of the figure was recorded at 100 mm/sec speed and the latter half at 25 mm/sec speed. *T*, time lines; *I*, *aVF*, and *V₁* surface EKG leads; *A*, atrial depolarization; *V*, ventricular depolarization; *RA*, high right atrium, *CSd*, recordings from the indicated electrodes from the distal coronary sinus using a decapolar catheter with 1-mm electrodes and 2-mm interelectrode separation; *Ap*, accessory pathway potential; *BP*, blood pressure; *LV (abl)*, ablation catheter in the LV against the mitral annulus.

potential was present from within the coronary sinus, whereas a similar potential was present at endocardial target sites in only one of the five patients. No complications or recurrences occurred in any of the five patients.

The next most common location of accessory pathways is the posteroseptal space, a large area including the os of the coronary sinus and spreading posteriorly in a triangular fashion to the posterior edges of the tricuspid and mitral valve annuli.[112] Accessory pathways in this area can be ablated most often from the atrial side around the os of the coronary sinus, but other patients require a ventricular approach along the tricuspid annulus, or from within the proximal coronary sinus itself. As mentioned above, pathways within the posteroseptal area can also be associated with a coronary sinus diverticulum.

Right free wall, midseptal, and anteroseptal pathways are less common locations for accessory pathways. Right free wall pathways are occasionally found in association with Ebstein's anomaly of the tricuspid valve. Unlike left-sided pathways, which can be mapped easily from the

coronary sinus, there is no venous structure available for mapping. However, some investigators have shown that the use of a mapping electrode placed in the right coronary artery is safe and beneficial, and one such electrode is now commercially available.[91, 113] The main problem with anteroseptal and midseptal pathway ablation is their close proximity to the AV node and His bundle and the accompanying risk of inducing heart block; nevertheless, with careful mapping to avoid sites with a His bundle potential, these pathways have been shown to be amenable to ablation without producing concomitant heart block.[114, 115]

Complete AV Node Ablation and AV Nodal Modification for AV Nodal Reentrant Tachycardia (AVNRT)

The modification of the AV node has been the other big success for radiofrequency ablation, by virtue of its frequency, the high success rate of RF ablation, and the

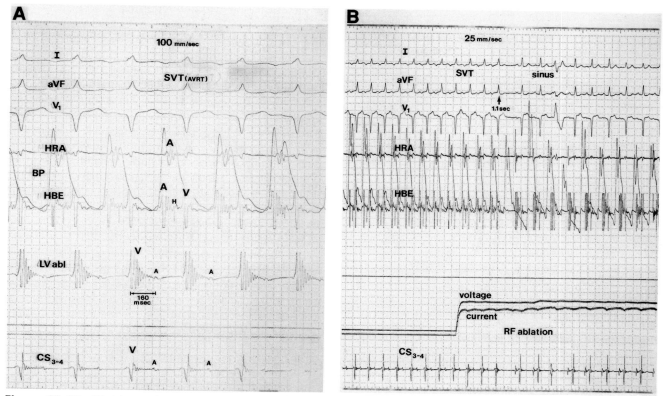

Figure 29-12. RF ablation of a left free wall pathway. **(A)** Preablation electrograms, recorded at 100 mm/sec speed during orthodromic AV reciprocating tachycardia, reveal a widely spaced V–A interval of 160 msec; nevertheless, this was the closest VA interval we were able to record (compare with the interval in the mid CS catheter from the closest recording poles). **(B)** (Recorded at 25 mm/sec speed). Following onset of ablation energy, SVT is broken and sinus rhythm is restored within 1.1 seconds (indicated by solid arrow), after which SVT remains noninducible with no evidence of accessory pathway conduction. This slide illustrates the variation in retrograde V–A intervals possible with accessory pathways. *AVRT,* AV reciprocating tachycardia; *HBE,* His bundle electrogram; *HRA,* high right atrium; *SVT,* supraventricular tachycardia. Remainder of abbreviations as in Figure 29-11.

insights into the nature of this arrhythmia gained by RF ablation.

Selective modification of the AV node developed from the ability of RF ablation to create complete AV block, first in animal studies, as described earlier,[7] and subsequently in humans (Fig. 29-14). The development of catheters with 4-mm-tip electrodes significantly increased the ease and success rate of this procedure.[13,62]

A prospective randomized comparison of DC and RF ablation of the AV junction was performed by Morady and associates.[116] Compared with RF energy, DC energy was less often effective, was associated with a significantly increased serum level of creatine kinase following the procedure, and resulted in an immediate post-ablation junctional escape rate that was much slower. In addition, one patient died suddenly 6 months following DC ablation. A similar conclusion was reached in the study of Olgin and Scheinman comparing DC and RF energy for AV junction ablation.[82]

This procedure has been demonstrated to be an effective alternative to drug therapy in the patient with refractory atrial fibrillation (or other atrial tachyarrhythmias that cannot be ablated directly). The usual approach to complete AV node ablation is from the right side of the heart, by positioning the ablation catheter to record a His bundle and then pulling it back into the atrium just a few millimeters to record a large atrial potential and a small His potential, at which position the distal AV node can be effectively ablated. Ablations performed from the site where a maximal His bundle potential can be recorded, on the other hand, tend to result only in right bundle branch block. With this technique, an 80% to 90% success rate has been recorded. An alternative left-sided approach has been developed for cases in which this right-sided approach is unsuccessful, namely, positioning the ablation catheter on the left ventricular septum just opposite to where the catheter records a His bundle potential from the right side of the heart. From this location, a His bundle

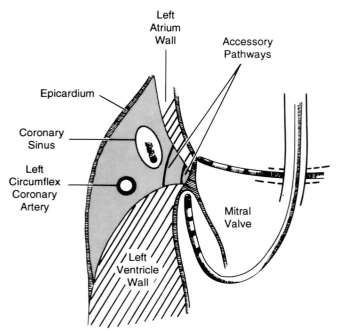

Figure 29-13. Schematic diagram of a longitudinal section of the left atrioventricular junction illustrating three approaches to ablation of a left free wall accessory pathway, namely, from the left ventricle with the catheter wedged underneath the mitral leaflet; from the left atrium (usually via the transseptal approach) with the catheter placed against the atrial aspect of the mitral annulus; and from within the coronary sinus. Accessory pathways, as illustrated in the figure, can run from the atrium to the ventricle either near the annulus or more subepicardially and nearer to the coronary sinus, in which case ablation may be difficult from any approach other than from within the coronary sinus.

potential can usually be recorded, and ablation at this site has been shown to be frequently successful, even when the right-side approach failed.[117–120] An alternative approach is ablation from the noncoronary cusp of the aortic valve, where a large His potential can also be recorded.[121]

A marker of success for either of these two approaches is the creation of flurries of accelerated junctional beats, presumably reflecting the creation of automaticity in the AV junction from the heating effects of the ablation catheter positioned against the AV node.[62, 122] All of these ablation procedures have in common, of course, the need for simultaneous placement of a permanent pacemaker, because the resulting escape rhythm, although often narrow complex, is felt to be too slow and too unstable to be relied upon without a pacemaker. An interesting case report used ablation directed at the posterior input into the AV node near the coronary sinus (an approach similar to that used for "slow pathway" AV nodal modification) to successfully target the fibers into the AV node with the shortest refractory period, thereby providing a nonpharmacologic alternative to medication for rate control of

atrial fibrillation without requiring a permanent pacemaker.[123]

The benefits of complete AV node ablation in certain patients can be quite significant. Although a variety of medications can be tried to control the rate of atrial fibrillation, they are often ineffective, particularly in situations where there is increased sympathetic tone or concomitant use of beta-adrenergic agonists (such as in asthma, chronic lung disease, or congestive heart failure), or in cases where the negative inotropic effects of drugs such as beta-blockers or calcium channel blockers are contraindicated. Furthermore, studies have shown that complete AV node ablation not only is symptomatically beneficial to patients but also increases left ventricular ejection fraction, presumably a reflection of improvement in tachycardia-related cardiomyopathy.[124, 125]

A significant improvement in this technique of complete AV node ablation has been the use of RF energy to modify the AV node for treatment of AV nodal reentrant tachycardia (AVNRT) without the need for permanent pacemaker insertion. The first technique, the so-called anterior or "fast-pathway" ablation, involves placing the

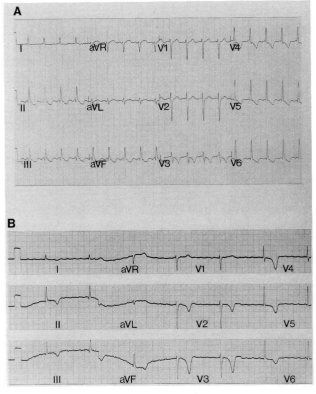

Figure 29-14. Twelve-lead electrocardiograms in a patient before (**A**) and after (**B**) RF catheter ablation of the AV junction. **A** shows atrial flutter with 2:1 ventricular response. **B** demonstrates rapid atrial flutter with complete AV block and a stable junctional escape rhythm after RF ablation.

ablation catheter slightly anterior and proximal to the site of the maximal His electrogram and delivering energy in such a fashion as to create PR prolongation of approximately 50% above the control value. When this is achieved, although the A-His interval is prolonged, 1:1 conduction through the AV node at normal heart rates remains intact while dual AV node curves are lost, suggesting that most conduction to the AV node is occurring over the slow AV nodal pathway (Figs. 29-15 through 29-17). In addition, retrograde AV node conduction over the retrograde fast AV nodal pathway is also significantly damaged or lost completely, providing another impediment to maintenance of AVNRT. This technique was shown to be feasible in animal models[126] and was subsequently shown to be successful in humans as well.[14, 18, 127, 128] The one drawback to this procedure is the inadvertent creation of enough AV nodal damage to cause complete heart block and necessitate permanent pacemaker implantation. Large series reported rates of 2% to 8% for unintentional complete heart block using this technique.[14, 18] However, a newer approach to this technique has been developed using a gradual increase in energy at the chosen site starting at 10 W and adding increments of 5 W until the desired PR prolongation is achieved. With this technique, no AV block was seen in a series of 38 consecutive patients.[129, 130] Similar to complete AV node ablation, success-

ful sites are usually heralded by flurries of junctional beats (Fig. 29-18).

An even more important advance in the use of catheter ablation for treatment of AVNRT has been the development of the "slow-pathway" approach to AV nodal modification. The ability to demonstrate longitudinal fractionation of the AV node during electrophysiologic testing[131] and the demonstration of two anatomically distinct pathways with different retrograde exits into the right atrium[132] provided the theoretic background for this technique. In 1990, Roman and associates first reported successful ablation of AVNRT by targeting the slow pathway along the lower tricuspid annulus near the os of the coronary sinus.[133] This technique was further defined by Jackman and colleagues, who demonstrated the existence of discrete potentials recordable during sinus rhythm shortly after the atrial electrogram which were markers for the site of successful ablation.[17] Using these potentials to choose ablation sites, they achieved successful selective slow pathway ablation in 55 patients with a median of only one ablation application. These potentials were postulated to represent potentials resulting from the atrial insertion of the slow AV nodal pathway, appearing shortly after the local atrial electrogram during sinus rhythm or typical ("slow–fast") AVNRT but before the atrial electrogram during retrograde activation of the slow pathway (i.e.,

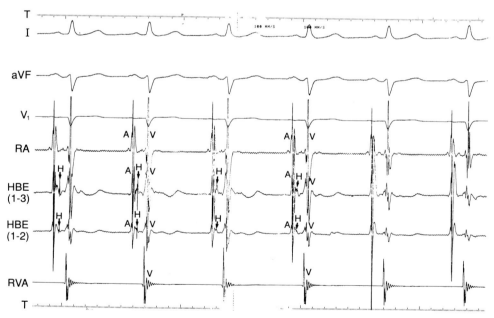

Figure 29-15. Demonstration of the withdrawal of the His bundle catheter (from left to right tracings) to the point where a small or barely visible His bundle potential with a relatively large atrial amplitude was recorded from the distal pair (electrodes #1 and #2) of the His bundle catheter (*HBE*) with an interelectrode distance of 10 mm. Tracings were recorded at 100 mm/sec paper speed. *H*, His bundle potential (indicated by an arrow): *RVA*, RV apex catheter. Other abbreviations as in Figure 29-11.

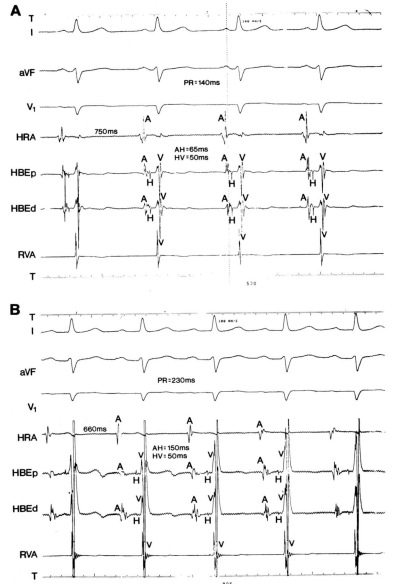

Figure 29-16. Simultaneous recordings (at 100 mm/sec paper speed) of the surface ECG and intracardiac electrograms in sinus rhythm before (**A**) and 3 months after (**B**) RF catheter modification of the AV node for cure of AV nodal reentrant tachycardia of the same patient shown in Figure 29-17. Note the prolongation of the PR interval (from 0.14 to 0.23 seconds) and the A-His interval (from 65 to 150 msec). The His-V interval and QRS complex remained unchanged. *HBEp* proximal His bundle electrograms; *HBEd*, distal His bundle electrograms. See Figures 29-11 and 29-15 for other abbreviations.

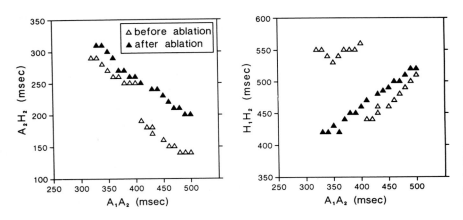

Figure 29-17. Graphic representation of the functional curves of the AV node before (*open triangles*) and 1 week after (*solid triangles*) RF catheter ablation of the patient in Figure 29-15.

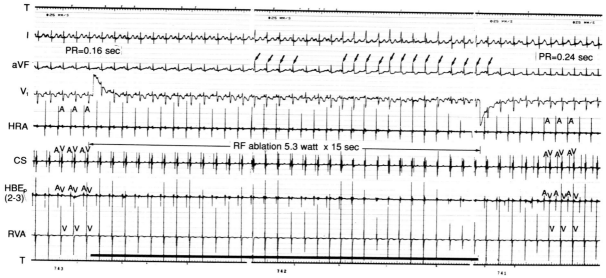

Figure 29-18. Simultaneous recordings of the surface ECG (leads *I*, *aVF*, and *V₁*) and intracardiac electrograms during RF catheter modification (anterior approach) of the AV node in a patient with refractory AV nodal reentrant tachycardia. An accelerated junctional rhythm with a cycle length of 450 msec (indicated by arrows) occurred during the latter portion of RF ablation. The PR interval increased from a baseline of 0.16 sec to 0.24 sec (50% increase) immediately after application of 79.5 J (5.3 W for 15 seconds) RF energy. Tracings were recorded at 25 mm/sec paper speed. Abbreviations as in Figures 29-11, 29-12, 29-15, and 29-16.

during atypical ["fast–slow"] AVNRT). They also tended to disappear, or at least diminish in amplitude, after successful ablation. The exact etiology of these potentials has been the subject of controversy, because other investigators have achieved nearly equivalent ablation results without targeting these potentials,[16, 134, 135] and because other investigators have also found them to be useful markers.[15]

Although many patients after ablation are left with electrophysiologic evidence of dual AV nodal pathways and isolated AV nodal echo beats, elimination of inducible tachycardia at the time of the study is usually enough to ensure absence of subsequent recurrence.[15, 17, 136] Other investigators, however, have suggested that persisting with ablation until there is complete elimination of slow pathway conduction results in a lower rate of recurrence, compared with accepting loss of inducible tachycardia alone as a therapeutic end point.[137, 138]

The presence of flurries of junctional tachycardia during application of the RF energy is almost ubiquitous at the ultimately successful ablation site[88] and presumably reflects the generation of automaticity induced by local heating, as discussed earlier (Fig. 29-19).[86] Although complete AV node ablation also is commonly associated with bursts of rapid junctional rhythm, the junctional rhythm associated with successful slow pathway ablation tends to be slower and is associated with retrograde conduction to the atrium after each junctional beat, whereas the junctional tachycardia resulting from complete AV node block usu-

ally has a faster rate and often does not exhibit retrograde atrial activation because both antegrade and retrograde conduction properties are destroyed simultaneously.[89]

Several studies have directly compared these two techniques of AV nodal modification, in general confirming that both techniques, in experienced hands, are safe and effective.[129, 134] The slow pathway technique does seem to offer a somewhat decreased incidence of complete heart block, decreased incidence of recurrence, and less alteration in normal AV node conduction. The anterior approach has also been associated with a risk of developing atypical AVNRT, using the slow pathway for retrograde conduction as a result of the damage to the retrograde fast pathway.[14, 139, 140] As a result, we and most other centers attempt the slow pathway approach first, and most centers report a greater than 90% success rate. Our approach is to advance the ablation catheter across the tricuspid valve, and then pull back to the valve while deflecting the tip toward the lower tricuspid annulus and toward the septum (Fig. 29-20). The desired electrogram usually reveals a small atrial depolarization and a large ventricular electrogram. The atrial electrogram usually is fractionated or exhibits a distinct second potential (Fig. 29-21), although in our experience successful ablation can occur without these features. If this location fails, the ablation catheter is deflected slightly more superiorly toward the His bundle catheter or moved slightly posteriorly toward the coronary sinus os, and ablation is attempted again. In our

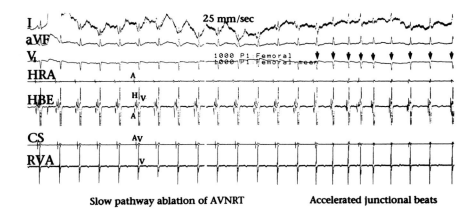

Slow pathway ablation of AVNRT   Accelerated junctional beats

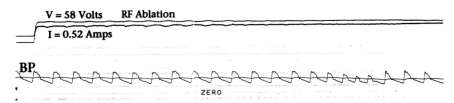

Figure 29-19. Demonstration of accelerated junctional beats (marked with solid arrows in the ECG) occurring during a successful slow pathway ablation in a patient with AVNRT. Note that the accelerated junctional beats are associated with 1:1 retrograde atrial activation in the high right atrial (*HRA*) tracing. Recording speed is 25 mm/sec. *I*, current in amps; *V*, volts. Other abbreviations as in Figures 29-11, 29-12, and 29-15.

Triangle of Koch

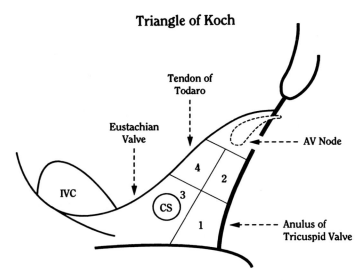

Figure 29-20. Diagram of the triangle of Koch. The triangle of Koch is bordered by the tendon of Todaro and the eustachian valve, the septal attachment of the tricuspid valve, and the orifice of the coronary sinus (CS). The compact AV node is located at the apex of this triangle near the central fibrous body. The successful location for most slow pathway ablations in our experience is site 1, anterior to the ostium of the coronary sinus and along the inferior border of the septal leaflet of the tricuspid annulus. Occasionally the successful sites are nearer to the coronary sinus (site 3) or more anterior, toward the His bundle and compact AV node (site 2). *IVC*, inferior vena cava.

experience, successful ablation sites are essentially always heralded by at least a few beats of junctional tachycardia. An example of the effect of slow pathway ablation on AV nodal function is shown in Figure 29-22.

A direct benefit of the development of the slow pathway approach to AV nodal modification has been a greatly enhanced understanding of the AV node and renewed interest in the controversy over the existence of an upper common pathway within the AV node in this arrhythmia. A related question is what exactly is this "slow pathway," the ablation of which clearly is successful in abolishing AVNRT (i.e., is it a distinct pathway, or is it an area of the AV node or the atrium that exhibits slow conduction, not by being a distinct pathway but instead by exhibiting anisotropic conduction properties). Histologic studies have shown the presence, in animal models, of preferential conduction tissue between the right atrium and the His bundle, which have been postulated to represent the equivalent of dual AV nodal pathways in humans.[141] Although anatomically discrete, the slow pathway can be viewed as part of the AV node, which would be supported by the presence of junctional automaticity produced during ablation at these sites. Keim and colleagues used intraoperative ice mapping to discover sites where the reentry circuit could be interrupted during AV nodal modification surgery, and they demonstrated discrete areas corresponding to the

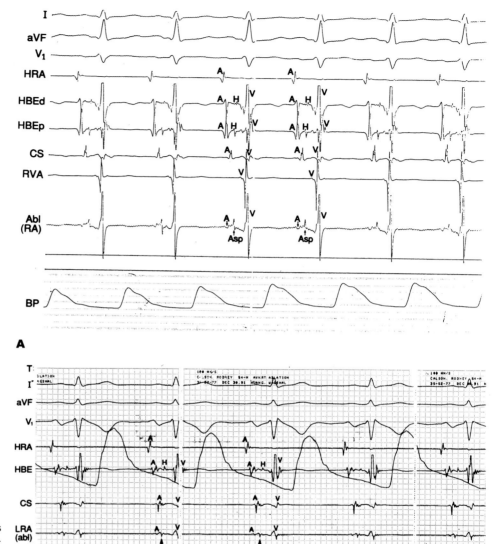

Figure 29-21. Typical potentials (labeled Asp or as solid arrows) recorded from the ablation catheter (*Abl*) along the lower septal leaflet of the tricuspid valve at the successful ablation sites of the slow AV nodal pathway in two patients (**A** and **B**). *LRA*, low right atrium; other abbreviations as in Figures 29-11, 29-12, 29-15, and 29-16.

fast and slow pathways; however, none of the intervening tissue between them was necessary for maintenance of the arrhythmia.[142] This suggests that these tissues are connected by either a broad band or multiple bands of tissue capable of completing the reentry circuit, rather than by a discrete pathway. This implies that instead of a defined upper common pathway within the AV node, the perinodal atrium as a whole is available to complete the circuit. Other evidence for this comes from the ability to demonstrate orthodromic capture of the atrial electrogram at the recording site of the His bundle potential from the proximal coronary sinus during entrainment, thereby strongly suggesting that this part of the atrium is within the reentry circuit, and thus that there is no intranodal upper common pathway.[143] The alternative view requires considering this entire area of tissue in the low right atrium as extended AV nodal "upper common pathway" tissue, dis-

Text continues on p. 930

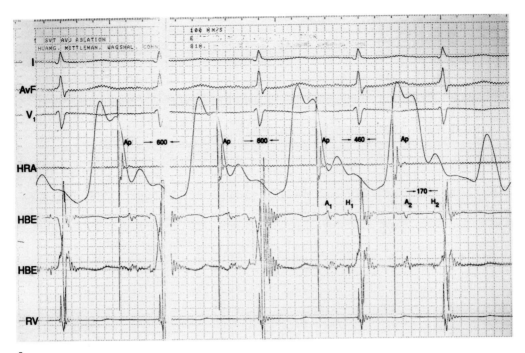

A

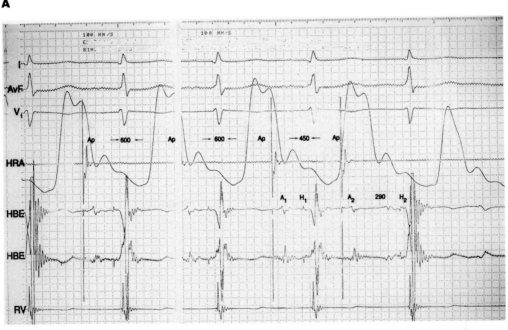

B

Figure 29-22. Illustration of the selective effects of the "slow pathway" ablation technique. Pre-ablation (**A** through **D**), the patient demonstrates obvious dual AV nodal physiology. In **A**, with an atrial pacing cycle length of 600 msec, an A_2 beat with a coupling interval of 460 msec conducts through the fast pathway with an A_2H_2 interval of 170 msec. In **B**, with the A_2 beat shortened by 10 msec to 450 msec, the premature beat now conducts through the slow pathway with an A_2H_2 interval of 290 msec, representing the effective refractory period of the fast AV nodal pathway at 450 msec.

(continued)

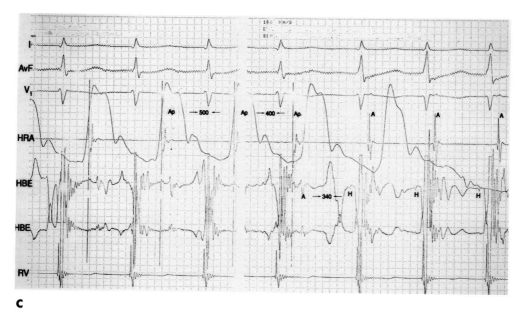

C

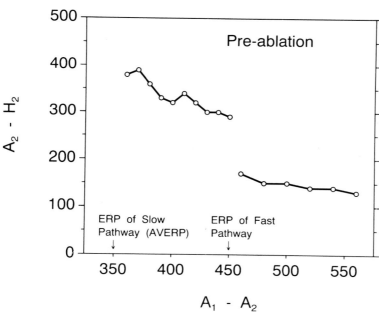

ERP = Effective Refractory Period

D

Figure 29-22. (*continued*) With an A_2H_2 coupling interval of 400 msec, the A_2H_2 interval is now 340 msec, and typical AV nodal reentry tachycardia is induced (**C**). Slow pathway conduction remains present until an A_1A_2 coupling interval of 350 msec, representing the effective refractory period of the slow AV nodal pathway (see the discontinuous preablation AV nodal function curves in **D**).

(*continued*)

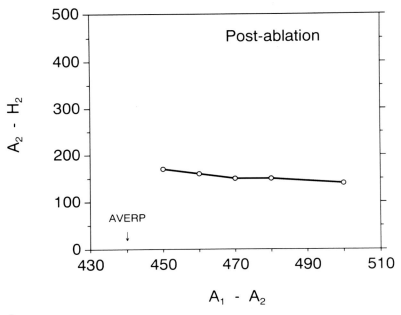

E

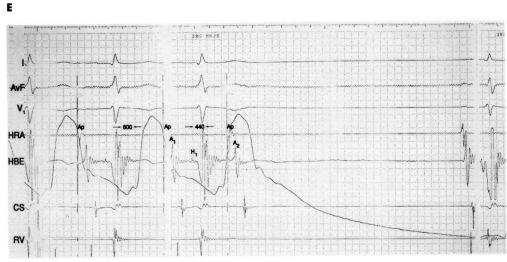

F

Figure 29-22. (*continued*) Following selective slow pathway ablation, an atrial premature beat with an A_1A_2 interval of 440 msec now fails to conduct (**E**). The postablation AV nodal function curve is shown in **F**. The A–H interval during the 600-msec straight atrial pacing drive train remained unchanged compared with its preablation value of 130 msec, illustrating unaffected fast-pathway function. Retrograde V–A conduction was also unchanged (VA Wenckebach cycle length was 360 msec preablation and 350 msec postablation). Thus, selective ablation of the slow pathway was achieved. Abbreviations as in Figures 29-11, 29-12, and 29-15.

crete from the surrounding atrium. This theory assumes that the fast and slow pathways and the tissue between them are all part of an extended AV node complex occupying most of Koch's triangle. This view is supported by the ability, in some patients, to transiently induce AVNRT without any evident atrial depolarization, as well as the ability to demonstrate atrial dissociation from the AVNRT with atrial pacing during the arrhythmia.[144, 145]

Atrial Flutter and Atrial Tachycardia

Several recent reports have documented successful use of RF energy for selective ablation of type I ("classical") atrial flutter, although widespread experience similar to that discussed above for AVNRT or accessory pathways has not yet been achieved. Successful ablation of type I atrial flutter evolved from the knowledge that this arrhythmia is due to reentry in the right atrium and that a defined area of slow conduction critical for the maintenance of this arrhythmia is present in the low posteroseptal right atrium, usually either just posterior or just inferior to the os of the coronary sinus.[146, 147] This area of slow conduction could be identified by prolonged low-amplitude fragmented electrical activity, early activation compared with the surface flutter waves during atrial flutter, and stimulus to P-wave intervals, when pacing from this site, that were fairly short (i.e., 20 to 40 msec), suggesting that the target was at the exit site from the area of slow conduction.[148] Feld and coworkers recently reported a series of 12 consecutive patients undergoing RF ablation for atrial flutter.[148] In 10 of the 12 patients (83%), RF energy (one to 14 applications) delivered at sites inferior or posterior to the coronary sinus ostium (identified as discussed above) resulted in termination and prevention of reinduction of atrial flutter. After a mean follow-up of 16 weeks, atrial flutter recurred in two patients, one of whom underwent repeat successful ablation; three patients developed self-limited infrequent recurrences of new atrial flutter or fibrillation. In another study involving nine patients, RF current terminated atrial flutter in all patients, although more than 50% of them had subsequent recurrences.[149] No complications were reported in either series.

With use of similar mapping techniques, a large degree of success has also been reported in several series of atrial tachycardia. Unlike type I atrial flutter, however, in this arrhythmia the ablation site can be anywhere in either the right or left atrium, and the arrhythmia mechanism can be either abnormal automaticity or reentry.[150–155] Approximately 10% to 15% of patients with atrial tachycardia have their tachycardia localized to the sinus node area (often called sinus node reentry tachycardia); this rhythm can also be successfully ablated with RF energy without (at least in the few patients described so far) damaging normal sinus node function.[152, 156]

Ventricular Tachycardia

RF ablation has had significant success in certain subsets of patients with ventricular tachycardia, although its application to large numbers of patients with ventricular tachycardia (VT) secondary to coronary artery disease is still unclear. Probably the first type of VT for which RF ablation has been particularly successful is bundle branch reentry tachycardia, in which the right bundle branch potential provides a particularly helpful guide for mapping. Although the usual patient with bundle branch reentry tachycardia has underlying idiopathic dilated cardiomyopathy,[157–159] it can be seen in any form of heart disease, and even in patients with conduction system disease as an isolated finding.[160] Several recent reports have highlighted the almost uniformly successful ability of ablation directed at the right bundle branch to cure this disease, making it important to rule out this easily treatable form of VT in any patient with this diagnosis.[157, 158]

Almost as successful has been the use of RF energy in so-called idiopathic left ventricular tachycardia (also referred to as exercise-induced tachycardia or verapamil-sensitive tachycardia) and right ventricular outflow tract tachycardia. Common to both of these disorders is the absence of any underlying heart disease; both arrhythmias are now felt to represent relatively small foci of reentry in either the lower septal portion of the left ventricle or the right ventricular outflow tract, respectively.[161–165] In some patients, triggered activity mediated by cyclic AMP has been implicated based on the patients' unique sensitivity to adenosine.[166, 167] Several recent reports have documented striking success for RF ablation in all of these entities, presumably on the basis of the rather small tachycardia zone, which in turn is composed of normal or near-normal tissue.[21, 166, 168] Mapping is usually performed with a combination of activation mapping during tachycardia and pace mapping morphology.

In contrast, in the much more common form of ventricular tachycardia related to coronary artery disease, catheter ablation has enjoyed much less success. The tachycardias are often faster and less stable, making mapping more difficult. Also, there are frequently multiple tachycardia morphologies in any particular patient. Animal studies and results of VT mapping in patients during surgery suggest that VT related to coronary disease can be complex and spread out over large areas of both the endocardial and epicardial surfaces of the heart.[169–174] As a result, the difficulty may lie in the fact that RF energy may not produce large enough lesions to reliably cure VT related to coronary artery disease. Alternatively, the limitation may be our scant understanding of this complex arrhythmia and thus our inability to localize the truly critical area that would be the best target for ablation. Nevertheless, Morady and colleagues published a series of 15 patients with 20 morphologies of VT related to coronary artery disease that were felt to be stable enough in the electrophysiology lab to allow mapping and ablation.[20] Sixteen of these 20 VT morphologies in 11 of the 15 patients were successfully ablated with no recurrences of the ablated VT morphologies during a mean of 9 months of follow-up. Appropriate target sites for ablation were selected on the basis of endocardial activation mapping (using the criterion of local endocardial activation time, relative to the onset of the QRS complex during VT, of at least -70 msec), identification of an isolated mid-diastolic potential, concealed entrainment, or pace mapping. Although these results will need to be confirmed in larger series of patients, they at least suggest that RF ablation may have a significant potential in this disorder as well.

CONCLUSIONS

On the basis of these exciting clinical results in many areas, it is clear why radiofrequency energy has become the technique of choice for catheter ablation and why DC energy is considered by some authors to be outmoded.[175] Over the past few years, the number of RF ablation procedures performed and the number of hospitals and electrophysiology laboratories performing them have increased dramatically.[176] These procedures not only improve the quality of life of affected patients (by changing a lifelong disease requiring expensive medications with potential side effects and often frequent relapses into a long-term cure free of medications) but also have been shown to be quite beneficial from a cost-effective view.[177, 178] Perhaps the greatest tribute to the benefits of RF energy is the realization that it took only about 5 years from the first animal studies using RF energy for catheter ablation (discussed at the beginning of this chapter) for RF energy catheter ablation to be established as the "procedure of choice" for many arrhythmias.[80, 179]

References

1. D'Arsonval M: Action physiologique des courants alternatifs. Comp Rend Soc De Biol 1891;43:283.
2. McLean A: The Bovie electrosurgical current generator. Arch Surg 1929;18:1863.
3. Fox J: Experimental relationship of radiofrequency electrical current and lesion size for application to percutaneous cordotomy. J Neurosurg 1970;33:415.
4. Organ LW: Electrophysiologic principles of radiofrequency lesion making. Appl Neurophysiol 1976;39:69.
5. Dickson JA, Calderwood SK: Temperature range and selective sensitivity of tumors to hyperthermia: a critical review. Ann NY Acad Sci 1980;335:180.
6. Pawl PP: Percutaneous radiofrequency electrocoagulation in the control of chronic pain. Surg Clin North Am 1975; 55:167.
7. Huang SKS, Bharati S, Graham AR, Lev M, Marcus FI, Odell RS: Closed chest catheter desiccation of the atrioventricular junction using radiofrequency energy—A new method of catheter ablation. J Am Coll Cardiol 1987;9:349.
8. Hoyt RH, Huang SKS, Marcus FI, Odell RS: Factors influencing trans-catheter radiofrequency ablation of the myocardium. J Appl Cardiol 1986;1:469.
9. Huang SKS, Bharati S, Lev M, Marcus FI: Electrophysiologic and histologic observations of chronic atrioventricular block induced by closed-chest catheter desiccation with radiofrequency energy. Pacing Clin Electrophysiol 1987;10:805.
10. Ring ME, Huang SKS, Graham AR, Gorman G, Bharati S, Lev M: Catheter ablation of the ventricular septum with radiofrequency energy. Am Heart J 1989;117:1233.
11. Huang SKS, Graham AR, Wharton K: Radiofrequency catheter ablation of the left and right ventricles: anatomic and electrophysiologic observations. Pacing Clin Electrophysiol 1988;11:449.
12. Langberg JJ, Chin MC, Rosenqvist M, et al: Catheter ablation of the atrioventricular junction with radiofrequency energy. Circulation 1989;80:1527.
13. Jackman WM, Wang X, Friday KJ, et al: Catheter ablation of atrioventricular junction using radiofrequency current in 17 patients: comparison of standard and large-tip catheter electrodes. Circulation 1991;83:1562.
14. Lee MA, Morady F, Kadish A, et al: Catheter modification of the atrioventricular junction with radiofrequency energy for control of atrioventricular nodal reentry tachycardia. Circulation 1991;83:827.
15. Haissaguerre M, Gaita F, Fischer B, et al: Elimination of atrioventricular nodal reentrant tachycardia using discrete slow potentials to guide application of radiofrequency energy. Circulation 1992;85:2162.
16. Kay GN, Epstein AE, Dailey SM, Plumb VJ: Selective radiofrequency ablation of the slow pathway for the treatment of atrioventricular nodal reentrant tachycardia: evidence for involvement of perinodal myocardium within the reentrant circuit. Circulation 1992;85:1675.
17. Jackman WM, Beckman KJ, McClelland JH, et al: Treatment of supraventricular tachycardia due to atrioventricular nodal reentry by radiofrequency catheter ablation of slow-pathway conduction. N Engl J Med 1992;327:313.
18. Calkins H, Sousa J, El-Atassi R, et al: Diagnosis and cure of the Wolff-Parkinson-White syndrome or paroxysmal supraventricular tachycardias during a single electrophysiologic test. N Engl J Med 1991;324:1612.
19. Jackman WM, Xunzhang W, Friday KJ, et al: Catheter ablation of accessory atrioventricular pathways (Wolff-Parkinson-White syndrome) by radiofrequency current. N Engl J Med 1991;324:1605.
20. Morady F, Harvey M, Kalbfleisch SJ, El-Atassi R, Calkins H, Langberg JJ: Radiofrequency catheter ablation of ventricular tachycardia in patients with coronary artery disease. Circulation 1993;87:363.
21. Klein LS, Shih HT, Hackett FK, Zipes DP, Miles WM: Radiofrequency catheter ablation of ventricular tachycardia in patients without structural heart disease. Circulation 1992;85:1666.
22. Gedes LA, Baker LE, Moore AG, Coulter TW: Hazards in the use of low frequencies for the measurement of physiological events by impedance. Med Biol Eng 1969;7:289.
23. Moore EN, Schaefer W, Kadish A, Hanich RF, Spear JF, Levine JH: Electrophysiological studies on cardiac catheter ablation. Pacing Clin Electrophysiol 1989;12:150.
24. Fisher JD, Kim SG, Matos JA, Waspe LE, Brodman R, Meray A: Complications of catheter ablation of tachyarrhythmias: occurrence, protection, prevention. Clin Prog Electrophysiol Pacing 1985;3:292.
25. Jones JL, Lepeschkin E, Jones RE, Rush S: Response of cultured myocardial cells to countershock-type electric field stimulation. Am J Physiol 1978;235:214.
26. Bardy GH, Ivey T, Coltori F, Stewart RB, Johnson G, Greene L: Developments, complications, and limitations of catheter-mediated electrical ablation of posterior accessory atrioventricular pathways. Am J Cardiol 1988;61:1309.

27. Fisher JD, Brodman R, Kim SG, et al: Attempted nonsurgical ablation of accessory pathways via the coronary sinus in the Wolff-Parkinson-White syndrome. J Am Coll Cardiol 1984; 4:685.

28. Brodman R, Fisher JD: Evaluation of catheter technique for ablation of accessory pathways near the coronary sinus using a canine model. Circulation 1983;67:923.

29. Lemery R, Leung TK, Lavallee E, et al: In vitro and in vivo effects within the coronary sinus of nonarcing and arcing shocks using a new system of low-energy DC ablation. Circulation 1991;83:279.

30. Linker NJ, Ward DE, Davies MJ, Camm AJ: Fatal coronary sinus rupture following attempted catheter ablation of an accessory pathway. J Electrophysiol 1989;3:2.

31. Feld M, Fisher J, Brodman R, Gollier F: Coronary sinus rupture complicating catheter ablation of atrioventricular junction. J Electrophysiol 1987;1:257.

32. Alberts WW, Wright EW, Feinstein V: Sensory responses elicited by subcortical high frequency electrical stimulation in man. J Neurosurg 1972;36:80.

33. Haines DE, Watson DD: Tissue heating during radiofrequency catheter ablation: a thermodynamic model and observations in isolated perfused and superfused canine right ventricular free wall. Pacing Clin Electrophysiol 1989; 12:962.

34. Twidale N, Wang X, Beckman KJ, et al: Factors associated with recurrence of accessory pathway conduction after radiofrequency catheter ablation. Pacing Clin Electrophysiol 1991;14:2042.

35. Haverkamp W, Hindricks G, Gulker H, et al: Coagulation of ventricular myocardium using radiofrequency alternating current: biophysical aspects and experimental findings. Pacing Clin Electrophysiol 1989;12:1.

36. Haines DE: Determinants of lesion size during radiofrequency catheter ablation: the role of electrode–tissue contact pressure and duration of energy delivery. J Cardiovasc Electrophysiol 1991;2:509.

37. Whayne JG, Nath S, Haines DE: What is the isotherm and time course of lesion formation in microwave versus radiofrequency catheter ablation? Circulation [Abstract] 1992; 86(suppl I):783.

38. Hindricks G, Haverkamp W, Gulker H: Radiofrequency coagulation of ventricular myocardium: improved prediction of lesion size by monitoring catheter tip temperature. Eur Heart J 1989;10:972.

39. Roti JL, Laszlo A: The effects of hyperthermia on cellular macromolecules. In: Urano M, Douple E, eds. Hyperthermia and Oncology, vol 1: Thermal Effects on Cells and Tissues. Utrecht, The Netherlands: VSP, 1988:13.

40. Raaphorst GP: Fundamental aspects of hyperthermic biology. In: Field SB, Hand JW, eds. An Introduction to the Practical Aspects of Clinical Hyperthermia. London: Taylor and Francis, 1990:10.

41. Wittkampf FH, Hauer RNW, Robles de Medina EO: Control of radiofrequency lesion size by power regulation. Circulation 1989;80:962.

42. Jackman WM, Kuck K-H, Naccarelli GV, Carmen L, Pitha J: Radiofrequency current directed across the mitral annulus with a bipolar epicardial-endocardial catheter electrode configuration in dogs. Circulation 1988;78:1288.

43. Langberg J, Griffin JC, Herre JM, et al: Catheter ablation of accessory pathways using radiofrequency energy in the canine coronary sinus. J Am Coll Cardiol 1989;13:491.

44. Grogan EW, Subramanian R, Whitesell LF, Nellis SH: Catheter ablation in the canine coronary sinus using radiofrequency energy. J Electrophysiol 1989;3:135.

45. Lee MA, Huang SK, Graham AR, Gorman G, Bharati S, Lev M: Radiofrequency catheter ablation of the canine atrium and tricuspid annulus. Circulation 1987;76(IV):405.

46. Jackman WM, Kuck K-H, Naccarelli GV, Pitha J, Carmen L: Catheter ablation at the tricuspid annulus using radiofrequency current in canines. J Am Coll Cardiol 1987;9:99.

47. Huang SK, Graham AR, Hoyt RH, Odell RC: Transcatheter desiccation of the canine left ventricle using radiofrequency energy: a pilot study. Am Heart J 1987;114:42.

48. Naccarelli GV, Kuck K-H, Pitha JV, Carmen L, Jackman WM: Catheter ablation of canine ventricular myocardium utilizing radiofrequency current. J Electrophysiol 1989;3:223.

49. Huang SKS, Graham AR, Lee MA, Ring ME, Gorman GD, Schiffman R: Comparison of catheter ablation using radiofrequency versus direct current energy: biophysical, electrophysiologic and pathologic observations. J Am Coll Cardiol 1991;18:1091.

50. Hauer RNW, de Bakker JMT, de Wilde AAM, et al: Ventricular tachycardia after in vivo DC shock ablation in dogs: electrophysiologic and histologic correlation. Circulation 1991; 84:267.

51. Levine J, Spear J, Weisman H, et al: The cellular electrophysiologic changes induced by high-energy electrical ablation in canine myocardium. Circulation 1986;73:818.

52. Haines DE, Watson DD, Verow AF: Electrode radius predicts radius during radiofrequency energy heating. Circ Res 1990;67:124.

53. Ring ME, Huang SK, Gorman G, et al: Determinants of impedance rise during catheter ablation of bovine myocardium with radiofrequency energy. Pacing Clin Electrophysiol 1989;12:1502.

54. Langberg JJ, Lee MA, Chin MC, et al: Radiofrequency catheter ablation: the effect of electrode size on lesion volume in vivo. Pacing Clin Electrophysiol 1990;13:1242.

55. Langberg JJ, Gallagher M, Strickberger SA, Amirana O: Temperature-guided radiofrequency catheter ablation with very large distal electrodes. Circulation 1993;88:245.

56. Wittkampf FH, Hauer RN, Robles de Medina EO: Radiofrequency ablation with a cooled porous electrode catheter. J Am Coll Cardiol [Abstract] 1988;11(2):17.

57. Huang SKS, Cuenoud H, Tandeguzman W: Increase in the lesion size and decrease in the impedance rise with a saline infusion electrode catheter for radiofrequency catheter ablation. Circulation [Abstract] 1989;80(4):II.

58. Oeff M, Langberg JJ, Chin MC, Finkbeiner WE, Scheinman MM: Ablation of ventricular tachycardia using multiple sequential transcatheter application of radiofrequency energy. Pacing Clin Electrophysiol 1992;15:1167.

59. Desai J, Nyo H, Vera Z, Tesluk H: Two phase radiofrequency catheter ablation of isolated ventricular endomyocardium. Pacing Clin Electrophysiol 1991;14:1179.

60. Coggins D, Chin M, Wonnell T, Stauffer P, Scheinman M, Langberg J: Efficacy of microwave energy for ventricular ablation. Pacing Clin Electrophysiol [Abstract] 1991; 14(II):703.

61. Gadhoke A, Aronovitz M, Zebede J, Manolis A, Estes NAM III: Are tissue contact and catheter orientation important variables in microwave ablation? Circulation [Abstract] 1992; 86(I):191.

62. Langberg JJ, Wonnell T, Chin MC, Finkbeiner W, Scheinman M, Stauffer P: Catheter ablation of the atrioventricular junction using a helical microwave antenna: a novel means of coupling energy to the endocardium. Pacing Clin Electrophysiol 1991;14:2105.

63. Wagshal AB, Huang SKS, Lin JC, et al: Use of a newly-designed microwave antenna for catheter ablation of the atrioventricular junction. J Am Coll Cardiol [Abstract] 1994;23:82A.

64. Blouin LT, Marcus FI, Lampe L: Assessment of effects of a radiofrequency energy field and thermistor location in an electrode catheter on the accuracy of temperature measurement. Pacing Clin Electrophysiol 1991;14:807.

65. Haines DE, Verow AF: Observations on electrode–tissue interface temperature and effect on electrical impedance during radiofrequency ablation of ventricular myocardium. Circulation 1990;82:1034.

66. Frohmer KJ, Podczeck A, Hief C, et al: Thermal catheter disruption during closed-chest radiofrequency ablation of the atrioventricular conduction system. Pacing Clin Electrophysiol 1990;13:719.

67. Pires LA, Huang SKS, Wagshal AB, Mittleman RS, Rittman WJ: Temperature-guided radiofrequency catheter ablation of closed-chest ventricular myocardium with a novel thermistor-tipped catheter. Am Heart J 1994;127:1614.

68. Haines DE, Watson DD, Halperin C: Monitoring electrode tip temperature during radiofrequency fulguration of ventricular myocardium is strongly predictive of lesion size. Circulation [Abstract] 1987;76(suppl IV):406.

69. Langberg JJ, Calkins H, El-Atassi R, et al: Temperature monitoring during radiofrequency catheter ablation of accessory pathways. Circulation 1992;86:1469.

70. Calkins H, Prystowsky E, Carlson D, et al: Site-dependent variability of electrode temperature during radiofrequency catheter ablation procedure. J Am Coll Cardiol [Abstract] 1994;23:276A.

71. Chen X, Borggrefe M, Hindricks G, et al: Radiofrequency ablation of accessory pathways; characteristics of transiently and permanently effective pulses. Pacing Clin Electrophysiol 1992;15:1122.

72. Langberg JJ, Calkins H, Kim Y, et al: Recurrence of conduction in accessory atrioventricular connections after initially successful radiofrequency catheter ablation. J Am Coll Cardiol 1992;19:1588.

73. Leitch JW, Klein GJ, Yee R, Leather RA, Kim YH: Does delayed loss of preexcitation after unsuccessful radiofrequency catheter ablation of accessory pathways result in permanent cure? Am J Cardiol 1992;70:830.

74. Wagshal AB, Pires LA, Mittleman RS, Cuello C, Bonavita GJ, Huang SKS: Early recurrence of accessory pathways after radiofrequency ablation does not preclude long-term cure. Am J Cardiol 1993;72:843.

75. Langberg JJ, Borganelli SM, Kalbfleisch SJ, Strickberger SA, Calkins H, Morady F: Delayed effects of radiofrequency energy on accessory atrioventricular connections. Pacing Clin Electrophysiol 1993;16:1001.

76. Dick M II, Dorostkar PC, Serwer G, Leroy S, Armstrong B: Delayed response to radiofrequency ablation of accessory connections. Pacing Clin Electrophysiol 1993;16:2143.

77. Stein KM, Lerman BB: Delayed success following radiofrequency catheter ablation. Pacing Clin Electrophysiol 1993;16:698.

78. Nath S, Whayne JG, Kaul S, et al: Effects of radiofrequency catheter ablation on regional myocardial blood flow: possible mechanism for late electrophysiological outcome. Circulation 1994;89:2672.

79. Delacey WA, Nath S, Haines DE, et al: Adenosine and verapamil-sensitive ventricular tachycardia originating from the left ventricle: radiofrequency catheter ablation. Pacing Clin Electrophysiol 1992;15:2240.

80. Scheinman MM: NASPE Policy Statement: Catheter ablation for cardiac arrhythmias, personnel, and facilities. Pacing Clin Electrophysiol 1992;15:715.

81. Greene TO, Pires LA, Cuello C, et al: Cardiovascular complications following radiofrequency catheter ablation of supraventricular tachyarrhythmias. Pacing Clin Electrophysiol [Abstract] 1993;16(II):946.

82. Olgin JE, Scheinman MM: Comparison of high energy direct current and radiofrequency catheter ablation of the atrioventricular junction. J Am Coll Cardiol 1993;21:557.

83. Chiang CE, Chen SA, Wang DC, et al: Arrhythmogenicity of catheter ablation in supraventricular tachycardia. Am Heart J 1993;125:388.

84. Twidale N, Beckman KJ, Hazlitt HA, et al: Radiofrequency catheter ablation of accessory pathways: are the ventricular lesions arrhythmogenic? Circulation [Abstract] 1991;84 (II):710.

85. Mittleman RS, Greene TO, Pires LA, et al: New atrial tachycardia occurring early after radiofrequency ablation of the slow pathway for AV nodal reentrant tachycardia. Circulation [Abstract] 1993;88(I):492.

86. Nath S, Lynch C, Whayne JG, Haines DE: Cellular electrophysiologic effects of hyperthermia on isolated guinea pig papillary muscle: implications for catheter ablation. Circulation 1993;88:1826.

87. Moulton K, Miller B, Scott J, Woods WT: Radiofrequency catheter ablation for AV nodal reentry: a technique for rapid transection of the slow AV nodal pathway. Pacing Clin Electrophysiol 1993;16:760.

88. Wang X, McClelland JH, Beckman KJ, et al: Accelerated junctional rhythm during slow pathway ablation. Circulation [Abstract] 1991;84(II):583.

89. Thakur RK, Klein GJ, Yee R, Stites W: Junctional tachycardia: a useful marker during radiofrequency ablation for atrioventricular node reentrant tachycardia. J Am Coll Cardiol 1993;22:1706.

90. Ge YZ, Shao PZ, Goldberger J, Kadish A: Cellular electrophysiologic changes induced in vitro by radiofrequency current: comparison with high energy electrical ablation. Pacing Clin Electrophysiol (In press)

91. Lesh MD, Van Hare GF, Schamp DJ, et al: Curative percutaneous catheter ablation using radiofrequency energy for ac-

cessory pathways in all locations: results in 100 consecutive patients. J Am Coll Cardiol 1992;19:1303.

92. Pires LA, Wagshal AB, Yong PG, et al: Clinical utility of 2-D echocardiography after uncomplicated radiofrequency catheter ablation—a prospective multicenter study. Circulation [Abstract] 1993;88(I):61.

93. Strickberger SA, Okishige K, Meyerovitz M, et al: Evaluation of possible long-term adverse consequences of radiofrequency ablation of accessory pathways. Am J Cardiol 1993; 71:473.

94. Solomon AJ, Tracy CM, Swartz JF, et al: Effect on coronary artery anatomy of radiofrequency catheter ablation of atrial insertion sites of accessory pathways. J Am Coll Cardiol 1993;21:1440.

95. Brodman R: Catheter ablation: a former arrhythmia surgeon's view. Pacing Clin Electrophysiol 1992;15:1231.

96. Calkins H, Niklason L, Sousa J, et al: Radiation exposure during radiofrequency catheter ablation of accessory atrioventricular connections. Circulation 1991;84:2376.

97. Lindsay BD, Eichling J, Dieter HD, et al: Radiation exposure to patients and physicians during radiofrequency catheter ablation for supraventricular tachycardias. Circulation [Abstract] 1991;84:II-646.

98. Kay GN, Epstein AE, Dailey SM, Plumb VJ: Role of radiofrequency ablation in the management of supraventricular arrhythmias: experience in 760 consecutive patients. J Cardiovasc Electrophysiol 1993;4:371.

99. Schluter M, Geiger M, Siebels J, Duckeck W, Kuck K-H: Catheter ablation using radiofrequency current to cure symptomatic patients with tachyarrhythmias related to an accessory atrioventricular pathway. Circulation 1991;84:1644.

100. Calkins H, Langberg JJ, Sousa J, et al: Radiofrequency catheter ablation of accessory atrioventricular connections in 250 patients: abbreviated therapeutic approach to Wolff-Parkinson-White syndrome. Circulation 1992;85:1137.

101. Silka MJ, Kron J, Halperin BD, et al: Analysis of local electrogram characteristics correlated with successful radiofrequency catheter ablation of accessory atrioventricular pathways. Pacing Clin Electrophysiol 1992;15:1000.

102. Chen X, Borggrefe M, Shenasa M, Haverkamp W, Hindricks G, Breithard G: Characteristics of local electrogram predicting successful transcatheter radiofrequency ablation of left-sided accessory pathways. J Am Coll Cardiol 1992;20:656.

103. Calkins H, Kim Y, Schmaltz S, et al: Electrogram criteria for identification of appropriate target sites for radiofrequency catheter ablation of accessory atrioventricular connections. Circulation 1992;85:565.

104. Jackman WM, Friday KJ, Scherlag BJ, et al: Direct endocardial recording from an accessory atrioventricular pathway: localization of the site of block, effect of antiarrhythmic drugs, and attempt at nonsurgical ablation. Circulation 1983;68:906.

105. Jackman WM, Friday KJ, Yeung-Lai-Wah JA, et al: New catheter technique for recording left free-wall accessory atrioventricular pathway activation: identification of pathway fiber orientation. Circulation 1988;78:598.

106. Lesh MD, Van Hare GF, Scheinman MM, Ports TA, Epstein LA: Comparison of the retrograde and transseptal methods for ablation of left free wall accessory pathways. J Am Coll Cardiol 1993;22:542.

107. Saul JP, Hulse E, De W, et al: Catheter ablation of accessory atrioventricular pathways in young patients: use of long vascular sheaths, the transseptal approach and a retrograde left posterior parallel approach. J Am Coll Cardiol 1993; 21:571.

108. Swartz JF, Tracy CM, Fletcher RD: Radiofrequency endocardial catheter ablation of accessory atrioventricular pathway atrial insertion sites. Circulation 1993;87:487.

109. Guiraudon GM, Guiraudon CM, Klein GJ, et al: The coronary sinus diverticulum: a pathologic entity associated with the Wolff-Parkinson-White syndrome. Am J Cardiol 1988;62: 733.

110. Lesh MD, Van Hare G, Kao AK, Scheinman MM: Radiofrequency catheter ablation for Wolff-Parkinson-White syndrome associated with a coronary sinus diverticulum. Pacing Clin Electrophysiol 1991;14:1479.

111. Langberg JJ, Man KC, Vorperian VR, et al: Recognition and catheter ablation of subepicardial accessory pathways. J Am Coll Cardiol 1993;22:1100.

112. Davis LM, Byth K, Ellis P, et al: Dimensions of the human posterior septal space and coronary sinus. Am J Cardiol 1991;68:621.

113. Lesh MD, Van Hare GF, Chien WW, Scheinman MM: Mapping in the right coronary artery as an aid to radiofrequency ablation of right-sided accessory pathways. Pacing Clin Electrophysiol [Abstract] 1991;14(II):671.

114. Schlüter M, Kuck K-H: Catheter ablation from right atrium of anteroseptal accessory pathways using radiofrequency current. J Am Coll Cardiol 1992;19:663.

115. Kuck K-H, Schlüter M, Gursoy S: Preservation of atrioventricular nodal conduction during radiofrequency current catheter ablation of midseptal accessory pathways. Circulation 1992;86:1743.

116. Morady F, Calkins H, Langberg JJ, et al: A prospective randomized comparison of direct current and radiofrequency ablation of the atrioventricular junction. J Am Coll Cardiol 1993;21:102.

117. Sousa J, El-Atassi R, Rosenheck S, et al: Radiofrequency catheter ablation of the atrioventricular junction from the left ventricle. Circulation 1991;84:567.

118. Trohman RG, Simmons TW, Moore SL, et al: Catheter ablation of the atrioventricular junction using radiofrequency energy and a bilateral cardiac approach. Am J Cardiol 1992; 70:1438.

119. Souza O, Gursoy S, Simonis F, et al: Right-sided vs left-sided radiofrequency ablation of the His bundle. Pacing Clin Electrophysiol 1992;15:1454.

120. Kalbfleisch SJ, Hummel JD, Man C, et al: A prospective randomized comparison of right vs left-sided radiofrequency ablation of the atrioventricular junction. Pacing Clin Electrophysiol [Abstract] 1992;16(II):93.

121. Cuello C, Huang SKS, Wagshal AB, Pires LA, Mittleman RS, Bonavita GJ: Radiofrequency catheter ablation of the atrioventricular junction by a supravalvular noncoronary aortic cusp approach. Pacing Clin Electrophysiol 1994;17:1182.

122. Huang SKS: Predictors of successful catheter ablation of the atrioventricular junction with radiofrequency energy. Pacing Clin Electrophysiol 1989;12:675.

123. Fleck RP, Chen P-S, Boyce K, Ross R, Dittrich HC, Feld GK: Radiofrequency modification of atrioventricular conduction by selective ablation of the low posterior septal right atrium

in a patient with atrial fibrillation and a rapid ventricular response. Pacing Clin Electrophysiol 1993;16:377.

124. Gillette PC, Smith RT, Garson A, et al: Chronic supraventricular tachycardia: a curable cause of congestive heart failure. JAMA 1985;253:391.

125. Rodriguez LM, Smeets LRM, Xie B, et al: Improvement in left ventricular function by ablation of atrioventricular nodal conduction in selected patients with lone atrial fibrillation. Am J Cardiol 1993;72:1137.

126. Huang SKS, Bharati S, Graham AR, Gorman G, Lev M: Chronic incomplete atrioventricular block induced by radiofrequency catheter ablation. Circulation 1989;80:951.

127. Haissaguerre M, Warin JF, Lemetayer P, Saoudi N, Guillem JP, Blanchot P: Closed-chest ablation of retrograde conduction in patients with atrioventricular nodal reentrant tachycardia. N Engl J Med 1989;320:426.

128. Goy JJ, Fromer M, Schlaepfer J, et al: Clinical efficacy of radiofrequency current in the treatment of patients with atrioventricular node reentrant tachycardia. J Am Coll Cardiol 1990;16:418.

129. Langberg JJ, Leon A, Borganelli M, et al: A randomized, prospective comparison of anterior and posterior approaches to radiofrequency catheter ablation of atrioventricular nodal reentry tachycardia. Circulation 1993;87:1551.

130. Langberg JJ, Harvey M, Calkins H, El-Atassi R, Kalbfleisch SJ, Morady F: Titration of power output during radiofrequency catheter ablation of atrioventricular nodal reentrant tachycardia. Pacing Clin Electrophysiol 1993;16:465.

131. Denes P, Wu D, Dhingra RC, Chuquimia R, Rosen KM: Demonstration of dual A-V nodal pathways in patients with paroxysmal supraventricular tachycardia. Circulation 1973; 48:549.

132. Sung RJ, Waxman HL, Saksena S, Juma Z: Sequence of retrograde atrial activation in patients with dual atrioventricular nodal pathways. Circulation 1981;64:1059.

133. Roman C, Wang X, Friday K, et al: Catheter technique for selective ablation of slow pathway in AV nodal reentrant tachycardia. Pacing Clin Electrophysiol [Abstract] 1990;13:498.

134. Mitrani RD, Klein LS, Hackett FK, Zipes DP, Miles WM: Radiofrequency ablation for atrioventricular node reentrant tachycardia: comparison between fast (anterior) and slow (posterior) pathway ablation. J Am Coll Cardiol 1993;21:432.

135. Jazayeri MR, Hempe SL, Sra JS, et al: Selective transcatheter ablation of the fast and slow pathways using radiofrequency energy in patients with atrioventricular nodal reentrant tachycardia. Circulation 1992;85:1318.

136. Lindsay BD, Chung MK, Gamache C, et al: Therapeutic end points for the treatment of atrioventricular node reentrant tachycardia by catheter-guided radiofrequency current. J Am Coll Cardiol 1993;22:733.

137. Baker JH, Plumb VJ, Epstein AE, Kay GN: Selective ablation of the slow AV nodal pathway: predictors of recurrent AV nodal reentrant tachycardia. Circulation [Abstract] 1992;86(suppl I):521.

138. Li HG, Klein GJ, Stites HW, et al: Elimination of slow pathway conduction: an accurate indicator of clinical success after radiofrequency atrioventricular node modification. J Am Coll Cardiol 1993;22:1849.

139. Goldberger J, Brooks R, Kadish A: Physiology of atypical atrioventricular junctional reentrant tachycardia occurring following radiofrequency catheter modification of the atrioventricular node. Pacing Clin Electrophysiol 1992; 15:2270.

140. Langberg JJ, Kim Y, Goyal R, et al: Conversion of typical to "atypical" atrioventricular nodal reentrant tachycardia after radiofrequency catheter modification of the atrioventricular junction. Am J Cardiol 1992;65:503.

141. Racker DK: Sinoventricular transmission in 10 mM K+ by the canine atrioventricular inputs, the superior atrionodal bundle and the proximal atrioventricular bundle. Circulation 1991;83:1745.

142. Keim S, Werner P, Jazayeri M, Akhtar M, Tchou P: Localization of the fast and slow pathways in atrioventricular nodal reentrant tachycardia by intraoperative ice mapping. Circulation 1992;86:919.

143. Satoh M, Miyajima S, Koyama S, Ishiguro J, Okabe M: Orthodromic capture of the atrial electrogram during transient entrainment of atrioventricular nodal reentrant tachycardia. Circulation 1993;88(I):2329.

144. Josephson ME, Miller JM: Atrioventricular nodal reentry: evidence supporting an intranodal location. Pacing Clin Electrophysiol 1993;16(II):599.

145. Wu D, Yeh S-J, Wang C-C, Wen M-S, Chang H-J, Lin F-C: Nature of dual atrioventricular node pathways and the tachycardia circuit as defined by radiofrequency ablation technique. J Am Coll Cardiol 1992;20:884.

146. Cosio FG, Arribas F, Palacios J, Tascon J, Lopez-Gil M: Fragmented electrograms and continuous electrical activity in atrial flutter. Am J Cardiol 1986;57:1309.

147. Olshansky B, Okumura K, Hess PG, Waldo AL: Demonstration of an area of slow conduction in human atrial flutter. J Am Coll Cardiol 1990;16:1639.

148. Feld GF, Fleck RP, Chen P-S, et al: Radiofrequency catheter ablation for the treatment of human type I atrial flutter: identification of a critical zone in the reentrant circuit by endocardial mapping techniques. Circulation 1992;86:1233.

149. Cosio FG, Lopez-Gil M, Goicolea A, Arribas F, Barroso JL: Radiofrequency ablation of the inferior vena cava–tricuspid valve isthmus in common atrial flutter. Am J Cardiol 1993; 71:705.

150. Tracy CM, Swartz JF, Fletcher RD: Radiofrequency catheter ablation of ectopic atrial tachycardia using paced activation sequence mapping. J Am Coll Cardiol 1993;21:910.

151. Wen M-S, Yeh S-J, Wang C-C, Lin F-C, Wu D: Radiofrequency ablation therapy in three patients with paroxysmal atrial tachycardia. Pacing Clin Electrophysiol 1993;16:2146.

152. Kay GN, Chong F, Epstein AE, et al: Radiofrequency ablation for treatment of primary atrial tachycardias. J Am Coll Cardiol 1993;21:901.

153. Walsh EP, Saul JP, Hulse JE, et al: Transcatheter ablation of ectopic atrial tachycardia in young patients using radiofrequency current. Circulation 1992;86:1138.

154. Goldberger J, Kall J, Ehlert F, et al: Effectiveness of radiofrequency catheter ablation for treatment of atrial tachycardia. Am J Cardiol 1993;72:787.

155. Chen S-A, Chaing C-E, Yang C-J, et al: Radiofrequency catheter ablation of sustained intra-atrial reentrant tachycardia in

adult patients: identification of electrophysiological characteristics and endocardial mapping techniques. Circulation 1993;88:578.

156. Sperry RE, Ellenbogen KA, Wood MA, Belz MK, Stambler BS: Radiofrequency catheter ablation of sinus node reentrant tachycardia. Pacing Clin Electrophysiol 1993;16:2202.

157. Cohen TJ, Chien WW, Lurie KG, et al: Radiofrequency catheter ablation for treatment of bundle branch reentrant ventricular tachycardia: results and long-term follow-up. J Am Coll Cardiol 1991;18:1767.

158. Blanck Z, Dhala A, Deshpande S, Sra J, Jazayeri M, Akhtar M: Bundle branch reentrant ventricular tachycardia: cumulative experience in 48 patients. J Cardiovasc Electrophysiol 1993;4:253.

159. Akhtar M, Damato AN, Batsford WP, Ruskin JN, Ogunkelu JB, Vargas G: Demonstration of re-entry within the His-Purkinje system in man. Circulation 1974;50:1150.

160. Blanck Z, Jazayeri M, Dhala A, Deshpande S, Sra J, Akhtar M: Bundle branch reentry: a mechanism of ventricular tachycardia in the absence of myocardial or valvular dysfunction. J Am Coll Cardiol 1993;22:1718.

161. Sung RJ, Huycke EC, Lai W-T, Tseng C-D, Chu H, Keung EC: Clinical and electrophysiologic mechanisms of exercise-induced ventricular tachyarrhythmias. Pacing Clin Electrophysiol 1988;11:1347.

162. Ohe T, Shimomura K, Aihara N, et al: Idiopathic sustained left ventricular tachycardia: clinical and electrophysiologic characteristics. Circulation 1988;77:560.

163. Okumura K, Matsuyama K, Miyagi H, Tsuchiya T, Yasue H: Entrainment of idiopathic ventricular tachycardia of left ventricular origin with evidence for reentry with an area of slow conduction and effect of verapamil. Am J Cardiol 1988; 62:727.

164. Aizawa Y, Naitoh N, Kitazawa H, et al: Frequency of presumed reentry with an excitable gap in sustained ventricular tachycardia unassociated with coronary artery disease. Am J Cardiol 1993;72:916.

165. Buxton AE, Waxman HL, Marchlinski FE, Simson MB, Cassidy D, Josephson ME: Right ventricular tachycardia: clinical and electrophysiologic characteristics. Circulation 1983; 68:917.

166. Wilber DJ, Baerman J, Olshansky B, Kall J, Kopp D: Adenosine-sensitive ventricular tachycardia: clinical characteristics and response to catheter ablation. Circulation 1993;87:126.

167. Lerman BB, Belardinelli L, West GA, Berne RM, DiMarco JP: Adenosine-sensitive ventricular tachycardia: evidence suggesting cyclic AMP-mediated triggered activity. Circulation 1986;74:270.

168. Page RL, Shenasa H, Evans JJ, Sorrentino RA, Wharton JM, Prystowsky EN: Radiofrequency catheter ablation of idiopathic recurrent ventricular tachycardia with right bundle branch block, left axis morphology. Pacing Clin Electrophysiol 1993;16:327.

169. Kaltenbrunner W, Cardinal R, Dubuc M, et al: Epicardial and endocardial mapping of ventricular tachycardia in patients with myocardial infarction: Is the origin of the tachycardia always subendocardially localized? Circulation 1991;84:1058.

170. El-Sherif N, Gough WV, Restivo M: Reentrant ventricular arrhythmias in the late myocardial infarction period; mechanism of resetting, entrainment, acceleration, or termination of reentrant tachycardia by programmed electrical stimulation. Pacing Clin Electrophysiol 1987;10:341.

171. Downar E, Harris L, Mickleborough LL, Shaikh NN, Parson ID: Endocardial mapping of ventricular tachycardia in the intact human heart: evidence for reentrant mechanisms. J Am Coll Cardiol 1988;11:783.

172. deBakker JM, van Capelle F, Janse M, et al: Macroreentry in the infarcted human heart: the mechanism of ventricular tachycardias with a "focal" activation pattern. J Am Coll Cardiol 1991;18:1005.

173. Fitzgerald DM, Friday KJ, Yeung-Lai-Wah JA, Bowman AJ, Lazzara R, Jackman WM: Myocardial regions of slow conduction participating in the reentrant circuit of multiple ventricular tachycardias: report on ten patients. J Cardiovasc Electrophysiol 1991;2:193.

174. Stevenson WG, Weiss JN, Wiener I, Nadamanee K: Slow conduction in the infarct scar: relevance to the occurrence, detection, and ablation of ventricular reentry circuits resulting from myocardial infarction. Am Heart J 1989;117:452.

175. Cunningham D: High-energy catheter ablation of cardiac arrhythmias: an outmoded technique in the 1990's. Clin Cardiol 1991;14:595.

176. Scheinman MM: North American Society of Pacing and Electrophysiology (NASPE) survey on radiofrequency catheter ablation: implications for clinicians, third party insurers, and government regulatory agencies. Pacing Clin Electrophysiol 1992;15:2228.

177. Buitler JD, Sousa J, Bolling SF, et al: Reduction in medical care cost associated with radiofrequency catheter ablation of accessory pathways. Am J Cardiol 1991;68:1656.

178. Kalbfleisch SJ, El-Atassi R, Calkins H, Langberg JJ, Morady F: Safety, feasibility, and cost of outpatient radiofrequency catheter ablation of accessory atrioventricular connections. J Am Coll Cardiol 1993;21:567.

179. DiMarco JP, Prystowsky EN, Ellenbogen KA, et al: AHA Subcommittee on Electrocardiography and Electrophysiology: catheter ablation in patients with cardiac arrhythmias (letter). Circulation 1992;85:390.

Cardiac Arrhythmias, 3rd edition, edited by William J. Mandel.
J. B. Lippincott Company, Philadelphia © 1995.

30

Michel Haissaguerre • Bruno Fischer
Frank Marcus • Jacques Clémenty

Role of Catheter Ablation for Treatment of Supraventricular Tachyarrhythmias

Curative treatment of supraventricular tachycardias was first performed using surgical procedures; more recently, catheter ablation has been used successfully. The energy source first used for catheter ablation was high-energy direct current, which was introduced in 1982 for interruption of atrioventricular (AV) conduction. The technique was then applied to all types of organized arrhythmias. From 1987, radiofrequency (RF) energy progressively replaced direct current (DC) energy because of its several advantages—particularly the better control of amount of energy delivered, the ability to direct the energy to a localized area, and the absence of barotrauma with resultant lesions that are more focal and homogenous.

We review the status of catheter ablation of supraventricular arrhythmias (excluding atrial fibrillation and His-bundle ablation) based on the literature as well as our experience of 921 patients using RF energy.

ATRIAL FLUTTER

The common type of atrial flutter, also sometimes referred to as type I, is almost unique among atrial arrhythmias because of the consistency of the atrial rate and the "saw-tooth" morphology of the flutter wave in the inferior leads. If it is often encountered as an acute or transitory arrhythmia; it may be chronic, paroxysmal, repetitive, or even permanent; the ventricular response may jump from 4:1 (75/min) to 2:1 (150/min) spontaneously or during exertion. As suggested by Puech and coworkers, this type of atrial flutter is a reentrant arrhythmia that depends on a circuit that is in the right atrium.[1-6] In a study by Klein and coworkers of three patients, preoperative endocardial mapping showed "early potentials" in reference to the negative portion of the F wave in the coronary sinus orifice region.[4] During preoperative epicardial mapping, there was a clustering of isochrones in the posteroseptal region, further suggesting that this area bounded by tricuspid anulus, coronary sinus ostium, and inferior vena cava orifice is a zone of slow conduction that may be critical to the circuit and may be interrupted by cryoablation of this area. Saumarez and associates, using computerized endocardial mapping of the AV node region, showed that atrial myocardial activation during type I atrial flutter begins at the inferior region and traverses the triangle of Koch, slowing as it does so in a region measuring about 8 × 3 mm that extends from the tricuspid anulus to the middle of the triangle and encompasses the area lateral to the coronary sinus.[6] The conduction velocity then increases rapidly near the apex of the triangle, activating the septum coincident with the negative portion of the surface electrocardiographic F wave while sweeping around the coronary sinus to fuse with the slower conducted activation wavefront in the middle of the triangle. In almost all the published reports, tachycardia endocardial mapping permits recording of fragmented potentials in the area of the inferior and posterior right atrial septum that has been suspected of being the critical slow conduction area of the reentrant circuit.[5,7-11] This led to attempted direct ablation of this area in 1987, using DC energy targeted on recording of fragmented potentials.[7,8] In our department, 27 patients underwent the fulguration procedure. As of their last follow-up visit (3 to 6 years), atrial flutter recurrences were prevented in only 9 patients (33%), and 12 (44%) had experienced episodes of paroxysmal atrial fibrillation. Nunain and associates also report successful ablation of atrial flutter in seven patients, using low-energy DC shocks delivered to the area of the coronary sinus ostium, without paying special attention to the recording of the local electrogram.[11] In this series, success may partly have been the result of the large number of shocks (up to 15) that were delivered and to the resulting relatively wide area that was ablated.

Ablation Using Radiofrequency Energy

The potential hazards of DC fulguration and its moderate long-term success in preventing late flutter recurrences led several investigators to use RF current for this indication.[12-18] The results appear to be better than those observed with fulguration. Other developments that may contribute to improvements in ablative treatment for atrial flutter include better-targeted sites for ablation. Based on their extensive experience in atrial flutter mapping, Cosio and colleagues proposed to ablate the area located between the tricuspid anulus and the inferior vena cava.[12] They proposed that the wavefront of atrial flutter is tunneled between the orifice of the inferior vena cava and the tricuspid ring. Delivery of RF energy to this area acutely terminates atrial flutter in almost all cases. Another approach reported by Feld and colleagues uses a combination of anatomic and electrophysiologic criteria.[13] Pacing at a rate slightly faster than the tachycardia rate and without changed morphology of the surface F wave (transient entrainment) and with early electrograms in reference to the surface F wave served as a target for ablation. In addition, the absence of any discernible delay between the pacing spike and the resulting electrograms was required, supporting the concept of ablation at the exit site from the area of slow conduction. Although flutter could not be terminated in all patients, short-term prevention of clinical atrial flutter recurrences was obtained in 10 of 12 patients. A third approach is the result of the observation of an association between induced AV nodal reentry tachycardia (AVNRT) and induced atrial flutter.[14] Based on the hypothesis of a shared common pathway between these arrhythmias, Interian and associates delivered RF pulses at the slow-pathway site and found that this prevented inducibility of both arrhythmias during an 8-month follow-up.[14] Finally, based on mapping studies, Nakagawa and coworkers suggested that a line of conduction block extends from the inferior vena cava to the coronary sinus

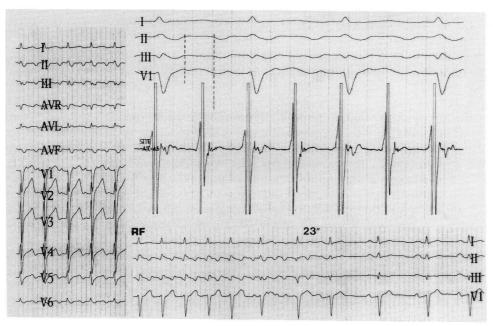

Figure 30-1. (*Left*) Twelve-lead electrogram of common atrial flutter. (*Top right*) Electrograms occurring at the middle of the plateau phase (*dotted lines*). They are recorded at the inferior vena cava–tricuspid isthmus in a stable position, evidenced by lack of beat-to-beat fluctuation of their amplitude. (Bottom right) A single radiofrequency application interrupted the atrial flutter at the 23rd second.

ostium, therefore suggesting that two isthmuses may be involved in flutter. One, as emphasized by Cosio, is between the tricuspid ring and the inferior vena cava, and the second is between the tricuspid anulus and the coronary sinus orifice.[15,16] Ablation at the first (n = 1 [number of patients]) or second (n = 7) site prevented atrial flutter recurrences in seven of eight cases after a 1-year mean follow-up.[16] Lastly, Lesh and associates reported high success rates (94%) in 18 patients by severing a critical isthmus of slow conduction bounded by anatomic or structural (including an atriotomy scar) obstacles.[18] From these experiences and those of our group, it appears clear that RF applications that terminate atrial flutter are more effective than fulguration. Figure 30-1 shows termination of tachycardia during RF-pulse delivery at the tricuspid anulus–inferior vena cava isthmus. Usually at this site, electrograms are narrow, although they have been found to also show a double spike or a fragmented aspect.

Our experience with ablation of atrial flutter includes 95 patients.[17] In the first 50 patients, RF energy was delivered during permanent or induced typical atrial flutter at sites where the electrograms occurred during the plateau phase. It is essential that the catheter position is stable, as evidenced by lack of beat-to-beat fluctuation of the amplitude of the electrogram. Three areas or isthmuses were targeted but not in any particular sequence: (1) from the tricuspid anulus to the inferior vena cava orifice, where electrograms were narrow and occurred during the first half of plateau phase; (2) from the tricuspid anulus to the coronary sinus ostium, where electrograms were narrow or sometimes dual; and (3) from the coronary sinus os to the inferior vena cava orifice, where electrograms showed a double spike or fragmented pattern. The end point was interruption of the atrial flutter and its non-inducibility. Atrial flutter was terminated in 43 patients, with six failures occurring in the first 12 patients. Figure 30-2 shows the areas where atrial flutter was interrupted and the timing of electrograms relative to the onset of F wave at the final successful sites. In a second group of 30 patients, we assessed the effects of a single line of RF lesions performed at each area described above in subgroups of 10 consecutive patients. Radiofrequency energy interrupted atrial flutter in seven of 10 patients at area 1, four of 10 patients at area 2, and one of 10 patients at area 3. In patients in whom the single RF line failed, other RF applications were delivered, either at the same or other areas, interrupting atrial flutter in 29 of 30 patients. Therefore, the highest success rate of ablation was at the isthmus between the tricuspid valve and the inferior vena cava orifice, which is the first-targeted area in our department. It is important to note that RF lesions applied at both areas 2 and 3 were not associated with as high a success rate as those applied only at area 1. This may be because of preservation of conduction in atrial fibers surrounding the proximal coronary

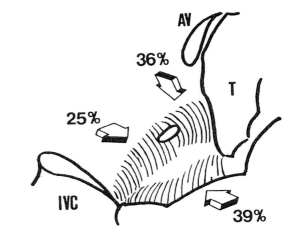

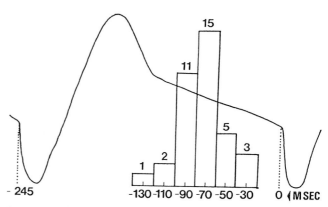

Figure 30-2. (*Top*) Sites of atrial flutter interruption (expressed as % from a group of 43 patients) between the tricuspid annulus (*T*), the coronary sinus ostium, and the inferior vena cava (*IVC*). *AV* indicates the atrioventricular nodal region. (*Bottom*) Timing of electrograms relative to the onset of F wave at the final successful sites in the first 37 successful cases.

sinus that may require RF application within the coronary sinus.

Figure 30-3 summarizes our overall results during a mean follow-up of 20 ± 8 months: 82% of patients have remained free of atrial flutter and atrial fibrillation. Atrial flutter recurred in 16 of 95 patients (17%), of whom 12 underwent a successful second and third ablation. Most importantly, interruption and noninducibility of common atrial flutter was accomplished in virtually 100% of patients, comparable with the success rate of either accessory pathways (APs) or AV nodal reentrant tachycardia. Refinement in the technique to prevent recurrences requires further understanding of the tachycardia circuit in addition to technological development in catheter design or energy sources to allow destruction of wider areas of atrial myocardium.

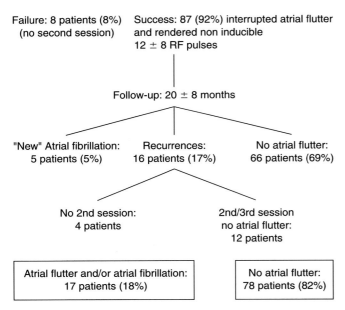

Figure 30-3. Results of radiofrequency ablation in 95 patients with common atrial flutter.

ATRIAL TACHYCARDIAS

Experience using RF ablation for atrial tachycardia is rapidly growing. The mechanism of atrial tachycardias appears to be more heterogenous than that of common atrial flutter, including reentry, abnormal automaticity, or triggered activity. In contrast to atrial flutter, these tachycardias may arise in various regions of both atria. Results using RF energy indicate a higher efficacy than for DC fulguration.[18, 20–33] Atrial tachycardia–mapping techniques generally use one or two fixed and stable intracardiac references (e.g., either the His bundle or a coronary sinus atrial electrogram or both) and two moving ablation catheters. The ablation catheters are then moved to the region that appears to be earliest in reference to the surface tachycardia P wave. Fine tuning is either by comparison with the intracardiac reference electrogram or electrograms or preferably by the second ablation catheter, which is moved around the first in search of even earlier atrial potentials. At times, fragmentation or double atrial spikes may be observed. Various pacing techniques (e.g., pace mapping during sinus rhythm to reproduce tachycardia P-wave morphology and entrainment tachycardia pace mapping) have been used to help identify the optimal ablation site but their specificity is questionable. In addition to the standard anteroposterior projection, the use of oblique views is highly recommended for better localization of the spatial catheter position. We favor the use of the projection that shows the greatest motion of the catheter tip for minimal change in position. If required, left atrial mapping may be performed through a patent foramen ovale or by transeptal catheterization.

If tachycardia is not present during mapping, it may be induced by pacing techniques or by infusion of isoproterenol or atropine. In some reports, atrial arrhythmias are classified according to their basic mechanism: arrhythmias due to (1) automaticity, (2) reentry arising in the sinus node area, (3) reentry arising outside the sinus node, and (4) enhanced sinus node automaticity.[19, 20, 23, 24]

Automatic atrial tachycardia mostly occur in children who have structurally normal atria. P-wave morphology is usually different from that observed during sinus rhythm. Neither AV block nor vagal maneuvers affect tachycardia.[19] Typically, during the electrophysiologic study, they cannot be initiated nor terminated with atrial premature depolarizations or rapid (burst or ramp) pacing. Spontaneous tachycardia initiation may exhibit a gradual increase in rate; also, transient pacing initiated during tachycardia may be followed by post-overdrive suppression.

Sinoatrial and intraatrial reentrant tachycardia are typically found in adults who have pathologic atria. They are initiated and terminated by timely premature beats or rapid pacing, and AV block does not affect the tachycardia. In intraatrial reentry, premature beats result in intraatrial conduction delay before tachycardia initiation, whereas they do not in sinoatrial reentry. In sinoatrial reentry, the P-wave morphology and activation sequence are identical to that of sinus beats, whereas they differ in reentry remote from sinus node.[24] It is noteworthy that in sinoatrial tachycardia, the area needing ablation may be wide and variable, extending from the base of the right atrial appendage to the mid-posterior atrial wall. Table 30-1 summarizes the results of ablation from different studies, including the mean or median number of pulses delivered, recurrence rate, and success rate. Our experience is summarized in Table 30-2, and one successful case is illustrated in Figure 30-4. The overall success rate is between 80% and 100%, whatever the mechanism of the atrial tachycardia, and the technique has been shown to be safe in the short term, despite the thinness of the atrial wall. Before drawing definite conclusions regarding long-term efficacy, however, we should recall from surgical experience that there are other potential sites for reentry in 25% of the cases, allowing recurrences after prolonged periods such as 1 year.[28] At the moment, we do not perform catheter ablation as first-line therapy for atrial tachycardias but recommend the procedure in patients who are symptomatic and drug-resistant or drug-intolerant or in the context of a tachycardia-induced cardiomyopathy.

In patients with inappropriate and symptomatic sinus node tachycardia that is not due to a curable cause and that is resistant to drug therapy including beta blockade, sinus node rate modification by RF ablation has been attempted. The successful site of ablation is located either anatomically at the lateral junction of the superior vena cava and the right atrium or guided electrophysiologically at the earliest site of atrial activation. In most patients, sinus node

TABLE 30-1. Radiofrequency Ablation Results in Atrial Tachycardias: Review of Literature

Study	Patients (n)	Reentry/Foci	Location RA	Location LA	Mean (m) or Median (M) Pulses	Success	Recurrence
Walsh, et al (22)	12	0/12	5	7	—	11 (92%)	—
Tracy, et al (31)	10	0/10	8	2	6 (m)	8 (80%)	2 (25%)
Kay, et al (30)	15	4/11	14	1	11 (m)	15 (100%)	3 (20%)
Chen, et al (32)	7	7	6	1	8 (m)	7 (100%)	0
Weiss (26)	10		8	2	4 (M)	8 (80%)	2 (25%)
Sanders, et al (24)	10	10/0	10	—	4 (m)	10 (100%)	0
Lesh, et al (18)	23	11/12	18	5	6 (m)	21 (91%)	2 (9%)

LA, left atrium; RA, right atrium.

function was modified, with a reduction in resting heart rate requiring permanent pacing.[34]

Ablation in Atrioventricular Nodal Reentrant Tachycardia

In patients with disabling drug-refractory AVNRT, catheter ablation has evolved rapidly from a last-resort treatment in the form of interruption of AV conduction to selective modification of AV nodal function as an ideal treatment. The anatomy of the involved reentrant circuit has been a matter of great controversy over the years. Limitation of the reentrant circuit to the AV node is mainly a problem of definition, depending on whether one is referring to the electrophysiologic AV node (which includes the atrial approaches of the transitional zone) or the anatomic compact AV node. Indeed, the different atrial approaches (anterior versus posterior) probably represent the substratum of the so-called "fast" and "slow" pathways involved in the tachycardia circuit. Catheter ablation in AV nodal reentrant tachycardia was introduced in 1986, using DC shocks applied to the retrograde fast pathway a few millimeters from the His bundle.[35] The risk of AV block targeting the fast pathway was 12% but has decreased to 2% to 7% with the use of RF current.[36,37] This risk, how-

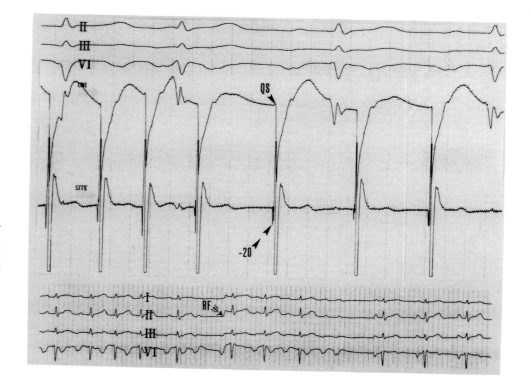

Figure 30-4. (*Top*) Unipolar (*uni*) and bipolar (*site*) electrograms at the successful ablation site of an atrial tachycardia. The unipolar electrogram shows a QS pattern. The first bipolar potential occurs 20 milliseconds before the onset of the P wave. (Bottom) Interruption of atrial tachycardia within 2 seconds of radiofrequency delivery.

TABLE 30-2. Radiofrequency Ablation Results in Patients With Atrial Tachycardia

Gender/Age	Clinical Presentation	Structural Heart Disease	Reentry (R) or Focus (F)	Location	Earliest Electrogram Relative to P-wave Onset (milliseconds)	Duration of Local Electrogram (milliseconds)	Pulses (n)	Success (S) or Failure (F)	Duration (mos)	Event
M/43	Incessant	—	F	CS OS	20	—	5	S	48	—
M/40	Chronic	DM	F	Post LA	—	—	6	F	48	—
F/23	Incessant	—	R	Sept paraHis	15	25	13	S	43	His-bundle ablation
F/42	Incessant	—	?	Multiple	—	—	25	F	43	—
F/29	Incessant	—	F	CS OS	35	40	1	S	34	—
M/57	Chronic	DM	R	Sept paraHis	50	50	4	S	31	—
M/37	Incessant	—	F	CS OS	35	—	5	S	19	Flutter
F/42	Chronic	IAD	R	Lat RA	Continuous activity		1	S	18	—
M/22	Incessant	DM	R	Lat RA	75	15	1	S	12	—
F/78	Paroxystic	—	R	Sinus node	40	85	1	S	12	—
F/44	Incessant	—	?	Post LA	45	—	18	S	11	—
F/26	Chronic	—	F	Ant RA	40	30	1	S	10	—
F/38	Incessant	Diverticulum	F	Sinus node	70	80	7	S	6	—
F/90	Chronic	MR	R	Multiple	—	—	7	F	5	His-bundle ablation
F/28	Paroxystic	—	F	Post RA	30	50	3	S	4	Other atrial tachycardia
F/16	Paroxystic	Ebstein's	R	Lat RA–Low RA	50	50	15	S	4	Other atrial tachycardia
M/42	Paroxystic	Ebstein's	R	Ant RA	70	75	1	S	4	—
F/31	Incessant	—	F	RA appendage	Mechanical block		2	S	2	—
M/23	Chronic	DM	F	Post LA	70	100	32	S	2	—
M/25	Paroxystic	—	F	Lat RA	25	40	1	S	1	—
12 F, 8 M 39 ± 18 year	—		10F – 8R		45 ± 19	53 ± 26	7 ± 9	17S – 3F	18 ± 17	

CSOS, coronary sinus ostium; DM, dilated cardiomyopathy; IAD, interatrial defect; LA, left atrium; RA, right atrium; MR, mitral regurgitation.

ever, is greater than that of using RF ablation to target the slow pathway, in which energy is applied 10 to 20 mm posterior to the His bundle, with a 3% or less incidence of AV block.[38–55] The techniques of selective fast- and slow-pathway ablation with RF energy depend on the positioning of catheters in specific locations: anterior para-Hissian and mid-posteroseptal, respectively.

Ablation of Fast Pathway

For fast-pathway ablation, the catheter is initially placed along the His bundle. The catheter is then withdrawn to obtain a large atrial but a small or no His-bundle potential. We believe that the site showing the shortest atrial-to-His (AH) interval must be sought. RF energy is applied to this region while monitoring the PR interval. Any prolongation should be followed by testing the retrograde conduction. The end point is elimination of retrograde conduction over the fast pathway and noninducibility of AV nodal reentry.

In our experience, the withdrawal of the catheter from the His-bundle site makes it possible to record unusual potentials if sustained attention is paid to recordings and high amplification is used. A slow potential can be recorded bridging the small interval between the large atrial and the small His potential. This slow potential disappears or decreases with atrial pacing that prolongs the PR interval. Frequently, spontaneous movement of the

catheter at that point produces junctional (Hissian) extra-systoles, with a reversal of the local activation sequence. Thus, the sequence His→slow potential→atrium allows exclusion of an atrial repolarization wave as the origin of the slow potentials. As in the posteroseptal region, we believe that this slow potential represents transitional tissue interfaced between atrial tissue and Hissian fibers, possibly supporting the so-called fast pathway on the anteroseptal region. In some patients, the local mechanical pressure of the catheter yields a sudden and prolonged PR interval consistent with transient interruption of the fast pathway. Lastly, RF delivery of low energy (5 W) produces a junctional rhythm, whereas higher power prolongs the PR interval and eliminates retrograde fast-pathway conduction. Figure 30-5 illustrates these findings.

Ablation of Slow Pathway

There is great controversy regarding the best technique to ablate the so-called slow pathway. Different approaches have been described. In one approach, electrogram patterns are used to identify the ablation site, whereas in the other approach, the ablating site is selected by anatomic criteria.[38–55]

ANATOMIC APPROACH. This technique involves multiple RF current applications in the posteroinferior interatrial septum. From the His-bundle region position, the catheter is

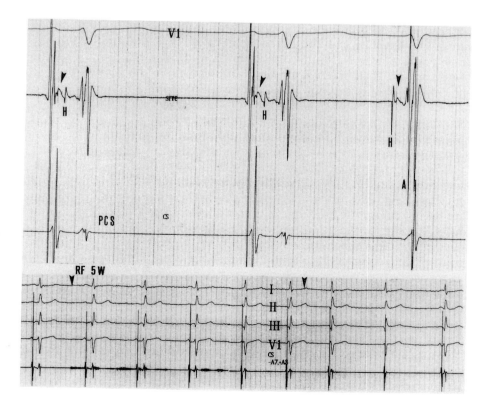

Figure 30-5. (*Top*) Presence of a slow potential (*arrows*) bridging the AH interval at the fast-pathway insertion site. The mechanical action of the catheter produces a junctional beat, with a reversal of the local activation sequence. (*Bottom*) Radiofrequency (*RF*) delivery of 5 W for 4 seconds immediately yields a junctional rhythm. We believe that such slow potentials may also represent the activation of the fast pathway.

withdrawn along the tricuspid septal anulus to the most posteroinferior aspect of the interatrial septum, adjacent to the coronary sinus ostium. One electrogram criterion is used by all authors to select target sites (i.e., an atrial ventricular electrogram ratio 0.5 or less).

One or usually two subsequent applications of RF energy are applied and the inducibility of AVNRT is assessed. If the tachycardia is still inducible, new RF applications are delivered at another site—either at the same posterior level but more atrially by withdrawing the catheter or more cephalad toward the mid-septum. Serial RF applications are delivered until either the tachycardia is noninducible or there is a total elimination of slow-pathway conduction.

The results from published studies demonstrate that the success rate is high (88% to 100%) but requires a median or mean number of five to 20 RF applications. Fast-pathway conduction is simultaneously modified in 8% to 13% of cases and the prevalence of AV block is low (0% to 3%). Recurrence of tachycardias is observed in 0% to 29% of patients, usually between 9% to 14%.[38–50]

ELECTROPHYSIOLOGIC APPROACH. This technique is based on three different types of electrophysiologic criteria: retrograde slow-pathway mapping, spike potentials, and slow potentials.[38,39,41,48]

Retrograde Slow-Pathway Mapping. Whereas retrograde fast pathway activity can be nearly always mapped to guide ablation, sustained retrograde slow-pathway conduction is present in only a fraction of patients during either ventricular stimulation or atypical fast–slow tachycardia. In a study by Jazayeri and coworkers, the retrograde conduction over the slow pathway was located in 24 of 106 patients.[48] This criterion appeared to be an impressive marker for slow-pathway ablation because 100% of patients were cured after a single RF application. Based on this result, the development of electrophysiologic or pharmacologic maneuvers facilitating a sustained retrograde slow-pathway conduction would be of great interest.

In four of six patients having the fast–slow or slow–slow form of AVNRT, we observed an interesting occurrence by using unfiltered unipolar recordings. The earliest site of atrial activity at the successful ablation site showed a double atrial potential, with an activation sequence reversed relative to that in sinus rhythm. The first atrial potential occurred 35 to 50 milliseconds before the P-wave onset in tachycardia, suggesting the exit of the slow pathway. It was, however, associated with an unipolar diphasic potential (Fig. 30-6) instead of the expected QS pattern. Later activities were recorded at more posterior sites, with a QS pattern of the unipolar potential. Therefore, this indicates that in slow–slow tachycardias, the earliest atrial activity during retrograde slow-pathway conduction reflects a type of pathway or bundle-transmitting

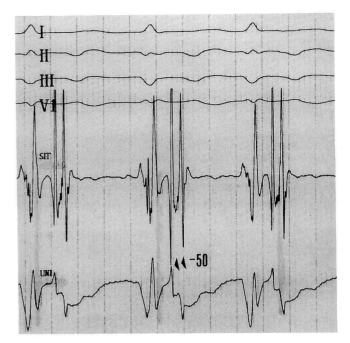

Figure 30-6. Earliest atrial activity (*double arrow*) during slow-slow form of AVNRT. The first bipolar potential occurs 50 milliseconds before the onset of the P wave. It was associated with a unipolar (*uni*) diphasic potential instead of the expected QS pattern, clearly demonstrating that the potential is not at the "exit" of the slow pathway. It may express a nodal bypass tract.

activation at more posterior sites, which may represent a nodal bypass tract. Ablation was successfully accomplished at this site with elimination of retrograde conduction.

In the absence of retrograde slow-pathway conduction, ablation can be guided by recordings of either spike potentials or slow potentials. Their value for slow-pathway mapping was assessed by MacGuire and colleagues using a grid of 60 electrodes during preoperative retrograde slow-pathway mapping in five patients.[54] In all patients, a slow potential was observed within the first 3 milliseconds of retrograde slow-pathway activation, and a spike potential was found in four of five patients. The highest slow potential was found at the slow-pathway insertion site, whereas the highest spike potential was usually found at some distance away. Therefore, this study demonstrates the constant presence of complex potentials at the slow-pathway insertion site but shows also their nonspecificity because they could be recorded in an area 13 mm in diameter.

Spike Potentials. Jackman and coworkers were the first to demonstrate the feasibility of RF catheter ablation of the slow pathway. Initially, these investigators used retrograde slow-pathway activation mapping and were then guided by a spike potential that is described as the activity of the slow-pathway atrial insertion.[38]

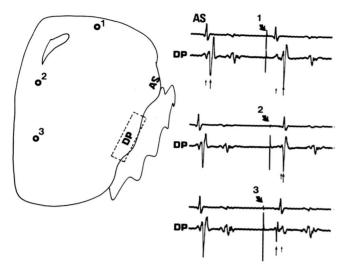

Figure 30-7. Presence of a double atrial potential (DP) at the mid- and posteroseptal region in a "normal" patient without atrioventricular nodal reentrant tachycardia. Three right atrial sites (stars) are paced. Pacing of site 2 below the sinus node region shortens the DP interval by anticipation of the second atrial potential (middle tracing). Pacing of site 3 anticipates even more the second atrial potential, leading to a reversal in the DP activation sequence (bottom tracing). Pacing of site 1 (roof of the right atrium) anticipates the first atrial potential and produces a widening of the DP sequence (top tracing). This suggests the functional linking of each atrial potential with different inputs; the first atrial potential is activated from the interatrial septum (as shown by its strict correlation with the timing of anteroseptal [AS] region), whereas the second atrial potential is activated from the posteroinferior right atrium.

During sinus rhythm, dual potentials were recorded in the posteroseptal region around or within the coronary sinus ostium. The first, a small atrial potential, was followed by a large second potential 10 to 40 milliseconds later. During fast–slow AVNRT, the large potential preceded the smaller atrial potential. An atrial extrastimulus during fast–slow tachycardia advanced the timing of atrial activation without altering the large potential. The target site for slow-pathway ablation was selected on the recording of the largest, sharpest, and latest second potential during sinus rhythm.[38] In 80 patients, Jackman and associates eliminated AVNRT in all (slow pathway in 78, fast pathway in two) using a median of two RF pulses. No clinical recurrence of AVNRT was observed. The experience of these authors includes 137 patients, with 100% success and a recurrence rate of 2%.

In a previous study, we found a similar dual potential in 11 normal patients. The temporal relation between the two potentials A_1 and A_2 was found to depend on the site of atrial pacing. Pacing at the sinus node region did not alter the A_1–A_2 morphology and sequence. In eight patients, pacing the lateral right atrium a few millimeters below the sinus node anticipated the A_2 potential, thus reducing the A_1–A_2 interval (Figs. 30-7 and 30-8). The lower the site of pacing, the greater the anticipation of A_2, leading to a fusion of A_1–A_2 and then a reversal in their activation sequence. In five patients, pacing the roof of the right atrium produced a widening of the A_1–A_2 sequence (see Fig. 30-7). This study clearly indicates the functional disso-

Figure 30-8. Radiogram in a left anterior oblique 60° view shows the usual recording site of slow potentials (top) and spike potential (bottom) marked in two frames. The spike potential region lies more posteriorly than the slow potentials region but both overlap considerably. On the left are recordings of double potentials (1, 2) during sinus rhythm. The end of spike potential 2 is prolonged by a slow potential (small arrow); this becomes evident (large arrow) with lateral atrial pacing stimulation (LRA). Note that LRA pacing stimulation produces a fusion of potentials 1 and 2, thus shortening the double potential sequence.

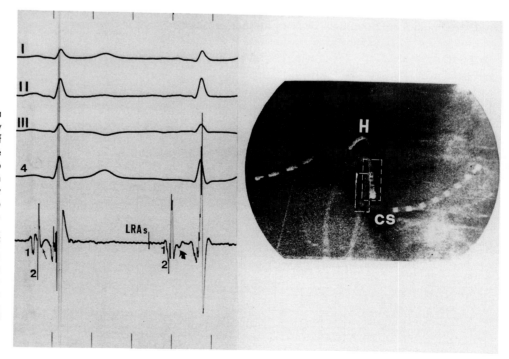

ciation of two atrial potentials. Because an opposite effect on the sequence of dual potential is observed below or above the sinus node region, a functional linking of each potential with atrionodal pathways originating from the sinus node may be suggested.

Slow Potentials. Slow potentials are defined as a low-amplitude activity (0.05 to 0.5 mV) that can be recorded in most humans along a band from the His bundle to the mid- and posterior part of the septum near the tricuspid anulus. Consistent slow potential activity cannot be found in 15% of patients, probably because their amplitude is too low. The region where slow potentials are recorded is generally more anterior than that of spike potentials but there is considerable overlap (see Fig. 30-8). Slow potentials are better separated from preceding atrial electrograms at the mid-septum than at the posterior septum, where they are prolonged or even included at the end of the atrial electrogram. The atrial electrograms are often slurred and fractionated, particularly in close proximity to the AV anulus (suggested by a low A/V electrogram ratio). In addition to high-gain amplification, atrial pacing maneuvers are mandatory to provide evidence of slow potentials. Indeed, their most specific pattern is their response to increasing atrial rates, which result in (1) a separation from preceding atrial electrograms (themselves unaltered by pacing rate), (2) a decline in amplitude and slope, and (3) an increase in duration until, frequently, the disappearance of any consistent activity. In some patients, however, microactivity persists, particularly during the first half of diastole in tachycardia, which may represent the last step in the rate disintegration of slow potentials. Atrial stimulation can reverse the polarity of potentials. Only atrial pacing makes

it possible to evidence either slow potentials concealed within the atrial potential (see Fig. 30-8) or slow potentials mimicking a sharp atrial potential, particularly in the form of multicomponent atrial potentials, which nearly always included slow potentials. We have previously shown that slow potentials do not represent atrial repolarization or Hissian activity. The extreme sensitivity of slow potentials relative to atrial rate is illustrated in Figure 30-9. Lastly, at the mid-septum, slow potentials with a significant His-bundle potential can be recorded. Although atrial pacing separates them from preceding atrial electrograms, these potentials remain unaltered before the QRS complex, occurring at the second half of diastole at long AH intervals. We believe these potentials represent the activity of the compact AV node.

The first ablation site is selected as that which shows a prominent slow potential in the posteroseptal region. The absence of a significant (more than 0.1 mV) His-bundle potential is checked by atrial pacing, prolonging the AV interval. In our experience, slow potentials with an amplitude of more than 0.05 mV are present in 89% and multiple or fractionated atrial potentials in 93% of successful ablation sites, with their combination being the most predictive electrogram. The likelihood of successful slow-pathway ablation is low in the absence of such complex potentials. Results in our experience of 243 patients are as follows. Fast pathway was deliberately or inadvertently ablated in 12 patients. High-degree AV block occurred in two patients during deliberate ablation of the fast pathway. Ablation of the slow pathway was achieved in 241 (99%) and failed in two young patients. During the ablation procedure, we decided that the risk of AV block was too high in the latter two patients and stopped the procedure.

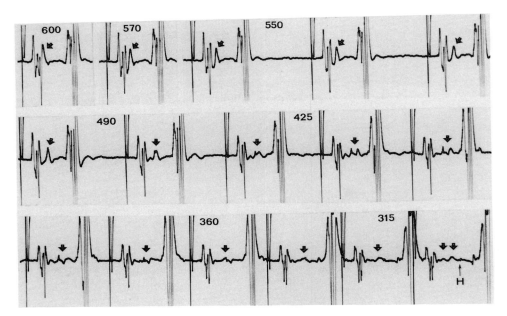

Figure 30-9. Slow potential (*arrows*) occurring just at the end of the atrial electrogram at an atrial cycle length of 600 milliseconds. Atrial pacing from 570 to 310 milliseconds result in a separation of slow potential from preceding atrial electrograms and a progressive disintegration of its morphology. Note the presence of a tiny His bundle potential (H).

Slow pathway was ablated or modified using an overall median of two RF pulses (one pulse in the last 100 patients). The time required for the therapeutic component was 41 ± 38 minutes and fluoroscopic time was 14 ± 14 minutes. During a follow-up period of 1 to 33 months, only nine patients (3.7%) had a clinical recurrence of tachycardias 1 to 8 weeks after ablation, which required a second successful session.

Determining the Better Approach

Analysis of the published data shows similar success rates with both approaches. More RF pulses, however, are required when using the anatomic approach to achieve slow-pathway ablation (five to 24 versus one to two). In contrast, slow pathway can be ablated with only one RF lesion in almost half the cases, using either spike or slow potential recordings, which argues against the need for a critical amount of tissue to be destroyed to prevent reentry. Whatever the approach, it appears not to affect the incidence of AV block. Furthermore, a higher rate of AVNRT recurrence has been reported in reports using the anatomic approach (9% to 14%) than those using the electrophysiologic approach (2% to 4%). Theoretically, this may be because of a lesser degree of accuracy in targeting the slow pathway. Kalbfleisch and colleagues presented a study comparing prospectively both approaches for ablating the slow pathway.[44] Both approaches were comparable in efficacy and duration but there were significantly more complex atrial electrograms at successful target sites versus unsuccessful ones. This suggests the superiority of electrogram mapping over anatomically defined targets to guide slow-pathway ablation.

The common feature in the electrophysiologic approaches is the use of multicomponent electrograms. Two types of components—ordinary atrial potentials and slow potentials—are to be differentiated and this requires two study conditions: high-gain amplification (50 to 100 mm/mV) and atrial pacing techniques. The main electrophysiologic difference is the sensitivity of slow potentials to atrial rate in contrast with preceding atrial potentials. Complex atrial potentials probably reflect multiple atrial fibers passing near or inserting at the transitional zone of the AV node. Our experience using retrograde slow-pathway mapping (see Fig. 30-6) suggests that in some cases these fibers act as a bundle. Slow potentials originate in a more specific tissue, termed "proximal AV bundle" by Racker or "subendocardially located transitional fibers" by de Bakker and associates and MacGuire and coworkers.[51, 53–55] An ongoing study using microelectrodes placed on slow potential sites shows characteristics of nodal potentials, which make slow potentials ideal candidates for the slow pathway.[53–55] That no activation wavefront can be followed during the anterograde slow part of

AVNRT is consistent with the disintegration of slow potentials at high atrial rates, which prevents their activation being followed by usual recordings. Finally, slow potentials at localized sites on the anterior septum suggests fewer transitional fibers anteriorly than posteriorly, which may explain partly the fastest conduction time in the anterior atrio-Hissian region. These hypotheses suggest a major role in the involvement of slow potentials and transitional fibers in both fast and slow AV conduction and AVNRT but do not exclude participation of atrial fibers.

Ablation of Accessory Pathways

Curative treatment for patients with tachycardia related to an AP initially was by surgery and by catheter ablation.[56–145] The first catheter fulguration of an AP was performed by Weber and Schmitz in 1983.[60] In 1984, Morady and Scheinman described a technique suitable for ablation of posteroseptal APs, in which DC shocks were delivered exclusively at the site related to an anatomic landmark—the coronary sinus ostium.[61] A definite improvement in AP catheter ablation was accomplished in 1986 by the ability to map along the different sites of AV rings using endocardial (particularly ventricular) electrograms, thus making it possible to consistently ablate AP in any location.[65, 68] The tricuspid anulus was mapped using the venous approach. The mitral anulus was mapped through a patent foramen oval, transseptal puncture, or by retrograde transaortic catheterization. The same technique of directly mapping the AV ring continues to be used to select the target site for ablation.

Determination of Ablation Site

Several parameters can be used to determine the optimal target site.

ACCESSORY PATHWAY POTENTIAL. Direct recording of the AP potential was initially used to localize the site for effective ablation. Differentiating this potential from atrial and ventricular depolarizations is difficult, however, and time-consuming. Although we believe that it is relatively easy to separate the AP from the atrial potential, it is extremely difficult to dissociate it from ventricular activation. Furthermore, it is necessary to study this site both under anterograde and retrograde conduction to demonstrate block at the atrial-Kent and Kent-ventricle interface, which frequently alters the pattern of the AP potential. Finally, Kuck and associates showed that in most patients, the site of AP block in anterograde and retrograde conductions appears consistently at the same interface (atrial or ventricular).[81] This implies that this potential may be separated from the atrial or ventricular activity in only a minority of patients. Therefore, the AP potential is usually referred to as being possible or probable, and it is not surprising that the use of this criterion by itself has a relatively low predictive value for successful ablation in some studies.[90,91]

To circumvent the problem of ascribing a non-atrial potential to the AP or the ventricular activation, we studied another means of validation based on the properties of unipolar recordings. Spach and colleagues demonstrated that unipolar polyphasic waveforms result from the superposition of potentials from different strands excited asynchronously, whereas a single (healthy) myocardial component must produce a uniphasic waveform.[72] Therefore, when we compare simultaneous bipolar and unipolar recordings, we assume that the first non-atrial potential (shown by atrial stimulation) is of ventricular origin if its timing is included *within* the unipolar uniphasic ventricular waveform and that it is the AP potential if its timing occurred *before* the intrinsic deflection of a QS-type ventricular waveform (Figs. 30-10 and 30-11). Although the AP potential is best seen in bipolar recordings, it appears in the unipolar recording as either a notch or a diphasic or negative deflection, with a different slope preceding the intrinsic deflection. In an ongoing prospective study, this criterion was found to be an excellent marker for successful ablation, with a positive predictive value of 85% in left lateral AP and a median of one RF application (see Fig. 30-11).

VENTRICULAR INSERTION SITE. This criterion is defined as the earliest onset of the ventricular electrogram in relation to the onset of delta wave.[68] It is generally associated with the shortest AV conduction time during preexcitation and is a reliable criterion for guiding ablation. It is essential, however, to note that the true local activation timing is ambiguous when using the wide recording electrodes needed for ablation and can only be reliably defined (Fig. 30-12) by using either unipolar intrinsic deflection or closely spaced bipolar electrograms.[72,106] The degree of prematurity of ventricular electrograms depends on AP location and varies from patient to patient.[87]

UNFILTERED UNIPOLAR RECORDINGS. In addition to the use of the intrinsic deflection for defining local activation timing, the morphology of the unfiltered ventricular wave provides direct information on the proximity of the catheter to the origin of the ventricular activation.[72] An initial unipolar ventricular R wave indicates an initial incoming wavefront through intervening myocardial tissue between the catheter and the site of preexcitation onset. The higher or the broader the R wave, the farther is the origin of ventricular excitation; therefore, it is less likely to be a successful ablation site. In contrast, a QS wave indicates proximity of the ventricular activation origin.

ATRIAL INSERTION SITE. This criterion—defined as the shortest VA time—is considered by some to be an impor-

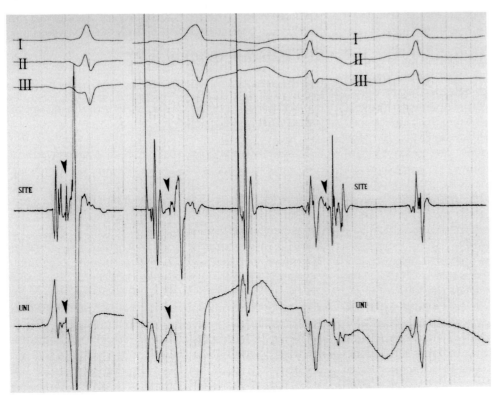

Figure 30-10. Demonstration of an accessory pathway (AP) potential (*arrows*) by exclusion of both atrial and ventricular activation. Atrial pacing produces a progressive separation of atrial and AP potential; block then occurs between ventricular potential and AP potential on the second narrow QRS. Note the sharpness and amplitude (0.1 mV) of AP potential (similar to His-bundle potential) and its unipolar diphasic morphology.

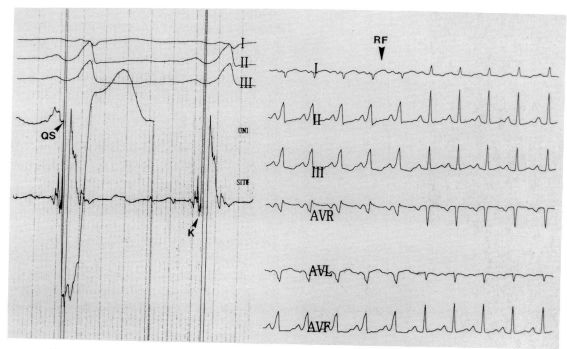

Figure 30-11. Example of bipolar and unipolar electrograms at successful ablation site for left lateral AP. A sharp and tiny accessory pathway (AP) potential (*K*) is present between atrial and ventricular potentials and occurs before the QS pattern of the unipolar ventricular potential. A single pulse eliminated AP conduction.

tant marker for successful ablation. In our experience and that of Calkins and colleagues, this criterion is only useful if continuous retrograde electric activity is recorded.[87,90] A more accurate identification of the atrial insertion site for left-sided AP has been proposed, using the atrial electrogram polarity reversal.

EFFECTS OF MICROENERGY AS A PRE-TEST FOR SUCCESSFUL ABLATION. The use of subthreshold stimulation has been introduced to pre-test the site of successful ablation.[110] This is particularly useful for evaluation of concealed AP during reciprocating tachycardia. Its high positive predictive value may prevent the delivery of multiple unneeded pulses. Further developments of this technique may prove important as a guide to accurate localization of the AP.

PACE MAPPING. Pace mapping can be used as an additional criterion for identifying the ablation site because it lacks accuracy if used alone. The A/V electrogram ratio obtained by catheters placed near the AV ring does not play any significant role in predicting a successful outcome. Ratio values varying from 0.05 to 6 have been found at successful ablation sites.

OPTIMAL CATHETER-TISSUE INTERFACE. It should be emphasized that catheter stability and a good tissue contact at the

target site are of paramount importance for successful ablation. Catheter stability can be better tested by observing whether the electrograms are stable than by the degree of catheter excursion on fluoroscopy. In addition, a high ST-segment elevation (more than 2 mV) on unipolar waveforms indicates excessive catheter contact with the myocardium, which may result in an impedance rise and subsequent complications.

In summary, the ablation site for manifest AP can be approached by finding the shortest AV interval. The earliest ventricular potential relative to delta wave onset must then be sought, ideally confirming the latter by the use of unipolar intrinsic deflection. A ventricular potential synchronous with the delta-wave onset is acceptable for a target site in left-sided preexcitations, whereas earlier values are sought to locate the optimal ablation site for right-sided preexcitations. A deflection preceding the main ventricular potential (suggesting an AP potential) is an additional favorable criterion.

Evaluation of Different Electrogram Criteria for Accessory Pathway Ablation

Despite different approaches, there is no significant difference in the reported success rate in AP ablation (which is more than 90%), suggesting that no mapping technique is

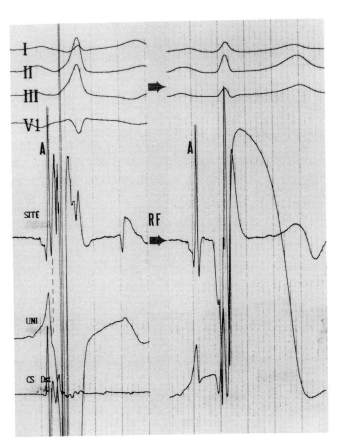

Figure 30-12. Electrograms at the successful ablation site of a left lateral accessory pathway (AP) before (*left panel*) and after radiofrequency (RF) ablation (*right panel*). The bipolar ventricular potential is complex, with multiple components and a peak potential occurring after the delta-wave onset. The unipolar (*uni*) ventricular waveform is uniphasic with a QS pattern and on intrinsic deflection, occurring just at the onset of the bipolar ventricular potential. This suggests that (1) the local ventricular timing is earlier than that expected from determination of the peak potential, and (2) the first bipolar ventricular potential is not an AP potential because it is included within a unipolar uniphasic ventricular waveform. After ablation, note the repolarization wave consistent with local atrial and ventricular lesions.

clearly superior to any other. Indeed, success rates obtained using either ventricular activation mapping, atrial mapping, or recording AP potentials are similar. The number of RF pulses needed to achieve ablation, however, appears to differ significantly (see Table 30-3). This is because of a different interpretation and lack of resolution of conventional electrograms and the difficulty in determining the exact onset of the delta wave. Minimizing the number of unneeded RF pulses requires using criteria that have a higher positive predictive value. Estimation of not only the timing but also the direction of the activation wavefront, as provided by unfiltered unipolar electrogram morphology or by atrial electrogram polarity reversal, may improve the accuracy of mapping. In our experience, ablation must not be attempted when a significant (more than 0.1 mV) R wave is seen in the unipolar ventricular wave recordings. Furthermore, we firmly believe that a more stringent and specific criterion for bipolar AP potential is accomplished by a comparison with both morphology and timing of unipolar recordings, dramatically enhancing the probability of success for an RF application. Particularly, it allows the ablation of left lateral AP, using a median of one pulse. Additional predictive accuracy may be expected using the effects of subthreshold stimulation on AP conduction in addition to the shortest retrograde VA time for ablating concealed AP.

SPECIFIC CONSIDERATIONS

Left lateral Accessory Pathway. The anteroposterior, right anterior oblique, or ideally, 60° left anterior oblique views are used for mapping. A catheter is inserted in the coronary sinus for localization of the AP atrial insertion using the shortest retrograde VA time, and for use as a radiographic reference. The site of the earliest ventricular activation can be determined if large ventricular electrograms are recorded. In addition, this catheter serves other functions: (1) because the coronary sinus is an epicardial structure, it can show earlier electrograms than those recorded from the endocardium, suggesting an epicardial course of the AP; and (2) if several RF pulses are delivered, the ablated sites can be referenced to the coronary sinus electrodes to prevent delivery of energy to similar sites. Some workers use a single catheter for mapping and ablation.[83] In some centers, the ablation catheter is introduced using the transseptal technique but most prefer the retrograde aortic approach to avoid the potential complications of transseptal catheterization. Both techniques are complementary, however.[69, 94, 112] In the transseptal approach, the ablation catheter must be held during ablation to insure contact with the atrial side of the mitral anulus, whereas a catheter introduced retrograde is usually positioned underneath the valve and has better stability and tissue contact. Unipolar ST-segment elevation suggests that the catheter pressure is too great and the catheter should be slightly withdrawn.

Right Anteroseptal Accessory Pathway. Radiographic anteroposterior or 30° right anterior oblique views are used for mapping. These pathways can be approached from underneath the tricuspid valve, as suggested by Jackman and coworkers, but this approach may be associated with a higher risk of inducing right bundle branch block.[82] The ablation catheter can be also introduced through a femoral vein and placed parallel to the His-bundle catheter. A superior atrial approach is more frequently used.[68, 113] A subclavian or jugular catheter is directed toward the atrial side of the tricuspid valve, usually 5 to 10 mm *anterior* and above the His-bundle catheter. The anterior position, well seen in oblique views, often requires that the catheter be twisted firmly in a clockwise direction throughout RF delivery. Although a tiny His-bundle potential is frequent, a significant (more than 0.1 mV) His-bundle potential must not be present at the ablation site. A catheter positioned at the His area guards against encroachment of the ablation catheter on this region throughout RF delivery. As a rule, the ventricular potentials should precede the delta-wave onset by a mean of 18 ± 10 milliseconds (i.e., occurring within the P wave). As in right lateral AP, the earliest-onset delta wave is recorded in the V_1–V_3 leads rather than in standard leads I, II, or III.

The major problem and challenge is to ablate AP while preserving AV conduction. In the ablation registries, complete AV block occurred mainly during ablation of right anteroseptal AP. This risk should be reduced with increased operator experience. Indeed, previous surgical and fulguration procedures, both causing large ablative lesions, showed a low incidence of AV block because these APs have an anterior rather than septal location.[68,114] We had only one patient who developed AV block during anteroseptal ablation using fulguration (at the atrial side of the anulus) in 25 patients. Therefore, AV block should be exceptional when focal lesions are caused by RF energy. In our opinion, AV conduction can be always preserved by (1) minimizing the number of RF pulses by using the maximum predictive criteria (if there is some doubt as to which target sites to choose, apply the first pulse at the most anterior site); (2) checking for the absence of a significant His-bundle potential by induction of narrow QRS complexes; (3) applying RF energy for 10 seconds or less if the pathway has not been changed; (4) stopping RF delivery immediately in the event of a sustained junctional rhythm because it is a constant marker, heralding the occurrence of AV block.

Right Lateral Accessory Pathway. Both oblique radiographic views are suitable for mapping. Subclavian or femoral vein approaches can be used. Like anteroseptal AP, extremely short or even virtually simultaneous AV times and early ventricular potentials are to be sought. These pathways may be difficult to ablate because of catheter instability and poor tissue contact. Higher energy outputs are usually necessary to achieve the same temperature as that achieved in left-sided AP.[115] Better catheter designs, such as those with long distal curves or the use of long sheaths, may be helpful to minimize this instability and improve tissue contact. Some workers recommend the use of a catheter introduced in the right coronary artery to serve as a reference.[116] This does not solve the problem of endocardial catheter instability, however, and

there is a risk of coronary spasm or endothelial abrasion, which may be potentially atherogenic. The site of the pathway can be easily recognized during catheter mapping and marked on the fluoroscopy screen, or a halo-shaped electrode can be inserted and place around the ring to locate the AP.

Mahaim Fibers. In our experience of 20 patients, we observed three types of decremental conducting AP. One patient had a true Mahaim nodoventricular AP. Four patients had a short (para-annular) AV AP, and 15 had a long AV AP. Therefore, most of these APs with anterograde decremental conduction properties are long pathways with a right lateral proximal insertion that can include AV node–type cells and a distal fascicular–right ventricular insertion.[117–120] Some of these APs may be ectopic nodal AV pathways. Although these pathways are not thought of as having retrograde conduction, in one case we found that conduction can occur from the ventricle through the AP but may be blocked at its proximal insertion.[121] Different approaches for ablation can be used: (1) ventricular insertion mapping, guided by the earliest ventricular potential relative to preexcitation onset; (2) atrial insertion mapping, using the shortest atrial stimulus-to-delta wave interval (the approximate location of the pathway can be also found by delivering late atrial extrastimuli during antidromic tachycardia and identifying the paratricuspid pacing site that results in the greatest advance in the timing of the next ventricular complex); and (3) direct recording of AP potentials, either at the atrial or ventricular insertion or along the pathway.[122–126] When we used the first technique, we found that most patients had both an arborization of the distal insertion and seven had a myocardial gap between this insertion and the right bundle branch system, suggesting a ventricular (not fascicular) distal insertion. The distal AP insertion was ablated in 13 patients, with only one case of right bundle branch block.[125] The ideal site for ablation is the proximal or middle part of the pathway because it is a narrow and insulated bundle-type structure. A spike originates from this bundle but its recording may be difficult because of the instability of the catheter. In seven of 15 cases, we observed a mechanical block of the AP at this site—a phenomenon also reported by Cappato and associates.[126]

Posteroseptal Accessory Pathway. Ablation of posteroseptal AP may be difficult because of the complex three-dimensional anatomy of the posterior space.[82,84,85,127,130] The effective ablation sites are (1) the tricuspid anulus or the margin of the coronary sinus ostium, (2) the coronary sinus or a venous branch, or (3) the mitral anulus. In some patients, RF pulses must be applied to both sides of the septum to achieve complete elimination of anterograde and retrograde AP conduction. Changes in the preexcitation pattern, either spontaneous or induced by pacing, are a reasonable indication that there is a wide insertion of AP fibers, requiring a greater number of maximum (both time and amount of energy delivered) applications of RF energy.

Right or left posteroseptal APs are conventionally defined by their ventricular insertion site, which gives (respectively) a predominant negative or positive maximally preexcited QRS complex in the V_1 lead. This simple differentiation is corroborated by the effects of functional bundle branch block on the ventriculoatrial interval during orthodromic reciprocating tachycardia.[129] In patients with prominent positive preexcitation in V_1, the occurrence of right bundle branch block prolonged the ventriculoatrial interval in only one of 18 patients, whereas left bundle branch block prolonged it in 14 of 19 patients (74%). In patients with prominent negative preexcitation in V_1, the occurrence of left bundle branch block during tachycardia did not increase the ventriculoatrial interval except in one of 12 patients (8%), whereas right bundle branch block increased the ventriculoatrial interval in two of 11 patients. In all cases, attempts to map and ablate from a right approach should be made either on the endocardial septum or in the proximal coronary sinus. It is important to remember that the left AP ventricular potentials are not as early as those on the right side. When the favorable site (based on anterograde and retrograde parameters) appears more than 15 mm inside the coronary sinus, left septal mapping is recommended. A 60° left anterior oblique view is optimal for AP ablation with a right-sided approach because it shows the maximal amplitude of catheter movements. Furthermore, the respective position of the septum, tricuspid, and mitral anulus are clearly differentiated in this position, and the ablation sites of right or left AP are usually directed toward the left or right side of the fluoroscopic screen, respectively.

In our experience, all posteroseptal AP with prominent negative preexcited complexes in V_1 were ablated from the right side (i.e., right endocardium [88%] or proximal coronary sinus [12%]). Right posteroseptal AP with negative delta-wave polarity in V_1 requires fewer RF applications than those with an isoelectric or positive initial vector (4 ± 3 versus 8 ± 6; $p < .05$). Posteroseptal AP with prominent positive preexcited complexes in V_1 were ablated at the right endocardium, the proximal coronary sinus, or the left endocardium in 55%, 27%, and 18% of cases, respectively. The high prevalence of APs related to the coronary sinus appears to be clearly related to a bias in the referral of patients who underwent prior unsuccessful ablation attempts; a similar prevalence was reported also by others.[127,130] In patients with left posteroseptal AP, some electrocardiogram parameters have a valuable though imperfect predictive accuracy for the side of approach. A QRS complex predominantly positive in aV_R had a 73% predic-

tive value for left endocardial or coronary sinus approach. A delta wave of more than 45° in V_1 lead had a 70% predictive value for a right endocardial approach. The association of a negative delta wave steeper than 45° in lead II, and a positive complex in aV_R yielded a 75% predictive value for a coronary sinus approach.

Mid-Septal Accessory Pathway. Mid-septal AP is described as AP located in the zone between the His bundle and the coronary sinus. Applying this definition, most APs have been ablated just above the coronary sinus; therefore, the approach is not different from that for the conventional posteroseptal AP.[132-134] True mid-septal APs are those that are adjacent to the His bundle (para-Hissian) or immediately posterior to the His bundle, close to the AV node (paranodal). This differentiation is of clinical importance because ablation of the APs that are close to the AV conducting system clearly involves the risk of developing AV block. We have encountered five paranodal AP and eight para-Hissian APs. The para-Hissian AP had an anteroseptal-type preexcitation pattern (positive delta wave in leads I, II, and AVF) but a QS pattern in V_1 and V_2. These criteria yielded an 82% predictive value for para-Hissian AP. Despite a local His-bundle potential measuring 0.10 to 0.4 mV, all were ablated without creating AV block, using low energy (10 to 15 W).

Permanent Junctional Reciprocating Tachycardia. This tachycardia is associated with APs having retrograde decremental conduction properties. Although typically described in the posteroseptal location, other AP locations have been recognized.[80] Our experience includes 28 patients with APs in the following locations: posteroseptal, 22 (79%); mid-septal, three (11%); right lateral, one (4%); and left lateral, two (7%). Guided by the shortest VA time and a QS pattern of the unipolar atrial wave during tachycardia, ablation was performed in all mid- or posteroseptal cases using a right-sided approach: right endocardial septum in 16 patients and proximal coronary sinus in nine patients (including one in the middle cardiac vein). In six of the latter cases, mapping the left endocardial septum showed less favorable electrograms than within the coronary sinus. Six of the nine patients ablated through the coronary sinus had an initially negative P wave in D_1 during tachycardia, versus six of the other 16 septal APs. This criterion yields a predictive value of 48% for this approach. The electrogram at the successful sites (see Fig. 30-9) showed earlier activation than the coronary sinus reference (subclavian catheter) in 24 out of 28 patients and was synchronous in four. A new finding was fractionated dual or multiple atrial electrograms at the successful site in 24 of 28 patients (86%), whereas this pattern was absent or less marked in most cases, either at the contiguous sites in tachycardia or at the same site in sinus rhythm. The duration of this local atrial electrogram was 52 ± 15 milliseconds. The complex electrogram was presumed to be related either to the complexity of the AP–atrial interface or the presence of an AP potential.

Management of Resistant Accessory Pathway

When electrograms are not favorable, a variety of different catheters from superior or femoral approaches must be tried. In some patients, ablation is unsuccessful despite apparently favorable electrograms, catheter stability, and adequate temperature delivery at target sites.[136] Under these circumstances, the following suggestions may be helpful.

1. Changing the site of ablation to the side of the anulus opposite to that where initial RF pulses were applied. In right-sided AP, a new catheter introduced from a superior vein may allow the catheter to be positioned beneath the tricuspid leaflet. In posteroseptal AP, we select sites showing a high A/V ratio instead of initially low ratios or vice versa. In left-sided AP (particularly posterior ones) that could not be ablated from beneath the leaflet, the catheter is advanced retrogradely into the left atrium and is then progressively withdrawn to ablate the atrial side of the mitral anulus, using the same anterograde parameters. Otherwise, a transseptal approach must be considered.

2. Changing the mapping criterion. Switching from the earliest anterograde to the earliest retrograde activation site is useful in posteroseptal or left lateral AP, in which an oblique course has been encountered relatively frequently. In five of our 14 posteroseptal AP patients (36%) ablated in the proximal coronary sinus or afferent branches, the local retrograde ventriculoatrial time was short despite a relatively long AV time during preexcitation. It should be emphasized that the mere positioning of the ablation catheter at the atrial or ventricular side of the anulus (as reflected by high or low A/V electrogram ratio) is to be distinguished from mapping of the atrial or ventricular insertion of the AP.

3. Seeking an AP potential. This may be self-evident but is a criteria that must be used, particularly when previous multiple RF applications guided by atrial or ventricular insertion mapping were unsuccessful. Accessory pathway potential is frequently present at a low amplitude between atrial and ventricular potentials that are separated more than usual, suggesting that previous ablations have altered a part of AP insertions.

4. Using a longer duration of RF pulse. Limiting unsuc-

cessful pulse duration to 10 seconds may miss a successful (possibly deep) site, which would require longer energy delivery. This applies to posteroseptal AP and also to presumed wide AP, for which the use of short pulses, although at appropriate sites, would not create significant confluent lesions for effective ablation.

5. Excluding structural abnormalities. Some posteroseptal APs are associated with a coronary sinus diverticulum or aneurysm. In these cases, the AP is usually found at the neck of the diverticulum. The presence of the minor forms of these structural abnormalities can be visualized only by direct angiography, as shown by Kuck and associates.[130]

6. Epicardially located AP. In 5% of our left lateral AP patients, the AP could not be ablated endocardially, and ablation inside the mid-distal coronary sinus was successful in 11 of 13 patients.[137] In seven of the 11 patients, the coronary sinus electrograms were more favorable than the endocardial, whereas they were comparable in the other four patients. In 10% and 27% of our right and left posteroseptal AP patients, respectively, ablation was required in the proximal coronary sinus or the middle cardiac vein. The energy used in the coronary sinus was only 8 to 20 W.

7. Using bipolar transseptal RF pulses. This technique has been proposed to ablate posteroseptal AP that cannot be ablated by unipolar pulses applied on either side of the septum.[134]

8. Sequential applications of RF energy or other sources of more penetrating energy. This can be used as the last resort to cover a wider area or to attain deeper tissue injury. The sequential ablation is supported by the fact that "successful" sites show less favorable electrograms than "unsuccessful" sites.[87, 136] In these situations, we think that previous applications guided on the shortest times have altered a part of AP insertions, leaving some fibers with longer conduction times, which can be ablated with additional applications. Furthermore, some cases suggested that scar tissue due to transiently successful ablation of AP limited heat transmission and effectiveness of subsequent RF pulses. These rare inadequacies of RF ablation applied through usual catheters can be circumvented either by the use of higher frequencies or possibly by the use of RF energy through new types of electrodes.[138–141]

Results

Table 30-3 summarizes the results of RF ablation in different studies, including the mean or median number of

TABLE 30-3. Literature Review of Accessory Pathway Ablation Using Radiofrequency Energy*

Study	Patients (n)	Accessory Pathways (n)	Mean (m) or Median (M)	Mean Fluoroscopy Time (min)	Recurrences (%)	Success (%)
Kuck, et al (83, 85)	105	111	9 (M)	53	3	89
	430	453	6 (M)		8	95
Jackman, et al (82)	166	177	3 (M)	—	9	99
Calkins, et al (84)	250	267	6 (M)	47	7	94
Miles, et al (98)	28	30	10 (m)	—	4	86
Lesh, et al (93)	100	109	8 (M)	66	10	89
Chen, et al (95)	57	60	6 (M)	—	—	80
Silka, et al (91)	100	107	6 (M)	—	—	87
Leather, et al (92)	75	84	5–14 (m)	33–63	0	71–90
Natale, et al (94)	80	82	6 (m)	34–42	4	92.5
Chen, et al (94)	142	166	10 (m)	50–67	10	96
Swartz, et al (96)	114	122	4 (M) 6 (m)	31–63	9	95

*Some reports are preliminary and do not reflect current results.

applications delivered, the fluoroscopy time, the total recurrence rate, and the success rate.

Since 1990, 555 patients were referred to our center for RF ablation of APs. Sixty-seven were children younger than 17 years of age (13 ± 8 years). Sixty-seven (12%) had previously had an unsuccessful attempt at catheter ablation of AP. Twenty-six had multiple APs (two APs, 23; three APs, three). Successful ablation was achieved in 545 patients (98%). The remaining 10 patients (2%) failed repeated RF ablation procedures; of these, seven had posteroseptal AP, two had left lateral AP, and one had right lateral AP. Direct-current fulguration successfully ablated five of the APs that could not be ablated with RF energy, markedly depressed AP conduction in a sixth, but failed in the other four patients. Table 30-4 summarizes our results. The results are divided into categories of success and failure. The failures were subdivided: those secondary to AP recurrence and refusal for reablation and those that failed repeated ablation attempts.

With a mean follow-up period of 14 ± 11 months, recurrences occurred in 8% of all APs: 42% of recurrences occurred at day 1, 12% at day 2 or 3, and 46% after day 7. The recurrence rate was higher in overt AP (12%) than in concealed AP (3%). In addition, the recurrence rate was significantly higher in patients with right anteroseptal or right lateral AP (14% to 19%), compared with those with posteroseptal (9%) or left lateral (4%) AP. In 15 patients, AP conduction recurred at day 1 to 3, then spontaneously disappeared until discharge. Recurrence was observed, however, in 11 of these 15 patients (73%). All but five patients with recurrences underwent a second or third successful ablation procedure.

Complications

The incidence of complications in multicenter reports was 3.8% in 787 patients reported by Scheinman and colleagues and 4.4% in a total of 2222 patients by Hindricks reporting from the European registry MERFS.[142,143] Complications reported in MERFS were arrhythmias, 0.81%; perforation–tamponade, 0.72%; AV block, 0.63%; pericardial effusion, 0.54%; pulmonary or cerebral embolism, 0.58%; vascular thrombosis, 0.36%; and other, 0.76%.[89] The incidence of severe complications, including complete AV block, embolic events, and cardiac tamponade, was 2.3%. Whether cardiac tamponade was due to either mechanical perforation or RF-induced perforation was not specified. This complication may be reduced by using lower power and avoiding unwarranted pressure contact, as reflected by high ST-segment elevation on unipolar waveforms. Embolic events occurred in 0.6% of patients. It is not clear whether heparin anticoagulation during the procedure prevents embolic event. Anticoagulation with heparin after the procedure is recommended for both right- and left-sided ablation. Maintenance with aspirin is also recommended for left-sided ablation. Although the relation of embolic events with an impedance rise is not proved, it is desirable to avoid this impedance change. In the future, this should be accomplished by the use of devices equipped with temperature or impedance monitoring and automatic energy control.

No major complication, including death, tamponade, or AV block, occurred in our series. Side effects related to the introduction or manipulation of catheters occurred in a total of 11 patients (2%): peripheral vascular damage,

TABLE 30-4. Radiofrequency Ablation Results in Patients With Accessory Pathway

| Accessory Pathway Location | Accessory Pathways (n) | Median Number of RF Pulses | Duration (min) | | Recurrences | Long-Term Follow-up | | |
			Ablation	Fluoroscopy		Success	Failures	Recurrences (non-ablated)
Overt RAS	37	4	54 ± 38	14 ± 12	7 (19%)	36	—	1
Overt R LAT	35	6	118 ± 157	50 ± 74	5 (14%)	33	1	1
Concealed RAS or R LAT	10	6	54 ± 32	19 ± 15	1 (10%)	10	—	—
Mahaim fibers	20	5	59 ± 51	19 ± 14	1 (5%)	20	—	—
Overt RPS	63	3	59 ± 58	24 ± 23	6 (9%)	60	3	—
Overt LPS	65	4	79 ± 69	38 ± 29	6 (9%)	61	3	1
Concealed PS	20	4	57 ± 38	21 ± 11	0	19	1	—
PJRT	28	3	62 ± 32	25 ± 8	4 (14%)	27	—	1
Overt L LAT	207	2	51 ± 42	19 ± 12	10 (5%)	203	2	2
Concealed LLAT	97	4	45 ± 30	17 ± 8	3 (3%)	97	—	—
TOTAL	582	3	58 ± 49	23 ± 21	40 (8%)	566 (97%)	10 (1.7%)	6 (1.3%)

RF, radiofrequency; RAS, right anteroseptal; RPS, right posteroseptal; LPS, left posteroseptal; PS, posteroseptal; PJRT, permanent form of recipolating tachycardia; LAT, lateral.

957

seven; pneumothorax, two; sepsis, one; and permanent mechanically induced left bundle branch block, one. Complications related to RF applications occurred in 11 patients (2%): right bundle branch block, mural thrombus in the coronary sinus, and distal right coronary artery spasm during RF delivery in the proximal coronary sinus.[1-3] A transient unilateral impairment of vision was observed in five patients at days 2, 2, 3, 5, and 12, respectively, presumably due to microemboli. Despite not using heparin during the procedure, this incidence is similar to that reported in groups using full heparinization. Conversely, heparinization not performed during the procedure may explain the absence of tamponade in our series.

Indications

Radiofrequency-energy catheter ablation is used as the procedure of choice for AP ablation. It is highly effective in eliminating AP conduction with a low risk. Therefore, it has been proposed as treatment for patients with drug-refractory AP-mediated tachycardias and even for symptomatic patients who refuse lifelong dependence on drug therapy. In asymptomatic patients with Wolff-Parkinson-White syndrome, the decision to ablate AP must be individualized and based on the electrophysiologic data, occupation or physical activities of the patient, and other personal factors.

Radiofrequency ablation in children warrants special consideration, particularly in younger children who have smaller cardiac structures, compared with adults. In experimental studies, RF lesions induced at the atrial and ventricular tissue bordering the AV anuli appear to increase in size as young animals mature to adults.[144] Lastly, the significant radiation exposure is associated with an increased lifetime risk of developing genetic disorders or malignancy. Given these uncertainties, we believe that catheter ablation techniques should be reserved for children with either drug-refractory or life-threatening tachycardias.

CONCLUSION

Radiofrequency-energy catheter ablation is used widely and successfully to treat a variety of supraventricular arrhythmias. Future research to further improve the efficacy and safety of the technique as well as to extend its use to other arrhythmias such as atrial fibrillation must include the design of catheters that ensure stable electrode-tissue contact, particularly for right-sided AP and catheters with multiple active electrodes. In addition, more precise location techniques and use of temperature-guided devices or other energy sources should improve the safety of these procedures. Lastly, follow-up surveillance of patients undergoing catheter ablation is needed to assess long-term safety.

Acknowledgements

Thanks to Joëlle Bassibey for assistance in writing this manuscript.

References

1. Puech P, Latour H, Grolleau R: Le flutter et ses limites. Arch Mal Coeur 1970;61:116.
2. Waldo AL, MacLean WAH, Karp RB, Kouchoukos NT, James RM: Entrainment and interruption of atrial flutter with atrial pacing. Studies in man following open heart surgery. Circulation 1977;56:737.
3. Chauvin M, Brechenmacher C, Voegtlin JR: Application de la cartographie endocavitaire à l'étude du flutter auriculaire. Arch Mal Coeur 1983;76:1020.
4. Klein GJ, Guiraudon GM, Sharma AD, Milstein S: Demonstration of macroreentry and feasibility of operative therapy in the common type of atrial flutter. Am J Cardiol 1986; 57:587.
5. Cosio FG, Arribas F, Palacias J, Tascon J, Lopez Gil M: Fragmented electrograms and continous electrical activity in atrial flutter. Am J Cardiol 1986;57:1309.
6. Saumarez RC, Parker J, Camm J: Geometrically accurate activation mapping of the atrioventricular node region during surgery; J Am Coll Cardiol 1992;19:601.
7. Saoudi N, Mouton Schleiffer D, Letac B: Direct catheter fulguration of atrial flutter. Lancet 1987;II:558.
8. Chauvin M, Brechenmacher C: Endocardial catheter fulguration for treatment of atrial flutter. Am J Cardiol 1988; 61:471.
9. Stevenson WG, Weiss JN, Wiener I, et al: Fractionated endocardial electrograms are associated with slow conduction in humans: evidence from pace mapping. J Am Coll Cardiol 1989;13:369.
10. Saoudi N, Atallah G, Kirkorian G, Touboul P: Catheter fulguration of the atrial myocardium in human type I atrial flutter. Circulation 1990;81:762.
11. Nunain SO, Linker NJ, Sneddon JF, Debbas NMG, Camm AJ, Ward DE: Catheter ablation by low energy DC shocks for successful management of atrial flutter. Br Heart J 1992; 67:67.
12. Cosio FG, Lopez Gil M, Goicolea A, Arribas F, Barroso JL: Radiofrequency ablation of the inferior vena cava-tricuspid valve Isthmus in common atrial flutter. Am J Cardiol 1993; 71:705.
13. Feld G, Fleck P, Chen PS, et al: Radiofrequency catheter ablation for the treatment of human type I atrial flutter: identification of a critical zone in the reentrant circuit by endocardial mapping techniques. Circulation 1992;86:1233.
14. Interian A, Cox MM, Jimenez R, et al: A shared pathway in atrioventricular nodal reentrant tachycardia and atrial flutter: implications for pathophysiology and therapy. Am J Cardiol 1993;71:297.

15. Nakagawa H, Wang X, McLelland J, et al: Line of conduction block extends from inferior vena cava to coronary sinus ostium in common atrial flutter. Pacing Clin Electrophysiol 1993;16(4):881.

16. Nakagawa H, McLelland J, Beckman K, et al: Radiofrequency ablation of common type atrial flutter. Pacing Clin Electrophysiol 1993;16(4):850.

17. Fischer B, Haissaguerre M, Le Metayer Ph, Egloff Ph, Warin JF: Radiofrequency catheter ablation of common atrial flutter. Pacing Clin Electrophysiol 1993;16:1099.

18. Lesh MD, Van Hare GF, Epstein LM, et al: Radiofrequency catheter ablation of atrial arrhythmias. Results and mechanisms. Circulation 1994;89:1074.

19. Josephson M: Supraventricular tachycardias. In: Clinical cardiac electrophysiology: techniques and interpretations. Josephson M, ed. Philadelphia: Lea & Feibiger, 1993:181.

20. Gillette P, Wampler D, Garson A, Zinner A, Ott D, Cooley D: Treatment of atrial automatic tachycardia by ablation procedures. J Am Coll Cardiol 1985;6:405.

21. Haissaguerre M, Warin JF, Le Metayer Ph: Fulguration des foyers de tachycardie atriales de l'adulte. Ann Cardiol Angeiol 1988;37:293.

22. Walsh EP, Saul JP, Hulse H, et al: Transcatheter ablation of ectopic atrial tachycardia in young patients using radio frequency current. Circulation 1992;86:1138.

23. Gossinger H, Wang X, Beckman K, et al: Radiofrequency catheter ablation of atrial tachycardias in the region of the sinus node. Pacing Clin Electrophysiol 1993;16(4):850.

24. Sanders WE, Sorrentino RA, Greenfield RA, Shenasa H, Hamer ME, Wharton MJ: Catheter ablation of sinoatrial node reentrant tachycardia. J Am Coll Cardiol 1994;23(4):926.

25. Shenasa H, Sanders W, Pressley J, et al: Safety and efficacy of radiofrequency catheter ablation of ectopic atrial tachycardia. Pacing Clin Electrophysiol 1993;16(4):850.

26. Weiss C, Hatala R, Cappato R, Schlüter M, Kuck KH: The encircling mapping technique—a simplified approach to ablation of ectopic atrial tachycardia. J Am Coll Cardiol 1994;23(2):82A.

27. Machell CH, Charlotte K: Management of primary atrial tachycardia with radiofrequency catheter ablation. J Am Coll Cardiol 1993;21(2):50A.

28. Ott DA, Gillette PC, Garson A, Cooley DA, Reul GJ, McNamara D: Surgical management of refractory supraventricular tachycardia in infants and children. J Am Coll Cardiol 1985;5:124.

29. Gillette PC: Successful transcatheter ablation of ectopic atrial tachycardia in young patients using radiofrequency current. Circulation 1992;86(4):1339.

30. Kay GN, Chong F, Epstein AE, Dailey SM, Plumb VJ: Radiofrequency ablation for treatment of primary atrial tachycardias. J Am Coll Cardiol 1993;21(4):901.

31. Tracy CM, Swartz JF, Fletcher RD, et al: Radiofrequency catheter ablation of ectopic atrial tachycardia using paced activation sequence mapping. J Am Coll Cardiol 1993;21 (4):910.

32. Chen SA, Chiang CE, Yang CJ, et al: Radiofrequency catheter ablation of sustained intra-atrial reentrant tachycardia in adult patients. Identification of electrophysiological characteristics and endocardial mapping techniques. Circulation 1993;88(2):578.

33. Poty H, Haissaguerre M, Warin JF, Saoudi N, Letac B: Radiofrequency catheter ablation of atrial tachycardias. Cardiostim 94, Nice, 15–18 juin 1994. Abstract.

34. Grogan EW, De Buitler M, Musser G: Radiofrequency modification of the sinus node for inappropriate sinus tachycardia. J Am Coll Cardiol 1992;19(3):270A.

35. Haissaguerre M, Warin JF, Lemetayer P, Saoudi N, Guillem JP, Blanchot P: Closed-chest ablation of retrograde conduction in patients with atrioventricular nodal reentrant tachycardia. N Engl J Med 1989;320:426.

36. Goy JJ, Fromer M, Schlaepfer J, et al: Clinical efficacy of radiofrequency current in the treatment of patients with atrioventricular node reentrant tachycardia. J Am Coll Cardiol 1990;6:418.

37. Lee MA, Morady F, Kadish A, et al: Catheter modification of the atrioventricular junction with radiofrequency energy for control of atrioventricular nodal reentry tachycardia. Circulation 1991;83:827.

38. Jackman WM, Beckman KJ, McClelland JH, et al: Treatment of supraventricular tachycardia due to atrioventricular nodal reentry by radiofrequency catheter ablation of slow-pathway conduction. N Engl J Med 1992;327:313.

39. Jazayeri MR, Hempe SL, Sra JS, et al: Selective transcatheter ablation of the fast and slow pathways using radiofrequency energy in patients with atrioventricular nodal reentrant tachycardia. Circulation 1992;85:1318.

40. Kay GN, Epstein AE, Dailey SM, Plumb VJ: Selective radiofrequency ablation of the slow pathway for the treatment of AV reentrant tachycardia. Evidence for involvement of perinodal myocardium within the reentrant circuit. Circulation 1992;85:1675.

41. Haissaguerre M, Gaita F, Fischer B, et al: Elimination of atrioventricular nodal reentrant tachycardia using discrete slow potentials to guide application of radiofrequency energy. Circulation 1992;85:2162.

42. Wathen M, Natale A, Wolfe K, Yee R, Newman D, Klein G: An anatomically guided approach to atrioventricular node slow pathway ablation. Am J Cardiol 1992;70:886.

43. Langberg JJ, Leon A, Borganelli M, et al: A randomized, prospective comparison of anterior and posterior approaches to radiofrequency catheter ablation of atrioventricular nodal reentry tachycardia. Circulation 1993;87:1551.

44. Kalbfleisch SJ, Strickberger A, Williamson B, et al: Randomized comparison of anatomic and electrogram mapping approaches to ablation of the slow pathway of atrioventricular nodal reentrant tachycardia. J Am Coll Cardiol 1994; 23:716.

45. Wu D, Yeh SJ, Wang CC, Wen MS, Lin FC: A simple technique for selective radiofrequency ablation of the slow pathway in atrioventricular node reentrant tachycardia. J Am Coll Cardiol 1993;21:1612.

46. Mitrani RD, Klein LS, Hackett FK, Zipes DP, Miles WM: Radiofrequency ablation for atrioventricular node reentrant tachycardia: comparison between fast (anterior) and slow (posterior) pathway ablation. J Am Coll Cardiol 1993;21:432.

47. Li HG, Klein GJ, Stites HW, et al: Elimination of slow pathway conduction: an accurate indicator of clinical success after radiofrequency AV node modification. J Am Coll Cardiol 1993;22:1849.

48. Jazayeri MR, Sra JS, Akhtar M: Transcatheter modification of the atrioventricular node using radiofrequency energy. Herz 1992;3:143.

49. Akhtar M, Jazayeri MR, Sra J, Blanck Z, Deshpande S, Dhala A: Atrioventricular nodal reentry. Clinical, electrophysiological and therapeutic considerations. Circulation 1993;88:282.

50. Moulton K, Miller B, Scott J, Woods WT: Radiofrequency catheter ablation for AV nodal reentry: a technique for rapid transection of the slow AV nodal pathway. Pacing Clin Electrophysiol 1993;16I:760.

51. Racker DK: Sinoventricular transmission in 10 mM K+ by canine atrioventricular nodal inputs: superior atrionodal bundle and proximal atrioventricular bundle. Circulation 1991;83:1738.

52. Haissaguerre M, Fischer B, Le Métayer Ph, Egloff Ph, Warin JF: Double potentials recorded during sinus rhythm in the triangle of Koch—evidence for functional dissociation from pacing of various right atrial sites. Pacing Clin Electrophysiol 1993;16(Pt II):1101.

53. De Bakker JMT, Coronel R, MacGuire MA, et al: Slow potentials in the AV-junctional area of patients operated on for atrioventricular node tachycardias and in isolated porcine hearts. J Am Coll Cardiol 1994;23:709.

54. MacGuire M, Bourke JP, Robotin MC, et al: High resolution mapping of Koch's triangle using sixty electrodes in humans with atrioventricular junctional (AV nodal) reentrant tachycardia. Circulation 1983;88:2315.

55. MacGuire MA, de Bakker JMT, Vermeulen JT, Opthof T, Becker AE, Janse MJ: The origin of "slow pathway" potentials. Correlation of extracellular potentials, intracellular potentials and histology. Pacing Clin Electrophysiol 1994;17II:749. Abstract.

56. Wellens HJJ, Brugada P: Value of programmed stimulation of the heart in patients with the Wolff-Parkinson-White syndrome. In: Josephson ME, Wellens HJJ, eds. Tachycardias. Philadelphia: Lea & Febiger, 1984:199.

57. Gallagher JJ, Pritchett ELC, Sealy WC, et al: The preexcitation syndromes. Prog Cardiovasc Dis 1978;20:285.

58. Scheinman MM, Morady F, Hess DS, et al: Catheter-induced ablation of the atrioventricular junction to control refractory supraventricular arrhythmias. JAMA 1982;248:851.

59. Gallagher JJ, Svenson R, Kasell J, et al: Catheter techniques for closed-chest ablation of the atrio-ventricular conduction system. A therapeutic alternative for the treatment of refractory supraventricular tachycardia. N Engl J Med 1982;306:194.

60. Weber H, Schmitz L: Catheter technique for closed-chest ablation of an accessory pathway. N Engl J Med 1983;308:654.

61. Morady F, Scheinman MM: Transvenous catheter ablation of posteroseptal accessory pathway in a patient with the Wolff-Parkinson-White syndrome. N Engl J Med 1984;310:705.

62. Critelli G, Gallagher JJ, Perticone F, et al: Transvenous catheter ablation of the accessory pathway in the permanent form of junctional reciprocating tachycardia. Am J Cardiol 1985;55:1639.

63. Fisher JD, Brodman R, Kim SG, et al: Attempted non-surgical ablation of accessory pathways via the coronary sinus in the Wolff-Parkinson-White Syndrome. J Am Coll Cardiol 1984;4:685.

64. Ward DE, Camm AJ: Treatment of tachycardias associated with the Wolff-Parkinson-White syndrome by transvenous electrical ablation of accessory pathways. Br Heart J 1985;53:64.

65. Haissaguerre M, Warin JF, Regaudie JJ, et al: Fulguration après enregistrement électrique direct de la voie de Kent. Arch Mal Coeur 1986;79:1072.

66. Bardy GH, Ivey T, Coltorti F, et al: Developments complications and limitations of catheter-mediated electrical atrioventricular pathways. Am J Cardiol 1988;61:1309.

67. Ruder MA, Hardwin Mead R, Gaudiani V, et al: Transvenous catheter ablation of extranodal accessory pathways. J Am Coll Cardiol 1988;11:1245.

68. Warin JF, Haissaguerre M, Le Metayer Ph, et al: Catheter ablation of accessory pathways with a direct approach. Circulation 1988;78:800.

69. Haissaguerre M, Warin JF: Closed-chest ablation of left lateral atrio-ventricular accessory pathways. Eur Heart J 1989;10:602.

70. Morady F, Scheinman MM, Kow WH, et al: Long-term results of catheter ablation of a posteroseptal accessory atrioventricular connection in 48 patients. Circulation 1989;79:1160.

71. Warin JF, Haissaguerre M, d'Ivernois Ch, et al: Catheter ablation of accessory pathways: technique and results in 248 patients. Pacing Clin Electrophysiol 1990;13:1609.

72. Haissaguerre M, Dartigues JF, Warin JF, et al: Electrogram patterns predictive of successful catheter ablation of accessory pathways. Value of unipolar recording mode. Circulation 1991;84:188.

73. Marcus FI: The use of radiofrequency energy for intracardiac ablation: historical perspective and results of experiments in animals. In: Breithardt G, Borggrefe M, Zipes DP, eds. Non pharmacological therapy of tachyarrhythmias. Mt. Kisco, NY: Futura Publishing, 1987:213.

74. Huang SK, Bharati S, Graham AR, et al: Closed-chest catheter dessication of the atrioventricular junction using radiofrequency energy; a new method of catheter-ablation. J Am Coll Cardiol 1987;9:349.

75. Borggrefe M, Budde T, Podczeck A, et al: High frequency alternating current ablation of an accessory pathway in humans. J Am Coll Cardiol 1987;10:576.

76. Borggrefe M, Hindricks G, Haverkamps W, et al: Radiofrequency ablation. In: Zipes DP, Jalife J, eds. Cardiac electrophysiology: from cell to bedside. Philadelphia: WB Saunders, 1990:997.

77. Lavergne T, Guize L, Le Heuzey J-Y, et al: Transvenous ablation of the atrioventricular junction in human with high-frequency energy. J Am Coll Cardiol 1987;9(Suppl):99A. Abstract.

78. Jackman WM, Kuck KH, Naccarelli GV, et al: Radiofrequency current directed across the mitral anulus with a bipolar epicardial-endocardial catheter electrode configuration in dogs. Circulation 1988;78:1288.

79. Jackman WM, Friday KJ, Yeung-Lai-Wah JA, et al: New catheter technique for recording left free-wall accessory atrioventricular pathway activation: identification of pathway fiber orientation. Circulation 1988;78:598.

80. Langberg JJ, Chin MC, Rosenqvist M, et al: Catheter ablation of the atrioventricular junction with radiofrequency energy. Circulation 1989;80:1527.

81. Kuck KH, Friday KJ, Kunze KP, et al: Sites of conduction block in accessory atrioventricular pathways; basis for concealed accessory pathways. Circulation 1990;82:407.

82. Jackman WM, Wang W, Friday KJ, et al: Catheter ablation of accessory atrioventricular pathways (Wolff-Parkinson-White syndrome) by radiofrequency current. N Engl J Med 1991; 324:1605.

83. Kuck KH, Schluter M: Single-catheter approach to radiofrequency ablation of left-side accessory pathways in patients with Wolff-Parkinson-White syndrome. Circulation 1991; 84:2366.

84. Calkins H, Souza J, El-Atassi R, et al: Diagnosis and cure of the Wolff-Parkinson-White syndrome of paroxysmal supraventricular tachycardias during a single electrophysiologic test. N Engl J Med 1991;324:1612.

85. Schluter M, Geiger M, Siebles J, et al: Catheter ablation using radio-frequency current to cure symptomatic patients with tachyarrhythmias related to an accessory atrio-ventricular pathway. Circulation 1991;84:1644.

86. Huang SKS: Radiofrequency catheter ablation of cardiac arrhythmias: appraisal of an evolving therapeutic modality. Am Heart J 1989;118:1317.

87. Haissaguerre M, Fischer B, Warin JF, et al: Electrogram patterns predictive of successful radiofrequency catheter ablation of accessory pathways. Pacing Clin Electrophysiol 1992;15(II):2138.

88. Prystowsky EN, Browne KF, Zipes DP: Intracardiac recording by catheter electrode of accessory pathway depolarization. J Am Coll Cardiol 1983;1:463.

89. Jackman WM, Friday KJ, Scherlag BJ, et al: Direct endocardial recording from an atrioventricular pathway: localization of the site of block effect of antiarrhythmic drugs and attempt at non surgical ablation at non surgical ablation. Circulation 1983;5:906.

90. Calkins H, Kim Y, Schmaltz S, et al: Electrogram criteria for identification of appropriate target sites for radiofrequency catheter ablation of accessory pathways. Circulation 1992; 85:565.

91. Silka MJ, Kron J, Halperin BD, et al: Analysis of local electrogram characteristics correlates with successful radiofrequency ablation of accessory pathways. Pacing Clin Electrophysiol 1992;15:1000.

92. Leather RA, Leitch JW, Klein GJ, et al: Radiofrequency catheter ablation of accessory pathways: A learning experience. Am J Cardiol 1991;68:1651.

93. Lesh MD, Van Hare GF, Schamp DJ, et al: Curative percutaneous catheter ablation using radiofrequency energy for accessory pathways in all locations: results in 100 consecutive patients. Am J Cardiol 1992;19:1303.

94. Natale A, Wathen M, Yee R, et al: Atrial and ventricular approaches for radiofrequency catheter ablation of left-sided accessory pathways. Am J Cardiol 1992;70:114.

95. Chen XU, Borggrefe M, Hindricks G, et al: Radiofrequency ablation of accessory pathways: characteristics of transiently and permanently effective pulses. Pacing Clin Electrophysiol 1992;15:1122.

96. Swartz JF, Tracy CM, Fletcher RD. Radiofrequency endocardial catheter ablation of accessory atrioventricular pathway atrial insertion sites. Circulation 1993;87:487.

97. Chen SA, Chiang CE, Tsang WP, et al: Recurrent conduction in accessory pathway and possible new arrhythmias after radiofrequency catheter ablation. Am Heart J 1993;125: 381.

98. Miles WM, Klein LS, Gering LE, et al: Efficacy and safety of catheter ablation using radiofrequency energy in patients with accessory pathways. J Am Coll Cardiol 1991;17:232A. Abstract.

99. Wittkampf FHM, Simmers TA, Hauer RNW: Repeated radiofrequency catheter ablation: effect of a bonus pulse on myocardial temperature. Eur Heart J 1994;14:256. Abstract.

100. Simmers TA, Hauer RN, Wittkampf FH, et al: Radiofrequency catheter ablation of accessory pathways: prediction of ablation outcome by unipolar electrogram characteristics. Pacing Clin Electrophysiol 1993;16(II):866.

101. Smeets J, Allessie M, Kirchlof CH, et al: High resolution mapping of ventriculoatrial conduction over the accessory pathway in patients with the Wolff Parkinson White syndrome. Eur Heart J 1990;11:1. Abstract.

102. Becker AE, Anderson RH, Durrer D, et al: The anatomic substrates of Wolff Parkinson White. A clinicopathologic correlation in seven patients. Circulation 1978;57:870.

103. Frank R, Brechenmacher C, Fontaine G. Apport de l'histologie dans l'étude des syndromes de préexcitation ventriculaire. Coeur Med Int 1976;15:337.

104. Fisher WG, Swartz JF: Three dimensional electrogram mapping improves ablation of left-sided AP. Pacing Clin Electrophysiol 1992;15:2344.

105. Farre J, Grande A, Martinelli J, et al: Atrial unipolar waveform analysis during retrograde conduction over left sided accessory atrioventricular pathways. In: Brugada P, Wellens HJJ. eds. Cardiac arrhythmias: where to go from here. Mt. Kisco, NY: Futura Publishing, 1987:243.

106. Kuck HH, Schluter M: The split-tip electrode catheter improvement in AP potential recording. J Am Coll Cardiol 1993;21:173A.

107. Kadish AH, Childs K, Schmaltz S, et al: Differences in QRS configuration during unipolar from adjacent sites: implications for the spatial resolution of pace-mapping. J Am Coll Cardiol 1991;17:143.

108. Dubuc M, Nadeau RN, Tremblay G, et al: Pace mapping using body surface potential maps to guide catheter ablation of accessory pathways in patients with Wolff Parkinson White syndrome. Circulation 1993;87:135.

109. Beckman K, Wang X, McClelland J, et al: Importance of recording accessory pathways potentials in patients undergoing repeat RF catheter ablation after failed initial procedure. Pacing Clin Electrophysiol 1993;16(II):865. Abstract.

110. Willems S, Hindricks G, Shenasa M, et al: Termination of orthodromic tachycardia using direct current sub-threshold stimulation in patients with concealed accessory pathways. Eur Heart J 1993;14:294. Abstract.

111. Iwa T, Borgreffe M, Shenasa M, et al: Prediction of exact energy delivery by unipolar electrocardiogram. Pacing Clin Electrophysiol 1992;15:590.

112. Lesh MD, Vanthare GF, Scheinman MM et al: Comparison of the retrograde and transseptal methods for ablation of left free wall accessory pathways. J Am Coll Cardiol 1993;22:542.

113. Schluter M, Kuck H: Catheter ablation from right atrium of

anteroseptal accessory pathways using radiofrequency current. J Am Coll Cardiol 1992;19:663.

114. Guiraudon GM, Klein GJ, Sharma AD, et al: Surgical approach to anterior septal accessory pathways in 20 patients with the Wolff Parkinson White syndrome. Eur J Cardiothorac Surg 1988;2:201.

115. Langberg JJ, Calkins H, El-Atassi R, et al: Temperature monitoring during radiofrequency catheter ablation of accessory pathways. Circulation 1992;86:1469.

116. Swartz JF, Cohen AI, Fletcher RD, et al: Right coronary epicardial mapping improves accessory pathway catheter ablation success. Circulation 1989;80:432. Abstract.

117. Inoue H, Matsuo H, Takayanagi K, Ishimitsu T, Murao S: Antidromic reciprocating tachycardia via a slow Kent bundle in Ebstein's anomaly. Am Heart J 1983;106:147.

118. Klein GJ, Guiraudon GM, Kerr CR, et al: "Nodoventricular" accessory pathway: evidence for distinct accessory atrioventricular pathway with atrioventricular node-like properties. J Am Coll Cardiol 1988;11:1035.

119. Tchou P, Lehmann MH, Jazayeri M, et al: Atriofascicular connection or a nodoventricular Mahaim fiber? Electrophysiological elucidation of the pathway and associated reentrant circuit. Circulation 1988;77:837.

120. Guiraudon CM, Guiraudon GM, Klein GJ: "Nodal ventricular" Mahaim pathway: histologic evidence for an accessory atrioventricular pathway with an AV node-like morphology. Circulation 1988;78(II):40.

121. Haissaguerre M, Warin JF, Le Metayer P, et al: Apport de l'enregistrement du potentiel spécifique dans l'expression des voies accessoires. Arch Mal Coeur 1988;81:293.

122. Haissaguerre M, Warin JF, Le Metayer Ph, et al: Catheter ablation of Mahaim fibers with preservation of atrioventricular nodal conduction. Circulation 1990;82:418.

123. McClelland J, Jackman W, Beckman K, et al: Direct recordings of right atriofascicular accessory pathway (Mahaim) potentials at the tricuspid anulus. Pacing Clin Electrophysiol 1992;15:547. Abstract.

124. Klein LS, Hackett FK, Zipes DP, et al: Radiofrequency catheter ablation of Mahaim fibers at the tricuspid anulus. Circulation 1993;87:738.

125. Haissaguerre M, Fischer B, Le Metayer Ph, et al: Nature of the distal insertion site of Mahaim fibers as defined by catheter ablation. Eur Heart J 1993;14:33. Abstract.

126. Cappato R, Hebe J, Schlüter M, et al: Observations on accessory connections with decremental conduction properties during radiofrequency current ablation. J Am Coll Cardiol 1993;21:50A. Abstract.

127. Wang X, Jackman WM, McClelland J, et al: Sites of successful radiofrequency ablation of posteroseptal accessory pathways. Pacing Clin Electrophysiol 1992;15:II 535. Abstract.

128. Dhala A, Sra J, Deshpande S, et al: Successful radiofrequency catheter ablation of left-sided posteroseptal accessory pathways using right atrial approach: left-sided or right-sided pathways? Circulation 1992;86:I 722. Abstract.

129. Haissaguerre M, Montserrat P, Warin JF, et al: Catheter abla-

tion of left posteroseptal accessory pathways and of long RP' tachycardias with a right endocardial approach. Eur Heart J 1991;12:845.

130. Kuck KH, Weiss C, Mietzko R, et al: Accessory AV-pathways related to the middle cardiac vein or to a coronary sinus diverticulum. Circulation 1993;87(I):295. Abstract.

131. Arruda M, Wang X, McClelland J, et al: ECG algorithm for predicting sites of successful RF ablation of accessory pathways. Pacing Clin Electrophysiol 1993;16:865. Abstract.

132. Kuck KH, Schluter M, Gursoy M: Preservation of atrioventricular nodal conduction during radiofrequency current catheter ablation of midseptal accessory pathways. Circulation 1992;86:1743.

133. Scheinman MM, Wang Y, Van Hare GF, et al: Electrocardiographic and electrophysiologic characteristics of anterior, midseptal and right anterior free wall accessory pathways. J Am Coll Cardiol 1992;20:1220.

134. Heald SC, Bashir Y, O'Nunain S, et al: Radiofrequency ablation of intermediate septal pathways using a bipolar LV-RV electrode configuration. J Am Coll Cardiol 1992;19:26A. Abstract.

135. Ticho BS, Saul JP, Hulse JE, et al: Variable location of accessory pathways associated with the permanent form of junctional reciprocating tachycardia and confirmation with radiofrequency ablation. Am J Cardiol 1992;70:1559.

136. Norris JF, Klein LS, Hackett K, et al: Why does radiofrequency catheter ablation fail when electrograms are ideal and tissue temperature is adequate? Pacing Clin Electrophysiol 1993; 16:865. Abstract.

137. Haissaguerre M, Gaita F, Fischer B, et al: Radiofrequency catheter ablation of left lateral accessory pathways via the coronary sinus. Circulation 1992;86(5):1464.

138. Rowland E, Cunningham D, Ahsan A, et al: Transvenous ablation of atrioventricular junction with a low energy power source. Br Heart J 1989;62:361.

139. Lemery R, Talajic M, Roy D, et al: Success, safety, and late electrophysiological outcome of low-energy direct-current ablation in patients with the Wolff Parkinson White syndrome. Circulation 1992;85:957.

140. Langberg JJ, Diehl K, Gallagher M, et al: Catheter modification of the AV junction using a microwave antenna. J Am Coll Cardiol 1992;19:26A. Abstract.

141. Langberg JJ, Gallagher M, Strickberger SA, et al: Temperature-guided radiofrequency catheter ablation with very large distal electrodes. Circulation 1993;88:245.

142. Scheinman MM: Catheter ablation for cardiac arrhythmias, personnel and facilities. Pacing Clin Electrophysiol 1992; 15:715.

143. Hindricks G, Haverkamp W: The Multicenter European Radiofrequency Survey: summary of the results—complications of radiofrequency catheter ablation of cardiac arrhythmias in 4372 patients. Eur Heart J 1993;14:256. Abstract.

144. Friedman RA, Hamra M, Fenrich A: Radiofrequency ablation of immature myocardium: damage further than the eye can see. Circulation 1992;86(I):239.

Cardiac Arrhythmias, 3rd edition, edited by William J. Mandel.
J. B. Lippincott Company, Philadelphia © 1995.

31

G. Fontaine • R. Frank • Y. Gallais • J. Elias Neto
J. Tonet • G. Lascault • P. Aouate • F. Poulain

Fulguration of Ventricular Tachycardia: A 10-Year Experience

Endocardial fulguration, also called high-energy direct-current (DC) ablation, is based on the delivery of a strong electric shock from the tip of an endocardial catheter, at the arrhythmogenic substrate. This therapeutic approach was originally used for the treatment of supraventricular tachycardia. It was applied to the treatment of ventricular tachycardia for the first time in 1982 by Hartzler and by Puech and coworkers.[1,2]

This technique has been used by our group for more than 10 years to treat ventricular tachycardia that is refractory to antiarrhythmic drugs. In our center, it has replaced surgical treatment in patients who do not have other indications for cardiac surgery. This approach has been successful, regardless of the etiology of the ventricular tachycardia.[3] Endocardial fulguration, however, has been replaced by radiofrequency ablation, and high-energy DC ablation is used only in patients resistant to radiofrequency ablation.[4]

CLINICAL SERIES

This chapter focuses on the results of fulguration in a series of 87 consecutive cases treated with fulguration alone or in association with antiarrhythmic drugs for the treatment of chronic ventricular tachycardia. This group was selected from a series of 350 consecutive cases admitted to Jean Rostand Hospital for the treatment of chronic recurrent ventricular tachycardia. Patients were not excluded from the series because of age, clinical condition, or other factors.

Most of these patients were referred from other cardiac centers, where they were considered resistant to drug therapy. Before being selected for fulguration, they were restudied with antiarrhythmic drugs according to our protocols. Only patients resistant to amiodarone alone or in combination with class Ic antiarrhythmic agents, beta-blocking agents, or both were considered candidates for fulguration. This chapter updates our experience, which has previously been reported elsewhere.[5-9]

The etiology of ventricular tachycardia includes 36 patients having chronic coronary ischemic heart disease with chronic ischemia that occurred 10 years or more after myocardial infarction, 23 patients with arrhythmogenic right ventricular dysplasia (ARVD), 11 patients with verapamil sensitive ventricular tachycardia, 10 patients with idiopathic dilated cardiomyopathy, and 4 patients with a previously operated congenital anomaly. In one of the three who had tetralogy of Fallot, ventricular tachycardia occurred 7 years after infundibular resection and one patient had ventricular tachycardia associated with Ebstein's malformation. There were also three additional patients who had idiopathic infundibular ventricular tachycardia.

In the present series, the classification of the etiology is different from that previously reported from our hospital. This is because of clarification of the etiology of the disease in patients previously classed as having ARVD or idiopathic dilated cardiomyopathy based on their long-term evolution. In addition, one patient who had a dilated right ventricle with ventricular tachycardia originally classified as ARVD developed cardiac insufficiency and had cardiac transplantation. The pathology of the heart showed a typical pattern of dysplasia in the right ventricle as well as diffuse ischemic heart disease, with multiple zones of fibrous tissue typical of coronary artery disease in the high septum. This patient was the only patient previously classified as ARVD who had fulguration in the left ventricle. The ventricular tachycardia was actually due to myocardial ischemia. This case has been reclassified in the group of patients with ventricular tachycardia complicating chronic myocardial infarction.

EQUIPMENT

Many of the techniques used in our hospital were originally developed for the surgical treatment of Wolff-Parkinson-White syndrome and ventricular tachycardia. They have evolved over the years and have been published elsewhere.[10] In this chapter, we outline the main steps of the technical protocol used.

Catheters, generally tri- or quadripolar USCI 7-F (Bard Electrophysiology, Billerica, MA), are selected after an in vitro electric nondestructive test using voltages similar to those applied during fulguration shocks.[11] These catheters are introduced through veins or arteries and are guided under fluoroscopy to the right or left ventricular cavities. In some patients, the catheters were introduced in the left ventricle through a plastic sheath originally used for endocardial biopsy.

The DC energy source is a Fulgucor (ODAM Company, Wissembourg, France) and is based on our design. The delivered energy ranged from 160 to 320 J. This generator incorporates two independent high-voltage generators: one is used for the fulguration procedure, which delivers a long pulse of about 7 milliseconds and relatively low peak voltage, and the other is used for cardioversion or defibrillation. This can be used for ablation, either immediately after the fulguration shocks or during programmed pacing in case of deterioration of ventricular tachycardia.

Two tape recorders are used. The first records the fluoroscopic events on videotape. The second records the electrocardiogram (ECG) tracings from four surface leads as well as endocardial signals. Comments by five investigators who wear microphones and headsets are also recorded on the same tape. This proved to be of great value to determine the causes of complications.

The radial blood pressure is continuously monitored during the procedure, and a Swan-Ganz catheter is used to record the pulmonary arterial and wedge pressure and to perform cardiac output measurements by thermodilution techniques. Monitoring of oxygen saturation of blood in the coronary sinus was instituted and appears to be an excellent indication of patient tolerance of the procedure.[12] On-line monitoring of coagulation parameters is performed during the procedure, starting as soon as catheters are introduced inside the left ventricle. Activation times are measured on an Electronic for Medicine VR12 recorder. After each fulguration shock, the voltage and current are displayed on the memory screen of a two-channel digital Tektronix 5116 oscilloscope. Therefore, it is possible to determine (1) whether the energy of each shock has been correctly delivered, and (2) that there is no damage to the catheter, which may be used for the next shock if necessary.

Before fulguration, class I antiarrhythmic drugs are discontinued for at least five half-lives of the drug. Amiodarone is continued. A preliminary electrophysiologic study was frequently performed at the beginning of our experience to determine the ease of induction of ventricular tachycardia, the hemodynamic effects of the arrhythmia, and the number of morphologies of the clinical and nonclinical ventricular tachycardias. Only sustained monomorphic tachycardias are considered for ablation. Fulguration is performed under general anesthesia because it is usually necessary to deliver several shocks during each session. When ventricular tachycardia is not present at the beginning of the procedure, tachycardia is induced by programmed pacing.

In the past, delivery of the shock was guided by mapping the so-called site of origin of ventricular tachycardia, but this is used only to guide the catheter to the approximate site for ablation. The technique of pace-mapping is used and should reproduce a QRS complex that is identical to that of the 12-lead QRS of the spontaneous ventricular tachycardia. Pace-mapping is best achieved by overdriving the ventricular tachycardia at a slightly higher rate, using the same catheter that will deliver the electric shocks. In addition, the same ventricular tachycardia morphology should be present at the interruption of pacing. We give particular attention to the area of slow conduction, which is frequently represented by fragmented potentials located between two ventricular QRS complexes. Additional features identify the zone of slow conduction, which is a necessary link for perpetuation of the arrhythmia.[13,14]

When the checklist is completed a countdown is started, during which relevant equipment is put into action. The shock is synchronized on the QRS complexes and is delivered between the distal electrode (as the anode) and an indifferent return electrode of large surface covered by a conductive jelly located in the back. From one to 17 shocks (mean, 3.5) are delivered during each session. Just after the shock, transient complete atrioventricular block may be observed and ventricular pacing is initiated by a catheter previously located at the apex of the right ventricle. The pacing catheter should be located at least 3 cm from the fulgurating electrode. If rapid ventricular tachycardia is induced or if ventricular tachycardia degenerates into ventricular fibrillation, a cardioversion shock is delivered to an anterior patch electrode. The posterior patch is the same electrode as that used during fulguration. This shock is delivered by the safety defibrillator, which is a part of the Fulgucor. Therefore, it is not necessary to uncover the chest or to move the x-ray equipment. Low energy in the range of 40 to 160 J is generally sufficient to convert ventricular tachycardia or ventricular fibrillation.

After delivering the fulgurating shock, the patient is given a rest period of 10 minutes, provided that he or she is in sinus rhythm. This is necessary to restore myocardial electric and hemodynamic balance. Programmed pacing is then resumed in an attempt to reinduce ventricular tachycardia. The procedure is ended when it is no longer possible to induce ventricular tachycardia, when the tachycardia has been modified so that only transient ventricular tachycardia is induced, or when the ventricular tachycardia is slow and well tolerated. The session is also interrupted when episodes of ventricular fibrillation or unstable ventricular tachycardia are induced or for technical reasons.

In four cases (three of ARVD and one patient who had previous surgery for tetralogy of Fallot), a different technique was used: two underwent radiofrequency ablation and two underwent fulgutronisation. This was DC energy; however, the waveform has been modified so that it is longer and of lower voltage to avoid barotrauma.

IMMEDIATE FOLLOW-UP

The in-hospital follow-up period consists of monitoring the radial blood pressure and central venous pressure for 24 hours. A subclavian electrode catheter located at the apex of the right ventricle is left in place for 1 to 10 days. During this time, a repeat electrophysiologic study may be performed, generally at the bedside, to determine whether the tachycardia is reinducible. During this immediate follow-up period, the ECG is monitored by telemetry

using computerized Hewlett-Packard monitoring equipment with the Nadia software.

Effectiveness of fulguration is generally reassessed before discharge by 24-hour ambulatory ECG recording, stress testing, and programmed pacing, including the use of up to three extrastimuli at a cycle length of 600, 500, and 400 milliseconds.

DEFINITION OF RESULTS

The patient is classified as a *success* when drugs are no longer needed or when patients who are noninducible after fulguration continue to take these medicines for safety reasons (very rapid ventricular tachycardia or ventricular fibrillation before fulguration) or to treat ventricular or supraventricular extrasystoles. In addition, the follow-up period should be at least equal to the longest interval between spontaneous consecutive attacks observed in the months preceding the ablation.

When the same dosage and drugs as before the fulguration procedure are effective, the patient is classified as a *partial success* because it may prevent ventricular arrhythmias after fulguration by modifying the arrhythmogenic substrate. The patient is classified as having *modified ventricular tachycardia* when the tachycardias with or without additional drug treatment are still present but at a slow rate and well tolerated. Patients in whom antiarrhythmic treatment different from that used before fulguration led to the control of ventricular tachycardia are considered as having *uninterpretable* results. In this group are also included patients who died after a follow-up that was too short to ascertain arrhythmia control. When ventricular tachycardia identical or similar to that present before ablation in rate and morphology occurs spontaneously or is inducible after ablation, the result is classified as a *failure* and pharmacologic attempts are made to prevent the arrhythmia.

The *fulguration efficacy* consists of the sum of *success*, *partial success*, and *modified ventricular tachycardia*. The *clinical efficacy* incorporates the cases of operative death considered as a clinical failure.

The final classification is made at the end of the follow-up period.

FOLLOW-UP AFTER HOSPITAL DISCHARGE

After hospital discharge, the follow-up of these patients is aided by a computer system, using a DEC PDP 11/23 + and specialized software developed at our institution. The follow-up consists of discussion with the general practitioner, the cardiologist, and the referring hospital in addition to direct phone calls to the patient or his family members. Duration of follow-up is the time interval between the first fulguration procedure and the last information obtained for each patient.

RESULTS

Results are calculated by microcomputer software developed by Fontaine using dBase IV programming language, version 1.5. Graphs are made with Statistica for Windows, version 4.3. Calculation of results is determined based on each ablation session. The time interval between two sessions is used if it is longer than 1 month. Patients who required a repeat ablation session were censored at the time of the repeat ablation session if they were treated with radiofrequency energy or fulgutronisation at that session, provided that the follow-up period is longer than the spontaneous duration of the longest interval between two consecutive attacks observed in the months preceding the ablation. The final classification of each case is made at the time of the last information. For those patients who had a heart transplant because of congestive heart failure, the data are censored at the date of transplant.

Some patients had their classification changed over time because of spontaneous improvement or worsening of their condition. Therefore, their classification at the end of the follow-up may be different when compared with their classification after their last ablation session.

Procedure-related death are included in the calculation of global clinical efficacy but are excluded in the study of fulguration efficacy. This is done to determine the effect of fulguration per se on the treatment of ventricular tachycardia. A hemodynamic death during the procedure does not indicate whether the patient was or was not controlled by the ablation.

Ischemic Heart Disease

The series of 36 patients who had ventricular tachycardia after myocardial infarction consists of 33 males and 3 females (Tables 31-1 and 31-2). The mean age was 60 years old, ranging from 29 to 76 years (Fig. 31-1). The distribution of the mean ejection fraction is presented in Figure 31-2. Eight patients had incessant ventricular tachycardia. The longest episode between consecutive attacks was 1 day in two patients, 1 week in seven, 1 month in 19, and 1 year in eight patients. Nineteen patients had a history of having more than 20 separate episodes of ventricular tachycardia. In nine patients, ventricular tachycardia was monomorphic; in 12, two morphologies were observed. Twelve patients had three morphologies and three patients had more than three morphologies. Eleven patients required two sessions, three had three sessions, and two had four sessions. In five cases, shocks were delivered only in the right ventricle and in both ventricles in five additional patients.

After the first procedure, success was obtained in eight patients, nine had a partial success, and there were 12 failures (Table 31-3). Two patients died during the procedure. The fulguration efficacy of a single session was 58.6% and clinical efficacy was 54.8%. In 11 of the 12 patients who failed the first session, repeat sessions were undertaken. This was performed in less than 1 month in eight patients or after 2, 7, and 21 months, respectively, in three patients. This new session led to success in three, to

TABLE 31-1. Clinical Characteristics of Ventricular Tachycardia Classified by Etiology

Etiology	N (m)	Age	EF	INC	>20 ep	1M	2M	3M	>3M	Shocks (n)
MI	36 (33)	60.8 ± 9.9 (29–76)	30.8 ± 11.2 (12–65)	8	19	9	12	12	3	1–10
ARVD	23 (14)	40.1 ± 14.4 (21–74)	57.4 ± 5.6 (48–69)	3	11	15	4	3	1	1–8
VSVT	11 (9)	32.5 ± 11.2 (17–51)	64.4 ± 6.6 (47–72)	2	8	11	—	—	—	1–7
IDC	10 (9)	34.7 ± 16.8 (14–70)	23.1 ± 5.3 (15–30)	6	7	6	2	1	1	1–12
OCA	4 (4)	21.5 ± 4.6 (15–28)	60.3 ± 6.1 (50–65)	1	1	2	0	1	1	2–10
IVT	3 (0)	36.3 ± 11.9 (26–53)	62 ± 11.2 (50–77)	2	3	3	—	—	—	1–6

The statistical results are indicated with the mean value, standard deviation, and the range in brackets.
MI, myocardial infarction; ARVD, arrhythmogenic right ventricular dysplasia; VSVT, verapamil-sensitive ventricular tachycardia; IDC, idiopathic dilated cardiomyopathy; OCA, operated congenital anomalies; IVT, idiopathic ventricular tachycardia; N (m), number of cases (males); EF, left ventricular ejection fraction; INC, incessant ventricular tachycardia; >20 ep, more than 20 different episodes of VT; 1 M, 2 M, 3 M, 1, 2, 3 morphologies; >3 M, more than 3 morphologies.

TABLE 31-2. Follow-Up Results of Table 31-1

Etiology	Complications	Follow-Up Survey	Follow-Up LD	Follow-Up Failures
MI	7 (24%)	12: 69 ± 34 (21–119)	17: 31 ± 28 (1–107)	1: 21
ARVD	3 (14%)	22: 71 ± 36 (1–122)	—	3: 71 ± 24 (49–104)
VSVT	1 (9%)	11: 54 ± 27 (6–96)	—	—
IDC	2 (25%)	1: 40	5: 17 ± 7 (2–24)	—
OCA	—	3: 36 ± 13 (33–54)	1: 87	—

Complications, complications observed for any session; follow-up surv, follow-up of survivals; follow-up LD, follow-up of late deaths; follow-up failures, follow-up of patients who failed the procedure.

partial success in three, and there were five failures. Thus, a 54.5% fulguration efficacy was obtained after the second session. The patient who did not have a second session had an arrhythmic death 21 months after having multiple episodes of ventricular tachycardia not controlled by drugs.

In three of the five patients who failed the second session, a third session was performed and led to a modified ventricular tachycardia in one and failure in two. In the two remaining patients, there was late improvement, leading to a success at the end of the follow-up in one and a partial success in the other.

In the two remaining cases who failed the third session, a fourth fulguration session was performed (6 months later in one patient), leading to a partial success in both. Five patients (13.9%) had uninterpretable results. Therefore, fulguration efficacy of 96.6% was obtained, with the clinical efficacy being 90.3%. A synthesis of these results is schematically depicted in Table 31-2 and graphically presented on Figure 31-3.

EARLY DEATHS. Four cases of early death (defined as death within 30 days of the fulguration procedure) include two peroperative and two postoperative deaths. Death was procedure-related in two: one patient had tamponade due to the fulguration before modification of the protocol and the other death was not directly related to the delivery of

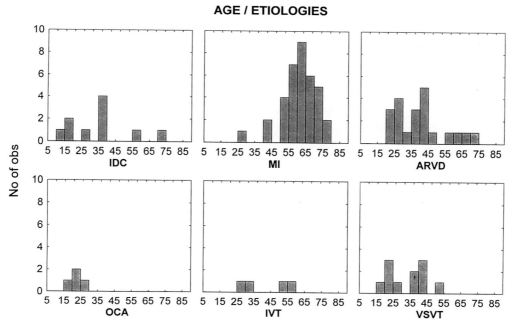

Figure 31-1. Histogram of age versus etiologies of ventricular tachycardia. *IDC*, idiopathic dilated cardiomyopathy; *MI*, myocardial infarction; *ARVD*, arrhythmogenic right ventricular dysplasia; *OCA*, operated congenital anomaly; *IVT*, idiopathic infundibular ventricular tachycardia; *VSVT*, verapamil-sensitive ventricular tachycardia.

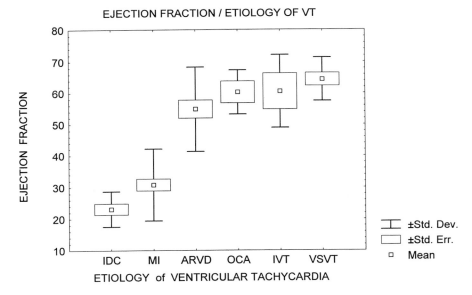

Figure 31-2. Ejection fraction versus etiologies. Abbreviations are the same as in Figure 31-1.

the shock. The two postoperative deaths were due to sepsis present before the ablative session in one and to cerebral ischemia resulting from inappropriate anesthesia in the other.

LATE DEATHS. Seventeen late deaths occurred in this series during a follow-up ranging from 21 to 119 months. A histogram of follow-up is presented in Figure 31-4. Fifteen patients died of cardiac disease—five due to sudden death that was preceded in three by warning symptoms (palpitations), nine due to congestive heart failure, one of a new acute myocardial infarction, and one of a stroke.

COMPLICATIONS. Other complications consisted of transient pulmonary edema during or just after the procedure in four cases. There was one case of hemopericardium.

One patient developed an elevation of the MB fraction of creatinekinase (CKMB) after inadvertent manipulation of the catheter in the anterior descending coronary artery. This minor complication has not been added to those of the other VT etiologies and is presented in Fig. 31-5.

Arrhythmogenic Right Ventricular Dysplasia

The 23 patients with ARVD consisted of 14 males and nine females. Their mean age was 40 years and the range was 21 to 74 years. Their mean left ejection fraction was 30% or more in all. Three patients had incessant ventricular tachycardia. The longest intervals between two consecutive episodes of ventricular tachycardia were 1 day in one, 1 month in 15, and 1 year in seven cases. Eleven cases had

more than 20 episodes. Ventricular tachycardia was monomorphic in 15 patients, had two morphologies in four, three morphologies in three, and four morphologies in one. Fourteen patients had two sessions and three had three sessions. All shocks were delivered to the right ventricle.

A successful outcome was observed after the first session in five cases, partial success in five, and failure occurred in 12 cases. Therefore, the fulguration efficacy was 45.5% after the first session. Eleven of these 12 patients who failed, in addition to two who had a partial success, and one who was classified as uninterpretable because of a too short follow-up time had repeat sessions within 1 month or 5, 6, 7, 8, 32, and 66 months later. This led to success in three, partial success in four, failure in six cases, and one operative death. The fulguration efficacy was 53.8% and clinical efficacy of this session was 50%. Three of these six patients who failed the second session had a third session within 1 month, leading to success in one and partial success in two. Two patients who also failed the second session were finally controlled by drug treatment. The last patient had surgery because of a congenital anomaly. At surgery, a simple ventriculotomy ablated the arrhythmogenic focus. Therefore, the overall fulguration efficacy was 86.4%. The clinical efficacy was 82.6%.

EARLY DEATHS. There was one death due to low output failure during the second session that occurred at the beginning of our experience before hemodynamic monitoring during the procedure was established.

LATE DEATHS. No late deaths have been observed in this series during the follow-up ranging from 1 to 122 months.

TABLE 31-3. Results of The Fulguration Procedure

	N	Success	Partial S.	Mod.	Failure	Op Dth	Ful Eff (%)	Clin Eff (%)
CHRONIC ISCHEMIC HEART DISEASE								
FI	36	8 (25.8)	9 (29)	0	12 (38.7)	2 (5.6)	58.6	54.8
FII	11	3 (27.3)	3 (27.3)	0	5 (45.5)	0	54.5	54.5
FIII	3	0	0	1 (33.3)	2 (66.7)	0	33.3	33.3
FIV	2	0	2 (100)	0	0	0	100	100
Fin Res	36	14 (45.2)	13 (41.9)	1 (3.2)	1 (3.2)	2 (5.6)	96.6	90.3
ARRHYTHMOGENIC RIGHT VENTRICULAR DYSPLASIA								
FI	23	5 (22.7)	5 (22.7)	0	12 (54.5)	0	45.5	45.5
FII	14	3 (21.4)	4 (28.6)	0	6 (42.9)	1 (7.1)	53.8	50
FIII	3	1 (33.3)	2 (66.7)	0	0	0	100	100
Fin Res	23	10 (43.5)	9 (39.1)	0	3 (13)	1 (4.3)	86.4	82.6
VERAPAMIL-SENSITIVE VENTRICULAR TACHYCARDIA								
FI	11	6 (54.5)	1 (9.1)	1 (9.1)	3 (27.3)	0	72.7	72.7
FII	4	3 (75)	0	1 (25)	0	0	100	100
FIII	1	1 (9.1)	0	0	0	0	100	100
Fin Res	11	9 (81.8)	2 (18.2)	0	0	0	100	100
IDIOPATHIC DILATED CARDIOMYOPATHY								
FI	10	2 (20)	1 (10)	1 (10)	5 (50)	1 (10)	44.4	40
FII	5	2 (40)	1 (20)	0	1 (20)	1 (20)	75	60
FIII	1	0	0	0	1 (100)	0	0	0
Fin Res	10	5 (50)	3 (30)	0	0	2 (20)	100	80
OPERATED CONGENITAL ANOMALIES								
FI	3	3 (75)	0	0	1 (25)	0	75	75
FII	1	0	1 (100)	0	0	0	100	100
FIII	1	1 (25)	0	0	0	0	100	100
Fin Res	4	4 (100)	0	0	0	0	100	100
IDIOPATHIC VENTRICULAR TACHYCARDIA								
FI	3	1 (33.3)	0	0	2 (66.7)	0	33.3	33.3
FII	1	1 (100)	0	0	0	0	100	100
Fin Res	3	2 (66.7)	0	0	1 (33.3)	0	66.7	66.7

Percentages are in brackets.
N, number of cases at the beginning of the study; Op Dth, operative deaths; FI, FII, FIII . . . , 1st session, 2nd session, 3rd session . . . ; Fin Res, Final results: results obtained after the follow-up. Partial S, Partial success; Mod, modified ventricular tachycardia; Ful Eff, fulguration efficacy; Clin Eff, clinical efficacy. Because of cases of spontaneous improvement or worsening, final results may be different from those recorded at the end of one or several procedures.

COMPLICATIONS. One case of hemopericardium occurred. In one patient, a clot in the infundibulum was found at routine follow-up by two-dimensional echocardiography and disappeared in few days after anticoagulant therapy.

Fascicular Tachycardia

Eleven patients had fascicular tachycardia, also called verapamil-sensitive ventricular tachycardia. Their mean age was 32 years old, ranging from 17 to 51 years. There were nine males and two females. Their mean ejection fraction was 64%, ranging from 47% to 72%. Two patients had incessant ventricular tachycardia. The longest intervals between two consecutive episodes of ventricular tachycardia were 1 week in one, 1 month in eight, and 1 year in two cases. Eight patients had a history of more than 20 episodes. All but one had monomorphic ventricular tachycardia with a right bundle branch block–left axis deviation pattern. Four patients required two sessions and one had three. In all but one of these patients, fulguration was delivered in the left ventricle; in one case, it was delivered at the apex of the right ventricle.

Success was obtained after a first session in six cases,

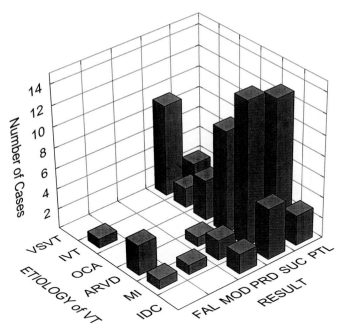

Figure 31-3. Graphic representation of the results versus the etiologies of ventricular tachycardia (VT). *FAL*, failure of the procedure; *MOD*, modified VT; *PRD*, operative death; *SUC*, success; *PTL*, partial success. Other abbreviations are the same as in Figure 31-1.

partial success in one, and one had a modified ventricular tachycardia. Three failures were observed, leading to a fulguration efficacy and clinical efficacy of 72.7% after the first session. Repeat sessions were performed after periods of 2, 5, and 25 months in the three cases who failed and in the patient who had the modified ventricular tachycardia after the first session. This led to three successes. The status of one patient who previously failed was changed to modified. This particular patient finally had a third successful session, leading to an overall fulguration efficacy and clinical efficacy of 100% (nine successes, two partial successes).

DEATHS. No case of early or late death occurred in this series during the study period ranging from 6 to 96 months.

COMPLICATIONS. One patient had hemopericardium.

Idiopathic Dilated Cardiomyopathy

The series of 10 patients with idiopathic dilated cardiomyopathy consisted of nine males and one female. Their mean age was 35 years, in the range of 14 to 70 years. Their

FOLLOW-UP

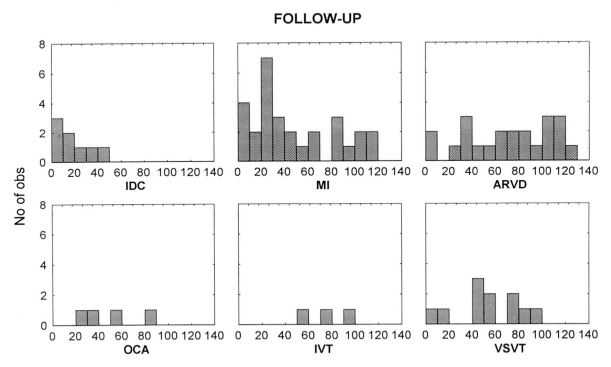

Figure 31-4. The shortest follow-up is observed in patients with idiopathic dilated cardiomyopathy because of the rapid attrition rate observed in this series. X axis, months; Y axis, number of cases. Abbreviations are the same as in Figure 31-1.

COMPLICATIONS

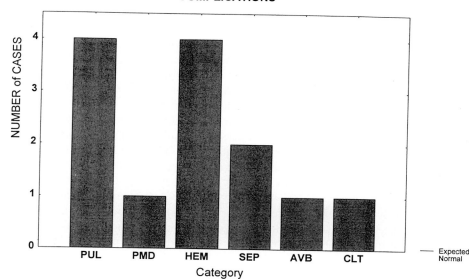

Figure 31-5. Presentation of total complications observed during or after the procedures. *PUL*, pulmonary edema; *PMD*, pacemaker dysfunction; *HEM*, hemopericardium; *SEP*, sepsis; *AVB*, third-degree atrioventricular block; *CLT*, clot formation.

mean ejection fraction was 23%, ranging from 15% to 30%. Six patients had incessant ventricular tachycardia. The longest intervals between two consecutive attacks were 1 day in one, 1 month in five, and 1 year in four patients. Seven patients had a history of more than 20 episodes. Ventricular tachycardia was monomorphic in six, two patients had two morphologies, one had three morphologies, and one had four morphologies. Five patients had two sessions. Shocks were delivered in the right ventricle in four cases.

A successful outcome was obtained in two patients, partial success in one, and one patient had a modified ventricular tachycardia after the first session. Five failures occurred. One patient died during the procedure. Therefore, the fulguration efficacy was 44.4% and the clinical efficacy was 40% after the first session. A second procedure was performed in five cases—within 1 month in three of these. The other patients had a second session after 2 and 9 months, respectively. This second session led to success in two, partial success in one, and failure in one case. One patient died during the second session. The patient who failed the second session had a third unsuccessful session, after which no further clinical recurrence was observed during the follow-up of 40 months and he was finally classified as a success. One patient, however, who was classified as a success after the second session developed new episodes of a different ventricular tachycardia 15 months later. He had a third session and was then classified as a success. The fulguration efficacy after the follow-up period was therefore 100% and the clinical efficacy was 80%.

EARLY DEATHS. One early death occurred in a patient who developed sepsis, leading to hyperkalemia and death the day after the fulguration procedure. The reason for this sequence of events was not evident.

A second patient who was in New York Heart Association Functional Class III died during the procedure due to low output. At autopsy, he had a moderate hemopericardium, probably related to the use of a catheter with a stiff guiding stylet. The hemopericardium may have played a role in his death.

One patient who had major pulmonary infection and incessant ventricular tachycardia had a successful fulguration but died of pulmonary infection.

LATE DEATHS. Five late deaths occurred in this series during the follow-up ranging from 2 to 40 months. Three had congestive heart failure, one patient died suddenly, and one had a noncardiac death.

COMPLICATIONS. One patient developed a complete atrioventricular block and required an implanted pacemaker.

Operated Congenital Heart Disease

There were four males having a mean age of 21.5 years old, ranging from 15 to 28 years. Their mean left ejection fraction was 60.3%, with a range of 50% to 65%. One patient had incessant ventricular tachycardia. The longest intervals between two consecutive attacks were 1 day in one, 1 week in one, 1 month in one, and 1 year in one case.

One patient had a history of more than 20 episodes. Two patients had monomorphic ventricular tachycardia, one had three, and one had four morphologies. One patient had two sessions and one had three. In all these patients, fulguration was delivered in the right ventricle.

After the first fulguration session, three complete success and one failure were observed, giving a fulguration efficacy and clinical efficacy of 75% after the first session. A second session was performed in the patient who failed and was classified as partial success; success was finally obtained after the third session, performed after 13 months. An overall fulguration efficacy and clinical efficacy of 100% was therefore obtained in this series.

DEATH. No early but one late sudden death preceded by ventricular arrhythmias occurred in another institution after 87 months in one case of tetralogy of Fallot during the overall follow-up, which ranged from 23 to 87 months.

Infundibular Idiopathic Ventricular Tachycardia

The three male patients with infundibular idiopathic ventricular tachycardia had a mean age of 36 years, ranging from 26 to 53 years. Their mean ejection fraction was 62%, with a range of 50% to 77%. One patient had incessant ventricular tachycardia. The longest intervals between two consecutive attacks were 1 day in one, 1 month in one, and 1 year in one patient. All had a history of more than 20 episodes and all had monomorphic ventricular tachycardia. One patient required two sessions. In all these patients, fulguration was delivered in the right ventricle.

In patients with infundibular idiopathic ventricular tachycardia, success was obtained in only one patient and two failures were observed after the first session. A second session was performed 9 days later in one case, leading to complete success. Final fulguration efficacy and clinical efficacy were therefore 66.7%. The last patient, who did not want a second session, was finally treated by drugs and pacemaker implantation. His follow-up was 75 months.

General Observations

Episodes of rapid ventricular tachycardia or ventricular fibrillation were observed just after the fulguration shock but were easily treated by DC defibrillation. Ventricular extrasystoles were also observed in the first days of the period of follow-up but did not require any other form of therapy.[15]

All the pacemaker patients had some transient modifications (a few seconds or minutes) of either programmed pacing functions or a change in their pacemaker program but only one in whom the shock was delivered in the right ventricular cavity close to the indwelling pacemaker catheter required pacemaker replacement.[16]

DISCUSSION

These results indicate that most of the patients who underwent DC fulguration for ventricular tachycardia had a successful outcome. Obvious differences in success and safety of the procedure are observed in patients with a good left ventricular function (e.g., verapamil-sensitive ventricular tachycardia, ARVD, outflow tract tachycardia, or operated congenital anomaly). It should be emphasized that all these patients were refractory to antiarrhythmic drugs, including amiodarone alone or in combination. It is not possible to say that the same technique could be extended to others with the same results after the learning curve.[17-19] This procedure requires special experience in terms of knowledge of the effects of high-voltage electric discharge in a saline medium.[20-26] It also requires special equipment, including a specifically chosen or modified DC defibrillator, proper drug management before the procedure, and strict programmed pacing protocols before discharge to ascertain arrhythmia control and eventual guidance of additional drug treatment.[17,27] For example, hemodynamically unstable ventricular tachycardias (or cases with inducible ventricular fibrillation) are difficult or even impossible to map. Appropriate use of amiodarone, including proper loading doses, makes the arrhythmia mappable in most cases.

Early Deaths

The eight early deaths, which represent 9.2% of the series, occurred mostly during the learning phase and only in the patients with poor left ventricular function (Figs. 31-6 and 31-7). Six of these eight early deaths were observed in patients who had an ejection fraction lower than or equal to 25%. This emphasizes that in this patient population, the procedure is not without risk. The mortality must be interpreted in view of these extremely ill patients who underwent the procedure as a last salvage effort. It should be noted that five patients were moribund when the fulguration procedure was performed and two were unconscious. This result is clearly better than the outcome obtained with previous ablative techniques, especially when we consider that many cases in whom fulguration was attempted would not have been candidates for surgery.[28-30] Study of the magnetic tape recordings of the endocardial and electrocardiographic signals and of the videotapes remote from the fatal event demonstrates that

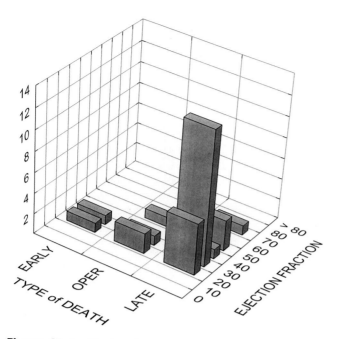

Figure 31-6. Bivariate histogram relating type of death and value of the left ventricular ejection fraction. *EARLY*, early operative death observed within 1 month after the procedure; *OPER*, operative death; *LATE*, late death.

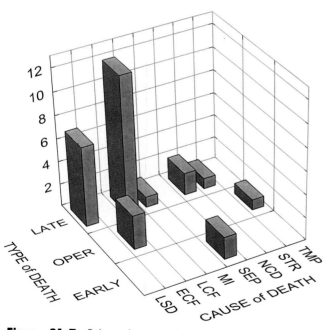

Figure 31-7. Relation between the type of death (early, operative, or late), as opposed to the cause of death. *TMP*, tamponade; *STR*, stroke; *NCD*, noncardiac death; *SEP*, sepsis; *MI*, myocardial infarction; *LCF*, low cardiac failure; *ECF*, early cardiac failure; *LSD*, late sudden death.

there was a learning curve up to case 23 and that in most cases, the protocols could be modified to avoid or prevent related deaths. These include:

- Monitoring the hemodynamics during the entire procedure
- Avoiding the use of high-energy (300 J) shock in patients with an ejection fraction below 20%
- Not delivering more than one high-energy shock (more than 160 J) in the same place *in the right ventricle*
- Avoiding the use of a too stiff catheter
- Using proper general anesthetic protocols
- Using cathodal instead of anodal shocks but repeating the shocks at the same place in the left ventricle if necessary

After each modification of the protocol, a new event of the same kind was not observed thereafter.

There were three cases of noncardiac deaths, all of them due to sepsis. One was the result of the procedure (the reason for this remains obscure); in two, sepsis was present before the procedure.

Late Sudden Deaths

The cases of sudden death in patients considered to be well controlled (three cases of success and three of partial success) were observed after 4, 14, 22, 30, 87, and 107 months, respectively, and may be considered a long-term failure of the technique. In the six patients who died suddenly, the time of follow-up ranged from 16 to 400 times the longest interval between two spontaneous consecutive attacks of ventricular tachycardia observed before ablation. In no case was the ECG recorded at the time of death; therefore, it was not possible to know whether the terminal event was the result of relapse of the previously fulgurated ventricular tachycardia or due to spontaneous occurrence of a different ventricular tachycardia. Conversely, two patients (with the shortest survival) experienced palpitations a few days or weeks before death and had an episode of sustained monomorphic tachycardia and asymptomatic episodes of ventricular tachycardia at 110 beats per minute recorded during Holter monitoring.

These six patients who were classified as successful or partially successful but had late sudden death suggest that the arrhythmogenic substrate is still present after ablation and may lead to new or recurrent fatal ventricular arrhythmia. This may be attributed to the progression of the disease or to a new ischemic event. No clear reason for sudden death was identified in the patient who had repair of a congenital anomaly and died suddenly 87 months after ablation.

Late Non–Sudden Deaths

In all cases except three, late non–sudden deaths were related to a cardiac mechanism. All but one of these deaths were due to congestive heart failure, with one due to acute myocardial infarction 82 months after ablation. In the eleven patients who had an ejection fraction equal to or less than 30%, the survival time exceeds 3 years in only 22% of the cases. All the patients who died had a history of myocardial infarction or idiopathic dilated cardiomyopathy (Fig. 31-8). Generally, all forms of death were mostly observed in the oldest population (Fig. 31-9).

Favorable Evolution

A success has been observed with a follow-up of 76 months after the last procedure in a patient originally classified as a partial success after four sessions. Before the first ablation, the longest interval between two attacks was 1 month. Success has been also observed in one patient who had three sessions for ventricular tachycardias related to idiopathic dilated cardiomyopathy (which was classified as failure) and who developed no further episodes of ventricular tachycardia during a follow-up period of 13 months after the last session. He experienced multiple episodes of ventricular tachycardia before the procedure. When the arrhythmia was first noted, the longest interval between attacks was 1 year. One patient with ARVD who

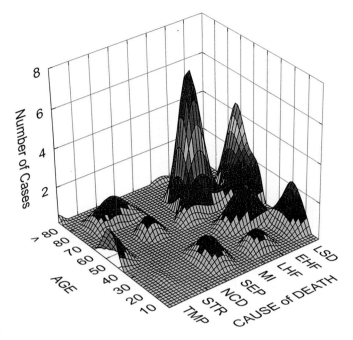

Figure 31-9. Bivariate three-dimensional histogram relating age and cause of death and stressing two peaks for late sudden death (*LSD*) and low heart output failure (*LHF*). These two events are mostly observed in the oldest population.

was classified as a partial success is no longer taking drugs after a follow-up period of 88 months. In this patient, ventricular tachycardia was incessant before the first ablation session. One case of ventricular tachycardia after myocardial infarction that was classified as failure after two sessions did not need drug therapy within a follow-up period of 44 months. The longest interval between attacks was 1 month in this patient before ablation therapy. Finally, three patients with either myocardial infarction, ARVD, or verapamil-sensitive tachycardia classified as partial success or failure (in the last case, at the time of discharge) proved to be successful, with a follow-up ranging from 6 to 38 months. The time without attacks after successful ablation was at least three times the longest interval observed before ablation.

In addition, one case of ventricular tachycardia classified as failure after two sessions is considered as partial success after 101 months of follow-up, and one case of ventricular tachycardia after myocardial infarction moved from failure to partial success with a follow-up of 22 months. He experienced incessant ventricular tachycardia before ablation.

These cases of improvement may be due to a late effect of modification of electrophysiologic properties of the arrhythmogenic substrate. This may be due to long-term retraction of the scar tissue resulting from the abla-

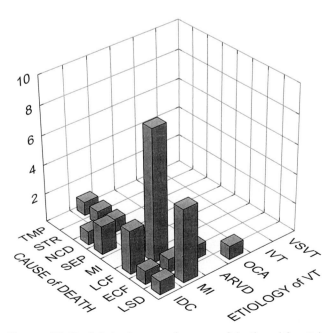

Figure 31-8. Relation between the cause of death and the etiology of ventricular tachycardia. Abbreviations are the same as those in Figures 31-3 and 31-7.

tion procedure or spontaneous favorable evolution of their disease.

Unfavorable Evolution

The long-term evolution is considered to be unfavorable if the patient developed relapses leading to a new session 2 months or longer after the patient was discharged from the hospital. The distribution of these intervals varies greatly, from 2 to 108 months as presented on the histogram of Figure 31-10. It demonstrates a consistent group up to 40 months, with three outlyers of longer than 60 months. In all these patients except one, ARVD and ventricular tachycardia was the result of the development of a new arrhythmia. Interpretation is less clear for patients who developed new attacks after 40 months and in whom other mechanisms could be postulated, such as partial modification of the arrhythmogenic substrate.

Ventricular Tachycardia Ablation Failures

One patient had an old myocardial infarction, an ejection fraction of 23%, and failed the procedure. For technical reasons, he underwent only a single session. He died suddenly after multiple episodes of ventricular tachycardia 21 months after ablation, illustrating the risks of this arrhythmia even if the tachycardias are relatively well tolerated.

The four other patients who failed one or two sessions with a follow-up ranging from 49 to 104 months had ARVD or infundibular ventricular tachycardia. All had a good left ventricular ejection fraction (50% to 65%) and their arrhythmias were finally controlled by drugs, with the exception of one patient who had surgery for ventricular

tachycardia. It may be that there was a late favorable effect of the procedure.

During the period of the study, techniques of mapping changed. It is probable that ablation performed in the area of slow conduction would improve the effectiveness of the procedure.[13, 14, 31–34]

Hemopericardium

A retrospective analysis showed that hemopericardium was due to injury from the catheter during its manipulation except in one case, in which it was probably the result of contraction of the parietal muscles during the shock when the catheter was located at the apex of the right ventricle. The resulting transmural puncture of the myocardial wall led to compressive hemopericardium, requiring urgent pericardiocentesis. In no case was it necessary to surgically repair rupture of the myocardial wall. This event, which was not observed before by our group (except in one case that was probably related to the use of a catheter with a guiding stylet), occurred in almost successive cases. It was observed with female patients and may have been due to manipulation of catheters by a relatively inexperienced investigator.

Efficacy Related to Etiology of Ventricular Tachycardia

Our results are presented according to the etiology. They demonstrate that this parameter is an important factor. For example, the fulguration procedure is the most effective in the group of patients who had verapamil-sensitive ventricular tachycardia.[35–37] Despite these ventricular tachycardias not being life-threatening, they are sometimes

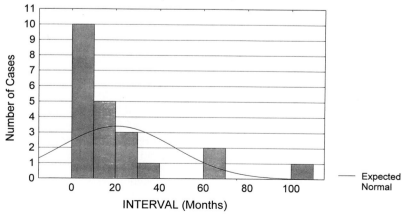

Figure 31-10. Distribution of the intervals between two sessions longer than 2 months, showing a decreasing frequency from 0 to 40 months, no requirement for urgent ablation between 40 and 60 months, and three cases after 60 months. These isolated three cases suggests the development of a new focus of ventricular tachycardia, except in one. These three patients had arrhythmogenic right ventricular dysplasia.

INTERVAL BETWEEN SESSIONS
K-S d=.26894, p<.10 ; Lilliefors p<.01

Number of Cases

INTERVAL (Months)

— Expected Normal

resistant to drug therapy and can be completely incapacitating. They usually occur in young patients who are in the most productive part of their life. Because an efficacy of 100% was achieved in this series, without the need for antiarrhythmic therapy, fulguration should be considered for treatment when radiofrequency ablation fails. This result is in agreement with that observed in patients with bundle branch ventricular tachycardia wherein the target structure is a relatively small piece of myocardium.[38,39]

In contrast, fulguration is least effective in patients with idiopathic ventricular tachycardia originating in the infundibular area or deep in the septum. This may be related to the quality of contact between catheter and the myocardial wall or to the depth of the arrhythmogenic tissue. We believe that ventricular tachycardia originating deep in the septum is the most difficult to ablate.

The remaining cases may be classified in two subgroups: those who have a good ejection fraction (e.g., verapamil-sensitive ventricular tachycardia and ARVD) and those having ventricular tachycardia with myocardial infarction or idiopathic dilated cardiomyopathy. In these two groups, the effectiveness ranges between 85% and 100%, but the long-term prognosis may mainly depend on the underlying myocardium. The graph in Figure 31-11 represents the surviving curve of patients with VT after myocardial infarction treated by the fulguration preocedure, indicating a survival rate of approximately 30% after 5 years. There are, however, striking anecdotal experiences, such as that of a 73-year-old physician who had repeated episodes of ventricular tachycardia 10 years after myocardial infarction. He had an ejection fraction of 22% and was moribund during a period of 5 days because of repetitive episodes of incessant ventricular tachycardia. He required two fulguration sessions, he is still alive after 10 years, and takes only low-dosage antiarrhythmic drug therapy.*

Adherence to Drug Therapy

In one case of ARVD, ventricular tachycardia was controlled for several years after fulguration and antiarrhythmic drug therapy. The antiarrhythmic treatment was changed without referring the patient back to our center and without electrophysiologic guidance. This patient developed a syncopal episode of ventricular tachycardia and was successfully resuscitated after cardiac arrest. He then had antiarrhythmic drug reevaluation at our center. This patient had no new episodes of ventricular tachycardia during a follow-up of 24 months. This demonstrates that at least in some patients, the arrhythmogenic substrate can

---

*Since the preparation of this manuscript, this patient in NYHA Functional Class III died suddenly. This sudden death was not preceded by warning symptoms.

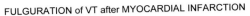

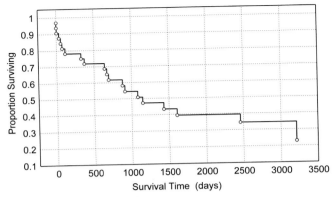

Figure 31-11. Survival curve of patients with VT after myocardial infarction treated by the fulguration procedure. This curve is well fitted on a decreasing exponential. The number of cases is too small to make valuable assumptions if the curve is broken in sub-groups based on ejection fraction, sudden death or other factors.

be stable for several years and that any modification of a correctly controlled antiarrhythmic treatment should be performed only by physicians skilled in electrophysiology.

Alternative Forms of Therapy

In our center, because of our selection of cases, ventricular tachycardia was particularly difficult to treat and frequent. In 55 patients (63.2%), the attacks were equal to or more frequent than one attack a month. This suggests that these patients would not have been good candidates for the implantation of an implantable cardioverter defibrillator before the ablation procedure.[40]

CKMB as a Marker of Success

In this series, CKMB was low (in the range of 37 ± 17 international units), suggesting that fulguration generally leads to a limited alteration of the arrhythmogenic substrate.[41] This hypothesis is suggested by the observation that in the subgroup of patients with dysplasia, the successful outcome was nonassociated with the highest CKMB measurement.[42]

Efficacy is also related to the number of morphologies of ventricular tachycardia. In three of our cases, in whom four to six different morphologies of monomorphic ventricular tachycardia were observed, it was necessary to deliver a mean of 12 shocks per patient during one or several sessions, as opposed to a mean value of 3.6 shocks per patient to control ventricular tachycardia in a series of 10 patients in whom only a single form of morphology required ablation.

CONCLUSION

Fulguration for the treatment of ventricular tachycardia is effective and in experienced hands should be associated with low morbidity and mortality. With this method, it is possible to obtain arrhythmia control for a long time. The fact that multiple sessions may be necessary to obtain a successful result in many patients suggests that fulguration is not an ideal energy source. Alternatively, mapping of the ventricular tachycardia needs to be improved.

It is also evident that it is difficult to predict the long-term evolution of arrhythmias after fulguration. It is easy to evaluate the results of this procedure in patients with incessant ventricular tachycardia. In other cases, however, in which ventricular tachycardia is relatively unfrequent, assessment of long-term efficacy is difficult and somewhat uncertain. Clinical evaluation after successful ablation of ventricular tachycardia may be dominated by the development of congestive heart failure in patients with structural heart disease, mostly after myocardial infarction or idiopathic dilated cardiomyopathy. Surprisingly good long-term results have been observed, however, even in patients with poor cardiac function. There is the risk that sudden death may occur in some patients during long-term follow-up.

To further improve short- and long-term results of ablation for ventricular tachycardia, other energy sources need to be explored. In addition, better techniques for mapping are needed.

Acknowledgement

Acknowledgements to Mrs. Nicole Proust for her assistance in the preparation of the manuscript.

References

1. Hartzler GO: Electrode catheter ablation of refractory focal ventricular tachycardia. J Am Coll Cardiol 1983;2:107.
2. Puech P, Gallay P, Grolleau R, Koliopoulos N: Traitement par electrofulguration endocavitaire d'une tachycardie ventriculaire recidivante par dysplasie ventriculaire droite. Arch Mal Coeur 1984;77:826.
3. Tonet JL, Fontaine G, Frank R, Grosgogeat Y: Treatment of ventricular tachycardias by endocardial catheter fulguration: further experience and long-term follow-up. Circulation 1988;78(uppl-II):306. Abstract.
4. Klein LS, Shih HT, Hackett K, Zipes DP, Miles WM: Radiofrequency catheter ablation of ventricular tachycardia in patients without structural heart disease. Circulation 1992; 85:1666.
5. Fontaine G, Frank R, Tonet JL, et al: Treatment of resistant ventricular tachycardia with endocavitary fulguration and antiarrhythmic therapy, compared to antiarrhythmic therapy alone: experience in 111 consecutive cases with a mean follow-up of 18 months. Tex Heart Inst J 1986;13:401.
6. Fontaine G, Tonet JL, Frank R, Rougier I: Electrode catheter ablation of ventricular tachycardia by fulguration and antiarrhythmic therapy. Experience of 43 patients with a mean follow-up of 29 months. Chest 1989;95:785.
7. Fontaine G, Tonet JL, Frank R, et al: Treatment of resistant ventricular tachycardia by endocavitary fulguration associated with antiarrhythmic therapy. Eur Heart J 1987;8 (Suppl D):133.
8. Fontaine G, Tonet JL, Frank R, et al: Traitement des tachycardies ventriculaires rebelles par fulguration endocavitaire associee aux anti-arythmiques. Arch Mal Coeur 1986;79:1152.
9. Frank R, Tonet J, Gallais Y, Lazraq S, Fellat R, Fontaine G: Le traitement des tachycardies ventriculaires par la fulguration endocavitaire. A propos de 86 cas. Arch Mal Coeur 1993; 86:1317.
10. Fontaine G, Cansell A, Tonet JL, et al: Techniques and methods for catheter endocardial fulguration. Pacing Clin Electrophysiol 1988;11:592.
11. Fontaine G, Cansell A, Lampe L, et al: Endocavitary fulguration (electrode catheter ablation): equipment-related problems. In: Fontaine G, Scheinman MM, eds. Ablation in cardiac arrhythmias. Mt. Kisco, NY: Futura Publishing, 1987:85.
12. Gallais Y, Lascault G, Tonet J, et al: Continuous measurement of coronary sinus oxygen saturation during ventricular tachycardia. Eur Heart J 1993;14(Suppl):368. Abstract.
13. Fontaine G: Du lieu d'origine a la zone a conduction lente. Application au traitement de la tachycardie ventriculaire. Arch Mal Coeur 1988;81:145
14. Frank R, Tonet JL, Kounde S, Farenq G, Fontaine G: Localization of the area of slow conduction during ventricular tachycardia. In: Brugada P, Wellens HJJ, eds. Cardiac arrhythmias: where to go from here? Mr. Kisco, NY: Futura Publishing, 1987:191.
15. Baraka M, Tonet J, Fontaine G, et al: Les troubles du rythme et de la conduction au decours immediat de la fulguration ventriculaire. Arch Mal Coeur 1988;81:269.
16. Fontaine G, Lemoine B, Frank R, Tonet JL, Maendely R, Grosgogeat Y: Effects of fulguration on the permanent pacemaker. In: Fontaine G, Scheinman MM, eds. Ablation in cardiac arrhythmias. Mt. Kisco, NY: Futura Publishing, 1987: 367.
17. Morady F, Scheinman MM, DiCarlo LA Jr, et al: Catheter ablation of ventricular tachycardia with intracardiac shocks: results in 33 patients. Circulation 1987;75:1037.
18. Touboul P, Atallah G, Kirkorian G, et al: Fulguration for refractory ventricular tachycardia: determinants of success. In: Fontaine G, Scheinman MM, eds. Ablation in cardiac arrhythmias. Mt. Kisco, NY: Futura Publishing, 1987:337.
19. Haissaguerre M, Warin JF, Le Metayer P, Guillem JP, Blanchot P: Traitement des tachycardies ventriculaires rebelles par fulguration utilisant de hautes energies cumulees. Arch Mal Coeur 1988;81:879.
20. Holt PM, Boyd EGCA: Physical and experimental aspects of ablation with direct-current schocks. In: Saksena S, Goldschlager N, eds. Electrical therapy for cardiac arrhythmias. Pacing, antitachycardia devices, catheter ablation. Philadelphia: WB Saunders, 1990:619.

21. Bardy GH, Coltorti F, Ivey TD, Yerkovich D, Greene HL: Effect of damped sine-wave shocks on catheter dielectric strength. Am J Cardiol 1985;56:769.

22. Fontaine G, Volmer W, Nienaltowska E, Aaddaj S, Cansell A, Grosgogeat Y: Approach to the physics of fulguration. In: Fontaine G, Scheinman MM, eds. Ablation in cardiac arrhythmias. Mt. Kisco, NY: Futura Publishing, 1987:101.

23. Fontaine G, Aldakar M, Iwa T Jr, Mrdja S, Grosgogeat Y: Aspects physiques et biophysiques des decharges electriques intracardiaques a haute energie. I. La bulle de fulguration. Ann Cardiol Angeiol (Paris) 1990;39:319.

24. Fontaine G, Aldakar M, Iwa T Jr, Mrdja S, Grosgogeat Y: Aspects physiques et biophysiques des decharges electriques intracardiaques a haute energie. II. Correlation entre les effets physiques et electriques pour des chocs liminaires et infraliminaires. Ann Cardiol Angeiol (Paris) 1990;39:389.

25. Fontaine G, Aldakar M, Iwa T Jr, Grosgogeat Y: Aspects physiques et biophysiques des decharges electriques intracardiaques a haute energie. III. Correlation entre les effets physiques et electriques pour des chocs supraliminaires. Ann Cardiol Angeiol (Paris) 1990;39:449.

26. Fontaine G, Umemura J, Iwa T, Aldakar M, Grosgogeat Y: Aspects physiques et biophysiques des decharges electriques intracardiaques a haute energie. IV. Effets des bulles de fulguration en milieu diphasique isotrope. Ann Cardiol Angeiol (Paris) 1991;40:515.

27. Borggrefe M, Breithardt G, Podczeck A, Rohner D, Budde TH, Martinez-Rubio A: Catheter ablation of ventricular tachycardia using defibrillator pulses: electrophysiological findings and long-term results. Eur Heart J 1989;10:591.

28. Fontaine G, Shantha N, Frank R, Tonet JL, Cansell A, Grosgogeat Y: New approaches in the electrophysiological determination of optimal treatment of recurrent tachyarrhythmias. In: Greenberg HM, Kulbertus HE, Moss AJ, Schwartz PJ, eds. Clinical aspects of life-threatening arrhythmias. Ann NY Acad Sci 1984;427:67.

29. Yee ES, Scheinman MM, Griffin JC, Ebert PA: Surgical options for treating ventricular tachyarrhythmia and sudden death. J Thorac Cardiovasc Surg 1987;94:866.

30. Borggrefe M, Podczeck A, Ostermeyer J, Breithardt G: The surgical ablation registry long term results of electrophysiologically guided antitachycardia surgery in ventricular tachyarrhythmias: a collaborative report on 665 patients. In: Breithardt G, Borggrefe M, Zipes DP, eds. Non-pharmacological therapy of tachyarrhythmias. Mt. Kisco, NY: Futura Publishing, 1987:109.

31. Fontaine G, Frank R, Tonet J, Grosgogeat Y: Identification of a zone of slow conduction appropriate for VT ablation. Theoretical and practical considerations. Pacing Clin Electrophysiol 1989;12(Pt II):262.

32. Morady F, Frank R, Kou WH, et al: Identification and catheter ablation of a zone of slow conduction in the reentry circuit of ventricular tachycardias in humans. J Am Coll Cardiol 1988;11:775.

33. Borggrefe M, Martinez-Rubio A, Karbenn U, Breithardt G: Pacing-interventions at the site of VT. Improvement of results of catheter ablation. Circulation 1989;80:4:223.

34. Klein HO, Schroder E, Trappe HJ, Kuhn E: Catheter ablation of ventricular tachycardia. how to define the area of ablation. Pacing Clin Electrophysiol 1988;11:911. Abstract.

35. Belhassen B, Rotmensch HH, Laniado S: Response of recurrent sustained ventricular tachycardia to verapamil. Br Heart J 1981;46:679.

36. Ohe T, Shimomura K, Aihara N, et al: Idiopathic sustained left ventricular tachycardia: clinical and electrophysiologic characteristics. Circulation 1988;77:560.

37. Ruffy R, Kim SS, Lal R: Paroxysmal fascicular tachycardia: electrophysiologic characteristics and treatment by catheter ablation. J Am Coll Cardiol 1985;5:1008.

38. Touboul P, Kirkorian G, Atallah G, et al: Bundle branch reentrant tachycardia treated by electrical ablation of the right bundle branch. J Am Coll Cardiol 1986;7:1404.

39. Akhtar M, Caceres J, Dongas J, Jazayeri M, Tchou P: Catheter ablation of right bundle branch: a highly effective technique for control of bundle branch reentrant ventricular tachycardia. In: Fourth symposium on the ablative techniques—Cardiostim 88. Monte-Carlo, Juin 1988. Abstract.

40. Gross JN, Song SL, Buckingham TA, Furman S: The Bilitch registry group influence of clinical characteristics and shock occurrence on ICD patient outcome: a multicenter report. Pacing Clin Electrophysiol 1991;14:1881.

41. Konttinen A, Somer H: Determination of serum creatine kinase isoenzymes in myocardial infarction. Am J Cardiol 1972;29:817.

42. Fontaine G, Frank R, Rougier I, et al: Electrode catheter ablation of resistant ventricular tachycardia in arrhythmogenic right ventricular dysplasia. Experience of 13 patients with a mean follow-up of 45 months. Eur Heart J 1989;10(Suppl D):74.

Cardiac Arrhythmias, 3rd edition, edited by William J. Mandel.
J. B. Lippincott Company, Philadelphia © 1995.

32

Leon Resnekov • Peng-Sheng Chen • WJ Mandel

High-Energy Electrical Current in the Management of Cardiac Dysrhythmias

The pharmacologic management of patients with cardiac rhythm disturbances, although time honored, may have the following serious limitations when used clinically:

1. There is no standard dose for any specific drug. The amounts given usually vary among patients.

2. The margin between therapeutic and toxic dosages is often small.

3. Because it is necessary to titrate the dose given against the effects obtained, the patient must be observed closely throughout pharmacologic therapy, which may last several days.

4. Many of the drugs used have important negative inotropic effects that may further compromise disturbed heart action. In addition, important dromotropic effects may emerge.

5. The toxic effects of a drug may be more serious than the effects of the rhythm disturbance.

6. Many drugs may suppress the normal sinus mechanism and inhibit reversion to sinus rhythm.

7. Proarrhythmic effects of drugs must be considered.

In contrast, an electrical shock terminates the ectopic rhythm and permits the sinus node to be reestablished as the pacemaker of the heart (Fig. 32-1). Such treatment is now known to be both successful and safe, provided careful adherence to detail is maintained.

HISTORIC HIGHLIGHTS

Ventricular fibrillation was described first by Hoffa and Ludwig in 1850.[1] Shortly thereafter, fatalities as a result of electrocution were reported, but the realization that an electrical shock could also terminate ventricular fibrillation came about only many years thereafter. In 1898, Prevost and Battelli[2] observed that a direct current (DC) shock across a dog's heart in ventricular fibrillation caused sinus rhythm to return. This important fact was ignored or unrecognized until the effects of electrical current on the heart were restudied by Kouwenhoven and colleagues in a series of experiments over many years[3] and by Ferris and coworkers[4] at almost the same time. Between 1927 and

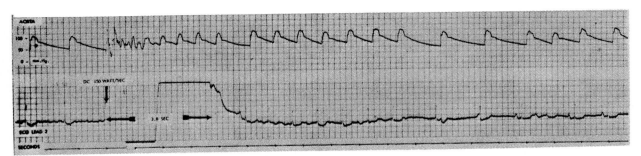

Figure 32-1. Electroversion of atrial fibrillation. Shown are central aortic pressure (*top*) and lead II of the electrocardiogram (*bottom*). Immediately following delivery of 150 watt-sec (J), atrial fibrillation is followed by ectopic beats recorded on the aortic tracing when electrical interference causes the electrocardiographic signal to be lost for 3.8 seconds. Subsequently, sinus rhythm with a prolonged PR interval and junctional beats are recorded before sinus rhythm is established.

1935, the following important conclusions on the effects of electricity on the heart were drawn:

1. Current rather than voltage is the proper criterion for shock intensity.

2. Ventricular fibrillation may be caused by the passage of an electrical current across the heart even in the absence of recognizable myocardial damage.

3. Ventricular fibrillation will cause death within a few minutes unless it is treated successfully by a second shock of appropriate intensity.

Not all electrical shocks will produce ventricular fibrillation, and King was able to show that those shocks delivered close to the apex of the T wave of the electrocardiogram were more likely to do so.[5]

Pioneer work using direct current electrical discharge clinically was undertaken by scientists in the U.S.S.R.[6] These early attempts are regarded as an important inspiration for later investigators, including Peleǎka (Czechoslovakia), Tsukerman (U.S.S.R.), and Lown and coworkers (United States).[7]

ELECTRICAL DEFIBRILLATION OF THE HEART

A high-energy impulse of short duration is delivered between two concave paddles applied closely to the heart (internal defibrillation) or through the chest wall using two flat paddles (external defibrillation).

External defibrillation for both direct and alternating currents depends on not only the electrical current used but also the resistance of the heart, of the bony cage, and of the skin. A current of at least 1 A is needed to bring all heart fibers instantaneously to the same refractory point.[8] To achieve a current of 1 A across the myocardium, 100 V at a

power of 100 W is usually required. The usual duration for an *alternating current* shock for defibrillation is 200 msec; thus, the energy needed for internal defibrillation is about 20 J. Because of the increased resistance, external AC defibrillation requires a sixfold increase in current and voltage rating, 1800 W for 0.2 seconds, producing 500 J. Note that the waveform for AC defibrillation is standard and is produced at the electrical generating station as a sinusoidal impulse with a frequency of 60 Hz.

Direct current defibrillators discharge a single capacitor or a bank of capacitors that have been charged previously for 2 to 10 seconds by line current and a step-up transformer. The duration of the delivered impulse is much shorter than for AC defibrillators, usually being in the range of 1.5 to 4 msec. An infinite variety of waveforms is obtained following a capacitor discharge. When unmodified, a spike discharge with a very abrupt rise in voltage and current to a sharp peak, followed by an exponential decay to the baseline, is obtained. This unmodified waveform can be shaped by adding varying amounts of inductance to the circuit. Experimental evidence has shown that defibrillation is safer and more likely to succeed when an inductance-modified waveform is used.[9] Inductance reduces the rate of rise of the current and voltage waveform to round off the peak and to prolong the down slope. As more inductance is introduced into the circuit, undesirable oscillations in the tail of the waveform occur. Many commercial DC defibrillators produce a monophasic, slightly underdamped current and voltage waveform, obtained by charging a capacitor of 16 μf to a maximum of 7000 V and discharging it across an inductance of 100 mh. The average duration of the waveform is 3.5 msec, and when maximally charged, 329 J of electrical energy is delivered. The current is about 19 A, and the power is 133,000 W. The waveform is shown in Figure 32-2.

Important variables relating to the safe clinical use of direct current shock are the capacitance of the conductors

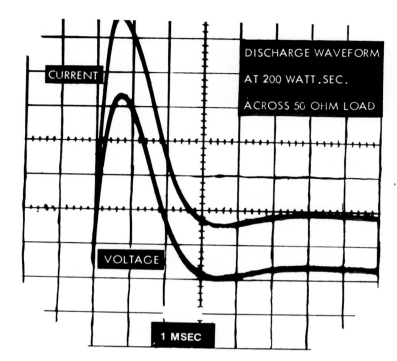

DISCHARGE WAVEFORM AT 200 WATT.SEC. ACROSS 50 OHM LOAD

CURRENT

VOLTAGE

1 MSEC

Figure 32-2. Monophasic, slightly underdamped waveform obtained when a capacitor of 16μf charged to 5 kV is discharged across an inductance of 100 mh and a 50-v̇ load. (Resnekov L, McDonald L: Appraisal of electroconversion in treatment of cardiac dysrhythmias. Br Heart J 1968;30:786.)

and the inductance of the circuit. The rise time of the waveform should not exceed 500 μsec, and absence of ringing of its tail should be ensured. Many different waveforms have been investigated, and the two that are most used in clinical practice are the damped sinusoidal (see Fig. 32-2) and the trapezoidal.

Many waveforms have been tested for defibrillation.[10] Recent studies have identified the importance of a biphasic configuration (reversal of polarity during the shock), which will result in a significant increase in efficiency. At present, the "ideal" biphasic waveform consists of asymmetric waveforms with the amplitude of the second waveforms smaller than that of the first, and a second waveform that is shorter or equal in duration to the first waveform.[11–16] The possible explanations for the increased efficiency of a biphasic waveform include decreased impedance; reactivation of the sodium channels by the first phase, allowing the second phase to excite the cells; and shortening of the refractory period by hyperpolarization by the first phase.[16–18] Of importance is that a very high energy shock may be able to induce ventricular fibrillation at *any* time during the cardiac cycle. This appears due to myocardial damage caused by a large shock field, leading to loss of cellular potassium, decreased contraction, prolonged depolarization, stimulation of adrenergic and cholinergic fibers, inhibition of pacemaker cells, and a decrease in cardiac functions secondary to myocardial necrosis.[18,19]

Note that the energy setting on the moving-coil meter of the defibrillator apparatus reflects the energy delivered to the skin. The true energy delivered to the heart muscle, however, is influenced by the resistance of the skin and deeper tissues. Nevertheless, a short-duration DC monophasic pulse allows the transmyocardial passage of 1.5 A or more. Shaping the electrical pulse by using an inductor in series permits the electrical energy to be delivered to the heart muscle without causing undue damage.

Alternating or Direct Current

Although direct current develops many times the power of alternating current (AC), less energy is delivered because the shock persists only for 3 to 4 msec. Alternating current shocks are more harmful to the myocardium and cause greater deterioration in ventricular function.[20]

Beck and colleagues were the first to defibrillate a human heart electrically using an AC discharge, and for many years thereafter, AC defibrillation was the standard method.[21] The waveforms of DC discharges are so dissimilar as to make any true comparison difficult. Why, then, did DC discharge become the preferred method? Two important clinical observations stimulated its use:

1. Alternating current frequently failed to defibrillate the heart in the presence of acute myocardial infarction.

2. Electrical conversion of rhythms other than ventricular fibrillation was needed.

A certain amount of experience had already been obtained in treating organized atrial and ventricular dysrhythmias with electrical current,[22] and although this was occasionally successful, alternating current used in this way could precipitate ventricular fibrillation and even death.[23] Nachlas and coworkers were able to demonstrate that direct current was unmistakably superior, even in terminating ventricular fibrillation.[24] Therefore, it seems reasonable to conclude from the above that alternating current is feasible and successful for treating ventricular fibrillation in the clinical setting but that direct current is more effective. However, under no circumstances should alternating current be used for treating atrial rhythm disturbances or ventricular tachycardia because of the high risk of precipitating ventricular fibrillation.

Is Synchronization Needed?

Despite the use of electrical circuits that produce acceptable waveforms, a transmyocardial or transthoracic DC shock occasionally precipitates ventricular fibrillation. For many years, a vulnerable period of ventricular excitability has been postulated in a wide variety of animals.[25] Wiggers and Wegria showed this period to be 27 msec before the end of ventricular systole in the dog,[26] and a similar period of vulnerability has also been demonstrated for the atrium.[27] The vulnerable period of the ventricle occurs just before the apex of the T wave of the electrocardiogram, at which time recovery from the refractory state is not uniform, thus allowing reentry of the depolarization wave, which favors self-sustained activity. The fact that a similar phenomenon also occurs in the human heart has been demonstrated by Castellanos and colleagues.[28] The time relationship of vulnerability in the ventricle and atrium for both alternating and direct current shocks is shown in Figure 32-3.

One can conclude, therefore, that in the treatment of rhythm disturbances other than ventricular fibrillation, the risk of inducing ventricular fibrillation is lessened by timing the DC shock to avoid the apex of the T wave. It is almost impossible to avoid the ventricular phase of vulnerability when AC shocks are used (see Fig. 32-3), and most DC defibrillators incorporate a synchronizer that permits triggering of the shock by the R or S wave of the electrocardiogram. When ventricular fibrillation is treated, the synchronizer should be switched out of the circuit. The chance of ventricular fibrillation following randomized unsynchronized shocks is approximately 2%.[29] Kreus and colleagues deliberately did not use a synchronizer in clinical practice, without dire consequences.[30] When a synchronizer is not used, sufficient energy must be delivered so that a current of at least 1.5 to 2 A flows across the heart; smaller energies may cause ventricular fibrillation and are dangerous. Therefore,

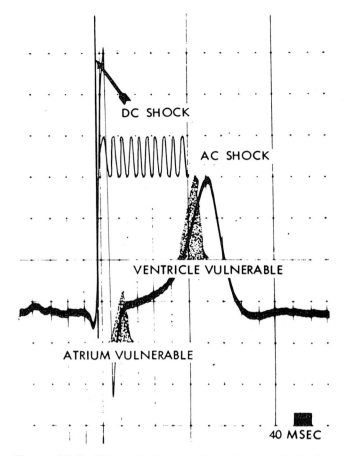

Figure 32-3. Vulnerable phases of the cardiac cycle for fibrillation of the atrium and ventricle. R-wave synchronization of a 3-msec direct current (DC) shock avoids the phases of vulnerability. Alternate current (AC) shocks, which persist for 100 to 250 msec, cannot be safely phased in this way. (Resnekov L, McDonald L: Appraisal of electroconversion in treatment of cardiac dysrhythmias. Br Heart J 1968;30:786.)

when no synchronizer is used, increased levels of energy settings are mandatory.

PHYSIOLOGY OF ELECTROVERSION

There is as yet no general agreement on the mechanism of ventricular fibrillation, and it is small wonder that the mechanism of electrical defibrillation remains in doubt. The subject has been reviewed by Antoni.[31] If a circus movement or reentry mechanism is assumed to be the cause of the fibrillation, the main effect of the DC defibrillation pulse might be synchronous stimulation of a normally refractory myocardium. If, on the other hand, defibrillation is thought to reduce the activity of a heterotopic focus, some other mode of action must be assumed (e.g., direct inhibition of the heterotopic pacemaker).

Wiggers in 1940 felt that defibrillation halted all the activation fronts in the ventricles during ventricular fibrillation ("total extinction" hypothesis).[32] This view was altered by Zipes and coworkers, who postulated that activation wavefronts must be altered only within a critical mass of myocardium (i.e., approximately 75% of the ventricular mass ["critical mass" hypothesis]).[33] Recently, Chen and colleagues proposed the "upper limit of vulnerability" hypothesis for defibrillation.[34–38] The hypothesis asserts that unsuccessful shocks slightly weaker than necessary to defibrillate halt all activation fronts during ventricular fibrillation. However, because the same shock also stimulates regions of the myocardium during their vulnerable period, it gives rise to new activation fronts that reinitiate ventricular fibrillation. To successfully defibrillate, the shock strength must reach or exceed the upper limit of vulnerability.

Multiple wavefronts occur in the myocardium continuously during ventricular fibrillation, which, according to Moe and colleagues, appears to be due to multiple shifting reentrant circuits.[39,40] This prediction was recently confirmed by multichannel computerized mapping studies, which showed that circulating reentrant wavefronts are present both at the onset[41,42] and 20 seconds after the initiation[36] of ventricular fibrillation.

The defibrillation threshold is not a single value but relates success to shock strength in a sigmoidal relationship.[43] Nevertheless, defibrillation thresholds are usually described as the lowest energy that consistently results in successful defibrillation. However, there is not an all-or-none phenomenon that can be established for defibrillation energies.

In contrast to energies that successfully defibrillate the heart, there is a point *below* a critical energy at which a delivered synchronized shock can *induce* ventricular fibrillation. The lowest value of energy delivered that fails to initiate ventricular fibrillation has been termed the upper limit of vulnerability.[44] Lower energy shocks that induce ventricular fibrillation may be due to subthreshold defibrillatory shocks that initiate new activation fronts by stimulating vulnerable tissue. The major importance of the concept of the upper limit of vulnerability relates to the high correlation with the defibrillation threshold.[38,44] This correlation has great potential for simplifying testing during implantation of automatic defibrillators (see Chapter 43).[38]

Experimental findings on isolated myocardial preparations have shed some light on the mechanism of ventricular fibrillation.[45] Both the above mechanisms (circus movement [reentry] or a heterotopic focus) seem important in DC defibrillation, but a significantly higher electri-cal energy is needed to cause transient inhibition of the heterotopic focus, allowing the sinus node to resume its normal role as pacemaker.

CLINICAL USE OF ELECTROVERSION

Capacitor discharge with inductance in series was first used clinically by Lown and coworkers to treat patients with refractory ventricular tachycardia.[7] The technique has sometimes been called *countershock*[46] or *cardioversion*,[7] although some have preferred the term *electroversion*.[47] Innumerable patients have now been treated successfully for both atrial and ventricular dysrhythmias, and the combined experience has completely justified the high initial hopes for, and confidence in, the method. The overall success rate for terminating atrial and ventricular rhythm disturbances is 90%.[48,49] It has also been shown that there is a success rate of more than 85% even when determined efforts at pharmacologic conversion of dysrhythmias have failed.[50] The correct choice of patients and meticulous attention to detail, including correction of electrolyte imbalance if present, postponing treatment in the presence of overdigitalization, proper synchronization, and the choice of antidysrhythmic agents immediately before and following treatment ensure both immediate success and the absence of a high incidence of complications.[48,51] The importance of meticulous attention to detail, however, cannot be overemphasized and is summarized below.

Technique

The Apparatus

Up to 7000 V may be needed to charge the capacitors to deliver 400 J. Furthermore, commercial apparatuses are either "isolated" or "nonisolated." In the former case, the output is isolated from earth (ground); with the nonisolated type, one paddle is grounded. The following monthly checks of the apparatus must be made:

1. A general examination for electrical safety
2. The waveform produced should be inspected critically following discharge across a 50-J load in the laboratory
3. The actual electrical energy of the discharge should be measured and compared with the setting on the apparatus. Most apparatuses provide a moving-coil meter that is calibrated in joules (watt-seconds), but models are still in use in which the desired energy is

obtained by depressing a labeled switch, a highly undesirable feature.

During the shock, it is most important that assisting personnel do not touch the patient or the bed, because with both isolated and nonisolated circuits, a large electrical field is created that results in a shock to any person in contact. In addition, the nonisolated unit has an added risk: if the paddle on the patient's chest conducts poorly, there is an electrical pathway between the "hot" paddle and the electrocardiographic electrode at earth potential (right leg), and an electrical burn may result.

Synchronization Test

Synchronization is a safety feature that should be used routinely unless ventricular fibrillation is being treated. Defibrillators now provide visual demonstration of synchronization by a superimposed "blip" on the electrocardiographic signal being monitored on the oscilloscope. Synchronization should always be tested before administering the first shock to the patient by charging the capacitor to a low energy (5 J), attaching the electrocardiographic cables to the patient, and then discharging the capacitor, holding the two paddles in close apposition away from the patient while the connecting lead of the electrocardiogram is applied to the two cables from the paddles. In this way, a "blip" is induced on the electrocardiogram and can be easily recorded on any electrocardiogram that is being used to monitor the electroversion (Fig. 32-4).

Paddles

Paddles of adequate size should always be used, because during ventricular fibrillation the heart is subdivided into a large number of fibrillating segments. To be successful, defibrillation must simultaneously depolarize the majority of myocardial fibers. It can be shown that the current density is 20 times greater between the paddles than at the margins of the heart when small electrodes are used, and this can produce myocardial damage because of a high interelectrode current density.[52] In addition, defibrillation may well fail because of the inadequate myocardial effect at some distance from the paddles. In contrast, when large-sized paddles are used, even the cardiac margins receive up to 42% of the total current discharge, and the risk of myocardial damage is less and the chance of successful defibrillation is greater. A diameter of 9.5 cm is recommended for adults, and a diameter of 4.5 cm is recommended for children. For both adults and children, spoon-shaped paddles of appropriate size are available for internal defibrillation. When an external DC shock is used, two anterior paddles or, alternatively, an anterior and a posterior paddle may be employed. The latter method is more convenient because the patient lies on the flat posterior paddle, and it is only the anterior paddle that must

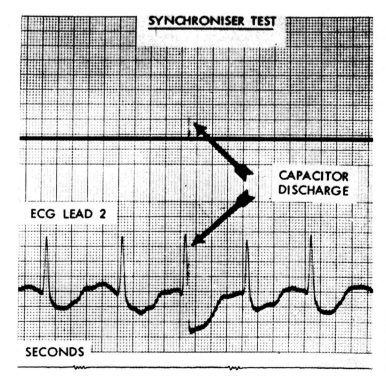

Figure 32-4. Test of synchronization. Note the small spike (upper tracing) superimposed on the electrocardiographic recording of lead II (lower tracing). See text for details. (Resnekov L, McDonald L: Appraisal of electroconversion in treatment of cardiac dysrhythmias. Br Heart J 1968;30:786.)

be held by the operator (an important safety measure, especially when an apparatus in which one paddle is grounded is being used). Lown and co-workers reported that using the anterior–posterior paddle position significantly lowered the energy required for electroversion,[53] but others could not confirm this finding.[49] Indeed, experimental work[24] has shown that the anterior positioning of the paddles, as originally suggested by Kouwenhoven,[54] results in delivering 2.5 times more current to the heart. It is likely that failure to note more striking clinical differences with variations in paddle placement results from the excess amounts of electrical energy that are consistently used to achieve electroversion. This being the case, the added safety of a flat posterior paddle, untouched by the operator and supported only by the weight of the patient, is advantageous, and the anteroposterior position is therefore recommended.

Self-adhesive electropads for defibrillation have been suggested.[55, 56] These obviate many of the disadvantages of traditional hand-held paddle-shaped electrodes applied to the skin's surface with electrocardiographic gel or saline-soaked pads. If the coupling agent inadvertently spreads across the chest, less electrical energy will be delivered to the heart. In addition, hand-held electrodes are often incorrectly placed, particularly when speed is needed (e.g., in treating ventricular fibrillation). Incorrect paddle placement was noted in 35% of patients treated for ventricular fibrillation.[57] The self-adhesive electropads could have a high electrical impedance, because no pressure is applied to them; indeed, in animal studies this was found to be the case.[58] A clinical study using the self-adhesive pads in 80 patients, however, demonstrated that the transthoracic impedance was $75 \pm 21 \Omega$, which compared very favorably with the expected transthoracic impedance of $67 \pm 36 \Omega$ with standard hand-held electrode paddles.[59] The advantage of not having to hold the paddles during the electrical discharge of the shock is obvious, and self-adhesive electrodes can be recommended.

Drugs

If at all possible, digoxin or any other digitalis preparation should be withheld for 24 to 48 hours before treatment. When treatment cannot be postponed and must be undertaken in the presence of heavy digitalization, the initial energy setting should be markedly reduced (5 to 10 J), and an intravenous injection of 100 mg of lidocaine should precede the shock. Many physicians use quinidine or some other antidysrhythmic agent orally, intramuscularly, or even intravenously routinely before direct current shock,[60] but the efficacy of these drugs in reducing energy requirements or in helping to maintain sinus rhythm thereafter is questionable.[49] It is possible, however, that an antidysrhythmic drug such as quinidine could help in

preventing premature beats immediately following DC shock,[61] which could precipitate a return to the dysrhythmia immediately after successful electroversion (see below).

Anticoagulants

The incidence of embolism following electroversion varies from 1.4% to 2.4%, a figure quite similar to that following the quinidine conversion of cardiac dysrhythmia.[62] The major risk of embolism associated with cardioversion occurs in patients with atrial fibrillation. There are now multiple studies in progress trying to identify the best method of therapy to prevent embolism associated with atrial fibrillation. These studies include:

1. The Boston Area Anticoagulation Trial for Atrial Fibrillation (BAATAF Study)
2. The Stroke Prevention and Atrial Fibrillation Study (SPAF)
3. The Danish Trial (AFASAK).[63–65]

These studies pointed out a clear advantage of Coumadin over placebo in preventing stroke in chronic atrial fibrillation of all causes. Pretreatment with Coumadin should be given for 3 weeks prior to cardioversion.

The need for anticoagulant protection was the subject of much debate in the absence of any well-controlled study, but such a study has now been reported,[66] and a statistically significant benefit in the group of patients who received electroversion under anticoagulant control has been shown. When there is a clear risk of embolism or thrombosis, as in patients with recent myocardial infarction, coronary heart disease, mitral valve disease, cardiomyopathy, prosthetic heart valves, or a previous history of embolism, prior anticoagulant therapy with a warfarin derivative should be given or heparin used when the need for DC shock is urgent. Because the risk of reverting to the rhythm disturbance is highest during the first month of treatment (see Figs. 32-9 and 32-10), anticoagulant therapy should be maintained for at least 4 weeks even after successful DC shock, after which it may be discontinued unless the underlying heart disease requires its continuance.

Anesthesia

General anesthesia is not required,[67, 68] but amnesia, which follows an intravenous injection of 5 to 10 mg of diazepam, is recommended.[69] Muscle relaxants, especially halothane, which is known to predispose to ventricular rhythm disturbances, should not be used with electroversion.[70] Although diazepam is a reasonably safe drug, it must be given cautiously to those patients with congestive cardiac failure. Because diazepam is safe and has a rapid action, the skilled help of an anesthesiologist is not mandatory, nor is elaborate anesthetic equipment needed. Other agents have gained popularity, including midazolam and Fentanyl. These agents have a more rapid onset of action and clear more quickly. These features are of potential significant value to the patient. The anesthesia for DC shock has been reviewed by Gilston and colleagues.[71]

The Treatment Room

Electroversion should be undertaken only in an area fully equipped for cardiac monitoring and resuscitation, if needed, including emergency pacemaking. The heart rate should be displayed throughout on a tachometer, if available. A technically satisfactory electrocardiographic lead should be clearly visible on an oscilloscope throughout, and provision should be made for recording the electrocardiogram in several leads as needed.

Routine Preparation

The method of treatment should be carefully explained to the patient and any anxiety relieved. For subsequent comparison, a short strip of lead V_1 of the electrocardiogram should be recorded just before the shock, because P waves can be difficult to detect immediately after DC shock, even when the patient is in sinus rhythm. The skin of the chest should be carefully prepared by liberally applying electrocardiogram paste, which should be rubbed in well to reduce electrical resistance and to prevent painful superficial skin burns. It is important that no conductive material be allowed to run between the two paddles, because current, which takes the path of least resistance, will be diverted away from the heart, possibly resulting in failure of treatment.

Electrical Energies

Small energies should be used first, and if these are unsuccessful, repeated shocks can be given at an increased energy-level setting. For an adult, an initial setting of 25 to 50 J is satisfactory, increasing the setting in 25- to 50-J increments. If heavy digitalization is present, an initial setting of 5 to 10 J is appropriate. If extrasystoles follow the first shock, and as a routine before treating a patient known to be heavily digitalized, 100 mg of lidocaine should be given intravenously before continuing to a higher energy setting. The initial setting for a child is 5 to 10 J delivered across appropriately sized pediatric paddles; this is then increased in 5- to 10-J increments. There should be great reluctance to exceed an energy setting of 300 J in an adult being treated for a chronic rhythm disturbance. However, when an acute dysrhythmia causes serious hemodynamic effects, maximum energies (400 J)

should be used if needed. The initial setting for ventricular fibrillation (no synchronizer in circuit) is 200 J, increasing thereafter to 300- or 400-J settings if needed. Energy settings for internal defibrillation (internal paddles) are 20 to 100 J in 20-J increments.

There are data to suggest that the initial shock for defibrillation should not exceed 200 J, because higher energies did not increase efficiency.[72, 73] There may be some benefit in keeping the second shock also at 200 J, because the transthoracic impedance is lowered by the first shock, and total energies greater than 425 J result in myocardial necrosis.[74, 75]

Current delivered by the defibrillator is inversely related to the impedance across the thorax.[74, 76] Therefore, optimizing impedance is beneficial and can be accomplished by: using a highly conductive interface between the paddles and the chest, increasing paddle size (a maximum of 13 cm), increasing the energy, using successive shocks to decrease impedance when delivered at short intervals, and decreasing the distance between the chest electrodes (expiration versus inspiration).[74, 77–81]

Antiarrhythmic drugs can alter the defibrillation threshold, including drugs that appear to increase (amiodarone, encainide) or decrease (bretylium) the energy requirements.[82, 83] This may be of great importance in the setting of implantable defibrillators.

Immediately After the Shock

With the reinstitution of sinus rhythm, or if sinus rhythm fails to occur after optional energies have been delivered, the amnesic drug is discontinued and a 12-lead electrocardiogram recorded. The electrocardiogram should be monitored on an oscilloscope for the next 24 hours or longer if needed, records of the blood pressure should be taken every half hour until the control value before the shock is regained, and serum enzyme levels should be obtained routinely 8 hours after the shock and repeated at appropriate intervals if the initial values are raised.

Specific Rhythm Disturbances

Atrial Fibrillation

Atrial fibrillation remains the most common rhythm disturbance treated by electroversion, and its cause is frequently rheumatic or coronary heart disease. Among other causes of atrial fibrillation, the lone or idiopathic variety requires special mention because the success rate of its electroversion is low, the incidence of complications is high, and the length of time during which sinus rhythm persists is disappointingly short.[84] For atrial fibrillation resulting from rheumatic heart disease, the initial success rate of treatment by electroversion is 90%, but for idiopathic atrial fibrillation it is less than 75%.[49, 51]

Success of electroversion is not related to the patients age or sex, the type of heart disease (idiopathic atrial fibrillation excepted), or even overall body size. However, an important factor is the duration of the rhythm disturbance.[51] When atrial fibrillation has been present for 5 years or longer, the rate of success is only 50% (Fig. 32-5). The overall size of the heart and selective enlargement of the left atrium also lessen the chance of success.[51]

Every patient with chronic atrial fibrillation requires individual assessment to determine whether treatment is really worthwhile. Despite this, there is no doubt that hemodynamic benefit can be achieved by successful electroversion.[85] Certain patients can be maintained free of cardiac failure only by repeated electrical termination of atrial fibrillation because their ventricular function requires the booster action of atrial systole to achieve an optimal output.

Although it is usually easy to achieve open-chest electroversion at heart surgery, reversion to atrial fibrillation in the immediate postoperative period is almost universal. Atrial fibrillation with the ventricular rate controlled by digoxin is preferred to rapidly changing cardiac rhythms in the postoperative state, and it is therefore recommended that the electroversion of these patients be postponed until they are convalescent following open- or closed-heart valve surgery.[51, 86]

The following groups of patients are, in general, unsuitable for electroversion unless special circumstances exist:

1. Patients with idiopathic or lone atrial fibrillation
2. Patients with coronary heart disease and atrial fibrillation with a slow ventricular response even in the absence of digoxin
3. Patients unable to maintain sinus rhythm for more than a brief period even when receiving suitable antidysrhythmic drugs
4. Patients presenting with atrial rhythm disturbances in rapid succession
5. Patients in the tachycardic phase of the tachycardia–bradycardia syndrome unless emergency pacemaking is at hand, because dangerous asystole may well follow a transmyocardial shock in this condition
6. Patients with long-standing atrial fibrillation (more than 5 years) with considerable enlargement of the heart (cardiothoracic ratio of more than 50%), unless successful cardiac surgery has been performed
7. Patients with atrial fibrillation in association with conduction disturbances

Atrial Flutter

A 95% success rate for converting atrial flutter is common.[51] The electrical energy setting needed is much lower than for atrial fibrillation, the average being 50 J. In contrast to idiopathic atrial fibrillation, atrial flutter not associated with a detectable heart disease may still be successfully reverted by DC shock with low-energy settings, and sinus rhythm may even be maintained for significantly long periods.[85]

Paroxysmal Atrial Tachycardia

The rate of successful electroversion of paroxysmal atrial tachycardia varies from 75% to 80% and depends on the underlying cause; even so, electrical reversion is preferable to pharmacologic therapy.[51] Direct current should not be used for digitalis-induced supraventricular or junctional tachycardia, except under the most unusual circumstances, because of the very high risk of precipitating ventricular fibrillation.[87]

Ventricular Tachycardia

The initial success rate for electroversion of ventricular tachycardia exceeds 97%, and electrical energies needed are low.[51] Direct current shock should be avoided if ventricular tachycardia is induced by digitalis, except under unusual circumstances.

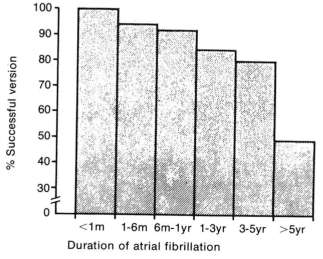

Figure 32-5. Percentage of successful electroversion and duration of atrial fibrillation in 147 patients before treatment (idiopathic atrial fibrillation excluded). m, month; yr, year. (Resnekov L, McDonald L: Appraisal of electroconversion in treatment of cardiac dysrhythmias. Br Heart J 1968;30:786.)

Ventricular Fibrillation

Experimental animal studies have shown the superiority of DC electrical defibrillation over AC electrical defibrillation for the treatment of patients with ventricular fibrillation.[24] In clinical practice, successful resuscitation, as judged by the patient's leaving the hospital, can be achieved in some 60% of patients using DC shock and well-conducted principles of resuscitation.[88] However, without meticulous attention to the latter, electrical defibrillation universally fails.

COMPLICATIONS OF ELECTROVERSION

Complications following electroversion are not as rare as initially predicted, nor do they relate only to drugs given to maintain sinus rhythm.[89] The incidence of complications among 220 patients treated with electroversion has been reported to be 14.5%.[47] (These do not include minor complications such as superficial burns due to poor preparation of the skin or transient rhythm disturbances immediately after shock.)

Complications are related to the energy-level settings used (Fig. 32-6). When a setting of 150 J was employed, there was a 6% incidence of complications, which increased to more than 30% at 400 J.[47] It is frequently patients being treated for atrial fibrillation who require higher energy-level settings, particularly when the dysrhythmia has persisted for more than 3 years and when the patient has a rhythm disturbance associated with cardio-myopathy or coronary heart disease. Similarly, patients with idiopathic atrial fibrillation require high energy-level settings.

From these facts, one can conclude that to prevent unnecessary complications, there rarely is an indication for exceeding settings of 300 J in patients who present with long-standing atrial fibrillation, and great caution must be advised in treating those patients who are heavily digitalized, those whose dysrhythmia is due to cardiomyopathy or coronary heart disease, and those whose atrial fibrillation is of the lone or idiopathic variety.

The origin of the raised serum enzyme levels following electroversion is still debated, and many consider damage to skeletal muscle to be the cause.[90] Other signs of myocardial damage frequently coexist,[51] suggesting that some of the elevation is due to release of enzymes from the damaged myocardium into the general circulation.[91]

The incidence of raised levels of serum enzymes is 10%.

Hypotension

Following electroversion, a fall in blood pressure not related to the anesthetic is more common when higher electrical energies are used. Hypotension may persist for several hours but usually requires no particular therapeutic intervention. Patients should, however, be carefully monitored until the control blood pressure level is regained.

The incidence of hypotension following electroversion is 3%.

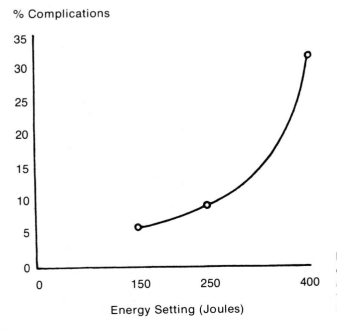

Energy Setting (Joules)		No. of Patients (220)
<	150	108
=	250	55
	400	37

Figure 32-6. Percentage of complications in 220 patients treated by electroversion related to the maximal energy settings used. (Resnekov L, McDonald L: Complications in 220 patients with cardiac dysrhythmias treated by phased direct current shock and indications for electroconversion. Br Heart J 1967;29:926.)

Electrocardiographic Evidence of Myocardial Damage

Electrocardiographic changes following electroversion may be recorded even in the absence of any untoward symptoms (Fig. 32-7). Patterns of myocardial infarction may persist for several months and are most common following treatment at higher energy-level settings.

The incidence of electrocardiographic evidence of myocardial damage following electroversion is 3%.

Pulmonary and Systemic Emboli

Embolism following electroversion indicates the need for prior anticoagulant administration (see above). The incidence of this complication is 1.4%.

Ventricular Dysrhythmia

Following electroversion, ventricular rhythm disturbances are common at low-energy settings if the patient is digitalized, and at high energies even in the absence of digoxin. Their emergence requires an intravenous antidysrhythmic drug before the energy-level setting is increased for a further shock.

Increase in Heart Size and Pulmonary Edema

Increase in heart size and pulmonary edema (Fig. 32-8), when they occur, are seen within 1 to 3 hours of electroversion, and these complications are unlike all others in that they are found only in patients successfully converted

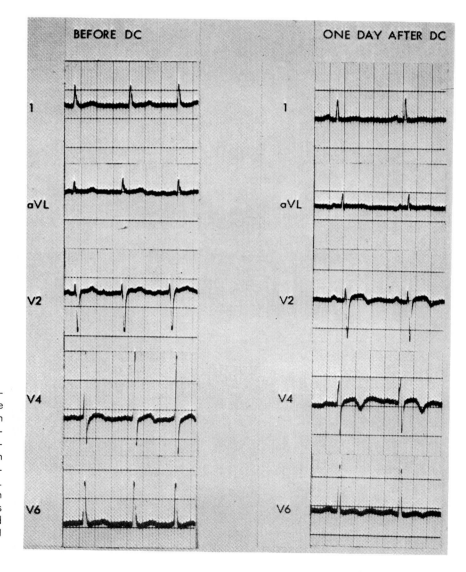

Figure 32-7. Electrocardiogram immediately before (left) and 1 day after (right) the electroversion of idiopathic atrial fibrillation using 300 J. In sinus rhythm, a pattern of nontransmural infarction is shown, which was associated with a diagnostic elevation of serum enzymes. The electrocardiographic abnormalities persisted for more than 6 months. (Resnekov L, McDonald L: Complications in 220 patients with cardiac dysrhythmias treated by phased direct current shock and indications for electroconversion. Br Heart J 1967;29:926.)

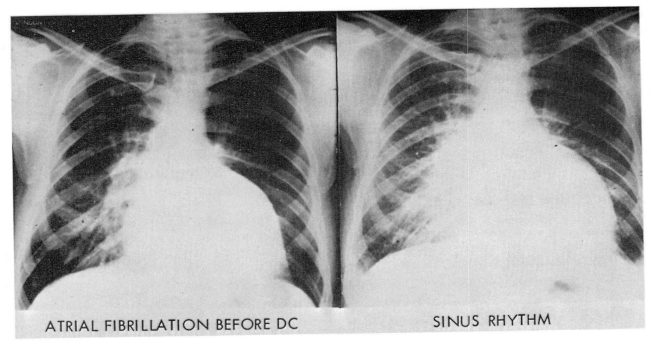

ATRIAL FIBRILLATION BEFORE DC   SINUS RHYTHM

Figure 32-8. Chest radiograph (posteroanterior) immediately before (left) and 12 hours after (right) the electroversion of atrial fibrillation (200 J) in a patient with corrected transposition of the great vessels. Note the marked increase in size of the heart and obvious pulmonary edema in sinus rhythm. (Resnekov L, McDonald L: Complications in 220 patients with cardiac dysrhythmias treated by phased direct current shock and indications for electroconversion. Br Heart J 1967;29:926.)

to sinus rhythm. (Their usual incidence is 3%.) Although Lown considered pulmonary emboli as the cause,[48] others believe that following electroversion there is considerable depression of mechanical function of the heart,[92] which in the presence of any additional obstruction to flow across the mitral valve or associated left ventricular dysfunction may result in pulmonary edema. As with the other complications, the incidence of these two findings is greatest following higher energy-level settings.

Pacemaker Dysfunction

Defibrillation does not appear to result in permanent damage unless the shock is delivered directly over the generator. It is appropriate to place the paddle at least 10 cm from the pulse generator and to check serially pacemaker function and pacemaker threshold for up to 6 weeks following transthoracic defibrillation.[93]

FOLLOW-UP STUDIES

Electroversion is very successful in the treatment of rhythm disturbances, but the number of patients remaining in sinus rhythm is disappointingly small, particularly

when patients with atrial fibrillation are treated.[49, 51] A 36-month follow-up study involving 183 patients who were successfully brought into sinus rhythm shows that less than 30% remained in sinus rhythm.[49] The highest incidence of reverting occurs by the end of the first month of the treatment (Fig. 32-9), but the incidence is actually highest within the first 24 hours of successful electroversion (Fig. 32-10). Patients with significant underlying heart disease and radiographic evidence of cardiac enlargement are particularly prone to revert to the original rhythm disturbance,[49, 51] and in any patient in whom atrial fibrillation is of long duration (3 years or longer), a 70% chance of reverting to that rhythm can be expected (Fig. 32-11).

PHARMACOLOGIC THERAPY AND ELECTROVERSION

Digitalis Preparation

Lown and coworkers found that in the presence of heavy digitalization, the DC threshold for ventricular tachycardia in the dog fell by some 2000%, to 0.2 J.[94] The importance of this observation in clinical practice is that although dig-

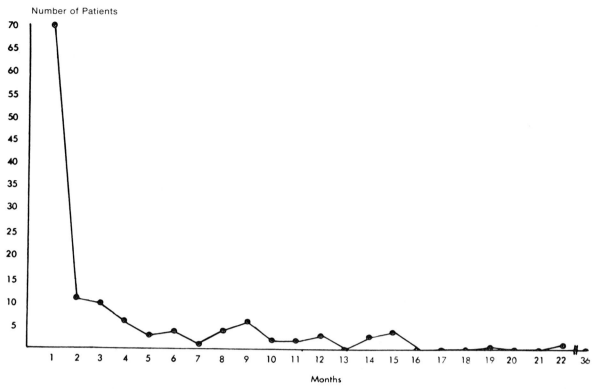

Figure 32-9. A 36-month follow-up study of 183 patients whose atrial fibrillation was successfully converted to sinus rhythm. Of the 183 patients, 131 (72%) reverted to atrial fibrillation, 70 within the first month. (See also Fig. 32-10.) (Resnekov L, McDonald L: Appraisal of electroconversion in treatment of cardiac dysrhythmias. Br Heart J 1968;30:786.)

italis effects may not be clinically apparent, they can be unmasked by an electrical shock, and any associated myocardial cell potassium deficit enhances this effect. Conversely, the administration of potassium may reverse the undesirable effects. The higher the electrical energy used, the higher the risk of emergence of serious ventricular dysrhythmias, and death has been reported as a result.[95] As already indicated, electroversion should rarely be used for the management of a known digitalis-induced rhythm disturbance. Despite the occasional reported success,[96] fatal ventricular fibrillation may follow even when the shock is properly synchronized.[87] If electroversion is needed in a patient known to be heavily digitalized, an intravenous injection of an antidysrhythmic drug should always precede the shock, and the energy-level setting should be significantly reduced, as previously indicated.

Propranolol may be helpful in reducing the dangerous myocardial sensitivity to a high energy level of electrical current. If used, however, it should be combined with intravenous atropine[97] to protect the patient against cardiac arrest, which may follow DC shock in patients primed with propranolol.[98]

Drugs to Maintain Sinus Rhythm

For sinus rhythm to follow cardioversion, the sinoatrial node must function adequately and must not be diseased or fibrosed. Ectopic beats should be kept to a minimum immediately after a shock.[69] Excess electrical energies can be harmful, and any interruption of the rhythm disturbance by the DC shock is good evidence that depolarization of the heart did occur and that the level of electrical energy used was adequate. If sinus rhythm fails to emerge or is short lived despite adequate electrical energies, it is likely that either the sinus node cannot function as the pacemaker or the ectopic rhythms were precipitated by a vagal surge or by a sudden release of catecholamine following the electrical discharge.

To improve pacemaker function following DC shock, atropine, 1 to 2 mg intravenously, should be routinely administered to patients in whom atrial fibrillation has been present for 5 years or longer, although the chance of these chronic dysrhythmic patients converting easily or maintaining sinus rhythm for any length of time thereafter is small.[49] Similarly, any bradycardia after DC shock will

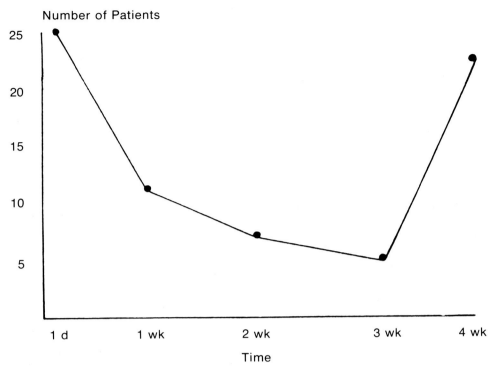

Figure 32-10. Of the 70 patients who reverted to atrial fibrillation within the first 4 weeks (see Fig. 32-9), 25 did so within the first day of electroversion. d, day; wk, week. (Resnekov L, McDonald L: Complications in 220 patients with cardiac dysrhythmias treated by phased direct current shock and indications for electroconversion. Br Heart J 1967;29:926.)

enhance the likelihood of atrial ventricular premature beats.[48] Note that although they are successful in suppressing ectopic beats, antidysrhythmic drugs such as quinidine, procainamide, lidocaine, and propranolol may depress pacemaker function. Furthermore, because there is already a likelihood of intense parasympathetic stimulation immediately after DC shock,[99] the *routine* use of these drugs is not advised because they may well precipitate dangerous asystole.

Isolated ventricular premature beats or ventricular tachycardia immediately after DC shock frequently results from overdigitalization, from the effects on the heart of the shock itself, and from a lowered myocardial potassium content. As previously indicated, such patients should be protected by postponing treatment if possible, by ensuring an adequate serum and myocardial potassium level, and by using antidysrhythmic drugs immediately before the shock, which should be delivered at a reduced energy-level setting.

Unfortunately, there is little evidence that any antidysrhythmic agent presently available, either alone or in combination with other agents, can maintain sinus rhythm when sinoatrial function is at fault, when serious underlying myocardial or valvular heart disease is present, or when atrial fibrillation has existed for 5 years or longer.

Nevertheless, sinus rhythm may be hemodynamically important in certain patients. Under these circumstances, antiarrhythmic agents may be used in an attempt to maintain sinus rhythm over a prolonged period. If cardiac failure is not too severe, it may be possible to maintain sinus rhythm by a combination of quinidine and propranolol,[100] which will permit reducing the dose of quinidine and thus lessening the chance of toxicity.

GENERAL ASPECTS OF THE USE OF HIGH-ENERGY ELECTRICAL CURRENT

The refinement of high-energy electrical current has been a very great advance in the management of cardiac dysrhythmias. Provided meticulous attention to detail is adhered to, the method is efficient, successful, and relatively free of complications. Nevertheless, important questions about its actual use in clinical practice remain, particularly regarding the possibility of causing myocardial damage. Closely allied is the level of energy to be used and its recommended upper limit, beyond which complication rates become forbiddingly high.

Complications following synchronized DC shock are often multiple.[47] Changes in the levels of serum enzymes

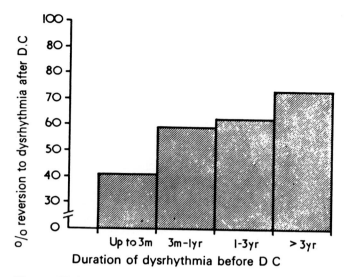

Figure 32-11. Percentage of patients who reverted to atrial fibrillation related to the duration of the dysrhythmia before electroversion (excluding idiopathic atrial fibrillation). m, month; yr, year; DC, direct current. (Resnekov L, McDonald L: Complications in 220 patients with cardiac dysrhythmias treated by phased direct current shock and indications for electroconversion. Br Heart J 1967;29:926.)

are the most common complication reported, and Ehsani and colleagues were able to show that in patients suffering acute myocardial infarction, high-energy electrical current discharge to the heart was followed by a release of creatine phosphokinase (CPK) into the peripheral blood, with a substantial rise in the MB, or cardiac fraction.[100] In patients without acute myocardial infarction, the same energy-level setting resulted in an increase in total CPK made up almost entirely of the MM, or skeletal muscle fraction. Earlier work by Dahl and coworkers showed that myocardial damage was caused by DC shock, particularly at high energy-level settings.[101] Myocardial damage is related to the energy level delivered, the size of the electrodes, and the time between shocks: careful attention to all of these factors should help minimize its occurrence.

In 1961, Peleǎka showed that myocardial damage could result from capacitor discharge.[102] The important electrical variables that relate to the safe clinical use of high-energy electrical current include the capacitance of the condensers, the value of inductance of the circuit, the resistance between the patient electrodes, and the rise time of the current waveform. If a defibrillation apparatus is considered in terms of a DC-resistive circuit, the resistance between the inductance and the body may alter significantly because of a change in total body impedance, and this may well be responsible for changes in the discharge-current waveform flowing across the heart.

Using trapezoidal current waveforms for external ventricular defibrillation, Tacker and associates reported that the effectiveness of treatment decreased as body weight

increased.[103] At present, there is a regrettable lack of certainty regarding the optimal characteristics for duration, peak current, and other parameters needed for effective and safe defibrillation. Nevertheless, high-output defibrillators have already been designed and are being recommended.[104] Much of the present argument regarding the need for higher-energy defibrillators in clinical use relates particularly to animal studies,[105] backed by as yet inadequate clinical investigations.[106]

In an attempt to resolve this question, Pantridge and associates undertook a prospective study in patients weighing 50 kg or more, particularly those in the 90-kg range.[107] A low energy of between 150 and 165 J was delivered to these subjects, and success in defibrillating the ventricle was good. Similar conclusions have been published by other investigators.[51, 108] Ventricular defibrillation depends for its success on not only delivering an efficient electrical shock to the myocardium but also observing the principles of cardiopulmonary resuscitation.

Cardiac damage due to electrical current and energy is associated with morphologic changes that are easily seen by light microscopy and ultrastructural observations.[109] There is a distinct morphologic pattern when a delivered dose exceeds 1 A/kg of body weight in an experimental animal using trapezoidal current waveforms. The higher the electrical amperage delivered, the more severe and extensive the damage. Davis and colleagues showed that such cardiac lesions are discrete and are found beneath the epicardium, but they may even be transmural in their extent.[110] There is disruption of myofilaments and of the mitochondria, which often contain lipid droplets. Areas of the myocardium that may be irreversibly damaged are replaced by fibrous scar tissue; if this is extensive, abnormal cardiac function could result. The clinical correlate of these extensive areas of myocardial damage is profound electrocardiographic changes, suggesting infarction (see Fig. 32-7),[49] and such patterns may persist for many months. In addition, they are associated with increases in serum enzyme levels.

More recently, the intravenous administration of 1 mg/kg of verapamil before delivering shocks was studied in animals to see whether less myocardial damage was caused when 4000 J was passed across the chest of dogs. Prior administration of verapamil reduced the amount of damage caused, whereas propranolol, 0.4 mg/kg intravenously, had no such beneficial effect. Also demonstrated during this study was the fact that more damage was caused when the electrical energy was divided among 10 shocks than when it was applied in 20 or 40 shocks at 0.5-minute intervals. The beneficial effects of verapamil provide further evidence for the role of calcium accumulation in cardiac necrosis after high-energy electrical shocks.[111]

Thus, much more study is needed before recommending that higher-energy DC defibrillators be universally available, lest their widespread use be associated with an increasing number of potentially serious cardiac complications following attempts at ventricular defibrillation using energy-level settings over 400 J when lower energy-level settings may well suffice.

References

1. Hoffa M, Luăwig C: Einige neue Versuche über Herzbewegung. Z Ration Med 1850;9:107.
2. Prevost JL, Battelli F: Quelques effets des décharges electriques sur le coeur des mammifrères. J Physiol Pathol Gen (Paris) 1900;2:40.
3. Kouwenhoven WB, Hooker DR, Langworthy OR: The current flowing through the heart under conditions of electric shock. Am J Physiol 1932;100:344.
4. Ferris LP, King BG, Spence PW, Williams HB: Effects of electrical shock on the heart. Elec Engineer 1936;55:498.
5. King BG: The effect of electric shock on heart action with special reference to varying susceptibility in different parts of the cardiac cycle. Aberdeen, Scotland: The Aberdeen University Press, 1934.
6. Gurvich NL, Yunyev GS: O vosstanovlenii normalnoi deyatel'nosti fibrilliruyuschego serdtsa teplokrovnikh possedstvom kondensatornogo razryada. Biull Eksp Biol Med 1939;8:55.
7. Lown B, Amarasingham R, Neuman J: New method for terminating cardiac arrhythmias. Use of synchronized capacitor discharge. JAMA 1962;182:548.
8. Hooker DR, Kouwenhoven WB, Langworthy OR: The effect of alternating electrical currents on the heart. Am J Physiol 1933;103:444.
9. Kouwenhoven WB, Milnor WR: Treatment of ventricular fibrillation using a capacitor discharge. J Appl Physiol 1954; 7:253.
10. Tacker WA Jr, Geddes LA: Electrical Defibrillation. Boca Raton, Florida: CRC Press, 1980:59.
11. Schuder JC, Stoeckle H, Dolan AM: Transthoracic ventricular defibrillation with square-wave stimuli: one-half cycle, one cycle, and multicycle waveforms. Circ Res 1964;15:258.
12. Jones JL, Jones RE: Improved defibrillator waveform safety factor with biphasic waveforms. Am J Physiol 1983;245:H60.
13. Schuder JC, McDaniel WC, Stoeckle H: Defibrillation of 100-kg calves with asymmetrical, bidirectional, rectangular pulses. Cardiovasc Res 1984;18:419.
14. Jones JL, Jones RE: Decreased defibrillator-induced dysfunction with biphasic rectangular waveforms. Am J Physiol 1984;247:H792.
15. Dixon EG, Tang ASL, Wolf PD, et al: Improved defibrillation thresholds with large contoured epicardial electrodes and biphasic waveforms. Circulation 1987;76:1176.
16. Tang ASL, Yabe S, Wharton JM, et al: Ventricular defibrillation using biphasic waveforms: the importance of phasic duration. J Am Coll Cardiol 1989;13:207.
17. Jones JL, Jones RE, Balasky G: Improved cardiac cell excitation with symmetrical biphasic defibrillator waveforms. Am J Physiol 1987;253:H1418.
18. Cranefield PF, Hoffman BF: Propagated repolarization in heart muscle. J Gen Physiol 1958;41:633.
19. Jones JL, Proskauer CC, Paull WK, et al: Ultrastructural injury to chick myocardial cells in vitro following "electric countershock." Circ Res 1980;46:387.
20. Yarbrough R, Ussery G, Whitley J: A comparison of the effects of A.C. and D.C. countershock on ventricular function in thoracotomized dogs. Am J Cardiol 1964;14:504.
21. Beck ES, Pritchard WH, Feil HS: Ventricular fibrillation of long duration abolished by electric shock. JAMA 1947; 135:985.
22. McDonald L, Resnekov L, Ross D: Resistant ventricular tachycardia a year after surgical correction of Fallot's tetralogy treated by external electric countershock. Lancet 1963; 2:708.
23. Zoll PM, Linenthal AJ: Termination of refractory tachycardia by external countershock. Circulation 1962;25:596.
24. Nachlas MM, Bix HH, Mower MM, Sieband MP: Observations on defibrillation and synchronized countershock. Prog Cardiovasc Dis 1966;9:64.
25. de Boer S: On the fibrillation of the heart. J Physiol (Lond) 1921;54:400.
26. Wiggers CJ, Wegria R: Ventricular fibrillation due to single, localized induction and condenser shocks applied during vulnerable phase of ventricular systole. Am J Physiol 1940; 128:500.
27. Andrus EC, Carter EP, Wheeler HA: Refractory period of the normally beating dog's auricle, with a note on the occurrence of auricular fibrillation following a single stimulus. J Exp Med 1930;51:357.
28. Castellanos A Jr, Lemberg L, Berkovits BV: Repetitive firing during synchronized ventricular stimulation. Am J Cardiol [Abstract] 1966;17:119.
29. Balagot RC, Bandelin VR: Comparative evaluation of some DC cardiac defibrillators. Am Heart J 1969;77:489.
30. Kreus KE, Salokannel SJ, Waris EK: Non-synchronised and synchronised direct-current countershock in cardiac arrhythmias. Lancet 1966;2:405.
31. Antoni H: Physiologische Grundlagen der elektrischen Defibrillation des Herzens. Verh Dtsch Ges Kreislaufforsch 1969;35:106.
32. Wiggers CJ: The physiologic basis for cardiac resuscitation from ventricular fibrillation—Method for serial defibrillation. Am Heart J 1940;20:413.
33. Zipes DP, Fischer J, King RM, et al: Termination of ventricular fibrillation in dogs by depolarizing a critical amount of myocardium. Am J Cardiol 1975;36:37.
34. Chen P-S, Shibata N, Wolf P, et al: Activation during successful and unsuccessful ventricular defibrillation in open chest dogs: evidence of complete cessation and regeneration of ventricular fibrillation after unsuccessful shocks. J Clin Invest 1986;77:810.
35. Chen P-S, Shibata N, Dixon EG, Martin RO, Ideker RE: Comparison of defibrillation threshold and the upper limit of ventricular vulnerability. Circulation 1986;73:1022.
36. Chen P-S, Wolf PD, Melnick SD, Danieley ND, Smith WM, Ideker RE: Comparison of activation during ventricular fibrillation and following unsuccessful defibrillation shocks in open chest dogs. Circ Res 1990;66:1544.
37. Chen P-S, Wolf PD, Ideker RE: The mechanism of cardiac defibrillation: a different point of view. Circulation 1991; 84:913.

38. Chen P-S, Feld GK, Kriett JM, et al: The relation between upper limit of vulnerability and defibrillation threshold in humans. Circulation 1993;88:186.

39. Ideker RE, Klein GJ, Harrison L, et al: The transition to ventricular fibrillation induced by reperfusion following acute ischemia in the dog: a period of organized epicardial activation. Circulation 1981;63:1371.

40. Moe GK, Rheinboldt WC, Abildskov JA: A computer model of atrial fibrillation. Am Heart J 1964;67:200.

41. Chen P-S, Wolf PD, Dixon WE, et al: Mechanism of ventricular vulnerability to single premature stimuli in open-chest dogs. Circ Res 1988;62:1191.

42. Frazier DW, Wolf PD, Wharton JM, Tang ASL, Smith WM, Ideker RE: Stimulus-induced critical point: mechanism for electrical initiation of reentry in normal canine myocardium. J Clin Invest 1989;83:1039.

43. Davy J-M, Fain ES, Dorian P, et al: The relationship between successful defibrillation and delivered energy in open-chest dogs: reappraisal of the "defibrillation threshold" concept. Am Heart J 1987;113:77.

44. Chen P-S, Shibata N, Dixon EG, et al: Comparison of the defibrillation threshold and the upper limit of ventricular vulnerability. Circulation 1986;73:1022.

45. Coraboeuf E, Suekane K, Breton D: Some effects of strong stimulations on the electrical and mechanical properties of isolated heart. In: Electrophysiology of the Heart. New York: Oxford Medical Publications, 1964.

46. Zoll PM, Linenthal AJ, Gibson W, et al: Termination of ventricular fibrillation in man by externally applied countershock. N Engl J Med 1956;254:727.

47. Resnekov L, McDonald L: Complications in 220 patients with cardiac dysrhythmias treated by phased direct current shock and indications for electroconversion. Br Heart J 1967;29:926.

48. Lown B: Electrical reversion of cardiac arrhythmias. Br Heart J 1967;29:469.

49. Resnekov L, McDonald L: Appraisal of electroconversion in treatment of cardiac dysrhythmias. Br Heart J 1968;30:786.

50. McDonald L, Resnekov L, O'Brien K: Direct current shock in treatment of drug resistant arrhythmias. Br Med J 1964;1:1468.

51. Resnekov L: Synchronized capacitor discharge in the management of cardiac arrhythmias with particular reference to the haemodynamic significance of atrial systole. M.D. Thesis, University of Cape Town, Cape Town, South Africa, 1965.

52. Peleǎka B: A high voltage defibrillator and the theory of high-voltage defibrillation. In: Proceedings of the Third International Conference of Medical Electronics. Springfield, IL: Charles C Thomas, 1960:265.

53. Lown B, Kleiger R, Wolff G: The technique of cardioversion. Am Heart J 1964;67:282.

54. Kouwenhoven WB, Jude JR, Knickerbocker GG, Chestnut WR: Closed chest defibrillation of the heart. Surgery 1957;42:550.

55. Zoll RH, Zoll PM, Frank HA, Belgard AH: New defibrillation electrodes. Med Instrument [Abstract] 1978;2:56.

56. Kerber RE, Martins KB, Kelly KJ, et al: Self-adhesive preapplied electrode pads for defibrillation and cardioversion. J Am Coll Cardiol 1984;3:815.

57. De Silva RA, Margolis B, Lown B: Determinants of success during in hospital defibrillation. Cited in Crampton RA: Accepted, controversial and speculative aspects of ventricular defibrillation. Prog Cardiovasc Dis 1980;23:167.

58. Ewy GA, Horan WJ, Ewy MD: Disposable defibrillator electrodes. Heart Lung 1977;6:127.

59. Kerber RE, Martins JB, Kelly KJ, et al: Self-adhesive preapplied electrode pads for defibrillation and cardioversion. Am J Cardiol 1977;6:127.

60. Rossi M, Lown B: The use of quinidine in cardioversion. Am J Cardiol 1966;19:234.

61. Resnekov L: Drug therapy before and after the electroversion of cardiac dysrhythmias. Prog Cardiovasc Dis 1974;16:531.

62. Goldman J: The management of chronic atrial fibrillation: indications for and method of conversion to sinus rhythm. Prog Cardiovasc Dis 1959–1960;2:465.

63. The Boston Area Anticoagulation Trial for Atrial Fibrillation Investigators. The effect of low-dose warfarin on the risk of stroke in patients with non-rheumatic atrial fibrillation. N Engl J Med 1990;323:1505.

64. Stroke Prevention in Atrial Fibrillation Study Group Investigators. Preliminary report of the stroke prevention in atrial fibrillation study. N Engl J Med 1990;322:863.

65. Petersen P, Kastrup J, Helweg-Larsen S, Boysen G, Godtfredsen J: Risk factors for thromboembolic complications in chronic atrial fibrillation. The Copenhagen AFASAK Study. Arch Intern Med 1990;150:819.

66. Storstein D: Cardioversion session 18. In Sandöe E, Flensted-Jensen E, Olesen K II, eds. Symposium on Cardiac Arrhythmias. Södertälje, Sweden: Astra, 1970:418.

67. Stock RJ: Cardioversion without anesthesia. N Engl J Med 1963;269:534.

68. Lown B: Cardioversion without anesthesia. N Engl J Med 1963;269:535.

69. Kahler RI, Burrow GN, Felig P: Diazepam induced amnesia for cardioversion. JAMA 1967;200:997.

70. Johnstone M, Nisbet HIA: Ventricular arrhythmia during halothane anaesthesia. Br J Anaesthesiol 1961;33:9.

71. Gilston A, Fordham R, Resnekov L: Anaesthesia for direct-current shock in the treatment of cardiac dysrhythmias. Br J Anaesthesiol 1965;37:533.

72. Kerber RE, Jensen SR, Gascho JA, et al: Determinants of defibrillation: prospective analysis of 183 patients. Am J Cardiol 1983;52:739.

73. Weaver WD, Cobb LA, Kopass MK, et al: Ventricular defibrillation—A comparative trial using 175J and 320J shocks. N Engl J Med 1983;307:1101.

74. Kerber RE, Grayzel J, Hoyt R, et al: Transthoracic resistance in human defibrillation. Influence of body weight, chest size, serial shocks, paddle size and paddle contact pressure. Circulation 1981;63:676.

75. Kerber RE: Energy requirements for defibrillation. Circulation 1986;74(suppl IV):IV-117.

76. Ewy GA, Ewy MD, Silverman J: Determinants of human transthoracic resistance to direct current discharge. Circulation 1972;46(suppl II):II-150.

77. Connell PN, Ewy GA, Dahl CF, et al: Transthoracic impedance to defibrillation discharge: effect of electrode size and electrode–chest wall interface. J Electrocardiol 1973;6:313.

78. Kerber RE, Jensen SR, Grayzel J, et al: Elective cardioversion:

influence of paddle-electrode location and size on success rates and energy requirements. N Engl J Med 1981;305:658.

79. Geddes LA, Tacker WA, Cabler DP, et al: Decrease in transthoracic resistance during successive ventricular defibrillation trials. Med Instrument 1975;9:179.

80. Hoyt R, Grayzel J, Kerber RE: Determinants of intracardiac current in defibrillation. Experimental studies in dogs. Circulation 1981;64:818.

81. Ewy GA, Hellman DA, McClung S, et al: Influence of ventilation phase on transthoracic impedance and defibrillation effectiveness. Crit Care Med 1980;8:164.

82. Babbs CF, Yim GKW, Whistler SJ, et al: Elevation of ventricular defibrillation threshold in dogs by antiarrhythmic agents. Am Heart J 1979;98:345.

83. Troup PJ, Chapman PD, Olinger GN, et al: The implanted defibrillator: relation of defibrillating lead configuration and clinical variables to defibrillation threshold. J Am Coll Cardiol 1985;6:1315.

84. Resnekov L, McDonald L: Electroversion of lone atrial fibrillation and flutter including haemodynamic studies at rest and on exercise. Br Heart J 1971;33:339.

85. Resnekov L: Haemodynamic studies before and after electrical conversion of atrial fibrillation and flutter to sinus rhythm. Br Heart J 1967;29:700.

86. Yang SS, Maranhao V, Monheit R, et al: Cardioversion following open-heart valvular surgery. Br Heart J 1966;28:309.

87. Rabbino MD, Likoff W, Dreifus L: Complications and limitations of direct-current countershock. JAMA 1964;190:417.

88. Gilston A, Resnekov L: Cardio-Respiratory Resuscitation. London: William Heinemann, 1971.

89. Lown B: Cardioversion of arrhythmias. II. Mod Concepts Cardiovasc Dis 1964;33:869.

90. Mandecki T, Giec L, Kargal W: Serum enzyme activities after cardioversion. Br Heart J 1970;32:600.

91. Ehsani A, Ewy GA, Sobel BE: Effects of electrical countershock on serum creatine phosphokinase (CPK) isoenzyme activity. Am J Cardiol 1976;37:12.

92. Logan WFWE, Rowlands DJ, Howitt G, Holmes AM: Left atrial activity following cardioversion. Lancet 1965;2:471.

93. Levine PA, Barold SS, Fletcher RD, et al: Adverse acute and chronic effects of electrical defibrillation and cardioversion on implanted unipolar cardiac pacing systems. J Am Coll Cardiol 1983;1:1413.

94. Lown B, Kleiger R, Williams J: Cardioversion and digitalis drugs: changed threshold to electric shock in digitalized animals. Circ Res 1965;17:519.

95. Gilbert R, Cuddy RP: Digitalis intoxication following conversion to sinus rhythm. Circulation 1965;32:58.

96. Corwin ND, Klein MJ, Friedberg CK: Countershock conversion of digitalis associated paroxysmal tachycardia with block. Am Heart J 1963;66:804.

97. Sloman G, Robinson JS, McClean K: Propranolol in persistent ventricular fibrillation. Br Med J 1965;1:895.

98. Lown B: In: Julian DG, Oliver MF, eds. Acute Myocardial Infarction. Edinburgh: Churchill Livingstone, 1968.

99. Childers RW, Rothbaum D, Arnsdorf M: The effects of DC shock on the electrical properties of the heart. Circulation [Abstract] 1967;36(suppl):II-85.

100. Byrne-Quinn E, Wing AJ: Maintenance of sinus rhythm after DC reversion of atrial fibrillation. A double-blind controlled trial of long-acting quinidine bisulphate. Br Heart J 1970; 32:370.

101. Dahl CF, Ewy GA, Warner ED, Thomas ED: Myocardial necrosis from direct current countershock. Effect of paddle electrode size and true interval between discharges. Circulation 1974;50:956.

102. Peleăka B: Cardiac arrhythmias following condenser discharges and their dependence upon strength of current and phase of cardiac cycle. Circ Res 1963;13:21.

103. Tacker WA Jr, Geddes LA, Rosborough JP, et al: Transchest ventricular defibrillation of heavy subjects using trapezoidal current waveforms. J Electrocardiol 1975;8:237.

104. Geddes LA, Bourland JD, Coulter TW, et al: A megawatt defibrillator for trans-chest defibrillation of heavy subjects. Med Electron Biol Engineer 1973;11:747.

105. Geddes LA, Tacker WA, Rosborough J, et al: Electrical dose for ventricular defibrillation of large and small animals using precordial electrodes. J Clin Invest 1974;53:310.

106. Tacker WA, Galiato F, Giuliani E, et al: Energy dosage for human transchest electrical ventricular defibrillation. N Engl J Med 1974;290:214.

107. Pantridge J, Adgey AAJ, Webb SW: Electrical requirements for ventricular defibrillation. Br Med J 1975;2:313.

108. Morgan MT, McElroy CR: Letter. Transchest electrical ventricular defibrillation. Am Heart J 1976;92:674.

109. Tedeschi CG, White CW Jr: A morphologic study of canine hearts subjected to fibrillation, electrical defibrillation and manual compression. Circulation 1954;9:916.

110. David JS, Lie JT, Bentinck DC, et al: Cardiac damage due to electrical current and energy. Light microscopic and ultrastructural observations of acute and delayed myocardial cellular injuries. In: Proceedings of Cardiac Defibrillation Conference. West Lafayette, IN: Purdue University, 1975:27.

111. Patton JN, Allen JD, Pantridge JF: The effects of shock energy, propranolol and verapamil on cardiac damage caused by transthoracic countershock. Circulation 1984;69:357.

Cardiac Arrhythmias, 3rd edition, edited by William J. Mandel.
J. B. Lippincott Company, Philadelphia © 1995.

33

John D. Gallagher

Anesthesia and Cardiac Arrhythmias

Drugs that produce general anesthesia perturb membrane lipids in the brain with subsequent alterations in the function of membrane spanning proteins.[1] It is not surprising that the complex effects of anesthetics on cell membranes and ionic channels of the central nervous system should extend to the channels of cardiac tissue and produce direct effects on cardiac cells.[2] Likewise, anesthetics are expected to interfere with the reflex regulation of the cardiovascular system, inhibiting peripheral and central components of the autonomic nervous system.

Although not intended to be encyclopedic, it is hoped that this review will highlight the diverse electrophysiologic effects of anesthetics and the potential for interaction between anesthetics and other cardiac drugs, and improve understanding of the patient who develops arrhythmias during anesthesia.

INCIDENCE OF ARRHYTHMIAS DURING SURGERY

Cardiac arrhythmias occur during anesthesia and surgery in as many as 60% of patients.[3] This prevalence must be considered, however, in light of the frequent occurrence of atrial and ventricular ectopy in 50% to 60% of presumably healthy men and women.[4,5]

In an early study of intraoperative arrhythmias using continuous electrocardiographic recording, Kuner and colleagues in 1967 studied 154 patients and found that 61.7% had one or more abnormal cardiac rhythms, excluding sinus tachycardia.[3] In order of frequency, wandering pacemaker (28%), isorhythmic atrioventricular dissociation (22%), nodal rhythm (19%), premature ventricular systoles (18%), sinus bradycardia (14%), premature atrial extrasystoles (14%), supraventricular tachycardia, (3%) and ventricular tachycardia (3%) were recorded. Six percent of patients displayed other arrhythmias, including atrial fibrillation, idioventricular rhythm, and block. There was no relationship between arrhythmias and age, preexisting general medical condition, sex, type of anesthesia (general versus regional or local), or, surprisingly, heart disease and existence of preoperative arrhythmias. Patients undergoing prolonged operations and neurosurgical and thoracic procedures had a higher incidence of arrhythmias, as did patients whose tracheae were intubated (72.2% versus 43.9%). Bertrand and associates, in 1971, found an 84% incidence of arrhythmias in 100 patients undergoing a variety of procedures, excluding thoracic surgery.[6] Ventricular rhythm disturbances were more frequent in patients with heart disease (60% versus 37%), in contrast to the findings of Kuner and colleagues.[3]

In demonstrating that patients with asymptomatic chronic hypokalemia were not at increased risk of perioperative arrhythmias, Vitez and coworkers serendipitously provided data on arrhythmia incidence in the contemporary general surgical population.[7] Of 150 patients reported in 1985, 18% of whom had preoperative arrhythmias noted, 43% developed arrhythmias intraoperatively. Premature atrial and ventricular contractions were noted in 12% and 19%, respectively, bigeminy in 3%, and junctional rhythm in 17%. Hirsch and colleagues, in 1988, described continuous electrocardiograms from 447 patients undergoing major cardiac or vascular procedures.[8] Monitoring was discontinued before atrial cannulation in cardiac procedures (83% of total). Frequent or life-threatening ventricular arrhythmias (Lown classes 2–4[9]) were noted in 21% of patients. Congestive heart failure, ventricular aneurysm, a history of chronic digoxin therapy, and existence of the arrhythmia on a preoperative ECG were associated with higher incidences of complex ventricular arrhythmias.

Of 230 males, 46% of whom had known coronary artery disease, major ventricular arrhythmias occurred perioperatively in 44% but increased in severity intraoperatively in only 2%. Smokers, those with a history of congestive heart failure, and those with electrocardiographic evidence of myocardial ischemia were at higher risk.[10]

Although 24 of 249 children aged 2 years or older developed premature atrial or ventricular beats or a ventricular bigeminal rhythm, none of 153 infants younger than 2 years of age had an episode of arrhythmia.[11] Arrhythmias appeared more frequently in children ventilated by mask who became hypercarbic, and in association with light anesthesia. The incidence during halothane anesthesia (11.6%) was greater than during all other techniques (2.0%).[11]

A selection of incidence studies (including several dealing with specific age groups, surgical procedures, or comparisons of anesthetics) in which continuous electrocardiogram recording was used is provided in Table 33-1.

TABLE 33-1. Incidence of Intraoperative Arrhythmias

Surgery (#patients)	Age (years)	Arrhythmias	Comments
None (50)[5]	22–28	APB, 64%; VPB, 54%; 2°AVB, 2%	Healthy young women without heart disease
None (50)[4]	23–27	APB, 56%; VPB, 50%; 2°AVB, 6%	Healthy men
General, noncardiac (154)[3]	6 wk–86	Total, 61.7%; SV arrhythmias, 60% V arrhythmias, 43%; both, 19%	Incidence highest in neurosurgical and thoracic; higher in intubated patients (see text)
General, nonthoracotomy (100)[6]	18–90	Total, 84%	Highest in those with cardiac disease. Highest during intubation and extubation (see text)
General, noncardiac (150)[7]	62 ± 12	Total, 43%	Highest in those with preexisting arrhythmias. Not related to serum K⁺ (see text)
Cardiac, vascular (447)[8]	51% > 60	None, 63%; mild, 16%; severe, 21%	Higher incidence: congestive failure, LV aneurysm, digoxin. Serum K⁺ not related (see text)
Adenoidectomy (48)[203]	5 ± 2.3	SV arrhythmias: Hal, 50% Enf/Iso, 0% V arrhythmias: Hal, 18% Enf/Iso, 0%	Suggestive of halothane catecholamine interaction[13]
Adenoidectomy, myringotomy (167)[204]	1–12	Total: Hal, 86.6% Enf, 38.9% V arrhythmias: Hal, 41.3% Enf, 2.8%	During halothane, VPB in 6 children, multifocal VPB in 5, VT in 8
Gynecologic laparoscopy (86)[177]	34.2	Placebo: SV arrhythmias, 42% VPB, 47% Nadolol: SV arrhythmias, 15% VPB, 3%	Thiopental, halothane, nitrous oxide, succinylcholine. Marked reduction following single-dose β-blockade
Oral surgery (100)[205]	10–60	Total: Hal, 22% Enf, 4% VPB: Hal, 14% Enf, 0%	
Oral surgery (50)[206]	23 ± 4.4	APB≥1 min⁻¹: Hal, 10% Iso, 4% VPB ≥ 1 min⁻¹: Hal, 16% Iso, 4%	Crossover study, highest incidence when halothane given on first operated side

APB, VPB, atrial and ventricular premature beats; AVB, atrioventricular block; SV, V arrhythmias, supraventricular, ventricular arrhythmias; LV, left ventricle; VT, ventricular tachycardia; Hal, halothane; Enf, enflurane; Iso, isoflurane

ELECTROPHYSIOLOGIC EFFECTS OF GENERAL ANESTHETICS

Despite waning clinical popularity due to problems of hepatotoxicity[12] and cardiac arrhythmias,[13,14] halothane remains the prototype for in vitro studies of the electrophysiologic effects of anesthetics. Fortunately, the effects of enflurane, isoflurane, and desflurane, the other clinically used inhaled anesthetics, and even model anesthetic alcohols, are similar enough to allow generalizations.

The most prominent membrane effects of halothane are marked alterations of myocardial calcium fluxes. Halothane abolishes Ca^{2+}-dependent action potentials[15] and decreases intracellular Ca^{2+} transients (Fig. 33-1).[16] Halothane and enflurane, but not isoflurane, inhibit release of Ca^{2+} from sarcoplasmic reticulum.[17-20] Halothane, isoflurane, enflurane, and heptanol reversibly reduce the amplitude of i_{si}, the slow inward calcium current,[2, 21-26] and the fast Na^+ current.[27] Both L- and T-type calcium currents are depressed to a similar extent by halothane, isoflurane, and enflurane.[28] The effects of anesthetics on potassium currents are somewhat controversial. Niggli and associates found that n-alkanols and halothane reduced both inward and outward rectifying K^+ currents.[2] In contrast, Hirota and colleagues found that halothane had no effect on the inward rectifier (i_{K1}).[29]

The effects of the intravenous anesthetics ketamine, methohexital, and propofol on the delayed rectifier (i_K) and inward rectifier (i_{K1}) have recently been reported.[30] Ketamine depressed i_{K1} but had no effect on i_K. Propofol, in contrast, depressed i_K but not i_{K1}. Methohexital had no effects on either current.

In microelectrode recordings of Purkinje fiber action potentials, halothane shortens the plateau phase and decreases action potential duration at 50% repolarization (APD_{50}).[31, 34-36] Although this may relate to the effects on plateau phase currents described above, inactivation of the persistent "window" sodium current by halothane and isoflurane may contribute.[37] Reductions in APD_{90} have been noted as well,[31,35] but not consistently.[34,36] The effective refractory period is reduced,[31,35] but an increase in functional refractoriness has been noted.[31] Halothane has little effect on resting membrane potential, action potential amplitude, or $\dot{V}_{max}$ in canine Purkinje fibers (Fig. 33-2).[31,34,36] Anesthetics slow conduction,[31,36] especially at the Purkinje fiber–ventricular muscle junction,[38] presumably by increasing intracellular or gap junction resistance.[39]

Halothane, isoflurane, and enflurane, the three currently used inhalational anesthetics, slow the rate of sinoatrial pacemaker discharge by both direct and indirect effects on sinoatrial node function (Fig. 33-3).[24, 40] In man, all three anesthetics have been variously reported to increase, decrease, or not change heart rate.[41] Isoflurane, however, most consistently produces an increase in heart rate.[41-43] Nitrous oxide, commonly used as an adjuvant during general anesthesia, usually produces no change or

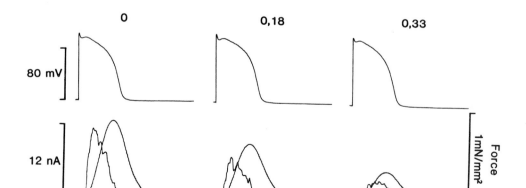

Figure 33-1. Effects of halothane on intracellular calcium transients in cat papillary muscle. Action potentials (upper trace), Ca^{2+} transients, represented by the calcium-sensitive aequorin dye signal expressed as photomultiplier current (lower trace, left), and developed tension (lower trace, right) are shown in the presence of increasing halothane dose. A marked reduction in aequorin signal, reflecting reductions in intracellular Ca^{2+} transients, and equivalent reduction in developed tension are noted. Action potential duration to 50% repolarization (APD_{50}) was shortened by halothane. (Bosnjak ZJ, Kampine JP: Effects of halothane on transmembrane potentials, Ca^{2+} transients, and papillary muscle tension in the cat. Am J Physiol 1986;251:H374.)

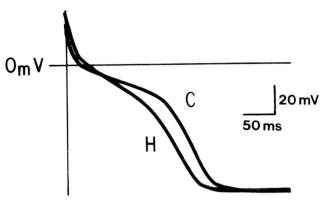

Figure 33-2. Effects of halothane on canine Purkinje fiber action potentials. Action potentials from Purkinje fibers before and after halothane 1% are superimposed. Halothane clearly shortens the plateau phase. The zero mV level, time, and amplitude calibrations are shown. Paced rate was 2 Hz. (Gallagher JD, unpublished data.)

a decrease in heart rate, but tachycardia has been seen in healthy volunteers.[44]

In the intact animal, halothane, enflurane, and isoflurane all slow conduction through the atrioventricular (AV) node, His bundle, and ventricle through a combination of direct actions and, more important, depression of sympathetic outflow during anesthesia (Fig. 33-4).[45] Isoflurane appears to be the least depressant.[45, 46] The atrial functional refractory period (FRP) is prolonged by halothane, enflurane, and isoflurane,[47–50] whereas the atrial effective refractory period (ERP) is consistently prolonged only by enflurane and isoflurane.[48–50] AV node FRP appears to be prolonged by all three agents,[48] but recent data suggest that in animals with intact autonomic nervous systems, halothane has minimal effects on AV node FRP.[50] In man, noninvasive His bundle recording during halothane anesthesia has shown a small but significant decrease in atrial–His (A–H) interval and no change in His-ventricular (H-V) interval.[51] It is unlikely that any clinically used anesthetic will produce high-grade heart block in the absence of intrinsic disease of the conduction system.

Halothane, enflurane, and isoflurane increase ventricular ERP,[52–54] but FRP may be shortened by halothane.[55] Although effects on conduction are common in in vitro preparations,[31] in vivo effects have been minimal,[52, 53] except for a report that halothane slowed ventricular activation time (His bundle-onset of epicardial electrogram).[55]

Table 33-2 summarizes the effects of various induction agents on heart rate.[56, 57] The chronotropic effects of commonly used narcotics are usually minimal, but bradycardia due to stimulation of vagal preganglionic neurons in the medulla oblongata, or direct depression of the sinus node, has been produced by morphine and fentanyl.[58] Meperidine, a weak anticholinergic, produces tachycardia at higher doses.[59]

Indirect Electrophysiologic Effects of Anesthetics

In addition to direct effects, anesthetics impair homeostatic regulatory mechanisms of the cardiovascular system by depression of baseline cardiovascular function and by alteration of reflex control of the cardiovascular system.

Halothane, enflurane, and isoflurane produce dose-dependent decreases in the myocardial inotropic state that correlate with decreases in transmembrane calcium transients.[16] Cardiac output decreases with the former two, but isoflurane spares cardiac output because of a marked reduction in peripheral resistance and afterload, coupled with a reflex increase in heart rate.[41]

Reflex regulation of the cardiovascular system, typified by the baroreceptor reflex, is also depressed by anesthetics. Halothane, enflurane, and isoflurane attenuate both pressor and depressor limbs of the baroreceptor reflex in man, with both halothane and enflurane more depressant than isoflurane.[60–63] This depression occurs at

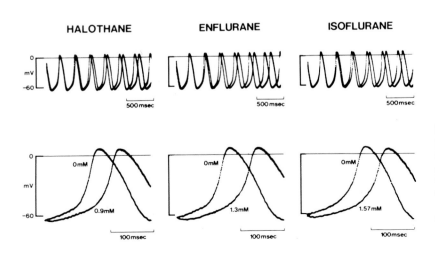

Figure 33-3. Effects of anesthetics on the guinea pig sinus node. Action potential tracings of spontaneously active cells in the guinea pig sinus node region are shown before and after 5-minute exposures to anesthetics at two different speeds and magnifications. Note the slowing caused by each anesthetic. (Bosnjak Z, Kampine J: Effects of halothane, enflurane and isoflurane on the SA node. Anesthesiology 1983;58:314.)

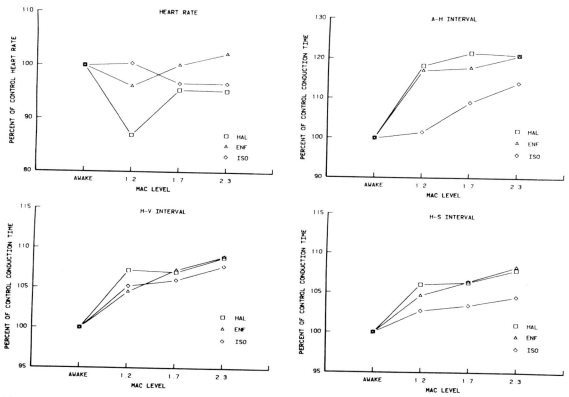

Figure 33-4. Effects of anesthetics on heart rate, atrioventricular node, and ventricular conduction. Note dose-dependent increases in A–H, H–V, and H–S intervals in autonomically intact, chronically instrumented dogs. MAC, the minimum alveolar concentration required to prevent movement, is an index of anesthetic potency. (Atlee JL, Brownlee SW, Burstrom RE: Conscious-state comparisons of the effects of inhalation anesthetics on specialized atrioventricular conduction times in dogs. Anesthesiology 1986;64:703.)

both peripheral and central sites. Seagard and colleagues studied carotid sinus afferent nerve activity and found that halothane sensitized the baroreceptor, a calcium-dependent peripheral effect due to both a change in sinus wall tension and a direct effect on the baroreceptor.[64] Involvement of central nervous system sites is suggested by de-

TABLE 33-2. Effects of Induction Agents on Heart Rate[56,57]

Anesthetic	Heart Rate Change
Thiopental	0–+36
Methohexital	+40–+50
Diazepam	−9–+13
Midazolam	−14–+21
Etomidate	0–+22
Ketamine	0–+59
Althesin	+11–+50
Propanidid	+40–+100
Propofol	0–+15

pression of baseline and reflex changes in preganglionic sympathetic nerve activity (Fig. 33-5).[65,66] Additional anesthetic actions appear to be ganglionic blockade by halothane and isoflurane,[65–67] and a blunting of the cardiac response to direct stimulation of cardiac sympathetic or parasympathetic nerves (Fig. 33-6).[65,66]

Halothane and isoflurane also depress vagal efferent activity.[42,68] Relatively greater suppression of parasympathetic versus sympathetic activity by isoflurane could explain the tachycardia often produced by the drug.[42]

The effects of several other anesthetic agents on baroreceptor control of heart rate have also been reported. Ebert studied the effect of nitrous oxide on baroreceptor-mediated changes in heart rate and vascular muscle efferent sympathetic nerve activity.[69] Nitrous oxide produced a 59% increase in baseline sympathetic nerve activity, yet a 39% decrease in the slope of the baroreceptor response was noted. Thus, nitrous oxide activates vascular sympathetic nerves while decreasing baroreflex-mediated changes in heart rate.

Priano and coworkers studied the effects of anesthetic induction agents on cardiovascular neuroregulation in

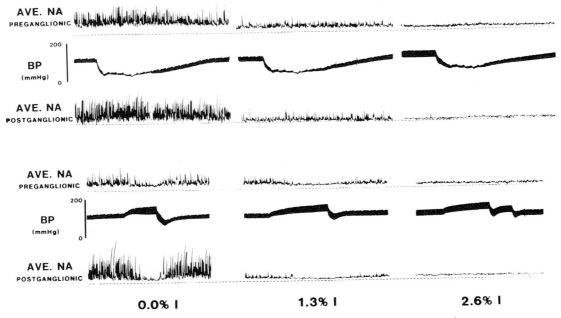

Figure 33-5. Effects of increasing isoflurane concentrations in response of preganglionic and post-ganglionic sympathetic nerve activities (*AVE. NA*) to changes in blood pressure. Note depression of both baseline activity and reflex response, especially to hypertension in the lower panels. The greater depression of postganglionic activity compared with preganglionic activity provides evidence for ganglionic blockade by isoflurane. (Seagard JL, Elegbe EO, Hopp FA, et al: Effects of isoflurane on the baroreceptor reflex. Anesthesiology 1983;59:511.)

dogs.[70] Occluders around the aorta and vena cava were used to produce hypotension or hypertension, and changes in R-R interval were recorded. Thiopental (20 mg/kg) and ketamine (5 mg/kg) reduced the slope of the R-R interval to systolic blood pressure relationship by 70% for a 10-minute period after injection. Diazepam (2 mg/kg) blunted the slope only at 3 minutes after administration, whereas etomidate had no effect on these reflexes.

The baroreflex control of heart rate by morphine, diazepam, and nitrous oxide anesthesia was studied by Kotrly and associates.[71] The pressor, depressor, and neck suction baroreflex slopes declined significantly, similar to the depression seen with potent inhaled agents.

Etomidate, known for its ability to induce anesthesia while minimally altering hemodynamics, maintained baseline sympathetic outflow and altered neither baro-

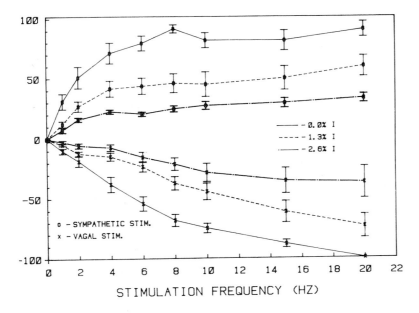

Figure 33-6. Effects of isoflurane on chronotropic response to vagal and sympathetic efferent stimulation. Dose-dependent attenuation of chronotropic response to nerve stimulation shows a depression of end-organ (i.e., cardiac) responsiveness. (Seagard JL, Elegbe EO, Hopp FA, et al: Effects of isoflurane on the baroreceptor reflex. Anesthesiology 1983;59:511.)

reflex regulation of cardiac rate nor sympathetic outflow.[72]

Propofol, in contrast, reduced basal sympathetic outflow by 76% and impaired baroreflex responses, especially the response to hypotension. Hypotension commonly occurred in propofol-treated patients.[72]

Regional Anesthesia and Local Anesthetics

Epidural anesthesia reduces postoperative complications in patients undergoing high-risk surgery[73] but may have serious electrophysiologic consequences, both from the direct effects of local anesthetics and from alterations in autonomic tone.[74] In dogs, thoracic epidural anesthesia slows heart rate, prolongs AV nodal conduction time and refractoriness, and prolongs ventricular refractoriness and action potential duration,[75] and in rats it reduces the incidence of ventricular arrhythmias during coronary artery ligation.[76]

The direct effects of local anesthetics are those of type 1B antiarrhythmics, although particular concern with the agents bupivacaine and etidocaine was raised when cases of sudden and prolonged cardiovascular collapse occurred after inadvertent intravenous injection, especially in parturients.[77] Morishima and colleagues found that the dose of bupivacaine required to produce cardiovascular collapse in sheep was half that of lidocaine, and that pregnant sheep were more susceptible than nonpregnant ewes.[78] In cats, de Jong and associates showed that bupivacaine, in contrast to lidocaine, produced ventricular arrhythmias at subconvulsant doses.[79] Clarkson and Hondeghem demonstrated more rapid, avid binding of bupivacaine, compared with lidocaine, to inactivated Na^+ channels.[80] Slow dissociation from the receptor by bupivacaine resulted in progressive block.[80] In isolated rabbit heart, bupivacaine blocked conduction at the Purkinje fiber–ventricular muscle junction in 100% of preparations, whereas lidocaine produced such block in only one of 10 experiments.[81]

Bupivacaine-induced K^+ channel blockade and the resultant prolongation of action potential duration increases the number of inactivated Na^+ channels and further contributes to toxicity. In isolated guinea pig hearts, ATP-sensitive K^+ channel agonists attenuate bupivacaine-induced atrioventricular block.[82]

An alternative hypothesis suggests that central nervous system effects are responsible for bupivacaine cardiotoxicity. Injection of bupivacaine into the cerebral ventricles in cats (but not intravenously) caused ventricular arrhythmias.[83] In rats, injection of bupivacaine, but not lidocaine, at the nucleus tractus solitarius produced lethal ventricular arrhythmias in 25% of animals.[84]

Controversy concerning the treatment of bupivacaine cardiotoxicity has been reviewed.[24] Prolonged resuscitation attempts should be anticipated, with administration of bretylium for ventricular tachycardia and epinephrine and atropine for electromechanical dissociation.[85, 86]

Neuromuscular Blocking Drugs

In guinea pig papillary muscle, pancuronium prolongs action potential duration, hyperpolarizes resting potential, augments action potential amplitude and $\dot{V}_{max}$ of phase 0, and enhances automaticity.[87] In halothane-anesthetized dogs, pancuronium shortened the A-H interval.[88] Clinically, pancuronium increases heart rate by 20% to 50%[89] through a vagolytic effect on cardiac muscarinic receptors[90] and stimulation of cardiac sympathetic ganglia.[91, 92]

The depolarizing neuromuscular blocker succinylcholine is useful because of the rapid onset and short duration of profound muscle relaxation it provides. Succinylcholine has, however, produced severe cardiac arrhythmias, most notably hyperkalemic cardiac arrest in patients with burns, trauma, or neuromuscular disease.[93] Succinylcholine most commonly causes pronounced bradycardia in children, but also in adults, especially after a second dose.[93] Whether this relates to stimulation of afferent vagal receptors, a central vagal effect, or sensitization by the choline metabolite of succinylcholine to further doses of succinylcholine has not been determined.[94] Succinylcholine may, in addition, produce sympathetic stimulation,[95, 96] accounting for the prevalence of ventricular ectopy. Yasuda and colleagues concluded that succinylcholine is a positive chronotrope, causing catecholamine release from canine cardiac adrenergic terminals, whereas the metabolite succinylmonocholine produces bradycardia through excitation of cholinergic receptors in the sinus node.[94]

Succinylcholine-induced atrial arrhythmias may be attenuated by prior administration of thiopental, atropine, ganglionic blocking drugs, or small doses of nondepolarizing relaxants.[93]

The more recently introduced neuromuscular blockers vecuronium and atracurium have few cardiovascular effects.[93]

DRUG INTERACTIONS

Aminophylline

Halothane is often chosen for asthmatic patients because of its bronchodilating properties.[97] Concurrent administration of aminophylline, however, may result in severe ventricular arrhythmias.[98] Stirt and Sullivan have summarized data suggesting that aminophylline has cardiac effects due to either phosphodiesterase inhibition, catecholamine release, or release of calcium from sarcoplasmic reticulum.[99] As halothane or theophylline concentrations increase, the likelihood of tachycardia and ventricular arrhythmias analogous to those produced by epinephrine increases. Isoflurane, in contrast, appears to be safe when administered with aminophylline.[100]

Tricyclic Antidepressants

Tricyclic antidepressants initially increase, but ultimately decrease, noradrenergic synaptic transmission.[101] Edwards and coworkers administered pancuronium and halothane or enflurane to dogs acutely or chronically treated with imipramine. Acute administration produced sinus tachycardia. After chronic administration (15 days), pancuronium produced ventricular ectopy, in halothane-anesthetized dogs but not enflurane-anesthetized dogs, that progressed to fibrillation in several dogs. Each dog that fibrillated had elevated serum norepinephrine concentrations, consistent with imipramine-induced blockade of catecholamine reuptake.[102] Spiss and associates presented somewhat contradictory evidence that 6 weeks of imipramine administration did not change adrenergic responsiveness or the arrhythmic dose of epinephrine in halothane-anesthetized dogs.[103] The authors suggested that chronic compensatory mechanisms reverted the hyperresponsive state to normal.[103] Caution is indicated when patients taking imipramine are anesthetized.

Amiodarone

Since the 1981 report of perioperative atropine- and isoproterenol-resistant bradycardia, low peripheral resistance, heart block, and depressed myocardial contractility in a patient treated with amiodarone,[104] several reports of perianesthetic problems in patients treated with amiodarone have appeared. A greater incidence of intraoperative cardiac rhythm disturbances (including atropine-resistant bradycardia, slow nodal rhythm, complete heart block, and pacemaker dependency) and increased requirements for perioperative circulatory and respiratory support have been documented in patients receiving amiodarone.[105, 106]

SPECIAL CONSIDERATIONS

Wolff-Parkinson-White and Preexcitation Syndromes

Given the recent trend toward elimination of "routine" preoperative testing, and an incidence of up to three per 1000 persons,[107] the initial presentation of Wolff-Parkin-

son-White syndrome may be intraoperative tachyarrhythmias.[108, 109] During anesthesia, with cardiovascular depression and a diminution of homeostatic reflexes, heart rates that may have been tolerated when awake can cause severe hypotension and require urgent cardioversion.

Although several investigators have reported the successful management of patients with Wolff-Parkinson-White syndrome,[108, 110, 111] few have investigated the properties of the accessory pathway during anesthesia. Gomez-Arnau and colleagues studied various anesthetic drugs in 18 patients scheduled for operative section of accessory pathways.[112] Fentanyl, in doses up to 50 μg/kg, and diazepam, 250 μg/kg, produced no change in the antegrade refractory period of the accessory pathway, whereas droperidol, in doses from 200 to 600 μg/kg, markedly prolonged the antegrade effective refractory period. Retrograde refractory period of the accessory pathway also increased significantly after droperidol (Fig. 33-7). Patients anesthetized with halothane and fentanyl demonstrated no important variations in either antegrade or retrograde refractoriness of the accessory pathway.[112] Sufentanil–lorazepam anesthesia mildly prolonged the effective refractory period of the accessory pathway in 21 patients undergoing surgical ablation.[113] These effects were clinically insignificant.[113] The inhaled agents, enflurane most, isoflurane next, and halothane least, increased refractoriness within the accessory pathway.[113]

Principles for the management of patients with Wolff-Parkinson-White syndrome have changed little since outlined by Sadowski and Moyers.[110] Whether the technique chosen is nitrous oxide–narcotic based,[110] high-dose nar-

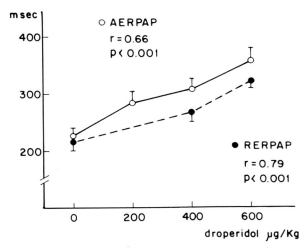

Figure 33-7. Effects of droperidol on antegrade and retrograde effective refractory period of accessory pathways in patients with Wolff-Parkinson-White syndrome. Increases in refractoriness after successive doses of droperidol are clearly seen. (Gomez-Arnau J, Marquez-Montes J, Avello F: Fentanyl and droperidol effects on the refractoriness of the accessory pathway in the Wolff-Parkinson-White syndrome. Anesthesiology 1983;58:307.)

cotic,[112] neuroleptanalgesia,[108] or deep inhalational anesthesia,[114] hemodynamic stability with prevention of sympathetic stimulation is essential. Anticholinergic block with atropine, and the use of tachycardia-inducing agents such as pancuronium, though discouraged by some,[108,110] have been used routinely by others with success.[110,112] Administration of volatile anesthetics during ablative surgery may confound interpretation of postablative studies.[113] In patients with preexcitation syndromes requiring anesthesia for nonablative surgery, volatile agents, especially enflurane, may reduce the risk of tachyarrhythmias through their effects on accessory pathway refractoriness.[113] Successful management of the patient with Wolff-Parkinson-White syndrome or one of its variants requires an understanding of the electrophysiologic manifestations of the syndrome, careful anesthetic management, and prompt therapy of life-threatening arrhythmias that may develop.

Pacemakers and the Implanted Cardioverter/Defibrillator

The ever-increasing sophistication of modern pacemakers has created a situation in which the perioperative management of patients with implanted pacemakers is increasingly marked more by ignorance and luck than by knowledgeable preparation. Domino underscored the need for such preparation when she described a patient with an implanted Medtronic Xyrel generator upon which a magnet was placed to convert the unit to a ventricular asynchronous pacing (VOO) mode during surgery.[115] Fortunately, Domino recognized that during electrocautery, the pacer was being randomly reprogrammed, and the magnet had opened the programming channel.[115] Extensive lists of available pacers, including magnet reversion rate, expected response to electrocautery (interference mode), and risk of random reprogramming, are available to hopefully prevent such a problem.[116] However, intro-

duction of newer models will quickly outdate these sources.

Because the simplistic approach of magnet conversion is untenable, thorough preparation is needed. The type of pacer, indications for pacing, programmed parameters, and current pacer function need to be assessed. An electrocardiogram and evaluation of the patient's underlying rhythm are helpful.

If electrocautery will be used intraoperatively, concerns about inhibition of the pacer (in sensing modes), reprogramming,[115] or interference-induced reversion to a VOO mode at a preprogrammed or factory-set rate must be considered, even if the recommendations of Simon are followed.[118] These include the use of short bursts of electrocautery, remote placement of the electrosurgery unit's ground plate, and use of as low a current as practical.[118]

Patients with cardiomyopathy may do poorly without dual chamber (DDD) pacing, and "interference mode" VOO rates after electrocautery or magnet reversion may generate inadequate cardiac output in certain patients. In contrast, generators with magnet reversion rates approaching 100 beats/minute, such as the Siemens-Elema 668, exist.[116] This degree of tachycardia could induce ischemia in certain patients. Finally, induction of ventricular tachycardia by VOO pacing has been demonstrated (Fig. 33-8).[119]

The potential for interactions between new technologies introduced into the operating room and pacemakers must always be considered. A situation of particular interest is extracorporeal shock wave lithotripsy. Although synchronous ventricular (VVI) pacers are generally safe, dual-chamber pacers may be doubled-counted by the lithotriptor, and activity-sensing, rate-responsive pacers may be damaged or accelerated.[120] Cooper and colleagues recommend converting to the VVI mode and avoiding lithotripsy in patients with abdominally implanted generators containing piezoelectric elements.[120]

In a patient with a DDD pacer undergoing stabilization of fractured cervical vertebrae, somatosensory

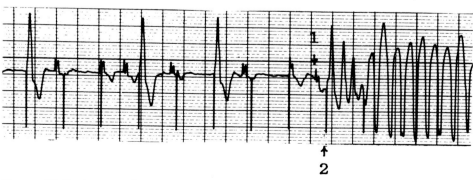

2

Figure 33-8. Initiation of ventricular tachycardia during VOO pacing. Arrow 1 is an intrinsic QRS complex and arrow 2 is a pacing impulse occurring on a T wave. (Zaidan JR: Pacemakers. Anesthesiology 1984;60:319.)

evoked potential (SEP) monitoring of the median nerve was performed to evaluate spinal cord function.[121] The SEP procedure consisted of repetitive transcutaneous electrical stimulation at intervals of 300 msec with recording of cortical responses.[121] When SEP testing was initiated, the pacemaker mistakenly interpreted the SEP stimulus as an atrial event.[121] The result was a pacemaker-mediated ventricular tachycardia that produced hypotension until the cessation of SEP current delivery.[121]

Samain and coworkers described pacemaker-mediated tachycardia in a patient anesthetized with isoflurane and fentanyl. Alterations in the electrophysiologic milieu, coupled with the appearance of premature atrial contractions, allowed ventriculoatrial conduction with a 330-msec interval, greater than the programmed 280-msec postventricular atrial refractory period. The resulting pacemaker-induced ventricular tachycardia at a rate of 117 beats/minute produced serious hypotension in the 71-year-old patient.[122]

Adequate understanding of modern pacemaker function can provide imaginative solutions to unexpected problems. During anesthesia, as sinus rate slows, a demand ventricular pacemaker may initiate ventricular pacing and, by abolishing atrial augmentation of stroke volume, produce hypotension. Reprogramming of hysteresis parameters is appropriate, but the VVI pacemaker may be suppressed by a peripheral nerve stimulator set to a 2-Hz frequency[123] or a transcutaneous pacing device set to a rate greater than the VVI pacemaker's inhibition rate and a current amplitude insufficient to capture the ventricle.[124] This allows emergence of underlying sinus bradycardia and restoration of blood pressure, albeit at heart rates less than the normal VVI rate. Caution is essential, however, because a patient reported by Kemnitz and Peters became asystolic with underlying 3° atrioventricular block when similar suppression was attempted.[124]

Rate-responsive pacing[125] creates new potential for perioperative misadventure. Myopotentials generated by electrocautery in the absence of neuromuscular blockade may result in inhibition or reversion to an interference mode, as documented in awake patients.[126] Pacemaker-induced tachycardia due to an inappropriate response of a respiratory-driven, rate-responsive pacer to controlled ventilation during general anesthesia has already been reported.[127] Sensed parameters such as QT interval,[128] pre-ejection period,[129] and depolarization gradient[130] may be affected by anesthetics.[131] Inadvertent hypothermia, perioperative stress, and uncoupling of oxygen consumption from the variables proposed for use as biosensors,[132] due to peripheral and pulmonary shunting under anesthesia, can all potentially affect algorithms used in rate-responsive pacing.

Only through consideration of the patient and his or her medical condition, the pulse generator, and the pulse generator's programmed parameters and response to predictable perioperative events can a rational approach to the management of the surgical patient with a pacemaker be undertaken. Choice of anesthetic agents does not appear to affect the pacing stimulation threshold in man.[133] Whether the pacer should be left to revert to an interference mode during electrocautery, whether it should be converted to a VOO mode by a magnet, or whether it should be reprogrammed (VOO, DOO, rate-responsiveness, and antitachycardia features eliminated, and so forth) is determined on an individual basis. All those caring for the patient must be involved in this decision.

Once a management scheme is chosen, continuous monitoring must include modalities not affected by electrocautery. In the case reported by Domino, use of a stethoscope and pulse palpation were essential for the diagnosis of random reprogramming during a time when the electrocardiogram was obscured in electromagnetic interference.[115] Direct arterial pressure monitoring and transesophageal echocardiography offer two alternative monitoring modalities of particular use when major surgery is undertaken, because each allows evaluation of the effects of atrioventricular synchrony, and each is minimally affected by electrocautery.

The automatic implantable cardioverter/defibrillator has proved to be of remarkable utility in preventing sudden death.[134-136] Although advances may ultimately eliminate the need for application of epicardial patches and electrodes,[137,138] a median sternotomy, or a lateral or subxiphoid thoracotomy, may be required for insertion. Although implantation during thoracic epidural anesthesia has been described,[139] general anesthesia is most commonly provided. The need for a general anesthetic and the occurrence of periods of circulatory arrest during intraoperative testing suggest a need for invasive monitoring in the majority of these patients, who may have abysmal underlying ventricular performance,[135] often compounded by antiarrhythmics that can be potent myocardial depressants.[104,140] Procaine can be substituted for lidocaine to provide anesthesia during placement of invasive monitors (if lidocaine is suspected to interfere with arrhythmia induction in certain patients), and isoproterenol may be required to facilitate arrhythmia induction.[141]

Patients with implanted defibrillators may present for emergent noncardiac surgery. Because electrocautery could initiate a spurious discharge from the unit, the automatic defibrillator should be inactivated during surgery. Deactivation of the Ventak unit (Cardiac Pacemakers, Inc.), for example, is accomplished by moving a specific magnet perpendicular to the device until it rests on the upper right corner of the generator. For 30 seconds, R-wave synchronous tones will be heard, indicating that the unit is activated. When the pulsed tones cease, a continuous tone is heard, indicating deactivation. The magnet is slowly removed, perpendicular to the unit. Premature magnet removal invokes a test discharge into the unit, wasting a potentially lifesaving discharge. Reactivation after surgery is accomplished by placing the magnet over the upper right corner until R-wave synchronous tones are again heard (approximately 30 seconds). The magnet is removed in a perpendicular direction and stored away from the patient. Gaba and associates caution that this is not always effective, and they describe an obese patient in whom a magnet would not deactivate the unit.[141] Electrocautery initiated a discharge in this patient. In addition to the risk of a spurious discharge inducing ventricular tachyarrhythmias in the patient, personnel in contact with the patient may receive a shock.[141, 142]

Because a lithotriptor may trigger discharge, implanted defibrillators should be deactivated before starting the procedure.[143] More important, shock waves may damage piezoelectric crystals in the generator.[143] Long and Venditti reported that taping Styrofoam board over the device while ensuring that the device was not in the direct path of the shock wave prevented damage.[143] Clearly, a physician familiar with the device and the management of patients receiving less common antiarrhythmics should be consulted immediately, but this cannot be allowed to delay urgent surgery.

ANESTHESIA AND ARRHYTHMIAS

Oculocardiac Reflex

Manipulation of the globe or extraocular muscles, especially the medial and lateral recti, may produce vagal affects on the heart via a trigeminal–vagal nerve reflex arc.[144] Most commonly, sinus bradycardia or arrest is noted, but a variety of arrhythmias, including rapid multifocal ventricular tachycardia, have been observed.[145] Children undergoing strabismus correction, due to heightened vagal tone, are particularly vulnerable, and up to 90% may exhibit the oculocardiac reflex.[144, 145] Fatigue of the reflex with repeated stimulation has been noted,[146] but prevention or attenuation with retrobulbar block or atropine (intravenous, intramuscular, or oral) appears effective.[144, 145] However, Katz cautions that although the incidence of the reflex was decreased from 72% to 30% with atropine pretreatment, arrhythmias that did occur were more prolonged and severe.[144] Thus, many choose observation with elimination of traction at the earliest sign of arrhythmia.[144, 145] Treatment with atropine or lidocaine, as appropriate, is proper for severe arrhythmias and those that do not fatigue.[146]

Sensitization to Catecholamines by Inhaled Anesthetics

Sensitization of the heart by halogenated hydrocarbon general anesthetics to the arrhythmogenic actions of catecholamines is a well-known but poorly understood phenomenon.[13] Johnston and coworkers determined the arrhythmia-producing dose of epinephrine in anesthetized adults undergoing transsphenoidal hypophysectomy including submucosal injection of epinephrine.[147] The ED_{50} was 2.1 µg/kg of epinephrine for halothane, 10.9 µg/kg for enflurane, and 6.7 µg/kg for isoflurane (Fig. 33-9). The dose–response curve for enflurane was less steep and the standard deviation larger, implying unpredictability when epinephrine is injected during an enflurane anesthetic.[147] Arrhythmogenic doses of epinephrine are similar during desflurane and isoflurane anesthesia.[149] Children appear to be less susceptible to epinephrine than adults.[148] When ventilation was carefully controlled to avoid hypercarbia, epinephrine doses of up to 15.7 µg/kg could be administered during halothane anesthesia without inducing ventricular arrhythmias.[148]

Thiopental,[150] nitrous oxide,[151] propofol,[152] and ketamine[153] potentiate halothane–epinephrine-induced ventricular arrhythmias. Neither pancuronium nor curare affects the arrhythmogenic dose of epinephrine,[154] but succinylcholine potentiates epinephrine effects.[155] The addition of 0.5% lidocaine,[147] or other amide local anes-

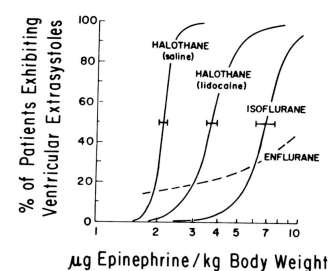

Figure 33-9. Comparative sensitizing activity of inhaled anesthetics. Abscissa shows amount of epinephrine required to evoke three or more premature ventricular contractions. Ordinate displays percentage of patients exhibiting the arrhythmia. (Johnston RR, Eger EI, Wilson C: A comparative interaction of epinephrine with enflurane, isoflurane and halothane in man. Anesth Analg 1976; 55:709.)

thetics,[156] to the epinephrine solution significantly increased the ED_{50}.

Availability of selective adrenergic receptor blockers has allowed the determination that both α_1-adrenergic and, to a lesser extent, β_1-adrenergic receptor stimulation by catecholamines are responsible.[157,158]

Despite decades of study, the electrophysiologic mechanism for sensitization has not been determined with certainty.[13] Using cultured heart cells, Miletich and colleagues showed that halothane and epinephrine induced arrhythmias that could be abolished by quinidine but not verapamil.[159] In contrast, Zuckerman and Wheeler produced three types of sympathomimetic-induced arrhythmogenic activity in single ventricular cells from rats.[160] Halothane inhibited both early and late aftercontractions and nonstimulated extrasystoles. Others suggest that arrhythmias result from a complex interplay of effects on supraventricular pacemakers, intraventricular conduction, and refractoriness, and elevation of left ventricular systolic pressure.[13,14]

In intact animals or isolated hearts, epinephrine produces sinus tachycardia, but when halothane is added, an atrioventricular junctional rhythm develops.[161,162] Presumably, this initial step in the sensitizing process reflects a greater susceptibility of the sinoatrial node to the depressant effects of halothane.[162] If left ventricular pressure is subsequently elevated, ventricular arrhythmias appear.[161] The elevated pressure and stretch may enhance automaticity of latent pacemakers, induce triggered activity, or slow conduction, facilitating reentry.[163] The origin site of bigeminal rhythms produced under these conditions appears to be the interventricular septum.[164]

Therapy with lidocaine, α_1-adrenergic blockers, or β-adrenergic antagonists, especially β_1 antagonists,[165] should be effective.[116] Dexmedetomidine, acting as an agonist at central α_2-adrenoceptors, tripled the arrhythmogenic dose for epinephrine in halothane-anesthetized dogs.[117] Kapur and Flacke found that verapamil raised the dose of epinephrine required to elicit ventricular arrhythmias during halothane anesthesia, but produced vasodilation and myocardial depression and slowed atrioventricular conduction.[166] Atlee and colleagues described hypotension, Wenckebach-type AV block, and sinus arrest when verapamil and any anesthetic agent, but especially enflurane, were given to dogs.[167] Diltiazem was less problematic.[167] The particularly profound interaction between verapamil and enflurane has been noted by others.[174] Administration of calcium chloride before verapamil has prevented hypotension without compromising antiarrhythmic efficacy in patients with supraventricular tachycardia,[175] but the effectiveness of this combination has not been verified in anesthetized patients.

A recent study compared the efficacy of lidocaine, verapamil, flecainide, E-4031 (K^+ channel blocker), and amiodarone on the duration of epinephrine-induced arrhythmias in halothane-anesthetized rats.[176] The authors emphasized the importance of K^+ channel blockade in addition to Ca^{2+} channel blockade in reducing arrhythmia duration. The effectiveness of drugs studied was amiodarone > verapamil > E-4031 = flecainide > lidocaine = saline.

Effects of Anesthetics on Arrhythmia Mechanisms

Despite the widespread view of halothane as an agent likely to cause arrhythmias,[147,177] recent data suggest that halothane and other volatile anesthetics may have antiarrhythmic actions.

Inhaled anesthetics increase atrial and atrioventricular nodal refractoriness, conditions that should not be conducive to supraventricular tachycardia caused by atrial or atrioventricular nodal reentry.[50] Invariably, inhaled anesthetics abolish sinus node reentry during programmed stimulation in dogs.[50,167]

Supraventricular arrhythmias occur commonly during anesthesia and may cause significant hemodynamic compromise. Yet only recently has a series of publications detailed the effects of anesthetics on the mechanisms of atrial arrhythmogenesis, and on the automaticity of dominant and subsidiary pacemakers in the atrium and Purkinje fibers.

In excised Purkinje fibers made to fire automatically by superfusion with epinephrine, the volatile anesthetics halothane, enflurane, and isoflurane increased spontaneous rate by accelerating phase 4 depolarization. Recovery from overdrive suppression was enhanced by enflurane but not affected by the other agents.[168]

Halothane alone or with epinephrine did not shift the site of earliest activation from the sinoatrial node in isolated canine atrium, whereas epinephrine produced shifts to subsidiary atrial pacemaker sites.[169] Interestingly, neither ouabain nor halothane tended to move the site of earliest atrial activation from the sinoatrial node region to subsidiary atrial sites. The combination of the two, however, caused a significant shift to subsidiary sites and, in several preparations, caused total atrial arrest.[170] Dissimilar to halothane, isoflurane, though not shifting the site of earliest activation itself, enhanced subsidiary pacemakers when combined with epinephrine. Thus, isoflurane, but not halothane, acted synergistically with epinephrine to increase arrhythmogenic potential in atrial tissue.[171]

In intact chronically instrumented dogs, Woehlck and colleagues detected pacemaker shifts from the sinus node to subsidiary atrial sites when halothane was administered with epinephrine.[172] However, parasympathetic blockade abolished these changes.[172] Both atropine and halothane facilitated His-bundle beats during exposure to epinephrine,[172] consistent with the results in isolated atrial tissue[169] and Purkinje fibers.[168] In a companion study, enflurane directly depressed sinoatrial node automaticity and increased automaticity of subsidiary atrial pacemakers. Enflurane sensitized the atrium to epinephrine-induced arrhythmias in the presence of muscarinic blockade. Isoflurane did not sensitize the atrium, and epinephrine-induced pacemaker shifts during isoflurane inhalation were caused by reflex-induced vagal suppression of the sinus node with escape of subsidiary pacemakers.[173]

The antiarrhythmic effects of anesthetics have been evaluated in a variety of models of ventricular tachycardia (VT) presumed to be caused by different electrophysiologic mechanisms.[178] Acute reperfusion arrhythmias that occur following coronary thrombolysis, emergent surgical revascularization, or balloon angioplasty depend on alterations of intracellular calcium handling.[179] Following acute coronary artery occlusion and reperfusion in dogs, halothane, enflurane, and isoflurane each reduced the incidence of reperfusion-induced ventricular fibrillation (VF).[179]

Twenty-four hours after two-stage ligation of the anterior descending coronary artery in dogs,[180] incessant ectopic ventricular activity is found.[181] This arrhythmia is generally thought to be caused by abnormal activity of partially depolarized, subendocardial Purkinje fibers that survived the infarct,[182] although triggered activity has also been observed.[182-184] Logic and associates in 1969 noted that halothane suppressed "idioventricular tachycardia" in each of nine dogs 24 to 72 hours after coronary artery ligation (Fig. 33-10).[185] Turner and colleagues, using an in vitro preparation 1 day after coronary artery ligation,

found that halothane slowed the rate of firing in those preparations in which abnormal automaticity was observed.[31]

One week after ligation of the anterior descending coronary artery in dogs, programmed stimulation induces reentrant VT within the surviving epicardial layer.[186, 187] In seven in vitro preparations, Turner and coworkers found that halothane prolonged functional refractoriness, but not absolute refractoriness (ERP), and slowed conduction of premature impulses.[31] The result in five of seven specimens was a widening of the zone of premature extrastimuli that induced reentrant responses. The authors suggested that this represented a proarrhythmic effect of halothane.[31]

Halothane, enflurane, and isoflurane increased the disparity between repolarization times of ischemic and nonischemic regions in this model, conditions that may facilitate reentry.[32, 33]

In dogs studied by programmed stimulation several days after infarction, halothane has been a predominantly antiarrhythmic drug. Induction of VT is prevented in association with an increase in ventricular ERP,[52-54, 131] without changing ventricular conduction[52, 53] or QRS duration.[53] Denniss and colleagues found that halothane 2% was antiarrhythmic in 47% of dogs with inducible VT.[53] A proarrhythmic effect of halothane, defined as the appearance of inducible VT or VF, was observed in 10% of the dogs with infarction but no inducible arrhythmias. Hunt and Ross noted that halothane 2% prevented induction of ventricular tachycardia in five of 10 dogs with previously inducible VT.[54] Deutsch and associates also found a 50% antiarrhythmic incidence when halothane was administered to dogs after occlusion–reperfusion infarction (Fig.

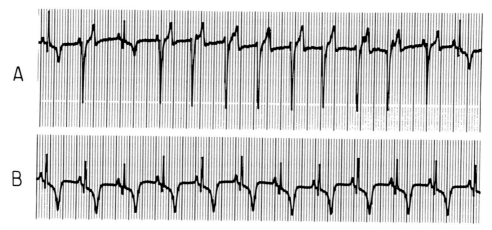

Figure 33-10. Effects of halothane on ventricular tachycardia in dogs 24 hours after myocardial infarction. (**A**) One day after ligation of the anterior descending coronary artery, a predominantly ventricular rhythm due to abnormal automaticity is seen. (**B**) After halothane 1%, sinus rhythm appears. Ventricular tachycardia reappeared after halothane was discontinued. (Gallagher JD, McClernan CA: The effects of halothane on ventricular tachycardia in intact dogs. Anesthesiology 1991;75:866.)

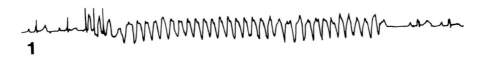

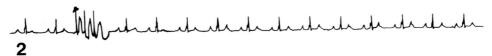

Figure 33-11. Effects of halothane on inducible reentrant ventricular tachycardia in dogs. One week after occlusion and reperfusion infarction of the anterior descending coronary artery, triple premature extrastimuli during sinus rhythm evoke sustained ventricular tachycardia (panel 1). After halothane, no arrhythmia can be induced (panel 2). (Courtesy of N. Deutsch, MD.)

33-11).[52] In three of 19 anesthetics administered to dogs without inducible VT, a proarrhythmic effect was observed. Proarrhythmic exacerbation of reentrant VT by antiarrhythmics is well known,[188] and the incidence reported for halothane is similar to that for other antiarrhythmics (Table 33-3).[189]

Delayed afterdepolarizations have been produced by toxic doses of cardiac glycosides, catecholamines or hypercalcemia, found in infarcted tissue, atrial tissue, canine coronary sinus, and simian mitral value tissue.[190] Halothane increases the dose of digitalis glycosides required to produce ventricular ectopy or sudden death in dogs,[191] and it abolishes tachyarrhythmias in ouabain-toxic Purkinje fibers.[34] The mechanism for the reduction of ouabain-induced triggered dysrhythmias appears to be a reduction in the amplitude of delayed afterdepolarizations.[192] In infarcted ventricles, examples of halothane abolishing delayed afterdepolarization-induced triggered activity have also been reported (Fig. 33-12).[31]

Prolongation of the QT interval is associated with the appearance of triggered automaticity due to early afterdepolarizations.[193] Although halothane may block ionic currents suggested to be responsible for early afterdepolarizations,[2,25,27,194,195] halothane, isoflurane, and enflurane prolong the QT interval.[131,196,197] Gallagher and colleagues evaluated the effects of halothane and quinidine in dogs.[199] QT interval prolongation was noted, and three of 20 dogs developed torsades de pointes.

The antiarrhythmic effects of halothane vary depending on the mechanisms responsible for VT. Those mechanisms dependent primarily on Ca^{2+} influx, abnormal automaticity[184,200] and delayed afterdepolarization-induced triggered activity,[190] are antagonized by halothane. In the models of reentrant ventricular tachycardia studied, in-

TABLE 33-3. Effects of General Anesthetics on Inducibility of Ventricular Arrhythmias

Investigator	Model	No. of Dogs	Inducibility	Proarrhythmia	Electrophysiologic Effects
Hunt[54]	LAD ligation	15	Control, 100%VT Hal, 50%VT Pento, 60%VT/30%VF F-D-N₂0, 90%VT	Not reported	Hal, PR↑; VERP↑ Pento, PR↑; QT↑ F-D-N₂0, no changes
Denniss[53]	LAD ligation	75	Control, 45%VT/VF Hal, 29%VT/VF	Hal, 4/41(10%)VT/VF; previously noninducible	Hal, PR↑; VERP↑
Deutsch[52]	LAD occlusion–reperfusion	18	Control, 12*/18 (67%) Hal, 6/12*(50%) Iso, 9/12*(75%) Enf, 4/11*(36%) all VT/VF	3/19 anesthetics (Hal, Enf, Iso) in 2 of 6 dogs previously noninducible	Normal zone: Hal, Enf, Iso—VERP↑; VRRP↑ Ischemic zone: Hal, ENF—VERP↑; VRRP↑ Iso, no change

*Halothane and enflurane, but not isoflurane, significantly reduced inducibility.

LAD, left anterior descending coronary artery; VT, ventricular tachycardia; VF, ventricular fibrillation; Hal, halothane; Pento, pentobarbital; F-D-N₂0, fentanyl, droperidol, nitrous oxide; Iso, isoflurane; Enf, enflurane; VERP↑, ventricular effective refractory period increased; PR and QT intervals determined from ECG recordings.

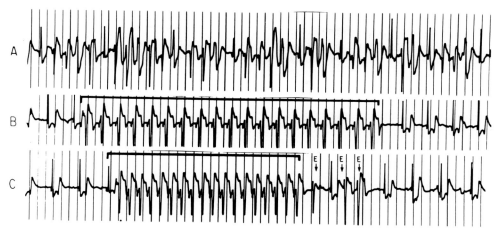

Figure 33-12. Effects of halothane on ouabain-induced ventricular tachycardia. Ouabain was infused into a dog until the ventricular arrhythmia seen in **A** appeared. After halothane, sinus rhythm appeared. Pacing for 20 beats at a cycle length of 400 mseconds (**B**) is unremarkable, but a train of paced ventricular beats at a 250-mseconds cycle length (**C**) triggers extrasystoles (*E*), characteristic of triggered activity. (Gallagher JD, McClernan CA: The effects of halothane on ventricular tachycardia in intact dogs. Anesthesiology 1991;75:866.)

haled anesthetics showed occasional proarrhythmia. Clinically, the effects of halothane will depend on the etiology of the arrhythmia. In the majority of ventricular arrhythmias seen in man, which are presumably reentrant in origin,[201] inhalation anesthetics may be beneficial but, like all other antiarrhythmics studied,[189] could be proarrhythmic. Avoidance of high doses of inhaled anesthetics (especially halothane and enflurane)[52] when induction of ventricular tachycardia is desired (e.g., during intraoperative mapping[202] or, occasionally, automatic defibrillator implantation)[134] would seem prudent.

References

1. Miller K: Specific and nonspecific actions of general anesthetics. In: Covino B, Fozzard H, Rehder K, Strichartz G, eds. Effects of anesthesia. Bethesda, MD: American Physiological Society, 1985:29–37.
2. Niggli E, Maurer R, Weingart R: Effects of general anesthetics on current flow across membranes in guinea pig myocytes. Am J Physiol 1989;256:C273.
3. Kuner J, Enescu V, Utsu F, Boszormenyi E, Bernstein H, Corday E: Cardiac arrhythmias during anesthesia. Dis Chest 1967;52:580.
4. Brodsky M, Wu D, Kanakis C, Rosen KM: Arrhythmias documented by continuous electrocardiographic monitoring in 50 male medical students without apparent heart disease. Am J Cardiol 1977;39:390.
5. Sobotka A, Mayer JH, Bauernfeind RA, Kanakis CJ, Rosen KM: Arrhythmias documented by 24-hour continuous ambulatory electrocardiographic monitoring in young women without apparent heart disease. Am J Cardiol 1981;101:753.
6. Bertrand CA, Steiner NV, Jameson AG, Lopez M: Disturbances of cardiac rhythm during anesthesia and surgery. JAMA 1971;216:1615.
7. Vitez TS, Soper LE, Wong KC, Soper P: Chronic hypokalemia and intraoperative dysrhythmias. Anesthesiology 1985;63:130.
8. Hirsch IA, Tomlinson DL, Slogoff S, Keats AS: The overstated risk of preoperative hypokalemia. Anesth Analg 1988;67:131.
9. Lown B, Wolf M: Approaches to sudden death from coronary heart disease. Circulation 1971;54:130.
10. O'Kelly B, Browner WS, Massie B, Tubau J, Ngo L, Mangano DT: Ventricular arrhythmias in patients undergoing noncardiac surgery. JAMA 1992;268:217.
11. Rolf N, Coté CJ: Persistent cardiac arrhythmias in pediatric patients: effects of age, expired carbon dioxide values, depth of anesthesia, and airway management. Anesth Analg 1991;73:720.
12. Vergani DP, Mieli-Vergani G, Alberti A, et al: Antibodies to the surface of halothane-altered rabbit hepatocytes in patients with severe halothane-associated hepatitis. N Engl J Med 1980;303:66.
13. Reynolds AK: On the mechanism of myocardial sensitization to catecholamines by hydrocarbon anesthetics. Can J Physiol Pharmacol 1984;62:183.
14. Bosnjak ZJ, Turner LA: Halothane, catecholamines, and cardiac conduction: anything new? Anesth Analg 1991;72:1.
15. Lynch C, Vogel S, Sperelakis N: Halothane depression of myocardial slow action potentials. Anesthesiology 1981;55:360.
16. Bosnjak ZJ, Kampine JP: Effects of halothane on transmembrane potentials, Ca^{2+} transients, and papillary muscle tension in the cat. Am J Physiol 1986;251:H374.
17. Komai H, Rusy BF: Negative inotropic effects of isoflurane and halothane in rabbit papillary muscles. Anesth Analg 1987;66:29.
18. Komai H, Rusy BF: Direct effect of halothane and isoflurane on the function of the sarcoplasmic reticulum in intact rabbit atria. Anesthesiology 1990;72:694.

19. DeTraglia MC, Komai H, Rusy BF: Differential effects of inhalation anesthetics on myocardial potentiated-state contractions in vitro. Anesthesiology 1988;68:534.

20. DeTraglia MC, Komai H, Redon D, Rusy BF: Isoflurane and halothane inhibit tetanic contractions in rabbit myocardium in vitro. Anesthesiology 1989;70:837.

21. Terrar D, Victory J: Influence of halothane on electrical coupling in cell pairs isolated from guinea pig ventricle. Br J Pharmacol 1988;94:509.

22. Terrar D, Victory J: Effects of halothane on membrane currents associated with contraction in single myocytes isolated from guinea pig ventricle. Br J Pharmacol 1988;94:500.

23. Terrar D, Victory J: Isoflurane depresses membrane currents associated with contraction in myocytes isolated from guinea-pig ventricle. Anesthesiology 1988;69:742.

24. Atlee JL, Bosnjak ZJ: Mechanisms for cardiac dysrhythmias during anesthesia. Anesthesiology 1990;72:347.

25. Ikemoto Y, Yatani A, Arimura H, Yoshitake J: Reduction of the slow inward current of isolated rat ventricular cells by thiamylal and halothane. Acta Anaesthesiol Scand 1985;29:583.

26. Bosnjak ZJ, Aggarwal A, Turner LA, Kampine JM, Kampine JP: Differential effects of halothane, enflurane, and isoflurane on Ca^{2+} transients and papillary muscle tension in guinea pigs. Anesthesiology 1992;76:123.

27. Ikemoto Y, Yatani A, Imoto Y, Arimura H: Reduction in the myocardial sodium current by halothane and thiamylal. Jpn J Physiol 1986;36:107.

28. Eskinder H, Rusch NJ, Supan FD, Kampine JP, Bosnjak ZJ: The effects of volatile anesthetics on L- and T-type calcium channel currents in canine cardiac Purkinje cells. Anesthesiology 1991;74:919.

29. Hirota K, Momose Y, Takeda R, Nakanishi S, Ito Y: Prolongation of the action potential and reduction of the delayed outward K^+ current by halothane in single frog atrial cells. Eur J Pharmacol 1986;126:293.

30. Baum VC: Distinctive effects of three intravenous anesthetics on the inward rectifier (I_{K1}) and the delayed rectifier (I_K) potassium currents in myocardium: implications for the mechanism of action. Anesth Analg 1993;76:18.

31. Turner LA, Bosnjak ZJ, Kampine JP: Actions of halothane on the electrical activity of Purkinje fibers derived from normal and infarcted canine hearts. Anesthesiology 1987;17:619.

32. Turner LA, Polic S, Hoffmann RG, Kampine JP, Bosnjak ZJ: Actions of volatile anesthetics on ischemic and nonischemic Purkinje fibers in the infarcted canine heart: regional action potential characteristics. Anesth Analg 1993;76:726.

33. Turner LA, Polic S, Hoffmann RG, Kampine JP, Bosnjak ZJ: Actions of halothane and isoflurane on Purkinje fibers in the infarcted canine heart: conduction, regional refractoriness, and reentry. Anesth Analg 1993;76:718.

34. Reynolds AK, Chiz JF, Pasquet AF: Halothane and methoxyflurane—A comparison of their effects on cardiac pacemaker fibers. Anesthesiology 1970;33:602.

35. Hauswirth O: The effects of halothane on single atrial ventricular and Purkinje fibers. Circ Res 1969;24:745.

36. Gallagher JD, Gessman LJ, Moura P, Kerns D: Electrophysiologic effects of halothane and quinidine on canine Purkinje fibers: evidence for a synergistic interaction. Anesthesiology 1986;65:278.

37. Eskinder H, Supan FD, Turner LA, Kampine JP, Bosnjak ZJ: The effects of halothane and isoflurane on slowly inactivating sodium current in canine cardiac Purkinje cells. Anesth Analg 1993;77:32.

38. Joyner RW, Overholt ED: Effects of octanol on canine subendocardial Purkinje-to-ventricular transmission. Am J Physiol 1985;249:H1228.

39. Burt JM, Spray DC: Volatile anesthetics block intercellular communication between neonatal rat myocardial cells. Circ Res 1989;65:829.

40. Bosnjak Z, Kampine J: Effects of halothane, enflurane and isoflurane on the SA node. Anesthesiology 1983;58:314.

41. Seagard JL, Bosnjak ZJ, Hopp FAJ, Kotrly KJ, Ebert TJ, Kampine JP: Cardiovascular effects of general anesthesia. In: Covino B, Fozzard H, Rehder K, Strichartz G, eds. Effects of anesthesia. Bethesda, MD: American Physiological Society, 1985:149–177.

42. Skovsted P, Sapthavichaikul S: The effects of isoflurane on arterial pressure, pulse rate, autonomic nervous activity, and barostatic reflexes. Can Anaesth Soc J 1977;24:304.

43. Stevens WC, Cromwell TH, Halsey MJ, Eger El, Shakespeare TF, Bahlman SH: The cardiovascular effects of a new inhalation anesthetic, Forane, in human volunteers at constant arterial carbon dioxide tension. Anesthesiology 1971;35:8.

44. Curling PE, Noback CR: Inhalational anesthetics: isoflurane and nitrous oxide. In: Kaplan JA, ed. Cardiac anesthesia. New York: Grune & Stratton, 1983:95–141.

45. Atlee JL, Brownlee SW, Burstrom RE: Conscious-state comparisons of the effects of inhalation anesthetics on specialized atrioventricular conduction times in dogs. Anesthesiology 1986;64:703.

46. Blitt CD, Raessler KL, Wightman MA, Groves BM, Wall CL, Geha DG: Atrioventricular conduction in dogs during anesthesia with isoflurane. Anesthesiology 1979;50:210.

47. Atlee JL, Alexander SC: Halothane effects on conductivity of the AV node and His-Purkinje system in the dog. Anesth Analg 1977;56:378.

48. Atlee JL, Rusy BF, Kreul JF, Eby T: Supraventricular excitability in dogs during anesthesia with halothane and enflurane. Anesthesiology 1978;49:407.

49. Ammendrup P, Atlee JL: Mechanical hyperventilation: effect on specialized atrioventricular conduction, supraventricular refractoriness, and experimental atrial arrhythmias in dogs anesthetized with pentobarbital or pentobarbital–halothane. Anesth Analg 1980;59:839.

50. Atlee JL, Yeager T: Electrophysiologic assessment of the effects of enflurane, halothane, and isoflurane on properties affecting supraventricular re-entry in chronically instrumented dogs. Anesthesiology 1989;71:941.

51. Scheffer GJ, Jonges R, Holley HS, et al: Effects of halothane on the conduction system of the heart in humans. Anesth Analg 1989;69:721.

52. Deutsch N, Hantler CB, Tait AR, Uprichard A, Schork MA, Knight PR: Suppression of ventricular arrhythmias by volatile anesthetics in a canine model of chronic myocardial infarction. Anesthesiology 1990;72:1012.

53. Denniss AR, Richards DA, Taylor AT, Uther JB: Halothane anesthesia reduces inducibility of ventricular tachyarrhythmias in chronic canine myocardial infarction. Basic Res Cardiol 1989;84:5.

54. Hunt GB, Ross DL: Comparison of effects of three anesthetic

agents on induction of ventricular tachycardia in a canine model of myocardial infarction. Circulation 1988;78:221.

55. Turner LA, Zuperka EJ, Purtock RV, Kampine JP: In vivo changes in canine ventricular conduction during halothane anesthesia. Anesth Analg 1980;59:327.

56. Reves JG, Kissin I: Intravenous anesthetics. In: Kaplan JA, ed. Cardiac anesthesia. New York: Grune & Stratton, 1983:3–30.

57. Fragen RJ, Shanks CA: Anesthetic induction characteristics of Diprivan (propofol) emulsion. Semin Anesth 1988;7:103.

58. Rosow CE: Cardiovascular effects of narcotics. In: Covino B, Fozzard H, Rehder K, Strichartz G, eds. Effects of anesthesia. Bethesda, MD: American Physiological Society, 1985: 195–205.

59. Patschke D, Eberlein HJ, Hess W, Oser G, Tarnow J, Zimmerman G: Haemodynamik, koronardurchblutung und myocardialer sauerstoffverbrauch unter hohen morphine-, pethidin-, fentanyl- und piritramiddosen. Anaesthetist 1977; 26:236.

60. Kotrly KJ, Ebert TJ, Vucins E, Igler FO, Barney JA, Kampine JP: Baroreceptor reflex control of heart rate during isoflurane anesthesia in humans. Anesthesiology 1984;60:173.

61. Morton M, Duke PC, Ong B: Baroreflex control of heart rate in man awake and during enflurane and enflurane–nitrous oxide anesthesia. Anesthesiology 1980;52:221.

62. Duke PC, Fownes D, Wade G: Halothane depresses baroreflex control of heart rate in man. Anesthesiology 1977; 46:184.

63. Bristow JD, Prys-Roberts C, Fischer A, Pickering TG, Sleight P: Effects of anesthesia on baroreflex control of heart rate in man. Anesthesiology 1969;57:422.

64. Seagard JL, Hopp FA, Bosnjak ZJ, Elegbe EO, Kampine JP: Extent and mechanism of halothane sensitization of the carotid sinus baroreceptors. Anesthesiology 1983;58:432.

65. Seagard JL, Elegbe EO, Hopp FA, et al: Effects of isoflurane on the baroreceptor reflex. Anesthesiology 1983;59:511.

66. Seagard JL, Hopp FA, Donegan JH, Kalbfleisch JH, Kampine JP: Halothane and the carotid sinus reflex: evidence for multiple sites of action. Anesthesiology 1982;57:191.

67. Bosnjak ZJ, Seagard JL, Wu A, Kampine JP: The effects of halothane on sympathetic ganglion transmission. Anesthesiology 1982;57:473.

68. Price HL, Linde HW, Morse HT: Central nervous actions in halothane affecting the systemic circulation. Anesthesiology 1963;24:770.

69. Ebert TJ: Differential effects of nitrous oxide on baroreflex control of heart rate and peripheral sympathetic nerve activity in humans. Anesthesiology 1990;72:16.

70. Priano LL, Bernards C, Marrone B: Effect of anesthetic induction agents on cardiovascular neuroregulation in dogs. Anesth Analg 1989;68:344.

71. Kotrly KJ, Ebert TJ, Vucins EJ, Roerig DL, Kampine JP: Baroceptor reflex control of heart rate during morphine sulfate, diazepam, N_2O/O_2 anesthesia in humans. Anesthesiology 1984;61:558.

72. Ebert TJ, Muzi M, Berens R, Goff D, Kampine JP: Sympathetic responses to induction of anesthesia in humans with propofol or etomidate. Anesthesiology 1992;76:725.

73. Yeager MP, Glass DD, Neff RK, Brinck-Johnsen T: Epidural anesthesia and analgesia in high-risk surgical patients. Anesthesiology 1987;66:729.

74. Covino BG: Cardiovascular effects of regional anesthesia. In: Covino B, Fozzard H, Rehder K, Strichartz G, eds. Effects of anesthesia. Bethesda, MD: American Physiological Society, 1985:207–215.

75. Hotvedt R, Platou ES, Refsum H: Electrophysiologic effects of thoracic epidural blockade in the dog heart in situ. Cardiovasc Res 1983;17:259.

76. Blomberg S, Ricksten S-E: Thoracic epidural anaesthesia decreases the incidence of ventricular arrhythmias during acute myocardial ischaemia in the anaesthetized rat. Acta Anaesthesiol Scand 1988;32:173.

77. Albright GA: Cardiac arrest following regional anesthesia with etidocaine or bupivacaine. Anesthesiology 1979;51: 285.

78. Morishima HO, Pedersen H, Finster M, et al: Bupivacaine toxicity in pregnant and nonpregnant ewes. Anesthesiology 1985;63:134.

79. de Jong RH, Ronfeld RA, DeRosa RA: Cardiovascular effects of convulsant and supraconvulsant doses of amide local anesthetics. Anesth Analg 1982;61:3.

80. Clarkson CW, Hondeghem LM: Mechanisms for bupivacaine depression of cardiac conduction: fast block of sodium channels during the action potential with slow recovery from block during diastole. Anesthesiology 1985;62:396.

81. Moller RA, Covino BG: Cardiac electrophysiologic effects of lidocaine and bupivacaine. Anesth Analg 1988;67:107.

82. Boban M, Stowe DF, Gross GJ, Pieper GM, Kampine JP, Bosnjak ZJ: Potassium channel openers attenuate atrioventricular block by bupivacaine in isolated hearts. Anesth Analg 1993;76:1259.

83. Heavner JE: Cardiac dysrhythmias induced by infusion of local anesthetics into the lateral cerebral ventricle of cats. Anesth Analg 1986;65:133.

84. Thomas RD, Behbehani MM, Coyle DE, Denson DD: Cardiovascular toxicity of local anesthetics; an alternative hypothesis. Anesth Analg 1986;65:444.

85. Kasten GW, Martin ST: Successful cardiovascular resuscitation after massive intravenous bupivacaine overdosage in anesthetized dogs. Anesth Analg 1985;64:491.

86. Kasten GW, Martin ST: Bupivacaine cardiovascular toxicity, comparison of treatment with bretylium and lidocaine. Anesth Analg 1985;64:911.

87. Jacobs HK, Lim S, Salem MR, Rao TLK, Mathru M, Smith BD: Cardiac electrophysiologic effects of pancuronium. Anesth Analg 1985;64:693.

88. Geha DG, Rozelle BC, Raessler KL, Groves BM, Wightman MA, Blitt CD: Pancuronium bromide enhances atrioventricular conduction in halothane-anesthetized dogs. Anesthesiology 1977;46:342.

89. Miller RD, Eger EI, Stevens WC, Gibbons R: Pancuronium-induced tachycardia in relation to alveolar halothane, dose of pancuronium, and prior atropine. Anesthesiology 1975; 42:352.

90. Hughes R, Chapple DJ: Effects of non-depolarizing neuromuscular blocking agents on autonomic mechanisms in cats. Br J Anaesth 1976;48:59.

91. Gardier RW, Tsevdos EJ, Jackson DB: Effects of gallamine and pancuronium on inhibitory transmission in cat sympathetic ganglion. J Pharmacol Exp Ther 1978;204:46.

92. Vercruysse P, Hanegreefs G, Vanhoutte PM: Influence of

skeletal muscle relaxants on the prejunctional effects of acetylcholine in adrenergically-innervated blood vessels. Arch Int Pharmacodyn Ther 1978;232:350.

93. Miller RD, Savarese JJ: Pharmacology of muscle relaxants and their antagonists. In: Miller RD, ed. Anesthesia. New York: Churchill Livingstone, 1986:889–943.

94. Yasuda I, Hirano T, Amaha K, Fudeta H, Obara S: Chronotropic effects of succinylcholine and succinylmonocholine on the sinoatrial node. Anesthesiology 1982;57:289.

95. Leiman BC, Katz J, Butler BD: Mechanisms of succinylcholine-induced arrhythmias in hypoxic or hypoxic: hypercarbic dogs. Anesth Analg 1987;66:1292.

96. Saegusa K, Furukawa Y, Takeda M, Chiba S: Tyramine-like action of succinylcholine in the isolated, blood-perfused canine atrium. Anesth Analg 1993;75:989.

97. Shnider SM, Papper EM: Anesthesia for the asthmatic patient. Anesthesiology 1961;22:886.

98. Roizen MF, Stevens WC: Multiform ventricular tachycardia due to the interaction of aminophylline and halothane. Anesth Analg 1978;57:738.

99. Stirt JA, Sullivan SF: Aminophylline. Anesth Analg 1981;60:587.

100. Stirt JA, Berger JM, Sullivan SF: Lack of arrhythmogenicity of isoflurane following administration of aminophylline in dogs. Anesth Analg 1983;62:568.

101. Moyer JA, Greenberg LH, Frazer A, Brunswick DJ, Mendels J, Weiss B: Opposite effects of acute and repeated administration of desmethylimipramine on adrenergic responsiveness in rat pineal gland. Life Sci 1979;2:2237.

102. Edwards RP, Miller RD, Roizen MF, et al: Cardiac responses to imipramine and pancuronium during anesthesia with halothane or enflurane. Anesthesiology 1979;50:421.

103. Spiss CK, Smith CM, Maze M: Halothane–epinephrine arrhythmias and adrenergic responsiveness after chronic imipramine administration in dogs. Anesth Analg 1984;63:825.

104. Gallagher JD, Lieberman RL, Meranze J, Spielman SR, Ellison N: Amiodarone-induced complications during cardiac surgery. Anesthesiology 1981;55:186.

105. Feinberg BI, LaMantia KR, Levy WJ: Amiodarone and general anesthesia—A retrospective analysis [Abstract]. Eighth Annual Meeting of the Society of Cardiovascular Anesthesiologists, 1986:137.

106. Liberman BA, Teasdale SJ: Anaesthesia and amiodarone. Can Anaesth Soc J 1985;32:629.

107. Wellens HJJ, Brugada P, Penn OC: The management of pre-excitation syndromes. JAMA 1987;257:2325.

108. van der Starre PJA: Wolff-Parkinson-White syndrome during anesthesia. Anesthesiology 1978;48:369.

109. Lubarsky D, Kaufman B, Turndorf H: Anesthesia unmasking benign Wolff-Parkinson-White syndrome. Anesth Analg 1989;68:172.

110. Sadowski AR, Moyers JR: Anesthetic management of the Wolff-Parkinson-White syndrome. Anesthesiology 1979;51:553.

111. Richmond MN, Conroy PT: Anesthetic management of a neonate born prematurely with Wolff Parkinson White syndrome. Anesth Analg 1988;67:477.

112. Gomez-Arnau J, Marquez-Montes J, Avello F: Fentanyl and droperidol effects on the refractoriness of the accessory pathway in the Wolff-Parkinson-White syndrome. Anesthesiology 1983;58:307.

113. Sharpe MD, Dobkowski WB, Murkin JM, Klein G, Guiraudon G, Yee R: The electrophysiologic effects of volatile anesthetics and sufentanil on the normal atrioventricular and accessory pathways in Wolff-Parkinson-White syndrome. Anesthesiology 1994;80:63.

114. Kumazawa T: Wolff-Parkinson-White syndrome during anesthesia. Masui 1970;23:68.

115. Domino KB, Smith TC: Electrocautery-induced reprogramming of a pacemaker using a precordial magnet. Anesth Analg 1983;62:609.

116. Atlee JL: Perioperative cardiac dysrhythmias: mechanisms, recognition, management. Chicago: Year Book Medical Publishers, 1985:362–367.

117. Hayashi Y, Sumikawa K, Maze M, et al: Dexmedetomidine prevents epinephrine-induced arrhythmias through stimulation of central α_2 adrenoceptors in halothane-anesthetized dogs. Anesthesiology 1991;75:113.

118. Simon AB: Perioperative management of the pacemaker patient. Anesthesiology 1977;46:127.

119. Zaidan JR: Pacemakers. Anesthesiology 1984;60:319.

120. Cooper D, Wilkoff B, Masterson M, et al: Effects of extracorporeal shock wave lithotripsy on cardiac pacemakers and its safety in patients with implanted cardiac pacemakers. PACE Pacing Clin Electrophysiol 1988;11:1607.

121. Merritt WT, Brinker JA, Beattie C: Pacemaker-mediated tachycardia induced by intraoperative somatosensory evoked potential stimuli. Anesthesiology 1988;69:766.

122. Samain E, Marty J, Dupont H, Mouton E, Desmonts JM: Intraoperative pacemaker-mediated tachycardia: a complication of dual-chamber cardiac pacemakers. Anesthesiology 1993;78:376.

123. Ducey JP, Fincher CW, Baysinger CL: Therapeutic suppression of a permanent ventricular pacemaker using a peripheral nerve stimulator. Anesthesiology 1991;75:533.

124. Kemnitz J, Peters J: Pacemaker interactions with transcutaneous cardiac pacing. Anesthesiology 1993;79:390.

125. Tyers GF: Current status of sensor-modulated rate-adaptive cardiac pacing. J Am Coll Cardiol 1990;15:412.

126. Lau CP, Linker NJ, Butrous GS, Ward DE, Camm AJ: Myopotential interference in unipolar rate responsive pacemakers. PACE Pacing Clin Electrophysiol 1989;12:1324.

127. Madsen GM, Andersen C: Pacemaker-induced tachycardia during general anaesthesia: a case report. Br J Anaesth 1989;63:360.

128. Boute W, Gebhardt U, Begemann MJ: Introduction of an automatic QT interval driven rate responsive pacemaker. PACE Pacing Clin Electrophysiol 1988;11:1804.

129. Chirife R: Physiologic principles of a new method for rate responsive pacing using the pre-ejection interval. PACE Pacing Clin Electrophysiol 1988;11:1545.

130. Paul V, Garratt C, Ward DE, Camm AJ: Closed loop control of rate adaptive pacing: clinical assessment of a system analyzing the ventricular depolarization gradient. PACE Pacing Clin Electrophysiol 1989;12:1896.

131. Deutsch N, Hantler CB, Tait AR: QT interval lengthening with halothane, enflurane, and isoflurane in dogs with recent myocardial infarction [Abstract]. Ninth Annual Meeting of the Society of Cardiovascular Anesthesiologists, 1989.

132. Stangl K, Wirtzfeld A, Heinze R, Laule M, Seitz K, Gobl G: A new multisensor pacing system using stroke volume, respiratory rate, mixed venous oxygen saturation, and temperature, right atrial pressure, right ventricular pressure, and dP/dt. PACE Pacing Clin Electrophysiol 1988;11:712.

133. Zaidan JR, Curling PE, Craver JM: Effect of enflurane, isoflurane, and halothane on pacing stimulation thresholds in man. PACE Pacing Clin Electrophysiol 1985;8:32.

134. Mirowski M, Mower MM, Reid PR, Watkins L, Langer A: The automatic implantable defibrillator: new modality for treatment of life-threatening ventricular arrhythmias. PACE Pacing Clin Electrophysiol 1982;5:384.

135. Winkle RA, Mead RH, Ruder MA, et al: Long-term outcome with the automatic implantable cardioverter-defibrillator. J Am Coll Cardiol 1989;13:1353.

136. Manolis AS, Rastegar H, Estes NAM: Automatic implantable cardioverter defibrillator current status. JAMA 1989;262:1362.

137. Saksena S, Parsonnet V: Implantation of a cardioverter/defibrillator without thoracotomy using a triple electrode system. JAMA 1988;259:69.

138. Saksena S, Tullo NG, Krol RB, Mauro AM: Initial clinical experience with endocardial defibrillation using an implantable cardioverter/defibrillator with a triple-electrode system. Arch Intern Med 1989;149:2333.

139. Gilbert TB, Kent JL, Foster AH, Gold MR: Implantable cardioverter/defibrillator placement in a patient with amiodarone pulmonary toxicity under thoracic epidural anesthesia. Anesthesiology 1993;79:608.

140. de Paola AA, Horowitz LN, Morganroth J, et al: Influence of left ventricular dysfunction on flecainide therapy. J Am Coll Cardiol 1987;9:163.

141. Gaba DM, Wyner J, Fish KJ: Anesthesia and the automatic implantable cardioveter/defibrillator. Anesthesiology 1985;62:786.

142. Marinchak RA, Friehling TD, Kline RA, Stohler J, Kowey PR: Effect of antiarrhythmic drugs on defibrillation threshold: case report of an adverse effect of mexiletine and review of the literature. PACE Pacing Clin Electrophysiol 1988;11:7.

143. Long AL, Venditti FJ Jr. Lithotripsy in a patient with an automatic implantable cardioverter defibrillator. Anesthesiology 1991;74:937.

144. Katz RL, Bigger JT: Cardiac arrhythmias during anesthesia and operation. Anesthesiology 1970;33:193.

145. France NK: Anesthesia for pediatric ophthalmologic surgery. In: Gregory GA, ed. Pediatric anesthesia. New York: Churchill Livingstone, 1983:778.

146. Moonie GT, Reese DL, Elton D: The oculocardiac reflex during strabismus surgery. Can Anaesth Soc J 1964;11:621.

147. Johnston RR, Eger EI, Wilson C: A comparative interaction of epinephrine with enflurane, isoflurane and halothane in man. Anesth Analg 1976;55:709.

148. Karl HW, Swedlow DB, Lee KW, Downes JJ: Epinephrine–halothane interactions in children. Anesthesiology 1983;58:142.

149. Moore MA, Weiskopf RB, Eger EI II, Wilson C, Lu G: Arrhythmogenic doses of epinephrine are similar during desflurane or isoflurane anesthesia in humans. Anesthesiology 1993;79:943.

150. Atlee JL, Malkinson CE: Potentiation by thiopental of halothane–epinephrine-induced arrhythmias in dogs. Anesthesiology 1982;57:285.

151. Liu W-S, Wong KC, Port JD, Andriano KP: Epinephrine-induced arrhythmias during halothane anesthesia with the addition of nitrous oxide, nitrogen, or helium in dogs. Anesth Analg 1982;61:414.

152. Kamibayashi T, Hayashi Y, Sumikawa K, Yamatodani A, Kawabata K, Yoshiya I: Enhancement by propofol of epinephrine-induced arrhythmias in dogs. Anesthesiology 1991;75:1035.

153. Koehntop DE, Liao JC, Van Bergen FH: Effects of pharmacologic alterations of adrenergic mechanisms by cocaine, tropolone, aminophylline, and ketamine on epinephrine-induced arrhythmias during halothane–nitrous oxide anesthesia. Anesthesiology 1977;46:83.

154. Schick LM, Chapin JC, Munson ES, Kushins LG: Pancuronium, d-tubocurarine, and epinephrine-induced arrhythmias during halothane anesthesia in dogs. Anesthesiology 1980;52:207.

155. Tucker WK, Munson ES: Effects of succinylcholine and d-tubocurarine on epinephrine-induced arrhythmias during halothane anesthesia in dogs. Anesthesiology 1975;42:41.

156. Chapin JC, Kushins LG, Munson ES, Schick LM: Lidocaine, bupivacaine, etidocaine and epinephrine-induced arrhythmias during halothane anesthesia in dogs. Anesthesiology 1980;52:23.

157. Hayashi Y, Sumikawa K, Tashiro C, Yoshiya I: Synergistic interaction of α_1- and β-adrenoceptor agonists on induction arrhythmias during halothane anesthesia in dogs. Anesthesiology 1988;68:902.

158. Maze M, Smith CM: Identification of receptor mechanism mediating epinephrine-induced arrhythmias during halothane anesthesia in the dog. Anesthesiology 1983;59:322.

159. Miletich DJ, Khan A, Albrecht RF, Jozefiak A: Use of heart cell cultures as a tool for the evaluation of halothane arrhythmia. Toxicol Appl Pharmacol 1983;70:181.

160. Zuckerman RL, Wheeler DM: Effect of halothane on arrhythmogenic responses induced by sympathomimetic agents in single rat heart cells. Anesth Analg 1991;72:596.

161. Reynolds AK: Cardiac arrhythmias in sensitized hearts—primary mechanisms involved. Res Commun Chem Pathol Pharmacol 1983;40:3.

162. Reynolds AK, Chiz JF, Tanikella T: On the mechanism of coupling in adrenaline-induced bigeminy in sensitized hearts. Can J Physiol Pharmacol 1975;53:1158.

163. Cranefield PF: The conduction of the cardiac impulse. Mount Kisco, NY: Futura, 1975:191.

164. Smith ER, Dresel PE: Site of origin of halothane–epinephrine arrhythmia determined by direct and echocardiographic recordings. Anesthesiology 1982;57:98.

165. Hayashi Y, Sumikawa K, Kuro M, Fukumitsu K, Tashiro C, Yoshiya I: Roles of β_1- and β_2-adrenoceptors in the mechanism of halothane myocardial sensitization in dogs. Anesth Analg 1991;72:435.

166. Kapur PA, Flacke WE: Epinephrine-induced arrhythmias and cardiovascular function after verapamil during halothane anesthesia in the dog. Anesthesiology 1981;55:218.

167. Atlee JL, Bosnjak ZJ, Yeager TS: Effects of diltiazem, verapamil, and inhalation anesthetics on electrophysiologic

properties affecting reentrant supraventricular tachycardia in chronically instrumented dogs. Anesthesiology 1990; 72:889.

168. Laszlo A, Polic S, Atlee JL III, Kampine JP, Bosnjak ZJ: Anesthetics and automaticity in latent pacemaker fibers: I. Effects of halothane, enflurane, and isoflurane in automaticity and recovery of automaticity from overdrive suppression in Purkinje fibers derived from canine hearts. Anesthesiology 1991;75:98.

169. Polic S, Atlee JL III, Laszlo A, Kampine JP, Bosnjak ZJ: Anesthetics and automaticity in latent pacemaker fibers: II. Effects of halothane and epinephrine or norepinephrine on automaticity of dominant and subsidiary atrial pacemakers in the canine heart. Anesthesiology 1991;75:298.

170. Polic S, Atlee JL III, Laszlo A, Kampine JP, Bosnjak ZJ: Anesthetics and automaticity in latent pacemaker fibers: III. Effects of halothane and ouabain on automaticity of the SA node and subsidiary atrial pacemakers in the canine heart. Anesthesiology 1991;75:305.

171. Boban M, Atlee JL III, Vicenzi M, Kampine JP, Bosnjak ZJ: Anesthetics and automaticity in latent pacemaker fibers: IV. Effects of isoflurane and epinephrine or norepinephrine on automaticity of dominant and subsidiary atrial pacemakers in the canine heart. Anesthesiology 1993;79:555.

172. Woehlck HJ, Vicenzi MN, Bosnjak ZJ, Atlee JL III: Anesthetics and automaticity of dominant and latent pacemakers in chronically instrumented dogs: I. Methodology, conscious state, and halothane anesthesia: comparison with and without muscarinic blockade during exposure to epinephrine. Anesthesiology 1993;79:1304.

173. Vicenzi MN, Woehlck HJ, Bosnjak ZJ, Atlee JL III: Anesthetics and automaticity of dominant and latent pacemakers in chronically instrumented dogs: II. Effects of enflurane and isoflurane during exposure to epinephrine with and without muscarinic blockade. Anesthesiology 1993;79:1316.

174. Marijic J, Bosnjak ZJ, Stowe DF, Kampine JP: Effects and interaction of verapamil and volatile anesthetics on isolated perfused guinea pig heart. Anesthesiology 1988;69:914.

175. Haft JI, Habbab MA: Treatment of atrial arrhythmias: effectiveness of verapamil when preceded by calcium infusion. Arch Intern Med 1986;146:1085.

176. Takada K, Sumikawa K, Kamibayashi T, et al: Comparative efficacy of antiarrhythmic agents in preventing halothane–epinephrine arrhythmias in rats. Anesthesiology 1993;79:563.

177. Burns JMA, Hart DM, Hughes RL, Kelman AW, Hillis WS: Effects of nadolol on arrhythmias during laparoscopy performed under general anaesthesia. Br J Anaesth 1988;61:345.

178. Rosen MR, Ilevento JP, Binah O, LeMarec H: The use of matrices of pharmacological agents in the diagnosis of arrhythmogenic mechanisms. J Electrophysiol 1987;1:30.

179. Kroll DA, Knight PR: Antifibrillatory effects of volatile anesthetics in acute occlusion/reperfusion arrhythmias. Anesthesiology 1984;61:657.

180. Harris AS: Delayed development of ventricular ectopic rhythms following experimental coronary occlusion. Circulation 1950;1:1318.

181. Lazzara R, El-Sherif N, Scherlag BJ: Electrophysiological properties of canine Purkinje cells in one-day-old myocardial infarction. Circ Res 1973;33:722.

182. LeMarec H, Dangman KH, Danilo PJ, Rosen MR: An evaluation of automaticity and triggered activity in the canine heart one to four days after myocardial infarction. Circulation 1985;71:1224.

183. El-Sherif N, Gough WB, Zeiler RH, Mehra R: Triggered ventricular rhythm in one-day-old myocardial infarction in the dog. Circ Res 1983;52:566.

184. Dangman KH, Dresdner DPJ, Zaim S: Automatic and triggered impulse initiation in canine subepicardial ventricular muscle cells from border zones of 24-hour transmural infarcts: new mechanisms for malignant cardiac arrhythmias? Circulation 1988;78:1020.

185. Logic JR, Morrow DH, Gatz RN: Idioventricular tachycardia complicating experimental myocardial infarction. Dis Chest 1969;56:477.

186. El-Sherif N, Mehra R, Gough WB, Zeiler RH: Reentrant ventricular arrhythmias in the late myocardial infarction period. Circulation 1983;68:644.

187. Mehra R, Zeiler RH, Gough WB, El-Sherif N: Reentrant ventricular arrhythmias in the late myocardial infarction period. A electrophysiologic–anatomic correlation of reentrant circuits. Circulation 1983;67:11.

188. Levine JH, Morganroth J, Kadish AH: Mechanisms and risk factors for proarrhythmia with type 1a compared with 1c antiarrhythmic drug therapy. Circulation 1989;80:1063.

189. Velebit V, Podrid P, Lown B, Cohen BH, Graboys TB: Aggravation and provocation of ventricular arrhythmias by antiarrhythmic drugs. Circulation 1982;65:886.

190. Cranefield P: Action potentials, afterpotentials, and arrhythmias. Circ Res 1977;41:415.

191. Reynolds AK, Horne ML: Studies on the cardiotoxicity of ouabain. Can J Physiol Pharmacol 1969;47:165.

192. Gallagher JD, Bianchi JJ, Gessman LJ: Halothane antagonizes digitalis toxicity in canine Purkinje fibers. Anesthesiology 1989;71:695.

193. Moss AJ: Prolonged QT-interval syndromes. JAMA 1986; 256:2985.

194. January CT, Riddle JM: Early afterdepolarizations: mechanism of induction and block. Circ Res 1989;64:977.

195. Coulombe A, Coraboeuf E, Malecot C, Deroubaix E: Role of the "Na window" current and other ionic currents in triggering early after-depolarizations and resulting re-excitations in Purkinje fibers. In: Zipes DP, Jalife J, eds. Cardiac electrophysiology and arrhythmias. Orlando, FL: Grune & Stratton, 1985:43–49.

196. Riley DC, Schmeling WT, Al-Wathiqui MH, Kampine JP, Warltier DC: Prolongation of the QT interval by volatile anesthetics in chronically instrumented dogs. Anesth Analg 1988;67:741.

197. Lindgren L: E.C.G. changes during halothane and enflurane anesthesia for E.N.T. surgery in children. Br J Anaesth 1981; 53:653.

198. Schmeling WT, Warltier DC, McDonald DJ, Madsen KE, Atlee JL, Kampine JP: Prolongation of the QT interval by enflurane, isoflurane, and halothane in humans. Anesth Analg 1991; 72:137.

199. Gallagher JD: Effects of halothane and quinidine on intracardiac conduction and QT$_c$ interval in pentobarbital-anesthetized dogs. Anesth Analg 1992;75:688.

200. Escande D, Coraboeuf E, Planche C: Abnormal pacemaking

is modulated by sarcoplasmic reticulum in partially-depolarized myocardium from dilated right atria in humans. J Mol Cell Cardiol 1987;19:231.

201. Mason JW, Stinson EB, Winkle RA, Oyer PE: Mechanisms of ventricular tachycardia: wide complex ignorance. Am Heart J 1981;6:1083.

202. Horowitz LN, Harken AH, Kastor JA, Josephson ME: Ventricular resection guided by epicardial and endocardial mapping for treatment of recurrent ventricular tachycardia. N Engl J Med 1980;302:589.

203. Johannesson GP, Lindahl SGE, Sigurdsson GH, Norden NE: Halothane, enflurane and isoflurane anaesthesia for ade-noidectomy in children, using two different premedications. Acta Anaesthesiol Scand 1987;31:233.

204. Sigurdsson GH, Carlsson C, Lindahl S, Werner O: Cardiac arrhythmias in non-intubated children during adenoidectomy. A comparison between enflurane and halothane anaesthesia. Acta Anaesthesiol Scand 1983;27:75.

205. Barker GL, Briscoe CE: The pathfinder high-speed E.C.G. analysis system: use in detection of arrhythmias during oral surgery. Br J Anaesth 1981;53:1079.

206. Hutchison GL, Davies CA, Main G, Gray IG: Incidence of arrhythmias in dental anaesthesia; a cross-over comparison of halothane and isoflurane. Br J Anaesth 1989;62:518.

Cardiac Arrhythmias, 3rd edition, edited by William J. Mandel.
J. B. Lippincott Company, Philadelphia © 1995.

34

Richard J. Gray

Diagnosis and Management of Arrhythmias in Post–Cardiac Surgical Patients

The high prevalence of certain arrhythmias following open-heart surgery has long been appreciated.[1,2] This occurrence is in addition to any preoperative arrhythmia tendencies that the patient may have. Although uncommonly life-threatening, they definitely add to postoperative morbidity and complicate patient management. Interestingly, the spectrum of atrial and ventricular arrhythmias does not appear to have significantly changed in recent years, despite dramatic increases in patient age, changes in etiology of disease and surgical indications, and improvements in surgical technique and postoperative management.

ATRIAL ARRHYTHMIAS

Frequency and Natural History

Supraventricular tachyarrhythmias occur in 30% of patients following coronary bypass and are even more prevalent in valve procedures, especially in elderly patients undergoing aortic valve replacement for calcific aortic stenosis; in the latter patients the incidence has been reported to be as high as 60%.[3] Atrial fibrillation is the most common of these, followed by atrial flutter, paroxysmal atrial tachycardia, and various junctional rhythms.

Although they can occur at any time during the first 2 or 3 weeks of convalescence,[4] atrial arrhythmias usually appear within the first five postoperative days, with a peak incidence on days 2 and 3.[5] On the basis of ambulatory Holter recordings, postoperative atrial fibrillation may recur during convalescence but rarely does so after 3 weeks and does not presage chronic atrial fibrillation.[6] Certain aspects of the surgical procedure itself are associated with atrial fibrillation, such as anesthesia induction, cannulation of the heart for cardiopulmonary bypass, and attempts to wean from cardiopulmonary bypass. Atrial fibrillation may also occur during rewarming from hypothermia, but at this time the ventricular response rate is usually slower, often in the range of 100 to 120 beats per minute, and most patients will exhibit spontaneous conversion to sinus rhythm without therapy.

The clinical consequences of postoperative atrial tachyarrhythmias vary tremendously. Many patients are asymptomatic with no hemodynamic embarrassment, especially if this problem occurs 4 or 5 days postoperatively. Palpitations may be present, and blood pressure and cardiac output are often maintained at only slightly lower levels than usual while at bed rest. More dramatic physiologic consequences, such as reduction in blood pressure or cardiac output, are seen mostly in patients with tenuous cardiac reserve, which may have depended heavily upon the atrial contribution to cardiac filling. Such is more often the case when atrial fibrillation occurs in the operating room. The patient with partial or incomplete coronary revascularization after coronary bypass surgery is also likely to tolerate atrial fibrillation poorly and experience ischemic chest pain because of the reduction in diastolic coronary filling time associated with the increase in myocardial oxygen consumption. Although stroke is relatively rare after coronary bypass, there appears to be an association with postoperative atrial fibrillation. In a recent study of 453 consecutive patients having coronary artery bypass, stroke or transient ischemic attack occurred in 10 patients (2.2%); postoperative atrial fibrillation occurred in 6 of these 10 (60%), but it was present in only 80 of the 443 (18%) patients who did not have stroke or transient ischemic attack.[7] A similar three- to fourfold increase in risk of stroke associated with postoperative atrial fibrillation was demonstrated by Reed and colleagues,[8] and an approximately twofold increase in stroke rate was reported by Fuller and associates.[5]

Etiology and Electrophysiology

The original circus movement theory (as proposed by Mayer[9] and subsequently Lewis,[10] along with Moe and his colleagues[11]) responsible for the "multiple wavelet" concept remains one of the leading hypotheses explaining atrial fibrillation. Heterogeneity of atrial depolarization results from multiple, small advancing wavefronts of electrical activity surrounding numerous small islands of refractory tissue. Allessie and colleagues provided confirmation and refinement of this concept by demonstrating that multiple wavelets due to intra-atrial reentry of the leading-circle type produce the continuity of impulse conduction during atrial fibrillation.[12] This would suggest that an enlarged atrial size and smaller atrial refractory period increase the likelihood of atrial fibrillation.[13] This has been confirmed in a canine model, where surgically induced atrial enlargement increased the susceptibility to induced atrial tachyarrhythmias.[14] Additional theories include the theory of multiple reentry, the theory of unifocal impulse formation, and the theory of multifocal impulse formation. Electrophysiologic changes in postoperative atrial fibrillation have been well reviewed by Lauer and associates.[15] The electrophysiologic properties of right atrial biopsy tissue were studied in patients undergoing surgery for aortic stenosis. In this study, postoperative atrial fibrillation correlated with abnormal phase 4 depolarization, conduction velocities, and transmembrane action potentials in patients 40 years of age and older.[16]

Four electrophysiologically distinct types of atrial fibrillation were recognized with the use of bipolar atrial recordings in 34 postoperative patients.[17] Type I atrial fibrillation was characterized by discrete atrial complexes and an isoelectric baseline. Type II had discrete complexes that were interspersed with a nonisoelectric baseline. Type III had completely chaotic patterns, and type IV was characterized by a combination of type III with either type I or type II; considerable pattern variability was noted in one half of the patients. It is interesting to speculate that this electrophysiologic nonhomogeneity may explain some of the variability of clinical correlation and the variable response to prophylactic treatment.

The mechanism of atrial flutter may well be similar or identical to that of atrial fibrillation and may well be a circus-movement tachycardia, based upon a dominance of experimental and clinical evidence. Postoperative atrial flutter (and fibrillation) has been succinctly reviewed by Waldo, who has demonstrated the ability to entrain and interrupt atrial flutter.[18] This also provides strong evidence of the intra-atrial reentrant properties of atrial flutter.[19]

In search of a possible cause of postoperative supraventricular tachyarrhythmias, various preoperative and intraoperative variables have been analyzed for possible clinical correlates. In one study, myocardial ischemic time appeared to be related to atrial fibrillation, but advanced age, sex, type and severity of preoperative symptoms, the presence of cardiomegaly, congestive heart failure, previous myocardial infarction, and number of bypass grafts were not significantly related.[20] In another study, however, patients older than 70 years of age who were undergoing aortic valve replacement for aortic stenosis were at more risk for atrial fibrillation, as were those with coexistence of mitral regurgitation or stenosis with significantly elevated pulmonary artery pressures.[3]

More recent studies have confirmed the importance of advanced age as a risk factor. Fuller and coworkers found that in a study of 1666 patients, atrial fibrillation developed in 28.4% of patients, and of all other pre- and postoperative variables, age was the dominant risk factor.[5] Interestingly, postoperative β-blocker therapy tended to offer less protection to the elderly in this series (Fig. 34-1).

Leitch and colleagues examined the records of 5807 patients having isolated coronary bypass and reported that the prevalence of atrial fibrillation (17.2% overall) was directly related to age at operation, varying from 3.7% in patients younger than 40 years of age to 27.7% in those older than 70 years of age.[21] After multivariate analysis, age remained the most important independent predictor of atrial fibrillation. Other important predictors were chronic airflow limitation, preoperative β-blocker use, and chronic renal failure, but not history of previous myocardial infarction, heart size on chest radiograph, or operative factors. In another study of 418 bypass patients,

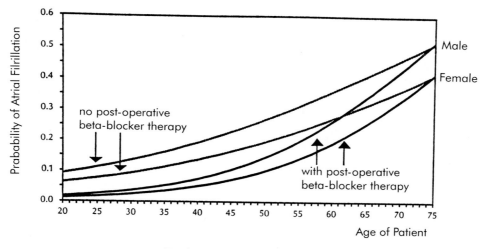

Logistic regression analysis

From Fuller, Adams, Buxton, "Atrial Fibrillation," *Journal of Thoracic and Cardiovascular Surgery*, June 1989

Figure 34-1. Logistic regression analysis in 473 patients showing the relationship of age, gender, and postoperative β-blocker therapy to the development of postoperative atrial fibrillation. This analysis suggests an increasing occurrence of atrial fibrillation with age ($p = 0.0001$), a negative relationship with β-blocker therapy ($p = 0.001$), and an increased occurrence in men ($p = 0.02$). There also appears to be a declining effectiveness of β-blocker therapy with older age ($p = 0.04$). (Fuller JA, Adams GG, Buxton B: Atrial fibrillation after coronary artery bypass grafting. J Thorac Cardiovasc Surg 1989:97:821.)

supraventricular tachyarrhythmias developed in 29% (85% of which were atrial fibrillation). Age was a significant factor, because those with supraventricular tachyarrhythmia were, on average, older (65 ± 8 years) than those without this arrhythmia (61 ± 11 years).[22] This is similar to the long-known age-associated risk of nonsurgical atrial fibrillation.[23, 24] Unfortunately, the age differences of those with and those without atrial fibrillation are narrow, and a logistic model using age is a poor predictor of postoperative atrial fibrillation.[5] The surgical use of the internal thoracic artery is not associated with a lower incidence of atrial fibrillation. In fact, Salem and associates found a higher incidence of postoperative atrial fibrillation associated with male smokers and a greater incidence of pericarditis in a group having myocardial revascularization with the internal thoracic artery compared with a population having revascularization with all saphenous vein grafts.[25]

Quantification of atrial fibrillation risk using three simple preoperative factors is provided in another, very useful study. Compared with control patients, the relative risk of atrial fibrillation is 1.91 in those over 60 years, 2.39 with the addition of cardiomegaly, and 3.47 in those over 60 years with cardiomegaly and left atrial enlargement.[26]

An innovative approach to the identification of those at risk for postoperative atrial fibrillation has been suggested by Lowe and colleagues. They conducted bipolar mid-right atrial alternating current stimulation of 25 μA, increasing until atrial fibrillation was induced (up to a maximum of 200 μA) intraoperatively, before bypass in 50 patients. Postoperative atrial fibrillation occurred in 18 (36%), 17 of whom had inducible atrial fibrillation (sensitivity, 94%). Of the 32 atrial fibrillation–free patients, 13 were not inducible (specificity, 41%).[27] The predictive value of a positive test is high, but the ability to discriminate those at low risk was limited. Such a test may be useful to identify those patients at higher risk of atrial fibrillation to target for aggressive prophylactic treatment.

An increase in postoperative adrenergic tone, as reflected by increases in 24-hour urine epinephrine and norepinephrine excretion[28] and serum levels,[29] coupled in some instances with β-blocker withdrawal, provides an environment most suitable for catecholamine-sensitive tachyarrhythmias. Salazar[30] and White[31] have observed a several-fold increase in atrial tachyarrhythmia incidence in patients in whom β-blockers were discontinued compared with those in whom preoperative β-blockers were continued postoperatively. The mechanism for these observations could be linked to the effects of β-blocker withdrawal on adrenergic tone and β-adrenergic receptor density.[32–34] Although the prophylactic benefits of β-blockers in this setting are somewhat variable, as discussed in a subsequent section of this chapter, their beneficial nature[35, 36] tends to support the pathophysiologic role of increased adrenergic tone in postoperative supraventricular tachyarrhythmias.

Postoperative pericarditis parallels the incidence of atrial tachyarrhythmias temporally and has long been a suspected cause, although the association of nonsurgical atrial fibrillation with pericarditis implies additional cardiac disease.[37]

During cardiopulmonary bypass, preservation of cardiac integrity is heavily dependent upon hypothermia. Atrial hypothermia is more difficult to achieve during cardiopulmonary bypass and has been suspected as a cause of postoperative atrial fibrillation.[38] In an animal model, experimentally produced ischemic injury of the supraventricular conduction system during hypothermic cardiopulmonary bypass has been associated with conduction delay within the atrioventricular (AV) node. Better hypothermia with use of intracavitary and special topical cooling techniques was able to prevent this type of conduction defect.[39] In other animal studies, investigators have corroborated the inadequacy of atrial preservation by demonstration of persistent electrical activity within the AV junctional area, and improvement of the likelihood of early postoperative sinus rhythm in animals, in which persistent electrical activity was abolished with special efforts to cool the right atrioventricular junction area.[40]

The occurrence of frequent premature atrial complexes is an excellent predictor of the development of atrial fibrillation or flutter. Also, when asked to recall an event that may have triggered the atrial fibrillation, patients may remember an episode of coughing, sneezing, or respiratory therapy. Inhalation therapy with or without the use of bronchodilators has been suspected as a factor in the development of atrial fibrillation but has never been confirmed because both occurrences are so common after surgery.

Prophylaxis

Preoperative digitalization (1 to 1.5 mg orally beginning 2 to 3 days prior to surgery) resulted in a much lower incidence of supraventricular tachyarrhythmias (5.5%) than in a control group (26%) in one study.[41] A similar reduction in the incidence of supraventricular tachyarrhythmia was noted in another study using postoperative digitalization (2% versus 15%).[42] Others using preoperative digitalization were unable to confirm this benefit; in fact, one study demonstrated a higher incidence of postoperative tachyarrhythmia in the treated group (27.8%) versus that of the untreated group (11.4%).[43]

Many other attempts at prevention of postoperative atrial arrhythmias have included various beta-blocking agents. The benefits of propranolol in postoperative atrial tachycardias were appreciated more than two decades ago.[44] There have been numerous studies demonstrating successful prevention of postoperative supraventricular tachyarrhythmias using propranolol begun postoperatively,[35,36,45,46] and one study using preoperative administration of propranolol.[47] The results and doses used are summarized in Table 34-1.[48] This otherwise successful picture is clouded somewhat by the finding, in one double-blind randomized study, that 80 mg daily of propranolol was not effective in reducing the incidence of supraventricular tachyarrhythmia.[48] The dose employed in this latter study was larger than that in the other studies demonstrating efficacy of propranolol. Another study using propranolol 10 mg t.i.d. after surgery also demonstrated no improvement over control patients.[49] Protection against atrial arrhythmias was demonstrated for timolol (0.5 mg intravenously twice daily),[50] as well as acebutolol, a cardioselective beta blocker,[51] nadolol,[52] metoprolol, and sotalol.[53,54] Combinations of postoperative digoxin and propranolol were also found to be effective in reducing the incidence of postoperative supraventricular tachyarrhythmia in two studies.[55,56]

Verapamil 40 mg three times daily begun postoperatively was not successful in prevention of supraventricular arrhythmias,[20] and in a separate study, 80 mg every 6 hours was beneficial in slowing the ventricular response but did not prevent atrial fibrillation and resulted in an unacceptably high incidence of hypotension, pulmonary edema, or cardiogenic shock.[57]

Flecainide (300 to 400 mg/day) was successful alone or when given with amiodarone in 32 of 40 nonsurgical patients with resistant, paroxysmal atrial fibrillation.[58] Also, in nonsurgical patients, others have found that flecainide is beneficial in preventing atrial fibrillation or flutter recurrence in 50% to 65% of patients for 3 to 9

TABLE 34-1. Summary of Effects of Propranolol on Postoperative SVT

Drug	Time Started	Incidence of SVT (%)	
		Control Group	Treatment Group
Propranolol (40 mg)	18 hr postop	18	8
Propranolol (20–40 mg)	6 hr postop	40	5
Propranolol (60 mg)	2 days postop	28	2.2
Digoxin	1 day preop		

SVT, supraventricular tachycardia.
Modified from Ivey MF, Ivey TD, Bailey WW, et al: Influence of propranolol on supraventricular tachycardia early after coronary artery revascularization. J Thorac Cardiovasc Surg 1983;85:214.

months provided they are able to tolerate the drug.[59, 60] This may have been due to an increase in the fibrillation threshold resulting from flecainide.[61] In any case, the future role of this drug is uncertain based on excessive cardiac deaths associated with this agent when used to treat post–myocardial infarction ventricular ectopia, as reported in the Cardiac Arrhythmia Survival Trial (CAST).[62]

Perioperative treatment with magnesium appears to lessen the incidence of postoperative atrial fibrillation. In a group of patients given magnesium sulfate intravenously (4 mEq/hour for the first 24 hours and 1 mEq/hour up to 96 hours), using a randomized, placebo-controlled protocol, atrial fibrillation was noted in approximately one half as many patients, and the total number of episodes was reduced to approximately one fourth compared with that associated with placebo treatment.[63]

Alinidine has demonstrated dramatic effectiveness in prevention of postoperative atrial fibrillation in a small, randomized, prospective study.[64] A derivative of clonidine, this agent has a selective bradycardic effect on the sinus node, independent of beta-adrenergic properties.

The majority of studies favor the use of small doses of propranolol or another beta blocker, preferably started before surgery, for prophylaxis of supraventricular arrhythmias in the postoperative cardiovascular surgical patient. This is especially true in individuals taking beta-blocking agents preoperatively. The author's experience with arrhythmia prophylaxis using both pre- and postoperative digitalization regimens, as well as postoperative propranolol, has been disappointing. Consequently, it is my policy to begin medical therapy at the development of the arrhythmia or at the appearance of frequent atrial premature complexes. Another useful approach would be to limit prophylaxis to those at highest risk on the basis of age, cardiomegaly, and left atrial enlargement.

Medical Management

Digitalization is the first line of therapy and is indicated at the time of appearance of frequent atrial premature complexes or the development of atrial tachyarrhythmias if the ventricular response rate is faster than 100 beats per minute. The dosing regimen depends on initial heart rate, clinical tolerance of the arrhythmia, patient age, body size, and renal function. With moderately rapid ventricular response rates (130–150 beats per minute) in a patient aged 60 to 70 years with normal renal function, 1.0 to 1.5 mg administered over 24 hours is often successful. During the loading phase, the intravenous route is recommended to ensure rapid and complete absorption. By the end of the loading phase, conversion to sinus rhythm usually has occurred, but if not, additional incremental doses of di-

goxin (total 0.5 mg) can be administered up to a total of 2.0 mg in 36 hours. The end point of digoxin administration, in addition to return to sinus rhythm, will be to control heart rate (i.e., 100–110 beats per minute or less). Additional supplementation with intravenous propranolol in 1-mg doses is occasionally needed for more complete slowing of the heart rate. Intravenous verapamil in a dose of 5 to 10 mg is effective in slowing the ventricular response rate in most patients and is associated with return to sinus rhythm in approximately 20% of patients.[65] Intravenous verapamil has occasionally been associated with hypotension, which can be lessened by a slower infusion rate and can be aborted by previous administration of calcium chloride.[66] Diltiazem has also demonstrated efficacy in reduction of the ventricular response rate in atrial tachyarrhythmias via inhibition of AV node conduction.[67]

Esmolol, an ultrashort-acting I.V. beta-blocking agent, has demonstrated effectiveness in controlling the heart rate during postoperative supraventricular tachyarrhythmia.[68] The incidence of conversion to sinus rhythm with esmolol is better than that with placebo and possibly superior to that with other agents such as verapamil and diltiazem.

If return to sinus rhythm has not occurred after these measures have been used, the next step is selection of a type I antiarrhythmic, such as quinidine sulfate or procainamide hydrochloride. Oral quinidine sulfate 200 to 300 mg every 2 to 6 hours has been a traditional approach to the medical conversion of supraventricular tachyarrhythmias. Intravenous procainamide hydrochloride has demonstrated effectiveness in acute termination of atrial fibrillation and flutter when given as a loading dose of 10 to 20 mg/kg followed by a maintenance infusion of 2 to 4 mg/minute.[69]

In one study, intravenous propafenone (2 mg/kg) slowed the ventricular response rate and resulted in conversion to sinus rhythm in 43% of patients, in contrast to placebo, which resulted in no conversion.[70]

In a nonsurgical population, flecainide also resulted in conversion to sinus rhythm in 71% of patients studied.[71]

Amiodarone, popular in Europe but often reserved for life-threatening ventricular arrhythmias in the United States, has demonstrated its efficacy in conversion of resistant chronic atrial fibrillation and maintenance of sinus rhythm, with success rates of 53% to 97%.[72–79]

In surgical patients, intravenous amiodarone in a dose of 2.5 to 5 mg/kg (via central I.V.) has been moderately successful in conversion to sinus rhythm or slowing of the ventricular response rate.[80] However, the slow onset of action of this important agent will limit its use to the more resistant cases in this clinical setting.

The above comments apply to the management of atrial fibrillation, whereas therapy directed toward control of atrial flutter may require a different response. Digoxin remains indicated as the drug of first choice; however, doses effective for atrial fibrillation may not appreciably increase AV blockade. The initial AV conduction ratio is commonly 2:1, resulting in a typical ventricular response of 150 beats per minute. In the presence of AV nodal conduction abnormalities or pretreatment with digoxin, the ventricular rate may be slower as a result of a 3:1 or 4:1 conduction ratio. Loading doses of digoxin varying from 1.5 to 2.0 mg are often necessary and even then may result in unpredictable and often disappointingly minor slowing of ventricular response rate. By the time AV blockade occurs, patients may exhibit signs or symptoms suggestive of digoxin toxicity. Consequently, beta blockers such as esmolol and calcium channel blockers such as verapamil and diltiazem have an important role in slowing the ventricular response. Once an arbitrary initial digitalization dose has been reached (generally 1.5 to 2.0 mg), or when the clinical picture suggests digoxin toxicity, esmolol at a dose of 0.5 mg/kg over 1 minute with a titrated maintenance infusion, or beta blockade using I.V. propranolol (0.05 to 0.10 mg/kg) given in increments of 1 mg by slow intravenous bolus injection, may also slow the ventricular response rate. Verapamil at a dose of 5 to 10 mg given intravenously over 1 minute is indicated; verapamil may also be used as a constant infusion. These pharmacologic maneuvers are usually successful in rapidly slowing the ventricular response rate. The results may be transient, thereby requiring repeat administration or constant infusion. Moreover, conversion to sinus rhythm occurs in a relative minority of cases.

Paroxysmal atrial tachycardia related to AV nodal reentry and ectopic atrial rhythms are much less common. Traditionally, the first steps include sedation, if the patient is agitated, often followed by carotid sinus massage. In the absence of preexcitation or AV nodal bypass tract–associated tachyarrhythmia, such as Wolff-Parkinson-White syndrome, as in the nonsurgical variety, management usually includes I.V. verapamil or digitalization, or both, which results in a high likelihood of conversion to sinus rhythm. Experience with intravenous adenosine triphosphate has been very successful, making it one of the most popular agents for reentrant AV nodal tachycardia in the nonsurgical population. This naturally occurring high-energy phosphate, when given as a rapid bolus of 20 mg intravenously, blocked the antegrade slow pathway through the AV node, rapidly terminating paroxysmal atrial tachycardia in all patients tested.[81, 82]

Elective Cardioversion

This treatment is reserved for drug treatment failures. It is uncommon for post–coronary bypass patients with no previous history of atrial arrhythmias to require this mo-dality. Cardioversion is more commonly used in patients undergoing valve surgery, especially mitral valve replacement, where atrial fibrillation, once established, becomes difficult to revert medically.

If atrial fibrillation is chronic and has been established for more than one year preoperatively, aggressive attempts, including cardioversion, are not generally recommended because of the high likelihood of relapse. An exception to this is the patient who exhibits several hours of sinus rhythm immediately after return from the operating room. Elective cardioversion may be used if aggressive medical measures fail, including digoxin (if indicated by the presence of a rapid ventricular response rate) and quinidine or Pronestyl. The principal risk of cardioversion, thromboembolism, is approximately 0.5%.

At the author's institution, this procedure is performed in a unit that is equipped for bedside electrocardiographic monitoring. That morning's digoxin dose is held and, if toxicity is clinically suspected, a serum digoxin level is obtained. A serum potassium level should be obtained the morning of cardioversion, and the patient should be kept at NPO for at least 6 hours prior to the procedure. A well-running intravenous line is essential. Oxygen, 4–6 L by mask, is used, and a "crash cart" with intubation equipment and ambu bag is in the patient's room. I prefer the extremely short-acting effects of Brevital, and arrange to have the patient's anesthesiologist available for administration of the sedative/analgesic and management of the airway. The safety factor thus provided more than outweighs the small added inconvenience of arranging for an additional physician. Anterior and posterior paddles (placed just beneath the tip of the left scapula) are preferred for atrial fibrillation. Premedication with I.V. lidocaine (50–100 mg) is available but not routinely given. Atropine is available for immediate use. The synchronization function is carefully checked.

Direct current shock is then delivered and increased in a stepwise fashion if needed. Initial shocks are in the low range (i.e., 25–50 W) to assess possible induction of ventricular arrhythmias. If atrial fibrillation does not convert at maximum power setting, anterior paddles are then used at maximum power setting.

Anticoagulation for cardioversion to terminate a brief period (3 to 4 days) of postoperative atrial fibrillation is not routinely practiced.

Overdrive Pacing

Atrial flutter and paroxysmal supraventricular tachycardia (PSVT) are often readily terminated by rapid stimulation of the atrium, using surgically implanted epicardial pacemaker wires. Atrial flutter must be differentiated from atrial fibrillation, which is not amenable to overdrive pacing. As discussed above, four types of atrial fibrillation can be recognized by atrial bipolar electrocardiograms. It is possible that type I atrial fibrillation with discrete but irregular atrial activity on epicardial right atrial bipolar recordings, with an isoelectric baseline interspersed between them, could be confused with flutter. Type II fibrillation has similar discrete atrial activity but with no isoelectric portion. Atrial flutter–fibrillation usually refers to atrial flutter waves on the surface electrocardiogram, but with irregular ventricular conduction as opposed to a predictable conduction ratio (2:1, 3:1, or 4:1) in typical atrial flutter. Flutter–fibrillation is not amenable to overdrive pacing; it represents either a form of type I or type II atrial fibrillation or, as has been witnessed in the operating room and in the experimental animal, flutter of the right atrium and fibrillation of the left atrium. Other variations of flutter include "atrial impure" flutter with faster atrial rates (>350) and coarse atrial fibrillation with atrial flutter rates (>400).[83] Both have slightly irregular flutter cycles and represent atypical atrial flutter, which is not usually amenable to overdrive pacing.

Overdrive pacing should always be performed with a bedside monitor and with a rhythm strip (multiple leads if possible, i.e., I, AVF, V_1) to determine the success of atrial capture and arrhythmia termination.

A pacing rate is selected just below the spontaneous rate and is increased at increments of 10 beats per minute until capture is obtained. This usually requires a rate 10 beats faster than the spontaneous atrial rate, and successful entrainment of the flutter rhythm requires a gradual increase in rate until the flutter waves become positive in orientation, as monitored in standard ECG lead II (Fig. 34-2).[84] Once atrial flutter has been entrained, sinus rhythm will ensue following abrupt cessation of pacing. If atrial flutter has been intermittently recurrent, control of the atrial mechanism may require short-term continuous atrial pacing, which can be achieved by gradual reduction of the atrial pacing rate to the appropriate physiologic level for that patient. Continuous atrial pacing in this mode over several hours may prevent the recurrence of atrial flutter or even fibrillation.

Failure to convert atrial flutter can be due to a number of factors. First, if the ventricular response rate is irregular, the diagnosis is not typical atrial flutter, and overdrive pacing usually will not succeed. A broken pacemaker wire or loss of contact with the epicardial surface will also result in failure, but if only one such wire is broken, unipolar pacing can be attempted using an electrode patch close to the functional wire exit on the skin surface as an indifferent lead. Insufficient stimulus strength is occasionally a problem because the threshold for capture may have risen to high levels, especially several days after surgery. The threshold will occasionally be above 20 mA, which is above the capacity of most commercially available pace-

Atrial Electrograms

Bipolar

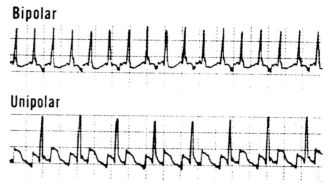

Unipolar

Figure 34-2. ECG leads II and III recorded from a patient with atrial flutter exhibiting 2:1 AV conduction. The atrial rate is 300 beats/minute. The black dots mark the onset of atrial pacing at the rate of 305 beats/minute. The atrial complexes become positive with nothing indicating capture. In panel B, the circle indicates termination of 30 seconds of rapid atrial pacing, allowing resumption of normal sinus rhythm. (MacLean, et al. Cardiovasc Med 1978;3:965.)

makers. A standard commercially available rapid atrial stimulator (i.e., Medtronics model 5375/2312) can be modified to deliver 25 to 28 mA. It should be noted that stimulus strength above 20 mA almost always results in symptomatic awareness, although it is usually tolerable for brief periods of time once the rationale has been explained to the patient. Finally, a weak pacemaker battery or inadequate contact between the leads and pacemaker must also be excluded.

Successful transvenous overdrive pacing of the right atrium for conversion of postoperative atrial flutter was reported in 21 of 25 patients who did not have functional epicardial atrial pacing wires.[85]

Often, additional dosing with digoxin, quinidine, or procainamide, or simply the passage of time, will ensure greater success. Consequently, repeated attempts at overdrive pacing should be tried until successful. The atrial arrhythmia will likely continue or recur as long as the stimulus responsible for it continues. Thus, it is almost always necessary to continue therapy with digoxin, and occasionally with beta blockers or type I antiarrhythmics as well, despite the success or failure of overdrive pacing.

Rapid atrial overdrive may occasionally precipitate atrial fibrillation. Because the ventricular response rate is often slower than in atrial flutter, this may be a desirable alternative and can usually be achieved by pacing the atria at rates of 450 beats per minute or higher for 10 to 20 seconds. Atrial overdrive can be used to reduce the ventricular response in atrial flutter despite failure to reach sinus rhythm. With rapid overdrive pacing at 400 beats per minute, for instance, the atrial conduction may be reduced from 2:1 at 150 beats per minute (atrial rate 300 beats per minute) to 4:1 at 100 beats per minute.

Bipolar atrial electrograms can be recorded by attaching one epicardial lead to each of the two arm leads of the ECG patient cable using an alligator clip. By recording standard lead I on the lead selector, the bipolar atrial electrogram is recorded, because standard lead I records between right and left arm leads. By selecting lead II or III, unipolar atrial electrograms can be recorded. Similarly, unipolar electrograms can be recorded by attaching the patient cables to the appropriate limbs, but attaching the atrial electrodes to the precordial patient lead and recording with the selector in the V lead. Because bipolar atrial electrograms record electrical activity only within the tissue subtended between their placement on the heart, limited or no ventricular activity will be seen in such a recording. Because the unipolar technique records the potential difference between a single atrial electrode and an indifferent electrode distant from the heart, both atrial and ventricular electrical activity will be recorded. This type of recording is useful when the relationship between atrial and ventricular events is important. The bipolar electrogram technique, however, when viewed with a simultaneous surface electrocardiogram, is actually the preferred technique because it allows clear-cut differentiation of the atrial and ventricular origins of signals and their relationship with each other (Fig. 34-3).[86]

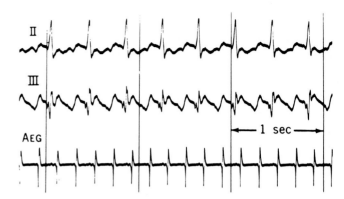

Figure 34-3. Simultaneous bipolar and unipolar atrial electrogram recording in patients with atrial flutter at a rate of 280 beats/minute and 2:1 AV conduction. The right and left arm leads are each attached to one of the atrial electrodes. To record a bipolar tracing from a single channel recording, standard lead I is selected; to record unipolar tracing, standard lead II or III is selected. (Waldo AL, MacLean WAH, eds. Diagnosis and treatment of cardiac arrhythmias following open heart surgery. Mount Kisco, NY: Futura, 1980:25.)

VENTRICULAR ARRHYTHMIAS

Ventricular ectopia, including nonsustained ventricular tachycardia, requiring at least a short course of therapy is seen early during convalescence in up to 50% of patients after open-heart surgery. This pattern occurs, paradoxically enough, despite apparent correction of myocardial ischemia, which is believed to be a trigger for ectopia. As with atrial tachyarrhythmias, the incidence is particularly high in the operating room during induction of anesthesia, during cannulation for cardiopulmonary bypass, with early weaning from bypass, and during the rewarming period. An especially high incidence is also noted beginning the third and fourth postoperative day. The reported incidence varies with the intensity of monitoring employed; with continuous ambulatory monitoring, a 57% incidence of complex ventricular arrhythmias (Lown grades 4 and 5) was detected in one study.[87] Although the mechanism and prognosis of postoperative ventricular arrhythmias are not well understood, those occurring in the setting of ischemic heart disease and coronary bypass surgery have been studied to a slightly greater degree.

In a given patient, ventricular arrhythmias are more frequent after surgery, at least within the first 6 or 8 weeks,

than they were preoperatively. Furthermore, exercise-induced ventricular ectopia is not reduced, and opinion is divided about whether there is an actual increase in such arrhythmias, despite successful revascularization.[88–90] Exercise ventricular ectopia has been linked to extensive coronary disease, a lower resting ejection fraction, and more than 2 mm of ischemic sinus tachycardia (ST) depression.[91] Continuation or new appearance of exercise-induced ventricular arrhythmias, when noted after successful revascularization, is associated with severe wall motion abnormalities and residual postoperative ischemic ST depression.[91]

Potential mechanisms that must be considered include the impact of elevated catecholamine levels, which are known to persist for several days after surgery, the occurrence of clinical or subclinical myocardial necrosis, and the effects of electrolyte abnormalities and postoperative digitalis administration. Surprisingly, serum magnesium levels are no lower in the presence of postoperative ventricular ectopia[92] or resumption of sinus rhythm immediately after cardiopulmonary bypass.[93] An intriguing finding is the suggestion that atrial and ventricular arrhythmias are associated with reduced red blood cell deformability as a result of cardiopulmonary bypass.[94]

Natural History

Studies on the natural history of postoperative ventricular ectopia are conflicting. One study found that even single premature ventricular contractions (PVCs) on a resting electrocardiogram were a prediction of poor outcome after bypass,[95] whereas a more recent study showed no difference in survival based on the presence or absence of complex ventricular ectopia on ambulatory monitoring in a postbypass population highly selected for normal preoperative ventricular function.[87]

Low-amplitude electrical activity at the terminus of the QRS (late potentials), as detected by signal-averaged electrocardiography, appears to have prognostic value regarding future risk of serious ventricular arrhythmia in the nonsurgical patient.[96] For instance, such findings are seen less often after successful thrombolysis treatment in acute myocardial infarction (MI).[97]

Until more conclusive data emerge, a responsible approach to treatment should be based on lessons learned from a nonsurgical population and individualized on the basis of known or suspected risk factors and the patient's past medical history. For instance, high-grade ventricular ectopia in the presence of ventricular dysfunction or segmental wall motion defects, recent MI, or recent appearance of ectopia would suggest a higher risk of untoward outcome, especially when late potentials are present. Similarly, a history of sudden cardiac death, sustained ventricular tachycardia, or fibrillation would impose higher risk and warrant more aggressive therapy.

Persistent frequent ventricular ectopia of ≥ 6 per minute should begin to arouse concern. This activity can often be suppressed by atrial pacing. This is accomplished by progressively increasing the pacing rate until the desired level of suppression is seen. However, it is rare to see benefits with pacing rates of >110 beats per minute.

With the new appearance of ventricular ectopia, surveillance for a metabolic or other inciting cause should be routine and initiated promptly. This would include, at minimum, measurement of serum potassium, blood count, and assessment of oxygenation status, using either arterial blood gas or noninvasive oximetry. The yield in this search will likely be low, but it should be kept in mind that in comparison with the nonsurgical patient, such abnormalities are much more common and are more poorly tolerated in the post–cardiac surgical patient, and the potential risk of missing such eminently treatable metabolic abnormalities can be high.

Management

Prophylactic treatment with lidocaine may reduce the incidence of nonsustained ventricular tachycardia, but there were no significant differences in other forms of ventricular ectopia, morbidity, or mortality in a small randomized, blinded trial in post–coronary bypass patients.[98]

The decision to initiate intravenous treatment is usually based on the occurrence of frequent or high-grade ventricular ectopia (usually >6 PVCs per minute, R-on-T phenomenon, frequent couplets, or multiform ectopia) or

when therapy is likely to be needed for only a short duration. For instance, even in the absence of metabolic factors, brief periods of high-grade ventricular ectopia may occur during the first 4 or 5 days after surgery. Intravenous therapy for as little as 12 hours may be followed by complete freedom from serious ventricular ectopia for the remainder of the hospital course.

Initiation of intravenous lidocaine with changeover to an oral agent is indicated when ventricular ectopia persists despite continued lidocaine, or when preoperative high-grade ectopia returns, and reinstitution of therapy with an oral agent alone is not sufficiently prompt.

Lidocaine is traditionally administered as a bolus (1 mg/kg) followed by a maintenance infusion of 2 to 4 mg/minute, although higher bolus doses of 2 to 3 mg/kg have been used intraoperatively. Dosing and pharmacology are basically similar to those of the nonsurgical patient. The principal side effects of disorientation and agitation are typically seen in older individuals and those with diminished liver function, usually in the setting of low cardiac output and diminished liver blood flow, and they do not appear to be more frequent in the postoperative patient.

As an alternative, or in addition to lidocaine when it alone is not successful in ectopia suppression, intravenous Pronestyl hydrochloride can also be used. An initial loading dose of 5 to 10 mg/kg (30–50 mg/minute infusion rate) is followed by a maintenance infusion of 2 to 3 mg/minute.

Initiation of therapy with an oral agent alone is indicated when the initial presentation is noncomplex ectopia, such as frequent singular ectopics or bigeminy, and when therapy is likely to be long term, such as with a history of preoperative arrhythmia. For patients in whom antiarrhythmic therapy had been used prior to surgery, it is wise to restart the same agent as long as it was well tolerated and seemingly effective. Although many newer agents are now available for oral use, procainamide and quinidine preparations remain extremely popular. Table 34-2 summarizes prescribing indications, dosages, and side effects of these and newer antiarrhythmics.[99] It should be noted that amiodarone, because of its potential serious side effects, is usually reserved for life-threatening arrhythmias refractory to other agents.

Treatment of ventricular tachycardia is often initiated with lidocaine, especially if it is nonsustained. Sustained ventricular tachycardia will also respond, and lidocaine can be used as long as relative hemodynamic stability is maintained. If resistant or recurrent ventricular tachycardia occurs despite lidocaine, bretylium may be used. Therapy is begun with a loading dose of 5 to 10 mg/kg given over 30 minutes, followed by an infusion of 1 to 4 mg/minute. As with Pronestyl hydrochloride, hypotension is the major side effect, in this case resulting from the vasodilating properties of bretylium. Polymorphous ventricular tachycardia, a particularly resistant form of ventricular

TABLE 34-2. Indications, Dosages, and Side Effects of Antiarrhythmic Drugs

Drug	Dose	Effective Serum Concentration	Side Effects	Route of Metabolism
Quinidine sulfate	200–700 mg every 6 hr	2–6 µg/mL	Diarrhea, cramps, thrombocytopenia, fever, CNS depression, proarrhythmia	Hepatic primary, renal secondary
Quinidine gluconate	330–660 mg every 6–8 hr	2–6 µg/mL	Similar to quinidine sulfate	Hepatic primary, renal secondary
Procainamide	250–1000 mg every 4 hr	4–10 µg/mL	Gastric upset, fever, arthralgias, lupus-like syndrome, proarrhythmia agranulocytosis	Hepatic primary, renal secondary
Procan SR	500–2000 mg every 6 hr	4–10 mg/100 mL	Similar to procainamide, agranulocytosis	Hepatic primary, renal secondary
Mexiletine	150–300 mg every 8 hr	0.5–2.0 mg/100 mL	Gastric upset, confusion, agitation, CNS depression, nausea	Hepatic
Tocainide	200–800 mg every 8 hr	3.5–10 mg/100 mL	Gastric upset, confusion, CNS depression, nausea	Renal primary, hepatic secondary
Flecainide	50–200 mg every 12 hr	200–1000 mg/mL	Blood dyscrasias, bone marrow depression	—
Amiodarone	200-800 mg per day	1.0–2.5 mg/100 mL	Pulmonary fibrosis, hypo- and hyperthyroidism, skin pigmentation, corneal deposits, myocardial depression, neurologic symptoms	Unknown

Modified from Gray R, Mandel W: Management of common postoperative arrhythmias. In: Gray R, Matloff J, eds. Medical management of the cardiac surgical patient. Baltimore: Williams & Wilkins, 1990.

tachycardia known as torsades de pointes, is characterized by a QRS pattern that meanders above and below the baseline. It is occasionally seen after surgery and is most commonly the result of toxicity or adverse reaction to a drug, usually an antiarrhythmic such as quinidine sulfate or procainamide. The initial approach is to stop any offending medication. The usual therapy for ventricular tachycardia is suggested but may be ineffective. Ventricular pacing at a rapid rate is most often helpful, and the addition of intravenous isoproterenol infusion is also indicated if other therapy fails. Bolus injection of I.V. magnesium sulfate (500–1000 mg) has become routine and may be helpful.

Therapy for ventricular fibrillation begins with rapid defibrillation followed by CPR measures if needed.

Conduction Disturbances

Intraventricular (Fascicular) Conduction Defects

The early postoperative appearance of fascicular conduction defects, including right bundle branch block, left anterior superior fascicular block (and combinations of the two), left bundle branch block, and interventricular conduction delay of unspecified type, occurs with moderate frequency (3%–5%). Although an adverse long-term prognosis is ascribed to left bundle branch block and nonspecific interventricular conduction delay, postoperative bundle branch block has no immediate clinical impact, and specific treatment is not needed.

Heart Block

Sinus Node Exit Block

Sinus node exit block is an uncommon inability of the electrical impulse to reach the atrium despite normal formation within the sinus node. This is recognized by failure of the P wave to appear at the anticipated time, resulting in a dropped P wave. This may occur in either a random manner or a recurring pattern. Observation of a dropped P wave is consistent with sinoatrial (SA) block if the P-to-P interval is a multiple of the P-P wave in normal sinus rhythm. For instance, a pause of exactly twice the usual P-to-P interval identifies a 2:1 SA exit block. Wenckebach periodicity of sinus node exit block may also occur. This is also identified by the dropping of the P wave with progressively shortening P-P intervals preceding the longest P-to-P interval, which includes the dropped P wave. Possible causes of this condition include intrinsic disease of the sinus node, traumatic injury of this region during surgery, increased vagal tone, excessive drug effect due to digoxin, beta-blocker, and calcium channel blocker therapy, and type I antiarrhythmic agents. If these drugs are present, blood level assessment is indicated. Treatment consists of reduction in dosage or discontinuation, if possible, of any offending agents. Epicardial atrial pacing is needed only in the unlikely event of frequent dropped beats; permanent pacemaker implantation is rarely needed.

Atrioventricular Conduction Disturbances

First-Degree Block

This is identified when the PR interval exceeds the upper limits of normal, which for adults is 0.20 seconds. Possible causes include internodal delay, AV node delay, and delay through the bundle of His. These changes can be due to fibrosis of the AV node, or toxicity or excessive effect with agents such as digoxin, beta-blocking, and calcium channel blocking agents, as well as quinidine and Pronestyl. Following cardiac surgery, it occurs transiently after valve replacement because of edema of the AV node region and is rarely the result of the surgical anatomic disruption.

Second-Degree AV Block

Mobitz type I, or Wenckebach AV, block is recognized as progressive prolongation of the PR interval until AV conduction fails, resulting in the absence of a QRS following a normal P wave, following which the PR interval is again short with repetition of the same sequence. This repetitious process can be recognized by a pattern of QRS appearance referred to as "group beating." Although the PR interval progressively lengthens, the R-to-R interval decreases, resulting in the shortest R-to-R interval just preceding the dropped ventricular beat.

Mobitz Type II Block

This refers to the failure of electrical impulse conduction through the AV node not preceded by a progressive lengthening of the PR interval. This may be represented by sporadic dropped single beats or a predictable pattern of AV block in which the dropped beats occur as a multiple of the atrial rate (e.g., 2:1, 3:1, or 4:1). Neither Mobitz type I nor type II AV block is rare in the immediate postoperative period, especially following valve replacement. It is extremely common to see all forms of AV blockade in the minutes following intraoperative washout of hyperkalemic myocardial preservation solution.

A vigorous search for offending drug effects or toxicity is in order with discontinuation of any but the most essential ones. Depending on the degree of AV blockade and the consequent heart rate, as well as the potential adequacy of lower escape rhythms, pacing may be needed. Because the condition is often transient, this is an ideal indication for epicardial ventricular pacing.

Complete AV Block

This condition is recognized by atrial activity that is faster than ventricular activity, in the absence of any predictable relationship between the two. As noted above, this is the expected consequence of cardioplegia washout during the first postoperative minutes, and occasionally is the consequence of antiarrhythmic drug therapy or toxicity. When noted as a specific result of the surgical procedure itself, it most often follows valve replacement, but it is transient in a majority of such patients. When due to the trauma of surgical manipulation in the area of the AV node or bundle of His, the condition may be temporary but often lasts several days. Inadvertent surgical transection of conduction tissue during valve excision and repair is also a well-known complication, obviously leading to permanent AV blockade.

Varying degrees of AV block are more common after aortic valve replacement than with other types of cardiac surgery. The initial observation reported complete heart block in 13% of patients.[100] A clinicopathologic study of these cases demonstrated that because of the proximity of the main bundle of His, a "danger zone" exists in the region of the noncoronary cusp and its adjacent portion of right coronary above the junction of the membranous and muscular septum below. Calcium debridement or deep suture placement in this zone was more likely to produce complete heart block.[100] On a more positive side, improvement in preoperative AV blockade after aortic valve replacement has also been described in over 20% of patients.[101] Improvement seen as late as 18 months after surgery is largely associated with improvement in left ventricular performance, implying that stretching of conduction tissue may have been an important mechanism.[101] Another important cause is inadequate atrial preservation during cardiopulmonary bypass. This has been suggested by the finding in animals of conduction delay, primarily in the AV node area, reversed by careful atrial preservation.

As with incomplete AV block, therapy depends on the underlying heart rate and adequacy of ventricular escape mechanism (a narrow complex rapid rate being preferable to a wide complex slower rate). Discontinuation of all potentially offending drugs, including digitalis, even when used in small, nontoxic doses, is suggested. Epicardial ventricular pacing is usually instituted when pacing wires are present if the underlying heart rate is inadequate.

The need for a permanent pacemaker is predicated upon the severity and permanence of any surgical trauma to the conduction system. The likelihood of recovering sinus rhythm is difficult to predict, but factors weighing against recovery include a heavily calcified AV node or aortic valve ring with extension into the septum, the appearance of AV block hours (or days) after surgery, and, to a lesser degree, a significant preoperative conduction defect. In the absence of excessive calcification, optimism is usually warranted, especially if the escape rhythm exhibits a narrow QRS complex with good rate. Under these conditions it is realistic to wait for up to 2 weeks before implanting a permanent pacemaker.

EPICARDIAL PACEMAKER ELECTRODES

Operative insertion of commercially available temporary epicardial pacemaker electrodes is a commonly used technique. Paired placement on the right atrium and right ventricle enhances diagnostic capability and allows pacing of any type of hemodynamically important bradycardia, as well as performance of overdrive atrial pacing. When their value is fully appreciated, they are used often enough to warrant routine use in all cases, especially in valve replacement, where they can be life-saving.

Care and Handling

Although electrical hazard remains a potential problem with epicardial pacemaking wires, in the author's experience with over 6000 such patients, this has never actually been identified as a complication. When unused, they are kept wrapped in a clean, dry, electrically isolated dressing, using the cap from a hypodermic needle.

Removal is usually planned for the day prior to discharge and is accomplished with gentle, steady traction. Resistance to removal is often overcome by leaving the wire on gentle traction for 1 to 2 hours. On the occasions where removal is not possible, the wire is pulled as far outward as possible and under sterile conditions is cut and allowed to retract deeply beneath the skin. Rare instances of late, recurrent infection due to a retained electrode have been identified as a consequence of incomplete retraction.

When the patient is on Coumadin, cessation of therapy to allow the prothrombin time to reach 50% activity prior to wire removal is suggested. All patients should be kept at bed rest for 2 hours after removal.

References

1. MacCuish RK: Cardiac arrhythmias following mitral valvulotomy. Acta Med Scand 1958;160:125.
2. Burback B, Schwedel JB, Young D: The role of digitalis in mitral valvuloplasty. Am Heart J 1957;54:863.
3. Douglas P, Hirshfeld JW, Edmunds LH: Clinical correlates of postoperative atrial fibrillation. Circulation 1984;70(4) (suppl II):ii165.
4. Smith EEJ, Shore DF, Monro JJ, et al: Oral verapamil fails to prevent supraventricular tachycardia following coronary artery surgery. Int J Cardiol 1985;9:37.
5. Fuller JA, Adams GG, Buxton B: Atrial fibrillation after coronary artery bypass grafting. J Thorac Cardiovasc Surg 1989; 97:821.
6. Landymore R, Howell F: Recurrent atrial arrhythmias following treatment for postoperative atrial fibrillation after coronary bypass operations. Eur J Cardiothorac Surg 1991; 5(8):436.
7. Taylor GJ, Malik SA, Colliver JA, et al: Usefulness of atrial fibrillation as a predictor of stroke after isolated coronary artery bypass grafting. Am J Cardiol 1987;60:905.
8. Reed GL, Singer DE, Picard EH, et al: Stroke following coronary-artery bypass surgery: a case-control estimate of the risk from carotid bruits. N Engl J Med 1988;319:246.
9. Mayer A: Rhythmical pulsation in scyphomedusae. Papers from Turtugas Laboratory, Washington. 1908;1:115.
10. Lewis T, Drury A, Iliescu C: Circus movement in clinical flutter of auricles. Heart 1921;8:341.
11. Moe GK, Abildskov JA: Atrial fibrillation as a self-sustaining arrhythmia independent of focal discharge. Am Heart J 1959;58:59.
12. Allessie MA, Bonke FM, Schopman FG: Circus movement and rapid atrial muscle as a mechanism of tachycardia. III. The "leading circle" concept: a new model of circus movement in cardiac tissue without the involvement of an anatomic obstacle. Circ Res 1977;41:9.
13. Wolf PA, Kannel WB, McGee DL, et al: Duration of atrial fibrillation and imminence of stroke: The Framingham Study. Stroke 1983;14:664.
14. Boyden PA, Hoffman BF: The effects on atrial physiology and structure of surgically induced right atrial enlargement in dogs. Circ Res 1981;49:1319.
15. Lauer MS, Eagle KA, Buckley MJ, DeSanctis RW: Atrial fibrillation following coronary artery bypass surgery. Prog Cardiovasc Dis 1989;31(5):367.
16. Bush HL, Gelband H, Hoffman BF, et al: Electrophysiologic basis for supraventricular arrhythmias following surgical procedures for aortic stenosis. Arch Surg 1971;103:620.
17. Wells JL, Karp RB, Kouchoukos NT, et al: Characterization of atrial fibrillation in man: studies following open heart surgery. PACE Pacing Clin Electrophysiol 1978;1:426.
18. Waldo AL: Mechanisms of atrial fibrillation, atrial flutter, and ectopic atrial tachycardia—a brief review. Circulation 1987; 75(suppl III):37.
19. Waldo AL, MacLean WH, Karp RB, et al: Entrainment and interruption of atrial flutter with atrial pacing: studies in man following open heart surgery. Circulation 1977;56:737.
20. Ormerod OJM, McGregor CGA, Stone DL, et al: Arrhythmias after coronary bypass surgery. Br Heart J 1984;51:618.
21. Leitch JW, Thomson D, Baird D, Harris P: The importance of age as a predictor of atrial fibrillation and flutter after coronary artery bypass grafting. J Thorac Cardiovasc Surg 1990; 100(3):338.
22. Crosby L, Pifalo W, Woll K, Burkholder J: Risk factors for atrial

fibrillation after coronary artery bypass grafting. Am J Cardiol 1990;66:1520.

23. Cameron A, Schwartz MJ, Kronmal RA, Kosinski AS: Prevalence and significance of atrial fibrillation in coronary artery disease (CASS Registry). Am J Cardiol 1988;61:714.

24. Kannel WB, Abbott RD, Savage DD, McNamara PM: Epidemiological features of chronic atrial fibrillation: The Framingham Study. N Engl J Med 1982;306:1018.

25. Salem B, Chaudhry A, Haikal M, et al: Sustained supraventricular tachyarrhythmias following coronary artery bypass surgery comparing mammary versus saphenous vein grafts. J Vasc Dis 1991;441.

26. Dixon EF, Genton E, Vacek JL, Moore CB, Landry J: Factors predisposing to supraventricular tachyarrhythmias after coronary artery bypass grafting. Am J Cardiol 1986;58:476.

27. Lowe J, Hendry P, Hendrickson S, Wells R: Intraoperative identification of cardiac patients at risk to develop postoperative atrial fibrillation. Ann Surg 1990;213(5):388.

28. Boudalas H, Snyder GL, Lewis RP, et al: Safety and rationale for continuation of propranolol therapy during coronary bypass operation. Ann Thorac Surg 1978;26:222.

29. Engelman RM, Haag B, Lemeshow S, et al: Mechanism of plasma catecholamine increases during coronary artery bypass and valve procedures. J Thorac Cardiovasc Surg 1983;86:608.

30. Salazar C, Frishman W, Friedman S, et al: B-blockade therapy for supraventricular tachyarrhythmias after coronary surgery: a propranolol withdrawal syndrome? Angiology 1979;30:816.

31. White HD, Antman GM, Glynn MA, et al: Efficacy and safety of timolol for prevention of supraventricular tachyarrhythmias after coronary artery bypass surgery. Circulation 1984;70:479.

32. Leftkowitz RJ, Caron MG, Stiles GL: Mechanisms of membrane receptor regulation. Biochemical, physiological and clinical insights derived from studies of the adrenergic receptors. N Engl J Med 1984;310:1570.

33. Miller RR, Olson HG, Amsterdam EA, et al: Propranolol-withdrawal rebound phenomenon. Exacerbation of coronary events after abrupt cessation of anti-anginal therapy. N Engl J Med 1975;293:416.

34. Aarons RD, Nies AS, Gal J, et al: Elevation of B-adrenergic receptor density in human lymphocytes after propranolol administration. J Clin Invest 1980;65:949.

35. Mohr R, Smolinsky A, Goor DA: Prevention of supraventricular tachyarrhythmia with low-dose propranolol after coronary bypass. J Thorac Cardiovasc Surg 1981;81:840.

36. Matangi MF, Neutze JM, Graham KJ, et al: Arrhythmia prophylaxis after aorto-coronary bypass. J Thorac Cardiovasc Surg 1985;89:439.

37. Spodick D: Frequency of arrhythmias in acute pericarditis determined by Holter monitoring. Am J Cardiol 1984;53:842.

38. Smith PK, Buhrman WC, Levett JM, et al: Supraventricular conduction abnormalities following cardiac operations. J Thorac Cardiovasc Surg 1983;85:105.

39. Smith PK, Buhrman BA, Ferguson TB, et al: Conduction block after cardioplegic arrest: prevention by augmented atrial hypothermia. Circulation 1983;68(suppl II):41.

40. Magilligan DL, Vij D, Peper W, et al: Failure of standard cardioplegic techniques to protect the conducting systems. Ann Thorac Surg 1985;39:403.

41. Johnson LW, Dickstein RA, Fruehan T, et al: Prophylactic digitalization for coronary artery bypass surgery. Circulation 1976;53:819.

42. Csicsko JF, Schatzlein MH, King RD: Immediate postoperative digitalization in the prophylaxis of supraventricular arrhythmias following coronary artery bypass. J Thorac Cardiovasc Surg 1981;81:419.

43. Tyras DH, Stothert JC, Kaiser GC, et al: Supraventricular tachyarrhythmias after myocardial revascularization: a randomized trial of prophylactic digitalization. J Thorac Cardiovasc Surg 1979;77:310.

44. Matloff JM, Solfson S, Gorlin R, et al: Control of postcardiac surgical tachycardias with propranolol. Circulation 1968;37 (suppl II):133.

45. Stephenson LW, MacVaugh H, Tomasello DN, et al: Propranolol for prevention of postoperative cardiac arrhythmias: a randomized study. Ann Thorac Surg 1980;29:113.

46. Williams J, Stephenson LW, Holford FD, et al: Arrhythmia prophylaxis using propranolol after coronary artery surgery. Ann Thorac Surg 1982;34:435.

47. Hammon JW, Wood AJJ, Prager RL, et al: Perioperative beta blockade and propranolol: reduction in myocardial oxygen demands and incidence of atrial and ventricular arrhythmias. Ann Thorac Surg 1984;38:363.

48. Ivey MF, Ivey TD, Bailey WW, et al: Influence of propranolol on supraventricular tachycardia early after coronary artery revascularization. J Thorac Cardiovasc Surg 1983;85:214.

49. Shafei H, Nashef SAM, Turner MA, Bain WH: Does low-dose propranolol reduce the incidence of supraventricular tachyarrhythmias following myocardial revascularisation?—A clinical study. Thorac Cardiovasc Surg 1988;36:202.

50. White HD, Antman EM, Glynn MA: Efficacy and safety of timolol for prevention of supraventricular tachyarrhythmias after coronary artery bypass surgery. Circulation 1984;70:479.

51. Daudon P, Gandjbakhch I, Corcos T, et al: Prevention of atrial arrhythmias after coronary bypass surgery by acebutolol, a cardioselective beta-blocker. J Am Coll Cardiol 1985;5(suppl):437.

52. Shukri F, Nsidinanya O, Josa M, et al: Efficacy of nadolol in preventing supraventricular tachycardia after coronary artery bypass grafting. Am J Cardiol 1987;60:51D.

53. Janssen J, Loomans L, Harink J, et al: Prevention and treatment of supraventricular tachycardia shortly after coronary artery bypass grafting: a randomized open trial. J Vasc Dis 1986;601.

54. Nystrom U, Edvardsson N, Berggren H, et al: Oral sotalol reduces the incidence of atrial fibrillation after coronary artery bypass surgery. Thorac Cardiovasc Surg 1993;41(1):3407.

55. Roffman JA, Fieldman A: Digoxin and propranolol in the prophylaxis of supraventricular tachydysrhythmias after coronary artery bypass surgery. Ann Thorac Surg 1981;31:496.

56. Mills SA, Poole GV, Breyer RH, et al: Digoxin and propranolol in the prophylaxis of dysrhythmias after coronary artery bypass grafting. Circulation 1982;68(suppl II):222.

57. Davison R, Hartz R, Kaplan K, et al: Prophylaxis of supraventricular tachyarrhythmia after coronary bypass surgery with oral verapamil: a randomized, double-blind trial. Ann Thorac Surg 1985;39:336.

58. Chouty F, Coumel P: Oral flecainide for prophylaxis of paroxysmal atrial fibrillation. Am J Cardiol 1988;62:35D.

59. Pietersen A, Hellemann H: Usefulness of flecainide for prevention of paroxysmal atrial fibrillation and flutter. Am J Cardiol 1991;67:713.

60. Clementy J, Dulhoste M, Laiter C, et al: Flecainide acetate in the prevention of paroxysmal atrial fibrillation: a nine-month follow-up of more than 500 patients. Am J Cardiol 1992;70:44A.

61. Van Gelder IC, Crrijns H, Van Gilst WH, De Langen CDJ, Van Wijk LM, Lie KI: Effects of flecainide on the atrial defibrillation threshold. Am J Cardiol 1989;63:112.

62. The Cardiac Arrhythmia Suppression Trial (CAST): Preliminary report: effect of encainide and flecainide on mortality in a randomized trial of arrhythmia suppression after myocardial infarction. N Engl J Med 1989;406.

63. Fanning W, Thomas C, Roach A, et al: Prophylaxis of atrial fibrillation with magnesium sulfate after coronary artery bypass grafting. Soc Thorac Surg 1991;52:529.

64. Kleinpeter UM, Iversen S, Tesch A, Schmiedt W, Mayer E, Oelert H: Prevention of supraventricular tachyarrhythmias post coronary artery bypass surgery. Eur Soc Cardiol 1987; 8:137.

65. Gray R, Conklin C, Sethna D, et al: The role of intravenous verapamil in supraventricular tachyarrhythmias after open-heart surgery. Am Heart J 1982;104(4):799.

66. Haft JI, Habbab MA: Treatment of atrial arrhythmias. Arch Intern Med 1986;146:1085.

67. Betriu A, Chaitman BR, Bourassa MG, et al: Beneficial effect of intravenous diltiazem in the acute management of paroxysmal supraventricular tachyarrhythmias. Circulation 1983; 67(I):88.

68. Gray RJ, Bateman TM, Czer LSC, et al: Esmolol: a new ultra-short-acting beta-adrenergic blocking agent for rapid control of heart rate in postoperative supraventricular tachyarrhythmias. J Am Coll Cardiol 1985;5:1451.

69. Halpern S, Ellrodt AG, Singh BN, et al: Efficacy of intravenous procainamide infusion in converting atrial fibrillation to sinus rhythm. Relation to left atrial size. Br Heart J 1980;44:589.

70. Connolly SJ, Mulji AS, Hoffert DL, Davis C, Shragge BW: Randomized placebo-controlled trial of propafenone for treatment of atrial tachyarrhythmias after cardiac surgery. J Am Coll Cardiol 1987;5:1145.

71. Goy J, Kaufmann R, Kappenberger L, Sigwart U: Restoration of sinus rhythm with flecainide in patients with atrial fibrillation. Am J Cardiol 1988;62:38D.

72. Horowitz L, Spielman S, Greenspan A, et al: Use of amiodarone in the treatment of persistent and paroxysmal atrial fibrillation resistant to quinidine therapy. J Am Coll Cardiol 1985;6:1402.

73. Graboys T, Podrid P, Lown B: Efficacy of amiodarone for refractory supraventricular tachyarrhythmias. Am Heart J 1983;206:870.

74. Gold R, Haffajee C, Charos G, et al: Amiodarone for refractory atrial fibrillation. Am J Cardiol 1987;57:124.

75. Blevins R, Kerin N, Benaderet D, et al: Amiodarone in the management of refractory atrial fibrillation. Arch Intern Med 1987;147:1401.

76. Rosenbaum M, Chiale P, Halpern M, et al. Clinical efficacy of amiodarone as an antiarrhythmic agent. Am J Cardiol 1976; 38:934.

77. Ward D, Camm A, Spurrell R: Clinical antiarrhythmic effects of amiodarone in patients with resistant paroxysmal tachycardias. Br Heart J 1980;44:91.

78. Haffajee C, Love J, Canada A, et al: Clinical pharmacokinetics and efficacy of amiodarone for refractory tachyarrhythmias. Circulation 1983;67:1347.

79. Gosselink T, Harry J, Crijns G, et al: Low-dose amiodarone for maintenance of sinus rhythm after cardioversion of atrial fibrillation or flutter. 1992;267(24):3289.

80. Installe E, Schoevaerdts JC, Gadisseux PH, et al: Intravenous amiodarone in the treatment of various arrhythmias following cardiac operations. J Thorac Cardiovasc Surg 1981; 81:302.

81. Dimarco JP, Sellers D, Belardinelli L: Rapid termination of supraventricular tachycardia by intravenous adenosine 999. Circulation 1983;68(suppl III):358.

82. Belhassen B, Pelleg A, Shoshani D, et al: Electrophysiologic effects of adenosine triphosphate in AV reentrant tachycardia. Circulation 1983;68(suppl III):358.

83. Atrial arrhythmias. In: Chung E, ed. Principles of cardiac arrhythmias. 4th ed. Baltimore: Williams & Wilkins, 1989: 124.

84. Cooper TB, MacLean WAH, Waldo AL: Overdrive pacing for supraventricular tachycardia. A review of theoretical implications and therapeutic techniques. PACE Pacing Clin Electrophysiol 1978;1:196.

85. Amsel B, Walter B: Salvage transvenous rapid atrial pacing to terminate atrial flutter after cardiac operations. Soc Thorac Surg 1992;53:648.

86. Waldo, MacLean, eds. Diagnosis and treatment of cardiac arrhythmias following open-heart surgery. New York: Futura, 1980:25.

87. Rubin DA, Nieminski KE, Monteferrante JC, et al: Ventricular arrhythmias after coronary artery bypass surgery: incidence, risk factors and long-term prognosis. J Am Coll Cardiol 1985;6:307.

88. Huikuri HV, Korhonen UR, Takkunen T: Ventricular arrhythmias induced by dynamic and static exercise in relation to coronary artery bypass grafting. Am J Cardiol 1985;55:948.

89. Anastassiades LC, Antonopoulos AG, Petsas AA: The effect of coronary revascularization on exercise-induced ventricular ectopic activity. Eur Soc Cardiol 1987;8:75.

90. Rasmussen, Lunde PI, Lie M: Coronary bypass surgery in exercise-induced ventricular tachycardia. Eur Soc Cardiol 1987;8:444.

91. Weiner DA, Levine SR, Klein MD, et al: Ventricular arrhythmias during exercise testing: mechanism, response to coronary bypass surgery and prognostic significance. Am J Cardiol 1984;53:1553.

92. Bunton RW: Value of serum magnesium estimation in diag-

nosing myocardial infarction and predicting dysrhythmias after coronary artery bypass grafting. Thorax 1983;38:946.

93. Hecker BR, Lake CL, Kron IL, et al: Influence of magnesium ion on human ventricular defibrillation after aortocoronary bypass surgery. Am J Cardiol 1985;55:61.

94. Hirayama T, Roberts D, Allers M, Belbout A, Al-Khaja N, Olsson GW: Association between arrhythmias and reduced red cell deformability following cardiopulmonary bypass. Scand J Thorac Cardiovasc Surg 1988;22:179.

95. Hammermeister KE, DeRouen TA, Dodge HT: Viables predictive of survival in patients with coronary disease. Circulation 1979;59:421.

96. Marcus NH, Falcone RA, Harken AH, et al: Body surface late potentials: effects of endocardial resection in patients with ventricular tachycardia. Circulation 1984;70:632.

97. Gang ES, Lew AS, Hong M, et al: Decreased incidence of ventricular late potentials after successful thrombolytic therapy for acute myocardial infarction. N Engl J Med 1989; 321:712.

98. Johnson R, Goldberger A, Thurer R: Lidocaine prophylaxis in coronary revascularization patients: a randomized, prospective trial. Soc Thorac Surg 1993;55:1180.

99. Gray R, Mandel W: Management of common postoperative arrhythmias. In: Gray R, Matloff J, eds. Medical management of the cardiac surgical patient. Baltimore: Williams & Wilkins, 1990:217.

100. Gannon PG, Sellers RD, Kanjuh VI, et al: Complete heart block following replacement of the aortic valve. Circulation 1966;(suppl I):33:I:152.

101. Thompson R, Mitchell A, Ahmed M, et al: Conduction defects in aortic valve disease. Am Heart J 1979;98:3.

Cardiac Arrhythmias, 3rd edition, edited by William J. Mandel.
J. B. Lippincott Company, Philadelphia © 1995.

35

Manfred Zehender • Thomas Meinertz
Annette Geibel • Hanjörg Just

Cardiac Arrhythmias and Sudden Death in Sports

Sport activities produce a variety of functional and morphologic changes in the human heart, the clinical and prognostic importance of which is a matter of discussion.[1-3] Sports-related bradycardic and tachycardic rhythm disturbances,[4-9] usually known as a complicating feature of a variety of heart diseases, has gained interest due to their relation to the occurrence of sudden cardiac death.[1,10-16] Approximately 5% of all sudden deaths in the United States in individuals younger than 40 years of age are sports-related.[17] This is particularly important due to an increased interest in competitive sports in a broad segment of the population, while at the same time high-performance sports represent a shift to more extreme values of human performance.

The intentions of this article are to describe the prevalence, severity, and prognostic relevance of bradycardic and tachycardic arrhythmias among the sports-performing population and competition-oriented athletes, to identify risk factors and conditions under which rhythm disturbances may aggravate and occasionally induce tachyarrhythmic sudden death, and to discuss diagnostic and therapeutic guidelines for arrhythmia detection and treatment, as well as the consequences of bradycardic and tachycardic arrhythmia findings for the type and extent of sports recommended for a particular athlete.

SPORTS-RELATED PHYSIOLOGIC CHANGES OF THE HEART

The heart reacts to acute physical stress with a rapid increase in heart rate and a secondary increase in contractility. By contrast, regular physical training results in a permanent adaptation process in the heart that is not immediately reversible. This process can be described as follows[18]: elevated pressure stress in the left heart, such as occurs in isometric types of sports, leads primarily to hypertrophy of the free and septal muscle segments to maintain normal mural tension.[4,19-22] The end-diastolic diameter of the heart is particularly enlarged in chronic volume overload, observed usually in endurance sports.[14,23-25] Both adaptation processes of the heart are relative when the body surface is considered,[19,20] and both result in absolute enlargement of the heart, although the different pathophysiologic changes must be taken into consideration. Unlike the situation in heart failure, which makes use of the same basic pressure–volume regulation mechanisms as the athletic heart for compensation, the sports-induced adaptation process in the heart is assessed as a physiologic and reversible extreme variant because of the lack of permanent damage. A training-dependent[7,25-28] vagotonic and compensatory decrease in heart rate at rest and under exercise[29-36] is also found as another adaptation process in all athletes. These adaption processes guarantee optimum ventricular filling and keep the loss of energy not converted to contractile force at high heart rates from increasing overproportionally.[37]

BRADYCARDIC ARRHYTHMIAS OF THE SINUS NODE

Sinus bradycardia in the surface ECG is found in the majority of athletes trained for isotonic exercise.[29,31-36,38,39] It is clearly correlated to training level[7,27,28,40] and results in exception cases to resting heart rates down to less than 25 beats per minutes.[30] Sinus pauses lasting more than 2 seconds are found in more than one third of the athletes and are certainly no cause for implantation of a pacemaker.[4] Pathophysiologically, this is a condition elicited by reduced sympathetic and elevated vagal tonus.[41-44] In addition, functional changes are postulated for the pacemaker cells of the sinus node.[45,46] Both factors appear to be responsible for an increased incidence of sinus arrhythmias and so-called wandering pacemakers in 13.5% to 69% of athletes,[47-52] compared with the normal population (up to 20%).[51,53] The different statements, ranging from 14% among 3,158 cyclists,[54] 42% among 30 ballet dancers,[31] and up to 69% in 42 basketball players,[34] can be traced to methodical and, to a lesser extent, exercise-related differences in recording such arrhythmias.

BRADYCARDIC ARRHYTHMIAS OF THE ATRIOVENTRICULAR NODE

The incidence of first-degree atrioventricular (AV) block is calculated at about 0.65%, second-degree AV block at 0.003% (type I or II), and third-degree AV block at 0.0002% in the general population. AV block is a common finding in competitive athletes and is closely related to the training condition. First-degree AV block is observed in 10% to 33% of athletes,[18,34,36,50,52,55-61] and about the same number had borderline PQ times in the surface.[29,35,36,47] Under adequate stress, there is a normalization of the PQ interval.[34,35,60,62] Nakamoto and colleagues observed a second-degree Wenckebach AV block in 10% of marathon runners clearly depending on training condition but which was documented only at rest.[60] Meytes and associates found the incidence in another 126 endurance athletes to be 2.4% in the resting ECG.[50] The frequency increases to more than 23% to 40% (normal population: 6%) when long-term electrocardiographic examinations are performed.[4,8,24]

According to the same investigators, the frequency of second-degree Mobitz AV block in endurance athletes was up to 8%.[9,24,63] The general incidence of third-degree AV block is 0.017% in athletes[9,55] and thus 100-fold that of the general population. However, a permanent[64] or transient third-degree AV block[2,65,66] does not rule out high levels of physical performance over longer periods.[67-70] Nevertheless, when a third-degree AV block is present, careful clinical evaluation to exclude underlying heart disease is recommended (Figs. 35-1). Similarly, in severe sinus node–induced bradycardia, the presence of binodal disease, as well as the high, transient vagal tone, may result in severe AV block. Figure 35-2 shows this phenomenon in an athlete after atrial pacemaker implantation.

Interestingly, in the early 1980s, Zeppilli and colleagues[61] and Fenici and associates[55] independently pointed out the reversibility of all of the above AV node changes when observed in athletes and when an organic heart disease is excluded. Zeppilli was able to offset this in seven of 10 endurance athletes with second-degree AV block by means of a Valsalva maneuver, in nine of 10 athletes by exercise, and in all athletes by the administration of atropine.[61] Of the total 12,000 athletes examined by Fenici, five presented with a second-degree AV block and two presented with a third-degree AV block. AV conduction normalized in all of these individuals with physical exercise and after discontinuing high-performance sports in a 9-year observation period.[55]

SUPRAVENTRICULAR TACHYARRHYTHMIAS

Unlike the bradycardic supraventricular forms of arrhythmia, paroxysmal atrial or AV nodal tachycardias are not found more frequently in athletes than in the general population.[6,71] Contrary to this, the incidence of atrial fibrillation is elevated in competitive athletes. It is found in long-term electrocardiographic examinations on an average of 0% to 0.063%[30,50,52,54,72] and is thus considerably higher than in the normal population of the same age (0.004%).[53] The pathophysiologic explanation is the more functional character of atrial fibrillation (such as vegetative imbalance), whereas supraventricular tachycardia requires a congenital or acquired anatomic substrate (e.g., reentry circus current). An incessant type of supraventricular tachycardia is very rare and seems to be restricted to patients with organic heart disease (Fig. 35-3).

The exercise dependence of supraventricular forms of arrhythmia was studied by Pantano and colleagues. A clear increase under exercise was found for all arrhythmias, despite low absolute incidence.[6] A prognostic relevance of these arrhythmias is assumed when they are associated with either hypertrophic cardiomyopathy (Fig. 35-4) or Wolff-Parkinson-White syndrome (Fig. 35-5). In hyper-

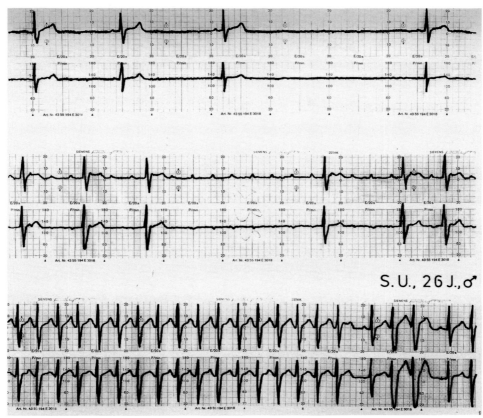

S.U., 26 J., ♂

Figure 35-1. A 24-year-old competitive cyclist complained of bradycardic–tachycardic phases following exercise with a recent episode of syncope. A history of recurrent infections of the upper respiratory tract was present. Seventy-two-hour Holter monitoring and repetitive exercise tests were required to document severe sinoatrial block at night (upper part) and AV nodal block (during paroxysmal atrial tachycardia) after exercising (middle part). The lower part of the figure shows a frequent sinus rhythm during exercising, which is conducted 1:1 to the ventricle. No organic lesion was observed during diagnostic evaluation. The patient underwent pacemaker implantation (DDD mode), is still active in competitive sports, and has been asymptomatic for 32 months.

trophic cardiomyopathy, it is assumed that the increased incidence of sudden cardiac death usually observed under exercise is an expression of ischemia in the hypertrophied muscle segment coupled with diastolic relaxation impairment, such as may occur in ventricular or supraventricular tachycardia.[16,73] A definite statement cannot yet be made, but such patients should not participate in high-performance sports.

The Wolff-Parkinson-White (WPW) syndrome cited above is also of particular importance in this regard. Contrary to earlier reports,[74,75] a more frequent occurrence of WPW syndrome in athletes (0.15%–2%)[3,30,50,76] compared with the general population (0.1%–0.15%) cannot be certain for methodologic reasons. First, the two groups of athletes and patients compared in the earlier tests differed in age; second, the sports–medical examinations with incidental documentation of preexcitation were performed more frequently than similar medical examina-

tions in the age-matched general population; and last, the sports-related vagal tone may have led to demasking of preexcitation.[3] This methodologically created "selection process," which frequently excludes symptomatic persons primarily from performance athletics, is important for the low incidence of WPW arrhythmias among athletes.[3,74] It is evident that the danger of hemodynamically unstable situations arising from the so-called AV-junctional tachycardia or WPW tachycardia is extremely rare, because the AV node usually limits the maximum rate of this type of reentry tachycardia to <220 beats per minute. In individual cases, however, the occurrence of secondary ventricular fibrillation following a paroxysmal WPW tachycardia has been reported. In these athletes, the coincidence of arrhythmia with massive acidosis and hypokalemia under extreme sports activities has been stressed to result in the fatal event.[77,78] By contrast, ventricular rates up to 300 beats per minute and more are possible during atrial

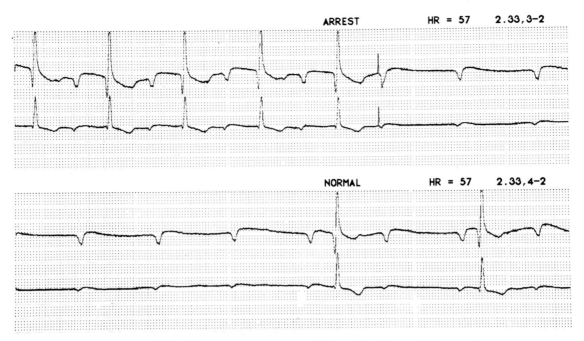

Figure 35-2. A 21-year-old female swimmer was examined 13 months after an AAI pacemaker was implanted to treat documented episodes of syncopal sinus arrest. At this time, no major conduction abnormalities of the AV node were observed. After pacemaker implantation, she stopped swimming for more than half a year, and then she started competitive swimming again. With increasing training level, she experienced an increasing number of episodes with slight dizziness and presyncope. During subsequent Holter recording, one episode of dizziness was documented in the postexercise phase. When heart rate dropped slightly below 60 beats/minute, a single atrial pacemaker beat induced an episode of severe AV block lasting for >6 seconds. The patient was subsequently treated with a DDD pacemaker.

fibrillation with rapid antegrade conduction via the accessory pathway, and they may induce ventricular fibrillation.[79] As described in the literature, therefore, athletes with WPW syndrome and documented, symptomatic arrhythmias should not participate in high-performance activities, unless persistent disappearance of preexcitation (blocking of the accessory pathway) can be proved in the exercise ECG at a heart rate <220 beats per minute, or, more reliable, a maximum AV conduction rate of <220 beats per minute can be proved by simple pacing in the right atrium. In our opinion, and contrary to the views of other authors,[3,35a,80] this also holds true for previously asymptomatic athletes with WPW syndrome, because the lack of tachycardia or atrial fibrillation episodes does not offer any conclusions regarding the absence of a fast conduction pathway.

VENTRICULAR TACHYARRHYTHMIAS

A so-called accelerated idioventricular rhythm is found most often in trained athletes as a consequence of a low sinus rate or supraventricular pauses. This rhythm, which usually originates from tertiary pacemaker centers, depends on training level and vagal tone,[46] usually occurs at a rate of 40 to 100 beats per minute, and is of no prognostic importance. The incidence is generally up to 7% among athletes,[30,47,76] increases to about 20% when long-term electrocardiographic examinations are considered,[4] and thus is 100-fold higher than in healthy nonathletes of comparable age.[81-84]

Ectopic ventricular forms of arrhythmia are apparently not more frequent among trained athletes with healthy hearts than in the general population.[4,9,79,85-88]

Figure 35-3. A 62-year-old competitive runner (15–20 km/day) presented with an asymptomatic, incessant type of tachycardia (**A**). During surface EKG, the patient had incomplete right bundle branch block (110 msec). Intracardiac leads (**B**, lower part) and programmed electrical stimulation proved an etcopic atrial tachycardia (each QRS complex is preceded by atrial activation originating from the high left atrium). The patient was not treated and remained asymptomatic for a follow-up of 52 months. ▶

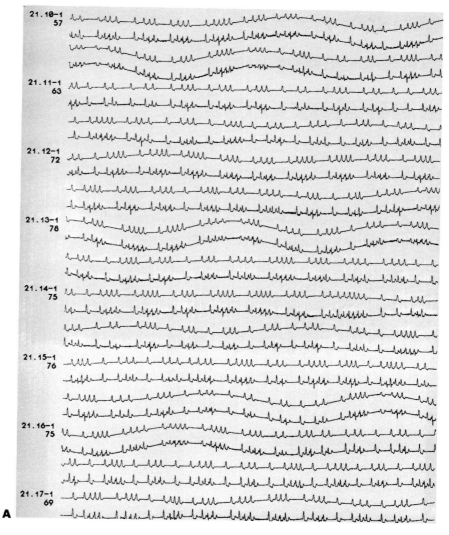

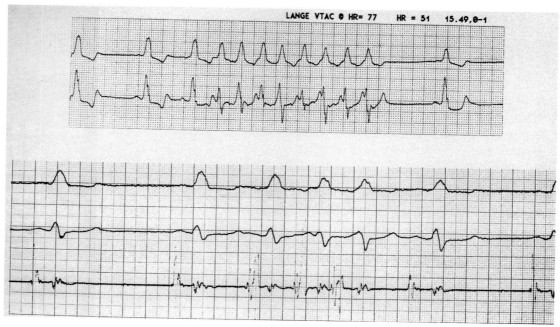

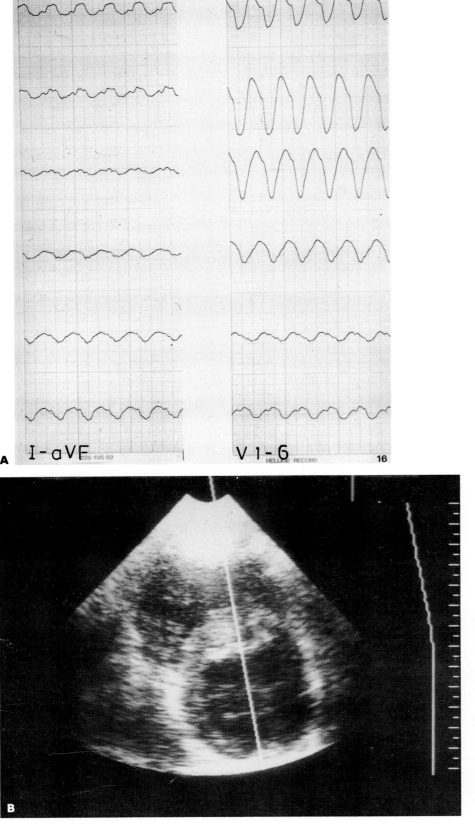

A

I–aVF

R

V 1–6

16

B

Figure 35-4. During competition, a 23-year-old tennis player experienced an episode of ventricular tachycardia (rate, 200 beats/minute, left axis deviation, left bundle branch block, **A**) and was successfully resuscitated. Echocardiographic findings indicated a marked septal hypertrophy with an outflow tract obstruction (gradient: 45 mmHg) **B**, (2-D echocardiogram). Competitive sport was stopped by the patient, who refused surgical intervention. When treated by beta-blocking agents and calcium channel blocking agents, the patient remained asymptomatic for 34 months.

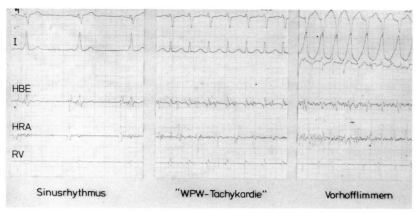

Sinusrhythmus   "WPW-Tachykardie"   Vorhofflimmern

Figure 35-5. A 24-year-old cyclist with known Wolff-Parkinson-White (WPW) syndrome (surface ECG, left part) presented with the first episode of WPW tachycardia with a rate of 170 beats/minute at his general physical examination. Because the patient was only slightly symptomatic, he was not treated. Thirteen months later, he experienced an episode of irregular palpitations. Subsequent programmed electrical stimulation (extracardial ECG [V_1,] and intracardial ECG (HBE, bundle of His; HRA, high right atrium; RV, right ventricle) demonstrated during atrial fibrillation a maximal AV conduction rate over the bypass tract >40 beats/minute higher than during WPW tachycardia. Sotalol reduced the maximal AV conduction rate during atrial fibrillation to 160 beats/minute and prevented reinduction of the WPW tachycardia. The patient agreed to this medication but stopped competitive sports 6 months later and remained event-free for 16 months.

Ventricular premature beats are reported in the literature in about one third of the athletes examined by long-term electrocardiography. In some studies the incidence increases to 70%, compared with 55% in a corresponding control group.[5] Pantano did not find an incidence of more than five ventricular extrasystoles per hour in any of 60 competitive athletes.[6] Furlanello and colleagues described the presence of nonsustained ventricular tachycardia in every third athlete who presented with symptomatic ventricular arrhythmias.[79] Northcote and associates observed an increased incidence of ventricular couplets and salvos in the 24-hour ECG of 21 highly trained squash players during and after training and during competition, but the frequency did not differ from that of an age-matched control group.[87] Interestingly, the arrhythmias observed in athletes during training and competition could rarely be reproduced by a normal exercise ECG, in spite of an adequate increase in rate. Pilcher and colleagues found no correlation between the long-term electrocardiographic occurrence of ventricular arrhythmias and training status of 80 endurance athletes. In this group, repetitive forms of ventricular arrhythmias were infrequent and occurred only during exercise.[88] Pantano investigated the exercise dependence of ventricular arrhythmias. Although only one standardized exercise ECG was compared with a 24-hour long-term ECG in this study of 60 long-distance athletes, the incidence of simple arrhythmias was more than doubled during exercise, complex arrhythmias increased fivefold, and ventricular tachycardia was observed with an incidence of 6%.[4] Analogous findings were described by Viitasalo and Talan in the early 1980s,[8,9] but individual figures on the frequency of complex arrhythmias extend to 25%.[5] At the same time, neither electro- nor echocardiographic parameters that predict the occurrence or severity of ventricular arrhythmias could be identified, in spite of a significant hypertrophy-dependent QT prolongation.[5,89] An R-on-T phenomenon was observed in only one of the 40 athletes examined.[5]

According to these findings, proof of tachycardic ventricular arrhythmia in competitive athletes should be reason enough for mandatory cardiologic examination as a precautionary measure (Fig. 35-6). Autopsy examinations in athletes who died suddenly during the performance of competitive sports indicated that organic abnormalities of the heart are very common (Table 35-1).

ATHLETIC ACTIVITY AND SUDDEN CARDIAC DEATH

According to The Framingham Study, the annual incidence of sudden cardiac death increases in nonathletes (depending on age) from 3/10,000 persons between 35 and 44 years of age to more than 25/10,000 persons ages 55 to 64 years.[90] By contrast, Koplan in the late 1970s estimated a

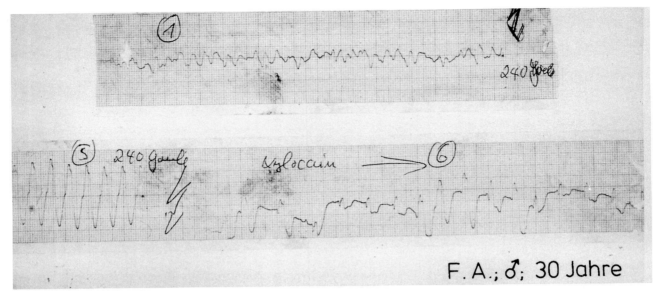

F. A.; ♂; 30 Jahre

A

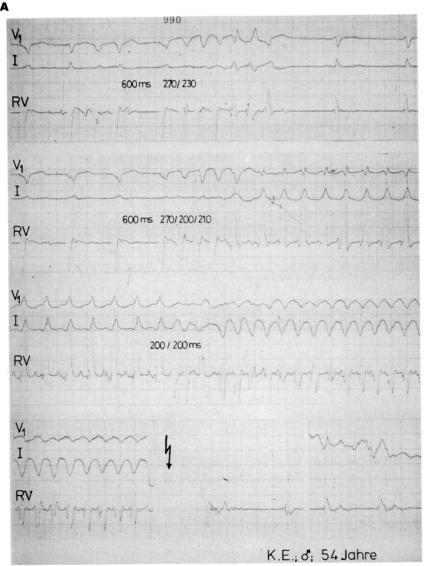

990

V₁
I

600 ms   270/230

RV

V₁
I

600 ms   270/200/210

RV

V₁
I

200/200 ms

RV

V₁
I

RV

K.E.; ♂; 54 Jahre

B

Figure 35-6. A 30-year-old, well-trained surfer experienced an episode of syncopal tachyarrhythmia. The first ECG registration during cardipulmonary resuscitation is shown in **A**. A subsequent diagnostic workup indicated a beginning dilated cardiomyopathy (ejection fraction: 44%). (**B**) Repetitive responses were induced (first row) during programmed electrical stimulation at basic pacing with 100 beats/minute and two premature stimuli (coupling intervals are given). Further shortening of the coupling interval of the premature beats resulted in induction of a sustained monomorphic ventricular tachycardia (second row). During an attempt to terminate the ventricular tachycardia by two premature beats, a new and faster type of tachycardia occurred (third row), which required DC countershock for termination. The patient was treated by amiodarone but continued competitive sports. Despite therapeutic plasma levels of amiodarone at 6 and 12 months of control, he died suddenly 14 months after the first event while jogging.

TABLE 35-1. Sudden Cardiac Death in Athletes

	James et al. Ann Intern Med 1967	Opie et al. Lancet 1975	Noakes et al. N Engl J Med 1979	Thompson et al. JAMA 1979	Morales et al. Circulation 1980	Maron et al. Circulation 1980
No. of athletes	2	21	5	18	3	3
Age (yrs)	15/18	17/58	27–44	42–60	17–54	17–54
Death during competition, training	+ +	+ +	+ +	+ +	+ +	+ +
Prodromal symptoms	1/2	9/21	1/5	6/18	—	—
Pathologic findings	2	—	4	14	3	27
Organic changes	0	—	0	0	0	14
HCM	0	—	1	13	0	3
CAD	0	—	0	0	3	3
Coronary anomaly / CAB	0	—	0	0	0	5
Hypertrophy + + +	2	—	0	0	0	0
Abn. conduction system	0	—	0	1	0	0
Myocarditis						
Compelling suspicion of CAD		18/21				

	Waller et al. Am J Cardiol 1980	Virmani et al. Am J Med 1982	Northcote et al. Lancet 1984	Corrado et al. Am J Med 1990	Burke et al. Am Heart J 1991	Furianello et al. PACE 1992
No. of athletes	5	30	30	22	34	8
Age (yrs)	40–53	18–57	35–60	11–35	14–40	14–40
Death during competition, training	+ +	(+)	+ +	18/22	+ +	7/8
Prodromal symptoms	1/5	?	22/30	12/22	?	?
Pathologic findings	5	26	27	22	34	8
Organic changes	0	0	1	0	8	0
HCM	5	22	23	4	9	3
CAD	0	0	0	2	6	0
Coronary anomaly / CAB	0	3	0	0	3	0
Hypertrophy + + +	0	0	0	3	0	1
Abn. conduction system	0	0	0	0	2	1
Myocarditis						
Compelling suspicion of CAD						

HCM, hypertrophic cardiomyopathy; CAD, coronary artery disease; CAB, coronary artery bridging

frequency of sudden cardiac death of 3/10,000 persons in 4 million long-distance runners between 20 and 59 years of age with a daily training period of at least 1 hour.[91] Thompson and Stern[92] and Siscovick and colleagues[93] described a higher incidence of sudden death in high-performance sports but also pointed out the importance of further subspecification. The retrospective study of Siscovick and associates on 133 recreational and competitive athletes who died suddenly during physical exercise showed that at a low level of training, peak exercise is associated with a 56-fold risk of sudden cardiac death compared with exercise-free periods. By contrast, at a high training level, the risk of sudden cardiac death under extreme physical stress was elevated only fivefold.[93] These findings argue against a close relation between sudden

cardiac death and high-performance sports and raise the question of other factors that may be of importance for an increased risk of sudden cardiac death.

In competing athletes, the incidence of sudden cardiac death increases by more than twofold when the athlete is older than 35 years of age (Table 35-2).[94] In the group of younger athletes, squash and jogging carry the highest risk of sudden cardiac death (see Table 35-2).[95] In athletes older than 35 years of age, jogging and tennis are most frequently associated with sudden cardiac death (see Table 35-2).[94] However, postmortem findings in athletes with sudden cardiac death indicate that an underlying, previously unknown heart disease is dominant over all of the above-mentioned risk factors.

The incidence of an underlying heart disease was

TABLE 35-2. Sudden Death During Different Types of Sports

Types of Sport	Sudden Death per 100,000 Athletes (age <35 years)	Total Number (age <35 years)
Jogging	4.3 (1.1)	27 (7)
Tennis	3.2 (0.2)	17 (1)
Soccer	2.6 (1.4)	49 (25)
Other ball games	1.6 (0.8)	28 (14)
Leisure sport activities	0.4 (0.2)	25 (10)

Type of Sport	Death During Recreational Sports (n)	Mean Age (yrs)
Golf	19	59
Jogging	16	48
Swimming	9	52
Bowling	5	50
Tennis	5	50
Basketball	4	36
Handball	3	50

Pool J: Sudden death and sports. In: Fagard R, Bekaert J. Sports cardiology. Kluwer Academic Publishers, 1986:223; Ragosta M, Crabtree J, Sturner W, Thompson P: Death during recreational exercise in the state of Rhode Island. Med Sci Sports Exerc 1984;16:339.

above 70% in all postmortem studies that included competitive athletes (see Table 35-1 and Fig. 35-6).[12a, 28a, 44, 77, 88a, 96–101] In younger athletes (<40 years of age), hypertrophic cardiomyopathy predominates (see Table 35-1).[13] This heart disease can be best diagnosed by echocardiography, although it is sometimes difficult to separate abnormal hypertrophy from physiologic, training-induced, and frequently septal-dominant muscle hypertrophy.[102,103] The concomitant occurrence of tachycardic arrhythmias and ischemia in the hypertrophied myocardium and a diastolic relaxation impairment ("myocardial stiffness") at high heart rates is held responsible for sudden cardiac death in hypertrophic cardiomyopathy. An unphysiologically strong (muscle weight 420–530 g, maximum wall thickness 16–23 mm) but symmetrical muscle hypertrophy and an impaired diastolic relaxation were recognized in a small group of endangered athletes.[13] In these patients, prognosis is considered to be good when muscle texture is normal and genetic abnormalities are not present. In the study by Burke and associates, when eight patients with hypertrophic cardiomyopathy were evaluated (mean heart weight: 543 g), all patients showed myofiber disarray as determined microscopically.[17] When these patients were compared with a matched group of patients with non–sports-related sudden cardiac death, hypertrophic

cardiomyopathy as the underlying heart disease was found eight times as often. However, in contrast to the usual risk stratification in patients with hypertrophic cardiomyopathy, none of these sudden death victims who experienced the fatal event during sports had a history of syncope or a known family history of cardiac problems.[17]

Congenital malformations are also common in younger athletes who die unexpectedly. In this group, anomalies of the coronary arteries and so-called muscular bridges are most common (see Table 35-1). They have increasingly been held responsible for the occurrence of sudden cardiac death. In cases of anomalous origin of the left coronary artery from the right sinus of Valsalva, the angle of origin at the aortic root increases with increased physical exercise; with the origin of the right coronary artery out of the left sinus of Valsalva, this shifts under exercise more sharply to the right. Both mechanisms may result in acute myocardial ischemia.[13, 17, 96] Thus, anomalous coronary arteries are found 10 times more often in exercise-related than in non–exercise-related sudden cardiac death.[17] Likewise, muscular bridges have been reported in victims of exercise-related sudden death and may also induce ischemia under exercise. However, such bridges are also observed in up to 20% of the general population.[13, 104] In a recent study by Burke and colleagues, muscular bridges showed a borderline significantly higher incidence in exercise-related than in non-exercise-related sudden death.[17] Although myocardial ischemia due to atherosclerosis is less common in younger patients with exercise-related sudden death, this diagnosis is established in every fifth patient.[17,96] In these patients, stenotic lesions are very common (>75%), whereas the presence of myocardial infarction and multiple vessel disease ranges from 0% to 50% of these patients in newer studies.[17,96,105] In a small group of patients, anabolic steroids have been reported to induce atherosclerotic lesions, myocardial infarction, and sudden death.[50a, 106] Vasospastic angina has also been reported in rare cases to induce syncope and sudden death.[107] Acute aortic rupture (most common in patients with Marfan syndrome), right ventricular cardiomyopathy, and inflammatory abnormalities are less frequently observed when young athletes die suddenly (see Table 35-1).

The racial and sexual differences in patients with underlying heart disease experiencing exercise-related sudden death have been addressed in only a few studies.[17] Except for sudden death from severe atherosclerosis (ratio, 0.57:1), no difference was observed between men and women. Blacks were more likely to suffer exercise-related sudden death due to hypertrophic cardiomyopathy (3:1), whereas whites were more likely to die from severe atherosclerosis (9:1).

Of particular interest, prodromal symptoms are reported in one third of younger athletes prior to the occurrence of sudden cardiac death.[13, 108] In the study reported by Thompson and associates, these symptoms even occurred immediately prior to cardiac death but did not result in cessation of exercise.[92]

In the group of athletes older than 40 years of age, the cause of sudden cardiac death shifts increasingly toward coronary heart disease. Vuori and colleagues described 10 cases of sudden cardiac death during sports activities in a long-term study of more than 1 million trained cross-country skiers older than 40 years of age. Eight of these individuals had coronary heart disease.[109] In another study by the same authors on 68,000 active persons followed for a 16-year observation period, 339 died during sports activities; 81% of these had coronary heart disease. Munschek reported on autopsy findings of 67 out of 124 competitive athletes (54%) who died suddenly of a basic cardiac disease during athletic activities; 59 had coronary heart disease.[14] Waller reported on five competitive athletes between 40 and 53 years of age who died suddenly during athletic competition; in each case, >75% coronary arterial stenosis was observed.[110] Opie, reporting on 10 athletes in this age group who died suddenly, found compelling evidence of coronary heart disease.[108] Electrical instability caused by chronic coronary heart disease appears to be just as important as the occurrence of acute myocardial ischemia or myocardial infarction.[111] Other field studies summarized in the article by Haskell support these findings in a total of more than 1 million competitive and recreational athletes.[1] Interestingly, the majority of the moderately trained or medium-trained athletes who died suddenly in this study had experienced short- or medium-term prodromal symptoms.[92, 109] Whether the incidence of sudden cardiac death events can be reduced in these patients by closer and more extensive medical supervision is still uncertain.[35a, 112, 113]

SUMMARY

High-performance sports are frequently associated with a variety of bradycardic, and rarely tachycardic, arrhythmias, of which some are training-related and others the result of an underlying heart disease. Especially in the presence of an underlying heart disease, the presence of tachyarrhythmias, rather than bradycardic arrhythmias, carries an increased risk of sudden cardiac death. The following recommendations are made in accordance with previous attempts[114–116] to identify high-risk candidates for sudden cardiac death among competitive and non-competitive athletes and among persons who perform medium- or high-level recreational exercise.

1. Sinus bradycardia and AV block are very common in athletes but do not require attention as long as they are asymptomatic or do not produce pauses >4 seconds. Competitive sports should not be recommended when first-degree AV block worsens during exercise or is associated with underlying heart disease.

   Persistent, rather than transient, second-degree AV block, Mobitz type II block, and third-degree AV block are extremely unusual findings, even in athletes, and should be considered a sign of organic lesions until the contrary is proved. Athletes who have an abnormal heart rate and whose arrhythmias disappear with exercise without marked sinus slowing or worsening of the type I second-degree heart block during or after exercise may be permitted to participate with caution in competitive sports. In the presence of congenital heart block, and especially when associated with an abnormal heart rate, symptomatic persons (e.g., those with ventricular arrhythmias or symptoms of fatigue) should have an atrial synchronous pacemaker inserted before participating in competitive sports.

2. Supraventricular and AV node ectopias are not more frequent in athletes than in the general population—except for atrial fibrillation. Premature atrial complexes create no limitation for competitive sports. In the presence of supraventricular tachycardia, especially when it is exercise-induced, effective prevention of recurrence is recommended before one participates in competitive sports. When there is a history of syncopal or presyncopal supraventricular tachycardia, competitive sports should be considered only after there has been adequate treatment preventing recurrence for at least 6 months. The same recommendations can be given for atrial fibrillation in the absence of an underlying heart disease. Athletes with AV junctional reentrant tachycardia can participate in all competitive sports when ventricular rate is controlled (e.g., when ventricular rate during tachycardia is lower than ventricular rate during exercise at maximal sinus rate).

   WPW syndrome is of particular importance because rapid conduction to the ventricle via the accessory AV pathway is possible, especially if atrial fibrillation is likely to occur. In younger and in symptomatic athletes, a more in-depth evaluation may be recommended before participation in moderate- to high-intensity sports. Athletes whose shortest R-R interval during atrial fibrillation is less than 300 milliseconds or whose accessory pathway refractory period is less than 250 milliseconds have the threat of very rapid ventricular rates and should not participate in competitive sports. When treatment is effective to lengthen these values, low-intensity sports activity is possible. Likewise, caution is required in athletes with hypertrophic cardiomyopathy. Here, hemodynamic deterioration must be anticipated with the occurrence of supraventricular tachycardia.

3. Premature ventricular beats occur among athletes with the same incidence as in the general population. Usually, they disappear under exercise and thus do not limit sports activities. When premature ventricular beats occur only during exercise, or increase in frequency and in complexity during exercise, only low-intensity competitive sports are recommended. Caution is indicated before allowing full participation in moderate- to high-intensity competitive sports. When any heart disease, especially congenital or idiopathic prolonged QT interval, is present, high- and moderate-intensity competitive sports are contraindicated. When premature ventricular beats in the presence of an underlying heart disease (except QT syndrome) are suppressed by medical therapy, low-intensity sports activity is possible.

4. The occurrence of repetitive ventricular forms of arrhythmia should always prompt cardiologic examination in search of underlying cardiac disease, particularly hypertrophic or dilated cardiomyopathy. When presyncope, syncope, and an underlying heart disease are excluded, an individual presenting with non-sustained ventricular tachycardia of uniform configuration that does not exceed 150 beats per minute during maximal exercise may participate with caution in all competitive sports. When a structural heart disease or a history of presyncope or syncope is present, the person with ventricular tachycardia exceeding 150 beats per minute during exertion, or with the long QT syndrome, may not engage in any competitive sports. Effective antiarrhythmic therapy preventing tachycardia recurrence for >6 months is required to permit participation in low-intensity competitive sports. Regardless of treatment, ventricular tachycardia associated with a long QT syndrome excludes the patient from competitive sports.

5. Any arrhythmias that once resulted in cardiac arrest (e.g., ventricular flutter or fibrillation) in the presence or absence of structural heart disease should exclude the patient from competitive sports. Selected patients who have been appropriately evaluated and treated may engage in low-intensity competitive sports.

6. Exercise-induced, sudden cardiac death in athletes is unusual without preexisting heart disease. The cause of sudden cardiac death among athletes younger than 40 years of age can be predominantly ascribed to congenital heart diseases (such as hypertrophic cardiomyopathy, coronary anomalies). In athletes older than 40 years of age and with increasing age, coronary heart disease is the most frequent autopsy finding. A

corresponding risk stratification should take these partial dangers into account.

References

1. Haskell WL: Sudden cardiac death during vigorous exercise. Int J Sports Med 1982;3:45.
2. Rost B, Hollmann W: Athlete's heart—A review of its historical assessment and new aspects. Int J Sports Med 1983;4:147.
3. Rost R, Hollmann W: Sportmedizinische Aspekte des WPW-Syndroms. Deutsche Zeitschr Sportmed 1978;X:273.
4. Hanne-Paparo N, Kellermann JJ: Long-term Holter ECG monitoring of athletes. Med Sci Sports Exerc 1981;13:294.
5. Palatini P, Maraglino G, Sperti G, et al: Prevalence and possible mechanisms of ventricular arrhythmias in athletes. Am Heart J 1985;110(3):561.
6. Pantano JA, Oriel RJ: Prevalence and nature of cardiac arrhythmias in apparently normal well-trained runners. Am Heart J 1982;104:762.
7. Rerych SK, Scholz PM, Sabiston DC Jr, Jones RH: Effects of exercise training on left ventricular function in normal subjects: a longitudinal study by radionuclide angiography. Am J Cardiol 1980;45:244.
8. Talan DA, Bauernfeind RA, Ashley WW, Kanakis C, Rosen KM: Twenty-four hour continuous ECG recordings in long distance runners. Chest 1982;19:24.
9. Viitasalo MT, Kala R, Eisalo A: Ambulatory electrocardiographic recording in endurance athletes. Br Heart J 1982;47:213.
10. Billmann G, Schartz P, Stone H: The effects of daily exercise on susceptibility to sudden cardiac death. Circulation 1984;69:1182.
11. Bruegmann U, Hopf R, Kaltenbach U: Ploetzlicher Herztod bei sportlicher Betaetigung. Deutsches Ärzteblatt 1987;84(17):808.
12. Cantwell JD, Fletcher GF: Sudden death and jogging. Physicals and Sports Medicine 1978;1:94.
12a. Burke AP, Farb A, Virmani R: Causes of sudden death in athletes. Cardiol Clin 1992;10:303.
13. Maron BJ, Roberts WC, Edwards JE, McAllister HA, Epstein SE: Sudden death in patients with hypertrophic cardiomyopathy: characterisation of 26 patients without functional limitations. Am J Cardiol 1978;41:803.
14. Munschek H: Ursachen des akuten Todes beim Sport in der Bundesrepublik. Sportarzt und Sportmedizin 1977;5:133.
15. Noakes TD, Opie LH: Autopsy-proved coronary atherosclerosis in marathon runners. N Engl J Med 1979;301:86.
16. Noakes TD, Rose G, Opie LH: Hypertrophic cardiomyopathy associated with sudden death during marathon racing. Br Heart J 1979;41:624.
17. Burke AP, Farb A, Virmani R, Goodin J, Smialek E: Sports-related and non-sports-related sudden cardiac death in young adults. Am Heart J 1991;121,(2)1:568.
18. Huston TP, Puffer JC, MacMillan DE, Rodney WM: The athletic heart syndrome. N Engl J Med 1985;313:24.
19. Keul J, Dickhuth H, Lehmann M, Staiger J: The athlete's heart—hemodynamics and structure. Int Sports Med 1982;3:33.

20. Keul J, Dickhuth H, Simon G, Lehmann M: Effect of static and dynamic exercise on heart volume, contractility and left ventricular dimensions. Circ Res 1981;48:162.

21. Morganroth J, Maron BJ, Henry WL, Epstein SE: Comparative left ventricular dimensions in trained athletes. Ann Intern Med 1975;82:521.

22. Snoeckx LHEH, Abeling HFM, Lambregts JAC, Schmitz JJF, Verstapen FTJ, Reneman RS: Echocardiographic dimensions in athletes in relation to their training programs. Med Sci Sports Exerc 1982;14:428.

23. Ikäheimo MJ, Palatsi IJ, Takkunen JT: Noninvasive evaluation of the athletic heart: sprinters versus endurance runners. Am J Cardiol 1979;44:24.

24. Underwood RH, Schwade JL: Noninvasive analysis of cardiac function of elite distance runners—echocardiography, vectorcardiography, and cardiac intervals. Ann NY Acad Sci 1977;301:297.

25. Wieling W, Borghols EAM, Hollander AP, Danner SA, Dunning AJ: Echocardiographic dimensions and maximal oxygen uptake in oarsmen during training. Br Heart J 1981; 46:190.

26. Adams TD, Yanowitz FG, Fisher AG, et al: Noninvasive evaluation of exercise training in college-age men. Circulation 1981;64:958.

27. De Maria AN, Neumann A, Lee G, Fowler W, Mason DT: Alterations in ventricular mass and performance induced by exercise training in man evaluated by echocardiography. Circulation 1978;57:237.

28. Ehsani AA, Hagberg JM, Hickson RC: Rapid changes in left ventricular dimensions and mass in response to physical conditioning and deconditioning. Am J Cardiol 1978;42:52.

28a. Gregoire JM, Caminiti G, Message R: Sudden death in athletes. Rev Med Brux 1990;11:272.

29. Attina DA, Falorni PL, Pieri A, Iannizzotto C, De Saint Pierre G: The electrocardiogram of the middle-aged men who practice physical activity outside of their normal work-time. In: Lubich T, Venerando A, eds. Sports cardiology. Bologna: Aulo Gaggi, 1980:257.

30. Chapman JH: Profound sinus bradycardia in the athletic heart syndrome. J Sports Med Phys Fitness 1982;22:45.

31. Cohen JL, Gupta PK, Lichtstein E, Chadda KD: The heart of a dancer: noninvasive cardiac evaluation of professional ballet dancers. Am J Cardiol 1980;45:959.

32. Hanne-Paparo N, Drory Y, Schoenfeld Y, Shapira Y, Kellermann JJ: Common ECG changes in athletes. Cardiology 1976;61:267.

33. Parker BM, Londeree BR, Cupp GV, Dubiel JP: The noninvasive cardiac evaluation of long-distance runners. Chest 1978;73:376.

34. Roeske WR, O'Rourke RA, Klein A, Leopold G, Karliner JS: Noninvasive evaluation of ventricular hypertrophy in professional athletes. Circulation 1976;53:286.

35. Van Ganse W, Versee L, Eylenbosch W, Vuylsteek K: The electrocardiogram of athletes: comparison with untrained subjects. Br Heart J 1970;32:160.

35a. Hergenroeder AC, Bricker JT: Pre-season cardiovascular examination: a review. J Adolesc Health Care 1990;11:379.

36. Venerando A, Rulli V: Frequency, morphology and meaning of the electrocardiographic anomalies found in olympic marathon runners and walkers. J Sports Med 1964;3: 135.

37. Astrand P, Rodohl K: Textbook of work physiology. New York: McGraw-Hill, 1977:176.

38. Bruns D: Muskelarbeit und Herzgrösse. Verh. 4. Dtsch Sportärztetagung. Berlin: Jena, 1927:91.

39. Ferrer M. The sick sinus syndrome. Circulation 1973;47:635.

40. Ward OC: A new familiar cardiac syndrome in children. J Ir Med Assoc 1964;54:103.

41. Dighton D: Sinuatrial block. Autonomic influences and clinical assessment. Br Heart J 1974;36:791.

42. Lin Y-C, Horvath SM: Autonomic nervous control of cardiac frequency in the exercise-trained rat. J Appl Physiol 1972; 33:796.

43. Scheuer J, Penpargkul S, Bhan AK: Experimental observations on the effects of physical training upon intrinsic cardiac physiology and biochemistry. Am J Cardiol 1974;33:744.

44. Williams RS, Eden RS, Moll ME, Lester RM, Wallace AG: Autonomic mechanisms of training bradycardia: β-adrenergic receptors in humans. J Appl Physiol 1981;51:1232.

45. Badeer HS: Cardiovascular adaptations in the trained athlete. In: Lubich T, Venerando A, eds. Sports cardiology. Bologna: Aulo Gaggi, 1980:3.

46. Ordway GA, Charles JB, Randall DC, Billman GE, Wekstein DR: Heart rate adaptation to exercise training in cardiac-denervated dogs. J Appl Physiol 1982;52:1586.

47. Beckner GL, Winsor T: Cardiovascular adaptations to prolonged physical effort. Circulation 1954;9:835.

48. Ford LE: Heart size. Circ Res 1976;39:297.

49. Hanne-Paparo N: Long term ECG monitoring of a sportsman with a second degree A-V block. In: Lubich T, Venerando A, eds. Sports cardiology. Bologna: Aula Gaggi, 1980:559.

50. Meytes I, Kaplinsky E, Yahini JH, Hanne-Paparo N, Neufeld HN: Wenckebach A-V block: a frequent feature following heavy physical training. Am Heart J 1975;90:426.

50a. Luke JL, Farb A, Virmani R, Sample RH: Sudden cardiac death during exercise in a weight lifter using anabolic androgenic steroids: Pathological and toxicological findings. J Forensic Sci 1990;35:1441.

51. Rossi F, Todaro A, Venerando A, Pigorini F: An investigation of pulmonary vascularization in endurance athletes. In: Lubich T, Venerando A, eds. Sports cardiology. Bologna: Aulo Gaggi, 1980:351.

52. Smith WG, Cullen KJ, Thorburn IO: Electrocardiograms of marathon runners in 1962 Commonwealth Games. Br Heart J 1964;26:469.

53. Hiss RG, Lamb LE: Electrocardiographic findings in 122,043 individuals. Circulation 1962;25:947.

54. Minamitani K, Miyagawa M, Konco M, Kitamura K: The electrocardiogram of professional cyclists. In: Lubich T, Venerando A, eds. Sports cardiology. Bologna: Aulo Gaggi, 1980:315.

55. Fenici R, Caselli G, Zeppilli P, Piovano G: High degree A-V block in 17 well-trained endurance athletes. In: Lubich T, Venerando A, eds. Sports cardiology. Bologna: Aulo Gaggi, 1980:523.

56. Holmgrenn A, Karlberg P, Pernow B: Circulatory adaptation at rest and during muscular work in patients with complete heart block. Acta Med Scand 1959;164:119.

57. Kambara H, Phillips J: Long-term evaluation of early repolarization syndrome (normal variant RS-T segment elevation). Am J Cardiol 1976;38:156.

58. Lengyel M, Gyárfás I: The importance of echocardiography in the assessment of left ventricular hypertrophy in trained and untrained schoolchildren. Acta Cardiol 1979;34:63.

59. Levy AM, Camm AJ, Keane JF: Multiple arrhythmias detected during nocturnal monitoring in patients with congenital complete heart block. Circulation 1977;55:247.

60. Nakamoto K: Electrocardiograms of 25 marathon runners before and after 100 meter dash. Jpn Circ J 1969;33:105.

61. Zeppilli P, Fenici R, Sassara M, Pirrami MM, Caselli G: Wenckebach second-degree A-V block in top-ranking athletes: an old problem revisited. Am Heart J 1980;100:281.

62. Gibbons LW, Cooper KH, Martin RP, Pollock ML: Medical examination and electrocardiographic analysis of elite distance runners. Ann NY Acad Sci 1977;301:283.

63. Young D, Eisenberg R, Fish B, Fisher JD: Wenckebach atrioventricular block (Mobitz I) in children and adolescents. Am J Cardiol 1977;40:393.

64. Turner LB: Asymptomatic congenital complete heart block in an Army Air Force pilot. Am Heart J 1947;34:426.

65. Venerando A: Electrocardiography in sports medicine. J Sports Med Phys Fitness 1979;19:107.

66. Wolffe JB: Intermittent heart block in athletes. Proceedings of the Sixteenth Congress of Sports Medicine, Hannover, Germany 1966:213.

67. Manning GW: Electrocardiography in the selection of Royal Canadian Air Force aircrew. Circulation 1964;10:401.

68. Paul MH, Rudolph AM, Nadas AS: Congenital complete atrioventricular block: problems of clinical assessment. Circulation 1958;18:183.

69. Thoren C, Herin P, Vavra J: Studies of submaximal and maximal exercise in congenital complete heart block. Acta Paediatr Belg 1974;28:132.

70. Winkler RB, Freed M, Nadas A: Exercise induced ventricular ectopy in children and young adults with complete heart block. Am Heart J 1980;99(1):87.

71. Crawford MH, O'Rourke RA: The athlete's heart. Adv Intern Med 1979;24:311.

72. Coelho A, Palileo E, Ashley W: Tachyarrhythmias in young athletes. J Am Coll Cardiol (in press)

73. Epstein SE, Maron B: Hypertrophic cardiomyopathy: an overview. In: Kaltenbach M, Epstein SE, eds. Hypertrophic cardiomyopathy. Berlin, Heidelberg, New York: Springer-Verlag, 1982:5.

74. Butschenko LA: Das Ruhe- und Belastungs-EKG bei Sportlern. Leipzig: Johannes Ambrosius Verlag, 1967.

75. So CS: Wolff-Parkinson-White-syndrom. Münch Med Wschr 1967;113:11.

76. Hanne-Paparo N, Wendkos MH, Brunner DT: T wave abnormalities in electrocardiograms of top-ranking athletes without demonstrating organic heart disease. Am Heart J 1971; 81:743.

77. Hejtmanick MR, Herrman GR: The electrocardiographic syndrome of short PR-interval and broad QRS complexes. Am Heart J 1957;54:708.

78. Holzmann M: Neue diagnostische und therapeutische Entwicklungen beim Syndrom von Wolff, Parkinson and White. Schweiz Med Wochenschr 1971;101:494.

79. Furlanello F, Bertoldi A, Bettini R, Dallago M, Vergara G: Life-threatening tachyarrhythmias in athletes. PACE Pacing Clin Electrophysiol 1992;15(9):1403.

80. Heinecker R: Die Bedeutung des WPW-Syndroms. Dtsch Med Wochenschr 1968;93:357.

81. Betghe KP, Meiners G, Lichtlen PR: Incidence and prognostic significance of ventricular arrhythmias in individuals without detectable heart disease. Eur Heart J 1983;4:338.

82. Brodsky M, Wu D, Denes P, Kanakis C, Rosen KM: Arrhythmias documented by 24-hour continuous electrocardiographic monitoring in 50 male students without apparent heart disease. Am J Cardiol 1977;39:390.

83. Karpman VL, Kukolevskiy GM, eds. The heart and sports. Moscow: Meditsina Press, 1968:106.

84. Sobotka PA, Mayer JH, Bauernfeind RA, Kanakis C, Rosen KM: Arrhythmias documented by 24-hour continuous ambulatory electrocardiographic monitoring in young women without apparent heart disease. Am Heart J 1981;101:753.

85. Freggiaro V, Morelloni S, Pareti G, et al: Prevalence of hyperkinetic ventricular arrhythmias in an ambulatory population of nonprofessional athletes. A study controlled by ambulatory electrocardiography. Clin Ther 1990;134(3):217.

86. Furlanello F, Bettini R, Bertoldi A, et al: Stable ventricular tachycardia in arrhythmogenic dysplasia of the right ventricle in sportsmen. Cardiologia 1990;30:82.

87. Northcote RJ, MacFarlane P, Ballantayne D: Ambulatory electrocardiography in squash players. Br Heart J 1983;50:372.

88. Pilcher GF, Cook A-J, Johnston BL, Fletcher GF: Twenty-four-hour continuous electrocardiography during exercise and free activity in 80 apparently healthy runners. Am J Cardiol 1983;52:859.

88a. Van Camp PA: Sudden death. Clin Sports Med 1992;11:273.

89. Browne KF, Prystowsky EN, Heger JJ, Cerimele BJ, Fineberg N, Zipes DP: Prolongation of the QT-interval induced by probucol: Demonstration of a method for determining QT interval change induced by a drug. Am Heart J 1984;107:680.

90. Kauller LH: Sudden death/definition and epidemiologic considerations. Prog Cardiovasc Dis 1980;23:114.

91. Koplan JP: Cardiovascular death while running. JAMA 1979; 23:114.

92. Thompson PD, Stern MP: Death during jogging or running. JAMA 1979;242:1265.

93. Siscovick D, Weiss N, Fletcher R, Lasky T: The incidence of primary cardiac arrest during vigorous exercise. N Engl J Med 1984;311:874.

94. Pool J: Sudden death and sports. In: Fagard R, Bekaert J. Sports cardiology. Amsterdam, Kluwer Academic Publishers, 1986:223.

95. Montpetit RR: Applied physiology of squash. Sports Med 1990;10(1):31.

96. Corrado D, Thiene G, Nava A, Rossi L, Pennelli N: Sudden death in young competitive athletes: clinicopathologic correlation in 22 cases. Am J Med 1990;89(5):588.

97. Johnson RJ: Sudden death during exercise. A cruel turn of events. Postgrad Med 1992;92(2):195.

98. Kenny A, Shapiro LM: Sudden cardiac death in athletes. Br Med Bull 1992;48(3):534.

99. La Harpe R, Rostan A, Fryc O: Sudden death during performance of sport: forensic medicine elucidation. Schweiz Z Sportmed 1992;40(2):65.

100. Sternon J, Stoupel E: Sudden death in young athletes. Rev Med Brux 1990;11(5):156.
101. Wesslen L, Pahlsen C, Friman G, Fohlman J, Lindquist O, Johansson C: Myocarditis caused by *Chlamydia pneumoniae* and sudden unexpected death in Swedish elite orienteer. Lancet 1992;340:427.
102. Menapace FJ, Hammer WJ, Rityer TF: Left ventricular size in competitive weight lifters: an echocardiographic study. Med Sci Sports Exerc 1982;3:141.
103. Simons SM, Moriarity J: Hypertrophic cardiomyopathy in a college athlete. Med Sci Sports Exerc 1992;24(12):1321.
104. Morales AR, Romanelli R, Boucek RJ: The neural LAD coronary artery, strenuous exercise and sudden death. Circulation 1980;62:230.
105. Minutiello L: Ischemic cardiomyopathy in young athletes. Description of 3 cases. Minerva Cardioangiol 1990;38 (11):505.
106. Lynberg KK: Myocardial infarction and death of a body builder after using anabolic steroids. Ugeskr Laeger 1991; 153(8):587.
107. Salerno JA, Guasti L, Panciroli C, Chimienti M, Previtali M, Bobba P: Syncope and sudden death due to vasospastic myocardial ischemia in young sportsmen. Cardiologia 1990;35(1):69.
108. Opie LH: Sudden death and sports. Lancet 1975,3:263.
109. Vuori I, Makarainen M, Jasselainen A: Sudden death and physical activity. Cardiology 1978;63:287.
110. Waller BF, Roberts WC: Sudden death while running in conditioned runners aged 40 years or more. Am J Cardiol 1980;45:1292.
111. Friedman M, Manwaring JH, Roseman RH: Instantaneous exercise and sudden deaths. JAMA 1972;225:1319.
112. Ali T: Sudden death in athletes in Trinidad and Tobago. West Indian Med J 1991;40(4):192.
113. Gibbons LW, Cooper KH, Meyer BM, Ellison C: The acute cardiac risk of strenuous exercise. JAMA 1980;244:1799.
114. Desseigne P, Tabib A, Loire R: Sudden death of the sportsman. Apropos of 23 cases with autopsy. Ann Cardiol Angeiol (Paris) 1991;40(4):175.
115. Jaeger M: Sudden death during sport activities. How can the incidence be reduced?. Ann Cardiol Angeiol (Paris) 1990; 39(10):565.
116. Zipes D, Cobb LA, Garson A, et al: Task Force VI: Arrhythmias. J Am Coll Cardiol 1985;6(6):1225.

Cardiac Arrhythmias, 3rd edition, edited by William J. Mandel.
J. B. Lippincott Company, Philadelphia © 1995.

36

Elliott M. Antman • Thomas W. Smith

Digitalis Toxicity: An Overview of Mechanisms, Manifestations, and Management

This chapter addresses our current understanding of clinically relevant aspects of the pharmacology of digitalis, with emphasis on digitalis toxicity and its management. Clinicians are aware that many patients on maintenance digoxin will derive little benefit from the drug beyond an improvement of cardiac function during periods of stress. Other patients, including some in sinus rhythm, continue to derive significant benefit from long-term digitalis administration. Because of the relatively narrow therapeutic window for digitalis glycosides, the continuing clinical challenge is to identify those patients having a favorable risk/benefit ratio for digitalis use, to recognize signs and symptoms of digitalis toxicity promptly when they develop, and to treat toxicity appropriately.

MECHANISM OF ACTION

It is now agreed that the positive inotropic effects of digitalis glycosides result from altered excitation–contraction coupling. Calcium ions constitute the trigger that couples electrical depolarization of the sarcolemma to mechanical contractile events. Several major structural elements in the cardiac cell are involved in the control of the free intracellular calcium ion concentration. Sarcolemmal membrane structures (Fig. 36-1) that regulate entry of calcium into the cell include the slow calcium channel, the sodium–calcium exchanger, and (indirectly) sodium and potassium–activated adenosine triphosphatase (NaK-ATPase) and the sodium–hydrogen exchanger. After decades of controversy, a consensus had emerged that the inotropic effects of digitalis glycosides result from binding to and inhibition of NaK-ATPase.[1]

Inhibition of NaK-ATPase pumps initiates a chain of events that alters excitation–contraction coupling by making more calcium available to contractile elements, thus enhancing the force of myocardial contraction (Fig. 36-2). The alpha subunit of NaK-ATPase that faces the outside of the cell is the only site identified in cardiac tissue with the binding properties required of the "digitalis receptor." Cardiac glycosides bind with high affinity and specificity to this site, resulting in the complete blockade of sodium and potassium transport by that enzyme unit. This observation has focused attention on the link between inhibition of sodium and potassium transport across the sarcolemmal membrane and alteration of calcium handling and the cardiac contractile state (Fig. 36-3).

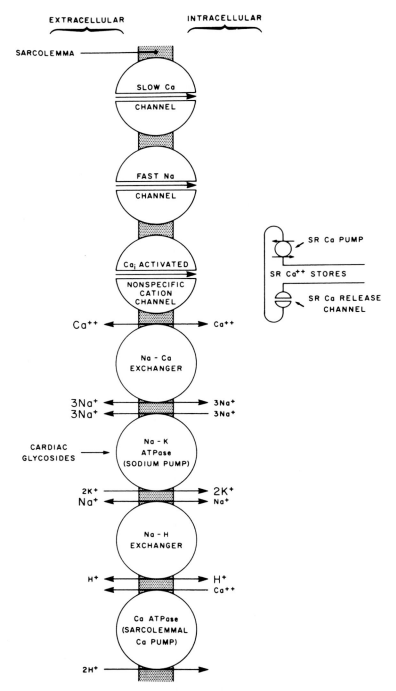

Figure 36-1. Selected components regulating cellular calcium homeostasis in myocardium. (1) The slow calcium channel, a voltage-sensitive protein complex that carries the slow inward calcium current during phase 2 of the cardiac action potential, provides the pulse of intracellular calcium $[Ca^{++}]_i$ that triggers calcium-induced release of a much larger amount of activator calcium from stores in the sarcoplasmic reticulum (SR). The arrow indicates the principal direction of ion movement when the channel is activated. (2) The fast sodium channel, another voltage-sensitive structure, mediates the upstroke of the cardiac action potential; this depolarization event results in activation of the slow calcium channel. (3) A putative intracellular calcium-activated nonspecific cation channel, less well characterized than the preceding components, could account for the transient depolarizing (and hence arrhythmogenic) inward current that occurs in response to toxic doses of cardiac glycosides (see text). (*continued*)

This link is now recognized to be the sodium–calcium exchanger that mediates the transsarcolemmal movement of calcium ion in exchange for sodium ion (see Fig. 36-1).[2,3] This process is electrogenic because a net movement of charge occurs (exchange of an estimated three sodium ions for each calcium ion); hence, it is sensitive to the membrane potential.[4] An increase in the intracellular concentration of sodium (as, for example, in response to digitalis-induced inhibition of sodium extrusion) favors increased calcium entry and also reduced calcium extrusion through sodium–calcium exchange.[5] Pivotal in establishing the role of sodium pump inhibition in the positive inotropic effect of digitalis has been the demonstration by Eisner and colleagues of the very steep dependence of tension development on the intracellular sodium concentration.[6] An increase in the intracellular sodium concentration of only 1 mmol, from 6 to 7 mmol, in response to sodium-pump inhibition resulted in a doubling of tension development in sheep cardiac Purkinje fibers. This explains why earlier workers, using less sensitive methods, had difficulty in demonstrating sodium-pump inhibition at subtoxic but positively inotropic concentrations of digitalis.

Additional cellular mechanisms are worthy of mention in relation to the positive inotropic effects of digitalis. It has been proposed that a small increase in the intracellular calcium ion concentration due to the previously mentioned sodium–calcium exchange mechanism acts as a positive feedback signal to increase calcium entry through slow calcium channels.[7] It is important to note, however, that positive inotropic effects can still be documented under appropriate experimental conditions in the absence of an increase in inward calcium movement through calcium channels.[7] Stimulation of the release and blockade of reuptake of norepinephrine from adrenergic nerve terminals in intact myocardium is another mecha-

nism by which digitalis can modulate myocardial contractile force, at least under experimental conditions in vitro (see Fig. 36-2). Studies of the sodium–hydrogen exchange process in cardiac myocytes have revealed yet another mechanism by which sodium-pump inhibition affects the contractile state. A digitalis-induced increase in the intracellular calcium ion concentration is accompanied by an increase in the intracellular concentration of hydrogen ion (a fall in the intracellular pH). This leads, in turn, to inward transsarcolemmal movement of sodium ion and outward movement of hydrogen ion through sodium–hydrogen exchange. Thus, the sequence of events outlined in Figure 36-2 includes a positive feedback signal on intracellular sodium concentration to increase it further and a negative feedback signal on intracellular pH to slow the rate of intracellular acidification, mediated in both cases by sodium–hydrogen exchange.

CARDIAC ELECTROPHYSIOLOGY

Woodbury and colleagues in the early 1950s found that exposure to digitalis first prolonged and then accelerated repolarization and decreased the amplitude of the action potential with little short-term effect on the resting potential (Fig. 36-4).[8,9] Numerous studies have subsequently dealt with the effects of digitalis glycosides on the various segments of the cardiac conducting system. Decreased membrane potentials have been noted in atrioventricular (AV) nodal cells, Purkinje fibers, and atrial and ventricular myocardial cells after exposure to toxic concentrations of digitalis glycosides. These findings are associated with decreases in action potential amplitude and upstroke velocity (V_{max}), and repolarization is accelerated in all cardiac cell types studied. Perhaps the most profound effect of toxic doses of digitalis compounds identified has been

Figure 36-1. (continued)
(4) The sodium–calcium exchanger is a membrane component that mediates the facilitated, bidirectional exchange of sodium for calcium across the sarcolemmal membrane. This process is sensitive to membrane potential because of the asymmetry of charge movement inherent in the stoichiometry of the process (three sodium ions for every calcium ion). Sodium–calcium exchange current may cause or contribute to oscillatory afterpotentials occurring as a result of digitalis toxicity. (5) The NaK-ATPase, or sodium pump. The cardiac glycoside-binding site is located on the outward-facing surface of the alpha subunit of this enzyme, which mediates the active transport of sodium and potassium ions against their respective concentration gradients. (6) The sodium–hydrogen exchanger, an amiloride-sensitive protein, mediates the electroneutral exchange of sodium for hydrogen ions and helps to facilitate the accumulation of intracellular sodium (and hence intracellular calcium) in response to cardiac glycosides. (7) The sarcolemmal calcium pump is a relatively low-capacity but high-affinity ATP-dependent ion-transport protein that extrudes calcium from cardiac cells against a large electrochemical gradient and helps to maintain the low levels of intracellular calcium ions that prevail during diastole. To the right of the sarcolemmal membrane are represented (8) the sarcoplasmic reticulum ATP-dependent calcium pump that is responsible for diastolic relaxation by rapid sequestration of calcium at end systole, and (9) the ryanodine-sensitive sarcoplasmic reticulum calcium-release channel that accounts for calcium-induced release of most of the calcium that activates contractile proteins in mammalian myocardium. (Smith, TW: Digitalis. Mechanisms of action and clinical use. N Eng J Med 1988;318:358.)

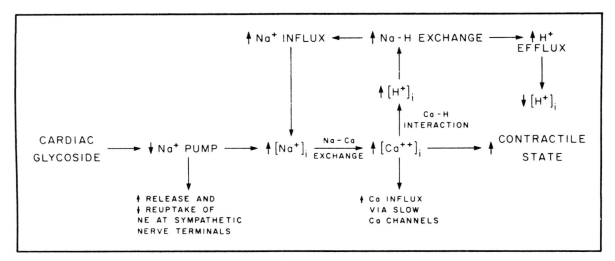

Figure 36-2. Mechanisms of modulation of myocardial function by cardiac glycosides. In addition to the horizontal sequence leading from cardiac glycoside–induced inhibition of the sodium pump to the enhancced myocardial contractile state, three ancillary processes are shown: enhanced norepinephrine (NE) release and reduced reuptake at cardiac sympathetic nerve terminals, which may occur in experimental circumstances but has doubtful clinical relevance; an enhanced slow inward calcium current with increased calcium influx through slow calcium channels in response to an increased concentration of intracellular calcium ions over a limited range of values for these ions; and decreased intracellular pH (increased $[H^+]_i$) in response to increased intracellular calcium, leading to enhanced sodium–hydrogen exchange and hence augmentation of the rise in intracellular sodium ($[Na^+]_i$) caused by sodium-pump inhibition. (Smith TW: Digitalis. Mechanisms of action and clinical use. N Engl J Med 1988;318:358.)

the development or acceleration of spontaneous phase 4 depolarization (Fig. 36-5). This is readily seen in AV nodal and Purkinje fibers because the conducting system tends to be more sensitive to the drug than is myocardial tissue. Finally, if exposure to toxic doses of digitalis is prolonged, electrical quiescence occurs.[10–13]

The cellular mechanism by which toxic doses of digitalis produce such effects is presumed to be related to the loss of intracellular potassium and accumulation of extracellular potassium, with a concomitant rise in intracellular sodium ion concentration, due to the inhibition of NaK-ATPase.[14] Elevated extracellular potassium augments

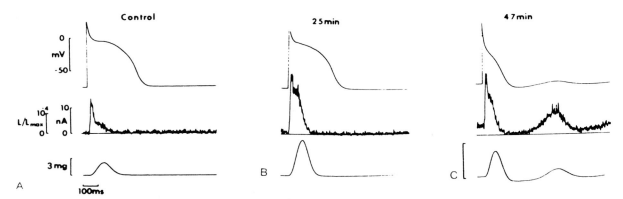

Figure 36-3. Calcium transients measured with aequorin during exposure to digitalis. Simultaneous signal-averaged recordings of membrane potential (top curve), signals from the calcium-activated bioluminescent protein aequorin (middle curve), and tension in a canine cardiac Purkinje fiber (bottom curve) before (**A**) and during (**B**, at 25 minutes, and **C**, at 47 minutes) exposure to 10^{-7}M ouabain. Note the delayed afterdepolarization in **C**, accompanying in an aequorin signal and a mechanical aftercontraction, both of which reflect a transient increase in the intracellular calcium–ion concentration. (Wier WG, Hess P: Excitation–contraction coupling in cardiac Purkinje fibers: effects of cardiotonic steroids on the intracellular $[Ca^{2+}]$ transient, membrane potential, and contraction. J Gen Physiol 1984;83:395.)

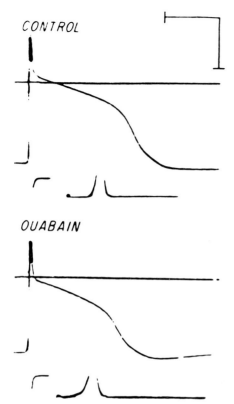

Figure 36-4. Typical effects of exposure to toxic concentrations of digitalis on a canine Purkinje fiber action potential. Note: (1) decrease in resting potential, (2) decrease in amplitude, (3) acceleration of voltage–time course of repolarization, (4) decrease in V_{max}, and (5) increase in phase 4 slope. (Rosen MR: Cellular electrophysiology of digitalis toxicity. J Amer Coll Cardiol 1985;5:22A.)

membrane conductance of potassium, accelerating repolarization and depressing the plateau of the action potential (phase 2). Action potential upstroke velocity and amplitude are depressed, resulting in a slowing of or block in conduction. Digitalis, along with its ability to enhance acetylcholine release (see below), causes a more notice-

able depression in conduction in tissues more sensitive to parasympathetic influence (i.e., the sinoatrial [SA] and AV nodes as well as the atrium). Tachyarrhythmias due to digitalis excess may in some cases be related to an increase in the slope of phase 4 depolarization (see Fig. 36-5 and Table 36-1).[11-13] To some degree, this enhancement of phase 4 depolarization may be augmented by increased efferent sympathetic traffic to the heart due to central nervous system actions of digitalis.

In addition to altering phase 4 depolarization, digitalis can induce oscillatory activity, resulting from delayed afterdepolarization and oscillatory afterpotentials (Fig. 36-6 and Table 36-1).[13,15] These delayed afterdepolarizations arise as a consequence of a sequence of events initiated by inhibition of the NaK-ATPase system. The resulting increase in intracellular calcium through Na–Ca exchange appears to trigger a transient inward current (I_{ti}) that may flow through a tetrodotoxin-insensitive channel (i.e., a channel different from the fast sodium channel)[16] or may represent an inward current resulting from the Na–Ca exchange process itself. Detailed electrophysiologic studies in isolated tissues suggest that calcium overload and delayed afterdepolarizations are likely mechanisms underlying many tachyarrhythmias associated with digitalis toxicity (see Table 36-1).

Alterations in extracellular potassium concentration modify the electrophysiologic events occurring in digitalis intoxication. Low extracellular potassium concentrations enhance the likelihood that digitalis will bind to myocardial receptor sites and also enhance the development of spontaneous phase 4 depolarization and automatic rhythms. In contrast, as extracellular potassium increases, cardiac glycoside binding to the NaK-ATPase system diminishes. At levels above the upper limit of normal, however, elevated extracellular potassium accelerates repolarization and decreases the resting potential and the amplitude and upstroke velocity of the action potential. This ultimately reduces conduction velocity significantly.[13] Any shift from the normal range of extracellular potassium

TABLE 36-1. Comparison of Digitalis-Induced Repetitive Ventricular Responses in Intact Animals and Delayed Afterdepolarizations in Isolated Tissues

Repetitive Ventricular Responses	Delayed Afterdepolarizations
Initiated by premature beat during T wave (after vulnerable period) or early diastole	Initiated most readily at short drive cycle lengths or by premature depolarizations occurring at short coupling intervals
With increasing degree of digitalis toxicity, the electrical current needed to induce repetitive ventricular responses decreases	With increasing degree of digitalis toxicity, the electrical current required to bring delayed afterdepolarizations to threshold potential decreases
With increasing digitalis toxicity, there is a greater likelihood of longer trains of repetitive ventricular responses	With increasing digitalis toxicity, the trains of tachyarrhythmias induced by delayed afterdepolarizations tend to get longer

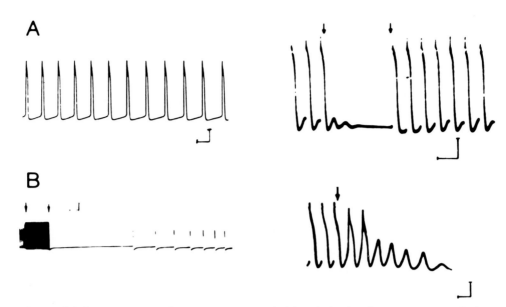

Figure 36-5. Comparison of automatic activity with delayed afterdepolarization in canine Purkinje fiber. In **A**, an automatic fiber with phase 4 depolarization (left) is compared with a fiber exposed to toxic concentrations of digitalis. After the first arrow, the drive is stopped, and a series of oscillations is seen. Drive is resumed at the second arrow, and several beats are needed before the delayed afterdepolarizations achieve full amplitude. In **B**, the panel to the left shows the effect of overdrive on an automatic rhythm. Rapid pacing starts at the first arrow and stops at the second arrow. Hyperpolarization occurs with overdrive. After overdrive, a long pause is observed before automatic firing resumes. At the right of **B**, pacing is stopped after three cycles, and two action potentials follow secondary to delayed afterdepolarizations reaching threshold. Subsequently, nonthreshold afterdepolarizations occur until they also cease. (Rosen MR: Cellular electrophysiology of digitalis toxicity. J Amer Coll Cardiol 1985;5:22A.)

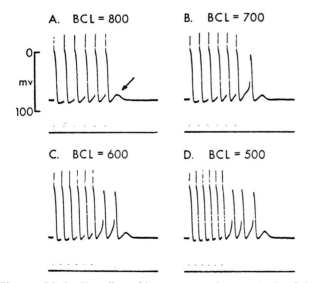

Figure 36-6. The effect of heart rate on the magnitude of delayed afterdepolarizations and triggered automaticity in canine Purkinje fibers exposed to toxic doses of digitalis. The bottom portion of each panel shows a train of six stimuli. Note that as the cycle length (BCL) decreases, the number of suprathreshold afterdepolarizations increases, therefore increasing the number of triggered action potentials. (Ferreir GR, Saunders JH, Mendez C: A cellular mechanism for the generation of ventricular arrhythmias by acetylstrophanthidin. Circ Res 1973;32:600.)

concentration, in association with digitalis excess, may provoke or exacerbate conduction disturbances and promote the appearance of ectopic activity in the atria, ventricles, or both.

Elevations in extracellular calcium can also reduce the threshold potential and, perhaps more important, augment the transient inward current associated with delayed afterdepolarizations. In contrast, a reduction in extracellular calcium tends to increase the threshold potential and thus augment excitability.[13]

Therefore, abnormal extracellular concentrations of potassium and calcium ions (and magnesium) can produce detrimental effects when administering digitalis. Vigorous efforts to maintain normal levels of these electrolytes are vital principles of clinical management in patients receiving digitalis glycosides.

Age appears to modify the electrophysiologic effects of digitalis. In neonatal hearts of some species, higher concentrations of digitalis are required to produce the typical effects of digitalis excess, whereas in heart preparations from older animals, such digitalis effects are seen more readily at lower concentrations.[17] The recognition and characterization of alpha subunit isoforms of NaK-ATPase with differing cardiac glycoside affinity and hence sensitivity promise to enhance our understanding of these developmental changes in digitalis sensitivity. Finally, the diseased myocardium appears to be especially sensitive to digitalis glycosides, and toxicity develops more easily.[18]

AUTONOMIC NERVOUS SYSTEM

Important effects of cardiac glycosides stem from their multifaceted influence on the autonomic nervous system.[19,20] In the parasympathetic system, digitalis glycosides have both central and peripheral effects. Afferent as well as efferent activity is altered, as is primary central nervous system processing of impulses (possibly resulting from inhibition of monovalent cation transport at related neural loci). The afferent impulses seem to be related predominantly to baroreceptors and chemoreceptors, especially in the carotid sinus and aortic arch.[19,20] The myocardium also appears to have receptors that mediate increases in afferent impulses in the presence of digitalis. Efferent activity is enhanced after digitalis administration, possibly as a result of enhanced ganglionic transmission. Of additional importance is the fact that digitalis potentiates cardiac vagal responses, especially in the SA and AV nodes.[21]

The influence of digitalis on the sympathetic nervous system under clinical circumstances remains to be elucidated but probably is clinically significant only at higher serum levels of glycoside. First, efferent sympathetic activity is affected generally in association with clearly toxic doses of digitalis. Second, digitalis, in excess, appears to cause the release of catecholamines from sympathetic nerve terminals or to prevent catecholamine uptake. Catecholamine release may potentiate digitalis toxicity (probably as a result of increasing automaticity of ectopic pacemakers), at least in part by increasing the magnitude of delayed afterdepolarizations.

PHARMACOKINETICS AND BIOAVAILABILITY OF DIGITALIS GLYCOSIDES

Clinically useful cardiac glycoside preparations are derived from the leaves and seeds of plants in the genera *Digitalis* and *Strophanthus*. The basic structure of each cardiac glycoside consists of a combination of an aglycone (or genin) with one to four glycoside moieties attached at the C-3 position of the steroid ring.[22] Although pharmacologic activity resides in the aglycone, water solubility and pharmacokinetic properties are determined to a large extent by the sugar moieties attached to the aglycone.[22] Figure 36-7 illustrates the derivation of clinically relevant digitalis preparations.

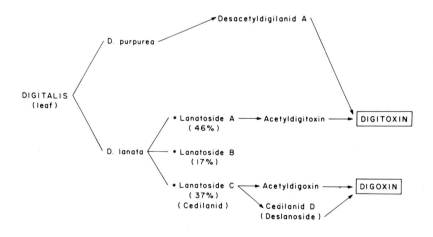

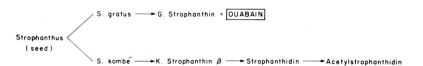

Figure 36-7. Schematic diagram of the derivation of digoxin, digitoxin, and ouabain. (Smith TW, Antman EM, Friedman PL, Blatt CM, Marsh JD: Digitalis glycosides: mechanisms and manifestations of toxicity. Prog Cardiovasc Dis 1984;26:413.)

Digoxin

Its flexibility of route of administration, intermediate duration of action, and readily available techniques for assay of serum levels make digoxin the cardiac glycoside used most frequently in hospital and office practice in both Europe and the United States.[23] In addition, digoxin may be administered intravenously, intramuscularly, or orally (in tablet, elixir, or encapsulated gel form). The intramuscular route of administration should not be used because of pain at the site of injection and unreliable absorption.

Approximately 37% of total body stores of digoxin is removed daily in patients without renal impairment. When renal function is normal, digoxin is excreted exponentially with an average half-life of 36 hours, irrespective of the route of administration (Fig. 36-8).[24] In older patients, a half-life of 48 hours is probably a better estimate, because they have a reduced glomerular filtration rate even in the presence of normal blood urea nitrogen (BUN) and creatinine levels. Renal excretion of digoxin is generally proportional to the glomerular filtration rate.[25,26] It is important, however, to realize that renal tubular reabsorption of digoxin may increase at low urinary flow rates and that vasodilator therapy in patients with congestive heart failure may enhance tubular secretion of digoxin.[27,28]

Although digoxin is excreted predominantly in unchanged form, in about 10% of individuals the drug is metabolized in the gut to digoxin reduction products such as dihydrodigoxin and dihydrodigoxigenin.[29,30] Thus, in those 10% of individuals receiving digoxin who form large amounts of reduction products, antibiotic therapy that alters gut flora can result in important increases in effective dose and body (and myocardial) digoxin content.[31]

Pharmacokinetic studies indicate that in the case of digoxin, steady-state plateau concentrations occur after about 7 days in patients with normal renal function.[32] When prompt onset of action is required, a loading dose should be given followed by daily maintenance therapy. Because digoxin pharmacokinetics are the same before and after the loss of large amounts of adipose tissue, lean body mass should be used when calculating dosage.[33,34] Only the unbound drug is active, but protein binding of digoxin is a minor pharmacokinetic factor (which stands in contrast to digitoxin).[35]

Bioavailability

Drug formulations that meet chemical and physical standards established by regulatory agencies are termed chemically equivalent. Biologic equivalence refers to the fact that the administration of two preparations results in similar concentrations of the drug in blood and tissues. Therapeutic equivalence indicates that such preparations show equal therapeutic benefit in clinical trials. Those preparations that are chemically equivalent but lack bio-

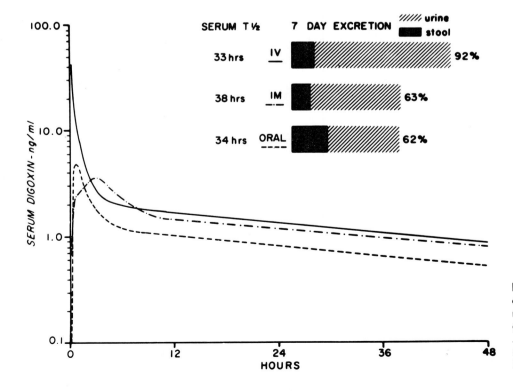

Figure 36-8. Pharmacokinetic comparison of intravenous, intramuscular, and orally administered digoxin. (Doherty JE, deSoyza N, Kane JJ, et al: Clinical pharmacokinetics of digitalis glycosides. Prog Cardiovasc Dis 1978;21:141.)

logic or therapeutic equivalence are said to differ in bioavailability. Previous studies have indicated that although tablets may contain chemically equivalent amounts of digoxin, disparities in dissolution rates coupled with variations among patients and circumstances of drug administration may lead to considerable inconsistency in digoxin bioavailability.[36,37] To minimize this clinical problem, the FDA has constructed guidelines for dissolution rates for all digoxin tablets marketed in the United States.[35]

Drug Interactions With Cardiac Glycosides

Drug interactions involving digitalis glycosides are predominantly of either the pharmacokinetic or the pharmacodynamic type. The multitude of drug interactions that have been reported to date have been summarized in several recent reviews. Table 36-2 outlines many of the established pharmacokinetic drug interactions and indicates suggested dosage modifications when needed.

PHARMACODYNAMIC INTERACTIONS

Corticosteroid therapy, insulin and glucose therapy, diuretic therapy, or a potassium-depleted diet may cause hypokalemia, increasing the cardiac effects of digitalis glycosides and enhancing the potential for digitalis toxicity. As noted above, myocardial binding of digoxin increases in the presence of hypokalemia, and the toxic electrophysiologic effects of digitalis glycosides are further enhanced when potassium levels are low.[38] Because many of the cardiac effects of digitalis are mediated indirectly through enhanced vagal tone, circumstances that augment vagal tone or reduce sympathetic nervous activity may exacerbate the electrophysiologic effects of the glycosides on cardiac tissue.

TABLE 36-2. Pharmacokinetic Drug Interactions with Digoxin

Drug	Mechanism of Interaction: Effect on Digoxin	Mean Magnitude of Interaction (%)	Suggested Intervention
Cholestyramine	Adsorption of digoxin	↓ 25	1. Give digoxin 8 hours before cholestyramine 2. Use solution or capsule form of digoxin
Antacids	Unclear	↓ 25	Temporal separation of time of administration
Kaolin-pectate	Adsorption of digoxin	?	1. Give digoxin 2 hours before kaolin-pectate 2. ? Use solution or capsule form of digoxin
Bran	Adsorption of digoxin	↓ 20	Temporal separation of time of administration
Neomycin Sulfasalazine PAS	Unknown	↓ 28 ↓ 18 ↓ 22	Increase dose of digoxin
Erythromycin Tetracycline (in <10% of subjects)	↑ Bioavailability by ↑ intestinal metabolism of digoxin by certain gut flora	↑ 43–116	1. Measure serum digoxin concentration 2. Decrease digoxin dose 3. Use solution or capsule form of digoxin
Quinidine	? ↓ Bioavailability ↓ volume of distribution, ↓ renal and nonrenal clearance	↓ 100	1. Decrease dose by 50% 2. Measure serum digoxin concentration
Amiodarone	↓ Renal and nonrenal clearance	↑ 70–100	Same as for quinidine
Verapamil	↓ Renal and nonrenal clearance	↑ 70–100	Same as for quinidine
Diltiazem	? ↓ Renal clearance	↑ 22	None
Nicardipine	Unknown	↑ 15	None
Tiapamil	Unknown	↑ 60	Same as for quinidine
Spironolactone	↓ Renal and nonrenal clearance	↑ 30	Measure serum digoxin concentration
Triamterene	↓ Nonrenal clearance	↑ 20	Measure serum digoxin concentration
Indomethacin (preterm infants)	? ↓ Renal clearance	↑ 50	Decrease dose by 25%

MEASUREMENT OF CARDIAC GLYCOSIDE CONCENTRATIONS: CLINICAL USE AND MISUSE

Inappropriate use or interpretations of serum digoxin concentrations can lead to suboptimal decisions and patient management. Several studies have defined the relationship between serum cardiac glycoside concentration and clinical responses (Table 36-3). From these data, which represent clinical experience in over 1000 patients, it is apparent that the concentrations of digoxin in patients believed clinically to be exhibiting digitalis toxicity and in those believed to be free of clinical evidence of toxicity overlap significantly.

In the case of an individual patient, no specific serum level can be identified to cleanly separate toxic from nontoxic states. A variety of causes of altered responsiveness to cardiac glycosides, resulting in either digitalis resistance or digitalis sensitivity, have been identified and are summarized in Table 36-4. When a patient on digoxin develops clinical symptoms suggestive of toxicity, a toxic response should be suspected, and it is appropriate to measure the serum digoxin level. However, certain metabolic abnormalities such as hypokalemia, hypomagnesemia, hypercalcemia, and severe acid–base imbalance predispose patients to digitalis toxicity even when the level of digoxin is found to be in the "therapeutic" range. Skepticism is appropriate when a laboratory result conflicts with clinical

TABLE 36-3. Serum or Plasma Concentrations—Patients With and Without Toxicity

Source	Mean Concentration (ng/mL)		Source	Mean Concentration (ng/mL)	
	Patients Without Toxicity	Patients With Toxicity		Patients Without Toxicity	Patients With Toxicity
Aronson et al	1.60	2.60	Lader et al	1.10	2.20
Beller et al	1.00	2.30	Lehmann et al		
Bernabei et al	1.00	2.90	Normokalaemic patients	N.S.‖	2.73
Bertler and Redfors*	0.90	2.40	Hypokalaemic patients	N.S.‖	1.76
Bertler et al*	1.40	3.10	Lichey et al	1.20	2.50
Booker and Jelliffe†	1.40	3.10	Loes et al	1.10	4.90
Burnett and Conklin	1.20	5.70	McCredie et al		
Carruthers et al‡	1.21	2.76	Infants	3.45	—
Chamberlain et al	1.40	3.10	Children	1.41	3.81
Doering et al	1.02	3.07	Morrison et al¶	0.76	3.35
Evered and Chapman	1.38	3.36	Oliver et al	1.60	3.00
Fogelman et al§	1.40	1.70	Park et al	1.10	3.80
Follath et al	1.20	3.20	Ritzmann et al*	1.20	5.50‖
Grahame-Smith and Everest*	2.40	5.70	Shapiro		
Hayes et al			Normokalaemic patients	N.S.‖	3.68
Infants	2.80	4.40	Hypokalaemic patients	N.S.‖	1.13
Children	1.30	3.40	Schermann and Bourdon	1.37	4.58
Hoeschen and Proveda	0.80–1.30	2.80	Singh et al	2.91	4.79
Howard et al§	0.97	0.91	Smith et al	1.30	3.30
Huffman et al	1.49	3.32	Smith and Haber	1.40	3.70
Iisalo et al	1.20	3.10	Suzuki and Ogawa	1.20	3.20
Johnston et al	1.00	3.15	Waldorff and Buch	1.00	2.30
Krasula et al			Weissel et al	1.38	2.97
Infants	1.70	3.60	Whiting et al	1.40	3.50
Children	1.10	2.90	Zeegers et al	1.60	4.40

Radioimmunoassay used in all instances except as noted:
*Rb update.　†Enzymatic displacement.　‡ATPase inhibition.
§Differences in mean concentration were statistically significant ([P<0.05] in all series except these.)
‖N.S., not stated. ¶Statistical significance not stated.
Smith T, Antman E, Friedman P, Blatt C, Marsh J: Digitalis glycosides: mechanisms and manifestations of toxicity. Prog Cardiovasc Dis 1984;26:433.

TABLE 36-4. Causes of Altered Responsiveness to Cardiac Glycosides

DIGITALIS RESISTANCE

Apparent:
    Tablets not taken as prescribed
    Inadequate bioavailability of tablets
    Inadequate intestinal absorption
    Increased metabolic degradation (e.g., by gut flora)
True end-organ resistance:
    With respect to control of ventricular response in the presence of atrial fibrillation or atrial flutter:
      a. Fever
      b. Elevated sympathetic tone from all causes, including uncontrolled congestive heart failure
      c. Hyperthyroidism

DIGITALIS SENSITIVITY

Apparent:
    Unsuspected use of digitalis
    Change from poorly absorbed tablets to well-absorbed tablets
    Decreased renal excretion
    Drug–drug interactions (e.g., quinidine)
True end-organ sensitivity to toxic effects:
    Advanced myocardial disease
    Active myocardial ischaemia
    Electrolyte imbalance (especially hypoklaemia)
    Acid–base imbalance
    Concomitant drug administration (e.g., catecholamines)
    Hypothyroidism
    Hypoxemia (especially in setting of acute respiratory failure)
    Altered autonomic tone (e.g., vagotonic states)

Smith T, Antman E, Friedman P, Blatt C, Marsh J: Digitalis glycosides: mechanisms and management. Prog Cardiovasc Dis 1984;26:437.

judgment. Measurement of serum digoxin levels should never be viewed as a substitute for clinical judgment, and therefore it is imprudent to use an isolated value as the sole criterion of the presence or absence of digitalis toxicity.

DIGITALIS TOXICITY

Epidemiology

In the late 1960s and early 1970s it was estimated that 15% to 30% of hospitalized patients receiving digitalis glycosides showed clinical or electrocardiographic evidence of toxicity. Since then, however, the incidence of definite or possible digitalis toxicity appears to have dropped significantly to 5% of hospitalized patients receiving cardiac glycosides.[38a] This has resulted from improved consistency in the bioavailability of marketed tablet preparations, development of the radioimmunoassay for serum digoxin concentrations, and continued improvements in clinical understanding of the clinical spectrum of symp-

toms and electrocardiographic manifestations of digitalis toxicity.[38b]

In contrast with earlier reports, recent reviews of digoxin intoxication in hospitalized patients reveal a lower incidence of significant hypokalemia (i.e., <3.7 mEq/L). This appears to have contributed to the current estimate of only a 5% mortality risk (compared with prior rates of 40%) in patients with definite toxicity.[38a, 38b]

Clinical Manifestations of Digitalis Toxicity

In 1970, a large-scale intoxication with cardiac glycosides occurred. A pharmaceutical firm in the Netherlands prepared one lot of digitalis tablets that contained 0.20 mg of digitoxin and 0.05 mg of digoxin instead of the intended 0.25 mg of digoxin with no digitoxin. Lely and VanEnter catalogued the various signs and symptoms exhibited by 179 patients who manifested digitalis toxicity as a result of this error (Table 36-5).[39] Nausea and vomiting, characteristic manifestations of digitalis toxicity, appear to be caused by a direct effect of the drug on the chemoreceptor trigger zone in the area postrema of the medulla of the brain stem.[40] This region of the central nervous system is devoid of a blood–brain barrier and may be the source of many of the neuroexcitatory effects of digitalis glycosides. A wide array of neurologic symptoms have been ascribed to digitalis toxicity.[41] A particularly dramatic neurotoxic symptom is visual disturbance, especially of color vision (halos around lights and augmented perception of yellow and green colors).

TABLE 36-5. Signs and Symptoms of Digitalis Toxicity

Manifestation	Prevalence (%)
Fatigue	95
Visual symptoms	95
Weakness	82
Nausea	81
Anorexia	80
Psychic complaints	65
Abdominal pain	65
Dizziness	59
Abnormal dreams	54
Headache	45
Diarrhea	41
Vomiting	40

Modified from Lely A, VanEnter C: Large-scale digitoxin intoxication. Br Med J 1970;3:737.

Electrocardiographic Manifestations of Digitalis Toxicity

Disturbances of Sinus Impulse Formation and Conduction

In the presence of ventricular contractile dysfunction, therapeutic concentrations of digitalis may cause slowing of the sinus rate via a positive inotropic effect and resultant withdrawal of sympathetic tone. However, when digitalis is administered to patients with normal ventricular performance, either no change in sinus rate occurs or only minor slowing is seen.[42, 43] Thus, the finding of isolated sinus bradycardia in digitalized patients should not be considered evidence of intoxication. Although pooled data from several series suggest that sinus bradycardia may be due to digitalis toxicity in 5% to 10% of cases, it is difficult to find evidence in the literature to support these estimates.

Because digitalis prolongs the effective refractory period of the sinoatrial junction, a variety of conduction blocks may be seen in that region (Fig. 36-9).[44] First-degree block between the sinus node and atrium results in a prolongation of sinoatrial conduction time. This cannot be diagnosed on the surface ECG because the one-to-one relationship between the sinus node and atrium persists. Second-degree sinoatrial block due to digitalis intoxication occurs either as 2-to-1 block (manifested as a doubling of the P-P interval) or as Wenckebach-type block (progressive decrease in the P-P interval before the dropped beat). Mobitz type II sinoatrial block (unexpected dropping of the P wave producing a P-P interval that is a multiple of the basic P-P cycle) can also be the result of digitalis intoxication. In contrast, Mobitz type II second-degree atrioventricular (AV) block has never been confirmed to be due to digitalis intoxication. Complete sinoatrial block (total absence of P waves, often followed by the emergence of an accelerated AV nodal rhythm) is

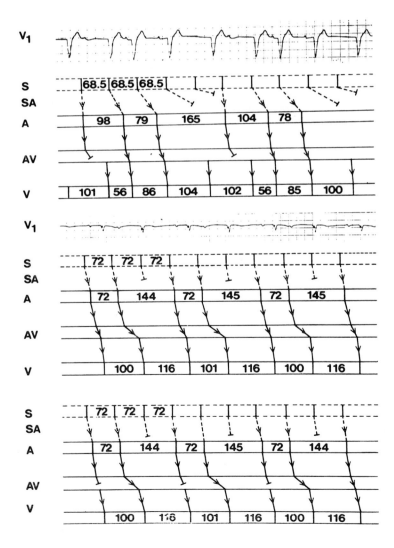

Figure 36-9. Wenckebach type (upper EKG) and Mobitz type II (lower ECG) second-degree sinoatrial (SA) block during digitalis excess. The upper EKG shows progressive shortening in P–P intervals prior to the blocked sinus impulse, which, as indicated in the diagram, is compatible with a Wenckebach type of conduction in the SA junction. QRS complexes result from both accelerated AV junctional escape beats (QRS complexes 1, 2, 5, 6, and 9) and conducted sinus beats. The latter show increasing conduction delay in the AV node following successive P waves. The lower EKG shows 3:1 Mobitz type II SA block. Two successive P waves are followed by QRS complexes with different P–R intervals. As shown in the diagram, this can be explained by either an increased delay in AV junctional conduction following two successive P waves or a sequence of a conducted P wave followed by an (accelerated) AV junctional escape beat. (Wellens HJJ: The electrocardiogram in digitalis intoxication. In: Yu PN, Goodwin JF, eds). Progress in cardiology. Philadelphia: Lea & Febiger, 1976:271.)

difficult to distinguish from prolonged sinus arrest. Brief periods of sinus arrest, however, can be detected by the presence of a pause in P waves that is not a multiple of the basic P-P cycle and the absence of the premonitory features of Mobitz type I second-degree sinoatrial block.

In most cases, digitalis glycosides can be administered safely even in the presence of preexisting sinus node dysfunction. Rather than withholding the potentially beneficial inotropic effects of cardiac glycosides, it seems reasonable to evaluate the electrophysiologic impact of digitalis in a given individual when sinus bradycardia or sinoatrial block is seen.[43] In certain instances, demand cardiac pacing may allow the beneficial hemodynamic effects of digitalis but reduce the risk of bradyarrhythmias.

Atrial Flutter

Atrial flutter probably occurs as an electrocardiographic manifestation of digitalis intoxication in less than 1% of patients with toxicity.[45, 46] However, although the underlying atrial rhythm is flutter, disturbances of AV conduction, including high-grade AV block and accelerated AV nodal rhythms, may develop in the presence of digitalis intoxication.

Atrial Fibrillation

Slowing of the ventricular response is the classic electrophysiologic effect of digitalis in the presence of atrial fibrillation. This occurs as a consequence of prolongation of AV nodal refractoriness and possibly by enhancement of concealed conduction in the AV node due to an increase in the atrial fibrillatory rate.[47] Evidence of digitalis intoxication is often subtle but should be suspected when the patient's heart rhythm demonstrates unexpected regularity or a regular irregularity.[44, 48] In addition, ventricular ectopic impulses may increase in frequency.

As the electrophysiologic effects of digitalis on AV conduction increase, progressively fewer impulses are transmitted through the AV node and progressively longer pauses are seen between QRS complexes. These pauses may be terminated by escape beats that originate in the AV junction, His bundle, or proximal portions of the left bundle branch.[47] The rate of these escape beats is usually between 45 and 55 beats per minute, and they may show an incomplete right bundle branch configuration. When digitalis toxicity is more advanced, there may be an increased rate of junctional escape beats and the progressive development of nonparoxysmal AV junctional tachycardia.[47-49] This is characterized by a regular AV junctional rhythm in the range of 70 to 100 beats per minute and is not significantly different from nonparoxysmal AV junctional tachycardia seen in acute inferior myocardial infarction, in myocarditis, and following cardiac surgical pro-

cedures such as mitral valve replacement (Fig. 36-10). Nonparoxysmal AV junctional tachycardia in the presence of atrial fibrillation may be accompanied by complex forms of exit block from the AV junction, pointing to the need for careful electrocardiographic analysis. A more advanced stage of digitalis intoxication in the presence of atrial fibrillation is characterized by the development of

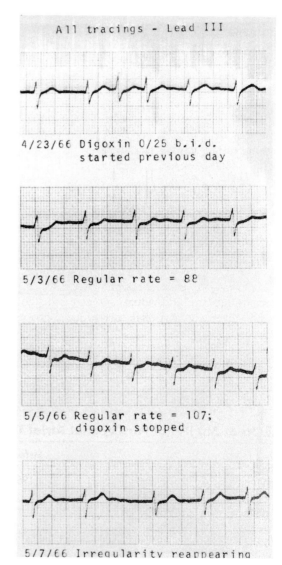

All tracings - Lead III

4/23/66 Digoxin 0/25 b.i.d. started previous day

5/3/66 Regular rate = 88

5/5/66 Regular rate = 107; digoxin stopped

5/7/66 Irregularity reappearing

Figure 36-10. Nonparoxysmal junctional tachycardia. Electrocardiograms of a 64-year-old woman after mitral valve replacement. The first strip shows an irregular response to atrial fibrillation. Ten days later, junctional tachycardia at a rate of 88 beats/minute with a high degree of entrance block had become established. Because the arrhythmia was unrecognized, digoxin continued to be administered, and 48 hours later the tachycardia rate was 107 beats/minute. The drug was then stopped, with reappearance of the usual irregular ventricular response to atrial fibrillation. (Kastor JA: Digitalis intoxication in patients with atrial fibrillation. Circulation 1973;47:888.)

potentially fatal hemodynamically compromising ventricular arrhythmias.

Atrial Tachycardia

The term paroxysmal atrial tachycardia (PAT) is reserved for that form of automatic atrial tachycardia in which the atrial rate is usually between 120 and 250 beats per minute and the P-wave morphology is different from that of sinus P waves; the atrial rate may be regular or irregular, and a warm-up phenomenon may be evident. AV block may or may not be present, producing average ventricular rates between 75 and 200 beats per minute. Paroxysmal atrial tachycardia may or may not be digitalis-induced. The more frequently encountered forms of supraventricular tachycardia, caused by a variety of mechanisms, are referred to as paroxysmal supraventricular tachycardia (PSVT). Table 36-6 summarizes the findings of four clinical studies of paroxysmal atrial tachycardia carried out between 1953 and 1972.[45–52] It may be estimated that the incidence of PAT per recorded ECG in hospitalized patients is about 0.1%. In 50% of 211 episodes of PAT, the rhythm disturbance was felt to be digitalis-induced; in 43% the arrhythmia was found not to be digitalis-induced; in 7% of episodes it was doubtful whether digitalis induced the arrhythmia. Thus, when one encounters an ECG showing PAT, the chance that it is due to digitalis toxicity is about 50%. However, the chances increase if the patient population includes a large number of digitalized individuals subjected to significant metabolic shifts (e.g., hypokalemia) during procedures such as dialysis.[45,53]

The rhythm most often confused with PAT is atrial flutter. Guidelines useful for differentiating digitalis-induced PAT from "common" atrial flutter (presumed to

originate low in the right atrium and to circulate in a caudal to cranial fashion, thus inscribing predominantly negative complexes in the inferior leads) are listed in Table 36-7 and illustrated in Figure 36-11.[45,53] In the presence of "uncommon" flutter (with predominantly positive complexes in the inferior leads), such distinctions become somewhat blurred. This confusion may occur in diseased atria with inherently slow flutter rates or during therapy with antiarrhythmic agents such as quinidine, which slow the flutter rate, or sympathomimetic agents such as theophylline, which speed the atrial rate in PAT. Analysis of the ECG, the clinical context, comparison with serial electrocardiograms, and withdrawal of digitalis along with supplemental potassium therapy remain important diagnostic as well as therapeutic tools.

AV Block

First-degree AV block is a common manifestation of digitalis effect, and it remains arguable whether such an observation indicates impending toxicity. In contrast, the appearance of second-degree or third-degree AV block in a patient receiving digitalis should be interpreted as probable evidence of digitalis toxicity.[44] Second-degree AV block in the presence of digitalis intoxication usually demonstrates Wenckebach periodicity (Fig. 36-12), but not infrequently one may observe periods of high-grade, second-degree AV block characterized by AV conduction ratios of 2:1, 3:1, or 4:1, with or without accompanying periods of Wenckebach conduction. It should be recalled that type II second-degree AV block has never been reported as a manifestation of digitalis intoxication. More advanced stages of digitalis toxicity can produce complete AV block. Recognizing third-degree AV block in sinus

TABLE 36-6. Studies of Paroxysmal Atrial Tachycardia

	Reference 50	Reference 45	Reference 51	Reference 52
Years studied	1953–1956	1942–1954	1960–1961	1969–1972
No. of ECGs screened	16,481	51,722	18,884	
No. of patients screened	8,147			
Incidence per ECG	1/412 = 0.2%	1/462 = 0.2%	1/1259 = 0.07%	
No. of episodes of PAT with block	40	112	(15)*	44
No. of patients with PAT with block	39	88	15	31
No. of episodes of digitalis-toxic PAT	16/40 = 40%	83/112 = 74%	(6)*	0
No. of patients with digitalis-toxic PAT		64/88 = 73%	6/15 = 40%	
No. of episodes of possible digitalis-toxic PAT		16/112 = 14%		
No. of patients with possible digitalis-toxic PAT		11/88 = 13%		
No. of episodes of non–digitalis-toxic PAT	24/40 = 60%	13/112 = 12%	(9)*	44 = 100%
No. of patients with non–digitalis-toxic PAT		13/88 = 15%	9/15 = 60%	31 = 100%

*Assumes one episode per patient for calculation.

TABLE 36-7. ECG Features of Digitalis-Induced PAT With Block Compared With Common Atrial Flutter

	PAT With Block	Common Atrial flutter
Usual atrial rate	150–250 bpm	Over 200 bpm
P-P baseline	Isoelectric	"Sawtooth"
AV response	1:1, 2:1, variable	Usually 2:1
P wave (limb leads)	Upright and diminutive	Inverted in leads II and III ("common flutter")
P-P interval	Regular or irregular	Regular
Ventricular premature beats	In 40% of cases	In 20% of cases
Carotid sinus pressure	AV block increased; atrial rate unchanged	AV block increased; atrial rate unchanged or accelerated
Onset and offset	Gradual change in rate; abrupt change in P wave	Abrupt
Potassium administration	Characteristic response (slowing of tachycardia and eventual reversion to sinus rhythm)	No effect

Modified from Lown B, Levin HD: Atrial arrhythmias, digitalis, and potassium. New York: Landsberger Medical Books, 1958.

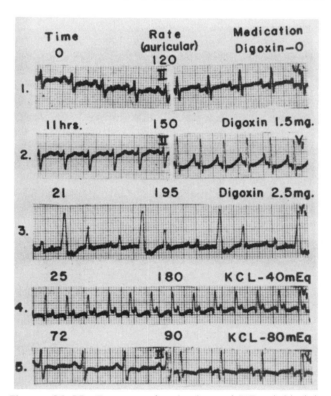

Figure 36-11. Evocation of early phase of PAT with block by intravenous digitalization with 1.5 mg of digoxin in a 17-year-old boy with myocarditis (strip 2). The nature of the arrhythmia was unrecognized; an additional 1.0 mg of digoxin was given for increasing pulmonary edema (strip 3). Although the patient was apparently moribund (strip 4), uneventful recovery followed the administration of 80 mEq of potassium chloride (strip 5). Note 1:1 response phase in strip 4. (Lown B, Wyatt NF, Levine HD: Paroxysmal atrial tachycardia with block. Circulation 1960;21:129.)

rhythm is comparatively easy because of complete dissociation between P waves and QRS complexes (usually being driven from an AV junctional pacemaker focus). In the presence of atrial fibrillation, the development of non-paroxysmal AV junctional tachycardia indicates digitalis toxicity. During atrial flutter, therapeutic doses of digitalis will increase the degree of block in the AV node, resulting in patterns of 4:1, 5:1, or 6:1 conduction rather than the customary 2:1 AV conduction. Importantly, there will be preservation of a fixed time relationship between flutter waves and QRS complexes. When such a relationship is lost, high-grade AV block should be suspected (Fig. 36-13).[44]

Ventricular Arrhythmias

Over 50% of digitalis-intoxicated patients exhibit ventricular premature depolarizations (VPDs).[44, 46] Such ectopic impulses are particularly common in the presence of structural heart disease, and it is often a clinical dilemma to determine whether or not the ventricular arrhythmia is a result of the patient's underlying heart disease or should be considered a manifestation of digitalis toxicity. VPDs of new onset occurring early in the course of digitalis therapy, after the dose of digitalis is increased, or during periods of electrolyte or acid–base shifts should raise the suspicion of digitalis intoxication. In addition, VPDs that appear in a bigeminal or trigeminal fashion or have a fixed coupling relationship to the preceding sinus beat and ventricular bigeminy with fixed coupling in which the VPDs alternatively show right and left axis deviation are suggestive of digitalis toxicity. Aberrant intraventricular conduction of supraventricular complexes during atrial

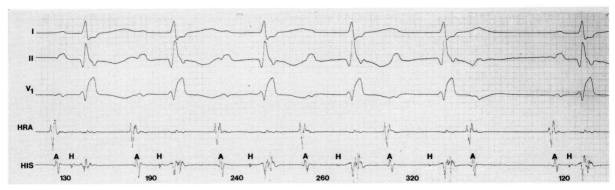

Figure 36-12. Surface electrocardiographic leads I, II, and V₁ recorded simultaneously with bipolar electrograms from the high right atrium (*HRA*) and His bundle region (*HIS*) in a patient with digitalis toxicity. The surface electrocardiogram reveals right bundle branch block as well as 6:5 type I second-degree AV block. Note progressive lengthening of the P–R interval prior to the nonconducted P wave. The His bundle electrogram reveals progressive lengthening of the A–H interval prior to the nonconducted P wave, thus localizing the site of block to the AV node. (Friedman PL, Antman EM: Electrocardiographic manifestations of digitalis toxicity. In Smith TW, ed. Digitalis glycosides. Orlando: Grune & Stratton, 1986:241.)

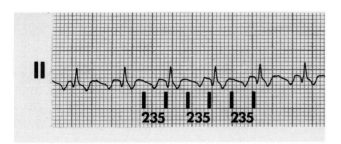

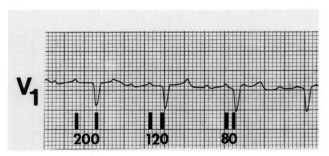

Figure 36-13. Top Panel: Surface electrocardiographic lead II from a patient with atrial flutter being treated with nontoxic doses of digoxin. There is 2:1 AV conduction. Note fixed time intervals of 235 msec between flutter waves and the QRS complexes that follow them. The R–R intervals are exactly twice the flutter cycle length. Bottom panel: Surface electrocardiographic lead V₁ in a different patient with atrial flutter and digitalis toxicity. Note lack of fixed time relations between flutter waves and QRS complexes. The R–R intervals are constant but unrelated to the flutter cycle length, suggesting complete AV block during flutter with emergence of an accelerated AV junctional rhythm. (Friedman PL, Antman EM: Electrocardiographic manifestations of digitalis toxicity. In: Smith TW, ed. Digitalis glycosides. Orlando: Grune & Stratton, 1986:241.)

fibrillation (Ashman's phenomenon) can also be difficult to differentiate from VPDs. One should recall that aberrantly conducted supraventricular beats during atrial fibrillation usually have the same or similar QRS morphology, have varying coupling with the preceding QRS, and occur sporadically. Also, right bundle branch block aberration is seen more frequently than left bundle branch block aberration. Digitalis-induced VPDs during atrial fibrillation characteristically manifest a fixed coupling to the preceding QRS and are usually seen in a bigeminal pattern. Multiform or repetitive ventricular premature depolarizations during atrial fibrillation are especially suggestive of digitalis toxicity.[44, 48]

Digitalis-induced ventricular tachycardia, accounting for only 10% of digitalis-induced arrhythmias, typically has a rate of between 150 and 180 beats per minute and may be characterized by QRS complexes of uniform morphology that are narrow.[54] This suggests a focus high in the intraventricular conduction system (Fig. 36-14). Bidirectional tachycardia, a particularly characteristic form of ventricular tachycardia, is seen almost exclusively in the setting of digitalis intoxication. This dysrhythmia typically exhibits QRS complexes with a right bundle branch block morphology in lead V₁, with frontal plane QRS complexes alternating between right and left axis deviation (Fig. 36-15).

Ventricular fibrillation (VF) may develop as the consequence of failure to recognize earlier digitalis-induced arrhythmias or to initiate appropriate therapy.[44, 55] In the presence of overwhelming toxicity due to suicidal or accidental ingestion of large amounts of cardiac glycoside, VF is often extremely difficult to reverse.

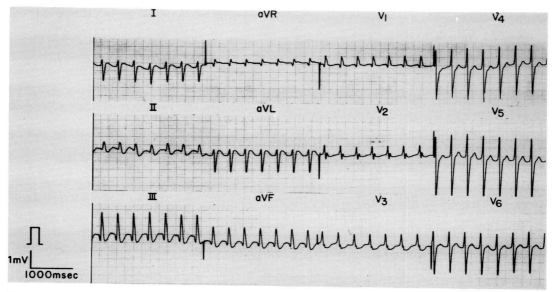

Figure 36-14. Twelve-lead electrocardiogram of ventricular tachycardia in a digitalis-intoxicated patient. Note relatively narrow QRS complexes. The pattern of right bundle branch block and marked right axis deviation suggests a site of origin in or near the anterior fascicle of the left bundle branch. (Friedman PL, Antman EM: Electrocardiographic manifestations of digitalis toxicity. In: Smith TW, ed. Digitalis glycosides. Orlando: Grune & Stratton, 1986:241.)

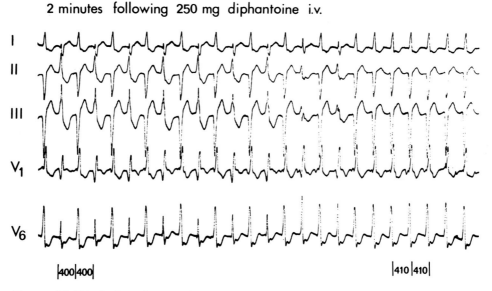

Figure 36-15. Surface electrocardiographic leads I, II, III, V₁ and V₆ during phenytoin infusion in a digitalis-intoxicated patient. Bidirectional tachycardia is present on the left. Note right bundle branch block pattern in V₁ with alternating left and right axis deviation. In the presence of phenytoin, this rhythm converted to ventricular tachycardia, characterized by a slower rate and uniform QRS morphology (*right*). (Wellens HJJ: The electrocardiogram in digitalis intoxication. In: Yu PN, Goodwin JF, eds. Progress in cardiology. Philadelphia: Lea & Febiger, 1976:271.)

Complex Arrhythmias

The cardiac arrhythmias resulting from digitalis intoxication include those caused by enhanced impulse generation or impaired conduction. On occasion, cardiac arrhythmias exhibiting varying degrees of both types of electrophysiologic abnormalities may be present simultaneously in a digitalis-intoxicated patient and should alert the clinician to a high probability of this etiology. An example of such complex arrhythmias can be seen in Figure 36-16.

Management of Digitalis Toxicity

No ECG pattern unequivocally indicates that a rhythm is digitalis-toxic in origin, although cardiac rhythm disturbances that demonstrate increased automaticity of ectopic pacemakers and failure of impulse conduction are highly suggestive. Early recognition of a potentially digitalis-toxic arrhythmia is critical to successful clinical management. Important general principles include the following:

1. Evaluate the rhythm disturbance and its potential risk to the patient. Serious rhythm disturbances such as complex ventricular arrhythmias necessitate admission to an intensive care unit; less worrisome arrhythmias can be managed adequately on a general hospital ward, assuming ECG monitoring is available.

2. Discontinue administration of cardiac glycosides.

3. Initiate potassium repletion unless the serum po-

tassium level is elevated when the patient is seen initially (e.g., >5.0 mEq/L), severe renal failure is present, AV conduction is markedly prolonged, or the patient has taken a massive overdose of digitalis (in which case serum potassium may rise to dangerously high levels).

4. Bradycardic rhythms that compromise hemodynamic function are best treated with a brief trial of intravenous atropine. A temporary demand pacemaker should be promptly inserted if atropine fails to resolve the situation. Infusion of drugs such as isoproterenol is best avoided because of the risk of provoking more serious ectopic arrhythmias.

5. Cardiac arrhythmias indicating enhanced automaticity may require suppressive antiarrhythmic therapy along with potassium supplementation.

6. Massive cardiac glycoside ingestion associated with potentially life-threatening arrhythmias or hyperkalemia that does not respond promptly to conventional measures should be treated with digoxin-specific antibody (Fab fragment) therapy.

One of the important elements of conventional treatment for digitalis toxicity involves potassium repletion.[56] However, this should be undertaken under carefully monitored conditions because of the potential for provoking more severe rhythm disturbances and even death. Potassium repletion may be accomplished via either the intravenous or the oral route, but the rate of intravenous infusion of potassium should not exceed 0.5 to 1.0 mEq/

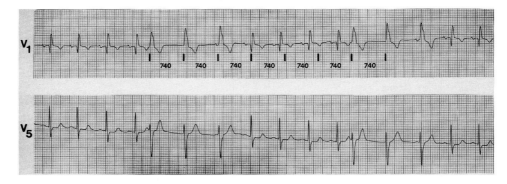

Figure 36-16. Complex arrhythmia in a patient with digitalis toxicity. Surface electrocardiographic leads V₁ and V₅ are shown. After four beats of sinus rhythm conducted with right bundle branch block aberrancy, an accelerated AV junctional rhythm emerges with a cycle length of 740 msec. This rhythm probably arises as a result of digitalis-induced enhanced impulse initiation below the AV node. AV dissociation is present during the accelerated junctional rhythm. The 8th QRS complex is a supraventricular capture beat, following which AV conduction of the sinus P waves is reestablished. Although the accelerated junctional focus is no longer apparent, it continues to depolarize at its own intrinsic cycle length, being protected by entrance block. Activity of the junctional focus during this period is concealed in the ECG. However, the junctional focus re-emerges when its time of depolarization fortuitously falls outside of the ventricular refractory period following a conducted P wave (12th QRS complex). (Friedman PL, Antman EM: Electrocardiographic manifestations of digitalis toxicity. In: Smith TW, ed. Digitalis glycosides. Orlando: Grune & Stratton, 1986:241.)

minute. Potassium solutions are best prepared in either saline or glucose but should not exceed a concentration of 120 to 160 mEq/L. If potassium is repleted orally, doses of 40 mEq every 1 to 4 hours may be given, provided acidosis is not present and renal function is adequate.[46] Regardless of the route used, a 12-lead electrocardiogram should be reviewed every 15 minutes to detect early evidence of impending potassium overdose, and serum potassium levels should be determined every 30 to 60 minutes.[57] When severe potassium depletion is present, it is probably best to administer intravenous potassium in saline rather than glucose solutions because of the possible complications of paradoxical worsening of hypokalemia with the latter.[58]

Suppressive antiarrhythmic therapy is traditionally attempted with lidocaine or phenytoin. Lidocaine is administered via serial intravenous 100-mg boluses every 3 to 5 minutes (not to exceed a total dose of 300 mg) until either a therapeutic effect occurs or lidocaine toxicity ensues.[57] This may then be followed by continuous infusion of 15 to 50 μg/kg of body weight/minute as required to maintain control of the rhythm disturbances. Potential adverse effects of lidocaine may occur commonly and generally involve the central nervous system (feelings of dissociation, agitation, or frank convulsions).

Phenytoin administration is best achieved by slow intravenous infusion of 100 mg every 5 minutes until the onset of toxicity (nystagmus, vertigo, ataxia, or nausea) or control of the arrhythmia. Oral maintenance doses of 400 to 600 mg/day are used if control of the arrhythmia has been achieved. Whereas 600 to 1000 mg of phenytoin may be needed to control ventricular arrhythmias not of digitalis-toxic origin, smaller doses (e.g., 200–400 mg) and low plasma concentrations have been found to be effective against digitalis-induced ventricular arrhythmias.[57] The likelihood of cardiac toxicity (both electrophysiologic and hemodynamic) is too great to consider beta-adrenergic blocking agents, quinidine, or procainamide the initial pharmacologic agents of choice to suppress digitalis-induced arrhythmias.

Clinical data are insufficient to evaluate the efficacy of newer antiarrhythmic drugs in comparison with the standard agents, and information about these new drugs should be considered preliminary. Of potential interest is verapamil, for which there is experimental evidence indicating that it is useful for treatment of triggered automaticity, but its use could be harmful in the presence of bradyarrhythmias or conduction disturbances.[41, 59]

Cardioversion

There is a widely held clinical impression that direct-current (DC) cardioversion can be hazardous in patients receiving cardiac glycosides, based on earlier clinical studies reporting that electrical shock provoked serious ventricular arrhythmias.[60–63] It is worth noting, however, that transthoracic DC shocks in undigitalized animals can also provoke ventricular arrhythmias that are related to the dose of electrical energy used.[64, 65] Although near-toxic doses of digitalis glycosides can lower the threshold for postshock ventricular arrhythmias, therapeutic levels of these drugs have not increased the risk of postshock ventricular arrhythmias in recent experimental and clinical studies.[66–68] Thus, the risk of arrhythmias does not appear to be increased when transthoracic shocks are delivered in the absence of digitalis toxicity.

The following guidelines are useful when considering DC cardioversion in digitalized patients:

1. If there is overt electrocardiographic evidence of digitalis excess, elective DC cardioversion should not be performed.

2. Energy titrations starting with 25 to 50 watt-seconds with subsequent increments as needed are used to deliver the smallest amount of energy that is likely to be effective.

3. Electrolyte imbalance, fever, hypoxia, and anxiety should all be prevented. All of these disturbances by themselves and apart from an interaction with digitalis can decrease the likelihood of successful cardioversion and increase the chance of provoking serious ventricular arrhythmias.

Digoxin-Specific Antibody for Resistant Toxicity

More aggressive measures sometimes deserve consideration when severe and resistant toxicity is encountered clinically (e.g., after accidental overdosage or suicidal ingestion). The clinical findings after massive digitalis ingestion are notable for hyperkalemia and ventricular tachyarrhythmias. Although hemodialysis and hemoperfusion may help to control hyperkalemia, they are unable to deal rapidly with the extensive tissue binding of digoxin and are therefore of limited value in the acute reversal of advanced, life-threatening toxicity.

Highly specific antibodies with a high affinity for digoxin have been raised in animals (e.g., sheep) and are used in radioimmunoassay measurements of serum digoxin concentration. The concept of antibody therapy for digitalis toxicity was developed in the 1970s; experience has now accumulated in more than 2000 cases treated. The intact digoxin-specific IgG molecule (150,000 d) presents certain problems that limit its usefulness in clinical practice, including the possibility of hypersensitivity and its long half-life of elimination (approximately 60 hours). Purified digoxin-specific antibody fragments (Fab) with a molecular weight of 50,000 have been developed to provide an intravenous form of treatment for severe digitalis toxicity. The smaller size of the Fab fragment permits a more rapid onset of action because of enhanced diffusion into the interstitial space. Furthermore, in patients with normal renal function, the digoxin-bound Fab fragments are excreted in the urine relatively rapidly with a half-life of about 16 hours. This minimizes the chance of late release of bound digoxin and reemergence of toxicity.

The proposed sequence of events that occurs after injection of digoxin-specific Fab fragments is as follows:

1. Intravascular digoxin is rapidly bound.

2. Fab fragments diffuse into the interstitial space and bind free interstitial digoxin.

3. The decreased extracellular free digoxin concentration promotes egress of free intracellular digoxin into the extracellular fluid where it is also rapidly bound.

4. Free digoxin molecules that dissociate from membrane receptors are rapidly bound and cannot reassociate with the alpha subunit of NaK-ATPase. This is the slowest but most important step in the reversal of digitalis toxicity.

5. The total extracellular digoxin concentration rises dramatically, but this digoxin is pharmacologically inactive because only the unbound form can bind to myocardial receptor sites. Measurement of serum digoxin concentrations by conventional immunoassay techniques following administration of Fab fragments is not helpful because the assay results are unreliable and often misleading (Fig. 36-17).

When administering digoxin-specific Fab fragments for management of serious digitalis toxicity, one attempts to deliver a stoichiometrically equivalent dose of Fab designed to neutralize the entire body load of digoxin. The formulas used are illustrated in Table 36-8, and their use is exemplified in the case described in Figure 36-18. Because the Fab fragments are excreted via the kidney, individuals with diminished renal function should be monitored particularly carefully. Although exacerbation of congestive heart failure may occur following removal of the inotropic support of digitalis, this has been encountered infrequently and remains at most a theoretic concern. Furthermore, "back titration" with the desired amount of digoxin can be performed in those rare patients in whom it is deemed important to restore the therapeutic benefits of digoxin after reversal of the toxic arrhythmia. In usual practice, however, other therapeutic avenues should be pursued, and redigitalization should be avoided until the antibody fragments have been eliminated. This may take as long as 1 week in persons with normal renal function and proportionately longer in persons with depressed renal function.

Serious advanced digitalis toxicity refractory to con-

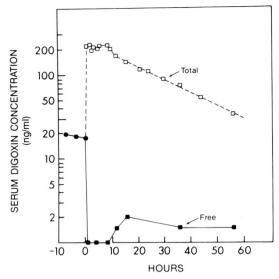

Figure 36-17. Time course of digoxin concentrations before (*filled circles*) and after treatment with digoxine-specific Fab fragments begun at 0 hours (total digoxin, empty squares; free digoxin, filled squares). (Smith TW, Haber E, Yeatman L, Butler VP Jr: Reversal of advanced digoxin intoxication with Fab fragments of digoxin-specific antibodies. N Engl J Med 1976;294:797.)

ventional measures was successfully reversed with Fab fragments in 90% of 150 patients in a multicenter experience between 1974 and 1986.[69] Some additional patients succumbed to irreversible cardiogenic shock or central nervous system damage despite initial improvement in the cardiac rhythm disturbances. Another patient who was initially stabilized died later from an overwhelming ingestion of digoxin that could not be treated fully because of an inadequate Fab supply. Others among the 10% who did not respond were, in most instances, believed to be suffering from cardiac arrhythmias resulting from underlying disease rather than from overt digitalis toxicity. These findings were confirmed by workers in Germany and China. Purified digoxin-specific Fab fragments are now

TABLE 36-8. Calculation of Equimolar Dose of Digoxin Specific Fab Fragments

I. Calculation of body load
   A. Ingested amount (mg) × 0.80
   B. $\dfrac{\text{Serum digoxin concentration} \times 5.6 \times \text{weight in kg}}{1000}$

II. Calculation of Digibind dose
   A. $\dfrac{\text{MW Fab} = 50{,}000}{\text{MW digoxin} = 781} = 64 \times \text{body load (mg)}$
      $= \text{Digibind dose (mg)}$
   B. $\dfrac{\text{Body load of digoxin (mg)}}{0.6 \text{ mg neutralized/40 mg vial}} = \text{Digibind dose in \# vials}$

MW, molecular weight; #, number of.

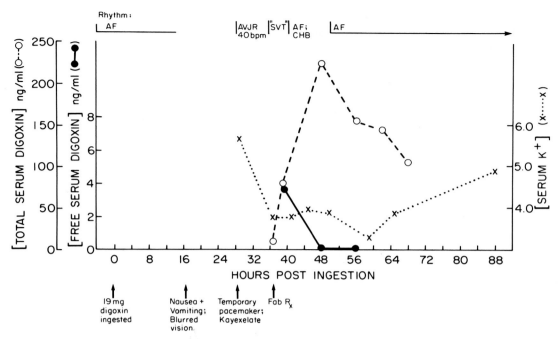

Figure 36-18. Flow diagram illustrating temporal relationships between recorded cardiac rhythms, ingestion of suicidal overdose of digoxin (superimposed on maintenance digoxin therapy), and results of treatment with digoxin-specific Fab fragments. This 60-year-old woman with rheumatic heart disease underwent mitral valve replacement for mitral stenosis. Her underlying rhythm was chronic atrial fibrillation (AF), and she was receiving digoxin 0.125 mg daily for control of the ventricular rate. At time 0 she ingested 19 mg of digoxin in a suicidal gesture and subsequently developed an accelerated atrioventricular junctional rhythm (AVJR). At about 40 hours post-ingestion, her rhythm changed to that shown in Figure 36-14, and this was erroneously interpreted as supraventricular tachycardia (SVT) at her referring hospital. When it was correctly identified as fascicular tachycardia, she was treated with 26 vials of Digibind designed to neutralize 15 mg of digoxin (80% of ingested load), as described in Table 36-8. Within 30 minutes, her rhythm once again became AF coincident with a dramatic rise in total (Fab bound) digoxin and fall in free digoxin. After 1 week, the patient was started back on her maintenance dose of digoxin 0.125 mg, in anticipation that a new steady state would be obtained in approximately 7 to 10 days. (Antman EM, Smith TW: Management of digitalis toxicity. Cardiac Impulse 1987;8:1.)

widely available in the United States and abroad for the treatment of advanced digoxin or digitoxin intoxication. An initial response to Fab is typically observed in <60 minutes, and complete reversal of toxicity is evident within 4 hours in those patients receiving adequate doses of Fab fragments.

Following publication of the multicenter trial, an observational surveillance report covering the first 2 years of postmarketing experience and reflecting data on about 15% of all treatments with Fab fragments in adults was published.[69a] Once again, the rapid time course of reversal of glycoside toxicity (initially within 1 hour and nearly complete by 4 hours) was seen. The rates of nonresponse to Fab treatment were 14% in patients developing suspected toxicity while on maintenance digoxin, 20% in those receiving loading doses or those who were hospitalized during therapy, and 15% in those with organic heart disease who ingested a single large oral dose. Failure

of response to Fab fragments was due to a combination of moribund clinical condition, error in diagnosis, and inadequate dosage. Allergic reactions occurred in 0.8% of patients, and recrudescence of toxicity (characteristically within 72 hours) occurred in 2.8% of patients.

Further research efforts should yield preparations of Fab fragments with even less (or absent) potential immunogenicity in humans. Removal of even the small potential immunologic hazard associated with Fab administration could extend the indications for this modality considerably. For example, it would be helpful to reverse digitalis effects rapidly to determine whether a given rhythm disturbance is the result of digitalis toxicity—in effect, a "reverse acetylstrophanthidin tolerance test," in which digitalis excess would be suggested by the disappearance of or improvement in a rhythm disturbance rather than exacerbation of the arrhythmia. Any clinical problems arising from withdrawal of the digitalis effect by Fab administration could be treated by giving additional increments of cardiac glycoside in excess of the antibody dose to restore therapeutic levels of unbound glycoside.

Monoclonal digoxin-specific antibodies have been developed using hybridoma techniques.[70] Reduced immunogenicity in humans could be created by recombining the variable regions of the light and heavy immunoglobulin chains to form a 23,000-d Fv fragment that could be engrafted on a framework region with human immune specificity.[41] Such measures could lead the way to antibody reversal of toxicity from other drugs or endogenous substances in the future.

References

1. Marban E, Smith T: Digitalis. In: Fozzard H, Haber E, Jennings R, Katz A, Morgan H, eds. The heart and cardiovascular system. New York: Raven Press, 1986:1573.
2. Eisner D, Lederer W: Na-Ca exchange: stoichiometry and electrogenicity. Am J Physiol 1985;248:C189.
3. Barry W, Biedert S, Miura D, Smith T: Changes in cellular Na^+, K^+ and Ca^{2+} contents, monovalent cation transport rate, and contractile state during washout of cardiac glycosides from cultured chick heart cells. Circ Res 1981; 9:141.
4. Mullins L: An electrogenic saga: consequences of sodium–calcium exchange in cardiac muscle. In: Blaustein M, Liberman M, eds. Electrogenic transport: fundamental principles and physiological implications. New York: Raven Press, 1984:161.
5. Smith T: Digitalis—mechanisms of action and clinical use. N Engl J Med 1988;318:358.
6. Eisner D, Lederer W, Vaughan-Jones R: The quantitative relationship between twitch tension and intracellular sodium activity in sheep cardiac Purkinje fibers. J Physiol (Lond) 1984;355:251.
7. Marban E, Tsien R: Enhancement of calcium current during digitalis inotropy in mammalian heart: positive feed-back regulation by intracellular calcium? J Physiol (Lond) 1982; 29:589.
8. Fingl E, Woodbury L, Hecht H: Effects of innervation and drugs upon direct membrane potentials of embryonic chick myocardium. J Pharmacol Exp Ther 1951;104:103.
9. Woodbury L, Hecht H: Effects of cardiac glycosides upon the electrical activity of single ventricular fibers of the frog heart, and their relation to the digitalis effect on the electrocardiogram. Circulation 1952;6:172.
10. Watanabe Y, Dreifus L: Electrophysiologic effects of digitalis on A-V transmission. Am J Physiol 1966;211:1461.
11. Vassalle M, Karis J, Hoffman B: Toxic effects of ouabain on Purkinje fibers and ventricular muscle fibers. Am J Physiol 1962;203:433.
12. Hoffman B, Singer D: Effects of digitalis on electrical activity of cardiac fibers. Prog Cardiovasc Dis 1964;7:226.
13. Rosen M: Cellular electrophysiology of digitalis toxicity. J Am Coll Cardiol 1985;5:22A.
14. Lin C, Vassalle M: Role of sodium in strophanthidin toxicity of Purkinje fibers. Am J Physiol 1978;234:H477.
15. Ferrier G, Saunders J, Mendez C: A cellular mechanism for the generation of ventricular arrhythmias by acetylstrophanthidin. Circ Res 1973;32:600.
16. Tsien R, Kass R, Weingart R: Cellular and subcellular mechanism of cardiac pacemaker oscillations. J Exp Biol 1979; 81:205.
17. Rosen M, Hordof A, Hodess A, et al: Ouabain induced changes in electrophysiologic properties of neonatal, young, and adult canine cardiac Purkinje fibers. J Pharmacol Exp Ther 1973;194:255.
18. Brennan J, Bonn J: Effects of ouabain on the electrophysiological properties of subendocardial Purkinje fibers surviving in regions of acute myocardial infarction. Am Heart J 1980;100:201.
19. Watanabe A: Digitalis and the autonomic nervous system. J Am Coll Cardiol 1985;5:35A.
20. Gillis R, Quest J: The role of the nervous system in the cardiovascular effects of digitalis. Pharmacol Rev 1980;31:19.
21. Toda N, West T: The influence of ouabain on cholinergic responses in the sinoatrial node. J Pharmacol Exp Ther 1966;153:104.
22. Hoffman B, Bigger JT, Jr: Digitalis and allied cardiac glycosides. In: Gilman A, Goodman L, Goodman A, eds. The pharmacological basis of therapeutics. New York: Macmillan, 1980:729.
23. Smith T, Braunwald E: The management of heart failure. In: Braunwald E, ed. Heart disease: a textbook of cardiovascular medicine. Philadelphia: W.B. Saunders, 1980:509.
24. Smith T: Drug therapy: digitalis glycosides. N Engl J Med 1973;288:719, 942.
25. Marcus F: Metabolic factors determining digitalis dosage in man. In: Marks B, Weissler A, eds. Basic and clinical pharmacology of digitalis. Springfield, IL: Charles C Thomas, 1972: 243.
26. Bissett J, Doherty J, Glanigan W, et al: Tritiated digoxin XIX. Turnover studies in diabetes insipidus. Am J Cardiol 1973; 31:327.
27. Cogan JJ, Humphreys M, Carlson C, et al: Acute vasodilator therapy increases renal clearance of digoxin in patients with congestive heart failure. Circulation 1981;64:973.
28. Steiness E: Renal tubular secretion of digoxin. Circulation 1974;50:103.
29. Luchi R, Gruber J: Unusually large digitalis requirements: a study of altered digoxin metabolism. Am J Med 1968;45:322.
30. Peters U, Falk L, Kalman S: Digoxin metabolism in patients. Arch Intern Med 1978;138:1074.
31. Lindenbaum J, Fund D, Butler V, et al: Inactivation of digoxin by the gut flora: reversal by antibiotic therapy. N Engl J Med 1981;305:789.
32. Marcus F, Burkhalter L, Curccia C, et al: Administration of tritiated digoxin with and without a loading dose: a metabolic study. Circulation 1966;34:865.
33. Abernathy D, Greenblatt D, Smith T: Digoxin disposition in obesity: clinical pharmacokinetic investigation. Am Heart J 1981;102:740.
34. Ewy G, Groves B, Ball M, et al: Digoxin metabolism in obesity. Circulation 1971;44:810.
35. Smith T, Antman E, Friedman P, Blatt C, Marsh J: Digitalis glycosides: mechanisms and manifestations of toxicity. Prog Cardiovasc Dis 1984;26:413.

36. Goldfinger S: Dissimilarities of digoxin. N Engl J Med 1971; 285:1376.

37. Koch-Weser J: Bioavailability of drugs. N Engl J Med 1974; 291:223, 503.

38. Hall R, Gelbart A, Silverman M, et al: Studies on digitalis-induced arrhythmias in glucose- and insulin-induced hypokalemia. J Pharmacol Exp Ther 1977;201:711.

38a. Mahdyoon H, Battilana G, Rosman H, Goldstein S, Gheorghiade M: The evolving pattern of digoxin intoxication: observations at a large urban hospital from 1980 to 1988. Am Heart J 1990;120:1189.

38b. Kelly R, Smith T: Recognition and management of digitalis toxicity. Am J Cardiol 1992;69:108G.

39. Lely A, VanEnter C: Larce-scale digitoxin intoxication. Br Med J 1970;3:737.

40. Somberg J, Kuhlman J, Smith T: Localization of the neurally mediated coronary vasoconstrictor properties of digitalis in the cat. Circ Res 1981;49:226.

41. Smith T, Antman E, Friedman P, Blatt C, Marsh J: Digitalis glycosides: mechanisms and manifestations of toxicity. Prog Cardiovasc Dis 1984;27:21.

42. Dhingra R, Amat-y-Leon F, Wyndham C, et al: The electrophysiologic effects of ouabain on sinus node and atrium in man. J Clin Invest 1975;56:555.

43. Reiffel J, Bigger J, Cramer M: Effects of digoxin on sinus nodal function before and after vagal blockade in patients with sinus nodal dysfunction. Am J Cardiol 1979;43:983.

44. Wellens H: The electrocardiogram in digitalis intoxication. In: Yu P, ed. Progress in cardiology. Philadelphia: Lea and Febiger, 1976:271.

45. Lown B, Wyatt N, Levine H: Paroxysmal atrial tachycardia with block. Circulation 1960;21:129.

46. Fisch C, Stone J: Recognition and treatment of digitalis toxicity. In: Fisch C, Surawicz B, eds. Digitalis. New York: Grune & Strattton, 1969:162.

47. Kastor J: Digitalis intoxication in patients with atrial fibrillation. Circulation 1973;47:888.

48. Fisch C, Zipes D, Noble R: Digitalis toxicity: mechanism and recognition. In: Yu P, Goodwin J, eds. Progress in cardiology. Philadelphia: Lea and Febiger, 1975:37.

49. Pick A, Domingues P: Nonparoxysmal AV nodal tachycardia. Circulation 1957;16:1022.

50. Freiermuth L, Jick S: Paroxysmal atrial tachycardia with atrioventricular block. Am J Cardiol 1958;1:584.

51. Morgan W, Breneman G: Atrial tachycardia with block treated with digitalis. Circulation 1962;25:787.

52. Storstein O, Rasmussen K: Digitalis and atrial tachycardia with block. Br Heart J 1974;36:171.

53. Lown B, Marcus F, Levine H: Digitalis and atrial tachycardia with block. A year's experience. N Engl J Med 1959;260:301.

54. Chung E: Digitalization and digitalis-induced cardiac arrhythmias. In: Chung E, ed. Principles of cardiac arrhythmias. Baltimore: Williams & Wilkins, 1983:648.

55. VonCappeller D, Copeland G, Stern T: Digitalis intoxication: a clinical report of 148 cases. Ann Intern Med 1959;5:869.

56. Bettinger J, Surawicz B, Bryfogle JW, et al: The effect of intravenous administration of potassium chloride on ectopic rhythms, ectopic beats and disturbances of A-V conduction. Am J Med 1956;21:521.

57. Bigger J Jr, Strauss H: Digitalis toxicity: drug interactions promoting toxicity and the management of toxicity. Semin Drug Treatment 1972;2:147.

58. Kunin A, Surawicz B, Sims E: Decrease in serum potassium concentrations and appearance of cardiac arrhythmias during infusion of potassium with glucose in potassium-depleted patients. N Engl J Med 1962;266:228.

59. Cranefield P: Action potentials, afterpotentials and arrhythmias. Circ Res 1977;41:415.

60. Rabbino W, Likoff W, Dreifus LS: Complications and limitations of direct current countershock. JAMA 1964;190:417.

61. Gilbert R, Cuddy R: Digitalis intoxication following conversion to sinus rhythm. Circulation 1965;32:58.

62. Lown B, Kleiger R, Williams J: Cardioversion and digitalis drugs: changed threshold to electric shock in digitalized animals. Circ Res 1965;17:519.

63. Robinson H, Wagner J: DC cardioversion causing ventricular fibrillation. Am J Med Sci 1965;249:300.

64. Peleska B: Cardiac arrhythmias following condenser discharges led through an inductance: comparison with effects of pure condenser discharges. Circ Res 1965;16:11.

65. Babbs C, Tacker W, Van Vleet JF, Bourland J, Geddes L: Therapeutic indices for transchest defibrillator shocks: effective, damaging and lethal electric doses. Am Heart J 1980;99:734.

66. Ditchey R, Karliner J: Safety of electrical cardioversion in patients without digitalis toxicity. Ann Intern Med 1971; 95:676.

67. Ditchey R, Curtis G: Effects of apparently nontoxic doses of digoxin on ventricular ectopy following direct-current electrical shocks in dogs. J Pharmacol Exp Ther 1981;218:212.

68. Mann D, Maisel A, Atwood J, Engler R, LeWinter M: Absence of cardioversion-induced ventricular arrhythmias in patients with therapeutic digoxin levels. J Am Coll Cardiol 1985;5:882.

69. Antman E, Wenger T, Butler V, Haber E, Smith T: Treatment of 150 cases of life-threatening digitalis intoxication with digoxin-specific Fab antibody fragments: final report of a multicenter study. Circulation 1990;81:1774.

69a. Hickey A, Wenger T, Carpenter V, et al: Digoxin immune Fab therapy in the management of digitalis intoxication: safety and efficacy results of an observational surveillance study. J Am Coll Cardiol 1991;17:590.

70. Lechat P, Mudgett-Hunter M, Margolies M, Haber E, Smith T: Reversal of lethal digoxin toxicity in guinea pigs using monoclonal antibodies and Fab fragments. J Pharmacol Exp Ther 1984;229:210.

Cardiac Arrhythmias, 3rd edition, edited by William J. Mandel.
J. B. Lippincott Company, Philadelphia © 1995.

37

Agustin Castellanos • Pedro R. Fernandez
Alberto Interian Jr. • Robert J. Myerburg

Pacemaker-Induced Arrhythmias

Many medical, technological, and geopolitical changes have occurred in the years since the first edition of this book was published. Therefore, a drastic revision of this chapter is mandatory. In 1980, the pulse generator used most often was the VVI pacemaker.[1] Thereafter, DVI pacemakers became popular. Later, they were superseded by other more sophisticated dual-chamber devices (DDD pacemakers). Finally, rate-adaptive (VVIR or DDDR) pacemakers arrived and are here to stay. Although we think the DDD devices should be the pacemakers of choice (except when specific contraindications exist), VVI pacing is also described here, mainly for didactic purposes. Moreover, various factors (e.g., cost, availability, locality, and modifications such as VVIR pacing) make it necessary for some physicians to use or follow-up patients having single-chamber devices. Therefore, this chapter discusses the arrhythmias produced by both single- and dual-chamber pacemakers. The term arrhythmia refers to any rhythm produced (initiated and sustained) by the pacemakers when they are functioning as predetermined by the respective manufacturer.

Although redundant, it should be emphasized that because in 1994 all pacemakers used in the United States are programmable, the mode and parameters may differ not only in devices from various manufacturers but in different generations of pacemakers made by the same manufacturer. Moreover, so-called eccentricities exist; this and rapid advances in the pacemaker field make it essential for the interpreter to check the brochure supplied by the manufacturer when attempting to interpret the electrocardiographic manifestations of pacemaker arrhythmias. This chapter has a general didactic orientation useful for physicians as well as for the multiple specialized pacemaker nurses. Generally, any parameter given is supplied as an example because some or all of the prototype descriptions may not apply (having been superseded by newer generations) at the time this book appears in print.

VVI PACEMAKERS

Pacemaker Intervals

The automatic interval is that between two consecutive spikes while the pacemaker is functioning in its VVI mode.[2] Classically, the escape interval is the interval between a natural beat and the subsequent spike.[2] Escape intervals conventionally are measured from the beginning of a sensed ventricular complex (or other electric signal)

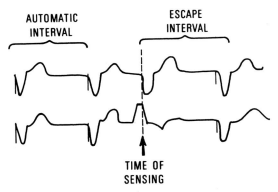

Figure 37-1. Diagrams of the duration of escape intervals in a patient with an implanted VVI pacemaker whose leads were properly positioned in the right ventricular apex. Escape intervals after right and left ventricular extrasystoles are shown in the top and bottom diagrams, respectively. The escape intervals measured from the beginning of the QRS complex in surface lead V₁ are similar (*top diagram*) and longer (*bottom diagram*) than the automatic interval. Nevertheless, the actual (electronic) time of sensing (*arrow* pointing to vertical broken line) was the same within the pulse generator.

to the subsequent spike.[3] Theoretically, the escape interval should equal the automatic interval.[2,3] This can be determined when ectopic right ventricular beats arise close to the sensing electrodes (Fig. 37-1, *top diagram*).

Actually, most escape intervals appear to be longer (when measured from the beginning of the QRS complexes) than the automatic intervals; sensing does not occur at the onset of the QRS complex recorded at the body surface but depends on the various factors that influence the signals perceived by the sensing electrodes. The moment of arrival of excitation at the sensing electrodes (in relation to the onset of the QRS complex) also plays a role.[2–7] This is well illustrated in patients having sinus rhythm and complete right bundle branch block or left ventricular ectopic beats when arrival of excitation at the right ventricular apical–sensing electrodes occurs at least 50 milliseconds after the onset of ventricular depolarization (see Fig. 37-1, *bottom diagram*). This interval, which represents the minimal left septal to right ventricular apex conduction time, can even be longer (up to 120 milliseconds) when ectopic beats originate in the posterosuperior wall of the left ventricle. In addition, escape intervals may be (by design) significantly longer than automatic intervals. This feature, called rate hysteresis, is shown in Figure 37-2.[8]

Escape intervals can be shorter than the automatic intervals. According to Barold and Keller, the term partial sensing implies that electric signals appearing at any moment of the cycle produce escape intervals shorter than automatic intervals (Fig. 37-3).[9] This phenomenon is attributed to signals of borderline amplitude or poor slew rate. Conversely, the term partial recycling is used when

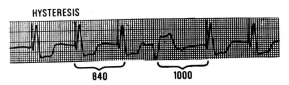

Figure 37-2. Rate hysteresis. Note that the escape interval was programmed to be significantly longer than the automatic interval.

the sorter escape intervals are related to the timing of the electric signals. Partial recycling is usually produced by spikes falling during the relative refractory period of the pacemaker, which occurs at the end of the absolute refractory period (Fig. 37-4). Except when it is a programmed eccentricity, partial sensing of implanted pacemakers is almost invariably due to malfunction of the pacing system (frequently, electrode displacement). Partial recycling, however, used to be a normal electronic feature of some early VVI pacemakers.[9]

Pacemaker Refractory Periods

The delivery refractory period follows the emission of a spike, and the sensing refractory period follows the spontaneous beat or a signal generated by external chest wall stimulation.[9] The duration of the sensing and delivery refractory periods can differ in some pulse generators.[9]

Many of the early pacemakers had an absolute and a relative refractory period. During the absolute refractory period, electric signals occurring early in the cycle (after a paced or a sensed beat) were not sensed. This does not imply pacemaker system malfunction. Thus, the clinician must know the duration of the refractory period of each pulse generator to differentiate between non-sensing due to normal pacemaker refractoriness and non-sensing related to malfunction. The relative refractory period, occurring after the absolute refractory period, had two electrocardiographic expressions. First, in some units, early sensing required a larger signal than later sensing. If signals of normal or slightly greater than normal amplitude were not sensed because of pacemaker relative refractoriness, the pacemaker absolute refractory period ap-

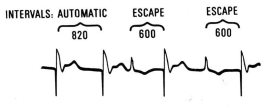

Figure 37-3. Partial sensing (shorter-than-normal escape intervals occurring after natural ventricular beats and falling in different moments of the cycle) in a patient with a VVI pacemaker.

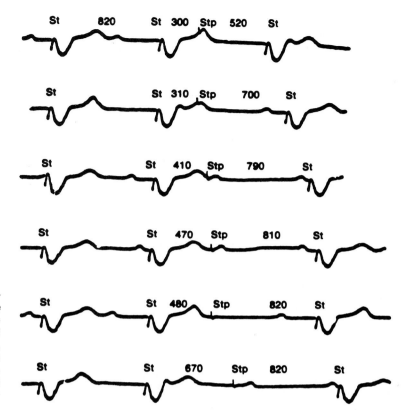

Figure 37-4. Partial recycling of VVI pacemaker exposed by premature external chest wall stimuli (*Stp*). The automatic interval measured 820 milliseconds. In the second, third, and fourth strips, premature chest wall stimuli with coupling intervals of 310, 410, and 470 milliseconds, respectively, caused partial pacemaker recycling, in which the escape intervals (700, 790, and 810 milliseconds, respectively) were shorter than the automatic interval (820 milliseconds). *ST*, automatic stimuli.

peared to be abnormally prolonged—thus falsely suggesting pacing system malfunction. Second, in other units, signals with the same amplitude resulted in full (normal) recycling later in the cycle, producing partial recycling (escape intervals of shorter than normal duration) during the pacemaker relative refractory period.[9,10]

Because the initial VVI pacemakers were sensitive to myopotential inhibition, refractory periods were usually followed by an interval in which a sensed event was defined as noise, which may result in an emission of a pacemaker spike at the end of the escape (or some other predetermined) interval.

Ventricular Fusion and Pseudofusion Beats

True fusion beats occur when the ventricles are activated, partly by the natural complex and partly by the pacemaker-initiated ventricular depolarization (Fig. 37-5). Pseudofusion beats result from the superimposition (on the surface electrocardiogram) of an ineffective ventricular spike on a QRS complex (see Fig. 37-5).[7] They occur because the initial part of the QRS complex (recorded at the body surface) may be inscribed before the moment of sensing.

VOO Pacing

Few pacemakers are implanted to provide VOO pacing. This mode of stimulation is most frequently produced when the physician or nurse, usually attempting to evaluate pacemaker function, applies an external magnet over the pulse generator. Spontaneous VOO stimulation is seen in the presence of electromagnetic interference whenever the pacemaker reverts to its noise rate or interference mode. The latter does not imply pacing system malfunction. Spontaneous VOO stimulation is seen when pacing system malfunction characterized by persistent failure to sense occurs.

Electromagnetic Interference

Electromagnetic interference arose when sensing circuits—required to avoid the competition that occurred with VOO pacemakers—were developed. VVI pacemakers, however, can be inhibited not only by natural electric activity but also by electromagnetic influences from other sources, either extrinsic (environmental) or intrinsic (skeletal muscle potentials; Fig. 37-6). Because of this potential hazard, manufacturers introduced various effective remedial changes, including shielding, filtration

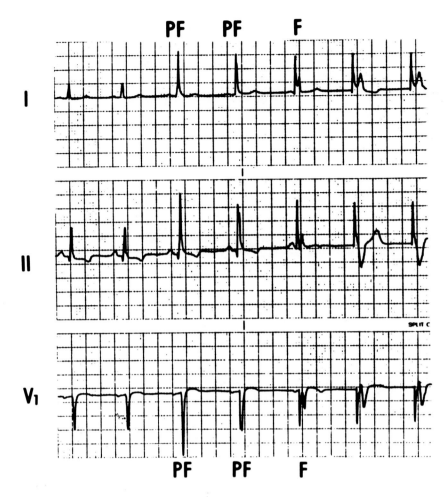

Figure 37-5. Fusion (*F*) and pseudofusion (*PF*) beats produced by normally functioning VVI pacemaker. The three leads were recorded simultaneously.

of extraneous signals, and incorporation of a noise rate or interference mode, during which the pacemaker reverted to a continuous asynchronous mode (Fig. 37-7).[11-20] Despite these changes, absolute protection may not be possible, especially if technological advances in fields other than medicine continue at the present rate.

In an early study examining the manner in which VVI pacemakers responded to simulated electromagnetic interference, we observed the expected reversion to VOO pacing in addition to an irregular and erratic ventricular stimulation mode.[21] Although electromagnetic inter-ference can still occur, myopotential inhibition (though less frequent than a decade ago) is still the major source of electromagnetic interference affecting VVI pacemakers. This problem has been encountered mainly with unipolar VVI pacemakers. A unipolar pacemaker is subject to myopotential inhibition because of the difference in voltage between the indifferent electrode (plate of the pulse generator) and the intracardiac electrodes, which are located on opposite sites of contracting muscle.[19] Also, myopotentials undergo low-pass filtering in the body, making the pacemaker more prone to them. Furthermore, amplitude

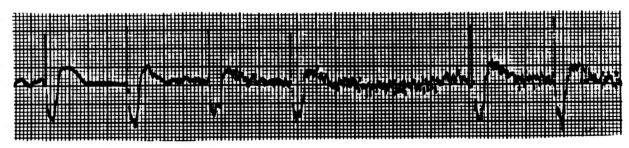

Figure 37-6. Myopotential inhibition of normally functioning VVI pacemaker.

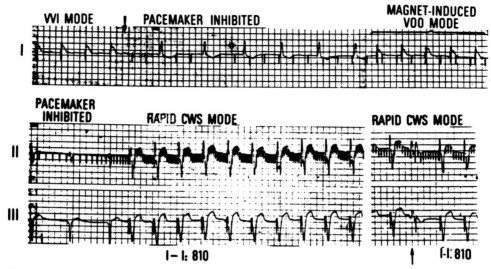

Figure 37-7. Normally functioning VVI pacemaker. Control-VVI mode of operation (beginning of *upper strip*), temporary inhibition by slow external chest wall stimulation (*arrow* in upper strip), and magnet-induced VOO mode of operation (*end* of upper strip). Note that the duration of the automatic interstimulus intervals (I-I) of the implanted pacemaker is designed to be the same (810 milliseconds) during both VVI and magnet-induced VOO modes of operation. The lower two simultaneously recorded strips show reversion to the electromagnetic-interference mode, which in this case equal rapid external chest wall stimulation (*CWS*). That the latter mode was VOO could be corroborated by noting that a premature QRS complex (*arrow*) did not recycle the pacemaker. Note that external stimuli did not distort QRS complexes in lead III. This shows that electromagnetic interference is best seen when simultaneous leads are recorded.

and frequency analysis of skeletal muscle potentials from the pectoral muscles reveals large enough amplitudes (and maximal derivatives) to inhibit pacemaker function.[19] Although their amplitude usually does not exceed 4 mV, the amplitude of the natural intraventricular electrogram is generally around 10 mV. Hence, several authors state that using 4 mV as the lowest sensitivity should reduce the incidence of myopotential inhibition without creating a significant risk of undersensing of the natural intraventricular electrograms.[19]

Though rare, years ago, myopotential inhibition occurred with bipolar electric systems.[14, 19, 22–25] In many cases, this may have been because of defective insulation of the catheter electrodes or penetration (or perforation), which in turn could have allowed myopotentials from the diaphragm to be picked up by the sensing electrodes. The latter implies pacing system malfunction.

Changes in the Electric Axis of the Pacemaker Spike

Although a change in amplitude and polarity of a pacemaker spike can be seen normally in a single lead when the spike is perpendicular to the lead, a change in more than one lead initially was considered to be a sign of pacing system malfunction (e.g., partial electrode fracture,

defective electrode insulation, or short-circuiting of bipolar electrodes). A spatial (three-lead) change, however, resulting in variations in the electric axis (in standard leads), amplitude, and polarity (in all leads) of the spike may be produced factitiously by a digital electrocardiographic machine, especially when pacing is unipolar.[26] The phenomenon illustrated in Figure 37-8 is an electrocardiographic artifact due to the digital "rollover" effect. In digital numeric systems, the largest possible positive number and largest negative number are adjacent. Hence, if the amplitude of the input signal exceeds the maximum positive value, a negative number may be recorded. Conversely, if the input is greater than the negative value, a positive number may be recorded. In Figure 37-8, the amplitude of the pacemaker spike (large when measured by oscilloscope) caused intermittent digital rollover that produced variations in spike polarity. Furthermore, beat-to-beat differences in the point from which the spike was sampled resulted in marked variability in pulse amplitude. Recording the same signal, using not only an oscilloscope but also a conventional (analog) electrocardiographic machine, confirmed the artifactual nature of the varying spatial orientation of the ventricular spike.[26] With widespread use of bipolar pacing (permanent and temporary), the major problem with pacemaker electrocardiography seems to be failure to detect small bipolar spikes (Fig. 37-9). Inspection of multiple leads (especially V_3 and V_4) is

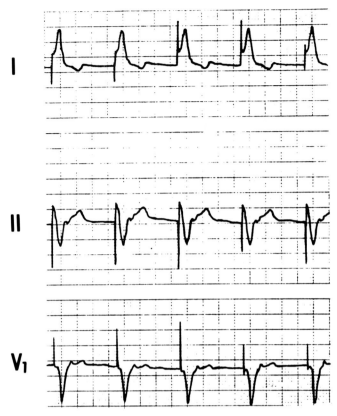

Figure 37-8. Spatial (three-lead) artifactual alternation of electrical axis, amplitude, and polarity of the unipolar pacemaker spikes.

frequently required to determine that the QRS complexes are indeed paced (as in lead II of Fig. 37-9).

VVIR PACEMAKERS

Technological progress has allowed the development of implantable pacemakers that use signals other than intracardiac electrograms to control the rate of stimulation.[27-32] Multiple sensors have been evaluated to perform rate-adaptive pacing: (1) using a standard pacing lead: activity and minute ventilation (the two most used, thus the only ones dealt with in this chapter); respiratory rate; QT interval; and paced depolarization integral; and (2) using a special pacing lead: central venous pH, central venous O_2 saturation, central venous temperature, right ventricular dP/dt, and right ventricular stroke volume.[27]

At first the most widely implanted single-chamber rate-responsive (VVIR) pacemakers were those that provided the capacity to increase heart rate in response to physical activity (Fig. 37-10).[33-38] In patients having abnormal sinoatrial function (chronotropic insufficiency) or

chronic atrial arrhythmias and after intentional or accidental complete atrioventricular (AV) block due to catheter ablation of the His bundle, a parameter other than atrial activity must be used to provide changes in heart rate appropriate to metabolic needs. Apparently, on a worldwide basis, activity sensor–based rate-adaptive pacing systems are the most frequently implanted units that use signals other than intracardiac electrograms to control the pacing rates. These pacemakers also can be subject to myopotential inhibition, in which case marked irregularities in the interspike intervals can be seen (Fig. 37-11). Initial generations of these pacemakers had eccentricities (i.e., normal modes of operation that could be interpreted as resulting from malfunction; Fig. 37-12).[37] Although most reports evaluating rate-adaptive (VVIR and DDDR) pacemakers have emphasized the response to controlled exercise (using a treadmill for relatively short periods of time), we believe that Holter monitoring also provides a good indication of their performance during the patient's daily activities (see Figs. 37-10 and 37-11). Less known is that pacemakers can also be used to analyze the validity of Holter monitoring. For example, Figure 37-13 was obtained from a patient with a VVI (not VVIR) device who was pacemaker-dependent and who had no ventricular arrhythmias. The graph of average, maximum, and minimal hourly ventricular rates shows that the rate was *not* consistently 70 per milliseconds (as programmed). Rates ranging from 67 to 82 were seen. Full disclosure revealed that this was because of interpretation by the Holter equipment of artifacts as ventricular beats. At first glance, the

SMALL SPIKES

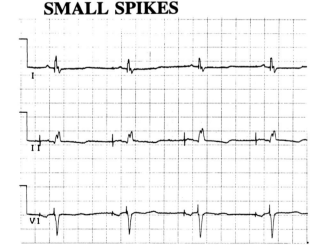

Figure 37-9. Almost invisible (small) bipolar spikes (simultaneously recorded leads I, II and V_1). During atrioventricular sequential pacing at normal standardization, atrial spikes are hardly visible in lead I, whereas ventricular spikes can be seen only with great difficulty in lead II.

VVIR

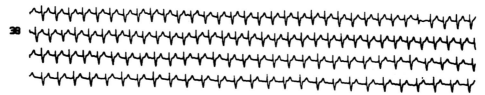

Figure 37-10. Holter-monitor recordings obtained at a slow paper speed (each strip representing 20 seconds) from a patient with VVIR pacemaker, showing the expected variations in rate during activity.

VVIR

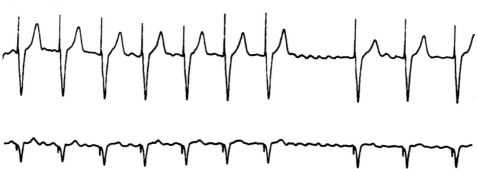

Figure 37-11. Myopotential inhibition of VVIR pacemaker (Holter-monitor recordings), showing erratic variations of the interspike intervals (simultaneously recorded monitoring leads equivalent to II and V₁).

Figure 37-12. Eccentricity of initial generator of Medtronic Activitrax (VVIR) pacemaker. Whereas **A** depicts normal recycling after a premature ventricular contraction, **B** shows the non–malfunction-related eccentricity: partial recycling, with escape interval (*EI*) equaling programmed upper cycle length of 480 milliseconds. *ML₂*, monitoring lead equivalent to standard II.

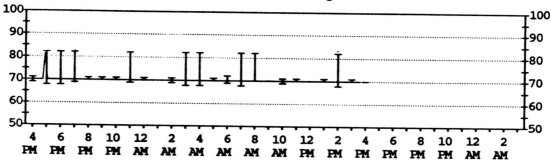

Figure 37-13. Evaluation of Holter monitoring, using a VVI pacemaker. In this pacemaker-dependent patient, the device was stimulating the ventricles at a constant rate of 70/minute. The graph displaying average minimum and maximum heart rates shows variability of the latter two. Real-time disclosure of the corresponding hours at which this occurred revealed that the Holter monitor had interpreted and counted artifacts as paced beats.

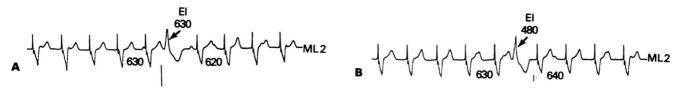

graph could have been interpreted as being that of a patient with a VVIR rather than a VVI pacemaker.

Rapid Recharge Function of Pacemakers After Sensing

Some pacemakers have contained rapid recharge circuits that operate after delivery of pacemaker stimuli.[39] Others are also designed with a rapid discharge circuit that is operative after sensing. The corresponding rhythm strips exhibit unusually clear, smaller-than-normal electrocardiographic artifacts, which are due to the rapid recharge effect after sensing. A similar phenomenon was observed in several patients who had Activitrax pacemakers (Medtronic, Minneapolis, MN).[33] In these cases, however, what appeared to be recharged artifacts were myopotential artifacts, causing pacemaker resetting.

DDD PACEMAKERS

Although DDD pacemakers (whether unipolar or bipolar) may be programmed to multiple modes, the following discussion applies to the "classic" DDD mode, which is the most versatile.[40–50] DDD pacemakers from different manufacturers do not operate in exactly the same way; moreover, even pacemakers from the same manufacturer may change as needs dictate. Further modifications will probably occur between the writing and publication of this edition. To reiterate—at the risk of being repetitious and redundant—physicians and paramedical personnel should routinely consult brochures supplied by the manufacturers to determine the parameters of the specific device used.

PACEMAKER ESCAPE INTERVALS

The atrial escape interval is that time elapsing between a ventricular spike or sensed ventricular beat and subsequent atrial spike (Fig. 37-14).[50,51] If no events are sensed in either chamber during the atrial escape interval, an atrial spike is delivered at its end, which then initiates the AV interval and its subintervals.

Fusion and pseudofusion beats are seen not only in patients with VVI pacemakers but also in those with DDD pacemakers. In addition, pseudo-pseudofusion beats can occur when an ineffective atrial spike falls on a QRS complex.[50] In a DDD pacemaker, the latter is an indication of malfunction if it occurs when a P wave is non-sensed.

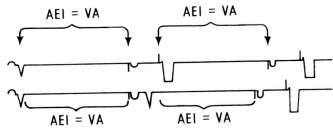

Figure 37-14. Diagram of atrial escape intervals (*AEI*) of a DDD pacemaker after natural-sensed and paced-ventricular QRS complexes. *VA,* the interval between the moment of at which the AEI began and that at which the atrial spike was emitted.

PACEMAKER ATRIOVENTRICULAR INTERVALS

Generally, five possible timing cycles exist during DDD pacing: (1) atrial pacing, with conduction through the normal (natural) AV pathway; (2) atrial and ventricular (sequential) pacing (Fig. 37-15, *right*); (3) atrial sensing and ventricular pacing (see Fig. 37-15, *left*); (4) atrial sensing and ventricular sensing (when the natural AV conduction time is shorter than the artificial AV conduction time); and (5) atrial pacing or atrial sensing, with AV conduction through the normal pathway, *and* ventricular pacing occurring after the beginning of the QRS complex but before the moment at which ventricular sensing occurs.[50]

During atrial and ventricular pacing, the AV interval is broken into several subintervals, from atrial to ventricular spike:

1. A short blanking subinterval, during which the atrial spike cannot inhibit the ventricular spike (thus avoiding the so-called cross-talk)
2. A safety-pacing subinterval, during which any sensed event (either an atrial stimulus, a ventricular ectopic beat, or noise) produces a "semi-committed" stimulus about 100 milliseconds later (Fig. 37-16)
3. An alert subinterval, during which a sensed event results in pacemaker recycling[31]

Short interspike intervals also occur during magnet-induced DOO pacing (Fig. 37-17).

The pure, natural AV interval is the time elapsing between a sensed P wave and a ventricular beat sensed before the ventricular spike is expected to occur. The interval between a sensed P wave and a ventricular spike need not be equal to that between an atrial and a ventricular spike because atrial sensing does not necessarily occur at the onset of the P wave. Artificial and natural AV intervals coexist when the ventricular spike—if emitted after the onset of a ventricular beat but before sensing—

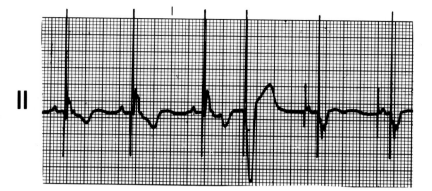

Figure 37-15. DDD pacemaker, providing P-wave–triggered pacing (*left*) and atrioventricular sequential pacing (*right*). The QRS complexes show different degrees of fusion, as can be determined when they were compared with the morphology of the pure (ventricular) paced QRS complex triggered by a premature atrial beat.

II

occurs within the QRS complexes recorded at the body surface.

CROSS-TALK

Usually, cross-talk occurs when the output of the atrial channel is sensed by the ventricular channel, so that a ventricular spike is not emitted.[31] In patients with complete AV block, cross-talk can lead to asystole. This phe-

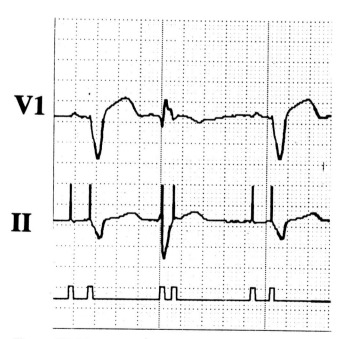

Figure 37-16. DDD pacemaker, providing atrioventricular (AV) sequential pacing, with the programmed AV intervals of 200 milliseconds (*left* and *right*) and the shorter artificial AV interval of 100 milliseconds (when a premature ventricular complex was sensed very soon after the atrial spike) resulting from the so-called safety pacing (*middle*).

nomenon is more frequently due to misplacement of the atrial lead (generally during temporary pacing) but can also occur with properly anchored atrial leads if pacing is unipolar or rarely, during bipolar stimulation with high output.

ATRIOVENTRICULAR SEQUENTIAL AND P-WAVE–TRIGGERED PACING

Atrioventricular sequential pacing occurs when the natural atrial rates are *below* the programmed lower rate (see Fig. 37-15, *right*).[50] In contrast, when the natural atrial rates range *between* the programmed lower rate and the programmed upper rate, the pacemaker provides P-wave–triggered pacing (see Fig. 37-15, *left*).[50]

The function of this pacemaker when the atrial rate is *above* the programmed upper rate is described subsequently.

ATRIAL REFRACTORY PERIODS

The atrial refractory period which starts with a ventricular event is called the postventricular refractory atrial refractory period.[50, 51] The total atrial refractory period, however, is usually composed of two parts: the AV interval and the postventricular atrial refractory period. As discussed below, in some models after a ventricular extrasystole, the postventricular atrial refractory period is automatically extended for variable periods, regardless of the programmed setting.[51] Early published specifications were slightly confusing because some brochures referred to the atrial refractory period as the total duration of the atrial refractory period after an atrial event, whereas others referred only to the postventricular atrial refractory period.[50]

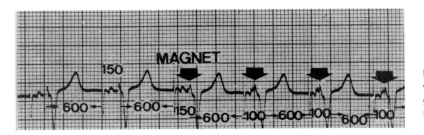

Figure 37-17. DDD pacemaker, providing atrioventricular (AV) sequential pacing, with the programmed AV interval of 150 milliseconds and with the shorter 100-millisecond AV intervals resulting from the DOO mode induced by magnet application.

MODES OF OPERATION WHEN SPONTANEOUS ATRIAL RATES ARE FASTER THAN PROGRAMMED UPPER VENTRICULAR RATES

If the atrial rate increases so that the PP intervals are significantly shorter than the atrial refractory period, only every other P wave is sensed, causing an abrupt halving of the ventricular rate (Fig. 37-18).[50]

The fastest ventricular rate possible is determined by the programmed upper rate.[50] Regardless of how early a P wave is sensed and regardless of the AV interval, the ventricular spike will not be emitted until after the end of the programmed upper cycle length. For example, in Figure 37-19, the atrial rate was slightly faster (130 beats/minute; cycle length, 460 milliseconds) than the programmed upper rate (125 beats/minute; cycle length, 460 milliseconds). Under these circumstances, the atrial refractory period, although always ending 155 milliseconds after a ventricular spike, was gradually extended because of the progressive increase in AV intervals. Note that because of the previously mentioned difference in atrial and ventricular rates, P waves two through eight yielded progressively longer AV intervals but coexisted

with constant ventricular VV intervals. Finally, P wave eight occurred close to the ventricular spike, thus falling within the atrial refractory period. It thus did not trigger a ventricular spike and the Wenckebach-like period ended. Thereafter, the pacemaker synchronized its output to the next sensed P wave (nine) at the programmed AV interval.

The differences between the natural AV nodal Wenckebach and the artificial Wenckebach-like periods are as follows: (1) the VV intervals are not constant, tending generally to decrease as the cycles progress, and (2) the nonconducted P wave is blocked because of the refractory period of the AV node, not of the atrium.[53]

When those pacemaker generations were introduced that had programmable atrial refractory periods capable of being increased for variable intervals after a sensed ventricular event, an unexpected event occurred: Wenckebach-like periods became less frequent.[52] This happened because the relation between the duration of the total atrial refractory period and the programmed upper cycle length determined whether the upper rate response would be 2:1 or Wenckebach-like AV block. Simply stated, (1) if the total atrial refractory period (AV interval plus postventricular atrial refractory period) is greater than the programmed upper rate, the response

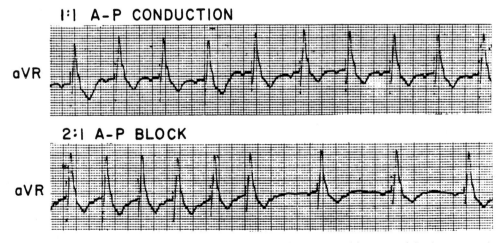

Figure 37-18. One-to-one P-wave–triggered pacing (*top strip* and first part of the *bottom strip*) with sudden onset of 2:1 block (end of *bottom strip*).

1 WENCKEBACH-LIKE AV RESPONSCE
2 SINUS P WAVES ARE NEGATIVE BECAUSE THE
   RECORDING LEAD WAS aVR

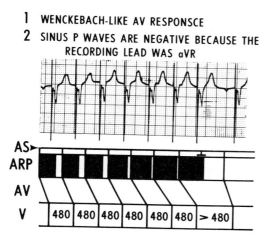

Figure 37-19. Eight-to-seven Wenckebach-like period, occurring during the normal function of a DDD pacemaker. *AS* indicates the moment that atrial sensing occurs. Black squares at the atrial refractory period (*ARP*) level represent pacemaker total ARP. *Oblique lines* at the atrioventricular (*AV*) level show an association between a P wave and a ventricular spike. Numbers (480 milliseconds) between vertical lines at the *V* level correspond to the programmed upper-cycle length.

is AV block; and (2) if the total atrial refractory period is less than the programmed upper cycle length, some degree of Wenckebach-like activity results, with the maximal prolongation of the AV interval (over control values) being the difference between the total atrial refractory period and the programmed upper cycle length.

Some pacemakers prevent abrupt changes while sinus or atrial tachycardia is present by converting to the fallback rate. The latter is the programmed rate to which ventricular stimulation falls decrementally when the natural atrial rate exceeds the programmed maximum ventricular rate for a given value.[30] The fallback mechanism can be accomplished by a shift to VVI or VVIR pacing, with the rate decreasing progressively to a given value without synchronization to atrial activity. Once the true fallback rate is reached, atrial synchronicity is resumed. An interesting option is rate-smoothing introduced by Cardiac Pacemakers, Inc. (CPI), which tends to eliminate large cycle-to-cycle changes by preventing the paced rate from changing more than a certain percentage (which can be

3%, 6%, 12%, and so on) from one paced VV interval to the next.[30] This option eliminates large fluctuations in rate during 2:1 block or Wenckebach-like behavior that occurs at the upper rate limit.

ENDLESS-LOOP TACHYCARDIA

The duration of the atrial refractory period of DDD pacemakers varies, depending on the manufacturer and on the programmed interval after sensed sinus or ectopic ventricular beats. If a retrograde P wave from an ectopic ventricular beat is sensed by the atrial amplifier, it initiates an AV delay.[31, 45, 46, 54, 55] Consequently, a ventricular spike is emitted at an interval that cannot exceed the programmed upper cycle length. If the paced ventricular beat also has retrograde conduction and the corresponding P wave is sensed, the process repeats itself. This arrhythmia was called endless-loop tachycardia by Furman and Fisher, in an analogy to a computer program that repeats itself ad infinitum.[45] Although it can be initiated by a spontaneous or paced impulse, it is always sustained by pacemaker participation (Figs. 37-20 through 37-22). Once started, the pacemaker limits the maximum rate but not its duration.[45–49, 55] Termination requires external intervention or spontaneous variability of natural conduction; therefore, efforts have been made to prevent its induction. This arrhythmia, the occurrence of which was predicted in 1969, can also be seen in patients with implanted atrial synchronous–ventricular inhibited pacemakers.[54, 56–58]

Endless-loop tachycardia requires not only retrograde conduction through a natural AV pathway but also a VA conduction time greater than the postventricular atrial refractory period. Thus, programming of the latter has decreased the frequency of this arrhythmia. In different generations of DDD pacemakers, endless-loop tachycardia has been variously initiated by (1) premature ventricular contractions with VA conduction; (2) ventricular escape beats with VA conduction; (3) premature atrial contractions triggering a ventricular spike after a long delay, with the corresponding paced ventricular beat having retrograde atrial conduction; and (4) magnet-induced DOO pacing, with the first atrial spike falling in the atrial refrac-

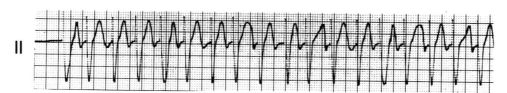

Figure 37-20. "Endless-loop" tachycardia, which was initiated by the retrograde conduction to the atria of a ventricular ectopic beat without an antecedent P wave (not shown).

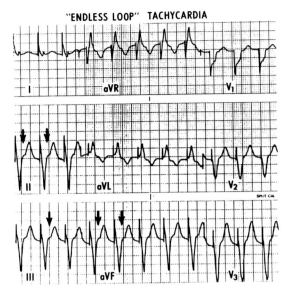

Figure 37-21. Twelve-lead electrocardiogram in a patient with an "endless-loop" tachycardia. *Arrows* indicate retrograde P waves.

tory period, so that the first ventricular spike can produce a QRS complex with retrograde conduction. Abolishment of endless-loop tachycardia requires spontaneous occurrence of VA block or external intervention such as carotid sinus massage. Magnet application, producing DOO pacing, can abruptly inhibit atrial sensing, thus interrupting the arrhythmia. Prevention is the best approach for the problems created by the occurrence of endless-loop tach-

ycardia. Extension of the atrial refractory period (in beats other than extrasystolic) limits the programmed upper rate. If the latter is too low (e.g., 100 beats/minute), it may not be ideal for a younger patient, who may need faster atrial rates with 1:1 AV conduction. One possible solution would be to have the pacemaker discriminate between sinus and retrograde P waves. Because a perfect solution does not yet exist, the following approaches have been tried:

1. A tachycardia termination algorithm.[59] This approach detects continued pacing at the ventricular rate, allowing it to proceed for 15 consecutive paced events, inhibiting the 16th ventricular output pulse, thus breaking the reentry loop.

2. The "fallback" response.[60] In this approach, if the atrial rate exceeds the programmed upper rate, up to four P-wave–triggered pacing pulses are allowed. After a pause, there is a shift to VVI pacing for about 36 seconds or until the programmed fallback rate is achieved. If an atrial rate below the programmed upper rate is apparent, this mode of response is discontinued so that P-wave–triggered pacing can be resumed.[60]

3. Atrial stimulation synchronous with a premature ventricular beat.[61] It appears that prophylaxis lies in the ability to extend the postventricular atrial refractory period (through programming) beyond the VA conduction time. Automatic extension of the postventricular atrial refractory period after a ventricular

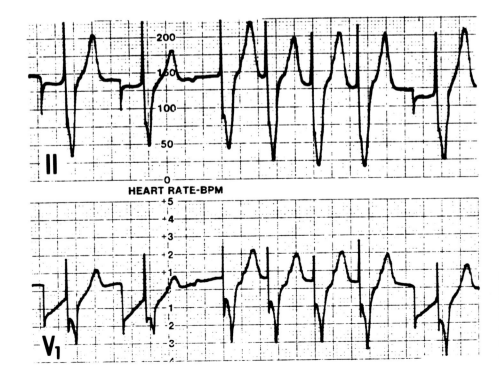

Figure 37-22. A premature atrial beat triggered a ventricular spike after a long artificial atrioventricular delay. The resulting paced ventricular beat had retrograde conduction to the atria and initiated short runs of "endless-loop" tachycardia.

extrasystole has been most helpful in this respect. Conceptual extension to infinity may be associated with the obligatory delivery of an AV sequentially paced beat.

It is possible for endless-loop tachycardia to occur with VV rates below the upper rate limit.[31] Of importance, this will overpower the tachycardia-terminating algorithms, depending on sustained ventricular pacing precisely at the upper rate limit and on decision-making algorithms that use a specific event (in this case the upper rate) as an absolute determinant of the tachycardia. The cycle length of the so-called "balanced" endless-loop tachycardia is determined by the sum of the VA conduction time and the AV interval.[31] When an endless-loop tachycardia has a rate that is below the upper rate, VA can be determined by subtracting the AV interval from the VV cycle length. In contrast, the VA cannot be determined by this method with an upper rate endless-loop tachycardia because by design, the AV interval may have been extended to maintain the selected upper rate limit.[31]

PSEUDO–ENDLESS-LOOP TACHYCARDIA

The term pseudo–endless-loop tachycardia was first used by Amikam and colleagues to refer to electrocardiographic findings that at first glance appeared to result from endless-loop tachycardia; in further evaluations, it was found to have mimicked the latter.[62] This arrhythmia resembled endless-loop tachycardia because it appeared after a premature ventricular contraction, its rate approached the upper rate limit, and the P wave was difficult to discern. A careful analysis revealed that the mechanism of this arrhythmia was different than that of endless-loop tachycardia because regular sinus P waves continued at their own rate. There was a combination of interference by a ventricular extrasystole of the regular sequence of normally conducted ventricular complexes and pace-

maker commitment to maintain an upper rate limit by prolonging the artificial AV interval. In summary, because retrograde conduction from the extrasystole did not exist, "true" endless-loop tachycardia did not occur.[62]

In our experience, however, the most frequent pseudo–endless-loop tachycardia is due to the occurrence of an ectopic atrial tachycardia. This diagnosis is easy when the ectopic rhythm produces positive P waves (Fig. 37-23) but when P waves are negative, the distinction between ectopic atrial and true endless-loop tachycardia may be extremely difficult from static tracings.

Atrial flutter may also produce what at first glance seems to be endless-loop tachycardia. In the presence of this arrhythmia, the response of DDD pacemakers depends on many factors—foremost of which are the duration of the pacemaker refractory periods, the AV delay, and the atrial rate of the flutter. Intermittent sensing of atrial flutter waves may result in erratic DDD pacing. When the relation between the factors mentioned above are appropriate, however, a regular pacemaker tachycardia (at the programmed upper rate or below it) can occur. For example, in Figure 37-24 a pacemaker ventricular rate of 100 beats per minute occurs because there is 3:1 atrio-pacemaker block. Figures 37-24 and 37-25 depict what happened when the pacemaker was manually programmed to the VVI mode. The usefulness of automatic mode switching (obviating manual handling of the device) incorporated in some DDDR pacemakers is obvious in this and other paroxysmal or intermittent supraventricular tachyarrhythmias.

ELECTROMAGNETIC INTERFERENCE

The presence of two sensing (atrial and ventricular) circuits in the unipolar DDD pacemakers enhances the possibility of interference between myopotentials and pacemaker.[32, 63] Whenever sensing of myopotential by the atrial

ATRIAL TACHY

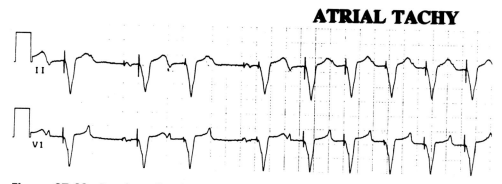

Figure 37-23. Pseudo–endless-loop tachycardia, occurring when an ectopic atrial tachycardia provided P-wave–triggered pacing at the programmed upper rate.

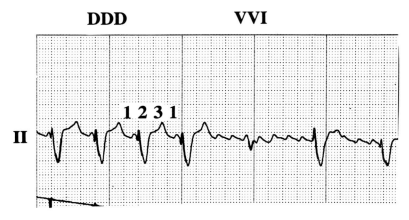

Figure 37-24. Pseudo–endless-loop tachycardia due to atrial flutter, with persistent 3:1 atrio-pacemaker block (*left*). For example, atrial beat 1 triggered the ventricular spike, whereas beats 2 and 3 occurred during the pacemaker refractory period. Atrial flutter waves became evident when the pacemaker was reprogrammed to the VVI mode. Whereas the first QRS complex after reprogramming is a natural beat, the second and third are paced beats.

channel is interpreted as intrinsic atrial activity, the ventricular rate increases to the programmed upper rate (Fig. 37-26). The resulting arrhythmia can also be considered as pseudo–endless-loop tachycardia. In these cases, careful analysis reveals the absence of retrograde P waves, without which endless-loop tachycardia cannot be present.[62, 63] Interestingly, Smyth and colleagues reported rapid firing of an atrial synchronous ventricular pacemaker induced by the electromagnetic field generated by a weapons detector.[64] Conversely, when myopotentials are interpreted by the ventricular channel as ventricular signals, ventricular input is inhibited, so that atrial spikes are not followed by ventricular spikes. Reversion to continuous asynchronous mode (DOO) may also occur.[32]

These phenomena are not rare during atrial unipolar pacing, but a study performed by Furman showed no evidence of myopotential interference at any sensitivity setting in the bipolar configuration in any pacemaker tested.[31] It should be remembered that technological advances are expected to occur in medicine, even at the dawn of healthcare reforms. Optimistically, these must be dealt with by advances in pacemaker technology.

Although the response of pacemakers to electromagnetic interference depends on the source, pacing mode, and pacing polarity, the greatest concern should be the pacemaker-dependent patient.[32] The following are some potential sources of interference: myopotentials, electrocauterization, cardioversion, defibrillation, electroshock therapy, diathermy, magnetic resonance imaging, extracorporeal shock-wave lithotripsy, transcutaneous nerve stimulation, therapeutic radiation, radiofrequency ablation, and close proximity to some heavy motors such as internal combustion engines or arc welding.[32]

Device–device interaction should be considered in a chapter of automatic implantable defibrillator. A priori knowledge that these effects can occur generally suffices. Again, devices from different manufacturers respond differently to electromagnetic interference.

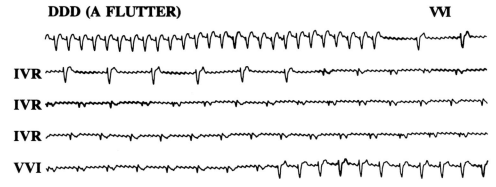

Figure 37-25. (Same patient as in Figure 37-24 but with recordings being performed at a slower paper speed.) Holter-monitor recordings (continuous strips), showing atrial flutter with 3:1 atrio-pacemaker block (*top left*). Reprogramming to VVI pacing with a slow rate resulted initially in pacemaker escape and thereafter in a slightly faster, natural idioventricular rhythm (*IVR*). Finally, in the right part of the *bottom strip*, the pacemaker was reprogrammed to the desired (*VVI*) rate.

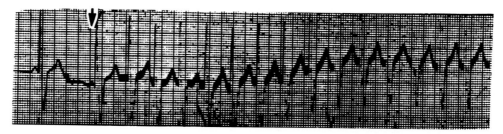

Figure 37-26. Myopotential interference, causing pseudo–endless loop tachycardia.

DDDR PACEMAKERS

The function of these pacemakers is not described as extensively as it would be in a book dealing exclusively with cardiac pacing. For a more extensive discussion on this subject, publications by Sgarbossa et al and Hayes should be consulted.[28,30]

In DDDR pacemakers, the programmed upper rate may be achieved by either P-wave tracking or sensor-driven pacing. The latter may be programmed to a higher rate than the former or vice versa, or both rates may be about the same. Consequently, at the upper rate limit this pacemaker can provide (1) Wenckebach-like block, (2) 2:1 block, (3) AV sequential pacing, (4) P-wave–triggered pacing, and (5) a combination of the above. In addition, there may be other upper rate behavior unique to DDDR pacemaker of certain manufacturers.

If the patient does not have chronotropic insufficiency and the tracking rate is higher than the sensor pacing rate, sensor-driven pacing may not occur. Consequently, DDDR function will be equal to DDD function. The Wenckebach-like and 2:1 block are seen only when this relation exists.

Conversely, sensor pacing occurs when the patient has chronotropic insufficiency or when the sensor pacing rate is higher than the P-wave tracking rate. Programming of DDDR pacemakers is best performed by the appropriate interplay of these rates. This can be accomplished by promoting a smooth (in contrast to abrupt) transition between the two types of pacing.[30] This transition has been described as being sensor-driven rate-smoothing in contrast to the rate-smoothing previously described.[30]

The two major types of sensors in use are activity sensors and minute ventilation sensors.[28] Activity-based rate-adaptive pacing seems to be the most used method. Our experience with these sensors is mainly with the first- and second-generation Medtronic units (Synergist and Legend; Figs. 37-27 and 37-28).

The minute ventilation type (i.e., the product of respiratory rate and tidal volume) is also a good sensor (Telectronics, META DDDR models).[28] Transthoracic impedance increases with respiration and decreases with expiration. The amplitude is used to represent tidal volume and the cyclic pattern represents respiratory rate.

The programmed upper rates are achieved by auto-

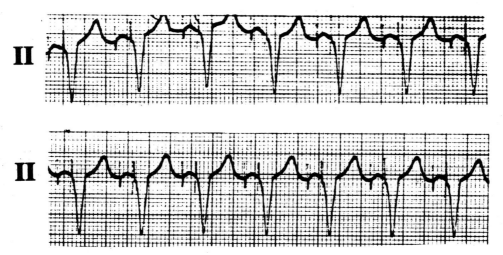

Figure 37-27. DDDR pacemaker, showing variations in rate (during atrioventricular sequential pacing) while the patient was performing slight exercise.

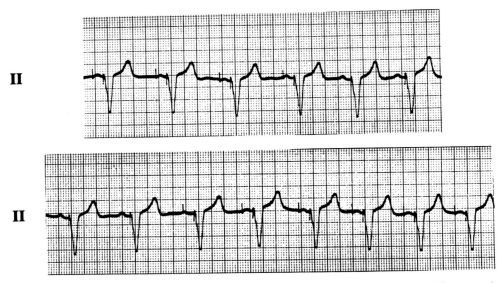

Figure 37-28. DDDR pacemaker. The *top strip* shows a response that could not be differentiated from that of a dual-chamber device pacemaker: atrioventricular (AV) sequential pacing at the programmed lower rate followed by P wave-triggered pacing when the sinus node fired at a slightly higher rate. The *bottom strip* shows a classic DDDR mode of pacing occurring during exercise: AV sequential pacing at a rate faster than that at which P-wave–triggered pacing was occurring.

matic shortening of the AV delay and postventricular atrial refractory period with increasing atrial rates. Furthermore, sensing of the atrial electrogram during the refractory period can lead to automatic reversion to the VVIR mode (Figs. 37-29 and 37-30).[28] This is an important feature for patients with intermittent atrial tachyarrhythmias.

Patients in whom clinically significant slow rates alternate with paroxysmal or intermittent atrial tachyarrhythmias used to pose a real challenge in terms of selecting an optimal pacing mode that could also provide atrial pacing. Automatic mode switching is available in some devices. Barold has not only reviewed this subject but has classified the various fallback mechanisms.[65] For example, a DDD pacemaker with a retriggerable atrial refractory period can switch automatically to the DVI mode when

DDDR

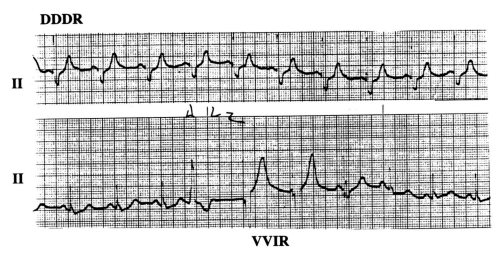

VVIR

Figure 37-29. Rate-adaptive dual-chamber device pacemaker, using minute ventilation as a sensor. The *top strip* shows P-wave–triggered pacing. Presumably, in the *bottom strip* a retrograde P wave was sensed during the refractory period (after a ventricular extrasystole). This caused temporary revision to VVIR mode.

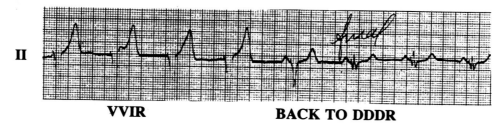

Figure 37-30. (Same patient as in figure 37-29.) After another episode of VVIR pacing, the pacemaker again reverts to the rate-adaptive dual-chamber device mode.

sensing a fast ectopic atrial rate (as previously stated, DDD pacemakers can switch to the DOO mode when subjected to interference).

It appears that most devices that can switch modes automatically when intermittent or paroxysmal supraventricular tachyarrhythmias occur convert to a DDIR (or rarely to VDIR) mode.[30,65–68] Even more intelligent pacemakers that implement algorithms to use information from atria and one or more sensors appear to be in the process of development. According to Barold, they may be expected to possess extensive programmability of the fallback mechanisms and the advanced technology will allow automatic mode switching and fallback functions to be customized according to the changing needs of the individual patient.[65] We agree.

References

1. Parsonnet V, Furman S, Smyth NPD, Bilitch M: Optimal resources for implantable cardiac pacemakers. Circulation 1983;68:227.
2. Barold SS, Gaidula JJ: Evaluation of normal and abnormal sensing function of demand pacemakers. Am J Cardiol 1971;28:201.
3. Lemberg L, Castellanos A, Berkovits B: Pacing on demand in A-V block. JAMA 1965;191:12.
4. Kastor JA, Berkovits BV, DeSanctis R: Variations in discharge rate of demand pacemaker not due to malfunction. Am J Cardiol 1970;25:344.
5. Vera Z, Mason D, Awan NA, et al: Lack of sensing by demand pacemakers due to intraventricular conduction defects. Circulation 1975;51:815.
6. Furman S, Hurzeler D, DeCaprio V: Cardiac pacing and pacemakers. III. Sensing the cardiac electrogram. Am Heart J 1977;93:794.
7. Barold SS: Fusion, pseudo fusion and confusion beats. St. Paul, MN, Impulse, Cardiac Pacemaker, Inc., 1972;1:1.
8. Castellanos A Jr, Lemberg L: Pacemaker arrhythmias and electrocardiographic recognition of pacemakers. Circulation 1973;47:1382.
9. Barold SS, Keller JW: Sensing problems with demand pacemakers. In: Samet P, ed. Cardiac pacing. New York: Grune & Stratton, 1973.
10. Sung, RJ, Castellanos A, Thurer RJ, Myerburg RJ: Partial pacemaker recycling of implanted QRS-inhibited pulse generators. Pacing Clin Electrophysiol 1978;1:189.
11. Parker B, Furman S, Escher DJW: Input signals to pacemakers in a hospital environment. Ann NY Acad Sci 1969;167:823.
12. Chatterjee K, Harris A, Leatham A: The risk of pacing after infarction, and current recommendations. Lancet 1969;2:1061.
13. Wirtzfeld A, Lampadius M, Ruprecht EO: Unterdruckung von Demand-Schrittmachern durch Muskelpotensiale. Dtsch Med Wochenschr 1972;97:61.
14. Mymin D, Cuddy TW, Sinha SN, et al: Inhibition of demand pacemakers by skeletal muscle potentials. JAMA 1973;223:527.
15. Piller LW, Kennelly BM: Myopotential inhibition of demand pacemakers. Chest 1974;66:418.
16. Ohm O-J, Hammer E, Morkrid L: Biological signals and their characteristics as a cause of pacemaker malfunction. In: Watanabe Y, ed. Cardiac pacing. Amsterdam: Excerpta Medica, 1976:401.
17. Ohm O-J, Brulnov DH, Pedersin OM, et al.: Interference effect of myopotentials on function of unipolar demand pacemakers. Br Heart J 1974;36:77.
18. Anderson ST, Pitt A, Whitford JA, et al.: Interference with function of unipolar pacemaker due to muscle potentials. J Thorac Cardiovasc Surg 1976;71:698.
19. Breivik K, Ohm O-J: Myopotential inhibited (VVI) pacemakers assessed by ambulatory Holter monitoring of the electrocardiogram. Pacing Clin Electrophysiol 1980;3:470.
20. Berger R, Jacobs W: Myopotential inhibition of demand pacemakers: Etiologic, diagnostic and therapeutic conclusions. Pacing Clin Electrophysiol 1979;2:596.
21. Castellanos A, Bloom MG, Sung RJ, et al: Modes of operations induced by rapid external chest wall stimulation in patients with normally functioning QRS inhibited (VVI) pacemakers. Pacing Clin Electrophysiol 1979;2:2.
22. Widlandsky S, Zipes DP: Suppression of a ventricular inhibited bipolar pacemaker by skeletal muscle activity. J Electrocardiol 1974;7:371.
23. Barold SS, Ong LS, Falkoff MD, et al: Inhibition of bipolar demand pacemaker by diaphragmatic myopotentials. Circulation 1977;56:679.
24. Amikam S, Peleg H, Lemer J, et al: Myopotential inhibition of a bipolar pacemaker caused by electrode insulation defect. Br Heart J 1977;39:1279.

25. El Gamal M, Van Gelder B: Suppression of an external demand pacemaker by diaphragmatic myopotentials: a sign of electrode perforation? Pacing Clin Electrophysiol 1979; 2:191.

26. Engler RL, Goldberger AL, Bhargava V, Kapelusznik D: Pacemaker spike alternans: an artifact of digital signal processing. Pacing Clin Electrophysiol 1982;5:748.

27. Mond HG: Do we really need multiple sensors for optimal rate-adaptive pacing? In: Barold SS, Mugica J, eds. New perspectives in cardiac pacing. Mt. Kisco, NY: Futura Publishing, 1993:305.

28. Sgarbossa EB, Pinski SL, Ching E, Maloney JD: Adverse effects and limitations of rate-adaptive pacing. In: Barold SS, Mugica J, eds. New perspectives in cardiac pacing. Mt. Kisco, NY: Futura Publishing, 1993:383.

29. Furman S: Rate modulated pacing. In: Furman S, Hayes DL, Holmes DR Jr, eds. A practice of cardiac pacing. Mt. Kisco, NY: Futura Publishing, 1993:401.

30. Hayes DL: Pacemaker electrocardiography. In: Furman S, Hayes DL, Homes DR Jr, eds. A practice of cardiac pacing. Mt. Kisco, NY: Futura Publishing, 1993:309.

31. Furman S: Sensing and timing the cardiac electrogram. In: Furman S, Hayes DL, Homes DR Jr, eds. A practice of cardiac pacing. Mt. Kisco, NY: Futura Publishing, 1993:89.

32. Hayes DL: Electromagnetic interference, drug-device interactions, and other practical considerations. In: Furman S, Hayes DL, Homes DR Jr, eds. A practice of cardiac pacing. Mt. Kisco, NY: Futura Publishing, 1993:665.

33. Castellanos A, Fernandez P, Thurer RJ, et al: Eccentricities of Activitrax pulse generators. Am J Cardiol 1989;63:874.

34. Ryden L, Smedgard P, Kruse I, Anderson K: Rate responsive pacing by means of activity sensing. Stimucoeur 1984;12:181.

35. Botella Solana S, Morel Cabedo S, Sanjuan Manez R, et al: Partial re-cycling in Activitrax pacemakers ECG's. Stimucoeur 1987;15:188.

36. Den Dulk K, Bouwels L, Lindemans F, et al: The Activitrax rate responsive pacemaker system. Am J Cardiol 1988;61:107.

37. Furman S: Pacemaker eccentricity. Pacing Clin Electrophysiol 1981;4:261.

38. Activitrax Multiprogrammable Rate Response (Activity) Pulse Generator. Models 8400/8402/8403. Technical Manual. 1st ed., 1986; 2nd ed., 1987. Minneapolis, MN: Medtronic.

39. Barold SS, Kulkarni H, Thawani AJ, et al: Electrocardiographic manifestations of the rapid recharge function of pulse generators after sensing. Pacing Clin Electrophysiol 1988;11:1215.

40. Funke HD: Une experience clinique de frois annes avec la stimulation sequentielle optimisee du coeur. Stimucoeur 1981;9:26.

41. Redd R, Messenger J, Castellanet M: Early experience with DDD pacing (Medtronic SP 0060). Clin Res 1982;30:18A.

42. Versatrav II Model 7000A Universal AV pacemaker. Minneapolis, MN: Medtronic, 1981.

43. Parsonnet V, Bernstein AD: Pseudomalfunctions of dual chamber pacemakers. Pacing Clin Electrophysiol 1983;6: 376.

44. Furman S: Arrhythmias of dual chamber pacemakers. Pacing Clin Electrophysiol 1982;5:469.

45. Furman S, Fisher JD: Endless loop tachycardia in an A-V universal (DDD) pacemaker. Pacing Clin Electrophysiol 1982;5:486.

46. Dendulk K, Lindemans FW, Bar FW, Wellens HJJ: Pacemaker related tachycardia. Pacing Clin Electrophysiol 1982;5:476.

47. Hauser RG: The electrocardiography of A-V universal DDD pacemakers. Pacing Clin Electrophysiol 1983;6:399.

48. Luceri RM, Castellanos A, Zaman L, Myerburg RJ: The arrhythmias of dual-chamber cardiac pacemakers and their management. Ann Intern Med 1983;99:354.

49. Funke HD: Cardiac pacing with the universal DDD pulse generator. Technological and electrophysiological considerations. In: Barold SS, ed. The third decade of cardiac pacing. Mt. Kisco, NY: Futura Publishing, 1982:191.

50. Barold SS, Falkoff MD, Ong LS, Heinle RA: Function and electrocardiography of DDD pacemakers. In: Barold SS, ed. Modern cardiac pacing. Mt. Kisco, NY: Futura Publishing, 1985:645.

51. Levine P: Postventricular atrial refractory periods and pacemaker medicated tachycardias. Clin Prog Pacing Electrophys 1:394 1983.

52. Furman S: Retreat from Wenckebach. Pacing Clin Electrophysiol 1984;7:1.

53. Castellanos A, Medina-Ravell V, Berkovits BV, et al: Atrial demand and AV sequential pacemakers. In: Dreifus LS, ed. Pacemaker therapy. Cardiovascular Clinics. Philadelphia: FA Davis. 1983:149.

54. Castellanos A, Lemberg L: Electrophysiology of pacing and cardioversion. New York: Appleton-Century Crofts, 1969:76.

55. Johnson CD: AV Universal (DDD) pacemaker-mediated reentrant endless loop tachycardia initiated by a reciprocal beat of atrial origin. Pacing Clin Electrophysiol 1984;7: 29.

56. Tolentino AO, Javier RP, Byrd C, Samet D: Pacemaker induced tachycardia associated with an atrial synchronous ventricular inhibited (ASVIP) pulse generator. Pacing Clin Electrophysiol 1982;5:251.

57. Freedman RA, Rothman MT, Mason JW: Recurrent ventricular tachycardia induced by an atrial synchronous ventricular-inhibited pacemaker. Pacing Clin Electrophysiol 1982; 5:490.

58. Bathen J, Gundersen T, Forfang K: Tachycardias related to atrial synchronous ventricular pacing. Pacing Clin Electrophysiol 1982;5:471.

59. Gelder LM, El-Gamal MIH, Baker R, Sanders RS: Tachycardia-termination algorithm: a valuable feature for interruption of pacemaker mediated tachycardia. Pacing Clin Electrophysiol 1984;7:283.

60. Van Mechelen R, Hagemeijrer F, De Jong J, De Boer H: Responses of an AV Universal (DDD) pulse generator (Cordis 233D) to programmed single ventricular extrastimuli. Pacing Clin Electrophysiol 1984;7:215.

61. Elmgvist H: Reply. Pacing Clin Electrophysiol 1984;7:304. Letters to the Editor.

62. Amikam S, Andrews C, Furman S: "Pseudo-endless loop" tachycardia in an AV Universal (DDD) pacemaker. Pacing Clin Electrophysiol 1984;7:129.

63. Quintal R, Dhurandhar RW, Jain RK: Myopotential inter-

ference with a DDD pacemaker—report of a case. Pacing Clin Electrophysiol 1984;7:737.

64. Smyth NPP, et al: Effect of an active magnetometer on permanently implanted pacemakers. JAMA 1972;221:162.

65. Barold SS: Automatic mode switching during antibradycardia pacing in patients without supraventricular tachyarrhythmias. In: Barold SS, Mugica J, eds. New perspectives in cardiac pacing. Mt. Kisco, NY: Futura Publishing, 1993:455.

66. Barold SS: The DDI mode of cardiac pacing. Pacing Clin Electrophysiol 1987;10:488.

67. Vitatron: DIAMOND DDDR. Extension des indications de la stimulation double chambre par la commutation adaptative de mode. Stimucoeur 1993;21:246.

68. Cardiac Pacemakers, Inc. (CPI): VIGOR DDD/DR: Reponse aux tachycardies atriales (RTA). Stimucoeur 1993;21:250.

Cardiac Arrhythmias, 3rd edition, edited by William J. Mandel.
J. B. Lippincott Company, Philadelphia © 1995.

38

James D. Maloney • Gabriel Vanerio
Sergio L. Pinski • Dirar S. Khoury

Chronic Pacing for the Management of Tachyarrhythmias: Basic and Clinical Aspects

HISTORY

It has been more than 30 years since the treatment of tachyarrhythmias by pacing was first proposed. In 1960, Zoll and coworkers reported the use of closed-chest ventricular pacing to treat ventricular tachyarrhythmias in patients with complete heart block.[1] In 1964, Sowton and associates reported suppression of ventricular arrhythmias by pacing in patients without heart block, and in 1967, Cohen and colleagues found ventricular pacing useful in the treatment of patients with supraventricular arrhythmias associated with the sick sinus syndrome.[2,3] Atrial pacing for the successful termination of reciprocating tachycardias and atrial flutter was reported in 1967 almost simultaneously by Massumi and coworkers, Haft and associates, and Durrer and colleagues.[4-6] Many other reports on the use of pacing for the prevention and termination of tachyarrhythmias soon followed.[7-12] The first *permanent* tachycardia-terminating pacemaker was implanted in 1967 by Ryan and coworkers in a patient with drug-refractory Wolff-Parkinson-White (WPW) syndrome and innumerable prior cardioversions.[13,14] During a severely symptomatic episode of orthodromic reciprocating tachycardia, a temporary ventricular lead was positioned

in the right ventricle with the hope of terminating the tachycardia by mechanically induced ventricular extrasystoles. Thereafter, it could be demonstrated that the supraventricular tachycardia (SVT) was easily terminated by ventricular competitive pacing at a rate of 75 beats per minute, and a permanent VVI pacemaker was implanted. When activated with a magnet by either a physician or the patient, the system would deliver asynchronous underdrive ventricular pacing capable of terminating the arrhythmia by a critically timed ventricular-paced beat.

Although the potential value of antitachycardia pacemakers (ATPM) in the management of supraventricular and ventricular arrhythmias is well documented, the proportion of new pacemakers that are implanted for the treatment of tachyarrhythmias remains negligible. This limited use is the result of both intrinsic drawbacks of antitachycardia pacing and of the potential advantages of competing treatment modalities. Arrhythmia surgery and catheter ablation reduced the potential growth of antitachycardia pacing, particularly for supraventricular arrhythmias. In addition, in the early 1980s, the implantable cardioverter-defibrillators (ICDs) displaced almost completely antitachycardia pacing as a treatment for ventricular tachycardia (VT) treatment. Antitachycardia pacing for ventricular tachyarrhythmias, however, is enjoying a resurgence in the 1990s because of the development of devices that combine cardioverter-defibrillator and anti-tachycardia-pacing modalities in tiered algorithms.

PACING TO PREVENT TACHYCARDIA ONSET

Basic Aspects

Clearly, the most desirable approach to tachyarrhythmia control would be that capable of preventing arrhythmias from occurring. This is particularly true for patients with rapid SVTs or VTs who experience syncope before the tachycardia is terminated. Four permanent-pacing techniques are effective in suppressing the onset of certain tachycardias in selected patients:

1. Rate support to prevent bradycardic events that may lead to tachycardias. Patients experiencing slow heart rates as a result of the sick sinus syndrome or complete atrioventricular (AV) block may exhibit rapid "escape" rhythms due to the bradycardia. Permanent atrial or ventricular pacing at conventional rates prevents the bradycardia and is effective in minimizing tachyarrhythmic episodes. Specifically, prevention of atrial bradycardia could decrease dispersion of repolarization and prevent the emergence of reentrant arrhythmias. This fact might be one of the reasons that in patients with sinus node dysfunction, atrial or dual-chamber pacing is associated with a lower incidence of chronic atrial fibrillation than is ventricular pacing.[15-17]

2. Moderately high rate suppression to prevent emergence of tachycardia. There is generally a relation between heart rate and ventricular premature beats or ventricular tachycardia. In many patients, a "window" of optimal antiarrhythmic rates can be determined.[18] Short-term pacing at rates slightly higher than the spontaneous rhythm (overdrive suppression) can suppress arrhythmias, probably by reducing the number of premature beats that cause tachycardia.[19] Analysis of spontaneous episodes of ventricular tachycardia or fibrillation shows that they are frequently preceded by a long RR cycle.[20] Therefore, it should be possible to prevent the arrhythmia by simple VVI pacing that avoids long RR cycles. Although the concept of preventing ventricular arrhythmias by overdrive pacing is attractive, it has narrow clinical applications. Ventricular pacing acts only on some of the determinants of these arrhythmias and generally, it does not prevent all the episodes. The relatively high rates (over 80 beats per minute) frequently

needed are not well tolerated in the long-term. Furthermore, ventricular pacing loses efficacy over time in many patients who respond to it acutely. Therefore, chronic pacing alone is rarely able to prevent clinical ventricular arrhythmias, and it is not recommended unless there is clear clinical evidence that it is effective over a long period.[21]

3. Dual-chamber pacing to inhibit reentry. Programmed extrastimuli in response to spontaneous atrial extrasystoles may prevent the establishment of AV nodal reentrant tachycardia.[22-27] In this technique, a ventricular stimulus is delivered immediately after a spontaneous atrial depolarization, avoiding activation of the ventricle through the slow pathway. Because the technique entails premature ventricular pacing in response to a premature atrial depolarization, it is called "preexcitation pacing."

4. Subthreshold stimulation. Subthreshold stimulation consists of the introduction of a train of subthreshold (not capable of producing a propagated ventricular response) conditioning stimuli, beginning at about half of the ventricular effective refractory period.[28,29] Limited studies in humans suggest that properly timed and located subthreshold stimuli, by altering local tissue refractoriness near the tachycardia focus, may prevent or terminate supraventricular or ventricular tachycardias.[30-31]

Clinical Applications

In some patients, tachyarrhythmias can be controlled pharmacologically or eliminated by catheter or surgical ablative procedures but bradycardia is a side effect. In those patients, conventional pacemakers, either single- or dual-chamber, are conveniently used to restore an appropriate rate.

A spectrum of tachyarrhythmias has been recognized in patients with chronic bradycardia. Because many of these arrhythmias seem to require a substrate of bradycardia, they have been termed bradycardia- or pause-dependent. In many instances, they can be prevented by cardiac pacing. The potential prevention of atrial tachyarrhythmias by atrial or dual-chamber pacing (mediated partly by the avoidance of atrial bradycardia) in patients with the sick sinus syndrome has already been mentioned. Patients with congenital heart disease and bradycardia-mediated supraventricular and ventricular arrhythmias seem to especially benefit from chronic pacing in the AAI or DDD modes.[32]

Paroxysmal atrial flutter and fibrillation of vagal origin are rare forms of atrial arrhythmia.[33,34] Episodes are variable in frequency and duration; frequently occur at rest, during sleeping or postprandially; last from minutes to several hours; and often end in the morning. Progressive sinus bradycardia and atrial bigeminy or trigeminy precede the attacks. Permanent atrial pacing at rates of 80 to 90 beats per minute prevents attacks in patients with drug-resistant or markedly symptomatic episodes of vagal atrial arrhythmias.[33,34]

The efficacy of transitory cardiac pacing in preventing episodes of torsades de pointes in the acquired (or pause-dependent) forms of the long-QTU syndrome is well known.[35] In the congenital forms of the syndrome, ventricular arrhythmias are often precipitated by sudden and intense sympathetic stimulation. These adrenergic-dependent arrhythmias are also facilitated by pauses, suggesting that both factors are operative.[36] Furthermore, a relatively high incidence of sinus node dysfunction and AV block seems to be present in children with congenital long-QT syndrome.[37,38,39] It is thus not surprising that permanent pacing has been reported as an effective treatment in combination with left cervical sympathectomy, beta blockers, or both.[40-42] Selection of pacing rates (ranging from 70 to 90 beats per minute) was guided by the magnitude of QT shortening after full beta blockade. Although the number of patients thus treated and reported to date is small, the results are so encouraging that permanent cardiac pacing should probably be considered in the treatment of all patients with congenital QTU syndrome and severe arrhythmias.

PACING FOR HEMODYNAMIC OR TACHYCARDIA RATE CONTROL

Temporary pacing has been used in patients with incessant tachycardias that are poorly tolerated and that recur immediately after cardioversion. To facilitate the control of the ventricular response, induction and maintenance of atrial fibrillation by rapid atrial pacing has been occasionally used in patients with atrial tachycardia or atrial flutter.[43,44] Widespread availability, however, of ablation techniques for the AV junction has almost completely eliminated the need for that approach.

The use of the AVT pacing mode to produce a perfectly timed atrial contraction during ventricular tachycardia is reported to transiently improve the hemodynamic status, but the long-term applicability of this technique seems to be minimal.[45,46]

PACING TO TERMINATE TACHYCARDIAS

Although it is clinically more desirable to prevent tachycardias, most research has been performed in the field of tachycardia termination by pacing. The following discus-sion is focused mainly on ventricular tachycardia but many of the mechanisms and concepts also apply to reentrant supraventricular arrhythmias such as AV reentry, AV nodal reentry, and atrial flutter.

Either reentry or triggered automaticity can be responsible for tachycardias that are reliably initiated or terminated by pacing techniques.[47] There is a substantial body of basic and clinical information suggesting that most clinically occurring recurrent tachyarrhythmias at both the supraventricular and ventricular level are of reentrant origin.[48] Reentry in the ventricular muscle, with or without contribution from specialized tissue, constitutes the most common mechanism of ventricular tachycardia, particularly in patients with coronary artery disease.[49,50] Reentry differs from automaticity in that a new wave of depolarization does not arise de novo but is initiated by propagation from an area excited by the previous wave of depolarization. It can only occur when an excitable tissue is activated late and is able to excite areas that were previously activated and have already recovered excitability.[47]

El-Sherif and coworkers propose the figure-eight as a representative model of reentry for ventricular tachycardia in the human ventricle.[51] This reentrant circuit has two circulating wavefronts around arcs of functional conduction block that coalesce into a slow common reentrant wavefront (Fig. 38-1). Four components can be discerned in the circuit:

1. An area of slow conduction, which may or may not have an excitable point of entry and one or more exit points and is protected laterally by anatomic or functional boundaries

2. Areas of orthodromic activation

3. The excitable gap (the time between the recovery of excitability and the arrival of the next impulse)—the width of which depends on the duration of the refractory period within the circuit, the length of the circuit, and the conduction velocity of the circulating impulse

4. A connection between the reentrant circuit and the rest of the ventricle

The whole reentrant circuit and the exit point have a dynamic behavior, with marked heterogeneity in conduction velocity and refractory periods. They are also strongly influenced by changes in the autonomic tone.[52] In the presence of an excitable gap, a correctly timed impulse from outside the circuit is theoretically able to invade and create bidirectional block in the circuit, thereby terminating the arrhythmia.

A single paced impulse will be able to enter a reentrant circuit only if the cycle length of the tachycardia is longer than the refractory period at the stimulation site plus the conduction time from the stimulation site to the site of origin of the tachycardia.[53,54,60,61] Subsequent paced beats are able to enter the tachycardia circuit only if

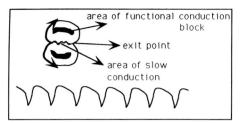
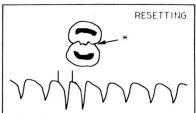
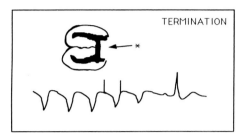
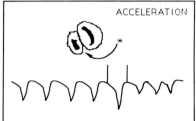

Figure 38-1. Diagram of a reentrant circuit and its different responses to programmed stimulation. (**A**) Figure-eight, with two circulating waveforms around areas of functional block coalescing into a slow conduction area. (**B**) The resetting phenomenon. The second stimuli collides with the area of slow conduction but penetrates the other part of the circuit, advancing it in time or "resetting" the tachycardia. (**C**) Tachycardia termination with two paced beats. The second stimuli enlarges the area of functional block, slicing the reentrant circuit. (**D**) Tachycardia acceleration. The second stimulus changes the circuit morphology, decreasing the revolution time with subsequent acceleration. The different morphology of the ventricular tachycardia is due to the different exit point of the impulse from the circuit. (Modified with permission from El-Sherif N: Mechanisms of resetting, entrainment, acceleration, or termination of reentrant ventricular tachycardia by programmed electrical stimulation. In: Breithardt G, Borggrefe M, Zipes DP, eds. Nonpharmacological therapy of tachyarrhythmias. Mt. Kisco, NY: Futura Publishing, 1987:341)

the tachycardia cycle length is longer than the sum of the refractory period of the preceding paced beat and the conduction time from the stimulation site to the tachycardia circuit. The introduction of multiple extrastimuli decreases the refractory periods of the surrounding myocardium (peeling back of refractoriness), allowing the impulse to reach the reentrant circuit at the appropriate time.

Fewer extrastimuli are needed, however, when the stimulation is applied to the normal zone close to the proximal side of the slow zone than to the distal side of the figure-eight model.[49–51]

From the above discussion, it can be inferred that cycle length of stimulation, number of stimuli, and site of stimulation are the three main factors that determine whether the delivered stimuli during antitachycardia pacing could reach the reentrant circuit in time to produce conduction block and therefore terminate the tachycardia.[49–51,53,54]

Numerous studies also emphasize the role of tachycardia cycle length in determining successful termination.[49–51,53,55] When the tachycardia cycle length is longer than 350 milliseconds (170 beats/minute), 60% to 80% of the episodes might be terminated successfully by using two stimuli or burst pacing, whereas only 20% to 40% of ventricular tachycardia episodes with rates equal to or shorter than 300 milliseconds (200 beats/minute) can be terminated in that manner. Antiarrhythmic therapy sometimes improves the chances of successful termination by decreasing the ventricular tachycardia rate.[55]

Possible explanations for the failure to terminate a reentrant arrhythmia by pacing include entrance block (delivered impulses are unable to enter a protected reentrant circuit) and tachycardia termination with reinitiation by subsequent extrastimuli.

Resetting and Entrainment

If an impulse is delivered at a relatively long coupling interval, it may enter the excitable gap, collide with the previous wavefront in the retrograde direction, and depolarize the circuit in the anterograde direction. In this way, the tachycardia is not terminated but its cycle length is advanced (see Fig. 38-1). This phenomenon is called "resetting." Most tachycardia terminated by pacing are usually reset at coupling intervals or paced intervals longer than those resulting in tachycardia termination.[56–58] Therefore, coupling intervals that reset the tachycardia suggest that shorter intervals may terminate it.

"Transient entrainment" is an electrophysiologic phenomenon that can usually be observed when pacing slightly above the tachycardia rate for longer periods (more than 15 beats).[59] Basically, entrainment can be defined as continuous resetting of the tachycardia by pacing.[60-63] Four criteria have been proposed to demonstrate transient entrainment. Demonstration of transient entrainment is generally regarded as a specific marker for reentrant arrhythmias with an excitable gap.[64-66]

Acceleration

Tachycardia acceleration or precipitation of ventricular fibrillation is a major limiting factor for ventricular antitachycardia pacing. It is reported to occur during 30% to 50% of attempts.[50, 53, 55, 67, 68] The efficacy and safety of antitachycardia pacing techniques are inversely related (Figs. 38-2 and 38-3). A higher incidence of tachycardia termination can be achieved with more aggressive protocols (more extrastimuli, shorter coupling intervals) but often only at the price of an unacceptable incidence of acceleration.

Several mechanisms may be responsible for acceleration of ventricular tachycardia. El-Sherif and associates report that tachycardia acceleration by overdrive stimulation is the result of the interruption of the original reentrant circuit by the first or first few stimulated beats.[51] The subsequent stimulated beats create a different circuit with a shorter revolution time. Degeneration into ventricular fibrillation can result from the fracturation of a regular figure-eight reentrant pattern into multiple asynchronous wavefronts.

Brugada and colleagues suggest that acceleration may also be the consequence of the induction of two waves circulating simultaneously in the same direction and using the same circuit.[69, 70]

TACHYCARDIA TERMINATION TECHNIQUES

Attempts to increase efficacy and decrease the dangers of termination techniques have spawned a long list of stimulation patterns.[71, 72] Unfortunately, there is no complete agreement on nomenclature. Different manufacturers often use different names for similar techniques available in their devices.[73, 74]

Termination techniques can be broadly classified into single- and multiple-capture techniques.

Single-capture techniques are only effective in relatively slow tachycardias. At rates above 160 beats per minute, the success rate is low unless the stimulus is delivered close to the reentrant circuit. Single-capture can be easily achieved by underdrive competitive pacing at a rate slower than that of the tachycardia. A pacemaker can be activated to deliver asynchronous pacing manually (by placing a magnet over the unit) or automatically (dual-demand or upside-down units).

Multiple-capture techniques require pacing at rates above the tachycardia. This is generally named overdrive pacing. If no more than three or four stimuli are used, it is known as programmed stimulation. Burst pacing is reserved for protocols using more than three or four stimuli.

The coupling interval of the first stimulus in a sequence can be fixed (programmed in milliseconds) or it can be programmed to occur at some fraction of the tachycardia cycle length (adaptive or orthoarrhythmic pacing, generally used at 65% to 85% of the tachycardia cycle length).

Coupling intervals within a burst may be constant or variable. Autodecremental pacing (all the coupling intervals within a sequence progressively decreasing by a fixed amount) is a feature in many ATPMs.[75] The problem of termination and reinitiation seems to be lessened with autodecremental bursts. More complex sequences (changing ramps, burst plus programmed stimulation) are also described.

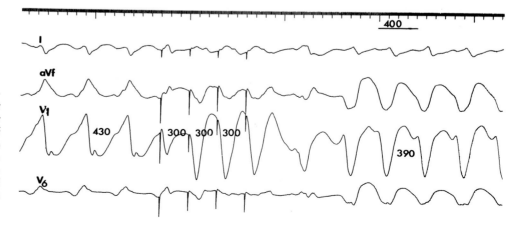

Figure 38-2. Tachycardia acceleration by burst pacing. A right bundle–right axis ventricular tachycardia with a cycle length of 430 milliseconds is accelerated to a different and faster (40 milliseconds shorter) ventricular tachycardia, with a burst sequence of four beats at 300 milliseconds each.

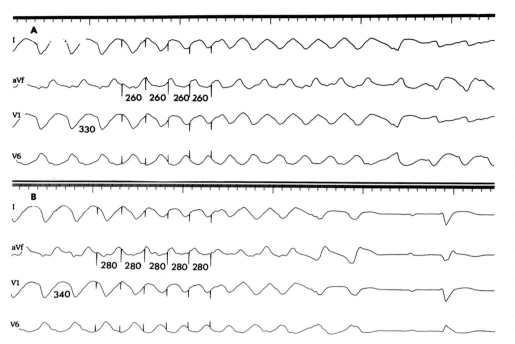

Figure 38-3. Acceleration and termination of ventricular tachycardia with burst pacing. (**A**) After five stimuli, the ventricular tachycardia is accelerated to a different ventricular tachycardia (cycle length, 280 milliseconds) and afterward slows down to the same interval as the previous arrhythmia but with other morphology. (**B**) The same tachycardia is successfully terminated with a burst-pacing sequence of five stimuli at 280 milliseconds. The tachycardia is transiently accelerated (as in *A*) for four beats before termination occurs.

Generally, ATPMs are programmed to recycle their sequences if they fail in their first attempt to terminate a tachycardia (Fig. 38-4). The total number of allowed attempts is dictated by the hemodynamic tolerance during tachycardia. Subsequent sequences may be similar to the first or more commonly, programmed to scan over a range of cycle lengths. Scanning is generally programmed to shorter cycle lengths but other algorithms (centrifugal scanning, self-searching scanning) can also be used with some devices.[76,77] Risk of acceleration is the shortcoming of scanning algorithms; a minimum pacing interval should also be programmed to avoid pacing at short cycle lengths and in this way diminish the risks of tachycardia acceleration.

The universal antitachycardia pacing mode described by den Dulk and colleagues is an example of an adaptive scanning algorithm, consisting of a stepwise decrease in the cycle length of stimulation combined with a stepwise increase of the number of paced beats in each attempt (Fig. 38-5).[78] Some devices allow two or more modalities of treatment. The secondary modalities are delivered after the primary has failed and are generally more aggressive. They can safely be used in the ventricle when there is backup defibrillation capability.

Figure 38-6 illustrates a practical approach to the selection of an antitachycardia pacing algorithm. It may need to be adapted to the specific characteristics of each pacing device.

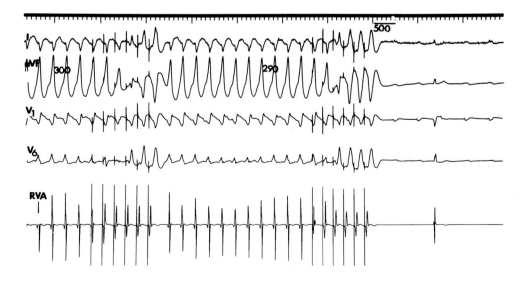

Figure 38-4. Scanning-burst pacing. Two sequences of burst pacing are shown. The first starts at 85% of the tachycardia cycle length (260 milliseconds) but does not terminate it. In the next sequence, the coupling intervals have a 10-millisecond decrement, enabling termination of the arrhythmia. *RVA,* right ventricular apex.

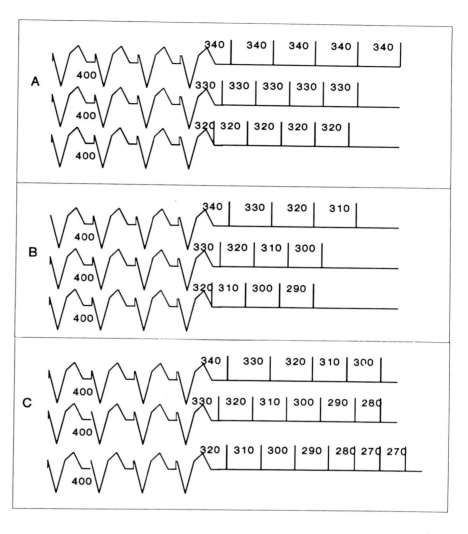

Figure 38-5. Three different termination algorithms, in which the paced interval is decreased by 10 milliseconds in subsequent attempts. The diagram represents a ventricular tachycardia with a cycle length of 400 milliseconds. (**A**) Burst pacing, with three attempts. Five stimuli are delivered at 85% of the tachycardia cycle length; the following attempts have shorter coupling intervals, which stay equal within each sequence. (**B**) Autodecremental pacing, with three attempts. In the first, the first coupling interval is delivered at 85% of the tachycardia cycle length; subsequent intervals are decremented by 10 milliseconds. In the following sequences, the first coupling interval is 10 milliseconds shorter than in the first sequence. (**C**) Autodecremental pacing, with a stepwise increase in the number of paced beats. The stimuli are decremented until a minimum interval is reached—in this example, 270 milliseconds.

Tachycardia Recognition

Effective tachyarrhythmia termination is only one aspect of correct functioning of antitachycardia devices. The importance of reliable tachycardia recognition capabilities in an ATPM is obvious. The ideal tachycardia recognition system should be reliable, technically simple, fast, sensitive (capable of detecting all episodes of the target arrhythmia), and specific (capable of discriminating between the target arrhythmia and other arrhythmias such as sinus tachycardia or atrial fibrillation). Although numerous tachycardia recognition techniques have been proposed, none has achieved all those goals.[79,80]

The first ATPMs were not automatic but manually activated.[81,82] This technique is useful only if the patient can recognize the tachycardia and remains hemodynamically stable during its course. This allowed him or her the use of an external triggering device at home or, if the possibility of arrhythmia acceleration existed, in the presence of a physician at the emergency room.[92] It is evident that the clinical feasibility of this approach is restricted to patients with infrequent and relatively benign arrhythmic episodes. Therefore, it has been almost completely abandoned.

Automatic tachycardia recognition systems can be classified as those that use either electric or hemodynamic criteria (Table 38-1.) Measurement of heart rate is the simplest automatic method of tachycardia recognition. As long as the sensing system accurately detects cardiac depolarization, a 100% sensitivity for tachycardias above the programmed rate cutoff can be achieved. Optimal sensing is crucial to the correct functioning of these algorithms. Some devices have mechanisms of automatic gain control to ensure continuous sensing when the intracardiac signal decreases in amplitude (e.g., ventricular fibrillation). It should be noted that rate criteria can sometimes be satisfied by myopotentials, oversensing of pacemaker spikes, T or P waves, or electromagnetic interference, with subsequent device intervention. The major drawback of rate-only detection is its poor specificity. As a result of rate

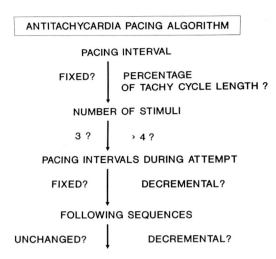

Figure 38-6. Practical approach to antitachycardia pacing algorithms.

overlap, atrial fibrillation or sinus tachycardia often cannot be differentiated from the target arrhythmia. Furthermore, rate-only devices fail to detect tachycardias below the rate cutoff (Fig. 38-7).

Rate stability and sudden onset are additional rate-related criteria that can be used to improve appropriate recognition of pathologic tachycardias. Rate stability is especially useful to differentiate atrial fibrillation from target arrhythmias. Only successive cycle lengths that fulfill the programmed interval stability criterion are counted as tachycardias. Stability parameters must be cho-

TABLE 38-1. Tachycardia Recognition Criteria

Electric	Hemodynamic
High-rate criteria	Mean right atrial pressure
Rate-related criteria	Right ventricular impedance
Rate stability	Right ventricular systolic
Sudden onset	pressure
Electrogram Characteristics	
Template matching	Right ventricular systolic pulse
Fourier analysis	pressure
Gradient pattern detection	Intraventricular Doppler
Intrinsic deflection time	ultrasound
Area under the electrogram	Pressure-volume loops
Magnitude-square	Stroke volume
coherence	Oxygen saturation
Analysis of Activation	
Sequence	
Av sequence	
Multiple activation	
sequence	
Effect of atrial stimuli	

AV, atrioventricular.

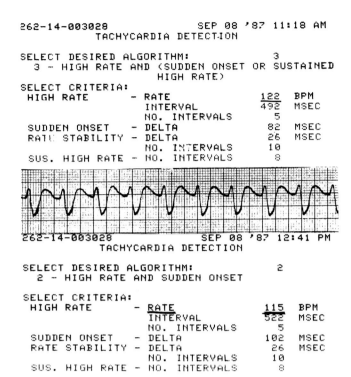

Figure 38-7. Detection problems with "slow" tachycardias. A patient with an antitachycardia pacemaker (ATPM) and an implantable cardioverter-defibrillator presented after 2 hours of rapid heart beats. Electrocardiogram showed sustained ventricular tachycardia at 118 beats per minute (bpm; below the programmed detection rate of 122 bpm). Detection rate was reprogrammed to 115 bpm. The ATPM immediately recognized and terminated the tachycardia (not shown). Antiarrhythmic drugs given to suppress frequent tachycardia episodes often slow them. Device functioning should be retested when changing antiarrhythmic drug regimen.

sen carefully because even sustained ventricular tachycardia may show some variability in RR intervals.

The rapid onset criterion is aimed to detect and reject sinus tachycardia. Rapid onset is typically associated with pathologic tachycardias, whereas sinus tachycardia is characterized by gradual acceleration (Fig. 38-8). This algorithm only detects tachycardia if the initial interval is shorter than a programmed percentage of the average of the previous intervals. Although useful, the algorithm is not completely specific. In some patients, there is overlap between the sudden onset of sinus and pathologic tachycardias.[83] Furthermore, atrial fibrillation has usually a sudden onset.

A variety of techniques rely on the analysis of electrogram characteristics as a way to differentiate between morphologically abnormal and normal rhythms.[84,85] Although they are generally effective in discriminating narrow supraventricular rhythms from ventricular tachycardia, they fail to recognize supraventricular arrhythmias with aberrancy. Furthermore, some of these techniques

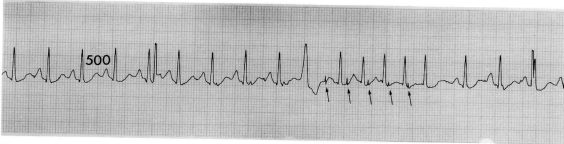

Figure 38-8. Limitations of current detection algorithms. Antitachycardia pacing is delivered in the atria during an exercise stress test in a patient having an Intertach for supraventricular tachycardia. Although the sudden onset criterion was programmed "on," it was overridden by the sustained high-rate criterion. Beta-blocking agents are frequently necessary to blunt sinus rates when there is overlap between sinus and tachycardia rates.

have considerable requirements of computation time and memory and are thus unsuitable for implementation in implantable devices. Probability density function is the only one of these techniques that is clinically available as a programmable option in AICD Ventak devices (CPI Inc., St. Paul, MN). The percentage of time that the electrogram recorded from the defibrillating electrodes spends away from baseline is analyzed and compared in normal and abnormal rhythms. During wide complex tachycardias (particularly ventricular fibrillation), the time that the electrogram spends at baseline is markedly decreased. This technique seems to be more accurate for ventricular fibrillation than for ventricular tachycardia. In one study, probability density function was found useful in patients without bundle branch block and with small QRS signals.[86] Template matching, Fourier analysis, gradient pattern detection, intrinsic deflection timing, magnitude-square coherence, and measurement of the area under the electrogram curve are techniques that basically consist of real-time digitizing, processing, and comparison of the signal with a "normal" reference beat.[84,85] Clinical experience with all of them is preliminary.

Analysis of activation sequences through the use of multiple electrodes could differentiate between sinus and ectopic beats.[87] Analysis of the AV sequence consists of the determination of the synchrony and timing of activation between the upper and lower chambers of the heart. The major problem with this approach is the differentiation between SVT and ventricular tachycardia with 1:1 retrograde conduction. Multiple activation sequence analysis, a further development of the approach in which multiple electrodes are placed in the ventricles and atrium, seems to detect differences in activation timing during sinus tachycardia, SVT, and VT. The potential problems of employing three or more permanent electrodes in the heart have not yet been investigated.

Hemodynamic sensors, which detect changes in physiologic parameters and theoretically determine the hemodynamic significance of a tachycardia, are under active investigation.[89] Examples are shown in Table 38-1. The major limitations of these approaches are the complexity and the uncertain long-term stability of the implanted sensors.

The determination of changes in right ventricular volume by measuring the electric impedance in the cavity is useful in differentiating hemodynamically stable from unstable arrhythmias.[89] Pressure changes in the cardiovascular system have also been studied as potential markers of the hemodynamic significance of tachyarrhythmias. Mean right atrial pressure, mean right ventricular systolic pressure, right ventricular pulse pressure, and mean arterial pressure are significantly different during ventricular tachycardia or ventricular fibrillation and 30 seconds after termination when compared with baseline.[90,01] In addition, mean atrial pressure significantly increases during rapid ventricular pacing when compared with baseline or rapid atrial pacing.[92] Analysis of pressure–volume loops are also described as being a useful technique in distinguishing stable monomorphic ventricular tachycardia from sustained SVT and atrial fibrillation.[93] Continuous assessment of cardiac output by intracavitary-echo Doppler ultrasound is also proposed as an approach to the hemodynamic recognition of significant tachycardias.[94]

It is likely that one or more of these hemodynamic sensors will soon be available in antitachycardia devices. Algorithms using a combination of hemodynamic and electric data will certainly be optimal for accurate detection and cataloging of a variety of tachyarrhythmias.

Clinical Experience With Antitachycardia Pacing

A variety of ATPMs are available, either commercially or under clinical investigation trials. Characteristics of some of those devices are depicted in Table 38-2.

TABLE 38-2. Antitachycardia Pacemakers Referenced in Recent Literature

Model (mfr)	Backup	Detection	Therapy	Telemetry	NIPS
Symbios 7008 (Medtronic)	DDD-M DVI-M VVI-M	Rate	VOO dual-demand DOO dual demand Atrial burst	Programmed settings Tachy event (1) Marker channel Intracardiac ECG	No
Orthocor II 284 (Cordis)	SSI-M SST-M	Rate	PES, burst Fixed, scan memory	Programmed settings Tachy log Short & long term	Yes
Intertach II 262-18 (Intermedics)	SSI-M SST-M OSO-M OSO-T	Rate Rate increase Rate stability Sustained high rate	PES, burst Fixed, scan Adaptive Autodecremental Memory	Measured values Programmed settings System efficacy Diagnostic data Intracardiac electrocardiogram	Yes
Tachylog II P-56 (Siemens-Pacesetter)	SSI-M	Rate Rate increase	PES, burst Fixed, self-search Memory	Programmed settings Tachy log System efficacy Holter function	Yes

mfr: manufacturer; PES: programmed extraestimuli.

Chronic Antitachycardia Pacing for Supraventricular Tachycardia

Patients with AV nodal reentry (Fig. 38-9) and AV reentry tachycardia are excellent candidates theoretically for chronic antitachycardia pacing. Selected patients with atrial flutter and intraatrial reentrant tachycardia (Fig. 38-10) can also be effectively treated by this therapeutic approach. Only patients with WPW and rapidly conducting accessory pathways should be excluded from consideration. In these cases, the accidental induction of atrial fibrillation during pacing attempts at SVT conversion may have catastrophic consequences.[95] In all other circumstances, the potential of harm is low, and clinical benefits are likely. Despite this and despite several ATPMs being approved for general use in SVT, few patients are receiving them; this number is not expected to grow substantially. Antitachycardia pacing for SVTs remains a tertiary therapy. This is not only a consequence of its intrinsic limitations but also of the attractiveness of other therapeutic modalities. Curative approaches such as surgical or catheter ablation of accessory pathways and modification of the AV node in patients with AV nodal reentry are preferred in many situations.[96,97,98] Even catheter ablation of the AV junction, with permanent implantation of an antibradycardia pacemaker, may be a valid option in patients with recalcitrant SVT.[99] Antitachycardia pacemakers are reserved for patients refractory or intolerant to drugs and

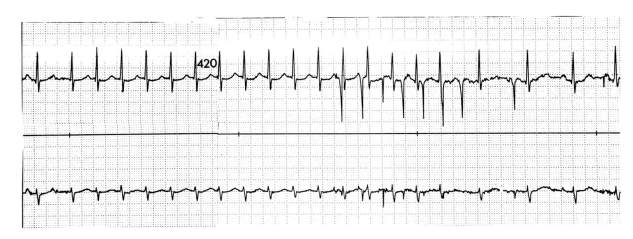

Figure 38-9. Holter-monitor recording showing termination of atrioventricular nodal reentry tachycardia by a burst of antitachycardia pacing.

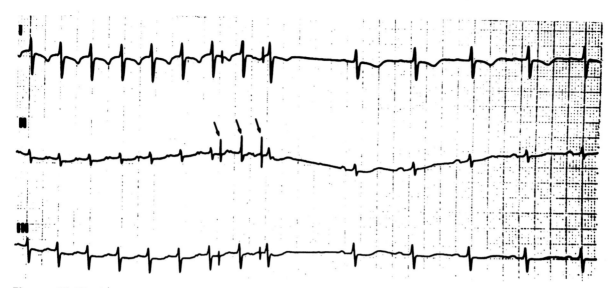

Figure 38-10. Termination of an intraatrial reentrant tachycardia by three atrial extrastimuli.

those who are not candidates for or refuse the above-mentioned ablative procedures.

Careful investigation of the properties of the clinical tachyarrhythmia and of its response to programmed stimulation is mandatory before considering chronic pacing as therapy for patients with SVT. In a study in the electrophysiologic laboratory (comprising 453 attempts to terminate SVTs in 111 patients), atrial fibrillation or atrial flutter was initiated in 9% of attempts, and it was more frequent with atrial (12%) than with ventricular (2%) pacing. It is noteworthy that in six patients, tachycardias could only be terminated by inducing another arrhythmia.[100]

Antitachycardia pacing from the right ventricle may be the only effective modality in some patients with tachycardias related to accessory pathways; it is also useful in patients in whom pacing in the atrium frequently induces atrial fibrillation. Nevertheless, it should be used with caution. In an early report, two patients with WPW and an ATPM in the right ventricle died suddenly.[101] If chronic antitachycardia pacing from the right ventricle is elected in patients with SVT, the programmed stimulation protocol (which should not be aggressive) must be extensively tested to ensure that it does not induce ventricular arrhythmias. It should be noted that patients with ischemic heart disease are less-than-ideal candidates for this approach.

There is no agreement on the number of test trials necessary before implant of a permanent ATPM for SVT. Supraventricular tachycardias are sensitive to changes in autonomic tone and antiarrhythmic-drug plasma levels. The tachycardia cycle length is significantly shorter in the upright than in the supine position, and it may further accelerate during exertion. As the overall tachycardia cycle length shortens, the window for tachycardia termination

also shortens.[102, 103] Ideally, testing should be done under all these physiologic circumstances. Early protocols aimed for at least 100 successful trials but this type of testing might be tedious and time-consuming.

Adaptive pacing modes save time during testing and tailoring of the pacing protocol because they can generally terminate tachycardias, irrespective of rate or body position. Den Dulk and coworkers point out also the advantages of adaptive protocols in patients with more than one tachycardia circuit (e.g., those with junctional reciprocating tachycardia and atrial flutter).[104] When correctly programmed, adaptive protocols easily cope with additional reentrant tachycardias. This makes ATPMs an attractive alternative for patients with multiple tachycardias.

Follow-up of patients with ATPMs for supraventricular arrhythmias has been thoroughly described by Griffin.[105] Only guidelines are provided here. Such care is most easily delivered in a setting in which facilities and personnel are focused on this problem. Evaluation encounters take longer than those for patients with antibradycardia pacemakers. Careful interrogation of the device is vital to assess appropriate function of the system or detect device failures. Determination of sensing and pacing thresholds during sinus rhythm and during tachycardia is also essential (Fig. 38-11). Finally, some episodes of SVT should be induced (through asynchronous pacing or the noninvasive programmed stimulation capabilities of newer devices) and the programmed settings observed for their ability to terminate the tachycardia efficiently. Adjustments should be made until the device is able to terminate induced episodes consistently with one or two bursts of pacing.

Complete withdrawal of antiarrhythmic drugs is a

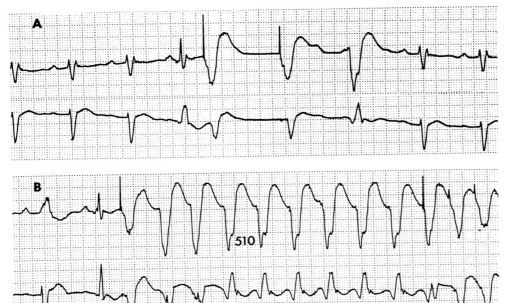

Figure 38-11. (**A**) Perils of undersensing with antitachycardia pacemakers (ATPMs). In a patient with an ATPM for ventricular tachycardia, there was consistent undersensing of ventricular premature complexes, with subsequent antibradycardia pacing at the programmed rate of 50. (**B**) The first delivered stimulus induces ventricular tachycardia, which the ATPM tries to convert (end of the strip). To avoid these events, the antibradycardia function should be cancelled (OVO or OAO modes) when possible.

desirable but not always attainable goal in patients with ATPMs for SVT. About 50% require antiarrhythmic drugs to reduce the incidence of episodes, slow the rate of tachycardias (to facilitate termination or improve hemodynamic tolerance), prevent the induction of atrial fibrillation during atrial pacing, or treat concomitant arrhythmias. In carefully selected patients, the quality of their life significantly improves with ATPMs. Previously prolonged episodes of SVT are rapidly terminated in an almost imperceptible way, and the patient is spared frequent hospital admissions.

Table 38-3 summarizes the published experience with ATPMs in SVT. Only those reporting more than five patients and providing reasonably complete information on follow-up are included in the analysis.[81,82,104–118] The distinction between "excellent" and "good" results is sometimes subjective. Generally, results are only fair in the long-term. In one study, efficacy dropped from 93% at 1-year follow-up to 68% at 8-year follow-up.[111] Development of chronic atrial fibrillation or precipitation of atrial fibrillation during attempts at tachycardia termination was the main complication. Reports dealing with latest models (Intertach II, Tachylog II) are encouraging. Whether the improved versatility of these models can overcome the long-term limitations of their predecessors is yet to be proved.

It remains to be seen whether catheter ablation techniques are truly successful for long-term management of atrial flutter and atrial fibrillation. It appears that paroxysmal supraventricular tachycardia (PSVT) due to atrioventricular nodal reentrant tachycardia (AVNRT), atrioventricular reentrant tachycardia, and probably focal atrial tachycardia are best managed by catheter ablation.

Chronic Antitachycardia Pacing for Ventricular Tachycardia

Beginning in the 1970s, a few patients received implantable ATPMs for the treatment of ventricular tachycardia. The early literature on the use of ATPMs for ventricular tachycardia has been thoroughly reviewed by Fisher and associates.[119] The reports, although generally promising, frequently failed to meet high standards of scientific validity.[120] Specifically, objectification of long-term patient outcome and of the number of patients who might benefit from each device or technique were often lacking. From that early experience, it can be concluded that although ventricular tachycardia can often be successfully terminated on a chronic basis, its occasional, sporadic, and unpredictable instance of acceleration or degeneration into ventricular fibrillation represents an insurmountable drawback of antitachycardia pacing for ventricular tachycardia (no fail-safe back-up). Consequently, ATPMs never achieved widespread acceptance as the sole treatment of ventricular tachycardia.

The wide clinical availability of implantable defibrillators renewed interest in pacing for ventricular tachycardia. A consensus was reached that "because pacing for ven-

TABLE 38-3. Implantable Pacemakers to Terminate Supraventricular Tachycardia

Study	Patients (n)	Model	Antiarrhythmic Drugs (%)	Follow-Up (mos)	Results Excellent	Results Good	Results Poor
Kahn, et al*[81]	12	Medtronic 5998 RF	67	15–36	10	—	—
Waxman, et al[82]	9	Medtronic 5998 RF	67	12–72	9	0	0
Spurrel, et al[106]	21	PASAR 4151 PASAR 4171	38	2–40	16	—	—
Sowton[107]	16	Tachylog	20	12 5–19	14	0	2
Griffin, et al*[108]	91	Cybertach-60	—	>21	69	—	—
Bertholet, et al[109]	13	PASAR 4151 Medtronic 5000	39	21 5–30	7	3	3
Peters, et al[110]	10	Medtronic 5998 RF	40	24–60	6	1	3
Fisher, et al[111]	16	Miscellaneous	100	6–177	12	4	0
Moller, et al[112]	13	PASAR 4171	61	16 4–53	8	4	1
Schnittger, et al[113]	11	Cybertach-60	36	84 64–108	4	2	5
Kappenberg, et al*[114]	63	Tachylog	49	30 2–100	47	12	4
Occheta, et al[115]	7	Orthocor II	71	20 2–30	7	0	0
Den Dulk, et al[104]	38	Miscellaneous	42	38	32	8	0
McComb, et al[116]	22	Intertach 262-12; 262-16	23	15 1–37	16	6	0
Sulke, et al[117]	10	Tachylog II	10	>12	9	1	0
Fromer, et al[118]	14	Intertach 262-12	29	31 6–49	8	4	2

*Multicenter trial.

tricular tachycardia may accelerate the tachycardia or produce ventricular flutter or ventricular fibrillation and because the primary arrhythmia may be a rapid ventricular tachycardia that cannot be terminated by pacing, or may be ventricular flutter or fibrillation, devices must be able to both convert and defibrillate."[121]

Beginning in 1986, investigators worldwide reported on the combined use of separate ATPMs and ICDs in patients with ventricular tachycardia.[122–123] At the same time, several manufacturers began the development and testing of devices capable of providing antitachycardia pacing and cardioverter-defibrillator modalities in a tiered or hierarchical algorithm. The availability of antitachycardia pacing with backup defibrillation has widened the applicability of chronic device therapy to subsets of patients who are not suitable candidates for earlier-generation ICDs. In patients with relatively slow well-tolerated (but nevertheless symptomatic) ventricular tachycardia, conventional ICD therapy exposes them to painful discharges. In patients with frequent tachycardia episodes despite drug therapy, conventional ICD therapy was un-

comfortable and had the likelihood of early battery depletion (Fig. 38-12). Patients with both slow well-tolerated tachycardias and occasional episodes of rapid tachycardia or fibrillation were only partially addressed with earlier ICDs. These limitations have been largely overcome by the low energy requirements and essentially imperceptible characteristics of antitachycardia pacing, with the fail-safe backup of defibrillation. A desirable goal of device therapy is the complete prevention of arrhythmic sudden death, with a minimum of high-energy defibrillation shocks and no or low-dose antiarrhythmic drug therapy.[126]

Lessons From Combined Use of Separate Antitachycardia Pacemakers and Implantable Cardioverter-Defibrillators

Insights gained from reports of combining separate ATPMs and ICDs apply to those patients with hemodynamic need for a dual-chamber bradycardia pacemaker; these same

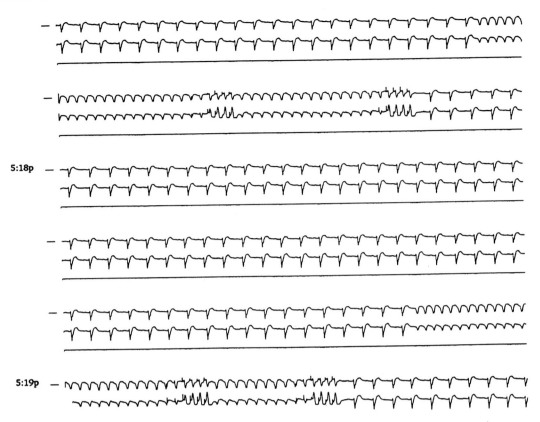

Figure 38-12. Frequent episodes of ventricular tachycardia adequately terminated by a tiered-therapy device. During a 2-minute period, two episodes of ventricular tachycardia are terminated by the scanning algorithm (both in the second attempt). The patient remained completely asymptomatic.

lessons are likely to be applicable to the atrial ICDs of the future.

The combined use of an independent ATPM and an ICD is cumbersome. The primary design of each device fails to consider that of the other, so that the potential for deleterious device-to-device interactions is always present. Many of these interactions may also occur when ICDs are used in combination with standard antibradycardia pacemakers (Fig. 38-).[127–130] Concomitant use of antiarrhythmic drugs may be a further source of interactions. Specifically, ICD discharges can adversely affect telemetry function and pacemaker capture and sensing thresholds. At the same time, pacing may seriously impair normal ICD function. If ventricular fibrillation is not sensed by the ATPM and antibradycardia pacing is consequently initiated, the arrhythmia may be not recognized as a result of "oversensing" of pacemaker stimuli as being QRS complexes by the ICD (Fig. 38-13). Double-counting (spike plus complex) may result in false-positive shocks (Fig. 38-14). Furthermore, antitachycardia pacing, alone or combined with the underlying rhythm, can trigger ICD

discharges. Finally, the ICD can be influenced during magnet testing of the antitachycardia pacing and vice versa, and even device programs may interact.[131, 132]

Despite these limitations, this combined therapy is clinically feasible in selected patients.[122–125] Ideally, the decision to implant both devices should be made preoperatively to facilitate the avoidance of interactions. There are, however, patients in whom the need for the ATPM is apparent only after ICD implantation (e.g., those with an increased number of ventricular tachycardia episodes after ICD implant or those in whom antiarrhythmic drugs given to decrease the number of ICD discharges markedly slow the rate of ventricular tachycardia).

The following rules are useful in avoiding deleterious interactions between two independent devices:

1. Pacing electrodes and rate-counting ICD electrodes must be bipolar and distanced as far as possible from each other (ideally, in different ventricular chambers). The ICD detection leads should record a minimal signal from the pacing leads and a latency be-

Figure 38-13. Possible deleterious interaction between an antitachycardia pacemaker (ATPM) and an implantable cardioverter-defibrillator (ICD). The ATPM tries to terminate a ventricular tachycardia below the detection rate of the ICD. After the second attempt, the tachycardia is accelerated over the ICD detection rate. The ATPM ceases to sense the faster tachycardia and delivers antibradycardia pacing at 50 beats per minute. Because of its "automatic gain control," the ICD could theoretically interpret the pacemaker spikes as QRS and ignore the ventricular tachycardia but the possibility of that event was adequately explored and ruled out during implant in this patient. After capacitor charging, a shock is delivered, with restoration of a paced rhythm.

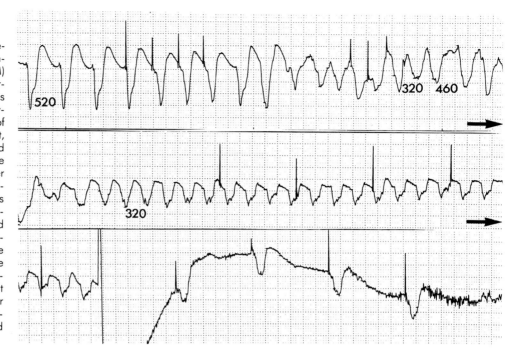

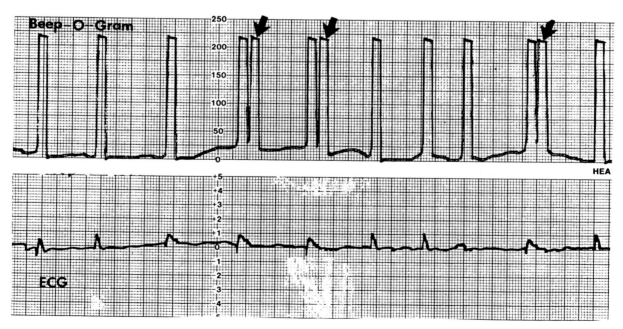

Figure 38-14. Deleterious interaction between a pacemaker and the implantable cardioverter-defibrillator (ICD). As shown in this "beep-o-gram," ventricular paced beats were frequently double-counted (*arrows*). This could eventually trigger an ICD discharge if the cutoff rate is reached.

tween the pace stimulus and the local electrogram of less than the refractory period of the ICD.

2. Pacing and sensing parameters should be optimized.

3. Special testing must be done at implantation, with awareness of the idiosyncrasies of each device.[122]

With the contemporary ICD devices, special consideration should be given to two features: automatic gain control (autosensitivity), which may be responsible for tachycardia nonrecognition during loss of pacemaker inhibition (see Fig. 38-13), and committed discharge characteristic, which is responsible for the short time frame available for successful combined device therapy (Fig. 38-15).

Tiered-Therapy Devices

There is ongoing active clinical use of and research with devices capable of delivering tiered therapy for ventricular arrhythmias. Characteristics of some devices released for clinical practice in the United States are depicted in Table 38-4.

They are all similar in a remarkable number of characteristics, including their antibradycardia- and antitachycardia-pacing capabilities, the presence of cardioversion and defibrillation options, and the capability to perform noninvasive programmed stimulation. Tiered-therapy devices are able to discriminate between two or more pathologic tachycardias (based on different rates) and deliver the programmed therapy for each one (Fig. 38-16). They differ in the availability of some ancillary features. Some devices

deliver not only monophasic shocks but also biphasic and sequential discharges. These modified discharges seem to improve the efficiency of defibrillation.[133, 134] Devices also differ in their diagnostic capabilities. Some of them store the actual electrograms of the arrhythmias that triggered the device intervention. The ability to retrieve and analyze those electrograms seems to be of great clinical value (Fig. 38-17).[135]

Because of their newness, there is rapidly expanding clinical experience with tiered-therapy devices. Preliminary data indicate an improved capability of these new devices to deal effectively with malignant ventricular arrhythmias.[136–138]

The tiered-therapy devices should result in increased numbers of patients who benefit from electric therapy of their ventricular arrhythmias. Nevertheless, the proper role of these devices in the therapeutic armamentarium is not yet clear. Several issues need to be answered regarding their cost-effectiveness and their comparison with the simpler but effective and available defibrillators. Several randomized trials are addressing ICD impact on total mortality. Potential drawbacks of the new devices should be noted. Their programming is time-consuming and requires considerable knowledge of the device's capabilities and limitations and of the patients clinical and inducible tachyarrhythmias. There is also concern about the safety and clinical usefulness of low-energy shocks.[139]

Conversely, several improvements of these devices over those of the first- and second-generation merit mention. Their noncommitted nature will allow their use in patients with frequent nonsustained arrhythmias and will make the use of concomitant antiarrhythmic therapy to

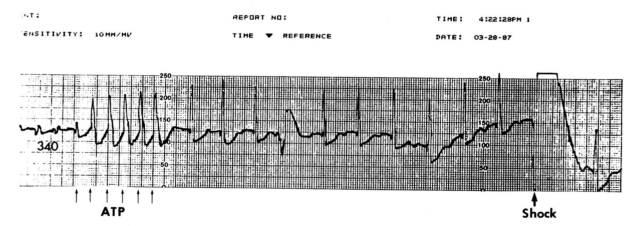

Figure 38-15. Deleterious interaction between an antitachycardia pacemaker and the committed implantable cardioverter-defibrillator (ICD). A ventricular tachycardia (three last beats) is effectively terminated by a burst of antitachycardia pacing (*ATP, arrows*). Nevertheless, the ICD begins charging, and a shock is delivered during sinus rhythm (without consequences). Noncommitted devices reconfirm the presence of the tachycardia immediately before delivering a shock and abort discharges for nonsustained arrhythmias. The noncommitted systems usually charge the device and then internally discharge the device. This may result in rapid battery depletion.

TABLE 38-4. Characteristics of Tiered-Therapy Devices

Model (Manufacturer)	Maximal Programmable Output (J)	Shock Waveform	Sensing	Tachycardia Zones	Diagnostic Capabilities
Cadence V=100 (Ventitrex)	40	Monophasic/biphasic	Automatic gain control	3	Event counters, therapy history, stored electrograms (2 m)
Guardian ATP 4210 (Telectronics)	30	Monophasic	Fixed (programmable)	3	Event counters, therapy history, snapshot electrograms
PCD 7217 B (Medtronic)	34	Monophasic; single/sequential	Autoadjusting sensitivity threshold	2	Event counters, therapy history
PRX 1700 (CPI)	32	Monophasic	Automatic gain control	3	Event counters, therapy history
Res-Q 102-01/02 (Intermedics)	40	Monophasic/biphasic	Automatic gain control	3	Event counters, therapy history

suppress those arrhythmias less necessary. Their diagnostic capabilities will improve the management of patients with asymptomatic discharges. Although none of them will have an incorporated hemodynamic sensor, their more versatile arrhythmia detection algorithms should make easier the distinction between sinus tachycardia or atrial fibrillation and ventricular tachycardia. Finally, the capability to perform noninvasive programmed stimulation will permit more frequent assessment of device function whenever antiarrhythmic drugs are changed or the patient's clinical status varies. The impact of the transvenous lead system coupled with the tiered ICD is beyond the scope of this chapter; however, its less traumatic and equally successful defibrillation efficacy is an obvious advancement. The availability of four or more ICD devices from various manufacturers and a more limited choice of nonthoracotomy lead systems has spawned clinical and regulatory issues regulating "mixing and matching" of one company's ICD device and other companies' transvenous leads.

These devices will be increasingly used in the next few years. Meanwhile, patients who have relative contraindications for available ICDs and those who require replacement of a first- or second-generation ICD and who have had multiple discharges in the past seem to be the most suitable candidates for tiered-therapy devices. Depending on the results of ongoing clinical trials, however, there is potential for expanding device indications.[140] Ultimately, detailed risk stratification of patients and the identification of those more likely to benefit from each of the several therapeutic modalities available will be crucial to optimize antiarrhythmic therapy in patients with ventricular arrhythmias.[141]

FUTURE DIRECTIONS

Atrial fibrillation is one of the most common sustained cardiac arrhythmias. It affects more than 1.5 million people in the United States alone and is associated with sig-

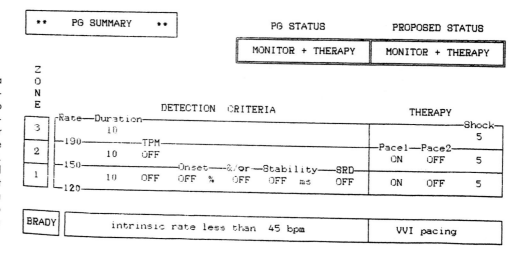

Figure 38-16. Telemetered data for a CPI PRX tiered-therapy device. The device is programmed to detect tachycardia in three different rate zones. Tachycardias over 190 beats per minute (bpm) are treated with high-energy shocks. Those with rates between 120 and 149 and 150 and 189 bpm are first treated with the antitachycardia pacing algorithm. The device also delivers antibradycardia pacing at 45 bpm.

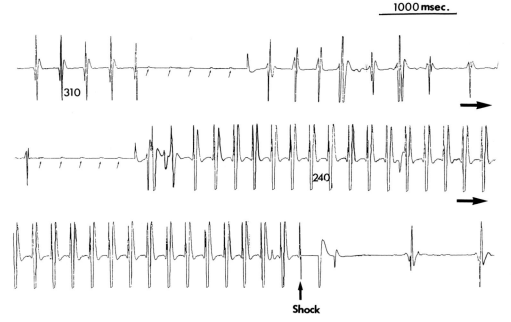

Figure 38-17. Usefulness of stored electrograms. Patient received a shock (preceded by palpitations) while at home. Electrograms retrieved from the Cadence device showed ventricular tachycardia (cycle length, 310 milliseconds). After a second attempt at antitachycardia pacing (*small arrows*), it is accelerated, satisfying the ventricular fibrillation criteria. A high-energy shock is delivered, with restoration of sinus rhythm. Note the difference in electrogram morphology between sinus rhythm and ventricular tachycardia.

nificant morbidity and increased mortality.[142] Evidence suggests that persistence of atrial fibrillation causes progressive shortening of the atrial refractory period and consequently enhances the transition to chronic atrial fibrillation. The development of the ICD for management of ventricular tachycardia and fibrillation has lead to efforts in adapting similar technology for the management of atrial fibrillation.[143,144] The potential benefits associated with such a device include (1) prompt arrhythmia termination, (2) combination with atrial pacing algorithms, (3) possible avoidance of anticoagulation, (3) hemodynamic improvement, (4) delay in progress of atrial disease, and (5) serving as a synergistic therapy as well as a backup to drug therapy. To defibrillate, an applied electric shock must halt the many automatous wavefronts of myocardial activation yet not introduce new activation fronts that reinduce fibrillation. Factors affecting the success of an atrial defibrillation shock to convert atrial fibrillation to normal sinus rhythm include (1) defibrillating electrode configuration, (2) defibrillating waveform morphology, (3) size of the left atrium, and (4) previous history of defibrillating shocks.

The role of atrial ATPM alone or in combination with an atrial defibrillator will depend on future studies. The patient definitely benefits from prevention and rapid conversion of atrial fibrillation relative to mortality, congestive heart failure, quality of life, and cost.[145,146] It is easy to visualize the universal arrhythmia management device that prevents, pace terminates, and, if necessary, facilitates defibrillation of atrial or ventricular arrhythmias. Technically, a universal arrhythmia-management system is feasible. It would include a dual-chamber pacing system and a dual-chamber defibrillating system. It is somewhat more difficult to implement, however. In the year 1995, it appears that the negative social and economic forces will make this type of progress more difficult in the near future.

References

1. Zoll PM, Linenthal AJ, Zarsky LRN: Ventricular fibrillation: treatment and prevention by external electric currents. N Engl J Med 1960;262:105.
2. Sowton E, Leatham A, Carson P: The suppression of arrhythmias by artificial pacing. Lancet 1964;2:1098.
3. Cohen HE, Kahn M, Donoso E: Treatment of supraventricular tachycardias with catether and permanent pacemakers. Am J Cardiol 1967;20:735.
4. Massumi RA, Kistin AD, Tawakkol AA: Termination of reciprocating tachycardia by atrial stimulation. Circulation 1967; 36:637.
5. Haft J, Kosowsky BD, Law SH, Stein E, Damato AN: Termination of atrial flutter by rapid electrical pacing of the atrium. Am J Cardiol 1967;20:239.
6. Durrer D, Schoo L, Schuilenburg RM, Wellens HJJ: The role of premature beats in the initiation and the termination of supraventricular tachycardia in the Wolff-Parkinson-White syndrome. Circulation 1967;36:644.
7. Zipes DP, Festoff B, Schaal SF, et al: Treatment of ventricular arrhythmia by permanent atrial pacemaker and cardiac sympathectomy. Ann Intern Med 1968;68:591.
8. Escher DJW: The treatment of tachyarrhythmias by artificial pacing. Am Heart J 1969;78:829.
9. DeSanctis RW, Kastor JA: Rapid intracardiac pacing for treatment of recurrent ventricular tachyarrhythmias in the absence of complete heart block. Am Heart J 1968;76:168.

10. Johnson RA, Hutter AM, DeSanctis RW, et al: Chronic overdrive pacing in the control of refractory ventricular arrhythmias. Ann Intern Med 1974;80:380.

11. Moss AJ, Rivers RJ: Termination and inhibition of recurrent tachycardias by implanted pervenous pacemakers. Circulation 1974;50:942.

12. Dreifus LS, Berkovits BV, Kimibiris D, et al: Use of atrial and bifocal cardiac pacemakers for treating resistant dysrhythmias. Eur J Cardiol 1975;3:257.

13. Ryan G, Easley PM, Zaroff LI, et al: Paradoxical use of a demand pacemaker in the treatment of supraventricular tachycardia due to Wolff-Parkinson-White syndrome. Circulation 1968;38:1037.

14. Barold SS, Ryan GF, Goldstein S: The first implanted tachycardia-terminating pacemaker. Pacing Clin Electrophysiol 1989;12:870.

15. Attuel P, Pellerin D, Mugica J, et al: DDD pacing: an effective treatment for recurrent atrial arrhythmias. Pacing Clin Electrophysiol 1988;11:1647.

16. Rosenqvist M, Brandt J, Schuller H: Long-term pacing in sinus node disease: effects of stimulation mode on cardiovascular morbidity and mortality. Am Heart J 1988;116:16.

17. Feuer J, Shandling A, Messenger J: Influence of cardiac pacing mode on the long-term development of atrial fibrillation. Am J Cardiol 1989;64:1376.

18. Zimmermann M, Maisonblanche P, Cauchemez B, et al: Determinants of the spontaneous ectopic activity in repetitive monomorphic idiopathic ventricular tachycardia. J Am Coll Cardiol 1986;7:1219.

19. Fisher JD, Teichman S, Ferrick A, et al: Antiarrhythmic effects of VVI pacing at physiologic rates: A crossover controlled evaluation. Pacing Clin Electrophysiol 1987;10:822.

20. Bayes de Luna A, Coumel P, Leclercq JF: Ambulatory sudden cardiac death: mechanisms of production of fatal arrhythmias on the basis of data from 157 cases. Am Heart J 1989;117:151.

21. Kowey PR, Engel TR: Overdrive pacing for ventricular tachyarrhythmias: a reassessment. Ann Intern Med 1983;99:651.

22. Spurrell RAJ, Sowton E: An implanted atrial synchronus pacemaker with a short atrioventricular delay for the prevention of paroxysmal supraventricular tachycardias. J Electrocardiol 1976;9:89.

23. Akhtar M, Gilbert CJ, Al-Nouri M, et al: Electrophysiologic mechanisms for modification and abolition of atrioventricular junctional tachycardia with simultaneous and sequential atrial and ventricular pacing. Circulation 1979;60:1443.

24. Sung RJ, Styperek JL, Castellanos A: Complete abolition of the reentrant SVT zone using a new modality of cardiac pacing with simultaneous atrioventricular stimulation. Am J Cardiol 1980;45:72.

25. Kuck KH, Kunze KP, Schluter M, et al: Tachycardia prevention by programmed stimulation. Am J Cardiol 1984;54:550.

26. Davies DW, Butrous GS, Spurrell RAJ, Camm AJ: Pacing techniques in the prophylaxis of junctional rentry tachycardia. Pacing Clin Electrophysiol 1987;10:519.

27. Begemann MJS, Bennekers JH, Kingma JH, et al: Prevention of tachycardia initiation by programmed stimulation. J Electrophysiol 1987;4:350.

28. Prystowsky EN, Zipes DP: Inhibition in the human heart. Circulation 1983;68:707.

29. Skale BT, Kallock MJ, Prystowsky EN, Gill RM, Zipes DP: Inhibition of premature ventricular extrastimuli by subthreshold conditioning stimuli. J Am Coll Cardiol 1985;6:133.

30. Gang ES, Peter T, Nalos PC, et al: Subthreshold atrial pacing in patients with a left-sided accesory pathway: an effective new method for terminating reciprocating tachycardia. J Am Coll Cardiol 1988;11:515.

31. Shenasa M, Cardinal R, Kus T, et al: Termination of sustained ventricular by ultrarapid subthreshold stimulation in humans. Circulation 1988;78:1135.

32. Silka MJ, Manwill JR, Kron J, et al: Bradycardia-mediated tachyarrhythmias in congenital heart disease and responses to chronic pacing at physiologic rates. Am J Cardiol 1990;65:483.

33. Coumel PH, Attuel P, Lavallee JP, Flammang D, Leclercq JF, Slama R: Syndrome d'arythmie auriculaire d'origine vagale. Arch Mal Coeur 1978;71:645.

34. Coumel PH, Friocourt P, Mugica J, Attuel P, Leclercq JF: Long-term prevention of vagal arrhythmia by atrial pacing at 90/min: experience with 6 cases. Pacing Clin Electrophysiol 1983;6:552.

35. Jackman WM, Friday KJ, Anderson JL, Alliot EM, Clark M, Lazzara R: The long QT syndromes: a critical review, new clinical observations and a unifying hypothesis. Prog Cardiovasc Dis 1988;31:115.

36. Jackman WM, Szabo B, Friday KJ, et al: Ventricular tachyarrhythmias related to early afterdepolarizations and triggered firing: relationship to QT interval prolongation and potential therapeutic role from calcium channel blockers. J Cardiovasc Electrophysiol 1991;1:170.

37. Kugler JD, Gerken KA: Sinus nodal dysfunction in young patients with long QT syndrome. Pacing Clin Electrophysiol 1991;14:159. Abstract

38. Scott WA, Dick M: Two:one atrioventricular block in infants with congenital long QT syndrome. Am J Cardiol 1987;60:1409.

39. Van Hare GF, Franz MR, Roge C, Scheinman MM: Persistent functional atrioventricular block in two patients with prolonged QT intervals: elucidation of the mechanism of block. Pacing Clin Electrophysiol 1990;13:608.

40. Wilmer CI, Stein B, Morris DC: Atrioventricular pacemaker placement in Romano-Ward syndrome and recurrent torsades de pointes. Am J Cardiol 1987;59:171.

41. Eldar M, Griffin JC, Abbott JA, et al: Permanent cardiac pacing in patients with the long QT syndrome. J Am Coll Cardiol 1987;10:600.

42. Weintraub RG, Gow ER, Wilkinson JL: The congenital long QT syndromes in childhood. J Am Coll Cardiol 1990;16:674.

43. Waldo AL, MacLean WAH, Karp RB, et al: Continuous atrial pacing to control recurrent or sustained supraventricular tachycardias following open heart surgery. Circulation 1976;54:245.

44. Moreira DAR, Shepard RB, Waldo AL: Chronic rapid atrial pacing to maintain atrial fibrillation: use to permit control of ventricular rate in order to treat tachycardia induced cardiomyopathy. Pacing Clin Electrophysiol 1989;12:761.

45. Hamer AW, Zaher CA, Rubin SA, et al: Hemodynamic benefits of synchronized 1:1 atrial pacing during sustained ventricular tachycardia with severely depressed ventricular function in coronary heart disease. Am J Cardiol 1985;55: 990.

46. Fisher JD, Kim SG, Mercando AD: Electrical devices for the treatment of arrhythmias. Am J Cardiol 1988;61:45A.

47. Frame LH, Hoffman BF: Mechanisms of tachycardia. In: Surawicz B, Reddy CP, Prystowsky EN, eds. Tachycardias. Boston: Martinus Niehaus, 1984:7.

48. Akhtar M, Tchou PJ, Jazayeri M: Mechanisms of clinical tachycardias. Am J Cardiol 1989;61:9A.

49. Wellens HJJ, Duren DR, Lie KI: Observations on mechanisms of ventricular tachycardia in man. Circulation 1976;54:237.

50. Josephson ME, Gotlieb CD: Ventricular tachycardias associated with coronary artery disease. In: Zipes DP, Jalife J, eds. Cardiac electrophysiology: from cell to bedside. Philadelphia: WB Saunders, 1990:571.

51. El-Sherif N, Cough WB, Restivo M: Reentrant ventricular arrhythmias in the late ventricular infarction period. 14: Mechanism of resetting, entrainment, acceleration, or termination of reentrant ventricular tachycardia by programmed electrical stimulation. Pacing Clin Electrophysiol 1987;10: 341.

52. Zipes DP, Miyazaki T: The autonomic nervous systen and the heart: basis for understanding interactions and effects on arrhythmia development. In: Zipes DP, Jalife J, eds. Cardiac electrophysiology: from cell to bedside. Philadelphia: WB Saunders, 1990:312.

53. Fisher JD, Mehra R, Furman S: Termination of ventricular tachycardia with bursts of ventricular pacing. Am J Cardiol 1978;41:94.

54. Fisher JD, Kim SG, Waspe LE, Matos JA: Mechanisms for the success and failure of pacing for termination of ventricular tachycardia: clinical and hypothetical considerations. Pacing Clin Electrophysiol 1983;6:1094.

55. Nacarelli GV, Zipes DP, Rahilly GT, et al: Influence of tachycardia cycle length and antiarrhythmic drugs on pacing termination and acceleration of ventricular tachycardia. Am Heart J 1983;105:1.

56. Almendral JM, Stamato NJ, Rosenthal ME, Marchlinski FE, Miller JM, Josephson ME: Reseting response patterns during sustained ventricular tachycardia: relationship to the excitable gap. Circulation 1986;74:722.

57. Almendral JM, Rosenthal ME, Stamato NJ, et al: Analysis of the resetting phenomenon in sustained uniform ventricular tachycardia; incidence and relation to termination. J Am Coll Cardiol 1986;8:294.

58. Stevenson W, Weiss JN, Weiner I, et al: Resetting of ventricular tachycardia: Implications for localizing the area of slow conduction. J Am Coll Cardiol 1988;11:522.

59. Waldo AL, MacLean WAH, Karp RB, et al: Entrainment and interruption of atrial flutter with atrial pacing. Studies in the man following open heart surgery. Circulation 1977;56:737.

60. MacLean WAH, Plumb VJ, Waldo AL: Transient entrainment and interruption of ventricular tachycardia. Pacing Clin Electrophysiol 1981;4:358.

61. Anderson KP, Swerdlow CD, Mason JW: Entrainment of ventricular tachycardia. Am J Cardiol 1983;53:335.

62. Waldo AL, Henthorn RW, Plumb VJ, et al: Demonstration of the mechanism of transient entrainment and interruption of ventricular tachycardia with rapid atrial pacing. J Am Coll Cardiol 1984;3:422.

63. Brugada P, Wellens HJJ: Entrainment as an electrophysiological phenomenon. J Am Coll Cardiol 1984;3:451.

64. Okumura K, Henthorn RW, Epstein AE, et al: Further observations on transient entrainment: importance of pacing site and properties of the components of the reentrant circuit. Circulation 1985;72:1293.

65. Mann DE, Lawrie GM, Luck JC, et al: Importance of the pacing site in entrainment of ventricular tachycardia. J Am Coll Cardiol 1985;5:781.

66. Henthorn RW, Okumura K, Olshansky B, et al: A fourth criterion for transient entrainment: the electrogram equivalent of progressive fusion. Circulation 1988;77:1003.

67. Waldecker B, Brugada P, Zehender M, Stevenson W, Den Dulk K, Wellens HJJ: Importance of modes of electrical termination of ventricular tachycardia for the selection of implantable antitachycardia devices. Am J Cardiol 1986; 57:150.

68. Jantzer JH, Hoffman RM: Acceleration of ventricular tachycardia by rapid overdrive pacing combined with extrastimuli. Pacing Clin Electrophysiol 1984;7:922.

69. Brugada J, Brugada P, Boersma L, et al: Observations on the mechanisms of ventricular tachycardia acceleration during programmed electrical stimulation. Pacing Clin Electrophysiol 1990;13:563. Abstract.

70. Brugada J, Boersma L, Kirchhhof C, et al: Double-wave reentry as a mechanism of acceleration of ventricular tachycardia. Circulation 1990;81:1633.

71. Fisher JD, Johnston DR, Kim SG, Furman S, Mercando AD: Implantable pacers for tachycardia termination: stimulation techniques and long-term efficacy. Pacing Clin Electrophysiol 1986;9:1325.

72. De Belder MA, Malik M, Ward DE, Camm AJ: Pacing modalities for tachycardia termination. Pacing Clin Electrophysiol 1990;13:231.

73. Bertholet M, Kulbertus HE: Antitachycardia pacing: available systems and related problems. In: Breithardt G, Borggrefe M, Zipes DG, eds. Nonpharmacological therapy of tachyarrhythmias. Mt. Kisco, NY: Futura Publishing, 1987:409.

74. Saksena S: Antiarrhythmic devices: in search of a common parlance. Pacing Clin Electrophysiol 1989;12:1579.

75. Charos GS, Haffajee CI, Gold RL, Bishop RL, Berkovits BV, Alpert JS: A theoretically and practically more effective method for interruption of ventricular tachycardia: self-adapting autodecremental overdrive pacing. Circulation 1986;73:309.

76. Nathan AW, Camm AJ, Bexton RS, et al: Initial experience with a fully implantable, programmable, scanning, extrastimulus pacemaker for tachycardia termination. Clin Cardiol 1982;5:22.

77. Holt P, Crick JCP, Sowton E: Antitachycardia pacing: a comparison of burst overdrive, self-searching and adaptive table scanning programs. Pacing Clin Electrophysiol 1986;9:490.

78. den Dulk K, Kersschot IE, Brugada P, Wellens HJJ: Is there a universal antitachycardia pacing? Am J Cardiol 1986;57:950.

79. Pannizzo F, Mercando AD, Fisher JD, Furman S: Automatic

methods for detection of tachyarrhythmias by antitachycardia devices. J Am Coll Cardiol 1988;11:308.

80. Haluska EA, Adler S, Calfee RV: Detection algorhithm selection in a tiered-therapy arrhythmia control device: a rationale for guiding programming. Pacing Clin Electrophysiol 1990;13:1196. Abstract.

81. Kahn A, Morris JJ, Citron P: Patient-initiated rapid atrial pacing to manage supraventricular tachycardia. Am J Cardiol 1976;38:200.

82. Waxman RW, Bonet JF, Sharma AD, et al: Patient initiated rapid atrial stimulation for treatment of paroxysmal supraventricular tachycardia. In: Meere C, ed. Proceedings of the VIth World Symposium on Cardiac Pacing. Montreal: Pacesymp, 1979, Chap 9, 1.

83. Mercando AD, Gableman G, Fisher JD, Furman S: Comparison of the rate of tachycardia development in patients: pathologic vs. sinus tachycardias. Pacing Clin Electrophysiol 1988;11:516. Abstract.

84. Davies DW, Tooley MA, Cochrane T, Camm AJ: Real-time automatic diagnosis and treatment of pathological tachycardia by analysis of electrogram morphology. In: Breithardt G, Borggrefe M, Zipes DG, eds. Nonpharmacological therapy of tachyarrhythmias. Mt. Kisco, NY: Futura Publishing, 1987: 421.

85. Ropella KM, Baerman JM, Sahakian AV, Swiryn S: Differentiation of ventricular tachycardias. Circulation 1990;82:2035.

86. Hemmer W, Weismuller P, Welz A, Lass M, Hannekum A: Reliability of PDF for tachycardia detection. Pacing Clin Electrophysiol 1990;13:1198. Abstract.

87. Mercando AD, Furman S: Measurement of differences in timing and sequence between two ventricular electrodes as a means of tachycardia differentiation. Pacing Clin Electrophysiol 1986;9:1069.

88. Stangl K, Laule M, Heinze R, Erhardt W, Wirtzfield A, Blomer H: Hemodynamic tachycardia detection: what parameters can be used? Pacing Clin Electrophysiol 1990;13:1212. Abstract.

89. Khoury D, McCalister H, Wilkoff B, et al: Continous RV volume assessment by catheter measurement of impedance for antitachycardia system control. Pacing Clin Electrophysiol 1989;12:1918.

90. Wood M, Ellenbogen KA, Lu B, Valenta H: A prospective study of right ventricular pressure and dP/dT to discriminant-induced ventricular tachycardia from supraventricular and sinus tachycardia in man. Pacing Clin Electrophysiol 1990;13:1148.

91. Sharma AD, Bennett T, Ericson M, Yee R, Klein GJ: Differentiation of hemodynamically stable from unstable ventricular tachycardia using right ventricular pressure parameters. J Am Coll Cardiol 1990;15:61A. Abstract.

92. Beauregard LAM, Volosin KJ, Waxman HL: Differentiation of arrhythmias by measurement of intracardiac pressures in man. Pacing Clin Electrophysiol 1991;14:161.

93. Auricchio A, Klein H, Trappe HJ, Troster J, Salo R, Shapland E: Pressure-volume loops during supraventricular and ventricular tachycardia. A new discriminating criterion. Pacing Clin Electrophysiol 1990;13:1190. Abstract.

94. Laule M, Stangl K, Heinze R, Erhardt W, Wirtzfield A, Schamlfeldt B: Evaluation of intracavitary echo-Doppler

95. measurement as equivalent for stroke volume and contractility. Pacing Clin Electrophysiol 1990;13:1201. Abstract.

95. Waldo AL, Akhtar M, Benditt DG, et al: Appropriate electrophysiologic study and treatment of patients with the Wolff-Parkinson-White syndrome. Pacing Clin Electrophysiol 1988;11:536.

96. Ferguson TB, Cox JL: Surgical therapy for patients with supraventricular tachycardia. Cardiol Clin 1990;8:535.

97. Morady F: Catheter ablation of accessory pathways. Cardiol Clin 1990;8:557.

98. Lee MA, Morady F, Kadish, et al: Catheter modification of the atrioventricular junction with radiofrequency energy for control of atrioventricular nodal reentry tachycardia. Circulation 1991;83:827.

99. Rosenquist M, Lee MA, Mouliner L, et al: Long-term follow-up of patients after transcatheter direct current ablation of the atrioventricular junction. J Am Coll Cardiol 1990;16:1467.

100. Waldecker B, Brugada P, Den Dulk K, Zehender M, Wellens HJJ: Arrhythmias induced during termination of supraventricular tachycardia. Am J Cardiol 1985;55:412.

101. Lau CP, Cornu E, Camm AJ: Fatal and nonfatal cardiac arrest in patients with an implanted antitachycardia device for treatment of supraventricular tachycardia. Am J Cardiol 1988;61:919.

102. Frank R, Fontaine G, Tonet JL: Changing modes with posture and exercise in antitachycardia pacing: Atrial pacing in orthodromic tachycardia. In: Breithard G, Borggrefe M, Zipes DP, eds. Nonpharmacological therapy of tachyarrhythmias. Mt. Kisco, NY: Futura Publishing, 1987:429.

103. Reiter MJ, Mann DE: Effects of upright posture on atrioventricular accessory pathway conduction. Am J Cardiol 1990; 65:623.

104. Den Dulk K, Brugada P, Smeets JL, Wellens HJJ: Long-term antitachycardia pacing experience for supraventricular tachycardia. Pacing Clin Electrophysiol 1990;13:1020.

105. Griffin JC: Follow-up techniques for patients with implanted antitachycardia devices. In: Saksena S, Goldschlager, eds. Electrical therapy for cardiac arrhythmias. Philadelphia: WB Saunders, 1990:516.

106. Spurrell RAJ, Nathan AW, Camm AJ: Clinical experience with implantable scanning tachycardia reversion pacemakers. Pacing Clin Electrophysiol 1984;7:1296.

107. Sowton E: Clinical results with the tachylog antitachycardia pacemaker. Pacing Clin Electrophysiol 1984;7:1313.

108. Griffin JC, Sweeney M: The management of paroxysmal tachycardias using the Cybertach-60. Pacing Clin Electrophysiol 1984;7:1291.

109. Bertholet M, Demoulin JC, Waleffe A, et al: Programmable extrstimulus pacing for long-term management of ventricular and supraventricular tachycardias: clinical experience in 16 patients. Am Heart J 1985;110:582.

110. Peters RW, Scheinman MM, Morady F, et al: Long-term management of recurrent paroxysmal tachycardia by cardiac burst pacing. Pacing Clin Electrophysiol 1985;8:335.

111. Fisher JD, Johnston DR, Furman S, Mercando AD, Kim SG: Long-term efficacy of antitachycardia pacing for supraventricular and ventricular tachycardias. Am J Cardiol 1987;60:1311.

112. Moller M, Simonsen E, Ing PA, Oxhoj H: Long-term follow-up

of patients treated with automatic scanning antitachycardia pacemaker. Pacing Clin Electrophysiol 1989;12:425.

113. Schnittger I, Lee JT, Hargis J, et al: Long-term results of antitachycardia pacing in patients with supraventricular tachycardia. Pacing Clin Electrophysiol 1989;12:936.

114. Kappenberger L, Valin H, Sowton E: Multicenter long-term results of antitachycardia pacing for supraventricular tachycardias. Am J Cardiol 1989;64:191.

115. Occhetta E, Bolognese L, Magnani A, et al: Clinical experience with Orthocor II antitachycardia pacing system for recurrent tachyarrhyhtmia termination. J Electrophysiol 1989;3:289.

116. McComb JM, Jameson S, Bexton RS: Atrial antitachycardia pacing in patients with supraventricular tachycardia: clinical experience with the Intertach pacemaker. Pacing Clin Electrophysiol 1990;13:1948.

117. Sulke AN, Bucknall CA, Sowton E: Supraventricular tachycardia control with Tachylog II: long term follow-up. Pacing Clin Electrophysiol 1990;13:1960.

118. Fromer M, Gloor H, Kus T, Shenasa M: Clinical experience with a new software-based antitachycardia pacemaker for recurrent supraventricular and ventricular tachycardias. Pacing Clin Electrophysiol 1990;13:890.

119. Fisher JD, Kim SG, Mercando AD: Electrical devices for treatment of arrhythmias. Am J Cardiol 1988;61:45A.

120. Fisher JD: Antitachycardia devices: minimum report standards. Pacing Clin Electrophysiol 1988;11:2.

121. Zipes DP, Akhtar M, Denes P, et al: Guidelines for clinical inracardiac electrophysiologic studies. A report of the American College of Cardiology/American Heart Association task force on assessment of diagnostic and therapeutic cardiovascular procedures. J Am Coll Cardiol 1989;14:1827.

122. Manz M, Gerckens U, Funke HD, Kirchhoff PG, Luderitz B: Combination of antitachycardia pacemaker and automatic implantable cardioverter/defibrillator for ventricular tachycardia. Pacing Clin Electrophysiol 1986;9:676.

123. Masterson M, Pinski SL, Wilkoff B, et al: Pacemaker and defibrillator combination therapy for recurrent ventricular tachycardia. Cleve Clin J Med 1990;57:330.

124. Newman DM, Lee MA, Herre JM, Langberg JJ, Scheinman M, Griffin JC: Permanent antitachycardia pacemaker therapy for ventricular tachycardia. Pacing Clin Electrophysiol 1989; 12:1387.

125. Ahern TS, Nydegger C, McCormick DJ, et al: Device interaction: antitachycardia pacemakers and defibrillators for sustained ventricular tachycardia. Pacing Clin Electrophysiol 1991;14:302.

126. Leitch JW, Gillis AM, Wyse G, et al: Reduction in defibrillation shocks with a device combining antitachycardia pacing, cardioversion and defibrillation. J Am Coll Cardiol 1991; 17:128A. Abstract.

127. Epstein AE, Kay N, Plumb VJ, Shepard RB, Kirklin JK: Combined automatic implantable cardioverter-defibrillator and pacemaker systems: implantation techniques and follow-up. J Am Coll Cardiol 1989;13:121.

128. Cohen AI, Wish MG, Fletcher RD, et al: The use and interaction of permanent pacemakers and the automatic implantable cardioverter defibrillator. Pacing Clin Electrophysiol 1988;11:704.

129. Singer I, Guarnieri T, Kupersmith J: Implanted automatic defibrillators: effects of drugs and pacemakers. Pacing Clin Electrophysiol 1988;11:2250.

130. Luderitz B: The impact of antitachycardia pacing with defibrillation. Pacing Clin Electrophysiol 1991:14:312.

131. Kim SG, Furman S, Matos JA, et al: Automatic implantable cardioverter/defibrillator: inadvertent discharges during permanent pacemaker magnet tests. Pacing Clin Electrophysiol 1987;10:579.

132. Rogers R, Ellenbogen KA: Letter to the editor. Pacing Clin Electrophysiol 1990;13:1687.

133. Winkle RA, Mead RH, Ruder MA, et al: Improved low energy defibrillation in man with the use of a biphasic truncated exponential waveform. Am Heart J 1989;117:122.

134. Bardy GH, Stewart RB, Ivey TD, et al: Intraoperative comparison of sequential-pulse and single-pulse defibrillation in candidates for automatic implantable defibrillators. Am J Cardiol 1987; 60:618.

135. Hook BG, Marchlinski FE: Value of ventricular electrogram recordings in the diagnosis of arrhythmias precipitating electrical device shock therapy. J Am Coll Cardiol 1991; 17:985.

136. Bardy GH, Troutman C, Johnson G, et al: A multiprogrammable antiarrhytmia device for the treatment of patients with ventricular tachycardia and ventricular fibrillation. J Am Coll Cardiol 1991;17:343A. Abstract.

137. Newman D, Hardy J, Thorne S, et al: Single centre experience with a combination antitachycardia pacemaker and defibrillator. J Am Coll Cardiol 1991;17:129A. Abstract.

138. Troster J, Trappe HJ, Siclari F, Wenzlaff P, Klein H, Auricchio A: Clinical evaluation of patients with a programmable defibrillator. Circulation 1990; 82:III. Abstract.

139. Siebels J, Geiger M, Schneider MAE, Kuck KH: The automatic implantable cardioverter/defibrillator: does low energy cardioversion offer any advantage over antitachycardia pacing in patients with ventricular tachycardia. J Am Coll Cardiol 1991;17:129A. Abstract.

140. Bigger JT: Prophylactic use of implantable cardioverter defibrillators: medical, technical, economic considerations. Pacing Clin Electrophysiol 1991;14:376.

141. Wellens HJJ, Brugada P: Treatment of cardiac arrhythmias: when, how, and where? J Am Coll Cardiol 1989;14:1417.

142. Kannel WB, Wokf PA: Epidemiology of atrial fibrillation. In: Falk RH, Podrid PJ, eds. Atrial fibrillation—mechanisms and management. New York: 1993:81.

143. Cooper RAS, Alferness CA, Smith WM, et al: Internal defibrillation of atrial fibrillation in sheep. Circulation 1993; 87:1673.

144. Kalman JM, Power JM, Chen JM, et al: Importance of electrode design, lead configuration and impedance for successful low energy transcatheter atrial defibrillation in dogs. J Am Coll Cardiol 1993;22:1199.

145. Sgarbossa EB, Pinski SL, Maloney JD, et al: Chronic atrial fibrillation and stroke in paced patients with sick sinus syndrome. Relevance of clinical characteristics and pacing modalities. Circulation 1993;88:1045.

146. Sgarbossa EB, Pinski SL, Maloney JD: The role of pacing modality in determining long-term survival in the sick sinus syndrome. Ann Intern Med 1993;119:359.

Cardiac Arrhythmias, 3rd edition, edited by William J. Mandel.
J. B. Lippincott Company, Philadelphia © 1995.

39

Eli S. Gang

Surgical Alternatives in the Management of Patients With Refractory Supraventricular Tachyarrhythmias Not Related to Preexcitation

Most patients with supraventricular tachyarrhythmias that require therapeutic intervention are readily treatable with pharmacologic agents. The end point of pharmacologic therapy can be empirically chosen when symptomatic relief is obtained or more precisely defined in the electrophysiology laboratory when the tachycardia is no longer provokable.[1] Indeed, new pharmacologic agents such as amiodarone, flecainide, and propafenone are effective in the management of supraventricular tachyarrhythmias.[2-5] Nonetheless, frequently patients are encountered who suffer from recurrent troublesome tachyarrhythmias unrelated to one of the preexcitation syndromes who are poorly controlled, unwilling, or unable to take pharmacologic agents. In such patients, nonpharmacologic alternatives must be considered, primarily for relief of symptoms but also because uncontrolled prolonged atrial tachycardias can cause severe hemodynamic derangement, even in young patients. Chronic atrial tachycardia can lead to salt and water retention, pericardial effusion, ascites, peripheral edema, and cardiomegaly. These abnormalities are frequently reversible after elim-

ination of the tachycardia.[6] Nonpharmacologic therapeutic modalities such as catheter ablation or modification of the atrioventricular (AV) junction or of ectopic atrial foci are reviewed elsewhere in this text. Similarly, antitachycardia permanent pacemakers are also discussed in another section. This chapter reviews contemporary advances in the surgical approaches to the treatment of refractory supraventricular arrhythmias that are not related to ventricular preexcitation.

The surgical therapy of tachycardias related to the various preexcitation syndromes is discussed later. For patients with poorly responsive supraventricular tachyarrhythmias not related to preexcitation and for whom pacemaker therapy is inappropriate, several surgical methods have been devised: (1) interruption of AV conduction by destruction or transection of the AV node–His-bundle conduction pathways, (2) modification of AV junctional conduction properties by direct incisional or cryoablative approaches, (3) excision or cryoablation of an arrhythmogenic region in the atria, (4) surgical exclusion of an atrial arrhythmogenic area, (5) isolation of the right or left atrium, and (6) complex multiple incisions in the atria, designed to eliminate the recurrence of atrial fibrillation.

INTERRUPTION OF ATRIOVENTRICULAR CONDUCTION

Interruption of AV conduction has been the most frequently employed surgical technique, presumably because of its relative simplicity and because historically it was among the first operations designed for control of refractory supraventricular tachyarrhythmias.[7–13] This type of surgery has been performed in patients having a variety of supraventricular tachyarrhythmias; namely, those with (1) known Kent bundles, in whom division of the pathway is unsuccessful or inadvisable; (2) drug-resistant atrial fibrillation or flutter and a rapid ventricular response; (3) an ectopic atrial pacemaking focus; (4) paroxysmal tachycardia secondary to reentry within the AV node; and (5) a junctional ectopic pacemaker.

Surgical techniques for interrupting AV conduction include suture ligation, electrocauterization, simple surgical transection, and cryoablation of the AV node–His-bundle region.[9,10] Intraoperative localization of the His bundle can be performed by recording the characteristic His-bundle electrogram, using a hand-held probe (Fig. 39-1). Sealy advises that the incision be made across the floor of the right atrium, anterior to the os of the coronary

sinus and above the tricuspid anulus.[8] The surgeon should also divide the right side of the atrial septum at its insertion into the right fibrous trigone. This approach is designed to interrupt AV conduction at the junction of the common bundle of His and the AV node, thereby preserving most of the His bundle and permitting the emergence of a stable junctional rhythm. Permanent demand electronic pacemakers are nonetheless implanted in all patients at the time of operation.

The preferred method for interrupting impulse conduction in the AV conduction system is by cryoablation of the AV node and upper portion of the bundle of His.[7,8,11–13] Mapping of the His bundle is performed, and the area producing the most prominent His deflection is then cooled with a cryoprobe (about 0.5 cm in diameter) to about 0°C for 30 seconds. Complete temporary heart block is thereby produced, which is easily reversible with rewarming. If this test cooling does not produce satisfactory AV block, the area is mapped again for an even greater His-bundle deflection preceded by a prominent atrial deflection. When satisfactory AV block is achieved, irreversible ablation is produced by cooling the area to −60°C for 2 to 3 minutes. One or two additional freeze lesions may be produced several millimeters proximal to the first lesion and nearer to the coronary sinus. Crysosurgical ablation of AV conduction offers several advantages over other surgical methods: first, it is reversible, so that permanent damage to atrial structures does not occur until conduction has been definitely interrupted; second, the "ice balls" produced by cryosurgery are small (about 1 cm in diameter), discrete, and not arrhythmogenic; finally, these lesions do not rupture, nor do they form aneurysms.[12]

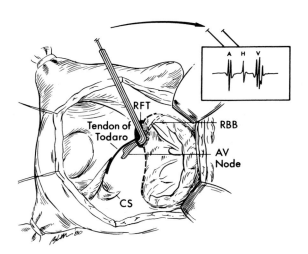

Figure 39-1. Intraoperative localization of the His bundle. A hand-held probe electrode is positioned over the His bundle. The *inset* illustrates a prominent His-bundle deflection on a His-bundle electrogram. The *dotted line* shows the site of incision for interruption of atrioventricular conduction. When cryosurgery is performed, the cryoprobe is placed in the same position as the probe. *RFT,* right fibrous trigone; *RBB,* right bundle branch; *CS,* coronary sinus. (Sealy WC: When is surgery indicated for control of supraventricular tachycardia? Am J Surg 1983;145:711.)

SURGICAL DISSECTION AND CRYOABLATION IN THE TREATMENT OF ATRIOVENTRICULAR NODAL REENTRANT TACHYCARDIA

A surgical approach directed specifically at arrhythmogenic atrial foci has become a viable therapeutic alternative, largely because of the experience gained by clinical electrophysiologists in the techniques of intraoperative and electrode catheter mapping. Precise localization of macroeentrant or microeentrant circuits and automatic atrial foci has enabled the cardiologist to direct the surgeon to the atrial site that requires surgical excision, section, or cryoablation.

A surgical approach has been described in a few patients having AV junctional reentrant tachycardia, in whom the tachycardia was surgically abolished but anterograde AV conduction was either unaffected or only slightly modified.[13–18] In the first case report, the cure of the tachycardia was actually fortuitous inasmuch as the surgical goal had been to produce complete AV block using the dissection and mapping techniques described above.[13] Postoperatively, however, the patient maintained AV conduction (albeit with a slightly prolonged PR interval) and was free of tachycardia. Presumably, conduction in one of the limbs of the AV nodal reentrant circuit was sufficiently damaged by the operative dissection to prevent subsequent reentry within the AV node. In the second patient, careful preoperative and intraoperative endocardial mapping showed earliest right atrial activation during right ventricular pacing to be low in the interatrial septum, anterior to the ostium of the coronary sinus. Selective atriotomy abolished ventriculoatrial conduction while preserving anterograde conduction (again, with slight PR interval prolongation).[14] These preliminary results suggested that partial or total interruption of an AV nodal reentrant circuit at its atrionodal junction may be possible in selected patients.

A similar surgical approach was prospectively evaluated by Ross and colleagues in a series of 10 patients who had troublesome AV junctional reciprocating tachycardia.[15,16] At the preoperative electrophysiologic study, these patients were divided into two groups: those with a ventriculoatrial (VA) interval of 40 milliseconds or less (seven patients) were designated as type A, and those with a ventriculoatrial (VA) interval greater than 40 milliseconds were designated type B. All seven type A patients demonstrated earliest atrial activation during tachycardia in the His-bundle lead; in six of seven patients, earliest atrial activation occurred before or at the onset of the QRS complex, suggesting short conduction time in the retrograde limb of the tachycardia. In contrast, earliest atrial activation in two of the three type B patients was recorded at the proximal region of the coronary sinus. Intraoperative endocardial mapping performed during tachycardia (eight patients) or during ventricular pacing (two patients) confirmed the preoperative observations that earliest atrial activation recorded in type A patients was anterior or anteromedial to the AV node, whereas in those with type B tachycardia, earliest atrial activation was posterior to the AV node, near the orifice of the coronary sinus (Fig. 39-2).

Surgical dissection was performed in all patients and included (1) exposure of the wall of the left atrium, AV nodal artery, central fibrous body, and tendon of Todaro; (2) dissection of the medial and anteromedial approaches to the AV node in type A patients (the posterior approaches to the AV node were preserved in this group of patients); and (3) dissection of the inferior wall of the coronary sinus, with preservation of the medial approaches to the AV node in type B patients. At a mean postoperative follow-up of 8 months, no recurrences of the tachycardia were observed. Anterograde AV conduction was normal (albeit

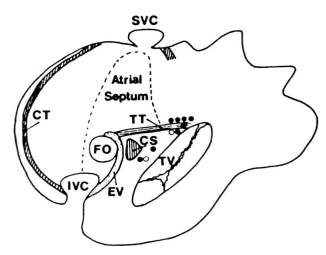

Figure 39-2. Earliest atrial activation sites obtained with right atrial endocardial intraoperative mapping. The *black dots* represent earliest atrial activation during tachycardia, and the *unfilled circles* represent earliest activation during ventricular pacing in two patients without inducible supraventricular tachycardia in the operating room. Earliest atrial sites from the type A patients were clustered at a site anterior or anteromedial to the atrioventricular node, whereas in the three type B patients, earliest atrial activation was clustered near the coronary sinus. *CS,* coronary sinus; *CT,* crista terminalis; *EV,* eustachian valve; *FO,* foramen ovale; *IVC,* inferior vena cava; *SVC,* superior vena cava; *TT,* tendon of Todaro; *TV,* tricuspid valve. (Ross DL, Johnson DC, Denniss R, et al: Curative surgery for atrioventricular junctional [AV nodal] reentrant tachycardia. J Am Coll Cardiol 1985;6:1383.)

with a slightly longer AH interval) in all patients; conduction over the anterograde "slow" pathway was abolished in five. In addition, retrograde VA conduction was preserved in the type A patients, although a prolongation of the retrograde His-to-atrium interval was documented in four of seven patients. In contrast, VA conduction was interrupted in two of three type B patients and significantly modified in the third.

The encouraging results of these preliminary reports were extended in a subsequent report from the same Australian group, portending a possible curative surgical option to patients with troublesome AV junctional reciprocating tachycardia.[16] These expectations were confirmed in later reports.[17,18] Cox and colleagues describe an elegant cryosurgical approach to the treatment of AV nodal reciprocating tachycardia.[17] This approach was based on experimental animal work, which had previously demonstrated that discrete cryolesions placed around the triangle of Koch were capable of prolonging AV conduction without creating complete heart block.[19] Experimental animal studies had also shown that discrete cryosurgical lesions were capable of selectively ablating only one of the pathways of conduction in animals having dual AV nodal pathways, thereby leaving AV conduction intact while interrupting the electrophysiologic milieu for reciprocating tachycardia.[20]

All of the eight patients described by Cox and associates had readily inducible tachycardia, which met the conventional electrophysiologic criteria for AV nodal reentrant tachycardia. Intraoperative electrophysiologic techniques differ from those of Ross and coworkers because no electrophysiologic mapping is performed in this operation. Instead, after normothermic cardiopulmonary bypass is instituted and a right atriotomy performed, the His bundle is identified and atrial pacing is instituted and the AV interval constantly monitored. Cryothermia is applied to about nine sites (Fig. 39-3), starting with the tendon of Todaro at the upper edge of the os of the coronary sinus. In this study, prolongation of the AV interval usually occurred during application of cryothermia at sites 7 or 8, at which time a linear prolongation of the AV interval is recorded and cryothermia is promptly terminated at the inception of complete heart block. The AV block thus produced is temporary and cryothermia is repeated at a slightly more peripheral site. After encircling the AV node with the 9 cryolesion sites, cryolesions are also placed within the triangle of Koch, again avoiding the creation of complete heart block. Thus, the objective of the operation is to cryoablate as much of the perinodal tissue as possible without causing permanent AV conduction block.[17]

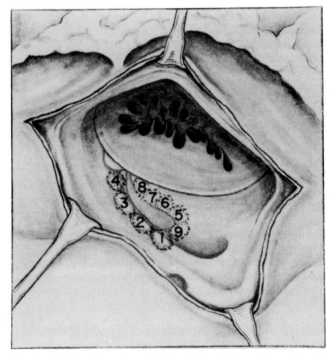

Figure 39-3. Sites of application of cryolesions. (From Cox JL, Holman WL, Cain ME: Cryosurgical treatment of atrioventricular node reentrant tachycardia. Circulation 1987;76:1329.)

This surgical approach effected a permanent cure of the tachycardia in all eight patients. Postoperative electrophysiologic measurements revealed no significant changes in anterograde AV conduction and the abolition of the typical discontinuous AV conduction curves seen before surgery. Moreover, VA conduction was eliminated in two patients but was essentially unchanged in the remaining six patients. Most importantly, none of the patients developed complete heart block or required permanent pacing.

The electrophysiologic data available from this study suggest that the cryosurgery eliminated anterograde conduction over the slow pathway in all patients and also eliminated "fast" retrograde conduction in the two patients who post-operatively had absent retrograde VA conduction. The anatomic correlates to the electrophysiologic observations of Cox and colleagues and Ross and associates are not yet definitive and are possibly contradictory. For example, if the fast pathway is the more anterior of the two (as suggested by Ross and coworkers and by preliminary catheter ablative reports), why was retrograde conduction eliminated by *posterior* dissection in two thirds of the patients in Ross and associates' study? Similarly, if cryolesions eliminated only the anterograde slow pathway in Cox and colleagues' study, why were both retrograde pathways eliminated in two of the patients (i.e., are the anterograde and retrograde atrial insertions of these pathways separate?). Although neither study can answer these kinds of questions, the pioneering results of Ross and coworkers and Cox and associates certainly suggest that perinodal atrial tissue is likely to be critical for the initiation and perpetuation of AV nodal reciprocating tachycardia.

EXCISION OR CRYOABLATION OF ARRHYTHMOGENIC ATRIAL FOCI

One of the earliest successful surgical series of excision or cryoablation of atrial tissue responsible for medically refractory atrial tachycardia was reported by Gillette and coworkers in 1981.[21] Three children with automatic ectopic atrial tachycardia were treated in this study. The diagnosis of "automatic" tachycardia was based on conventional clinical electrophysiologic definitions that included the inability to initiate or terminate the tachycardia with programmed electric stimulation, "resetting" of the tachycardia after atrial premature extrastimuli, and observation of a "warm-up" phenomenon at the onset of a paroxysm of the tachycardia. Preoperative and intraoperative mapping localized two of these tachycardias to the left atrium and one to the right atrial appendage. The left atrial foci were ablated with endocardial and epicardial application of a cryoprobe during cardiopulmonary bypass; the right atrial tachycardia was cured with excision of the anterior third of the right atrial appendage and cryoblation of the surgical margins. Cardiopulmonary bypass was not needed during the surgery performed on the right atrial tachycardia.

Wyndham and associates report the surgical treatment of a patient with drug-resistant atrial tachycardia that appeared to have a reentrant mechanism because induction and termination of the tachycardia could reliably perform in the electrophysiology laboratory.[22] Endocardial and epicardial mapping performed in the operating room localized the site of origin of the atrial tachycardia to the posterolateral lip of the right atrial appendage. This region was excised, and the atrial tachycardia was no longer inducible. Interestingly, microelectrode studies of the atrial tissue removed during surgery demonstrated a low resting membrane potential and after the application of electric stimuli, delayed afterdepolarization. The latter was large enough to attain threshold and produced a sustained rhythm that was terminated with electric stimuli. This may have been the first clinical observation of triggered automaticity in humans and points to the difficulty of assigning an electrophysiologic mechanism to a tachycardia by its response to programmed electric stimulation.

Still another example of surgical excision of an atrial tachycardia (probably automatic in mechanism) is reported by Josephson and colleagues.[23] The site of origin of this tachycardia was at the posterior lip of the fossa ovalis (Fig. 39-4) and necessitated resection of part of the atrial

septum in addition to placement of a Dacron patch. Interestingly, the excised tissue contained a proliferation of mesenchymal cells, suggesting that a mesenchymal atrial tumor may have been responsible for the clinical tachycardia.

Newer surgical reports have been published that attest to the efficacy of direct surgical treatment of drug refractory atrial focal tachycardia.[16,18,24] The site of origin of the tachycardias appears to be almost always in the right atrium. In the series of eight patients reported by Seals and coworkers, seven of eight patients had an arrhythmia that was initiated with programmed atrial stimulation and was therefore assumed to be reentrant in mechanism.[24] Curiously, all were drug-refractory.

Other studies support the preponderance of right atrial focal tachycardias. For example, the clinical and electrophysiologic characteristics of sustained intraatrial reentrant tachycardia is described by Haines and colleagues.[25] The diagnosis of reentry was based on the ability to terminate the tachycardia with pacing in all patients and to initiate it in eight of 19 patients. In contrast to the surgical series, drug suppression of the tachycardia was achieved in 17 of 19 patients, and catheter-induced high-grade AV block was performed in the remaining two. As in the surgical series, the site of tachycardia was almost always in the right atrium (14 of 15 patients in whom a site was determined). A likely conclusion from these data is that the clinical spectrum of response to antiarrhythmic drugs in patients with atrial tachycardias (particularly

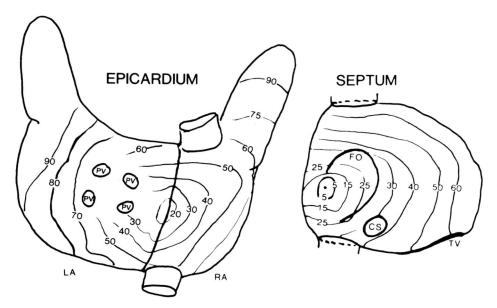

Figure 39-4. Epicardial and endocardial activation maps in an arrhythmia possibly caused by an atrial tumor. *CS*, coronary sinus; *FO*, fossa ovalis; *LA*, left atrium; *PV*, pulmonary veins; *RA*, right atrium; *TV*, tricuspid valve. (Josephson ME, Spear JF, Harken AH, et al: Surgical excision of automatic atrial tachycardia. Am Heart J 1982;104:1076.)

when reentrant in mechanism) is wide; furthermore, physicians probably emphasize the newest modality of therapy available to them (whether it be surgery or catheter ablation), particularly when faced with the prospect of offering long-term antiarrhythmic drug therapy to young patients.

The surgical procedures used in the treatment of patients with focal atrial tachycardia depend on the location and number of arrhythmic foci. For example, Lawrie and associates describe techniques that include simple direct surgical excision of right atrial muscle without cardiopulmonary bypass (Fig. 39-5) and epicardial cryoablation of atrial tissue in the normothermic atrium, again without bypass.[18] Of the four patients who had epicardial cryoablation *alone*, however, two required reoperation because of recurrence of the arrhythmia. These authors also describe wide excision of right atrial muscle under cardiopulmonary bypass and replacement of atrial tissue by Gore-Tex patch grafts (Fig. 39-6).

Several important conclusions can be drawn from the works of the authors cited above. First, subtotal right atrial resection is hemodynamically well-tolerated and offers good long-term results. Second, epicardial cryoablation appears to be relatively unreliable as the sole surgical treatment; therefore, the surgical procedure should include extensive atrial excision in most cases. Finally, focal atrial tachycardia frequently involves more than one arrhythmogenic focus and may be associated with several arrhythmia mechanisms (e.g., accessory pathways or AV nodal reciprocating tachycardia), thus necessitating careful preoperative and intraoperative electrophysiologic studies to eliminate all potential tachycardias.

Surgical therapy has also been applied to a relatively unusual variant of ectopic atrial tachycardia, namely, sino-atrial reentrant tachycardia. Kerr and associates describe a 42-year-old woman who had a chronic tachycardia that was shown at electrophysiologic study to originate in the high anterolateral right atrium.[26] Intraoperative epicardial mapping confirmed that earliest atrial activation was at the junction of the high right atrium and superior vena cava (i.e., near the anatomic location of the sinus node). A series of cryosurgical lesions was applied to the sites of earliest atrial activation, forming a cuff around the region of the sinus node and effecting essentially the exclusion of the sinus node region from the remainders of the right atrium. A similar operation was described by Lawrie and colleagues and is shown in Figure 39-7.[18] In our experience, a useful intraoperative mapping maneuver in such cases is the search for the sinus node electrogram during epicardial mapping, which allows precise localization of the sinus node during normal sinus rhythm.[27]

Postoperatively, the patient described by Kerr and coworkers had a stable atrial rhythm originating in the low right atrium. This is consistent with our experience and that of others who have found that after surgical exclusion or excision of the sinus node, a relatively stable low right atrial rhythm is likely to emerge and assume a dominant pacemaking role.[28–30] Although usually reliable and responsive to autonomic changes, this new focus may occasionally fail, as was evidenced by Kerr's patient, who at 12 months after surgery required insertion of a permanent atrial pacemaker because of symptomatic intermittent pauses in atrial rhythm.

Resectable atrial tachycardias may also arise from sites of previous cardiac surgery. We have performed intraoperative epicardial mapping in a patient 60 years of age, referred because of drug-refractory recurrent supraventricular tachycardia. Twenty-five years before the hos-

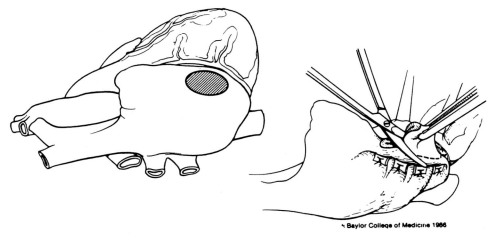

↖ Baylor College of Medicine 1986

Figure 39-5. Localization and excision of right atrial tachycardia focus. Note that the excision is performed in the closed heart. (From Lawrie GM, Lin HT, Wyndham CRC, DeBakey ME: Surgical treatment of supraventricular arrhythmias. Ann Surg 1987;205:700.)

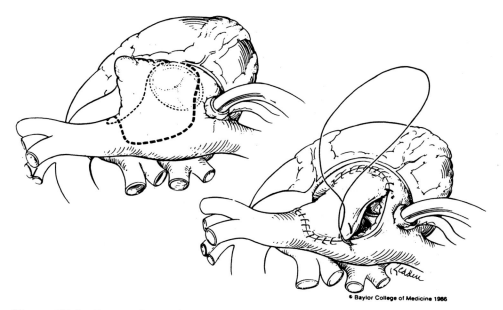

Figure 39-6. Excision of upper half of the right atrium in a patient with multiple tachycardia foci. *Light dashed line* represents intraatrial incision. *Heavy line* represents atrial free wall excision. A Gore-Tex patch is used to replace excised tissue. (From Lawrie GM, Lin HT, Wyndham CRC, DeBakey ME: Surgical treatment of supraventricular arrhythmias. Ann Surg 1987;205:700.)

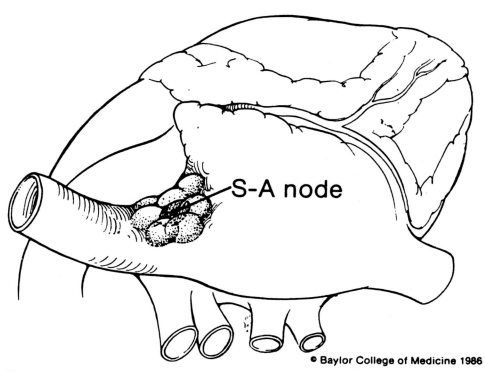

Figure 39-7. Cryothermic technique can be applied to patients with sinoatrial reentrant rhythms. The sinus node region is surrounded by cryolesions and becomes electrically excluded. (From Lawrie GM, Lin HT, Wyndham CRC, DeBakey ME: Surgical treatment of supraventricular arrhythmias. Ann Surg 1987;205:700.)

pital admission for this procedure, the patient had undergone repair of an atrial septal defect. The patient's poor response to all available antiarrhythmic medications (including amiodarone), coupled with demonstration of a moderate-sized septal defect, prompted surgical intervention. Intraoperative epicardial mapping during the patient's atrial tachycardia suggested a macroreentrant circuit around the superior vena cava (Fig. 39-8). Unidirectional conduction block appeared to occur at the lateral margin of the right atrium, immediately adjacent to the earliest site of atrial activation during tachycardia, and corresponded to the site of extensive scarring from the previous atriotomy. Cryoblation was performed at the sites of earliest and latest activation. Postoperatively, the patient has had no recurrences of the atrial tachycardia, although episodes of atrial fibrillation have been recorded.

SURGICAL EXCLUSION OF ATRIAL TACHYCARDIA

Atrial tachyarrhythmias are occasionally encountered that are located in parts of the atria that are not resectable (e.g., the left atrium near one of the pulmonary veins). Also, as noted, right atrial tachycardias may be multifocal in origin and not amenable to isolated cryolesions or multiple excision maneuvers. Work performed by Williams and colleagues in dogs suggests that the left atrium can be safely excluded surgically.[31] While the left atrium is thereby electrically isolated from the rest of the heart (and remains either electrically silent or develops a slow intrinsic rhythm), normal AV conduction is maintained from the right atrium and no adverse hemodynamic effects are associated with loss of a synchronous left atrial contraction.

Similar reasoning led to the development of a right atrial isolation surgical technique.[32] This technique results in the electrical isolation of the body of the right atrium but with maintenance of continuity between a normally functioning sinus node and the left atrium and preservation of normal atrioventricular conduction. The procedure involves a posterolateral right atriotomy that encircles the upper right atrium but excludes the sinus node region. The incision is extended anteromedially to the tricuspid valve anulus and inferiorly just posterior to the the os of the coronary sinus. Postoperative stimulation of atrial tachycardia shows confinement of the tachycardia to the isolated right atrium, without propagation to the left atrium or to the ventricles (Fig. 39-9). Postoperative hemodynamic measurements also demonstrate that the right atrial isolation procedure does not adversely affect cardiac hemodynamics, despite the loss of synchronous right atrial contraction during sinus rhythm.[33] Actually, during simulated (paced) right atrial tachycardia, cardiac performance was superior when the involved atrial segment was isolated, compared with when it was in continuity with the rest of the heart.

These experimental surgical principles were applied by Anderson and associates to a patient having a paroxysmal atrial tachycardia localized to the junction of the right superior pulmonary vein and left atrium.[34] Surgical isolation of the portion of the left atrium containing the point of earliest atrial activation and both right pulmonary veins was effected by an encircling incision, with the edges then being reapproximated.

Postoperatively, the patient had a sinus rhythm (sinus tachycardia) with 1:1 AV conduction, whereas the isolated left atrial tissue had a slow independent rate that was not conducted to the right atrium or to the ventricles.

LONG-TERM FOLLOW-UP AFTER SURGERY FOR ECTOPIC ATRIAL RHYTHMS

Because the surgical techniques described above are new and the number of patients few, "long-term" follow-up is a relative descriptor. As such, the largest series of patients with surgically treated ectopic atrial tachycardias followed-

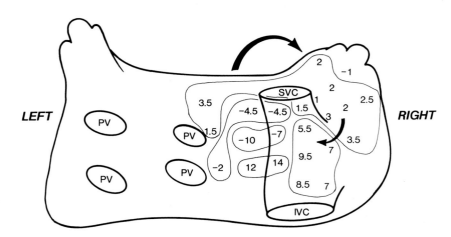

Figure 39-8. Epicardial activation map obtained during atrial tachycardia, showing a posterior unfolded view of the atria. Local epicardial activation times are shown in milliseconds. Earliest epicardial activation was 10 milliseconds before activation of the right atrial reference electrode and was located at the posterolateral right atrium. Unidirectional block appears to occur at the recording sites caudal to the earliest site; atrial activation follows the clockwise sequence shown. Extensive atrial scarring from previous surgery was noted along the lateral margin of the right atrium. *PV*, pulmonary veins; *SVC*, superior vena cava; *IVC*, inferior vena cava.

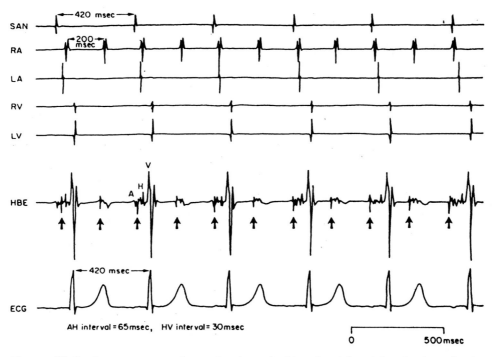

Figure 39-9. Postoperative simulation of tachycardia. Note that right atrial pacing is confined to right atrium and does not affect sinus rhythm or normal conduction. *SAN*, sinus node; *RA*, right atrium; *LA*, left atrium; *RV* and *LV*, right and left ventricles; *HBE*; His bundle electrogram. (From Williams JM, Ungerieder RM, Loftland GK, et al: Left atrial isolated, new technique for the treatment of supraventricular arrhythmias. J Thorac Cardiovasc Surg 1980;80:373.)

up for the longest period after operative therapy was published.[35] Of 15 patients with these tachycardias, 10 were sent to surgery because an effective antiarrhythmic regimen could not be identified. In the operating room, computer-aided mapping was performed and focal ablation (including excision and cryoablation) was performed in four patients; six patients underwent atrial isolation procedures. At a mean follow-up period of 4 years, ectopic atrial tachycardia recurred in only one patient. Two patients also required permanent pacemaker insertion because of severe sinus node dysfunction. In contrast, ectopic atrial tachycardia recurred in three of the five patients treated medically during a mean follow-up period of about 6 years. Certainly in the hands of this surgical team, surgery was an effective long-term option for those patients having atrial arrhythmias difficult to treat with antiarrhythmic medications.

SURGERY FOR ATRIAL FIBRILLATION

A most innovative approach to an exceedingly common clinical problem was developed during the past several years by a most innovative surgeon, James Cox.[36–40] Atrial fibrillation has been estimated to occur in about 0.4% of the population of the United States.[35] Epidemiologic studies performed before the widespread use of aspirin or warfarin in patients with atrial fibrillation indicate that the yearly incidence of significant cerebroembolic events in the United States is about 150,000.[41] Clearly this is a problem of enormous clinical magnitude. To date, the usual medical approach has consisted of antiarrhythmic drug administration and some form of anticoagulation therapy. Advances in catheter ablative therapy have also allowed control of rapid heart rate by the nonsurgical creation of complete heart block, with subsequent dependence (to variable degrees) on a permanent pacemaker.

Previous surgical approaches devised for the control of atrial fibrillation were somewhat limited and did not gain a significant following. The first, a left atrial isolation procedure described above, has the disadvantage of leaving the patient prone to thromboembolic events because the left atrium continues to either fibrillate or remains electrically silent.[31]

A second surgical approach to the treatment of atrial fibrillation was first described by Guiraudon and colleagues and dubbed the "atrial corridor" technique.[42] A long-term follow-up study (average, 20 months) was provided by the same group and affords a basis for evaluation of this technique.[43] The surgery consists of two essential maneuvers: (1) disconnection of the left atrial free wall from its attachment to the atrial septum, and (2) the creation of an electrically isolated right atrial strip (corridor), connecting the sinus node region to the region of the AV node (anterior to the orifice of the coronary sinus).

Although the authors were justifiably pleased with their results—seven of nine patients remained free of symptomatic atrial fibrillation at follow-up—attention must be drawn to several significant drawbacks to this technique. First, at predischarge electrophysiologic study, the electrically excluded left atria were still fibrillating in five of the nine patients. Second, permanent ventricular pacemakers were implanted in four patients who manifested severe sinus node dysfunction postoperatively. Finally, hemodynamic data or descriptions of the presence or absence of atrial contraction in nonfibrillating atria were not provided. Therefore, it may be concluded that the corridor procedure may leave the left atria fibrillating, with all of the attendant thromboembolic and hemodynamic consequences unaltered; it may also significantly alter sinus node function, thereby requiring permanent ventricular pacing. Inasmuch as similar results can be achieved by simple catheter ablation of the AV nodal region with catheter ablative techniques without thoracotomy, this technique appears to have relatively little appeal for most patients.

The shortcomings of the existing medical and surgical alternatives to the treatment of atrial fibrillation led to the development of the "maze procedure" by Cox and colleagues.[36–40,44] Based on extensive animal and human intraoperative mapping experiments, it was concluded that atrial flutter usually is caused by a single relatively large reentrant circuit and that atrial fibrillation may also occasionally be caused by a single reentrant circuit as well as by multiple reentrant loops. Furthermore, as had been previously proposed by others, anatomic obstacles such as the pulmonary veins and the inferior and superior vena cava were involved in some circuits; in other cases, reentry occurred in the absence of anatomic barriers and was presumably due to functional conduction blocks, which may be caused by chemically produced inhomogeneity in local refractory periods, for example.

The maze procedure has earned this sobriquet because it is based on the concept of creating multiple blind alleys for the electric impulse to traverse, thus preserving atrial myocardial contraction and transport but at the same time interrupting the conduction routes of the most common reentrant pathways and generally making it impossible for large macroreentrant circuits to exist. The procedure is schematically illustrated in Figures 39-10 and 39-11. As shown, both appendages are excised and the pulmonary veins are surgically isolated. The sinoatrial nodal impulse propagates posteriorly and inferiorly and then traverses the right atrium anteriorly. Propagation to the left atrium follows, with concomitant penetration of the septum in an anteroposterior direction beneath the septal portion of the incision. The left atrial wavefront continues around the base of the lateral left atrium onto the posterior surface of the left atrium, whereon it is blocked from further propagation by the left atrial incisions. Concomitantly, the septal impulse spreads to the posterior surfaces of the left and right atria and is also blocked from further propagation.

The first seven patients to undergo the maze procedure had good clinical outcomes; all patients were free of atrial fibrillation at follow-up periods ranging from 2 months to 2.5 years.[39] The series was expanded to 22

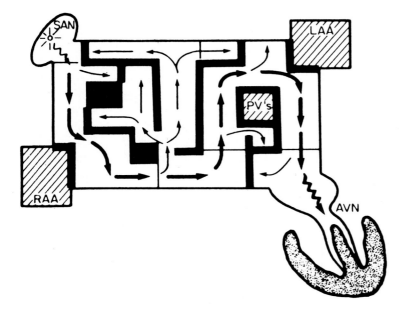

Figure 39-10. Schematic description of maze procedure. *RAA*, right atrial appendage; *LAA*, left atrial appendage; *SAN*, sinoatrial node; *AVN*, atrioventricular node. (From Cox JL, Schuessler RB, D'Agostino HJ, et al: The surgical treatment of atrial fibrillation. III. Development of a definitive surgical procedure. J Thorac Cardiovasc Surg 1991;101:569.)

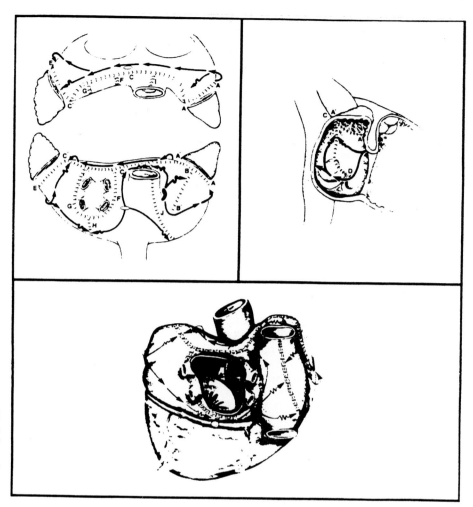

Figure 39-11. Two-dimensional and three-dimensional representations of the maze procedure. (From Cox JL, Schuessler RB, D'Agostino HJ, et al: The surgical treatment of atrial fibrillation. III. Development of a definitive surgical procedure. J Thorac Cardiovasc Surg 1991;101:569.)

patients and subsequently also reported.[44] All patients survived the surgery, with three having late occurrences of atrial flutter at 5, 6 and 15 months postoperatively. The atrial flutter proved responsive to a single antiarrhythmic agent. Echocardiographic studies have been performed in all patients and atrial transport function appears to have been preserved in all. Nine of these[22] patients required implantation of permanent pacemakers before hospital discharge. In the remainder, normal AV conduction appears to have been maintained.

This surgery appears to hold great promise for the treatment of patients who are particularly troubled by recurrent atrial fibrillation or by thromboembolic episodes related to this arrhythmia. It has the added advantage of not requiring intraoperative mapping and localization of an arrhythmogenic circuit or focus because the procedure is performed in the same manner in each patient. The obvious drawbacks of the procedure are its relative complexity and the need for a surgical sophistication and temperament that may not be possessed by many

surgeons other than the creator of the procedure. Within the next several years, the true role of this type of surgery in the management of patients with atrial fibrillation will become evident.

CONCLUSION

Important strides have been made in the surgical treatment of recalcitrant supraventricular tachyarrhythmias that are not related to the preexcitation syndromes. Many of the new surgical procedures offer the patient the prospect of surgical cure and freedom from troublesome and frequently dangerous pharmacologic agents.

The burgeoning catheter ablative option is likely to make the number of patients referred for surgical therapy of atrial arrhythmias smaller each year. Nonetheless, it remains likely that the surgical approach will continue to play a role in the management of at least some patients who have particularly obdurate atrial tachyarrhythmias.

References

1. Bauernfeind RA, Wyndham CR, Dhingra RC, et al: Serial electrophysiologic testing of multiple drugs in patients with atrioventricular nodal reentrant paroxysmal tachycardia. Circulation 1980;62:1341.

2. Marcus FI, Fontaine GH, Frank R, Grosgoeat Y: Clinical pharmacology and therapeutic applications of the antiarrhythmic agent, amiodarone. Am Heart J 1981;101:480.

3. Haffajee CI, Love JC, Canada AT, et al: Clinical pharmacokinetics and efficacy of amiodarone for refractory tachyarrhythmias. Circulation 1983;67:1347.

4. Roden DM, Woosley RL: Flecainide. N Engl J Med 1986; 315:36.

5. Funk-Brentano C, Kroemer HK, Lee JT, Roden DM: Propafenone. N Engl J Med 1990;322:518.

6. Bigger JT: Effect of atrial tachyarrhythmias and atrial pacing on supraventricular tissues. Pacing Clin Electrophysiol 1984;7:483.

7. Sealy WC, Gallagher JJ, Kasell J: His bundle interruption of control of inappropriate ventricular responses to atrial arrhythmias. Ann Thorac Surg 1981;32:429.

8. Sealy WC: When is surgery indicated for control of supraventricular tachycardia? Am J Surg 1983;145:711.

9. Garcia R, Arciniegas E: Recurrent atrial flutter: treatment with a surgically induced atrioventricular block and ventricular pacing. Arch Intern Med 1973;132:754.

10. Gooch AS, Jan MA, Fernandez J, et al: Uncontrolled tachycardia in atrial fibrillation. Management by surgical ligature of AV bundle and pacemaker. Ann Thorac Surg 1974;17:181.

11. Harrison L, Gallagher JJ, Kasell J, et al: Cryosurgical ablation of the AV node-His bundle, a new method for producing AV block. Circulation 1977;55:463.

12. Klein GJ, Sealy WC, Pritchett ELC, et al: Cryosurgical ablation of the atrioventricular node-His bundle: long-term follow-up and properties of the juntional pacemaker. Circulation 1980;61:8.

13. Pritchett ELC, Anderson RW, Benditt DG, et al: Reentry within the atrioventricular node: surgical cure with the atrioventricular conduction. Circulation 1979;60:440.

14. Marquez-Montes J, Rufilanchas JJ, Esteve JJ, et al: Paroxysmal nodal reentrant tachycardia, surgical cure. Chest 1983; 83:690.

15. Ross DL, Johnson DC, Denniss R, et al: Curative surgery for atrioventricular junctional (AV nodal) reentrant tachycardia. J Am Coll Cardiolol 1985;6:1383.

16. Johnson DC, Nunn GR, Richards DA, Uther JB, Ross DL: Surgical therapy for supraventricular tachycardia, a potentially curable disorder. J Thorac Cardiovasc Surg 1987; 93:913.

17. Cox JL, Holman WL, Cain ME: Cryosurgical treatment of atrioventricular node reentrant tachycardia. Circulation 1987;76:1329.

18. Lawrie GM, Lin HT, Wyndham CRC, DeBakey ME: Surgical treatment of supraventricular arrhythmias. Ann Surg 1987; 205:700.

19. Holman WL, Ikeshita M, Lease JG, Smith PK, Ferguson TB, Cox JL: Elective prolongation of AV conduction by multiple cryolesions. J Thorac Cardiovasc Surg 1982;84:554.

20. Holman WL, Ikeshita M, Lease JG, Smith PK, Lofland GK, Cox JL: Cryosurgical modification of retrograde atrioventricular conduction. Implications for the surgical treatment of atrioventricular nodal reentrant tachycardia. J Thorac Cardiovasc Surg 1986;91:826.

21. Gillette PC, Garson A, Hesslien PS, et al: Successful surgical treatment of atrial, junctional and ventricular tachycardia unassociated with accessory connections in infants and children. Am Heart J 1981;102:984.

22. Wyndham CRC, Arnsdorf MF, Levitsky S, et al: Successful surgical excision of focal paroxysmal atrial tachycardia, observations in vivo and in vitro. Circulation 1980;62:1365.

23. Josephson ME, Spear JF, Harken AH, et al: Surgical excision of automatic atrial tachycardia. Am Heart J 1982;104:1076.

24. Seals AA, Lawrie GM, Magro S, et al: Surgical treatment of right atrial focal tachycardia in adults. J Am Coll Cardiol 1988;11:1111.

25. Haines DE, DiMarco JP: Sustained intraatrial reentrant tachycardia: clinical, electrocardiographic and electrophysiologic characteristics and log-term follow-up. J Am Coll Cardiol 1990;15:1345.

26. Kerr CR, Klein GG, Guiraudon GM, Webb JG: Surgical therapy for sinoatrial reentrant tachycardia. Pacing Clin Electrophysiol 1988;11:776.

27. Reiffel JA, Gang ES, Gliklich J, et al: The human sinus node electrogram: a transvenous catheter technique and comparison of directly measured and indirectly estimated sinoatrial conduction time in adults. Circulation 1980;62:1324.

28. Sealy WC, Seabber AV: Cardiac rhythm following exclusion the sinoatrial node and most of the right atrium form the remainder of the heart. J Thorac Cardiovasc Surg 1979; 77:436.

29. Sealy WC, Seaber AV: Surgical isolation of the atrial septum from the atria: Identification of an atrial septal pacemaker. J Thorac Cardiovasc Surg 1980;80:742.

30. Randall WC, Wehrmacher WH, Jones SB: Hierarchy of supraventricular pacemaker. J Thorac Cardiovasc Surg 1981; 82:797.

31. Williams JM, Ungerieder RM, Loftland GK, et al: Left atrial isolated, new technique for the treatment of supraventricular arrhythmias. J Thorac Cardiovasc Surg 1980;80:373.

32. Harada A, D'Agostino HJ, Schuessler RB, Boineau JP, Cox JL: Right atrial isolation: a new surgical treatment for supraventricular tachycardia (I). J Thorac Cardiovasc Surg 1988; 95:643.

33. Harada A, D'Agostino HJ, Boineau JP, Cox JL: Right atrial isolation etc. (II). J Thorac Cardiovasc Surg 1988;95:651.

34. Anderson KP, Stinson EB, Mason JW: Surgical exclusion of focal paroxysmal atrial tachycardia. Am J Cardiol 1982; 49:869.

35. Prager NA, Cox JL, Lindsay BD, Ferguson TB, Osborn JL, Cain ME: Long-term effectiveness of surgical treatment of ectopic atrial tachycardia. J Am Coll Cardiol 1993;22:85.

36. Cox JL, Schuessler RB, Cain ME, et al: Surgery for atrial fibrillation. Semin Thorac Cardiovasc Surg 1989;1(1):67.

37. Cox JL, Schuessler RB, Boineau JP: The surgical treatment of atrial fibrillation. I. Summary of the current concepts of the mechanisms of atrial flutter and atrial fibrillation. J Thorac Cardiovasc Surg 1991;101:402.

38. Cox JL, Canavan TE, Schuessler RB, et al: The surgical treatment of atrial fibrillation II. Intraoperative electrophysiologic mapping and description of the electrophysiologic basis of atrial flutter and atrial fibrillation. J Thorac Cardiovasc Surg 1991;101:406.

39. Cox JL, Schuessler RB, D'Agostino HJ, et al: The surgical treatment of atrial fibrillation. III. Development of a definitive surgical procedure. J Thorac Cardiovasc Surg 1991; 101:569.

40. Cox JL: The surgical treatment of atrial fibrillation IV. Surgical technique. J Thorac Cardiovasc Surg 1991;101:584.

41. Fisher CM: Embolism in atrial fibrillation. In: Kulbertus HE, Olsson SB, Schlepper M, eds. Atrial Fibrillation. Molndal, Sweden: AB Hassle, 1982:192.

42. Guiraudon GM, Campbell CS, Jones DL, et al: Combined sino-atrial node atrio-ventricular node isolation: a surgical alternative to His bundle ablation in patients with atrial fibrillation. Circulation 1985;72:III.

43. Leitch JW, Klein G, Yee R, Guiraudon G: Sinus node-atrioventricular node isolation: long-term results with the "corridor" operation for atrial fibrillation. J Am Coll Cardiol 1991;17:970.

44. Cox JL, Boineau JP, Schessler RB, et al: Successful surgical treatment of atrial fibrillation: review and clinical update. JAMA 1991;266:1976.

Cardiac Arrhythmias, 3rd edition, edited by William J. Mandel.
J. B. Lippincott Company, Philadelphia © 1995.

40

T. Bruce Ferguson Jr. • James L. Cox

Surgical Management of the Wolff-Parkinson-White Syndrome

The development of the surgical techniques for ablation of accessory atrioventricular (AV) pathways responsible for the AV tachycardias associated with the Wolff-Parkinson-White (WPW) syndrome represents a milestone in the history of cardiac surgery. Without the 25 years of experience, insight, and knowledge gained by the surgical treatment of this arrhythmia, it is doubtful that the developments that resulted in the radiofrequency ablation techniques that are first-line therapy for this arrhythmia could have occurred. Knowledge of these historical, anatomic, and electrophysiologic developments should serve as points of reference well into the future—for radiofrequency ablation techniques and results and for those few patients who still require definitive surgical intervention for this problem.

This chapter is designed to provide the reader with a basic understanding of the surgical electrophysiology and techniques that have been and are being used in the surgical treatment of WPW syndrome.

HISTORICAL ASPECTS

Kent first demonstrated muscular connections between the atria and the ventricles of mammals in 1893 and erroneously concluded that those connections were multiple,

always located on the right side of the heart, and represented the normal pathways of AV conduction.[1] In 1906, Tawara, working in Aschoff's laboratory, described the true anatomy and physiology of the specialized conduction system of the heart by identifying and characterizing the AV node, His bundle, bundle branches, and the Purkinje system.[2] In the same year, Keith and Flack identified the sinoatrial node as the heart's normal pacemaker, thus completing the elucidation of the normal conduction system as we know it.[3]

During the 1920s, Paul Dudley White, one of the great teachers and clinical cardiologists of this century, noted that a small group of young, apparently normal patients with ventricular preexcitation on their standard electrocardiograms (ECGs) had frequent bouts of paroxysmal tachycardia. During a trip to London, he discovered that John Parkinson, an English physician, had collected a similar series of patients. White suggested that Louis Wolff, one of White's fellows, combine his and Parkinson's series of patients and report their observations, which Wolff did in 1930.[4] Although the authors did not understand the anatomic basis of the abnormal ECG in these patients, they pointed out that such ECG abnormalities were frequently associated with sudden bouts of tachycardia. It remained for Wolferth and Wood to suggest in 1933 and prove in 1943 that the ECG patterns in patients with WPW syndrome were due to accessory anatomic connections between the atrium and ventricle similar to those previously described by Kent.[5,6]

Despite the observations of Wolferth and Wood, the electrophysiologic basis for WPW syndrome remained controversial for several decades, even though Durrer and Roos demonstrated eccentric electric conduction across the AV groove by intraoperative mapping of a patient with WPW syndrome in 1967.[7] Final confirmation of the anatomic–electrophysiologic basis for WPW syndrome was provided in the late 1960s. Boineau and Moore performed epicardial mapping in animals with WPW syndrome and documented the presence of an anatomic accessory AV connection located at the precise site of ventricular preexcitation.[8] Subsequently, Burchell and colleagues temporarily ameliorated WPW syndrome at the time of surgery by injecting procainamide into the AV groove at the site of ventricular preexcitation in a patient undergoing surgery for an atrial septal defect.[9] Although conduction across the accessory AV connection resumed postoperatively, Burchell's experience confirmed that surgical intervention in these patients was feasible. Shortly thereafter, Sealy and associates successfully divided an accessory pathway in a patient with WPW syndrome and thereby initiated the new field of cardiac arrhythmia surgery.[10]

Since Sealy's original operative success, the surgical techniques for the treatment of WPW syndrome have continued to evolve into the two primary contemporary surgical techniques: the endocardial approach and the epicardial approach.

ANATOMIC AND ELECTROPHYSIOLOGIC BASIS FOR THE WOLFF-PARKINSON-WHITE SYNDROME

Anatomic Considerations

Histologically, the accessory AV connections (accessory pathways) characteristic of WPW syndrome have the appearance of normal atrial muscle; specifically, they do not resemble either the specialized conduction system or nerve tissue. Embryologically, they are thought to represent aberrant persistence of AV ring tissue that connects the atria to the ventricles across the AV groove in the developing heart and for a short period after birth, normally regressing during the maturation process of the fibrous skeleton of the heart.[11] Accessory pathways may be located anywhere in the AV groove around the base of the heart except that region between the left fibrous trigone and the right fibrous trigone (Fig. 40-1). Because this region of the fibrous skeleton of the heart represents the site where the anterior leaflet of the mitral valve is contiguous with the aortic valve anulus, there is no ventricular myocardium immediately beneath the mitral anulus in this

region. Thus, it is impossible for accessory AV connections to be located in this position.

Traditionally, the location of accessory pathways in WPW syndrome has been based on the site of insertion of the ventricular end of the pathway. This arbitrary classification of accessory pathway locations into left free wall, posteroseptal, right free wall, and anteroseptal (in decreasing order of frequency) has proved to be advantageous, not only because of the dissimilarities of the electrophysiologic manifestations of pathways in each of these four areas but also because the surgical approach to each of these four spaces is unique. The four anatomic spaces in which a given accessory pathway may reside are identified by viewing the AV groove in the *horizontal* plane (see Fig. 40-1). Both the preoperative catheter electrophysiologic study and the intraoperative mapping procedure are directed toward localizing an accessory pathway to one of these four anatomic spaces.

In addition, however, an appreciation of the potential for accessory pathways to be located at different depths in the *vertical* plane of the AV groove is necessary to understand many of the important principles that guide successful surgery for WPW syndrome.[11] Because of the anatomic limitations imposed by the valve anulus and the epicardium overlying the AV groove externally (Fig. 40-2), all accessory pathways must connect to the atrium somewhere between the valve anulus and the epicardial reflection off the atrium, and they must connect to the ventricle somewhere between the valve anulus and the epicardial reflection off the ventricle.[12] Thus, accessory pathways are confined (in the vertical plane) to locations (1) near the valve anulus, (2) within the fat pad of the AV groove, or (3) just beneath the epicardium overlying the AV groove. Success with radiofrequency ablation techniques indicates that at least on the left side, most accessory pathway connections are probably juxtaanular. The increased difficulty in ablating right-sided pathways (particularly free wall pathways) is because of the anatomic variance on the right side of the heart, both on the free wall and in the posteroseptal space.

Finally, these accessory connections can exist as broad bands of tissue, which may conduct only preferentially over a small portion of that broad band. This concept, confirmed by computerized intraoperative mapping studies, has led to wide anatomically based dissections for WPW syndrome to ablate all possible accessory AV conduction tissue during the initial operative procedure.[13,14]

Electrophysiologic Considerations

During sinus rhythm in a patient with WPW syndrome, AV conduction occurs through both the normal conduction system and the accessory pathway (Fig. 40-3A through D). Because accessory pathways do not usually exhibit the

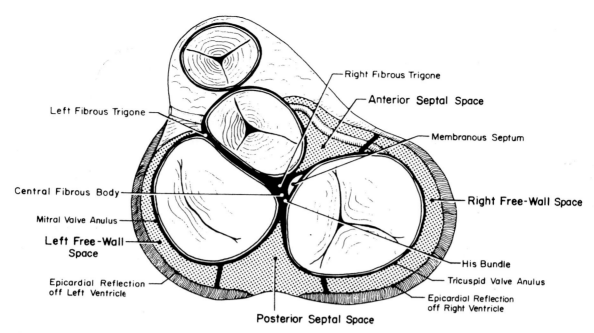

Figure 40-1. Diagram of the superior view of the heart with the atria cut away, demonstrating the boundaries of each of the four anatomic areas where accessory pathways can occur in the Wolff-Parkinson-White syndrome. The boundaries of the *left free wall* space of the mitral valve anulus and the ventricular epicardial reflection extend from the left fibrous trigone to the posterior septum. The boundaries of the *posterior septal* space are the tricuspid value anulus, the mitral value anulus, the posterior superior process of the left ventricle, and the ventricular epicardial reflection. The boundaries of the *right free wall* space are the tricuspid value anulus and the epicardial reflection, extending from the posterior septum to the anterior septum. The boundaries of the *anterior septal* space are the tricuspid value anulus, the membranous portion of the interatrial septum, and the ventricular epicardial reflection. All accessory atrioventricular connections must insert into the ventricle somewhere within these anatomic boundaries. (Modified from Cox JL, et al: Experience with 118 consecutive patients undergoing surgery for Wolff-Parkinson-White syndrome. J Thorac Cardiovasc Surg 1985;90:490)

conduction delay characteristic of the AV node, the atrial impulse reaches the ventricle first, across the accessory pathway. Thus, the earliest site of ventricular activation during normal sinus rhythm in patients with WPW syndrome is at the site of insertion of the accessory pathway into the ventricular myocardium. On the standard limb-lead ECG, this preexcitation of the ventricle causes an early deflection off the isoelectric line, the so-called delta wave. Thus, the rapid antegrade conduction across an accessory pathway with ventricular preexcitation is responsible for the three ECG findings first described by Wolff, Parkinson, and White in 1930: a short PR interval, a wide QRS complex, and a delta wave (Fig. 40-4).

Supraventricular tachycardia develops in patients with WPW syndrome when an antegrade conduction block occurs in the accessory pathway (see Fig. 40-3E). Antegrade conduction still occurs normally through the AV node–His-bundle complex, and the QRS complex on the standard ECG, for that beat is normal. As the electric impulse activates the ventricles from the apex to the base, it encounters the ventricular end of the accessory pathway,

which has not been activated. The electric impulse thus continues to propagate in a retrograde direction across the accessory pathway to reactivate the atrium. This retrograde atrial activation proceeds back into the AV node–His-bundle complex in an antegrade fashion and the reentrant circuit is completed (see Fig. 40-3F).

The most common form of tachycardia associated with WPW syndrome (reciprocating tachycardia) is that just described, in which antegrade conduction occurs through the AV node–His-bundle complex and retrograde conduction occurs across the accessory pathway. This type of reciprocating tachycardia is called orthodromic supraventricular tachycardia and is found in more than 90% of the reciprocating tachycardias associated with WPW syndrome (Fig. 40-5). Infrequently, reciprocating tachycardia may occur in patients in whom antegrade conduction occurs across accessory pathways with retrograde conduction through the AV node-His bundle complex. This reciprocating tachycardia is referred to as antidromic supraventricular tachycardia and occurs in fewer than 10% of patients with WPW syndrome.

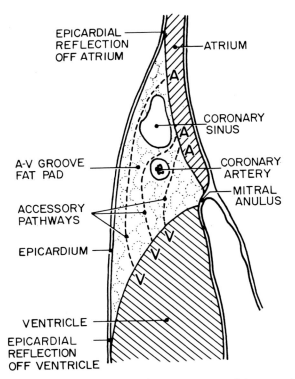

Figure 40-2. Representation of a cross-section of the posterior left heart, showing the different depths that left free wall pathways can be located in relation to the mitral anulus and the epicardium overlying the atrioventricular (AV) groove. Note that regardless of the depth of the accessory pathway in the vertical plane of the AV groove, the atrial end of the accessory pathway must attach to the atrium somewhere between the mitral valve anulus and the epicardial reflection off the atrium. Likewise, the ventricular end of the accessory pathway must connect to the ventricle somewhere between the mitral value anulus and the epicardial reflection off the ventricle. (From Cox JL, Ferguson TB Jr: Surgery for the Wolff-Parkinson-White syndrome: the endocardial approach. Semin Thorac Cardiovasc Surg 1989;1:34)

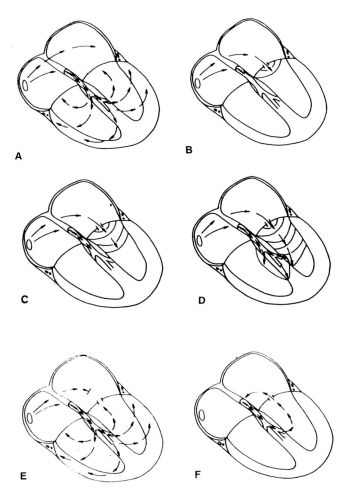

Figure 40-3. (**A**) Normal spread of electric activation in heart during sinus rhythm. Electric impulse is delayed approximately 100 milliseconds in atrioventricular node. (**B** through **D**) Spread of electric activation during sinus rhythm in Wolff-Parkinson-White syndrome, with an accessory pathway in left free wall position. (**E**) Antegrade block in the left free wall accessory pathway results in normal ventricular depolarization but permits retrograde activation of the accessory pathway. (**F**) Typical orthodromic reciprocating tachycardia in patient with Wolff-Parkinson-White syndrome. (Modified from Cox JL: The surgical management of cardiac arrhythmias. In: Sabiston DC, Spencer FC, eds. Gibbon's surgery of the chest, 5th ed Philadelphia: WB Saunders 1990)

Atrial flutter or fibrillation occurs in about 30% of patients with WPW syndrome. Depending on the conduction characteristics of the accessory pathway, the association of atrial fibrillation with WPW syndrome may be a lethal combination. If the antegrade refractory period of the accessory pathway is less than 220 milliseconds, the accessory pathway is capable of conducting the chaotic atrial electric impulses directly to the ventricles, resulting in ventricular fibrillation.[15,16] During this potentially lethal form of the WPW syndrome, the accessory pathway is activated passively and is not a direct component of the arrhythmia.

Finally, accessory pathways are classified as being either "manifest" or "concealed." Manifest pathways such as those described above are capable of conducting in both antegrade and retrograde directions. Thus, during normal sinus rhythm, the ECG is abnormal because of antegrade conduction across the accessory pathway (which preexcites the ventricles); during atrial fibrillation, the ventricles may also be vulnerable to fibrillation. Concealed accessory pathways conduct in only the retrograde (ventricular to atrial) direction. Therefore, the QRS morphology during sinus rhythm is normal; during atrial fibrillation, AV conduction occurs exclusively through the AV node–His-bundle complex. Thus, the ventricular rate response to atrial fibrillation in WPW patients with concealed accessory pathways is similar to that of patients without accessory pathways. Concealed accessory pathways comprise the retrograde limb of the reentrant circuit during orthodromic supraventricular tachycardia. In addi-

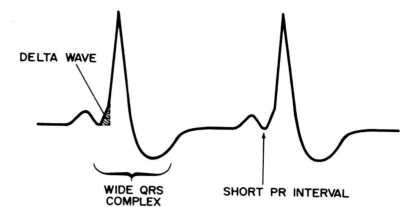

Figure 40-4. Schematic of the electrocardiogram findings in a patient with Wolff-Parkinson-White syndrome during normal sinus rhythm. (From Cox JL: Surgery for the Wolff-Parkinson-White Syndrome; the endocardial approach. Semin Thorac Cardiovasc Surg 1989;1:34)

tion, rarely they may serve as the retrograde limb during pathways.[17]

Preoperative Electrophysiologic Evaluation

All patients slated for surgery for WPW syndrome must first undergo a preoperative catheter endocardial electrophysiology study.[18] These studies should be performed by a clinical electrophysiologist, with adequate support personnel in a general electrophysiologic laboratory specially equipped for electrophysiologic studies. The recording and amplification system should be able to process both multiple intracardiac electrograms and surface ECG leads. The intracardiac signals range in amplitude from 0.50 to 20 mV; with most of the principal frequencies between 10 and 10,000 Hz, bandpass filtering and amplification are required. Multiple types of stimulators are available for programmed stimulation of the heart. A variety of cathe-

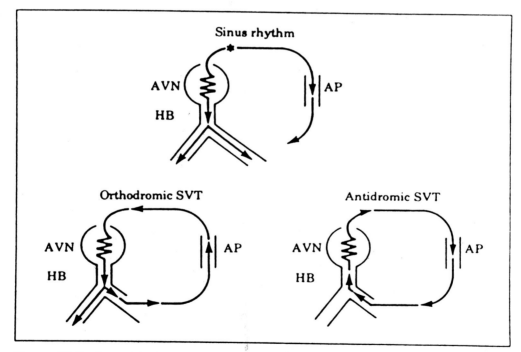

Figure 40-5. Atrioventricular conduction in Wolff-Parkinson-White syndrome. During sinus rhythm, anterograde conduction occurs over both the atrioventricular node (*AVN*) and the accessory pathway (*AP*). During orthodromic supraventricular (*SVT*), the AVN comprises the anterograde limb, and the AP comprises the retrograde limb of the reentrant circuit. During antidromic SVT, the AP comprises the anterograde limb, and the AVN comprises the retrograde limb of reentry. (From Lindsay B: Cardiac arrhythmias: recognition and management. In: Dunagan WC, Ridner ML, eds. Manual, Department of Medicine, Washington University School of Medicine. 26th ed. Boston: Little Brown Publishers, 1988:140)

ters with multiple poles (range, 3 to 12) are available in sizes 6 to 7 French for adults and 3 to 5 French for children, with interelectrode distances of 5 to 10 mm.

The goals of the preoperative electrophysiology study are to (1) document the arrhythmia as being supraventricular in origin, (2) evaluate the response of the supraventricular tachycardia to programmed electrical stimulation to determine whether it is reentrant or automatic in nature, (3) establish the conduction properties of the normal specialized conduction system, (4) document that the etiology of the arrhythmia is WPW syndrome, and (5) to define the location of the accessory pathway responsible for WPW syndrome.

Electrocardiographic features during sinus rhythm of WPW syndrome include a short PR interval (less than 120 milliseconds); an initial slurring of the QRS complex, giving rise to the delta wave; an abnormally wide QRS complex (more than 120 milliseconds) due to fusion of the ventricular activation by depolarization of the ventricle down both the normal AV node–His bundle and the accessory pathway; and secondary ST- and T-wave changes. Delta-wave polarity, QRS axis in the frontal plane, and precordial R-wave transition can often be relied on to regionalize the ventricular insertion to the left lateral (Fig. 40-6), left posterior (Fig. 40-7), posteroseptal (Fig. 40-8), right free wall (Fig. 40-9) and anteroseptal (Fig. 40-10) regions of the atrioventricular groove (Table 40-1).[19] The 12-lead ECG during orthodromic supraventricular tachy-

cardia demonstrates a normal QRS morphology in the absence of aberration in the His-Purkinje system. The relation of the P wave to the QRS complex is a more reliable criterion for distinguishing orthodromic supraventricular tachycardia from AV nodal reentrant tachycardia; during orthodromic tachycardia, atrial activation begins 70 to 100 milliseconds after the onset of the QRS complex and requires 50 to 60 milliseconds to complete (Fig. 40-11). Thus, the P wave most frequently occurs after the QRS complexes and distorts the ST segment in the first half of the RR interval. The 12-lead ECG recorded during antidromic tachycardia shows maximal preexcitation, with a pattern that is characteristic of the accessory pathway location (Fig. 40-12). When evident, retrograde P waves have a 1:1 relation with ventricular activation, because AV or ventriculo-atrial (VA) block would terminate the tachycardia. Atrioventricular dissociation suggests that the tachycardia is ventricular in origin.

During atrial fibrillation, the ventricles may be activated through the AV node–His-Purkinje system, the accessory pathway, or both, depending on the intrinsic electrophysiologic properties of each. Accordingly, the QRS morphology during atrial fibrillation varies with the contribution of conduction through the normal and anomalous AV pathways to ventricular activation (Fig. 40-13). In patients with accessory pathways having short refractory periods, ventricular activation occurs predominantly through the accessory pathway, the QRS reflects maximal

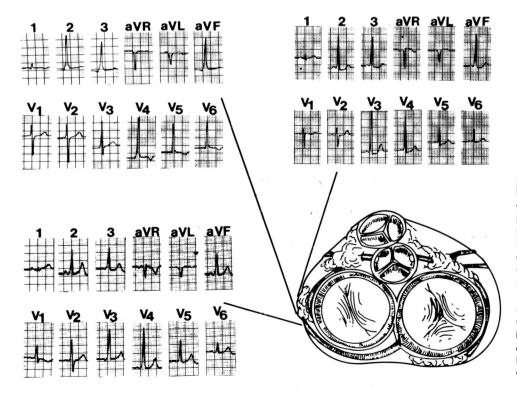

Figure 40-6. Representative 12-lead electrocardiograms recorded during sinus rhythm from three patients with left-lateral accessory pathways. Characteristic features include negative delta waves in aV$_L$ and frequently lead I, a normal QRS axis in the frontal plane, and early precordial R-wave transition. (From Lindsay BD, Crossen KJ, Cain ME: Concordance of distinguishing electrocardiographic features during sinus rhythm with the location of accessory pathways in the Wolff-Parkinson-White syndrome. Am J Cardiol 1987;59:1093)

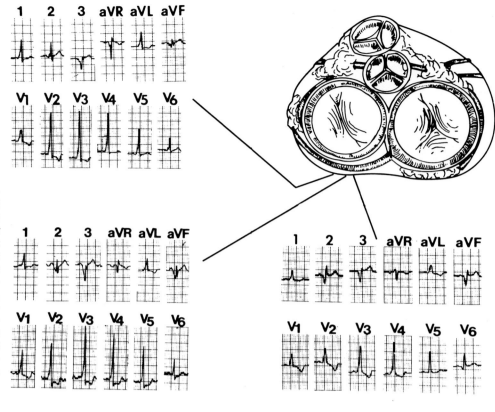

Figure 40-7. Representative 12-lead electrocardiograms recorded during normal sinus rhythm from three patients with left posterior accessory pathways. Characteristic features include negative delta waves in the inferior leads and a prominent R wave in V_1 (R:S ratio > 1). (From Lindsay BD, Crossen KJ, Cain ME: Concordance of distinguishing electrocardiographic features during sinus rhythm with the location of accessory pathways in the Wolff-Parkinson-White syndrome. Am J Cardiol 1987;59:1093)

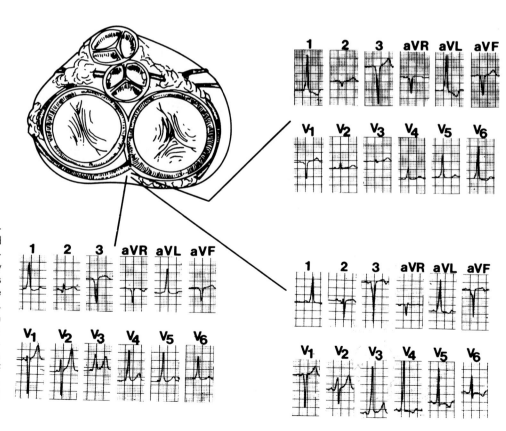

Figure 40-8. Representative 12-lead electrocardiograms recorded during sinus rhythm from three patients with posteroseptal accessory pathways. Characteristic features include negative delta waves in the inferior leads, left superior QRS axis, and an R:S ratio < 1 in V_1. (From Lindsay BD, Crossen KJ, Cain ME: Concordance of distinguishing electrocardiographic features during sinus rhythm with the location of accessory pathways in the Wolff-Parkinson-White syndrome. Am J Cardiol 1987;59:1093)

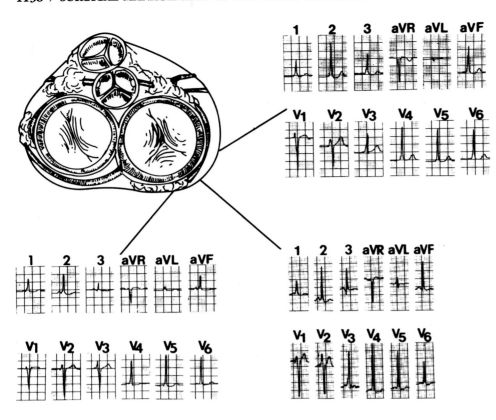

Figure 40-9. Representative 12-lead electrocardiograms recorded during normal sinus rhythm from three patients with right free wall accessory pathways. Characteristic features include a negative delta wave in lead aV_R, normal QRS axis, and precordial R-wave transition in V_3–V_5. (From Lindsay BD, Crossen KJ, Cain ME: Concordance of distinguishing electrocardiographic features during sinus rhythm with the location of accessory pathways in the Wolff-Parkinson-White syndrome. Am J Cardiol 1987;59: 1093)

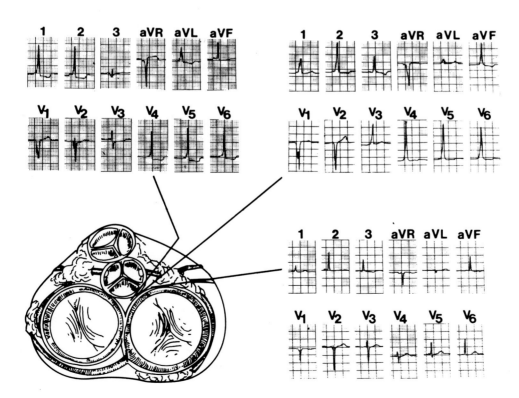

Figure 40-10. Representative 12-lead electrocardiograms recorded during sinus rhythm from three patients with anteroseptal accessory pathways. Characteristic features include negative delta waves in V_1 and V_2, normal QRS axis, and precordial R-wave transition in V_3–V_5. (From Lindsay BD, Crossen KJ, Cain ME: Concordance of distinguishing electrocardiographic features during sinus rhythm with the location of accessory pathways in the Wolff-Parkinson-White syndrome. Am J Cardiol 1987;59:1093)

TABLE 40-1. Characteristic Electrocardiogram Patterns of Accessory Pathways in Specific Regions

Region	Negative Delta Wave	QRS Axis in Frontal Plane	R > S
Left lateral	I and/or aV$_L$	Normal	V$_1$–V$_3$
Left posterior	III and aV$_F$	−75 to +75	V$_1$
Posteroseptal	III and aV$_F$	0 to −90	V$_2$–V$_4$
Right free wall	aV$_R$	Normal	V$_3$–V$_5$
Anteroseptal	V$_1$ and V$_2$	Normal	V$_3$–V$_5$

R > S, precordial R-wave transition.

Adapted from Lindsay BD, Crossen KL, Cain ME: Concordance of distinguishing electrocardiographic features during sinus rhythm with the location of accessory pathways in the Wolff-Parkinson-White syndrome. Am J Cardiol 1987;59:1093

preexcitation, and ventricular rates may exceed 250 beats per minute.

Patients are routinely studied while fasting and in the absence of antiarrhythmic drugs, with sedation used if necessary. Femoral, antecubital, subclavian, or jugular approaches can be used for venous access, whereas femoral or brachial arterial cannulation is necessary for a left-heart catheterization. To obtain data from the left atrium, indirect recording from the coronary sinus is most commonly used, unless the patient has a patent foramen ovale or atrial septal defect. Multiple catheters are positioned for routine electrophysiologic evaluation of patients with WPW syndrome. Routinely, four multipolar catheters are inserted transvenously, with two each positioned in the right atrium and right ventricle.

A quadripolar or tripolar catheter is positioned at the AV junction to record the His-bundle potential, and a decapolar catheter is positioned in the coronary sinus (Fig. 40-14).

Assessment of Anterograde Ventricular Activation

Analysis of anterograde ventricular activation is performed during sinus rhythm, incremental atrial pacing from the right and left atria, programmed atrial extrastimuli from the right and left atria, and during orthodromic supraventricular tachycardia and spontaneous junctional beats. The coronary sinus can be partitioned into anterolateral, lateral, posterolateral, posterior, paraseptal, and septal

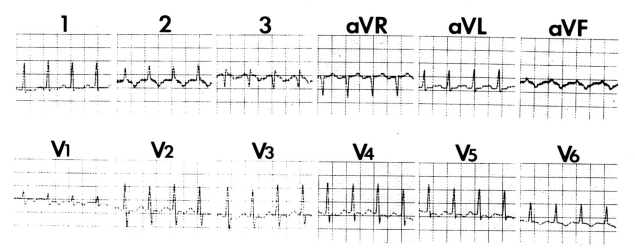

Figure 40-11. Twelve-lead electrocardiogram during orthodromic supraventricular tachycardia (SVT). The QRS complex is normal in the absence of aberration in the His-Purkinje system or other underlying cardiac abnormalities. During SVT, atrial activation begins 70 to 110 milliseconds after the onset of the QRS complex and requires 50 to 60 milliseconds for completion. Consequently, the P wave occurs after the QRS complex and typically distorts the ST segment in the first half of the RR interval. (From Cain ME, Lindsay BD: The preoperative electrophysiologic study. In: Cox JL, ed. Cardiac surgery: state of the art reviews. Philadelphia: Hanley & Belfus, 1990)

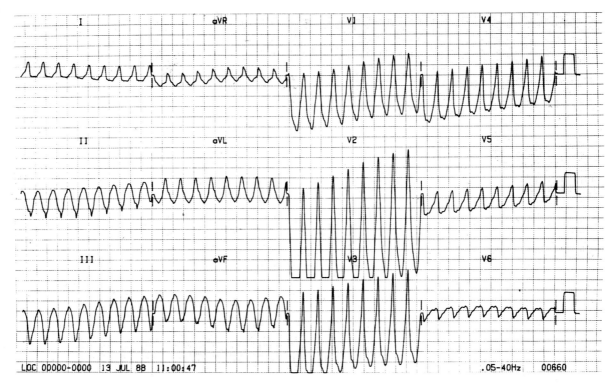

Figure 40-12. Twelve-lead electrocardiogram during antidromic supraventricular tachycardia (SVT). Maximal preexcitation is evident. Retrograde P waves may be detectable during the first half of the RR interval. (From Cain ME, Lindsay BD: The preoperative electrophysiologic study. In: Cox JL, ed. Cardiac surgery: state of the art reviews. Philadelphia: Hanley & Belfus, 1990)

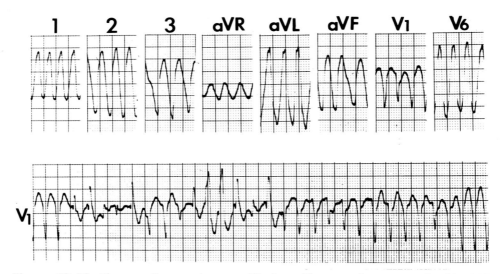

Figure 40-13. Electrocardiograms during atrial fibrillation. The ventricular rate is rapid and the QRS morphologies are varied because of fusion through the accessory pathway and normal atrioventricular conduction system and exclusive conduction through the accessory pathway. (From Cain ME, Lindsay BD: The preoperative electrophysiologic study. In: Cox JL, ed. Cardiac surgery: state of the art reviews. Philadelphia: Hanley & Belfus, 1990)

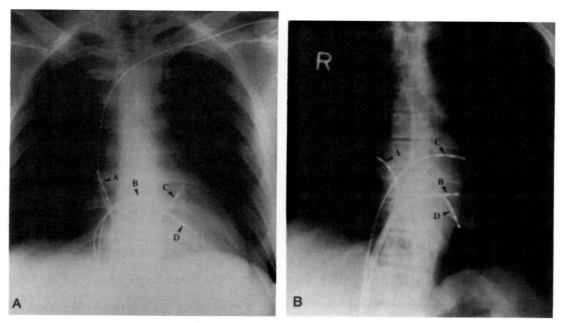

Figure 40-14. Catheter positioning for patients undergoing electrophysiologic study for supra-ventricular tachycardia. (**A**) Coronary sinus catheter (*C*) is inserted through the left subclavian vein. Other catheters are inserted through the femoral approach. (**B**) Left atrial catheter (*C*), advanced across a patient foramen ovale, is used in place of a coronary sinus catheter. *A*, high right atrial catheter; *B*, His-bundle catheter; *D*, right ventricular catheter. (From Platia EV: The electrophysiologic study. In Platia EV, ed. Management of cardiac arrhythmias: the nonpharmacologic approach. Philadelphia: JB Lippincott, 1987)

segments; often, however, it is necessary to map the coronary sinus in two stages. Anterograde ventricular activation times are recorded by measuring the interval between the onset of the delta wave on the surface ECG and local ventricular electrograms (delta-V interval). Incremental pacing is performed, beginning at a cycle length of 600 milliseconds, and the paced cycle length is reduced in 50-millisecond decrements to 300 milliseconds. Ventricular preexcitation is usually more pronounced at faster-paced cycle lengths because of decremental AV nodal conduction and selective ventricular activation by the accessory pathway. Alternating or varying patterns of ventricular preexcitation suggest a second accessory pathway. In patients with single pathways, the delta-V interval at the site showing the shortest activation time remains constant during perturbations that facilitate anterograde conduction over the accessory pathway. During maximal preexcitation, local activation times at the site of the ventricular insertion of the accessory pathway typically show ventricular electrograms coincident with or preceding the onset of the delta wave on the surface ECG (Fig. 40-15). The remainder of the ventricle activates radially from this early site.

Single atrial extrastimuli are introduced at paced cycle lengths of 600 and 400 milliseconds, beginning at a

coupling interval 40 milliseconds less than the paced cycle length, then reducing this interval in 10-millisecond increments; the purpose of programmed atrial extrastimuli is to evaluate patterns of ventricular preexcitation and to determine whether dual AV nodal physiology is present. Multiple accessory pathways are present when changes are detected during incremental atrial pacing, atrial premature extrastimuli, or pacing from multiple atrial sites.

Assessment of Retrograde Conduction

The site of the atrial insertion of the accessory pathway is defined by the pattern of retrograde activation during orthodromic supraventricular tachycardia or ventricular pacing at a cycle length associated with exclusive retrograde conduction over the accessory pathway. Moreover, in patients with concealed accessory pathways, assessment of retrograde atrial activation during orthodromic supraventricular tachycardia is the only definitive way to localize toe accessory pathway. In this part of the preoperative study, retrograde atrial activation times during incremental ventricular pacing, programmed ventricular extrastimuli, and orthodromic supraventricular tachycardia are assessed and expressed as ventricular-atrial (VA) intervals, measured from the onset of the QRS complex in the ECG

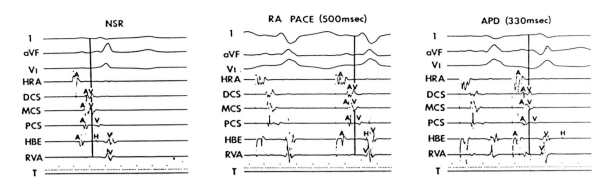

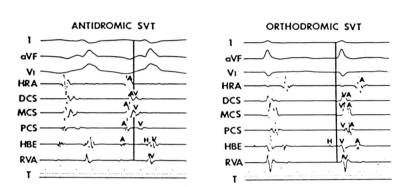

Figure 40-15. Comparison of atrial and ventricular activation patterns from a patient with a single, left free wall accessory pathway during sinus rhythm (*NSR*), pacing from the right atrium (*RA PACE*) at 500 milliseconds, an atrial premature depolarization (*APD*), *antidromic* supraventricular tachycardia (*SVT*), and *orthodromic SVT*. Each panel is organized from top to bottom, with electrocardiogram leads I, aV$_F$, and V$_1$ intracardiac recordings from the high right atrium (*HRA*); distal (*DCS*), mid-(*MCS*), and proximal coronary sinus (*PCS*); His-bundle (*HBE*); right ventricular apex (*RVA*); and time lines (*T*). The *solid vertical line* demarcates the onset of the delta wave in the QRS complex and serves as a reference for measuring local delta-to-V, QRS-to-V, or QRS-to-A activation times. During sinus rhythm and perturbations facilitating anterograde conduction through the accessory pathway, the shortest delta-to-V interval is located consistently at the DCS and MS recording sites. Other ventricular sites are activated later. During orthodromic SVT, anterograde conduction is through the normal atrioventricular conduction system. Retrograde conduction occurs exclusively through the accessory pathway capable of anterograde and retrograde conduction. (From Cain ME, Cox JL: Surgical treatment of supraventricular arrhythmias. In: Platia EV, ed. Management of cardiac arrhythmias: the nonpharmacologic approach. Philadelphia: JB Lippincott, 1987:304)

to the first major rapid deflection in the local atrial electrogram. Frequently, mapping with a standard 6 French quadripolar catheter of additional atrial sites around the tricuspid anulus is necessary. The earliest retrograde atrial activation recorded during orthodromic tachycardia is generally 80 to 110 milliseconds after the onset of the QRS complex (see Fig. 40-15). Longer VA activation times indicate that the catheter is not near the accessory pathway.

Confirming evidence of a free wall pathway is the effect of bundle branch block during orthodromic supraventricular tachycardia on VA conduction times and cycle length of the tachycardia.[20] Prolongation of the tachycardia cycle length and more importantly, the VA conduction by more than 25 milliseconds with development of bundle

branch block is diagnostic of a free wall accessory pathway ipsilateral with the conduction delay; this phenomenon results because bundle branch block ipsilateral to the accessory pathway enlarges the macroreentrant circuit. Anterograde activation must proceed to the contralateral ventricle before reaching the accessory pathway by slow muscle-to-muscle conduction. Failure of both right and left bundle branch block to alter the cycle length of the arrhythmia or VA conduction time suggests the presence of a septal or paraseptal accessory pathway.

Because septal accessory pathways may be close to the normal conduction system, pathways in this location constitute a more difficult diagnostic preoperative problem. Septal pathways are suspected when earliest retrograde atrial activation during orthodromic supraventricular tachycardia is recorded from the proximal coronary sinus or low right atrial septum.[18] Comprehensive atrial mapping is required to identify definitively a septal pathway and to distinguish posterior from anterior locations. The findings of more than one early atrial activation site during orthodromic reciprocating tachycardia suggest multiple accessory pathways. In addition, the assessment of retrograde atrial activation patterns during incremental ventricular pacing, programmed ventricular extrastimuli, and inducible antidromic reciprocating tachycardia often yields confirmatory information.

Role of the Accessory Pathway in the Genesis of Clinical Arrhythmias

Preoperative electrophysiologic study findings that indicate participation of the accessory pathway or pathways in a clinical arrhythmia include:

1. Lack of disparate AV nodal refractory curves with initiation of supraventricular tachycardia (e.g., does not depend on a critical AH delay)
2. Eccentric retrograde atrial activation
3. VA conduction identical to that during ventricular pacing at a similar rate
4. Prolongation of VA conduction and cycle length of the tachycardia during development of bundle branch block ipsilateral to the accessory pathway
5. Inability to initiate or sustain supraventricular tachycardia in the presence of AV block
6. Ability to preexcite the atria during supraventricular tachycardia at a time when the His bundle is refractory
7. Termination of supraventricular tachycardia in the absence of atrial activation by a ventricular extrastimulus delivered when the His bundle is refractory to retrograde penetration

In the case of septal pathways, confirmation that an accessory pathway participates in the supraventricular tachycardia relies predominantly on demonstrating continuous AV nodal refractory curves, initiation of supraventricular tachycardia not critically dependent on AH delay, demonstration that early programmed ventricular extrastimuli can conduct retrogradely to the atria with a septal activation pattern without intervening conduction over the AV node–His bundle (i.e., retrograde His appears after atrial depolarization), and preexcitation of the atria by a ventricular extrastimulus delivered during supraventricular tachycardia at a time when the His bundle is refractory.

Finally, demonstration of passive participation of the accessory pathway during atrial fibrillation or flutter or other atrial arrhythmias is confirmed by the presence of the typical preexcited QRS complex, which may be even more bizarre because of an increased degree of anterograde AV nodal conduction delay, resulting in a greater degree of ventricular activation through the accessory pathway.

Additional Preoperative Studies

The preoperative evaluation should also include an echocardiogram to exclude valvular heart disease or impaired ventricular function. The need for cardiac catheterization is determined by age, history of symptoms suggestive of myocardial ischemia, or knowledge of a preexisting cardiac problem in addition to the supraventricular tachycardia. At Washington University, preoperative cardiac catheterization is routinely obtained in all patients older than age 50 years.

Risks and Complications of Preoperative Electrophysiologic Evaluation

Preoperative electrophysiologic studies are associated with low morbidity and mortality rates.[21] Reported complications in one large series include deep venous thrombosis in 0.4%, pulmonary emboli in 0.6%, local or systemic infections in 0.6%, and pneumothorax in 0.5%.[22] Other reported complications include ventricular perforation, with tamponade.[17] As performed by experienced electrophysiologists, however, the risks are low and the expected yield of the studies is excellent; in our institution, intraoperative mapping provides information not obtained on the preoperative study in only about 5% of cases.

SURGICAL INDICATIONS AND CONTRAINDICATIONS

The major indication for surgical intervention in WPW syndrome is medical refractoriness.[23-27] Other common indicators are patient intolerance to drug therapy, detrimental side effects of antiarrhythmic agents, and poor patient compliance. Major additions to these surgical indications include (1) recurrent supraventricular tachycardia in young, otherwise healthy patients, and (2) spontaneous atrial fibrillation that conducts rapidly enough antegrade across the accessory pathway to allow the induction of ventricular fibrillation from the atrium. The inclusion of young patients whose arrhythmias might be controllable with antiarrhythmic agents represents a liberalization of previous surgical indications.[28] Surgery for WPW syndrome is no longer an experimental procedure and due to its safety and curative nature, many consider it to be the conservative alternative to a lifetime of dependence on antiarrhythmic drugs.

ANESTHETIC CONSIDERATIONS FOR CARDIAC ARRHYTHMIA SURGERY

Surgical therapy for WPW syndrome can be performed with little or no accompanying anesthetic risk. Factors that must be considered include (1) avoidance of halothane anesthesia because of the myocardial depressant effects; (2) a smooth sedative synthetic-narcotic nitrous-oxide anesthetic technique to permit early extubation postoperatively in these otherwise healthy young patients; (3) central venous catheterization without advancement of a Swan-Ganz catheter beyond the inferior vena cava–right atrial junction to meticulously avoid catheter damage to the bypass tracts on the right side of the heart (whether manifest or concealed); (4) avoidance of antiarrhythmic drugs and standard forms of perianesthetic treatments for arrhythmias; (5) prompt cardioversion for hemodynamically unstable arrhythmias; and (6) close cooperation with the surgeon and electrophysiologist to optimize conditions in the operating room for inducing the clinical tachyarrhythmia to permit intraoperative mapping.

INTRAOPERATIVE ELECTROPHYSIOLOGIC MAPPING

The availability of computerized mapping systems has obviated the need to use cardiopulmonary bypass for the intraoperative mapping of patients with WPW syndrome.[29,30] After safe induction of general orotracheal anesthesia, a median sternotomy is performed; this is our standard incision for all arrhythmia procedures requiring cardiopulmonary bypass. The heart is suspended in a pericardial cradle, and the ascending aorta is cannulated in standard fashion for cardiopulmonary bypass. The right atrial appendage is cannulated, with a right-angled cannula placed into the superior vena cava for venous return; the inferior vena cava is not cannulated until after completion of all presurgical intraoperative mapping to avoid iatrogenic "bumping" of the manifest or concealed accessory pathway with temporary interruption of conduction over the pathway.

Epicardial pacing and sensing electrodes are sutured onto the atrium and ventricle near the suspected site of the accessory pathway. We employ an elastic band containing 16 bipolar electrodes for simultaneous multipoint mapping (Fig. 40-16)[31] The band electrode is first placed around the ventricular side of the AV groove and electro-

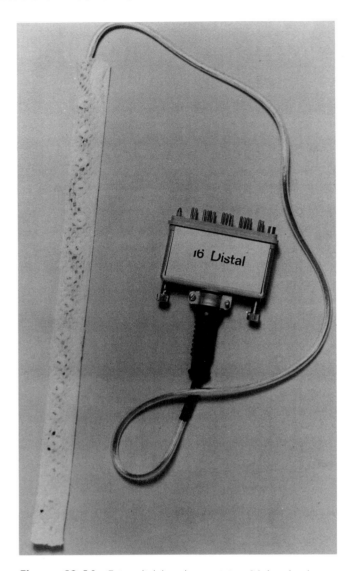

Figure 40-16. Epicardial band containing 16 bipolar button electrodes. (From Kramer JB, Corr PB, Cox JL, et al: Arrhythmia and conduction disturbances: simultaneous computer mapping to facilitate intraoperative localization of accessory pathways in patients with Wolff-Parkinson-White syndrome. Am J Cardiol 1985;56:571)

grams are recorded simultaneously from the 16 bipolar electrodes during normal sinus rhythm and during atrial pacing (Fig. 40-17). The digitized data are then displayed on a color graphics terminal in the operating theater, and a window of activation encompassing the preexcited ventricular depolarization is selected (Fig. 40-18). The computer system then automatically selects the activation times. The electrogram recorded from the electrode located nearest the site of ventricular insertion of the accessory pathway shows the earliest activation (Fig. 40-19). This multipolar mapping system is particularly helpful in detecting the presence of multiple accessory pathways during ventricular pacing. Because retrograde conduction is faster across the accessory pathway than through the AV node–His-bundle complex, the atrium still activates earliest at the site of atrial insertion of the accessory pathway.

These antegrade and retrograde epicardial mapping studies are capable of detecting not only free wall pathways but also anteroseptal and posteroseptal accessory pathways (Fig. 40-24). If, however, a septal pathway is detected during the epicardial mapping procedure, the patient is placed on cardiopulmonary bypass, a right atriotomy is performed, and endocardial mapping of the right atrium and atrial septum is completed, using a hand-held single-point mapping system, before proceeding with surgical dissection. This endocardial procedure further localizes the septal pathways in preparation for surgical dissection of either the antero- or posteroseptal space.

Finally, use of a computerized multipoint mapping system allows accurate accessory pathway localization from a single preexcited beat when preexcitation is intermittent (Fig. 40-25).

SURGICAL TECHNIQUES

The objective of surgery for WPW syndrome is to divide the accessory pathway or pathways responsible for the syndrome. There are two surgical approaches that are commonly used to divide these accessory pathways (Fig.

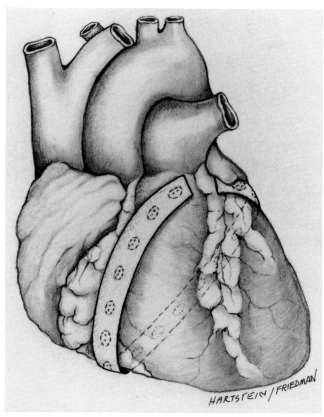

Figure 40-17. Placement of band electrode around ventricular side of atrioventricular groove in patient with Wolff-Parkinson-White syndrome during stable antegrade preexcitation. (From Cox JL: Intraoperative computerized mapping techniques. In: Brugada P, Wellens HJJ, eds. Cardiac arrhythmias: where to go from here? Mt. Kisco, NY: Futura Publishing, 1987)

that are capable of conducting in the antegrade direction (Fig. 40-20).

The band electrode is then moved to the atrial side of the AV groove (Fig. 40-21) and reciprocating tachycardia is induced with programmed electrical stimulation. Only a few cycles of tachycardia are allowed to occur because hemodynamic compromise is common and the patients are not on cardiopulmonary bypass. Atrial electrograms are recorded from the bipolar electrodes on the band and the digitized data are again displayed on the graphics terminal (Fig. 40-22). The activation times are determined by the computer, and the earliest site of retrograde atrial activity during the tachycardia is displayed (Fig. 40-23). These retrograde atrial maps are especially important because they may demonstrate previously unsuspected concealed accessory pathways that would have gone undetected if only an antegrade map had been performed. If reciprocating tachycardia cannot be induced intraoperatively, the retrograde atrial mapping is performed

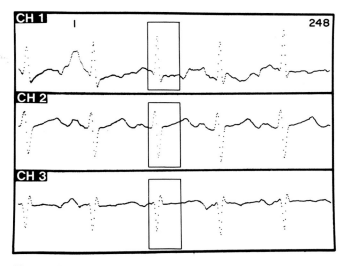

Figure 40-18. Hard copy of color-graphics terminal display of three digitized standard electrocardiogram leads used to select desired preexcited QRS complex (*inside window*). Window can be narrowed or enlarged, and it can be moved to any portion of QRS complex. (From Cox JL: Intraoperative computerized mapping techniques. In: Brugada P, Wellens HJJ, eds. Cardiac arrhythmias: where to go from here? Mt. Kisco, NY: Futura Publishing, 1987)

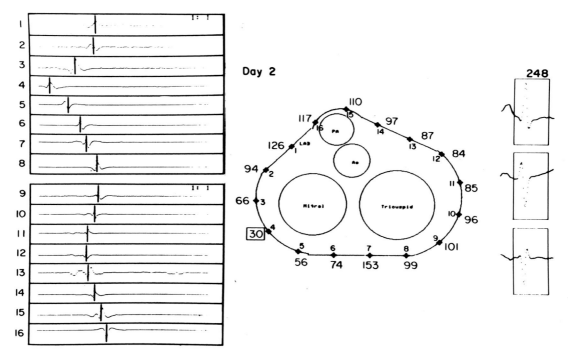

Figure 40-19. (**Left**) Hard copy of color-graphics terminal display, showing activation sequence of 16 electrodes contained in band. Because this is antegrade ventricular reexcitation, the map and band are placed on ventricular side of the atrioventricular groove and the electrode showing earliest activation (electrode 4) is located at the site of ventricular insertion of accessory pathway. (**Right**) Hard copy of color-graphics terminal display, showing activation sequence of base of ventricles during stable antegrade preexcitation. Designated window is displayed on right side of screen and the activation sequence is related to the diagrammatic sketch of the base of the heart, with the earliest site of ventricular activity during stable antegrade preexcitation being enclosed in box. (Modified from Cox JL: Intraoperative computerized mapping techniques. In: Brugada P, Wellens HJJ, eds. Cardiac arrhythmias: where to go from here? Mt. Kisco, NY: Futura Publishing, 1987)

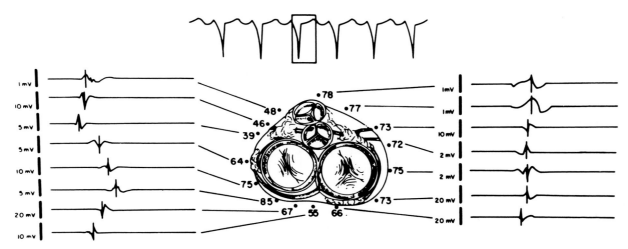

Figure 40-20. Anterograde ventricular epicardial activation, demonstrating two distinct accessory pathways: left anterolateral and posteroseptal (activation times are 39 and 55 milliseconds, respectively). (From Kramer JB, Corr PB, Cox JL, et al: Arrhythmia and conduction disturbances: Simultaneous computer mapping to facilitate intraoperative localization of accessory pathways in patients with Wolff-Parkinson-White syndrome. Am J Cardiol 1985;56:571)

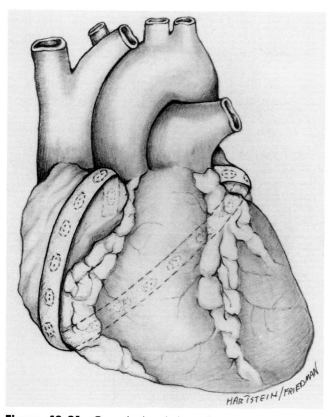

Figure 40-21. Once the band electrode is moved to the atrial side of atrioventricular groove, reciprocating tachycardia is induced and retrograde atrial map is performed. (From Cox JL: Intraoperative computerized mapping techniques. In Brugada P, Wellens HJJ, eds. Cardiac arrhythmias: where to go from here? Mt. Kisco, NY: Futura Publishing, 1987)

40-26). The endocardial technique is designed to divide the ventricular end of the accessory pathway, and the epicardial technique is directed toward division of the atrial end of the pathway.[12, 18, 19, 23, 24, 31] Although the epicardial technique has been described as a closed-heart cryosurgical technique, it is neither closed-heart nor cryosurgery-dependent in most patients.[18] At our institution, we prefer to employ the endocardial technique for all accessory pathways, regardless of location.

LEFT FREE WALL ACCESSORY PATHWAYS

If the *endocardial* technique is employed, accessory pathways on the left side of the heart are approached through a left atriotomy after the heart has been arrested with cold crystalloid potassium cardioplegic solution. A supraanular incision is placed 2 mm above the mitral valve anulus, extending from the left fibrous trigone to the posterior

septum (Fig. 40-27*A* and *B*). The entire space is dissected completely in every patient, regardless of the precise location of the accessory pathway within that space. After placing the supraanular incision, a plane of dissection is established between the underlying AV groove fat pad and the top of the left ventricle throughout the length of the supraanular incision (see Fig. 40-27*C* and *D*). It is important to carry this plane of dissection all the way to the epicardial reflection off the posterior left ventricle to be certain to divide any accessory pathway that might be located in the subepicardial position in the AV groove. After this dissection, it is still theoretically possible for an accessory pathway located immediately adjacent to the valve anulus to remain intact unless the anulus has been cleaned meticulously with a sharp nerve hook or knife. To preclude this possibility, the two ends of the supraanular incision are then "squared off" to the level of the mitral anulus prior to closure of this incision (see Fig. 40-27*E*). Even if such a juxtaanular pathway survived the previous dissection, the small rim of atrial tissue to which it would be attached are isolated from the remainder of the heart; therefore, the potential conduction circuit would be interrupted (Fig. 40-28). This dissection exposes the entire left free wall space and each of its boundaries. Therefore, there is no other site in this space where an accessory pathway could insert into the ventricle.

The *epicardial* approach to left free wall accessory pathways, as originally described, incorporates dissection from the atrial side of the AV groove (Fig. 40-29). The epicardial reflection off the atrium is opened and a plane

Text continues on p. 1150

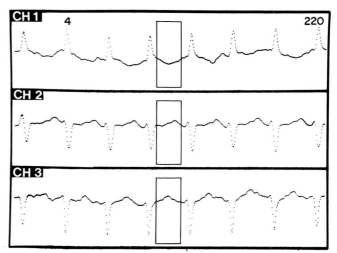

Figure 40-22. Hard copy of color-graphics terminal display, showing window centered over suspected site of retrograde P wave (after QRS complex) during reciprocating tachycardia. (From Cox JL: Intraoperative computerized mapping techniques. In: Brugada P, Wellens HJJ, eds. Cardiac arrhythmias: where to go from here? Mt. Kisco, NY: Futura Publishing, 1987)

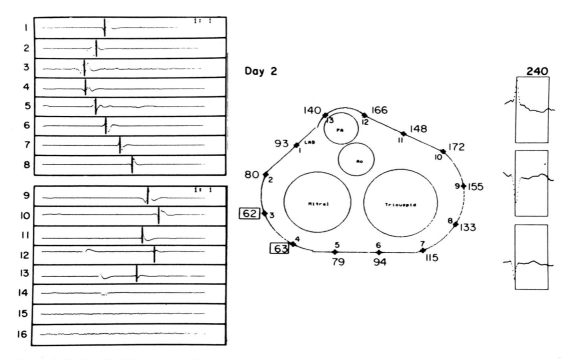

Figure 40-23. (**Left**) Hard copy of color-graphics terminal display, showing activation sequence of base of atrium during reciprocating tachycardia, as determined by band electrode array. Distal three electrograms were not in contact with heart and are therefore to be ignored. (**Right**) Hard copy of color-graphic terminal display, showing retrograde atrial activation sequence of base of atrium during reciprocating tachycardia superimposed on diagrammatic sketch of base of heart. Electrodes 3 and 4 activate almost simultaneously, indicating that insertion of atrial end of accessory pathway is located midway between these two electrodes. *Aø*, aorta; *PA*, pulmonary artery; *LAD*, left anterior descending artery. (Modified from Cox JL: Intraoperative computerized mapping techniques. In: Brugada P, Wellens HJJ, eds. Cardiac arrhythmias: where to go from here? Mt. Kisco, NY: Futura Publishing, 1987)

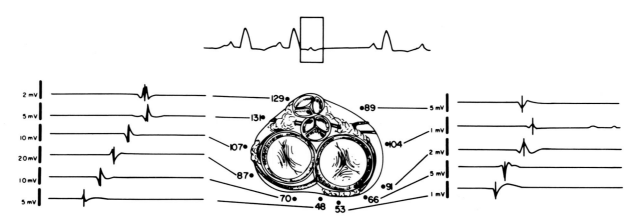

Figure 40-24. Retrograde atrial epicardial activation times during single atrioventricular echo beat. Accessory pathway is located in posterior septum, where activation time is 48 milliseconds. (From Kramer JB, Corr PB, Cox JL, et al: Arrhythmia and conduction disturbances: Simultaneous computer mapping to facilitate intraoperative localization of accessory pathways in patients with Wolff-Parkinson-White syndrome. Am J Cardiol 1985;56:571)

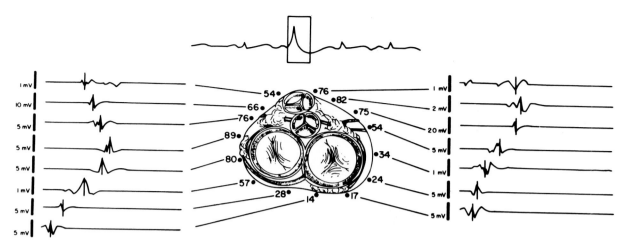

Figure 40-25. Anterograde ventricular epicardial activation times during intermittent ventricular preexcitation. Electrogram demonstrates a single preexcited beat. Activation map indicates presence of right paraseptal accessory pathway, where activation time is 14 milliseconds. (From Kramer JB, Corr PB, Cox JL, et al: Arrhythmia and conduction disturbances: simultaneous computer mapping to facilitate intraoperative localization of accessory pathways in patients with Wolff-Parkinson-White syndrome. Am J Cardiol 1985;56:571)

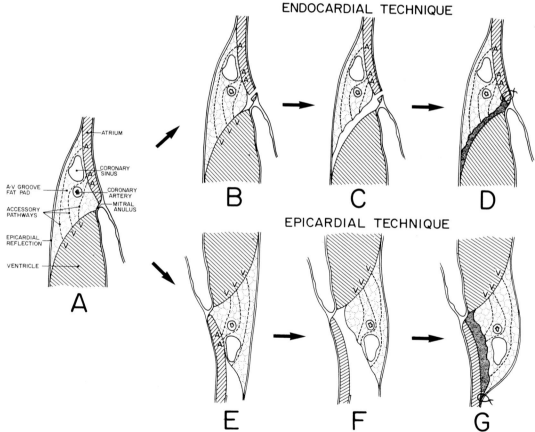

Figure 40-26. Representation of a cross-section of the posterior left heart, showing the different depths that left free wall pathways can be located in relation to the mitral anulus and epicardial reflection (A). The endocardial surgical technique is depicted in **B** through **D** and the epicardial technique in **E** through **G**. (From Cox JL: The surgical management of cardiac arrhythmias. In: Sabiston DC, Spencer FC, eds. Surgery of the chest. 5th ed. Philadelphia: WB Saunders, 1990:1861)

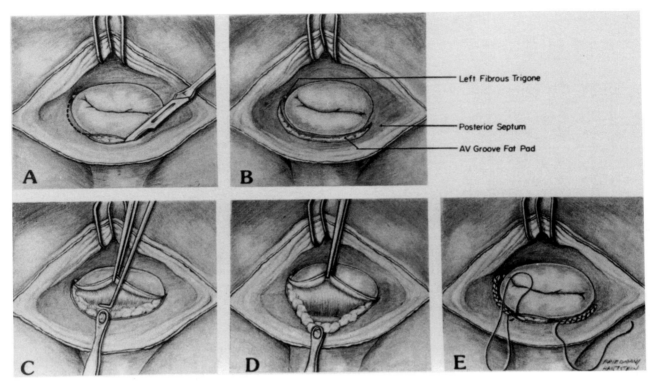

Figure 40-27. Surgeon's view of endocardial technique for dividing left free wall accessory pathways in Wolff-Parkinson-White syndrome. (Modified from Cox JL, Gallagher JJ, Cain, ME: Experience with 118 consecutive patients undergoing surgery for the Wolff-Parkinson-White syndrome. J Thorac Cardiovasc Surg 1985;90:490)

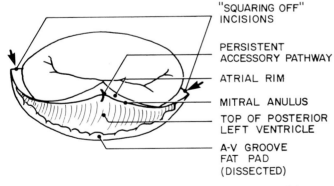

Figure 40-28. The adjunctive procedure of squaring-off the two ends of the supraanular incision when using the endocardial technique for the treatment of the Wolff-Parkinson-White (WPW) syndrome. This squaring-off maneuver is employed to isolate the rim of atrial tissue above the mitral valve anulus in case there is a persistent juxtaanular accessory pathway that has been missed after completion of the dissection of the left free wall space. Because the atrial rim of tissue is isolated by this squaring-off maneuver, even if there is a persistent accessory pathway immediately adjacent to the mitral anulus, it no longer connects to the left atrium; therefore, the WPW syndrome cannot recur because of the presence of this juxtaanular accessory pathway. (From Cox JL, Ferguson TB Jr: Surgery for the Wolff-Parkinson-White syndrome: the endocardial approach. Semin Thorac Cardiovasc Surg 1989;1:34)

of dissection is established between the AV groove fat pad and the atrial wall. The plane of dissection is extended to the level of the posterior mitral valve anulus and carried slightly onto the top of the posterior left ventricle. This dissection divides the atrial end of all accessory pathways in this region except those that are located immediately adjacent to the mitral valve anulus. A cryosurgical lesion is placed at the level of the mitral anulus to interrupt juxtaanular pathways that might have been missed during the prior surgical dissection (Fig. 40-30). The atrial epicardial reflection is then reapproximated. To expose the atrial side of the AV groove on the left side of the heart for the epicardial approach, it is necessary to elevate the apex of the heart out of the pericardium. This maneuver causes hypotension in most patients to such an extent that cardiopulmonary bypass must be instituted to maintain stable hemodynamics.[18,31]

The advocates of the epicardial approach state that the ventricular preexcitation caused by antegrade conduction across the accessory pathway disappears in virtually every case during this dissection, indicating that the pathway has been divided by the surgical dissection.[18] Despite this observation, they recommend placement of one or more cryolesions at the level of the mitral valve anulus to destroy

The epicardial dissection technique has been modified to a so-called direct approach.[32] The AV junction is exposed by a direct incision of the fat pad along the *ventricular* wall. The epicardium of the fat pad is incised longitudinally along the left ventricular edge anterior to the coronary sinus in the inferior segment of the coronary sulcus (Fig. 40-31). For most cases, cardiopulmonary bypass is still required. A plane of cleavage is found over the left ventricular wall, and the AV junction is identified. This technique requires (1) identification, ligation, and division of the obtuse margin cardiac vein, and (2) dissection of the obtuse marginal coronary artery and other ventricular branches of the circumflex coronary system over a 1- to 2-cm segment; the long-term effects of this skeletonization are not known. Finally, the great cardiac vein and the AV groove fat pad, including the left circumflex coronary artery, is mobilized and isolated on a large-stay suture, exposing the entire left free wall space, except the region near the left fibrous trigone; this area cannot be adequately exposed from either of these epicardial approaches and requires either closed-heart endocardial cryoablation of this region (which is near the origin of the left main coronary artery) or an endocardial dissection. After completion of the direct epicardial dissection, epicardial mapping is performed with a hand-held electrode and cryolesions are placed along the AV groove.[32] We have

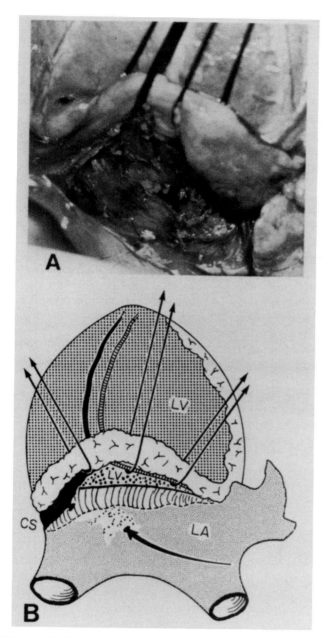

Figure 40-29. The epicardial approach to left free wall accessory pathways. (**A**) A schematic of the left ventricle, as viewed from an operative position. (**B**) The fat pad is mobilized and the atrioventricular junction exposed. (From Guiraudon GM, et al: Surgery for the Wolff-Parkinson-White syndrome: the epicardial approach. Semi Thorac Cardiovasc Surg 1989;1:21)

any accessory pathways located immediately adjacent to the valve anulus that might have survived the dissection. Although the cryosurgery is unnecessary if the pathway has already been divided by the dissection (i.e., the ventricular preexcitation has disappeared), this technique has nevertheless been labeled a cryosurgical technique by its advocates.

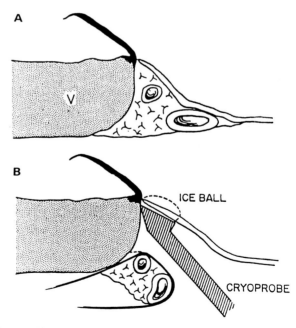

Figure 40-30. Rationale of the epicardial approach. (**A**) Cross-section of the left atrioventricular sulcus. (**B**) Exposure of the atrioventricular sulcus by mobilizing the fat pad en bloc and epicardial cryoablation of the atrioventricular junction are shown. (From Guiraudon GM, et al: Surgery for the Wolff-Parkinson-White syndrome: the epicardial approach. Semin Thorac Cardiovasc Surg 1989:1:21)

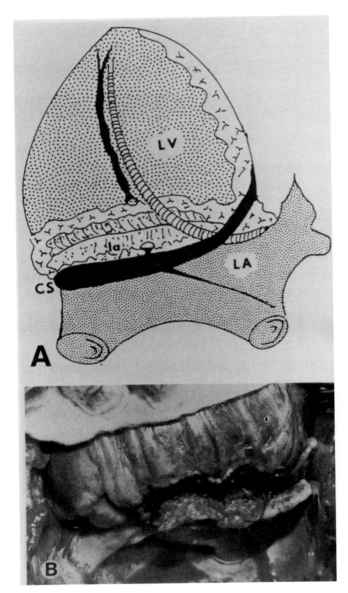

Figure 40-31. Direct prevenous left ventricular wall approach. (**A**) Schematic depiction of the direct "incision" of the fat pad and exposure of the atrioventricular junction. (**B**) An operative view. (From Guiraudon GM, et al: Surgery for the Wolff-Parkinson-White syndrome: the epicardial approach. Semin Thorac Cardiovasc Surg 1989;1:21)

adopted this approach to decrease the incidence of injury to the coronary sinus and the amount of tension placed on the posterior left atrium; this excessive tension has produced tears in the atrial tissue at the AV junction in a few patients in the past.[18] Thus, this newer direct approach divides the ventricular end of the accessory AV connection just as the endocardial approach does.

POSTEROSEPTAL ACCESSORY PATHWAYS

With the *endocardial* approach to posteroseptal accessory pathways, normothermic cardiopulmonary bypass is instituted and a right atriotomy is performed after conventional epicardial mapping. After completing the endocardial mapping described above, a supraanular incision is placed 2 mm above the posteromedial tricuspid valve anulus, beginning at least 1 cm posterior to the His bundle (localized in Fig. 40-32A) beneath the coronary sinus (see Fig. 40-32B). The supraanular incision is extended in a counterclockwise direction, well onto the free wall of the posterior right atrium (see Fig. 40-32C). This latter extension is important for two reasons: (1) it provides a larger incision for better exposure in the depths of the posteroseptal space near the posterosuperior process of the left ventricle, and (2) it simplifies identification of the epicardial reflection off the posterior right ventricle, a landmark that is to be followed across the crux of the heart to the posterior left ventricle during dissection of the posteroseptal space. Once the fat pad occupying the posteroseptal space has been identified through the supraanular incision, a plane of dissection is established between the fat pad and the top of the posterior ventricular septum (see Fig. 40-32D and E). Before instituting cardioplegic arrest, this plane is developed in the anterior portion of the posteroseptal space closest to the His bundle, approaching the central fibrous body from the posterior aspect. The junction of the posteromedial mitral and tricuspid valve anuli forms an inverted "V" at the posterior edge of the central fibrous body and the fat pad comes to a point at the apex of that "V" (see Fig. 40-32F). The apex of the "V" is always posterior to the His bundle, although the distance between the apex of the "V" and the penetration of the bundle through the central fibrous body is variable.[33] As long as the dissection in this region remains posterior to the central fibrous body, the His bundle will not be damaged. Once the anterior point of the fat pad is gently dissected away from the apex of the "V" (i.e., away from the posterior edge of the central fibrous body), the mitral valve anulus comes into view at the point where it joins the tricuspid valve to form the central fibrous body. The heart is usually arrested with cold crystalloid cardioplegia at this point but it is not absolutely necessary to do so. If the plane of dissection is relatively bloodless and easily identified, the entire posteroseptal space can be dissected with the heart beating. Conversely, if the plane is extremely vascular from the beginning, it is acceptable to perform the entire dissection under cardioplegic arrest.

Because the epicardial reflection off the posterior right ventricle has already been identified, visualization of the mitral valve anulus in the anterior portion of the posteroseptal space completes the identification of the

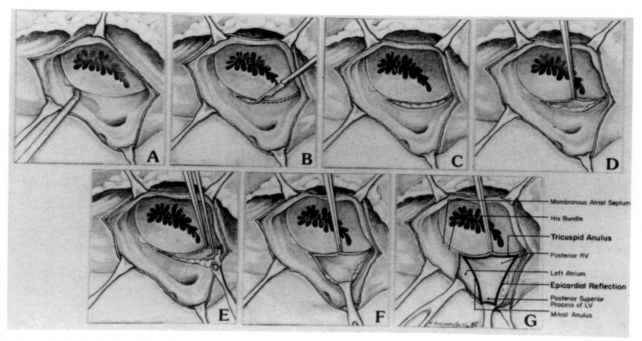

Figure 40-32. Endocardial technique for surgical division of posterior septal accessory pathways in Wolff-Parkinson-White syndrome. *RV*, right ventricle; *LV*, left ventricle. (Modified from Cox JL, Gallagher JJ, Cain ME: Experience with 118 consecutive patients undergoing surgery for the Wolff-Parkinson-White syndrome. J Thorac Cardiovasc Surg 1985;90:490)

boundaries of dissection of the space. The plane of dissection between the fat pad and the top of the posterior ventricular septum is developed completely by following the mitral anulus over to the posterosuperior process of the left ventricle and by following the epicardial reflection from the posterior right ventricle, across the posterior crux, onto the posterior left ventricle (see Fig. 40-32G). It is absolutely essential to divide all structures, penetrating the posterior ventricular septum and the posteroseptal space, including, if necessary, the AV node artery. We have found that the AV node artery leaves the posterior ventricular septum to enter the fat pad within the posteroseptal space in about 50% of patients with posteroseptal accessory pathways.[16] In every case, we have ligated it and have never experienced any AV node dysfunction as a result.

If the *epicardial* approach is used for posteroseptal pathways, the posteroseptal region, the adjacent inferior right ventricular region, and the left posterior paraseptal region are all dissected from the atrial epicardial aspect (Fig. 40-33).[32] The inferior AV groove fat pad is mobilized en bloc and the inferior right ventricular wall–AV junction is exposed. The right coronary artery and its branches are identified. The mid-cardiac vein is ligated and divided. The right atrial–left ventricular fat pad is mobilized and

the posterosuperior process of the left ventricle is exposed. Complete exposure requires cauterization of small arteries and veins coursing over the ventricular process, including the AV node artery. The pericardium is incised anterior to the coronary sinus and the left AV junction and the left posteroseptal region is exposed. The right and the left AV junctions are dissected, especially in the posteroseptal region, to expose the whitish AV lamina. Ablation of epicardial pathways is secured by epicardial cryoablation of the exposed AV junction, using overlapping applications of a cryoprobe while monitoring antegrade AV nodal conduction. If preexcitation exists after placement of these cryolesions, blind endocardial cryoablation is necessary with a cryoprobe placed into the right atrium through a small pursestring suture in the right atrial appendage. This epicardial dissection is performed without cardiopulmonary bypass, with the heart retracted by a large suture passed through a sterile piece of cardboard and the acute margin of the heart. Occasionally, the posterolateral branch of the right coronary must be divided to obtain adequate exposure and complete mobilization of the coronary sinus. If a left paraseptal pathway is present, cardiopulmonary bypass is necessary to connect the left free wall and posteroseptal epicardial dissections.

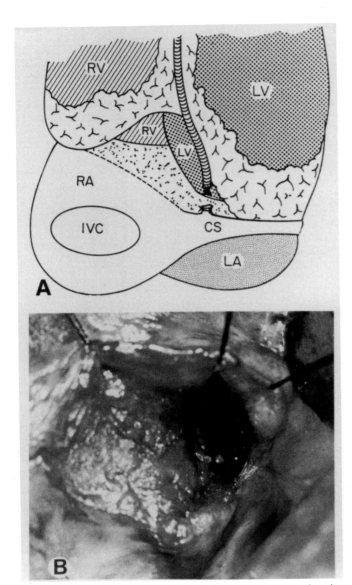

Figure 40-33. The epicardial approach to posteroseptal pathways. (**A**) Schematic showing the mobilization of the fat pad and exposure of the RA–LA sulcus. (**B**) Operative view. (From Guiraudon GM, et al: Surgery for the Wolff-Parkinson-White syndrome: the epicardial approach. Semin Thorac Cardiovasc Surg 1989;1:21)

Right Free Wall Accessory Pathways

In our opinion, this is the one circumstance in which the epicardial technique without cardioplegic arrest is probably as easy to perform technically as the *endocardial* technique with cardioplegic arrest. The epicardial technique can usually be applied in these patients without cardiopulmonary bypass, making it a true closed-heart procedure. We prefer to open the right atrium to perform

endocardial mapping, however, because there is frequently a large amount of fat in the AV groove on the right side, making the epicardial mapping less than optimal. After localizing the accessory pathway, the heart is arrested with crystalloid cardioplegia and a supraanular incision is placed 2 mm above the tricuspid valve anulus, extending around the entire right free wall. A plane of dissection is established between the underlying AV groove fat pad and the top of the right ventricle throughout the length of the supraanular incision. This dissection plane is developed all the way to the epicardial reflection off the ventricle so that the entire right ventricular free wall that is in contact with the AV groove fat pad is free of any penetrating fibers from the fat pad.

When employing the *epicardial* approach for right free wall pathways, an incision is made in the epicardium at the site of its reflection off the atrium to cover the AV groove fat pad of the right atrial free wall (Fig. 40-34). A plane of dissection is established between the external right atrial wall and the AV groove fat pad, downward to the level of the tricuspid valve anulus. This plane of dissection is established throughout the entire length of the right atrial free wall. Numerous anterior cardiac veins frequently open into the right atrium over the anterior portion of the right free wall, making hemostasis difficult, which in turn makes precise anatomic dissection even more difficult. Nevertheless, the epicardial approach to right free wall pathways can be safely and effectively accomplished in most patients.

There is an additional problem with right free wall dissections (regardless of the surgical approach employed) that is not encountered on the left side.[12] The atrium and ventricle tend to fold over on each other at the tricuspid anulus more than they do on the left side at the level of the mitral anulus (Fig. 40-35). This condition results in right-sided pathways appearing to be located in a more endocardial position than those on the left side, but they are not. Because of the folding over of the right atrial and ventricular walls at the anular level, the AV groove fat pad does not actually touch the true tricuspid valve anulus, as it does the mitral anulus on the left. Therefore, when the fat pad is dissected away from the tricuspid anulus using the epicardial technique, the ventricular preexcitation usually does not disappear. This observation has been reported on several occasions by advocates of the epicardial technique, who erroneously attribute it to an endocardial accessory pathway.[25,31] As in the case on the left, right-sided accessory pathways must connect to the atrium somewhere between the valve anulus and the atrial epicardial reflection and to the ventricle somewhere between the valve anulus and the ventricular epicardial reflection. Unlike the left side, the folded-over anatomy of the tricuspid anulus precludes the division of accessory pathways located adjacent to the anulus by the casual dissection

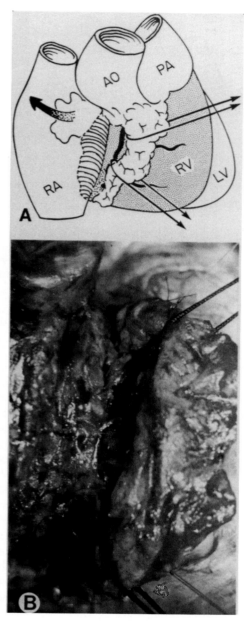

Figure 40-34. Right ventricular free wall approach. (**A**) Schematic of the exposure of the right coronary fossa and anterior right ventricular atrioventricular sulcus. (**B**) Operative view. (From Guiraudon GM, et al: Surgery for the Wolff-Parkinson-White syndrome: the epicardial approach. Semin Thorac Cardiovasc Surg 1989;1:21)

of the fat pad away from the heart. To interrupt right free wall accessory pathways that reside too close to the valve anulus to be divided by routine dissection, one of three adjunctive measures must be added to the dissection: (1) mechanical unfolding of the atrium and ventricle, so that the true valve anulus can be seen and freed of any adjacent

fibers connecting the atrium and ventricle (applicable to both the epicardial and endocardial techniques); (2) application of a cryolesion to the tissues near the valve anulus to destroy the juxtaanular accessory pathway (applicable to both techniques); or (3) squaring off of the supraanular incision at both ends to isolate the atrial rim of tissue to which a juxtaanular accessory pathway would connect (applicable to the endocardial technique). This "folding over" of the atrium and ventricle at the level of the tricuspid anulus is more pronounced in patients with Ebstein's anomaly, a condition present in 11% of the patients in our surgical series.[34] This is true whether the patient has the classic Ebstein's anomaly or only the mild form of the disease. If adjunctive cryosurgery is used in the epicardial dissection technique, both epicardial and endocardial cryolesions are often necessary to ablate the accessory AV connection.

Anteroseptal Accessory Pathways

Epicardial mapping is excellent for documenting an anteroseptal, but it does not localize these pathways precisely because of the large fat pad covering both the atrium and ventricle and the anteroseptal space. Therefore, we feel that endocardial mapping is especially important in these patients, particularly because in our experience, these pathways are more frequently located adjacent to the His bundle (anteriorly) than are posteroseptal pathways (posteriorly).[30] To perform the *endocardial* dissection, after performing retrograde endocardial mapping through a right atriotomy with the patient on cardiopulmonary bypass, a supraanular incision is placed just anterior to the His bundle, 2 mm above the tricuspid anulus, and extended in a clockwise direction well onto the right anterior free wall. The initial endocardial incision frequently abolishes ventricular preexcitation, but whether or not preexcitation persists, the entire anteroseptal space should be dissected. After the initial supraanular incision is completed, a plane of dissection is established between the fat pad occupying the anteroseptal space and the top of the right ventricle. This plane of dissection is developed completely—to the aorta medially and to the epicardial reflection off the ventricle anteriorly. During this dissection, the fat pad must be retracted gently to avoid injury to the proximal right coronary artery, which courses through the fat pad before entering the AV groove of the anterior right free wall (see Fig. 40-1). In addition, when the anteromedial portion of the anteroseptal space is being dissected, extreme care should be taken to avoid injury to the aorta. This is actually the external surface of the right coronary sinus of Valsalva beneath the orifice of the right coronary artery, and it is therefore thin.

Although the *epicardial* approach has been at-

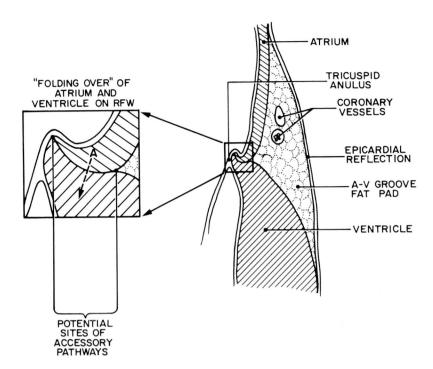

Figure 40-35. "Folding over" of the right atrium and right ventricle near the tricuspid anulus on the right free wall. Note that simple dissection of the atrioventricular groove fat pad away from the ventricle (endocardial technique) or atrium (epicardial technique) does not divide accessory pathways connecting the atrium and ventricle if they are near the tricuspid anulus. This is a common location for right free wall accessory pathways, explaining the erroneous concept that they are "endocardial" pathways. (From Cox JL: The surgical management of cardia arrhythmias, In: Sabiston DC Jr, Spencer FC, eds. Surgery of the chest. 5th ed. Philadelphia: WB Saunders, 1990:1861)

tempted for anteroseptal pathways, poor surgical results have caused the advocates of the epicardial technique to switch to the endocardial approach for these pathways.[25,32]

Special Circumstances: Nodoventricular and Nodofascicular Accessory Connections, Ebstein's Anomaly, and Coronary Sinus Diverticula and Aneurysms; Surgical Intervention After Radiofrequency Ablation

Nodofascicular and fasciculoventricular connections, as described by Mahaim,[11] are present between the nodal and fascicular components of the nodal bundle axis and the ventricular septum. Classically, these fibers are depicted as originating from the atrioventricular node or penetrating (His) bundle, then perforating the central fibrous body to insert into the ventricular myocardium. The electrocarpdiographic pattern depends largely on the site of origin of the fibers (Fig. 40-36)[35,36] but rate-dependent prolongation of conduction time and a low right ventricular insertion site can usually be demonstrated on the preoperative electrophysiologic study. In addition, the ECG demonstrates a left bundle branch configuration during preexcitation. The appropriateness of schematically picturing these accessory pathways as being nodoventricular has been questioned. Tchou and coworkers

suggest that such pathways represent atriofascicular connections, with decremental conduction properties without direct anatomic connection to the AV nodal tissue.[37] Klein and associates suggest that typical nodoventricular connections may be atypical AV accessory connections, with decremental conduction properties and a distal right ventricular insertion site.[38] It is worth noting that these so-called Mahaim connections are regularly found in otherwise normal hearts without arrhythmias.[39] Whatever the exact electrophysiologic substrate, from a surgical point of view, Mahaim fibers may connect the His bundle to the ventricular septum by traversing the posteroseptal space region or they may traverse the anteroseptal space, in which case the Mahaim connection is anterior to the His bundle.[40-42] In addition, right free wall AV connections with typical Mahaim-like characteristics preoperatively and intraoperatively have been reported, and left-sided nodoventricular connections have also been described.[43,44]

Depending on the spatial separation of the Mahaim fiber and the His bundle, these accessory connections can be interrupted, using standard endocardial surgical dissection techniques in combination with cryosurgery. The operation performed depends on the location of the accessory connection, which is determined by preoperative and intraoperative mapping. When the posteroseptal space is involved, a combination of discrete cryosurgery and a posteroseptal space dissection is required in some patients; in others, cryosurgery alone is sufficient to interrupt

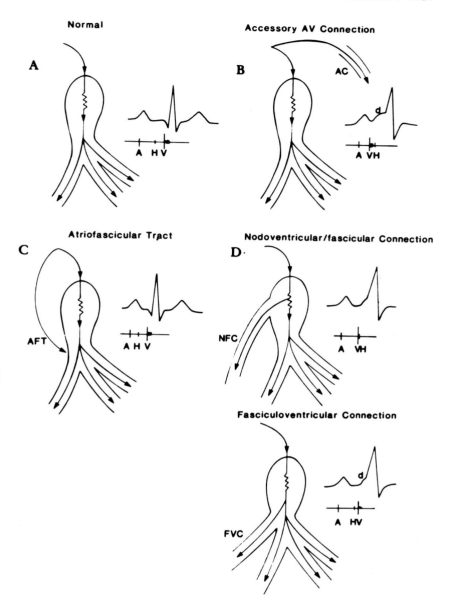

Figure 40-36. Configurations presumed responsible for the observed electrocardiogram patterns in preexcitation. The electrocardiogram, His-bundle electrogram, and schematic of the conduction system as occurs normally (**A**); with an accessory atrioventricular (AV) connection (**B**); and atriofascicular tract (**C**) and nodoventricular/fascicular and fasciculoventricular connections (**D**). *A,* atrial electrogram; *H,* His-bundle electrogram; *V,* ventricular electrogram; *d,* delta wave; *AC,* accessory AV connection; *AFT,* atriofascicular tract; *NFC,* nodoventricular/fascicular connection; and *FVC,* fasciculoventricular connection. (From Gornick CC, Benson DW Jr: Electrocardiographic aspects of the preexcitation syndromes. In: Benditt DG, Benson DW, eds. Cardiac preexcitation syndromes: Origins, evaluation, and treatment. Boston: Martinus Nijhoff, 1986)

the pathway.[45] In still others, a combination of cryosurgery and both antero- and posteroseptal dissections is necessary. Finally, a subset of patients have what should be truly classified as para-Hisian connections because despite all of these maneuvers, the accessory connection is so closely juxtaposed to the His bundle that it cannot be separated, and cryosurgical ablation of the entire His bundle is the only therapeutic alternative that remains to provide control of the arrhythmia.[46]

Ebstein's anomaly is a congenital malformation in which the origins of the septal or posterior leaflets (or both) of the tricuspid valve are displaced downward into the right ventricle.[47] These two leaflets of the valve are usually deformed and the anterosuperior leaflet is usually larger than normal. The septal and posterior leaflets are attached to the right ventricular wall rather than to the atrioventricular ring (Fig. 40-37). In addition, there is an accentuation of the normal infolding of the atrial and ventricular muscle at the level of the true anulus.

There is a wide spectrum of variability, with many patients having the mild form of this disease.[48] In the severest forms, the proximal portion of the right ventricle is atrialized and may be so thin as to appear aneurysmal. The right atrium may be dilated, and an atrial septal defect of any type may be present.[49]

The position of the AV node and conduction bundles in patients with Ebstein's malformation is normal, although the right bundle branch may be compressed by

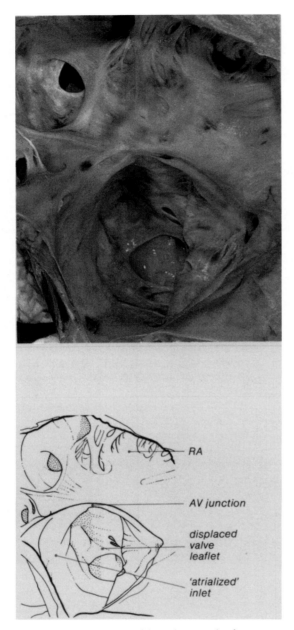

Figure 40-37. Inlet aspect of the right ventricle of a severe example of Ebstein's malformation. (From Becker AE, Anderson RH: Cardiac pathology. New York: Raven press, 1983)

thickened endocardium.[50] The incidence of arrhythmias and conduction disturbances in this patient population is high, and about 5% of these patients have accessory AV connections responsible for WPW syndrome. An additional undetermined percentage of patients with WPW syndrome have the mild form of Ebstein's malformation.

In our experience, a distinct association between patients with Ebstein's anomaly and the specific location of the accessory pathways exists. Most commonly, patients with this anomaly have posteroseptal accessory AV connections. In our series, however, most patients with Ebstein's malformation or the mild form of the disease had a combination of right free wall and posteroseptal accessory pathways at the time of intraoperative mapping. This correlation is so high that if a patient is found to have this combination of pathways on the preoperative electrophysiologic study, a cardiac echocardiogram is indicated to determine the status of the tricuspid valve.

In patients with Ebstein's anomaly, it is frequently difficult to define the true location of the tricuspid anulus. This is best accomplished by first identifying the AV groove fat pad on the right free wall epicardially. This fat pad is always located in the plane of the true tricuspid anulus. Therefore, an endocardial incision is placed exactly opposite the AV groove fat pad on the right atrial free wall and extended clockwise in that same plane into the posteroseptal space. Because the conduction tissue lies in the normal location in patients with Ebstein's anomaly, the endocardial incision is stopped beneath the os of the coronary sinus in a fashion similar to that in non-Ebstein's patients (see Fig. 40-32). Once the supraanular incision is made, the remainder of the operative procedure is identical to that described above for posteroseptal pathways. If valve replacement or placement of an anuloplasty ring is necessary for severe Ebstein's malformation, the valve or anuloplasty ring should be placed *below* the coronary sinus by sutures placed through the true tricuspid anulus. Plication of the atrialized ventricle may or may not be necessary.[51]

The entity that his been termed the "anomalous coronary sinus," with or without a "coronary sinus diverticulum," is usually associated with accessory pathways in the posteroseptal space. The coronary sinus is the portion of the cardiac venous system that begins at the origin of the oblique vein of Marshall (that part of the cardiac venous system that drains the left atrium) and ends at the ostium of the coronary sinus in the right atrium. The great cardiac vein of Galen, the posterior vein of the left ventricle, and the marginal, middle, and small cardiac veins all drain into the coronary sinus in the normal anatomic configuration (Fig. 40-38).[52] The coronary sinus is normally contained within the posterior epicardial AV groove fat pad and does not come in contact with the top of the ventricular septum. For this reason, it can be readily separated from the top of the ventricle during dissection of the posteroseptal space. Frequently, however, the coronary sinus is covered by a thin band of atrial muscle and if an accessory AV connection is present, it is usually intimately associated with the coronary sinus and its venous branches.[53]

The anomalous coronary sinus is a rare congenital abnormality that probably results from a malformation of the confluence of the middle cardiac vein and the sinus. Abnormalities of the proximal sinus itself are even more

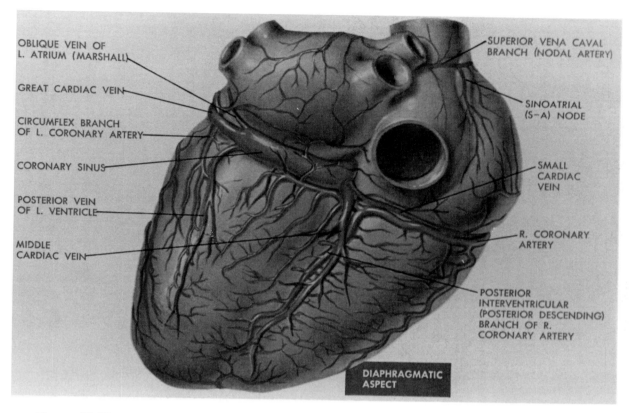

OBLIQUE VEIN OF
L. ATRIUM (MARSHALL)

GREAT CARDIAC VEIN

CIRCUMFLEX BRANCH
OF L. CORONARY ARTERY

CORONARY SINUS

POSTERIOR VEIN
OF L. VENTRICLE

MIDDLE
CARDIAC VEIN

SUPERIOR VENA CAVAL
BRANCH (NODAL ARTERY)

SINOATRIAL
(S–A) NODE

SMALL
CARDIAC
VEIN

R. CORONARY
ARTERY

POSTERIOR
INTERVENTRICULAR
(POSTERIOR DESCENDING)
BRANCH OF R.
CORONARY ARTERY

DIAPHRAGMATIC
ASPECT

Figure 40-38. Arterial and venous anatomy, viewed from the posterior (diaphragmatic) aspect. (From Netter, FH: A complication of paintings on the normal and pathologic anatomy and physiology, embryology, and diseases of the heart. Vol. 5. In: Yonkman FF, ed. The CIBA collection of medical illustrations 1969.)

uncommon and usually result in a diverticulum. Malformation of the os of the coronary sinus may accompany this entity, including gross enlargement of the opening of the coronary sinus or the presence of two channels within the os (one representing the true coronary sinus draining the posterior left heart and the second representing a greatly enlarged and separate great vein) (Fig. 40-39). In these instances, the tight adherence of the inferior wall of the coronary sinus abnormality to the posterosuperior process of the left ventricle and the posterior interventricular septum constitutes the problem that is encountered during arrhythmia surgery. Guiraudon describes six patients with true diverticula of the coronary sinus in this region, with the diverticulum being a round or oval structure with a narrow mouth that drains into the sinus.[54] The body of the diverticulum is within the epicardial layers of the posterior left ventricle at the septoparietal junction. The epicardial surface is covered by the epicardial reflection, and the diverticulum may occupy most of the posteroseptal space when viewed from the outside of the heart (Fig. 40-40).

To ablate accessory pathways associated with these

abnormalities, modification of the standard endocardial technique is necessary. In patients with an anomalous coronary sinus or coronary sinus diverticulum, the inferior wall of the sinus or diverticulum is fused with the posterior interventricular septum, with no intervening fat pad. Because the coronary sinus itself can be intimately associated with the accessory AV connections, the coronary sinus must be isolated in some way from the ventricular surface to interrupt the accessory pathway in these patients. In dissecting the coronary sinus off the septum, a small rim of the inferior coronary sinus wall must be left attached to the posterior septum. Although this maneuver interrupts the accessory connection in most instances of this anomaly, complete dissection of the entire posteroseptal space is still performed. Closure of the endocardial incision is performed in the standard fashion, as described above. The coronary sinus drainage is unimpeded because the defect quickly becomes re-adherent to the ventricular surface of the dissection. Closure of the defect in the coronary sinus is neither necessary nor advisable.

Surgical intervention after radiofrequency ablation is most often for right-sided lesions because they are associ-

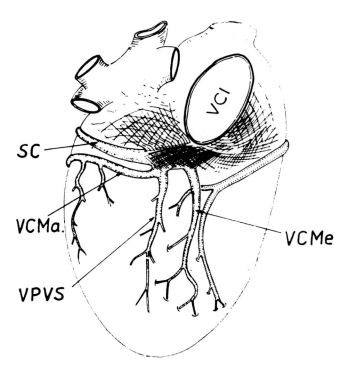

Figure 40-39. Unusual configuration of the coronary sinus (SC). VCMₐ—passing parallel to SC—unites with the posterior descending vein (VPVS) in a common trunk provided with a single orifice in coronary sinus. (From Maros TN, Racz L, Plugor S, Maros TG: Contributions to the morphology of the human coronary sinus. Anat Anz 1983;154:133)

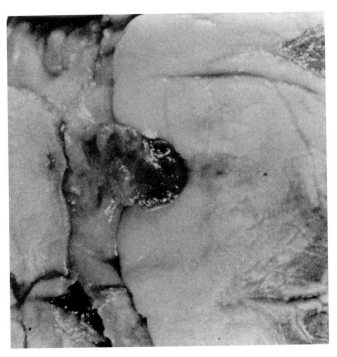

Figure 40-40. Photograph of an aneurysm of the human coronary sins. The mouth of this saccular aneurysm was 6 mm and was located in the distal portion of the coronary sinus near the ostium. (From Silver MA, Rowley NE: The functional anatomy of the human coronary sinus. Am Heart J 1988;115:1080)

ated with (1) more complex anatomy, (2) more anatomic variability, and (3) a higher failure rate than left-sided lesions. Generally, the surgical approaches used are the same as those described above. At the time of surgery, the previously applied radiofrequency lesions may or may not be apparent, depending in part on the number of lesions and the amount of radiofrequency energy used.

When the amount of energy applied becomes excessive, however, problems can arise at the time of subsequent surgical intervention. In these circumstances, the radiofrequency energy coagulates the subendocardial tissues, obliterating the normal planes of surgical dissection. This is true whether the endocardial or epicardial approach is used. In these instances, the surgical interruption of the accessory becomes considerably more difficult, if not impossible. It is apparent that the most prudent course of action after reasonable attempts at radiofrequency ablation by an experienced electrophysiologist is to consider surgical intervention on the assumption that an anatomic abnormality exists that obviates successful radiofrequency therapy. This recognition and decision should be made before application of excessive amounts of radiofrequency energy, with the potential of complications related to further surgical therapy.

SURGICAL RESULTS AND COMPLICATIONS

Several factors complicate the analysis of the results, surgical mortality, and complication rates after surgery to interrupt accessory AV connections. The operative techniques have been almost in continual evolution since Sealy's pioneering work in 1968,[10] with technical advances being made by multiple surgeons on multiple continents. The indications for surgical intervention have changed as greater success has been achieved with operation. As mentioned earlier, a greater understanding of the electrophysiologic and anatomic principles on which these operations are based laid the foundation for the technical advances that followed. Finally, different authors have used different methods to analyze and report their results.

In the available literature, surgical success is defined as (1) interruption of the accessory connection or connections in a single operation, with confirmation on the intraoperative postsurgical electrophysiologic study and no evidence of recurrence in the follow-up period; (2) interruption of the pathway in a single operation, with confirmation but with recurrence of the arrhythmia in the follow-up period; this arrhythmia is adequately controlled and tolerated in the absence of drug therapy or on drug therapy to which the patient was previously unresponsive; (3) failure of interruption of the pathway in the initial operative procedure but with successful interruption during a second or third operative procedure; and (4) failure to interrupt the pathway despite one or more surgical procedures but with treatment by iatrogenic His-bundle ablation, insertion of a pacemaker, and a satisfactory clinical result. Regarding the reporting of mortality and complication rates in these series, operative mortality has generally been reported as in-hospital mortality and not 30-day mortality, and the complications reported have been generally perioperative in nature.

Several large series, many of them personal, have been published and these encompass a variety of surgical techniques. As described above, the *endocardial* ap-proach, originally reported by Iwa and colleagues, in-volves cardiopulmonary bypass, an atriotomy, and in many instances a period of cardioplegic arrest.[55,56] The *epicardial* approach involves cardiopulmonary bypass in most cases, does not require an atriotomy except in certain cases, and uses a combination of surgical dissection and cryoablation to interrupt the pathway. Other authors have reported modifications of these two basic approaches.

Representative data from the literature are summa-rized in Tables 40-2 and 40-3. Presented are the number of patients, the number and location of the pathways, concur-rent arrhythmias and cardiac diseases, and the results and complications of surgery, as reported in publications re-lating to each of the seven largest series in the litera-ture.[23-25,57-63] A direct comparison of results is probably not valid because these series encompass different time

TABLE 40-2. Surgical Results Associated With Division of Accessory Pathways

Study	Gallagher, et al[24]	Cox, et al[23]	Lawrie, et al[59]	Iwa, et al[58]	Johnson, et al[57]	Guiraudon, et al[63]	Ott, et al[60]
Patients (n)	267	118	57	277	118	316	79
Pathways (n)	304	149	91	301	134	339	82
PATHWAY LOCATION (N)							
LFW	143	86	55	134	81	204	41
RFW	53	19	14	68	17	32	25
PS	81	36	18	25*	33	75	13
AS	27	8	4	-	3	28	3
Multiple	40	24	21	28	19	23	3
ASSOCIATED DISEASES							
Cardiac/oprn	74/NR	56/20	11/NR	57/NR	18/NR	22/NR	4/3
Arrhyth/oprn	NR	40/11	NR	NR	9/0†	NR	NR
SURGICAL RESULTS (N)							
I	212 (79.4%)	110 (93.2%)	49 (85.9%)	236 (85.1%)	110 (93.2%)	302 (95.5%)	70 (88.6%)
II	7	1	0	16	6	3	3
III	20	0	4	6	0	10	4
IV	0	0	0	1	0	0	0
MORTALITY (N)							
Total	11	6	2	11	1	0	1
Complicated‡	6	5	2	10	0	0	0

*Combined number of septal pathways in this series.

†All nine patients had atrioventricular node reentry.

‡Complicated; additional cardiac procedure performed during operation.

LFW, left free wall; RFW, right free wall; PS, posteroseptal; AS, anteroseptal; arrhyth, other arrhythmia; oprn, operation; NR, not reported; I, number of patients surviving first operation, with successful division of the path-way(s); II, number of patients surviving first operation, with recurrence of the arrhythmia but with adequate arrhythmia control on medication alone; III, number of patients surviving first operation, with recurrence, and surviving second or third reoperation, with successful division of the pathway(s); IV, number of patients surviving one or more successful operations without heart block/pacemaker therapy and poor medical control post-operatively.

From Ferguson TB Jr, Cox JL: Management of complications related to electrophysiologic surgery. In: Waldhausen JA, Orringer MB, eds. Management of complication in cardiothoracic surgery. Chicago, IL: Year Book Medical Publishers 1991;303.

TABLE 40-3. Surgical Complications Associated With Accessory Pathways

Study	Gallagher, et al[24]	Cox, et al[23]	Lawrie, et al[59]	Iwa, et al[58]	Johnson, et al[57]	Guiraudon, et al[63]	Ott, et al[60]
INTRAOPERATIVE COMPLICATIONS							
Heart Block							
Pacemaker (n)							
Elective	8	0	1	7*	0	0	1
Iatrogenic	17	1	1	–	1	1	0
Transient	NR	3	3	9	NR	NR	NR
Surgical (n)							
Left atrial tear	0	0	0	0	0	4	0
Coronary sinus injury	0	0	0	0	0	3	0
Intraoperative coagulopathy	0	0	0	0	0	1	0
Iatrogenic mitral insufficiency	0	0	0	0	1	0	0
POSTOPERATIVE COMPLICATIONS							
New postoperative pathways (n)	2	0	0	0	3	3	1
Total recurrence (n)	35 (11.5%)	1 (0.6%)	5 (5.5%)	23‡ (7.6%)	9 (6.7%)	16 (4.7%)	9 (10.9%)
Postcardiotomy syndrome (n)	+†	8	NR	NR	1	1	NR
Right ventricular dysfunction(n)	1	7	NR	NR	NR	1	NR
Left ventricular dysfunction (n)	1	5	NR	NR	NR	2	NR
Supraventricular arrhythmias (n)	NR	5	NR	NR	NR	0	NR
Hemorrhage (n)	NR	1	1	NR	3	5	NR
Infection (n)	NR	0	1	NR	4	NR	NR
Pulmonary embolus (n)	NR	NR	NR	NR	2	NR	NR
Pneumonia (n)	NR	NR	NR	NR	4	NR	NR
Stroke (n)	NR	NR	NR	NR	NR	1	NR

* Both elective and iatrogenic.

† Mentioned but number not stated.

‡ Assumes all cases of heart block are iatrogenic.

Pacemaker—elective, insertion after His-bundle ablation because of failure to interrupt the pathway and persistent tachycardia; pacemaker—iatrogenic, inadvertent creation of heart block at time of surgery; transient, temporary heart block postoperatively not requiring permanent pacemaker insertion; new postoperative pathways, "nonmanifest" or "concealed" pathways present but appearing clinically only in the postoperative period; total recurrence, sum of the number of pathways (1) missed at the original operation, (2) necessitating iatrogenic pacemaker insertion, and (3) that are new postoperative pathways.

From Ferguson TB Jr, Cox JL: Management of complications related to electrophysiologic surgery. In: Waldhausen JA, Orringer MB, eds. Management of complication in cardiothoracic surgery. Chicago, IL: Year Book Medical Publishers 1991;303.

intervals and surgical techniques; nevertheless the results illustrate the experiences of these authors, the overall results, and the types of complications associated with surgery for this congenital anomaly.

Gallagher and associates report their experience with the first 267 patients operated on for WPW syndrome at Duke University during the years 1968 through 1982.[24] During this time, considerable modifications in the surgical techniques were made. Virtually all patients were operated on using an endocardial approach, however. The complications reported include missed (those not divided at the initial operative procedure but successfully reoperated on, those not found at the initial operative procedure but successfully reoperated on, or those incompletely divided at the initial operative procedure but with an arrhythmia controlled postoperatively, with or without medication) pathways in 27 patients, iatrogenic heart block in 17 patients, and the elective creation of heart block in 8 patients because of inability to localize or divide the pathway coupled with uncontrollable arrhythmias. In this early series, 11 patients died; six of these were patients with associated cardiac problems or complications. The overall efficacy of the initial surgical intervention in this series was 212 of 267 (79.4%).

The surgical results have improved over time, with a decreasing mortality, increasing initial operation efficacy, and increasing overall success rate; this improvement has occurred in both infants and children as well as adults. Cox and coworkers and Johnson and associates report identical initial operation efficacy rates (see Table 40-2) of 93.2%.[23,57] In the former series, a total recurrence or total number of pathways rate (see Table 40-3) of 0.6% was achieved. In both these series, the endocardial approach was exclusively used. Iwa and associates in Japan and Lawrie and colleagues in this country report similar results using predominantly an endocardial technique.[58,59] Ott and associates achieved similar results in a series of infants and children with supraventricular tachycardias associated with accessory pathways.[60,61] Guiraudon has achieved an excellent initial operation efficacy with an epicardial dissection technique but at the expense of a significant intraoperative complication and reoperation rate.[25,31,32,62,63] The intraoperative complications reported with this technique include hemorrhage associated with separation of the left atrium from the left ventricle and injury to the coronary sinus in 3.8% of patients undergoing left free wall dissections. Some authors have expressed concern over the risk of this dissection from the epicardial approach.[26] This technique uses cryoablation of the dissected AV groove to obliterate pathways thought to be located near the anulus of the tricuspid or mitral valves; other authors have expressed concern regarding the risk of injury to the coronaries from adjacent cryoablation.[64] Mortality rates have approached zero and initial operation

efficacy has approached 100% for both endocardial and epicardial techniques. Interestingly, the mortality for patients without associated cardiac disease operated on using an endocardial-based approach had an operative mortality of 0.98% (9 of 916). The mortality in this group for those patients with associated cardiac disease was 3.5% (32 of 916); in most of these cases, a concomitant cardiac operative procedure was performed.

As illustrated in Table 40-3, the incidence of iatrogenic heart block has been reduced to zero with a greater understanding of the anatomy of the posteroseptal space.[56] Temporary heart block after surgical dissection of the posteroseptal space occasionally occurs but in most cases resolves in the operating room.

Postoperative complications that have been reported are listed in Table 40-3. These include postcardiotomy syndrome (more commonly associated with left free wall pathways), temporary right or left ventricular dysfunction, postoperative temporary atrial fibrillation, stroke, coagulopathy, postoperative hemorrhage, infection, and chylopericardium. The incidence of these complications is not significantly different from other forms of closed- and open-heart surgery.[65]

Surgical intervention after failed radiofrequency ablation should yield similar results, with the caveat that excessive applications of energy have not been applied to the tissues, as mentioned above.

SUMMARY

The incidence of successful surgical correction of WPW syndrome approaches 100%, with an operative mortality that ranges from 0% to 0.5%.[34] Complication rates after these operations are likewise extremely low. Both early and late recurrences after surgery, using either the endocardial or epicardial technique, are extremely unusual. The surgical treatment of WPW syndrome remains as the paradigm for effective cure of supraventricular arrhythmias.

References

1. Kent AFS: Researches on structure and function of the mammalian heart. J Physiol 1893;14:233.
2. Tawara S: Das Reizleitungssytem des Saugetierherzens. Jena: Gustav Fisher, 1906.
3. Keith A, Flack M: The form and nature of the muscular connections between the primary divisions of the vertebrate heart. J Anat Physiol 1907;41:172.
4. Wolff L, Parkinson J, White PD: Bundle branch block with short PR interval in healthy young people prone to paroxysmal tachycardia. Am Heart J 1930;5:685.
5. Wolferth CC, Wood FC: The mechanism of production of

short PR intervals and prolonged QRS complexes in patients with presumably undamaged hearts: hypothesis of an accessory pathway of auriculo-ventricular conduction (bundle of Kent). Am Heart J 1933;8:297.

6. Wood FC, Wolferth CC, Gaeckler GD: Histologic demonstration of accessory muscular connections between auricle and ventricle in a case of short PR interval and prolonged QRS complex. Am Heart J 1943;25:454.

7. Durrer D, Roos JP: Epicardial excitation of the ventricles in a patient with Wolff-Parkinson-White syndrome (type B). Circulation 1967;35:15.

8. Boineau JP, Moore EN: Evidence for propagation of activation across an accessory atrio-ventricular connection in types A and B pre-excitation. Circulation 1970;41:375.

9. Burchell HB, Frye RL, Anderson MW, et al: Atrial-ventricular and ventricular-atrial excitation in Wolff-Parkinson-White syndrome (type B): temporary ablation at surgery. Circulation 1967;36:663.

10. Cobb FR, Bluemschein SD, Sealy WC: Successful surgical interruption of the bundle of Kent in a patient with Wolff-Parkinson-White syndrome. Circulation 1968;38:1018.

11. Ferguson TB Jr: Anatomic and electrophysiologic principles in the surgical treatment of cardiac arrhythmias. In: Cox JL, ed. Cardiac arrhythmia surgery. Philadelphia: Hanley & Belfus, 1990:41.

12. Cox JL, Ferguson TB Jr: Surgery for the Wolff-Parkinson-White syndrome: the endocardial approach. Semin Thorac Cardiovasc Surg 1989;1:34.

13. Canavan TE, Schuessler RB, Boineau JP, Corr PB, Cain ME, Cox JL: Computerized global electrophysiological mapping of the atrium in patients with the Wolff-Parkinson-White Syndrome. Ann Thorac Surg 1989;46:223.

14. Ferguson TB Jr, Cox JL: Surgical therapy for patients with supraventricular tachycardian In: Scheinman MM, ed. Supraventricular tachycardia. Philadelphia: WB Saunders, 1990.

15. Benditt DG: Characteristics of atrioventricular conduction and the spectrum of arrhythmias in the Lown-Ganong-Levine syndrome. Circulation 1978;57:454.

16. Myerburg RJ, Sung RJ, Castellanos A: Ventricular tachycardia and ventricular fibrillation in patients with short PR intervals and narrow QRS complexes. Pacing Clin Electrophysiol 1979;2:568.

17. Cain ME, Cox JL: Surgical treatment of supraventricular tachyarrhythmias. In: Platia EV, ed. Management of cardiac arrhythmias: the nonpharmacologic approach. Philadelphia: JB Lippincott, 1987:304.

18. Cain ME, Lindsay BD: The preoperative electrophysiologic study. In: Cox JL, ed. Cardiac surgery: state of the art reviews. Philadelphia: Hanley & Belfus, 1990:1.

19. Lindsay BD, Crossen KJ, Cain ME: Condcordance of distinguishing electrocardiographic features during sinus rhythm with the location of accessory pathways in the Wolff-Parkinson-White syndrome. Am J Cardiol 1987;59:1093.

20. Coumel P, Attuel P: Reciprocating tachycardia in overt and latent preexcitation: influence of functional bundle branch block on the rate of the tachycardia. Eur J Cardiol 1974;1:423.

21. DiMarco JP, Garan H, Ruskin JN: Complications in patients undergoing cardiac electrophysiologic procedures. Ann Intern Med 1982;97:490.

22. Horowitz LN: Safety of electrophysiologic studies. Circulation 1986;73:II.

23. Cox JL, Gallagher JJ, Cain ME: Experience with 118 consecutive patients undergoing surgery for the Wolff-Parkinson-White syndrome. J Thorac Cardiovasc Surg 1985;90:490.

24. Gallagher JJ, Sealy WC, Cox JL, et al: Results of surgery for preexcitation caused by accessory atrioventricular pathways in 267 consecutive cases. In: Josephson ME, Wellens HJJ, eds. Tachycardias: mechanisms, diagnosis, treatment. Philadelphia: Lea & Febiger, 1984:259.

25. Guiraudon GM, Klein GJ, Sharma AD, et al: Closed-heart technique for Wolff-Parkinson-White syndrome: further experience and potential limitations. Ann Thorac Surg 1986;42:651.

26. Lowe JE: Surgical treatment of the Wolff-Parkinson-White syndrome and other supraventricular tachyarrhythmias. J Cardiac Surg 1986;1:117.

27. Mahomed Y, King RD, Zipes DP, et al: Surgical division of Wolff-Parkinson-White pathways utilizing the closed-heart technique2'q 2-year experience in 47 pati%nts. Ann Thorac Surg 1988;45:4y5.

28. Cox JL. Current Status of Cardiac Arrhythmia Surgery. Editorial. Circulation 1985;71:413.

29. Witkowski FX, Corr PB: An automated simultaneous transmural cardiac mapping system. Am J Physiol 1984;247:H661.

30. Cox JL, Ferguson TB Jr: Cardiac arrhythmia surgery. In: Wells SA, ed. Current problems in surgery. Chicago: Year Book Medical Publishers, 1989:193.

31. Guiraudon GM, Klein GJ, Gulamhusein S, et al: Surgical repair of Wolff-Parkinson-White syndrome: a new closed-heart technique. Ann Thorac Surg 1984;37:67.

32. Guiraudon GM, Klein GJ, Sharma AD, et al: Surgery for the Wolff-Parkinson-White syndrome: the epicardial approach. Semin Thorac Cardiovasc Surg 1989;1:21.

33. Kurosawa A, Becker AE: The conduction bundle at the atrioventricular junction. An anatomical study. Eur J Cardiothorac Surg 1989;3:293.

34. Ferguson TB Jr, Cox JL: The surgical treatment of cardiac arrhythmias. In: Parmley WW, Chatterjee K, eds. Cardiology. hiladelphia: JB Lippincott, 1989:1.

35. Bardy GH, Fedor JM, German LD, Packer DL, Gallagher JJ: Surface electrocardiographic clues suggesting presence of a nodofascicular Mahaim fiber. J Am Coll Cardiol 1984;3:1161.

36. Ellenbogen KA, Ramirez NM, Packer DL, et al: Accessory nodoventricular (Mahaim) fibers: a clinical review. Pacing Clin Electrophysiol 1986;9:868.

37. Tchou P, Lehmann MJ, Jazayeri M, Akhtar M: Atriofascicular connection or a nodoventricular Mahaim fiber? Electrophysiologic elucidation of the pathway and associated reentrant circuit. Circulation 1988;44:837.

38. Klein GJ, Guiraudon GM, Sharma AD, et al: Surgical treatment of tachycardias: indications and electrophysiological assessment. In: Yu PN, Goodwin JF, eds. Progress in cardiology. Philadelphia: Lea & Febiger, 1986:139.

39. Davies MJ, Anderson RH, Becker AE: Morphological basis for pre-excitation. In: The conduction system of the heart. London: Butterworths, 1983:181.

40. Gallagher JJ, Selle JG, Sealy WC, et al: Surgical interruption of

nodoventricular Mahaim fibers with preservation of normal A-V conduction. J Am Coll Cardiol 1986;7:133A. Abstract.

41. Schechtmann N, Botvinick EH, Dae M, et al: The scintigraphic characteristics of ventricular pre-excitation through Mahaim fibers with the use of phase analysis. J Am Coll Cardiol 1989;13:882.

42. Gillette PC, Garson A, Cooley DA, McNamara DG: Prolonged and decremental antegrade conduction properties in right anterior accessory connections: wide QRS antidromic tachycardia of left bundle branch pattern without Wolff-Parkinson-White configuration in sinus rhythm. Am Heart J 1982; 103:66.

43. Klein GJ, Guiraudon GM, Kerr CR, et al: "Nodoventricular" accessory pathway: evidence for a distinct accessory atrioventricular pathway with atrioventricular node-like properties. J Am Coll Cardiol 1988;11:1035.

44. Abbott JA, Scheinman MM, Morady F, et al: Coexistent Mahaim and Kent accessory connections: diagnostic and therapeutic implications. J Am Coll Cardiol 1987;10:364.

45. Cox JL, Ferguson TB Jr, Lindsay BD, Cain ME: Peri-nodal cryosurgery for AV nodal reentrant tachycardia in 23 patients. J Thorac Cardiovasc Surg 1990;99:440.

46. Klein GJ, Sealy WC, Pritchett ELC, et al: Cryosurgical ablation of the atrioventricular node-His bundle: long-term followup and properties of the junctional pacemaker. Circulation 1980;61:8.

47. Kirklin JW, Barratt-Boyes BG: Ebstein's malformation. In: Cardiac surgery. New York: John Wiley & Sons, 1986:889.

48. Sealy WC: The cause of the hemodynamic disturbances in Ebstein's anomaly based on observations at operation. Ann Thorac Surg 1979;27:536.

49. Becker AE, Becker MJ, Edwards JE: Pathologic spectrum of dysplasia of the tricuspid valve: features in common with Ebstein's malformation. Arch Pathol 1971;91:167.

50. Lev M, Liberthson RR, Joseph RH, et al: The pathologic anatomy of Ebstein's disease. Arch Pathol 1970;90:334.

51. Timmis HH, Hardy JD, Watson DG: The surgical management of Ebstein's anomaly. The combined use of tricuspid valve replacement, atrioventricular plication, and atrioplasty. J Thorac Cardiovasc Surg 1967;53:385.

52. Stamato N, Goodwin M, Foy B: Diagnosis of coronary sinus diverticulum in Wolff-Parkinson-White syndrome using coronary angiography. Pacing Clin Electrophysiol 1989;12:1589.

53. Maros TN, Racz L, Plugor S, Maros TG: Contributions to the morphology of the human coronary sinus. Anat Anz 1983; 154:133.

54. Guiraudon GM, Guiraudon CM, Klein GJ, Sharma AD, Yee R: The coronary sinus diverticulum: a pathologic entity associated with the Wolff-Parkinson-White Syndrome. Am J Cardiol 1988;62:733.

55. Iwa T, Kazui T, Sugii S, Wada J: Surgical treatment of Wolff-Parkinson-White Syndrome. Kyobu Geka 1970;23:513.

56. Ferguson TB Jr, Cox JL: Surgical Treatment for the Wolff-Parkinson-White syndrome: the endocardial approach. In: Zipes DP, Jalife J, eds. Cardiac electrophysiology. Philadelphia: WB Saunders 1990;892.

57. Johnson DC, Nunn GR, Richards DA, Uther JB, Ross DL: Surgical therapy for supraventricular tachycardia, a potentially curable disorder. J Thorac Cardiovasc Surg 1987;93: 913.

58. Iwa T, Mikai D, Misaki T, Mitsui T, Matsunaga Y: Surgical management of the Wolff-Parkinson-White syndrome. In: Iwa T, Fontaine G, eds. Cardiac arrhythmias: recent progress in investigation and management. Amsterdam: Elsevier, 1988.

59. Lawrie GM, Lin H, Wyndham CRC, DeBakey ME: Surgical treatment of supraventricular arrhythmias-results in 67 patients. Ann Surg 1987;205:700.

60. Ott DA, Garson A, Cooley DA, McNamara DG: Definitive operation for refractory cardiac tachyarrhythmias in children. J Thorac Cardiovasc Surg 1985;90:681.

61. Ott DA, Garson A, Cooley DA, Smith RT, Moak J: Cryoablative techniques in the treatment of cardiac tachyarrhythmias. Ann Thorac Surg 1987;43:138. .

62. Guiraudon GM, Klein GJ, Sharma AD, Jones DL, McLellan DG: Surgical ablation of posterior septal accessory pathways in the Wolff-Parkinson-White syndrome by a closed heart technique. J Thorac Cardiovasc Surg 1986;92:406.

63. Guiraudon GM, Klein GJ, Sharma AD, Yee R, McLellan DG: Surgery for the Wolff-Parkinson-White syndrome: the epicardial approach. Presented at Clinical Updates and Advancements in Cardiovascular Diagnosis and Therapy; Jan. 9-12, 1989; Acapulco, Mexico.

64. Kirklin JW, Barratt-Boyes BG: Tachycardias. In: Kirklin JW, Barratt-Boyes BG, eds. Cardiac surgery. New York: John Wiley & Sons, 1986:1359.

65. Kirklin JW, Barratt-Boyes BG: Postoperative care. In: Kirklin JW, Barratt-Boyes BG, eds. Cardiac surgery. New York: John Wiley & Sons, 1986:139.

Cardiac Arrhythmias, 3rd edition, edited by William J. Mandel.
J. B. Lippincott Company, Philadelphia © 1995.

41

A. John Camm • M.H. Anderson

Surgery for Ventricular Tachycardia

Ventricular tachycardias can cause dramatic symptoms, such as presyncope and syncope. Recurrent sustained ventricular tachycardias are associated with a first-year mortality of more than 40% and therefore require aggressive management.[1] A broad spectrum of therapies are available for ventricular tachycardia, including antiarrhythmic drugs, the implantable defibrillator, arrhythmia surgery, and catheter ablation. The techniques of surgery for ventricular tachycardia have developed dramatically over the last 40 years, following initial reports of relief of ventricular arrhythmias after ventricular aneurysmectomy.[2] Surgical strategies have included indirect methods (e.g., sympathectomy, coronary revascularization, and cardiac transplantation) and other approaqhes that aim to directly interfere with the substrate for the arrhythmia, including ventriculotomy, endocardial resection, cryoablation, and laser ablation. Steady refinement of surgical technique and identification of markers of lower surgical risk have resulted in a fall in operative mortality. The place of ventricular tachycardia surgery among the armamentarium of antiarrhythmic therapies has been threatened by the development of transvenous lead systems for the implantable defibrillator. The implant-related mortality associated with these systems is probably fivefold lower than that of surgery for ventricular tachycardia and referrals for sur-

gery have fallen. In this chapter, we consider the historical development of ventricular tachycardia surgery, mapping techniques, and its role in relation to other therapies.

HISTORY

In 1959, Couch reported the case of a woman aged 54 years who developed drug-resistant ventricular tachycardia after suffering an anterolateral myocardial infarction.[2] She had undergone a ventriculoplasty (i.e., excision of aneurysm) in 1956 and during follow-up, she suffered no further episodes of ventricular tachycardia despite not taking antiarrhythmic drugs. Couch drew attention to the association between ventricular aneurysm and ventricular arrhythmias and suggested that aneurysmectomy was successful because the irritable focus was excised with the aneurysm. There followed a host of case reports and small series of patients testifying to the relief of ventricular tachycardia after resection of aneurysms.[3-6] Buda and colleagues reported a large series of 203 left ventricular aneurysmectomies; in 49 instances, the surgery was performed for refractory life-threatening ventricular arrhythmias.[7] There was a high operative mortality (20%), predominantly due to surgery soon after an acute myocardial infarction. Thirty-five of the patients who underwent operative procedures for ventricular arrhythmias survived for a mean follow-up of 41 months; of these, 13 had no recurrence of arrhythmias. With longer follow-up, however, it became clear that even when combined with coronary revascularization, aneurysmectomy was generally ineffective at abolishing ventricular arrhythmias. For example, in the report from Ricks and colleagues, 21 patients underwent a combination of aneurysmectomy, aneurysm plication, or coronary grafting for the control of life-threatening arrhythmias; 14 survived to leave the hospital.[8] There was one additional late death, three patients had recurrent documented ventricular arrhythmias, and six others had persistent troublesome palpitations. Thus, only four of the original 21 patients survived symptom-free. Another study that drew attention to the inadequacy of aneurysmectomy in controlling ventricular tachyarrhythmias was that reported by Sami and colleagues.[9] Ten patients who underwent aneurysmectomy in an attempt to abolish arrhythmias were followed-up by ambulatory monitoring and exercise testing. Two died suddenly, and runs of ventricular tachycardia were noted in three others. The remaining five patients all had frequent multifocal extrasystoles. Similar results have been noted by other groups.[10–13]

INDIRECT SURGICAL METHODS

Sympathectomy

Although bilateral sympathectomy was employed as a form of management of refractory ventricular arrhythmias associated with coronary and other forms of heart disease, the technique was not particularly successful.[14, 15] The advent of a wide variety of beta blockers has virtually eliminated the need for this form of surgery. The idiopathic long-QT syndrome is associated with an imbalance in the sympathetic innervation of the heart, and there were early reports of reduced incidence of syncope and sudden death after left stellectomy.[16] Schwartz and colleagues reported the outcome of 86 patients with long-QT syndrome treated by left sympathectomy from their world registry of long-QT syndrome patients.[17] Beta-blocking therapy was continued in 84% of patients. Sympathectomy was performed either by left stellectomy, left cervicothoracic sympathectomy, or by high thoracic left sympathectomy (which has the advantage of avoiding Horner's syndrome). The incidence of symptomatic arrhythmic episodes was dramatically reduced after surgery and 5-year mortality was 6%, compared with 35% in 126 patients not treated with anti-adrenergic interventions.[18]

Not all reports suggest that left sympathectomy is efficacious for long-QT syndrome. Bhandari and coworkers report 10 patients, of whom eight developed recurrent symptoms (syncope in four, presyncope in six, and cardiac arrest in three).[19] The authors suggest that concomitant drug treatment, more extensive surgery, pacing, or implantation of an automatic defibrillator should be considered for such patients.

Mitral Valve Replacement

A handful of reports address the value of mitral valve replacement for the management of documented ventricular tachyarrhythmias occurring in association with mitral valve prolapse.[20–22] In most instances, ventricular ectopy persisted after mitral valve replacement but symptoms attributable to malignant ventricular arrhythmias did not. Additional antiarrhythmic therapy—sometimes unsuccessful, although not always tried before surgery—was often necessary after surgery. Sustained tachyarrhythmias were not provoked before or at surgery and therefore were not usually mapped. In one instance, Cobbs and King mapped spontaneously occurring ventricular ectopic beats and discovered that the apparent epicardial origin was close to the base of the posterior papillary muscle.[20] Pressure at this point prevented the ectopic activity. Based on such data and the morphologic characteristics of the ventricular tachycardia, most reports agree that the likely mechanisms of these arrhythmias in mitral valve prolapse is stretching of the mitral subvalvar structures, especially the posterior papillary muscle.

Coronary Revascularization

Coronary revascularization is associated with a reduction in the incidence of sudden cardiac death from 4.7% to 2.5% over a 5-year follow-up.[23] This effect is particularly marked in patients with impaired left ventricular function and extensive coronary disease. Coronary revascularization is also associated with a reduction of 33% in inducibility of arrhythmias in patients with a preoperative inducible arrhythmia.[24] The failure to abolish a greater proportion of ventricular arrhythmias occurs because the arrhythmias are not due to acute ischemia but to chronic ischemic damage and infarction that has produced the arrhythmic substrate. Because of the severity of obstructive coronary disease in victims of sudden unexpected cardiac death, it was hoped that coronary revascularization would reduce the incidence of recurrent malignant ventricular arrhythmias in such patients. Some evidence for this hypothesis comes from the observation of Levine and coworkers that the time to delivery of first implantable defibrillator therapy is longer in patients who undergo coronary artery bypass grafting.[25]

In some patients with exercise-induced sustained ventricular tachycardia, the relief of severe proximal coronary stenoses undoubtedly abolishes the arrhythmia, as assessed by long-term follow-up study and electrophysiologic testing.[26–28] It is difficult, however, to predict which patients will benefit in this way. Certainly, preoperative angiography is not helpful but the development of ventricular tachyarrhythmias only in the presence of ischemic repolarization changes on the electrocardiogram may be a helpful indicator, especially if the arrhythmias appear to arise from the ischemic territory.

Cardiac Transplantation

The development of cardiac transplantation offers another mode of treatment for patients with intractable ventricular tachycardia.[29] For patients with seriously impaired left ventricular function and a refractory arrhythmia, which renders them a poor risk for conventional ventricular tachycardia surgery, transplantation may offer the best long-term chance of survival. It is also appropriate therapy for patients with intractable ventricular tachycardia resistant to all other approaches. The limited supply of donor organs restricts the more widespread use of this therapy, and survival figures for good-risk patients undergoing conventional antiarrhythmic surgery are better than those for cardiac transplantation. Patients also avoid the detrimental effects of long-term immunosuppression. Cardiac autotransplantation, which avoids these problems, has been used to denervate the heart in a patient with the long-QT syndrome.[30] This produced only a temporary remission of the patients torsades de pointes tachycardia.

SURGICAL TECHNIQUES

Intraoperative Mapping

Epicardial and endocardial mapping techniques during normal rhythms and induced arrhythmias have been used for a variety of clinical and experimental purposes since 1913.[31,32] Operative mapping has developed concurrently with modern surgical techniques, with the realization that better surgical management of patients with ventricular tachycardia can be obtained by employing various methods of mapping to localize the origin or likely origin of the arrhythmia. Five different forms of mapping the ventricle are in use:

1. Electrogram mapping during tachycardia (endocardial, epicardial, and transmural exploration) to obtain an activation or potential distribution map and define the earliest activity during tachycardia or the course of a reentrant pathway critical to the perpetuation of tachycardia

2. Electrogram mapping during sinus rhythm (endocardial, epicardial, and transmural exploration) to identify those areas of late or abnormal activation that could form the substrate for reentrant ventricular tachycardia

3. Cryothermal mapping during tachycardia (epicardial and endocardial exploration) to localize a point at which freezing terminates tachycardia

4. Pace mapping (epicardial and endocardial exploration) to identify a point at which artificial ventricular pacing produces a QRS complex identical to that occurring during ventricular tachycardia

5. Visual inspection mapping to locate abnormal tissue that may provide a substrate for tachycardia

Electrogram recording to construct activation maps during tachycardia and cryothermal tachycardia termination mapping require that tachycardia be stimulated and sustained in the operating room. Most coronary-related and idiopathic tachycardias can be provoked by programmed stimulation.[33] In the presence of anesthetic drugs and after surgery, particularly after a ventriculotomy, it may prove difficult to induce ventricular tachycardia. Elevating the blood temperature to 38°C or infusing isoprenaline may help to provoke and sustain the arrhythmia. Rapid tachycardias may degenerate quickly to sinus rhythm. Intravenous procainamide or ajmaline may slow the tachycardia sufficiently to prevent degeneration and allow accurate mapping.[34] The induction and maintenance of tachycardia during open-chest and open-heart procedures does not seem to produce significant cardiac damage, provided that the total duration of normothermic cardiopulmonary bypass with the beating heart is kept to a minimum, preferably less than 45 minutes. Some investigators have sought to minimize potential subendocardial damage during surgery by intraaortic balloon counterpulsation during the induced arrhythmia.

Electrogram Mapping During Tachycardia

In 1974, Fontaine and colleagues reported the use of epicardial mapping to determine the site of transmural ventriculotomy in three cases of resistant ventricular tachycardia.[35] The patients were free of their arrhythmia after 8, 7, and 5 months of follow-up. This report suggests that electrophysiologic guidance of tissue resection may improve the poor rate of success with blind aneurysmectomy. In the following year, Wittig and Boineau reported from their experience of the surgical treatment of three patients with ventricular tachycardia and from experimental evidence with ischemic arrhythmias in dogs that epicardial, endocardial, and transmural mapping was necessary to locate the focus of irritability.[36] Spielman and colleagues investigated the relative value of epicardial and endocardial mapping and demonstrated that epicardial mapping alone would have missed many of the tachycardias that were correctly located with endocardial mapping.[37]

The technique of activation mapping is as follows:

1. Stationary electrodes are fixed on the ventricle of interest or on both ventricles.

2. By pacing through one of these electrodes, tachycardia is stimulated.

3. A roving hand-held or fingertip electrode is moved over the surface of the heart, using a grid reference system. This so-called mapping electrode is usually a triangular bipolar arrangement to ensure that the direction of depolarization cannot be perpendicular to all three electrode pairs.[38]

4. Electrograms are usually bipolar band-pass, filtered between about 50 and 500 Hz and amplified to achieve 1 cm/mV when recorded on paper at speeds of at least 100 mm/second.

5. Electrograms from the mapping electrode are recorded together with several surface electrocardiographic leads and electrograms from at least one stationary electrode.

6. Each electrogram is timed in relation to a constant reference, usually the electrogram from a stationary electrode pair, and the timing is adjusted relative to the onset of the QRS complex.

7. The timing of the electrogram is related to the position from which it was recorded using a stylized grid. At this stage, isochrone (equal time) contours may be calculated and drawn. The latter step is rarely necessary.

8. After the epicardial map has been performed, the relevant ventricle is opened, preferably through scar tissue, and the endocardial surface is mapped during tachycardia (Fig. 41-1).

Since 1974, some comparisons between blind aneurysmectomy and electrophysiologically guided surgical therapy have been published.[39–42] All have clearly indicated that map-guided surgery is vastly superior because patients survive longer and suffer fewer recurrences of their ventricular arrhythmia. It is difficult, however, to make a proper comparison because the patients treated by electrophysiologically directed resection were mostly operated on at a later date than those treated with blind

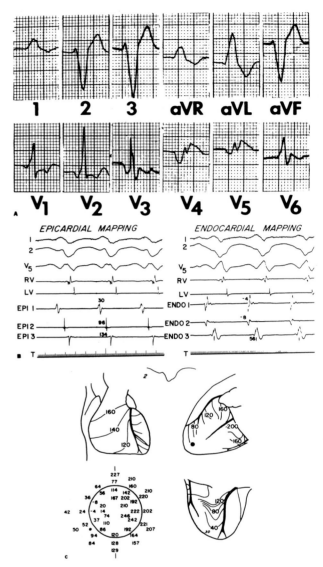

Figure 41-1. (**Top**) A 12-lead electrocardiogram during ventricular tachycardia. (**Middle panels,** *left*) Epicardial mapping and (*right*) endocardial mapping. (**Bottom**) An epicardial isochronic map (AP, lateral, posterior views) and an endocardial map, showing the earliest activation point (viewed from the feet toward the head). (With permission from Josephson ME, Harken AH, Horowitz, LN: Endocardial excision: a new surgical technique for the treatment of recurrent ventricular tachycardia. Circulation 1979;60:1430.)

aneurysmectomy, and there is no study in which patients were randomly allocated to one of the two treatment protocols. Nevertheless, the results are so convincing that this methodologic inadequacy can probably be ignored.

To construct an activation map of the endocardial or epicardial surface, electrograms must be recorded from between 50 and 100 points. Using a roving hand-held electrode, this requires at least 5 to 10 minutes and requires the rhythm to be stable during this period. Ventricular tachycardias often degenerate rapidly or several tachycardias with multiple morphologies may coexist. Therefore, it is sometimes necessary to map the ventricles quickly. Simultaneous recording of electrograms from multiple points may allow the collection of all data during just a few beats of tachycardia. A variety of ingenious electrode arrays and computer algorithms to collect and process the electrograms into activation maps have been developed (Fig. 41-2). Ideker and colleagues describe a triple array system.[42a] A flexible nylon mesh sock containing 27 electrodes was fitted over the epicardial surface of

the heart to obtain a general activation map from which to define an approximate origin for the tachycardia. A 3 × 3 cm plaque containing 25 electrodes was then placed over the region of interest to allow a more detailed map of this area. Finally, a needle array, consisting of five electrodes (each separated by 3 mm) was used to explore the transmural activation sequence. An electrode system designed to collect endocardial electrograms is reported by de Bakker and associates.[43] A balloon with 30 electrodes on its surface was inserted into the left ventricle through an incision usually made in aneurysmal or akinetic area. The balloon was then inflated to bring the terminals into con-

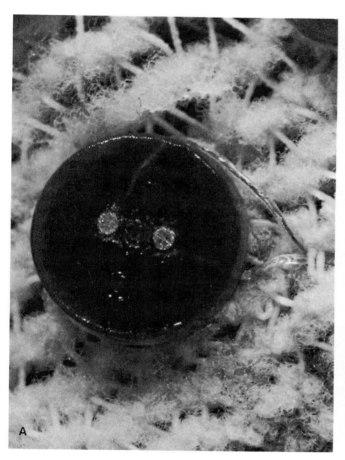

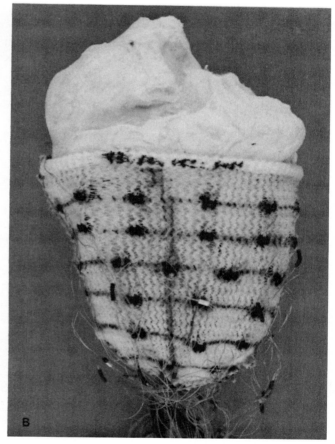

Figure 41-2. (**A**) Molded epoxy bipolar snap electrode attached to the woven sock. The electrode contacts are 0.7 mm in diameter and separated by 2 mm, measured center to center. The wires leading to the electrode contacts from the outside of the sock are visible to the right as they emerge from under the elastic cross-mesh fibers between two longitudinal nylon fibers. The small circular indentation on the face of the electrode at 7 o'clock is from a pin used to eject the hardened epoxy from the mold. (**B**) The sock electrode array applied to the latex mold of a human heart. The female snaps are sewn to the sock in six circumferential rows from base to apex. The female snaps are visible in the photograph as black circles. The top three rows have 12 snaps each, whereas the bottom three rows have eight snaps each. Each female snap supports a snap electrode on the inside of the sock. The line on the sock extending from apex to base is used to align the sock on the heart at the time of surgery. (From Worley SJ, Ideker RE, Mastrototaro I, et al: A new sock electrode for recording epicardial activation from the human heart: one size fits all. Pacing Clin Electrophysiol 1987;10:21)

tact with the endocardium. With this system, de Bakker and his group studied 32 patients with ventricular tachycardias and demonstrated that the endocardial site of origin of some ventricular tachycardias with identical surface QRS complexes could vary from beat to beat by up to 4 cm. Mickleborough and colleagues increased the number of electrodes mounted on the mapping balloon to 112.[44] The signals from this device are processed by computer to produce activation maps. Hauer and colleagues extended the role of the computer by developing a method whereby the site of origin of an arrhythmia in relation to anatomic landmarks can be accurately predicted from the results of preoperative catheter mapping.[45] They performed this analysis on eight ventricular tachycardias and computed the location of the arrhythmogenic site to within 1 cm of the site of origin determined by operative mapping in seven of the eight tachycardias. In the remaining case, the computed site of origin was less than 2 cm distant from the mapped origin of tachycardia.

The steady spread of computer-assisted mapping techniques will minimize the time taken to achieve a map and allow more accurate maps to be obtained, even when arrhythmias are not sustained. The ability to produce a moving image aids recognition of the region of slow conduction in the circuit. The future development of three-dimensional mapping may further assist in localization of the tachycardia.

Another approach to mapping during tachycardia has been developed. This is termed *potential distribution mapping* and uses an array of multiple electrodes in the ventricle, as does activation mapping. The electrograms recorded are unipolar, however, and the maps that are produced show absolute voltage. It is suggested that such technique may be superior to conventional activation mapping in ease and rapidity of interpretation, and it is less sensitive to minor separation of the recording electrodes from the endocardial surface.[46, 47] To date, this technique has been applied only to the mapping of induced septal ventricular tachycardias in dogs.

Electrogram Mapping During Sinus Rhythm

Ventricular tachycardia in association with chronic coronary artery disease is thought to be due to reentry phenomena. In such cases, electric activity should continue through systole and diastole. If diastolic activity is confined to a small mass of tissue, it may be possible to remove that tissue to prevent further tachycardia. Diastolic potentials have been described as "late" because they occur more than 100 milliseconds after the onset of the QRS complex

or occur entirely outside the QRS complex.[48, 49] Other abnormal potentials have been described in association with coronary disease. "Fractionated" potentials are continuous multicomponent electrograms longer than 50 milliseconds and less than 1 mV in amplitude (Fig. 41-3).[50] "Split" or double potentials have a distinct isoelectric segment between multiple discrete potentials. Wiener and colleagues demonstrated that such abnormal electrograms are often recorded from aneurysmal tissue and in some patients, particularly those with a history of ventricular tachycardia, they may also be recorded from an epicardial or endocardial border zone surrounding an aneurysm.[50] Klein and colleagues confirmed these findings in a larger group of 38 patients, of whom 21 had serious ventricular arrhythmias associated with either a left ventricular aneurysm or an akinetic area resulting from a myocardial infarction.[48] Although abnormal potentials could sometimes be recorded only from the endocardium, which was mapped in only 10 of the 38 with arrhythmias, Klein and associates found that in the 21 patients with arrhythmias, 20 had late potentials, 20 had fractionated potentials, and 13 had double potentials.[48] In the 17 patients who had no history of arrhythmia, only two had late potentials and one had both double and fractionated potentials. Thus in this study, abnormal potentials were sensitive and highly specific markers of ventricular tachycardia.

A different perspective emerged from the study reported by Kienzle and colleagues.[49] They studied 13 patients, all of whom had a history of recurrent sustained ventricular tachycardia associated with a previous extensive myocardial infarction. During sinus rhythm, fractionated endocardial electrograms were recorded in all but late potentials and were recorded only in four of 13 patients. Late electrograms were recorded from areas activated early during induced tachycardia more consistently than were fractionated or split potentials. These workers also noted that fractionated potentials were recorded from more sites (36%) than were late potentials (5%). They pointed out that if surgery were designed to remove all endocardium from which abnormal electrograms were recorded, a seemingly more extensive operation than indicated from tachycardia activation sequence mapping would be needed. Large areas of scarred endothelium may give rise to late potentials but in the absence of a suitable reentry circuit, this finding is of no consequence because the tissue behaves as "dead-end" substrate.

Bourke and colleagues assessed the use of intraoperative fragmentation mapping in patients whose tachycardia could not be mapped using conventional techniques, either because it was noninducible at the time of surgery or because of hemodynamic instability.[51] These patients represented a third of all their patients operated on for ventricular tachycardia. Perioperative mortality was 24%.

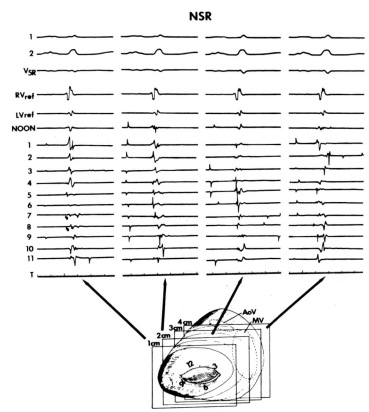

NSR

Figure 41-3. Multiple endocardial electrograms recorded during normothermic bypass during sinus rhythm. Note the marked fractionation and reduced amplitude of some of the left ventricular sites. (With permission from Kienzle MG, Miller J, Falcone RA, et al: Intraoperative endocardial mapping during sinus rhythm: relationship to site of origin of ventricular tachycardia. Circulation 1984;70:957)

Arrhythmia recurrence rate in the survivors was 19%, with one death. Thus, when conventional mapping fails, fragmentation mapping may offer a useful alternative.

Cryothermal Mapping

Reducing the temperature of the myocardium to 0°C produces conduction block, which is relieved when the temperature is allowed to rise again. Thus, if tissue that forms a critical part of the reentry circuit supporting the tachycardia is cooled, the tachycardia breaks and should not be reinducible until the tissue is rewarmed. Similarly, automatic mechanisms of tachycardia may be suppressed by local cooling. Therefore, cooling of the myocardium with a cryoprobe may be used to confirm the origin or pathway of an arrhythmia. This technique was first applied to the localization of the His bundle or atrioventricular (AV) node before attempted destruction of AV conduction.[52] Cryomapping has been successfully used to aid in the localization of ventricular tachycardia by Gallagher and colleagues and by Camm and associates.[53-55] The method requires that sustained and stable tachycardia can be initiated at surgery.

Pace Mapping

If a tachycardia with a distinct morphology cannot be initiated or sustained long enough for an adequate activation map, the technique of pace mapping may be employed.[56] This involves pacing the ventricle with a roving electrode and attempting to match the paced QRS complex with previously recorded QRS complexes of the ventricular tachycardia (Fig. 41-4). Such recordings may be made preoperatively or preferably during identical circumstances (e.g., chest open during normothermic cardiopulmonary bypass) perioperatively. Pacing the ventricle from different sites results in different QRS configurations; the technique of attempting to mimic tachycardia complexes by ventricular pacing can be applied to the identification of the origin of ventricular tachycardia and used as an aid in the direct surgical eradication of tachycardias.[57-59] Initially, epicardial pacing was advocated but because most coronary-related tachycardias arise from the endocardium, endocardial pacing was subsequently evaluated.[60,61] Although O'Keefe and coauthors were able to identify with epicardial pace mapping the tachycardia origin in a series of nine patients, it is probable that the source of some tachycardias is not accurately identified by

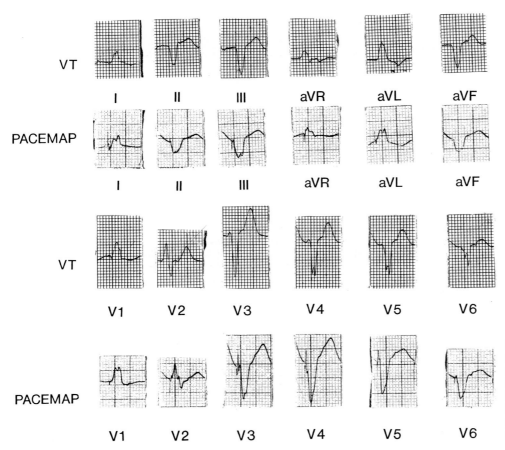

Figure 41-4. These traces taken during preoperative endocardial mapping show close concordance between the morphology of the patient's ventricular tachycardia and the electrocardiogram produced by pacing in the area of tachycardia origin.

epicardial pacing because the epicardial breakthrough point may be many centimeters away from the true endocardial origin.[62]

Endocardial pacing at the site of origin of ventricular tachycardia accurately simulates the tachycardia QRS complex but similar QRS complexes can be obtained by pacing at widely divergent points, and different QRS complexes can result from pacing at closely adjacent points.[61] It may therefore take a long time to locate the tachycardia focus using pace mapping. Apparently, the energy and rate of pacing do not seem to influence the resultant QRS complex. Ventricular pacing may engage, drive, and entrain a reentry circuit and closely reproduce the tachycardia QRS simply by being nearly "on circuit" rather than by pacing in a critical part of the circuit. Conversely, pacing from a point source may never reproduce the tachycardia QRS if it results from conduction over a long reentry circuit. Despite these theoretic limitations, pace mapping is useful if tachycardia cannot be initiated in the operating room. It should not, however, be used instead of activation mapping.

Visual Inspection

For a variety of reasons (which follow), several groups of investigators suggest that the endocardial surface of the heart should be visually inspected and that all abnormal endocardium likely to give rise to ventricular tachycardia should be removed:

1. It may not be possible to obtain an adequate activation map or cryothermal termination point because ventricular tachyarrhythmias may not be provoked at surgery or when successfully initiated may not be sustained or may degenerate into ventricular fibrillation.

2. Mapping during sinus rhythm is nonspecific because it generally reveals large areas from which abnormal electrograms are recorded. This necessitates excision of extensive areas of endocardium.

3. In some patients, the endocardium cannot be mapped during any rhythm because of adherent thrombi.

4. Polymorphic (multiple distinct QRS shapes) or

pleomorphic (continuously changing QRS shape) ventricular tachycardias and ventricular fibrillation are impossible to map without sophisticated multiple simultaneous recordings and computer-based algorithms to construct activation maps.

5. All mapping techniques take at least 15 minutes and may last as long as an hour.

6. Pace mapping may provide misleading information.

In patients with endocardial scars due to previous myocardial infarction, the abnormal (thick and white) endocardium can easily be seen. Except when the scar extends throughout the entire thickness of the free wall or septum or involves the papillary muscles or extends into the AV valve ring, it can easily and quickly be stripped away. Thus, visual inspection and extensive endocardial resection has been safely and effectively used to manage patients with ventricular tachycardias and ventricular fibrillation.

Comparison of Mapping Methods

Josephson and colleagues compared preoperative endocardial mapping with operative endocardial mapping in 18 patients undergoing surgery for the control of 24 tachycardias (right bundle branch block morphology in 12 and left bundle branch block in 12).[63] Catheter mapping accurately predicted the origin of tachycardia in all 24 cases. Tachycardia origins determined by the two techniques were within 4 to 8 cm of each other. In the same paper, endocardial preoperative mapping was compared with epicardial mapping. The origins of the 12 right bundle branch block morphology tachycardia were correctly localized to the left ventricle but 11 of the 12 left bundle branch block–morphology tachycardias were wrongly localized by epicardial mapping. One tachycardia that arose from the right ventricular outflow tract was accurately located by epicardial mapping. Otherwise, there was considerable discrepancy between epicardial breakthrough and endocardial origin because tachycardias arose from near the endocardium or within the septum. Thus, endocardial activity uniformly preceded the earliest epicardial electrogram, and in only one patient did epicardial activation coincide with the onset of the surface QRS. The endocardial origin was confirmed when excision of the earliest activated endocardial site led to eradication of the tachycardias. Spielman and colleagues, Wittig and Boineau, and Horowitz and associates also found that epicardial mapping was inaccurate, particularly when the tachycardias arose from the interventricular septum.[36,37,64]

The accuracy of endocardial pace mapping was evaluated against endocardial and epicardial activation mapping by Josephson and associates.[61] They found that the paced QRS complex tended to reflect the epicardial breakthrough point rather than the endocardial origin and that pace mapping could only be used to determine the gross region (e.g., anterior wall of the left ventricle) from which the tachycardia arose. They suggest that pace mapping either be corroborative or be used only when tachycardia could not be initiated at surgery.

Kienzle and colleagues compared endocardial mapping in sinus rhythm with endocardial activation mapping during ventricular tachycardia in 13 patients.[49] They note that fractionated, split, or late electrograms during sinus rhythm were seen over large areas and were not specific to the site of tachycardia origin. Similar results with endocavity catheter mapping during sinus rhythm are reported by Cassidy and associates.[65] Wiener and associates report excellent results using endocardial fragmentation mapping to identify areas for excision.[66]

Gessman and colleagues compared three methods of intraoperative mapping: tachycardia activation sequence, cryothermal termination mapping, and normal sinus rhythm late potential mapping in 14 patients undergoing surgery for the management of ventricular tachycardia.[67] The tachycardia was provoked and mapped in 10 patients and in eight of these, a cryothermal termination site was discovered. There was an excellent correspondence between the sites of origin identified by cryothermal and activation mapping. In all 14 patients, normal sinus rhythm late potential mapping was performed and in 13 patients, late potentials were identified. In eight patients, the late potentials were confined to the area from which the tachycardia arose. There was therefore a reasonable correlation between all three techniques, and they are obviously complimentary.

Development of a multi-electrode balloon endocardial mapping catheter has led to hopes of improved surgical results in patients with tachycardias that cannot be sustained at the time of intraoperative mapping. Mickleborough and colleagues compared 15 patients who underwent orthodox mapping techniques and 15 who underwent balloon electrode array, passed transatrially.[44] Ventricular tachycardia was successfully induced in all 30 patients. Endocardial maps were obtained in all 15 patients who underwent balloon transatrial mapping but in only 10 of the 15 patients mapped using conventional techniques. Balloon array mapping was markedly superior at mapping multimorphologic tachycardias with disparate sites of origin. At postoperative electrophysiologic study, 36% (5 of 14) patients mapped using the standard approach still had inducible ventricular tachycardia. In the transatrial balloon approach group, only 8% (1 of 12) still had inducible ventricular tachycardia. There was no significant difference in cardiopulmonary bypass time between the two groups.

DIRECT SURGICAL METHODS

Ventriculotomy

Fontaine and colleagues first described a condition known as arrhythmogenic right ventricular dysplasia, which is characterized by ventricular tachyarrhythmias associated with thinning, fatty infiltration, and aneurysmal dilation of the right ventricle, particularly in the apical, infundibular, and posterobasal regions.[68] Sustained ventricular arrhythmias emanate from the thinned or aneurysmal areas of the right ventricular free wall. A transmural incision through the area of epicardial breakthrough of these ventricular arrhythmias or through myocardium from which late potentials may be recorded terminates the arrhythmia, which cannot be reinduced. In a report of 12 cases of arrhythmogenic right ventricular dysplasia, Fontaine and associates found that a simple transmural ventriculotomy abolished medically refractory tachycardia in eight of the 12 patients.[69] The ventricular tachycardia recurred in four, and there were two deaths unrelated to arrhythmias.

In arrhythmogenic right ventricular dysplasia, epicardial mapping successfully locates the arrhythmogenic site, presumably because of the thin wall of the abnormal right ventricle. For similar reasons, reentrant activity (which supports tachycardia in arrhythmogenic right ventricular dysplasia) must conduct transversely through the myocardium rather than from endocardium to epicardium or vice versa. Thus, a simple ventriculotomy through the epicardial breakthrough point should abolish tachycardia in this condition. Conversely, in coronary patients, a simple transmural ventriculotomy based on epicardial mapping has only rarely been successful.[70]

There is often multiple tachycardia morphology in patients with arrhythmogenic right ventricular dysplasia. Therefore, multiple ventriculotomies may be required. Alternatively, an encircling transmural ventriculotomy may be used to isolate several sites of origin. Such an operation was developed by Boineau and Cox and successfully used in three patients.[71] In this operation, a full-thickness semicircular ventriculotomy is performed between two points of the tricuspid anulus.

Guiradon and colleagues describe an extensive encircling ventriculotomy to isolate the entire right ventricular free wall from the remainder of the heart.[72] This is accomplished by a full-thickness ventriculotomy that extends along the attachment of the right ventricular free wall to the interventricular septum. The moderator band connecting the free wall to the septum is also divided. The attachments of the free wall anteriorly to the aortic anulus and posteriorly to the tricuspid anulus are divided, using incision or cryoablation. The operation results in total electrical isolation of the right ventricular wall. The technique is described in two patients having arrhythmogenic right ventricular dysplasia initiating several morphologies of ventricular tachycardia and occurring from multiple sites in the right ventricular free wall. It was anticipated that a smaller exclusion procedure for discrete cryosurgery would not be sufficient because of the extensive arrhythmia substrate. The surgery was successful in the immediate postoperative period, and the patients were followed-up for 3 and 4 months after the operation. In one patient, the right ventricular tachycardia was almost incessant but was entirely confined to the right ventricle. Although paradoxical septal motion occurred in both patients, there was no significant hemodynamic impairment. The potential hemodynamic effects of right ventricular disarticulation have been investigated by Jones and colleagues.[73] They report a systematic investigation of the technique of right ventricular disconnection in the dog. No major hemodynamic disturbances were noted but a moderate reduction of left ventricular pressure and a reduced cardiac output occurred. This impairment of left ventricular function was almost reversed by stimulating the right ventricle synchronously with left ventricular activation. A series of 10 patients—nine of whom had right ventricular disarticulation—was reported by Nimkhedkar and coworkers. All manifested signs of right heart failure in the early postoperative period but after a mean follow-up of 3 years, all patients were alive and in New York Heart Association classes I or II.

This operation seem ideally suited for patients with arrhythmogenic right ventricular dysplasia. Initial experience has been encouraging but long-term experience is needed. In particular, the result of this operation on right ventricular diastolic function remains to be determined.

Boineau and Cox reported another extensive but successful exclusion procedure. The supracristal intraventricular septum was disarticulated from the remainder of the heart to isolate a tachycardia focus in a young girl who had suffered refractory ventricular tachycardia after an episode of coxsackievirus B5 myocarditis 6 years previously.[71]

Encircling Endocardial Ventriculotomy

Encircling endocardial ventriculotomy was introduced as a specific form of surgery to manage chronic ventricular tachycardia after myocardial infarction.[74] The aim of the surgery is to exclude the origin of tachycardia from the remainder of the heart. The technique involves entering the heart through the myocardial infarction scar or aneurysm and making a vertical incision from the endocardium that extends almost to the epicardium (Fig. 41-5). Theoretically, such an incision conserves the epicardial blood vessels and perpendicular penetrating branches. If the incision involves the septum, it is made about 1 cm deep or may even transect the septum completely.[74, 75] The incision is designed to encircle the entire scar or arrhythmogenic area. It is repaired in a conventional manner with Teflon buttresses and a running suture. When the incision heals, the fibrous tissue thus formed creates an insulating barrier to the spread of electric activation, which may effectively isolate an arrhythmia mechanism or interrupt part of a reentry circuit responsible for generating the arrhythmia.[76]

The first report describes five patients, all of whom were treated successfully with this operation between 1975 and 1978.[74] By 1980, 21 patients had been operated on by the group in Paris; the operation was successful in 18 patients.[77] A detailed report of the first 15 of these 22 patients reveals that many of them had had other procedures as part of their operation (e.g., aneurysmectomy in six patients and right coronary bypass grafting in one patient).[78] It is therefore difficult to be sure how critical the endocardial ventriculotomy was in these patients but because other procedures do not usually abolish arrhythmias, the additional specific surgery was probably responsible for the good results. In 1982, Fontaine and coworkers again updated the series.[79] By then, 27 patients had undergone operation, with a 1-month recurrence rate of 8% and a mortality rate of 15%. At 5 years after the operation, there was a 24% recurrence rate and a mortality rate of 33%. Both the mortality and the recurrence rate were substan-

tially lower for the 16 patients operated on after December 1978; although the original operation did not rely on perioperative electrophysiologic mapping, it was employed for later operations.

Other groups report their experience with encircling endocardial ventriculotomy. For example Cox and colleagues report that nine patients underwent encircling endocardial ventriculotomy at Duke University.[75] There were three operative deaths from low output and two late deaths. Overall, only four patients had a successful operation, and three of these had some endocardial resection as part of their surgery. In 1982, Ostermeyer and colleagues compared the efficacy of electrophysiologically guided encircling endocardial ventriculotomy (31 patients) with simple aneurysmectomy and appropriate coronary artery bypass grafting (10 patients).[80] Encircling endocardial ventriculotomy was clearly more effective but this was possibly because of the perioperative mapping associated with the encircling ventriculotomy rather than the nature of the surgery itself. In 1984, the same group detailed the results of 40 patients who had undergone some form of encircling endocardial ventriculotomy guided by mapping techniques.[81] The operation was combined with aneurysmectomy in 34 patients and coronary bypass grafting in 30 patients. There were three operative and six late deaths. Spontaneous recurrence of tachycardia occurred in only two patients during a mean follow-up period of almost 19 months. Postoperatively, programmed ventricular stimulation provoked ventricular tachycardia in only about a fourth of the patients.

When the operation was conceived, it was anticipated

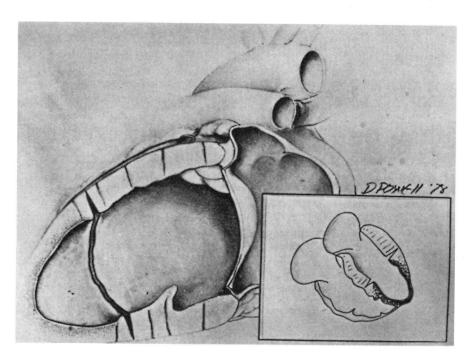

Figure 41-5. The incision used for the encircling endocardial ventriculotomy. The depth of the incision is shown, as well as the need for the incision to be done above the area of endocardial fibrosis. (From Guiraudon G, Fontaine G, Frank R, et al: Encircling endocardial ventriculotomy: a new surgical treatment for life-threatening ventricular tachycardias resistant to medical treatment following myocardial infarction. Ann Thorac Surg 1978;26:438)

that the blood supply to the myocardium enclosed within the ventriculotomy would not be impaired because the epicardial and penetrating coronary arteries would not be damaged by the incision. It was therefore hoped that myocardial function in the already scarred area surrounded by the ventriculotomy would not be further compromised. This was consistent with the clinical impressions noted in earlier reports but it soon became evident that encircling endocardial ventriculotomy was not appropriate for patients with an already badly damaged left ventricle because of further deterioration of left ventricular function after this form of surgery.[82] Ungerleider and colleagues investigated the effect of encircling endocardial ventriculotomy on left ventricular function in normal dogs and demonstrated a significant decrease in diastolic compliance in addition to reduced systolic pump function.[83] This was attributed to the severe fall of myocardial blood flow in the area surrounded by the ventriculotomy.[84]

A variety of modifications to the technique of encircling ventriculotomy have been proposed. For example, in two male patients without inducible tachycardia, Guiradon and colleagues have attempted to ablate all electric activity in the border zone around an infarct by a series of overlapping cryolesions.[85] Over a short follow-up period (4 months), these patients have done well, with no recurrences and no need for antiarrhythmic drugs. These workers have named this technique "encircling endocardial cryoablation."

Landymore and colleagues combine the concepts of encircling endocardial ventriculotomy and endocardial resection in an operation that they refer to as "encircling endocardial resection."[86] The authors describe a simple operation consisting of the removal of all visibly diseased endocardium from the border surrounding ventricular aneurysms. The operation was performed without electrophysiologic map guidance on 10 patients with drug-refractory ventricular tachycardia, combined with aneurysmectomy in eight patients and coronary artery bypass grafting in nine patients. The extensive nature of this operation is indicated by the need for partial reimplantation of the mitral valve apparatus in nine patients. No arrhythmias recurred after surgery but there were two late deaths.

Endocardial Resection

Josephson and associates and Harken and colleagues, from the University of Pennsylvania, introduced a surgical technique known as endocardial resection that was specifically designed to remove anatomic substrate for this type of ventricular tachycardia.[87,88] In patients with previous myocardial infarction, ventricular arrhythmias usually arise from the endocardium in the so-called twilight or border zone surrounding the infarct scar, where there are islands of apparently normal myocardial cells interspersed with infarcted or ischemic tissue. It was reasoned that the arrhythmia focus could be removed by excising the endocardium. To minimize the extent of the operation, electrophysiologic mapping techniques—particularly on the endocardial surface—are used to identify the site of origin of the arrhythmia. About 10 to 25 cm^2 of endocardium are peeled off the underlying ventricular muscle. The stripping may extend 2 to 3 cm away from the scar and involve up to 40% of its circumference (Fig. 41-6).

Numerous reports extol endocardial resection for the management of patients with drug-refractory tachyarrhythmias.[89–93] A group of 100 patients treated by the University of Pennsylvania group underwent this operation. Ninety of the 100 patients also underwent aneurysmectomy and in 61, an average of 1.6 coronary grafts were implanted. Ninety-one patients survived surgery and in this group, 200 morphologically distinct tachycardias were mapped preoperatively. Sixty-four patients and 171 tachycardias could not be induced after surgery and in 10 other patients, 13 further tachycardias were noninducible after antiarrhythmic drug treatment. Of the 89 patients who underwent postoperative electrophysiologic testing, 15 still had inducible tachycardias.

Cryoablation

Cryoablation of conduction tissue such as the His bundle or Kent pathway was reported in 1977.[52] A cryosurgical machine and probe are shown in Figure 41-7. In 1978, Gallagher and colleagues published a case report of the successful cryosurgical treatment of ventricular tachycardia associated with scleroderma.[53] A second success was reported in 1979 by Camm and colleagues.[54] Vermeulen and colleagues describe the use of cryosurgery for the treatment of persistent symptomatic ventricular bigeminy.[94] The patients were young and did not have previous ischemic heart disease. To avoid a ventriculotomy, with its potential arrhythmogenic properties and the possibility of further impairment of left ventricular function, the cryosurgery and mapping were performed through the aortic root.

The advantages of cryosurgery are summarized by Harrison and associates.[52] Cryolesions are histologically well-demarcated, with a sharp border between the scar and healthy myocardium. The scar is mechanically strong because fibrous tissue, collagen, and elastic tissue are not affected by the freezing process. Hemorrhage is not produced, and cryoablation of blood vessels does not lead to hemolysis, thrombosis, or embolization. Six months after the direct freezing of major epicardial canine coronary arteries, there is intimal hyperplasia in most instances but coronary vessel occlusion is not seen.[95]

The size of the cryolesion depends on the tempera-

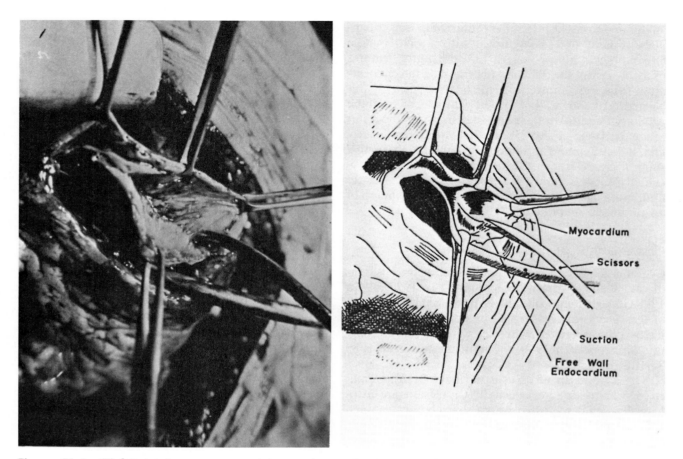

Figure 41-6. (**Right**) Artist's representation of the actual surgical technique. (**Left**) Note the section of the endocardium from the left ventricular wall. (From Harken AH, Josephson ME, Horowitz LN: Surgical endocardial resection for the treatment of malignant ventricular tachycardia. Ann Surg 1979;190:456)

ture of the cryoprobe, probe size, the duration of the freeze, and the number of cryoablations performed. It also depends on the temperature of the myocardium before application of the cryoprobe. Holman and colleagues[96] created cryolesions in the left ventricular free wall of dogs. When the animals were treated during hypothermic cardioplegic cardiac arrest (6° to 12°C), the lesions were significantly larger than those produced during normothermic arrest.

The sharp demarcation of the cryolesions from the untreated myocardium reduces the likelihood of an arrhythmia substrate being created by the cryolesion; however, Kerr and colleagues report a case of accelerated junctional tachycardia that appeared to arise from tissue adjacent to an area of ventricular tachycardia.[97] The arrhythmogenic potential of cryolesions has been systematically studied in dogs by Klein and associates.[98]

Programmed ventricular stimulation did not provoke any ventricular tachycardias. Only far-field or extrinsic electric signals were recorded from the cryoablated tissue. In most animals, frequent ventricular ectopic activity was observed in the first few days after creation of a cryolesion. These ectopic beats appear to arise from the edge of the cryolesion and may have a similar electrocardiographic morphology to the tachycardias treated by the cryoablation.

Laser Ablation

The use of an Nd:YAG laser in 12 patients with ischemic ventricular tachycardia was reported by Mesnildrey and colleagues in 1985.[99] The 10 survivors were arrhythmia-free after 8 months follow-up, and nine of them required no antiarrhythmic therapy. The Nd:YAG laser's properties of high power and coagulation necrosis without tissue sectioning make it particularly useful for antiarrhythmic surgery. Experience with other types of lasers has been widely reported. Saksena and colleagues used a 15-W argon laser to perform a ventriculotomy (Fig. 41-8) and

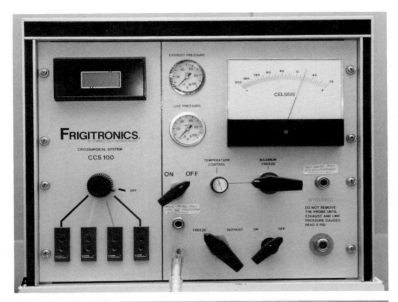

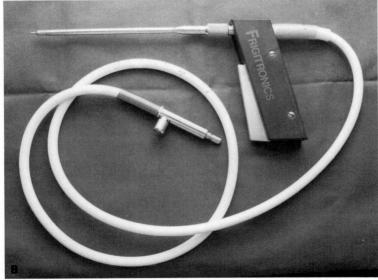

Figure 41-7. Cryosurgical machine and probe for use during arrhythmia surgery.

then proceeded to endocardial mapping.[100] Pulsed laser discharges were then used to vaporize endocardial scar in areas of presystolic activation. Aneurysmectomy was then performed. Seven ventricular tachycardia foci were treated in five patients. Five of the ventricular tachycardia foci had been deemed unresectable using conventional techniques. Postoperative studies revealed no inducible tachycardias in four of the five patients, and the fifth patient was responsive to a drug that had been ineffective preoperatively. Short-term follow-up over 3 to 5 months revealed no recurrence of symptomatic ventricular tachycardia. It is clear from this study that laser treatment of a limited area of endocardium is successful but exactly how much tissue must be destroyed to prevent tachycardia remains to be determined.

CO_2-laser ablation has also been used in conjunction with conventional subendocardial resection to ablate that portion of the endocardial scar involving the anterolateral papillary muscle, an area where the application of conventional treatment usually requires additional mitral valve replacement.[101] Thus, the application of laser ablation may maintain high operative success rates in more difficult cases.

CHOICE OF SURGICAL TECHNIQUE

A surgical ablation registry has been established by Borggrefe and others to collect data on patients undergoing surgery for ventricular tachyarrhythmias.[102] Although it is

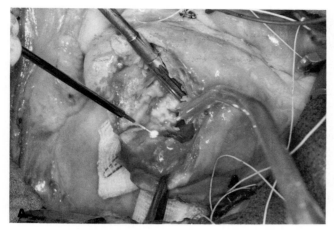

Pre-Ablation

Sustained VT Cycle Length - 330 ms

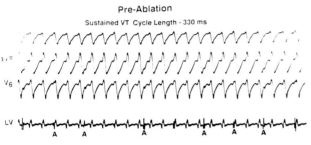

During Laser Irradiation

Sustained VT Cycle Length - 400-420 ms

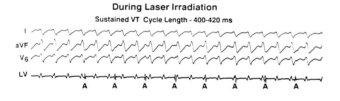

Sustained VT Cycle Length - 420 ms   Sinus Rhythm with A-V Block

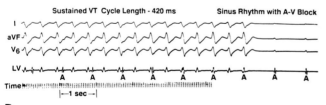

B

Figure 41-8. (A) Laser ablation of ventricular tachycardia. A 15-W argon laser catheter delivery system is used to irradiate the ventricular endocardium. **(B)** The electrocardiogram shows a stable ventricular tachycardia. Laser activation occurs at points marked *A*. Tachycardia initially slows and then terminates suddenly after laser activation. (From Krol RB, Saksena S: Laser ablation for supraventricular and ventricular tachycardia: present status and future promise. J Intervent Cardiol 1990;3:113.)

not comprehensive, a large pool of data has been collected on 665 patients. In this study, localized endocardial resection was performed in 33.2%, with the addition of cryosurgery in another 16.1%, partial encircling endocardial ventriculotomy in 16.8%, and complete encircling endocardial ventriculotomy in 9.3%. Cryosurgery alone

was performed in 7.4% and other therapies (e.g., coronary artery bypass grafting alone) in 12.5%. In addition to the specific therapies, 73% of patients underwent aneurysmectomy and 55% coronary artery bypass grafting.

Operative mortality data was as follows:

Complete endocardial encircling ventriculotomy, 13%
Partial endocardial encircling ventriculotomy, 8%
Localized endocardial resection, 10%
Localized endocardial resection with cryosurgery, 16%
Extended endocardial resection, 27%
Endocardial encircling ventriculotomy combined with
    endocardial resection, 23%
Cryosurgery alone, 8.5%

The more localized procedures, such as endocardial resection and cryosurgery, seem to be associated with a lower mortality.

Long-term survival in this study was similar to that for the endocardial resection, complete endocardial encircling ventriculotomy, and localized endocardial resection plus cryosurgery groups. The cryosurgery alone group had poorer long-term survival, and the partial endocardial encircling ventriculotomy group had better survival. These figures must be viewed as a simple observation, however, because this is not a randomized study.

SELECTION OF PATIENTS FOR SURGERY

Before submitting a patient to surgery for ventricular tachycardia, two important factors must be considered. The first is the risk of perioperative death associated with the proposed therapy; the second is the success rate in terms of long-term abolition of tachycardia.

OPERATIVE RISK

Operative risk is affected by the choice of surgical approach but clinical features of the patient are also important. Borggrefe and coworkers analyzed several variables for the 665 patients on the surgical ablation registry.[102] They found no significant association of operative risk with age, ejection fraction, cycle length of ventricular tachycardia, number of episodes of ventricular tachycardia, presence of coronary artery disease, triple vessel disease, or presence of incessant ventricular tachycardia. Only the severity of heart failure, as classified on clinical grounds (New York Heart Association functional class IV), was associated with a poor clinical outcome.

Because many of these patients have ventricular aneurysms, scoring left ventricular function based on overall ejection fraction may be ignoring the importance of the function of nonaneurysmal myocardium. This has been recognized by van Hemel and associates.[103] They divided the right oblique left ventricular angiogram into five segments and the left oblique angiogram into four segments. The angiograms were independently reported. Retrospective analysis of the 69 patients operated on from 1980 to 1986 showed that 13 (19%) had fewer than three left ventricular segments with normal motion or slight hypokinesia, whereas 55 (80%) had three or more contractile segments. In the group with fewer than three contractile segments, actuarial survival (including in-hospital mortality) was 46% at 1 year and 11% at 3 years follow-up. For the group with three or more contractile segments, these percentages were 64% and 53%, respectively.

Many patients who develop ventricular tachycardia do so after a myocardial infarction, and the timing of surgery after the myocardial infarction may be an important factor. Some reports suggest that surgery in the first 4 months postinfarction is associated with a poor outcome.[104, 105] Newer series, however, suggest that surgery in this group is a practical alternative, especially when the 1-year mortality in this group may be as high as 80% when treated medically.[106–108]

Patients with ventricular tachycardia of nonischemic origin may have better long-term survival than those with an ischemic origin. Lawrie and coworkers give a figure of 78% 5-year survival for nonischemic ventricular tachycardia patients against 48% for patients with ischemic heart disease.[109] The 14 patients they describe had ventricular tachycardia secondary to cardiomyopathy, acute myocarditis, arrhythmogenic right ventricular dysplasia, tumor, postoperative Tetralogy of Fallot, and acute bacterial endocarditis.[1–3] The remaining four cases were idiopathic. Preoperative or intraoperative mapping was successful in 13 cases.

VENTRICULAR TACHYCARDIA RECURRENCE RATE

A few factors have been identified that can predict the likelihood of surgical success preoperatively.

The anatomic site of origin has been identified as being important. Saksena and colleagues show a higher frequency of ventricular tachycardia inducibility postoperatively in patients with an inferior site of origin for their tachycardia.[110] They report that this is because of the difficulty of adequate endocardial resection in these patients. Hargrove and colleagues report using cryoablation

of the ventricular muscle between the basal end of the ventriculotomy and the mitral valve anulus (anular isthmus).[111] This improved the postoperative noninducibility rate from 56% to 93%.

Brandt and coworkers studied 33 patients who had had surgery for drug-resistant sustained ventricular tachycardia.[111a] Fourteen of these patients still had inducible ventricular tachycardia postoperatively. They found no difference between these patients and the 19 patients in whom ventricular tachycardia was noninducible in the following characteristics; previous syncope, cardiac arrest, number of drug trials, site of infarction, and ventricular tachycardia cycle length. Only the presence of three-vessel disease and a period of fewer than 3 months since myocardial infarction were associated with an unfavorable outcome. Mickleborough and associates show a reduced rate of recurrent ventricular tachycardia associated with successful mapping of the site or sites of origin.[44]

POSTOPERATIVE ASSESSMENT

Because surgery for ventricular tachycardia is not always successful, it is essential to assess whether tachycardia can still be induced postoperatively. Even if tachycardia can still be induced, patients often respond to drugs to which they were resistant before surgery.

The surgical ablation registry records data on 330 postoperative electrophysiologic studies.[102] Clinical ventricular tachycardia was induced in 17%. In an additional 74%, either no arrhythmia or nonsustained ventricular tachycardia was inducible. In the remaining 9%, a nonclinical ventricular tachycardia was induced. During follow-up, 12% of patients with noninducible ventricular tachycardia and 13% with inducible nonclinical ventricular tachycardia had an arrhythmic event, predicting a generally good prognosis for these patients. Of the patients with inducible clinical ventricular tachycardia, 41% had a recurrence of ventricular tachycardia.

A wide variety of stimulation protocols were used in collection of this data. The ideal postoperative stimulation protocol remains the subject of debate. Miller and colleagues report that cycle length of induced ventricular tachycardia can be useful in predicting the risk of spontaneous recurrent ventricular tachycardia.[112] When induced ventricular tachycardia had a cycle length of more than 30 milliseconds below that of the most rapid preoperative ventricular tachycardia, the risk of a subsequent spontaneous arrhythmic event was 25%. In patients who did not meet this criterion, recurrence rate was 77%. The presence or absence of ventricular ectopic beats has not been shown to be of predictive value.[113]

DOES ANTIARRHYTHMIA SURGERY STILL HAVE A ROLE IN THE MANAGEMENT OF PATIENTS WITH VENTRICULAR TACHYCARDIA?

It is clear that surgical techniques have developed tremendously over the last 20 years; with improved patient selection, this has contributed to a steady improvement in operative mortality and long-term outcome. Over the last 14 years, these developments have been paralleled by the rapid development of the implantable cardioverter defibrillator (ICD) after its first use in man in 1980.[114] Implantation of all of the early ICD systems required a thoracotomy, and implant-related mortality was at least 3%.[115] The development of transvenous electrode systems that avoid the need for thoracotomy has reduced this figure to less than 1%.[116] Even with continued refinement of surgical techniques and patient selection, it is unlikely that the operative mortality of arrhythmia surgery can be brought below this level. Many arrhythmia surgery centers have noticed a reduction in patients being referred for arrhythmia surgery, and it is likely that this is because of increased use of the ICD. With few exceptions, studies of the ICD suggest that patients have a sudden cardiac death rate of 2% per annum or less, which is at least comparable if not better with that in the surgical studies described above.[117-120] The only apparent advantage of surgery over the ICD is the ability to deliver a cure rather than palliation of the arrhythmia. Realistically, the final superiority of one therapy will only be established by a prospective randomized controlled trial. Although many trials of the ICD versus conventional antiarrhythmic drug therapy are planned or in progress, there have been no controlled trials of antiarrhythmia surgery.[121-123] To demonstrate a mortality benefit for either the ICD or surgery, such a trial would have to recruit thousands of patients, and it is unlikely ever to be conducted. The design of trials that use surrogate end points (such as ICD shock-therapy delivery and cost-efficacy) to compare two such different therapies is fraught with difficulty.

The role of surgery for the treatment of ventricular arrhythmias is being further eroded by the development of catheter ablation techniques. Ablation with direct-current shocks is associated with significant mortality, has a relatively low efficacy, and may be proarrhythmic.[124-126] Radiofrequency ablation appears safer, although its long-term efficacy remains to be identified.[127,128] Radiofrequency ablation may be particularly suited to the thinner-walled structure of the right ventricle.[129] Even if the recurrence rate of ventricular tachycardia is higher with radiofrequency ablation, the combination of this therapy with the ICD may achieve a low sudden death rate, with low arrhythmia recurrence rates.

Nonetheless, ventricular tachycardia still has a definite role to play in patients who have drug-resistant ventricular tachycardia with frequent recurrences that is resistant to therapy with ablation techniques. Social factors may also influence choice of therapy. In the United Kingdom, patients with an ICD are banned from driving any motor vehicle for life.[130] In young patients, this may grossly affect their employment prospects. They may elect to accept a higher operative mortality in return for freedom from such restriction. It is vital that the surgical skills to perform ventricular arrhythmia are maintained in a limited number of centers so that the best therapy can be offered to these patients. Such centers could also form the core for randomized study of ventricular tachycardia surgery versus the implantable defibrillator.

CONCLUSION

Electrophysiologically guided surgery is an effective treatment of ventricular tachycardia. Newer developments in mapping techniques have enabled effective treatment of less stable arrhythmias. Most perioperative deaths are due to heart failure and only in a few patients do truly refractory arrhythmias occur.

Because surgery carries a significant mortality, it is still not indicated as first-line therapy. The precise role of surgery in the treatment of ventricular tachycardia remains to be defined. The lack of controlled trials of this therapy and the perception that it is associated with a high operative mortality have resulted in a decline in its popularity. There remains a role for limited trials to evaluate the long-term outcome of patients treated with surgery versus the ICD.

References

1. Wilber DJ, Garan H, Finkelstein D, et al: Out-of hospital cardiac arrest. Use of electrophysiological testing in the prediction of long-term survival. N Engl J Med 1988;318:19.
2. Couch OA: Cardiac aneurysm with ventricular tachycardia and subsequent excision of aneurysm. Circulation 1959; 55:251.
3. Basta LL: Aneurysmectomy in treatment of ventricular and supraventricular tachyarrhythmias in patients with postinfarction and traumatic ventricular aneurysms. Am J Cardiol 1973;32:693.
4. Hunt D, Sloman G, Westlake G: Ventricular aneurysmectomy for recurrent tachycardia. Br Heart J 1969;31:264.
5. Magidson O: Resection of postmyocardial infarction ventricular aneurysms for recurrent tachycardia. Dis Chest 1969;56(3):211.
6. Wald RW, Waxman MB, Corey PN, Gunstensen J, Goldman BS: Management of intractable ventricular tachyarrhythmias after myocardial infarction. Am J Cardiol 1979;44:329.

7. Buda AJ, Stinson EB, Harrison DC: Surgery for life-threatening ventricular tachaarrhythmias. Am J Cardiol 1979;44:1171.

8. Ricks WB, Winkle RA, Shumway NE, Harrison DC: Surgical management of life-threatening ventricular arrhythmias in patients with coronary artery disease. Circulation 1977; 56:38.

9. Sami M, Chaitman BR, Bourassa MG, et al: Long term follow-up of aneurysmectomy for recurrent ventricular tachycardia or fibrillation. Am Heart J 1978;96:303.

10. Gallagher JJ, Oldham HN, Wallace AG, et al: Ventricular aneurysm with ventricular tachycardia. Am J Cardiol 1975; 35:696.

11. Geha AS, Farshidi A, Batsford WP, Hammond GL: Surgical treatment of ventricular aneurysms and arrhythmias associated with coronary arterial occlusive disease. Conn Med 1980;44:369.

12. Brawley RK, Magovern GJ, Gott VL, et al: Left ventricular aneurysmectomy. J Thorac Cardiovasc Surg 1983;85:712.

13. Loop FD, Effler DB, Navia JA, et al: Aneurysms of the left ventricle: survival and results of a ten-year surgical experience. Ann Surg 1973;178:399.

14. Ecker RR, Mullins CB, Grammer JC, et al: Control of intractable ventricular tachycardia by coronary revascularisation. Circulation 1971;44:666.

15. Ester EH, Iziar HL: Recurrent ventricular tachycardia: a case treated successfully by bilateral cardiac sympathectomy. Am J Med 1961;31:493.

16. Moss AJ, McDonald J: Unilateral cervicothoracic sympathetic ganglionectomy for the treatment of long QT interval syndrome. N Engl J Med 1971;285:903.

17. Schwartz PJ, Locati EH, Moss AJ, et al: Left cardiac sympathetic denervation in the therapy of congenital long QT syndrome. Circulation 1991;84:503.

18. Schwartz PJ, Locati E: The idiopathic long QT syndrome: pathogenetic mechanisms and therapy. Eur Heart J 1985; 6(Suppl D):103.

19. Bhandari AK, Scheinman MM, Morady R, et al: Efficacy of left cardiac sympathectomy in the treatment of patients with long QT syndrome. Circulation 1984;70:1018.

20. Cobbs BW, King SB: Ventricular buckling: a factor in the abnormal ventriculogram and peculiar hemodynamics associated with mitral valve prolapse. Am Heart J 1977;93:741.

21. Ross A, De Weese JA, Yu PN: Refractory ventricular arrhythmias in a patient with mitral valve prolapse. Successful control with mitral valve replacement. J Electrocardiol 1978;11:289.

22. Missotten A, Dotremont G, Goddeeris P, et al: Mitral valve replacement in a patient with mitral valve prolapse complicated by severe ventricular arrhythmias. Acta Cardiol 1980; 35:391.

23. Holmes DR, Davis K, Gersh BJ, et al: Risk factor profiles of patients with sudden cardiac death and death from other cardiac causes: a report from the coronary artery surgery study (CASS). J Am Coll Cardiol 1989;13:524.

24. Manolis AS, Rastegar H, Estes NA, et al: Effects of coronary artery bypass grafting on ventricular arrhythmias: results with electrophysiological testing and long-term follow-up. Pacing Clin Electrophysiol 1993;16:984.

25. Levine JH, Mellits D, Baumgardner RA, et al: Predictors of first discharge and subsequent survival in patients with automatic implantable cardioverter-defibrillators. Circulation 1991;84:558.

26. Codini MA, Sommerfeldt L, Ebel CE, et al: Efficacy of coronary bypass grafting in exercise-induced ventricular tachycardia. J Thorac Cardiovasc Surg 1981;81:502.

27. Garan H, Ruskin JN, Dimarco JP, et al: Electrophysiologic studies before and after myocardial revascularisation in patients with life-threatening ventricular arrhythmias. Am J Cardiol 1983;51:519.

28. Rasmussen K, Lunde PI, Lie M: Coronary bypass surgery in exercise-induced ventricular tachycardia. Eur Heart J 1987; 8:444.

29. Steinbeck G, Haberl R, Kemkes BM: Herztransplantation bei therapieresistenten, rezidivierenden Kammertachykardien und Kammerflimmern. (Heart transplantation in therapy-resistant, recurrent ventricular tachycardias and ventricular fibrillation). Z Kardiol 1987;76(8):479.

30. Till JA, Shinebourne EA, Pepper J, Camm AJ, Ward DW: Complete denervation of the heart in a child with congenital long QT and deafness. Am J Cardiol 1988;62:1319.

31. Rothberger CJ, Winterberg H: Studen uber die Bestimung des Ausgangspunktes ventricckularer extrasystolen mit Hilfe des electrokardiogramms. Pflugers Arch Physiol 1913; 154:571.

32. Rothschild LT: The excitatory process in the dog's heart. II. The ventricles. Proc Trans R Soc 1915;206:181.

33. Morady F, Scheinman MM, Hess DS, Sung RJ, Shen E, Shapiro W: Electrophysiological testing in the management of survivors of out-of-hospital cardiac arrest. Am J Cardiol 1983;51:85.

34. Fontaine G, Guiradon G, Frank R, et al: Intraoperative mapping and surgery for the prevention of lethal arrhythmias after myocardial infarction. Ann NY Acad Sci 1982;382:396.

35. Fontaine G, Frank R, Guiradon G, et al: Surgical treatment of resistant reentrant ventricular tachycardia by ventriculotomy: a new application of epicardial mapping. Circulation (Abstract) 1974;49(Suppl III):82.

36. Wittig JH, Boineau JP: Surgical treatment of ventricular arrhythmias using epicardial, transmural and endocardial mapping. Ann Thorac Surg 1975;20:117.

37. Spielman SR, Michelson EL, Horowitz LN, et al: The limitations of epicardial mapping as a guide to the surgical therapy of ventricular tachycardia. Circulation 1978;57:666.

38. Fontaine G, Guiradon G, Frank R, et al: Intraoperative mapping and surgery for the prevention of lethal arrhythmias after myocardial infarction. Ann NY Acad Sci 1982;382:396.

39. Harken AH, Horowitz LN, Josephson ME: Comparison of standard aneurysmectomy and aneurysmectomy with directed endocardial resection for treatment of recurrent sustained ventricular tachycardia. J Thorac Cardiovasc Surg 1980;8:527.

40. Mason JW, Stinson EB, Winkle RA, et al: Relative efficacy of blind left ventricular aneurysm resection for the treatment of recurrent ventricular tachycardia. Am J Cardiol 1982; 49:241.

41. Mason JW, Stinson EB, Winkle RA, et al: Surgery for ventricular tachycardia: efficacy of left ventricular aneurysm resection compared with operation guided by electrical activation mapping. Circulation 1982;65:1148.

42. Ostermeyer J, Breithardt G, Kolvenbach R, et al: The surgi-

cal treatment of ventricular tachycardias. Simple aneurysmectomy versus electrophysiologically guided procedures. J Thorac Cardiovasc Surg 1982;84:704.

42a. Ideker RE, Smith WM, Wallace AG, et al: A computerized method for the rapid display of ventricular actination during the intraoperative study of arrhythmias. Circulation 1979;59:449.

43. de Bakker JMT, Janse MJ, Van Capelle FJL, Durrer D: Endocardial mapping by simultaneous recording of endocardial electrograms during cardiac surgery for ventricular aneurysm. J Am Coll Cardiol 1983;2:947.

44. Mickleborough LL, Harris L, Downar E, Parson I, Gray G: A new intraoperative approach for endocardial mapping of ventricular tachycardia. J Thorac Cardiovasc Surg 1988; 95:271.

45. Hauer RN, de Zwart MT, De Bakker JM, et al: Wire skeleton method for representation of arrhythmogenic sites determined with catheter mapping, compared with intraoperative mapping. Circulation 1984;70:11.

46. Harada A, D'Agostino HJ, Schuessler RB, Boineau JP, Coc JL: Potential distribution mapping: new method for precise localisation of intramural septal origin of ventricular tachycardia. Circulation 1988;78(Suppl III):III-137.

47. Tweddell J, Branham BH, Harada A, et al: Potential mapping in septal tachycardia: evaluation of a new intraoperative mapping technique. Circulation 1989;80(Suppl I):1-97.

48. Klein H, Karp RB, Kouchoukos NT, et al: Intraoperative electrophysiologic mapping of the ventricles during sinus rhythm in patients with a previous myocardial infarction. Identification of the electrophysiologic substrate of ventricular arrhythmias. Circulation 1982;66:847.

49. Kienzle MG, Miller J, Falcone RA, et al: Intraoperative endocardial mapping during sinus rhythm: relationship to site of origin of ventricular tachycardia. Circulation 1984;70:957.

50. Wiener I, Mindich B, Pitchon R: Determinants of ventricular tachycardia in patients with ventricular aneurysms: results of intraoperative epicardial and endocardial mapping. Circulation 1982;65:856.

51. Bourke JP, Campbell RWF, Renzulli JM, et al: Surgery for ventricular tachyarrhythmias based on fragmentation mapping in sinus rhythm alone. Eur J Cardiothorac Surg 1989; 3:401.

52. Harrison L, Gallagher JJ, Kasell J: Cryosurgical ablation of the A-V node-His bundle. A new method for producing A-V block. Circulation 1977;55:463.

53. Gallagher JJ, Anderson RW, Kasell J: Cryoablation of drug-resistant tachycardia in patient with a variant of scleroderma. Circulation 1978;57:190.

54. Camm J, Ward DE, Cory-Pearce R, et al: The successful cryosurgical treatment of paroxysmal ventricular tachycardia. Chest 1979;75:621.

55. Camm J, Ward DE, Spurrell RAJ, Rees GM: Cryothermal mapping and cryoablation in the treatment of refractory cardiac arrhythmias. Circulation 1980;62:67.

56. Curry PVL, O'Keefe DB, Pitcher D, et al: Localisation of ventricular tachycardia by a new technique—pace-mapping. Circulation, 1979;60 (Suppl II):25. Abstract.

57. Lewis T: The mechanism and graphic registration of the heart beat. London: Shaw & Sons, 1925.

58. Kastor JA, Spear JF, Moore EN: Localisation of ventricular irritability by epicardial mapping: origin of digitalis induced unifocal tachycardia from left ventricular Purkinje tissue. Circulation 1972;45:952.

59. Horowitz LN, Spear JF, Moore EN: Subendocardial origin of ventricular arrhythmias in 24-hour-old experimental myocardial infarction. Circulation 1976;53:56.

60. Waxman HL, Josephson ME: Ventricular activation during ventricular endocardial pacing. I. Electrocardiographic patterns related to site of pacing. Am J Cardiol 1982;50:1.

61. Josephson ME, Waxman HL, Cain ME, et al: Ventricular activation during ventricular endocardial pacing. II. Role of pace-mapping to localize origin of ventricular tachycardia. Am J Cardiol 1982;50:11.

62. O'Keefe DN, Curry PVL, Prior AL, et al: Surgery for ventricular tachycardia using operative pace mapping. Proc Br Coll Surg 1980;43:116.

63. Josephson ME, Horowitz LN, Spielman SR, et al: Comparison of endocardial catheter mapping with intraoperative mapping of ventricular tachycardia. Circulation 1980;61:395.

64. Horowitz LN, Josephson ME, Harken AH: Epicardial and endocardial activation during sustained ventricular tachycardia in man. Circulation 1980;61:1227.

65. Cassidy DM, Vassallo JA, Buxton AE, et al: The value of catheter mapping during sinus rhythm to localise site of origin of ventricular tachycardia. Circulation 1984;69:1103.

66. Wiener I, Mindich B, Pitchon R: Fragmented endocardial electrical activity in patients with ventricular tachycardia: a new guide to surgical therapy. Am Heart J 1984;107:86.

67. Gessman LJ, Gallagher JD, Demorizi NM, et al: Comparison of intraoperative activation, cryothermal and normal sinus rhythm—late potential mapping of patients with ventricular tachycardia. Pacing Clin Electrophysiol 1985;8:312

68. Fontaine G, Guiradon G, Frank R, et al: Surgical management of ventricular tachycardia unrelated to myocardial ischaemia or infarction. Am J Cardiol 1982;49:397.

69. Fontaine G, Guiradon G, Frank R: Stimulation studies and epicardial mapping in ventricular tachycardia: study of mechanisms and selection for surgery. In: Kulbertus HE, ed. Reentrant arrhythmias. Baltimore: University Park Press, 1977:334.

70. Spurrell RAJ, Camm AJ: Surgical treatment of ventricular tachycardia. Br Heart J 1978;40:38.

71. Boineau JP, Cox JL: Rationale for a direct surgical approach to control ventricular arrhythmias. Relation of specific intraoperative techniques to mechanism and location of arrhythmic circuit. Am J Cardiol 1982;49:381.

72. Guiradon GM, Klein GJ, Gulamhusein SS, et al: Total disconnection of the right ventricular free wall. Surgical treatment of right ventricular tachycardia associated with right ventricular dysplasia. Circulation 1983;67:463.

73. Jones DL, Guiradon GM, Klein GJ: Total disconnection of the right ventricular free wall. Physiological consequences in the dog. Am Heart J 1984;107:1169.

74. Guiraudon G, Fontaine G, Frank R, et al: Encircling endocardial ventriculotomy: a new surgical treatment for life-threatening ventricular tachycardias resistant to medical treatment following myocardial infarction. Ann Thorac Surg 1978;26:438.

75. Cox JL, Gallagher JJ, Ungerleider RM: Encircling endocardial

ventriculotomy refractory ischaemic ventricular tachycardia. J Thorac Cardiovasc Surg 1982;83:865.

76. Ungerleider RM, Holman WL, Stanley TI III, et al: Encircling endocardial ventriculotomy for refractory ischaemic ventricular tachycardia. J Thorac Cardiovasc Surg 1982;83:840.

77. Fontaine G, Guiraudon G, Frank R: Ventricular resection for recurrent ventricular tachycardia. N Engl J Med 1980;303:339.

78. Fontaine G, Guiradon G, Frank R: Mechanism of ventricular tachycardia with and without associated chronic myocardial ischaemia. surgical management based on epicardial mapping. In: Narula OS, ed. Cardiac arrhythmias. Electrophysiology, diagnosis and management. Baltimore: Williams & Wilkins, 1979:516.

79. Fontaine G, Guiradon G, Frank R: Intraoperative mapping and surgery for the prevention of lethal arrhythmias after myocardial infarction. Ann NY Acad Sci 1982;382:396.

80. Ostermeyer J, Breithardt G, Kolvenbach R, et al: The surgical treatment of ventricular tachycardias. J Thorac Cardiovasc Surg 1982;84:704.

81. Ostermeyer J, Breithardt G, Borggrefe M, Godehardt C, Geipel L, Bircks W: Surgical treatment of ventricular tachycardias. Complete versus partial encircling endocardial ventriculotomy. J Thorac Cardiovasc Surg 1984;87:517.

82. Fontaine G: Surgery for ventricular tachycardia. The view from Paris. Int J Cardiol 1982;1:351.

83. Ungerleider RM, Holman WL, Calcagno D, et al: Encircling endocardial ventriculotomy for refractory ischaemic ventricular tachycardia. Pt I. J Thorac Cardiovasc Surg 1982; 83:850.

84. Ungerleider RM, Holman WL, Calcagno D, et al: Encircling endocardial ventriculotomy for refractory ischaemic ventricular tachycardia. Pt II. J Thorac Cardiovasc Surg 1982; 83:857.

85. Guiradon GM, Klein GJ, Vermeulen FE, et al: Encircling endocardial cryoablation: a technique for surgical treatment of ventricular tachycardia after myocardial infarction. Circulation 1983;68(III):176.

86. Landymore RW, Kinley CE, Gardner M: Encircling endocardial resection with complete removal of endocardial scar without intraoperative mapping for the ablation of drug-resistant ventricular tachycardia. J Thorac Cardiovasc Surg 1985;89:18.

87. Josephson ME, Harken AH, Horowitz LN: Endocardial excision: a new surgical technique for the treatment of recurrent ventricular tachycardia. Circulation 1979;60:1430.

88. Harken AH, Jodephson ME, Horowitz LN: Surgical endocardial resection for the treatment of malignant ventricular tachycardia. Ann Surg 1979;190:456.

89. Josephson ME, Horowitz LN, Harken AH: Surgery for recurrent sustained ventricular tachycardia associated with coronary artery disease: the role of subendocardial resection. Ann NY Acad Sci 1982;382:381.

90. Horowitz LN, Harken AH, Kastor JA, Josephson ME: Ventricular resection guided by epicardial and endocardial mapping for treatment of recurrent ventricular tachycardia. N Engl J Med 1980;302:589.

91. Moran JM, Kehoe RF, Loeb JM, et al: Operative therapy of malignant ventricular rhythm disturbances. Ann Surg 1983; 198;479.

92. Page PL, Arciniegas JG, Plumb VJ, et al: Value of early postoperative epicardial programmed ventricular stimulation after surgery for ventricular tachyarrhythmias. J Am Coll Cardiol 1983;2:1046.

93. Rothschild M, Moran J, Zheutlin T, et al: Post-operative programmed stimulation in predicting arrhythmic recurrence in patients undergoing endocardial resection. Circulation 1984;70:292.

94. Vermeulen FEE, van Hemel NM, Guiradon GM, et al: Cryosurgery for ventricular bigeminy using a transaortic closed ventricular approach. Eur Heart J 1988;9:979.

95. Holman WL, Ikeshita M, Ungerleider RM, et al: Cryosurgery for cardiac arrhythmias: acute and chronic effects on coronary arteries. Am J Cardiol 1983;51:149.

96. Holman WL, Ikeshita M, Douglas JM, et al: Cardiac cryosurgery: effects of myocardial temperature on cryolesion size. Surgery 1983;93:268.

97. Kerr CR, Gallagher JJ, Cox JL, et al: Accelerated junctional tachycardia at a rate of 190 beats/minute following cryosurgery and aneurysmectomy for ventricular tachycardia: a case report. Pacing Clin Electrophysiol 1982;5:442.

98. Klein GJ, Harrison L, Ideker RF, et al: Reaction of the myocardium to cryosurgery: electrophysiology and arrhythmogenic potential. Circulation 1979;59:364.

99. Mesnildrey P, Laborde F, Piwnice A: Laser et troubles du rhythme. Ann Cardiol Angeiol 1985;34:707.

100. Saksena S, Hussain M, Gielchinsky I, Gadhoke A, Pantopoulos D: Intraoperative mapping-guided argon laser ablation of malignant ventricular tachycardia. Am J Cardiol 1987;59:78.

101. Isner JM, Mark Estes NA, Payne DD, Rastegar H, Clarke RH, Cleveland RJ: Laser-assisted endocardiectomy for refractory ventricular tachyarrhythmias: preliminary intraoperative experience. Clin Cardiol 1987;10:201.

102. Borggrefe M, Podczeck A, Ostermeyer J, Breithardt G, the Surgical Ablation Registry: Long-term results of electrophysiologically guided antitachycardia surgery in ventricular tachyarrhythmias: a collaborative report on 665 patients. In: Breithardt G, Borggrefe M, Zipes DP, eds. Nonpharmacological therapy of tachyarrhythmias. Mt. Kisco, NY: Futura Publishing, 1987.

103. van Hemel NM, Vermeulen FFE, Kingma JH, Defauw JJAM, de Bakker JNI, Ascoop CAPL: Improved results of surgery for postinfarction ventricular tachycardia using the left ventricular segmental wall motion score as criterion for operability. (Submitted).

104. Wald RW, Waxman MB, Corey PN, et al: Management of intractable ventricular tachyarrhythmias after myocardial infarction. Am J Cardiol 1979;44:329.

105. Buda AJ, Stinson EB, Harrison DC: Surgery for life-threatening ventricular tachyarrhythmias. Am J Cardiol 1979;44:1171.

106. Miller JM, Marchlinski FE, Harken AH, et al: Subendocardial resection for sustained ventricular tachycardia in the early period after acute myocardial infarction. Am J Cardiol 1985;55:980.

107. Bourke JP, Tansuphaswadikul S, Cowan JC, Hilton JC, Campbell RWF: Role of surgical therapy for sustained ventricular tachycardia and fibrillation early after myocardial infarction. In: Breithardt G, Borggrefe M, Zipes DP, eds. Nonphar-

macological therapy of tachyarrhythmias. Mt. Kisco, NY: Futura Publishing, 1987.

108. Wellens HJJ, Bar FWH, Vanagt EJDM, et al: Medical treatment of ventricular tachycardia: consideration in the selection of patients for surgical treatment. Am J Cardiol 1982;49:186.

109. Lawrie GM, Pacific A, Kaushik R: Results of direct surgical ablation of tachycardia not due to ischemic heart disease. Ann Surg 1989;209(6):716.

110. Saksena S, Hussain SM, Wasty N, Gielchinsky I, Parsonnet V: Long-term efficacy of subendocardial resection in refractory ventricular tachycardia: relationship to site of arrhythmia origin. Ann Thorac Surg 1986;42:685.

111. Hargrove WC, Miller JM, Vassallo JA, Josephson ME: Improved results in the operative management of ventricular tachycardia related to inferior wall infarction. J Thorac Cardiovasc Surg 1986;92:726.

111a. Brandt B, Martins JB, Kienzle MG: Predictors of failure after endocardial resection for sustained ventricular tachycardia. J Thorac Cardiovasc Surg 1988;95:495.

112. Miller JM, Hargrove WC, Jospehson ME: Significance of "nonclinical" ventricular arrhythmias induced following surgery for ventricular tachyarrhythmias. In: Breithardt G, Borggrefe M, Zipes DP, eds. Nonpharmacological therapy of tachyarrhythmias. Mt. Kisco NY: Futura Publishing, 1987.

113. Herling IM, Horowitz LN, Josephson ME: Ventricular ectopic activity after medical or surgical treatment for recurrent sustained ventricular tachycardia. Am J Cardiol 1980;45:633.

114. Mirowski M, Reid PR, Mower MM, et al: Termination of malignant ventricular arrhythmias with an implanted automatic defibrillator in human beings. N Engl J Med 1980;303:322.

115. Nisam S, Mower M, Moser S: ICD clinical update: first decade, initial 10,000 patients. Pacing Clin Electrophysiol 1991;14:255.

116. Lindemans FW, van Binsbergen E, Connolly D: European PCD study patients with Transvene™ lead systems. Medtronic. Maastricht: Bakken Research Center, 1991.

117. Gross J, Zilo P, Ferrick K, Fisher JD, Furman S: Sudden death mortality in implantable cardioverter defibrillator patients. Pacing Clin Electrophysiol 1991(A);14:250.

118. Winkle RA, Mead RH, Ruder MA, et al: Long-term outcome with the automatic implantable cardioverter-defibrillator. J Am Coll Cardiol 1989(A);13:1353.

119. Winkle RA, Mead RH, Ruder MA, et al: Ten year experience with implantable defibrillators. Circulation 1991;84:II. Abstract.

120. Fogoros RN, Elson JJ, Bonnet CA: Actuarial incidence and pattern of occurrence of shocks following implantation of the automatic implantable cardioverter defibrillator. Pacing Clin Electrophysiol 1989;12:1465.

121. Bigger JT: Future studies with the implantable cardioverter-defibrillator. Pacing Clin Electrophysiol 1991;14:883.

122. Wever EFD, Hauer RNW: Cost-effectiveness considerations: the Dutch prospective study of the automatic implantable cardioverter defibrillator as first-choice therapy. Pacing Clin Electrophysiol 1992;15:690.

123. Cardiomyopathy Trial Investigators: Cardiomyopathy trial. Pacing Clin Electrophysiol 1993;16:576.

124. Evans GT, Scheinman MM, Zipes DP, et al: Catheter ablation for control of ventricular tachycardia: a report of the percutaneous cardiac mapping and ablation registry. Pacing Clin Electrophysiol 1986;9:1391.

125. Morady F, Scheinman MM, Griffin JC, et al: Results of catheter ablation of ventricular tachycardia using direct current shocks. Pacing Clin Electrophysiol 1989;12:252.

126. Hauer RN, Robles de Medina EO, Borst C: Proarrhythmic effects of ventricular electrical catheter ablation in dogs. J Am Coll Cardiol 1987;10:1350.

127. Gursoy S, Chiladakis I, Kuck KH: First lessons from radiofrequency catheter ablation in patients with ventricular tachycardia. Pacing Clin Electrophysiol 1993;16:687.

128. Morady F, Harvey M, Kalbfleisch SJ, et al: Radiofrequency catheter ablation of ventricular tachycardia in patients with coronary artery disease. Circulation 1993;87:363.

129. Aizawa Y, Chinushi M, Naitoh N, et al: Catheter ablation with radiofrequency current of ventricular tachycardia originating from the right ventricle. Am Heart J 1993;125:1269.

130. Gold R, Oliver M: Fitness to drive: updated guidance on cardiac conditions in holders of ordinary driving licenses. Health Trends 1990;22:31.

Cardiac Arrhythmias, 3rd edition, edited by William J. Mandel.
J. B. Lippincott Company, Philadelphia © 1995.

42

Melinda L. Marks • H. Leon Greene

Sudden Cardiac Death[*]

Sudden cardiac death is one of the major causes of premature mortality in the United States.[1] Estimates are difficult, but it is said that between 200,000 and 600,000 persons die each year of sudden cardiac death.[2] Overall mortality from cardiovascular disease in the United States has been decreasing, but sudden death remains a problem of enormous magnitude, causing substantial loss of life, economic hardship, and emotional and psychological distress for surviving family members.[3-5]

A precise definition of sudden cardiac death that is both widely accepted and easy to apply is difficult to formulate.[6-14] Most commonly, sudden cardiac death is regarded as demise from cardiovascular collapse within 1 hour of the onset of symptoms in patients in whom existing disease processes would not have been suspected to cause a mortal event were it not for a terminal arrhythmia.[10-14] This definition is difficult to apply to individual cases because nearly three fourths of all patients have had recognized cardiovascular disease before the event and many have chronic or recurrent symptoms obscuring precise classification.[15-20] Most difficult is the patient with chronic congestive heart failure in whom a change in symptoms may be difficult to interpret. An operational definition has been proposed for the Cardiac Arrhythmia Suppression Trial (CAST), one that addresses mechanism more specifically than timing.[14,21,22] Adaptation of the term sudden *arrhythmic* cardiac death makes the distinction easier by eliminating those deaths due to terminal congestive heart failure or shock, regardless of timing, and by excluding deaths that occur rapidly due to ischemic ventricular dysfunction, cardiogenic shock, or myocardial rupture. In the CAST study, patients were considered to have had a sudden arrhythmic cardiac death only if their underlying disease would have been expected to allow survival for at least 4 months.

Although many investigations have centered on identification of patients at high risk of developing an initial episode of sudden cardiac death before any major arrhythmic event, others have concentrated on patients in whom an episode of sudden cardiac death has been aborted.[15-20,23-33] In addition, a distinction must be made between patients who survive an episode of ventricular fibrillation and patients who develop recurrent sustained ventricular tachycardia.[34-36]

*Supported in part by grants from the Medic I Foundation, Seattle, WA; from the American Heart Association, Washington Affiliate; and grant RO1 HL31472 from the National Heart, Lung, and Blood Institute, Public Health Service, Department of Health and Human Services, Bethesda, MA.

MECHANISMS OF SUDDEN CARDIAC DEATH

The mechanism of sudden arrhythmic cardiac death has been defined both in the out-of-hospital and in-hospital setting.[15-16,18-20,37-44] Evaluation of electrocardiograms recorded immediately after sudden collapse shows three common rhythm disturbances associated with this event: ventricular fibrillation, asystole, and electromechanical dissociation. The relative proportion of these arrhythmias depends on the patient population studied and the time from collapse to first recording of an electrocardiogram. About a third to half of all patients attended promptly have ventricular fibrillation as the initial recorded rhythm.[45-49] Only rarely does a patient have collapse with loss of consciousness due to arrhythmias such as sustained ventricular tachycardia (without degeneration to ventricular fibrillation); atrial fibrillation or flutter (unless the patient has Wolff-Parkinson-White syndrome, wherein atrial fibrillation can induce ventricular fibrillation over an accessory atrioventricular bypass tract, an uncommon scenario); or other supraventricular arrhythmias.

Ambulatory electrocardiographic evaluations (Holter-monitor recordings) of patients during the development of sudden cardiac death show a higher incidence of ventricular tachyarrhythmias but these studies are difficult to interpret.[50-55] All of these patients were selected to have electrocardiographic monitoring by some combination of symptoms and signs. Commonly, these patients had previous episodes of palpitations, presyncope, or syncope, and the Holter-monitor recording was applied in an attempt to define the etiology of these symptoms. Many of these patients were treated with antiarrhythmic drugs, which might alter the characteristics of the initiating arrhythmia and the arrhythmia at the time of subsequent symptoms or collapse. Nevertheless, these Holter-monitor recordings suggest that ventricular tachycardia that rapidly degenerates to ventricular fibrillation is the most common cause of cardiovascular collapse and sudden cardiac death and may be implicated in up to 85% of all cardiac arrests.[54]

After prolonged ventricular fibrillation, the voltage of the signal decreases to fine ventricular fibrillation, then to a "flat line" or asystole, although a few patients have been documented to convert spontaneously to a slow idioventricular rhythm before asystole supervenes.

SUCCESS OF RESUSCITATION

Major advances have been made in the resuscitation of victims of sudden cardiovascular collapse. Rapid response medical systems have improved the survival rate of these victims over the past two decades.[50,61] Early application of cardiopulmonary resuscitation (CPR) before the arrival of the first responding medic unit has improved both cardio-

vascular and neurologic recovery. Bystander CPR after a witnessed collapse clearly yields improved results of resuscitation attempts.[37,56-76] The interval from the patient's collapse to the institution of CPR is vitally important.[37,58,70] Nearly half of patients who receive bystander CPR have purposeful activity at admission to the hospital, compared with 6% of patients who do not receive bystander CPR. Sixty-one percent of patients who receive bystander CPR are conscious 24 hours after their collapse, compared with 9% of patients who do not receive bystander CPR.[58] Thus, best results are obtained when the patient's collapse is witnessed and CPR is administered quickly. Institution of automatic defibrillators in the out-of-hospital setting has shortened the time from collapse to delivery of the first defibrillating shock. These devices have improved survival and neurologic recovery, and their use is becoming more widespread.[38,47,77-80]

In addition, other factors are identified with favorable recovery: high-amplitude ventricular fibrillation on the first recording of an electrocardiogram, short medic response time, short duration of CPR before defibrillation, and early treatment with rapid defibrillation.[61] Long-term survival is best in patients in whom the initial rhythm is ventricular fibrillation. Rarely does a patient with asystole or electromechanical dissociation survive.[37] In Seattle, about two thirds of all patients with cardiac arrest are successfully resuscitated, and about a fourth to a third of the total population of patients with cardiac arrest are ultimately discharged from the hospital alive and well.[15,37,61]

Whether advanced age of the patient in whom resuscitation is attempted influences survival is debated. Survival from cardiac arrest in elderly patients is significantly less than in younger patients (10% vs 24%, $p < .001$).[43] However, younger patients are more likely to have ventricular fibrillation as the initial rhythm at the time of cardiac arrest, associated with better resuscitation and survival rates.[43,44] The initial rhythm is a better predictor of survival ($p < .0001$) than patient age ($p < .005$).[43] In patients with ventricular fibrillation as the initial rhythm, the effect of age on survival does not become apparent until ≥80 years old.[44]

Patients who develop cardiac arrest while hospitalized are more likely to have a poor outcome, primarily because of the underlying disease processes, which are in themselves irreversible and responsible for the patient's in-hospital demise.[39-42]

EARLY TREATMENT OF THE SURVIVOR OF VENTRICULAR FIBRILLATION

Initial efforts should be directed toward stabilizing the patient after resuscitation from ventricular fibrillation. Initially, these patients may have recurrent arrhythmias and hemodynamic instability. Metabolic abnormalities may be quite profound during the first few minutes or hours after the resuscitation, and the initial attention should be directed toward correcting these metabolic abnormalities, particularly pH, potassium, pO_2, pCO_2, calcium, and magnesium.

Early rhythm instability can commonly be suppressed simply with correction of the metabolic abnormalities. Thereafter, treatment with lidocaine is often sufficient to suppress arrhythmias, although subsequent treatment with procainamide or bretylium tosylate as parenteral agents may be necessary. Although the initial few hours after an arrest may be punctuated by flurries of ventricular tachycardia or ventricular fibrillation, rhythm stability commonly is rapidly achieved.

Hemodynamic instability is another hallmark of the patient resuscitated from a cardiac arrest. Profound alterations in adrenergic tone can cause surges of blood pressure into the markedly hypertensive range (adrenergic storm), alternating with intermittent hypotension. Frequently these patients require invasive hemodynamic monitoring, with frequent adjustments of vasopressor and vasodilator drugs.

The first electrocardiograms may be quite abnormal simply because of the metabolic abnormalities associated with the resuscitation. It is quite common to have transient intraventricular conduction delays, bundle branch blocks, and some patients who are seen quickly after their initial arrest may have ST-segment elevations suggestive of acute transmural myocardial infarction or coronary spasm that resolve within minutes or hours without long-term evidence of myocardial infarction. In contrast, about a fifth of all patients develop new Q waves, and the myocardial infarction can also be documented with serial enzyme evaluations.[15] In these patients, the myocardial infarction is thought to be responsible for the arrhythmia that produced cardiovascular collapse. On the contrary, four fifths of patients with coronary artery disease do not have a new Q-wave myocardial infarction, although 38% of patients have elevated myocardial enzymes, consistent with myocardial damage.[15,81] In the era of thrombolytic therapy, it is difficult to refrain from giving thrombolytic agents to some of these patients who have profound ST-segment elevation. Because of the potential devastating neurologic consequences associated with giving a thrombolytic agent to someone having toxic or ischemic damage to the cerebral microcirculation after prolonged CPR, it is generally thought that thrombolytic agents should not be given. A better way to accomplish reperfusion in these patients is direct angioplasty, often a difficult logistic feat even in a tertiary medical center.

Neurologic recovery critically depends on the amount of time a patient has been without cerebral circulation.[70–74] Early bystander CPR, early arrival of the medics, and prompt defibrillation are essential to adequate neuro-

logic recovery. Many factors can be used to predict the likelihood of serious neurologic damage: the Glasgow coma scale on arrival of the patient at the hospital, the serum glucose measured soon after the cardiac arrest, and the progression of neurologic findings during the early hours after the resuscitation.[75,76,82,83] Unresponsiveness and flaccid paralysis with lack of cranial nerve function are all serious negative prognostic factors. Extensor posturing predicts a worse outcome than flexor posturing. Early return of responsiveness, the ability to follow commands, conjugate eye movements, and spontaneous cranial nerve function portend a better outcome. Evaluation of the cerebrospinal fluid enzyme creatinine kinase (the BB isoenzyme) at 48 to 72 hours also yields excellent prognostic information.[84] The likelihood of the patient awakening is inversely proportional to the elevation of cerebrospinal fluid creatinine kinase-BB. Likewise, the longer a patient remains unresponsive, the less likely that the patient will ultimately regain consciousness and satisfactory neurologic function. Many studies have attempted to improve neurologic recovery by interventions applied soon after cardiac arrest. Administration of barbiturates, calcium channel blocking drugs, or steroids has not consistently yielded better neurologic function.[85–88]

Other medical complications of resuscitation must be diligently sought: aspiration pneumonia, pneumothorax (including tension pneumothorax), ruptured or infarcted abdominal viscera, sepsis, gastrointestinal bleeding, and evidence for peripheral vascular insufficiency, aortic dissection, or embolization.

ETIOLOGY OF SUDDEN CARDIAC DEATH

The underlying disease responsible for the ventricular fibrillation in the United States is overwhelmingly coronary artery disease. Noncardiac causes of collapse without cardiac arrest must be excluded (e.g., vertebrobasilar insufficiency, subarachnoid bleeding, massive blood loss, pulmonary embolus, seizure disorder, or ruptured abdominal aortic aneurysm due to atherosclerosis, cystic medial necrosis, or Marfan's syndrome). About 75% of all patients with sudden cardiac death have coronary artery disease as the only identifiable pathology, with or without preexisting myocardial scar from prior myocardial infarction.[15] As noted, only 19% of patients with coronary artery disease have a new Q-wave myocardial infarction associated with the episode of ventricular fibrillation, whereas 38% of patients have enzymatic evidence of myocardial damage.[15,81] Other diseases contributing to sudden cardiac death include cardiomyopathy, both dilated and hypertrophic; valvular heart disease; congenital heart disease; electrolyte abnormalities; drug toxicity; long QT syndrome; and a variety of less common causes (Table

TABLE 42-1. Diseases and Conditions Associated with Sudden Cardiac Death

Coronary artery disease
  Acute ischemia/infarction
  Chronic coronary disease without recent infarction
  Ruptured myocardium
  Coronary arteritis
  Coronary spasm
  Myocardial bridge
Cardiomyopathy
  Dilated
  Hypertrophic
    Symmetric
    Asymmetric
Myocarditis
Infiltrative myocardial disease
Valvular heart disease
Congenital heart disease
  Coronary artery anomalies
  Valvular heart disease
  Tetralogy of Fallot
Long-QT syndromes
  Congenital
    Jervell-Lange-Nielsen syndrome
    Romano-Ward syndrome
  Acquired
    Drug toxicity
    Electrolyte abnormalities
Toxins (e.g., cocaine)
Proarrhythmic effects of antiarrhythmic drugs
Electrolyte abnormalities
Wolff-Parkinson-White syndrome
Mitral valve prolapse
Right ventricular dysplasia
Cardiac tumors
Pulmonary hypertension
Cardiac trauma
Primary electrical disease

42-1). Only a small percentage of patients have no identifiable structural heart disease. These patients may have either a primary electric disorder or a myopathic process that is too subtle to be detected by echocardiography, angiography, or radionuclide ventriculography.

TYPICAL SURVIVOR OF VENTRICULAR FIBRILLATION

The typical ventricular fibrillation survivor is a male with an average age of about 60 years.[15, 17] Three fourths of patients have had prior evidence of cardiovascular disease: angina, congestive heart failure, prior myocardial infarction, or hypertension.[15] These histories do not identify which patients with coronary disease will develop ventricular fibrillation because many patients having these histories never develop sudden cardiovascular collapse. Most patients are neither taking antiarrhythmic drugs nor exercising vigorously at the time of their cardiovascular collapse. Although patients who develop a myocardial infarction at the time of the ventricular fibrillation may have chest pain as an antecedent symptom, most patients do not have distinct warning symptoms before the time of collapse. Most patients with coronary artery disease do not develop new Q waves on the electrocardiogram with the episode of ventricular fibrillation.[15] A third to half of all patients have enzymatic evidence for myocardial necrosis, however.

These findings suggest possible underlying mechanisms for the production of ventricular fibrillation. Although transient myocardial ischemia may produce serious arrhythmias, most patients do not have evidence for major coronary artery occlusion at the time of their episode of ventricular fibrillation. Many patients have had previous myocardial damage from remote myocardial infarction, providing the substrate for arrhythmias. The trigger mechanism for development of ventricular fibrillation is unknown. Transient myocardial ischemia produced by platelet aggregation, coronary vasospasm, or exercise-induced ischemia may play a role in some patients, although a uniform hypothesis for the mechanism of production of ventricular fibrillation is elusive. Although some patients may have minor degrees of hypokalemia, it is generally not thought that this abnormality is the etiology of the arrhythmia in most patients.[89–90]

One major goal is to identify patients at high risk of ventricular fibrillation before the time that they develop their first serious arrhythmia.[23–26] Studies have included exercise testing, signal-averaged electrocardiography, body potential surface mapping, heart rate variability, and the integration of multiple clinical risk factors.[23–26, 91–101] Ventricular premature depolarizations on Holter-monitor recording and left ventricular dysfunction measured by radionuclide ventriculography after a myocardial infarction were used in the CAST study but the risk of an arrhythmic event in this population even by today's standards was not high enough to warrant aggressive evaluation and treatment.[21, 22] To date, no individual technique has been identified with sufficient sensitivity and specificity to allow accurate prediction of events before the first episode.

COMPARISON OF PATIENTS HAVING RECURRENT SUSTAINED VENTRICULAR TACHYCARDIA WITH PATIENTS HAVING VENTRICULAR FIBRILLATION

Studies that have evaluated patients with serious ventricular arrhythmias often combined patients with recurrent sustained ventricular tachycardia and patients with ventricular fibrillation.[27-32, 102-109] Although many patients may have both arrhythmias, patients with recurrent sustained ventricular tachycardia may have a different underlying substrate.[33-36] These patients can tolerate recurrent sustained ventricular tachycardia for remarkable lengths of time, often hours or even days. Patients with recurrent sustained ventricular tachycardia more commonly have had a prior myocardial infarction, have a lower ejection fraction, and have a left ventricular aneurysm.[34] In patients with recurrent sustained ventricular tachycardia, signal-averaged electrocardiographic late potentials are more common, and the arrhythmia induced at electrophysiologic study is more likely to be sustained ventricular tachycardia than ventricular fibrillation.[33-36, 108, 110] Patients with a history of ventricular fibrillation more commonly have a polymorphic ventricular tachycardia induced or may even have only ventricular fibrillation induced at electrophysiologic study.[34, 108] Induced arrhythmias in patients resuscitated from ventricular fibrillation more commonly have a rapid rate and are more difficult to terminate with pacing, requiring cardioversion more frequently.[34] Patients with a history of ventricular fibrillation may respond to antiarrhythmic drugs differently from patients with recurrent sustained ventricular tachycardia. Likewise, the response to antiarrhythmic devices, particularly the ability of pacing therapies to terminate ventricular arrhythmias, may be quite different in these two patient populations.

EVALUATION OF THE SURVIVOR OF VENTRICULAR FIBRILLATION

The initial evaluation of the cardiac disease responsible for the cardiac arrest should include serial assessment of serum cardiac enzymes and electrocardiograms.

All patients should have a thorough evaluation for the presence of structural heart disease after neurologic recovery and achievement of hemodynamic and cardiac rhythm stability. Cardiac and coronary anatomy should be defined by cardiac catheterization and angiography. Many patients have a cardiac arrest associated with severe coronary artery disease and some have exercise-induced cardiac arrest, suggesting that transient myocardial ischemia played a role in the production of the ventricular fibrillation. Thus, exercise testing may be useful.[111]

In addition to establishing the anatomic diagnosis, both left and right ventricular function should be evaluated by echocardiography, radionuclide ventriculography, or contrast angiography. Often the only clue to the existence of unusual diseases such as right ventricular dysplasia is an enlarged right ventricle on echocardiography.[112-114] Right ventricular endomyocardial biopsy has been performed in patients who have ventricular tachycardia or ventricular fibrillation and no clinical evidence of

structural heart disease.[115] In our local experience, however, biopsy is rarely diagnostic or useful.

Most physicians additionally prefer to use (1) baseline drug-free Holter-monitor recording to assess the extent of ambient ectopy, and (2) baseline drug-free electrophysiologic study to determine whether inducible ventricular arrhythmias are present.

PREDICTORS OF RISK OF RECURRENCE OF VENTRICULAR FIBRILLATION

Most studies of the risk of recurrent cardiac arrest have examined patients with coronary artery disease.[15-20, 116-118] The most powerful predictor for recurrence of cardiac arrest is a history of congestive heart failure.[16, 119-122] Patients with congestive heart failure frequently have a history of remote myocardial infarction and evidence of left ventricular dysfunction measured by a low ejection fraction at radionuclide ventriculography.[120] In a study of 154 survivors of out-of-hospital ventricular fibrillation, resting radionuclide ventriculography was performed an average of 128 ± 74 days after resuscitation. Average follow-up for the patients was 37 ± 20 months, with an overall mortality of 35%. Those patients with a normal left ventricular ejection fraction (more than 0.50) had a low mortality rate of 4.5% at 4 years, whereas patients with a low ejection fraction (less than 0.35) had a mortality rate of 60%. In another study of 239 patients having sustained ventricular tachycardia or ventricular fibrillation and followed-up for 14.8 ± 13.9 months, a higher New York Heart Association functional class was an independent predictor of both sudden death and cardiac death on multivariate regression analysis.[105]

Another powerful predictor of recurrence of ventricular fibrillation includes the absence of a Q-wave myocardial infarction with the episode of ventricular fibrillation.[16, 119] A patient's risk of recurrence is highest if no myocardial infarction has occurred, documented by both normal cardiac isoenzymes and by electrocardiograms without new Q waves. At intermediate risk is the patient with enzymatic evidence of a myocardial infarction but without new Q waves. At lowest risk is the patient with both isoenzyme elevations and evolution of new Q waves. A patient with new Q waves developing coincidentally with the cardiac arrest has only a 2% likelihood of arrhythmia recurrence in 1 year, a risk so low that it cannot be satisfactorily modified by any antiarrhythmic therapy.[16] Male gender and a remote myocardial infarction before the episode of ventricular fibrillation also predicts a higher risk of recurrence.[16, 119]

Exercise treadmill testing may be useful in evaluation for myocardial ischemia or left ventricular dysfunction. In a study of 90 survivors of ventricular fibrillation, the development of angina or inability to elevate systolic arterial blood pressure with exercise significantly correlated with subsequent mortality.[111] Fifty-five percent of patients who developed angina on exercise treadmill testing developed subsequent cardiac arrest, compared with 16% of patients who did not develop angina. In patients who did not develop a systolic blood pressure rise of 10 mmHg or more during exercise testing, the survival rates over the first 4 years were 62% at 1 year, 46% at 2 years, 38% at 3 years and 31% at 4 years. In patients with normal blood pressure response, the survival rates were significantly higher: 82% at 1 year, 74% at 2 years, 68% at 3 years and 58% at 48 years ($p = .004$).

Other predictors of high risk of recurrent ventricular fibrillation include the presence of extensive coronary artery disease, advanced age, complex ectopy on Holter monitoring, inducibility at electrophysiologic study, and a history of cigarette smoking.[27–32, 121–124]

The risk of recurrence of ventricular fibrillation in patients with etiologies other than coronary artery disease is more difficult to predict in an individual patient because fewer of these patients are available in each clinical subgroup to develop statistically relevant predictors. The overall risk, however, of recurrence in patients with noncoronary etiologies is probably at least as high as the recurrence rate in patients with coronary disease. This finding probably reflects the more severely impaired left ventricular function found in the noncoronary patient population, which has a high prevalence of dilated cardiomyopathies.[125, 126]

Electrophysiologic testing is also useful in stratifying the risk for recurrent cardiac arrest in patients with recurrent sustained ventricular tachycardia or resuscitated sudden cardiac death, particularly after drug therapy. Wilbur and colleagues showed that left ventricular dysfunction and inducibility at electrophysiologic study are powerful additive factors in predicting a recurrence of cardiac arrest. Other studies show that patients who are noninducible at baseline electrophysiologic study still have a substantial risk of recurrent ventricular fibrillation, particularly if severe left ventricular dysfunction is present.[27–32] Patients with the best outcome are those with a high ejection fraction inducible at baseline electrophysiologic study and suppressed on antiarrhythmic drugs. Those who have a high ejection fraction and who are noninducible at baseline electrophysiologic study also have a reasonably good outcome. In a study of 241 survivors of out-of-hospital ventricular fibrillation by Poole and coworkers, however, the status of the left ventricular function was such a powerful predictor of recurrent cardiac arrest that other factors were not independently predictive of outcome.[109]

Signal-averaged electrocardiography has been used to evaluate the presence of low-amplitude high-frequency late potentials that are believed to represent areas of slow conduction within the myocardium and thus indicate a substrata for reentrant arrhythmias. Although late potentials are often present in patients with recurrent sustained ventricular tachycardia, correlation with inducibility has been inconsistent.[36, 127] Dolack and coworkers examined 71 subjects who had experienced sustained ventricular tachycardia (25 patients) or ventricular fibrillation (46 patients).[110] Late potentials were detected in 83% of patients with ventricular tachycardia and in 50% of patients with ventricular fibrillation, occurring in 65% of ventricular fibrillation patients with previous myocardial infarction. The presence of late potentials did not correlate with other clinical variables measured (age, presence of coronary artery disease, or left ventricular ejection fraction) and did not correlate with inducibility of sustained ventricular tachycardia or ventricular fibrillation at electrophysiologic testing.

Having estimated the risk of recurrence of ventricular fibrillation in the patient already resuscitated from the first episode of ventricular fibrillation, the physician can determine how aggressive the subsequent evaluation and therapy should be. Patients who have a low risk of recurrence of ventricular fibrillation have little to gain from any treatment program, whereas those patients with a high risk of recurrence should have extensive evaluation, treatment, and follow-up.

CORRECTING PRIMARY ABNORMALITIES

The first principle of the treatment of patients with aborted sudden cardiac death should be to correct the primary abnormality responsible for the arrhythmia. In some instances, cardiac arrest may be precipitated by metabolic abnormalities such as electrolyte disturbances, hypoxemia, acidosis, or the proarrhythmic effects of drugs. Electrolyte abnormalities and acid–base disturbances should first be corrected. Drugs that might have caused the cardiac arrest, including antiarrhythmic drugs that could have produced a proarrhythmic response in certain patients, should be discontinued. Most patients have identifiable structural heart disease, however.

Functionally significant anatomic abnormalities, such as valvular disease, coronary artery disease, and congenital abnormalities, should likewise be corrected. The ideal candidate for coronary artery bypass graft surgery or percutaneous transluminal coronary angioplasty is the patient who (1) is young with multivessel disease and good distal vessels, (2) has normal left ventricular function without evidence of old myocardial scar, (3) is otherwise healthy, without evidence for an acute myocardial infarction (either by enzymes or electrocardiographic changes) at the time of ventricular fibrillation, (4) has no ambient arrhythmias on ambulatory Holter-monitor recording, and (5) is noninducible on electrophysiologic study but has angina pectoris on exercise testing associated with either a fall in blood pressure, severe ST-segment depression, or exercise-induced arrhythmias. Clearly, such an ideal patient is uncommon and frequently a decision to perform revascularization surgery or angioplasty is difficult. Nevertheless, most physicians feel that complete revascularization should be attempted in these patients if possible.

THERAPY AND OUTCOME OF THE SURVIVOR OF VENTRICULAR FIBRILLATION

Many options are available for the treatment of patients who have survived an episode of out-of-hospital ventricular fibrillation. Drugs; surgery (coronary artery bypass grafting, directed arrhythmia surgery, valve replacement); antiarrhythmic devices; catheter or chemical ablation of arrhythmogenic foci; and combinations of these therapies have all been attempted.

Drugs

Antiarrhythmic drug therapy is often given to patients after cardiac arrest to prevent recurrent cardiac arrest. Empiric drug therapy with class I agents (without control by Holter-monitor recording or electrophysiologic testing) has not been shown to improve prognosis.[117]

Two major forms of arrhythmia assessment are possible in patients who have survived an episode of ventricular fibrillation. In one, noninvasive Holter-monitor ambulatory electrocardiographic recording is used to establish a baseline degree of ventricular ectopy, and repeat Holter-monitor recording is performed to assess the efficacy of drug therapy in suppressing spontaneous arrhythmias.[128,129] This technique has a high degree of day-to-day variability, even without therapy, and can be difficult to interpret.[130-134] The alternative method of assessment is invasive electrophysiologic testing, in which ventricular tachyarrhythmias are induced by programmed electrical stimulation, and the effect of drug therapy on inducibility is subsequently assessed. Suppression of inducibility corresponds to a good clinical outcome, particularly in patients with recurrent sustained ventricular tachycardia.[27-33,103-110]

Publication of the CAST study has raised questions about the Holter method of assessment of drug respon-

siveness.[21,22] The CAST study used Holter-monitor recordings to assess suppression of ventricular ectopy after a myocardial infarction in patients who had not yet suffered any serious cardiac arrhythmias. Patients treated with antiarrhythmic drugs had an increased risk of sudden cardiac death, compared with patients treated with placebo, despite ambient arrhythmias being well-suppressed on Holter-monitor recording. This finding has led to the hypothesis that patients who respond to antiarrhythmic drugs by suppression of ventricular ectopy may simply be healthier and less prone to serious ventricular arrhythmias, the so-called healthy responder phenomenon.[135] Because of these findings, similar questions have been raised about the responses to electrophysiologic testing. It is possible that patients whose inducibility is suppressed by an antiarrhythmic drug simply are less likely to develop serious ventricular arrhythmias because their underlying disease is less severe.

Wilbur and coworkers, examining 166 survivors of a cardiac arrest due to a ventricular tachyarrhythmia, found that persistently inducible ventricular tachycardia not suppressed with antiarrhythmic drug therapy was a highly significant predictor of recurrent cardiac arrest.[27] After a median follow-up of 21 months, the cumulative survival without cardiac arrest in 91 patients who were inducible and suppressed on antiarrhythmic drugs was 88%, compared with 67% in 36 patients who could not be suppressed on antiarrhythmic drug therapy and 87% in 35 patients who were initially noninducible. Thus, patients who had no inducible arrhythmias at initial electrophysiologic study had a survival comparable with patients who were inducible and suppressed. The risk of recurrent cardiac arrest can be further stratified based on left ventricular ejection fraction, with a relative risk of recurrent cardiac arrest in patients with poor left ventricular function (left ventricular ejection function 0.30 or less) compared with patients with good left ventricular function (left ventricular ejection function greater than 0.30) of 2.6.[136] In our series of 241 patients surviving out-of-hospital ventricular fibrillation, the long-term outcome was analyzed based on the rhythm induced at baseline drug-free electrophysiologic testing.[109] Arrhythmia-free survival at 2 years was significantly higher in patients without (81%) compared with those with (65%) inducible sustained ventricular tachycardia. Patients with inducible ventricular fibrillation had an arrhythmia-free survival of 71%, compared with 79% in patients with only inducible nonsustained ventricular tachycardia. In this study, suppression of inducible arrhythmias on antiarrhythmic drugs did not correlate to improved arrhythmia-free survival, perhaps because many (71%) of the patients in the nonsuppressed group were taking amiodarone and did not subsequently receive serial electrophysiologic evaluations. Left ventricular function was the most important determinant of outcome, especially in patients who did not have inducible ventricular arrhythmias on electrophysiologic study or who had inducible arrhythmias that were not suppressed by antiarrhythmic drugs. Other studies show that electrophysiologic testing is useful for identifying patients who have a low risk of recurrent sudden cardiac arrest.[29-33, 102-109]

An early small-scale randomized controlled clinical study compared Holter monitoring with electrophysiologic testing and suggested that electrophysiologic testing may be more useful in some subgroups.[136] Fifty-seven patients with ventricular tachyarrhythmias were studied (35 patients with sustained ventricular tachycardia, 15 patients with nonsustained ventricular tachycardia, and seven patients with ventricular fibrillation). They were initially evaluated by noninvasive tests, including 18-hour ambulatory Holter-monitor electrocardiographic recording, exercise treadmill testing, and electrophysiologic testing. Of 29 patients randomized to the noninvasive approach, recurrent symptomatic sustained ventricular tachycardia was seen in 13 patients (45%), compared with five of 28 patients (18%) randomized to antiarrhythmic drug therapy guided by electrophysiologic testing. The ESVEM study (Electrophysiologic Study Versus Electrocardiographic Monitoring) showed that both methods of guiding therapy were useful, although ambulatory monitoring more often predicted a successful drug regimen.[137-139]

Adverse effects of antiarrhythmic drugs have been highlighted by the publication of the CAST study.[21, 22] Although this trial specifically addressed a different patient population, concern has been raised that generally, antiarrhythmic drugs could be increasing mortality in other patient populations also. Response to an antiarrhythmic drug by suppression of spontaneous ventricular ectopic activity or suppression of inducibility at electrophysiologic study does not necessarily indicate that these drugs will improve survival. Proarrhythmic effects of antiarrhythmic drugs could also worsen the outcome in other clinical situations.[140-154] Quinidine may increase the risk of death for patients taking the drug, even for supraventricular arrhythmias. Furberg reviewed studies evaluating antiarrhythmic drug therapy in patients with ventricular arrhythmias.[153] His analysis also suggests that antiarrhythmic drugs may have no effect or even a deleterious effect in some patient populations. Such findings might also pertain to the population of survivors of ventricular fibrillation.

The CASCADE Study (Cardiac Arrest in Seattle: Conventional versus Amiodarone Drug Evaluation) compared amiodarone to conventional antiarrhythmic drugs in survivors of out-of-hospital ventricular fibrillation.[155] Amiodarone administered empirically was superior to conventional drugs guided by electrophysiologic testing or Holter-monitor recording.[156, 157] This study, however, did not have a comparison group treated with no antiarrhythmic drugs.

Surgery

Coronary artery bypass grafting has been shown to reduce the incidence of sudden cardiac death in patients with coronary artery disease.[158, 159] Two studies evaluated the efficacy of coronary artery bypass grafting in cardiac arrest survivors.[160, 161] Kelly and associates report 50 patients who had been resuscitated from out-of-hospital cardiac arrest who were undergoing coronary artery bypass graft surgery as the sole surgical intervention.[160] Patients were evaluated with electrophysiologic testing before and after coronary artery bypass grafting. Eighty percent of the patients with inducible ventricular tachycardia preoperatively continued to have inducible ventricular tachycardia or ventricular fibrillation when studied postoperatively. None of the 10 patients with inducible ventricular fibrillation at preoperative electrophysiologic study had inducible ventricular tachycardia or ventricular fibrillation at the study after surgery. Therefore, there was reduction in inducible sustained ventricular arrhythmias with isolated coronary artery bypass grafting, which was due mainly to the reduction in inducible ventricular fibrillation. The patients were followed-up for a mean of 39 ± 29 months. Two patients had recurrent cardiac arrest not associated with acute myocardial infarction, both of whom retained inducible monomorphic ventricular tachycardia postoperatively. A third patient had sustained monomorphic ventricular tachycardia without cardiac arrest, and this patient was noninducible on postoperative electrophysiologic testing. Therefore, inducibility on electrophysiologic testing postoperatively was not significantly predictive of arrhythmia recurrence or sudden death. Cobb and coworkers evaluated 39 survivors of out-of-hospital ventricular fibrillation using a case-control method, comparing medical treatment with isolated coronary artery bypass grafting.[161] Mortality for the medically treated group was 41%, and for surgically treated patients it was 21%, including one operative death. Recurrent sudden cardiac death was seen in 17% of medically treated patients and 3% of surgically treated patients at 2 years ($p = .02$). Therefore, there is evidence that coronary revascularization alone may benefit a selected group of cardiac arrest survivors; however, the role of electrophysiologic testing is unclear for predicting which patients are adequately treated with coronary bypass grafting alone.

In many patients, coronary artery bypass grafting alone is not effective in reducing the risk for recurrent cardiac arrest. Previous myocardial infarction or ventricular aneurysm provides the substrate for reentry, and in patients with monomorphic ventricular tachycardia, primary arrhythmia surgery may be beneficial. Electrophysiologic testing may also be useful in caring for these cardiac arrest survivors by mapping the site of origin of induced ventricular tachycardia, providing data to direct surgical therapy for the ventricular tachycardia.[162,163] Several techniques have been used to surgically ablate ventricular tachycardia, including resection of diseased subendocardium, aneurysmectomy, and cryoablation of ventricular tachycardia foci. These techniques have been used both with and without intraoperative mapping of the site of ventricular tachycardia origin. Generally, because they are associated with an operative mortality of 5% to 21%, these techniques are used for arrhythmias. Operative mortality is greatest in patients with depressed left ventricular function and an origin of ventricular tachycardia in the posterior left ventricle. Inducibility of ventricular arrhythmias postoperatively by programmed stimulation is found in 2% to 32% of cases, and long-term survival at 5 years varies from 33% to 70%.[164–167]

Antiarrhythmic Devices

The first automatic implantable cardioverter–defibrillator was implanted in February 1980. This device is useful in the treatment of life-threatening ventricular arrhythmias, although strictly controlled studies are lacking.[168–175] Initial experience suggested that this device was useful in patients who had already suffered at least one episode of cardiac arrest, and tens of thousands of them have been implanted around the world.[170] The outcome of these patients seems improved, compared with historical controls, and studies attributing device success whenever a shock is delivered to a patient suggest the devices are useful in prolonging life.[176] The arrhythmic death rate in patients with the implantable cardioverter–defibrillator has been reported to be 2% at 1 year and 4% at 2 years.[170] Lehmann and colleagues suggest that the automatic implantable cardioverter–defibrillator is the treatment of choice for survivors of cardiac arrest.[172] These studies are not controlled, however, and distinction between non–sudden cardiac death and sudden arrhythmic cardiac death can be difficult.[14] Several ongoing studies are comparing antiarrhythmic drug therapy with the implantable defibrillator in patients with sustained ventricular tachycardia or ventricular fibrillation.[177–179]

Catheter Ablation

Catheter ablation for ventricular arrhythmias has been used almost exclusively for patients with recurrent sustained monomorphic ventricular tachycardia.[180] This technique is limited in prevention of sudden cardiac death, primarily because patients frequently have more than one type of ventricular tachycardia. In addition, patients who have been resuscitated from ventricular fibrillation often cannot undergo mapping studies because the induced arrhythmias are polymorphic or hemodynamically unstable. Techniques for these procedures include the use of a percutaneous catheter placed in the ventricle to deliver either direct current or radiofrequency energy at the site of origin of ventricular tachycardia. Evans and coworkers report the results of the percutaneous cardiac mapping and ablation registry; clinical improvement is limited.[181]

Several investigators have evaluated the role of transcoronary chemical ablation of ventricular tachycardia with ethanol.[182,183] The initial report consisted of 3 patients with successful results when treated with ethanol injected in the coronary artery branch supplying the arrhythmogenic focus.

Combination Therapy

Frequently, patients undergo therapy with combination approaches. Treatment with both an antiarrhythmic drug and implantation of the automatic implantable cardioverter–defibrillator is common. In some centers, however, addition of drug therapy is reserved for patients with frequent episodes that require termination by the automatic implantable cardioverter–defibrillator. The incidence of proarrhythmic effects of antiarrhythmic drugs may be minimized by limiting the use of the drugs to patients in which the implantable cardioverter–defibrillator repeatedly discharges.

Ongoing studies will assess the effects of antiarrhythmic drug therapy and therapy with the implantable cardioverter–defibrillator before the time that a patient suffers a cardiac arrest.[184] The goal of such investigations is to identify high-risk patients before their initial cardiac arrest. Patient-risk stratification before a first cardiac arrest, however, is not yet sufficiently sophisticated to identify high-risk patients accurately enough to warrant widespread use of potentially toxic drugs or the implantation of expensive devices.

References

1. Gordon T, Kannel WB: Premature mortality from coronary heart disease: the Framingham Study. JAMA 1971;215:1617.
2. National Center for Health Statistics: Advance report, final mortality statistics, 1981. Monthly Vital Stat Rep 1981;33 (Suppl DHHS):4.
3. Gordon T, Thom T: The recent decrease in CHD mortality. Prev Med 1975;4:115.
4. Goldberg RJ: Declining out-of-hospital sudden coronary death rates. Additional pieces of the epidemiologic puzzle. Circulation 1989;79:1369.
5. Gillum RF: Sudden coronary death in the United States. 1980–1985. Circulation 1989;79:756.

6. Hinkle LE Jr, Thaler HT: Clinical classification of cardiac deaths. Circulation 1982;65:457.

7. Goldstein S, Friedman L, Hutchinson R, et al: Timing, mechanism and clinical setting of witnessed deaths in postmyocardial infarction patients. J Am Coll Cardiol 1984;3:1111.

8. Block G, Wickland B: "Sudden death"—what are we talking about? Circulation 1972;45:256.

9. Friedman M, Manwaring JH, Rosenman RH, Donlon G, Ortega P, Grube SM: Instantaneous and sudden deaths. Clinical and pathological differentiation in coronary artery disease. JAMA 1973;225:1319.

10. WHO Scientific Group: The pathological diagnosis of acute ischemic heart disease. World Health Organ Techn Rep Ser 1970;441:5.

11. Goldstein S: The necessity of a uniform definition of sudden coronary death: witnessed death within 1 hour of the onset of acute symptoms. Am Heart J 1982;103:156.

12. Joint International Society and Federation of Cardiology/World Health Organization Task Force on Standardization of Clinical Nomenclature: Report. Nomenclature and criteria for diagnosis of ischemic heart disease. Circulation 1979;59:607.

13. Marcus FL, Cobb LA, Edwards JE, et al: Mechanism of death and prevalence of myocardial ischemic symptoms in the terminal event after myocardial infarction. Am J Cardiol 1988;61:8.

14. Greene HL, Richardson DW, Barker AH, et al: Classification of deaths after myocardial infarction as arrhythmic or nonarrhythmic (the Cardiac Arrhythmia Pilot Study). Am J Cardiol 1989;63:1.

15. Cobb LA, Werner JA, Trobaugh GB: Sudden cardiac death: I. A decade's experience with out-of-hospital resuscitation. Mod Concepts Cardiovasc Dis 1980;49:31.

16. Cobb LA, Werner JA, Trobaugh GB: Sudden cardiac death: II. Outcome of resuscitation, management, and future directions. Mod Concepts Cardiovasc Dis 1980;49:37.

17. Greene HL: The ventricular fibrillation survivor: when and how to treat. Mod Med 1985;53:64.

18. Baum RS, Alvarez H III, Cobb LA: Survival after resuscitation from out-of-hospital ventricular fibrillation. Circulation 1974;50:1231.

19. Schaffer WA, Cobb LA: Recurrent ventricular fibrillation and modes of death in survivors of out-of-hospital ventricular fibrillation. N Engl J Med 1975;293:260.

20. Cobb LA, Baum RS, Alvarez H III, Schaffer WA: Resuscitation from out-of-hospital ventricular fibrillation: 4 years follow-up. Circulation 1975;51:III-223.

21. Echt DS, Liebson PR, Mitchell LB, et al: Mortality and morbidity in patients receiving encainide, flecainide or placebo. The Cardiac Arrhythmia Suppression Trial. N Engl J Med 1991;324:781.

22. Cardiac Arrhythmia Suppression Trial II Investigators: Effect of the antiarrhythmic agent moricizine on survival after myocardial infarction. N Engl J Med 1992;327:227.

23. Buxton AE, Simson MB, Falcone RA, Marchlinski FE, Doherty JU, Josephson ME: Results of signal-averaged electrocardiography and electrophysiologic study in patients with nonsustained ventricular tachycardia after healing of acute myocardial infarction. Am J Cardiol 1987;60:80.

24. Kuchar DL, Thorburn CW, Sammel NL: Prediction of serious arrhythmic events after myocardial infarction: signal-averaged electrocardiogram, Holter monitoring and radionuclide ventriculography. J Am Coll Cardiol 1987;9:531.

25. Denniss AR, Richard DA, Cody DV, et al: Prognostic significance of ventricular tachycardia and fibrillation induced at programmed stimulation and delayed potentials detected on the signal-averaged electrocardiograms of survivors of acute myocardial infarction. Circulation 1986;74:731.

26. Gomes JA, Winters SL, Stewart D, Horowitz S, Milner M, Barreca P: A new noninvasive index to predict sustained ventricular tachycardia and sudden death in the first year after myocardial infarction: based on signal-averaged electrocardiogram, radionuclide ejection fraction and Holter monitoring. J Am Coll Cardiol 1987;10:349.

27. Wilbur DJ, Garan H, Finkelstein D, et al: Out-of-hospital cardiac arrest. Use of electrophysiologic testing in the prediction of long-term outcome. N Engl J Med 1988;318:19.

28. Swerdlow CD, Freedman RA, Peterson J, Clay D: Determinants of prognosis in ventricular tachyarrhythmia patients without induced sustained arrhythmias. Am Heart J 1986;111:433.

29. Roy D, Waxman HL, Kienzle MC, Buxton AE, Marchlinski FE, Josephson ME: Clinical characteristics and long-term follow-up in 119 survivors of cardiac arrest: relation to inducibility at electrophysiologic testing. Am J Cardiol 1983;52:969.

30. Freedman RA, Swerdlow CD, Soderholm-Difatte V, Mason JW: Prognostic significance of arrhythmia inducibility or noninducibility at initial electrophysiologic study in survivors of cardiac arrest. Am J Cardiol 1988;61:578.

31. Zheutlin TA, Steinman RT, Mattioni TA, Kehoe RF: Long-term arrhythmic outcome in survivors of ventricular fibrillation with absence of inducible ventricular tachycardia. Am J Cardiol 1988;62:1213.

32. Morady F, DiCarlo L, Winston S, Davis JL, Scheinman MM: Clinical features and prognosis of patients with out-of-hospital cardiac arrest and a normal electrophysiologic study. J Am Coll Cardiol 1984;4:39.

33. Swerdlow CD, Bardy GH, McAnulty J, et al: Determinants of induced sustained arrhythmias in survivors of out-of-hospital ventricular fibrillation. Circulation 1987;76:1053.

34. Adhar GC, Larson LW, Bardy GH, Greene HL: Sustained ventricular arrhythmias: differences between survivors of cardiac arrest and patients with recurrent sustained ventricular tachycardia. J Am Coll Cardiol 1988;12:159.

35. Denniss AR, Ross DL, Richards DA, et al: Differences between patients with ventricular tachycardia and ventricular fibrillation as assessed by signal-averaged electrocardiogram, radionuclide ventriculography and cardiac mapping. J Am Coll Cardiol 1988;11:276.

36. Freedman RA, Gillis AM, Keren A, Soderholm-Difatte V, Mason JW: Signal-averaged electrocardiographic late potentials in patients with ventricular fibrillation or tachycardia: correlation with clinical arrhythmia and electrophysiologic study. Am J Cardiol 1985;55:1350.

37. Weaver WD, Cobb LA, Hallstrom AP, et al: Considerations for improving survival from out-of-hospital cardiac arrest. Ann Emerg Med 1986;15:1181.

38. Weaver WD, Hill D, Fahrenbruch CE, et al: Use of the auto-

matic external defibrillator in the management of out-of-hospital cardiac arrest. N Engl J Med 1988;319:661.

39. Bedell SE, Delbanco TL, Cook EF, Epstein FH: Survival after cardiopulmonary resuscitation in the hospital. N Engl J Med 1983;309:569.

40. Youngner SJ, Lewandowski W, McClish D, Jukmalis BW, Coulton C, Bartlett ET: "Do-not-resuscitate" orders: incidence and implications in a medical intensive care unit. JAMA 1985;253:54.

41. Rozenbaum EA, Shenkman L: Predicting outcome of inhospital cardiopulmonary resuscitation. Crit Care Med 1988;16:583.

42. Taffet GE, Teasdale TA, Luchi RJ: In-hospital cardiopulmonary resuscitation JAMA 1988;260:2069.

43. Tresch DD, Thakur RK, Hoffman RG, Aufderheide TP, Brooks HL: Comparison of outcome of paramedic-witnessed cardiac arrest in patients younger and older than 70 years. Am J Cardiol 1990;65:453.

44. Longstreth WT, Cobb LA, Fahrenbruch CE, Copass MK: Does age affect outcomes of out-of-hospital cardiopulmonary resuscitation? JAMA 1990;264:2109.

45. Weaver WD, Cobb LA, Hallstrom AP, et al: Considerations for improving survival from out-of-hospital cardiac arrest. Ann Emerg Med 1986;15:1181.

46. Eisenberg M, Bergner L, Hallstrom A: Paramedic programs and out-of-hospital cardiac arrest. I. Factors associated with successful resuscitation. Am J Public Health 1979;69:30.

47. Weaver WD, Hill D, Fahrenbruch CE, et al: Use of the automatic external defibrillator in the management of out-of-hospital cardiac arrest. N Engl J Med 1988;319:661.

48. Weaver WD, Hill DL, Fahrenbruch CE, et al: Automatic external defibrillators: importance of field testing to evaluate performance. J Am Coll Cardiol 1987;10:1259.

49. Weston CFM, Stephens MR, Organ P: Resuscitation by ambulance staff. Letter. Br Med J 1990;301:928.

50. Pratt CM, Francis MJ, Luck JC, Wyndham CR, Miller RR, Quinones MA: Analysis of ambulatory electrocardiograms in 15 patients during spontaneous ventricular fibrillation with special reference to preceding arrhythmic events. J Am Coll Cardiol 1983;2:789.

51. Panidis IP, Morganroth J: Sudden death in hospitalized patients: cardiac rhythm disturbances detected by ambulatory electrocardiographic monitoring. J Am Coll Cardiol 1983;2:798.

52. Kay GN, Plumb VJ, Arciniegas JB: Torsade de pointes: the long-short initiating sequence and other clinical features: observations in 32 patients. J Am Coll Cardiol 1983;2:806.

53. Milner PG, Platia EV, Reid PR, Griffith LSC: Ambulatory electrocardiographic recordings at the time of fatal cardiac arrest. Am J Cardiol 1985;56:588.

54. de Luna AB, Coumel P, Leclercq JF: Ambulatory sudden cardiac death: mechanisms of production of fatal arrhythmias on the basis of data from 157 cases. Am Heart J 1989;117:151.

55. Nikolic G, Bishop RL, Singh JB: Sudden death recorded during Holter monitoring. Circulation 1982;66:218.

56. Cobb LA: Prehospital cardiac care: does it make a difference? Am Heart J 1982;103:316.

57. Cobb LA, Alvarez Y III, Copass MK: A rapid response system for out-of-hospital cardiac emergencies. Med Clin North Am 1976;60:283.

58. Cobb LA, Hallstrom AP: Community-based cardiopulmonary resuscitation: what have we learned? Ann NY Acad Sci 1982;382:330.

59. Cobb LA, Hallstrom AP, Thompson RG, Mandel LP, Copass MK: Community cardiopulmonary resuscitation. Ann Rev Med 1980;31:453.

60. Mandel LP, Cobb LA: Initial and long-term competency of citizens trained in CPR. Emerg Health Serv Q 1982;1:49.

61. Greene HL: Sudden arrhythmic cardiac death—mechanisms, resuscitation and classification: the Seattle perspective. Am J Cardiol 1990;65:4B.

62. Alvarez H, Cobb LA: Experiences with CPR training of the general public. Proceedings of the National Conference on Standards for Cardiopulmonary Resuscitation and Emergency Cardiac Care, May 16–18, 1973, Dallas, TX. American Heart Association, 1975:33.

63. Thompson RG, Hallstrom AP, Cobb LA: Bystander-initiated cardiopulmonary resuscitation in the management of ventricular fibrillation. Ann Intern Med 1979;90:737.

64. Gillum RF, Feinleid M, Margolis JR, Fabsitz RR, Brasch RC: Delay in the prehospital phase of acute myocardial infarction. Arch Intern Med 1976;136:649.

65. Guzy PM, Pearce ML, Greenfield S: The survival benefit of bystander cardiopulmonary resuscitation in a paramedic served metropolitan area. Am J Public Health 1983;73:766.

66. Copley DP, Mantle JA, Rogers WJ, Russell RO Jr, Rackley CE: Improved outcome for prehospital cardiopulmonary collapse with resuscitation by bystanders. Circulation 1977;56:901.

67. Cummins RO, Eisenberg MS: Pre-hospital cardiopulmonary resuscitation: is it effective? JAMA 1985;253:2408.

68. Lund I, Skulberg A: Cardiopulmonary resuscitation by lay people. Lancet 1976;2:702.

69. Tweed WA, Bristow G, Donen N: Resuscitation from cardiac arrest: assessment of a system providing only basic life support outside of hospital. Can Med Assoc J 1980;122:297.

70. Weaver WD, Cobb LA, Hallstrom AP, Fahrenbruch CE, Copass MK, Ray R: Factors influencing survival after out-of-hospital cardiac arrest. J Am Cardiol 1986;7:752.

71. Hallstrom AP, Cobb LA, Swain M, Mensinger K: Predictors of hospital mortality after out-of-hospital cardiopulmonary resuscitation. Crit Care Med 1985;13:927.

72. Eisenberg MS, Cummins RO, Damon S, Larsen MP, Hearne TR: Survival rates from out-of-hospital cardiac arrest: recommendations for uniform definitions and data to report. Ann Emerg Med 1990;19:1249.

73. Cummins RO, Ornato JP, Thies WH, Pepe PE: Improving survival from sudden cardiac arrest: the "chain of survival" concept. Circulation 1991;83:1832.

74. Weaver WD, Copass MK, Bufi D, Ray R, Hallstrom AP, Cobb LA: Improved neurologic recovery and survival after early defibrillation. Circulation 1984;69:943.

75. Longstreth WT Jr, Diehr P, Cobb LA, Hanson RW, Blair AD: Neurologic outcome and blood glucose levels during out-of-hospital radiopulmonary resuscitation. Neurology 1986;36:1186.

76. Longstreth WT Jr, Inui TS, Cobb LA, Copass MK: Neurologic

recovery after out-of-hospital cardiac arrest. Ann Intern Med 1983;98:588.

77. Weaver WD, Copass MK, Hill DL, Fahrenbruch C, Hallstrom AP, Cobb LA: Cardiac arrest treated with a new automatic external defibrillator by out-of-hospital first responders. Am J Cardiol 1986;57:1017.

78. Eisenberg MS, Copass MK, Hallstrom AP, et al: Treatment of out-of-hospital cardiac arrests with rapid defibrillation by emergency medical technicians. N Engl J Med 1980;302:1379.

79. Cummins RO, Thies W, Paraskos J, et al: Encouraging early defibrillation: the American Heart Association and automated external defibrillators. Ann Emerg Med 1990;19:1245.

80. Cummins RO, Thies W: Automated external defibrillators and ACLS: a new initiative from the American Heart Association. Am J Emerg Med 1991;9:91.

81. Cobb LA, Hallstrom AP, Weaver WD, Copass MK, Haynes RE: Clinical predictors and characteristics of the sudden cardiac death syndrome. Proceedings of the USA/USSR First Joint Symposium on Sudden Death, October 3–5, 1977, Yalta, USSR. Department of Health, Education and Welfare. Publication NIH 78-1470, 1978:99.

82. Teasdale G, Jennett B: Assessment of coma and impaired consciousness. Lancet 1974;2:81.

83. Longstreth WT Jr, Diehr P, Inui TS: Prediction of awakening after out-of-hospital cardiac arrest. N Engl J Med 1983;308:1378.

84. Longstreth WT Jr, Clayson KJ, Chandler WL, Sumi SM: Cerebrospinal fluid creatine kinase activity and neurologic recovery after cardiac arrest. Neurology 1984;34:834.

85. Smith AL: Barbiturate protection in cerebral hypoxia. Anesthesiology 1977;47:285.

86. Brain Resuscitation Clinical Trial 1 Study Group: Randomized clinical study of thiopental loading in comatose survivors of cardiac arrest. N Engl J Med 1986;314:397.

87. Kirsch JR, Dean JM, Rogers MC: Current concepts in brain resuscitation. Arch Intern Med 1986;146:1413.

88. Grafton ST, Longstreth WT Jr: Steroids after cardiac arrest: a retrospective study with concurrent, nonrandomized controls. Neurology 1988;38:1315.

89. Salerno DM, Asinger RW, Elsperger J, Ruiz E, Hodges M: Frequency of hypokalemia in successfully resuscitated out-of-hospital cardiac arrest compared to that in acute transmural myocardial infarction. Am J Cardiol 1987;59:84.

90. Thompson RG, Cobb LA: Hypokalemia after resuscitation from out-of-hospital ventricular fibrillation. JAMA 1982;248:2860.

91. Krone RJ, Gillespie JA, Weld FM, Miller JP, Moss AJ, the Multicenter Postinfarction Research Group: Low-level exercise testing after myocardial infarction: usefulness in enhancing clinical risk stratification. Circulation 1985;71:80.

92. Tibbits PA, Evaul JE, Goldstein RE, et al: Serial acquisition of data to predict one-year mortality rate after acute myocardial infarction. Am J Cardiol 1987;60:451.

93. Fioretti P, Brower RW, Simoons ML, et al: Prediction of mortality during the first year after acute myocardial infarction from clinical variables and stress test at hospital discharge. Am J Cardiol 1985;55:1313.

94. Waters DD, Bosch X, Bouchard A, et al: Comparison of clinical variables and variables derived from a limited pre-discharge exercise test as predictors of early and late mortality after myocardial infarction. J Am Coll Cardiol 1985;5:1.

95. Debusk RF, Dennis CA: "Submaximal" pre-discharge exercise testing after acute myocardial infarction. Who needs it? Am J Cardiol 1985;55:299.

96. Nielsen JR, Mickley H, Damsgaard EM, Froland A: Predischarge maximal exercise test identifies risk for cardiac death in patients with acute myocardial infarction. Am J Cardiol 1990;65:149.

97. Haberl R, Jilge G, Pulter R, Steinbeck G: Comparison of frequency and time domain analysis or the signal-averaged electrocardiogram in patients with ventricular tachycardia and coronary artery disease: methodologic validation and clinical relevance. J Am Coll Cardiol 1988;12:150.

98. Gardner MJ, Montague TJ, Armstrong CS, Horacek BM, Smith ER: Vulnerability to ventricular arrhythmia: assessment by mapping of body surface potential. Circulation 1986;73:684.

99. Faugere G, Savard P, Nadeau RA, et al: Characterization of the spatial distribution of late ventricular potentials by body surface mapping in patients with ventricular tachycardia. Circulation 1986;74:1323.

100. Farrell TG, Bashir Y, Cripps T, et al: Risk stratification for arrhythmic events in postinfarction patients based on heart rate variability, ambulatory electrocardiographic variables and the signal-averaged electrocardiogram. J Am Coll Cardiol 1991;18:687.

101. Dreifus LS, Agarwal JB, Botvinick EH, et al: Heart rate variability for risk stratification of life-threatening arrhythmias. J Am Coll Cardiol 1993;22:948.

102. Ruskin JN, DiMarco JP, Garan H: Out-of-hospital cardiac arrest: electrophysiologic observations and selection of long-term antiarrhythmic therapy. N Engl J Med 1980;303:607.

103. Swerdlow CD, Gong G, Echt DS, et al: Clinical factors predicting successful electrophysiologic-pharmacologic study in patients with ventricular tachycardia. J Am Coll Cardiol 1983;1:409.

104. Ruskin JN: Primary ventricular fibrillation. N Engl J Med 1987;317:307.

105. Swerdlow CD, Winkle RA, Mason JW: Determinants of survival in patients with ventricular tachyarrhythmias. N Engl J Med 1983;308:1436.

106. Mason JW, Winkle RA: Accuracy of the ventricular tachycardia-induction study for predicting long-term efficacy and inefficacy of antiarrhythmic drugs. N Engl J Med 1980;303:1073.

107. Kuchar DL, Rottman J, Berger E, Freeman CS, Garan H, Ruskin JN: Prediction of successful suppression of sustained ventricular tachyarrhythmias by serial drug testing from data derived at the initial electrophysiologic study. J Am Coll Cardiol 1988;12:982.

108. Kuchar DL, Garan H, Ruskin JN: Electrophysiologic evaluation of antiarrhythmic therapy for ventricular tachyarrhythmias. Am J Cardiol 1988;62:39H.

109. Poole JE, Mathisen TL, Kudenchuk PJ, et al: Long-term outcome in patients who survive out-of-hospital ventricular fibrillation and undergo electrophysiologic studies: evaluation by electrophysiologic subgroups. J Am Coll Cardiol 1990;16:657.

110. Dolack GL, Callahan DB, Bardy GH, Greene HL: Signal-

averaged electrocardiographic late potentials in resuscitated survivors of out-of-hospital ventricular fibrillation. Am J Cardiol 1990;65:1102.

111. Weaver WD, Cobb LA, Hallstrom AP: Characteristics of survivors of exertion and nonexertion-related cardiac arrest: value of subsequent exercise testing. Am J Cardiol 1982;50: 671.

112. Manyari DE, Duff HJ, Kostuk WJ, et al: Usefulness of noninvasive studies for diagnosis of right ventricular dysplasia. Am J Cardiol 1986;57:1147.

113. Daubert C, Descaves C, Foulgoc J-L, Bourdonnec C, Laurent M, Gouffault J: Critical analysis of cineangiographic criteria for diagnosis of arrhythmogenic right ventricular dysplasia. Am Heart J 1988;115:448.

114. Robertson JH, Bardy GH, German LD, Gallagher JJ, Kisslo JA: Comparison of 2-dimensional echocardiographic and angiographic findings in arrhythmogenic right ventricular dysplasia. Am J Cardiol 1985;55:1506.

115. Strain JE, Grose RM, Factor SM, Fisher JD: Results of endomyocardial biopsy in patients with spontaneous ventricular tachycardia but without apparent structural heart disease. Circulation 1983;68:1171.

116. Goldstein S, Friedman L, Hutchinson R, et al: Timing, mechanism and clinical setting of witnessed deaths in postmyocardial infarction patients. J Am Coll Cardiol 1984;3:1111.

117. Moosvi AR, Goldstein S, VanderBrug S, et al: Effect of empiric antiarrhythmic therapy in resuscitated out-of-hospital cardiac arrest victims with coronary artery disease. Am J Cardiol 1990;65:1192.

118. Goldstein S, Landis JR, Leighton R, et al: Predictive survival models for resuscitated victims of out-of-hospital cardiac arrest with coronary artery disease. Circulation 1985;71:873.

119. Hallstrom AP, Cobb LA: Predicting risk of recurrence in sudden cardiac death syndrome. Emerg Health Serv Rev 1984;2:49.

120. Ritchie JL, Hallstrom AP, Trobaugh GB, Caldwell JH, Cobb LA: Out-of-hospital sudden coronary death: rest and exercise radionuclide left ventricular function in survivors. Am J Cardiol 1985;55:645.

121. Weaver WD, Lorch GS, Alvarez H III, Cobb LA: Angiographic findings and prognostic indicators in patients resuscitated from sudden cardiac death. Circulation 1976;54:895.

122. Eisenberg MS, Hallstrom AP, Berner L: Long-term survival after out-of-hospital cardiac arrest. N Engl J Med 1982;306: 1340.

123. Weaver WD, Cobb LA, Hallstrom AP: Ambulatory arrhythmias in resuscitated victims of cardiac arrest. Circulation 1982;66:212.

124. Hallstrom AP, Cobb LA, Ray R: Smoking as a risk factor for recurrence of sudden cardiac death. N Engl J Med 1986; 314:271.

125. Oseran DS, Speck SM, Weaver WD, Greene HL, Cobb LA: Ventricular fibrillation in patients with normal coronary arteries. Circulation 1983;68:III. Abstract.

126. Massie BM, Conway M: Survival of patients with congestive heart failure: past, present, and future prospects. Circulation 1987;75(Suppl IV):IV-11.

127. Borbola J, Ezri MD, Denes P: Correlation between the signal-averaged electrocardiogram and electrophysiologic study

findings in patients with coronary artery disease and sustained ventricular tachycardia. Am Heart J 1988;115:116.

128. Graboys TB, Lown B, Podrid PJ, DeSilva R: Long-term survival of patients with malignant ventricular arrhythmia treated with antiarrhythmic drugs. Am J Cardiol 1982;50:437.

129. Vlay SC, Kallman CH, Reid PR: Prognostic assessment of survivors of ventricular tachycardia and ventricular fibrillation with ambulatory monitoring. Am J Cardiol 1984;54:87.

130. Anderson JL, Anastasiou-Nana MI, Menlove RL, Moreno FL, Nanas JN, Barker AH: Spontaneous variability in ventricular ectopic activity during chronic antiarrhythmic therapy. Circulation 1990;82:830.

131. Winkle RA: Antiarrhythmic drug effect mimicked by spontaneous variability of ventricular ectopy. Circulation 1987; 57:1116.

132. Michelson EL, Morganroth J: Spontaneous variability of complex ventricular arrhythmias detected by long-term electrocardiographic recording. Circulation 1980;61:690.

133. Pratt CM, Slymen DJ, Wierman AM, et al: Analysis of the spontaneous variability of ventricular arrhythmias: consecutive ambulatory electrocardiographic recordings of ventricular tachycardia. Am J Cardiol 1985;56:67.

134. Pratt CM, Theroux P, Slymen D, et al: Spontaneous variability of ventricular arrhythmias in patients at increased risk for sudden death after acute myocardial infarction: consecutive ambulatory electrocardiographic recordings of 88 patients. Am J Cardiol 1987;59:278.

135. Hallstrom AP, Greene HL, Huther ML: The healthy responder phenomenon in nonrandomized clinical trials. Stat Med 1991;10:1621.

136. Mitchell LB, Duff HJ, Manyari DE, Wyse DG: A randomized clinical trial of the noninvasive and invasive approaches to drug therapy of ventricular tachycardia. N Engl J Med 1987; 317:1681.

137. The ESVEM Investigators: The ESVEM Trial. Electrophysiologic study versus electrocardiographic monitoring for selection of antiarrhythmic therapy of ventricular tachyarrhythmias. Circulation 1989;79:1354.

138. Mason JW, Electrophysiologic Study versus Electrocardiographic Monitoring Investigators: A comparison of electrophysiologic testing with Holter monitoring to predict antiarrhythmic-drug efficacy for ventricular tachyarrhythmias. N Engl J Med 1993;329:445.

139. Mason JW, Electrophysiologic Study versus Electrocardiographic Monitoring Investigators: A comparison of seven antiarrhythmic drugs in patients with ventricular tachyarrhythmias. N Engl J Med 1993;329:452.

140. Velebit V, Podrid P, Lown B, Cohen BH, Graboys TB: Aggravation and provocation of ventricular arrhythmias by antiarrhythmic drugs. Circulation 1982;65:886.

141. Morganroth J, Horowitz LN: Incidence of proarrhythmic effects from quinidine in the outpatient treatment of benign or potentially lethal ventricular arrhythmias. Am J Cardiol 1985;56:585.

142. Rae AP, Kay HR, Horowitz LN, Spielman SR, Greenspan AM: Proarrhythmic effects of antiarrhythmic drugs in patients with malignant ventricular arrhythmias evaluated by electrophysiologic testing. J Am Coll Cardiol 1988;12:131.

143. Koster RW, Wellens HJJ: Quinidine-induced ventricular flut-

ter and fibrillation without digitalis therapy. Am J Cardiol 1976;38:519.

144. Nguyen PT, Scheinman MM, Seger J: Polymorphous ventricular tachycardia: clinical characterization, therapy, and the QT interval. Circulation 1986;74:340.

145. Bigger JT Jr, Sahar DI: Clinical types of proarrhythmic response to antiarrhythmic drugs. Am J Cardiol 1987;59:2E.

146. Ruskin JN, McGovern B, Garan H, DiMarco JP, Kelly E: Antiarrhythmic drugs: a possible cause of out-of-hospital cardiac arrest. N Engl J Med 1983;309:1302.

147. Zipes DP: Proarrhythmic effects of antiarrhythmic drugs. Am J Cardiol 1987;59:26E.

148. Morganroth J: Risk factors for the development of proarrhythmic events. Am J Cardiol 1987;59:32E.

149. Podrid PJ, Lampert S, Graboys TB, Blatt CM, Lown B: Aggravation of arrhythmia by antiarrhythmic drugs-incidence and predictors. Am J Cardiol 1987;59:38E.

150. Horowitz LN, Greenspan AM, Rae AP, Kay HR, Spielman SR: Proarrhythmic responses during electrophysiologic testing. Am J Cardiol 1987;59:45E.

151. Roden DM, Woosley RL, Primm RK: Incidence and clinical features of the quinidine-associated long QT syndrome: implications for patient care. Am Heart J 1986;111:1088.

152. Coplen SE, Antmann EM, Berlin JA, Hewitt P, Chalmers TC: Efficacy and safety of quinidine therapy for maintenance of sinus rhythm after cardioversion. A meta-analysis of randomized control trials. Circulation 1990;82:1106.

153. Furberg CD: Effect of antiarrhythmic drugs on mortality after myocardial infarction. Am J Cardiol 1983;52:32C.

154. Wyse DG, Morganroth J, Ledingham R, et al: New insights into the definition and meaning of proarrhythmia during initiation of antiarrhythmic drug therapy from the Cardiac Arrhythmia Suppression Trial and Pilot study. J Am Coll Cardiol 1994;23:1130.

155. CASCADE Investigators: Cardiac arrest in Seattle: conventional versus amiodarone drug evaluation (the CASCADE study). Am J Cardiol 1991;67:578.

156. CASCADE Investigators: Randomized antiarrhythmic drug therapy in survivors of cardiac arrest (The CASCADE study). Am J Cardiol 1993;72:280.

157. Dolack GL, CASCADE Investigators: Clinical predictors of implantable cardioverter defibrillator shocks: results of the CASCADE Trial. Am J Cardiol 1994;73:237.

158. DeWood MA, Notske RN, Berg R Jr, et al: Medical and surgical management of early Q wave myocardial infarction. I. Effects of surgical reperfusion on survival, recurrent myocardial infarction, sudden death and functional class at 10 or more years of follow-up. J Am Coll Cardiol 1989;14:65.

159. Holmes DR Jr, Davis KB, Mock MB, et al: The effect of medical and surgical treatment on subsequent sudden cardiac death in patients with coronary artery disease: a report from the Coronary Artery Surgery Study. Circulation 1986; 73:1254.

160. Kelly P, Ruskin JN, Vlahakes GJ, Buckley MJ Jr, Freeman GS, Garan H: Surgical coronary revascularization in survivors of prehospital cardiac arrest: its effect on inducible ventricular arrhythmias and long-term survival. J Am Coll Cardiol 1990; 15:267.

161. Cobb LA, Hallstrom AP, Zia M, Trobaugh GB, Greene HL, Weaver WD: Influence of coronary revascularization on recurrent sudden cardiac death syndrome. J Am Coll Cardiol 1983;I(2):688. Abstract.

162. Horowitz LN, Harken AH, Kastor JA, Josephson ME: Ventricular resection guided by epicardial and endocardial mapping for treatment of recurrent ventricular tachycardia. N Engl J Med 1980;302:589.

163. Landymore RW, Gardner MA, McIntyre AJ, Barker RA: Surgical intervention for drug-resistant ventricular tachycardia. J Am Coll Cardiol 1990;16:37.

164. Cox JL: Patient selection criteria and results of surgery for refractory ischemic ventricular tachycardia. Circulation 1989;79(Suppl I):I-163.

165. Hargrove WC, Miller JM: Risk stratification and management of patients with recurrent ventricular tachycardia and other malignant ventricular arrhythmias. Circulation 1989;79 (Suppl I):1-178.

166. Zee-Cheng C, Kouchoukos NT, Connors JP, Ruffy R: Treatment of life threatening ventricular tachycardia with nonguided surgery supported by electrophysiologic testing and drug therapy. J Am Coll Cardiol 1989;13:153.

167. Ivey TD, Bardy GH, Misbach GA, Greene HL: Surgical management of refractory ventricular arrhythmias in patients with prior inferior myocardial infarction. J Thorac Cardiovasc Surg 1985;89:369.

168. Mirowski M, Reid PR, Mower MM, et al: Termination of malignant ventricular arrhythmias with an implanted automatic defibrillator in human beings. N Engl J Med 1980; 303:322.

169. Marchlinski FE, Flores BT, Buxton AE, et al: The automatic implantable cardioverter/defibrillator: efficacy, complications, and device failures. Ann Intern Med 1986;104:481.

170. Thomas AC, Moser SA, Smutka ML, Wilson PA: Implantable defibrillation: eight years clinical experience. Pacing Clin Electrophysiol 1988;11:2053.

171. Mirowski M, Reid PR, Winkle RA, et al: Mortality in patients with implanted automatic defibrillators. Ann Intern Med 1983;98:585.

172. Lehmann MH, Steinman RT, Schuger CD, Jackson K: The automatic implantable cardioverter defibrillator as antiarrhythmic treatment modality of choice for survivors of cardiac arrest unrelated to acute myocardial infarction. Am J Cardiol 1988;62:803.

173. Kim SG: Implantable defibrillator therapy: does it really prolong life? How can we prove it? Am J Cardiol 1993;71:1213.

174. Connolly SJ, Yusuf S: Evaluation of the implantable cardioverter defibrillator in survivors of cardiac arrest: the need for randomized trials. Am J Cardiol 1992;69:959.

175. Moss A: One randomized defibrillator trial is worth 1,000 descriptive reports. Pacing Clin Electrophysiol 1993;16:247.

176. Fogoros RN, Elson JJ, Bonnet CA: Actuarial incidence and pattern of occurrence of shocks following implantation of the automatic implantable cardioverter. Pacing Clin Electrophysiol 1989;12:1465.

177. Siebels J, Cappato R, Rüppel R, Schneider MAE, Kuck KH, CASH Investigators: Preliminary results of the Cardiac Arrest Study Hamburg (CASH). Am J Cardiol 1993;72:109F.

178. Connolly SJ, Gent M, Roberts RS, et al: Canadian Implantable Defibrillator Study (CIDS): study design and organization. Am J Cardiol 1993;72:103F.

179. Epstein AE: AVID necessity. Pacing Clin Electrophysiol 1993;16:1773.

180. Ward DE, Camm AJ: The current status of ablation of cardiac conduction tissue and ectopic myocardial foci by transvenous electrical discharges. Clin Cardiol 1986;9:237.

181. Evans GT, Scheinman MM, Executive Committee of the Percutaneous Cardiac Mapping and Ablation Registry, Catheter Ablation for Control of Ventricular Tachycardia: A report of the percutaneous cardiac mapping and ablation registry. Pacing Clin Electrophysiol 1986;9:1391.

182. Okishige K, Andrews TC, Friedman PL: Suppression of incessant polymorphic ventricular tachycardia by selective intracoronary ethanol infusion. Pacing Clin Electrophysiol 191;14:188.

183. Brugada P, deSwart H, Smeets JLRM, Wellens HJJ: Transcoronary chemical ablation of ventricular tachycardia. Circulation 1989;79:475.

184. Bigger JT Jr: Future studies with the implantable cardioverter defibrillator. Pacing Clin Electrophysiol 1991;14:883.

Cardiac Arrhythmias, 3rd edition, edited by William J. Mandel.
J. B. Lippincott Company, Philadelphia © 1995.

43

Morton M. Mower • Charles Swerdlow • William J. Mandel
C. Thomas Peter • Peng-Sheng Chen

Use of the Automatic Implantable Cardioverter–Defibrillator in the Treatment of Malignant Ventricular Tachyarrhythmias

The first clinical implantation of an automatic implantable cardioverter–defribrillator (ICD) was performed at Johns Hopkins Hospital in Baltimore on February 4, 1980.[1] The therapy has enjoyed accelerating growth, with more than 50,000 units implanted worldwide, using devices manufactured by six companies (Table 43-1). After review of the early work that led to this new therapeutic modality, this chapter centers on its current clinical use and the prospects of future developments.

RATIONALE FOR THE IMPLANTABLE CARDIOVERTER–DEFIBRILLATOR

Fully two thirds of the mortality from coronary artery disease is due to sudden cardiac death, a syndrome that also occurs in patients with heart disease of other etiologies. There are an estimated 400,000 victims annually in the United States, and the incidence is no less striking in other developed nations. It is generally accepted that sudden cardiac death usually reflects disturbances in cardiac electric activity, culminating in ventricular fibrillation and death. Management of patients who are subject to this disorder is fraught with almost unsurmountable diffi-

culties because most die within minutes of the onset of symptoms, long before they are able to reach a medical facility.

Because of clinicians' increased ability to identify many patients at high risk of dying suddenly, the latter part of the 1970s saw a significant increase in aggressive antiarrhythmic therapy, including drugs, antitachycardia pacemakers, cardiac surgery, and finally, the ICD. The basic idea behind the development of the ICD was to provide selected high-risk patients with the means of restoring normal heart rhythm within seconds, without the need for specialized medical personnel or additional equipment. Because the device could not prevent arrhythmias, it was intended to complement other treatments and serve as a backup or safety mechanism. The ICD could then be compared with implantable demand pacemakers, except ventricular tachyarrhythmias rather than asystole are sensed and the delivered discharges are a million times higher energy than pacemaker impulses.

Early Studies

The biologic and engineering feasibility of the ICD was demonstrated in 1969, when the first experimental model

TABLE 43-1. Implantable Cardioverter–Defibrillators Available or Under Investigation

Attribute	CPI VENTAK P	CPI PRX	CPI PRX$_2$	CPI P$_2$	Medtronic PCD	Medtronic PCD Jewel	Intermedics RES Q	Siemens Siecure	Telectronics A/P	Telectronics Guardian	Ventritex Cadence
Weight (g)	240	220	233	233	197	132	220	220	269	270	237
Programmable rate/energy	Yes	Yes	Yes	Yes	Yes	Yes	Yes	Yes	Yes	Yes	Yes
Bradycardia pacing	No	Yes	Yes	Yes	Yes	Yes	Yes	Yes	Yes	Yes	Yes
Anitachycardia pacing	No	Yes	Yes	No	Yes	Yes	Yes	Yes	Yes	No	Yes
Waveforms	M	M	B$_1$	B$_1$	M,S	M,B$_1$	B$_1$	N/A	M	M	M,B$_1$
Minimum energy (J)	0.1	0.1	0.1	0.1	0.2	0.2	0.1	2.5	0.5	3	0.1
Maximum energy (J)	30	32	34	34	34	34	40	40	30	30	38
Tiered therapy	No	Yes	Yes	Partial*	Yes	Yes	Yes	Yes	Yes	No	Yes
Committed	Yes	No	P VT VF	P VT VF	VT NO VF YES	VT NO VF Yes	Yes	Yes	No	No	No
Stored electrograms	No	No	Yes	Yes	No	Yes	No	N/A	Snapshot	No	Yes
Noninvasive EPS	No	Yes	Yes	Yes	Yes	Yes	Yes	Yes	Yes	No	Yes

M, monophasic; S, sequential; B$_1$, biphasic; N/A, not announced; P, programmable; VF, ventricular fibrillation; VT, ventricular tachycardia.
* No antitachycardia pacing.

was built and successfully tested in animals.[2] The initial prototype monitored pulsatile ventricular pressure, using a transducer mounted on the tip of a transvenous electrode catheter placed in the right ventricle. Ventricular fibrillation abolished the phasic nature of the pressure curve, which if longer than 6 seconds triggered the capacitor-charging cycle. When fully charged (about 20 seconds after onset of fibrillation), the device delivered an electric shock between the right ventricular electrode and another located more proximally on the catheter at the level of the superior vena cava. In the event of unsuccessful defibrillation, the device recycled and delivered additional shocks. If normal rhythm resumed, the counter-shock discharge was inhibited. Figure 43-1 shows one of the first experimental models, and Figure 43-2 displays its functional performance. In some more advanced models (Fig. 43-3), the sensing system monitored a cardiac contraction signal and the endocardial electrogram, requiring the absence of both signals to initiate a charging cycle.[3]

The single intravascular catheter, which was used in these initial systems, was capable of defibrillating dogs with 5 to 10 J and baboons with even less energy.[4-6] Figure 43-4 shows the induction of ventricular fibrillation in an anesthetized baboon and its termination with a catheter-delivered 0.5-J countershock. Clinical studies performed later during open-heart surgery for coronary bypass grafting demonstrated that catheter defibrillation was also feasible in humans, even under conditions of extreme myocardial ischemia and metabolic dysfunction.[7] The required energies ranged from 5 to 15 J, comparing favorably with those found in the animal studies.

The initial prototype systems were followed by more advanced models, characterized by greater miniaturization, progressive refinement of the electrode and sensing

systems, increased safety, and higher reliability. The size, weight, structural characteristics, and functional performance of the units at last met the stringent criteria for long-term implantation in humans.[6] Preclinical testing included analysis of the long-term bench performance of the defibrillator and the effects of exposure to various physical stresses, such as vacuum, pressure, temperature cycling, mechanical vibrations and shocks, and to electromagnetic interference. Many of the test conditions exceeded the standards required of implantable pacemakers. Anatomic effects of chronic electrode implantation and defibrillatory discharges were studied for up to 11 months and found to be minimal. Figure 43-5 shows selected frames from a film taken during a successful automatic fibrillation–defibrillation sequence in a fully conscious dog. The applied physics laboratory of the Johns Hopkins University also made an independent evaluation of basic device design, provocation challenges to the sensing system, analysis of components, manufacturing and quality control procedures, and review of the preclinical test data. On the basis of the examination, the device was found suitable for use in a clinical setting.[8,9]

First Clinical Model

The first sensing system that was used clinically was based on the analysis of the probability density function (PDF) and was specific for ventricular fibrillation. It identified the arrhythmia directly rather than by monitoring indirect parameters of cardiac activity, such as arterial pressure, R waves, or electric impedance.[10] The logic circuit measured the time spent by the input electrogram between two amplitude limits located near zero potential. In essence,

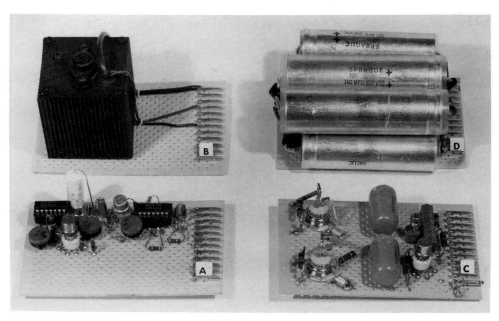

Figure 43-1. One of the first experimental prototypes of the automatic defibrillator on four 3- × 4-inch circuit boards. (**A**) Sensing circuit. (**B**) High-voltage converter. (**C**) Switching circuit. (**D**) Capacitor bank. The batteries, not shown, were as large as this entire array. (Mirowski M, Mower MM, Staewen WS, et al: Standby automatic defibrillator: an approach to prevention of sudden cardiac death. Arch Intern Med 1970;126:158.)

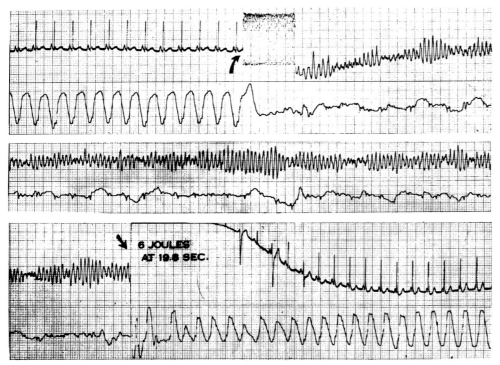

Figure 43-2. Simultaneous electrocardiographic and right ventricular pressure curves, recorded during operating cycle of the early prototype shown in Figure 43-1. Ventricular fibrillation is induced in a dog, with low-level alternating current (*top arrow*); 19.8 seconds later, an intracardiac catheter discharge of 6 J is automatically delivered (*bottom arrow*), causing sinus rhythm to resume. The strips are continuous. (Mirowski M, Mower MM, Staewen WS, et al: The development of the transvenous automatic defibrillator. Arch Intern Med 1972;129:773.)

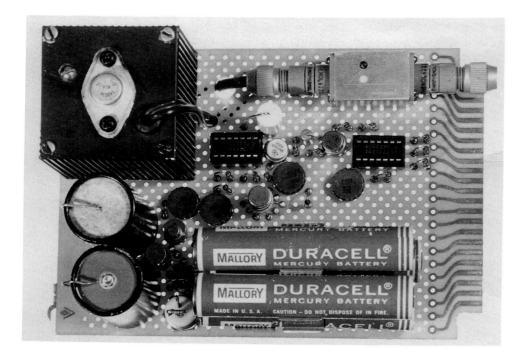

Figure 43-3. Single-circuit board model, with 10-J output capability. The 4.5- × 6.5-inch card contains a high-voltage DC–DC converter (*upper left*), the capacitor bank (*lower left*), the transducer connector and the balancing network (*upper right*), and two AA batteries (*lower right*). The remaining elements form the sensing and switching circuitry. (Mirowski M, Mower MM, Staewen WS, et al: The development of the transvenous automatic defibrillator. Arch Intern Med 1972;129:773.)

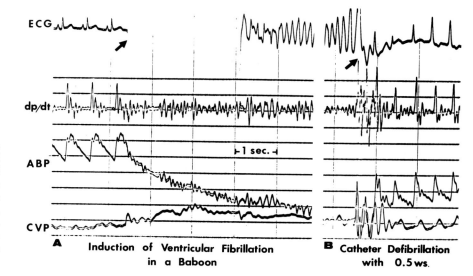

Figure 43-4. (**A**) Induction of ventricular fibrillation in a baboon, with low-level alternating current. (**B**) Restoration of normal rhythm with an 0.5-J catheter-delivered discharge. *ECG*, electrocardiogram; *ABP*, arterial blood pressure; *CVP*, central venous pressure. (Mirowski M, Mower MM, Reid PR, Watkins L Jr: Automatic implantable defibrillator. Cardiovasc Clin 1983;14:197.)

ventricular fibrillation is characterized by a striking absence of isoelectric potential segments (Fig. 43-6).[8]

Because the success of catheter defibrillation depended critically on maintaining proper position of the catheter tip in the apex of the right ventricle and because the exact energy requirements in humans were still un-

known, it was decided that the first clinical implants would use at least one electrode that could be precisely fixed in place surgically. Initially, this was a flexible cup and later was a rectangular patch containing titanium mesh. A titanium spring placed in the superior vena cava formed the second electrode (Fig. 43-7).

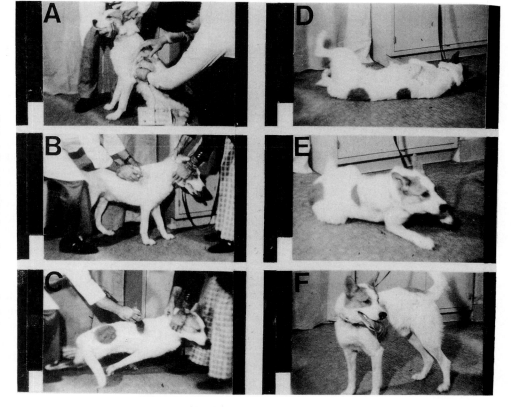

Figure 43-5. Selected frames from a motion picture of a typical automatic defibrillation episode. (**A**) Defibrillator testing procedure with the external analyzer. (**B**) Ventricular fibrillation is induced by magnetic activation of an implanted fibrillator. (**C**) Loss of consciousness secondary to the arrhythmia. (**D**) Delivery of the defibrillatory shock, 15 seconds after the onset of fibrillation. (**E** and **F**) The animal 5 and 15 seconds, respectively, after automatic defibrillation. (Mirowski M, Mower MM, Langer A: Miniaturized implantable automatic defibrillator for prevention of sudden death from ventricular fibrillation. Amsterdam, Excerpta Medical International Congress Series 1978;458:660.)

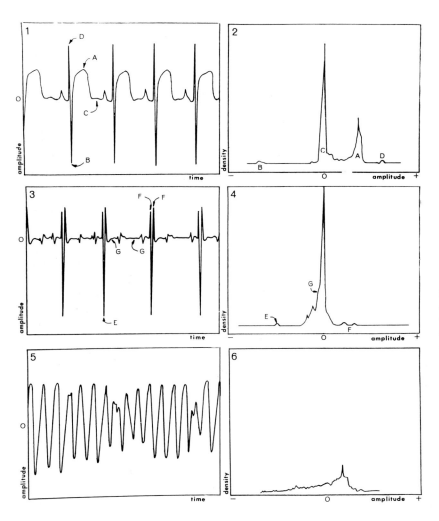

Figure 43-6. Selected input electrograms (**1, 3,** and **5**), with their corresponding probability density function graphs (**2, 4,** and **6**). (**1**) Normal input electrogram. (**2**) Peak at zero amplitude; *C* indicates that the signal spends considerable time near baseline. (**3**) Filtered input signal. (**4**) Filtering augments the peak at zero amplitude (*G*) and decreases the heights of secondary peaks. (**5**) Filtered ventricular fibrillation signal. (**6**) Absence of peak at zero amplitude reflects the short time the signal is near baseline and indicates the diagnosis of ventricular fibrillation. (Mirowski M, Mower MM, Langer A, Heilman MS: The automatic implantable defibrillator: a new avenue. In: Bircks W, Loogen F, Schulte HD, Seipel L, eds. Medical and surgical management of tachyarrhythmias. Berlin: Springer-Verlag, 1980:77.)

Truncated exponential discharges were used because they are simple to generate and, for a given defibrillation efficacy, require low peak voltage and current. A constant energy level was delivered by varying pulse duration between 3 and 8 milliseconds to compensate variations in heart-electrode resistance. Defibrillatory discharges of 25 J were delivered about 15 seconds after onset of an arrhythmia, and the device could recycle as many as three times during a single episode if needed. The strength of the third and fourth shocks was increased to as much as 45 J.

FURTHER DEVELOPMENTS OF THE IMPLANTABLE CARDIOVERTER–DEFIBRILLATOR

Early Units

Although the first clinical device was highly successful in terminating ventricular fibrillation and ultimately implanted in 32 patients, it soon became apparent that most

sudden cardiac death survivors who were referred for implantation suffered from hemodynamically unstable ventricular tachycardias rather than from ventricular fibrillation, which was observed only at a later stage. Consequently, significant modifications were implemented to make the system responsive to the entire range of ventricular tachyarrhythmias. The new unit monitored heart rate as well as the probability density function. A bipolar right ventricular electrode was added for precise rate determination, R-wave synchronization, and eventually for pacing. The original automatic defibrillator was thus transformed into an ICD. This unit was phased into the clinical study in April 1982.[11]

The automatic implantable cardioverter–defibrillator (AICD) was physically somewhat similar to the early pacemaker (Fig. 43-8). It measured 11.2 × 7.1 × 2.5 cm and weighed 292 g. An inner can housed the electronic package (consisting of more than 300 discrete components) and was located in the upper part of the device. Capacitors, lithium batteries, and a test-load resistor occupied the lower portion. The titanium outer can was hermetically

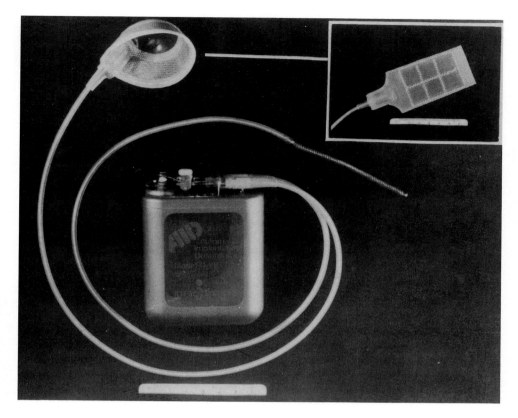

Figure 43-7. Automatic implantable defibrillator, with two defibrillating electrodes. (*Inset*) Patch electrode used as an alternative to the apical cup electrode. (Mirowski M, Mower MM, Reid PR: Treatment of malignant ventricular arrhythmias in man with an implanted automatic defibrillator. Crit Care Med 1981;9:388.)

sealed with a laser-beam weld. A piezoelectric crystal located near the center of the can emitted magnetically triggered coded audio signals, which could be used to check the sensing function and to 0determine whether the unit was active or inactive. If the device was active, the unit beeped synchronously with the QRS complexes, allowing one to easily ascertain that each QRS complex was being sensed and that there was no miscounting due to T-wave sensing.

A magnet also activated and deactivated the device as desired. Keeping it in place for 30 seconds caused the device to change its state and a different set of sounds to be emitted. In contrast to the beeping sounds of the active sensing unit, the deactivated unit had a solid or steady tone. With the help of an external monitoring device, the AIDCHECK-B, the battery strength and the cumulative number of pulses delivered through the leads to the patient could be determined. A transient application of the magnet triggered the testing cycle. As the batteries became depleted, the charge times telemetered out to the AIDCHECK-B were prolonged. When they remained elevated despite repeated testing, elective replacement was suggested. The magnet was also used to divert a pulse to the internal test-load resistor if it was desired that the shock *not* be given to the patient. The battery charger for the AIDCHECK-B was very useful during implantation as a source of low-level alternating current to induce malig-

nant arrhythmias for testing whether the units functioned properly.[12]

The original clinical trials with the first defibrillating device (the automatic implantable defibrillator or AID) and the subsequent improved AICD version (AID-B/BR) lasted from February 1980 through October 1985. At that time, the Food and Drug Administration (FDA) gave approval to the second-generation device and in March 1986 to an integrated circuit third generation unit, the VENTAK-C, also known as model 1500.

The VENTAK-C, although incorporating no additional functions, showed slight improvement in the PDF and automatic gain control circuitry. In addition and most importantly, it was highly manufacturable and required minimal soldering and other hand assembly. This added remarkably to its reliability.

The VENTAK-C proved to be acceptable as a clinical unit. Its parameters were set at the factory, however, and could not subsequently be changed. The VENTAK-P device (model 1600), which entered clinical trials in September 1988, is a multi-programmable integrated-circuit unit whose parameters can be changed as desired by the physician. This unit measures 10.1 cm × 7.6 cm × 2.0 cm and weighs 240 g. The VENTAK-P delivers discharges that can be individually set by the physician to vary from 0.1 to 30 J, with the final two shocks (if necessary) being 30 J. The low energy settings are designed to terminate ventricular tach-

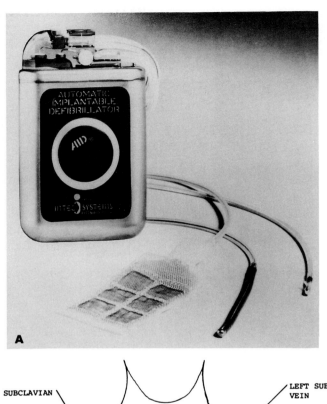

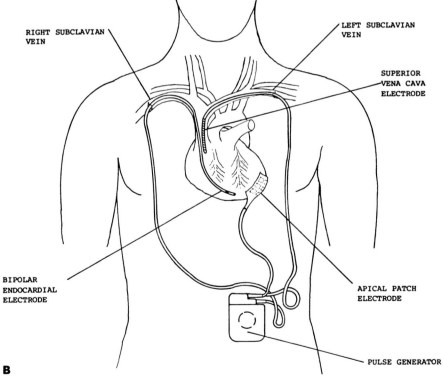

Figure 43-8. (**A**) The automatic implantable cardioverter–defibrillator, with (**B**) its superior vena cava, bipolar right ventricular, and apical patch electrodes. (Mirowski M, Reid PR, Mower MM, et al: Use of the automatic implantable cardioverter-defibrillator in the treatment of malignant ventricular tachyarrhythmias. Herz 1984;9:85.)

ycardia and the high energy settings to convert ventricular fibrillation. Programmability also allows the selection of any combination of available detection algorithms, thus eliminating the need for separate models. A delay in the shock delivery is also programmable.

Functional Performance of Early Units

In the electrophysiology laboratory, the diagnostic accuracy was 98% for both ventricular fibrillation and ventricular tachycardias, and the devices were highly effective in terminating abnormal rhythms during testing in the laboratory and for spontaneous rhythms afterward. The time from onset of induced arrhythmias until their termination ranged between 11.5 and 36 seconds, with a mean of 17 seconds. Figure 43-9 is an example of a malignant arrhythmia induced in the electrophysiology laboratory with alternating current, which was automatically reverted by the implanted device. Figure 43-10 is an example of a spontaneous arrhythmia recorded on a monitor, which was corrected automatically. Reversions were usually accomplished with a single internal discharge, although in some instances the device had to recycle once or even twice to achieve this. In another spontaneous arrhythmia (Fig. 43-11), the first discharge accelerated the rhythm but the device recycled twice and corrected it on the third shock.

PATIENT SELECTION

The initial patient selection criteria for ICD insertion were quite rigorous. The patient was required to have survived at least two episodes of cardiac arrest not in the context of acute myocardial infarction—one with electrocardiographic documentation and one occurring despite presumably adequate treatment. Most implantees had been unresponsive to many conventional and investigational drug regimens also. The average number of previous cardiac arrests in the group was four and the average number of drugs that failed was five.

The criteria was later relaxed to require only a single episode of arrhythmic cardiac arrest, with evidence of incomplete protection by medical treatment, as determined by continuing inducibility during electrophysiologic studies or stress testing.

The FDA has thus far defined two groups of patients at high risk of sudden death in whom this therapy is indicated. These are (1) patients who have survived at least one episode of cardiac arrest due to ventricular tachyarrhythmia not associated with acute myocardial infarction, and (2) those without previous arrest, who have inducible arrhythmias at electrophysiologic testing that cannot be suppressed by conventional antiarrhythmic therapy.

Even so, only a minority of patients from high-risk groups go on to receive an ICD or even electrophysiologic

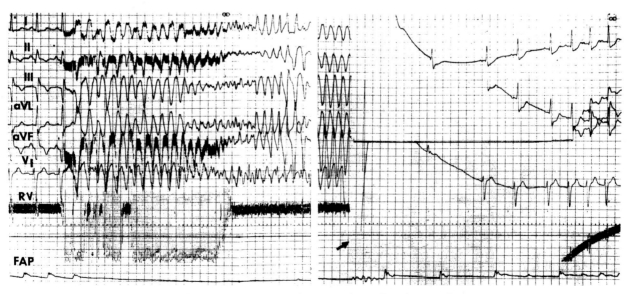

Figure 43-9. (**A**) Initiation of ventricular flutter/fibrillation during an electrophysiologic study, using alternating current. (**B,** *arrow*) Unit automatically reverses the arrhythmia to normal sinus rhythm. Leads I, II, III, a V_F, and V_1 are standard electrocardiographic leads. *RV,* right ventricular electrogram; *FAP,* femoral arterial pressure. (Mirowski M, Mower MM, Reid PR: The automatic implantable defibrillator. Am Heart J 1980;100:1089.)

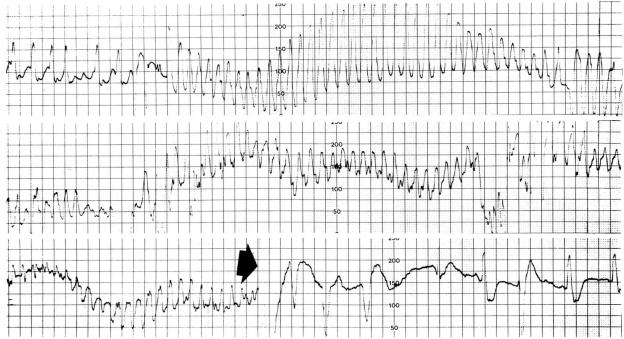

Figure 43-10. Electrocardiographic recording in a postoperative patient who developed a well-tolerated atrial flutter 28 minutes long, during which the implanted unit remained quiescent. The last few beats of this rhythm are seen in the *left* of the *upper strip*. Two spontaneous premature ventricular contractions then occur, followed by ventricular flutter/fibrillation; 23 seconds later (*arrow*), the malignant arrhythmia is automatically terminated by the 25-J discharge. The strips are continuous. (Mirowski M, Reid PR, Watkins L, et al: Clinical treatment of life-threatening ventricular arrhythmias with the automatic implantable defibrillator. Am Heart J 1981;102:265.)

testing. Most individuals continue to receive only empiric therapy, if any. Reasons for this are complex, but may include the general cardiologist being (1) unaware of the magnitude of the sudden cardiac death problem, (2) reluctant to lose his patient to a specialized center, and (3) unwilling to admit his own therapeutic defeat. As electrophysiology grows as a subspeciality and general medical attitudes change, the number of patients who present for study may be as many as several hundred thousand per year. Even by modestly increasing the number of patients who enter into appropriate testing, a marked effect on the eventual number of patients benefiting from this therapy should easily be seen. Moreover, it appears that the implant criteria, as they stand, are unduly restrictive. One area of contention is the requirement for inducibility. This dates back to 1985 when the Health Care Financing Administration adopted guidelines for Medicare, requiring arrhythmias to be inducible and unable to be suppressed by antiarrhythmics for ICD implantation to be reimbursed. Data now indicate that there are numerous noninducible patients with cardiac arrest or recurrent symptomatic ventricular tachycardia who are clearly at risk of sudden cardiac death. Some of these may have QT-interval syndrome (in both overt and concealed forms), mitral valve prolapse, or primary electric disease but many patients with coronary artery disease and nonischemic cardiomyopathy are also not inducible. In such patient groups, there are no therapeutic indices upon which to base treatment decisions.

The North American Society of Pacing and Electrophysiology (NASPE) has issued a consensus statement, covering their suggestions for patient selection criteria for ICD implantation (Table 43-2).

IMPLANTATION TECHNIQUES

Early in the clinical trials, the apical lead was always implanted through a left thoracotomy. This is still done in patients who have had previous chest surgery, to avoid dissection at a previously operated site. Also, because implantation has always been considered to be part of an overall comprehensive strategy to combat the malignant arrhythmias, (including new investigational drugs and antiarrhythmic surgery, as indicated), many of the patients

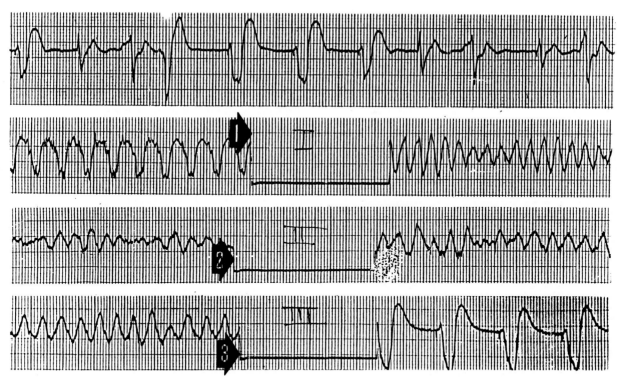

Figure 43-11. Automatic correction of accelerated rhythm. (*Upper strip*) Paced rhythm present before spontaneous ventricular tachycardia developed at a rate of 176 beats/min, shown on the left side of the second strip. The first discharge (*arrow 1*) accelerates the tachycardia to ventricular fibrillation. The device recycles, delivers a second discharge (*arrow 2, third strip*), which is ineffective; it recycles again, this time restoring the patient's initial rhythm (*lower strip*). The strips are not continuous. (Mirowski M, Reid PR, Mower MM, et al: Use of the automatic implantable cardioverter-defibrillator in the treatment of malignant ventricular tachyarrhythmias. Herz 1984;9:88.)

have undergone other cardiac surgical procedures (e.g., coronary artery bypass grafting, aneurysmectomy with endocardial resection, prosthetic valve replacement, and myectomy) at implantation. Median sternotomy has thus come to be preferred for many patients. It significantly shortens the implantation procedure and minimizes postoperative discomfort.[13] Subxyphoidal and left subcoastal techniques similar to pacemaker-lead insertion have been developed, further simplifying the procedure and representing a significant technical and clinical advance.[14,15] These later techniques reduced the morbidity and hospitalization associated with ICD implantation.

A new technique has been developed that allows the surgeon to use a thoracoscope to implant extrapericardial patches.[16] This methodology may be applicable to either first implants or problems with transvenous lead systems. Patches may be placed intra- or extrapericardial. The defibrillation thresholds may be higher with extrapericardial placement but the risk of vascular erosion is lessened. Alternatively, two patches are used for the transcardiac pair.

The patches come in two sizes: the smaller has a 13.5-cm^2 and the larger of 27-cm^2 surface area. Lower thresholds may often be achieved using larger electrodes, although they may also predispose to greater pericardial irritation and to a higher incidence of atrial arrhythmias. The rate channel can be provided by the right ventricular endocardial lead or by a screw-in lead alternative. Other combinations are also possible. In the event that an artificial pacemaker is implanted in addition to the cardioverter–defibrillator, the pacemaker must be bipolar rather than unipolar, and the pacing leads must be located as far away as possible for the rate-sensing leads.

The superior vena cava catheter electrode has a 7-cm^2 titanium spring. The rate lead consists of either a bipolar right ventricular endocardial catheter or two epicardial screw-in electrodes placed 1 cm apart in the left ventricle. The catheter electrode is passed percutaneously, using a 14-French peel-away introducer. Most often, the subclavian vein is chosen but the internal jugular vein also serves as the entry site.

Transvenous defibrillating leads (Endotak, CPI; and

TABLE 43-2. Patient Selection Criteria for Implantable Cardioverter–Defibrillator Implantation—North American Society of Pacing and Electrophysiology Consensus Statement

CLASS I

1. One or more episodes of spontaneous sustained ventricular tachycardia or ventricular fibrillation in a patient in whom electrophysiological testing and/or spontaneous ventricular arrhythmias cannot be used accurately to predict efficacy of other therapies.
2. Recurrent episodes of spontaneous sustained ventricular tachycardia or ventricular fibrillation in a patient despite antiarrhythmic drug therapy (guided by electrophysiological testing or noninvasive methods).
3. Spontaneous sustained ventricular tachycardia or ventricular fibrillation in a patient in whom antiarrhythmic drug therapy is limited by intolerance or noncompliance.
4. Persistent inducibility of clinically relevant sustained ventricular tachycardia or ventricular fibrillation at electrophysiological study, on best available drug therapy or despite surgical/catheter ablation, in a patient with spontaneous sustained ventricular tachycardia or ventricular fibrillation.

CLASS II

1. Syncope of undetermined etiology in a patient with clinically relevant sustained ventricular tachycardia or ventricular fibrillation induced at electrophysiological study in whom antiarrhythmic drug therapy is limited by inefficacy, intolerance, or noncompliance.

CLASS III

1. Sustained ventricular tachycardia or ventricular fibrillation mediated by acute ischemia/infarction or toxic/metabolic etiologies, amenable to correction or reversibility.
2. Recurrent syncope of undetermined etiology in a patient without inducible sustained ventricular tachyarrhythmias.
3. Incessant ventricular tachycardia or ventricular fibrillation.
4. Ventricular fibrillation secondary to atrial fibrillation in the Wolff-Parkinson-White syndrome in a patient whose bypass tract is amenable to surgical or catheter ablation.
5. Surgical, medical, or psychiatric contraindications.

Transvene, Medtronic) are implanted, similar to conventional pacemaker leads.[17-21] These systems also use a subcutaneous patch, which controls the directions of the shock given through this lead. Experience with the Endotak and Transvene lead systems permits the implantation of an ICD without thoracotomy.[17-22] These systems use one or more transvenous leads (right ventricle, superior vena cava, coronary sinus) generally with a subcutaneous patch electrode.[17-24]

The development of smaller size units permits the implanting physician to use a subpectoral approach in selected patients.[20,25] This implantation site is generally more palatable to the patient. Furthermore, the development of an "active" unit again simplifies the implantation procedure, eliminating the use of a subcutaneous patch electrode.

To assist in lead implantation, a number of measurements—including the energy requirements for defibrillation—are made at implantation. An external cardioverter–defibrillator (ECD) unit is connected to the implanted lead system, which has an output waveform similar to that of the implantable units and a deliverable energy-level adjustment from 0.1 to 40 J. The arrhythmia is provoked repeatedly and the amount of energy required to consistently revert it is determined. The unit most suitable for the patient can be selected, depending on the need for antitachycardia pacing or low-energy cardioversion, for example. The unit that is finally chosen for implantation is then attached to the leads with temporary lead wires, to allow continuous recordings of rate and transcardiac signals. The arrhythmia is then reinduced to ensure that the selected unit is able to recognize and correct it automatically. If so, the header lead wires are replaced with permanent nylon header caps containing O-rings to cover the set screws and seal the terminals, and the implantation procedure is then completed.

During the final stages of implantation, the device is often temporarily deactivated to avoid false triggering, especially when a cautery is being used. Sometimes, it is left off in the immediate postoperative period to minimize triggering of supraventricular arrhythmias, which are occasionally present at this time. For the long term, many patients receive the most suitable antiarrhythmic drug regimen that can be found for them.[26]

BASIC CONCEPTS

Defibrillation requires that a minimal current density or voltage gradient is achieved throughout all or nearly all of ventricular myocardium. Ideal defibrillation electrodes permit uniform myocardial current distribution to minimize the requirements for stored energy and to avoid unnecessarily high current densities, which may cause myocardial damage or induce arrhythmias. Non-uniform current distributions are an inevitable result of placing electrodes close to the heart, however.

Probability Function of Defibrillation

Defibrillation is NOT an all-or-none phenomenon. A sigmoidal relation exists between defibrillation success and the shock strength used. A minimum field strength of 6 V per centimeters appears to be needed for defibrillation using a monophasic truncated waveform and 3 to 4 V per centimeter for biphasic pulses. Increasing or decreasing the shock strength results in a success or failure rate, which can be expressed as sigmoidal relation (Fig. 43-12).[27]

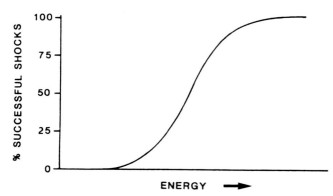

Figure 43-12. Defibrillation is not an all or none phenomenon. This diagram represents a plot of energy delivered versus percentage of successful defibrillation. Lower energies never defibrillate, whereas higher energies always defibrillate, but the intermediate energy delivered provides variable results. This may be expressed as a sinusoidal dose (energy) response (defibrillation) curve. (Kerber, RE, McPherson D, Charbonnier F, et al. Automated impedance—based energy adjustment for defibrillation: experimental studies. Circulation 1985;71:136.)

Defibrillation Waveforms and Pulses

Transthoracic defibrillators discharge capacitors through a series inductor, which produces a critically damped sinusoidal waveform. Because the inductor in these defibrillators weighs several kilograms, this waveform is impractical for implanted pulse generators.

Many different waveforms have been used for defibrillation. Implantable cardioverter–defibrillators generally use truncated, damped, exponential waveforms. The output capacitor is discharged through the resistive load between the anodal and cathodal electrodes, either for a predetermined time (fixed-duration pulse) or until the voltage has fallen to a predetermined value (fixed-tilt pulse). Multiple investigators have demonstrated the advantage of biphasic waveforms for defibrillation. A biphasic pulse is produced when the polarity of the pulse is reversed during delivery. Of additional importance is the observation that asymmetric biphasic waveforms are more efficient than symmetric biphasic defibrillation shocks. The asymmetric biphasic waveforms defibrillates at a lower energy and potentially leads to less post-shock hemodynamic dysfunction. The most commonly employed biphasic pulse is the asymmetric biphasic pulse, produced by reversing the polarity of the output of a single capacitor, so that the trailing-edge voltage of the first phase equals the leading-edge voltage of the second phase. Typically, the second phase is equal to or shorter than the first phase. Such asymmetric biphasic pulses generally have proved superior to monophasic pulses delivered over the same pathway. Furthermore, if the second phase of the biphasic waveform is of a shorter duration, the defibrilla-

tion threshold is lower. Biphasic waveforms that have a low-tilt first phase and a high-tilt second phase have a lower defibrillation threshold. Limited data suggest that a third phase may even be better than the biphasic shock waveforms (Fig. 43-14).[28–35]

Several reasons are cited for the potential benefit of biphasic waveforms, including:

1. Decreased impedance
2. Reactivation of the sodium channels by the first phase, allowing the second phase to excite the cells (i.e., the first phase acting as a conditioning pulse to hyperpolarize some of the myocardium and thereby reactive sodium channels, allowing the second phase to excite the cells)
3. Shortened refractoriness secondary to hyperpolarization of cells by the first phase.
4. The large voltage change between the end of the first and the beginning of the second phase, enhancing ability to stimulate the myocardium

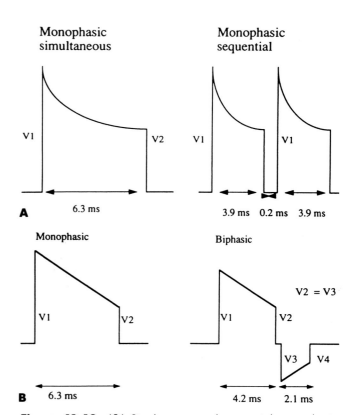

Figure 43-13. (A) Simultaneous and sequential monophasic waveforms with fixed pulse duration. Sequential pulses are generated by a dual capacitor system. **(B)** Monophasic and biphasic waveforms with fixed pulse duration. In the biphasic waveform the leading edge voltage of the second phase (V3) equals the trailing edge voltage (V2) of the first phase. (June W, Manz M, Moosdorf R, et al. Clinical efficacy of shock waveform and lead configurations for defibrillation. Am Ht J 1994;127:985.)

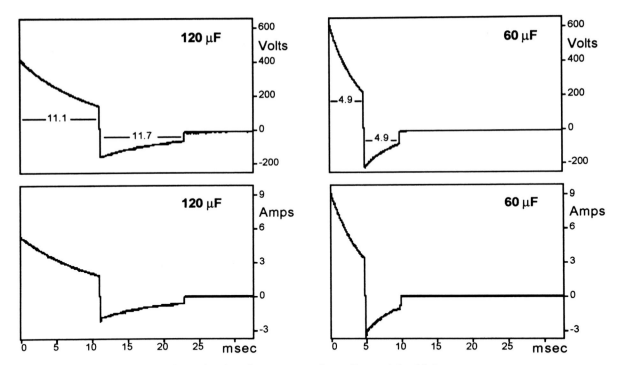

Figure 43-14. Voltage waveforms (*top*) and current waveforms (*bottom*) for 10-J asymmetric biphasic pulses, delivered from right ventricle to submuscular patch. Waveforms for 120-μF capacitors are shown on the left, and waveforms for 60-μF capacitors are shown on the right. Waveforms were digitized at 100 kHz and recorded on a Macintosh computer. The tilt of each phase is 65%. The trailing-edge voltage of the first phase equals the leading-edge voltage of the second phase. The phases are separated by 0.2 milliseconds. The programmed leading-edge voltage was 410 V for the 120-μF capacitor and 580 V for the 60-μF capacitor. The measured voltages are 420 and 611 V, and the corresponding calculated stored energies are 10.7 J and 11.5 J, respectively. The measured leading-edge current is 5.21 A for the 120-μF capacitor and 8.68 A for the 60-μF capacitor; the corresponding calculated pathway resistances are 81 Ω and 70 Ω, respectively. When monophasic pulses were used, only the first phase of each pulse was delivered (Reprints with permission from Swerdlow C, Kass RM, Chen P-S, et al: Effect of capacitor size and pathway resistance on defibrillator threshold for implantable defibrillators. Circulation 1994 [in press].)

5. The potential gradient for defibrillation being less with biphasic than with monophasic waveforms
6. Less-detrimental effects in regions of high potential gradient with biphasic, as compared with monophasic waveforms[27]

Clinical defibrillation configurations include two or three electrodes. Three-electrode systems may be used to deliver a shock between one electrode and the two remaining electrodes coupled together (simultaneous or bidirectional shock) or two shocks separated temporarily between the common electrode and each of the the two electrodes (sequential shocks). Most studies agree that the defibrillation threshold is lower for two-electrode systems when the cathode is placed closest to the greatest mass of myocardium.[36,37] In three-electrode systems, the common electrode is usually the cathode. When simultaneous bidirectional shocks are used, the field strength is weakest in the region between the two anodes. The anodes should

therefore be placed to minimize the amount of myocardium between the anodes. In contrast, equidistant electrode spacing is optimal for sequential shocks.[38] Even with epicardial electrodes, dramatic changes in defibrillation threshold may occur when the number of defibrillating electrodes is increased from two to three (Fig. 43-15).

Defibrillation Electrodes and Pathways

Defibrillating electrodes have a larger surface area and lower resistance than pacing electrodes. The relation between defibrillation threshold and electrode surface area has been studied systematically for epicardial patch electrodes. These studies show that the defibrillation threshold decreases as electrode surface area increases, until about half the epicardial surface is covered. Thereafter, the defibrillation threshold increases.[39] Because the current

TWO PATCH SYSTEM

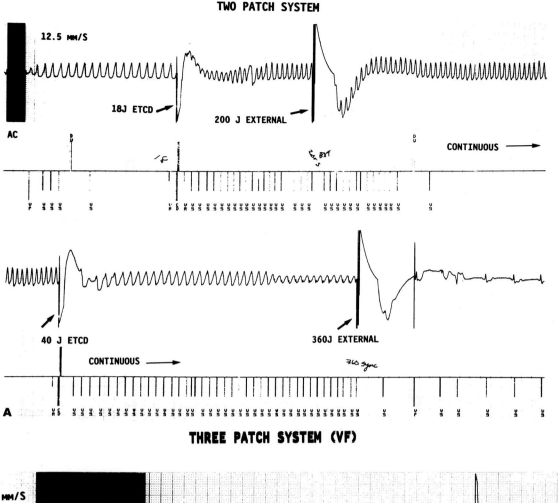

THREE PATCH SYSTEM (VF)

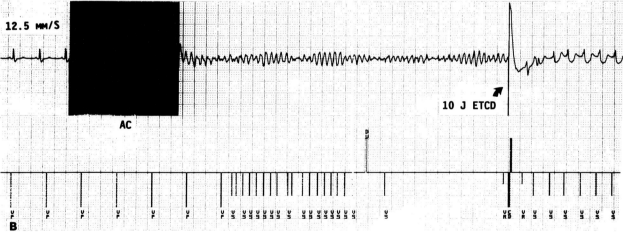

Figure 43-15. Effect of a third electrode on epicardial defibrillation threshold, using monophasic pulses. (**A**) Using two large patch electrodes, an 18-J synchronized shock from an external cardioverter–defibrillator that simulates the implantable cardioverter–defibrillator (*ETCD*, external tachyarrhythmia control device) accelerates monomorphic ventricular tachycardia. Both a 200-J external shock and a 40-J internal shock from the two patch electrodes fail to terminate the arrhythmia. (**B**) After addition of a third medium electrode, a 10-J sequential pulse shock, delivered from a posterior cathode to two equidistant anodes, terminates induced ventricular fibrillation.

density at the end of patch electrodes is higher than the current density in the middle, current shunts between the edges of closely spaced patch electrodes.[40] Furthermore, excessively large patches may decrease the efficacy of emergency transthoracic defibrillation by insulating the heart from transthoracic shocks.[41] The surface areas of transvenous electrodes are generally smaller than the surface areas of epicardial or subcutaneous patch electrodes.

When intrathoracic patch electrodes are placed epicardially or extrapericardially, relatively uniform fields can be achieved throughout much of the ventricular myocardium. In contrast, transvenous electrode placement is limited by anatomic considerations for electrode stability. Usually, at least one defibrillating coil electrode is on a catheter, in which the tip electrode is placed in the right ventricular apex and used for pacing. A second coil electrode may be placed on the same catheter, with spacing such that the proximal electrode lies near the junction of the right atrium and superior vena cava.

Alternatively, a second catheter may be used for a second coil electrode. Although this requires insertion of another electrode catheter, it provides the flexibility of positioning the two transvenous electrodes independently. The second coil may be positioned at the junction of the right atrium and superior vena cava, in the innominate vein, or in the coronary sinus.

When monophasic pulses are used, most nonthoracotomy electrode configurations require a subcutaneous or submuscular patch electrode to complete a three-electrode system.[42] When shocks are delivered from the common right ventricular electrode to the patch, the patch is usually positioned in the infraclavicular, high axillary, or retroscapular positions.[43, 44] Alternative patch locations may be preferable if the patch or coronary sinus electrode are common.

In contrast, pure transvenous two-electrode configurations are usually successful for biphasic pulses. The most commonly used electrode locations are right ventricle and superior vena cava or innominate vein. Excellent results have been reported for biphasic pulses, using a "unipolar" defibrillation configuration between a right ventricular electrode and the titanium shell of a new 80-cm³ ICD pulse generator in a subcutaneous left pectoral pocket (Figs. 43-16 and 43-17).[45]

TIERED-THERAPY IMPLANTABLE CARDIOVERTER–DEFIBRILLATORS

History

Tiered-therapy ICDs have evolved rapidly since the first human implants of an automatic defibrillator in 1980. The initial nonprogrammable 250-g device was implanted by

thoracotomy as a therapy of last resort for patients with primary ventricular fibrillation.[1] Current ICDs are one of several therapeutic alternatives for patients with various life-threatening ventricular tachyarrhythmias; they are implanted transvenously and weigh as little as 132 g.[46] Critical developments in the evolution of ICDs include the use of true bipolar sensing to permit therapy of rapid ventricular tachycardia, low-energy synchronized cardioversion, backup bradycardia pacing, tiered therapy, telemetry of stored electrograms, and transvenous implantation.[47–51] Examples of current ICD pulse generators are shown in Figure 43-18.

Pulse Generator

Implantable cardioverter–defibrillators must monitor the cardiac rhythm continuously, detect arrhythmias rapidly, select appropriate therapy, and assess the efficacy of delivered therapy. All ICDs include sensing electrodes, which transmit ventricular electric activity to the sense amplifier; signals from the sense amplifier are then fed into microprocessor-based control circuits. These logic circuits detect the cardiac rhythm and determine the ICDs response to that rhythm. The battery provides power to run the low-voltage sensing and control circuits, the high-voltage defibrillation circuits, and other functions, such as memory and telemetry. The low voltage stored by the battery is converted to high voltage by a direct-current to direct-current (DC/DC) transformer. This high voltage is stored on a high-voltage–output capacitor and then discharged across the high-voltage–output circuits and defibrillating electrodes (Fig. 43-19).

Battery

Implantable cardioverter–defibrillator batteries must be capable of supplying high currents to charge the high-voltage–output capacitors while providing stable noise-free power for the low-voltage components of the pulse generator. Lithium-silver-vanadium oxide batteries are used by contemporary defibrillators because they are energy-dense and provide high peak currents. They also have a close correlation between voltage during open-circuit or low-current operation and voltage during high-current charging of the output capacitors; thus, battery voltage can be used as a reliable measure of end of service. With an energy density of 1800 J/cm³, a typical 10-cm³ ICD battery stores enough energy for 600 30-J shocks. In practice, however, this capacity is reduced by losses in the DC/DC transformer and in the currents required for monitoring, bradycardia pacing, and electrogram storage.

Direct-Current to Direct-Current Transformer

To generate the high voltages required for defibrillation, the 3.2- to 6.4-V output of the battery is passed through an oscillator circuit and then into the primary coil of a step-up transformer. The oscillating high voltage induced on the secondary coil is then rectified, and the resultant DC charges the output capacitor to voltages of up to 750 V. This induced current creates electromagnetic interference, which complicates sensing of the cardiac signal during the charging process. Some ICD programmers measure the duration of this induced current, using a coil that acts as

the secondary coil of an air transformer. The duration of the charging process or "charge time" is used as an additional measure of end of service.

Capacitors

Capacitors, which are composed of two conducting surfaces separated by a dielectric, are used to store electric charge. Contemporary ICDs use aluminum electrolytic capacitors because of their high energy densities of about 1.5 J/cm³. They are similar to those used in photoflash units. A limitation of this technology is that the capacitor

Figure 43-16. Posteroanterior (*left*) and lateral (*right*) chest radiographs. (**A**) The posterior patch electrode of this two-patch epicardial system was noted to be crinkled at the time of elective pulse-generator replacement. The monophasic defibrillation threshold exceeded 30 J. A hybrid system using simultaneous pulse defibrillation from a coronary sinus cathode to right ventricular endocardial and anterior patch anodes reduced the defibrillation threshold to 12.5 J (Medtronic Transvene system). (**B**) Sequential pulse defibrillation from coronary sinus cathode to right ventricular and subcutaneous anodes (Medtronic Transvene system). True bipolar sensing is performed by tip and ring electrodes on right ventricular lead.

(*continued*)

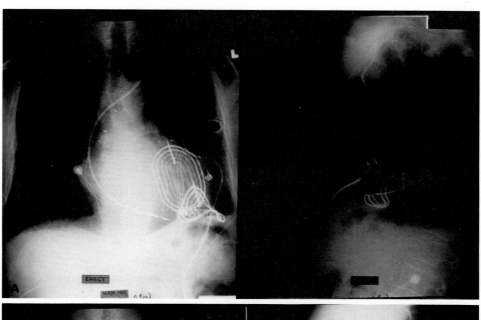
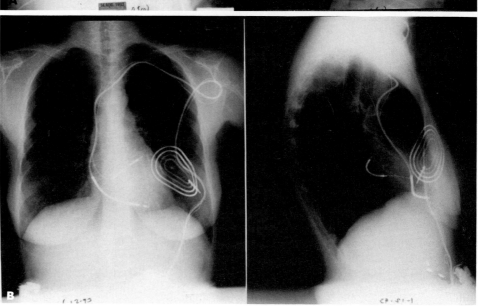

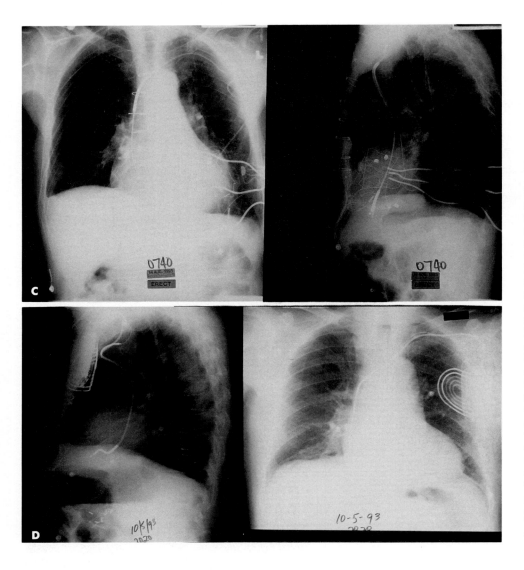

Figure 43-16. (*continued*)
(**C**) Simultaneous defibrillation from right ventricular cathode to superior vena cava and subcutaneous anodes using CPI Endotak electrode. The subcutaneous electrode is an array. Integrated bipolar sensing occurs between tip electrode and distal coil. Epicardial defibrillation patch electrodes and screw-in bipolar sensing electrodes are also present. The epicardial system had been implanted 8 years before. After the pulse-generator pocket became infected, as a result of a routine pulse-generator change for battery depletion, the pulse generator was explanted and the electrodes were cut off in the pocket. The transvenous system was implanted after a course of antibiotics. (**D**) The lateral chest radiograph is on the left. Unipolar defibrillation between right ventricular electrode and left retropectoral patch electrode. The 83-cm³ pulse generator (Medtronic 7219) is implanted superficial to the patch. (*continued*)

slowly loses its ability to store charge (deforms) unless it is charged (reformed) at periodic intervals. Alternative capacitor technologies may provide higher energy densities without the need for periodic reformation but have not yet proved practical.

The energy (E) stored in a capacitor of capacitance C, charged to a voltage V is expressed as:

$$E = \frac{CV^2}{2}.$$

The size of ICD pulse generators depends only weakly on capacitance but strongly on stored energy. Output capacitors in contemporary ICDs vary from 120 to 150F. Thus, delivery of a 30-J shock requires charging to 632 to 707 V. The size of output capacitors is constrained by the combined requirements to store sufficient energy to defibril-

late reliably and to operate below voltages at which components of the output circuit fail or myocardial damage occurs.[52–54] The output circuits of pulse generators can operate safely at voltages over 1000 V.[52, 55] There is substantial reason to believe that voltages higher than those used may be safe.[56, 57] Smaller capacitors may permit lower defibrillation thresholds and consequently, smaller pulse generators.[55, 58]

SENSING AND DETECTION OF TACHYARRHYTHMIAS

Sensing is the process by which an ICD determines the timing of each ventricular depolarization. Sensing of sequential depolarizations results in series of intervals

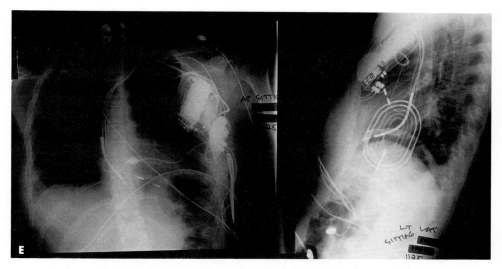

Figure 43-16. (*continued*) (**E**) In this patient with a prior DDD pacemaker who required atrio-ventricular sequential pacing, the tip of the implantable cardioverter–defibrillator (ICD) right ventricular defibrillating electrode was positioned in the inflow tract to avoid sensing interaction with either the atrial or ventricular channel of the pacemaker.

Fourth Generation ICD System

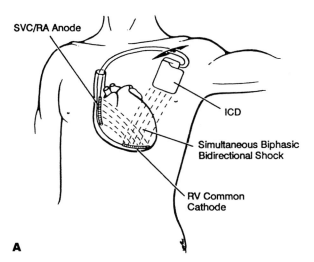

SVC/RA Anode

ICD

Simultaneous Biphasic
Bidirectional Shock

RV Common
Cathode

A

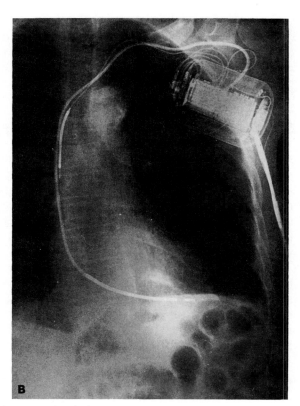

B

Figure 43-17. A fourth generation ICD with a single transvenous lead and a generator which acts as an "active" electrode for defibrillation. (**A**) A diagram with the defibrillation pathways outlined. (**B**) An x-ray of the implanted device.

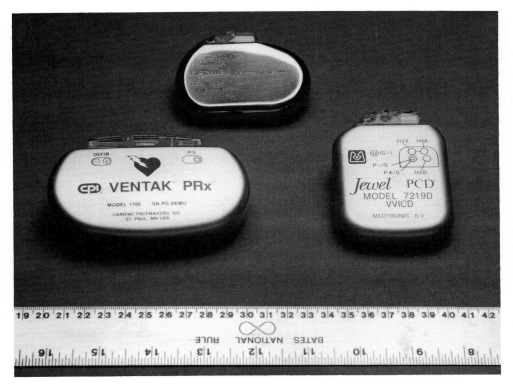

Figure 43-18. Tiered-therapy implantable cardioverter–defibrillator (ICD) pulse generators. (*Left to right*) CPI PRX 1700 (monophasic pulses, 81 cm³; for clinical use in the U.S.); Medtronic PCD 7219D tiered-therapy ICD (biphasic pulses and stored electrograms, 83 cm³; in U.S. clinical trials); Angelon Sentinel 2000 (biphasic pulses, 60 cm³; scheduled to begin U.S. clinical trials in 1995).

(cycle lengths). Detection is the process by which an ICD determines whether this series of sensed intervals corresponds to a sustained tachyarrhythmia that requires therapy.

Sensing

Although the earliest implanted defibrillator used the same large electrodes for sensing and defibrillating, subsequent ICDs use one or two small, separate sensing electrodes.[1] Implantable cardioverter–defibrillators may use true bipolar sensing from a pair of closely spaced epicardial electrodes or the tip and ring electrode of a right ventricular catheter.

Alternatively, they may use integrated bipolar sensing between a distal ring electrode and a right ventricular shocking coil. Although integrated bipolar sensing does not require a separate sensing ring electrode, it has been reported to cause failed redetection of ventricular fibrillation due to decreased signal amplitude after a shock.[59]

Sensing Circuit

The signal from the sensing electrodes first passes through a sensing amplifier. This amplifier must be able to recover rapidly after defibrillation shocks and pacing pulses. The amplified signal then passes through a band-pass filter, designed to reject low-frequency T waves and high-frequency electromagnetic interference and myopotentials. The signal is then rectified, so that the sensing threshold is not influenced by R-wave polarity. Finally, a threshold circuit compares the processed signal to a threshold voltage and senses an R wave when the signal exceeds the threshold (Fig. 43-20).

Automatic Gain Control and Autoadjusting Sensitivity

Reliable sensing of ventricular fibrillation is the principal sensing problem for ICDs. The electrogram amplitude during ventricular fibrillation is highly variable. It is generally lower than the amplitude during sinus rhythm or ventricular tachycardia and decreases as the duration of ventricular fibrillation increases. Fixed-gain sensing has proved to be unreliable, and most ICDs use either automatic gain control or autoadjusting sensitivity as feedback mechanisms to ensure reliable sensing of low-amplitude signals.[60] In the automatic gain control method, the amplifier gain is adjusted to keep the output of the amplifier constant, and a fixed threshold is used to sense R waves. In the autoadjusting-sensitivity method, amplification is constant, and sensing threshold is adjusted inversely in relation to the peak amplitude of the R wave. In each method,

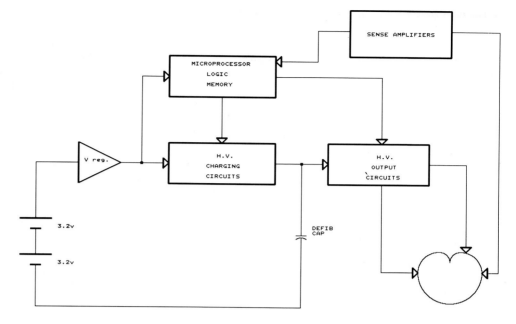

Figure 43-19. Implantable cardioverter–defibrillator block diagram. (Reprinted with permission from Mehra R: Tachyarrhythmia termination: lead systems and hardware design. In: Singer I (ed): Implantable cardioverter defibrillators. Mt Kisco, NY: Futura Publishing, 1994, in press)

there is a separate time constant for gain or threshold increases and for gain or threshold decreases.

The requirement for reliable sensing of variable- and low-amplitude electrograms during ventricular fibrillation creates an inherent conflict, which may result in undersensing of sinus rhythm or oversensing of T waves. The former may be proarrhythmic for ICDs that have bradycardia-pacing capability; the latter may result in inappropriate inhibition of bradycardia pacing, inappropriate therapy, or delivery of antitachycardia pacing at the wrong rate.[61]

Detection Algorithms

Although early algorithms for detection of ventricular fibrillation required fulfillment of both rate and morphology criteria, morphology criteria for detection of ventricular fibrillation are optional or absent in contemporary ICDs. Implantable cardioverter–defibrillator detection algorithms for ventricular fibrillation are highly sensitive, at the expense of being less specific because some undersensing is expected to occur. In most ICDs, ventricular

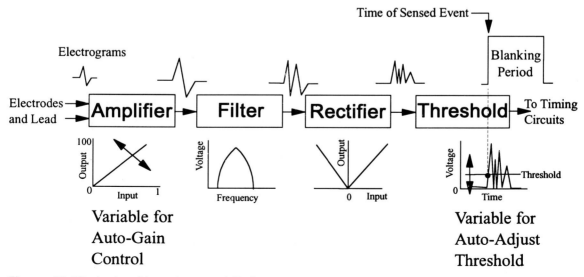

Figure 43-20. Implantable cardioverter–defibrillator detection circuit. (Reprinted with permission from Olson WH: Tachycardia sensing and detection. In: Singer I, ed. Implantable cardioverter defibrillators. Mt. Kisco, NY: Futura Publishing, 1994, in press.)

fibrillation is detected when a certain percentage of intervals in a sliding window (usually 10 to 24 intervals) fulfill the rate criterion for ventricular fibrillation.

In contrast to the generally similar "X of Y" counting used to detect ventricular fibrillation, ICDs differ in their approach to detection of ventricular tachycardia. One manufacturer uses an approach in which consecutive intervals must exceed the rate criterion for ventricular tachycardia. Other manufacturers use X of Y counting. The consecutive-interval scheme diminishes inappropriate detection of atrial fibrillation, without compromising sensitivity for detection of monomorphic ventricular tachycardia (Fig. 43-21).[62, 63]

Tachyarrhythmia Zones and Redetection

Tiered-therapy ICDs classify tachyarrhythmias into different zones, based on cycle length to deliver therapy appropriate for the specific arrhythmia. If the cycle length of a tachycardia varies around the boundary between these two zones, detection may be delayed. The maximum possible delay depends on the specific method used to increment or decrement the interval counters for each zone. Serious delays have been reported rarely.[58]

Redetection, distinct from initial detection, refers to detection after delivery of therapy to determine whether the arrhythmia has terminated, accelerated, or continued unchanged. A redetected arrhythmia may accelerate from one tachycardia zone to another or accelerate but remain within the same zone. Generally, redetection algorithms are more liberal than initial detection algorithms. Redetection may be delayed briefly after delivery of therapy to allow transient delays in arrhythmia termination after antitachycardia pacing or post-shock nonsustained ventricular tachycardia.

Stored Electrograms

A major limitation of earlier ICDs were the clinician's inability to ascertain the exact event that precipitated unit discharge. In the newest generation of ICDs, electrograms can be stored for later telemetry to allow review of the arrhythmia status at the time of discharge. This feature allows the clinician to evaluate (1) appropriateness of a shock; (2) atrial fibrillation that causes the unit to discharge; (3) inappropriate sensing; (4) reason for aborted shock (i.e., nonsustained ventricular tachycardia); (5) ventricular fibrillation or fast ventricular tachycardia induced by antitachycardia pacing therapy; and (6) delivery of asymptomatic therapies (Fig. 43-22).

Telemetry of these data allows the clinician to (1) reprogram the ICD to respond to the events recorded, (2) institute or change drug therapy, or (3) correct technical problems, such as lead fracture.[64–68]

ANTITACHYCARDIA PACING

In many instances, overdrive pacing using a variety of techniques can successfully terminate ventricular tachycardia. The major concern has been the possibility of acceleration of ventricular tachycardia or the precipitation of ventricular fibrillation. The ability to have backup defibrillation has enhanced the enthusiasm for pacing therapy to terminate ventricular tachycardia, especially in light of the patient's limited awareness of the event if therapy is successful (Fig. 43-23).

Antitachycardia pacing in tiered-therapy devices has generally used either burst or ramp techniques. Both of these modalities have been linked to rate adaptation, which initiates pacing as a percentage of the RR interval of

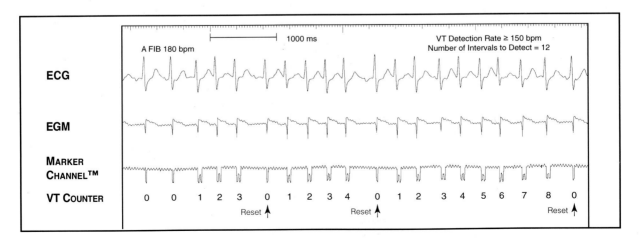

Figure 43-21. Discrimination of atrial fibrillation from ventricular tachycardia by consecutive interval counting.

the index ventricular tachycardia. Burst pacing delivers a series of pulses of identical RR interval. The pulse-train duration is programmable. In addition, the number of therapeutic trials is programmable. Furthermore, there is the option to program a progressive decrease in the RR intervals of each burst in a chain of burst therapies (i.e.,

adaptive burst at 81% of the ventricular tachycardia RR interval, with a serial decrement of 15 milliseconds in each of the subsequent attempts at burst pacing). Finally, a lower-limit RR interval for any burst can be programmed (i.e., no burst RR interval can be less than 250 milliseconds).

Ramp pacing is another mode of antitachycardia pac-

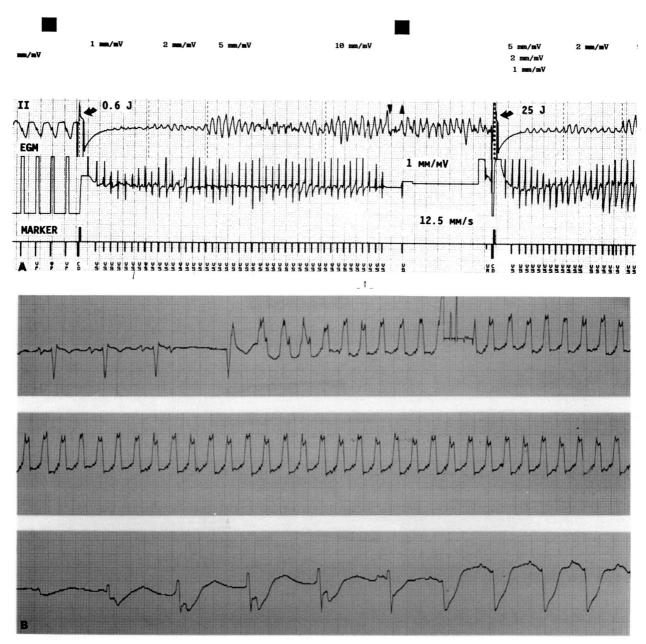

Figure 43-22. (**A**) Surface electrocardiographic lead II, telemetered bipolar right ventricular electrogram and the telemetered implantable cardioverter–defibrillator marker channel are shown (Medtronic PCD 7219). The gain for the telemetered electrogram is 1 mm/mV. Ventricular fibrillation is induced by a 0.6-J shock on the T wave during ventricular pacing at cycle length 500 milliseconds. After a failed 25-J monophasic shock, the amplitude of the true bipolar electrogram remains unchanged (**B and C**) Electrograms from a P₂ ICD (CPI) with an episode of ventricular tachycardia (**B**) and ventricular fibrillation (**C**). Note the clear difference between the sinus rhythm electrocardiogram and the electrograms during ventricular tachycardia and ventricular fibrillation.

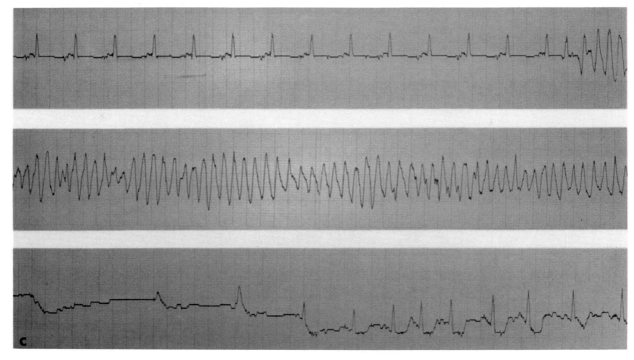

Figure 43-22. (continued)

ing. This too is programmable in the rate-adaptive mode but each ramp-pacing attempt has a programmed interval decrement, allowing progressive RR intervals in each ramp therapy to be decreased (i.e., by 5 milliseconds). Furthermore, subsequent ramp therapies, after the initial attempt, can be coupled to the last RR interval of the ventricular tachycardia by the rate-adaptive percentage (e.g., 81% minus a programmable number of milliseconds; i.e., 81% minus 10 milliseconds for each subsequent ramp therapy). The number of pulses of each ramp can be programmed, as can the shortest RR interval delivered any time (i.e., an RR interval will never be less than 250 milliseconds).[69–74]

LOW-ENERGY CARDIOVERSION

The advantages of low-energy shock delivery are immediate termination of tachycardia, combined with the lack of discomfort experienced by the patient when shocks of less than or equal to 0.75 J are used. This lack of discomfort, coupled with the advantage of extremely rapid charge times, reduces the time needed for shock delivery. The success of low-energy cardioversion has generally been 65% or less. The successful attempts at low-energy cardioversion generally have been related to higher energy (i.e., 2 to 10 J) and the presence of slower ventricular tachycardia rates (see Fig. 43-23A and 43-23E)

After low-energy cardioversion, atrial arrhythmias have been precipitated in up to 20% of patients. In addition, failure to convert with a low-energy shock has been associated with acceleration of the ventricular tachycardia rate in approximately 10% of patients.[69, 70, 74–78]

Risks and Complications

Perioperative Problems

The subjective reactions to internal discharges are variable, generally causing momentary discomfort but usually well-tolerated, even in a conscious state. The sensation most frequently described by the implantees is that of a moderate blow to the chest. Frequent discharges require deactivation of the device until some control of the frequency of the arrhythmia can be established. Because many of the patients have severe left ventricle dysfunction and because implantation may require extensive surgery, general anesthesia, and induction of multiple episodes of ventricular fibrillation, many perioperative and postoperative problems are expected to occur. Problems, however, have been relatively infrequent. Postoperatively, transient pericardial rubs are the rule. Infections occur in a small number of patients. Lead dislodgements occur, as does a small incidence of venous thrombosis, treatable with anticoagulants. In many patients, seroma formation usually resolves spontaneously; needle aspiration appears unwar-

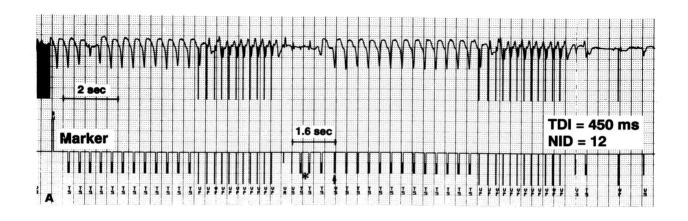

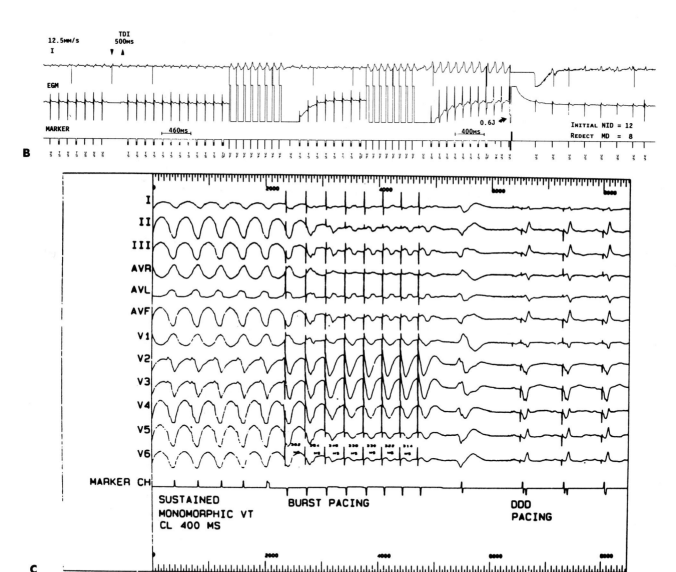

Figure 43-23. Tiered therapy. (**A**) A surface electrocardiographic lead and the telemetered implantable cardioverter–defibrillator (ICD) marker channel (Medtronic PCD 7217). During monomorphic ventricular tachycardia, an 11-pulse burst of antitachycardia pacing fails to terminate the arrhythmia. Reset of the ventricular tachycardia interval counter by the interval-stability criterion comparison of the interval denoted by an *arrow* with that denoted by an *asterisk* delayed redetection for 1.6 seconds. The second burst of antitachycardia pacing (12-pulse) terminates ventricular tachycardia. One bradycardia pacing pulse follows delivery of antitachycardia pacing. Intervals detected as ventricular tachycardia are denoted as *TS*; those sensed but not detected as ventricular tachycardia are denoted as *VS*. *VP*, pacing; *VR*, sensing in the posttherapy refractory period; *TDI*, ventricular tachycardia *(continued)*

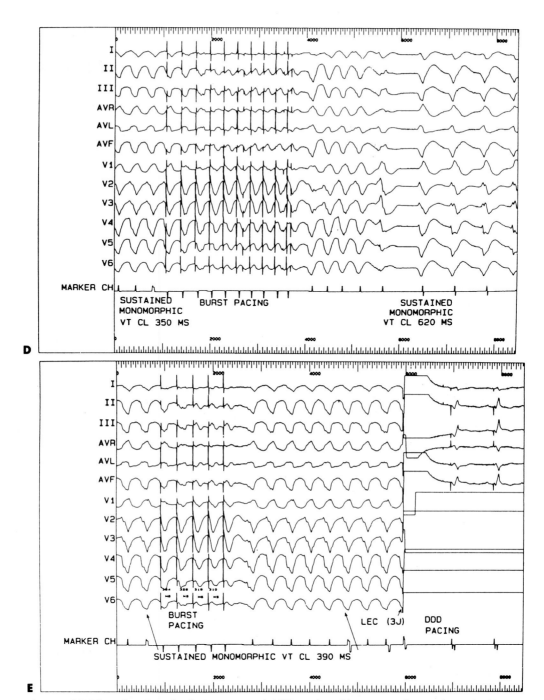

Figure 43-23. (*continued*) detection interval; *NID*, number of (consecutive) intervals required to detect ventricular tachycardia. (**B**) Surface electrocardiographic lead I, telemetered bipolar right ventricular electrogram and the telemetered ICD marker channel (Medtronic PCD 7219). (*Left*) The ventricular tachycardia cycle length exceeds the TDI of 450 milliseconds, that ventricular tachycardia is not detected. The *down* and *up arrowheads* denote reprogramming of the TDI to 500 milliseconds. Twelve consecutive intervals are detected, and the first antitachycardia pacing burst of eight pulses is unsuccessful. The second burst accelerates the tachycardia, which is then terminated by a 0.6-J cardioversion pulse. *TD* denotes detection of ventricular tachycardia. Other abbreviations as in **A**. (**C**) A 12-lead ECG with monomorphic VT (CL 400 msec). Burst pacing for 8 complexes with a decrement of 8 msec between each stimulus results in termination of VT and restoration of the basic rhythm (DDD pacing). (**D**) A 12-lead ECG during sustained monomorphic VT (CL 350 msec). Burst pacing for 10 complexes failed to terminate the tachycardia but ultimately converts the rhythm to a different morphology VT with a slower rate (CL 620). (**E**) A 12-lead ECG during sustained monomorphic VT (CL 390). Initial therapy with a 5-beat decremental burst (8 msec decrements) fails to terminate the episode. The second therapy with a 3J shock terminates the VT and the basic rhythm (DDD pacing) is restored. (**C–E** from Estes NAM III, Haugh CJ, Wang PJ, Manolis AS: Antitachycardia pacing and low-energy cardioversion for ventricular tachycardia termination: a clinical perspective. Am Heart J 1994 127:1038.)

ranted and potentially dangerous. Vascular complications, such as coronary vein or artery erosion, have been observed, especially with intrapericardial patches. Lead fractures or insulation breaks also have been observed. Skin erosion, constrictive pericarditis, and psychiatric problems have also been noted (Table 43-3).[79-88]

Failure to Redetect

Delivery of a shock by an ICD may result in a change in the amplitude of the endocardial electrograms for integrated bipolar sensing circuits, thereby potentially causing a failure of the ICD to redetect ongoing ventricular fibrillation. Studies have evaluated the effect of defibrillation shocks on the amplitude of endocardial electrograms.[89] Jung and colleagues systematically studied electrogram amplitudes in a small series of patients having an endocardial defibrillation system.[90] Their data identified that the endocardial sensing electrograms showed a significant decrease during ventricular fibrillation and a further drop after the initial defibrillation discharge; that is, 10.5 ± 3.8 mV (regular sinus rhythm); 6.3 ± 1.9 mV (initial ventricular fibrillation); and 2.2 ± 1.3 mV (during redection of ventricular fibrillation). After restitution of sinus rhythm, it took at least 30 seconds to restore electrograms to their baseline amplitude.[90]

Effects of Subthreshold Shocks

There is some controversy concerning the effects of unsuccessful (subthreshold) shocks on the ultimate energy requirement for successful defibrillation. There have been observations that have demonstrated an increase, no change, or a decrease in energy requirements for successful defibrillation with subsequent shocks.[91]

This area of controversy has not been fully resolved. Other factors may also play a role (e.g., changes in autonomic tone, potassium levels).

Aggravation of Arrhythmias After Implantation

Several groups have identified apparent significant increases in the frequency of ventricular tachycardia and ventricular fibrillation in the early follow-up period, post-ICD implantation. Earlier studies were performed exclusively with thoracotomy-based systems, whereas Bocker and colleagues compare their results using thoracotomy with transvenous systems.[92-94] The latter study found a similar incidence of aggravation of ventricular tachycardia and ventricular fibrillation, independent of the type of implantation. Incessant ventricular tachycardia was not observed in either group or patients, however.

An additional complicating feature was the develop-

TABLE 43-3. Complications of Implantable Cardioverter–Defibrillator Implantation

Early		Late	
Complications	**Estimated Incidence (%)**	**Complications**	**Estimated Incidence (%)**
Death (intra- or early postoperative)	<1–8	Infection	1–6
High defibrillation threshold—AICD not implanted	1–4	Lead migration†	10–40
		Early generation failure/malfunction	5–8
Vascular erosion	<1–2	Lead fracture/insulation break	<1–2
Arterial embolic events		Skin erosion	<1–3
Intraoperative myocardial infarction	<1–4	Need for acute psychiatric support	2–10
Vascular thrombosis (usually subclavian vein)*	2–10	Failure to sense VT above rate cutoff	<1–2
Infection	1–5	Constrictive pericarditis	<1
Atelectasis/pneumonia	<1–10		
Pneumothorax	<1–4		
Large symptomatic pleural effusion	<1–10		
Large seromas (generator pocket)	2–5		
Subcutaneous hematoma	1–2		
Bradycardia (post-shock), requiring pacing	<1–4		
Failure to terminate VT/VF during postoperative testing	3–6		
Early reoperation (change lead or generator)	<1–5		

*Seen exclusively with endovascular spring lead.
†Prior to use of Silastic anchor.
Modified from Marchlinski FE, Buxton AE, Flores B: The automatic implantable cardioverter defibrillator (AICD): follow-up and complicantions. In: El-Sherif N, Samet P, eds. Cardiac pacing and electrophysiology. Philadelphia: WB Saunders, 1991:743.
AICD, automatic cardioverter–defibrillator; VF, ventricular fibrillation; VT, ventricular tachycardia.

ment of atrial fibrillation, which occurred in the early postoperative period in 20% of thoracotomy-based ICD implants in one study.[93] This may lead to inappropriate shocks, even with adequate programming.

The increased incidence of ventricular tachycardia and ventricular fibrillation in the early post-implantation period may require initiation of antiarrhythmic drug therapy, which may have additional impact.

The mechanism for the increased incidence of ventricular tachycardia and ventricular fibrillation in the ICD recipients is not clear but increased levels of catecholamines may play an important role.[94]

Tired-therapy devices, when programmed initially to include low-energy cardioversion, have been observed to initiate ventricular fibrillation, especially in patients with poor left ventricle function.[95]

High Defibrillation Thresholds at Implantation

The incidence of high defibrillation thresholds (more than 25 J) at initial implantation is reported to be between 5% and 20%.[96,97] In one large series of 1946 patients, it was noted that 72% (65 of 90) of patients were on antiarrhythmic drugs, with 50% (45 of 90) being on amiodarone.[97]

Implantation criteria generally use a "safety margin" of 10 or more Joules above the measured defibrillation thresholds. If the patient initially is observed to have a high defibrillation threshold (e.g., more than 25 J), a variety of maneuvers are employed to obtain a satisfactory defibrillation threshold. For epicardial implants, these maneuvers include (1) using larger patches, (2) repositioning the patches, (3) using three patches, (4) changing extrapericardial to intrapericardial positioning of the patches, (5) using a transvenous spring electrode with the patches, (6) using a coronary sinus electrode, and (7) discontinuing antiarrhythmic drug therapy. The three-patch system is used in various combinations. Changes in polarity are also tested. If monophasic waveforms were initially used, a switch to bipolar waveforms appears to be essential.[96–98]

Chronic Rise in Defibrillation Thresholds

Follow-up testing of ICDs is considered mandatory by some investigators to select the best patient-specific form of therapy. The follow-up testing has generally been done at least 2 months after the initial implantation. Venditti and colleagues investigated the change in defibrillation thresholds in patients at 2 and 6 months post-implantation, using a transvenous lead system with a subcutaneous patch.[99] These authors observed a significant increase in defibrillation thresholds from implantation to the 2-month post-implantation test but no significant change

from the 2-month to the 6-month post-implantation test— 13.3 ± 4.3 J (initial implantation); 16.5 ± 4.7 J (2 months); 17.5 ± 5.4 J (6 months). Nevertheless, the chronic threshold still remained within the energy range that is acceptable for appropriate functioning of the ICD.

Of additional import is the observation that defibrillation thresholds can be significantly altered by antiarrhythmic drug therapy. Studies in the experimental laboratory and in man demonstrate variable results with a variety of agents.[100–102] Administration of antiarrhythmic agents after implantation must be considered, however, to exert a potentially negative influence on the defibrillation thresholds. There may, therefore, be a reason to recheck defibrillation thresholds in the steady-state setting of antiarrhythmic drug treatment.

Influence of Antiarrhythmic Agents on Implantable Cardioverter–Defibrillator Programming Parameters

In addition to potential changes in the defibrillation threshold, antiarrhythmic drug administration after initial implantation or adjustment in the dosage regime may significantly alter inducibility, cycle length, and the ability to terminate ventricular tachycardia using antitachycardia pacing. Furthermore, these drugs may convert sustained to nonsustained episodes of ventricular tachycardia of moderate length or slow the tachycardia rate below the cutoff for the device. It may therefore be necessary to reevaluate a variety of programming characteristics in these patients if there is a change in the antiarrhythmic drug regime. This requires in-hospital evaluation and potentially significant changes in programming characteristics of the tiered-therapy device.[11, 100, 101, 103]

Sensing Errors

Several centers have evaluated problems with tiered-therapy devices related to sensing problems, over and above concerns with device technology or programming errors. Many of these sensing problems, when recognized, were eliminated by reprogramming changes.

Prior studies in non–tiered-therapy devices identified sensing errors associated with distinguishing supraventricular arrhythmias from ventricular arrhythmias and lead problems.[104–109] Tiered-therapy devices have problems based on algorithm conflicts for bradycardia pacing and tachycardia sensing. In the absence of sensed complexes, does the device initiate bradypacing or adjust amplifier gain to detect ventricular fibrillation? Furthermore, in adjusting T-wave oversensing by raising the sensing threshold, reduction in the speed and accuracy of detecting ventricular fibrillation may occur. In addition, lengthening the post-pacing sensing refractory period to reduce T-wave oversensing may result in prevention or delay in detection of a tachycardia.

The sense amplifier continuously adjusts by either altering the gain or sense threshold after a fixed number of events of different amplitude or the passage of a fixed time period. In the setting of nonsustained ventricular tachycardia, the gain is decreased, with possible failure to sense subsequent signals. The device may then begin bradycardia pacing, with a possibility of initiation of ventricular tachycardia.[105] Furthermore, atrial premature complexes or ventricular premature complexes may lead to a sinus complex after the premature complex, which has a reduced or possibly non-sensed amplitude.[61] This may lead to inappropriate pacing, with potential for induction of ventricular tachyarrhythmias. Furthermore, T-wave oversensing may lead to double counting and initiation of therapy for a spurious "tachycardia."[61]

Inappropriate Detection of Supraventricular Tachyarrhythmias

Early ICDs (which detected tachyarrhythmias primarily by rate criteria) delivered inappropriate shocks for supraventricular arrhythmias that satisfied these criteria.[104–106] Inappropriate shocks for atrial fibrillation occur in up to 12% of these patients and in 25% of those with a history of atrial fibrillation.[104–109] Frequently, they are multiple and account for half of inappropriate shocks.[107, 108] Inappropriate shocks triggered by documented sinus tachycardia occur in up to 9% of patients[105, 107, 108] and many undocumented shocks during vigorous exercise are presumed to have been triggered by sinus tachycardia.[105, 107, 108, 110] In addition to causing pain, inappropriate shocks may be proarrhythmic and rarely fatal.[104, 111, 112]

Inappropriate detection of atrial fibrillation and sinus tachycardia by newer tiered-therapy cardioverter–defibrillators is a greater problem.[43, 113] The probability of rate overlap between the target ventricular tachycardia and supraventricular arrhythmias is greater; pacing therapies delivered during supraventricular arrhythmias may induce ventricular tachycardia, and cardioversion may induce atrial fibrillation, which may in turn be sensed as ventricular tachycardia and treated with pacing, reinitiating ventricular tachycardia.[104, 111]

For these reasons, tiered-therapy ICDs include algorithms to discriminate ventricular tachycardia from supraventricular arrhythmias. Interval stability (stability) algorithms are designed to distinguish ventricular tachycardia from atrial fibrillation by rejecting irregular arrhythmias that fulfill rate criteria. Onset algorithms are designed to distinguish sinus tachycardia from ventricular tachycardia by rejecting tachycardias in which the rate increases grad-

ually. One interval-stability algorithm has proved highly specific for rejecting atrial fibrillation with ventricular rates less than 170 per minute, while producing minimal delays in detection of monomorphic ventricular tachycardia.[58] Onset algorithms have proved less specific and occasionally compromise sensitivity for detection of ventricular tachycardia.[58] Some tiered-therapy devices include a "sustained high rate" criterion to prevent onset criteria from rejecting pathologic tachycardias. These criteria, however, further decrease specificity (Fig. 43-24).[114]

Inappropriate Therapy for Nonsustained Ventricular Tachycardia

Although antitachycardia pacing is delivered immediately after the detection criterion is met, shock therapy is delivered only after the output capacitor has been charged. In the noncommitted mode, ICDs confirm the persistence of ventricular tachycardia or ventricular fibrillation during or after completion of the charging process, to avoid shocks for nonsustained ventricular tachycardia. In the committed mode, such confirmation is not required. Most tiered-therapy ICDs have a noncommitted mode for ventricular tachycardia. Modes for ventricular fibrillation include committed, noncommitted, and programmable (see Table 43-1). Although noncommitted shocks prevent inappropriate therapies for nonsustained ventricular tachycardia, the rare failure to reconfirm the presence of a tachyarrhythmia results in withholding appropriate therapy (Fig. 43-25).[50, 58]

Lead Problems

Lead systems have been the source of significant problems. Generally, patients with lead failures have had inappropriate shocks or elevated pacing thresholds. In one large study, the endocardial lead systems were found to be more reliable than epicardial systems.[115] Stambler's cooperative study identified a 12% complication rate related to lead problems. At least a third of these complications were adapter-related.[115]

PACEMAKERS AND IMPLANTABLE CARDIOVERTER—DEFIBRILLATORS

Multiple problems have arisen in patients who need or will have permanent pacemakers. The implanting physician must take special care to have the ICD sensing leads as far from the pacing electrodes as possible, in an attempt to prevent double sensing. In addition, if the pacemaker fails to sense ventricular tachycardia or ventricular fibrillation,

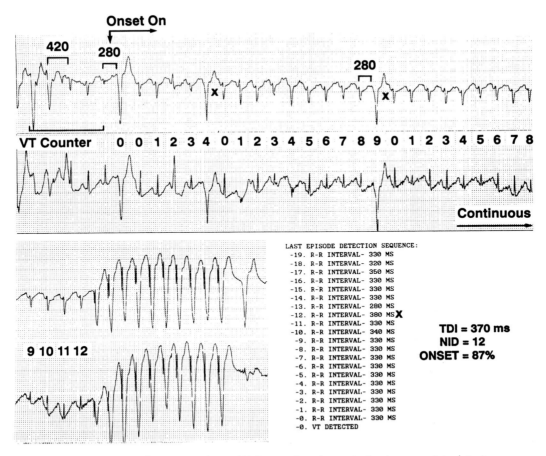

Figure 43-24. Tracing from a two-channel Holter monitor, demonstrating inappropriate detection of ventricular tachycardia caused by premature ventricular complexes during sinus tachycardia, despite use of an onset criterion. The onset criterion of the Medtronic PCD 7217 is designed to discriminate initiation of ventricular tachycardia (characterized by an abrupt increase in rate) from sinus tachycardia, in which the rate increases gradually. For any interval, the *calculated onset ratio* is the ratio of that interval to the mean of the four preceding baseline intervals. The *onset criterion* requires (1) that the calculated onset ratio for an interval be less than the *programmed onset ratio* and (2) that the second or third interval preceding that interval exceeds the ventricular tachycardia Detection interval. The ventricular tachycardia detection interval is 370 milliseconds the number of intervals to detect is 12, and the programmed onset ratio is 87%. The value of the ventricular tachycardia interval counter is shown between the upper and lower channels. The premature ventricular complex, with a coupling interval of 280 milliseconds (*top left*), fulfills the onset criterion: The preceding 420-millisecond pause that follows a run of nonsustained ventricular tachycardia provides the necessary interval, which exceeds the ventricular tachycardia detection interval; the onset ratio (calculated from measured intervals on the Holter recording) is approximately 78%. The ventricular tachycardia interval counter is reset twice by postextrasystolic pauses, denoted by *X* but the PCD onset criterion is not reset because this requires that two consecutive intervals exceed the ventricular tachycardia detection interval. The second *X* corresponds to interval 12 of the detection sequence. Interval 11 is the first of consecutive intervals that fulfill the interval criterion in the final detection sequence. When the ventricular tachycardia interval count reaches 12, inappropriate antitachycardia pacing is delivered.

it may continue to deliver pacing pulses asynchronously during these episodes. The ICD autogain or autoadjusting sensitivity may interpret the large pacing artifacts as a nontachycardia arrhythmia and filter out the baseline ventricular tachycardia or ventricular fibrillation signals. This causes the ICD NOT to deliver appropriate therapy. Furthermore, ICD shocks may cause reprogramming of or damage to the pacemaker generator (Fig. 43-26).[116–123]

Major points to be considered at the time of implantation include placing the sensing electrodes as far as possible from the pacing leads. Unipolar pacemakers generally need to be converted to a bipolar mode if possible or the

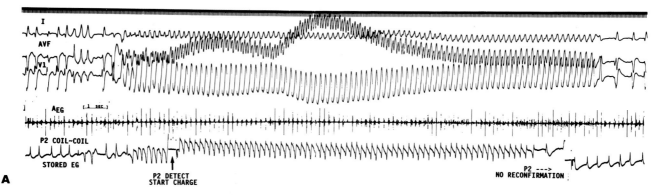

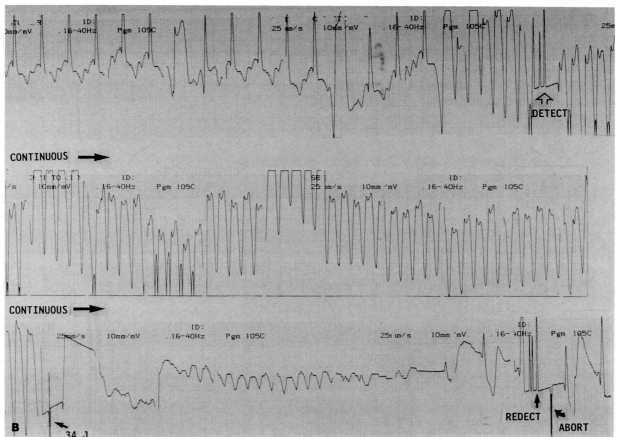

Figure 43-25. Value of aborted shock capability and stored electrograms. (**A**) Postoperative testing of CPI VentakP2 Model 1705. Spontaneous onset of self-terminating ventricular tachycardia during atrial fibrillation. Three surface electrocardiographic leads and bipolar atrial electrogram are shown in real time. The stored electrograms from the two coils of the Endotak Model 64 electrode were retrieved by telemetry and approximately time-aligned with the real-time recording. Ventricular tachycardia terminates during the charging cycle before delivery of the 34-J shock, so therapy was aborted. (**B**) Stored electrograms from a spontaneous episode of ventricular tachycardia in the same patient. After delivery of the 34-J shock, ventricular tachycardia continues at the same rate for about 6 seconds before termination. The quality of the electrogram deteriorates after the shock but the cycle length is unchanged. The implantable cardioverter–defibrillator (ICD) begins to redetect and then aborts the capacitor charge. Note that the ICD's rate-counting circuit uses an integrated bipolar signal from tip electrode to distal coil rather than the coil–coil signal. Similar degradation of the integrated bipolar signal has been reported after high-energy shocks, however.

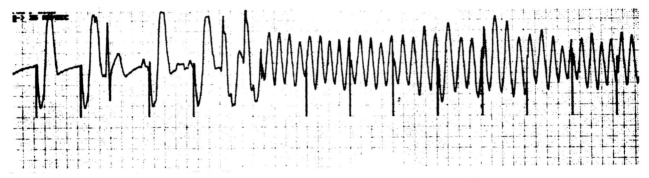

Figure 43-26. Ventricular fibrillation in a patient with a VVI pacemaker. Note the continued discharge of the VVI pacemaker which is detected by the ICD. The appropriate therapy is therefore not initiated. (Courtesy Medtronics, Inc., Minneapolis, Minn.)

unit and lead changed to bipolar unit. There is also a need for a dedicated bipolar unit to avoid post-shock power-on reset to unipolar mode.

At the time of final testing, the pacemaker should be programmed to maximum output and duration to check for possible oversensing.

Tiered-therapy ICDs avoid many of these problem with bradycardia pacing but some problems still exist because some patients still require dual-chamber pacing.[61, 115–116]

Routine pacemaker programming may result in alterations in the ICD when the programming wand or a magnet is applied to the pacemaker generator area. This may result in (1) deactivation of the ICD, (2) inappropriate discharge, or (3) some form of reprogramming of the ICD. It may be best to inactivate the ICD during pacemaker programming or reprogramming. Therefore, the ICD should be interrogated postpacemaker programming. The inactivation of an ICD can occur with any electromagnetic interference such as the programming wand. The interference, however, may need to exceed 30 seconds to produce inactivation.

Implantable cardioverter–defibrillator shocks can result in alteration of pacemaker function, with reversion to the VVI mode, or the generator mode may be changed to elective replacement indication or power-on reset mode.

AUTOMOBILE DRIVING AND IMPLANTABLE CARDIOVERTER–DEFIBRILLATORS

In the United States, state laws are not uniform regarding driving limitations in patients with arrhythmias; only a small number of states have any laws restricting driving. There are no laws specifically indicating guidelines for patients with ICDs. Furthermore, there appears to be no consensus among cardiologists relative to recommendations for these patients.

It has been suggested that patients with syncope with ICD shocks should not be allowed to drive.[124] Patients who receive only high-energy shocks for ventricular tachycardia or ventricular fibrillation seem to be at moderate risk for loss of consciousness with ICD shocks and probably should not be allowed to drive.

Two surveys have attempted to analyze the recommendations of physicians regarding driving in patients with ICDs.[125, 126] The recommendations were highly variable. Moreover, one survey of ICD patients' behavior in a group that was advised against driving indicates that 70% were driving within 8 months of implantation.[127]

Clearly, a uniform set of guidelines needs to be developed for use by all implanting physicians. It is expected that a combined policy statement from the ASPE and the American Heart Association will be forthcoming soon.

EFFECTIVENESS IN TREATING SUDDEN DEATH SURVIVORS AND PATIENTS WITH VENTRICULAR ARRHYTHMIAS

Enhanced Survival

Even the initial 52 patients who were implanted in Baltimore were shown by actuarial curves to have had markedly reduced mortality when Kaplan-Meier survival-curve analysis was performed for them (Fig. 43-27).[1] A hypothetical expected mortality statistic (indicating what would have occurred in the group of patients if the AICD had not been implanted) was constructed, using as end points either the patients' actual death or the first out-of-hospital resuscitation. Deaths were classified as sudden unless they were clearly otherwise. The 1-year mortality

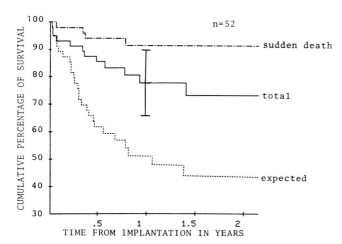

Figure 43-27. Life-table survival analysis of the initial 52 patients with defibrillators. The upper curve (*broken line*) includes patients whose deaths were unwitnessed and presumably sudden and arrhythmic. The middle curve (*solid line*) shows total mortality. The lower curve (*dotted line*) estimates the mortality that would have occurred in the same group of patients without a defibrillator. The difference between identical time points on the middle and lower curves is an estimate of the improvement in survival. The 95% confidence interval at 1 year for the total survival curve is shown. (Mirowski M, Reid PR, Winkle RA, et al: Mortality in patients with implanted defibrillators. Ann Intern Med 1983;98:585.)

VENTAK-C, this component was more than 99% at 1 year. Although it would be naive to believe that all of the increased survival is due to the device, to the exclusion of antiarrhythmic and any other concurrent therapy given the patients, there seems little doubt that the implanted units provide the major share of the benefit.

Worldwide, since the beginning of the use of these devices, survival rates have continued to be high. Figure 43-29 indicates actuarial data for 7000 patients in the CPI follow-up study.

Because there are many centers whose figures are being included and over which the manufacturer exerts little control over timely reporting, some of the figures have been criticized for possible under-reporting of deaths. Conversely, results from large single centers known to be providing excellent data follow-up show almost identical results. For example, Winkle and co-workers report that actuarial survival rates, incidence-free of sudden and total deaths, were 99% and 92% at 1 year and 96% and 74% at 5 years.[134, 135]

At present, it is clear that the ICD is able to prevent sudden cardiac death due to ventricular tachyarrhythmias. Data show that the sudden death rate is equal to or less than 5% at 3 years. Longer-term follow-up studies, however, demonstrate a less than expected incidence of sud-

from all causes was 22.9%, the sudden death mortality 8.5%, and the predicted mortality 48%.[128] These figures indicated a 52% decrease in total mortality and a corresponding significant reduction in the arrhythmic component during the initial year after device implantation.[129-133]

Another indication that these devices are effective is inferred from further improvements in the actuarial curves as successive models better able to perform their intended function are phased into clinical use. As more patients became enrolled, it is possible to compare the respective effectiveness of the first- and second-generation devices used in the study. Figure 43-28 displays survival curves for the first 99 patients implanted in Baltimore, divided into two groups according to the model they received. In each panel, the arrhythmic mortality is indicated by the upper curve and the total mortality by the lower curve. Patients whose early model was subsequently replaced with the AICD were withdrawn at that time from the AID population and entered into the AICD group. The curves indicate that at 1 year, the total mortality rates were 26% and 16.6%, whereas the mortality due to arrhythmias was 10.6% for the early model series and only 2% for the AICD series. Needless to say, the virtual abolition of arrhythmic mortality is extremely significant.

After the VENTAK-C was phased into clinical use, still further improvements were noted in the actuarial curves, especially regarding the arrhythmic survival. With the

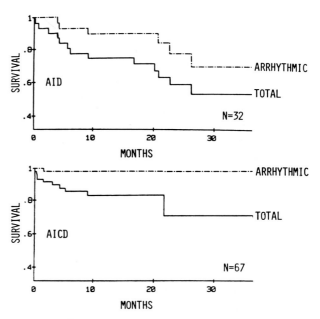

Figure 43-28. Comparison of arrhythmic rates and total mortality in patients treated with two different implanted models. Patients whose early automatic defibrillator unit (**A**) was subsequently replaced with an automatic implantable cardioverter–defibrillator (**B**) were withdrawn from the population in **A** at that time and entered into the automatic implantable cardioverter–defibrillator group in **B**. *AID*, automatic implantable defibrillator; *AICD*, automatic implantable cardioverter–defibrillator.

AICD PATIENT SURVIVAL FREE OF:	1 Yr	2 YR	3 YR	4 Yr	5 Yr
Sudden Death	98.4%	97.4%	96.6%	95.3%	94.8%
Cardiac death	96.5%	94.2%	91.9%	90.5%	88.3%
All death	92.2%	87.7%	83.8%	80.8%	77.2%

Figure 43-29. Actuarial survival, free of events in the overall automatic implantable cardioverter–defibrillator (AICD) implant cohort, numbering more than 7000 patients. Note virtual elimination of sudden deaths through the 5-year period, in addition to striking limitation of death from all causes.

den cardiac death, compared with predicted. Survival data from all-cause mortality was 19.8% at 3 years and 33.1% at 6 years follow-up in 1737 patients.[136] These late data indicate that although arrhythmia death is low, cardiac and all-cause mortality remains high. These data are the cause of significant medical and economic concerns regarding the real need of ICD implantation in some of these patients. These concerns have led to the development of multiple studies to ascertain the exact benefits of ICD implantation, with specific emphasis on patient selection, need for anti-arrhythmic drug therapy, impact of revascularization procedures, and other medical therapies. Arguments have been put forth suggesting that it has *not* been convincingly shown that ICD implantation prolongs life, compared with alternative therapy.[137–140] This point, associated with the cost and morbidity of device implantations, suggests that device implantation may not be justifiable in some patients. Furthermore, it is important to realize (1) that sudden cardiac death is only a fraction of total cardiac death, and (2) about 20% of sudden deaths are due to bradyarrhythmias or electric mechanical dissociation. It has been assumed, therefore, that if half of the post-arrest deaths are sudden and 80% of these are due to ventricular fibrillation–ventricular tachycardia, a reduction of 90% in sudden arrhythmic deaths leads to only a 36% maximum reduction in total cardiac mortality.[141] It is thought that many patients who are at high risk for arrhythmic deaths are also at high risk for nonarrhythmic cardiac deaths, secondary to progressive myocardial dysfunction.

Multiple studies with some significant methodologic limitations have provided strong (albeit somewhat circumstantial) data that ICD implantation prolongs survival in certain subsets of patients with life-threatening arrhythmias. In one subgroup with reasonable (greater than 40%) left ventricular ejection fraction and limited or no evidence of congestive heart failure, the benefit of ICD implantation compared with drug therapy may be evident only after years. In contrast, in patients with depressed left ventricular function (left ventricular ejection fraction less than 40%) and some evidence of congestive heart failure,

the benefit of ICD may be shown early but the total cardiac mortality may not be improved.[142–148] These observations resulted in the development of the following multiple prospective studies, to try to determine appropriate patient selection and benefits of ICD implantation.

CORONARY ARTERY BYPASS GRAFTING TRIAL. Retrospectively, data from 3200 coronary artery bypass grafting (CABG) operations were reviewed to evaluate the potential for prophylactic ICD implantation. In this analysis, 17% of the patients younger than 80 years old had a left ventricular ejection fraction of less than 36%. The mortality rate in this group was 28% in 24 months.

The study was designed to evaluate patients who do not have a history of ventricular tachycardia or ventricular fibrillation but have an abnormal signal-averaged electrogram (i.e., a filtered QRS duration greater than 114 milliseconds). Patients are to be randomized to ICD or no ICD therapy at the time of CABG, with an end point of total death or cardiac arrest.

MULTICENTER UNSUSTAINED TACHYCARDIA TRIAL. This study was designed to answer whether electrophysiologically guided therapy is able to reduce sudden cardiac death or sustained ventricular tachycardia. Patients are entered who have nonsustained ventricular tachycardia and an ejection fraction equal to or less than 40%. All patients undergo an electrophysiologic study. If sustained ventricular tachycardia is induced, patients are randomized to no antiarrhythmic drug therapy or electrophysiologically guided therapy. If electrophysiologically guided therapy is unsuccessful, an ICD is implanted. The primary end point is sudden cardiac death or cardiac arrest.

MULTICENTER AUTOMATIC DEFIBRILLATOR IMPLANT PATIENT TRIAL. Patients are to be evaluated if they have a history of myocardial infarction and left ventricular dysfunction (left ventricular ejection fraction equal to or less than 35% and nonsustained ventricular tachycardia). All patients are to undergo electrophysiologic study and must have sustained ventricular tachycardia not suppressible by intravenous procainamide. The patients are randomized to either conventional antiarrhythmic drug therapy or an ICD. The primary end point is arrhythmic death.

CARDIAC ARREST STUDY—HAMBURG. Patients who are survivors of sudden cardiac death, with documented ventricular tachycardia or ventricular fibrillation, are included. Patients are randomized to either antiarrhythmic drugs or ICD therapy. Extensive cardiac testing is performed, including electrophysiologic studies. Antiarrhythmic drug therapy includes amiodarone, metoprolol, and propafenone. The electrophysiologic study results do not influence treatment. The primary end point is total mortality, with secondary end points of recurrence of cardiac arrest, hemodynamically unstable ventricular tachycardia, or drug cessation because of side effects. To date, the propafenone arm has been discontinued because this therapy has been clearly inferior to ICD implantation.

ANTIARRHYTHMIC VERSUS IMPLANTABLE DEFIBRILLATOR STUDY. This study randomizes to the best drug treatment of an ICD patient who has either (1) been resuscitated from ventricular fibrillation, (2) sustained ventricular tachycardia with syncope, or (3) sustained ventricular tachycardia, with serious hemodynamic consequences, and has a left ventricular ejection fraction of equal to or less than 40%. Drug therapy is amiodarone or sotalol. The study initially intends to answer whether drugs are better than an ICD for a high-risk population.

CLINICAL ACCEPTANCE

Although these devices appear to be quite expensive, plus the added costs of surgical and hospital fees, preliminary data and more formal studies now underway indicate that in addition to the large reduction obtained in mortality, the cost-effectiveness of the therapy measured in terms of expenditure per life-year saved is higher than that of other antiarrhythmic modalities and well within the range of accepted treatment modalities for other disease processes. It appears that the need for frequent and expensive rehospitalizations for arrhythmic breakthroughs and for extensive serial drug testing—in itself expensive—may be appreciably diminished.

As a result, the acceptance of this treatment modality is impressive. Implantable cardioverter–defibrillator prescription, implantation, and follow-up are routine, and Medicare and third-party payors are reimbursing for the procedure. The therapy is no longer experimental and is even being considered the "gold standard" and the "treatment of choice" for patients with high arrhythmic risk.

FUTURE DEVELOPMENTS

The future promises several important advances in application of ICD therapy. Perhaps the most exciting relates to the possibility of estimating the defibrillation threshold accurately without multiple inductions of ventricular fibrillation. Most studies support the hypothesis that unsuccessful shocks that are slightly weaker than necessary to defibrillate fail because they fall into the vulnerable period of some ventricular tissue and thereby reinitiate ventricular fibrillation.[149–153] The shock strength above which ventricular fibrillation cannot be reinitiated, even when the shock falls into the vulnerable period, is known as the upper limit of vulnerability and should be the same as the defibrillation threshold.[150–154] A simplified method of measuring the upper limit of vulnerability is reported to predict the defibrillation threshold, with sufficient accuracy that it could be used as a clinical surrogate for the defibrillation threshold.[154]

In the future, detection algorithms will integrate dual-chamber sensing, detection of QRS width, and sensing of non-electrogram signals to provide information about hemodynamics. These methods may improve tachyarrhythmia discrimination. Use of improved defibrillation waveforms, optimal capacitor size, and new lead systems may lower defibrillation thresholds sufficiently to permit ICDs with lower output. This would permit smaller pulse generators and technically easier and cosmetically more acceptable pectoral implantation.

CONCLUSION

Implantable cardioverter–defibrillator therapy is a revolutionary advance in the prevention of sudden cardiac death. The ability of these devices to diagnose ventricular fibrillation and tachycardia and their ability to treat them has resulted in an impressive decrease in arrhythmic mortality. The potential risks and dangers observed with this new diagnostic–therapeutic system are acceptable under the circumstances and are steadily diminishing. Clinical benefits of these systems might be even greater and longer lasting for patients with less marked degrees of left ventricular dysfunction than those thus far implanted. As the clinical experience grows, the patient populations that can benefit from this intervention will most certainly be broadened.

References

1. Mirowski M, Reid PR, Mower MM, et al: Termination of malignant ventricular arrhythmias with an implanted automatic defibrillator in human beings. N Engl J Med 1980; 303:322.
2. Mirowski M, Mower MM, Staewen WS, et al: Standby auto-

matic defibrillator: an approach to prevention of sudden cardiac death. Arch Intern Med 1970;126:158.

3. Mirowski M, Mower MM, Staewen WS, et al: The development of the transvenous automatic defibrillator. Arch Intern Med 1972;129:773.

4. Mower MM, Mirowski M, Spear JF, Moore EN: Patterns of ventricular activity during catheter defibrillation. Circulation 1974;49:858.

5. Mirowski M, Mower MM, Reid PR, Watkins L Jr: Ventricular defibrillation through a single intravascular catheter electrode system. Clin Res 1971;19:328.

6. Mirowski M, Mower MM, Reid PR, Watkins L Jr: Automatic implantable defibrillator. In: Dreifus LS ed. Pacemaker therapy. Philadelphia: FA Davis, 1983:195.

7. Mirowski M, Mower MM, Gott VL, Brawley RK: Feasibility and effectiveness of low-energy catheter defibrillation in man. Circulation 1973;47:79.

8. Mirowski M, Mower MM, Langer A, et al: A chronically implanted system for automatic defibrillation in sudden death from ventricular fibrillation. Circulation 1978;58:90.

9. Mirowski M, Mower MM, Bhagavan BS, et al: Chronic animal and bench testing of the implantable automatic defibrillator. In: Meere C ed. Proceedings of the VIIth World Symposium on Cardiac Pacing. Montreal, Canada: Pacesymp, 1980.

10. Mirowski M, Mower MM, Langer A, Heilman MS: The automatic implantable defibrillator: a new avenue. In: Bircks W, Loogen F, Schulte HD, Seipel L, eds. Medical and surgical management of tachyarrhythmias. Springer-Verlag, 1980:71. Berlin.

11. Reid PR, Mirowski M, Mower MM, et al: Clinical evaluation of the internal automatic cardioverter-defibrillator in survivors of sudden cardiac death. Am J Cardiol 1983;51:1608.

12. Mower MM, Reid PR, Watkins L Jr, Mirowski M: Use of alternating current during diagnostic electrophysiologic studies. Circulation 1983;67:69.

13. Watkins L Jr, Mirowski M, Mower MM, et al: Automatic defibrillation in man: the initial surgical experience. J Thorac Cardiovasc Surg 1981;82:492.

14. Watkins L Jr, Mirowski M Mower MM, et al: Implantation of the automatic defibrillator: the sub-xyphoid approach. Ann Thorac Surg 1982;34:515.

15. Laurie GM, Morris GC Jr, Howell JF, et al: Left subcostal insertion of the sutureless myocardial electrode. Ann Thorac Surg 1976;21:350.

16. Bielefeld MR, Yano OJ, Cabreroza SE, Treat MR, et al: Thoracoscopic placement of implantable cardioverter-defibrillator patch leads in sheep. Circulation 1993;88(P 2):447.

17. McCowan R, Maloney J, Wilkoff B, et al: Automatic implantable cardioverter-defibrillator implantation without thoracotomy using an endocardial and submuscular patch system. J Am Coll Cardiol 1991;17:41.

18. Yee R, Klein GJ, Leitch JW, et al: A permanent transvenous lead system for an implantable pacemaker cardioverter-defibrillator: nonthoracotomy approach to implantation. Circulation 1992;85:196.

19. Hauser RG, Nisam S, McVeigh KC, Kurschinski DT: Worldwide experience with the endotak transvenous defibrillation lead. Xth International Congress (New Frontiers of Arrhythmias), Marillena, Italy 1992;69:75.

20. Bardy GH, Johnson G, Poole JE, et al: A simplified, single-lead unipolar transvenous cardioversion-defibrillation system. Circulation 1993;88:543.

21. Brooks R, Garan H, Torchiana D, et al: Determinants of successful nonthoracotomy cardioverter-defibrillator implantation: experience in 101 patients using two different lead systems. J Am Coll Cardiol 1993;22:1835.

22. Bardy GH, Hofer B, Johnson G, et al: Implantable transvenous cardioverter-defibrillators. Circulation 1993;87:1152.

23. Bardy GH, Allen MD, Mehra R, et al: Transvenous defibrillation in humans via the coronary sinus. Circulation 1990; 81:1252.

24. Kudenchuk PJ, Bardy GH, Dolack GL, et al: Efficacy of a single-lead unipolar transvenous defibrillator compared with a system employing an additional coronary sinus electrode. A prospective, randomized study. Circulation 1994; 89:2641.

25. Ip JH, Mehta D, Pe E, et al: Subpectoral implantation of cardioverter-defibrillator combined with a nonepicardial lead system: preliminary experience with a novel approach. Am J Cardiol 1993, 72:857.

26. Mower MM, Reid PR, Watkins L Jr, et al: Automatic implantable cardioverter-defibrillator: structural characteristics. Pacing Clin Electrophysiol 1984;7:1331.

27. Ideker RE, Tsang ASL, Frazier DW, Shibata N, Chen PS, Wharton JM: Ventricular defibrillation: basic concepts in cardiac pacing and electrophysiology. In: El-Sherif N, Samet P, eds. 3rd ed. Philadelphia: WB Saunders, 1991:713.

28. Fain ES, Sweeney MB, Franz MR: Improved internal defibrillation efficacy with a biphasic waveform. Am Heart J 1989;117:358.

29. Chapman PD, Vetter JW, Souza JJ, Wetherbee JN, Troup PJ: Comparison of monophasic with single and dual capacitor biphasic waveforms for nonthoracotomy canine internal defibrillation. J Am Coll Cardiol 1989;14:242.

30. Winkle RA, Mead RH, Ruder MA, et al: Improved low energy defibrillation efficacy in man with the use of a biphasic truncated exponential waveform. Am Heart J 1989;117:122.

31. Tang ASL, Yabe S, Wharton JM, Dolker M, et al: Ventricular defibrillation using biphasic waveforms: the importance of phasic duration. J Am Coll Cardiol 1989;13:207.

32. Kavanagh KM, Tang ASL, Rollins DL, et al: Comparison of the internal defibrillation thresholds for monophasic and double and single capacitor biphasic waveforms. J Am Coll Cardiol 1989;14:1343.

33. Saksena S, An H, Mehra R, et al: Prospective comparison of biphasic and monophasic shocks for implantable cardioverter-defibrillators using endocardial leads. Am J Cardiol 1992;70:304.

34. Swartz JF, Fletcher RD, Karasik PE: Optimization of biphasic waveforms for human nonthoracotomy defibrillation. Circulation 1993;88:2646.

35. Wyse DG, Kavanagh KM, Gillis AM, Mitchell LB, et al: Comparison of biphasic and monophasic shocks for defibrillation using a nonthoracotomy system. Am J Cardiol 1993;71:197.

36. Bardy G, Ivey T, Allen M, Johnson G, Greene H: Evaluation of electrode polarity on defibrillation efficacy. Am J Cardiol 1989;63:433.

37. O'Neill P, Boshene K, Lawrie G, Marvill L, Pacifico A: The automatic implantable cardioverter-defibrillator: effect of patch polarity on defibrillation threshold. J Am Coll Cardiol 1991;17:707.

38. Mehra R, Norenberg M, DeGroot P: Comparison of defibrillation thresholds with pulsing techniques requiring three epicardial electrodes. Pacing Clin Electrophysiol 1989;11:527. Abstract.

39. Mehra R, DeGroot P, Norenberg S: Three dimensional finite element model of the heart for analysis of epicardial defibrillation: effect of patch surface area. Pacing Clin Electrophysiol 1989;23:652A. Abstract.

40. Ideker R, Wolf P, Alferness C, Krawssowska W, Smith W: Current concepts for selecting the location, size, and shape of defibrillation electrodes. Pacing Clin Electrophysiol 1990;14:227.

41. Walls J, Schuder J, Curtis J, et al: Adverse effect of permanent cardiac internal defibrillator patches on external defibrillation. Am J Cardiol 1989;64:1144.

42. Hauser R, Knuchinsky D, McVeigh K, Thomas A, Mower M: Clinical results with nonthoracotomy ICD systems. Pacing Clin Electrophysiol 1993;16:141.

43. Bardy GH, Hoffer B, Johnson G, et al: Implantable transvenous cardioverter-defribrillators. Circulation 1993;87:1152.

44. Saksena S, Krol R, Mehta D, Raju R, DeGroot P, Mehra R: Optimal biphasic electrode location for cardioverter-defibrillators with endocardial defibrillation leads. Circulation 1992;86:I. Abstract.

45. Bardy G, Johnson G, Poole J, et al: A simplified, single-lead unipolar transvenous cardioverter-defibrillator system. Circulation 1993;88:543.

46. PCD jewel arrhythmia control device: technical manual. Minneapolis, MN. Medtronic, Inc. 1993.

47. Winkle R, Bach S, Echt D: The automatic implantable defibrillator. Local ventricular bipolar sensing to detect ventricular tachycardia and fibrillation. Am J Cardiol 1993;52:265.

48. Zipes D, Jackman W, IIeger J: Clinical transvenous cardioversion of recurrent life-threatening ventricular tachycarrhythmias: low energy synchronized cardioversion of ventricular tachycardia and termination of ventricular fibrillation in patients using a catheter electrode. Am Heart J 1982;103:789.

49. Haluska E, Whistler S, Cafee R: A hierarchical approach to the treatment of ventricular tachycardias. Pacing Clin Electrophysiol 1986;9:1320.

50. Hurwitz JL, Hook BG, Blores BT, Marchlinski FE: Importance of abortive shock capability with electrogram storage in cardioverter-defibrillator devices. J Am Coll Cardiol 1993;4:895.

51. Troup P: Implantable cardioverters and defibrillators. Curr Probl Cardiol 1989;14:679.

52. Mehra R: Tachyarrhythmia termination: lead systems and hardware design. In: Singer I, ed. Implantable cardioverter defibrillators. Mt. Kisco, NY: Futura Publishing, 1994. In press.

53. Peleska B: Cardiac arrhythmias following condenser discharges and their dependence upon strength of current and phase of cardiac cycle. Circ Res 1963;13:21.

54. Tacker WA, Geddes LA, McFarlane J, et al: Optimum current duration for capacitor-discharge defibrillation of canine ventricles. J Appl Physiol 1969:27:480.

55. Kroll M: A minimal model of the monophasic defibrillation pulse. Pacing Clin Electrophysiol 1993;16:769.

56. Chang M, Inoue H, Kallok M: Double and triple sequential shocks reduce ventricular defibrillation threshold in dogs with and without myocardial infarction. J Am Coll Cardiol 1986;8:1393.

57. Jones D, Klein G, Guiradon G: Internal cardiac defibrillation in man: Pronounced improvement with sequential pulse delivery to two different orientations. Circulation 1986;73:484.

58. Swerdlow C, Chen PS, Kass R, Allard J, Peter T: Discrimination of ventricular tachycardia from sinus tachycardia and atrial fibrillation in a tiered-therapy cardioverter-defibrillator. J Am Coll Cardiol 1994;23:1343.

59. Jung M, Manz M, Moosdorf R, Luderitz B: Failure of an implantable cardioverter-defibrillator to redetect ventricular fibrillation in patients with a nonthoracotomy lead system. Circulation 1992;86:1217.

60. Sperry R, Ellenbogen K, Wook M, Stambler B, DiMarco J, Haines D: Failure of a second and third generation implantable cardioverter defibrillator to sense ventricular tachycardia. Implications for fixed-gain sensing devices. Pacing Clin Electrophysiol 1992;15:749.

61. Callans D, Hook B, Kleiman R, Mitra R, Flores B, Marchlinski F: Unique sensing errors in third-generation implantable cardioverter-defibrillators. J Am Coll Cardiol 1993;22:1135.

62. Anderson M, Murgatroyd F, Hnalkova K, et al: Computer modeling of misdiagnosis of atrial fibrillation as ventricular tachycardia by algorithms used in the implantable defibrillator. Comput Cardiol 1993;847.

63. Transvene PCD clinical summary. Minneapolis, MN: Medtronic, Inc. 1993.

64. Hook BG, Marchlinski FE: Value of ventricular electrogram recordings in the diagnosis of arrhythmias precipitating electrical device shock therapy. J Am Coll Cardiol 1991;17:985.

65. Newman D, Dorian P, Downar E, et al: Use of telemetry functions in the assessment of implanted antitachycardia device efficacy. Am J Cardiol 1991;70:616.

66. Hurwitz JL, Hook BG, Flores BT, Marchlinski FE: Importance of abortive shock capability with electrogram storage in cardioverter-defibrillator devices. J Am Coll Cardiol 1993;21:895.

67. Grimm W, Flores BF, Marchlinski FE: Symptoms and electrocardiographically documented rhythm preceding spontaneous shocks in patients with implantable cardioverter-defibrillator. Am J Cardiol 1993;71:1415.

68. Hook BG, Callans DJ, Kleiman RB, Flores BT, Marchlinski FE: Implantable cardioverter-defibrillator therapy in the absence of significant symptoms. (Rhythm diagnosis and management aided by stored electrogram analysis). Circulation 1993;87:1897.

69. Leitch JW, Gillis AM, Wyse G, et al: Reduction in defibrillator shocks with an implantable device combining antitachycardia pacing and shock therapy. J Am Coll Cardiol 1991;18:145.

70. Bardy GH, Troutman C, Poole JE, et al: Clinical experience

with a tiered-therapy, multiprogrammable antiarrhythmia device. Circulation 1992;85:1689.

71. Wietholt D, Block M, Isbruch F, et al: Clinical experience with antitachycardia pacing and improved detection algorithms in a new implantable cardioverter-defibrillator. J Am Coll Cardiol 1993;21:885.

72. Gillis AM, Leitch JW, Sheldon S, et al: A prospective randomized comparison of autodecremental pacing to burst pacing in device therapy for chronic ventricular tachycardia secondary to coronary artery disease. Am J Cardiol 1993;72:1146.

73. Newman D, Dorian P, Hardy J: Randomized controlled comparison of antitachycardia pacing algorithms for termination of ventricular tachycardia. J Am Coll Cardiol 1993;21:1413.

74. Bardy GH, Poole JE, Kudenchuk PJ, Dolack GL, Kelso D, Mitchell R: A prospective randomized repeat-crossover comparison of antitachycardia pacing with low-energy cardioversion. Circulation 1993;87:1889.

75. Fromer M, Brachmann J, Block M, et al: Efficacy of automatic multimodal device therapy for ventricular tachyarrhythmias as delivered by a new implantable pacing cardioverter-defibrillator (Results of a European multicenter study of 102 implants). Circulation 1992;86:363.

76. Porterfield JG, Porterfield LM, Smith BA, Bray L: Experience with three different third-generation cardioverter-defibrillators in patients with coronary artery disease or cardiomyopathy. Am J Cardiol 1993;72:301.

77. Choue CW, Kim SG, Fisher JD, et al: Comparison of defibrillator therapy and other therapeutic modalities for sustained ventricular tachycardia or ventricular fibrillation associated with coronary artery disease. Am J Cardiol 1994;73:1075–1079.

78. The PCD Investigator Group: Clinical outcome of patients with malignant ventricular tachyarrhythmias and a multiprogrammable implantable cardioverter-defibrillator implanted with or without thoracotomy: an international multicenter study. J Am Coll Cardiol 1994;223:1521.

79. Marchlinski FE, Flores BT, Buxton AE, et al: The automatic implantable cardioverter-defibrillator. Efficacy, complications and device failures. Ann Intern Med 1986;104:481.

80. Lucern RM, Thurer RJ, Palatianos GM, et al: The automatic implantable cardioverter-defibrillator: results, observations and comments. Pacing Clin Electrophysiol 1986;9:1343.

81. Gabry MD, Brodman R, Johnston D, et al: Automatic implantable cardioverter defibrillator: patient survival, battery longevity and shock delivery analysis. J Am Coll Cardiol 1987;9:1349.

82. Borbola J, Denes P, Ezri MD, et al: The automatic implantable cardioverter defibrillator: clinical experience, complications and follow-up. Arch Intern Med 1988;148:70.

83. Platia EV, Veltri EP, Griffith LSC, et al: Post defibrillation bradycardia following implantable defibrillator discharge. J Am Coll Cardiol 1986;7:73A. Abstract.

84. Almassi GH, Chapman PD, Troup PJ, et al: Constrictive pericarditis associated with patch electrodes of the automatic implantable cardioverter-defibrillator. Chest 1987;92:369.

85. Kadri N, Niazi I, Elkhatib I, et al: Automatic implantable cardioverter defibrillator: Problems and complications. J Am Coll Cardiol 1987;9:142A. Abstract.

86. Cooper DK, Luceri RM, Thurer RJ, et al: The impact of the automatic implantable cardioverter defibrillator on quality of life. Clin Prog Electrophysiol Pacing 1986;4:306.

87. Mosteller RD, Lehmann MH, Thomas AC, Jackson K: Operative mortality with implantation of the automatic cardioverter-defibrillator. Am J Cardiol 1991;68:1340.

88. Marchlinski FE, Buxton AE, Flores B: The automatic implantable cardioverter defibrillator (AICD): follow-up and complications. In: El-Sherif N, Samet P, eds. Cardiac pacing and electrophysiology. Philadelphia: WB Saunders, 1991:743.

89. Bardy GH: Ensuring automatic detection of ventricular fibrillation. Circulation 1992;86:1634.

90. Jung W, Manz M, Moosdorf R, Luderitz B: Failure of an implantable cardioverter-defibrillator to redetect ventricular fibrillation in patients with a nonthoracotomy lead system. Circulation 1992;86:1217.

91. Murakawa Y, Gliner BE, Shankar B, Thakor NV: The effect of an unsuccessful subthreshold shock on the energy requirement for the subsequent defibrillation. Am Heart J 1989;117:1065.

92. Kim SG, Fisher JD, Furman S, et al: Exacerbation of ventricular arrhythmias during the postoperative period after implantation of an automatic defibrillator. J Am Coll Cardiol 1991;18:1200.

93. Gartman DM, Bardy GH, Allen M, Misbach GA, Ivery TD: Short term morbidity and mortality of implantation of automatic implantable cardioverter-defibrillator. J Thorac Cardiovasc Surg 1990;100:353.

94. Bocker D, Block M, Isbruch F, et al: Comparison of frequency of aggravation of ventricular tachyarrhythmias after implantation of automatic defibrillators using epicardial versus nonthoracotomy lead systems. Am J Cardiol 1993;71:1064.

95. Lauer MR, Young C, Liem B, et al: Ventricular fibrillation induced by low-energy shocks from programmable implantable cardioverter-defibrillators in patients with coronary artery disease. Am J Cardiol 1994;73:559.

96. Pinski SL, Vanerio G, Castle LW, et al: Patients with a high defibrillation threshold: clinical characteristics, management and outcome. Am Heart J 1991;122:89.

97. Epstein AE, Ellenbogen KA, Kirk KA, et al: Clinical characteristics and outcome of patients with high defibrillation thresholds: a multicenter study. Circulation 1992;86:1206.

98. Brooks R, Torchiana D, Vlahakes GJ, Ruskin JN, McGovern BA, Garan H: Successful implantation of cardioverter-defibrillator systems in patients with elevated defibrillation thresholds. J Am Coll Cardiol 1993;22:569.

99. Venditti FJ Jr, Martin DT, Vassolas G, Bower S: Rise in chronic defibrillation thresholds in nonthoracotomy implantable defibrillator. Circulation 1994;89:216.

100. Echt DS, Black JN, Barbey JT, Coxe DR, Cato E: Evaluation of antiarrhythmic drugs on defibrillation energy requirements in dogs. Sodium channel block and action potential prolongation. Circulation 1989;79:1106.

101. Huang SKS, Tan de Guzman WL, Chenarides JG, Okike NO, Vander Salm TJ: Effects of long-term amiodarone therapy on the defibrillation threshold and the rate of shocks of the implantable cardioverter-defibrillator. Am Heart J 1991;122:720.

102. Kadish AH, Marchlinski FE, Josephson ME, et al: Amiodarone: correlation of early and late electrophysiologic studies with outcome. Am Heart J 1986;112:1134–1140

103. DaTorre S, Bondke H, Brinker J, et al: Increased pacing threshold after an automatic defibrillator shock: effects of antiarrhythmic drugs. Circulation 1987;76:IV. Abstract.

104. Johnson NJ, Marchlinski FE: Arrhythmias induced by device antitachycardia therapy due to diagnostic nonspecificity. J Am Coll Cardiol 1991;18:1418.

105. Kelly PA, Cannom DS, Garan H, et al: The automatic implantable cardioverter-defibrillator; efficacy, complications and survival in patients with malignant ventricular arrhythmias. J Am Coll Cardiol 1991;11:1278.

106. Winkle R, Mead H, Ruder M, et al: Long term outcome with the automatic implantable cardioverter defibrillator. J Am Coll Cardiol 1989;13:1353.

107. Fogaros RN, Elson JJ, Bonnet CA: Actuarial incidence and pattern of occurrence of shocks following implantation of the automatic implantable cardioverter defibrillator. Pacing Clin Electrophysiol 1989;15:1667.

108. Grimm W, Flores BP, Marchlinski FE: Electrocardiographically documented unnecessary, spontaneous shocks in 241 patients with implantable cardioverter defibrillators. Pacing Clin Electrophysiol 1992;15:1667.

109. CEDARS Investigators: Comprehensive evaluation of defibrillators and resuscitative shocks (CEDARS) Study; Does atrial fibrillation increase the incidence of inappropriate shock by implanted defibrillators? J Am Coll Cardiol 1993; 21:278A. Abstract.

110. Meissner MD, Lehman MH, Steinman RT, et al: Ventricular fibrillation in patients without significant structural heart disease: a multicenter experience with implantable cardioverter-defibrillator therapy. J Am Coll Cardiol 1993;21:1406.

111. Birgersdotter-Green U, Rosenqvist M, Lindemans FW, Ryden L, Radegran K: Holter documented sudden death in a patient with an implanted defibrillator. Pacing Clin Electrophysiol 1991;15:1008.

112. Cohen TJ, Chien WW, Lurie KG, et al: Implantable cardioverter defibrillator proarrhythmia: case report and review of the literature. Pacing Clin Electrophysiol 1991;14:1326–1329

113. Bardy GH, Troutman C, Poole JE, et al: Clinical experience with a tiered-Therapy multiprogrammable antiarrhythmia device. Circulation 1992;85:1689.

114. Warren J, Martha RO: Clinical evaluation of automatic tachycardia diagnosis by an implanted device. Pacing Clin Electrophysiol 1986;9:1079.

115. Stambler BS, Wood MA, Damiano RJ, Greenway PS, Smutka ML, Ellenbogen KA: Sensing/pacing lead complications with a newer generation implantable cardioverter-defibrillator: worldwide experience from the Guardian ATP 4210 Clinical Trial. J Am Coll Cardiol 1994;23:123.

116. Kelly PA, Mann DE, Damle RS, Reiter MJ: Oversensing during ventricular pacing in patients with a third-generation implantable cardioverter-defibrillator. J Am Coll Cardiol 1994; 23:1531.

117. Epstein AE, Kay GN, Plumb VJ, Shepard RB, Kirklin JK: Combined automatic implantable cardioverter-defibrillator and pacemaker systems: implantation techniques and follow-up. J Am Coll Cardiol 1989;13:121.

118. Spotnitz HM, Ott GY, Bigger T Jr, Steinberg JS, Livelli F Jr: Methods of implantable cardioverter-defibrillator-pacemaker insertion to avoid interactions. Ann Thorac Surg 1992;53:253.

119. Cohen AI, Wish MH, Fletcher RD, et al: The use and interaction of permanent pacemakers and the automatic implantable cardioverter-defibrillator. PACE 1988;11:704.

120. Singer I, Guarnieri T, Kupersmith J: Implanted automatic defibrillators: effects of drugs and pacemakers. PACE 1988; 11:2250.

121. Singer I, Kupersmith J: AICD therapy: drug/pacemaker interactions and future directions. Primary Cardiology 1990: 16:7:67.

122. Calkins H, Brinker J, Veltri EP, Guarnieri T, Levine JH: Clinical interactions between pacemakers and automatic implantable cardioverter-defibrillators. J Am Coll Cardiol 1990;16:666.

123. Ahern TS, Nydegger C, McCormick DJ, Marinchak R, Kowey P, Horowitz LN, Worley S, Kutalek SP: Device interaction—antitachycardia pacemakers and defibrillators for sustained ventricular tachycardia. PACE Part II, 1991;14:302.

124. Kou WH, Calkins H, Lewis RR, et al: Incidence of loss of consciousness during automatic implantable cardioverter-defibrillator shocks. Ann Int Med 1991;115:942.

125. Strickberger SA, Cantillon CO, Friedman PL: When should patients with lethal ventricular arrhythmia resume driving? Ann Int Med 1991;115:560.

126. DiCarlo LA, Winston SA, Honoway S, Reed P: Driving restrictions advised by midwestern cardiologists implanting cardioverter defibrillators: present practices, criteria utilized and compatibility with existing state laws. PACE 1992; 15:1131.

127. Finch NJ, Leman RB, Kratz JM, Gillette PC: Driving safety among patients with automatic implantable cardioverter defibrillators. JAMA 1993;270:1587.

128. Mirowski M, Reid PR, Winkle RA, et al: Mortality in patients with implanted automatic defibrillators. Ann Int Med 1983; 98:585.

129. Liberthson RR, Nagel EL, Hirschman JC, Nussenfeld SR: Prehospital ventricular fibrillation: prognosis and follow-up course. N Engl J Med 1974;291:317.

130. Baum RS, Alvarez H III, Cobb LA: Survival after resuscitation from out-of-hospital ventricular fibrillation. Circulation 1974;50:1231.

131. Goldstein S, Landis JR, Leighton R, et al: Characteristics of the resuscitated out-of-hospital cardiac arrest victim with coronary heart disease. Circulation 1981;64:977.

132. Cobb LA, Baum RS, Alvarez H III, Schaffer WA: Resuscitation from out-of-hospital ventricular fibrillation: 4 years follow-up. Circulation 1975 (suppl III); III-223-III-228.

133. Schaffer WA, Cobb LA: Recurrent ventricular fibrillation and modes of death in survivors of out-of-hospital ventricular fibrillation. N Engl J Med 1975;293:259.

134. Winkle RA, Mead RH, Ruder MA, et al: Long-term outcome with the automatic implantable cardioverter-defibrillator. J Am Coll Cardiol 1989;16:1353.

135. Winkle RA, Mead RH, Ruder MA, et al: Ten year experience with implantable defibrillators (abstract). Circulation 1991; 84:II-416.

136. Song SL: The Bilitch Report. Performance of implantable cardiac rhythm management devices. PACE 1992;15:475.

137. Furman S: AICD benefit. PACE 1989;12:399.

138. Connolly SJ, Yusuf S: Evaluation of the implantable cardioverter defibrillator in survivors of cardiac arrest: the need for randomized trials. Am J Cardiol 1992;69:959.

139. Kim SG: Implantable defibrillator therapy: Does it really prolong life? How can we prove it? Am J Cardiol 1993; 71:1213.

140. Fogoros RN: The implantable defibrillator backlash. Am J Cardiol 1991;67:1424.

141. Sweeney MO, Ruskin JN: Mortality benefits and the implantable cardioverter-defibrillator. Circulation 1994;89:1851.

142. Fogoros RN, Fiedler SB, Elson JJ: The automatic implantable cardioverter-defibrillator in drug-refractory ventricular tachyarrhythmias. Ann Intern Med 1987;107:635.

143. Newman D, Suave MJ, Herre J, et al: Survival after implantation of the cardioverter defibrillator. Am J Cardiol 1992; 69:899.

144. Fogoros RN, Elson JJ, Bonnet CA, Fiedler SB, Burkholder JA: Efficacy of the automatic implantable cardioverter-defibrillator in prolonging survival in patients with severe underlying cardiac disease. J Am Coll Cardiol. 1990;16:381.

145. Myerburg RJ, Luceri RM, Thurer R, et al: Time to first shock and clinical outcome in patients receiving an automatic implantable cardioverter-defibrillator. J Am Coll Cardiol 1989;14:508.

146. Bocker D, Block M, Isbruch F, et al: Do patients with implantable defibrillators live longer? J Am Coll Cardiol 1993; 21:1638.

147. Levine JH, Mellits ED, Baumgardner RA, et al: Predictors of first discharge and subsequent survival in patients with automatic implantable cardioverter-defibrillators. Circulation 1991;84:558.

148. Mehta D, Saksena S, Krol R: Survival of implantable cardioverter-defibrillator recipients: role of left ventricular function and its relationship to device use. Am Heart J. 1992; 124:1608.

149. Chen P-S, Shibata N, Wolf P, et al: Activation during successful and unsuccessful ventricular fibrillation in open chest dogs: evidence of complete cessation and regeneration of ventricular fibrillation after unsuccessful shocks. J Clin Invest 1986;77:810.

150. Chen P-S, Shibata N, Dixon EG, Martin RO, Ideker RE: Comparison of the defibrillation threshold and the upper limit of ventricular vulnerability. Circulation 1986;255: 1022.

151. Chen P-S, Wolf PD, Melnick SD, Danieley ND, Smith WM, Ideker RE: Comparison of activation during ventricular fibrillation and following unsuccessful defibrillation shocks in open chest dogs. Cir Res 1990;66:1544.

152. Chen P-S, Wolf PD, Ideker RE: The mechanism of cardiac defibrillation: a different point of view. Circulation 1991; 84:913.

153. Chen P-S, Feld GK, Kriett JM, et al: Relation between upper limit of vulnerability and defibrillation threshold in humans. Circulation 1993;88:186.

154. Hwang C, Swerdlow CD, Kass RM, et al: The upper limit of vulnerability reliably predicts the defibrillation threshold in humans. Circulation 1994;90:2308.

Index

Note: Page numbers followed by *f* indicate figures; page numbers followed by *t* indicate tables.